a Lange medical book

CURRENT Surgical Diagnosis & Treatment

12th Edition

Edited by

Gerard M. Doherty, MD
N. W. Thompson Professor of Surgery
Chief, Division of Endocrine Surgery
Section Head, General Surgery
University of Michigan
Ann Arbor, Michigan

Lawrence W. Way, MD
Professor & Vice-Chair
Department of Surgery
University of California, San Francisco
San Francisco, California

Lange Medical Books/McGraw-Hill
Medical Publishing Division

New York Chicago San Francisco Lisbon London Madrid Mexico City
Milan New Delhi San Juan Seoul Singapore Sydney Toronto

The McGraw·Hill Companies

Current Surgical Diagnosis & Treatment, Twelfth Edition

1 2 3 4 5 6 7 8 9 0 DOC/DOC 0 9 8 7 6 5

ISBN: 0-07-142315-X
ISSN: 0894-2277

Notice

Medicine is an ever-changing science. As new research and clinical experience broaden our knowledge, changes in treatment and drug therapy are required. The authors and the publisher of this work have checked with sources believed to be reliable in their efforts to provide information that is complete and generally in accord with the standards accepted at the time of publication. However, in view of the possibility of human error or changes in medical sciences, neither the authors nor the publisher nor any other party who has been involved in the preparation or publication of this work warrants that the information contained herein is in every respect accurate or complete, and they disclaim all responsibility for any errors or omissions or for the results obtained from use of the information contained in this work. Readers are encouraged to confirm the information contained herein with other sources. For example and in particular, readers are advised to check the product information sheet included in the package of each drug they plan to administer to be certain that the information contained in this work is accurate and that changes have not been made in the recommended dose or in the contraindications for administration. This recommendation is of particular importance in connection with new or infrequently used drugs.

This book was set in Garamond by Silverchair Science + Communications, Inc.
The editors were Karen Edmondson and Karen Davis.
The production supervisor was Sherri Souffrance.
The cover designer was Mary McKeon.
The index was prepared by Marilyn J. Rowland.
RR Donnelley, Crawfordsville, was printer and binder.

This book is printed on acid-free paper.

International Edition ISBN 0-07-110510-7

Contents

Authors

Craig T. Albanese, MD
Professor & Chief of Pediatric Surgery
Stanford University School of Medicine
Stanford, California
calbanese@stanfordmed.org
Chapter 45: Pediatric Surgery

John T. Anderson, MD, FACS
Associate Professor
Department of Surgery
Division of Trauma & Emergency Surgery
University of California, Davis
Davis, California
Chapter 12: Shock & Acute Pulmonary Failure in Surgical Patients

Nicholas M. Barbaro, MD
Professor of Neurological Surgery
Residency Director
University of California, San Francisco
San Francisco, California
Chapter 37: Neurosurgery & Surgery of the Pituitary—Traumatic Peripheral Nerve Lesions; Tumors of Peripheral Nerves; Pain

Samuel W. Beenken, MD
Professor of Surgery
University of Alabama, Birmingham
Birmingham, Alabama
Chapter 15: Head & Neck Tumors

Mitchel S. Berger, MD
Professor & Chairman, Department of Neurological Surgery
Chair, Brain Tumor Research Center
University of California, San Francisco
San Francisco, California
Chapter 37: Neurosurgery & Surgery of the Pituitary—Brain Tumors

Sigurd Berven, MD
Assistant Professor
Department of Orthopedic Surgery
University of California, San Francisco
San Francisco, California
Chapter 42: Orthopedics

David S. Bradford, MD
Professor & Chair Emeritus, Department of Orthopedic Surgery
University of California, San Francisco
San Francisco, California
bradford@orthosurg.ucsf.edu
Chapter 42: Orthopedics

Daniel C. Brennan, MD
Associate Professor, Medicine
Division of Renal Diseases
Director, Transplant Nephrology
Medical Director, Pharmacoeconomic Transplant Research
Washington University School of Medicine
St. Louis, Missouri
Chapter 5: Special Medical Problems in Surgical Patients—Renal Disease & the Surgical Patient

Aaron B. Caughey, MD, MPP, MPH
Assistant Professor, Medical
Director, Diabetes and Pregnancy Program,
Department of Obstetrics, Gynecology and Reproductive Sciences
University of California, San Francisco
San Francisco, California
Chapter 5: Special Medical Problems in Surgical Patients—Pregnancy & the Surgical Patient

Marcelle I. Cedars, MD
Reproductive Endocrinology and Fertility
UCSF Women's Health-Mount Zion
San Francisco, California
Chapter 41: Gynecology—Correction of Infertility Due to Tubal Abnormalities; Endometriosis

George J. Chang, MD
Assistant Professor
Department of Surgical Oncology
M.D. Anderson Cancer Center
Houston, Texas
gchang@mdanderson.org
Chapter 29: Small Intestine
Chapter 30: Large Intestine
Chapter 31: Anorectum

Lee-May Chen, MD
Clinical Instructor of Obstetrics, Gynecology, and Reproductive Sciences
University of California, San Francisco
San Francisco, California
lee-may.chen@ucsfmedctr.org
Chapter 41: Gynecology—Gynecologic Malignancies

Orlo H. Clark, MD
Professor and Vice Chair
Department of Surgery
University of California, San Francisco
San Francisco, California
clarko@surgery.ucsf.edu
Chapter 16: Thyroid and Parathyroid

J. Perren Cobb, MD
Associate Professor
Department of Surgery
Director, Cellular Injury & Adaption Laboratory
Washington University School of Medicine
St. Louis, Missouri
cobb@msnotes.wustl.edu
Chapter 8: Inflammation, Infection, & Antimicrobial Therapy

William W. Colman, MD
Private Practice
Dutchess County, New York
Chapter 42: Orthopedics

Christopher S. Cooper, MD
Associate Professor of Pediatric Urology
Department of Urology
University of Iowa College of Medicine and Children's Hospital of Iowa
Iowa City, Iowa
christopher-cooper@uiowa.edu
Chapter 40: Urology

Philip D. Darney, MD
Professor of Obstetrics, Gynecology, and Reproductive Sciences
San Francisco General Hospital
University of California, San Francisco
San Francisco, California
Chapter 41: Gynecology—Contraception

K. Barrett Deatrick, MD
House Officer
Resident in Surgery
University of Michigan Hospitals
Ann Arbor, Michigan
Chapter 7: Power Sources in the Operating Room

Robert H. Demling, MD
Professor of Surgery
Harvard Medical School
Boston, Massachusetts
Director, Burn Center
Department of Surgery
Brigham & Women's Hospital
Boston, Massachusetts
rhdemling@partners.org
Chapter 14: Burns & Other Thermal Injuries

Karen E. Deveney, MD
Professor of Surgery
Oregon Health Sciences University
School of Medicine
Portland, Oregon
deveneyk@ohsu.edu
Chapter 32: Hernias and Other Lesions of the Abdominal Wall

Edward Diao, MD
Professor
Department of Orthopedic Surgery
University of California, San Francisco
San Francisco, California
diaoe@orthosurg.ucsf.edu
Chapter 42: Orthopedics

William P. Dillon, MD
Professor, Radiology, Neurology, Neurosurgery
Chief, Neuroradiology Section
Vice-Chairman, Department of Radiology
University of California, San Francisco
San Francisco, California
bill.dillon@radiology.ucsf.edu
Chapter 37: Neurosurgery & Surgery of the Pituitary—Neurodiagnostic Procedures

Gerard M. Doherty, MD
N.W. Thompson Professor of Surgery
Chief, Division of Endocrine Surgery
Section Head, General Surgery
University of Michigan
Ann Arbor, Michigan
gerardd@umich.edu
Chapter 2: Preoperative Care
Chapter 3: Postoperative Care
Chapter 4: Postoperative Complications
Chapter 5: Special Medical Problems in Surgical Patients—Endocrine Disease & the Surgical Patient
Chapter 7: Power Sources in the Operating Room
Chapter 8: Inflammation, Infection, & Antimicrobial Therapy
Chapter 9: Fluid & Electrolyte Management
Chapter 20: Esophagus & Diaphragm
Chapter 21: The Acute Abdomen
Chapter 22: Peritoneal Cavity
Chapter 23: Stomach & Duodenum
Chapter 25: Biliary Tract
Chapter 26: Pancreas

Robert Domush, MD
Obstetrics and Gynecology
UCSF Women's Health-Mount Zion
San Francisco, California
Chapter 41: Gynecology—Fistulas

Quan-Yang Duh, MD
Professor, Department of Surgery
University of California, San Francisco
San Francisco, California
quan-yang.duh@med.va.gov
Chapter 33: Adrenals

J. Englebert Dunphy, MD*
Formerly Professor of Surgery Emeritus
University of California, San Francisco
San Francisco, California
Chapter 1: Approach to the Surgical Patient

Charles Eichler, MD
Professor of Clinical Surgery
Division of Vascular Surgery
University of California, San Francisco
San Francisco, California
eichlerc@surgery.ucsf.edu
Chapter 34: Arteries

*Deceased.

Lisa Everson, MD
Associate Clinical Professor of Obstetrics, Gynecology, and Reproductive Sciences
University of California, San Francisco
San Francisco, California
eversonl@obgyn.ucsf.edu
Chapter 41: Gynecology—Adnexal Masses

Robert E. H. Ferguson, Jr., MD
Resident, Division of Plastic & Reconstructive Surgery
University of Kentucky, College of Medicine
Lexington, Kentucky
Chapter 43: Plastic and Reconstructive Surgery

Roger Fontes, Jr., MD
Private Practice
Henderson, Nevada
Chapter 42: Orthopedics

Douglas L. Fraker, MD, FACS
Jonathan E. Rhoads Associate Professor of Surgery
Vice-Chair, Clinical Affairs & Director, General Surgery
Chief, Division of Surgical Oncology
The University of Pennsylvania
Philadelphia, Pennsylvania
fraker@mail.med.upenn.edu
Chapter 27: Spleen

Elena A. Gates, MD
Professor of Obstetrics, Gynecology & Reproductive Sciences
Division Director, General Gynecology
University of California, San Francisco
San Francisco, California
gatese@obgyn.ucsf.edu
Chapter 41: Gynecology—Congenital Anomalies of the Female Reproductive System; Benign Tumors of the Vulva & Vagina

Armando E. Giuliano, MD
Director, Joyce Eisenberg Keefer Breast Center
Clinical Professor of Surgery
University of California, Los Angeles
Los Angeles, California
Chief of Surgical Oncology
John Wayne Cancer Institute
Santa Monica, California
giulianoa@jwci.org
Chapter 17: Breast

Sean C. Glasgow, MD
Resident
Department of Surgery
Washington University School of Medicine
St. Louis, Missouri
glasgows@wustl.edu
Chapter 10: Surgical Metabolism & Nutrition

Mindy Goldman, MD
Associate Clinical Professor of Obstetrics and Gynecology
University of California, San Francisco
San Francisco, California
Chapter 41: Gynecology—Ectopic Pregnancy

Stephen Gunther, MD
Private Practice
Willits, California
Chapter 42: Orthopedics

Nalin Gupta, MD, PhD
Bruce Dettmer Endowed Chair in Pediatric Neurosurgery
University of California, San Francisco
San Francisco, California
guptan@neurosurg.ucsf.edu
Chapter 37: Neurosurgery & Surgery of the Pituitary—Pediatric Neurosurgery

Scott L. Hansen, MD
Assistant Professor
Plastic and Reconstructive Surgery
University of California, San Francisco
San Francisco, California
Chapter 44: Hand Surgery

Mark R. Hemmila, MD
Assistant Professor
University of Michigan
Ann Arbor, Michigan
mhemmila@umich.edu
Chapter 13: Management of the Injured Patient

Virginia M. Herrmann, MD
Professor of Surgery
Memorial Health University Medical Center
Savannah, Georgia
Chapter 10: Surgical Metabolism & Nutrition

Robert F. Hickey, MD
Division of Pediatric Emergency Medicine
Children's Hospital of Pittsburgh
Pittsburgh, Pennsylvania
Chapter 5: Special Medical Problems in Surgical Patients—Respiratory Disease & the Surgical Patient

Edward C. Hill, MD
Professor Emeritus, Department of Obstetrics, Gynecology, & Reproductive Sciences
University of California, San Francisco
San Francisco, California
Chapter 5: Special Medical Problems in Surgical Patients—Pregnancy & the Surgical Patient
Chapter 41: Gynecology—Congenital Anomalies of the Female Reproductive System

Daniel B. Hinshaw, MD
Medical Director Palliative Care Consultation Team & Staff Surgeon
VA Ann Arbor Health Care System
Ann Arbor, Michigan
Professor of Surgery
University of Michigan
Ann Arbor, Michigan
hinshaw@umich.edu
Chapter 5: Special Medical Problems in Surgical Patients—Management of the Older Surgical Patient

Julian T. Hoff, MD
Professor and Chair, Department of Neurosurgery
University of Michigan
Ann Arbor, Michigan
jhoff@umich.edu
Chapter 37: Neurosurgery & Surgery of the Pituitary—Diagnosis & Management of Depressed States of Consciousness

James W. Holcroft, MD
Professor of Surgery
School of Medicine
University of California, Davis
Sacramento, California
jwholcroft@ucdavis.edu
Chapter 12: Shock & Acute Pulmonary Failure in Surgical Patients

Martin C. Holland, MD
Associate Professor of Neurological Surgery
University of California, San Francisco
San Francisco, California
Chapter 37: Neurosurgery & Surgery of the Pituitary—Craniocerebral Trauma

William Holmes, MD
Assistant Professor, Department of Orthopedic Surgery
University of California, San Francisco
San Francisco, California
holmesw@orthosurg.ucsf.edu
Chapter 42: Orthopedics

Serena S. Hu, MD
Professor of Clinical Orthopedics
University of California, San Francisco
San Francisco, California
hus@orthosurg.ucsf.edu
Chapter 42: Orthopedics

Michael H. Humphreys, MD
Professor of Medicine
University of California, San Francisco
Chief, Division of Nephrology
San Francisco General Hospital
San Francisco, California
mhhsfgh@itsa.ucsf.edu
Chapter 9: Fluid & Electrolyte Management

Thomas K. Hunt, MD
Professor Emeritus, Department of Surgery
University of California, San Francisco
San Francisco, California
wound@itsa.ucsf.edu
Chapter 6: Wound Healing

David Jablons, MD
Professor of Surgery
University of California, San Francisco
San Francisco, California
jablonsd@surgery.ucsf.edu
Chapter 18: Thoracic Wall Pleura, Mediastinum, & Lung

Alison Jacoby, MD
Obstetrics and Gynecology
UCSF Women's Health-Mount Zion
San Francisco, California
Chapter 41: Gynecology—Leiomyomas of the Uterus

William R. Jarnagin, MD
Associate Professor of Surgery
Weill Medical College of Cornell University
Attending Surgeon
Memorial Sloan-Kettering Cancer Center
New York, New York
jarnagiw@mskcc.org
Chapter 24: Liver & Portal Venous System

Stephen A. Kamenetzky, MD
Associate Professor of Clinical Ophthalmology & Visual Sciences
Department of Ophthalmology
Washington University School of Medicine
St. Louis, Missouri
kamenet@mindspring.com
Chapter 39: The Eye & Ocular Adnexa

Hubert T. Kim, MD, PhD
Assistant Professor
Department of Orthopedic Surgery
University of California, San Francisco
San Francisco, California
kim.hubert_t@sanfrancisco.va.gov
Chapter 42: Orthopedics

Sharon Knight, MD
Obstetrics and Gynecology
UCSF Women's Health-Mount Zion
San Francisco, California
Chapter 41: Gynecology—Pelvic Organ Prolapse & Urinary Incontinence

Matt J. Koch, MD
Assistant Professor, Medicine
Division of Renal Diseases
Washington University School of Medicine
St. Louis, Missouri
Chapter 5: Special Medical Problems in Surgical Patients—Renal Disease & the Surgical Patient

Abner Korn, MD
Obstetrics and Gynecology
UCSF Women's Health-Mount Zion
San Francisco, California
Chapter 41: Gynecology—Abnormal Uterine Bleeding

William C. Krupski, MD*
Formerly with The Permanente Medical Group
Kaiser Foundation Hospital
San Francisco, California
Clinical Professor of Surgery
University of California, San Francisco
San Francisco, California
Chapter 34: Arteries
Chapter 35: Amputation

Sandeep Kunwar, MD
Assistant Professor of Neurological Surgery
University of California, San Francisco
San Francisco, California
Chapter 37: Neurosurgery & Surgery of the Pituitary—Brain Tumors; Pituitary Tumors

Lisa Lattanza, MD
Assistant Clinical Professor
Department of Orthopedic Surgery
University of California, San Francisco
San Francisco, California
lattanza@orthosurg.ucsf.edu
Chapter 42: Orthopedics

Michael T. Lawton, MD
Assistant Professor of Neurological Surgery
University of California, San Francisco
San Francisco, California
Chapter 37: Neurosurgery & Surgery of the Pituitary—Intracranial Aneurysms; Arteriovenous Malformations

Lee Learman, MD, PhD
Department of Obstetrics, Gynecology, & Reproductive Sciences
University of California, San Francisco
San Francisco, California
Chapter 41: Gynecology—Chronic Pelvic Pain; Adenomyosis

Chienying Liu, MD
Staff Endocrinologist
Kaiser-Permanente
Santa Rosa, California
Chapter 33: Adrenals

*Deceased.

Mahesh Mankani, MD
Assistant Professor
Department of Surgery
University of California, San Francisco
San Francisco, California
mmankani@sfghsurg.ucsf.edu
Chapter 44: Hand Surgery

Geoffrey T. Manley, MD, PhD
Associate Professor of Neurological Surgery
University of California, San Francisco
San Francisco, California
Chapter 37: Neurosurgery & Surgery of the Pituitary—Spinal Cord Injury

Barry M. Massie, MD
Chief, Cardiology Division
Veterans Administration Hospital
San Francisco, California
barry.massie@med.va.gov
Chapter 5: Special Medical Problems in Surgical Patients—Heart Disease & the Surgical Patient

Michael W. McDermott, MD
Assistant Professor, Department of Neurological Surgery
University of California, San Francisco
San Francisco, California
mcdermottm@neuro.ucsf.edu
Chapter 37: Neurosurgery & Surgery of the Pituitary—Brain Tumors

Scot H. Merrick, MD
Professor of Clinical Surgery
University of California, San Francisco
San Francisco, California
merricks@surgery.ucsf.edu
Chapter 19: The Heart, Part I: Acquired Diseases

Louis M. Messina, MD
Professor and Chief
Division of Vascular Surgery
Edwin J. Wylie Chair in Surgery
University of California, San Francisco
San Francisco, California
messina@surgery.ucsf.edu
Chapter 34: Arteries
Chapter 36: Veins & Lymphatics

Ronald D. Miller, MD
Professor & Chairman
Department of Anesthesia
& Perioperative Care
Professor of Cellular
& Molecular Pharmacology
University of California, San Francisco
San Francisco, California
millerr@anesthesia.ucsf.edu
Chapter 11: Anesthesia

Linda M. Mundy, MD
University of Pennsylvania
Philadelphia, Pennsylvania
mundyl623@aol.com
Chapter 8: Inflammation, Infection, & Antimicrobial Therapy

Ashok Nambiar, MD
Clinical Fellow
Department of Transfusion Medicine
National Institutes of Health
Bethesda, Maryland
anambiar@mail.cc.nih.gov
Chapter 5: Special Medical Problems in Surgical Patients—Hematology Disease & the Surgical Patient

Alexander M. Papanastasio, MD
Department of Neurological Surgery
University of California, San Francisco
San Francisco, California
Chapter 37: Neurosurgery & Surgery of the Pituitary—Spinal Cord Injury

Warwick J. Peacock, MD
Professor Emeritus
University of California, San Francisco
San Francisco, California
Chapter 37: Neurosurgery & Surgery of the Pituitary—Pediatric Neurosurgery

Larry H. Pitts, MD
Professor of Neurological Surgery & Otolaryngology
University of California, San Francisco
San Francisco, California
Chapter 37: Neurosurgery & Surgery of the Pituitary—Spinal Cord Injury

Jeffrey D. Punch, MD
Associate Professor of Surgery
Chief, Division of Transplantation
University of Michigan
Ann Arbor, Michigan
jpunch@umich.edu
Chapter 47: Organ Transplantation

Joseph H. Rapp, MD
Professor of Surgery in Residence
University of California, San Francisco
Chief, Vascular Surgery Service
San Francisco Veterans Administration
Medical Center
San Francisco, California
Chapter 34: Arteries

Mark L. Rosenblum, MD
Chair, Department of Neurosurgery
Henry Ford Hospital
Detroit, Michigan
Chapter 37: Neurosurgery & Surgery of the Pituitary—Surgical Infections of the Central Nervous System

Guy Rosenthal, MD
Clinical Instructor
Clinical Research Center
University of California, San Francisco
San Francisco, California
Chapter 37: Neurosurgery & Surgery of the Pituitary—Spinal Cord Injury

Lee D. Rowe, MD
Private Practice
General Otolaryngology
Philadelphia, Pennsylvania
Chapter 38: Otolaryngology

Michael S. Sabel, MD, FACS
Assistant Professor of Surgery
University of Michigan
Ann Arbor, Michigan
msabel@umich.edu
Chapter 46: Oncology

Andrew A. Shelton, MD
Assistant Professor of Surgery (General Surgery)
Stanford University School of Medicine
Stanford, California
shelton@stanford.edu
Chapter 29: Small Intestine
Chapter 30: Large Intestine
Chapter 31: Anorectum

Philip A. Starr, MD, PhD
Associate Professor of Neurological Surgery
University of California, San Francisco
San Francisco, California
Chapter 37: Neurosurgery & Surgery of the Pituitary—Movement Disorders Responsive to Surgery

Karl G. Sylvester, MD
Assistant Professor of Surgery
Division of Pediatric Surgery
Stanford University Medical Center
Lucile Packard Children's Hospital
Stanford, California
Chapter 45: Pediatric Surgery

Bobby K-B Tay, MD
Assistant Professor
Department of Orthopedic Surgery
University of California, San Francisco
San Francisco, California
tayb@orthosurg.ucsf.edu
Chapter 42: Orthopedics

Pietro Tedesco, MD
Fellow in Gastrointestinal Surgery
Department of Surgery
University of California, San Francisco
San Francisco, California
Chapter 20: Esophagus & Diaphragm

Pierre R. Theodore, MD
Assistant Professor of Surgery
Division of Cardiothoracic Surgery
Department of Surgery
University of California, San Francisco
San Francisco, California
Chapter 18: Thoracic Wall, Pleura, Mediastinum, and Lung

Philip V. Theodosopoulos, MD
Director, Division of Skull Base Surgery
Assistant Professor
University of Cincinnati
Cincinnati, Ohio
Chapter 37: Neurosurgery & Surgery of the Pituitary—Intracranial Aneurysms

Pearl T.C.Y. Toy, MD
Professor
University of California, San Francisco
San Francisco, California
Chief, Blood Bank
Moffitt-Long/Mt. Zion Hospitals
San Francisco, California
pearl.toy@clinlab.ucsfmedctr.org
Chapter 5: Special Medical Problems in Surgical Patients—Hematology Disease & the Surgical Patient

Linda M. Tsai, MD
Instructor in Clinical Ophthalmology & Visual Sciences
Department of Ophthalmology
Washington University, School of Medicine
St. Louis, Missouri
Chapter 39: The Eye & Ocular Adnexa

J. Blake Tyrell, MD
Professor Emeritus
Division of Endocrinology
University of California, San Francisco
San Francisco, California
blaket@medicine.ucsf.edu
Chapter 33: Adrenals

Marshall M. Urist, MD
Professor & Vice-Chairman
Department of Surgery
Chief, Section of Surgical Oncology
University of Alabama, Birmingham
Birmingham, Alabama
mmurist@ccc.uab.edu
Chapter 15: Head & Neck Tumors

Henry C. Vasconez, MD
Professor & Chief
Division of Plastic & Reconstruction Surgery
Program Director, Plastic Surgery
University of Kentucky, College of Medicine
Lexington, Kentucky
hvasc@uky.edu
Chapter 43: Plastic & Reconstructive Surgery

Luis O. Vasconez, MD
Professor & Director
Division of Plastic Surgery
University of Alabama School of Medicine
Birmingham, Alabama
Chapter 43: Plastic & Reconstructive Surgery

G. Edward Vates, MD, PhD
Assistant Professor
School of Medicine and Dentistry
University of Rochester
Rochester, New York
gedward_vates@urmc.rochester.edu
Chapter 37: Neurosurgery & Surgery of the Pituitary—Intracranial Aneurysms

Edward Verrier, MD
Chief, Division of Cardiothoracic Surgery
Professor and Vice Chairman of Clinical Affairs
Department of Surgery
University of Washington
Seattle, Washington
edver@u.washington.edu
Chapter 19: The Heart, Part II: Congenital Heart Diseases

Cornelia S. von Koch, MD, PhD
Department of Neurological Surgery
University of California, San Francisco
San Francisco, California
Chapter 37: Neurosurgery & Surgery of the Pituitary—Diagnosis & Management of Depressed States of Consciousness, Surgical Infections of the Central Nervous System

Elaine Waetjen, MD
University of California, Davis
Davis, California
Chapter 41: Gynecology—Pelvic Organ Prolapse & Urinary Incontinence

Wendy L. Wahl, MD
Associate Professor of Surgery
Director, Trauma Burn Intensive Care Unit
University of Michigan
Ann Arbor, Michigan
wlwahl@umich.edu
Chapter 13: Management of the Injured Patient

Thomas W. Wakefield, MD
S. Martin Lindenauer Professor of Surgery
Section Head, Vascular Surgery
University of Michigan
Ann Arbor, Michigan
thomasww@umich.edu
Chapter 36: Veins & Lymphatics

Lawrence W. Way, MD
Professor & Vice-Chair
Department of Surgery
University of California, San Francisco
San Francisco, California
lwway@aol.com
Chapter 1: Approach to the Surgical Patient
Chapter 20: Esophagus & Diaphragm
Chapter 23: Stomach & Duodenum
Chapter 25: Biliary Tract
Chapter 26: Pancreas
Chapter 28: Appendix

Philip R. Weinstein, MD
Professor of Neurological Surgery
University of California, San Francisco
San Francisco, California
Chapter 37: Neurosurgery & Surgery of the Pituitary—Tumors of the Spinal Cord, Invertebral Disk Disease

Mark L. Welton, MD
Associate Professor & Chief
Section of Colon & Rectal Surgery
Department of Surgery
Stanford University School of Medicine
Stanford, California
mwelton@stanford.edu
Chapter 29: Small Intestine
Chapter 30: Large Intestine
Chapter 31: Anorectum

Richard D. Williams, MD
Rubin H. Flocks Chair & Professor
Department of Urology
University of Iowa College of Medicine
Iowa City, Iowa
richard-williams@uiowa.edu
Chapter 40: Urology

Charles B. Wilson, MD, DSc, MSHA
Professor Emeritus
Department of Neurological Surgery
University of California, San Francisco
San Francisco, California
Chapter 37: Neurosurgery & Surgery of the Pituitary—Tumors of Peripheral Nerves

Ronald K. Woods, MD, PhD
Pediatric Cardiothoracic Surgery
Mary Bridge Children's Hospital
Tacoma, Washington
Chapter 19: The Heart, Part II: Congenital Heart Diseases

Charles D. Yingling, PhD
Clinical Professor
Stanford University School of Medicine
Stanford, California
Chapter 37: Neurosurgery & Surgery of the Pituitary—Intraoperative Neurophysiologic Monitoring

David M. Young, MD
Assistant Professor of Surgery in Residence
Chief of Plastic Surgery
Director of Burn Service
San Francisco General Hospital
San Francisco, California
dyoung@sfghsurg.ucsf.edu
Chapter 44: Hand Surgery

Preface

Current Surgical Diagnosis & Treatment is intended to serve as a ready source of information about diseases managed by surgeons. Like other books in this Lange series, it emphasizes quick recall of major diagnostic features and brief descriptions of disease processes, followed by approaches for definitive diagnosis and treatment. Epidemiology, pathophysiology, and pathology are discussed to the extent that they contribute to the book's ultimate purpose, which is guidance for patient care. About one third of the book is focused on general medical and surgical topics important in the management of all patients.

The book also includes limited current references to journal literature for the reader who wishes to pursue specific additional detail. Because of the concise nature of this text, more focused exploration may be useful to gain detail in specific areas.

OUTSTANDING FEATURES

- To maintain currency of the information, this text is revised and updated frequently. The most recent edition was published in 2003. With each revision, particular subjects are completely, substantially, partially, or minimally rewritten as indicated by the progress in each field. New authors and chapters are introduced for the text as needed.
- Illustrations have been judiciously chosen to clarify anatomic and surgical concepts.
- Over 1000 diseases and disorders are covered.
- Thorough coverage is provided of the role of minimally invasive surgical procedures.

INTENDED AUDIENCE

- **Students** will find this book to be an authoritative introduction to surgery as it is taught and practiced at major teaching institutions.
- **House officers** will find many occasions to refer to the concise discussions of the diseases that they must deal with each day as well as the less common ones calling for quick study on the spot.
- **Medical practitioners** who must occasionally deal with surgical problems or who have occasion to counsel patients needing surgical referrals will have many uses for this book.
- **Practicing surgeons** will find it useful as a guide to the most current management strategies.

ORGANIZATION

This book is organized chiefly by organ system. Lists of subjects taken up in the longer chapters are presented in the Table of Contents, but for some users the more convenient portal of entry to the text will be the Index.

Early chapters provide general information about the relationship between surgeons and their patients (Chapter 1), preparation for surgery (Chapter 2), postoperative care (Chapter 3), and surgical complications (Chapter 4). Further chapters deal with the medical problems in patients who require surgery, wound healing, inflammation, infection, antibiotics, fluid and electrolyte management, and surgical metabolism and nutrition. The main series of body systems topics begins with the chapter on head and neck tumors and ends with the chapter on hand surgery. Further chapters on pediatric surgery, oncology, and organ transplantation complete the coverage.

NEW TO THIS EDITION

Along with the customary revision of all sections as called for by changing concepts in each field covered in this book, the following major changes have been made.

- This has been a particularly complete revision with extensive changes to most chapters to update the material.
- Several sections in Chapter 5 on special medical problems in surgical patients have been rewritten by new authors, including pregnancy in a surgical patient, and the management of the older surgical patient.
- The management of the injured patient, which details trauma care, has been completely revised by two new authors.
- Esophagus and Diaphragm has been extensively revised with the addition of a new lead author.
- Liver and Portal Venous System has been extensively updated and rewritten by a new lead author.
- Oncology has been written as a new chapter by a new lead author, with extensive coverage of lymphoma, melanoma, sarcoma, and systemic cancer therapy.
- Organ Transplantation has been rewritten by a new lead author.
- A new chapter on Power Sources in the Operating Room has been added.

ACKNOWLEDGMENTS

The editors and contributors continue to acknowledge their gratitude to the now deceased J. Englebert Dunphy, MD, for his inspiration and lifetime of service to the practice and teaching of surgery. We are also particularly grateful for the important contributions that the staff at McGraw-Hill has made to ensuring accurate, high quality text. We are also grateful to our colleagues and readers who have offered comments and criticisms for our guidance in preparing future editions. We hope that anyone with an idea, suggestion, or criticism regarding this book will contact us.

Finally, we would like to acknowledge the untimely death of one of our colleagues and co-authors. Dr. William Krupski was a long-time friend and supporter of each of us who has spent time at the University of California, San Francisco. His personal strengths and character will be missed in our community.

Gerard M. Doherty, MD
Lawrence W. Way, MD

Ann Arbor, Michigan, and San Francisco, California
September 2005

Approach to the Surgical Patient 1

J. Englebert Dunphy, MD, & Lawrence W. Way, MD*

The management of surgical disorders requires not only the application of technical skills and training in the basic sciences to the problems of diagnosis and treatment but also a genuine sympathy and indeed love for the patient. The surgeon must be a doctor in the old-fashioned sense, an applied scientist, an engineer, an artist, and a minister to his or her fellow human beings. Because life or death often depends upon the validity of surgical decisions, the surgeon's judgment must be matched by courage in action and by a high degree of technical proficiency.

THE HISTORY

At their first contact, the surgeon must gain the patient's confidence and convey the assurance that help is available and will be provided. The surgeon must demonstrate concern for the patient as a person who needs help and not just as a "case" to be processed. This is not always easy to do, and there are no rules of conduct except to be gentle and considerate. Most patients are eager to like and trust their doctors and respond gratefully to a sympathetic and understanding person. Some surgeons are able to establish a confident relationship with the first few words of greeting; others can only do so by means of a stylized and carefully acquired bedside manner. It does not matter how it is done, so long as an atmosphere of sympathy, personal interest, and understanding is created. Even under emergency circumstances, this subtle message of sympathetic concern must be conveyed.

Eventually, all histories must be formally structured, but much can be learned by letting the patient ramble a little. Discrepancies and omissions in the history are often due as much to overstructuring and leading questions as to the unreliability of the patient. The enthusiastic novice asks leading questions; the cooperative patient gives the answer that seems to be wanted; and the interview concludes on a note of mutual satisfaction with the wrong answer thus developed.

* Deceased.

BUILDING THE HISTORY

History taking is detective work. Preconceived ideas, snap judgments, and hasty conclusions have no place in this process. The diagnosis must be established by inductive reasoning. The interviewer must first determine the facts and then search for essential clues, realizing that the patient may conceal the most important symptom—eg, the passage of blood by rectum—in the hope (born of fear) that if it is not specifically inquired about or if nothing is found to account for it in the physical examination, it cannot be very serious.

Common symptoms of surgical conditions that require special emphasis in the history taking are discussed in the following paragraphs.

Pain

A careful analysis of the nature of pain is one of the most important features of a surgical history. The examiner must first ascertain how the pain began. Was it explosive in onset, rapid, or gradual? What is the precise character of the pain? Is it so severe that it cannot be relieved by medication? Is it constant or intermittent? Are there classic associations, such as the rhythmic pattern of small bowel obstruction or the onset of pain preceding the limp of intermittent claudication?

One of the most important aspects of pain is the patient's reaction to it. The overreactor's description of pain is often obviously inappropriate, and so is a description of "excruciating" pain offered in a casual or jovial manner. A patient who shrieks and thrashes about is either grossly overreacting or suffering from renal or biliary colic. Very severe pain—due to infection, inflammation, or vascular disease—usually forces the patient to restrict all movement as much as possible.

Moderate pain is made agonizing by fear and anxiety. Reassurance of a sort calculated to restore the patient's confidence in the care being given is often a more effective analgesic than an injection of morphine.

Vomiting

What did the patient vomit? How much? How often? What did the vomitus look like? Was vomiting projectile? It is especially helpful for the examiner to see the vomitus.

Change in Bowel Habits

A change in bowel habits is a common complaint that is often of no significance. However, when a person who has always had regular evacuations notices a distinct change, particularly toward intermittent alternations of constipation and diarrhea, colon cancer must be suspected. Too much emphasis is placed upon the size and shape of the stool—eg, many patients who normally have well-formed stools may complain of irregular small stools when their routine is disturbed by travel or a change in diet.

Hematemesis or Hematochezia

Bleeding from any orifice demands the most critical analysis and can never be dismissed as due to some immediately obvious cause. The most common error is to assume that bleeding from the rectum is attributable to hemorrhoids. The character of the blood can be of great significance. Does it clot? Is it bright or dark red? Is it changed in any way, as in the coffee-ground vomitus of slow gastric bleeding or the dark, tarry stool of upper gastrointestinal bleeding? The full details and variations cannot be included here but will be emphasized under separate headings elsewhere.

Trauma

Trauma occurs so commonly that it is often difficult to establish a relationship between the chief complaint and an episode of trauma. Children in particular are subject to all kinds of minor trauma, and the family may attribute the onset of an illness to a specific recent injury. On the other hand, children may be subjected to severe trauma though their parents are unaware of it. The possibility of trauma having been inflicted by a parent must not be overlooked.

When there is a history of trauma, the details must be established as precisely as possible. What was the patient's position when the accident occurred? Was consciousness lost? Retrograde amnesia (inability to remember events just preceding the accident) always indicates some degree of cerebral damage. If a patient can remember every detail of an accident, has not lost consciousness, and has no evidence of external injury to the head, brain damage can be excluded.

In the case of gunshot wounds and stab wounds, knowing the nature of the weapon, its size and shape, the probable trajectory, and the position of the patient when hit may be very helpful in evaluating the nature of the resultant injury.

The possibility that an accident might have been caused by preexisting disease such as epilepsy, diabetes, coronary artery disease, or hypoglycemia must be explored.

When all of the facts and essential clues have been gathered, the examiner is in a position to complete the study of the present illness. By this time, it may be possible to rule out (by inductive reasoning) all but a few diagnoses. A novice diagnostician asked to evaluate the causes of shoulder pain in a given patient might include ruptured ectopic pregnancy in the list of possibilities. The experienced physician will automatically exclude that possibility on the basis of gender or age.

Family History

The family history is of great significance in a number of surgical conditions. Polyposis of the colon is a classic example, but diabetes, Peutz-Jeghers syndrome, chronic pancreatitis, multiglandular syndromes, other endocrine abnormalities, and cancer are often better understood and better evaluated in the light of a careful family history.

Past History

The details of the past history may illuminate obscure areas of the present illness. It has been said that people who are well are almost never sick, and people who are sick are almost never well. It is true that a patient with a long and complicated history of diseases and injuries is likely to be a much poorer risk than even a very old patient experiencing a major surgical illness for the first time.

In order to make certain that important details of the past history will not be overlooked, the system review must be formalized and thorough. By always reviewing the past history in the same way, the experienced examiner never omits significant details. Many skilled examiners find it easy to review the past history by inquiring about each system as they perform the physical examination on that part of the body.

In reviewing the past history, it is important to consider the nutritional background of the patient. There is a clear awareness throughout the world that the underprivileged malnourished patient responds poorly to disease, injury, and operation. Malnourishment may not be obvious on physical examination and must be elicited by questioning.

Acute nutritional deficiencies, particularly fluid and electrolyte losses, can be understood only in the light of the total (including nutritional) history. For example, low serum sodium may be due to the use of diuretics or a sodium-restricted diet rather than to acute loss. In this connection, the use of any medications must be carefully recorded and interpreted.

A detailed history of acute losses by vomiting and diarrhea—and the nature of the losses—is helpful in estimating the probable trends in serum electrolytes. Thus, the patient who has been vomiting persistently with no evidence of bile in the vomitus is likely to have acute pyloric stenosis associated with benign ulcer, and hypochloremic alkalosis must be anticipated. Chronic vomiting without bile—and particularly with evidence of changed and previously digested food—is suggestive of chronic obstruction, and the possibility of carcinoma should be considered.

It is essential for the surgeon to think in terms of nutritional balance. It is often possible to begin therapy before the results of laboratory tests have been obtained, because the specific nature and probable extent of fluid and electrolyte losses can often be estimated on the basis of the history and the physician's clinical experience. Laboratory data should be obtained as soon as possible, but knowledge of the probable level of the obstruction and of the concentration of the electrolytes in the gastrointestinal fluids will provide sufficient grounds for the institution of appropriate immediate therapy.

The Patient's Emotional Background

Psychiatric consultation is seldom required in the management of surgical patients, but there are times when it is of great help. Emotionally and mentally disturbed patients require surgical operations as often as others, and full cooperation between psychiatrist and surgeon is essential. Furthermore, either before or after an operation, a patient may develop a major psychotic disturbance that is beyond the ability of the surgeon to appraise or manage. Prognosis, drug therapy, and overall management require the participation of a psychiatrist.

On the other hand, there are many situations in which the surgeon can and should deal with the emotional aspects of the patient's illness rather than resorting to psychiatric assistance. Most psychiatrists prefer not to be brought in to deal with minor anxiety states. As long as the surgeon accepts the responsibility for the care of the whole patient, such services are superfluous.

This is particularly true in the care of patients with malignant disease or those who must undergo mutilating operations such as amputation of an extremity, ileostomy, or colostomy. In these situations, the patient can be supported far more effectively by the surgeon and the surgical team than by a consulting psychiatrist.

Surgeons are increasingly aware of the importance of psychosocial factors in surgical convalescence. Recovery from a major operation is greatly enhanced if the patient is not worn down with worry about emotional, social, and economic problems that have nothing to do with the illness itself. Incorporation of these factors into the record contributes to better total care of the surgical patient.

THE PHYSICAL EXAMINATION

The complete examination of the surgical patient includes the physical examination, certain special procedures such as gastroscopy and esophagoscopy, laboratory tests, x-ray examination, and follow-up examination. In some cases, all of these may be necessary; in others, special examinations and laboratory tests can be kept to a minimum. It is just as poor practice to insist on unnecessary thoroughness as it is to overlook procedures that may contribute to the diagnosis. Painful, inconvenient, and costly procedures should not be ordered unless there is a reasonable chance that the information gained will be useful in making clinical decisions.

THE ELECTIVE PHYSICAL EXAMINATION

The elective physical examination should be done in an orderly and detailed fashion. One should acquire the habit of performing a complete examination in exactly the same sequence, so that no step is omitted. When the routine must be modified, as in an emergency, the examiner recalls without conscious effort what must be done to complete the examination later. The regular performance of complete examinations has the added advantage of familiarizing the beginner with what is normal so that what is abnormal can be more readily recognized.

All patients are sensitive and somewhat embarrassed at being examined. It is both courteous and clinically useful to put the patient at ease. The examining room and table should be comfortable, and drapes should be used if the patient is required to strip for the examination. Most patients will relax if they are allowed to talk a bit during the examination, which is another reason for taking the past history while the examination is being done.

A useful rule is to first observe the patient's general physique and habitus and then to carefully inspect the hands. Many systemic diseases show themselves in the hands (cirrhosis of the liver, hyperthyroidism, Raynaud's disease, pulmonary insufficiency, heart disease, and nutritional disorders).

Details of the examination cannot be included here. The beginner is urged to consult special texts.

Inspection, palpation, and auscultation are the time-honored essential steps in appraising both the normal and the abnormal. Comparison of the two sides of the body often suggests a specific abnormality. The slight droop of one eyelid characteristic of Horner's syndrome can only be recognized by comparison with the opposite side. Inspection of the female breasts, particularly as the patient raises and lowers her arms, will often reveal slight dimpling indicative of an infiltrating carcinoma barely detectable on palpation.

Successful palpation requires skill and gentleness. Spasm, tension, and anxiety caused by painful examination procedures may make an adequate examination almost impossible, particularly in children.

Another important feature of palpation is the laying on of hands that has been called part of the ministry of medicine. A disappointed and critical patient often will say of a doctor, "He hardly touched me." Careful, precise, and gentle palpation not only gives the physician the information being sought but also inspires confidence and trust.

When examining for areas of tenderness, it may be necessary to use only one finger in order to precisely localize the extent of the tenderness. This is of particular importance in examination of the acute abdomen.

Auscultation, once thought to be the exclusive province of the physician, is now more important in surgery than it is in medicine. Radiologic examinations, including cardiac catheterization, have relegated auscultation of the heart and lungs to the status of preliminary scanning procedures in medicine. In surgery, however, auscultation of the abdomen and peripheral vessels has become absolutely essential. The nature of ileus and the presence of a variety of vascular lesions are revealed by auscultation. Bizarre abdominal pain in a young woman can easily be ascribed to hysteria or anxiety on the basis of a negative physical examination and x-rays of the gastrointestinal tract. Auscultation of the epigastrium, however, may reveal a murmur due to obstruction of the celiac artery.

Examination of the Body Orifices

Complete examination of the ears, mouth, rectum, and pelvis is accepted as part of a complete examination. Palpation of the mouth and tongue is as essential as inspection. Every surgeon should acquire familiarity with the use of the ophthalmoscope and sigmoidoscope and should use them regularly in doing complete physical examinations.

THE EMERGENCY PHYSICAL EXAMINATION

In an emergency, the routine of the physical examination must be altered to fit the circumstances. The history may be limited to a single sentence, or there may be no history if the patient is unconscious and there are no other informants. Although the details of an accident or injury may be very useful in the total appraisal of the patient, they must be left for later consideration. The primary considerations are the following: Is the patient breathing? Is the airway open? Is there a palpable pulse? Is the heart beating? Is massive bleeding occurring?

If the patient is not breathing, airway obstruction must be ruled out by thrusting the fingers into the mouth and pulling the tongue forward. If the patient is unconscious, the respiratory tract should be intubated and mouth-to-mouth respiration started. If there is no pulse or heartbeat, start cardiac resuscitation.

Serious external loss of blood from an extremity can be controlled by elevation and pressure. Tourniquets are rarely required.

Every victim of major blunt trauma should be suspected of having a vertebral injury capable of causing damage to the spinal cord unless rough handling is avoided.

Some injuries are so life-threatening that action must be taken before even a limited physical examination is done. Penetrating wounds of the heart, large open sucking wounds of the chest, massive crush injuries with flail chest, and massive external bleeding all require emergency treatment before any further examination can be done.

In most emergencies, however, after it has been established that the airway is open, the heart is beating, and there is no massive external hemorrhage—and after antishock measures have been instituted, if necessary—a rapid survey examination must be done. Failure to perform such an examination can lead to serious mistakes in the care of the patient. It takes no more than 2 or 3 minutes to carefully examine the head, thorax, abdomen, extremities, genitalia (particularly in females), and back. If cervical cord damage has been ruled out, it is essential to turn the injured patient and carefully inspect the back, buttocks, and perineum.

Tension pneumothorax and cardiac tamponade may easily be overlooked if there are multiple injuries.

Upon completion of the survey examination, control of pain, splinting of fractured limbs, suturing of lacerations, and other types of emergency treatment can be started.

LABORATORY & OTHER EXAMINATIONS

Laboratory Examination

Laboratory examinations in surgical patients have the following objectives: (1) screening for asymptomatic disease that may affect the surgical result (eg, unsuspected anemia or diabetes); (2) appraisal of diseases that may contraindicate elective surgery or require treatment before surgery (eg, diabetes, heart failure); (3) diagnosis of disorders that require surgery (eg, hyperparathyroidism, pheochromocytoma); and (4) evaluation of the nature and extent of metabolic or septic complications.

Patients undergoing major surgery, even though they seem to be in excellent health except for their surgical disease, should have age-appropriate laboratory examination. A history of renal, hepatic, or heart disease requires detailed studies. Medical consultation may be helpful in the total preoperative appraisal of the surgical patient. It is essential, however, that the surgeon not become totally dependent upon a medical consultant for the preoperative evaluation and management of the patient. The total management must be the surgeon's responsibility and is not to be delegated. Moreover, the surgeon is the only one with the experience and background to interpret the meaning of laboratory tests in the light of other features of the case—particularly the history and physical findings.

Imaging Studies

Modern patient care calls for a variety of critical radiologic examinations. The closest cooperation between the radiologist and the surgeon is essential if serious mistakes are to be avoided. This means that the surgeon must not refer the patient to the radiologist, requesting a particular examination, without providing an adequate account of the history and physical findings. Particularly in emergency situations, review of the films and consultation are needed.

When the radiologic diagnosis is not definitive, the examinations must be repeated in the light of the history and physical examination. Despite the great accuracy of x-ray diagnosis, a negative gastrointestinal study still does not exclude either ulcer or a neoplasm; particularly in the right colon, small lesions are easily overlooked. At times, the history and physical findings are so clearly diagnostic that operation is justifiable despite negative imaging studies.

Special Examinations

Special examinations such as cystoscopy, gastroscopy, esophagoscopy, colonoscopy, angiography, and bronchoscopy are often required in the diagnostic appraisal of surgical disorders. The surgeon must be familiar with the indications and limitations of these procedures and be prepared to consult with colleagues in medicine and the surgical specialties as required.

Preoperative Care

2

Gerard M. Doherty, MD

The care of the patient with a major surgical problem commonly involves distinct phases of management that occur in the following sequence:

(1) Preoperative care
Diagnostic workup
Preoperative evaluation
Preoperative preparation
(2) Anesthesia and operation
(3) Postoperative care
Postanesthetic observation
Intensive care
Intermediate care
Convalescent care

DEFINITIONS & OBJECTIVES

Preoperative Care

The **diagnostic workup** is concerned primarily with determining the cause and extent of the present illness. **Preoperative evaluation** consists of an overall assessment of the patient's general health in order to identify significant abnormalities that might increase operative risk or adversely influence recovery. **Preoperative preparation** includes interventions dictated by the findings on diagnostic workup and preoperative evaluation, and by the nature of the expected operation.

Postoperative Care

The **postanesthetic observation** phase of management is the few hours immediately after operation during which the acute reaction to operation and the residual effects of anesthesia subside. A postanesthetic recovery unit with special staff and equipment is usually provided for this purpose. Patients who need continued cardiopulmonary support or continued invasive monitoring to avoid major morbidity and death should be transferred to an intensive care unit.

Intermediate care is usually provided on an inpatient nursing unit until the patient's recovery can continue at home during the convalescent phase.

The Continuum of Surgical Care

The continuum of surgical care has been represented above as progressing through a series of pre- and postoperative phases. In practice, these phases merge, overlap, and vary in relative importance from patient to patient. Complications, death, and the therapeutic end result in the surgical patient depend upon the competence with which each succeeding phase is managed. The rapid progression and severe episodic stress of major surgical illness leave small margin for errors in management. The care immediately preceding and following operation, which includes preoperative evaluation and preparation and postanesthetic observation and intensive care, is especially critical. The increased complexity of surgical critical care has resulted in a team approach to the ICU patient, with management directed by the primary surgeon and the critical care specialists in the ICU, whose role it is to maintain optimum care.

PREOPERATIVE EVALUATION

General Health Assessment

The initial diagnostic workup of the surgical patient is focused on the cause of the presenting complaints. Except in strictly minor surgical illness, this initial workup should be supplemented by a complete assessment of the patient's general health. This evaluation, which should be completed prior to all major operations, seeks to identify abnormalities that may influence operative risk or may have a bearing on the patient's future well-being. Preoperative evaluation includes at least a complete history and physical examination. The evaluation should initially focus on the clinical assessment of risk based on the patient's history and current symptoms. This assessment should guide the remainder of the evaluation. Bleeding tendencies, medications currently being taken, and allergies and reactions to antibiotics and other agents should be noted and prominently displayed on the chart.

The physical examination should be thorough and must include neurologic examination and assessment of peripheral arterial pulses (carotid, radial, femoral, popliteal, posterior tibial, and dorsalis pedis). The adequacy of circulating blood volume can be determined by the adequacy of peripheral perfusion, the fullness of neck veins in the supine and partially erect positions, and tests for orthostatic changes in blood pressure and pulse. Severe cardiovascular disease will make these parameters much more difficult to interpret. Patients who are prone to a hypovolemic state include those with significant weight loss as a result of cancer, gastrointestinal disease, or drugs such as diuretics. Peripheral vascular disease should be suspected if there is a history of transient ischemic attacks, claudication, or diabetes. If a carotid bruit is found, other studies may be indicated to specifically evaluate for stenosis. Rectal examination and pelvic examination should be performed as dictated by the patient's specific disease and health-maintenance examination schedule.

All significant complaints, physical findings, and test abnormalities should be adequately evaluated by appropriate further tests, examinations, and consultations. Practice in the United States has generally included a complete blood count and serum electrolyte measurements for patients over 40 and a chest x-ray and electrocardiogram for those over 50. Although these recommendations are simple to apply, they are not entirely supported by the medical literature and may result in more testing than is absolutely necessary. All test results must be interpreted in the context of the individual patient. For example, a hemoglobin of 8 g/dL is generally physiologically safe for tissue oxygen delivery but may be inadequate in the patient with reduced cardiac output. The adequacy of liver and kidney function should be tested if impairment is suspected, because each organ plays a major role in the response to and clearance of various anesthetic agents both preoperatively and intraoperatively. Selection of the ideal agent depends on recognition of liver or renal impairment in the preoperative period. Psychiatric consultation should be considered in patients with a history of significant mental disorder that may be exacerbated by operation and in patients whose complaints may have a psychoneurotic basis.

If the scheduled procedure will or may require blood replacement, the preoperative preparation should include planning for that possibility. Appropriate strategies may include storing autologous blood in the weeks prior to operation to allow reinfusion, directed-donor blood storage for transfusion, or phlebotomy and hemodilution immediately preoperatively with subsequent reinfusion.

In summary, the preoperative evaluation should be comprehensive to assess the patient's overall state of health, to determine the risk of the impending surgical treatment, and to guide the preoperative preparation.

Garcia-Miguel FJ, Serrano-Aguilar PG, Lopez-Bastida J: Preoperative assessment. Lancet 2003;362:1749.

Halaszynski TM, Juda R, Silverman DG: Optimizing postoperative outcomes with efficient preoperative assessment and management. Crit Care Med 2004;32:S76.

Specific Factors Affecting Operative Risk

A. The Compromised or Altered Host

Patients may be considered compromised or altered hosts if significant impairment of systems and tissues does not permit a normal response to operative trauma or infection. Preoperative recognition of an abnormal nutritional or immune state is of obvious importance.

1. Nutritional assessment—Malnutrition leads to a significant increase in the operative death rate. Weight loss of more than 20% caused by illness such as cancer or intestinal disease not only results in a higher death rate but also a greater than threefold increase in the postoperative infection rate. There is no one best way to determine nutritional status, but it is clear that dietary history is of major importance in the assessment, as is a working knowledge of the basic nutritional deficiencies associated with certain disease states, particularly vitamin deficiencies. Standard biochemical parameters that indicate impairment in the visceral protein mass include a serum albumin of less than 3 g/dL or a serum transferrin of less than 150 mg/dL.

Even when malnutrition is diagnosed, the utility of short-term (7–10 days) preoperative hyperalimentation is not clear. It is known that nutrition can improve wound healing and immune function. Current indications for supportive measures before elective surgery include a history of weight loss in excess of 10% of body weight or an anticipated prolonged postoperative recovery period during which the patient will not be fed orally.

2. Assessment of immune competence—Increased knowledge and appreciation of immune defenses have led to a greater awareness of the increased postoperative rates of complications and death due to infection in patients with immune deficiency disorders. Many immune deficiency states are linked to malnutrition. Total lymphocyte count and cell-mediated immunity measurement are the two most commonly performed tests. Anergy or impaired immunity is diagnosed if no response is noted to any of the skin tests, whereas a positive response (5 mm or more of induration at the test site) to one or more skin tests indicates normal lymphocyte activity. Anergy is associated with an increased susceptibility to infectious complications. Other more specific tests include neutrophil chemotaxis and measurements of specific lymphocyte populations. Patients at high risk for immune deficiency in whom this information is helpful include elderly patients and those with malnutrition, severe trauma or burns, or cancer.

3. Other factors leading to increased infection— Certain drugs may reduce the patient's resistance to infection by interfering with host defense mechanisms. Corticosteroids, immunosuppressive agents, cytotoxic drugs, and prolonged antibiotic therapy are associated with an increased incidence of invasion by fungi and other organisms not commonly encountered in infections. A high rate of wound, pulmonary, and other infections is observed in renal failure, presumably as a result of decreased host resistance. Granulocytopenia and diseases that may produce immunologic deficiency—eg, lymphomas, leukemias, and hypogammaglobulinemia—are frequently associated with septic complications. The uncontrolled diabetic patient is also more susceptible to infection (see Chapter 5).

B. Pulmonary Dysfunction

The patient with compromised preoperative pulmonary function is susceptible to postoperative pulmonary complications, including hypoxia, atelectasis, and pneumonia. Preoperative evaluation of the degree of respiratory impairment is necessary in patients at high risk for postoperative complications. This evaluation includes a history of heavy smoking and cough, obesity, advanced age, and known pulmonary disease, particularly before major intrathoracic or upper abdominal surgery. Pertinent factors in the history include the presence and character of cough and excessive sputum production, history of wheezing, and exercise tolerance. Pertinent physical findings include the presence of wheezing or prolonged expiration. A chest x-ray, ECG, blood gases, and some basic pulmonary function tests are useful preoperative studies in these patients. Although evaluation of arterial oxygen tension is helpful, the major reason for obtaining preoperative blood gases is to evaluate for CO_2 retention, which indicates severe pulmonary dysfunction. If surgery is necessary, supplemental oxygen must be used carefully in the postoperative period, because overuse may accentuate CO_2 retention and aggravate concomitant respiratory acidosis. The most helpful screening pulmonary function tests are forced vital capacity (FVC) and forced expiratory volume in 1 second (FEV_1). Values less than 50% of predicted, based on age and body size, indicate significant airway disease with a high risk for complications.

Preoperative pulmonary preparation for a period as short as 48 hours has been shown to significantly decrease postoperative complications. Even a few days of abstinence from smoking will decrease sputum production. Oral or inhaled bronchodilators along with twice-daily chest physical therapy and postural drainage will help clear inspissated secretions from the airway. Before operation, patients should be instructed in techniques of coughing, deep breathing, and use of one of the incentive spirometry devices that increase inspiratory effort.

C. Delayed Wound Healing

This problem can be anticipated in certain categories of patients whose tissue repair process may be compromised. Important factors include protein depletion, ascorbic acid deficiency, marked dehydration or edema, severe anemia, diabetes mellitus, and smoking. The most important component is maintenance of adequate blood volume and perfusion. Decreased perfusion results in a marked decrease in tissue oxygen tension, which in turn correlates with delayed wound healing or infection. Often the decrease is not clinically evident, but it can be expected to occur in patients receiving chronic diuretic therapy or those with underlying myocardial dysfunction. Large doses of corticosteroids depress wound healing in humans. Wounds in patients who have received appreciable doses of corticosteroids preoperatively should be closed with special care to prevent disruption and managed postoperatively as though healing will be delayed.

Operation can be required on a patient receiving cytotoxic chemotherapy for malignancy. These drugs usually interfere with cell proliferation and tend to decrease the tensile strength of the surgical wound. Although experimental evidence to support this assumption is equivocal, it is wise to manage wounds in patients receiving cytotoxic drugs as though healing will be slower than normal.

Decreased vascularity and other local changes occur after a few weeks or months in tissues that have been heavily irradiated. These are potential deterrents to wound healing; surgical incisions in patients who have been irradiated must be planned to avoid complications due to delayed healing in these areas if possible. Radiation therapy at levels of 3000 cGy or more are injurious to skin and to connective and vascular tissues. Chronic changes include scarring, damage to fibroblasts and collagen, and degenerative changes with subsequent hyalinization in the walls of blood vessels. Angiogenesis, observable as the capillary budding in granulation tissue and collagen formation, is inhibited when these changes are well established, so that surgical wounds in heavily irradiated tissues will heal slowly or may break down in the presence of infection. When radiation is given prior to operation, there is an optimal delay period (2–12 weeks) after completion of the radiation therapy before operation is performed in order to minimize wound complications. Technical problems in correctly timed operations for cancer are not usually increased by low-dosage (2000–4000 cGy) adjunctive radiotherapy. With radiation dosage in the therapeutic range (5000–6000 cGy), there is an increased incidence of wound complications, though this can be minimized by careful surgical technique and proper timing.

D. Drug Effects

Drug allergies, sensitivities, and incompatibilities and adverse drug effects that may be precipitated by operation must be foreseen and, if possible, prevented. A history of skin or other untoward reactions or sickness after injection, oral administration, or other use of any of the following substances should be noted so they can be avoided:

Penicillin or other antibiotic
Morphine, codeine, meperidine, or other opioid
Procaine or other anesthetic
Aspirin or other analgesic
Barbiturates
Sulfonamides
Tetanus antitoxin or other serum
Iodine, thimerosal (Merthiolate), or other germicide
Any other medication
Any foods such as eggs, milk, or chocolate
Adhesive tape

A personal or strong family history of asthma, hay fever, or other allergic disorder should alert the surgeon to possible hypersensitivity to drugs.

Drugs currently or recently taken by the patient may require continuation, dosage adjustment, or discontinuation. Medications such as digitalis, insulin, and corticosteroids must usually be maintained and their dosage carefully regulated during the operative and postoperative periods. Prolonged use of corticosteroids (even though discontinued 1 month or more preoperatively) may be associated with hypofunction of the adrenal cortex, which impairs the physiologic responses to the stress of anesthesia and operation. The standard stress dose of hydrocortisone (100 mg three times daily) is more than is required during surgical stress; however, such a patient should receive corticosteroids immediately before, during, and after operation. Anticoagulants should be discontinued for most patients and most operations. If the interval of anticoagulant discontinuation must be minimized, heparin can be used in the perioperative period.

The anesthesiologist must also be concerned with the long-term preoperative use of central nervous system depressants (eg, barbiturates, opioids, and alcohol), which may be associated with increased tolerance for anesthetic drugs; tranquilizers (eg, phenothiazine derivatives such as chlorpromazine); and antihypertensive agents, which may be associated with hypotension in response to anesthesia.

E. Risks of Thromboembolism

Increased risk factors for deep vein thrombophlebitis and pulmonary embolus include cancer, obesity, myocardial dysfunction, age over 45 years, and a prior history of thrombosis. Prophylaxis and treatment of venous thrombotic disease are discussed in Chapter 37.

F. The Elderly Patient

Operative risk should be judged on the basis of physiologic rather than chronologic age, and an elderly patient should not be denied a needed operation because of age alone. The hazard of the average major operation for the patient over age 60 years is increased only slightly provided there is no cardiovascular, renal, or other serious systemic disease. Assume that every patient over 60—even in the absence of symptoms and physical signs—has some generalized arteriosclerosis and potential limitation of myocardial and renal reserve. Accordingly, the preoperative evaluation should be comprehensive. Occult cancer is not infrequent in this age group; therefore, even minor gastrointestinal and other complaints should be thoroughly investigated by the physician.

Administer intravenous fluids with care so as not to overload the circulation. Monitoring of intake, output, body weight, serum electrolytes, and central venous pressure is important in evaluating cardiorenal response and tolerance in this age group.

Aged patients generally require smaller doses of strong narcotics and are frequently depressed by routine doses. Codeine is usually well tolerated. Sedative and hypnotic drugs often cause restlessness, mental confusion, and uncooperative behavior in the elderly and should be used cautiously. Preanesthetic medications should be limited to atropine or scopolamine in the debilitated elderly patient, and anesthetic agents should be administered in minimal amounts.

G. The Obese Patient

Obese patients have an increased frequency of concomitant disease and a high incidence of postoperative wound complications. A controlled preoperative weight loss program is often beneficial before elective procedures.

Halaszynski TM, Juda R, Silverman DG: Optimizing postoperative outcomes with efficient preoperative assessment and management. Crit Care Med 2004;32:S76.

Consultations

The opinion of a qualified consultant should be obtained when it may be of benefit to the patient, when requested by the patient or family members, or when it may be of medicolegal importance. The physician should take the initiative in arranging consultation when the treatment proposed is controversial or exceptionally risky, when dangerous complications occur, or when the physician senses that the patient or family members are unduly apprehensive regarding the plan of management or the course of events. Consultation with cardiac or other medical or surgical specialists preoperatively is important if the patient has abnormal findings in their fields of competence. It is also beneficial for the specialist consultant to become acquainted with the patient and the condition preoperatively when the possibility exists that the consultant will be called upon for advice later in connection with a postoperative complication or development.

Anesthesia consultation is always requested prior to major surgery. In poor-risk patients, this consultation should be requested several days in advance of operation if possible. The patient's prospects for a smooth and uncomplicated anesthetic experience are greatly improved by the anesthesiologist's preoperative evaluation and advice. The assessment classifies the patient as follows:

Class 1: Healthy
Class 2: Mild systemic disease
Class 3: Severe but not incapacitating disease
Class 4: Severe disease, constant threat to life
Class 5: Moribund patient not expected to survive for 24 hours

Preoperative Note

When the diagnostic workup and preoperative evaluation have been completed, all details should be reviewed and a preoperative note written in the chart. The note summarizes the pertinent findings and decisions, gives the indications for the operation proposed, and attests that there has been a discussion of the complications and risks of the operation between surgeon and patient (ie, informed consent has been obtained). This constitutes a final check on the adequacy of the analysis of the patient's problem, the need for treatment, and the patient's understanding of these facts.

PREOPERATIVE PREPARATION

Major operations create surgical wounds and cause severe stress, subjecting the patient to the hazard of infection and metabolic and other derangements. Appropriate preoperative preparation facilitates wound healing and systemic recovery by making certain that the patient's condition is optimal. Operation also results in psychic trauma to the patient and to family members and has significant medicolegal implications, all of which deserve special consideration preoperatively to avoid postoperative repercussions. In emergency conditions, time for preparation is limited but is usually sufficient to permit the principles of good surgical preparation to be followed. In elective operation, meticulous preoperative preparation is both possible and mandatory and includes the following steps.

Informing the Patient

Surgery is a frightening prospect for both patient and family. Their psychologic preparation and reassurance should begin at the initial contact with the surgeon. Appropriate explanation of the nature and purpose of preoperative studies and treatments establishes confidence. When all pertinent information has been gathered, it is the surgeon's responsibility to describe the planned surgical procedure and its risks and possible consequences in understandable terms to the patient and usually also to the next of kin. The potential need for blood transfusion must be addressed. This discussion must be documented in the chart. It is also very helpful to explain to the patient what will happen in the operating room before induction of anesthesia and in the recovery room. Similarly, prompt postoperative interpretation of pertinent findings and prospects to patient and family contributes to rapport and to cooperation during the recovery period.

Operative Permit

The patient or the patient's legal guardian must sign (in advance) a permit authorizing a major or minor operation. The nature, risk, and probable result of the operation or procedure must be made clear to the patient or a legally responsible relative or guardian so that the signed permit will constitute informed consent. A signed consent is not valid except for the specific operation or procedure for which it was obtained.

Emergency lifesaving operations or procedures may have to be done without a permit. In such cases, every effort should be made to obtain adequate consultation. The situation should be carefully documented in the chart.

Legal and institutional requirements regarding permits vary. It is essential that the physician understand and follow local regulations.

Asepsis & Antisepsis in the Prevention of Wound Infection

Protection of the surgical patient from infection is a primary consideration throughout the preoperative, operative, and postoperative phases of care. The factor of host resistance that influences the individual patient's susceptibility to infection has been discussed above. The incidence and severity of infection, particularly wound sepsis, are related also to the bacteriologic status of the hospital environment and to the care with which basic principles of asepsis, antisepsis, and surgical technique are implemented. The entire hospital environment must be protected from undue bacterial contamination in order to avoid colonization and cross-infection of surgical patients with virulent strains of bacteria that will invade surgical wounds in the operating room in spite of aseptic precautions taken during operation. Prevention of wound infection therefore involves both application of general concepts and techniques of antisepsis and asepsis in the hospital at large and the use of specific procedures in preparation for operation.

A. Sterilization

The only completely reliable methods of sterilization in wide current use for surgical instruments and supplies are (1) steam under pressure (autoclaving), (2) dry heat, and (3) ethylene oxide gas.

1. Autoclaving—Saturated steam at a pressure of 750 mm Hg (14.5 psi above atmospheric pressure) at a temperature of 120 °C destroys all vegetative bacteria and most resistant dry spores in 13 minutes. Sterilization time is markedly shortened by the high-vacuum or high-pressure autoclaves now widely used.

2. Dry heat—Exposure to continuous dry heat at 170 °C for 1 hour will sterilize articles that would be spoiled by moist heat or are more conveniently kept dry. If grease or oil is present on instruments, safe sterilization calls for a 4-hour exposure at 160 °C.

3. Gas sterilization—Liquid and gaseous ethylene oxide as a sterilizing agent will destroy bacteria, viruses, molds, pathogenic fungi, and spores. It is also flammable and toxic, and it will cause severe burns if it comes in contact with the skin. Gas sterilization with ethylene oxide is an excellent method for sterilization of most heat-sensitive materials, including telescopic instruments, plastic and rubber goods, sharp and delicate instruments, and miscellaneous items such as electric cords and sealed ampules. It has largely replaced soaking in antiseptics as a means of sterilizing materials that cannot withstand autoclaving. Gas sterilization is normally carried out in a pressure vessel (gas autoclave) at slightly elevated pressure and temperature. Following sterilization, a variable period of time is required for dissipation of the gas from the materials sterilized. Solid metal or glass items such as knives, drills, and thermometers may be used immediately following sterilization. Lensed instruments and packs including cloth, paper, rubber, and other porous items must usually be kept on the shelf exposed to air for 24–48 hours before use. Certain types of materials or complex instruments, such as a cardiac pacemaker, may require 7 days of exposure to air before use.

B. Skin Antiseptics

The most important applications of skin antiseptics are the hand scrub of the operating team and the preparation of the operative field.

1. Hand scrub routine—Although the duration of the hand scrub is not universally defined, a 5-minute scrub before the first case—provided a brush is used—appears to be sufficient. Greatest attention should be paid to the fingertips and nails, since these areas harbor the greatest numbers of bacteria. A 2-minute scrub is adequate between cases. Solutions containing chlorhexidine or one of the iodophors appear to be most effective. Other skin antisepsis techniques, such as the use of alcohol-based skin lotions applied to clean hands for 1 minute and allowed to dry on the skin, also are effective at decreasing skin colonization.

2. Preparation of the operative field—Initial preparation of the skin is usually done the afternoon or evening before operation. The area should be washed with soap and water, making sure that it is grossly quite clean. A shower is satisfactory. The type of soap used makes little difference. Soap is a weak antiseptic and is useful because of its nonirritating detergent action, especially when washing is combined with mechanical friction.

For elective operations involving areas with high levels of resident bacteria (eg, hands, feet) or likely to be irritated by strong antiseptics (eg, face, genitalia), preoperative degerming of the skin can be improved by repeated use of chlorhexidine gluconate (Hibiclens). Instruct the patient to wash the area several times daily with one of these preparations (and with nothing else) for 3–5 days before the scheduled day of operation. It has been established that shaving the surgical area the night before or within several hours before surgery increases the skin bacterial flora. Therefore, it is recommended that if necessary at all, shaving be performed immediately before the operation, preferably in an adjacent preparation area. Shaving may be eliminated if only fine hairs are present, as their presence has not been found to increase the incidence of infection.

3. In the operating room—A 1-minute skin preparation using either 70% alcohol or 2% iodine in 90% alcohol—followed by a polyester adherent wound drape—has been shown to be as effective in controlling wound infections as the more traditional 5- to 10-minute wound scrub with povidone-iodine.

Iodine is one of the most efficient skin antiseptics available. It rarely causes skin reactions in this concentration. Avoid streaming of iodine outside of the operative field. Do not use iodine on the perineum, genitalia, or face; on irritated or delicate skin (eg, small children); or when the patient has a history of iodine sensitivity. For iodine-sensitive patients, one can use 80% isopropyl or 70% ethyl alcohol. Apply to the skin with a gauze swab for 3 minutes and allow to dry before draping. Alternatively, tinted tincture of benzalkonium (1:750) may be used.

For sensitive areas (perineum, around the eyes, etc), apply iodophor, chlorhexidine, or 1:1000 aqueous benzalkonium solution.

Disease transmission to patients and health care workers—especially with the hepatitis virus and the AIDS virus—is a major problem in the operating room environment. Both can be transmitted to the patient and care providers by blood. Transmission to the surgeon or nurse via a needle or cut is of major concern because of the frequent occurrence of accidental punctures. Since the infected patient cannot readily be detected in the absence of a mandatory preoperative testing program, universal precautions are required, including the following:

- **a.** All health care workers should routinely use appropriate barrier precautions—gloves, masks, goggles, etc—to prevent skin and mucous membrane exposure when contact with blood or body fluids is anticipated.
- **b.** Immediate hand and other skin surface washing is necessary if contamination occurs.
- **c.** Special precautions must be taken to avoid accidental injuries, eg, needle punctures and cuts.
- **d.** Workers who have any open wounds should avoid direct patient contact.
- **e.** If a glove is torn, it should be removed and changed as promptly as patient safety permits and the needle or instrument removed from the sterile field.

C. Control of Hospital Environment

Hospital cross-infection with hemolytic, coagulase-positive *Staphylococcus aureus* and other organisms is always a potential problem. Strains endemic in hospitals are often resistant to many antimicrobial drugs as a consequence of the widespread use of these agents. Relaxation of aseptic precautions in the operating room and an unwarranted reliance on "prophylactic" antibiotics contribute to the development of resistant strains. The result may be a significant increase in the incidence of hospital-acquired wound infection, pneumonitis, and septicemia, the latter two complications especially affecting infants, the aged, and the debilitated.

Although pyogenic cocci are major offenders, enteric gram-negative bacteria (particularly the coliform and proteus groups and *Pseudomonas aeruginosa*) are increasingly prominent in hospital-acquired infections.

1. Hospital administration

- **a.** The surgical infection control program should be coordinated closely with that of other services through a hospital infection committee set up to promulgate and enforce regulations.
- **b.** All significant infections must be reported immediately. A clean wound infection rate of more than 1% indicates a need for more effective control measures. The wound infection rate should be continuously monitored on the surgical services.

2. Cultures—Obtain culture and antibiotic sensitivity studies on all significant infections.

3. Isolation—Isolate every patient with a significant source of communicable bacteria; every case of suspected communicable infection until the diagnosis has been ruled out; and every patient in whom cross-infection will be serious.

4. Aseptic technique

- **a.** The operating room should be considered an isolation zone that may be entered only by persons wearing clean operating attire (which may not be worn elsewhere).
- **b.** All open wounds should be aseptically dressed to protect them from cross-infection and to prevent heavy contamination of the environment. Eliminate dressing carts containing supplies and equipment for multiple bedside dressings.
- **c.** Hand washing before and after each contact with a patient is a simple but important routine measure in control of infection.

5. Antibiotics—Prophylactic antibiotics are indicated for clean contaminated or contaminated cases. Even for clean cases, prophylactic antibiotics may decrease the rate of infection for procedures at significant risk. When possible, antibiotic therapy should be based on sensitivity studies. Antibiotics should be given in adequate doses and discontinued as soon as it is appropriate to do so.

6. Epidemiology

- **a.** Personnel with active staphylococcal infections should be excluded from patient contact until they have recovered. Personnel carrying staphylococci in their nasal passages or gastrointestinal tracts must observe personal hygiene but need not be removed from duty unless they prove to be a focus of infection. The advisability of treatment of the carrier is uncertain, since the carrier state is frequently transient or recurrent in spite of treatment.
- **b.** Every significant infection acquired in the hospital should be investigated to determine its origin and spread, possible contacts and carriers, and whether improper techniques may have been responsible.

Association of periOperative Registered Nurses: Recommended practices for cleaning and caring for surgical instruments and powered equipment. AORN J 2002;75:627.

Association of periOperative Registered Nurses: Recommended practices for surgical hand antisepsis/hand scrubs. AORN J 2004;79:416.

Bolding B: Flash sterilization (steam). Canadian Operating Room Nursing J 2003;21:31.

Mangram AJ et al: Guideline for Prevention of Surgical Site Infection, 1999. Am J Infect Control 1999;27:97.

National Nosocomial Infections Surveillance (NNIS) System Report: Data summary from January 1992 through June 2003, issued August 2003. Am J Infect Control 2003;31:481.

Postoperative Care 3

Gerard M. Doherty, MD

The recovery from major surgery can be divided into three phases: (1) an immediate, or postanesthetic phase; (2) an intermediate phase, encompassing the hospitalization period; and (3) a convalescent phase. During the first two phases, care is principally directed at maintenance of homeostasis, treatment of pain, and prevention and early detection of complications. The convalescent phase is a transition period from the time of hospital discharge to full recovery. The trend toward earlier postoperative discharge after major surgery has shifted the venue of this period.

THE IMMEDIATE POSTOPERATIVE PERIOD

The major causes of early complications and death following major surgery are acute pulmonary, cardiovascular, and fluid derangements. The postanesthesia care unit (PACU) is staffed by specially trained personnel and provided with equipment for early detection and treatment of these problems. All patients should be monitored in this specialized unit initially following major procedures. While en route from the operating room to the PACU, the patient should be accompanied by a physician and other qualified attendants. In the PACU, the anesthesiology service generally exercises primary responsibility for cardiopulmonary function. The surgeon is responsible for the operative site and all other aspects of the care not directly related to the effects of anesthesia. The patient can be discharged from the recovery room when cardiovascular, pulmonary, and neurologic function have returned to baseline, which usually occurs 1–3 hours following operation. Patients who require continuing ventilatory or circulatory support or who have other conditions that require frequent monitoring are transferred to an intensive care unit. In this setting, nursing personnel specially trained in the management of respiratory and cardiovascular emergencies are available, and the staff to patient ratio is higher than it is on the wards. Monitoring equipment is available to enable early detection of cardiorespiratory derangements.

Postoperative Orders

Detailed treatment orders are necessary to direct postoperative care. The transfer of the patient from OR to PACU requires reiteration of any patient care orders. Unusual or particularly important orders should also be communicated to the nursing team orally. The nursing team must also be advised of the nature of the operation and the patient's condition. Postoperative orders should cover the following:

A. Monitoring

1. Vital signs—Blood pressure, pulse, and respiration should be recorded frequently until stable and then regularly until the patient is discharged from the recovery room. The frequency of vital sign measurements thereafter depends upon the nature of the operation and the course in the PACU. When an arterial catheter is in place, blood pressure and pulse should be monitored continuously. Continuous electrocardiographic monitoring is indicated for most patients in the PACU. Any major changes in vital signs should be communicated to the anesthesiologist and surgeon immediately.

2. Central venous pressure—Central venous pressure should be recorded periodically in the early postoperative period if the operation has entailed large blood losses or fluid shifts, and invasive monitoring is available. A Swan-Ganz catheter for measurement of pulmonary artery wedge pressure is indicated under these conditions if the patient has borderline cardiac or respiratory function.

3. Fluid balance—The anesthetic record includes all fluid administered as well as blood loss and urine output during the operation. This record should be continued in the postoperative period and should also include fluid losses from drains and stomas. This aids in assessing hydration and helps to guide intravenous fluid replacement. A bladder catheter can be placed for frequent measurement of urine output. In the absence of a bladder catheter, the surgeon should be notified if the patient is unable to void within 6–8 hours after operation.

4. Other types of monitoring—Depending on the nature of the operation and the patient's preexisting conditions, other types of monitoring may be necessary. Examples include measurement of intracranial pressure and level of consciousness following cranial surgery and monitoring of distal pulses following vascular surgery or in patients with casts.

B. Respiratory Care

In the early postoperative period, the patient may remain mechanically ventilated or treated with supplemental oxygen by mask or nasal prongs. These orders should be specified. For intubated patients, tracheal suctioning or other forms of respiratory therapy must be specified as required. Patients who are not intubated should do deep breathing exercises frequently to prevent atelectasis.

C. Position in Bed and Mobilization

The postoperative orders should describe any required special positioning of the patient. Unless doing so is contraindicated, the patient should be turned from side to side every 30 minutes until conscious and then hourly for the first 8–12 hours to minimize atelectasis. Early ambulation is encouraged to reduce venous stasis; the upright position helps to increase diaphragmatic excursion. Venous stasis may also be minimized by intermittent compression of the calf by pneumatic stockings.

D. Diet

Patients at risk for emesis and pulmonary aspiration should have nothing by mouth until some gastrointestinal function has returned (usually within 4 days). Most patients can tolerate liquids by mouth shortly after return to full consciousness.

E. Administration of Fluid and Electrolytes

Orders for postoperative intravenous fluids should be based on maintenance needs and the replacement of gastrointestinal losses from drains, fistulas, or stomas.

F. Drainage Tubes

Drain care should be included in the postoperative orders. Details such as type and pressure of suction, irrigation fluid and frequency, and skin exit site care should be specified. The surgeon should examine drains frequently, since the character or quantity of drain output may herald the development of postoperative complications such as bleeding or fistulas.

G. Medications

Orders should be written for antibiotics, analgesics, gastric acid suppression, deep vein thrombosis prophylaxis, and sedatives. If appropriate, preoperative medications should be reinstituted. Careful attention should be paid to replacement of corticosteroids in patients at risk, since postoperative adrenal insufficiency may be life-threatening. Other medications such as antipyretics, laxatives, and stool softeners should be used selectively as indicated.

H. Laboratory Examinations and Imaging

The use of postoperative laboratory and radiographic examinations should be to detect specific abnormalities in high-risk groups. The routine use of daily chest radiographs, blood counts, electrolytes, and renal or liver function panels is not useful.

THE INTERMEDIATE POSTOPERATIVE PERIOD

The intermediate phase starts with complete recovery from anesthesia and lasts for the rest of the hospital stay. During this time, the patient recovers most basic functions and becomes self-sufficient and able to continue convalescence at home.

Care of the Wound

Within hours after a wound is closed, the wound space fills with an inflammatory exudate. Epidermal cells at the edges of the wound begin to divide and migrate across the wound surface. By 48 hours after closure, deeper structures are completely sealed off from the external environment. Sterile dressings applied in the operating room provide protection during this period. Dressings over closed wounds should be removed on the third or fourth postoperative day. If the wound is dry, dressings need not be reapplied; this simplifies periodic inspection. Dressings should be removed earlier if they are wet, because soaked dressings increase bacterial contamination of the wound. Dressings should also be removed if the patient has manifestations of infection (such as fever or increasing wound pain). The wound should then be inspected and the adjacent area gently compressed. Any drainage from the wound should be examined by culture and Gram-stained smear. Removal of the dressing and handling of the wound during the first 24 hours should be done with aseptic technique. Medical personnel should wash their hands before and after caring for any surgical wound. Gloves should always be used when there is contact with open wounds or fresh wounds.

Generally, skin sutures or skin staples may be removed by the fifth postoperative day and replaced by tapes. Sutures should be left in longer (eg, for 2 weeks) in incisions that cross creases (eg, groin, popliteal area); for incisions closed under tension; for some incisions in the extremities (eg, the hand); and with incisions of any kind in debilitated patients. Sutures should be removed if suture tracts show signs of infection. If the incision is healing normally, the patient may be allowed to shower or bathe by the seventh postoperative day.

Fibroblasts proliferate in the wound space quickly, and by the end of the first postoperative week, new collagen is abundant in the wound. On palpation of the wound, connective tissue can be felt as a prominence (the healing ridge) and is evidence that healing is normal. Tensile strength is minimal for the first 5 days. It increases rapidly between the fifth and twentieth postoperative days and more slowly thereafter. Wounds continue to gain tensile strength slowly for about 2 years. In otherwise healthy patients, the wound should be subjected to only minor stress for 6–8 weeks. When wound healing is expected to be slower than normal (eg, in elderly or debilitated patients or those taking corticosteroids), activity should be delayed even further.

Adequate tissue perfusion is important for wound healing. In a patient with venous stasis, for example, tissue perfusion increases, and a wound of the lower extremity heals faster if the extremity is elevated and edema is eliminated. Oxygen tension has a profound effect on healing tissue. Indolent healing in an amputation stump may be substantially improved by increasing blood supply to the area by inflow procedures.

When a wound has been contaminated with bacteria during surgery, it is often best to leave the skin and subcutaneous tissues open and either to perform delayed primary closure or allow secondary closure to occur. The wound is loosely packed with fine-mesh gauze in the operating room and is left undisturbed for 4–5 days; the packing is then removed. If at this time the wound contains only serous fluid or a small amount of exudate, the skin edges can be approximated with tapes. If drainage is considerable or infection is present, the wound should be allowed to close by secondary intention. In this case, the wound should be packed with moist-to-dry dressings, which are changed once or twice daily. The patient can usually learn how to care for the wound and should be discharged as soon as his or her general condition permits. Most patients do not require visiting nurses to assist with wound care at home.

Wound healing is faster if the state of nutrition is normal and there are no specific nutritional deficits. For example, vitamin C deficiency interferes with collagen synthesis and vitamin A deficiency decreases the rate of epithelialization. Deficiencies of copper, magnesium, and other trace metals decrease the rate of scar formation. Supplemental vitamins and minerals should be given postoperatively when deficiencies are suspected, but wound healing cannot be accelerated beyond the normal rate by nutritional supplements.

Wound problems should be anticipated in patients taking corticosteroids, which inhibit the inflammatory response, fibroblast proliferation, and protein synthesis in the wound. Maturation of the scar and gain of tensile strength occur more slowly. Extra precautions include using nonabsorbable suture materials for fascial closure, delaying removal of skin stitches, and avoiding stress in the wound for 3–6 months.

Management of Drains

Drains are used either to prevent or to treat an unwanted accumulation of fluid such as pus, blood, or serum. Drains are also used to evacuate air from the pleural cavity so that the lungs can reexpand. When used prophylactically, drains are usually placed in a sterile location. Strict precautions must be taken to prevent bacteria from entering the body through the drainage tract in these situations. The external portion of the drain must be handled with aseptic technique, and the drain must be removed as soon as it is no longer useful. When drains have been placed in an infected area, there is a smaller risk of retrograde infection of the peritoneal cavity, since the infected area is usually walled off. Drains should usually be brought out through a separate incision, because drains through the operative wound increase the risk of wound infection. Closed drains connected to suction devices (Jackson-Pratt or Blake drains are two examples) are preferable to open drains (such as Penrose) that predispose to wound contamination. The quantity and quality of drainage should be recorded, and contamination minimized. When drains are no longer needed, they may be withdrawn entirely at one time if there has been little or no drainage or may be progressively withdrawn over a period of a few days.

Sump drains (such as Davol drains) have an airflow system that keeps the lumen of the drain open when fluid is not passing through it, and they must be attached to a suction device. Sump drains are especially useful when the amount of drainage is large or when drainage is likely to plug other kinds of drains. Some sump drains have an extra lumen through which saline solution can be infused to aid in keeping the tube clear. After infection has been controlled and the discharge is no longer purulent, the large-bore catheter is progressively replaced with smaller catheters, and the cavity eventually closes.

Postoperative Pulmonary Care

The changes in pulmonary function observed following anesthesia and surgery are principally the result of decreased vital capacity, functional residual capacity (FRC), and pulmonary edema. Vital capacity decreases to about 40% of the preoperative level within 1–4 hours after major intra-abdominal surgery. It remains at this level for 12–14 hours, slowly increases to 60–70% of the preoperative value by 7 days, and returns to the baseline level during the ensuing week. FRC is affected to a lesser extent. Immediately after surgery, FRC is near the preoperative level, but by 24 hours postoperatively it has decreased to about 70% of the preoperative level. It remains depressed for several days and then gradually returns to its preoperative value by the tenth day. These changes are accentuated in patients who are obese, who smoke heavily, or who have preexisting lung disease. Elderly patients are particularly vulnerable because they have decreased compliance, increased closing volume, increased residual volume, and increased dead space, all of which enhance the risk of postoperative atelectasis. In addition, reduced FEV_1 impairs the aged patient's ability to clear secretions and increases the chance of infection postoperatively.

The postoperative decrease in FRC is caused by a breathing pattern consisting of shallow tidal breaths without periodic maximal inflation. Normal human respiration includes inspiration to total lung capacity several times each hour. If these maximal inflations are eliminated, alveolar collapse begins to occur within a few hours and atelectasis with transpulmonary shunting is evident shortly thereafter. Pain is thought to be one of the main causes of shallow breathing postoperatively. Complete abolition of pain, however, does not completely restore pulmonary function. Neural reflexes, abdominal distention, obesity, and other factors that limit diaphragmatic excursion appear to be as important.

The principal means of minimizing atelectasis is deep inspiration. Periodic hyperinflation can be facilitated by using an incentive spirometer. This is particularly useful in patients with a higher risk of pulmonary complications (eg, elderly, debilitated, or markedly obese patients). Early mobilization, encouragement to take deep breaths (especially when standing), and good coaching by the nursing staff suffice for most patients.

Postoperative pulmonary edema is caused by high hydrostatic pressures (due to left ventricular failure, fluid overload, decreased oncotic pressure, etc), increased capillary permeability, or both. Edema of the lung parenchyma narrows small bronchi and increases resistance in the pulmonary vasculature. In addition, pulmonary edema may increase the risk of pulmonary infection. Adequate management of fluids postoperatively and early treatment of cardiac failure are important preventive measures.

Systemic sepsis increases capillary permeability and can lead to pulmonary edema. In the absence of deranged cardiac function or fluid overload, the development of pulmonary edema postoperatively should be regarded as evidence of sepsis.

RESPIRATORY FAILURE

Most patients tolerate the postoperative changes in pulmonary function described above and recover from them without difficulty. Patients who have marginal preoperative pulmonary function may be unable to maintain adequate ventilation in the immediate postoperative period and may develop respiratory failure. In these patients, the operative trauma and the effects of anesthesia reduce respiratory reserve below levels that can provide adequate gas exchange. In contrast to acute respiratory distress syndrome (see Chapter 13), early postoperative respiratory failure (which develops within 48 hours after the operation) is usually only a mechanical problem, ie, there are minimal alterations of the lung parenchyma. However, this problem is life-threatening and requires immediate attention.

Early respiratory failure develops most commonly in association with major operations (especially on the chest or upper abdomen), severe trauma, and preexisting lung disease. In most of these patients, respiratory failure develops over a short period (minutes to 1–2 hours) without evidence of a precipitating cause. By contrast, late postoperative respiratory failure (which develops beyond 48 hours after the operation) is usually triggered by an intercurrent event such as pulmonary embolism, abdominal distention, or opioid overdose.

Respiratory failure is manifested by tachypnea of 25–30 breaths per minute with a low tidal volume of less than 4 mL/kg. Laboratory indications are acute elevation of P_{CO_2} above 45 mm Hg, depression of P_{O_2} below 60 mm Hg, or evidence of low cardiac output. Treatment consists of immediate endotracheal intubation and ventilatory support to ensure adequate alveolar ventilation. As soon as the patient is intubated, it is important to determine whether there are any associated pulmonary problems such as atelectasis, pneumonia, or pneumothorax that require immediate treatment.

Prevention of respiratory failure requires careful postoperative pulmonary care. Atelectasis must be minimized using the techniques described above. Patients with preexisting pulmonary disease must be carefully hydrated to avoid hypovolemia. These patients must hyperventilate in order to compensate for the inefficiency of the lungs. This extra work causes greater evaporation of water and dehydration. Hypovolemia leads to dry secretions and thick sputum, which are difficult to clear from the airway. High F_{IO_2} in these patients removes the stabilizing gas N_2 from the alveoli, predisposing to alveolar collapse. In addition, it may impair the function of the respiratory center, which is driven by the relative hypoxemia, and thus further decrease ventilation. The use of epidural blocks or other methods of local analgesia in patients with COPD may prevent respiratory failure by relieving pain and permitting effective respiratory muscle function.

Postoperative Fluid & Electrolyte Management

Postoperative fluid replacement should be based on the following considerations: (1) maintenance requirements, (2) extra needs resulting from systemic factors (eg, fever, burns), (3) losses from drains, and (4) requirements resulting from tissue edema and ileus (third space losses). Daily maintenance requirements for sensible and insensible loss in the adult are about 1500–2500 mL depending on the patient's age, gender, weight, and body surface area. A rough estimate can be obtained by multiplying the patient's weight in kilograms times 30 (eg, 1800 mL/24 h in a 60-kg patient). Maintenance requirements are increased by fever, hyperventilation, and conditions that increase the catabolic rate.

For patients requiring intravenous fluid replacement for a short period (most postoperative patients), it is not necessary to measure serum electrolytes at any time during the postoperative period, but measurement is indicated in more complicated patients (those with extra fluid losses, sepsis, preexisting electrolyte abnormalities, or other factors). Assessment of the status of fluid balance requires accurate records of fluid intake and output and is aided by weighing the patient daily.

As a rule, 2000–2500 mL of 5% dextrose in normal saline or in lactated Ringer's solution is given daily. Potassium should usually not be added during the first 24 hours after surgery, because increased amounts of potassium enter the circulation during this time as a result of operative trauma and increased aldosterone activity.

In most patients, fluid loss through a nasogastric tube is less than 500 mL/d and can be replaced by increasing the infusion used for maintenance by a similar amount. About 20 meq of potassium should be added to every liter of fluid used to replace these losses. However, with the exception of urine, body fluids are isosmolar and if large volumes of gastric or intestinal juice are replaced with normal saline solution, electrolyte imbalance will eventually result. Whenever external losses from any site amount to 1500 mL/d or more, electrolyte concentrations in the fluid should be measured periodically, and the amount of replacement fluids should be adjusted to equal the amount lost. Table 3–1 lists the compositions of the most frequently used solutions.

Losses that result from fluid sequestration at the operative site are usually adequately replaced during operation, but in a patient with a large retroperitoneal dissection, severe pancreatitis, etc, third space losses may be substantial and should be considered when postoperative fluids are given.

Fluid requirements must be evaluated frequently. Intravenous orders should be rewritten every 24 hours or more often if indicated by special circumstances. Following an extensive operation, fluid needs on the first day should be reevaluated every 4–6 hours.

Postoperative Care of the Gastrointestinal Tract

Following laparotomy, gastrointestinal peristalsis temporarily decreases. Peristalsis returns in the small intestine within 24 hours, but gastric peristalsis may return more slowly. Function returns in the right colon by 48 hours and in the left colon by 72 hours. After operations on the stomach and upper intestine, propulsive activity of the upper gut can remain disorganized for 3–4 days. In the immediate postoperative period, the stomach may be decompressed with a nasogastric tube. Nasogastric intubation was once used in almost all patients undergoing laparotomy to avoid gastric distention and vomiting, but it is now recognized that routine nasogastric intubation is unnecessary and may cause postoperative atelectasis and pneumonia. For example, following cholecystectomy, pelvic operations, and colonic resections, nasogastric intubation is not needed in the average patient, and it is probably of marginal benefit following operations on the small bowel. On the other hand, nasogastric intubation is probably useful after esophageal and gastric resections and should always be used in patients with marked ileus or a very low level of consciousness (to avoid aspiration) and in patients who manifest acute gastric distention or vomiting postoperatively.

The nasogastric tube should be connected to low intermittent suction and irrigated frequently to ensure patency. The tube should be left in place for 2–3 days or until there is evidence that normal peristalsis has returned (eg, return of appetite, audible peristalsis, or passage of flatus). The nasogastric tube enhances gastroesophageal reflux, and if it is clamped overnight for assessment of residual volume, there is a slight risk of aspiration.

Table 3–1. Composition of frequently used intravenous solutions.

Solution	Glucose (g/dL)	Na^+ (meq/L)	Cl^- (meq/L)	HCO_3 (meq/L)	K^+ (meq/L)
Dextrose 5% in water	50	...	...	...	...
Dextrose 5% and sodium chloride 0.45%	50	77	77	...	...
Sodium chloride 0.9%	...	154	154	...	...
Sodium chloride 0.45%	...	77	77	...	...
Lactated Ringer's solution	...	130	109	28	4
Sodium chloride 3%	...	513	513	...	...

Once the nasogastric tube has been withdrawn, fasting is usually continued for another 24 hours, and the patient is then started on a liquid diet. Opioids may interfere with gastric motility and should be stopped in patients who have evidence of gastroparesis beyond the first postoperative week.

Gastrostomy and jejunostomy tubes should be connected to low intermittent suction or dependent drainage for the first 24 hours after surgery. Absorption of nutrients and fluids by the small intestine is not affected by laparotomy, and enteral nutrition through a jejunostomy feeding tube may therefore be started on the second postoperative day even if motility is not entirely normal. Gastrostomy or jejunostomy tubes should not be removed before the third postoperative week, because firm adhesions should be allowed to develop between the viscera and the parietal peritoneum.

After most operations in areas other than the peritoneal cavity, the patient may be allowed to resume a regular diet as soon as the effects of anesthesia have completely worn off.

Postoperative Pain

Severe pain is a common sequela of intrathoracic, intraabdominal, and major bone or joint procedures. About 60% of such patients perceive their pain to be severe, 25% moderate, and 15% mild. In contrast, following superficial operations on the head and neck, limbs, or abdominal wall, less than 15% of patients characterize their pain as severe. The factors responsible for these differences include duration of surgery, degree of operative trauma, type of incision, and magnitude of intraoperative retraction. Gentle handling of tissues, expedient operations, and good muscle relaxation help lessen the severity of postoperative pain.

While factors related to the nature of the operation influence postoperative pain, it is also true that the same operation produces different amounts of pain in different patients. This varies according to individual physical, emotional, and cultural characteristics. Much of the emotional aspect of pain can be traced to anxiety. Feelings such as helplessness, fear, and uncertainty contribute to anxiety and may heighten the patient's perception of pain.

It was once thought that anesthesia and analgesia in neonates and infants was too risky and that these young patients did not perceive pain. It is now known that reduction of pain with appropriate techniques actually decreases morbidity from major surgery in this age group.

The physiology of postoperative pain involves transmission of pain impulses via splanchnic (not vagal) afferent fibers to the central nervous system, where they initiate spinal, brain stem, and cortical reflexes. Spinal responses result from stimulation of neurons in the anterior horn, resulting in skeletal muscle spasm, vasospasm, and gastrointestinal ileus. Brain stem responses to pain include alterations in ventilation, blood pressure, and endocrine function. Cortical responses include voluntary movements and psychologic changes, such as fear and apprehension. These emotional responses facilitate nociceptive spinal transmission, lower the threshold for pain perception, and perpetuate the pain experience.

Postoperative pain serves no useful purpose and may cause alterations in pulmonary, circulatory, gastrointestinal, and skeletal muscle function that set the stage for postoperative complications. Pain following thoracic and upper abdominal operations, for example, causes voluntary and involuntary splinting of thoracic and abdominal muscles and the diaphragm. The patient may be reluctant to breathe deeply, promoting atelectasis. The limitation in motion due to pain sets the stage for venous stasis, thrombosis, and embolism. Release of catecholamines and other stress hormones by postoperative pain causes vasospasm and hypertension, which may in turn lead to complications such as stroke, myocardial infarction, and bleeding. Prevention of postoperative pain is thus important for reasons other than the pain itself. Effective pain control may improve the outcome of major operations.

A. Physician-Patient Communication

Close attention to the patient's needs, frequent reassurance, and genuine concern help minimize postoperative pain. Spending a few minutes with the patient every day in frank discussions of progress and any complications does more to relieve pain than many physicians realize.

B. Parenteral Opioids

Opioids are the mainstay of therapy for postoperative pain. Their analgesic effect is via two mechanisms: (1) a direct effect on opioid receptors and (2) stimulation of a descending brain stem system that contributes to pain inhibition. Although substantial relief of pain may be achieved with opioids, they do not modify reflex phenomena associated with pain, such as muscle spasm. Opioids administered intramuscularly, while convenient, result in wide variations in plasma concentrations. This, as well as the wide variations in dosage required for analgesia among patients, reduces analgesic efficacy. Physician and nurse attitudes reflect a persistent misunderstanding of the pharmacology and psychology of pain control. Frequently, the dose of opioid prescribed or administered is too small and too infrequent. When opioid usage is limited to temporary treatment of postoperative pain, drug addiction is extremely rare.

Morphine is the most widely used opioid for treatment of postoperative pain. Morphine may be administered intravenously, either intermittently or continuously. Except as discussed below in the section on patient-controlled analgesia, these last methods require close supervision and are impractical except in the PACU or intensive care unit. Side effects of morphine include respiratory depression, nausea and vomiting, and clouded sensorium. In the setting of severe postoperative pain, however, respiratory depression is rare, because pain itself is a powerful respiratory stimulant.

Meperidine is an opioid with about one-eighth the potency of morphine. It provides a similar quality of pain control with similar side effects. The duration of pain relief is somewhat shorter than with morphine. Like morphine, meperidine may be given intravenously, but the same requirements for monitoring apply.

Other opioids useful for postoperative analgesia include hydromorphone and methadone. Hydromorphone is usually administered in a dose of 1–2 mg intramuscularly every 2–3 hours. Methadone is given intramuscularly or orally in an average dose of 10 mg every 4–6 hours. The main advantage of methadone is its long half-life (6–10 hours) and its ability to prevent withdrawal symptoms in patients with morphine dependence.

C. Nonopioid Parenteral Analgesics

Ketorolac tromethamine is a nonsteroidal anti-inflammatory drug (NSAID) with potent analgesic and moderate anti-inflammatory activities. It is available in injectable form suitable for postoperative use. In controlled trials, ketorolac (30 mg) has demonstrated analgesic efficacy roughly equivalent to that of morphine (10 mg). A potential advantage over morphine is its lack of respiratory depression. Gastrointestinal ulceration, impaired coagulation, and reduced renal function—all potential complications of NSAID use—have not yet been reported with short-term perioperative use of ketorolac.

D. Oral Analgesics

Within several days following most abdominal surgical procedures, the severity of pain decreases to a point where oral analgesics suffice. Aspirin should be avoided as an analgesic postoperatively, since it interferes with platelet function, prolongs bleeding time, and interferes with the effects of anticoagulants. For most patients, a combination of acetaminophen with codeine (eg, Tylenol No. 3) or propoxyphene (Darvocet-N 50 or -N 100) suffices. Hydrocodone with acetaminophen (Vicodin) is a synthetic opioid with properties similar to those of codeine. For more severe pain, oxycodone is available in combination with aspirin (Percodan) or acetaminophen (Percocet, Tylox). Oxycodone is an opioid with slightly less potency than morphine. As with all opioids, tolerance develops with long-term use.

E. Patient-Controlled Analgesia

Patient-controlled analgesia (PCA) puts the frequency of analgesic administration under the patient's control but within safe limits. A device containing a timing unit, a pump, and the analgesic medication is connected to an intravenous line. By pressing a button, the patient delivers a predetermined dose of analgesic (usually morphine, 1–3 mg). The timing unit prevents overdosage by interposing an inactivation period (usually 6–8 minutes) between patient-initiated doses. The possibility of overdosage is also limited by the fact that the patient must be awake in order to search for and push the button that delivers the morphine. The dose and timing can be changed by medical personnel to accommodate the needs of the patient. This method appears to improve pain control and even reduces the total dose of opioid given in a 24-hour period. The addition of a background continuous infusion to the patient-directed administration of analgesic appears to offer no advantage over PCA alone.

F. Continuous Epidural Analgesia

Opioids are also effective when administered directly into the epidural space. Topical morphine does not depress proprioceptive pathways in the dorsal horn, but it does affect nociceptive pathways by interacting with opioid receptors. Therefore, epidural opioids produce intense, prolonged segmental analgesia with relatively less respiratory depression or sympathetic, motor, or other sensory disturbances. In comparison with parenteral administration, epidural administration requires similar dosage for control of pain, has a slightly delayed onset of action, provides substantially longer pain relief, and is associated with better preservation of pulmonary function. Epidural morphine is usually administered as a continuous infusion at a rate of 0.2–0.8 mg/h with or without the addition of 0.25% bupivacaine. Analgesia produced by this technique is superior to that of intravenous or intramuscular opioids. Patients managed in this way are more alert and have better gastrointestinal function. Side effects of continuous epidural administration of morphine include pruritus, nausea, and urinary retention. Respiratory depression may occur. Because the patient is unable to urinate, bladder catheterization is almost always required.

G. Intercostal Block

Intercostal block may be used to decrease pain following thoracic and abdominal operations. Since the block does not include the visceral afferents, it does not relieve pain completely, but it does eliminate muscle spasm induced by cutaneous pain and helps to restore respiratory function. It does not carry the risk of hypotension—as does continuous epidural analgesia—

and it produces analgesia for periods of 3–12 hours. The main disadvantage of intercostal blocks is the risk of pneumothorax and the need for repeated injections. These problems can be minimized by placing a catheter in the intercostal space or in the pleura through which a continuous infusion of bupivacaine 0.5% is delivered at a rate of 3–8 mL/h.

REFERENCES

Wound Healing

Clark MA, Plank LD, Hill GL: Wound healing associated with severe surgical illness. World J Surg 2000;24:648.

Hunt TK, Hopf HW: Wound healing and wound infection. What surgeons and anesthesiologists can do. Surg Clin North Am 1997;77:587.

Singer AJ, Clark RA: Cutaneous wound healing. N Engl J Med 1999;341:738.

Wilmore DW: Metabolic response to severe surgical illness: overview. World J Surg 2000;24:705.

Witte MB, Barbul A: General principles of wound healing. Surg Clin North Am 1997;77:509.

Fluid Therapy

Kim PK, Deutschman CS: Inflammatory responses and mediators. Surg Clin North Am 2000;80:885.

Plank LD, Hill GL: Sequential metabolic changes following induction of systemic inflammatory response in patients with severe sepsis or major blunt trauma. World J Surg 2000;24:630.

Rooke GA: Autonomic and cardiovascular function in the geriatric patient. Anesthesiol Clin North Am 2000;18:31.

Pain

Austrup ML, Korean G: Analgesic agents for the postoperative period. Opioids. Surg Clin North Am 1999;79:253.

Buggy DJ, Smith G: Epidural anaesthesia and analgesia: better outcome after major surgery? Growing evidence suggests so. BMJ 1999;319:530.

Etches RC: Patient-controlled analgesia. Surg Clin North Am 1999;79:297.

Grass JA: The role of epidural anesthesia and analgesia in postoperative outcome. Anesthesiol Clin North Am 2000;18:407.

Krauss B, Green SM: Sedation and analgesia for procedures in children. N Engl J Med 2000;342:938.

Power I, Barratt S: Analgesic agents for the postoperative period. Nonopioids. Surg Clin North Am 1999;79:275.

Rawal N: Epidural and spinal agents for postoperative analgesia. Surg Clin North Am 1999;79:313.

Sorkin LS, Wallace MS: Acute pain mechanisms. Surg Clin North Am 1999;79:213.

Wiklund RA, Rosenbaum SH: Anesthesiology. First of two parts. N Engl J Med 1997;337:1132.

Wiklund RA, Rosenbaum SH: Anesthesiology. Second of two parts. N Engl J Med 1997;337:1215.

Postoperative Complications*

4

Gerard M. Doherty, MD

Postoperative complications may result from the primary disease, the operation, or unrelated factors. Occasionally, one complication results from another previous one (eg, myocardial infarction following massive postoperative bleeding). The clinical signs of disease are often blurred in the postoperative period. Early detection of postoperative complications requires repeated evaluation of the patient by the operating surgeon and other team members.

Prevention of complications starts in the preoperative period with evaluation of the patient's disease and risk factors. Improving the health of the patient before surgery is one goal of the preoperative evaluation. For example, cessation of smoking for 6 weeks before surgery decreases the incidence of postoperative pulmonary complications from 50% to 10%. Correction of gross obesity decreases intra-abdominal pressure and the risk of wound and respiratory complications and improves ventilation postoperatively.

The surgeon should explain the operation and the expected postoperative course to the patient and family. The preoperative hospital stay, if one is necessary, should be as short as possible both to reduce costs and to minimize exposure to antibiotic-resistant microorganisms. Adequate training in respiratory exercises planned for the postoperative period substantially decreases the incidence of postoperative pulmonary complications.

Early mobilization, proper respiratory care, and careful attention to fluid and electrolyte needs are important. On the evening after surgery the patient should be encouraged to sit up, cough, breathe deeply, and walk, if possible. The upright position permits expansion of basilar lung segments, and walking increases the circulation of the lower extremities and lessens the danger of venous thromboembolism. In severely ill patients, continuous monitoring of systemic blood pressure and cardiac performance enables identification and correction of mild derangements before they become severe. Other aspects of prevention of complications are discussed in Chapters 3 and 5.

WOUND COMPLICATIONS

Hematoma

Wound hematoma, a collection of blood and clot in the wound, is one of the most common wound complications and is almost always caused by imperfect hemostasis. Patients receiving aspirin or low-dose heparin have a slightly higher risk of developing this complication. The risk is much higher in patients who have been given systemically effective doses of anticoagulants and those with preexisting coagulopathies. Vigorous coughing or marked arterial hypertension immediately after surgery may contribute to the formation of a wound hematoma.

Hematomas produce elevation and discoloration of the wound edges, discomfort, and swelling. Blood sometimes leaks through skin sutures. Neck hematomas following operations on the thyroid, parathyroid, or carotid artery are particularly dangerous, because they may expand rapidly and compromise the airway. Small hematomas may resorb, but they increase the incidence of wound infection. Treatment in most cases consists of evacuation of the clot under sterile conditions, ligation of bleeding vessels, and reclosure of the wound.

Seroma

A seroma is a fluid collection in the wound other than pus or blood. Seromas often follow operations that involve elevation of skin flaps and transection of numerous lymphatic channels (eg, mastectomy, operations in the groin). Seromas delay healing and increase the risk of wound infection. Those located under skin flaps can usually be evacuated by needle aspiration. Compression dressings should then be applied to seal lymphatic leaks and prevent reaccumulation. Small seromas that recur may be treated by repeated evacuation. Seromas of the groin, which are common after vascular operations, are best left to resorb without aspiration, since the risks of introducing a needle (infection, disruption of vascular structures, etc) are greater than the risk associated with the seroma itself. If seromas

* Coagulation disorders and postoperative renal failure are discussed in Chapter 5, postoperative wound infection and other aspects of wound sepsis in Chapter 9, acute respiratory distress syndrome in Chapter 13, and pulmonary embolism in Chapter 37.

persist—or if they start leaking through the wound—the wound should be explored in the operating room and the lymphatics ligated.

Wound Dehiscence

Wound dehiscence is partial or total disruption of any or all layers of the operative wound. Rupture of all layers of the abdominal wall and extrusion of abdominal viscera is evisceration. Wound dehiscence occurs in 1–3% of abdominal surgical procedures. Systemic and local factors contribute to the development of this complication.

A. Systemic Risk Factors

Dehiscence is rare in patients under age 30 but affects about 5% of patients over age 60 having laparotomy. It is more common in patients with diabetes mellitus, uremia, immunosuppression, jaundice, sepsis, hypoalbuminemia, and cancer; in obese patients; and in those receiving corticosteroids.

B. Local Risk Factors

The three most important local factors predisposing to wound dehiscence are inadequate closure, increased intra-abdominal pressure, and deficient wound healing. Dehiscence often results from a combination of these factors rather than from a single one. The type of incision (transverse, midline, etc) does not influence the incidence of dehiscence.

1. Adequacy of closure—This is the single most important factor. The fascial layers give strength to a closure, and when fascia disrupts, the wound separates. Accurate approximation of anatomic layers is essential for adequate wound closure. Most wounds that dehisce do so because the sutures tear through the fascia. Prevention of this problem includes performing a neat incision, avoiding devitalization of the fascial edges by careful handling of tissues during the operation, placing and tying sutures correctly, and selecting the proper suture material. Sutures must be placed 2–3 cm from the wound edge and about 1 cm apart. *Dehiscence is often the result of using too few stitches and placing them too close to the edge of the fascia.* It is unusual for dehiscence to recur following reclosure, implying that adequate closure was technically possible at the initial procedure. In patients with risk factors for dehiscence, the surgeon should "do the second closure at the first operation," ie, take extra care to prevent dehiscence. Modern synthetic suture materials (polyglycolic acid, polypropylene, and others) are clearly superior to catgut for fascial closure. In infected wounds, polypropylene sutures are more resistant to degradation than polyglycolic acid sutures and have lower rates of wound disruption. Wound complications are decreased by obliteration of dead space. Ostomies and drains should be brought out through separate incisions to reduce the rate of wound infection and disruption.

2. Intra-abdominal pressure—After most intra-abdominal operations, some degree of ileus exists, which may increase pressure by causing distention of the bowel. High abdominal pressures can also occur in patients with chronic obstructive pulmonary disease who use their abdominal muscles as accessory muscles of respiration. In addition, coughing produces sudden increases in intra-abdominal pressure. Other factors contributing to increased abdominal pressure are postoperative bowel obstruction, obesity, and cirrhosis with ascites formation. Extra precautions are necessary to avoid dehiscence in such patients.

3. Deficient wound healing—Infection is an associated factor in more than half of wounds that rupture. The presence of drains, seromas, and wound hematomas also delays healing. Normally, a "healing ridge" (a palpable thickening extending about 0.5 cm on each side of the incision) appears near the end of the first week after operation. The presence of this ridge is clinical evidence that healing is adequate, and it is invariably absent from wounds that rupture.

C. Diagnosis and Management

Although wound dehiscence may occur at any time following wound closure, it is most commonly observed between the fifth and eighth postoperative days, when the strength of the wound is at a minimum. Wound dehiscence may occasionally be the first manifestation of an intra-abdominal abscess. The first sign of dehiscence is discharge of serosanguineous fluid from the wound or, in some cases, sudden evisceration. The patient often describes a popping sensation associated with severe coughing or retching. Thoracic wounds, with the exception of sternal wounds, are much less prone to dehiscence than are abdominal wounds. When a thoracotomy closure ruptures, it is heralded by leakage of pleural fluid or air and paradoxic motion of the chest wall. Sternal dehiscences, which are almost always associated with infection, produce an unstable chest and require early treatment. If infection is not overwhelming and there is minimal osteomyelitis of the adjacent sternum, the patient may be returned to the operating room for reclosure. Continuous mediastinal irrigation through small tubes left at the time of closure appears to reduce the failure rate. In cases of overwhelming infection, the wound is best treated by debridement and closure with a pectoralis major muscle flap, which resists further infection by increasing vascular supply to the area.

Patients with dehiscence of a laparotomy wound and evisceration should be returned to bed and the wound covered with moist towels. With the patient under general anesthesia, any exposed bowel or omentum should be rinsed with lactated Ringer's solution containing antibiotics and then returned to the abdomen. After mechanical cleansing and copious irrigation of the wound, the previous sutures should be removed and the wound reclosed using additional measures to prevent recurrent dehiscence, such as full-thickness retention sutures of No. 22 wire or heavy nylon. Evisceration carries a 10% mortality rate due both to contributing factors (eg, sepsis and cancer) and to resulting local infection.

Wound dehiscence without evisceration is best managed by prompt elective reclosure of the incision. If a partial disruption (ie, the skin is intact) is stable and the patient is a poor operative risk, treatment may be delayed and the resulting incisional hernia accepted. It is important in these patients that skin stitches not be removed before the end of the second postoperative week and that the abdomen be wrapped with a binder or corset to prevent further enlargement of the fascial defect or sudden disruption of the covering skin. When partial dehiscence is discovered during treatment of a wound infection, repair should be delayed if possible until the infection has been controlled, the wound has healed, and 6–7 months have elapsed. In these cases, antibiotics specific for the organisms isolated from the previous wound infection must be given at the time of hernia repair.

Recurrence of evisceration after reclosure of disrupted wounds is rare, though incisional hernias are later found in about 20% of such patients—usually those with wound infection in addition to dehiscence.

Miscellaneous Problems of the Operative Wound

Every new operative wound is painful, but those subject to continuous motion (eg, incisions that cross the costal margin) may be more painful than others. In general, the pain of an operative wound decreases substantially during the first 4–6 postoperative days. Chronic pain localized to one portion of an apparently healed wound may indicate the presence of a stitch abscess, a granuloma, or an occult incisional hernia. Abnormalities on examination of the wound usually allow for easy diagnosis; when this is difficult, ultrasound scanning may help detect a fascial defect or a collection of fluid associated with granulomas or abscesses. Rarely, a neuroma in the wound is responsible for focal pain and tenderness late in the postoperative course. Persistent localized pain is best treated by exploring the area, usually under local anesthesia, and removing a stitch, draining an abscess, or closing a hernia defect. Small sinus tracts usually result from stitch abscesses. The infected stitch can usually be removed with a clamp or crochet hook passed down the tract. If drainage continues, it is occasionally necessary to reopen the skin for better exposure and to remove a series of infected stitches.

Patients with ascites are at risk of fluid leak through the wound. Left untreated, **ascitic leaks** increase the incidence of wound infection and, through retrograde contamination, may result in peritonitis. Prevention in susceptible patients involves closing at least one layer of the wound with a continuous suture and taking measures to avoid the accumulation of ascites postoperatively. If an ascitic leak develops, the wound should be explored and the fascial defect closed. The rest of the wound, including the skin, should also be closed.

RESPIRATORY COMPLICATIONS

Respiratory complications are the most common single cause of morbidity after major surgical procedures and the second most common cause of postoperative deaths in patients older than 60 years. Patients undergoing chest and upper abdominal operations are particularly prone to pulmonary complications. The incidence is lower after pelvic surgery and even lower after extremity or head and neck procedures. Pulmonary complications are more common after emergency operations. Special hazards are posed by preexisting chronic obstructive pulmonary disease (chronic bronchitis, emphysema, asthma, pulmonary fibrosis). Elderly patients are at much higher risk because they have decreased compliance, increased closing and residual volumes, and increased dead space, all of which predispose to atelectasis.

Atelectasis

Atelectasis, the most common pulmonary complication, affects 25% of patients who have abdominal surgery. It is more common in patients who are elderly or overweight and in those who smoke or have symptoms of respiratory disease. It appears most frequently in the first 48 hours after operation and is responsible for over 90% of febrile episodes during that period. In most cases, the course is self-limited and recovery uneventful.

The pathogenesis of atelectasis involves obstructive and nonobstructive factors. Obstruction may be caused by secretions resulting from chronic obstructive pulmonary disease, intubation, or anesthetic agents. Occasional cases may be due to blood clots or malposition of the endotracheal tube. In most instances, however, the cause is not obstruction but closure of the bronchioles. Small bronchioles ($\leq$ 1 mm) are prone to close when lung volume reaches a critical point ("closing volume"). Portions of the lung that are dependent or compressed are the first to experience bronchiole closure since their regional volume is less than that of nondependent portions. Shallow breathing and failure to periodically hyperinflate the lung result in small alveolar size and decreased volume. The closing volume is higher in older patients and in smokers owing to the loss of elastic recoil of the lung. Other nonobstructive factors contributing to atelectasis include decreased functional residual capacity and loss of pulmonary surfactant.

The air in the atelectatic portion of the lung is absorbed, and since there is minimal change in perfusion, a ventilation/perfusion mismatch results. The immediate effect of atelectasis is decreased oxygenation of blood; its clinical significance depends on the respiratory and cardiac reserve of the patient. A later effect is the propensity of the atelectatic segment to become infected. In general, if a pulmonary segment remains atelectatic for over 72 hours, pneumonia is almost certain to occur.

Atelectasis is usually manifested by fever (pathogenesis unknown), tachypnea, and tachycardia. Physical examination may show elevation of the diaphragm, scattered rales, and decreased breath sounds, but it is often normal. Postoperative atelectasis can be largely prevented by early mobilization, frequent changes in position, encouragement to cough, and use of an incentive spirometer. Preoperative teaching of respiratory exercises and postoperative execution of these exercises prevents atelectasis in patients without preexisting lung disease. Intermittent positive pressure breathing is expensive and less effective than these simpler exercises.

Treatment consists of clearing the airway by chest percussion, coughing, or nasotracheal suction. Bronchodilators and mucolytic agents given by nebulizer may help in patients with severe chronic obstructive pulmonary disease. Atelectasis from obstruction of a major airway may require intrabronchial suction through an endoscope, a procedure that can usually be performed at the bedside with mild sedation.

Pulmonary Aspiration

Aspiration of oropharyngeal and gastric contents is normally prevented by the gastroesophageal and pharyngoesophageal sphincters. Insertion of nasogastric and endotracheal tubes and depression of the central nervous system by drugs interfere with these defenses and predispose to aspiration. Other factors, such as gastroesophageal reflux, food in the stomach, or position of the patient, may play a role. Trauma victims are particularly likely to aspirate regurgitated gastric contents when consciousness is depressed. Patients with intestinal obstruction and pregnant women—who have increased intra-abdominal pressure and decreased gastric motility—are also at high risk of aspiration. Two-thirds of cases of aspiration follow thoracic or abdominal surgery, and of these, one-half result in pneumonia. The death rate for grossly evident aspiration and subsequent pneumonia is about 50%.

Minor amounts of aspiration are frequent during surgery and are apparently well tolerated. Methylene blue placed in the stomach of patients undergoing abdominal operations can be found in the trachea at completion of the procedure in 15% of cases. Radionuclide techniques have shown aspiration of gastric contents in 45% of normal volunteers during sleep.

The magnitude of pulmonary injury produced by aspiration of fluid, usually from gastric contents, is determined by the volume aspirated, its pH, and the frequency of the event. If the aspirate has a pH of 2.5 or less, it causes immediate chemical pneumonitis, which results in local edema and inflammation, changes that increase the risk of secondary infection. Aspiration of solid matter can produce airway obstruction. Obstruction of distal bronchi, though well tolerated initially, can lead to atelectasis and pulmonary abscess formation. The basal segments are affected most often. Tachypnea, rales, and hypoxia are usually present within hours; less frequently, cyanosis, wheezing, and apnea may appear. In patients with massive aspiration, hypovolemia caused by excessive fluid and colloid loss into the injured lung may lead to hypotension and shock.

Aspiration has been found in 80% of patients with tracheostomies and may account for the predisposition to pulmonary infection in this group. Patients who must remain intubated for long periods should have a low-pressure, high-volume type of cuff on their tube, as this helps to prevent aspiration and limits the risk of pressure necrosis of the trachea.

Aspiration can be prevented by preoperative fasting, proper positioning of the patient, and careful intubation. A single dose of cimetidine before induction of anesthesia may be of value in situations where the risk of aspiration is high. Treatment of aspiration involves reestablishing patency of the airway and preventing further damage to the lung. Endotracheal suction should be performed immediately, as this procedure confirms the diagnosis and stimulates coughing, which helps to clear the airway. Bronchoscopy may be required to remove solid matter. Fluid resuscitation should be undertaken concomitantly. Antibiotics are used initially when the aspirate is heavily contaminated; they are used later to treat pneumonia.

Postoperative Pneumonia

Pneumonia is the most common pulmonary complication among patients who die after surgery. It is directly responsible for death—or is a contributory factor—in more than half of these patients. Patients with peritoneal infection and those requiring prolonged ventilatory support are at highest risk for developing postoperative pneumonia. Atelectasis, aspiration, and copious secretions are important predisposing factors.

Host defenses against pneumonitis include the cough reflex, the mucociliary system, and the activity of alveolar macrophages. After surgery, cough is usually weak and may not effectively clear the bronchial tree. The mucociliary transport mechanism is damaged by endotracheal intubation, and the functional ability of the alveolar macrophage is compromised by a number of factors that may be present during and after surgery (oxygen, pulmonary edema, aspiration, corticosteroid therapy, etc). In addition, squamous metaplasia and loss of ciliary coordination further hamper antibacterial defenses. More than half of the pulmonary infections that follow surgery are caused by gram-negative bacilli. They are frequently polymicrobial and usually acquired by aspiration of oropharyngeal secretions. Although colonization of the oropharynx with gram-negative bacteria occurs in only 20% of normal individuals, it is frequent after major surgery as a result of impaired oropharyngeal clearing mechanisms. Aggravating factors are azotemia, prolonged endotracheal intubation, and severe associated infection.

Occasionally, infecting bacteria reach the lung by inhalation—eg, from respirators. *Pseudomonas aeruginosa* and klebsiella can survive in the moist reservoirs of these machines, and these pathogens have been the source of epidemic infections in intensive care units. Rarely, contamination of the lung may result from direct hematogenous spread from distant septic foci.

The clinical manifestations of postoperative pneumonia are fever, tachypnea, increased secretions, and physical changes suggestive of pulmonary consolidation. A chest x-ray usually shows localized parenchymal consolidation. Overall mortality rates for postoperative pneumonia vary from 20% to 40%. Rates are higher when pneumonia develops in patients who had emergency operations; are on respirators; or develop remote organ failure, positive blood cultures, or infection of the second lung.

Maintaining the airway clear of secretions is of paramount concern in the prevention of postoperative pneumonia. Respiratory exercises, deep breathing, and coughing help prevent atelectasis, which is a precursor of pneumonia. Although postoperative pain is thought to contribute to shallow breathing, neither intercostal blocks nor epidural narcotics prevent atelectasis and pneumonia when compared with traditional methods of postoperative pain control. The prophylactic use of antibiotics does not decrease the incidence of gram-negative colonization of the oropharynx or that of pneumonia. Treatment consists of measures to aid the clearing of secretions and administration of antibiotics. Sputum obtained directly from the trachea, usually by endotracheal suctioning, is required for specific identification of the infecting organism.

Postoperative Pleural Effusion & Pneumothorax

Formation of a very small pleural effusion is fairly common immediately after upper abdominal operations and is of no clinical significance. Patients with free peritoneal fluid at the time of surgery and those with postoperative atelectasis are more prone to develop effusions. In the absence of cardiac failure or a pulmonary lesion, appearance of a pleural effusion late in the postoperative course suggests the presence of subdiaphragmatic inflammation (subphrenic abscess, acute pancreatitis, etc). Effusions that do not compromise respiratory function should be left undisturbed. If there is a suspicion of infection, the effusion should be sampled by needle aspiration. When an effusion produces respiratory compromise, it should be drained with a thoracostomy tube.

Postoperative pneumothorax may follow insertion of a subclavian catheter or positive-pressure ventilation, but it sometimes appears after an operation during which the pleura has been injured (eg, nephrectomy or adrenalectomy). Pneumothorax should be treated with a thoracostomy tube.

FAT EMBOLISM

Fat embolism is relatively common but only rarely causes symptoms. Fat particles can be found in the pulmonary vascular bed in 90% of patients who have had fractures of long bones or joint replacements. Fat embolism can also be caused by exogenous sources of fat, such as blood transfusions, intravenous fat emulsion, or bone marrow transplantation. **Fat embolism syndrome** consists of neurologic dysfunction, respiratory insufficiency, and petechiae of the axillae, chest, and proximal arms. It was originally described in trauma victims—especially those with long bone fractures—and was thought to be a result of bone marrow embolization. However, the principal clinical manifestations of fat embolism are seen in other conditions. The existence of fat embolism as an entity distinct from posttraumatic pulmonary insufficiency has been questioned.

Fat embolism syndrome characteristically begins 12–72 hours after injury but may be delayed for several days. The diagnosis is clinical. The finding of fat droplets in sputum and urine is common after trauma and is not specific. Decreased hematocrit, thrombocytopenia, and other changes in coagulation parameters are usually seen.

Once symptoms develop, supportive treatment should be provided until respiratory insufficiency and central nervous system manifestations subside. Respiratory insufficiency is treated with positive end-expiratory pressure ventilation and diuretics. The prognosis is related to the severity of the pulmonary insufficiency.

CARDIAC COMPLICATIONS

Cardiac complications following surgery may be life-threatening. Their incidence is reduced by appropriate preoperative preparation.

Dysrhythmias, unstable angina, heart failure, or severe hypertension should be corrected before surgery whenever possible. Valvular disease—especially aortic stenosis—limits the ability of the heart to respond to increased demand during operation or in the immediate postoperative period. When aortic stenosis is recognized preoperatively—and assuming that the patient is monitored adequately (Swan-Ganz catheterization, central venous pressure, etc)—the incidence of major perioperative complications is small. Thus, patients with preexisting heart disease should be evaluated by a cardiologist preoperatively. Determination of cardiac function, including indirect evaluation of the left ventricular ejection fraction, identifies patients at higher risk for cardiac complications. Continuous electrocardiographic monitoring during the first 3–4 postoperative days detects episodes of ischemia or dysrhythmia in about a third of these patients. Oral anticoagulant drugs should be stopped 3–5 days before surgery, and the prothrombin time should be allowed to return to normal. Patients at high risk for thromboembolic disease should receive heparin until approximately 6 hours before the operation, when heparin should be stopped. If needed, heparin can be restarted 36–48 hours after surgery along with oral anticoagulation.

General anesthesia depresses the myocardium, and some anesthetic agents predispose to dysrhythmias by sensitizing the myocardium to catecholamines. Monitoring of cardiac activity and blood pressure during the operation detects dysrhythmias and hypotension early. In patients with a high cardiac risk, regional anesthesia may be safer than general anesthesia for procedures below the umbilicus.

The duration and urgency of the operation and uncontrolled bleeding with hypotension have been individually shown to correlate positively with the development of serious postoperative cardiac problems. In patients with pacemakers, the electrocautery current may be sensed by the intracardiac electrode, causing inappropriate pacemaker function.

Noncardiac complications may affect the development of cardiac complications by increasing cardiac demands in patients with a limited reserve. Postoperative sepsis and hypoxemia are foremost. Fluid overload can produce acute left ventricular failure. Patients with coronary artery disease, dysrhythmias, or low cardiac output should be monitored postoperatively in an intensive care unit.

Dysrhythmias

Most dysrhythmias appear during the operation or within the first 3 postoperative days. They are especially likely to occur after thoracic procedures.

A. Intraoperative Dysrhythmias

The overall incidence of intraoperative cardiac dysrhythmias is 20%; most are self-limited. The incidence is higher in patients with preexisting dysrhythmias and in those with known heart disease (35%). About one-third of dysrhythmias occur during induction of anesthesia. These dysrhythmias are usually related to anesthetic agents (eg, halothane, cyclopropane), sympathomimetic drugs, digitalis toxicity, and hypercapnia.

B. Postoperative Dysrhythmias

These dysrhythmias are generally related to reversible factors such as hypokalemia, hypoxemia, alkalosis, digitalis toxicity, and stress during emergence from anesthesia. Occasionally, postoperative dysrhythmias may be the first sign of myocardial infarction. Most postoperative dysrhythmias are asymptomatic, but occasionally the patient complains of chest pain, palpitations, or dyspnea.

Supraventricular dysrhythmias usually have few serious consequences but may decrease cardiac output and coronary blood flow. Patients with atrial flutter or fibrillation with a rapid ventricular response and who are in shock require cardioversion. If they are hemodynamically stable, they should have the heart rate controlled with digitalis, beta-blockers, or calcium channel blockers. Associated hypokalemia should be treated promptly.

Ventricular premature beats are often precipitated by hypercapnia, hypoxemia, pain, or fluid overload. They should be treated with oxygen, sedation, analgesia, and correction of fluid losses or electrolyte abnormalities. Ventricular dysrhythmias have a more profound effect on cardiac function than supraventricular dysrhythmias and may lead to fatal ventricular fibrillation. Immediate treatment is with lidocaine, 1 mg/kg intravenously as a bolus, repeated as necessary to a total dose of 250 mg, followed by a slow intravenous infusion at a rate of 1–2 mg/min. Higher doses of lidocaine may cause seizures.

Postoperative complete heart block is usually due to serious cardiac disease and calls for the immediate insertion of a pacemaker. First- or second-degree heart block is usually well tolerated.

Postoperative Myocardial Infarction

Approximately 0.4% of all patients undergoing an operation in the USA develop postoperative myocardial infarction. The incidence increases to 5–12% in patients undergoing operations for other manifestations of atherosclerosis (eg, carotid endarterectomy, aortoiliac graft). Other important risk factors include preoperative congestive heart failure, ischemia identified on dipyridamole-thallium scan or treadmill exercise test, and age over 70 years. In selected patients with angina, consideration should be given to coronary revascularization before proceeding with a major elective operation on another organ.

Postoperative myocardial infarction may be precipitated by factors such as hypotension or hypoxemia. Clinical manifestations include chest pain, hypotension, and cardiac dysrhythmias. Over half of postoperative myocardial infarctions, however, are asymptomatic. The absence of symptoms is thought to be due to the residual effects of anesthesia and to analgesics administered postoperatively.

Diagnosis is substantiated by electrocardiographic changes, elevated serum creatine kinase levels—especially the MB isoenzyme—and serum troponin I levels. The mortality rate of postoperative myocardial infarction is as high as 67% in high-risk groups. The prognosis is better if it is the first infarction and worse if there have been previous infarctions. Prevention of this complication includes postponing elective operations for 3 months or preferably 6 months after myocardial infarction, treating congestive heart failure preoperatively, and controlling hypertension perioperatively.

Patients with postoperative myocardial infarction should be monitored in the intensive care unit and provided with adequate oxygenation and precise fluid and electrolyte replacement. Anticoagulation, though not always feasible after major surgery, prevents the development of mural thrombosis and arterial embolism after myocardial infarction. Congestive heart failure should be treated with digitalis, diuretics, and vasodilators as needed.

Postoperative Cardiac Failure

Left ventricular failure and pulmonary edema appear in 4% of patients over age 40 undergoing general surgical procedures with general anesthesia. Fluid overload in patients with limited myocardial reserve is the most common cause. Postoperative myocardial infarction and dysrhythmias producing a high ventricular rate are other causes. Clinical manifestations are progressive dyspnea, hypoxemia with normal CO_2 tension, and diffuse congestion on chest x-ray.

Clinically inapparent ventricular failure is frequent, especially when other factors predisposing to pulmonary edema are present (massive trauma, multiple transfusions, sepsis, etc). The diagnosis may be suspected from a decreased PaO_2, abnormal chest x-ray, or elevated pulmonary artery wedge pressure. The treatment of left ventricular failure depends on the hemodynamic state of the patient. Those who are in shock require transfer to the intensive care unit, placement of a pulmonary artery line, monitoring of filling pressures, and immediate pre- and afterload reduction. Preload reduction is achieved by diuretics (and nitroglycerin if needed); afterload reduction, by administration of sodium nitroprusside. Patients who are not in shock may, instead, be digitalized. Rapid digitalization (eg, divided intravenous doses of digoxin to a total of 1–1.5 mg over 24 hours, with careful monitoring of the serum potassium level), fluid restriction, and diuretics may be enough in these cases. Fluids should be restricted, and diuretics may be given. Respiratory insufficiency calls for ventilatory support with endotracheal intubation and a mechanical respirator. Although pulmonary function may improve with the use of positive end-expiratory pressure, hemodynamic derangements and decreased myocardial reserve preclude it in most cases.

PERITONEAL COMPLICATIONS

Hemoperitoneum

Bleeding is the most common cause of shock in the first 24 hours after abdominal surgery. Postoperative hemoperitoneum—a rapidly evolving, life-threatening complication—is usually the result of a technical problem with hemostasis, but coagulation disorders may play a role. For example, many of these patients have experienced substantial intraoperative blood loss, and several transfusions have been already given. As a consequence, changes usually observed after transfusion, such as thrombocytopenia, may be present. Other causes of coagulopathy such as mismatched transfusion, administration of heparin, etc, should also be considered. In these cases, bleeding tends to be more generalized, occurring in the wound, venipuncture sites, etc.

Hemoperitoneum usually becomes apparent within 24 hours after the operation. Its manifestations are those of intravascular hypovolemia: tachycardia, decreased blood pressure, decreased urine output, and peripheral vasoconstriction. If bleeding continues, abdominal girth may increase. Changes in the hematocrit are usually not obvious for 4–6 hours and are of limited diagnostic help in patients who sustain rapid blood loss.

The manifestations may be so subtle that the diagnosis is overlooked. Only a high index of suspicion, frequent examination of patients at risk, and a systematic investigation of patients with postoperative hypotension will result in early recognition of the problem. Preexisting disease and drugs taken before surgery as well as those administered during the operation may cause hypotension. The differential diagnosis of immediate postoperative circulatory collapse also includes pulmonary embolism, cardiac dysrhythmias, pneumothorax, myocardial infarction, and severe allergic reactions. Infusions to expand the intravascular volume should be started as soon as other diseases have been ruled out. If hypotension or other signs of hypovolemia persist, one must reoperate promptly. At operation, bleeding should be stopped, clots evacuated, and the peritoneal cavity rinsed with saline solution.

Complications of Drains

Postoperative drainage of the peritoneal cavity is indicated to prevent fluid accumulation such as bile or pancreatic fluid or to treat established abscesses. Drains may be left to evacuate small amounts of blood, but drain output cannot be used to provide a reliable estimate of the rate of bleeding. The use of drains in operations not expected to have fluid leaks (such as cholecystectomy, splenectomy, and colectomy) increases the rate of postoperative intra-abdominal and wound infection. Latex Penrose drains, which were once popular, should be avoided because of the risk of introducing infection. Large rigid drains may erode into adjacent viscera or vessels and cause fistula formation or bleeding. This risk is lessened with the use of softer Silastic drains, and removing them as early as possible. Drains should not be left in contact with intestinal anastomoses, as they promote anastomotic leakage and fistula formation.

POSTOPERATIVE PAROTITIS

Postoperative parotitis—a rare but serious staphylococcal infection of the parotid gland—is limited almost entirely to elderly, debilitated, malnourished patients with poor oral hygiene. It appears in the second postoperative week and is associated with prolonged nasogastric intubation. The triggering factors are dehydration and poor oral hygiene, and the pathogenesis consists of a decrease in the secretory activity of the gland with inspissation of parotid secretions that become infected by staphylococci or gram-negative bacteria from the oral cavity. This results in inflammation, accumulation of cells that obstruct large and medium-sized ducts, and, eventually, formation of multiple small abscesses. These lobular abscesses, separated by fibrous bands, may dissect through the capsule and spread to the periglandular tissues to involve the auditory canal, the superficial skin, and the neck. If the disease is not treated at this stage, it may produce acute respiratory failure from tracheal obstruction.

Clinically, parotitis first appears as pain or tenderness at the angle of the jaw. With progression, high fever and leukocytosis develop, and there is swelling and redness in the parotid area. The parotid usually feels firm, and even after abscesses have formed, fluctuance is uncommon.

Prophylaxis includes adequate fluid intake, avoiding the use of anticholinergics, minimizing trauma during intubation, and, most importantly, good oral hygiene (frequent gargles, mouth irrigation, and other mouth cleansing and moistening measures). Stimulation of salivary flow with chewing gum, hard candy, etc, may also be useful. Routine observance of these simple preventive measures has virtually eliminated parotitis, which was once a common postoperative complication.

When signs of acute parotitis appear, fluid obtained from Stensen's duct by gentle compression of the gland should be cultured. Vancomycin should be started while the results of cultures are awaited. Warm moist packs and mouth irrigations may be helpful. In most instances, the disease responds promptly to these measures. If the disease progresses, the parotid must be surgically drained. The procedure consists of elevating a skin flap over the gland and making multiple small incisions parallel to the branches of the facial nerve. The wound is then packed open.

COMPLICATIONS CAUSED BY POSTOPERATIVE ALTERATIONS OF GASTROINTESTINAL MOTILITY

The presence, strength, and direction of normal peristalsis are governed by the enteric nervous system. Anesthesia and surgical manipulation result in a decrease of the normal propulsive activity of the gut, or postoperative ileus. Several factors worsen ileus or prolong its course. These include medications—especially opioids—electrolyte abnormalities, inflammatory conditions such as pancreatitis or peritonitis, and pain. The degree of ileus is related to the extent of operative manipulation.

Gastrointestinal peristalsis returns within 24 hours after most operations that do not involve the abdominal cavity. In general, laparoscopic approaches cause less ileus than open procedures. After laparotomy, gastric peristalsis returns in about 48 hours. Colonic activity returns after 48 hours, starting at the cecum and progressing caudally. The motility of the small intestine is affected to a lesser degree, except in patients who have had small bowel resection or who were operated on to relieve bowel obstruction. Normal postoperative ileus leads to slight abdominal distention and absent bowel sounds. Return of peristalsis is often noted by the patient as mild cramps, passage of flatus, and return of appetite. Feedings should be withheld until there is evidence of return of normal gastrointestinal motility. There is no specific therapy for postoperative ileus.

Gastric Dilation

Gastric dilation, a rare life-threatening complication, consists of massive distention of the stomach by gas and fluid. Predisposing factors include asthma, recent surgery, gastric outlet obstruction, and absence of the spleen. Infants and children in whom oxygen masks are used in the immediate postoperative period and adults subjected to forceful assisted respiration during resuscitation are also at risk. Occasionally, gastric dilation develops in patients with anorexia nervosa or during serious illnesses without a specific intercurrent event.

As the air-filled stomach grows larger, it hangs down across the duodenum, producing a mechanical gastric outlet obstruction that contributes further to the problem. The increased intragastric pressure produces venous obstruction of the mucosa, causing mucosal engorgement and bleeding and, if allowed to continue, ischemic necrosis and perforation. The distended stomach pushes the diaphragm upward, which causes collapse of the lower lobe of the left lung, rotation of the heart, and obstruction of the inferior vena cava. The acutely dilated stomach is also prone to undergo volvulus.

The patient appears ill, with abdominal distention and hiccups. Hypochloremia, hypokalemia, and alkalosis may result from fluid and electrolyte losses. When the problem is recognized early, treatment consists of gastric decompression with a nasogastric tube. In the late stage, gastric necrosis may require gastrectomy.

Bowel Obstruction

Failure of postoperative return of bowel function may be the result of paralytic ileus or mechanical obstruction. Mechanical obstruction is most often caused by postoperative adhesions or an internal (mesenteric) hernia. Most of these patients experience a short period of apparently normal intestinal function before manifestations of obstruction supervene. About half of cases of early postoperative small bowel obstruction follow colorectal surgery.

Diagnosis may be difficult because the symptoms are difficult to differentiate from those of paralytic ileus. If plain films of the abdomen show air-fluid levels in loops of small bowel, mechanical obstruction is a more likely diagnosis than ileus. Enteroclysis or an ordinary small bowel series with barium sulfate may aid diagnosis.

Strangulation is uncommon because the adhesive bands are broader and less rigid than is typical of late small bowel obstruction. The death rate is high (about 15%), however, probably because of delay in diagnosis and the postoperative state. Treatment consists of nasogastric suction for several days and, if the obstruction does not resolve spontaneously, laparotomy.

Small bowel intussusception is an uncommon cause of early postoperative obstruction in adults but accounts for 10% of cases in the pediatric age group. Ninety percent of postoperative intussusceptions occur during the first 2 postoperative weeks, and more than half in the first week. Unlike idiopathic ileocolic intussusception, most postoperative intussusceptions are ileoileal or jejunojejunal. They most often follow retroperitoneal and pelvic operations. The cause is unknown. The symptom complex is not typical, and x-ray studies are of limited help. The physician should be aware that intussusception is a possible explanation for vomiting, distention, and abdominal pain after laparotomy in children and that early reoperation will avoid the complications of perforation and peritonitis. Operation is the only treatment, and if the bowel is viable, reduction of the intussusception is all that is needed.

Postoperative Fecal Impaction

Fecal impaction after operative procedures is the result of colonic ileus and impaired perception of rectal fullness. It is principally a disease of the elderly but may occur in younger patients who have predisposing conditions such as megacolon or paraplegia. Postoperative ileus and the use of opioid analgesics and anticholinergic drugs are aggravating factors. Early manifestations are anorexia and obstipation or diarrhea. In advanced cases, marked distention may cause colonic perforation. The diagnosis of postoperative fecal impaction is made by rectal examination. The impaction should be manually removed, enemas given, and digital examination then repeated.

Barium remaining in the colon from an examination done before surgery may harden and produce barium impaction. This usually occurs in the right colon, where most of the water is absorbed, and is a more difficult management problem than fecal impaction. The clinical manifestations are those of bowel obstruction. Treatment includes enemas and purgation with polyethylene glycol-electrolyte solution (eg, CoLyte, GoLYTELY). Diatrizoate sodium (Hypaque), a hyperosmolar solution that stimulates peristalsis and increases intraluminal fluid, may be effective by enema if other solutions fail. Operation is rarely needed.

POSTOPERATIVE PANCREATITIS

Postoperative pancreatitis accounts for 10% of all cases of acute pancreatitis. It occurs in 1–3% of patients who have operations in the vicinity of the pancreas, and with higher frequency after operations on the biliary tract. For example, pancreatitis occurs in about 1% of patients undergoing cholecystectomy and in 8% of patients undergoing common bile duct exploration. In the latter cases, it does not appear to be related to the performance of intraoperative cholangiograms or choledochoscopy. Postoperative pancreatitis after biliary surgery is worse in patients who have had biliary pancreatitis preoperatively. Pancreatitis occasionally occurs following cardiopulmonary bypass, parathyroid surgery, and renal transplantation. Postoperative pancreatitis is frequently of the necrotizing type. Infected pancreatic necrosis and other complications of pancreatitis develop with a frequency three to four times greater than in biliary and alcoholic pancreatitis. The reason postoperative pancreatitis is so severe is unknown, but the mortality rate is 30–40%.

The pathogenesis in most cases appears to be mechanical trauma to the pancreas or its blood supply. Nevertheless, manipulation, biopsy, and partial resection of the pancreas are usually well tolerated, so the reasons that some patients develop pancreatitis are unclear. Prevention of this complication includes careful handling of the pancreas and avoidance of forceful dilation of the choledochal sphincter or obstruction of the pancreatic duct. The 2% incidence of pancreatitis following renal transplantation is probably related to special risk factors such as use of corticosteroids or azathioprine, secondary hyperparathyroidism, or viral infection. Acute changes in serum calcium are thought to be responsible for pancreatitis following parathyroid surgery. Hyperamylasemia develops in about half of patients undergoing heart surgery with extracorporeal bypass, but clinical evidence of pancreatitis is present in only 5% of these patients.

The diagnosis of postoperative pancreatitis may be difficult in patients who have recently had an abdominal operation. Hyperamylasemia may or may not be present. One must be alert to renal and respiratory complications and the consequences of necrotizing or hemorrhagic pancreatitis. Because of the high frequency with which complications develop, frequent monitoring of the pancreas and retroperitoneum with CT scans is useful.

POSTOPERATIVE HEPATIC DYSFUNCTION

Hepatic dysfunction, ranging from mild jaundice to life-threatening hepatic failure, follows 1% of surgical procedures performed under general anesthesia. The incidence is greater following pancreatectomy, biliary bypass operations, and portacaval shunt. Postoperative hyperbilirubinemia may be categorized as prehepatic jaundice, hepatocellular insufficiency, and posthepatic obstruction (Table 4–1).

Table 4–1. Causes of postoperative jaundice.

Prehepatic jaundice (bilirubin overload)
Hemolysis (drugs, transfusions, sickle cell crisis)
Reabsorption of hematomas
Hepatocellular insufficiency
Viral hepatitis
Drug-induced (anesthesia, others)
Ischemia (shock, hypoxia, low-output states)
Sepsis
Liver resection (loss of parenchyma)
Others (total parenteral nutrition, malnutrition)
Posthepatic obstruction (to bile flow)
Retained stones
Injury to ducts
Tumor (unrecognized or untreated)
Cholecystitis
Pancreatitis
Occlusion of biliary stents

Prehepatic Jaundice

Prehepatic jaundice is caused by bilirubin overload, most often from hemolysis or reabsorption of hematomas. Fasting, malnutrition, hepatotoxic drugs, and anesthesia are among the factors that impair the ability of the liver to excrete increased loads of bilirubin in the postoperative period.

Increased hemolysis may result from transfusion of incompatible blood but more often reflects destruction of fragile transfused red blood cells. Other causes include extracorporeal circulation, congenital hemolytic disease (eg, sickle cell disease), and effects of drugs.

Hepatocellular Insufficiency

Hepatocellular insufficiency, the most common cause of postoperative jaundice, occurs as a consequence of hepatic cell necrosis, inflammation, or massive hepatic resection. Drugs, hypotension, hypoxia, and sepsis are among the injurious factors. Although posttransfusion hepatitis is usually observed much later, this complication may occur as early as the third postoperative week.

Benign postoperative intrahepatic cholestasis is a vague term used to denote jaundice following operations that often involve hypotension and multiple transfusions. Serum bilirubin ranges from 2 to 20 mg/dL and serum alkaline phosphatase is usually high, but the patient is afebrile and postoperative convalescence is otherwise smooth. The diagnosis is one of exclusion. Jaundice clears by the third postoperative week.

Hepatocellular damage occasionally occurs after intestinal bypass procedures for morbid obesity. Cholestatic jaundice may develop in patients receiving total parenteral nutrition.

Posthepatic Obstruction

Posthepatic obstruction can be caused by direct surgical injury to the bile ducts, retained common duct stones, tumor obstruction of the bile duct, or pancreatitis. Acute postoperative cholecystitis is associated with jaundice in one-third of cases, though mechanical obstruction of the common duct is usually not apparent.

One must determine if a patient with postoperative jaundice has a correctable cause that requires treatment. This is particularly true for sepsis (when decreased liver function may sometimes be an early sign), lesions that obstruct the bile duct, and postoperative cholecystitis. Liver function tests are not helpful in determining the cause and do not usually reflect the severity of disease. Liver biopsy, ultrasound and CT scans, and transhepatic or endoscopic retrograde cholangiograms are the tests most likely to sort out the diagnostic possibilities. Renal function must be monitored closely, since renal failure may develop in these patients. Treatment is otherwise expectant.

POSTOPERATIVE CHOLECYSTITIS

Acute postoperative cholecystitis may follow any kind of operation but is more common after gastrointestinal procedures. Acute cholecystitis develops shortly after endoscopic sphincterotomy in 3–5% of patients. Chemical cholecystitis occurs in patients undergoing hepatic arterial chemotherapy with mitomycin and floxuridine with such frequency that cholecystectomy should always be performed before infusion of these agents is begun. Fulminant cholecystitis with gallbladder infarction may follow percutaneous embolization of the hepatic artery for malignant tumors of the liver or for arteriovenous malformation involving this artery.

Postoperative cholecystitis differs in several respects from the common form of acute cholecystitis: It is frequently acalculous (70–80%), more common in males (75%), progresses rapidly to gallbladder necrosis, and is not likely to respond to conservative therapy. The cause is clear in cases of chemical or ischemic cholecystitis but not in other forms. Factors thought to play a role include biliary stasis (with formation of sludge), biliary infection, and ischemia.

CLOSTRIDIUM DIFFICILE COLITIS

Postoperative diarrhea due to *Clostridium difficile* is a common nosocomial infection in surgical patients. The spectrum of illness ranges from asymptomatic colonization to—rarely—severe toxic colitis. Transmission from hospital personnel probably occurs. The main risk factor is perioperative antibiotic use. The diagnosis is established by identification of a specific cytopathic toxin in the stool or culture of the organism from stool samples or rectal swabs. In severely affected patients, colonoscopy reveals pseudomembranes. Prevention is accomplished by strict handwashing, enteric precautions, and minimizing antibiotic use. Treatment of established infection is with intravenous metronidazole or, for infections with resistant pathogens, oral vancomycin.

URINARY COMPLICATIONS

Postoperative Urinary Retention

Inability to void postoperatively is common, especially after pelvic and perineal operations or operations conducted under spinal anesthesia. Factors responsible for postoperative urinary retention are interference with the neural mechanisms responsible for normal emptying of the bladder and overdistention of the urinary bladder. When its normal capacity of approximately 500 mL is exceeded, bladder contraction is inhibited. Prophylactic bladder catheterization should be performed whenever an operation is likely to last 3 hours or longer or when large volumes of intravenous fluids are anticipated. The catheter can be removed at the end of the operation if the patient is expected to be able to ambulate within a few hours. When bladder catheterization is not performed, the patient should be encouraged to void immediately before coming to the operating room and as soon as possible after the operation. During abdominoperineal resection, operative trauma to the sacral plexus alters bladder function enough so that an indwelling catheter should be left in place for 4–5 days. Patients with inguinal hernia who strain to void as a manifestation of prostatic hypertrophy should have the prostate treated before the hernia.

The treatment of acute urinary retention is catheterization of the bladder. In the absence of factors that suggest the need for prolonged decompression, such as the presence of 1000 mL of urine or more, the catheter may be removed.

Urinary Tract Infection

Infection of the lower urinary tract is the most frequently acquired nosocomial infection. Preexisting contamination of the urinary tract, urinary retention, and instrumentation are the principal contributing factors. Bacteriuria is present in about 5% of patients who undergo short-term (< 48 hours) bladder catheterization, though clinical signs of urinary tract infection occur in only 1%. Cystitis is manifested by dysuria and mild fever and pyelonephritis by high fever, flank tenderness, and, occasionally, ileus. Diagnosis is made by examination of the urine and confirmed by cultures. Prevention involves treating urinary tract contamination before surgery, prevention or prompt treatment of urinary retention, and careful instrumentation when needed. Treatment includes adequate hydration, proper drainage of the bladder, and specific antibiotics.

CENTRAL NERVOUS SYSTEM COMPLICATIONS

Postoperative Cerebrovascular Accidents

Postoperative cerebrovascular accidents are almost always the result of ischemic neural damage due to poor perfusion. They often occur in elderly patients with severe atherosclerosis who become hypotensive during or after surgery (from sepsis, bleeding, cardiac arrest, etc). Normal regulatory mechanisms of the cerebral vasculature can maintain blood flow over a wide range of blood pressures down to a mean pressure of about 55 mm Hg. Abrupt hypotension, however, is less well tolerated than a more gradual pressure change. Irreversible brain damage occurs after about 4 minutes of total ischemia.

Strokes occur in 1–3% of patients after carotid endarterectomy and other reconstructive operations of the extracranial portion of the carotid system. Embolization from atherosclerotic plaques, ischemia during carotid clamping, and postoperative thrombosis at the site of the arteriotomy or of an intimal flap are usually responsible. Aspirin, which inhibits platelet aggregation, may prevent immediate postoperative thrombosis.

Open heart surgery using extracorporeal circulation or deep cooling is also occasionally followed by stroke. The pathogenesis of stroke is thought to be related to hypoxemia, emboli, or poor perfusion. The presence of a carotid bruit preoperatively increases the risk of postoperative stroke after coronary bypass by a factor of 4. Previous stroke or transient ischemic attacks and postoperative atrial fibrillation also increase the risk. For patients undergoing noncardiac, noncarotid surgery, the risk of stroke is about 0.2%. Predictors of risk in these patients are the presence of cerebrovascular, cardiac, or peripheral vascular disease and arterial hypertension.

Seizures

Epilepsy, metabolic derangements, and medications may lead to seizures in the postoperative period. For unknown reasons, patients with ulcerative colitis and Crohn's disease are peculiarly susceptible to seizures with loss of consciousness after surgery. Seizures should be treated as soon as possible to minimize their harmful effects.

PSYCHIATRIC COMPLICATIONS

Anxiety and fear are normal in patients undergoing surgery. The degree to which these emotions are experienced depends upon diverse cultural and psychologic variables. Underlying depression or a history of chronic pain may serve to exaggerate the patient's response to surgery. The boundary between the normal manifestations of stress and **postoperative psychosis** is difficult to establish, since the latter is not really a distinct clinical entity.

Postoperative psychosis (so-called) develops in about 0.5% of patients having abdominal operations. It is more common after thoracic surgery, in the elderly, and in those with chronic disease. About half of these patients suffer from mood disturbances (usually severe depression). Twenty percent have delirium. Drugs given in the postoperative period may play a role in the development of psychosis; meperidine, cimetidine, and corticosteroids are most commonly implicated. Patients who develop postoperative psychosis have higher plasma levels of β-endorphin and cortisol than those who do not. These patients also lose, temporarily, the normal circadian rhythms of β-endorphin and cortisol. Specific psychiatric syndromes may follow specific procedures, such as visual hallucinations and the "black patch syndrome" after ophthalmic surgery. Preexisting psychiatric disorders not apparent before the operation sometimes contribute to the motivation for surgery (eg, circumcision or cosmetic operations in schizophrenics).

Clinical manifestations are rare on the first postoperative day. During this period, patients appear emotionless and unconcerned about changes in the environment or in themselves. Most overt psychiatric derangements are observed after the third postoperative day. The symptoms are variable but often include confusion, fear, and disorientation as to time and place. Delirium presents as altered consciousness with cognitive impairment. These symptoms may not be readily apparent to the surgeon, as this problem usually occurs in sick patients whose other problems may mask the manifestations of psychosis. Early psychiatric consultation should be obtained when psychosis is suspected so that adequate and prompt assessment of consciousness and cognitive function can be done and treatment instituted. The earlier the psychosis is recognized, the easier it is to correct. Metabolic derangements or early sepsis (especially in burn patients) must be ruled out as the cause. Severe postoperative emotional disturbances may be avoided by appropriate preoperative counseling of the patient by the surgeon. This includes a thorough discussion of the operation and the expected outcome, acquainting the patient with the intensive care unit, etc. Postoperatively, the surgeon must attend to the patient's emotional needs, offering frequent reassurance, explaining the postoperative course, and discussing the prognosis and the outcome of the operation.

Special Psychiatric Problems

A. The ICU Syndrome

The continuous internal vigilance that results from pain and fear and the sleep deprivation from bright lights, monitoring equipment, and continuous noise causes a psychologic disorganization known as ICU psychosis. The patient whose level of consciousness is already decreased by illness and drugs is more susceptible than a normal individual, and the result is decreased ability to think, perceive, and remember. When the cognitive processes are thoroughly disorganized, delirium occurs. The manifestations include distorted visual, auditory, and tactile perception; confusion and restlessness; and inability to differentiate reality from fantasy. Prevention includes isolation from the environment, decreased noise levels, adequate sleep, and removal from the intensive care unit as soon as possible.

B. Postcardiotomy Delirium

Mental changes that occasionally follow open heart surgery include impairment of memory, attention, cognition, and perception and occasionally hysteria, depressive reaction, and anxiety crisis. The symptoms most often appear after the third postoperative day. The type of operation, the presence of organic brain disease, prolonged medical illness, and the length of time on extracorporeal circulation are related to the development of postcardiotomy psychosis. Mild sedation and measures to prevent the ICU syndrome may prevent this complication. In more severe cases, haloperidol (Haldol) in doses of 1–5 mg given orally, intramuscularly, or intravenously may be required. Haloperidol is preferred over phenothiazines in these patients because it is associated with a lower incidence of cardiovascular side effects.

C. Delirium Tremens

Delirium tremens occurs in alcoholics who stop drinking suddenly. Hyperventilation and metabolic alkalosis contribute to the development of the full-blown syndrome. Hypomagnesemia and hypokalemia secondary to alkalosis or nutritional deficits may precipitate seizures. Readaptation to ethanol-free metabolism requires about 2 weeks, and it is during this period that alcoholics are at greatest risk of developing delirium tremens.

The prodrome includes personality changes, anxiety, and tremor. The complete syndrome is characterized by agitation, hallucinations, restlessness, confusion, overactivity, and, occasionally, seizures and hyperthermia. The syndrome also causes a hyperdynamic cardiorespiratory and metabolic state. For example, cardiac index, oxygen delivery, and oxygen consumption double during delirium tremens and return to normal 24–48 hours after resolution. The wild behavior may precipitate dehiscence of a fresh laparotomy incision. Diaphoresis and dehydration are common, and exhaustion may herald death.

Withdrawal symptoms may be prevented by giving small amounts of alcohol, but benzodiazepines are the treatment of choice. Vitamin B_1 (thiamine) and magnesium sulfate should also be given.

The aims of treatment are to reduce agitation and anxiety as soon as possible and to prevent the development of other complications (eg, seizures, aspiration pneumonia). General measures should include frequent assessment of vital signs, restoration of nutrition, administration of vitamin B, correction of electrolyte imbalance or other metabolic derangements, and adequate hydration. Physical restraint, though necessary for seriously violent behavior, should be as limited as possible. With proper care, most patients improve within 72 hours.

D. Sexual Dysfunction

Sexual problems commonly occur after certain kinds of operations, such as prostatectomy, heart surgery, and aortic reconstruction. The pathogenesis is unclear. In abdominoperineal resection, severance of the peripheral branches of the sacral plexus may cause impotence. It is important to discuss this possibility with the patient before any operation with a risk of impotence is performed. When sexual dysfunction is psychogenic, reassurance is usually all that is needed. If psychogenic impotence persists beyond 4–6 weeks, psychiatric consultation is indicated.

COMPLICATIONS OF INTRAVENOUS THERAPY & HEMODYNAMIC MONITORING

Air Embolism

Air embolism may occur during or after insertion of a venous catheter or as a result of accidental introduction of air into the line. Intravenous air lodges in the right atrium, preventing adequate filling of the right heart. This is manifested by hypotension, jugular venous distention, and tachycardia. This complication can be avoided by placing the patient in the Trendelenburg position when a central venous line is inserted. Emergency treatment consists of aspiration of the air with a syringe. If this is unsuccessful, the patient should be positioned right side up and head down, which will help dislodge the air from the right atrium and return circulatory dynamics to normal.

Phlebitis

A needle or a catheter inserted into a vein and left in place will in time cause inflammation at the entry site. When this process involves the vein, it is called phlebitis. Factors determining the degree of inflammation are the nature of the cannula, the solution infused, bacterial infection, and venous thrombosis. Phlebitis is one of the most common causes of fever after the third postoperative day. The symptomatic triad of induration, edema, and tenderness is characteristic. Visible signs may be minimal. Prevention of phlebitis is best accomplished by observance of aseptic techniques during insertion of venous catheters, frequent change of tubing (ie, every 48–72 hours), and rotation of insertion sites (ie, every 4 days). Silastic catheters, which are the least reactive, should be used when the line must be left in for a long time. Hypertonic solutions should be infused only into veins with substantial flow, such as the subclavian, jugular, or vena cava. Venous catheters should be removed at the first sign of redness, induration, or edema. Because phlebitis is most frequent with cannulation of veins in the lower extremities, this route should be used only when upper extremity veins are unavailable. Removal of the catheter is adequate treatment.

Suppurative phlebitis may result from the presence of an infected thrombus around the indwelling catheter. Staphylococci are the most common causative organisms. Local signs of inflammation are present, and pus may be expressed from the venipuncture site. High fever and positive blood cultures are common. Treatment consists of excising the affected vein, extending the incision proximally to the first open collateral, and leaving the wound open.

Cardiopulmonary Complications

Perforation of the right atrium with cardiac tamponade has been associated with the use of central venous lines. This complication can be avoided by checking the position of the tip of the line, which should be in the superior vena cava, not the right atrium. Complications associated with the use of the flow-directed balloon-tipped (Swan-Ganz) catheter include cardiac perforation (usually of the right atrium), intracardiac knotting of the catheter, and cardiac dysrhythmias. Pulmonary hemorrhage may result from disruption of a branch of the pulmonary artery during balloon inflation and may be fatal in patients with pulmonary hypertension. Steps in prevention include careful placement, advancement under continuous pressure monitoring, and checking the position of the tip before inflating the balloon.

Ischemic Necrosis of the Finger

Continuous monitoring of arterial blood pressure during the operation and in the intensive care unit requires insertion of a radial or femoral arterial line. The hand receives its blood supply from the radial and ulnar arteries, and because of the anatomy of the palmar arches, patency of one of these vessels is usually enough to provide adequate blood flow through the hand. Occasionally, ischemic necrosis of the finger has followed use of an indwelling catheter in the radial artery. This serious complication can usually be avoided by evaluating the patency of the ulnar artery (Allen's test) before establishing the radial line and by changing arterial line sites every 3–4 days. After an arterial catheter is withdrawn, a pressure dressing should be applied to avoid formation of an arterial pseudoaneurysm.

POSTOPERATIVE FEVER

Fever occurs in about 40% of patients after major surgery. In most patients the temperature elevation resolves without specific treatment. However, postoperative fever may herald a serious infection, and it is therefore important to evaluate the patient clinically. Features often associated with an infectious origin of the fever include preoperative trauma, ASA class above 2, fever onset after the second postoperative day, an initial temperature elevation above 38.6 °C, a postoperative white blood cell count greater than 10,000/μL, and a postoperative serum urea nitrogen of 15 mg/dL or greater. If three or more of the above are present, the likelihood of associated bacterial infection is nearly 100%.

Fever within 48 hours after surgery is usually caused by atelectasis. Reexpansion of the lung causes body temperature to return to normal. Because laboratory and radiologic investigations are usually unrevealing, an extensive evaluation of early postoperative fever is rarely appropriate if the patient's convalescence is otherwise smooth.

When fever appears after the second postoperative day, atelectasis is a less likely explanation. The differential diagnosis of fever at this time includes catheter-related phlebitis, pneumonia, and urinary tract infection. A directed history and physical examination complemented by focused laboratory and radiologic studies usually determine the cause.

Patients without infection are rarely febrile after the fifth postoperative day. Fever this late suggests wound infection or, less often, anastomotic breakdown and intra-abdominal abscesses. A diagnostic workup directed to the detection of intra-abdominal sepsis is indicated in patients who have high temperatures (> 39 °C) and wounds without evidence of infection 5 or more days postoperatively. CT scan of the abdomen and pelvis is the test of choice and should be performed early, before overt organ failure occurs.

Fever is rare after the first week in patients who had a normal convalescence. Allergy to drugs, transfusion-related fever, septic pelvic vein thrombosis, and intra-abdominal abscesses should be considered.

Block BM et al: Efficacy of postoperative epidural analgesia: a meta-analysis. JAMA 2003;290:2455.

Eagle KA et al: Guidelines for perioperative cardiovascular evaluation for noncardiac surgery: an abridged version of the report of the American College of Cardiology/American Heart Association Task Force on Practice Guidelines. Mayo Clin Proc 1997;72:524.

McGuire BE et al: Intensive care unit syndrome: a dangerous misnomer. Arch Intern Med 2000;160:906.

Moller AM et al: Effect of preoperative smoking intervention on postoperative complications: a randomised clinical trial. Lancet 2002;359:114.

National Nosocomial Infections Surveillance (NNIS) System Report, data summary from January 1992 through June 2003, issued August 2003. Am J Infect Control 2003;31:481.

Rabinowitz RP, Caplan ES: Management of infections in the trauma patient. Surg Clin North Am 1999;79:1373.

Sitges-Serra A, Girvent M: Catheter-related bloodstream infections. World J Surg 1999;23:589.

van 't Riet M et al: Meta-analysis of techniques for closure of midline abdominal incisions. Br J Surg 2002;89:1350.

Special Medical Problems in Surgical Patients

5

ENDOCRINE DISEASE & THE SURGICAL PATIENT

Gerard M. Doherty, MD

DIABETES MELLITUS

Diabetic patients undergo more surgical procedures than do nondiabetics, and management of the diabetic patient before, during, and after surgery is an important responsibility of the surgeon. Fortunately, because close control of fluids, electrolytes, glucose, and insulin is now possible in the operating room, control of blood glucose levels during the perioperative period is usually relatively simple. Marked hyperglycemia should be avoided during surgery; the greater danger, however, is from severe unrecognized hypoglycemia.

Preoperative Workup

Blood glucose concentrations may be elevated in diabetic patients during the preoperative period. Physical trauma, if present, combined with the emotional and physiologic stress of the illness may cause epinephrine and cortisol levels to rise, in each case resulting in increased blood glucose levels. If exogenous cortisol is being administered (eg, to a renal or pancreatic transplant recipient), marked insulin resistance and elevations of blood glucose levels regularly result. Infections may also increase blood glucose concentrations, occasionally to dangerous levels. Inactivity in bedridden patients can increase blood glucose levels by causing insulin resistance. Hypokalemia—frequently the result of diuretic therapy but also of epinephrine release induced by trauma—may prevent B cells from secreting adequate amounts of insulin and may thereby raise blood glucose levels in patients with type 2 diabetes.

The preoperative workup of patients with diabetes mellitus includes a thorough physical examination, with special care to discover occult infections; an ECG to rule out myocardial infarction; and a chest x-ray to identify hidden pneumonia or pulmonary edema. A complete urinalysis can rule out urinary tract infection and proteinuria, the earliest signs of diabetic renal disease. Serum potassium levels are measured to check for hypokalemia or hyperkalemia, the latter usually resulting from hyporeninemic hypoaldosteronism, a relatively common syndrome in diabetics. Serum creatinine levels are used to assess renal function. The serum glucose concentration should ideally be between 100 and 200 mg/dL, but operation can be safely performed in patients whose serum glucose is as high as 350–400 mg/dL preoperatively.

Preoperative & Intraoperative Management of Diabetic Patients

A. Type 2 (Non-Insulin-Dependent) Diabetes Mellitus

Approximately 85% of diabetics over age 50 years have only a moderately decreased ability to produce and secrete insulin, and when at home they can usually be controlled by diet or by sulfonylureas. If the serum glucose level is below 250 mg/dL on the morning of surgery, sulfonylureas should be withheld; long-acting sulfonylurea drugs—glipizide, glyburide, and chlorpropamide—should be discontinued on the day before surgery; and 5% glucose solution should be administered intravenously at a rate of about 100 mL/h. This means that over a 10-hour period, only 50 g of glucose would be given; by contrast, during an average day, a diabetic on a normal diet would consume four to five times as much carbohydrate (ie, 200–250 g). During any but the most extensive surgery, the pancreas should be able to produce enough insulin to handle this modest glucose load and at the same time prevent undue gluconeogenesis.

If the fasting glucose level is above 250–300 mg/dL or if the patient is taking small doses of insulin but does not actually require insulin to prevent ketoacidosis, an alternative approach is to add 5 units of insulin directly to each liter of 5% glucose solution being given at 100 mL/h. If the operation is lengthy, blood glucose levels should be measured every 3–4 hours during surgery to ensure adequate glucose control. The goal is to maintain glucose levels between 100 and 200 mg/dL, but there is little immediate metabolic harm in allowing levels to go as high as 250 mg/dL.

B. Type 1 (Insulin-Dependent) Diabetes Mellitus

Type 1 patients require insulin during surgery. It can be administered by any of the following methods: (1) subcutaneous administration of long-acting insulin; (2) constant infusion of a mixture of glucose and insulin; or (3) separate infusions of glucose and insulin. Intravenous boluses of regular insulin are rarely, if ever, indicated. The effect of single boluses of insulin given intravenously typically lasts only minutes, leading to the danger of acute hypoglycemia followed shortly thereafter by recurrent hyperglycemia. With either technique, blood glucose levels should be monitored at least every 2 hours during the procedure to avoid hypoglycemia below 60 mg/dL and hyperglycemia above 250 mg/dL. Blood glucose levels can be measured rapidly during surgery with a portable electronic glucose analyzer.

1. Conventional procedure for insulin administration—The first and still most widely used method of controlling blood glucose levels during surgery is to administer subcutaneously, on the morning of the operation, one-third to one-half the patient's usual dose of long-acting insulin plus one-third to one-half of the usual dose of short-acting insulin. This is followed by intravenous infusion of 5% or even 10% glucose at a rate of 100 mL/h preoperatively and intraoperatively. If the operation is prolonged, potassium chloride should be added at a rate of 20 meq/h.

There are a number of disadvantages to this procedure, which results in giving the full day's insulin requirement preoperatively. First, after subcutaneous administration, the absorption of NPH and regular insulin varies greatly in individual patients, especially when they are inactive. Second, although surgeons may prefer that operations on diabetics be scheduled early in the day, often the procedure must be delayed until afternoon. The relatively small amounts of glucose being administered are then inadequate to compensate for the 18–20 hours the patient has been without food, with the result that the insulin causes severe afternoon hypoglycemia. In the average diabetic, the peak action of regular insulin occurs about 6 hours after its administration. Therefore, if regular insulin is given subcutaneously at 7 AM, its peak action in an average patient will occur at about 1 PM. As a result, following subcutaneous administration of regular insulin in the early morning, the patient's glucose concentration may be inadequately controlled early in the morning; and if surgery is delayed, the peak action of regular insulin in the early afternoon and of NPH insulin in the later afternoon may result in severe hypoglycemia. If surgery must be delayed, it is imperative that blood glucose levels be carefully monitored for hypoglycemia and additional glucose given as necessary.

2. Intravenous infusion of insulin in glucose solution—Another option is to treat type 1 diabetics undergoing surgery by giving an infusion of 5% or 10% glucose solution containing 5, 10, or even 15 units of insulin per liter, depending on the patient's initial blood glucose concentration. At an infusion rate of 100 mL/h, the insulin is administered at a rate of 0.5, 1, or 1.5 units/h, respectively. In patients receiving corticosteroids, as much as 20 units per liter of insulin may be required.

There are a number of advantages to this regimen. First, the problem of absorption of insulin is avoided, since it is given intravenously. As a result, instead of an average 6-hour lag for maximal response to regular insulin, the effect starts within 10–15 minutes and is relatively constant. Second, unlike the fixed insulin dose with subcutaneous administration, the insulin infusion can be changed at any time in response to changes in blood glucose levels. Third, the dangers of hypo- and hyperglycemia are minimized, because if the intravenous solution is stopped (if the needle is inadvertently removed or the tubing clamped), both the glucose and the insulin are discontinued simultaneously. Since only about 10% of insulin adsorbs to glass or plastic, the resulting reduction in dosage is of little therapeutic importance. A similar continuous intravenous infusion of insulin has also become a common way to treat diabetic ketoacidosis.

3. Use of insulin "piggy-backed" into the glucose infusion—Instead of mixing insulin in the same bottle as the glucose, an insulin solution is infused ("piggy-backed") into the tubing delivering the 5% or 10% glucose. Generally, 50 units of regular insulin are mixed with 500 mL of normal saline—a solution containing 1 unit of insulin per 10 mL of solution. The glucose solution is given at a rate of 100 mL/h, and the insulin infusion is adjusted (usually by IVAC pump) to deliver a total of 5 mL (0.5 units), 10 mL (1 unit), 30 mL (30 units) per hour, etc, depending on the results of blood glucose determinations obtained approximately hourly during the surgical procedure. Of the three techniques, this is the most flexible and allows the closest control of blood glucose levels. It requires careful monitoring of the pump delivery rate, because too rapid infusion of insulin will cause hypoglycemia. A number of simple algorithms have been recommended for adjusting the rate of insulin infusion according to the previous plasma glucose levels. This approach is especially useful during prolonged operations. The simplest and most practical procedure is to give no insulin if plasma glucose is less than 90 mg/dL. Above values of 90 mg/dL, the dosage of regular insulin in units per hour should equal 1% of the previous hour's plasma glucose (mg/dL)—eg, at a glucose level of 200 mg/dL, give 2 units/h; at 300 mg/dL, give 3 units/h, etc.

Postoperative Care

With either of the intravenous infusion techniques, it is best to continue the glucose-insulin infusion until the patient is eating. Hypoglycemia, the most common postoperative complication, most often follows the use of long-acting insulin given subcutaneously before surgery. Although hypoglycemia may also occur if the intravenous insulin infusion is excessive in relation to that of the glucose, an infusion of 1.5 units or less of insulin per hour, when given with 5% glucose, rarely results in hypoglycemia. Blood glucose levels should be measured every 2–4 hours and the patient monitored for signs and symptoms of hypoglycemia (eg, anxiety, tremulousness, profuse sweating without fever). When hypoglycemia is detected, the amount of glucose infused should be promptly increased and the insulin decreased. It is rarely advisable to stop the insulin infusion completely for mild hypoglycemia, since a smoother transition to euglycemia results if the insulin is continued but at a lower dose.

A marked increase in glucose and insulin requirements postoperatively suggests the presence of occult infection (eg, wound infection, cellulitis at the intravenous site, urinary tract infection, or unrecognized aspiration pneumonia).

Adjustments in the rate of glucose or insulin administration must be based on *blood* glucose levels.

Hyperosmolar Coma

Hyperosmolar coma, the result of severe dehydration, may occur in undiagnosed diabetics who have been given large amounts of glucose during surgery. The resulting osmotic diuresis leads to disproportionate water loss, dehydration, and hyperosmolarity. Hyperosmolar coma rarely occurs until the serum glucose level exceeds 800 mg/dL and the osmolarity exceeds 340 meq/L. Hyperosmolar coma is best avoided by monitoring fluid input and output, measuring blood glucose levels, and instituting treatment promptly if the value exceeds 400 mg/dL.

Golden SH et al: Perioperative glycemic control and the risk of infectious complications in a cohort of adults with diabetes. Diabetes Care 1999;22:1408.

Hirsch IB et al: Diabetes management in special situations. Endocrinol Metab Clin North Am 1997;26:631.

Kaufman FR et al: Perioperative management with prolonged intravenous insulin infusion versus subcutaneous insulin in children with type I diabetes mellitus. J Diabetes Complications 1996;10:6.

Vanhaeverbeek M: Peri-operative care: management of the diabetic patient. A novel controversy about tight glycemic control. Acta Clin Belg 1997;52:313.

THYROID DISEASE

Both hyper- and hypothyroidism represent serious problems for patients undergoing surgery. It may be difficult to establish an adequate airway in patients with large goiters. The hyperthyroid patient undergoing surgery is apt to develop hypertension, severe cardiac dysrhythmias, congestive heart failure, and hyperthermia.

Life-threatening thyrotoxicosis (thyroid storm) may be precipitated by any operation but especially by thyroidectomy, which accentuates thyroxine release. It is therefore preferable to bring hyperthyroid patients into a euthyroid state before surgery. This takes 1–6 weeks and is best accomplished by treatment with propylthiouracil, 800–1000 mg/d for about 1 week, followed by a maintenance dose of 200–400 mg/d. If emergency surgery is required, adequate sedation and potassium iodide plus a β-adrenergic blocking agent such as propranolol should be given in addition to propylthiouracil.

Hypothyroid patients are subject to acute hypotension, shock, and hypothermia during surgery; if the patient is allowed to breathe spontaneously, severe CO_2 retention may result from hypoventilation. **Myxedema coma** should be suspected in patients who fail to awaken promptly from anesthesia and who manifest CO_2 retention, even to the point of CO_2 narcosis, accompanied by hypothermia. Increased tissue friability, poor wound healing, and even wound dehiscence may also occur. It is highly advisable to treat myxedematous patients with levothyroxine before elective surgery. In an emergency (eg, severe myxedema requiring immediate surgery), treatment should consist of levothyroxine sodium, 500 μg (0.5 mg) intravenously, by nasogastric tube, or orally. If there is no emergency, the euthyroid state may be gradually restored with levothyroxine, 25 μg/d, with the dose increased over several weeks to a maintenance dose of 150–200 μg/d. It is also always advisable to obtain a baseline cortisol level before treatment of myxedema to rule out coexistent Addison's disease (Schmidt's syndrome), since levothyroxine therapy can precipitate addisonian crisis in this setting.

Attia J et al: Diagnosis of thyroid disease in hospitalized patients: a systematic review. Arch Intern Med 1999;159:658.

Cooper DS: Antithyroid drugs for the treatment of hyperthyroidism caused by Graves' disease. Emerg Med Clin North Am 1998;27:225.

Kahaly GJ et al: Cardiac risks of hyperthyroidism in the elderly. Thyroid 1998;8:1165.

Koutras DA: Subclinical hyperthyroidism. Thyroid 1999;9:311.

Ladenson PW et al: Complications of surgery in hypothyroid patients. Am J Med 1984;77:261.

ADRENAL INSUFFICIENCY

Patients with adrenal insufficiency undergoing the stress of operation are at risk of addisonian crisis, manifested by salt wastage, decreased blood volume, hypotension, shock, and death. For at least 2–3 days preoperatively, they should receive fluid and sodium chloride replacement intravenously (usually 1–3 L of normal saline per day) and cortisol therapy (20 mg each morning and 10 mg each afternoon). On the day of surgery, 100 mg of cortisol is administered intramuscularly or intravenously just before the operation, followed by 50–100 mg every 6 hours during surgery—a regimen that mimics the normal endogenous cortisol response to stress (up to 300 mg/d). Saline is continued postoperatively at a rate of at least 2–3 L/d, with careful monitoring of blood pressure, serum electrolyte concentrations, and urine output. In the absence of complications, the cortisol dosage can be decreased by half each day until the usual maintenance dose of about 30 mg/d is reached.

Patients receiving chronic corticosteroid therapy may present with severe hypokalemia and at times serious hypertension, both of which should be corrected before surgery. Stress doses of cortisol (approximately 300 mg/d) must be administered during surgery according to the protocol described for addisonian patients. If the patient is diabetic, large doses of insulin (eg, 3 units/h) may be required to control blood glucose levels during surgery. Postoperatively, slow wound healing and a predisposition to infection should be anticipated. Infections in these patients may occur without fever.

PITUITARY INSUFFICIENCY

Patients with **panhypopituitarism** must be treated for thyroid and adrenocorticosteroid insufficiency with the doses of levothyroxine and cortisol set forth in the preceding sections.

HEART DISEASE & THE SURGICAL PATIENT

Barry M. Massie, MD

Anesthesia and surgery present a finite risk to any patient, but this risk is increased in the patient with preexisting heart disease, whether clinically apparent or undiagnosed. Indeed, complications related to heart disease are the major cause of nonsurgical perioperative deaths.

Cardiac disease may be exacerbated by many of the physiologic changes accompanying surgery, including fluctuations in heart rate, blood pressure, blood volume, oxygenation, pH, and coagulability. These may lead to myocardial ischemia due to increased myocardial O_2 demand or reduced coronary blood flow, impaired myocardial contractility, and altered cardiac performance due to changes in preload or afterload. Increased circulating catecholamines or sympathetic nervous system activity may precipitate arrhythmias as well as increase heart rate and blood pressure. Anesthesia and medications such as vagolytics and muscle relaxants have direct effects on myocardial contractility, automaticity, and conduction.

While the operative period itself is stressful, intraoperative cardiac complications are in fact relatively uncommon as a result of careful monitoring and improved understanding of the risk of the accompanying hemodynamic alterations. The greatest risk occurs in the 72 hours following operation, when fluid volume shifts, fluctuations in heart rate and blood pressure, and medication changes are greatest and the ability to control them is compromised. The best approach to minimizing cardiac complications is to maintain one's awareness of the presence and severity of preexisting heart disease and of the risk of asymptomatic and unrecognized disease.

Given this information, the medical consultant, anesthesiologist, and surgeon can weigh the following key questions: (1) Is the operation urgent, essential but with elective timing, or optional? (2) Does the patient have heart disease, manifest or silent? (3) What additional risk does heart disease impose? (4) Can this risk be reduced by additional treatment or by delaying surgery? The answers to these questions will determine the appropriate management strategy. Urgent surgery must proceed, so the problem for the consultant and anesthesiologist is to minimize risk. Elective surgery may need to be delayed or canceled depending on the risk to benefit ratio.

Cardiac Conditions Masquerading as Surgical Illnesses

Cardiovascular diseases may occasionally produce symptoms that mimic surgical conditions, and this possibility must be considered before operation. Such presentations include the following:

(1) Myocardial infarction or angina pectoris presenting with epigastric pain, suggesting peptic ulcer, gallbladder disease, or other surgical abdominal disease.

(2) Right heart failure presenting as right upper quadrant pain due to hepatic congestion, suggesting gallbladder disease.

(3) Nonspecific gastrointestinal symptoms such as anorexia, nausea, early satiety, and weight loss due to severe heart failure, suggesting cancer or other abdominal surgical disease.

(4) Ascites due to heart failure or pericardial disease.

(5) Dysphagia due to left atrial enlargement or diseases of the aorta.

(6) Back and abdominal pain due to aortic dissection.

(7) Abdominal pain due to splenic, renal, or mesenteric emboli from infective endocarditis, emboli of cardiac origin, or atrial myxoma.

(8) Upper abdominal pain and even jaundice due to pulmonary infarction.

Most of these conditions are readily recognized if they are considered. More typical associated symptoms are usually present. The ECG should reveal evolving or recent infarction, and the physical examination and chest x-ray should demonstrate heart failure or signs of pericardial disease. Echocardiography will confirm the presence of left or right ventricular failure, valvular disease, and pericardial disease and may reveal a source of emboli.

Preoperative Evaluation of the Surgical Patient for Cardiovascular Disease

All patients should be evaluated for possible cardiovascular disease preoperatively. The extent of this evaluation will depend on the statistical likelihood of previously unrecognized disease if the patient is asymptomatic and the nature of the heart condition if the diagnosis is known. A careful history is the primary screening procedure. Key areas of inquiry include the presence of dyspnea, exercise tolerance (and what limits it), chest discomfort and other ischemic equivalents (epigastric, throat, shoulder, or arm discomfort), edema, syncope or presyncope, or a history of heart murmur, hypertension, or failing an employment or insurance physical examination. Patients with a family history of premature coronary disease or with associated peripheral vascular disease should be assumed to be at high risk for ischemic heart disease, as should patients with a long history of diabetes. Patients with hyperlipidemia or hypertension are also at increased risk.

The physical examination will occasionally demonstrate a previously unrecognized heart murmur, mitral valve prolapse, irregular heart rhythm, or hypertension. In patients with heart disease, it will reveal the severity and degree of compensation of heart failure and provide a guide to the severity of valvular disease.

Most patients should have a preoperative ECG, though the yield is low in young patients with negative histories and examinations. Important findings include abnormal rhythms and conduction, left ventricular hypertrophy, myocardial infarction, and "nonspecific" ST segment and T wave abnormalities. A routine preoperative chest x-ray has a low yield in healthy subjects but may be useful in patients with symptoms or an abnormal physical examination. Additional noninvasive tests or procedures that may be indicated to diagnose and define the severity of cardiac abnormalities include echocardiography, exercise testing, stress (exercise or dipyridamole) thallium scintigraphy, radionuclide ejection fraction measurements, and ambulatory monitoring. In some patients, cardiac catheterization and coronary arteriography are indicated to determine the severity of heart disease and the need for additional medical or other intervention before surgery.

The evaluation and management of specific cardiac diseases and abnormalities are discussed below.

Relative Contraindications to Surgery

There are no absolute contraindications to surgery, but a number of cardiac conditions substantially increase the risks and become relative contraindications. These include recent myocardial infarction, an unstable or progressive pattern of angina pectoris, decompensated heart failure, severe aortic or mitral stenosis, and severe hypertension. Most heart diseases do not themselves prohibitively increase the surgical risk, but when they are progressive, unstable, or decompensated, the level of risk rises abruptly.

Several approaches have been proposed for quantifying operative risk. The most widely used of these is the Goldman Index, which provides a point score for findings associated with additional risk:

Finding	Points
S_2 gallop or elevated venous pressure	11
Myocardial infarction in previous 6 months	10
More than five VPCs/min on any ECG	7
Nonsinus rhythm or APCs on last ECG	7
Age > 70 years	5
Emergency operation	4
Intrathoracic, intraperitoneal, or aortic surgery	3
Significant aortic stenosis	3
Poor general medical condition	3

The risk of cardiac death and life-threatening cardiac complications rises progressively with the total point score—from less than 1% when the score is 0–5 points, to 7% for 6–12 points, 13% (2% mortality rate) with 13–25 points, to 78% (including a 56% mortality rate) in patients with scores over 26 points.

Detsky has modified this multifactorial index to take into account the nature of the operation. However, it should be recognized that these indices serve two functions: to identify factors of risk and to provide probabilities for populations. In assessing the individual patient, the physician must make a judgment based upon the specific cardiac disease, its severity, and its stability.

Specific Cardiac Conditions

A. Coronary Artery Disease

Coronary artery disease is the most common cardiac disease and the major cause of morbidity and mortality in patients undergoing surgery. Several categories of patients must be considered: those with prior myocardial infarction, those with angina pectoris, and those with possible asymptomatic coronary disease. Virtually all patients who have had a myocardial infarction have coronary artery disease and are at risk for further ischemia or reinfarction. This risk is highest in patients in whom the infarction is most recent, declining from approximately 20–30% (or higher in earlier studies) in the first 3 months, to 10–15% after 4–6 months, and to 5% thereafter. With advances in medical therapy, better diagnostic testing, and improved perioperative management, these numbers are falling, but it is still preferable to delay elective surgery for 3–6 months after myocardial infarction. The propensity for ischemia and reinfarction are higher following nontransmural infarctions, in which the volume of residual ischemic myocardium is greater. If the infarction is recent, such patients should undergo stress testing with exercise or dipyridamole thallium scintigraphy to identify individuals with large areas of ischemia before major surgery; these patients should undergo coronary angiography and revascularization if indicated. It may be helpful to assess left ventricular function noninvasively in patients with anterior transmural infarctions, since they may have significantly decreased ejection fractions in the absence of symptomatic heart failure.

Angina pectoris also reflects underlying coronary artery disease and is just as important an indicator of risk as is prior infarction. When the pattern is progressive or unstable or the activity threshold is very low, operation should be postponed at least until the angina can be stabilized by medical therapy. If major noncardiac surgery is planned, coronary arteriography is usually indicated in patients with unstable or severely limiting angina to detect critical lesions.

Patients with *stable* mild to moderate angina pectoris, old myocardial infarctions, or multiple risk factors without overt coronary artery disease represent a group with intermediate perioperative risk. When major surgery (especially vascular procedures) is planned or if additional risk factors such as age over 70 years, diabetes mellitus, or heart failure are present, further evaluation may be warranted. Since exercise testing is often not feasible, pharmacologic stress with dipyridamole or adenosine in association with perfusion scintigraphy or echocardiography are usually employed. Individuals with demonstrable ischemia, especially when it involves multiple or large areas, are at increased risk; coronary arteriography or additional medical therapy may be indicated.

However, before additional noninvasive diagnostic procedures are performed, there are several things to consider. First, in *stable* patients with mild or even moderate symptoms, the risk of a major cardiac event (cardiac death, nonfatal infarction) as a complication of surgery averages just 2%, rising to only 5% with the most stressful (eg, vascular) operations. Consequently, myocardial revascularization by coronary artery bypass surgery or percutaneous transluminal angioplasty is rarely justified in such patients preoperatively. Although noninvasive imaging procedures could theoretically identify high-risk subgroups, experience has not been consistently good. Therefore, routine stress testing for risk stratification is not warranted, and imaging tests should generally be reserved for instances where the results are likely to alter management, such as to postpone surgery or change the planned procedure. Decisions concerning evaluation for coronary revascularization should be based upon the patient's symptoms or other accepted indications, such as multivessel disease in a patient with underlying left ventricular dysfunction, rather than specifically for decreasing perioperative risk. Therefore, all patients with cardiac risk factors who are undergoing major operations must be managed carefully during and after surgery whether or not noninvasive studies are normal. And there is no convincing evidence that preliminary coronary revascularization improves the outcome even in high-risk patients.

Patients with coronary artery disease or a high probability of coronary artery disease need to be managed carefully. Preoperative medications—including beta-blockers in particular but also nitrates and calcium-channel blockers—should be continued throughout the perioperative period. Aspirin should be continued unless concerns about hemostasis are overriding; addition of aspirin postoperatively may be useful, since many infarcts may be caused by a postoperative hypercoagulable state. Excessive tachycardia, hypertension, and hypotension should be avoided. Complications are most common in the second to fifth postoperative days, so vigilance must be maintained.

B. Congestive Heart Failure

Severe or decompensated congestive heart failure is an important risk factor for perioperative cardiac death. Surgery should be postponed until congestive heart failure is stable, pulmonary edema is absent, and excessive fluid is eliminated. A stable regimen of diuretics, angiotensin-converting enzyme inhibitors, and digoxin when indicated should be instituted. Underlying reversible causes (such as valvular lesions, ischemia, or uncontrolled hypertension) should be identified and treated. For major surgery, hemodynamic monitoring intraoperatively and postoperatively is essential. Decompensation is most common during and after the second postoperative day, when extravascular fluid begins to be mobilized. Weights, fluid balance, and oxygenation must be followed closely and diuretic therapy reinstituted early unless hypotension is present.

C. Valvular Heart Disease

Valvular heart disease in the absence of congestive heart failure is usually well tolerated during surgery. The exceptions are critical aortic stenosis and mitral stenosis. The former can be associated with hypotension and heart failure, while the latter often causes pulmonary edema when the heart rate increases, atrial fibrillation occurs, or excessive fluid volume is administered. Nonetheless, patients with moderate obstructions (eg, aortic valve area > 0.8 cm^2; mitral area > 1.2 cm^2) usually do well, and those with even more severe stenoses can be managed successfully with careful monitoring if the need for surgery is urgent. Mitral valve prolapse is an indication for antibiotic prophylaxis in nonsterile procedures but does not increase the risk of surgery.

D. Dysrhythmias and Conduction Abnormalities

Supraventricular arrhythmias can usually be managed with agents such as verapamil and esmolol as well as with digoxin. Frequent ventricular ectopy does indicate increased risk, but this usually reflects associated myocardial disease, which should be sought and evaluated. It is not necessary to suppress asymptomatic nonsustained ventricular arrhythmias preoperatively. Ventricular ectopy and ventricular tachycardia occurring during or after surgery often reflect arrhythmias that were present preoperatively. Treatment is required only when they result in symptoms or hemodynamic compromise. Electrolyte imbalance, hypoxia, and electrocardiographic evidence of bigeminy or infarction should be sought and treated. Prophylactic antiarrhythmic activity has not been shown to be beneficial.

Left bundle branch block or bifascicular block also indicates higher risk, since these findings often indicate myocardial disease. However, progression to advanced atrioventricular block during surgery is rare. Prolonged PR intervals, Mobitz I (Wenckebach) atrioventricular block, or sinus bradycardia (heart rate less than 45–50/min) often reflects excessive medication effect from digoxin, β-adrenergic blocking agents, and calcium channel-blocking agents. These dosages should be adjusted downward if possible. Higher degrees of atrioventricular blockade should usually be managed with temporary or permanent pacing.

E. Congenital Heart Disease

In general, if these lesions are associated with heart failure, severe pulmonary hypertension (systolic pulmonary pressure above 80 mm Hg), or hypoxemia, the risk of surgery is high.

F. Hypertension

Patients with uncomplicated and controlled hypertension usually tolerate surgery well. The presence of left ventricular hypertrophy with repolarization changes indicates mildly increased risk, perhaps because of a higher incidence of associated coronary artery disease. Indeed, untreated and suboptimally treated hypertension do not appear to significantly increase risk when the pressure is below 160/105 mm Hg, since it is relatively easy to reduce it with anesthesia and parenteral agents. When the pressure exceeds 180/110 mm Hg, the incidence of severe perioperative hypertension increases along with the need for prolonged parenteral treatment and observation as well as the risk of complications.

Antihypertensive medications should be continued to avoid withdrawal syndromes, especially when the patient is receiving central sympatholytics or beta-blockers. This can usually be accomplished with oral medication, but transdermal clonidine, sublingual nifedipine, and intravenous calcium-channel blockers (verapamil and diltiazem) and parenteral beta-blockers and converting enzyme inhibitors are available.

Special Issues Related to Monitoring & Anesthesia

A. Medications

It is feasible and desirable to continue most medications in the perioperative period. This is especially true with medications for coronary artery disease, congestive heart failure, and hypertension. If additional medications are needed, parenteral therapy is should be provided.

B. Hemodynamic Monitoring

Hemodynamic monitoring of high-risk patients during major surgical procedures has become routine. This is essential for patients with congestive heart failure, impaired left ventricular function (ejection fraction below 40%), critical valve disease, and recent myocardial infarction when the surgery is major. It probably is not necessary in patients at risk for ischemia with preserved left ventricular function except in the case of major vascular procedures. Perhaps the most valuable period for hemodynamic monitoring in high-risk patients is the immediate postoperative period, when appropriate parameters for fluid administration and blood pressure can be difficult to define.

C. Transesophageal Echocardiography

This technique is being increasingly used in the operating room. It permits excellent visualization of the left ventricle and can provide continuous monitoring of cavity size, contractile function, and segmental wall motion. In experienced hands, transesophageal echocardiography allows early detection of heart failure and myocardial ischemia, but its additional value beyond hemodynamic monitoring in noncardiac surgery has not been proved, and for that reason its routine use, even in high-risk patients, is not indicated.

D. Choice of Anesthetics

There is no conclusive evidence that the choice of anesthetics affects outcomes in patients with heart disease, and the selection of the route of anesthesia and the choice of agent are best left to the anesthesiologist. Epidural anesthesia may be preferable when a low spinal level is adequate for the procedure, but hypotension is a problem with higher levels. Narcotics have little myocardial depressant action and may be preferable to the volatile gases in patients with diminished contractility.

E. Antibiotic Prophylaxis

Patients with valvular heart disease and prosthetic heart valves require antibiotic prophylaxis for bacteremia, including genitourinary, gastrointestinal, oropharyngeal, and gallbladder surgery. The usual regimen is ampicillin, 2 g intravenously, plus gentamicin, 1.5 mg/kg intravenously 30 minutes before operation. This may be repeated after 8 hours. Vancomycin, 1 g intravenously over 60 minutes, can be substituted in patients allergic to penicillin.

F. Anticoagulation

Patients with prosthetic valves and other heart conditions may be receiving chronic anticoagulation. In the former case, interruption of anticoagulation should be as brief as possible. Such patients should have their warfarin withdrawn 5 days prior to surgery and be maintained on intravenous heparin from the time their prothrombin time falls below 1.5 times control until 6 hours before operation. Heparin can usually be resumed 12 hours postoperatively. Anticoagulation for other indications can usually be withdrawn safely for the perioperative period.

Abraham S et al: Coronary risk of noncardiac surgery. Prog Cardiovasc Dis 1991;34:205.

Ashton CM et al: Incidence of perioperative myocardial infarction in men undergoing noncardiac surgical procedures. Ann Intern Med 1993;118:504.

Baron J-F et al: Dipyridamole-thallium scintigraphy and gated radionuclide angiography to assess cardiac risk before abdominal aortic surgery. N Engl J Med 1994;330:663.

Massie BM et al: Assessment of perioperative risk: have we put the cart before the horse? J Am Coll Cardiol 1993;21:1353.

Wong T et al: Perioperative cardiac risk assessment for patients having peripheral vascular surgery. Ann Intern Med 1992;116:745.

RESPIRATORY DISEASE & THE SURGICAL PATIENT

Robert F. Hickey, MD

Risk Factors

The most common perioperative complications involve the pulmonary system. The relatively high incidence of pulmonary complications is associated with anesthesia and surgery, and the two primary determinants are the operative site and the presence of lung disease. The correlation between the site of surgical incision and the incidence of pulmonary complications—from high to low—is thoracotomy, upper abdomen, lower abdomen, and periphery. The introduction of laparoscopic surgery has altered this basic paradigm, introducing a possible technique for reducing postoperative respiratory complications in high-risk patients. However, in these same patients, the complexity of intraoperative management may be increased. Pulmonary complications occur least frequently in patients with normal lung function who are undergoing peripheral surgery.

Secondary determinants of perioperative pulmonary complications include a history of smoking, age, obesity, and cooperativeness of the patient in postoperative care. These factors probably facilitate the development of lung disease, decrease the ability of the patient to cooperate in common maneuvers used to prevent or treat pulmonary complications, and compromise laryngeal integrity.

Laparoscopic Surgery

The advantage of laparoscopic surgery is that the use of smaller incisions and reduction in surgical trauma results in less postoperative pain and earlier recovery of bowel function. Thus, the impact of laparoscopic surgery on postoperative respiratory function may be intermediate between that of peripheral surgery and a lower abdominal incision and thus reduce postoperative respiratory complications. The disadvantage of this technique is its impact on both circulation and ventilation intraoperatively. Laparoscopic surgery requires the introduction of a pneumoperitoneum, distending the abdomen (usually with carbon dioxide) to intra-abdominal pressures of 11–15 mm Hg. Measurements in relatively healthy patients have shown that this maneuver results in a reduction of lung volume, systemic hypercapnia, reduction in cardiac index, and an increase in cardiac filling pressures and systemic vascular resistance. In these healthy patients, it is recommended that ventilation be increased to normalize $PaCO_2$. In patients with serious lung disease, the impact of introduction of a pneumoperitoneum is unknown. Additionally, attempts to normalize $PaCO_2$ have the potential to introduce air trapping with resultant circulatory collapse. At present, we would recommend that in patients with severe lung disease laparoscopic surgery may require extensive intraoperative monitoring with the possibility of converting to an open procedure if so indicated.

Specific Diseases & Problems

A. Acute Upper Respiratory Tract Infections

Both anesthesia and surgery provide opportunities for the spread of infection because respiratory defense mechanisms are compromised and instrumentation of the airway may be required. Therefore, the presence of a cold, pharyngitis, or tonsillitis is a relative contraindication to elective surgery, since viral infections decrease defense mechanisms against bacterial infections. If surgery is necessary, the appropriate antibiotic should be administered and manipulation of the infected area avoided when possible. No studies document the rate of complications or the preferred anesthetic techniques applicable to this situation.

B. Acute Lower Respiratory Tract Infections (Tracheitis, Bronchitis, Pneumonia)

These infections are absolute contraindications to elective surgery. For emergency surgery, therapy includes humidification of inhaled gases, removal of lung secretions, and continued administration of bronchodilators and antibiotics. If surgery is not absolutely necessary, the course of action is uncertain because no information is available concerning the incidence and severity of pulmonary complications.

C. Chronic Obstructive Pulmonary Disease (COPD) (Bronchitis, Emphysema, Bronchiectasis)

In patients with chronic obstructive pulmonary disease, the well-documented increase in the incidence and severity of postoperative pulmonary complications is related to the degree of lung disease. Two studies have investigated the influence of preoperative treatment of lung disease on the incidence of postoperative pulmonary complications. In both studies, patients underwent upper abdominal or thoracic surgery, and lung disease was defined by pulmonary function testing. In one study, therapy lasted 1 week and consisted of cessation of smoking, administration of antibiotics for purulent sputum, administration of bronchodilators, and physical therapy. In the second study, therapy lasted for 2 days and consisted of administration of antibiotics and bronchodilators and physical therapy. Both studies reported marked reduction in the incidence and severity of complications. The 1-week study reported decreased length of hospitalization for its patients.

Two other studies demonstrated the interaction between lung disease and the surgical site. They suggest that in peripheral surgery, lung disease is not a factor in the production of pulmonary complications unless disease is very severe (eg, severe enough to result in elevated $PaCO_2$). However, both of these studies were performed on a limited number of patients.

The results of these four studies indicate that patients with lung disease who are scheduled for elective upper abdominal or thoracic surgery should have preoperative treatment. Treatment should decrease the incidence and severity of postoperative pulmonary complications and shorten the hospital stay. A minimum of 1 week of therapy should include cessation of smoking, administration of antibiotics for purulent sputum and bronchodilators when indicated, and physical therapy to help remove excess sputum. Therapy can be performed on an outpatient basis. While any patient with lung disease should be treated regardless of plans for surgery, the focus here is on the prevention of death and illness from pulmonary complications in the surgical patient along with reduction of hospital time required to recover from surgical procedures.

D. Bronchial Asthma

Retrospective studies indicate that patients with bronchial asthma who are undergoing surgery are at increased risk of pulmonary complications. Preoperative management includes adjustment of bronchodilator medication, cessation of smoking, and treatment of infection. Intraoperative bronchoconstriction from mechanical stimulation of the airway must be prevented so that appropriate anesthetics can be given in adequate concentrations. Since intraoperative use of bronchodilators may be necessary, adverse interactions between anesthetic agents and bronchodilators must be avoided. Many patients with bronchial asthma have been treated with corticosteroids and require corticosteroid therapy in the perioperative period.

E. Restrictive Lung Disease (Caused by Pulmonary Fibrosis or Obesity)

Little information exists on perioperative pulmonary complications secondary to restrictive lung disease. Restrictive lung disease reduces lung volumes and decreases arterial oxygen tension; the decrease in arterial oxygen tension is particularly noticeable with exercise. Preoperative preparation is similar to that for any other lung disease and consists of treatment of infection, removal of sputum, and discontinuance of smoking. When controlled ventilation is required for patients with pulmonary fibrosis, it may be necessary to use smaller tidal volumes and more rapid respiratory rates than normal.

The effects of obesity on the development of perioperative pulmonary complications are most easily demonstrated in the massively obese patient. Obesity exists when the body weight is 1.2 times the normal weight; in morbid obesity, the weight is at least twice the normal weight. Pulmonary compromise is mostly due to reduction in lung volumes, leading to hypoxemia, airway obstruction from encroaching soft tissues in the airway, and perhaps an increase in gastric contents and acidity. If the problems are recognized and evaluated preoperatively, complications can be minimized. The massively obese patient should be mobilized as soon as possible postoperatively.

Preoperative Evaluation of Pulmonary Function

The purpose of preoperative pulmonary evaluation is to assess the risk of perioperative lung complications. This information not only guides perioperative pulmonary care but also selects patients for specific preoperative treatment that will decrease the risk of pulmonary complications and the length of the hospital stay. Such evaluations should be made before hospital admission to allow time for treatment if indicated.

Ideally, pulmonary evaluation is performed by the referring physician or surgeon (or both) at the time surgery is proposed. The site of surgery is a major consideration in the decision to perform pulmonary function tests and institute treatment (see Risk Factors, above). Other indications for pulmonary function testing arise primarily from the patient's history and physical examination and include factors present in lung disease, such as exertional dyspnea, exercise tolerance, cough, production of sputum, history of smoking, previous pulmonary complications, asthma, age, and body weight. Patients with mild pulmonary compromise who are to undergo peripheral surgery (not abdominal or thoracic surgery) probably do not require pulmonary function testing. When testing is necessary, simple spirometry with measurement of forced expiratory airflow is usually all that is required. If airflow on forced expiration is reduced significantly, the response to bronchodilators should be measured and arterial blood gases determined. More extensive tests such as diffusing capacity, radioisotopic ventilation-perfusion scans, and pulmonary artery catheterization are usually necessary only in patients with pulmonary hypertension or life-threatening lung disease or in those who require thoracic surgery.

Many studies have been done to try to determine which pulmonary function tests are the most reliable indicators of surgical and anesthetic risk and which reveal the greatest risk. Specific tests are usually correlated with perioperative complications, but for the most part these studies are not definitive, and as yet there are no absolute criteria for "operability." Tests can provide guidelines but are not reliable predictors for the following reasons:

(1) Patients with normal pulmonary function may develop perioperative pulmonary complications, though the incidence is low.

(2) Criteria developed for one surgical procedure (eg, thoracotomy) may not be accurate for another procedure.

(3) Pulmonary function tests cannot take into account intangibles such as patient cooperativeness. Tests do not measure the amount of sputum produced or predict the likelihood of pulmonary aspiration.

In general, simple spirometry with some measurement of impairment of airflow provides the best and least expensive screening test. Patients undergoing thoracic surgery without lung resection are at increased risk if FEV_1 or maximum breathing capacity is less than 50% of normal. For peripheral surgery, these values are lower (about 30% of predicted normal values). $PaCO_2$ greater than 45 mm Hg in patients not receiving ventilatory depressant drugs who are undergoing abdominal surgery or thoracotomy without lung tissue rejection indicates potential life-threatening pulmonary complications. Surgery on these patients should proceed only after adequate consultation. In peripheral surgery as well, elevated $PaCO_2$ indicates a greater likelihood of pulmonary complications and the possible need for postoperative mechanical ventilation and special monitoring.

Bartlett RH: Pulmonary pathophysiology in surgical patients. Surg Clin North Am 1980;60:1323.

Celi BR et al: A controlled trial of intermittent positive pressure breathing, incentive spirometry, and deep breathing exercises in preventing pulmonary complications after abdominal surgery. Am Rev Respir Dis 1984;130:12.

Craig DB: Postoperative recovery of pulmonary function. Anesth Analg 1981;60:46.

Cunningham AJ et al: Laparoscopic cholecystectomy: anesthetic implications. Anesth Analg 1993;76:1120.

Ford GT et al: Toward prevention of postoperative pulmonary complications. (Editorial.) Am Rev Resp Dis 1984;130:4.

Joris JL et al: Hemodynamic changes during laparoscopic cholecystectomy. Anesth Analg 1993;76:1067.

Keagy BA et al: Correlation of preoperative pulmonary function testing with clinical course in patients after pneumonectomy. Ann Thorac Surg 1983;36:253.

Kimball WR et al: Dynamic hyperinflation and ventilator dependence in chronic obstructive pulmonary disease. Am Rev Respir Dis 1982;126:991.

Miller JI et al: Pulmonary function test criteria for operability and pulmonary resection. Surg Gynecol Obstet 1981;153: 893.

Odeberg S et al: Haemodynamic effects of pneumoperitoneum and the influence of posture during anesthesia for laparoscopic surgery. Acta Anaesth Scand 1994;38:276.

Okeson GC: Pulmonary dysfunction and surgical risk: how to assess and minimize the hazards. Postgrad Med 1983;74:75.

Poe RH et al: Small airway testing and smoking in predicting risk in surgical patients. Am J Med Sci 1982;283:57.

Shah DM et al: Prevention of pulmonary complications in high risk patients. Surg Clin North Am 1980;60:1359.

Tisi GM: Preoperative evaluation of pulmonary function: Validity, indications, and benefits. Am Rev Respir Dis 1979;119:293.

RENAL DISEASE & THE SURGICAL PATIENT

Daniel C. Brennan, MD, & Matt J. Koch, MD

The discussion of renal disease and the surgical patient is primarily concerned with two clinical situations: management of the surgical patient with preexisting renal disease and management of the surgical patient who develops renal complications perioperatively. To understand the management of patients with renal disease, it is first necessary to have a fundamental knowledge of the normal function of the kidney and the implications of various degrees of renal insufficiency.

NORMAL RENAL FUNCTION & ASSESSMENT OF RENAL DISEASE

The principal task of the kidney is to maintain physiologic homeostasis through regulation of body fluids, osmolarity, electrolyte concentration, and acidity. The kidney accomplishes this through filtration of blood, formation of a plasma ultrafiltrate, and processing of the ultrafiltrate via secretion, reabsorption, and excretion. The kidney controls regulation of salt, water, and body pH as well as the excretion of water-soluble metabolic end products, toxins, and drugs. It is responsible also for the production of several hormones, including renin, erythropoietin, and 1,25-dihydroxyvitamin D_3.

Renal disease manifests as a perturbation of these normal functions. It should be suspected if there is evidence of hypertension, volume dysregulation (edema or volume contraction), electrolyte disturbances, proteinuria, hypoalbuminemia, hematuria, pyuria, anemia, or an elevated serum urea nitrogen or creatinine. Initial evaluation of renal disease should include a comprehensive history and physical examination, urinalysis, and determination of serum electrolytes, including calcium, phosphorus, and magnesium, as well as uric acid, urea nitrogen, creatinine, and albumin and an assessment of renal function or glomerular filtration rate (GFR).

Utility of Urinalysis

Urinalysis of a freshly voided urine specimen includes (1) dipstick assessment of pH, specific gravity, glycosuria, proteinuria, hematuria, and pyuria; and (2) microscopic examination for cells, casts, or crystals. The physiologic urine pH ranges from 4.5–8.0. An alkaline pH should make one suspect the presence of a urinary tract infection with a nitrate-splitting bacterium such as proteus. The specific gravity may range from 1.001–1.035 and corresponds to osmolalities of 50–1000 mosm/kg. These represent roughly the minimum and maximum concentrating abilities of the kidney. A specific gravity of 1.010 denotes isosthenuria—ie, the urine osmolality matches the plasma osmolality. In the absence of proteinuria, glucosuria, or iodinated contrast administration, a specific gravity > 1.018 implies preserved concentrating ability. Measurement of the urine specific gravity is useful in differentiating between prerenal azotemia (high specific gravity) and acute tubular necrosis (ATN), which is associated with isosthenuria. The specific gravity also aids in the interpretation of proteinuria as detected on a dipstick. The normal protein excretion rate is less than 150 mg/d. It is important to realize that the dipstick detects the concentration of protein. Thus, detection of protein in a concentrated urine specimen may not represent overt proteinuria. Additionally, the acute development of significant proteinuria can occur in association with events such as a febrile illness or congestive heart failure. The proteinuria in this case will normalize with resolution of the underlying disorder. Glucose, cells, casts, and crystals are not normally observed on urinalysis. Glucosuria generally indicates uncontrolled diabetes or tubular dysfunction. White blood cells indicate infection or interstitial nephritis. Red blood cells may be of glomerular or nonglomerular origin and may indicate tumor, infection, trauma, stones, prostatitis, or primary renal disease. White cell casts indicate pyelonephritis; red cell casts indicate glomerulonephritis; and coarse-granular or "muddy-brown" casts indicate ATN.

Disturbances of electrolytes, difficulties with fluid regulation, and anemia are unusual until the GFR decreases to 20–40 mL/min. Thus, surgical management of patients with this level of renal insufficiency is similar to that of patients with normal renal function. Patients with GFRs below 20 mL/min require careful preoperative hydration and blood transfusion. Most patients with GFRs below 10 mL/min have end-stage renal disease (ESRD) and are on dialysis. Preoperative hydration should be avoided in these patients, and blood transfusions should be administered during hemodialysis to avoid volume overload. Erythropoietin (epoetin alfa) is not effective for the rapid correction of anemia in chronic renal failure and ESRD.

Use of Ultrasonography

Renal ultrasonography is noninvasive and commonly used to assess kidney size and rule out obstruction, vascular stenosis, or thrombosis. The normal kidney size is 10–13 cm in length. Small kidneys reflect chronic disease. Large kidneys are seen with diabetes, amyloidosis, multiple myeloma, human immunodeficiency virus (HIV), lymphoma, polycystic kidney disease, and renal vein thrombosis.

ACUTE RENAL FAILURE & OLIGURIA

The definition of acute renal failure varies, but can be thought of as a recent rise in serum creatinine levels greater than 0.5 mg/dL when the baseline serum creatinine is less than 3 mg/dL or at least a 1 mg/dL rise when the serum creatinine is greater than 3 mg/dL. A daily increase of this magnitude is referred to as an **anephric rise**. Patients with limited muscle mass can have significant acute or chronic renal failure without an impressive increase in serum creatinine. For this reason, an estimated creatinine clearance (CrCl) or GFR should be calculated in all patients at baseline. A patient with an anephric rise in serum creatinine should be considered to have a GFR < 10/mL/minute regardless of the calculated value. Calculations that estimate renal function include the easy-to-use Cockroft-Gault equation (Table 5–1) for CrCl. Any formula used to calculate CrCl or GFR, including a 24-hour urine collection, is only an estimate and has no validity in the setting of a changing serum creatinine level.

Renal failure may be oliguric (< 500 cc of urine/day) or nonoliguric (> 500 cc of urine/day). Oliguric renal failure is often representative of a more significant insult, and there is no known advantage in preserving renal function by using diuretics in an attempted conversion to a nonoliguric state. However, responsiveness to diuretics does make management of fluids and electrolytes much easier and may help avoid the need for dialysis.

If diuretics are used, furosemide should be given at a dose of 80–200 mg intravenously (IV). If there is no response to a 200-mg dose, a furosemide drip is unlikely to work, but occasionally will have an effect. A furosemide drip can be initiated after giving a moderate bolus and is usually run at a rate of 10–30 mg/h. Even if it there is no desire to produce a negative fluid balance, diuretics can be used in conjunction with replacement fluids to help mitigate electrolyte or acid/base disturbances. Patients can become refractory to loop diuretics after chronic use, and the addition of a thiazide diuretic to the regimen can sometimes produce a marked diuresis. When available, intravenous chlorothiazide at a dose of 250–500 mg can be used in conjunction with a loop diuretic. Oral agents such as hydrochlorothiazide can also be added, but the presence of bowel edema can significantly impair their absorption and effect. Metabolic alkalosis may result from repeated diuretic use. If the alkalosis is severe, or if the patient is refractory to continued diuresis, the addition of intravenous acetazolamide (125–250 mg) to a loop-and-thiazide diuretic combination may often assist the diuretic response as long as the serum bicarbonate is at a level above the normal renal threshold for excretion.

Table 5–1. Cockroft-Gault equation for creatinine clearance estimation.

$$\frac{(140 - \text{Age}) \times (\text{Weight in kg})}{72 \times \text{Serum creatinine in mg/dL}}$$

Multiply by 100% for ~ Creatinine clearance in mL/min

For females multiply × 0.85 to correct for less muscle mass

Dopamine was formerly used in an attempt to improve renal circulation and improve renal function in the setting of acute renal failure. However, in retrospective analysis it has shown no benefit and may in fact be harmful by potentiating arrhythmias; thus, the practice should be avoided.

Causes of Acute Renal Failure

Acute renal failure (ARF) in the surgical setting almost always falls into the category of ischemic ATN resulting from a prerenal etiology of hypovolemia, hypotension, sepsis, or otherwise decreased effective circulating volume. Timely correction of a prerenal etiology can prevent or lessen the severity of ATN. This and other possible causes of ARF in the surgical setting are discussed below.

A. Prerenal

Physical examination and laboratory data can often help distinguish a prerenal state from other potential causes of renal failure. When the etiology is not clear, often in the setting of poor cardiac function, central pressure monitoring may be indicated. As long as the cardiopulmonary status is not tenuous, the administration of normal saline is usually indicated as a diagnostic tool. An adequate fluid trial should be given, remembering that only 250 cc of each liter of normal saline administered remains in the intravascular compartment.

B. ATN

Any prolonged, severe cause of a prerenal etiology leads to acute tubular necrosis (ATN). Nephrotoxic agents, such as amphotericin, aminoglycoside antibiotics, and nonsteroidal anti-inflammatory agents, alone or in conjunction with additional insults, can also precipitate ATN. Several urinary studies may be helpful in differentiating a prerenal state from ATN as the cause of ARF in assessing the kidney's ability to appropriately conserve sodium and water (Table 5–2). These studies may be misleading in patients with preexisting renal insufficiency or after the use of diuretics and only have validity in the setting of oliguria. Recovery from ATN can require several days to several weeks.

Table 5–2. Urine studies: Prerenal vs. ATN.

Test	Prerenal	ATN
Urine osmolality (mosm/kg)	> 500	< 300
FeNa (UNa/PNa)/(Ucr/Pcr) × 100	< 1%	> 2%
UNa (mmol/L)	< 10	> 20
Urine specific gravity	> 1.018	< 1.015

FeNa = Fractional excretion of sodium
Pcr = Plasma creatinine mg/dL
PNa = Plasma sodium mmol/L
Ucr = Urinary creatinine mg/dL
UNa = Urinary sodium mmol/L

C. Obstructive Nephropathy

Prolonged obstructive uropathy can lead to renal damage. Complete unilateral obstruction can present with minimal laboratory or examination findings in the setting of preexisting normal renal function. Obstruction should be relieved as soon as possible to help prevent further damage and preserve renal function. In the setting of volume depletion, retroperitoneal fibrosis, or metastatic carcinoma, the classic radiologic signs of hydronephrosis may not be present and additional studies may be warranted in these settings. Bladder ultrasound or Foley catheter placement with documentation of postvoid residual, renal ultrasound, retrograde pyelography, and occasionally a Whitaker test may be necessary for the diagnosis of obstruction. Internal or percutaneous nephrostomy tube placement may be needed for urgent relief of obstruction. As with resolving ATN, relief of obstruction can result in a massive, appropriate diuresis. Orders to give intravenous fluid at a rate equal to urinary output can be counterproductive and falsely prolong the apparent state of diuresis.

D. Acute Renal Artery or Renal Vein Occlusion

The diagnosis of either of these scenarios requires a high index of suspicion. A unilateral event is most common, but rarely bilateral occlusion may occur. Appropriate institution dependent imaging studies should be obtained immediately and surgical or thrombolytic treatment is required urgently if the affected kidney is to be salvaged.

E. Interstitial Causes

Acute interstitial nephritis (AIN) from medications and bilateral pyelonephritis (or unilateral pyelonephritis in the setting of renal insufficiency) can also cause renal failure. AIN is a diagnosis of exclusion. The finding of urinary eosinophils is nonspecific and may be absent in AIN and present in the setting of many other causes of renal failure. The diagnosis of pyelonephritis is usually straightforward. Urinary white blood cells (WBCs) are not specific for infection, can be present in AIN and other renal diseases, and are routinely found in increasing numbers in the setting of chronic renal insufficiency.

F. Contrast Nephropathy

Direct nephrotoxic effects as well as a vasoconstrictive effect likely mitigate contrast nephropathy. Patients with diabetes or baseline renal insufficiency are at increased risk. The risk is decreased, but not eliminated, with the use of nonionic or lower osmolality media. Acute renal failure resulting from contrast nephropathy is usually apparent 1–2 days following the study, but sometimes is not evident for several days afterward. Prevention involves avoiding diuresis, hydrating with normal saline at 1 cc/kg/h for 12 hours before and after the procedure as cardiopulmonary status allows, and possibly, administering acetylcysteine.

G. Cholesterol Embolization

Cholesterol emboli (CE) can affect any vascular bed and most often occur after a vascular procedure but can also occur after trauma, in the setting of anticoagulation, or spontaneously. The syndrome can include fever, elevated WBCs (including eosinophilia), elevated amylase and lipase levels, elevated liver enzyme levels, and an elevated sedimentation rate, among other findings. The classic "blue toe" or other cutaneous findings such as livedo reticularis may be transient or not seen at all. When involving the renal vasculature, CE can result in severe ARF, but more commonly cause a stuttering progressive course.

Fluids & Electrolytes

A. Salt and Water

The development of hypernatremia or hyponatremia in the surgical setting is usually iatrogenic and results from fluid administration or free water restriction. The sodium value in mmol/L is a reflection of the ratio of free water to the sodium content. Hyponatremia can also result from fluid shifts in hyperosmolar states such as hyperglycemia. Occasionally, hyponatremia in the surgical setting is secondary to the syndrome of inappropriate antidiuretic hormone (SIADH). Nausea, pulmonary processes, and medications including opiates can cause SIADH. The urine osmolality will be inappropriately elevated at > 100 mosm/kg and the patient usually appears euvolemic. The syndrome of inappropriate antidiuretic hormone must be differentiated from disease states causing an ineffective circulating volume that also cause hyponatremia and present with a similar urine osmolality. Correction should be gradual (an increase in the serum sodium of < 8 mmol/L/day) unless the process is known to have occurred acutely or if the patient is having severe neurologic symptoms as a result. Correction involves limiting free water, increasing salt and protein administration, using loop diuretics if needed and rarely hypertonic saline. A formula to estimate the expected correction in the serum sodium with the administration of one liter of fluid is provided in Table 5–3.

Hypernatremia can result from the administration of hypertonic fluids, including sodium bicarbonate solution, as well as from inadequate free water. Osmotic diuresis in the setting of hyperglycemia, mannitol administration, or tube feeds can also lead to free water loss and hypernatremia. Ongoing losses, including insensible losses, need to be taken into account when correcting hypernatremia. Rapid correction of chronic hypernatremia is of less concern than rapid correction of hyponatremia, but decreasing the serum sodium by no more than 12 mmol/L/d is a reasonable goal unless the clinical situation dictates otherwise. The formula in Table 5–3 can be used to estimate the expected correction with 1 L of fluid administration in the setting of hyponatremia as well. As the dynamics are not static, it is extremely important to monitor the serum sodium closely for evidence of adequate treatment or for overcorrection. As the urine osmolality and hemodynamics change, so too will the rate of change of the serum sodium without a change in the infusion rate of the solution.

B. Potassium

Hyperkalemia is most commonly encountered in the setting of renal insufficiency. Hyperglycemia causes cellular shifts of potassium and is easily treated. Other causes include decreased effective circulating volume resulting in diminished renal tubular flow, and nonorganic acidosis. Many medications can cause hyperkalemia, and a careful review of the patient's medication list is in order. Chronic hyperkalemia in patients with ESRD is usually better tolerated than an acute rise in patients with ARF, and the threshold for urgent treatment should be adjusted. Likewise, electrocardiogram findings in chronic hyperkalemia may be minimal despite a marked elevation of the serum potassium. Urgent treatment for a potassium level < 6.0 mmol/L is seldom indicated in any patient. Electrocardiogram findings in hyperkalemia classically follow a progression of peaked and narrowed T waves, shortened QT interval, prolonged PR interval, and finally a widened QRS complex that can eventuate in ventricular fibrillation or asystole. Calcium gluconate administration immediately stabilizes the cell membrane and should be administered first if marked electrocardiogram changes or clinical signs consistent with documented hyperkalemia are present. Subsequent treatments are designed to shift potassium into the cells, but urinary or gastrointestinal elimination (or hemodialysis) is required to reduce the potassium burden (Table 5–4). If hemodialysis is necessary and readily available, predialysis treatment of the hyperkalemia should be limited to calcium gluconate, if necessary, and insulin with glucose. Using multiple modalities will often limit the effectiveness of hemodialysis, as much of the potassium will have been driven into the cells. Unless the patient is already hyperglycemic, insulin should be given with an amp of dextrose to avoid hypoglycemia. Acutely, sodium bicarbonate likely produces the majority of its effect via dilution and diuresis rather than by correction of acidosis and should be avoided in patients with volume overload or diminished urine output. The often-overused agent sodium polystyrene exchanges potassium for sodium in the gut. The product includes sorbitol, which presents a risk of bowel ischemia, especially if given in the postoperative setting. There is also a significant sodium load and a profound diarrhea associated with its use. When possible,

Table 5–3. Expected serum sodium value after fluid administration.

Expected Change in Serum Sodium after Administration of 1 Liter of Fluid

$$= \frac{\text{Infusate Na (mmol/L)} + \text{Infusate K (mmol/L)} - \text{Serum Na (mmol/L)}}{\text{Estimated Total Body Water (kg)} + 1}$$

Dividing the desired change in serum sodium by the expected change after infusion of 1 liter of solution gives the volume of that solution necessary to reach the desired serum sodium. Dividing the calculated volume by the desired time period gives the rate of infusion.

Normal saline (NS) =154 mmol/L Na
3% saline = 513 mmol/L Na
D5W = 0 mmol/L Na
(From Adrogué HJ, Madias NE: Hyponatremia. N Engl J Med 2000;342:1581.)

Table 5–4. Treatment of hyperkalemia.

Calcium gluconate 10%	10 cc IV over 2 minutes (repeat × 1 if needed)
Insulin combined with dextrose	10 units Regular Insulin IV with 50 g dextrose
Albuterol	10–20 mg via nebulizer or 0.5 mg IV
Sodium bicarbonate	50 meq IV over 2 minutes
Sodium polystyrene sulfonate	15 g in sorbitol orally 50 g in sorbitol and tap water rectally

restoration of renal perfusion with fluids and diuretics is the ultimate goal.

Hypokalemia usually results from diuresis or gastrointestinal losses. Hypomagnesemia should be ruled out as a contributing factor in refractory hypokalemia. The relationship between the serum potassium and the potassium deficit is unpredictable, but can be profound at levels less than 3 mmol/L. Potassium replacement should be given orally whenever possible. In patients with renal failure and hypokalemia, replacement should be cautious unless the deficit is thought to be severe.

Acid/Base Disorders

Acidemia and alkalemia are not uncommon findings in the surgical setting. Double or triple disorders involving combinations of metabolic or respiratory acidosis and alkalosis are seen frequently and a systematic approach to these entities should be routine. The laboratory evaluation should include an assessment of pH, serum bicarbonate and pCO_2 (with calculations for appropriateness of correction), and anion gap (with correction for low albumin levels if necessary). Additional testing for a potential underlying cause, such as lactic acidosis, should be based on the clinical concern and a review of the laboratory values. Reflex correction of acidemia or alkalemia is not warranted unless the pH is markedly abnormal, is worsening, or both. Bicarbonate should be cautiously administered in the setting of poor perfusion because increased generation of carbon dioxide can result and the acidosis can actually worsen. This effect may only be apparent on analysis of the venous blood gas and not on the arterial side. If bicarbonate is given, it is usually easiest to add three amps of sodium bicarbonate (50 meq each) to 1 L of D5W. Adjustment of a ventilator or the use of BiPAP to lower the pCO_2 in the presence of inadequate respiratory compensation for metabolic acidosis should be the first step. Patients with compromised respiratory function can "wear out" attempting to compensate for a metabolic acidosis and the pH can decrease rapidly in this setting. Treatment of the metabolic acidosis or mechanical assistance for respirations is often required.

Metabolic alkalosis is usually the result of diuresis or some other form of "contraction alkalosis." Restoring the intravascular volume status with sodium chloride solution as clinically appropriate is often all that is necessary. In patients with compromised pulmonary function, severe metabolic alkalosis can worsen the tendency for pCO_2 retention, and some correction of the underlying disorder may be mandated.

Dialysis Modalities

The need for acute dialysis in the surgical patient is often precipitated by volume overload that is refractory to diuretics, severe metabolic acidosis that cannot or should not be corrected by the administration of bicarbonate, or hyperkalemia and other electrolyte disorders. "Uremia" is an indication for dialysis and constitutes a syndrome of vomiting, anorexia, nausea, itching, listlessness, and asterixis associated with renal failure. Symptoms do not correlate directly with the degree of azotemia. Pericarditis and polyneuropathy from uremia are absolute indications for dialysis. Acute dialysis options include intermittent or continuous modalities. Currently there are no available data to support the routine use of one method over another in terms of outcomes. A continuous modality may be selected if rapid shifts in intravascular volume status are not likely to be tolerated. If intermittent hemodialysis is used, the frequency should be based on volume status, acid/base and electrolyte issues, and the overall catabolic state. Daily evaluation is necessary rather than a predetermined alternate-day schedule.

Transplant Recipients

Most renal transplant recipients are on a stable regimen of immunosuppressive medications, and this needs to be continued. "Stress dose" steroids are rarely needed and should not routinely be administered. Other medications can dramatically increase or decrease the levels of immunosuppressive agents, and vigilance in prescribing is warranted. All renal transplant recipients or potential renal transplant recipients should receive blood transfusions that have been leuko-poor filtered to reduce exposure to white cells that may sensitize patients to HLA (transplant) antigens or transmit viral diseases such as cytomegalovirus.

Medication Dosing in Renal Failure

In addition to avoiding nephrotoxic agents in the setting of acute renal failure, medications that are eliminated by the renal route require dosing adjustments. Accumulation of a drug or its metabolites can lead to severe central nervous system toxicity or other side effects. All agents, including maintenance medications and any new medications prescribed, need to be evaluated for the possibility of toxicity in the setting of renal failure. Further dosing adjustments are needed should the patient require hemodialysis, and these are dependent upon the estimated clearance provided by the modality selected.

Continued dosing with analgesics such as meperidine or morphine should be avoided. If chronic intravenous pain medication is required, hydromorphone should be used. Oxycodone is the favored oral agent. These agents are eliminated primarily by the hepatic route and do not result in the accumulation of significant metabolites.

Nutrition

Patients in ARF are usually catabolic and prolonged periods of inadequate nutrition are detrimental. Whether potassium, sodium, and phosphorus are given by oral, tube-feed, or intravenous route, limitations of these substances are often necessary. Protein intake should be adequate (1–1.2 g/kg/d), and the classic "renal diet" that is often automatically ordered predisposes to malnutrition and should be avoided. Adequate nutrition should not be avoided in an attempt to prevent the need for hemodialysis. Oral calcium carbonate can be used to help bind phosphorus in the diet. Short-term increases in the calcium and phosphorus product greater than that desired in the chronic setting are of little concern.

Adrogué HJ, Madias NE: Hypernatremia. N Engl J Med 2000;342:1493.

Adrogué HJ, Madias NE: Hyponatremia. N Engl J Med 2000;342:1581.

Aronoff G et al: *Drug Prescribing in Renal Failure: Dosing Guidelines for Adults,* 4th ed. American College of Physicians, 1999.

Aronson S et al: Perioperative renal dysfunction and cardiovascular anesthesia: concerns and controversies. J Cardiothorac Vasc Anesth 1998;12:567.

Ayus JC et al: Abnormalities of water metabolism in the elderly. Semin Nephrol 1996;16:277.

Conger JD: Interventions in clinical acute renal failure: what are the data? Am J Kidney Dis 1995;26:565.

Klahr S et al: Acute renal failure. N Engl J Med 1998;338:671.

Slapak M: Acute renal failure in general surgery. J R Soc Med 1996;89(Suppl 29):13.

Tepel M et al: Prevention of radiographic-contrast-agent-induced reductions in renal function by acetylcysteine. N Engl J Med 2000;343:180.

HEMATOLOGICAL DISEASE & THE SURGICAL PATIENT

Ashok Nambiar, MD, & Pearl T.C.Y. Toy, MD

PREOPERATIVE HEMOSTATIC EVALUATION

Surgery challenges hemostasis. A patient's risk of bleeding from surgery depends not only on any preexisting hemostatic defect but also on the extent, site, and type of surgical procedure being performed. All patients should be evaluated for their risk of bleeding based on the specific surgery being planned.

Preoperative hemostatic assessment begins with a comprehensive personal history for bleeding tendencies. This provides the basis for further diagnostic studies and helps assess the probability of future bleeding. Patients should be asked about epistaxis, gingival bleeding, bruising, ecchymoses, and menorrhagia. A history of mucocutaneous bleeding at these sites suggests von Willebrand disease (vWD), thrombocytopenia, or functional platelet disorders. Patients with hemophilia A or hemophilia B may recall spontaneous muscle or joint hemorrhages. A history of excessive bleeding during or following circumcision, tonsillectomy, tooth extraction, other surgeries, or during childbirth can be very helpful in uncovering a hemostatic disorder. When appropriate, obtain detailed reports of hospital visits for bleeding symptoms and previous hemostatic workup, as well as transfusions and other therapeutic interventions done to secure hemostasis.

The history should also rule out any underlying hepatic, renal, immunologic, or hematologic diseases. It is important to obtain an accurate history of drug intake, as medications like aspirin, nonsteroidal anti-inflammatory drugs (NSAIDs), clopidogrel, and warfarin impair hemostasis. Patients with hereditary bleeding disorders frequently give a history of bleeding tendency in other family members. The physical examination should focus on any evidence of ongoing mucocutaneous bleeding, splenomegaly, or other signs of systemic disease that may suggest an underlying hemostatic defect.

A hematology consultation is strongly suggested for all patients with a history of unexplained excessive bleeding. Several studies have shown that routine preoperative prothrombin time (PT) and activated partial thromboplastin time (aPTT) testing is unnecessary in patients scheduled for low-risk surgery, provided that a carefully obtained history failed to reveal a bleeding tendency or a risk for abnormal bleeding. Testing of coagulation function should be part of the preoperative workup in patients scheduled for high-risk surgery. Initial laboratory testing includes PT, aPTT, complete blood count (CBC), examination of the blood smear, and biochemical tests of hepatic and renal function. The bleeding time does not predict abnormal surgical bleeding and is not routinely recommended. If a screening test is positive, specific tests to rule out deficiencies of individual coagulation factors, von Willebrand factor (vWF), and platelet function defects are performed. vWD has a prevalence of approximately 1% in the general population. Most individuals with mild vWD and occasionally patients with other mild isolated factor deficiencies are undiagnosed. However, some may have significant bleeding during major surgery. Laboratory workup and diagnosis during the initial assessment allows for appropriate perioperative management.

Baker R: Pre-operative hemostatic assessment and management. Transfus Apheresis Sci 2002;27:45.

Seligsohn U, Coller BS: Classification, clinical manifestations and evaluation of disorders of hemostasis. In: *Williams Hematology,* 6th ed, p. 1471. Buetler E et al (editors.) McGraw-Hill, 2001.

APPROACH TO ANEMIA IN THE SURGICAL PATIENT

Preoperative Evaluation

Surgical patients with anemia should undergo a thorough workup to identify and treat the underlying cause before elective procedures are undertaken. A detailed history should be obtained to identify any symptoms of blood loss from the genitourinary and gastrointestinal tracts. A history of renal, hepatic, hematologic, or endocrinologic disorders and a medication history should be elicited. A history suggestive of hemolytic episodes or a family history of anemia may offer clues to the diagnosis. Signs of pallor, jaundice, lymphadenopathy, and organomegaly should be sought on physical examination.

A complete laboratory evaluation including CBC, reticulocyte count, peripheral smear, and stool guaiac test should be done. Iron studies, hemolysis workup, and bone marrow examination may be needed to distinguish anemia of impaired production or ineffective erythropoiesis from those resulting from hemoglobinopathies, peripheral destruction, or blood loss. Correctable causes of anemia, like deficiencies of iron, folate, and vitamin B_{12}, should be treated. Recombinant erythropoietin is indicated for chemotherapy-related anemia and the anemia of chronic renal failure. Preoperative red blood cell (RBC) transfusions are not routinely recommended, and the decision to transfuse should be based on the need to improve tissue oxygenation.

RBC Transfusions

There has been a dramatic decrease in the risk of transfusion-transmitted viral infections. Yet, other complications of transfusion like transfusion-related acute lung injury, bacterial contamination, and hemolytic reactions continue to cause significant morbidity and mortality. There are also concerns about risks from unknown infectious agents and questions regarding the availability and cost of blood products. Recent clinical trials compared restrictive strategies of transfusion with the use of more liberal transfusion "triggers" and found them to be equally effective. There is now a better understanding of the compensatory physiologic mechanisms operative in anemia. These developments have led to the formulation of guidelines for RBC transfusions in anemic patients and changes in transfusion practices in the perioperative setting.

The decision to transfuse RBCs should be made only after determination of the need to increase tissue oxygen delivery in patients unable to meet this requirement through normal cardiopulmonary mechanisms. The hemoglobin and hematocrit levels alone are no longer an acceptable trigger for transfusion; patients should be assessed individually for their risk of complications from inadequate oxygenation. In the perioperative setting, transfusions are rarely indicated when the hemoglobin level is more than 10 g/dL and are almost always needed when the hemoglobin falls below 7 g/dL. For patients with hemoglobin levels between 7 and 10 g/dL, the decision to transfuse should be based on an assessment of anticipated blood loss and the presence of any underlying organ dysfunction or hemostatic disorder. For example, surgical patients with cardiopulmonary disease should be transfused if the hemoglobin levels are less than 10 g/dL, while a hemoglobin level of 8 g/dL would be an appropriate threshold for transfusion for patients without risk factors for ischemia.

Blood should be transfused one unit at a time, followed by an assessment of benefit and further need. Excessive transfusions in critically ill patients are associated with poor outcomes. A large multicenter, randomized, controlled clinical trial involving critically ill patients compared a restrictive strategy of RBC transfusion with a liberal strategy. In the absence of coronary disease, the outcomes were equal or better in patients who were transfused when their hemoglobin dropped below 7 g/dL when compared with those who were transfused to keep their hemoglobin levels above 10 g/dL. Although adequately powered, controlled studies in surgical patients are not available, we now have a better understanding of the level of anemia at which RBC transfusions avoid adverse outcomes. Patients with symptoms of anemia should be transfused as needed.

In patients with sickle cell disease, routine preoperative transfusion therapy for minor procedures is unnecessary. For moderate- and high-risk procedures, preoperative transfusions decrease perioperative and postoperative complications. A multicenter study compared a conservative regimen of preoperative transfusions targeted only to achieve hemoglobin level greater than 10 g/dL with an aggressive regimen (preoperative transfusions combined with red cell exchange therapy, if needed) aimed at achieving both a preoperative hemoglobin level higher than 10 g/dL and hemoglobin S level below 30%. The conservative approach was shown to be as effective as the aggressive regimen in preventing perioperative complications and resulted in only half as many transfusion-related complications.

Hébert PC et al: A multicenter, randomized, controlled clinical trial of transfusion requirements in critical care. N Engl J Med 1999;340:409.

Practice guidelines for blood component therapy: a report by the American Society of Anesthesiologists Task Force on Blood Component Therapy. Anesthesiology 1996;84:732.

Vichinsky EP et al: A comparison of conservative and aggressive transfusion regimens in the perioperative management of sickle cell disease. N Engl J Med 1995;333:206.

SURGERY IN PATIENTS WITH DISORDERS OF HEMOSTASIS

Platelet Disorders

A. Thrombocytopenia

Surgical patients with thrombocytopenia should be evaluated by a hematologist. Low platelet counts can result from decreased production or increased peripheral destruction. Disorders of the bone marrow like aplastic anemia, myelodysplastic syndrome, drug toxicity, or neoplastic infiltration result in thrombocytopenia. Common disorders that lead to immune-mediated destruction of platelets include idiopathic thrombocytopenic purpura (ITP), systemic lupus erythematosus (SLE), chronic lymphocytic leukemia (CLL), lymphoma, and viral infections like cytomegalovirus (CMV) and HIV. Drug-dependent antibodies are an important cause of platelet destruction, and hence a complete medication history should be obtained to rule out agents like heparin, quinidine, phenytoin, sulphonamide, and thiazide. It is particularly important to rule out heparin-induced thrombocytopenia (HIT) as a cause of the thrombocytopenia, as continued exposure to heparin in the perioperative period can have disastrous consequences. Congestive splenomegaly and splenic involvement by lymphoma can also cause thrombocytopenia. In patients with underlying medical illnesses, nonimmune causes of platelet consumption like thrombotic thrombocytopenic purpura (TTP) and sepsis should also be considered.

B. Disorders of Platelet Function

Patients with a long history of mucocutaneous bleeding may have hereditary or acquired disorders of platelet function. Inherited disorders include Glanzmann thrombasthenia, Bernard-Soulier syndrome, and storage pool defects; consultation with a hematologist is recommended. However, acquired disorders of platelet function are much more common in clinical practice, and their preoperative recognition and management prevents surgical morbidity. Drugs like aspirin, NSAIDs, and high-dose penicillin and antiplatelet agents like ticlopidine, clopidogrel, and abciximab inhibit platelet function and contribute to an increase in surgical bleeding. Uremic patients develop a platelet function abnormality in addition to their mild thrombocytopenia and can present with mucocutaneous bleeding. Besides splenomegaly-induced thrombocytopenia, platelet function can also be abnormal in patients with liver disease. Platelet dysfunction is also commonly seen for several hours after cardiopulmonary bypass surgery.

Perioperative Management

Identification and treatment of the primary cause is recommended prior to elective surgery. In patients with decreased production of platelets, surgery should be deferred if possible until control or resolution of the underlying pathology and return of the counts to hemostatic levels. For invasive procedures, platelet transfusions are recommended if the platelet count is less than 50,000/μL. For patients undergoing major surgery, or surgery involving highly vascular sites, maintain a platelet count above 75,000/μL. For patients undergoing neurosurgery, the commonly used threshold for platelet transfusions is 100,000/μL.

Thrombocytopenia secondary to splenomegaly or immune-mediated platelet destruction is not improved by platelet transfusions, and routine prophylactic transfusions are not recommended. Platelet transfusions are not indicated in drug-induced thrombocytopenia if the drug is still present in the circulation. The management of HIT is described later. Thrombocytopenia of TTP responds to plasma exchange. Platelet transfusions are generally withheld, unless the patient is receiving plasma exchange and continues to be severely thrombocytopenic and at high risk for bleeding. Platelet transfusions are also withheld in type IIB vWD and HIT.

The management of platelet function disorders will depend upon the etiology. Patients with hereditary disorders of platelet function are usually managed with conservative measures; platelet transfusions are reserved for serious bleeding. Aspirin should be discontinued at least 7 days before surgery and NSAIDs should be withheld for 2–3 days. Ticlopidine and clopidogrel should ideally be withheld for 10 days before invasive procedures. In emergent situations, DDAVP has been given to reduce bleeding due to drug-induced platelet dysfunction; platelet transfusions may be needed to ensure hemostasis for high-risk procedures. The glycoprotein IIb/IIIa inhibitors have different mechanisms of action and the duration of their antiplatelet effect varies.

While platelet inhibition by abciximab, a large monoclonal antibody, lasts for several days, the antiplatelet effects of the synthetic small-molecule GP IIb/IIIa inhibitors, tirofiban and eptifibatide, resolve in a few hours. In patients on abciximab, platelets have been transfused to secure hemostasis during emergent surgical interventions.

In uremic patients, the correction of anemia has a beneficial effect on hemostasis. RBCs should be transfused to achieve a hematocrit of 30%. The platelet dysfunction seen in uremia improves after dialysis. In the absence of dialysis, platelet transfusions are not recommended, as donor platelets also become dysfunctional. Low-dose conjugated estrogens given daily for 4–5 days reduce bleeding in uremic patients and the effect lasts for 10–15 days. For more urgent reversal of the hemostatic defect, DDAVP is recommended. Cryoprecipitate can aid platelet aggregation and adhesion and decrease bleeding in uremic patients. The platelet dysfunction seen with cardiopulmonary bypass spontaneously corrects in 24–48 hours. If necessary, DDAVP can be used to control bleeding.

Platelet Dose

The usual dose is one unit of platelets per 10 kg of body weight. One unit of platelets increases the platelet count by 5000–10,000/μL in a 70-kg adult; a six-unit pool of random donor platelets (obtained from whole blood), or an equivalent dose of single donor platelets (collected by apheresis) can be expected to raise the platelet count by 30,000–60,000/μL.

Refractoriness to Platelet Transfusions

It is important to obtain a platelet count 15 minutes to 1 hour after a platelet transfusion to document an increase in the platelet count. A failure to achieve an adequate increment in platelet counts could be due to immunologic or nonimmunologic reasons. Patients with splenomegaly, sepsis, or fever or those on medications like amphotericin B may fail to respond to platelet transfusions. Alternatively, in chronically transfused patients or multiparous women, the refractoriness may be secondary to the development of HLA or antiplatelet antibodies. The diagnosis is established by HLA and platelet antibody assays. Coordination with the blood bank to obtain HLA-matched platelets or crossmatched platelets is necessary to successfully correct the thrombocytopenia prior to surgery.

Chun R et al: Platelet glycoprotein IIb/IIIa inhibitors: overview and implications for the anesthesiologist. Anesth Analg 2002;95:879.

Mannucci PM: Hemostatic drugs. N Engl J Med 1998;339:245.

Norfolk DR et al: Consensus conference on platelet transfusion, Royal College of Physicians of Edinburgh, 27–28 November 1997. Br J Haematol 1998;101:609.

COAGULATION FACTOR DEFICIENCIES

Patients with hereditary coagulation disorders can safely undergo surgical procedures, provided that a diagnosis of the defect is made prior to surgery. Coagulation factor replacement in the perioperative period reduces the risk of bleeding complications in these patients. A hematology consult is strongly recommended.

von Willebrand Disease

vWD is the most common hereditary coagulation disorder. vWF, a large multimeric protein synthesized in endothelial cells and platelets, plays a crucial role in hemostasis by supporting platelet-endothelial cell adhesion. vWF is also the carrier protein for factor VIII. The vWF:factor VIII complex stabilizes factor VIII and localizes it to the site of bleeding and platelet plug formation; activation of coagulation, thrombin generation, and fibrin clot formation ensue.

Quantitative or qualitative deficiencies of vWF can lead to a hemostatic defect that manifests with mucocutaneous bleeding, menorrhagia, or excessive surgical bleeding. Based on the underlying pathophysiology, vWD is classified into types I, II (A, B, M, and N), and III. Eighty percent of vWD patients have the type I form. These patients have a mild bleeding tendency resulting from the decreased production of vWF. Patients with type IIA vWD have a qualitative abnormality of vWF. Although their vWF levels may be normal, their plasma lacks the high- and intermediate-molecular-weight multimers of vWF. The type IIB variant results from a mutation that causes increased affinity of vWF for its platelet receptor, GP 1b. This heightened interaction leads to in vivo platelet aggregation and a rapid turnover of the highest molecular weight vWF multimers. Patients often have mild thrombocytopenia and their plasma shows an absence of the highest molecular weight multimers. The vWF in type IIN vWD has normal platelet adhesion function but binds defectively to factor VIII. This variant mimics hemophilia A, because uncomplexed factor VIII has a short half-life, and affected individuals have low levels of factor VIII. Type III vWD is a rare, severe form that results from very low levels of vWF and factor VIII.

The plasma levels or activity of the individual components of the vWF:factor VIII complex are measured in the laboratory using different assays. The vWF antigen (vWF:Ag) assay quantitates the plasma levels of vWF; ristocetin cofactor assay is the standard functional assay that measures plasma vWF activity and is the most sensitive and specific single test for vWD. Functional factor VIII coagulant activity is measured by one-stage clotting assays based on aPTT. Because factor VIII levels are variably reduced, screening tests like aPTT may not be abnormal in patients with mild vWD. The diagnosis is established by a combination of assays for vWF:Ag, vWF activity, vWF multimers, and factor VIII.

The coagulation abnormalities can be corrected by raising plasma levels of vWF and factor VIII. In most patients with type I vWD, the plasma concentration of vWF can be increased for several hours by the administration of DDAVP. At the time of diagnosis, a therapeutic test dose of DDAVP (0.3 μg/kg) is given by slow IV infusion and the response documented. In individuals who show a twofold to threefold increase in vWF activity and factor VIII levels, this dose given 15–30 minutes before surgery ensures hemostasis. Some type IIA patients may respond to DDAVP. This agent is ineffective in type III vWD. DDAVP is contraindicated in type IIB disease because the highest molecular weight vWF released from storage may induce spontaneous platelet aggregation and worsen the thrombocytopenia. Platelet transfusions are also contraindicated in type IIB for the same reason. Plasma products containing high-molecular-weight vWF multimers and factor VIII are used in the management of most patients with types II and III vWD. Optimal hemostasis can be assured by the twice-daily administration of virus-inactivated factor VIII concentrates that contain vWF during surgery and for 2–3 days postoperatively. Daily infusions are adequate for minor bleeding. Because of the residual risk of viral transmission, cryoprecipitate is no longer recommended for vWD.

Mannucci PM: How I treat patients with von Willebrand disease. Blood 2001;97:1915.

Hemophilia

Hemophilia A, a deficiency of factor VIII, and hemophilia B, a deficiency of factor IX, are X-linked recessive disorders. They are similar clinically and are divided into mild, moderate, and severe forms. Patients with mild hemophilia have factor VIII or IX levels that are > 5% of normal; they do not bleed spontaneously but may do so excessively during surgery. Factor levels are 1–5% of normal in individuals with moderate hemophilia. Trauma and surgery provoke excessive bleeding, and unlike the mild group, these patients may occasionally have spontaneous bleeding. Patients with severe hemophilia have factor levels that are < 1% of normal. Their clinical picture is one of frequent spontaneous hemorrhages, and they have a very high risk of bleeding from surgery or trauma.

In contrast to patients with vWD and platelet disorders, patients with hemophilia present with painful bleeding into the deep tissues and joints. Laboratory diagnosis is based on abnormal aPTT and decreased levels of factor VIII or IX. The therapeutic approach depends upon the severity of the disorder and the risk for bleeding. Patients with mild hemophilia A respond to the administration of DDAVP, which is adequate for minor trauma or prior to tooth extractions. Symptomatic patients with moderate or severe hemophilia are treated with plasma-derived factor VIII concentrates or recombinant factor VIII preparations. Mild hemarthrosis and superficial hematomas can be managed by raising the plasma levels of factor VIII to > 30% of normal; patients with CNS hemorrhage or severe retroperitoneal bleeding require therapeutic targets of 80–100% of normal activity.

Factor replacement to achieve 100% plasma levels should be initiated prior to major surgical procedures. One unit of factor VIII activity is the amount of factor VIII present in one mL of normal plasma. A dose of 1 U/kg body weight of factor VIII will raise levels by 2%. Infusions are given every 12 hours. A similar approach is adopted for patients with hemophilia B. High-purity factor IX concentrates or recombinant factor IX are available for replacement therapy. Factor IX has a larger volume of distribution; a dose of 1 U/kg body weight raises plasma levels only by 1%. However, factor IX has a longer half-life, and maintenance doses are needed only once every 18–24 hours. In the postoperative period, coagulation tests and factor levels should be monitored. Regardless of active bleeding, infusions are given to maintain factor levels above 30% of normal and are continued until wound healing is complete.

Replacement therapy is complicated by the development of inhibitors to factors VIII and IX in 10–25% of hemophilia A patients and 2–5% of hemophilia B patients. These patients are refractory to treatment with factor preparations. Factor VIIa can secure hemostasis by circumventing the need for factors VIII and IX. Recombinant factor VIIa is indicated in the surgical management of patients with high-titer inhibitors to factors VIII and IX.

SURGERY IN PATIENTS RECEIVING ANTICOAGULANTS

Heparins, Warfarin, & Newer Anticoagulants

Unfractionated heparin (UFH), a mixture of glycosaminoglycans, inhibits coagulation by enhancing the activity of antithrombin (AT), a naturally occurring anticoagulant. AT inhibits activated factors II, IX, X, XI, and the tissue factor:VIIa complex. Unlike UFH, low-molecular-weight heparin (LMWH) anticoagulant activity is achieved primarily through the inhibition of factor Xa. LMWH, however, has better bioavailability and a more predictable anticoagulant response. UFH has a half-life of 1 hour; LMWH has a longer half-life, ranging from

2–4 hours after IV administration to 3–6 hours after SC administration.

Lepirudin, bivalirudin, and argatroban are direct thrombin inhibitors. Lepirudin has a half-life of 80 minutes, and unlike argatroban (half-life, 50 minutes), its elimination is impaired in patients with renal insufficiency. Danaparoid sodium (half-life, 25 hours) has predominantly anti-Xa activity. Fondaparinux is a novel AT-dependent anticoagulant with anti-Xa activity. Warfarin is an orally active anticoagulant, which acts through inhibition of the vitamin K-dependent carboxylation step during the hepatic synthesis of coagulation factors II, VII, IX, and X.

The optimum management of anticoagulation in both the emergent and elective surgical setting requires an understanding of the pharmacokinetics of the rapidly expanding inventory of anticoagulant drugs. While warfarin and UFH have fairly predictable and distinct effects on PT and aPTT, respectively, some of the newer anticoagulants do not reliably prolong these assays, and are monitored differently. Since a normal PT and aPTT do not rule out concurrent use of anticoagulants, the patient's medication history should be diligently sought. This is all the more imperative if there is a high risk for bleeding, because specific inhibitors or antidotes are not available to neutralize some of the newer agents.

The risk of bleeding from a procedure has to be balanced against the risk of thrombosis from stopping anticoagulation before surgery. For most patients on warfarin (steady-state INR of 2.0–3.0), withholding medication for 4–5 days prior to surgery will allow their INR to decrease to a safe level of less than 1.5. For those with a higher starting INR, medications should be withheld for a longer period. In patients with a high risk for thrombosis (for example, those with mechanical heart valves), UFH can be substituted for warfarin, with cessation of the infusion 4 hours before surgery. Except following neurosurgical procedures, anticoagulation with heparin can generally be restarted as early as 12 hours after surgery.

Emergent reversal of anticoagulation may be required in some patients. For those on warfarin, this can be achieved in 24 hours by stopping warfarin and administering 2–4 mg of vitamin K, IV. If immediate reversal is required, the above measures should be combined with the administration of fresh frozen plasma (FFP). Recombinant factor VIIa has also been used successfully for the acute reversal of warfarin anticoagulation prior to invasive procedures or surgery.

For patients on heparin, emergent reversal of anticoagulation before surgery depends upon the heparin preparation. For patients receiving IV UFH, it is adequate to stop the drug 3–4 hours before the procedure; those on LMWH should have received their last dose not later than 10–12 hours before surgery. Protamine sulfate is used for the immediate reversal of heparin anticoagulation. Protamine is only partially effective against LMWH and is ineffective against fondaparinux, argatroban, lepirudin, or danaparoid. 1 mg of protamine neutralizes 100 U of UFH or LMWH. The dose is calculated based on the amount of heparin given over the previous 4 hours, with adjustments made for the longer half-life of LMWH. If spinal or epidural anesthesia is being planned, complete reversal of anticoagulation should be achieved prior to both the placement and removal of the needle or catheter.

Deveras RA, Kessler CM: Reversal of warfarin-induced excessive anticoagulation with recombinant human factor VIIa concentrate. Ann Intern Med 2002;137:884.

Spandorfer J: The management of anticoagulation before and after procedures. Med Clin North Am 2001;85:1109.

Warkentin TE, Crowther MA: Reversing anticoagulants both old and new. Can J Anesth 2002;49:S11.

Heparin-Induced Thrombocytopenia

HIT is an IgG-mediated syndrome, characterized by the formation of heparin-dependent antibodies that recognize heparin-platelet factor 4 complexes. The antigen-antibody interaction on the platelet surface activates platelets and the coagulation system, leading to thrombocytopenia and an increased risk for thrombotic complications.

Patients typically present with an unexplained, mild-moderate fall in their platelet counts, 5–10 days following exposure to either UFH or LMWH. Since the thrombocytopenia is severe in only a minority of patients, any decrease in the platelet count to below 50% of the baseline should be evaluated for HIT. The onset of thrombocytopenia after heparin reexposure can be abrupt in patients who have recently received heparin. Both venous and arterial thromboses can complicate HIT. The frequency of HIT varies widely based on the type of heparin and the length of exposure. Compared to LMWH, UFH is associated with a tenfold greater risk of HIT. Among orthopedic patients receiving UFH for 10–14 days, 3–5% have developed HIT, with 30–40% of them manifesting with thrombotic complications.

Early detection and management are critical to prevent thrombotic sequelae. Laboratory diagnosis is made by sensitive enzyme immune assays that detect HIT antibodies, or by the more specific platelet activation assays. All exposure to heparins (including heparin flushes and heparin-coated catheters) should cease in patients diagnosed with HIT. As HIT antibodies cross-react with LMWH, this drug is contraindicated in patients with HIT. Nonheparin anticoagulants like danaparoid, lepirudin, and argatroban are used to treat patients with HIT and thrombosis. Studies have shown that patients with isolated thrombocytopenia and no clinical evidence of thrombosis are at a higher risk for thrombosis. Therapy with lepirudin or argatroban is recommended in these patients until the platelet counts normalize.

A challenging situation develops when patients with HIT or a history of HIT require cardiac or vascular surgery. In patients with acute or recent HIT, the nonheparin anticoagulants danaparoid, lepirudin, and argatroban are used to achieve anticoagulation. These agents have their drawbacks; unlike heparin, they do not have an antidote and cannot be monitored with routine aPTT and ACT tests. Lepirudin has a shorter half-life (80 min) compared to danaparoid (25 h), can be monitored with the ecarin clotting time, and is preferred in patients with liver dysfunction. Argatroban is favored in patients with renal insufficiency. Given the disadvantages of nonheparin anticoagulants, some centers have combined full-dose UFH with antiplatelet agents like abciximab or tirofiban for emergent anticoagulation in the setting of acute HIT. HIT antibodies tend to be transient, disappearing in weeks to months after an occurrence of HIT. In patients with a remote history of HIT and negative antibody tests, UFH has been used safely.

Warkentin TE: Heparin-induced thrombocytopenia and the anesthesiologist. Can J Anesth 2002;49:S36.

DISSEMINATED INTRAVASCULAR COAGULATION (DIC)

DIC can be initiated by a number of diverse clinical situations, including septicemia, burns, trauma, liver disease, obstetric accidents, hemolytic transfusion reactions, malignancy, and envenomation. The entrance of tissue factor, a potent procoagulant, into the systemic circulation activates the coagulation system, leading to profound thrombin generation, fibrin formation, deposition of fibrin-platelet thrombi in the microvasculature, and end-organ damage. The consumption of coagulation factors and platelets leads to a hemorrhagic tendency, which is further compounded by the anticoagulant and antiplatelet effects of fibrin degradation products (FDP) generated by secondary fibrinolysis.

The underlying disease dominates the clinical picture. Diffuse mucocutaneous bleeding or localized bleeding from surgical wounds is the most common presentation. DIC may also present as digital gangrene or purpura fulminans. Laboratory findings include prolongation of PT, aPTT, and thrombin time (TT); thrombocytopenia; decreased fibrinogen and AT; and elevated levels of D-dimers and FDP. Schistocytes may be seen on the peripheral smear. Some of these findings may also be seen in severe liver disease, making it sometimes difficult to distinguish DIC from the severe coagulopathy of hepatic disease. Less frequently, a primary fibrinolytic syndrome should be ruled out. The laboratory findings in chronic DIC can be more subtle. More sophisticated tests for DIC, like assays for soluble fibrin and thrombin activation fragments F_{1+2}, are helpful but not routinely available.

The management of DIC should be individualized and directed at the aggressive treatment of the triggering disease process. A hematology consult should be obtained. There is no consensus regarding the use of anticoagulants, antifibrinolytics, and blood components in patients with DIC. In general, the approach will differ based on whether the clinical presentation is one of thrombotic complications or one of uncontrolled hemorrhage. In patients with active bleeding, abnormal coagulation tests, and hypofibrinogenemia, replacement of the consumed clotting factors with large volumes of FFP may be required to correct the defect. Cryoprecipitate is given to maintain fibrinogen levels above 100 mg/dL. Severe thrombocytopenia should be corrected with platelet transfusions. High levels of circulating FDP can cause a platelet function defect. If patients are not actively bleeding, blood products should not be infused prophylactically just to correct the coagulopathy of DIC. Heparin may exacerbate the bleeding in acute DIC. Conversely, patients with thrombotic complications like digital gangrene have been successfully treated with UFH or LMWH. Antifibrinolytic agents like EACA have been used in conjunction with heparin, in severely bleeding patients who have clear evidence of a primary or secondary hyperfibrinolytic process. Recombinant human activated protein C may have a therapeutic role in DIC associated with sepsis.

Bick RL: Disseminated intravascular coagulation: a review of etiology, pathophysiology, diagnosis and management: guidelines for care. Clin Appl Thrombosis/Hemostasis 2002;8:1.

HEMOSTASIS IN PATIENTS WITH LIVER DISEASE

Liver disease is associated with an increased risk of perioperative bleeding complications. Hepatic function tests, coagulation profiles, and imaging studies should be obtained to rule out underlying hepatic disease or to assess the degree of impairment. The liver synthesizes the majority of the coagulation factors, including factors II, V, VII, VIII, IX, X, XI, and XIII. Regulatory factors like protein C, protein S, and AT and components of the fibrinolytic pathway like plasminogen and antiplasmin are also produced in the liver. Besides, the liver is also the major site of clearance of activated clotting factors and FDP.

The hemostatic defects seen in liver disease are multifactorial. Decreased synthesis of clotting factors can lead to a coagulopathy. Dysfibrinogenemia is more common than severe hypofibrinogenemia and contributes to the coagulopathy. The accumulation of FDP can impair coagulation, and the decreased clearance of antiplasmin can lead to unchecked fibrinolysis. Thrombocytopenia resulting from splenomegaly worsens the bleeding tendency. A platelet function defect has also been described in patients with liver disease. Laboratory tests initially show an elevated PT; aPTT and TT become abnormal as the coagulopathy worsens. The levels of almost all clotting factors are decreased in patients with severe liver disease. Factor VIII and fibrinogen are acute-phase reactants and are decreased only in end-stage disease. Mild elevations of FDP and D-dimers may suggest an ongoing chronic DIC.

The approach to securing hemostasis in patients with significant hepatic dysfunction depends upon the urgency of the situation. For elective surgery, the initial approach is to administer vitamin K. Exogenous vitamin K will correct a deficiency arising from malabsorption or cholestasis but will not reverse a hepatic synthetic defect. FFP is recommended when patients do not respond to vitamin K or when emergent reversal of the coagulopathy is required. Patients with abnormal PTs that are prolonged by greater than 3 seconds benefit from FFP therapy. FFP is not recommended for patients with minimal elevations of PT. Cryoprecipitate is indicated for dysfibrinogenemia or marked hypofibrinogenemia. Severely thrombocytopenic patients should receive platelet transfusions. Fibrinolytic inhibitors like EACA have been used in liver disease complicated by systemic fibrinolysis. Some recent reports indicate that recombinant factor VIIa may be beneficial in the acute management of the coagulopathy of liver disease. While correction of the coagulopathy is very important, surgical outcomes are also dependent on the aggressive perioperative management of coexisting ascites, varices, renal dysfunction, and encephalopathy.

MASSIVE TRANSFUSION

Massive transfusion is the replacement in 24 hours of the entire blood volume of a patient. Patients who have rapidly received large volumes of crystalloids and blood components during the course of resuscitation face many complications and pose a considerable therapeutic challenge. Dilutional coagulopathy is an important complication of massive transfusion. Since whole blood is rarely available, the administration of large volumes of plasma-depleted RBC components results in a drop in the levels of plasma clotting factors. Plasma-depleted RBC includes packed RBCs, washed RBCs, and cell-saver salvaged RBCs. An elevation in PT and aPTT may be noted following replacement of more than one-half of the blood volume, although clinically significant increases in bleeding occur only when PT and aPTT are more than 1.5 times the control values. The concentration of fibrinogen falls below the critical level of 100 mg/dL and clotting factor levels fall below 20% of control values when 1.5–2 blood volumes are replaced. The coexistence of a consumptive process may, however, significantly alter these temporal correlations. Consumptive coagulopathy provoked by underlying tissue damage decreases the level of coagulation factors, and by activating fibrinolysis further impairs hemostatic pathways. Clinical coagulopathy may thus result much earlier in the course of a massive transfusion.

The coagulopathy manifests clinically as diffuse mucocutaneous bleeding and oozing from surgical wounds and catheter sites. Hypothermia impairs coagulation and platelet function and worsens the coagulopathy. The constant monitoring of body temperature, use of warming devices that can handle large volumes of blood and fluids, and additional appropriate rewarming methods are required to achieve normothermia. The results of coagulation tests done in the laboratory at standard temperatures may be misleading, as they may fail to correlate with the in vivo slowing of coagulation function seen in hypothermia. Although the dilution of plasma clotting factors occurs earlier, eventually a fall in platelet count to below the critical threshold of 50,000/μL occurs. Significant thrombocytopenia is seen after about 2 volumes are replaced in patients with normal baseline platelet counts and an intact spleen.

Anticipation of the hemostatic defects is the cornerstone to managing the coagulopathy of massive transfusion. Laboratory monitoring using PT, aPTT, TT, fibrinogen level, and platelet counts is recommended as replacement approaches one blood volume, with repetition of this panel of tests for every additional half blood volume that gets replaced. Patients with abnormal PT or aPTT and those at increased risk for consumptive coagulopathy develop dilutional coagulopathy earlier; monitoring should be more aggressive and preferably include a DIC screening panel. Laboratory tests may not always correlate with the clinical onset of coagulopathy; the decision to infuse blood components is based on a combination of clinical evidence of microvascular bleeding, alterations in coagulation parameters, and assessment of volume replacement. Generally, the finding of PT or aPTT that is greater than 1.5 times control values is an indication for infusing FFP. Supplementation with cryoprecipitate is done when the fibrinogen levels are below 100 mg/dL. Platelets should be transfused if the counts fall below 50,000–75,000/μL.

Massively transfused patients are also at risk for citrate toxicity from the infusion of large amounts of citrate in the anticoagulant preservative solution. Failure of the liver to rapidly metabolize this large load results in hypocalcemia and hypomagnesemia, which if profound can cause hemodynamic instability and worsen the coagulopathy. Profound alterations in acid-base balance are common in massively transfused patients. Although the plasma levels of potassium in stored blood are high, hyperkalemia following transfusion is generally not a problem owing to its rapid distribution in the extracellular fluid. However, critical hyperkalemia has occurred during the use of very rapid infusion devices. The correction of acid-base imbalance and electrolyte abnormalities is essential to the control of coagulopathy.

Drummond JC et al: The massively bleeding patient. Anesthesiol Clin North America 2001;19:633.

HEMATOLOGIC CONDITIONS THAT MIMIC ACUTE ABDOMINAL DISEASE

Sickle Cell Anemia

Sickle cell patients can present with a variety of intra-abdominal syndromes. Careful physical examination and clinical monitoring are important to make the distinction between conditions requiring medical management from those needing surgical intervention. Acute painful episodes or "crisis" can involve the abdomen. They usually last for a few days, varying in intensity from mild to severe, and may be precipitated by dehydration or infection. Symptoms usually resolve after adequate rehydration and provision of supplemental oxygen and medications for pain control. Antibiotic therapy for infection and RBC transfusions is sometimes required. Worsening signs and symptoms should raise concerns about complications like bowel infarction. Sickle cell patients are also at risk for cholelithiasis, acute splenic sequestration syndrome, and infectious intra-abdominal processes. Some patients may present with a hepatic ischemic syndrome, characterized by fever, abdominal pain, tender hepatomegaly, hyperbilirubinemia, leukocytosis, and deteriorating hepatic function. Appropriate laboratory and imaging studies should be done to arrive at the correct diagnosis.

Intra-Abdominal Vasculitis

Henoch-Schönlein purpura, SLE, rheumatoid vasculitis, Takayasu's arteritis, and polyarteritis nodosa are examples of systemic vasculitis that can present with severe abdominal symptoms. Patients with intra-abdominal vasculitis may present with colicky abdominal pain or major bleeding from the gastrointestinal tract. Intestinal obstruction, perforation, or intussusception may complicate the illness and represent a true surgical emergency. It is important to recognize the abdominal manifestations as part of a systemic process. For example, patients with Henoch-Schönlein purpura typically have other manifestations like migratory polyarthritis, palpable purpura on the extremities, or glomerulonephritis. Similarly, polyarthritis, rash, or renal involvement usually accompanies the abdominal involvement in SLE. Management is primarily directed at the underlying cause.

BLOOD CONSERVATION STRATEGIES

Preoperative Autologous Blood Donation (PABD)

Liberal PABD practices have now come under closer scientific and economic scrutiny. The collection of autologous blood is often carried too far; studies show that up to half the collections are discarded. Autologous blood donation is not without risks in patients with significant underlying cardiopulmonary disease. Complications like bacterial contamination and hemolytic transfusion reactions can also occur following autologous blood transfusions. Moreover, the estimated risk of contracting transfusion-transmitted diseases from allogeneic blood is now remarkably low. Certain advantages of autologous blood, however, remain, including prevention of red-cell alloimmunization and availability of compatible blood for patients with multiple alloantibodies.

In spite of adequate iron supplementation, anemia induced by the preoperative collection of blood is not fully corrected by compensatory erythropoiesis. While studies of PABD demonstrated a decrease in the risk of exposure to allogeneic blood, they also showed an increase in the exposure to any transfusion (allogeneic, autologous, or both). Selection of patients likely to benefit from PABD should be based on an assessment of their cardiopulmonary status, baseline hemoglobin levels, and anticipated surgical blood loss. In general, only patients undergoing procedures that are associated with substantial blood loss are likely to benefit from PABD. The number of units required should be estimated and collection planned to allow for compensatory erythropoiesis before surgery. Patients undergoing PABD should receive aggressive iron supplementation. The routine use of erythropoietin in the setting of PABD is not currently recommended.

Acute Normovolemic Hemodilution (ANH)

ANH requires the coordinated efforts of the anesthesiologists, nursing staff, and the blood bank service; it is now rarely performed in the United States. Criteria for patient selection include preoperative hemoglobin of at least 12 g/dL; anticipation of large blood loss; absence of significant underlying coronary, pulmonary, renal, or hepatic disease; and absence of severe hypertension or active infection.

During ANH, whole blood is removed from the patient immediately before surgery and stored in standard blood bags at room temperature. Simultaneously, crystalloid and colloid are infused to restore the blood volume. The hematocrit can safely be lowered to 20–25%, as compensatory hemodynamic changes such as decreased peripheral resistance and increased cardiac output ensure adequate tissue oxygenation. Once major blood loss has come to an end, the collected blood units are reinfused in the reverse order of collection. Platelets and coagulation factors in the collected blood (stored at room temperature for a maximum of 8 hours) are largely intact and functional and provide good hemostasis.

Studies comparing ANH to PABD in patients undergoing radical prostatectomy or total joint arthroplasty did not show a reduction in the need for allogeneic transfusions between the two groups. However, surgical blood loss for these procedures has decreased, and neither ANH nor PABD is necessary in many patients who undergo these procedures.

Intraoperative & Postoperative Blood Salvage

Intraoperative recovery of blood is cost effective if at least two units of blood can be recovered using the automated cell-washing devices. The shed blood is collected using microaggregate filters, mixed with anticoagulant, and washed; and the RBCs are resuspended in saline to a hematocrit of 50–60%. This is stored at room temperature and reinfused within 6 hours after collection. This procedure is contraindicated if the surgical site is grossly contaminated with bacteria or amniotic fluid. It is relatively contraindicated in those situations where there is a concern for possible contamination of autologous red cells with malignant cells.

Postoperative blood salvage refers to the recovery of blood from surgical drains. The collected blood is typically dilute, partially hemolyzed and defibrinated, and should be reinfused through a microaggregate filter within 6 hours of initiating the collection. The infusion of large volumes of unprocessed shed blood should be avoided.

Goodnough LT et al: Transfusion medicine, Second of Two Parts. N Engl J Med 1999;340:525.

INFECTIOUS RISKS OF TRANSFUSION

Viruses

Blood donations in the United States are tested for evidence of infection with HIV, human T-cell lymphotropic virus (HTLV), hepatitis B virus (HBV), hepatitis C virus (HCV), and West Nile virus (WNV), using serologic and nucleic acid assays. In spite of the sophisticated testing, rare cases of disease transmission from blood units collected during the window phase of a viral infection (ie, the early period when the donor is infected but the tests are still negative) may occur. It is estimated that in the United States, the current risks of viral transmission from a blood unit are as follows: HIV—1 in 2.14 million, HTLV—1 in 3 million, HBV—1 in 488,800, and HCV—1 in 1.94 million. Transfusion-transmission of WNV occurred in the United States in 2002. Nucleic acid testing to screen all blood donors for WNV infection was implemented in July 2003. Although hepatitis A virus, CMV, and parvovirus B19 can be transmitted by blood components, routine laboratory testing is not done for these viruses.

Bacteria

The risk of transfusing bacterially contaminated platelet products is estimated at 1 in 2000. With the introduction in March 2004 of mandatory bacterial testing of all platelet products in the USA, this risk should decrease substantially. Red blood cell transfusions have a much lower rate of bacterial infection.

Parasites

Malaria is the most common transfusion-transmitted parasitic infection in the USA. Transfusion-transmitted babesiosis and Chagas' disease have also been reported. Donor testing for these agents is not currently done.

Prions

Donors potentially infected with variant Creutzfeldt-Jakob disease (vCJD) are excluded from the US donor pool by screening for a history of travel and residence in Europe. No laboratory test for screening donors is available. A single case of possible transfusion-transmitted vCJD was recently reported from the United Kingdom.

Dodd RY et al: Current prevalence and incidence of infectious disease markers and estimated window-period risk in the American Red Cross blood donor population. Transfusion 2002;42:975.

Llewelyn CA et al: Possible transmission of variant Creutzfeldt-Jakob disease by blood transfusion. Lancet 2004;363:417.

TRANSFUSION THERAPY

Whole Blood

Whole blood is composed of 450–500 mL of donor blood, containing RBCs (hematocrit, 35–45%), plasma, clotting factors (reduced levels of labile factors V and VIII), and anticoagulant. Platelets and granulocytes are not functional. It is indicated for red cell replacement in massive blood loss with pronounced hypovolemia. However, it is not routinely available.

Red Blood Cells (RBCs)

RBCs are obtained by apheresis collection or prepared from whole blood by centrifugation and removal of plasma, followed by supplementation with 100 mL of adenine-containing red cell nutrient solution. The hematocrit is 55–60% and the volume is 300–350 mL. RBCs collected in CPDA-1 anticoagulant have a hematocrit of 65–80% and a storage volume of 250–300 mL. RBC transfusions are indicated to increase oxygen-carrying capacity in anemic patients. Hemoglobin levels of 7–9 g/dL are well tolerated by most asymptomatic patients. A transfusion trigger of 7g/dL is commonly used in most stable patients. Symptomatic patients with cardiac, pulmonary, or cerebrovascular disease may require RBC transfusions at higher hemoglobin levels. In a nonbleeding 70-kg recipient, transfusion of one unit of RBCs should increase hemoglobin level by 1 g/dL and the hematocrit by 3%.

Washed Red Blood Cells

RBCs are washed with saline to remove > 98% of plasma proteins and resuspended in approximately 180 mL of saline, at an approximate hematocrit of 75%. Anemic patients with recurrent or severe allergic reactions benefit from washed RBCs. Patients with severe IgA deficiency who test positive for anti-IgA antibodies should receive RBCs washed with 2–3 L of saline or receive blood collected from IgA-deficient donors.

Leukocyte-Reduced Red Blood Cells

Third-generation leukocyte reduction filters remove > 99.9% of the contaminating leukocytes, leaving $< 5 \times 10^6$ white blood cells per unit. Filtration done soon after collection (prestorage leukoreduction) is more effective than bedside filtration. Patients experiencing recurrent febrile nonhemolytic transfusion reactions (FNHTR) to RBCs or platelets should receive leukocyte-reduced products. The prophylactic use of leukoreduced RBCs and platelets in patients with long-term transfusion needs decreases the likelihood of HLA alloimmunization and protects from immune platelet refractoriness and recurrent FNHTR. Leukoreduction also decreases the risk of transmission of CMV infection in immunosuppressed CMV-seronegative patients.

Irradiated Red Blood Cells

RBCs are irradiated with 25 Gy of gamma irradiation. All cellular products should be irradiated for patients who are at risk for transfusion-associated graft versus host disease (TA-GVHD). Adult patients at risk for TA-GVHD include, but are not limited to, the following: those with congenital severe immunodeficiency, hematological malignancy receiving intensive chemo-radiotherapy, Hodgkin's and non-Hodgkin's lymphoma, certain solid tumors (neuroblastoma and sarcoma), peripheral blood stem cell and marrow transplants, or recipients of fludarabine-based chemotherapy and those receiving directed donations from blood relatives or HLA-matched platelets. Acellular products like fresh frozen plasma and cryoprecipitate are not irradiated. Leukoreduction is not an acceptable substitute for irradiation.

Frozen-Deglycerolized Red Blood Cells

RBCs frozen in glycerol are washed extensively in normal saline to remove the cryoprotectant, and then resuspended in saline at a hematocrit of approximately 75%. More than 99.9% of the plasma is removed and few leukocytes remain in the product. Patients who are alloimmunized to multiple antigens or those with antibodies against high-frequency antigens are supported with blood collected from donors with rare phenotypes. Most patients with severe IgA deficiency can safely receive RBCs washed with 2 L or more of saline. Frozen-deglycerolized RBCs are an equally safe and effective, albeit more cumbersome, alternative for these patients. Rarely, patients may require RBCs collected from IgA-deficient donors. A national rare donor program facilitates the collection and storage of rare blood types.

Platelets

Apheresis platelets are collected from single donors by apheresis and contain at least 3×10^{11} platelets in 250–300 mL plasma. Random-donor platelets (RDP) are platelet concentrates that are prepared from whole blood and contain 5.5×10^{10} platelets suspended in approximately 50 mL of plasma. Five to six units of RDP are pooled into a single pack to provide an adult dose. Platelet transfusions are indicated for the management of active bleeding in thrombocytopenic patients. Nonthrombocytopenic patients with congenital or acquired disorders of platelet function may also require platelets to stop bleeding manifestations. Platelet transfusions are also indicated prophylactically in patients requiring line placement or minor surgery when the platelet counts are < 50,000/μL and in patients undergoing major surgical procedures when the count falls below 75,000/μL. Patients scheduled for ophthalmic, upper airway, or neurosurgical procedures should have platelet counts above 100,000/μL. Platelets are not usually recommended for the correction of thrombocytopenia in patients with HIT, type IIB vWD, ITP, or TTP. The clinical indications for the use of washed, irradiated, and leukoreduced platelets are analogous to those described under RBCs. Patients with platelet refractoriness secondary to HLA alloimmunization should be supported with HLA-matched platelets.

Fresh Frozen Plasma

FFP is obtained by apheresis or prepared by centrifugation of whole blood and frozen within 8 hours of collection. It contains normal levels of all clotting factors, albumin, and fibrinogen. FFP is indicated for the replacement of coagulation factors in patients with deficiencies of multiple clotting factors as seen in the coagulopathy of liver disease, DIC, warfarin overdose, and massive transfusions. One mL of FFP contains one unit of coagulation factor activity; soon after the infusion of a 10–15 mL/kg dose, the activity of all coagulation factors increases by 20–30%. Coagulation tests should be monitored to determine efficacy and appropriate dosing intervals. FFP should be used only if the INR is > 1.5 or the PT/aPTT are elevated at least > 1.5 times the normal. Patients with liver disease who have minimally altered PT/aPTT and nominal bleeding should initially be managed with vitamin K replacement. Similarly, most patients with warfarin overdose can be managed by stopping warfarin for 48 hours and monitoring coagulation tests till they return to baseline levels. FFP is indicated only for active bleeding or if there is a risk for bleeding from an emergent procedure. FFP is the only replacement product currently available for patients with rare disorders like isolated factor deficiencies (V, X, XI) or C-1 esterase inhibitor deficiency. Patients with severe IgA deficiency should be supported with IgA-deficient plasma. FFP is the first choice for fluid replacement in patients with TTP undergoing therapeutic plasma exchange. FFP is not indicated for volume replacement, nutritional support, or replacement of immunoglobulins.

Cryoprecipitate

Cryoprecipitate is the cold-insoluble precipitate formed when FFP is thawed at 1–6 °C. This is then resuspended in 10–15 mL plasma. It contains > 150 mg fibrinogen, > 80 IU factor VIII, 40–70% of vWF, and 20–30% of factor XIII present in the initial unit of FFP, and 30–60 mg of fibronectin. Each unit (bag) of cryoprecipitate increases fibrinogen level by 5–10 mg/dL. Eight to 10 bags are pooled and infused as a single dose in a 70-kg adult. Cryoprecipitate is indicated for the correction of hypofibrinogenemia in dilutional coagulopathy and the hypofibrinogenemia/dysfibrinogenemias of liver disease and DIC. Cryoprecipitate improves platelet aggregation and adhesion and decreases bleeding in uremic patients. It has been used for the correction of factor XIII deficiency and it is the source of fibrinogen in the 2-component fibrin sealant (Tisseel). Cryoprecipitate is no longer used to treat patients with hemophilia A or vWD.

Granulocyte Transfusions

Granulocytes are collected by leukapheresis from donors stimulated with G-CSF and steroids to mobilize neutrophils from the marrow storage pool into peripheral blood. On average they contain $\geq 1 \times 10^{10}$ granulocytes suspended in 200–300 mL plasma. About $1–3 \times 10^{11}$ platelets and 10–30 mL RBCs are also present in the product. Granulocyte transfusions are indicated in severely neutropenic (absolute neutrophil count $< 0.5 \times 10^3/\mu L$) patients with bacterial sepsis who have not responded to optimum antibiotic therapy after 48–72 hours, provided there is a reasonable expectation of recovery of bone marrow function. Transfusions are given daily until clinical improvement or neutrophil recovery occurs.

Rh Immune Globulin (RhIG)

This is composed of high titer anti-D immunoglobulin derived from pooled human plasma and is available in 300-µg and 120-µg doses (IV) or 300-µg and 50-µg doses (IM). RhIG is used for prophylaxis against alloimmunization to Rh (D) antigen in Rh (D)-negative individuals, especially children and women of childbearing age who have been exposed to Rh (D)-positive RBCs via RBC, platelet, or granulocyte transfusions. A 300-µg dose of RHIG, administered within 72 hours of exposure, protects against up to 15 mL of Rh (D)-positive red cells. RHIG is routinely used for antenatal prophylaxis in Rh (D)-negative women and postpartum prophylaxis in Rh (D)-negative women with Rh (D)-positive infants.

Blood Substitutes

The development of a safe red cell substitute is much anticipated. It is unlikely that red cell substitutes will replace allogeneic blood. However, a product with demonstrated safety and efficacy could have an impressive clinical impact in the transfusion management of hemorrhagic shock in the setting of combat or trauma, or in patient subgroups like Jehovah's Witnesses or those with multiple red cell antibodies. Red cell substitutes are oxygen-carrying solutions that can expand the blood volume and oxygenate tissues. Three different classes of oxygen transporters—modified hemoglobin, liposome-encapsulated hemoglobin, and perfluorocarbons—are in different stages of development. Some products are in phase III trials and could be available for clinical use in a few years.

Free hemoglobin has several disadvantages, including its rapid dissociation into dimers and clearance by the kidney, scavenging of NO and vasoactivity, and impaired oxygen unloading capabilities. Hemoglobin should be chemically modified before it can be used for carrying oxygen. Bovine, human, and recombinant hemoglobin-based oxygen carriers have been developed. Some manufacturers have modified hemoglobins using intra- or inter-molecular cross-linking to yield cross-linked tetramers or polymerized tetramers. Others have obtained surface modification by means of conjugation to macromolecules like polyethylene glycol. Liposome-encapsulated hemoglobin is still in the early stages of development. Perfluorocarbon-based products transport oxygen in the dissolved state. However, they require very high inspired partial oxygen pressures to be as efficient as the hemoglobin-based systems in carrying oxygen. Several newer fluorocarbon compounds are currently undergoing trials as red cell substitutes.

Stowell CP et al: Progress in the development of RBC substitutes. Transfusion 2001;41:287.

TRANSFUSION REACTIONS

Acute reactions usually occur during the transfusion, but can present several hours after its completion. Those appearing after 24 hours are classified as delayed transfusion reactions. A careful clinical assessment and prompt laboratory workup are essential to detect and manage transfusion reactions and guide further transfusion support.

Acute Hemolytic Transfusion Reaction (AHTR)

The estimated risk of AHTR per unit transfused is 1 in 25,000. AHTR is immune-mediated and results from intravascular or extravascular hemolysis when donor red cells are lysed by RBC antibodies present in the recipient plasma. These may be naturally occurring isohemagglutinins (anti-A and anti-B) or alloantibodies (eg, anti-Jk^a, anti-Kell, and anti-Fy^a). AHTR can also result from the lysis of recipient red cells by incompatible antibodies present in plasma-containing products like FFP or platelets. Infrequently, interdonor incompatibility in patients receiving multiple units can cause RBC hemolysis. Infusion of ABO-incompatible blood is the leading cause of AHTR. A majority of errors occur during the administration of blood and from incorrect patient identification during phlebotomy. Errors occurring in the blood bank are responsible for about one-third of the deaths resulting from AHTR.

Nonimmune mediated hemolysis occurs when donor red cells are lysed by microbial contamination or by the addition of medications or hypotonic solutions to the blood bag. RBC in bags stored at inappropriate temperatures may undergo lysis. Donor red cells can also be lysed by thermal damage from malfunctioning blood warmers or by physical damage in the extracorporeal circuit. Recipient red cells can undergo nonimmune hemolysis following the administration of large amounts of hypotonic replacement fluids. Episodes of hemolysis as part of the underlying disease in patients with G6PD deficiency, hereditary spherocytosis, sickle cell disease, or paroxysmal nocturnal hemoglobinuria should be distinguished from transfusion reactions.

The formation of antigen-antibody complexes on the surface of targeted red cells leads to complement activation and intravascular lysis of red cells. The C3a and C5a anaphylatoxins, free hemoglobin, cytokines, and interleukins that are liberated mediate the hypotension, bronchospasm, renal ischemia, and activation of the coagulation cascade seen in AHTR. Common signs and symptoms include fever, rigors, severe anxiety, vomiting, and pain in the chest, abdomen, flank, or infusion site. Patients may develop dyspnea, hypotension, diffuse bleeding, and hemoglobinuria. The severity generally depends upon the volume and rate of infusion of incompatible red cells, and on the nature of the antigen and titers of antibody involved. In anesthetized patients, unexplained hypotension, diffuse bleeding, or hemoglobinuria may be the only clues of an ongoing AHTR.

AHTR can be fatal; early detection and aggressive management are warranted. The transfusion should be stopped immediately, the infusion set replaced, and the IV line kept open with normal saline. Cardiopulmonary status should be rapidly assessed and appropriate support provided. The blood bank should be notified, the patient's identity reconfirmed and checked with identifiers on the issued blood unit, and the remaining blood product along with the attached labels and infusion set returned to the blood bank. A fresh blood sample should be drawn and sent to the blood bank. Additionally, blood samples for CBC, plasma hemoglobin, bilirubin, LDH, haptoglobin, electrolytes, blood urea nitrogen, and creatinine should be sent. A fresh urine sample should be tested for hemoglobin. The blood bank works up a suspected hemolytic transfusion reaction by first carrying out a clerical check to verify that all labels on the blood unit match the recipient. The posttransfusion plasma sample is visually inspected for hemoglobinemia, and a direct antiglobulin test (direct Coombs' test) is done to look for evidence of antibody coating of transfused red cells. If positive, the eluate is examined to identify the coating antibody. Additional testing may include reconfirmation of the ABO and Rh type of the patient (using both pretransfusion and posttransfusion specimens) and of the donor unit. The antibody screen and crossmatch are also repeated to confirm donor-patient compatibility.

If AHTR is suspected, a hematology consult should be obtained. In general, following resuscitation, maintenance IV fluid infusions at 3000 $mL/m^2/d$ are given, paying careful attention to fluid balance and renal function. Brisk diuresis is achieved using IV furosemide, and the urine output is maintained at > 100 mL/h. Alkalinization with sodium bicarbonate is done to keep the urinary pH > 7.0. Close monitoring is done for signs of ongoing hemolysis or coagulopathy; dialysis therapy is initiated if renal function deteriorates. If blood bank tests are negative for an antibody-mediated AHTR, nonimmune hemolysis should be excluded.

Delayed Hemolytic Transfusion Reaction (DHTR)

These immune-mediated reactions result from the destruction of transfused red cells by either a newly formed alloantibody or an anamnestic increase in titer of a hitherto undetectable antibody. They are typically seen in patients who have been previously alloimmunized through transfusion or pregnancy and present 3–10 days after a serologically compatible red cell transfusion. Occasionally, a DHTR may present after a delay of several weeks. The implicated antibodies are commonly directed against the Rh and Kell system antigens, and rarely fix complement. Unlike AHTR, RBC destruction occurs primarily in the splenic and hepatic phagocytic compartments, and is accompanied by minimal cytokine release. The patient may be asymptomatic or present with fever, jaundice, or malaise. Rarely, patients may present with intravascular hemolysis and renal dysfunction. Progression of DHTR to renal failure and DIC is rare.

Laboratory investigation may show a drop in the hematocrit, reticulocytosis, hyperbilirubinemia, elevated LDH levels, and low haptoglobin. The antibody screen is repeated using a new blood sample. A direct antiglobulin test is done and the eluate examined to identify the responsible antibody. RBCs for future transfusions should be phenotypically negative for the antigen against which the patient developed an antibody.

Febrile Non-Hemolytic Transfusion Reaction (FNHTR)

This is characterized by a rise in temperature of 1 °C or more, typically with shaking chills, occurring during or up to 4 hours after a transfusion. The severity of FNHTR is dose-related, and with continued infusion, a rise in temperature of several degrees and debilitating symptoms may develop. FNHTR is a diagnosis of exclusion, and other causes of fever, including AHTR, bacterial contamination, and fever associated with underlying disease or medication, should be ruled out. The estimated frequency of FNHTR is 0.5% per unit transfused, with higher rates seen in frequently transfused patients and multiparous women. Patients whose plasma contains antibodies directed against HLA, platelet, or granulocyte antigens form antigen-antigen complexes on the surface of transfused platelets and leukocytes, leading to complement activation and release of complement components and inflammatory cytokines. Some FNHTRs are mediated by cytokines elaborated in vitro by the leukocytes present in the blood product.

If a reaction is suspected, the transfusion should be stopped, clerical checks performed, and the remaining product returned to the blood bank. The fever is usually self-limited and responds to antipyretics. Control of rigors may require meperidine, 25–50 mg IV. If AHTR or bacterial contamination is suspected, appropriate diagnostic workup should be performed. Individuals with FNHTR benefit from premedication with acetaminophen. Patients who have had two or more FNHTRs should receive prestorage, leukoreduced products.

Allergic Transfusion Reaction

These reactions occur in 1–3% of transfused patients. Like FNHTR, they are more frequent in chronically transfused patients. Reactions usually result from recipient hypersensitivity to plasma proteins in the donor plasma. The reactions can vary from mild uncomplicated urticaria to fatal anaphylaxis. Usually, the reactions are mild, limited to localized rash, pruritus, and flushing, and do not require a detailed workup. Infrequently, patients may present with systemic manifestations including severe bronchospasm, laryngeal swelling, hypotension, and shock.

Uncomplicated reactions are managed by stopping the transfusion and administering H_1-blocking antihistamines. The transfusion can be restarted if symptoms improve. However, if symptoms reappear and progress, the transfusion should be stopped. For future transfusions, the patient is premedicated with antihistamines. The addition of H_2 blockers and, if necessary, steroids may help patients with recurrent reactions. Saline-washed products are needed only for patients with severe reactions. Patients who develop anaphylactic transfusion reactions are resuscitated with fluids, vasopressors, bronchodilators, and respiratory support as needed. All anaphylactic reactions should be investigated to rule out severe IgA deficiency in the patient. If testing reveals the presence of anti-IgA antibodies in a patient with severe IgA deficiency, washed cellular products should be provided for future transfusions. It is recommended that RBCs be washed with higher volumes of saline (2–3 L) for satisfactory removal of IgA. Frozen deglycerolized RBCs are essentially free of IgA and are probably as safe as RBCs collected from IgA-deficient donors. Plasma products for these patients should be obtained only from confirmed IgA-deficient donors.

Transfusion-Associated Circulatory Overload

Circulatory overload is a frequently overlooked complication of transfusion, possibly occurring in up to 1% of transfusions in elderly patients. A rapid increase in the intravascular volume in elderly patients, in patients with severe chronic anemia, or in patients with compromised cardiopulmonary or renal function can precipitate acute pulmonary edema. The signs and symptoms develop during or soon after transfusion. Patients may present with dyspnea, cough, wheezing, tachycardia, hypoxemia, and elevated blood pressure. The transfusion should be stopped. IV diuresis should be initiated, the patient placed in an upright position, supplemental oxygen provided, and fluid balance reassessed. Diuretics can be given prophylactically if further transfusions are needed. Blood components may also have to be divided into smaller aliquots, and infused at a slower rate (1 mL/kg/h).

Transfusion-Related Acute Lung Injury (TRALI)

One in 5000 transfusions of plasma-containing components may be complicated by TRALI. All plasma-containing blood components (RBCs, platelets, FFP, cryoprecipitate, intravenous gammaglobulin and granulocytes) have been implicated. One model for TRALI proposes a primary role for leukoagglutinating antibodies. HLA class I and II antibodies and antineutrophil antibodies found in the donor plasma react with the patient's leukocytes. Less frequently, such antibodies in the recipient plasma form complexes with donor leukocytes. Antigen-antibody complex formation and complement activation lead to aggregation, margination, and sequestration of neutrophils in the pulmonary microvasculature. The release of lysosomal enzymes and free radicals from neutrophils causes vascular endothelial damage. The end result is a capillary leak syndrome with extravasation of fluid into the interstitium and alveolar spaces.

The two-hit model for TRALI proposes a priming event like sepsis or trauma, followed by transfusion, which is the second event. Neutrophils in the pulmonary vasculature are believed to undergo activation by lipid mediators in stored plasma, release destructive enzymes, and cause a capillary leak syndrome. Signs and symptoms occur during or within 6 hours of the transfusion and include fever, hypotension, and respiratory distress that can rapidly progress to severe hypoxemia and respiratory failure. Chest x-rays may show a bilateral extensive "white-out" pattern in florid cases. The central venous and pulmonary capillary wedge pressures are normal, indicating a noncardiogenic origin for the pulmonary edema. Rapid and intensive respiratory support, including intubation if needed, is the key to therapy. While most patients improve clinically and radiologically in 72–96 hours, TRALI is fatal in 5–8% of patients.

Popovsky MA: Transfusion-related acute lung injury. Curr Opin Hematol 2000;7:402.

BACTERIAL CONTAMINATION

Approximately 1 in 2000 platelet products is bacterially contaminated; only a smaller number have clinically significant septic reactions. Bacteria enter the donor unit, either during the collection process or during component preparation. Most reactions are reported with components (eg, platelets) that are stored at room temperature. These are commonly associated with gram-positive organisms like Staphylococcus, while RBC products stored at 4–6 °C are associated with gram-negative organisms like *Enterobacter, Yersinia, Pseudomonas,* and *Serratia.* Patients may rapidly develop high fever, chills, rigors, vomiting, diarrhea, dyspnea, hypotension, and shock, especially if endotoxin-producing gram-negative organisms are involved. The transfusion should be stopped and resuscitative measures instituted. Blood samples should be drawn, and along with the remaining blood product, sent for cultures. Broad-spectrum antibiotics should be started and the therapy modified based on culture results.

PREGNANCY & THE SURGICAL PATIENT

Aaron B. Caughey, MD, MPP, MPH, &
Edward C. Hill, MD

The incidence of surgical illness in pregnant and nonpregnant women of the same age group is similar and equals about 1:500 gestations. Pregnancy may alter or mask the signs and symptoms of the particular presentation or course of disease, so that diagnosis is made more difficult. Furthermore, the fetus and changes in maternal physiology and anatomy must be considered in the use of diagnostic tests, medical therapy, and the planning of surgical procedures. Any major operation represents a risk not only to the mother but to the fetus as well. One study based upon the Swedish Health Registry suggested an increase in both preterm delivery and growth restriction in infants that resulted from pregnancies that involved a surgical procedure.

Although there is no evidence that congenital anomalies are induced in the developing fetus by anesthesia, semielective procedures should be deferred until the second trimester of pregnancy, exercising the greatest precautions to prevent hypoxia and hypotension. Emergent surgical procedures should proceed as necessary; however, changes in maternal physiology—particularly in cardiac output and maternal blood volume—as well as of the size of the gravid uterus must be considered.

Radiologic Investigation

If possible, one should avoid diagnostic radiologic examinations of the lower abdomen and pelvis, especially during the first 6 weeks, when the fetus is particularly susceptible to irradiation. Radioactive isotopes pose a particular hazard to the fetus. Radioactive iodine or pertechnetate for thyroid scanning and bone scanning with radioactive strontium or calcium are contraindicated because these agents cross the placenta and are taken up by fetal tissues. Alternative modalities such as sonography and MRI are useful in many circumstances.

Laparoscopic Surgery

Laparoscopy for a variety of surgical problems, including diagnostic exploration, cholecystectomy, appendectomy, and ovarian cystectomy, has been used increasingly in the past 2 decades. Most of the evidence regarding safety of laparoscopy comes from case series, but common sense suggests guidelines about the use of laparoscopic surgery during pregnancy. The primary issues to consider when using laparoscopy in pregnancy are (1) placement of the initial trocar or Veress needle so as to avoid the uterus; (2) having adequate visualization to operate; (3) keeping CO_2 pressures as low as possible to preserve blood flow to and from the uterus; and (4) avoiding manipulation of the gravid uterus, which may induce preterm labor or cause uterine injury and kinking off the blood supply to the uterus. Placement of the initial trocar can be best managed by the open technique after the first trimester. Avoiding trocar injuries and preserving laparoscopic viewing angles is easiest prior to 18–20 weeks.

Medical Management

There are a variety of medications that are contraindicated in pregnancy and many whose use during pregnancy has not been studied. Furthermore, because of increases in the maternal blood volume, creatinine clearance, and hepatic metabolism, dosing regimens may need to be modified. Other than in the emergent setting, one should seek obstetric consultation before starting medical therapy of a pregnant patient with a surgical illness. Specialists in perinatology and maternal-fetal medicine are available for this purpose.

Doll DC et al: Management of cancer during pregnancy. Arch Intern Med 1988;148:2058.

Fatum M et al: Laparoscopic surgery during pregnancy. Obstet Gynecol Surv 2001;56:50.

Mazze RI et al: Reproductive outcome after anesthesia and operation during pregnancy: a registry study of 5,405 cases. Am J Obstet Gynecol 1989;161:1178.

Reedy MB et al: Laparoscopy during pregnancy: a study of laparoendoscopic surgeons. J Reprod Med 1997;42:33.

Reedy MB et al: Laparoscopy during pregnancy: a study of five fetal outcome parameters with use of the Swedish Health Registry. Am J Obstet Gynecol 1997;177:673.

SPECIFIC SURGICAL ISSUES IN PREGNANCY

1. Appendicitis

Acute appendicitis occurs about once in every 2000 pregnancies. The signs and symptoms are similar to those that occur in nonpregnant women, but they may be modified. First, the symptoms of early appendicitis may be disregarded because of the nausea, vomiting, and lower abdominal discomfort often present in the first and second trimesters of normal pregnancy. Moderate leukocytosis and sedimentation rate elevation are common during pregnancy. Moreover, the enlarging uterus often carries the appendix higher in the abdomen, so that McBurney's point can no longer be used. This can lead to misdiagnosis of appendicitis as cholecystitis, chorioamnionitis, or gastroenteritis. The differential diagnosis also includes ectopic pregnancy, ruptured corpus luteum cyst, adnexal torsion, round ligament syndrome, degenerating myoma, and pyelonephritis.

Peritoneal signs should only be seen with a ruptured cyst, ectopic pregnancy, or appendicitis. However, there may be relatively little rigidity associated with inflammation of the appendix, and rebound tenderness may be hard to define. Thus, the sensitivity of peritoneal signs for appendicitis is decreased, though specificity is still high. Adler's sign may be helpful. The pain is located while the patient is in the supine position. If the pain shifts to the left when she turns on her left side, the cause may be uterine or adnexal. If the pain remains in the same location, appendicitis should be suspected. A positive Bryan sign, indicative of acute appendicitis, is exacerbation of pain when the uterus is shifted to the right side. Ultrasonographic imaging of the appendix may be useful in confirming the diagnosis. If ultrasound is of no use and acute appendicitis is suspected, the risks of radiation exposure of a spiral CT to the fetus in the second and third trimester may be outweighed by the benefits of its diagnostic accuracy. However, early in pregnancy, if the physical signs are significant, then it is preferable to perform diagnostic laparoscopy.

The course of the disease may vary as well. In particular, the gravid uterus may effectively displace the omentum and loops of small intestine. Thus, rupture of the appendix is more often associated with widespread dissemination of infection, generalized peritonitis, and a higher mortality rate in gravid than in nongravid patients. If an abscess does form following perforation, the gravid uterus forms the medial wall of the abscess. The intense inflammatory process can initiate uterine contractions, resulting in loss of the fetus or preterm delivery.

The management of acute appendicitis during pregnancy is appendectomy. Because of the seriousness of perforation, aggressive management of suspected appendicitis is preferable. Perforation of the appendix occurs most commonly in the third trimester and is often associated with a delay in performing laparotomy. If generalized peritonitis exists, depending on the gestational age, delivery by cesarean section may be considered since the incidence of premature labor is high and fetal death in utero due to bacterial sepsis is not uncommon. Beyond 34 weeks of gestation, there is little to be gained by expectant management of the pregnancy; however, before 32–34 weeks, continuous fetal monitoring throughout the period of surgical management and postoperatively until the patient has defervesced will ensure continuation of the pregnancy.

Throughout the first trimester until about 18–20 weeks of gestation, a laparoscopic approach to appendectomy is reasonable. There are more than 20 laparoscopic appendectomies reported in the literature. The most common complication is spontaneous abortion, though it is difficult to estimate what percentage can actually be attributed to the operation itself as opposed to the infectious disease process. If an open approach is used, regional anesthesia is preferred, and the transverse or oblique muscle-splitting incision should be placed somewhat higher than would be the case in a nonpregnant patient.

Blaakaer J et al: Abruptio placentae as complication to acute appendicitis. Int J Gynaecol Obstet 1989;29:179.

Curet MJ et al: Laparoscopy during pregnancy. Arch Surg 1996;31:546.

Dornhoffer JL et al: Appendicitis complicating pregnancy. Kans Med 1988;89:139.

Masse RI et al: Appendectomy during pregnancy: a Swedish Registry study of 778 cases. Obstet Gynecol 1991;77:835.

2. Cholecystitis & Cholelithiasis

Acute cholecystitis in pregnancy occurs with a prevalence of about 1 in 3500–6500 pregnancies. However, the incidence of biliary colic is higher in pregnant than in nonpregnant patients (at least 1:1000 pregnancies). It is associated with gallstones in 50% of cases.

Sonographic studies show that the volume of the gallbladder is twice the normal size beyond 14 weeks of gestation, and both the rate of emptying and the percentage emptied are lower during pregnancy.

The symptoms are the same as in the nonpregnant patient, with an abrupt onset of right upper quadrant abdominal pain radiating to the right scapula, low-grade fever, and nausea and vomiting. Cholecystitis may be difficult to distinguish from acute appendicitis, with the high position of the appendix associated with the third trimester of pregnancy. Ultrasound may be helpful in diagnosis.

Unlike appendicitis, however, acute cholecystitis in the first trimester of pregnancy is best managed conservatively, with hospitalization, parenteral fluids, nasogastric suction, antispasmodics, analgesics, and broad-spectrum antibiotics. In three out of four patients treated conservatively, there will be improvement within 2 days, and a definitive surgical procedure can be deferred until the second trimester or the postpartum period. Surgery should be done whenever there is doubt regarding the differentiation from acute appendicitis or if there is no response to conservative therapy as manifested by an enlarging mass (empyema), jaundice (common duct obstruction), evidence of rupture, or associated pancreatitis. Gallstone-induced pancreatitis increases both fetal and maternal death rates. Cholecystectomy is the procedure of choice, but cholecystostomy may be performed if technical difficulties warrant it, gallbladder excision being delayed until the puerperium.

As with appendectomy, the laparoscopic approach is now commonly used in pregnant patients. One advantage over laparoscopic appendectomy is that the operative field is less likely to be obstructed by the gravid uterus before 20 weeks, so that manipulation of the uterus is less common. Conversely, surgeons are more likely to attempt laparoscopic cholecystectomy at later gestations because of the seemingly better exposure then achieved than with laparoscopic surgery in the lower abdomen and pelvis. A number of laparoscopic procedures in the third trimester have been reported, with the most common complications being preterm contractions and preterm labor. Rarely, uterine injury with Veress needle and trocar placement has been reported. In the third trimester, further consideration should be given to expectant management of cholecystitis with antibiotic therapy, and if surgical intervention is indicated an open procedure may be preferable to laparoscopy in most cases.

Baillie J et al: Endoscopic management of choledocholithiasis during pregnancy. Surg Gynecol Obstet 1990;171:1

Elderling SC: Laparoscopic cholecystectomy in pregnancy. Am J Surg 1993;165:625.

Gouldman JW et al: Laparoscopic cholecystectomy in pregnancy. Am Surg 1998;64:93.

Morrell DG et al: Laparoscopic cholecystectomy during pregnancy in symptomatic patients. Surgery 1992;112:856.

Steinbrook RA et al: Laparoscopic cholecystectomy during pregnancy. Surg Endosc 1996;10:511.

3. Intestinal Obstruction

Intestinal obstruction occurs infrequently during pregnancy. Adhesive bands are the most common cause of intestinal obstruction, and displacement of the intestine is most likely to occur when uterine growth carries the pregnancy into the abdomen around the fourth or fifth month of gestation; near term, when the fetus moves into the pelvis; or postpartum, with sudden reduction in the size of the uterus. Other causes during pregnancy are volvulus, intussusception, and large bowel cancer.

The symptoms and signs of intestinal obstruction are the same as those that occur in the nonpregnant woman, though the clinical picture may be obscured by the nausea and vomiting of early pregnancy, round ligament pain, and the abdominal distention already produced by the pregnancy. Radiologic investigation of the abdomen may be diagnostic and must be obtained. The gestational age and the benefit to the particular clinical situation of the diagnostic studies should be weighed.

Management of bowel obstruction is similar to that of the nonpregnant patient. If the patient has no signs of perforation or bowel necrosis, bowel rest (nothing by mouth) with or without nasogastric decompression can be used as first-line management, and many patients will recover with this conservative management. However, if this fails and exploratory surgery is indicated, it should be performed without delay. Consideration of gestational age can inform the surgical plan. Near term, a cesarean section may be required to obtain necessary exposure. If the fetus is undelivered, continuous fetal monitoring is indicated postoperatively until the patient has recovered.

Coleman MT et al: Nonobstetric emergencies in pregnancy: trauma and surgical conditions. Am J Obstet Gynecol 1997;177:497.

Lopez Carral JM et al: Volvulus of the right colon in pregnancy. Int J Clin Pract 1998;52:270.

Lord SA et al: Sigmoid volvulus in pregnancy. Am Surg 1996;62:380.

4. Hernias

Hiatal hernia is common during pregnancy; perhaps 15–20% of pregnant women develop this condition as a result of pressure against the stomach by the enlarging uterus. The principal symptom is reflux esophagitis, with severe heartburn aggravated by recumbency or ingestion of a large meal and relieved by an upright position or antacids. Very rarely, hematemesis may result from ulceration of the esophageal mucosa.

Elevation of the upper half of the body while reclining, frequent small meals, and antacids given liberally are usually effective treatment. The gastroesophageal reflux caused by the hiatal hernia may also be treated with H_2 blockers or proton pump antagonists. Most hiatal hernias disappear following the pregnancy. Surgical correction is required only for those that persist postpartum and remain symptomatic.

Umbilical, inguinal, and ventral hernias usually are accompanied by symptomatic exacerbations during pregnancy. The increase in abdominal pressure during pregnancy may make them more obvious to the patient or clinician, leading to their diagnosis. Repair can be done electively after delivery. Surgery during pregnancy is indicated only in the rare event of an incarcerated or strangulated hernia.

Firstenberg MS et al: Gastrointestinal surgery during pregnancy. Gastroenterol Clin North Am 1998;27:73.

Katz PO et al: Gastroesophageal reflux disease during pregnancy. Gastroenterol Clin North Am 1998;27:153.

Mayer IE et al: Abdominal pain during pregnancy. Gastroenterol Clin North Am 1998;27:1.

5. Cancer of the Breast

The rate of breast cancer during pregnancy has increased as a result of the increased average age of pregnant women. The rate was estimated to be 1:3000 pregnancies in the mid 1980s and has recently been estimated as high as 1:2000–1:1500. The breast changes that occur during gestation make detection of early breast carcinoma much more difficult. Since there may be considerable delay in diagnosis, many cases are advanced by the time the diagnosis is made. In one study, the rate of node-positive disease was 61% in pregnant or lactating patients versus 38% in nonpregnant patients.

Breast cancer in pregnancy is found on self-examination in the majority of cases. Diagnostic management is similar to that in nonpregnant patients, though the efficacy of mammography is reduced in pregnancy because of the increased radiographic density. Ultrasound is useful. Biopsy and appropriate surgical treatment should be undertaken as soon as cancer is suspected.

The overall cure rate for breast cancer developing during pregnancy or lactation is significantly lower than that of nonpregnant women of comparable age. This is most likely because delay in diagnosis results in more advanced disease. Cure rates of 90% have been achieved in pregnant patients with stage I disease. While the breast cancer itself does not seem to affect pregnancy outcome, management of the disease needs to consider the pregnancy.

Therapeutic abortion is not indicated in the patient with localized disease of a favorable microscopic type. Interruption of an early pregnancy as part of estrogen ablation may be of some palliative benefit to the woman with advanced disease, but there is no specific evidence to support this. Thus, the decision about pregnancy termination in the setting of breast cancer management needs to be made via a series of counseling sessions involving a team including a perinatologist and an oncologist.

The surgical management of breast cancer is not likely to affect the pregnancy other than exposure to anesthesia; thus, the resection (mastectomy or breast conservation) should proceed as indicated at any stage of gestation. However, chemotherapy and particularly radiation therapy may affect the fetus.

Finley JL et al: Fine-needle aspiration cytology of breast masses in pregnant and lactating women. Diagn Cytopathol 1989;5:255.

Gallenberg MM et al: Breast cancer and pregnancy. Semin Oncol 1989;16:369.

Higgins S et al: Pregnancy and lactation after breast-conserving therapy for early-stage breast cancer. Cancer 1994;73:2175.

Michels KB et al: Prospective assessment of breastfeeding and breast cancer incidence among 89,877 women. Lancet 1996;347:431.

Parente JT et al: Breast cancer associated with pregnancy. Obstet Gynecol 1988;71(Part 1):861.

Tretli S et al: Survival of breast cancer patients diagnosed during pregnancy or lactation. Br J Cancer 1988;58:382.

Zemlickis D et al: Maternal and fetal outcomes after breast cancer in pregnancy. Am J Obstet Gynecol 1992;166:781.

6. Ovarian Tumors & Ovarian Torsion

A cystic corpus luteum is the most frequent cause of ovarian enlargement during pregnancy. This structure rarely exceeds 6 cm in diameter and gradually diminishes in size as the pregnancy progresses. The corpus luteum is responsible for secreting the hormones that maintain the pregnancy until about 10 weeks of gestation. It is usually asymptomatic, and careful observation is required to distinguish it from a proliferative type of cystic enlargement. Adnexal masses that are not corpus luteum cysts are encountered in approximately 1:1000 pregnancies. Only 2–5% of these are actually ovarian cancer, making that incidence between 1:50,000 and 1:20,000 pregnancies.

Adnexal masses are often asymptomatic unless there is hemorrhage into the tumor, rupture of the cyst, or torsion of the pedicle—complications that are definitely increased during pregnancy (see Chapter 41). Thus, adnexal masses in pregnancy are most commonly identified either on initial examination or upon routine ultrasound. However, some are not found until the immediate postpartum period, when the uterine size no longer masks their presence and the abdominal wall is flaccid. When a pelvic mass separate from the uterus is identified in pregnancy, the next step in diagnosis is ultrasound. Whether seen on routine ultrasound or identified on physical examination, determining whether an ovarian lesion is malignant or benign is of the utmost importance.

Most ovarian neoplasms are cystic; solid tumors are quite rare. The cystic neoplasms most often seen during pregnancy are benign cystic teratomas (about 40% are of this variety), serous and mucinous cystadenomas, and endometrial cysts. Ovarian cancer is quite uncommon in pregnancy (< 1:20,000 pregnancies), but of the three major subtypes—epithelial, stromal, and germ cell—during pregnancy, germ cell tumors seem to be more common. Dysgerminoma is the most frequently encountered solid tumor. Serous and mucinous cystadenocarcinomas and endometrioid carcinomas are the most common histologic types.

Management of the asymptomatic adnexal mass in pregnancy is controversial. If there is no ultrasonographic evidence of malignancy, the mass can be followed expectantly during through the first trimester. Serial ultrasound examination is used to follow the growth or resolution of the adnexal mass. At any point, surgical management of the adnexal mass needs to be weighed against increased risk of complications of the pregnancy. In general, because of the increased risk of adnexal torsion, ovarian cysts and tumors larger than 6 cm are removed via cystectomy in the mid second trimester. Depending on the size of the mass, either laparotomy or laparoscopy can be used. It is important to evaluate the mass via ultrasound immediately before operation to reassess both the indication and the surgical approach.

If a true ovarian neoplasm is suspected, consultation with a gynecologic oncologist should be obtained, and a staging and diagnostic procedure can usually be performed in the second trimester. A conservative staging procedure has been described consisting of removal of the ovary containing the mass, peritoneal washings, and extensive pelvic and abdominal examination. Depending on the stage of disease, termination of the pregnancy should be considered.

An ovarian mass may be diagnosed when a patient presents with abdominal pain. Operation may be indicated if there is an acute abdominal emergency caused by ovarian torsion or rupture or hemorrhage of an ovarian cyst. Again, a laparoscopic approach is reasonable. If the pregnancy is early (less than 10 weeks gestation) and termination is not wanted, it is optimal to avoid cystectomy because of the contribution of the corpus luteum to the pregnancy. In the setting of ovarian torsion, untwisting the adnexa results in a viable ovary in most cases.

Bider D et al: Outcome of pregnancy after unwinding of ischemic hemorrhagic adnexum. Br J Obstet Gynaecol 1989;96:426.

Buller RE et al: Conservative surgical management of dysgerminoma concomitant with pregnancy. Obstet Gynecol 1992;79:887.

Busine A et al: Conservative laparoscopic treatment of adnexal torsion during pregnancy. J Obstet Biol Reprod 1994;23:918.

El Yahia AR et al: Ovarian tumors in pregnancy. Aust N Z J Obstet Gynecol 1991;31:327.

Farahmand SH et al: Case report: ovarian endodermal sinus tumor associated with pregnancy: review of the literature. Gynecol Oncol 1991;41:156.

Fleischer AC et al: Sonographic evaluation of maternal disorders during pregnancy. Radiol Clin North Am 1990;28:51.

Hess L et al: Adnexal mass occurring with intrauterine pregnancy: report of fifty-four patients requiring laparotomy for definitive management. Am J Obstet Gynecol 1996;174:1499.

Horbelt D et al: Mixed germ cell malignancy of the ovary concurrent with pregnancy. Obstet Gynecol 1994;84:662.

Malfetano JH et al: Cisplatinum combination chemotherapy during pregnancy for advanced epithelial ovarian carcinoma. Obstet Gynecol 1990;75:545.

Platek DN et al: The management of a persistent adnexal mass in pregnancy. Am J Obstet Gynecol 1995;173:123.

Soriano D et al: Laparoscopy versus laparotomy in the management of adnexal masses during pregnancy. Fertil Steril 1999;71: 955.

MANAGEMENT OF THE OLDER SURGICAL PATIENT

Daniel B. Hinshaw, MD

In 2000, 30.1% of all outpatient visits to general surgeons were made by individuals 65 years of age and older. As the population continues to age and perioperative care has become more sophisticated, surgeons are presented with ever-increasing numbers of older patients seeking surgical treatment. The operative rate per 1000 population for patients aged 65 years and older is more than twice that of the general population. Despite a 50% improvement in surgical mortality for this population since the 1960s, older patients account for about 70% of postoperative deaths and complications.

It is projected that between 2010 and 2030 the percentage of individuals aged 65 and over will increase from 13–20% of the US population. The fastest-growing segment of the population will be people aged 85 and over.

By 2050, life expectancy is projected to increase to ~86 years for women and ~80 years for men. Because of the increased longevity of women, the proportion of women to men living at age 65 and older in 1994 was 3:2. In those aged > 85 years it was a ratio of 5:2. This disproportionate relationship between aging women and men is expected to continue in the 21st century. A majority of older persons living alone will be women. Thus, the surgeon in the 21st century will encounter the elderly (more often female) with ever-increasing frequency in his or her practice.

More than the mere accumulation of years, aging represents the aggregated effect of often multiple chronic conditions (impairments) that lead to a narrowing of physiologic reserve known as homeostenosis. Actual chronological age is less important than the nature, extent, and chronicity of the impairment. An acute illness normally has a rapid onset and is often accompanied by severe symptoms that are usually of short duration. On the other hand, chronic illness persists over a long period of time (> 3 months) and affects the overall function of the organism at many levels, including intellectual, emotional, social, and spiritual, not just the physical level of function. Acute illnesses are typically encountered and managed as diseases, whereas chronic illnesses (conditions) are more often manifested as impaired function. Figure 5–1 illustrates the interplay between an acute problem (disease) and the chronic condition(s) (functional impairment) of each person seeking health care. Although this model has relevance for patients of all ages, it is particularly pertinent for the older surgical patient. The degree of functional impairment associated with an ever-increasing burden of chronic conditions and compounded by the challenge of polypharmacy puts the elderly at greater risk when confronted with the need for an operation. Unlike many younger patients who are less functionally impaired, the older surgical patient is not only struggling with some degree of functional impairment but is often further constrained by limited social support and the lack of other resources.

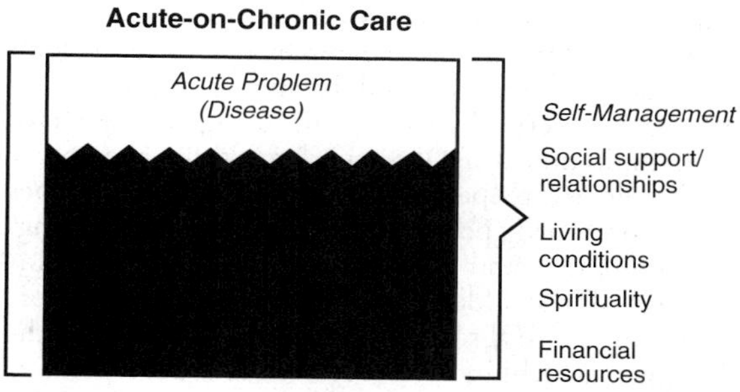

Figure 5–1. Acute-on-chronic care model. The interplay between chronic conditions that impair function and an acute illness secondary to a disease process is illustrated. Chronic conditions form the substrate upon which an acute disease process develops and is experienced. Medical management in the form of assessment, disease management, and referral for specialized services is in tension with self-management that includes social support/relationships, living conditions, spirituality, and financial resources. (Adapted from and courtesy of Dr Brent Williams, Division of General Medicine, University of Michigan, Ann Arbor, MI.)

The Importance of Functional Status

With increasing functional limitations from chronic illness, the older surgical patient may have difficulty performing even basic activities of daily living (ADLs) (Table 5–5). Approximately 23% of the elderly report

Table 5–5. Activities of daily living.

Feeding oneself
Bathing
Toileting (continence)
Transferring from bed to chair
Dressing
Grooming

some limitation of ADLs or instrumental ADLs (IADLs). IADLs are more complex tasks such as food preparation, shopping, and balancing a checkbook. Among the very old (85+ years of age), 53% have some limitation of ADLs. Fundamentally, the ability of the elderly to perform their ADLs often defines their continued potential for independent living. Hospitalization and especially surgery threaten maintenance of the older patient's independent performance of the ADLs because of the frequent deconditioning and debility that occur in the postoperative period. It is critical to assess the functional status of the prospective older candidate for surgery prior to scheduling an operation. Recognition of functional deficits prior to surgery will facilitate better assessment of operative risk and may identify the need for intensive rehabilitative interventions prior to and after the operation.

Diminished functional status should always be placed within the context of the support system available to the older surgical patient. The overall prospects for a good outcome in an older surgical patient with diminished functional status will be considerably different depending on the level of support available. For example, if the patient has a healthy spouse, other caregivers are available, and has a stable financial situation, the patient is much more likely to do well after discharge than an impoverished, homeless individual with limited social contacts who may otherwise have the same functional status. Discharge planning for the elderly surgical patient should begin prior to the operation. The level of social support available in combination with the degree of functional limitation experienced by the older surgical patient will determine whether discharge to home or to a skilled nursing facility will occur. A part of informed consent for the elderly surgical patient should include a discussion about potential changes (declines) in functional status and level of independent living that may occur after elective surgery.

Age-Related Changes in Organ Function

As a rule, organ function decreases with aging, though it usually remains adequate to meet the stress of surgery, and age as such is rarely a contraindication to operative management.

A. Pulmonary Function

Decreased pulmonary function due to aging should pose no risk to surgical candidates who are otherwise free of pulmonary disease. However, diminished pulmonary reserve may exaggerate conditions that would be better tolerated by younger patients, with attendant risk of postoperative hypoxia, atelectasis, and pneumonia. Pain, oversedation, infection, and intrathoracic or upper abdominal surgical procedures may increase this risk.

B. Cardiovascular Function

In healthy older persons, cardiac output rises in response to exercise well into the ninth decade. Since the maximal heart rate is diminished in the aged (220 – Age) and increased cardiac output depends upon stroke volume, cardiac performance is vulnerable to volume depletion (hemorrhage, dehydration, excessive diuresis).

Diminished sinus node activity and loss of cardiac conducting tissue increase the likelihood of arrhythmias. Decreased responsiveness to catecholamines, heightened vascular resistance, and reduced left ventricular compliance may limit the ability of the aging cardiovascular system to cope with stress. Blunted baroreceptor reflexes increase the risk of postural hypotension, especially during ambulation shortly after surgery.

A history of myocardial infarction or angina is a major risk factor. The prevalence of arteriosclerotic heart disease (often asymptomatic) in men aged 60 or older is about 20%, rising to 40% after age 80. Arrhythmias, heart failure, myocardial ischemia (often asymptomatic) and infarction, and thromboembolism are the most serious cardiovascular problems in older patients.

In addition to the classic findings, cardiac problems in the aged may be manifested as acute confusion, weakness and hypotension, severe fatigue, dyspnea, neurologic changes, arrhythmias, and pulmonary edema. Any of these states should be investigated (eg, by CK, serial ECGs, isotope studies) as possible signs of myocardial ischemia. The hours immediately after surgery are especially dangerous for patients with ischemic heart disease, and during this time the patient should be monitored with great care for pain, hypoxia, hypotension, and other conditions that may increase cardiac work

The risk of postoperative cardiac failure is increased in the presence of an S gallop or distended external jugular veins, a heart rate of less than 100/min after 2 minutes of stationary bicycle exercise in the supine position, or the presence of ischemic changes (which may occur in the absence of symptoms) on the ECG in the immediate postoperative period.

Patients at increased risk for postural hypotension often have elevated systolic blood pressures and may be identified by a drop of 20 mm Hg or more in systolic pressure after 2–3 minutes in the upright position following a 5-minute period in the supine position. If postural hypotension is detected, ambulation should be allowed with caution. Volume status and hypotensive drugs must be attended to in the immediate postoperative period.

Control of hypertension, arrhythmias, angina, and cardiac failure will reduce perioperative mortality and morbidity in older patients. Unless contraindicated, cardiac medications should be continued until the morning of surgery. Monitoring of cardiovascular status following surgery (eg, blood gases, Swan-Ganz line, ECGs) is often necessary and should be instituted earlier for suspected cardiac embarrassment in patients aged 65 and above.

Good management of pain decreases catecholamine release and arrhythmias, but it is equally important to guard against oversedation and hypoxia.

Early ambulation of older patients protects them against deconditioning, and together with low-dose heparin prophylaxis (5000 units every 8–12 hours) reduces the frequency of thromboembolism.

C. Renal Function

Most persons experience a decline in glomerular filtration rate (GFR) of at least 30% by the eighth decade, though one-third of older persons who are free of renal and cardiovascular disease have a well-preserved GFR as attested by serial creatinine clearance measurements. A reduction in GFR and renal blood flow may predispose geriatric patients to postoperative renal failure and toxicity from drugs cleared by the kidney. Impaired thirst perception, decreased urine concentration, and reduced renin response to volume contraction weaken the older patient's defense against hypotension when challenged by hemorrhage, nasogastric drainage, third-space sequestration of fluid, or dehydration.

Decreased dilutional capacity may lead to overhydration and hyponatremia after vigorous fluid administration, with serious cardiovascular (pulmonary edema) or central nervous system (cerebral edema) complications. Reduced NH_4^+ secretion impairs the aged patient's ability to correct acidosis.

A history of renal disease is present in a minority of patients who develop postoperative renal failure; detection of subclinical renal insufficiency in older surgical candidates is an important priority to protect them against this potentially catastrophic event.

Because muscle mass and creatinine production are much less in many older patients, serum creatinine levels may be normal despite a 60% or more decline in GFR. Nomograms and formulas that estimate creatinine clearance without the need for urine collections have proved unreliable. Therefore, if incipient renal failure is suspected, a 12- to 24-hour creatinine clearance determination should be obtained before nonemergent surgery.

A 50% or more reduction in GFR (< 50–60 mL/min) reflects an increased risk of postoperative renal failure. Operations lasting more than 3 hours or involving clamping of the aorta above the renal arteries are additional risk factors.

Avoiding volume depletion or overhydration, limiting the use of nephrotoxic drugs or drugs cleared by the kidney, monitoring acid-base status and urine output, and maintaining urine volume at 1 mL/min all help minimize renal complications postoperatively.

D. Central Nervous System Function

The aged brain has a diminished ability to maintain cerebral blood flow during hypotension and a decreased acetylcholine content in many areas of the cerebrum and associated structures.

Because autoregulatory control of cerebral blood flow is impaired in older patients, signs of cerebral ischemia may appear when mean arterial pressure (MAP) falls below 80 mm Hg.

$$\text{MAP} = 0.33 \times [\text{Systolic blood pressure} - \text{Diastolic blood pressure}] + \text{Diastolic blood pressure}$$

Geriatric surgical patients whose systolic blood pressure is 105 mm Hg or less should be closely monitored for cognitive impairment or confusion, and corrective action should be taken as appropriate (eg, decrease vasodilator therapy, improve volume status).

The risk of bladder obstruction in older men with enlarged prostates who receive anticholinergic drugs (eg, diphenhydramine, some antidepressants, opioids) is well known, but these drugs may lead to acute confusion in the elderly (especially those with Alzheimer's disease) as a consequence of age-related depletion of acetylcholine in the cerebrum and elsewhere in the central nervous system. Postoperatively, older patients receiving anticholinergics should be examined for acute confusion, and these drugs should be used only when absolutely required.

SPECIAL PROBLEMS OF OLDER PATIENTS

Altered Drug Disposition

Changes in body composition, renal function, hepatic function, and nutritional status may lead to increased risks when older surgical patients receive drugs. The great frequency of polypharmacy among the elderly adds the risk of multiple drug interactions.

A. Changes in Body Composition

Increased fat and decreased muscle mass in old age result in diminished total body water and contracted volume of distribution for water-soluble drugs such as nitrates, aminoglycosides, and some antihypertensive agents. To avoid overdosing with water-soluble drugs, therapy should begin at the low end of the dosage scale, with regular monitoring of drug levels in older subjects.

B. Diminished Renal Function

Diminished renal function is common in old age, and unless this is borne in mind patients may receive excessive doses of nephrotoxic agents (eg, nonsteroidal anti-inflammatory agents, aminoglycosides) or drugs cleared by the kidney (eg, digoxin, some calcium-channel blockers) that accumulate and cause side effects.

C. DECREASED LIVER FUNCTION

Hepatic mass and function decline by about 30% by the eighth decade. This poses little danger unless it is exacerbated by decreased blood flow (hypotension, volume contraction) or by drugs that inhibit hepatic enzymes (eg, cimetidine) or that reduce liver blood flow (eg, cimetidine, propranolol). In such cases, there is a risk of toxicity from drugs (eg, nitrates, propranolol, morphine) cleared by rapid hepatic inactivation.

D. MALNUTRITION

Malnutrition is present in 20% of hospitalized older patients, and decreased serum albumin levels associated with malnutrition (or with acute phase reactions to infection) may lead to an increase in the free serum levels of drugs that are highly protein-bound (eg, quinidine, warfarin, rifampin, propranolol), with attendant risks of toxicity. Patients with hypoalbuminemia who receive such drugs should be monitored closely for toxic side effects.

Pain

Several factors contribute to making control of postoperative pain a challenging problem in the elderly. At baseline, almost 50% of the elderly have some type of pain (most commonly musculoskeletal). Older individuals often underreport their pain. Due to cognitive and other factors, the standard means of assessing pain in most hospitals (numerical pain scale) is not particularly helpful in the elderly. Nonverbal cues are much more important signs of pain in the older patient than the young. Social withdrawal, decreased activity and movement, even confusion are subtle but important potential signs of poorly controlled pain. It is not uncommon to inquire about the pain of an older patient and receive an initial negative response: "I have no pain," although the nurses complain that the patient will not move in/out of bed. Only with further questioning does the qualifying statement come "… as long as I don't move!" Unfortunately, even the mildly cognitively impaired surgical patient may not be able to verbalize his or her pain, but will manifest it by being unable to get out of bed, deep breathe, and cough very effectively during the recovery process. The use of patient-controlled analgesia (PCA) in the elderly is also fraught with difficulties. The older patient is less apt to understand how to take full advantage of the self-administration capability of PCA. Quite often, PCA orders have not taken into account the older patient's chronic pain that would require a continuous dose of opiate as well as the demand dose required for the acute incisional pain.

As mentioned above, the decreased renal clearance of medications in the elderly impacts the choice of analgesics. Nonsteroidal anti-inflammatory agents should be used with caution and at lower doses in the elderly because of their associated renal and GI toxicity. Opiates should also be titrated cautiously to achieve pain relief with lower initial doses ("start low and go slow"). Doses of most opiates will need to be adjusted for renal insufficiency. Fentanyl and methadone are the two opiates that do not require adjustment in renal insufficiency because of their primary clearance through the liver.

Delirium

In the older surgical population (65+ years), the incidence of delirium may be as high as 60%. A key feature of delirium is an impaired ability to focus one's attention. A quick and very useful tool to screen for the risk of delirium is the measure of attention used in the Bedside Confusion Scale. The patient is asked as a test of attention to recite the months of the year backwards. Even some degree of hesitation with this test is a sensitive predictor of patients who are at increased risk for delirium. Since mortality rates for delirious inpatients can be from 2- to 20-fold higher than nondelirious subjects, this simple screening method may be extremely helpful in further defining preoperative risk.

When confronted with an apparently confused postoperative patient, a systematic approach to assessing for delirium is useful. The Confusion Assessment Method (CAM) is one such approach. In the Confusion Assessment Method, for a diagnosis of delirium to be made, three consistent features of delirium must be present: (1) the episode must represent an *acute* change in mental status; (2) the symptoms of confusion should *fluctuate* throughout the day; and (3) there should be *inattention* (difficulty focusing one's attention). Also, one of two variable features, either disorganized (incoherent) thinking or an altered level of consciousness (eg, hyperalert/agitated, lethargic, or stuporous), should be present.

The best approach to the management of delirium is its prevention. Thus, recognition of patients at risk preoperatively can be followed by preventive strategies implemented during the recovery period. Older individuals with multiple preexisting conditions including dementia, visual or auditory impairment, and renal insufficiency will be much more vulnerable to insults predisposing to delirium than younger individuals without these impairments. Relatively minor stressors (eg, change of environment, mild infection, mild hypoxia) may be sufficient to trigger delirium in the compromised elderly. Thus, the most important strategy for treating delirium is to reduce/eliminate the potential and real stressors that may have triggered the delirium. Vigorous and regular efforts to reorient the confused patient should be made by staff while providing easily visible cues to time, person, and place for self-orientation, as well. Sources of infection (particularly urinary tract) should be sought and treated. Medications should be reviewed and where possible, medications associated with delirium (especially benzodiazepines and those with anticholinergic properties, eg, diphenhydramine, opiate analgesics) should be minimized or eliminated. A history of prior substance abuse may be revealing in the confused and agitated patient who had his or her last drink of alcohol prior to admission or who has not continued to receive a chronically administered benzodiazepine since admission. Paradoxically, poorly controlled postoperative pain can also trigger or exacerbate delirium.

It is critical to assess the level of pain over time in the delirious patient prior to onset of the confusion to identify pain as a potential factor. In general, physical restraints are usually not as helpful as directed efforts to reorient the confused patient and may be dangerous. For the older, agitated patient with delirium, low doses of antipsychotic medications (eg, 0.25–0.5 mg orally or 0.125–0.25 mg parenterally of haloperidol; 0.25–1.0 mg risperidone orally) should be given.

Depression

Depression is quite common in the elderly. It has been identified in 17–37% of older primary care patients, with 30% of this population meeting criteria for major depression. The presentation of depression in the elderly can be different from that in younger patients. Older patients are more apt to emphasize somatic complaints (~65%) and deemphasize the presence of a depressed mood. They are more likely to have psychotic symptoms (eg, delusions centered on somatic complaints, guilt, persecution, etc). The challenge for the surgeon is that unrecognized depression may be a complicating factor postoperatively and may be difficult to differentiate from delirium and dementia. A quick effort to screen preoperatively for a past history of depression or treatment with antidepressants is important. Surveying the patient for common constitutional symptoms (eg, fatigue, hypersomnia or insomnia, weight loss or gain) as well as suicidal thoughts, depressed mood, and anhedonia will help identify the problem prior to scheduling for an operation. For elective surgery it is prudent to treat depression prior to the operation.

Dementia

Dementia refers to a significant reduction or decline in two or more areas of cognitive function. It is not a normal part of aging. Alzheimer's disease (AD) is the most common form of dementia, with vascular dementia the second most common type. Usually, dementia begins after age 60; survival is ~8–10 years after the appearance of symptoms. Approximately 30% of the population aged 85 and over has AD. Currently it affects ~4 million people in the USA and is projected to affect 14 million by 2040.

Dementia adds greatly to the challenges of perioperative care by reducing the ability of the patient to participate meaningfully in his or her treatment and process of recovery. Since AD is a terminal illness, it is important for the surgeon to be aware of its natural history prior to considering the appropriateness of an operative intervention (eg, a request for feeding tube placement). Although a more detailed screening tool (ie, Folstein Mini-Mental Status Exam) exists, a shorter, reliable test of cognitive function, the Mini-Cog, may be completed quickly in the pressured environment of the surgical clinic. In the Mini-Cog, the patient is told to remember 3 items and later recall them. Between hearing the 3 items and being asked to recall them, the patient is asked to draw a clock face with the time at 8:20. If the patient cannot recall any of the 3 items, this is suspicious for dementia. The clock-drawing task helps to clarify if dementia may be present when only 1 or 2 items are recalled correctly.

Falls

About one-third of those who are 65+ years of age fall, with an increasing percentage as age increases. Falls are a significant source of morbidity and mortality in the elderly; there are 1 million fractures a year. The fear of falling may limit a patient's ADLs and ability to cooperate during postoperative recovery. A number of problems may contribute to the etiology of falls: poor vision, incontinence, various medications (eg, opiates, antihypertensives, psychotropic agents, etc), altered vestibular function, and delirium. A quick and useful screening test for gait disturbance and fall risk is the "Get Up And Go" test. Each patient who has had a history of at least one fall will benefit from this screening test. The patient should be observed for posture while sitting in a straight-back chair without armrests. The patient is then asked to rise from the chair (preferably without using his or her arms) and then walk 10 feet, turn 180 degrees and return to the chair to sit down. Abnormalities in transfers, balance, or gait are good predictors of fall risk and should be followed up with a full geriatric evaluation.

Pressure Sores

The incidence of pressure sores varies depending on the venue and quality of care and the population being treated. Overall prevalence among hospitalized patients is in the range of 3–11%. Immobilization, urinary and fecal incontinence, and malnutrition expose aged patients to the development of pressure sores. Patients with predisposing factors should have daily inspection of pressure points for evidence of early skin ischemia (blanching erythema), stage I (nonblanching erythema), stage II (shallow ulcers), and stages III & IV (progressively deeper ulceration) pressure sores. Patients at high risk should be protected by being kept dry, by frequent turning (ideally every 2 hours) to relieve pressure, and by the use of air or foam mattresses. Treatment of skin ulcers involves wet-to-dry dressings to remove dead tissue and surgical debridement to remove more extensive areas of necrotic material. Hydrocolloid dressings may be useful in clean wounds with viable tissue present to help maintain a moist, less traumatic environment. Ultimately, skin grafting or flap coverage may be indicated for more extensive lesions.

Infection

Patients of advanced age who are infected in the perioperative period may have atypical or nonspecific manifestations, including failure to develop a fever. Often, the presenting picture is one of slowness to recover function after surgery, cognitive impairment (delirium), or persistent weakness. If infection is suspected, the triad of fever, leukocytosis, and elevated band count strongly support the diagnosis of bacterial invasion, and the absence of these indicators is good evidence against infection.

Aalami OO et al: Physiological features of aging persons. Arch Surg 2003:138:1068.

Clancy DJ et al: Dietary restriction in long-lived dwarf flies. Science 2002;296:319.

Flacker JM, Marcantonio ER: Delirium in the elderly: optimal management. Drugs & Aging 1998;13:119.

Gloth III FM: Principles of perioperative pain management in older adults. Clin Geriatr Med 2001;17:553.

Jonasson O, Kwakwa F: Aging of America: Implications for the surgical workforce. In: *Principles and Practice of Geriatric Surgery*, pp. 105–110. Rosenthal RA, Zenilman ME, Katlic MR (editors). Springer-Verlag, 2001.

Katz PR et al: *Geriatrics Syllabus for Specialists.* American Geriatrics Society, 2002.

Kim S: Molecular biology of aging. Arch Surg 2003;138:1051.

O'Neill GO, Patrick M: The health of older Americans. In: *The State of Aging and Health in America.* Merck Institute of Aging & Health and The Gerontological Society of America, 2002.

Sarhill N et al: Assessment of delirium in advanced cancer: the use of the Bedside Confusion Scale. Am J Hospice & Palliat Care 2001;18:335.

Wound Healing

6

Thomas K. Hunt, MD

Only a century ago, complicated and incomplete healing after injury was the rule rather than the exception. Surgeons had little choice but to accept draining wounds and invasive infections. The evolution of wound care and antisepsis in the 18th and 19th centuries changed surgery as dramatically as the discovery of anesthesia. Even so, poor healing, infection, and excessive scarring continue to be leading causes of disability and death. New means of aiding healing and preventing infections have been developed, and to use them efficiently, knowledge of the basic mechanisms of healing is required.

FORMS OF HEALING

Surgeons customarily divide types of wound healing into first and second "intention." **First intention (primary) healing** occurs when tissue is cleanly incised and reapproximated and repair occurs without complication. **Second intention (secondary) healing** occurs in open wounds through formation of granulation tissue* and eventual coverage of the defect by spontaneous migration of epithelial cells. Most infected wounds and burns heal in this manner. Primary healing is simpler and requires less time and material than secondary healing. It sometimes happens that primary healing is possible but there is insufficient vascular or nutritional reserve to support secondary healing. For example, an ischemic limb may heal primarily, but if the wound opens and becomes secondarily infected, it may not have the resources to granulate and epithelialize and may not heal. These two forms may be combined in **delayed primary closure,** when a wound is allowed to heal open under a carefully maintained, occlusive dressing for about 5 days and is then closed as if primarily. Such wounds are less likely to become infected than if closed immediately because their oxygen needs are better met.

THE NATURE OF REPAIR

The major components of repair are shown in Figure 6–1. The lines in the diagram indicate signaling processes that include growth factors, complement, classic inflammatory mediators, and metabolic signals such as hypoxia and accumulated lactate. Often several signals are capable of controlling any given step, showing that many wound healing mechanisms are redundant. The following describes the complex process of wound healing as a stepwise process proceeding from coagulation and inflammation through fibroplasia, matrix deposition, angiogenesis, epithelialization, collagen maturation, and finally wound contraction.

THE INITIAL RESPONSE: COAGULATION & INFLAMMATION

Immediately after injury, the coagulation products fibrin, fibrinopeptides, fibrin split products, and complement components begin to attract inflammatory cells—particularly macrophages—into the wound. Platelets activated by thrombin release IGF-1, TGFα, TGFβ, and PDGF, then attract leukocytes and fibroblasts into the wound. Damaged endothelial cells respond to a signal cascade involving complement product C5a, TNFα, IL-1, and IL-8 and express receptors for integrin molecules on the cell membranes of leukocytes. This allows circulating leukocytes to adhere to the endothelium and then migrate into the wounded tissue. Their interleukins and other inflammatory components, such as histamine, serotonin, and bradykinin, cause vessels first to constrict in aid of hemostasis, and later dilate, becoming so porous that blood plasma and leukocytes can move freely into the area.

The newly arrived inflammatory cells increase metabolic demand. Since the local microvasculature has been damaged, a local energy sink results, and PaO_2 falls while CO_2 accumulates. Lactate in particular plays a critical role, but its source is mainly aerobic, from activated and oxygenated levels.

These conditions persist throughout repair, and—together with other stimulants such as fibrin, foreign bodies, bacteria, etc—they direct leukocytes, particularly macrophages, to release a variety of cytokines, chemoattractants, and growth factors. New information leads to a picture of wound healing as a reaction to oxidative stress. These events trigger reparative processes and ensure their continuation, because macro-

* Granulation tissue is the red, granular, moist tissue that appears during healing of open wounds. Microscopically, it contains new collagen, new blood vessels, fibroblasts, and inflammatory cells, especially macrophages.

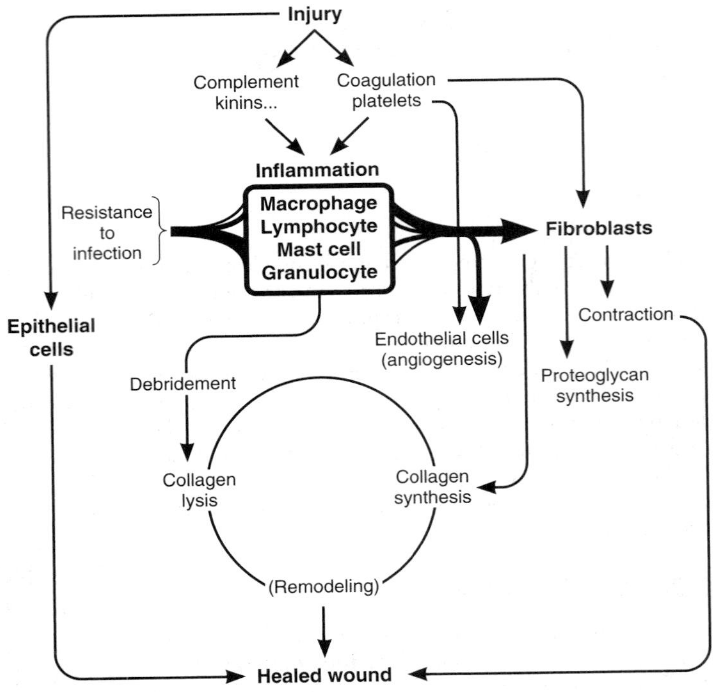

Figure 6–1. Schematic diagram of the sequence of events in wound healing. (Reprinted by permission of Thomas K. Hunt.)

phages, which secrete most of the growth-promoting products, assume the control of repair as the flood of coagulation-mediated growth substances begins to ebb. Furthermore, macrophages, stimulated by fibrin, release large quantities of lactate. Though hypoxia may contribute, this process continues even in the presence of oxygen, thereby maintaining the environment of injury. The environment causes them to release growth promoters and more lactate. Lactate acts as a "surrogate" of hypoxia, and by itself stimulates angiogenesis and collagen deposition through instigation of growth factors.

By the third or fourth day after injury, the reparative cells become arranged in a characteristic spatial relationship as shown in Figure 6–2. Wound cells proceed in orderly single file—leaders first, followers next. Unless the wound becomes infected, its granulocyte population, which dominated during the first days, diminishes. Macrophages now cover the cut surface. Immature fibroblasts, the product of growth signals, lie just beneath, mixed with buds of new vessels. More mature fibroblasts are scattered behind. The spatial relations of cells with respect to oxygen and lactate concentrations define zones of reparative activities. Recently, it has become apparent that stem cells contribute fibroblasts, but the extent of this contribution is unknown.

These spatial relationships show how macrophages condition an acidic, hypoxic, high-lactate growth-promoting environment that acts as a "growth center" synthesizing and depositing new collagen in an area still rich in lactate but better oxygenated as is required for collagen synthesis and deposition.

FIBROPLASIA & MATRIX DEPOSITION

Fibroplasia

During the course of healing, fibroplasia (replication of fibroblasts) is stimulated by multiple mechanisms, starting with PDGF, IGF-1, and TGFβ released by platelets and later by the continual release of numerous peptide growth factors from macrophages and fibroblasts within the wound. FGF, IGF-1, VEGF, IL-1, IL-2, IL-8, PDGF, TGFα, TGFβ, and TNFα all seem to be potential contributors.

Dividing fibroblasts are seen mainly near the wound edge, where they are exposed to the growth environment and to an oxygen tension of approximately 40 mm Hg in normally healing wounds. In cell culture, this PaO_2 is optimal for fibroblast replication.

Smooth muscle cells are likely progenitors because fibroblasts seem to stream from the adventitia and media of vessels. Lipocytes, pericytes, and others are also

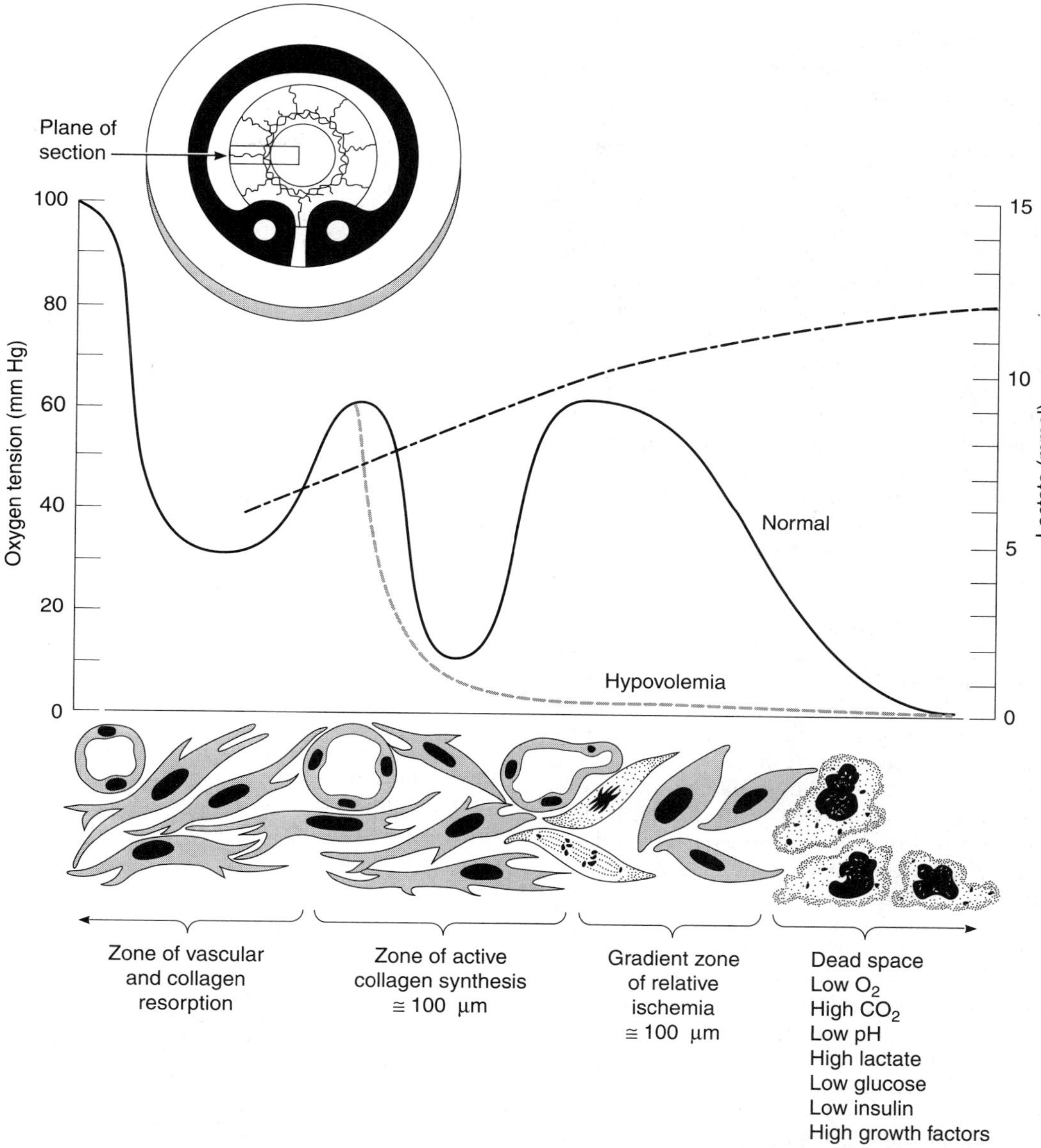

Figure 6–2. Diagram of oxygen tension and lactate concentration in a cross-section of a rabbit ear chamber wound. Macrophages lead into the dead space. Fibroblasts and new blood vessels follow. In hypovolemia (as shown by the dashed line) the distal capillaries shut down and the fragile leading edge of the wound literally becomes anoxic.

candidates. Perhaps all contribute. As noted, stem cells contribute.

Matrix Deposition

The fibroblasts secrete the collagen and proteoglycans of the connective tissue matrix that weld wound edges together. They assume high-molecular-weight polymeric forms and become the physical basis of wound strength.

Collagen synthesis is not a constitutive property of fibroblasts but must be stimulated. The mechanisms that regulate the stimulation and synthesis of collagen are not actively clear, except that they are multifactorial and include both growth factors and metabolic inputs such as lactate. The collagen gene promoter has binding sites to corticoids, TGFβ, and retinoids, which control collagen gene expression, whereas other growth factors regulate glycosaminoglycans, tissue inhibitors of metalloproteinase (TIMP), and fibronectin synthesis. A more basic observation, however, is that mere accumulation of lactate in the extracellular environment directly stimulates transcription of collagen genes as well as posttranslational processing of collagen peptide. This mechanism, which is not pH-dependent, rests on the size of the intracellular pool of adenosine diphosphoribose (ADPR), a key regulatory substance that normally inhibits collagen mRNA synthesis and other vital steps that facilitate collagen export from fibroblasts. ADPR results from the nicotinamide moiety being removed from NAD^+. Accumulation of lactate converts NAD^+ to NADH. As a consequence, less NAD^+ is available to be converted to ADPR. When ADPR in the nucleus is depleted for any reason—as it is when the NAD^+ pool is diminished—this inhibitory control is released, and more collagen mRNA is formed. The cause of decreased NAD^+ can be hypoxia, accumulation of lactate, excessive conversion of NAD^+ to ADPR, and probably others.

The increase in collagen mRNA leads to an increased procollagen peptide. This, however, is not sufficient to increase collagen deposition because procollagen peptide cannot be transported from the cell to the extracellular space until, in a posttranslational step, some of its prolines are hydroxylated. In this reaction, performed by the dioxygenase prolyl hydroxylase, an oxygen atom derived from dissolved O_2 is inserted (as a hydroxyl group) into selected collagen prolines in the presence of ascorbic acid, iron, and α-ketoglutarate. The activity of this enzyme is normally suppressed by cytoplasmic ADPR. Thus, accumulation of lactate—or any other process that decreases the NAD^+ pool—leads to production of collagen mRNAs, increased collagen peptide synthesis, and (provided enough ascorbate and oxygen is present) increased posttranslational modification and secretion of collagen monomers into the extracellular space.

Another dioxygenase, lysyl hydroxylase, hydroxylates many of the procollagen lysines and sets the stage for later lysyl to lysyl link between collagen molecules and fibers, thereby endowing them with considerable strength. It, too, requires adequate amounts of ascorbate and oxygen. These oxygenase reactions (and therefore collagen deposition) proceed only as fast as the local concentration of oxygen (PaO_2) will allow. The rates are half-maximal at about 20 mm Hg and maximal at about 200 mm Hg. They can be "forced" to supernormal rates by tissue hyperoxia. Collagen deposition, wound strength, and angiogenesis rates can vary clinically as much as threefold as tissue PO_2 is elevated.

ANGIOGENESIS

Angiogenesis is necessary for all but the most minor wound healing. It becomes visible about 4 days after injury but begins 2 or 3 days earlier when new capillaries sprout out of preexisting venules and grow toward the injury in response to chemoattractants released by platelets and macrophages. In primarily closed wounds, sprouting vessels soon meet and connect with counterparts migrating from the other side of the wound, thus establishing blood flow across the wound. In unclosed wounds or those not well closed, the new capillaries fuse only with neighbors migrating in the same direction, and granulation tissue is formed instead (Figure 6–3).

The regulation of wound angiogenesis is inducible in unwounded tissue by the addition of chemoattractants to endothelial cells. Examples found in wounds include PDGF (homodimer BB), FGF, TNFα, TGFβ, and VEGF.

Maintenance of the NAD^+ pool severely inhibits the process. Thus, either unmet metabolic needs or the appearance of them lead through a growth factor mechanism involving VEGF to an anatomic response probably of general biologic significance.

Numerous growth factors and cytokines are said to stimulate angiogenesis, but animal experiments indicate that the dominant angiogenic stimulants in wounds are derived first from platelets in response to coagulation and then from macrophages in response to hypoxia or high lactate, fibrin, etc. Given the aerobic origin of wound lactate, it alone can stimulate VEGF in the presence of oxygen. Added oxygen then supports collagen deposition.

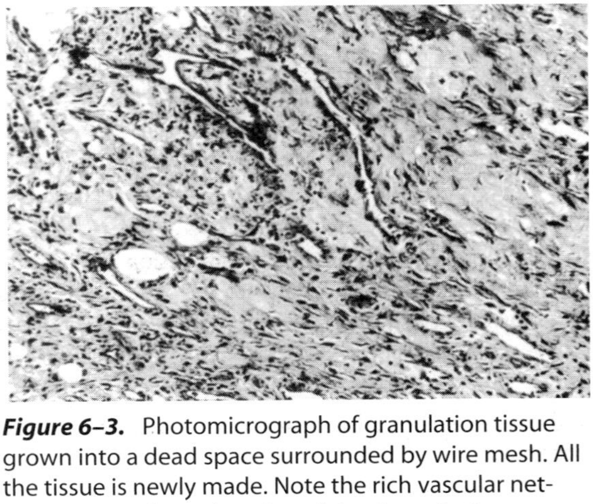

Figure 6–3. Photomicrograph of granulation tissue grown into a dead space surrounded by wire mesh. All the tissue is newly made. Note the rich vascular network, especially at the edge of the tissue in the upper left corner, where several open capillaries are leaking red cells into the wound.

EPITHELIALIZATION

Epithelial cells respond to many of the same stimuli as do fibroblasts and endothelial cells. A variety of growth factors regulate their replication. TGFβ, for instance, tends to keep epithelial cells from differentiating and thus may potentiate and perpetuate mitogenesis, though it is itself not a mitogen for these cells. TGFα and keratinocyte growth factor (KGF) are epithelial cell mitogens.

Mitoses appear in epithelium a few cells away from the wound edge. The new cells migrate over the cells at the edge and into the unhealed area and anchor to the first unepithelialized place that they encounter. The PaO_2 on the underside of the cell at the anchor point is likely to be low. Low PaO_2 stimulates squamous epithelial cells to produce TGFβ, presumably hindering terminal differentiation and favoring mitosis. This process repeats itself until the wound is closed.

Squamous epithelialization and differentiation proceed maximally when the local PaO_2 approaches about 700 mm Hg and when surface wounds are kept moist.

Contrary to classic thought, even short periods of drying can impair the process. Wounds should be kept moist. The exudate from acute, uninfected superficial wounds also contains growth factors and lactate and therefore recapitulates the growth environment found internally.

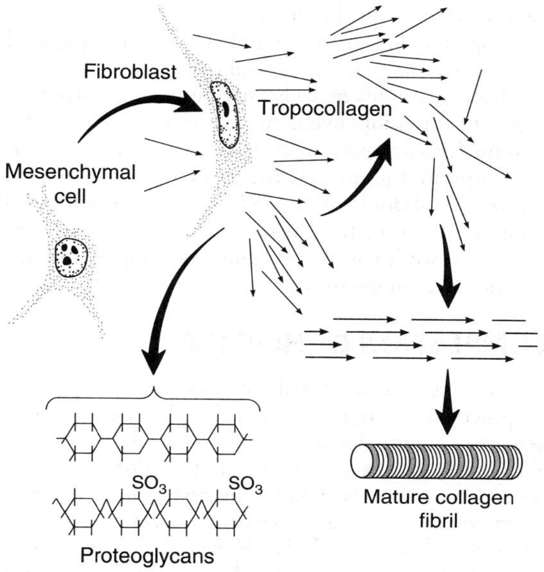

Figure 6–4. Schematic representation of collagen synthesis, deposition, and polymerization. The molecules polymerize with a "three-fourths stagger" overlap, which accounts for the cross banding visible on electron microscopy.

COLLAGEN FIBER MATURATION, LYSIS, & CONTRACTION

Replacement of an extracellular matrix is a complex process. First, fibroblasts replace the provisional fibrin extracellular matrix with collagen monomers. Extracellular enzymes, some of which are PaO_2-dependent, quickly polymerize these monomers but in a pattern that is much more random than normal, thus leaving young wounds weak and brittle. This brittleness is overcome when the first, hastily placed, matrix is replaced with a more mature one that contours larger, better organized, stronger, and more durable fibers (Figure 6–4).

Turnover and reorganization of new matrix is an important feature of healing, and fibroblasts and leukocytes secrete collagenases that ensure the lytic component. Turnover occurs rapidly at first and then more slowly. Even in simple wounds, increased turnover can be detected chemically for as long as 18 months. Healing is successful when a net excess of matrix is deposited despite concomitant lysis. Lysis, being destructive, is less dependent upon energy and nutrition. If synthesis is impaired, lysis weakens wounds. In some tissues (eg, colon), lysis unnecessarily weakens tissue structure, and inhibition of lysis with orally administrable agents leads to quicker gain of tensile strength. This is one of many features of healing that has not yet been clinically exploited.

During rapid turnover, wounds gain strength and durability but also are vulnerable to contraction and stretching. Fibroblasts exert the force for contraction. Fibroblasts attach to collagen and each other and pull the collagen network together when the cell membranes shorten as the fibroblasts migrate. The fibers are then fixed in the packed positions by a variety of cross-linking mechanisms. Both open and closed wounds tend to contract if not subjected to a superior counterforce. The phenomenon is best seen in surface wounds, which may close 90% or more by contraction alone in loose skin. For instance, the residual of a large open wound on the back of the neck may be only a small area of epithelialization. On the back, the buttock, or the neck, this is often a beneficial process, whereas in the face and about joints, the results may be disabling or disfiguring. This undesirable result is usually termed a contracture or a stricture. Skin grafts, especially thick ones, impede but do not totally stop the process. Dynamic splints, passive or active stretching, or insertion of flaps containing dermis and subdermis may be needed to counteract contraction. The force can be quite strong, but even severely contracted joints can usually be straightened with countertraction. Prevention of a stricture in a ureteric repair, for example, depends on ensuring that the opposing tissue edges are well perfused so that healing can proceed quickly to completion and contraction can stop. The longer the wound is open, the larger role that contraction plays in its final closure.

Healing wounds may also stretch during active turnover when tension overcomes contraction. This may account for the laxity of scars in ligaments of injured but unsplinted joints and the tendency for hernia formation in abdominal wounds of obese patients. If wounds are traumatized when passively stretched, contraction or weakness may continue for long periods and may become troublesome.

COMPLETION OF HEALING

Healing and growth of malignancies are strikingly similar processes. As opposed to their role in oncogenesis, however, growth factors in wound healing are more obedient to the basic controls, and healing stops at an appropriate point. Normally, the final stimuli to release of growth factors and cytokines seem to be local hypoxia and lactic acidosis. When these stimuli disappear as the new microcirculation matures, healing should stop. However, the reason for cessation of healing is debated.

Keloids, that is, local overgrowths of connective tissue, and hypertrophic scars, which occur particularly in pigmented skin, probably represent a loss of normal control over the healing process, but few facts are known. Hypertrophic scars are generally self-limited, are related to residual inflammation, and may regress after a year or so. The last areas of a burn to heal are the most often hypertrophic through traction, reinjury, and tension. Immune mechanisms may also contribute to scar. Prolonged inflammatory reactions potentiate scar. Therapy is another intralesional injection of anti-inflammatory steroids, dressing with thick layers of Silastic that raise the level temporarily and thereby increase the activity of lytic enzymes, or both.

ROLE OF TISSUE HYPOXIA

Impaired perfusion and oxygenation are the most frequent causes of healing failure. Oxygen is required for successful inflammation, bacterial-killing angiogenesis, epithelialization, and matrix (collagen) deposition. The critical oxygenases involved have Km values for oxygen of about 20 mm Hg and maximums of about 200 mm Hg, which means that their reaction rates are governed by PaO_2 and blood perfusion throughout the entire physiologic range. The PaO_2 of wound fluid in human incisional wounds is about 30–40 mm Hg, implying that these enzymes normally function just beyond half capacity. Wound PaO_2 is depressed by blood volume deficiency, catecholamine infusion, or cold. On the other hand, under ideal conditions, wound fluid PaO_2 can be raised above 100 mm Hg by improved perfusion and breathing of oxygen. Human healing is profoundly influenced by local blood supply, vasoconstriction, and all other factors that govern perfusion and blood oxygenation.

Cardiopulmonary diseases affect wound healing, but vasoconstriction due to sympathetic nervous system activity is the principal background clinical problem. Prevention or resolution of problems can be achieved by turning off sympathetic activity by correcting blood volume deficits, alleviating pain, and avoiding hypothermia. Wounds in highly vascularized tissues (eg, head, anus) heal rapidly and are remarkably resistant to infection.

IMPAIRED HEALING IN DISORDERS OF INFLAMMATION

The growth signals and lytic enzymes released by inflammatory cells are necessary for repair. Excessive and inadequate inflammatory responses can pose problems. Failure to heal is common in patients taking anti-inflammatory corticosteroids, immune suppressants, or cancer chemotherapeutic agents and whose inflammatory responses are blunted. Open wounds suffer more than primarily healing ones. The inhibiting effect of these agents diminishes as their effect on inflammation lessens. The clinical corollary is that administration is less harmful after the third day than on the first. Healing impaired by inadequate inflammation, especially that due to corticosteroids, can be accelerated by vitamin A systemically or locally. Experimentally, this appears to pertain to diabetics as well. In experiments, some of the growth factors have also had this effect. Both growth factors and vitamin A increase the number of inflammatory cells in the wound.

Inflammation may also be excessive. A major excess of inflammation (eg, in response to endotoxin) can excite inflammatory cells to produce cytolytic cytokines and excessive proteinases with the consequence of lysis of newly formed tissue. In gram-negative wound infections or septic shock, granulation tissue may not develop or it may even be lysed.

Massive injuries give rise to large inflammatory reactions, and cytokines from large but otherwise uncomplicated wounds can produce systemic symptoms. Extensive wounds can produce large amounts of lactate that must be reconverted to glucose in the liver—a process that contributes to the hypermetabolism of trauma. High levels of lactate also enhance oxidant production and loss of cell function.

Debridement of damaged tissue and early immobilization of fractures minimize the above effects. Stimulation of the reticuloendothelial system, major amounts of injured tissue, and failure to debride can produce the systemic inflammatory response syndrome (SIRS) even in the absence of infection.

EFFECT OF MALNUTRITION

Malnutrition impairs healing, since healing depends on cell replication, specific organ function (liver, heart, lungs), and matrix synthesis. Weight loss and protein depletion have been shown experimentally to be risk factors for poor healing. Nevertheless, healing may be normal in patients who have lost weight over a long period as opposed to a short but severe loss. Deficient healing is seen mainly in patients with acute malnutrition (ie, in the weeks just before or after an injury or operation). Even a few days of starvation measurably impairs healing, and an equally short period of repletion can reverse the deficit. Wound complications increase in severe malnutrition. A period of preoperative corrective nutrition is generally helpful for patients who have recently lost 10% or more of their body weight. This subject is covered in detail in Chapter 11.

HEALING OF SPECIALIZED TISSUES

Nerves

The brain heals largely through connective tissue scar formation in which glial and perivascular cells seem to differentiate into fibroblasts. When a peripheral nerve is severed, the distal nerve degenerates, leaving the axon sheaths to heal together by inosculation. The axon then regenerates from the nerve cell through the rejoined sheaths, advancing as much as 1 mm/d. Unfortunately, because individual neural sheaths have no means of seeking out their original distal ends, the axon sheaths reconnect randomly, and motor nerve axons may regenerate in vain into a sensory distal sheath and end organ. The functional result of neural regeneration, therefore, is more satisfactory in the purer peripheral nerves and in nerves rejoined by microscopic surgical techniques. Recent advances in stem cell and growth factor technology and the ischemic, hypoxic nature of wounds suggests that means may be devised to improve nerve regeneration. This is currently one of the forefronts of surgical research.

Intestine

The rate of repair varies from one part of the intestine to the other in proportion to vascularity. Anastomoses of the colon and esophagus are most precarious and most likely to leak, whereas leakage of stomach or small intestine anastomoses is rare. Intestinal anastomoses usually regain strength rapidly. By 1 week they resist bursting more strongly than the more normal surrounding intestine. However, the surrounding intestine also participates in the reaction to injury, loses a large portion of its collagen by lysis, and in adverse conditions may lose strength. For this reason, leakage is about as likely to occur a few millimeters from the anastomosis as it is in the anastomosis itself, especially at the site of excessively tight sutures or staples. Drugs such as fluorouracil limit lysis and in experimental conditions appear to prevent the early loss of strength in colonic wounds.

Any event that delays collagen synthesis or exaggerates collagen lysis is likely to increase the risk of perforation and leakage (Figure 6–5). The danger of leakage is greatest from the fourth to seventh days, when tensile strength normally would rise rapidly but is prevented from doing so by increased lysis or compromised collagen deposition. Local infection, which often occurs near esophageal and colonic anastomoses, promotes lysis and delays synthesis, thus increasing the likelihood of perforation.

Though the surgeon aims for primary healing in anastomoses, much of the healing actually occurs by second intention in both sutured and stapled anastomoses. Fine surgical technique is more likely to promote primary repair.

Adhesions are wrongly assumed to be an almost inevitable consequence of abdominal surgery. The most powerful stimuli to adhesions is ischemic tissue because ischemic tissues attract a new blood supply that takes the form of vascularized adhesions, abscesses, and foreign bodies. All attract nests of macrophages, which are activated to generate a fibrotic process.

Simple peritoneal defects are less likely to cause adhesions. When severe trauma, large defects, infection, ischemia, or foreign bodies are added, the process becomes more intense. Trauma and inflammation excite plasma leaks and deposition of fibrin. If allowed to remain, the fibrin increases the volume of ischemic tissue. Peritoneum normally produces plasminogen activator, which quickly leads to fibrin lysis. Exogenous plasminogen activator has decreased the occurrence of adhesions in experimental circumstances, but side effects discourage its clinical use.

Attempts to prevent adhesions by suturing peritoneal defects usually worsen the problem by causing local

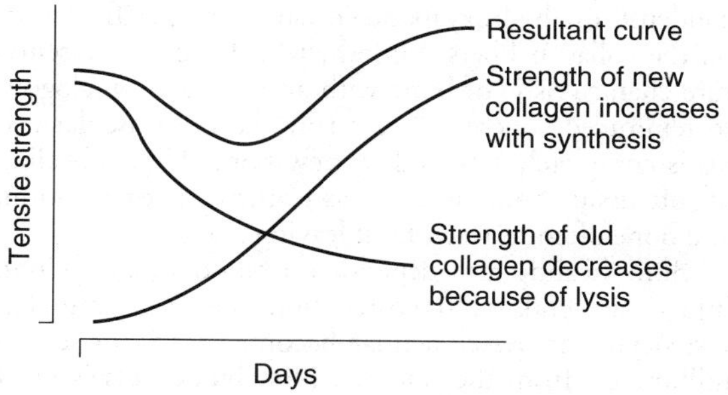

Figure 6–5. Tensile strength is the resultant between the strength of old collagen as affected by lysis and new collagen as affected by synthesis and lysis.

ischemia and suture granulomas. Starch powder used in most surgical gloves as a lubricant was a great improvement over talc, but severe peritoneal (as well as pericardial, pleural, and meningeal) inflammatory reactions due to starch and leading to adhesions are well documented. Evidence indicates that lymphocytes participate in healing more so in colon wounds than in wounds of other tissues. Immunologic contribution is proportionately greater.

Bone

Bone healing is controlled by many of the same mechanisms that control soft tissue healing. It, too, occurs in three morphologic stages: an inflammatory stage, a reparative stage, and a remodeling stage. The duration of each stage varies depending on the location and nature of the fracture.

Injury (fracture) leads to hematoma formation from the damaged blood vessels of the periosteum, endosteum, and surrounding tissues. Within hours, an inflammatory infiltrate of neutrophils and macrophages is recruited into the hematoma as in soft tissue injuries. Monocytes and granulocytes debride and digest necrotic tissue and debris, including bone, on the fracture surface. This process continues for days to weeks depending on the amount of necrotic tissue.

During the reparative stage, the hematoma is gradually replaced by specialized granulation tissue that has the power to form bone. This tissue, known as **callus,** develops from both sides of the fracture and is composed of fibroblasts, endothelial cells, and bone-forming cells (chondroblasts, osteoblasts). The extent to which callus forms from the medulla, the periosteum, or cortical bone depends upon the site of fracture, the degree of immobilization, and the type of bone injured. As macrophages (osteoclasts) phagocytose the hematoma and injured tissue, fibroblasts (osteocytes) deposit a collagenous matrix, and chondroblasts deposit proteoglycans in a process called enchondral bone formation. This step, prominent in some bones, is then converted to bone as osteoblasts condense on hydroxyapatite crystals on specific points on the collagen fibers. Endothelial cells form a vasculature characteristic of bone with an end result analogous to reinforced concrete. Eventually the fibrovascular callus is completely replaced by new bone. Unlike healing of soft tissue, bone healing has features of regeneration, and bone often heals without leaving a scar.

Bone healing also depends on blood supply. Upon injury, the ends of fractured bone become avascular. Osteocyte and vessel lacunae become vacant for several millimeters from the fracture. New blood vessels must sprout from preexisting ones and migrate into the area of injury. As new blood vessels cross the bone ends, they are preceded by osteoclasts just as macrophages precede them in soft tissue repair. In bone, this unit is called the "cutting cone" because it literally bores its way through bone in the process of connecting with other vessels. Excessive movement of the bone ends during this revascularization stage will break the delicate new vessels and delay healing.

Osteomyelitis originates most often in ischemic bone fragments. Hyperoxygenation hastens fracture healing and aids in the cure (and potentially the prevention) of osteomyelitis. Acute or chronic hypoxia slows bone repair. Applications of electrical currents maintain its progress.

Once the fracture has been bridged, the new bone remodels in response to the mechanical stresses upon it, with restoration to normal or near-normal strength. During this process, as in soft tissue, preexisting bone and its vascular network are simultaneously removed and replaced. Increased bone turnover may be detected as long as 6–9 years after injury. Although remodeling is exceptionally efficient, it cannot correct deformities of angulation or rotation in misaligned fractures. Careful fracture reduction is still useful.

Fibroblasts, chondroblasts, and osteoblasts in healing fractures are derived from surrounding primitive mesenchyme. The origin of the mesenchyme is less clear. It seems to arise from muscle, fascia, periosteum, endothelium, marrow, even from circulating stem cells, as well as directly from fibrous tissue. The differentiation of these mesenchymal cells into bone-forming cells appears to be governed by specific growth factors such as bone morphogenetic protein (BMP), TGFβ, IGF-1, GM-CSF, and PDGF, all of which stimulate proliferation and induce the differentiation of osteoblasts in cell culture. BMP (which belongs to the TGFβ supergene family) appears to be the most specific for bone and is found in large quantity in bone matrix. BMP induces ectopic bone formation in the absence of preexisting bone and induces cartilage formation in vivo.

Bone repair may occur through primary or secondary intention. Primary repair can occur only when the fracture is stable and aligned and its surfaces closely apposed. This is the goal of rigid plate fixation of fractures. When these conditions are met, capillaries can grow across the fracture and rapidly reestablish a vascular supply. Little or no callus forms. Secondary repair with callus formation is more common.

Bone repair can be manipulated. Electrical stimulation, growth factors, and distraction osteogenesis are three promising new tools for this purpose. Electrical currents applied directly (through implanted electrodes) or induced by external alternating electromagnetic fields accelerate repair by inducing new bone formation in much the same way as small piezoelectric currents produced by mechanical deformation of intact bone controls remodeling along lines of stress. The technique of electrical stimulation has been used successfully to treat nonunion of bone (where new bone formation between bone ends fails, often requiring long periods of bed rest). BMP-impregnated implants have accelerated bone healing in animals and have been used with encouraging results to treat large bony defects and nonunions.

The **Ilizarov technique,** linear distraction osteogenesis, can lengthen bones, stimulate bone growth across a defect, or correct defects of angulation. The Ilizarov device is an external fixator attached to the bones through metal pins or wires. A surgical break is created and then slowly pulled apart (1 mm/d) or slowly reangulated. The vascular supply and subsequent new bone formation migrate along with the moving segment of bone.

SUTURES

The ideal suture material would be flexible, strong, easily tied, and securely knotted. It would excite little tissue reaction and would not serve as a nidus for infection.

Stainless steel wire is inert and maintains strength for a long time. It is difficult to tie and may have to be removed late postoperatively because of pain. It does not harbor bacteria, and it can be left in granulating wounds, when necessary, and will be covered by granulation tissue without causing abscesses. However, sinuses due to motion are fairly common.

Silk is an animal protein but is relatively inert in human tissue. It is commonly used because of its favorable handling characteristics. It loses strength over long periods and is unsuitable for suturing arteries to plastic grafts or for insertion of prosthetic cardiac valves. Silk sutures are multifilament and provide a potential haven for bacteria. Occasionally, silk sutures form a focus for small abscesses that migrate and "spit" through the skin, forming small sinuses that will not heal until the suture is removed.

Catgut (made from the submucosa of bovine intestine) will eventually resorb, but the resorption time is highly variable. It excites considerable inflammatory reaction and tends to potentiate infections. Catgut also loses strength rapidly and unpredictably in the intestine and in infected wounds as a consequence of acid and enzyme hydrolysis. There is little need for catgut suture in modern surgery, though a considerable amount is still used.

Synthetic nonabsorbable sutures are generally inert and retain strength (do not fracture) longer than wire. However, their handling characteristics are not as good as those of silk, and they must usually be knotted at least four times, resulting in large amounts of retained foreign body. Multifilament plastic sutures are just as apt to become infected and migrate to the surface as silk sutures. Monofilament plastic, like wire, will not harbor bacteria. Nylon monofilament is extremely nonreactive, but it is difficult to tie. Monofilament polypropylene is intermediate in these properties. Plastic sutures are required for cardiovascular work because they are not absorbed. Vascular anastomoses to prosthetic vascular grafts rely indefinitely on the strength of sutures; therefore, use of absorbable sutures may lead to aneurysm formation. Even monofilament sutures will "spit." However, this disadvantage is generally confined to sizes of 00 and larger.

Synthetic absorbable sutures are strong, have predictable rates of loss of tensile strength, incite a minimal inflammatory reaction, and have special usefulness in gastrointestinal, urologic, and gynecologic surgery. Compared with catgut, polyglycolic acid and polyglactin retain tensile strength longer in gastrointestinal anastomoses. Polydioxanone sulfate and polyglycolate are monofilament and lose about half their strength in 50 days, thus solving the problem of premature breakage in fascial closures. Poliglecaprone 25 is a newer monofilament synthetic suture with faster reabsorption, retaining 50% tensile strength at 7 days, and 0% at 21 days. This suture is suitable for soft tissue approximation but is not intended for fascial closure.

Tapes are the skin closure of choice for clean or contaminated wounds. They minimize the probability of infection by not connecting the skin surface to the wound dead space. They cannot be used on actively bleeding wounds or wounds with complex surfaces, such as those in the perineum.

Staples, whether for internal use or skin closure, are mainly steel-tantalum alloys that incite a minimal tissue reaction. The technique of staple placement is different from that of sutures, but the same basic rules pertain. There are no real differences in the healing that follows suture or stapled closures. Stapling devices tend to minimize errors in technique, but at the same time they do not offer a feel for tissue and have limited ability to accommodate to exceptional circumstances. Staples are preferable to sutures for skin closure, since they do not provide a conduit for contaminating organisms. Staples are not, however, preferable to skin tapes.

IMPLANTABLE MATERIALS

Although prosthetic materials are constantly being improved, none are ideal in regard to tissue compatibility, permanent fixation, and resistance to infection. Two principles are paramount: biocompatibility and a fabric that is incorporated into tissue. Biocompatibility is the foremost consideration. Both specific and nonspecific immune mechanisms are involved in the inflammatory reaction to foreign materials. Highly incompatible materials, such as wood splinters, are rejected immediately with an acute inflammatory process that includes massive local release of proteolytic enzymes. Consequently, the foreign body is never incorporated and lies loosely in a fibrous pocket. Mechanical irritation may induce a similar reaction, which accounts for the occasional spontaneous rejection of large (usually larger than 00), stiff suture materials from soft tissue sites. In less severe incompatibility, rejection is not so vigorous and proteolysis not so prominent. Mononuclear cells and lymphocytes—the major components of wound inflammatory tissue—direct a response that creates a fibrous capsule which may be acceptable in a joint replacement but it may distort a breast reconstruction severely.

Most implants must become anchored to adjacent normal tissues by allowing ingrowth of fibrous tissue or bone. This requires biocompatibility and interstices large enough to incite ingrowth just as in a wound and to allow pedicles of vascularized tissue to enter and join similar units. In bone this imparts stability. In vascular grafts, the invading tissue supports neointima formation, which retards mural thrombosis and distal embolization. Soft tissue will grow into pores larger than about 50 μm in diameter and even faster into larger ones. Of the vascular prostheses, woven Dacron is best for tissue incorporation. In bone, sintered, porous metallic surfaces are best. Large-screen polypropylene mesh can be used to support the abdominal wall or chest even in the presence of infection and is usually well incorporated into the granulation tissue that penetrates the mesh. Microporous polytetrafluoroethylene (Teflon) sheets are often not well incorporated and are not suitable for use in infected tissues.

Unfortunately, when the mechanical properties of the implant do not match those of the host tissue, shear forces may overcome delicate biologic unions, with loosening of anchoring sites, especially with orthopedic prostheses.

The implantation space remains vulnerable to infection for years and is a particular problem in implants that cross the body surface. Mesh cuffs around vascular access devices that incite incorporation have successfully forestalled infection for months, but infections that arise from bacteria entering the body along "permanently" implanted foreign bodies, which traverse the skin surface, remain an unsolved problem.

Plastic implants are often chosen for texture and flexibility. Silastic materials are highly compatible, but fixation and material fatigue are problems. Cosmetic implants—particularly silicone breast implants—have a low but troublesome incidence of deforming fibrotic capsule formation. In addition to idiosyncratic healing responses, there is also the problem of toxic responses to trace components such as plasticizers and hardeners. Potential complications include cancers if materials such as asbestos are present even in small amounts. The case for systemic complications such as connective tissue diseases from Silastic implants has not been proved.

DECUBITUS & OTHER CHRONIC ULCERS

Decubitus Ulcers

Decubitus ulcers can be disastrous complications of immobilization. They result from prolonged pressure that robs tissue of its blood supply, irritative or contaminated injections, and prolonged contact with moisture, urine, and feces. Most patients who develop decubitus ulcers are also poorly nourished. Pressure ulcers are common in paraplegics, immobile elderly patients after orthopedic procedures, and drug addicts who take overdoses and lie immobile for hours. The ulcers vary in depth and often extend from skin to a bony pressure point such as the greater trochanter, the sacrum, or the head.

Most decubitus ulcers are preventable. Hospital-acquired ulcers are nearly always the result of inadequate nursing care, inappropriate positioning on operating tables, and ill-fitting casts or other orthopedic appliances.

Treatment is difficult and usually prolonged. The first important step is to incise and drain any infected spaces or necrotic tissue. Dead tissue is debrided until the exposed surfaces are viable. Many ulcers will then heal spontaneously. However, deep ulcers may require surgical closure, sometimes with removal of underlying bone. The defect may require closure by judicious movement of thick, well-vascularized tissue into the affected area. Musculocutaneous flaps are the treatment of choice when chronic infection and significant tissue loss are combined. However, recurrence is common because the flaps are usually insensate.

Chronic Wounds

Chronically unhealed wounds, especially on the lower extremity, are common in the setting of vascular, immunologic, and neurologic disease. Venous ulcers, largely of the lower leg, reflect poor perfusion and perivascular leakage of plasma into tissue. This is the result of venous hypertension produced by incompetent venous valves. Most venous ulcers will heal if the venous congestion and edema are relieved by bed rest, compression stockings, or surgical procedures that eliminate incompetent feeding vessels.

Arterial or ischemic ulcers, which tend to occur on the lateral ankle or foot, are best treated by revascularization. Hyperbaric oxygen, which provides a temporary source of enhanced oxygenation that stimulates angiogenesis, is an effective though expensive alternative when revascularization is not possible. Useful information can be obtained by transcutaneous oximetry.

Tissues with a low PaO_2 will not heal spontaneously. However, if oxygen tension can be raised into a relatively normal range by oxygen administration even intermittently, the lesion will probably respond to oxygen therapy.

Sensory loss, especially of the feet, leads to ulceration. Bony deformities due to fractures, the so-called Charcot deformity, are difficult problems. Ulcers in patients with diabetes mellitus may have two causes. Patients with neuropathic ulcers usually have good circulation, and their lesions will heal if protected from trauma by bed rest, special shoes, or splints. Recurrences are common, however. Diabetics with ischemic disease, whether they have neuropathy or not, are at risk for gangrene, and they frequently require amputation when revascularization is not possible. Insulin dressings have been advocated. More recently, intermittent warming has been helpful.

In pyoderma gangrenosum, granulomatous inflammation with or without arteritis kills skin and subcutaneous skin, possibly by a mechanism involving excess cytokine release. These ulcers are associated with inflammatory bowel disease and certain types of arthritis and chondritis. Corticosteroids or other anti-inflammatory drugs are helpful. However, anti-inflammatory corticosteroids can also contribute to poor healing by inhibiting cytokine release. In these cases, topical or systemic vitamin A restores the inflammatory mechanism and may induce healing of the lesions. Distinguishing between these possibilities in patients with inflammatory bowel disease may be difficult.

Infection may contribute to the lack of healing of chronic ulcers or may be a complication. The bacteria are usually mixed and staphylococci are commonly present. Antibiotics should be part of initial therapy in most cases. However, antibiotics are a secondary concern to enhanced vulnerability.

The first principle in managing chronic wounds is to diagnose and treat any underlying circulatory disease. The second principle is never to allow open wounds to dry (ie, use moist dressings). Moist dressings may also relieve pain. A third principle is to control any infection with systemic antibiotics. Topical barriers to infection are useful but not always necessary. A fourth principle is to recognize that chronically scarred tissue is usually poorly perfused. Debridement of unhealthy tissue, often followed by skin grafting, may be required for healing. A fifth principle is to reduce autonomic vasoconstriction by means of warmth, moisture, pain relief, or pharmacologic vasodilation medications.

A number of growth factors have been shown to accelerate healing of acute wounds in animals. They include FGFs, TGFβ, IGF-1, PDGF, and EGF, and the list is growing. However, in the setting of chronic human wounds, with the perfusion problems noted above, "proof" of efficacy has been difficult to develop, and no clear-cut advantage to any formulation has yet been convincingly demonstrated. The one exception is the recent randomized, prospective, double-blind, placebo-controlled, multicenter trial by the Diabetic Ulcer Study Group, which demonstrated that daily topical application of recombinant human PDGF-BB homodimer moderately accelerates healing and results in more wounds that heal completely. The effect, however, is small.

SURGICAL TECHNIQUE

The most important means of achieving optimal healing after operation is good surgical technique. Many cases of healing failure are due to technical errors. Tissue should be protected from drying and contamination. The surgeon should use fine instruments; should perform clean, sharp dissection; and should make minimal, skillful use of electrocautery, ligatures, and sutures. All of these precautions contribute to the most important goal of surgical technique—gentle handling of tissue. Even the best ligature or suture is a foreign body that may strangulate tissue if tied tightly. The skillful operator who uses sutures minimally and gently will be rewarded with the best results. Good hemostasis is a laudable objective, but excessive sponging, electrocautery, and tying of small vessels are traumatic and invite infection.

Wound Closure

As with many surgical techniques, the exact method of wound closure may be less important than how well it is performed. The tearing strength of sutures in fascia is no greater than 3–4 kg. There is little reason for use of sutures of greater strength than this. Excessively tight closure strangulates tissue and leads to hernia formation and infection.

If surgeons could foresee the future, dehiscence (undesired spontaneous separation of wound edges) would be none, since techniques to prevent it are well known. The surgeon can choose the techniques to meet the needs and risks of the individual wound (Figures 6–6 and 6–7). The most common technical causes of dehiscence are infection and excessively tight sutures.

The ideal closure for small wounds in healthy patients is with fine interrupted sutures placed loosely and conveniently close to the wound edge. In abdominal wounds, the peritoneum need not be sutured, but posterior and anterior fasciae are sutured with nonabsorbable or slowly absorbable sutures.

Unfortunately, surgeons often must operate on patients who have impaired wound healing. In these cases, closures must be stronger. A more secure closure begins with a running or mattress absorbable suture in

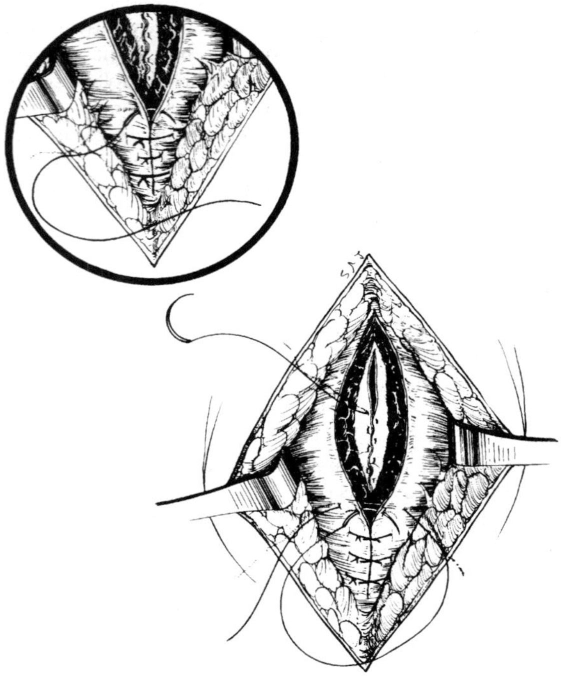

Figure 6–6. Closure of peritoneum with continuous sutures. Fascia closure with figure-of-eight sutures (top) and simple interrupted sutures (bottom) is illustrated. "Running" closures are also useful, and the suture "bites" should be similar to those illustrated, 1 and 1.5 cm apart and 1–1.5 cm apart.

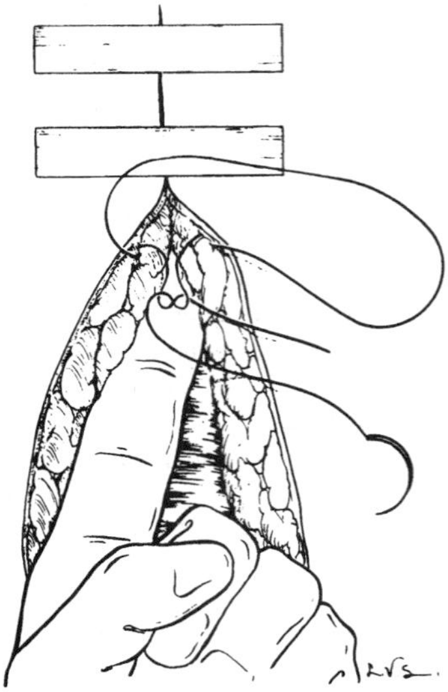

Figure 6–7. Skin closure with interrupted subdermal sutures and Steri-Strips.

the posterior sheath, joint capsule, or submucosa. The closure is continued with simple buried retention sutures through the fascia in which the farthest point of penetration is at least 1 cm from the wound edge. When the tension is placed this far back, the fascial fibers closer to the wound that become weakened by postinjury collagen lysis are not expected to provide critical support. The lytic effect extends for about 5 mm to each side of the wound edge. The skin is preferably closed with adhesive strips unless bleeding from the wound or an uneven surface makes adherence of the strips precarious, in which case staples are the next choice. With this fascial closure, the skin can easily be left open for delayed primary or secondary closure. Subcutaneous tissues rarely need to be sutured closed.

In all closures, sutures should be placed as far apart as possible consistent with approximation of tissue. Sutures placed too tightly and too close together obstruct blood supply to the wound. In most cases of dehiscence, suture material cuts through tissue. Broken or untied sutures are found less often.

It is useful to assess wound risk in advance, so that the proper choice of closure can be made easily (Table 6–1).

Delayed primary closure is a technique by which the subcutaneous portion of the wound is left open for 4–5 days and then closed with skin tapes. During the delay period, angiogenesis and healing start, and bacteria are cleared from the wound. The success of this method depends on the ability of the surgeon to detect minor signs of infection. Merely leaving the wound open for 4 days does not guarantee that it will not become infected. Some wounds (eg, fibrin-covered or inflamed wounds) should not be closed but should be left open for secondary closure.

POSTOPERATIVE CARE

The appearance of delayed wound infection—weeks to years after operation—emphasizes that all wounds are contaminated and that the line between apparent infection and apparent normal repair is a fine one. A minor setback such as a period of cardiac failure or of malnutrition will often allow infection to become established. Most frequently, however, poor tissue perfusion and oxygenation of the wound during the postoperative period weaken host resistance. Regulation of perfusion is due—more than anything—to sympathetic nervous activity. The instigators of vasoconstriction are cold, pain, hypovolemia, fear, beta-blockers, cigarette smoking, and hypoxemia. Recent tests show that special efforts to remove or limit these

Table 6–1. Controllable factors affecting healing.

Factors that decrease collagen synthesis
Smoking
Starvation (protein depletion)
Corticosteroids
Infection[1]
Hypoxemia and hypovolemia
Radiation injury
Trauma, including the operation itself
Uremia
Diabetes mellitus
Drugs: dactinomycin, fluorouracil, methotrexate, others
Advanced age
Operative factors
Tissue injury
Poor blood supply
Poor apposition of surrounding tissues (pelvic anastomosis, unreduced fracture, unclosed dead space)
Factors that increase collagen synthesis
Starvation
Severe trauma
Inflammation
Infection
Steroids

[1]Some infections may in time cause excess collagen deposition.

factors reduce the wound infection rate by more than half. Maintenance of normothermia and blood volume is particularly important. Appropriate assurance that peripheral perfusion is adequate is best obtained from peripheral tissues rather than urine output, central venous pressure, or wedge pressure—none of which correlate with peripheral wound tissue oxygenation. What does correlate with tissue oxygenation is the capillary refill time on the forehead or patella, which should be less than 2 seconds and 5 seconds, respectively; or true thirst and eye globe turgor (which should match the observer's). Collagen deposition is increased also by the addition of oxygen breathing (nasal prongs or light mask) but only in well-perfused patients. Unfortunately, there are as yet no convenient clinical means of measuring wound PaO_2 that can be done routinely.

Postoperative care of the wound also involves cleanliness, protection from trauma, and maximal support of the patient. Even closed wounds can be infected by surface contamination, particularly within the first 2–3 days. Bacteria gain entrance most easily through suture tracts. If a wound is likely to be traumatized or contaminated, it should be protected during this time. Such protection may require special dressings such as occlusive sprays or repeated cleansings as well as dressings.

Some mechanical stress enhances healing. Even fracture callus formation is greater if slight motion is allowed. Patients should move and stress their wounds a little. Early ambulation and return to normal activity are, in general, good for repair.

The ideal care of the wound begins in the preoperative period and ends only months later. The patient must be prepared so that optimal conditions exist when the wound is made. Surgical technique must be clean, gentle, and skillful. Postoperatively, wound care includes maintenance of nutrition, blood volume, and oxygenation. Although wound healing is in many ways a local phenomenon, ideal care of the wound is essentially ideal care of the patient.

DRAINS

Although localized collections in the chest and abdominal cavities often require drainage, wounds rarely do. Routine use of drains is more harmful than helpful. If drainage of reapproximated wounds that have been opened due to infection is needed, it should be done with vacuum-assisted techniques.

Allen DB et al: Wound hypoxia and acidosis limit neutrophil bacterial killing mechanisms. Arch Surg 1997;132:991.

Cho M et al: Hydrogen peroxide stimulates macrophage vascular endothelial growth factor release. Am J Physiol Heart Circ Physiol 2001;280:H2357.

Constant JS et al: Lactate elicits vascular endothelial growth factor from macrophages: a possible alternative to hypoxia. Wound Repair Regen 2000;8:353.

Demling RH et al: Micronutrients in critical illness. Crit Care Clin 1995;11:651.

Feng JJ et al: Angiogenesis in wound healing. J Surg Pathol 1998;3:1.

Greif R et al: Supplemental perioperative oxygen to reduce the incidence of surgical wound infection. N Engl J Med 2000;342:161.

Hartmann M et al: Effect of tissue perfusion and oxygenation on accumulation of collagen in healing wounds: randomized study in patients after major abdominal operations. Eur J Surg 1992;158:521.

Hopf H et al: Subcutaneous perfusion and oxygen during acute severe isovolemic hemodilution in healthy volunteers. Arch Surg 2000;135:1443.

Hopf HW et al: Wound tissue oxygen tension predicts the risk of wound infection in surgical patients. Arch Surg 1997;132:997.

Hunt TK et al: Wound healing and wound infection: what surgeons and anesthesiologists can do. Surg Clin North Am 1997;77:587.

Israelsson LA et al: Closure of midline laparotomy incisions with polydioxanone and nylon: the importance of suture technique. Br J Surg 1994;81:1606.

Rovee DT et al: *The Epidermis in Wound Healing.* CRC Press, 2004.

Sahota PS et al: Approaches to improve angiogenesis in tissue engineered skin. Wound Repair Regen 2004;12:635.

Schaffer M et al: Neuropeptides: mediators of inflammation and tissue repair? Arch Surg 1998;133:1107.

Steed DL: Clinical evaluation of recombinant human platelet-derived growth factor for the treatment of lower extremity diabetic ulcers. Diabetic Ulcer Study Group. J Vasc Surg 1995; 21:71.

Unemori EN et al: Relaxin induces vascular endothelial growth factor expression and angiogenesis selectively at wound sites. Wound Repair Regen 2000;8:361.

Wackenfors A et al: Effects of vacuum-assisted closure therapy on inguinal wound edge microvascular blood flow. Wound Repair Regen 2004;12:600.

Wicke C et al: Effects of steroids and retinoids on wound healing. Arch Surg 2000;135:1256.

Power Sources in Surgery

7

K. Barrett Deatrick, MD, & Gerard M. Doherty, MD

Modern surgery has been redefined by the presence of powered instruments, technological tools that in many ways have revolutionized the delicacy, precision, and accuracy of the various operations performed. Yet many people who use these implements every day have very little understanding of exactly how these tools work. A complete treatise on electromagnetic generation of heat and the physics of current generation are beyond the scope of this chapter (and are already available from other authors). This chapter will focus on some fundamental rules that govern the behavior of electrical currents and some relatively straightforward principles which, when understood, help guide the use of these technologies.

ELECTROSURGERY

Principles of Electricity

An electrical **circuit** is any pathway that allows the uninterrupted flow of electrons. Electrical **current** is the flow of electricity (the number of electrons) in a given circuit over a constant period of time and is measured in **amperes** (A). Current can be supplied either as direct current (DC) with constant positive and negative terminals or as alternating current (AC) with constantly reversing poles. The electromotive force, or **voltage**, is a measurement of the force that propels the current of electrons and is related to the difference in potential energy between two terminals. The **resistance** is the tendency of any component of a circuit to resist the flow of electrons; it applies to direct current (DC) circuits. The equivalent of this tendency in an alternating current (AC) circuit is known as **impedance**.

Any electromagnetic wave, from household electricity to radio broadcasts to visible light, can be described by three components: speed, frequency, and wavelength. Since all electromagnetic waves travel at the speed of light, which is a constant, these waves depend on the relationship between their frequency and wavelength. These three characteristics are defined by the equation

$$c = f\lambda$$

(where c is the speed of light, 2.998×10^8 m/s, and frequency [f] and wavelength [λ] are inversely related; that is, as frequency increases, wavelength decreases, and vice versa). The ability to pass high-frequency current through the human body without causing excess damage makes electrosurgery possible.

Electrocautery

Electrosurgery is often incorrectly termed electrocautery, which is a separate technique. **Electrocautery** is a closed-circuit DC device in which current is passed through an exposed wire offering resistance to the current (Figure 7–1). The resistance causes some of the electrical energy to be dissipated as heat, increasing the temperature of the wire, which then heats tissue. In true electrocautery, *no current passes through the patient.* This technique is primarily applied for microsurgery, such as ophthalmologic procedures, where a very small amount of heating will produce the desired effect, or where more heat or current may be dangerous.

1. Principles of Electrosurgery

True electrosurgery, colloquially referred to as the "Bovie" (following its inventor, William T. Bovie, engineer and collaborator of Harvey Cushing), is perhaps the most ubiquitous power source in surgery. Although the principle of using heat to cauterize bleeding wounds dates back to the third millennium BC, the directed use of electrical current to produce these effects is a far more recent development. Other scientists and engineers made significant contributions to the development of this new technology, but Bovie refined the electrical generator and made it practical and applicable to everyday surgery. At the most fundamental level, electrosurgery uses high-frequency (radiofrequency) electromagnetic waves to produce a localized heating of tissues, leading to localized tissue destruction. The effect produced (cutting vs. coagulation) depends on how this energy is supplied.

A useful exercise to understand the way electrosurgery works is to follow the flow of current from the power outlet as it travels through the patient and returns to the wall outlet. By convention, charge is depicted as moving from positive (cathode) to negative (anode) even though the particles that are actually moving are of course electrons, which have a negative charge. The following descriptions are based on that convention, following the flow of positive charge.

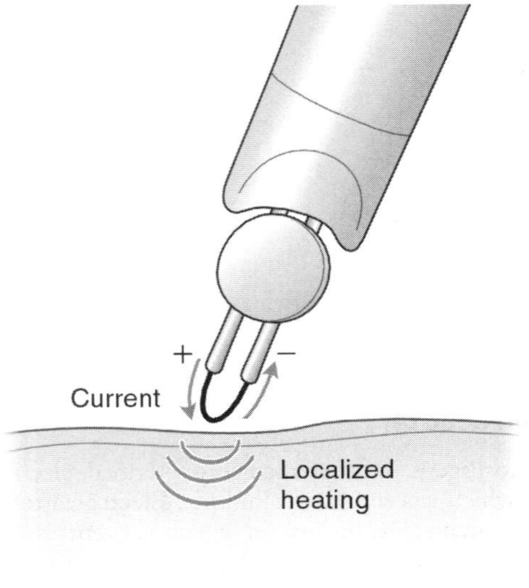

Figure 7–1. In electrocautery, current passes through a wire loop and heats it. This heat cauterizes tissue. No current passes through the patient.

Monopolar Circuits

The electrosurgical circuit consists of four primary parts: the electrosurgical generator, the active electrode, the patient, and the return electrode. Current flows from the electrosurgical generator after it is modulated to a high-frequency, short-wavelength current, and where multiple waveforms can be produced. (The importance of the waveform will be discussed in the following sections.) The current flows from the machine, through the handpiece, out the tip of the device, to the patient. If the patient were not connected in some way either to a negative terminal or to ground, no current would flow, as there would be no way to complete the circuit, hence nowhere for the charge to go. However, the patient is always connected to the electrosurgical generator by a return electrode. This allows the charge delivered by the electrosurgical probe to pass through the patient, exerting its effect and back to the generator, completing the circuit. In reality, the term "monopolar" circuit is incorrect, as there are in fact two poles (the active and return electrodes). However, monopolar electrosurgery (Figure 7–2A) is distinguished from bipolar electrosurgery, in which both electrodes are under the surgeon's direct control.

Bipolar Circuits

The essential components of the bipolar electrosurgical circuit are the same as those in the monopolar circuit; however, in this system, the active and return electrodes are in the same surgical instrument. In this technique, high-frequency current is passed through the active electrode and through the patient to heat and disrupt tissue. In this arrangement, however, the return electrode is included in the handpiece, as the opposite pole of the active electrode. This allows heating of only a discrete amount of tissue (Figure 7–2B).

The Electromagnetic Spectrum & Tissue Effects

The current that powers the electrosurgical generator is supplied at a frequency of 60 Hz. This type of electromagnetic energy can indeed cause very strong (potentially lethal) neuromuscular stimulation, making it unsuitable for use in its pure form. Muscle and nerve stimulation, however, ceases at around 100,000 cycles per second (100 kHz). Current with a frequency above this threshold can be delivered safely, without the risk of electrocution. The outputs of electrosurgical generators deliver current with a frequency greater than 200,000 cycles per second (200 kHz). Current at this frequency is known as **radiofrequency** (RF); it is in the same portion of the spectrum as some radio transmitters. This level of RF, released from a radio antenna, is capable of producing serious RF burns if the proper precautions are not taken.

Applying electrosurgical current to a patient produces localized tissue destruction via intense heat production, yet, barring a mishap, no other lesions are produced during application of this technique. The reason that the effect is exerted only at the site where the surgeon is operating—and not at the site of the return electrode—is that the surface area by which the charge is delivered is much smaller than that to which it returns. Thus, there is a far greater **density of charge** at the site of the handpiece ("active" electrode) contact than there is at the site of return. If there is another connection between the patient and ground, and if it also comprises a relatively small surface area, the patient could be in danger of suffering an electrosurgical burn, if this pathway offers less resistance to the flow of current. Similarly, if the return electrode were to be damaged, or if contact was not maintained, a burn could occur in this area. The possibility of a burn at the site of the return electrode is eliminated in most modern machines by the presence of a monitoring system. The monitoring system assesses the completeness of contact (by maintaining a smaller, secondary circuit) and automatically disables power if full contact of the pad (such as could be caused by tripping over a wire and tearing the return pad) is lost.

2. Types of Electrosurgery

All types of electrosurgery exert their effects via the localized production of heat and the resultant effects on the

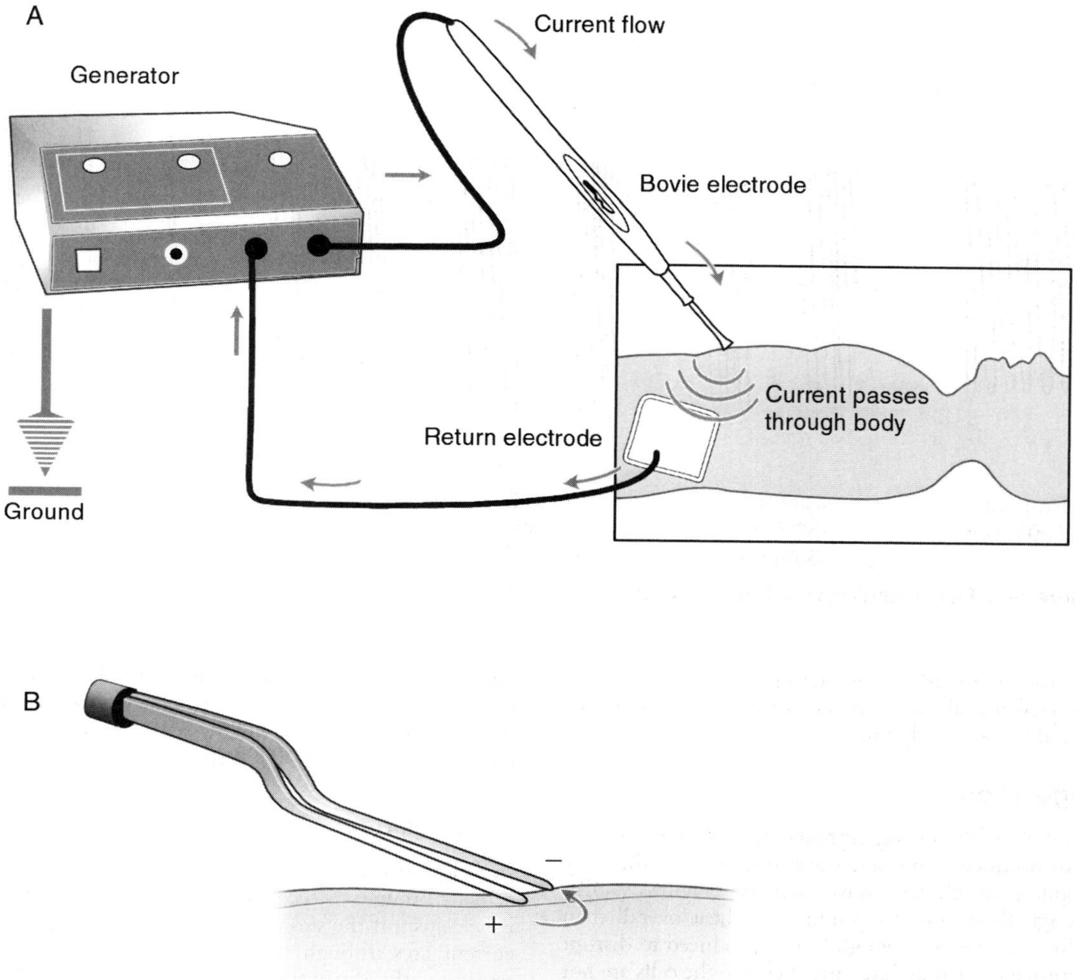

Figure 7–2. **A:** In monopolar electrosurgery, current from an electrosurgical generator passes from an active electrode (the "Bovie" tip) through the patient to a return electrode of greater area. **B:** In bipolar electrosurgery, the active and return electrodes are in the handpiece, and current only flows through the surgical site.

tissues subjected to it. Therefore, the different effects produced by electrosurgical instruments are created by altering the manner in which this heat is produced and delivered. Adjusting this heat is made possible by altering the wave pattern by which the current is delivered.

Cutting

Cutting depends on the production of a continuous sine wave of current (Figure 7–3A). Compared with coagulation current (discussed in the next section), cutting current has a relatively low voltage. It also has a relatively high crest factor, which is the ratio of the peak voltage to the mean (root-mean-square) voltage of the current. Additionally, it has a relatively high "duty cycle"—that is, once the current is applied, the current is actively flowing during the entire application.

In this technique, the tip of the electrode is held just slightly off the surface of the tissue. The flow of the high-frequency current through the resistance of the patient's tissue at a very small site produces intense heat, vaporizing water, exploding the cells in the immediate vicinity of the current. Thus, cutting occurs with minimal coagulum production, and consequentially, minimal hemostasis. A combination of coagulation and cutting can be produced by setting the electrosurgical

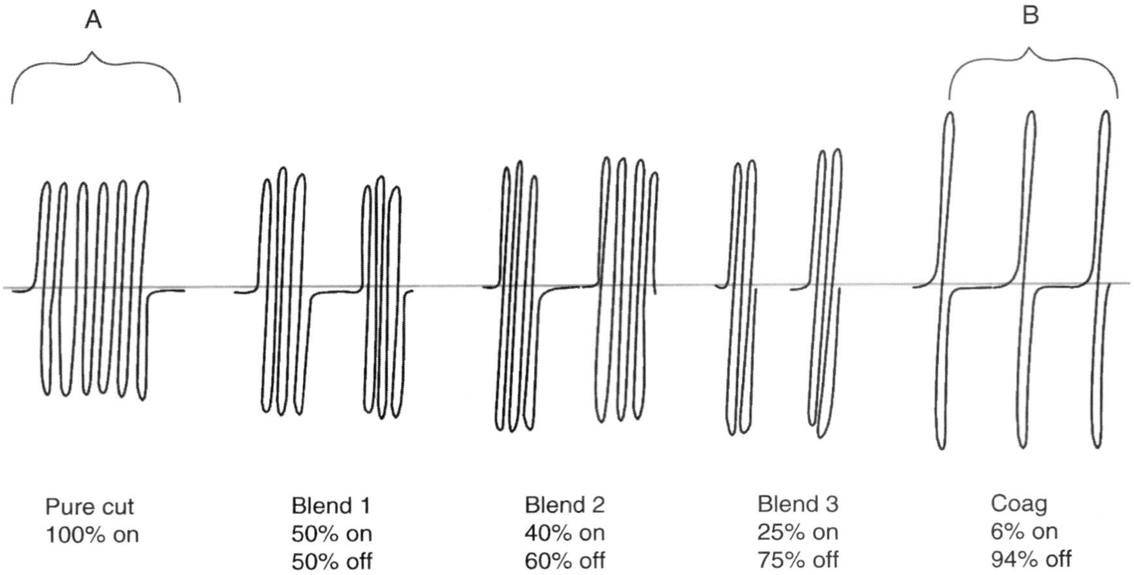

Figure 7–3. Electrosurgical waveforms. **A:** Cutting current. **B:** Coagulation current.

generator to "**blend**," which damps down a portion of the waveform, allowing greater formation of a coagulum and consequently more control of local bleeding.

Coagulation

In contrast with cutting currents, **coagulation** currents do not produce a constant waveform. Rather, they rely on spikes of electric wave activity (Figure 7–3B). Although these currents produce less heat overall than the direct sine wave, enough heat is produced to disrupt the normal cellular architecture. Because the cells are not instantly vaporized, however, the cellular debris remains associated with the edge of the wound, and the heat produced is enough to denature the cellular protein. This accounts for the formation of a coagulum, a protein-rich mixture that allows sealing of smaller blood vessels and control of local bleeding. Compared to cutting, coagulation currents have a higher crest factor and a shorter duty cycle (94% off, 6% on). In part, the increased voltage is necessary to overcome the impedance of air during the process of arcing current to the tissues.

Coagulation can be accomplished by using desiccation or fulguration.

A. Desiccation

With **desiccation** the conductive tip is placed in direct contact with the tissue. Direct contact of the electrode with tissue reduces the concentration of the current; less heat is generated and no cutting action occurs. A relatively low power setting is used, resulting in a limited area of tissue ablation with coagulation. Desiccation is achieved most efficiently with the "cutting" current. The cells dry out and form a coagulum rather than vaporize and explode.

B. Fulguration

In **fulguration**, the tip of the active electrode is not actually brought into contact with the tissues, but rather is held just off the surface and, following activation, the current arcs through the air to the target. Again this results in the disruption of normal cellular protein to form a coagulum and char the tissue, forming a black eschar at the site of operation. It is possible to "cut" with the coagulation current and, conversely, to coagulate with the cutting current by holding the electrode in direct contact with tissue. It may be necessary to adjust power settings and electrode size to achieve the desired surgical effect. The benefit of using the cutting current is that far less voltage is needed, an important consideration during minimally invasive procedures.

3. Variables Influencing Tissue Effect

Just as the power setting and the waveform affect the results of the current application, any change in the circuit that influences the impedance of the system will influence the tissue effect. These include the size of the electrode, the position of the electrode, the type of tissue, and the formation of eschar.

Size of the Electrode

The smaller the electrode, the higher the current concentration. Consequently, the same tissue effect can be achieved with a smaller electrode, even though the power setting is reduced. At any given setting, the longer the generator is activated, the more heat is produced. The greater the heat, the farther it will travel to adjacent tissue (thermal spread). (See various electrodes, Figure 7–4.)

Placement of the Electrode

Placement of the electrode can determine whether vaporization or coagulation occurs. This is a function of current density and the heat produced while sparking to tissue versus holding the electrode in direct contact.

Type of Tissue

Tissues vary widely in resistance.

Eschar

Eschar is relatively high in resistance to current. Electrodes should be kept clean and free of eschar, maintaining lower resistance within the surgical circuit.

4. Disadvantages & Potential Hazards

Alternate Site Burns

Early electrosurgical generators used a **ground referenced** circuit design. In this type of construction, grounded current from the wall outlet was directly modulated, and it was assumed that it would return to the generator via the return electrode. With this type of system, however, any path of low resistance to ground can complete the circuit, including metal instruments, ECG leads, and other wire and conductive surfaces. This situation presented a relatively high hazard for alternate site burns when current was not distributed over a great enough area to dissipate the current.

Modern electrosurgical units use isolated generator technology. The isolated generator separates the therapeutic current from ground by referencing it within the generator circuitry. In an isolated electrosurgical system, the circuit is completed by the generator, and electrosurgical current from isolated generators will not recognize grounded objects as pathways to complete the circuit. Isolated electrosurgical energy recognizes the patient return electrode as the preferred pathway back to the generator. Since the ground is not the reference for completion of the circuit, the potential for alternate site burns is greatly reduced. However, if the return electrode were to become partially disconnected, a burn at the site of the return electrode would be possible if the area was not great enough to distribute the current widely enough to prevent heating of the tissue, or if the impedance was too high. It is important to place the return electrode over a well-vascularized tissue mass (not over areas of vascular insufficiency) or over bony prominences where contact might be compromised. For this reason, some electrosurgical generators use a monitoring system that assesses the quality of the contact between the return electrode and the patient by monitoring impedance, which is related to surface area. Any loss of contact between this electrode and the generator results in interruption of this circuit and deactivation of the system.

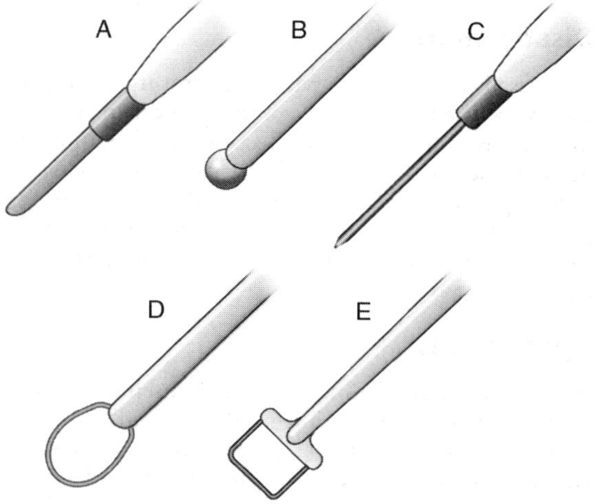

Figure 7–4. **A:** Knife electrode. **B:** Ball electrode. **C:** Needle electrode. **D:** Loop electrode. **E:** Wire electrode.

Surgical Fires

In any setting with high heat sources and an ample supply of oxygen, vigilance against combustion is essential. Potential risks for ignition include drapes, gowns, gas (particularly in bowel surgery or cases involving the upper airway), and hair. Careful application of electrosurgery and use of a protective holster to store the electrode while not in use are important to minimize these risks.

Minimally Invasive Surgery

Several safety concerns are unique to minimally invasive surgery, given the limited and relatively tight environment in which operations occur. One potential danger is that of direct coupling between the electrode and other conductive instruments, leading to inadvertent tissue damage. Additionally, with the use of high-voltage currents (especially those used for coagulation), there is a risk of breakdown in the insulation, resulting in arcing from an exposed conductor to adjacent tissue that may lead to unwanted tissue damage. The likelihood of such damage can be reduced by using cutting current to lower the voltage used.

One unique hazard is the potential for creating a capacitor with the cannulae used. A **capacitor** is any conductor separated from another conductor by a dielectric. The conductive electrode separated from either a metal cannula or the abdominal wall (both good conductors) can induce capacitance in either of these structures. For maximum safety, an all-metal cannula (by which current can escape to the rest of the body) rather than a combination of metal and plastic should be used, and vigilance must be maintained at all times.

5. Principal Applications for Electrosurgery

Electrosurgery is ubiquitous in its presence within the modern operating room. In its earliest use by Dr. Cushing, it allowed surgery on previously inoperable vascular tumors in neurosurgery. Today, electrosurgery is an essential component of all types of surgery. Applications include dissection in all types of general and vascular surgery, allowing tissue to be resected with minimal blood loss. Additionally, use in urology facilitates transurethral resection of the prostate and other procedures. In gynecologic practice, electrosurgical instruments are essential in cervical resections and biopsies.

6. Argon Beam Coagulation

Principles

Argon beam coagulation is closely related to basic application of electrosurgery. Argon beam coagulation uses a coaxial flow of argon gas to conduct monopolar RF current to the target tissue. Argon is an inert gas that is easily ionized by the application of an electrical current. When ionized, argon gas becomes far more conductive (less impedance) than normal air and provides a more efficient pathway for transmitting current from the electrode to tissues (Figure 7–5).

The current arcs along the pathway of the ionized gas, which is heavier than both oxygen and nitrogen, and thereby displaces air. Whereas current can sometimes follow unpredictable pathways while arcing through the air, the argon gas allows more accurate placement of current flow. Once the current arrives at the tissue, it produces its coagulating effect in the same manner as conventional electrosurgery. Argon beam coagulation devices can operate only in two modes: pinpoint coagulation and spray coagulation. They do not cut even the most delicate tissue.

Advantages

There are multiple advantages to this type of electrosurgical current delivery. First, it allows use of the coagulation mode without contact of the electrode. This prevents buildup of eschar, which diminishes electrode efficiency, on the electrode tip. Second, there is generally decreased smoke and a reduced odor from coagulating with this type of current. Third, there is decreased tissue loss and reduced tissue damage when the current is more accurately targeted. Fourth, because the argon gas is delivered at room temperature, there is less of a danger of the instrument igniting gowns or drapes. Finally, the beam of coagulation generally improves coagulation and reduces blood loss and the risk of rebleeding.

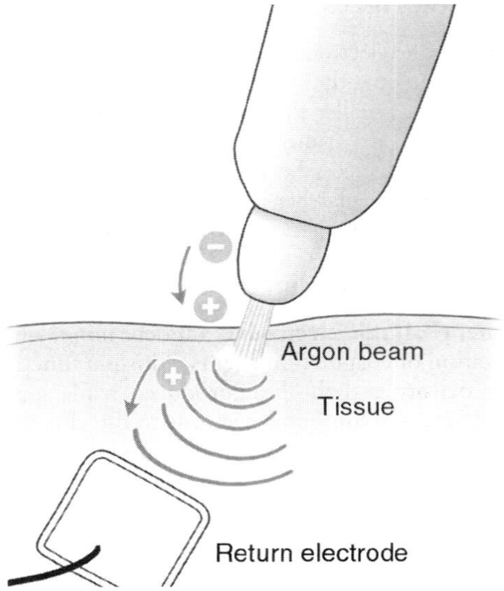

Figure 7–5. Ionized argon gas facilitates the flow of current from the handpiece to the tissue.

Disadvantages

One disadvantage of this type of electrosurgery is that it cannot be used to produce a cutting effect in the same manner as other types of electrosurgical equipment. Second, the nozzle for gas delivery can become clogged, reducing its efficiency, and just as with other electrosurgical instruments, if it is used for a prolonged period of time, it may overheat and then cause inadvertent damage when set aside.

Applications

Argon beam coagulation is especially useful for procedures in which the surgeon needs to rapidly and efficiently coagulate a wide area of tissue. It is especially suited to dissecting very vascular tissues and organs, such as the liver. Its efficiency at delivering a consistent current load and its inability to become occluded with eschar are advantageous when there is a significant risk of hemorrhage.

MECHANICAL (ULTRASONIC) TISSUE DISRUPTION

Apart from passing current through the patient to produce localized heating and tissue destruction (either cutting or coagulation), there are other means of transferring electrical potential energy into energy for surgery. Two of the most prominent of these technologies are dependent on the production of ultrasonic vibrations, although each produces its effect in a unique manner.

1. Ultrasonic Scalpels & Clamps

Principles

Several types of ultrasonic "scalpels" and clamps allow cutting and coagulation of tissue in a technique completely different from that employed in electrosurgery. In these instruments, electrical energy from a power source is transformed into ultrasonic vibrations by a transducer, a unit that expands and contracts in response to electrical current at a frequency of up to 55,500 cycles per second. This is amplified in the shaft of the instrument to magnify the vibrating distance of the blade, which moves longitudinally. The blade tip vibrates through an amplitude of around 200 μm. As the blade tip vibrates, it produces cellular friction and denatures proteins. These denatured proteins form a coagulum, which allows sealing of coapted blood vessels. When the instrument is left in place longer, secondary heat is produced, and larger blood vessels may be sealed. By producing cellular disruption in this fashion, the temperatures achieved are between 50 °C and 100 °C. In contrast, in conventional electrosurgery, tissues are subject to temperatures between 150 °C and 400 °C. Thus, using an ultrasonic device, tissues can be dissected without burning or oxidizing tissues, without producing an eschar, and there is less potential to disrupt the coagulum when removing the instrument. When one is cutting using the clamp portion of the instrument, energy is transferred to the tissue through the active blade under applied force, minimizing lateral spread. Additionally, the motion of the blade induces cavitation along the cell surfaces, whereby low pressure causes cell fluid to vaporize and rupture (Figure 7–6).

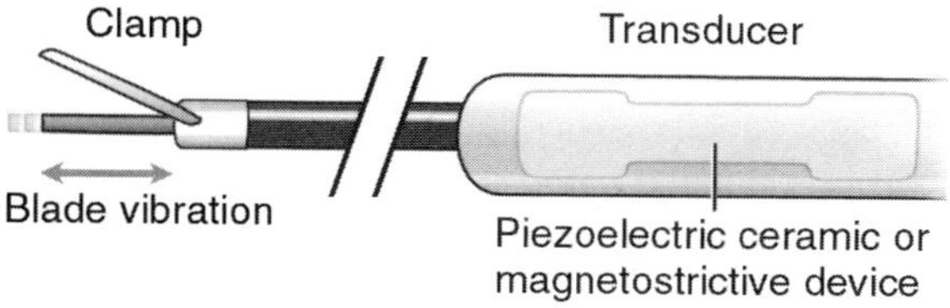

Figure 7–6. Ultrasonic scalpel.

Advantages

The advantages of an ultrasonic scalpel system are clearest when one is operating in tight spaces, with the attendant risks of damage to adjacent structures. This makes such instruments especially suited for laparoscopic and other types of minimally invasive procedures. Additionally, while the potential still exists for damaging adjacent tissue with an inadvertent contact of an active tip with tissue, there is no risk of current inadvertently arcing to adjacent structures, since the current is converted into mechanical energy in the handpiece. Further, there is no neuromuscular stimulation produced, since no current passes through the patient. Since the tissue effects are exerted through mechanical disruption of the cells, and coagulation occurs at much lower temperatures than used in conventional electrosurgery, lateral thermal tissue damage is minimized. Further, since the tissues are not heated to the point of combustion or carbonization of proteins, there is no eschar formation on the blade, and less smoke is produced.

Disadvantages

A primary disadvantage of this system is that the components are more expensive than those used for conventional electrosurgery, and with more mechanical parts, there are more potential areas of breakage. Further, whereas electrosurgery can be applied throughout an operation, ultrasonic scalpels are typically used for more controlled dissection around the site of interest.

Applications

The primary applications of ultrasonic instruments are found when traditional electrosurgery is unsuitable or not desirable. As mentioned above, they are particularly useful during minimally invasive procedures, due to the risks of running an active electrode through a cannula and into a body cavity. The lack of current flow mitigates this risk. Additionally, the reduced smoke production by instruments of this type is advantageous in this setting. In patients where there is a concern about current flow due to questions about electrophysiology (such as with implantable cardiac defibrillators or pacemakers), these instruments eliminate a source of concern by avoiding the hazard of passing current through the patient's body.

2. Cavitational Ultrasonic Surgical Aspiration

Principles

Cavitational ultrasonic surgical aspirators work on many of the same principles as the ultrasonic scalpels mentioned above. In the handpiece, current passes through a coil and induces a magnetic field. The magnetic field excites a transducer of a nickel alloy (either a piezoelectric or magnetostrictive device), expanding and contracting, resulting in an oscillating motion (vibration) in the longitudinal axis with a frequency of 23 or 36 kHz. These ultrasonic mechanical vibrations are magnified over the length of the handpiece. The amount of oscillation varies: With low frequency, there is greater amplitude, with high frequency, there is lower amplitude. The oscillating tip, when brought into contact with tissue, causes fragmentation of tissue via producing cavitation at the cell surface, with low pressure outside the cell leading to cellular disruption. This high-frequency vibration produces heat, which is reduced via a closed, recirculating cooling water system. This system maintains the temperature of the tip at approximately 40 °C.

As tissue is fragmented, the debris must be carried away, and this is another function of these instruments, as implied by their name. For irrigation, IV fluid (water or saline) is fed through tubing to the handpiece, where it irrigates the surgical site and suspends the fragmented tissue debris. Removal of this debris is possible because the instrument contains a vacuum pump that provides suction. Suction pulls irrigation fluid, fragmented tissue, and other material through the distal tip of the handpiece. The material is contained in a separate canister.

Some ultrasonic surgical aspirator instruments have technology that allows the surgeon to influence the selectivity of the disruption induced by the instrument itself. Some surgeons attempt to gain extra control by lowering the amplitude of the tip oscillations. Lowering amplitude in an attempt to gain greater selectivity when fragmenting tissue near critical structures, however, only results in a reduced speed of tissue removal. By using a mode in which on/off power intervals are supplied, the reserve power (which governs the tip response when encountering tissue) is reduced. The total amount of power in the oscillating hollow tip is determined by the amount of reserve power available. Reserve power maintains tip oscillation when a resistive load is placed on the tip, as occurs when it contacts tissue. As the resistance increases, more power is supplied to the tip (Figure 7–7).

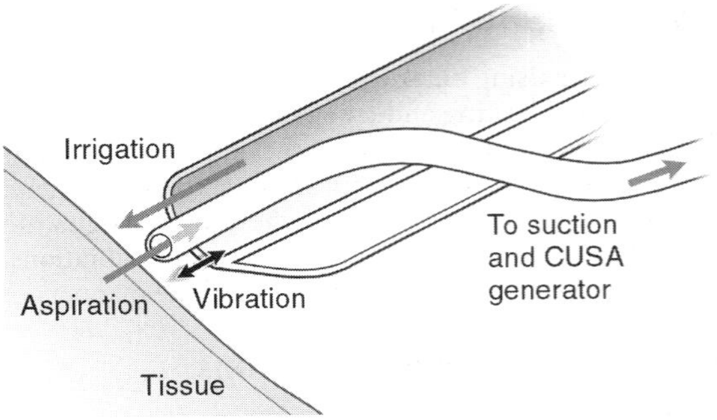

Figure 7–7. Cavitational ultrasonic surgical aspirator.

Applications

Ultrasonic surgical aspirator systems have their primary application in situations where fragmentation, emulsification, and aspiration of a significant amount of tissue is desirable. Since minimal additional hemostasis is provided, this instrument is not as versatile in its application to general surgery as electrosurgery or the more high-power ultrasonic scalpel. In general surgery, its primary application is in liver resection, where it can disrupt parenchyma while leaving major vasculature and the biliary ducts intact.

REFERENCES

ConMed: *Electrosurgical Generator + ABC Mode Operator's Manual.* Conmed Corporation, 1999.

Duffy S, Cobb GV: *Practical Electrosurgery,* 1st ed. Chapman & Hall Medical, 1995.

Pearce JA: *Electrosurgery.* Chapman & Hall, 1986.

Valleylab. *CUSA Excel System User's Guide.* Tyco Healthcare Group, 2000.

RELEVANT WEB SITES

[Johnson & Johnson Gateway, Technology Overview.]
http://www.jnjgateway.com

[Valleylab. Principles of Electrosurgery Online.]
http://www.valleylab.com/education/poes/index.html

Inflammation, Infection, & Antimicrobial Therapy

8

Linda M. Mundy, MD, Gerard M. Doherty, MD, & J. Perren Cobb, MD

INFLAMMATION & INFECTION

SURGICAL INFECTIONS

A surgical infection is an infection that (1) is unlikely to respond to nonsurgical treatment (it usually must be excised or drained) and occupies an unvascularized space in tissue or (2) occurs in an operated site. Common examples of the first group are appendicitis, empyema, gas gangrene, and most abscesses.

Surgeons are regrettably familiar with the vicious circle of operation or injury, infection, malnutrition, immunosuppression, organ failure, reoperation, further malnutrition, and further infection. One of the fine arts of surgery is to know when to intervene with excision, drainage, physiologic support, antibiotic therapy, and nutritional therapy. For infections arising in a space or in dead tissue, by far the most important aspect of treatment is to establish surgical drainage.

Pathogenesis

Three elements are common to surgical infections: (1) an infectious agent, (2) a susceptible host, and (3) a closed, unperfused space.

A. The Infectious Agent

Although a few pathogens cause most surgical infections, many organisms are capable of doing so. Among the aerobic organisms, streptococci may invade even minor breaks in the skin and spread through connective tissue planes and lymphatics. *Staphylococcus aureus* is the most common pathogen in wound infections and around foreign bodies. Klebsiella often invades the inner ear and enteric tissues as well as the lung. Enteric organisms, especially the Enterobacteriaceae and enterococci, are often found together with anaerobes. Among the anaerobes, bacteroides species and peptostreptococci are often present in surgical infections, and clostridium species are major pathogens in ischemic tissue.

Pseudomonas and serratia are usually nonpathogenic surface contaminants but may be opportunistic and even lethal invaders in critically ill or immunosuppressed patients. Some fungi (histoplasma, coccidioides) and yeasts (candida), along with nocardia and actinomyces, cause abscesses and sinus tracts, and even animal parasites (amebas and echinococcus) may cause abscesses, especially in the liver. Destructive granulomas, such as tuberculosis, once required excision, but antibiotic therapy has now superseded operation for this purpose in most cases. Other rare diseases such as cat-scratch fever, psittacosis, and tularemia may cause suppurative lymphadenitis and require drainage or excision.

Identification of the pathogen by smear and culture remains a cardinal step in therapeutic decision making. The surgeon must inform the microbiologist of peculiar circumstances associated with any given specimen, so that appropriate smears and cultures can be done; serious errors may otherwise result.

B. The Susceptible Host

Surgical infections such as appendicitis and furuncles occur in patients whose only defect in immunity is a closed space in tissue. However, patients with suppressed immune systems are being seen with increasing frequency, and their problems have become a major surgical challenge. **Immunosuppression** seems a simple concept but in fact usually represents a combination of defects of the multifaceted immune mechanism.

1. Specific immunity—The immune process that depends upon prior exposure to an antigen involves detection and processing of antigen by macrophages, mobilization of T and B lymphocytes, synthesis of specific antibody, and other functions. Its importance is illustrated in AIDS, transplant immunosuppression, and agammaglobulinemia, each of which is associated with only a slight increase in the frequency and severity of some surgical infections. Specific abnormalities of cell-mediated and humoral immunity have been reported in almost every imaginable form of surgical infection. For instance, severe injury in animals and patients is associated with a subsequent decrease in T cell-dependent immune cell function and thus depressed adaptive immunity. Unfortunately, the clinical significance of this and other isolated defects of specific immunity is obscure, and their clinical importance in the complex immune system is difficult to determine (see Systemic Inflammatory Response Syndrome, below). In general, isolated defects contribute little to the severity of ordinary surgical infections. Major defects contribute substantially to morbidity, mortality, and resource consumption.

2. Nonspecific immunity—Innate or nonspecific immunity serves to limit damage during the first few hours after infection. Despite the emphasis in the literature on specific immune mechanisms, nonspecific immunity, which depends on phagocytic leukocyte migration, ingestion, and cidal activity for microorganisms, is the principal means by which the host defends against abscess-forming and necrotizing infections.

a. Chemoattraction and phagocytosis—Invading microbes display molecular patterns that are shared among groups of pathogens. Examples include lipopolysaccharides (LPS) of gram-negative bacteria, lipoteichoic acid of gram-positive bacteria, mannans of yeast, and double-stranded RNA of certain viruses. To control infection, the host uses an array of pattern recognition receptors (complement, adhesins, collectins, bactericidal permeability-increasing protein [BPI], LPS-binding protein [LBP]) that bind to these molecular moieties, acting together with effector cells to eliminate them. Typically, granulocytes internalize these pattern-receptor complexes by engulfment into a phagocytic vacuole. The subsequent release of chemoattractants causes the movement (diapedesis) of leukocytes from the bloodstream to the tissue, increasing leukocyte numbers locally and the likelihood that the invading microbe will be destroyed. These steps require little or no oxygen, but chemotaxis is vulnerable to a number of disorders, particularly anti-inflammatory steroid hormones and malnutrition, which reduce the number of granulocytes that arrive at a contaminated site in a given time.

b. Killing mechanisms—Once the phagosome is formed, other cytoplasmic granules (lysosomes) fuse with it and release into it preformed and increasingly acidic proteolytic solutions that kill most bacteria and fungi.

A second process, termed "oxidative killing," is particularly important to the killing of organisms such as staphylococci, which are commonly responsible for surgical infections. This mechanism consumes and requires molecular oxygen, which it converts to superoxide anion. In this process, a membrane-bound NADPH oxidase is activated, and a burst of respiration (oxygen consumption) follows. Part of the consumed oxygen is converted to a series of oxygen radicals (including superoxide, hydroxyl radical, and hypochlorite), which are released into phagosomes and assist in bacterial killing. This process is progressively inhibited when extracellular oxygen tension falls below about 30 mm Hg. When oxygen tension is 0 mm Hg, the antibacterial capacity of normal granulocytes for *S aureus* and *E coli,* for instance, falls by half—to the same capacity observed in granulocytes taken from victims of chronic granulomatous disease, which results from the genetic absence of membrane-bound oxidase and which without aggressive antibiotic therapy is lethal in early childhood.

Whether a given inoculum will establish an infection and become invasive depends to a great extent on how well tissue perfusion—and therefore oxygenation—can meet the increased metabolic demands of the granulocytes. Inflammatory signals from complement factors and histamine, for instance, dilate vessels and help direct blood flow to infected areas, but if blood volume or regional vascular supply is so poor that tissue perfusion cannot increase, invasive infection ensues. Tissue oxygen supplies can often be raised by increasing blood volume and arterial PO_2 and are lowered by hypovolemia and pulmonary insufficiency. Tests in animals show that correcting arterial hypoxia aborts bacterial infections as effectively as does use of specific antibiotics and that antibiotics are far more effective when phagocytes have an adequate oxygen supply.

Patients with pulmonary disease, severe trauma, congestive heart failure, hypovolemia, or excessive levels of vasopressin, angiotensin, or catecholamines have hypoxic peripheral tissues and are unusually susceptible to infection. They are truly immunosuppressed. Support of the circulation is just as important to immune defense as is nutrition or antibiotic therapy.

3. Anergy—Anergy is defined as the lack of inflammatory response to skin test antigens. It characterizes a population of immunosuppressed patients who tend to develop infections and die from them. The skin tests used to diagnose anergy are those often used to test recall antigens and delayed hypersensitivity—but in fact they test much of the spectrum of antibacterial immunologic events, including antigen detection and processing by macrophages, release of lymphokines, antibody synthesis, and the inflammatory response, including leukocyte chemotaxis. One event they do not detect is, conspicuously, the final crucial step of actually killing bacteria. Anergy has many causes, including defective T and B lymphocytes, the presence of excess anti-inflammatory corticosteroids, defective antigen processing, and increased numbers of suppressor T cells. Among surgical patients, severe malnutrition, trauma, shock and sepsis suppress skin test responses, which become active again after resolution of the acute process.

4. Immunity in diabetes mellitus—Diabetes mellitus impairs immunity. Well-controlled diabetics resist infection normally except in tissues made ischemic by arterial disease, while uncontrolled diabetics do not. The mechanism is unknown, except that leukocytes from poorly controlled diabetics adhere, migrate, and kill bacteria poorly. They improve their performance when glucose control is regained. Leukocytes also function poorly without insulin, and insulin is consumed in wounds and other poorly perfused spaces, resulting in low ambient insulin levels.

C. The Closed Space

Most surgical infections start in a susceptible, usually poorly vascularized place in tissue such as a wound or a natural space. The common denominators are poor perfusion, local hypoxia, hypercapnia, and acidosis. Some natural spaces with narrow outlets, such as those of the appendix, gallbladder, ureters, and intestines, are especially prone to becoming obstructed and then infected.

The peritoneal and pleural cavities are potential spaces, and their surfaces slide over one another, thereby dispersing contaminating bacteria. Foreign bodies, dead tissue, and injuries interfere with this mechanism and predispose to infection. Fibrin inhibits the clearing of bacteria. It polymerizes around bacteria, trapping them; this encourages abscess formation but at the same time prevents dangerous spread of infection.

Foreign bodies may have spaces in which bacteria can reside. Infarcted tissue is markedly susceptible to infection. Thrombosed veins, for example, rarely become infected unless intravenous catheters enter them and act as entry points for bacteria.

Spread of Surgical Infections

Surgical infections usually originate as a single focus and become life-threatening by spreading and releasing toxins. Spreading occurs by several mechanisms.

A. Necrotizing Infections

Necrotizing infections tend to spread along anatomically defined paths. Necrotizing fasciitis spreads along poorly perfused fascial and subcutaneous planes, its toxins causing thrombosis even of large vessels ahead of the necrotic area, thus creating more ischemic and vulnerable tissue.

B. Abscesses

If not promptly drained, abscesses enlarge, killing more tissue in the process. Leukocytes contribute to necrosis by releasing lysosomal enzymes during phagocytosis. Natural boundaries can be breached; eg, intestinal cutaneous fistulas may form, or blood vessel walls may be penetrated.

C. Phlegmons and Superficial Infections

Phlegmons contain little pus but much edema. They spread along fat planes and by contiguous necrosis, combining features of both of the above kinds of spread. Retroperitoneal peripancreatic inflammation or infection is typical. Superficial infections may spread along skin not only by contiguous necrosis but also by metastasis.

D. Spread of Infection Via the Lymphatic System

Lymphangitis produces red streaks in the skin and travels proximally along major lymph vessels. However, it may also occur in hidden places such as the retroperitoneum in puerperal sepsis.

E. Spread of Infection Via the Bloodstream

Empyema and endocarditis caused by intravenously injected contaminated drugs are now common. Brain abscesses resulting from infections elsewhere in the body (especially the face) occur in infants and diabetics. Liver abscesses may complicate appendicitis and inflammatory bowel disease, sometimes as a result of suppurative phlebitis of the portal vein (pylephlebitis).

Complications

A. Fistulas and Sinus Tracts

Fistulas and sinus tracts often result when abdominal abscesses contiguous to bowel open to the skin. When tissue necrosis compounds the development of sinus tracts and erodes major blood vessels, severe bleeding may occur. This is most troublesome in irradiated tissue of nonhealing neck wounds and in infected groin wounds after vascular surgery.

Some intestinal fistulas originate in poorly fashioned or necrotic suture lines, and some result from contiguous abscesses that eventually penetrate both bowel and skin, often helped along by the surgeon who must drain the abscess.

B. Suppressed Wound Healing

Suppressed wound healing is a consequence of infection. The mechanism is probably stimulation by bacteria of cytokines, which in turn stimulates proteolysis, especially collagenase production.

C. Immunosuppression and Superinfection

Immunosuppression is a common consequence of injury, which includes surgery, trauma, shock, or infection or sepsis. Superinfection occurs when immunosuppression provides an opportunity for invasion by opportunistic, often antibiotic-resistant organisms.

D. Bacteremia

The term bacteremia denotes the presence of bacteria in blood. The significance of bacteremia is variable. Bacteremia that follows dental work is usually rapidly cleared and harmless, except in patients with damaged heart valves, cardiac, vascular, or orthopedic prostheses, or impaired immunity. It occurs predictably during instrumentation of the gastrointestinal tract or infected urinary tract. Patients in these groups are at increased risk and should receive an appropriate prophylactic antibiotic regimen.

E. Organ Dysfunction, Sepsis, and the Systemic Inflammatory Response Syndrome

Infection and tissue damage initiate the inflammatory response, a very tightly controlled, adaptive response to eliminate dead or infected tissue. At the site of injury, endothelial cells and leukocytes coordinate the local release of mediators of the inflammatory response, including cytokines (tumor necrosis factor-α), interleukins, interferons, leukotrienes, prostaglandins, nitric oxide, reactive oxygen species, and products of the classic inflammatory pathway (complement, histamine, and bradykinin) (Table 8–1). When localized to diseased tissue, these mediators are highly effective at recruiting and arming cells of the innate and adaptive immune systems to destroy invading organisms and elicit reparative mechanisms in wounded tissue. However, if the degree of the infectious or traumatic insult exceeds the ability of the host to contain it, the inflammatory response becomes systemic. The result is whole body activation of the inflammatory response, with resultant disruption of normal cellular metabolism and microcirculatory perfusion. This leads to clinical deterioration, manifested as dysfunction of the brain (delirium), lungs (hypoxia), heart and blood vessels (shock and edema), kidneys (oliguria), intestines (ileus), liver (hyperbilirubinemia), and the hematologic (coagulopathy, anemia) and immunologic systems (immunosuppression). This syndrome is referred to as **multiple organ dysfunction syndrome (MODS)**. The risks of organ failure in general are directly proportionate to the duration and severity of shock and inversely proportionate to the age and underlying health of the patient. It is frequently difficult or impossible to determine whether the cause of organ dysfunction in critically ill patients is severe infection or inflammation. Consensus definitions were therefore established in 1992. The term **sepsis** is used when the systemic response results from infection. In contrast, when the systemic response occurs in the absence of infection, as it does in severe burns, trauma, and pancreatitis, it is called **systemic inflammatory response syndrome (SIRS)**. The interrelationships between infection, bacteremia, sepsis, and SIRS are depicted in Figure 8–1.

Diagnosis

The aim of management is to detect and treat sepsis before it evolves into more advanced stages.

A. Physical Examination

Physical examination is the easiest way to localize a surgical infection. When infection is suspected but cannot be identified initially, repeated examination will often reveal subtle warmth, erythema, induration, tenderness, or splinting due to a developing abscess. Failure to repeat the physical examination is the most common reason for delayed diagnosis and therapy.

B. Laboratory Findings

1. General findings—Laboratory data are of limited value. Leukocytosis may give way to leukopenia when the infection is severe. Acidosis is helpful in diagnosis, and signs of disseminated intravascular coagulation are useful as well. Otherwise unexplained respiratory, hepatic, renal, and gastric (ie, stress ulcers) failure is strong evidence for sepsis.

2. Cultures—Positive cultures help to differentiate SIRS from sepsis even though 50% of cases of sepsis are culture-negative. If infection is suspected, cultures of blood, sputum, and urine are collected routinely initially, especially in hospitalized patients given the high frequency of nosocomial pneumonia and urinary tract infections (see below). This is particularly important because data from the Centers for Disease Control and Prevention (CDC) suggest that 70% of the bacteria causing hospital-associated infections are resistant to at least one of the drugs most commonly used to treat them. Other fluids such as cerebrospinal fluid, pleural and joint effusions, and ascites can be aspirated and cultured based upon signs or symptoms that specifically indicate these sites as potential sources of infection. In general, pus from abscesses should be cultured unless the causative organism is known. In rapidly advancing cases, two separate blood cultures should be taken within 15 minutes. In less urgent situations, cultures should be taken over a 24-hour period, and up to six cultures should be taken if the patient has enigmatic fevers and either a cardiac or joint prosthesis or vascular shunt. False-negative blood culture results occur in about 20% of cases. False-positive results are difficult to define, since skin commensals (even some diphtheroids and *Staphylococcus epidermidis*), regarded as contaminants in the past, have proved occasionally to be true pathogens. Arterial blood cultures may be necessary to detect fungal endocarditis.

Table 8–1. Cytokines and growth factors.

Peptide	Site of Synthesis	Regulation	Target Cells	Effects
G-CSF	Fibroblasts, monocytes	Induced by IL-1, LPS, IFN-α	Committed neutrophil progenitors (CFU-G, Gran)	Supports the proliferation of neutrophil-forming colonies. Stimulates respiratory burst.
GM-CSF (IL-3 has almost identical effects)	Endothelial cells, fibroblasts, macrophages, T lymphocytes, bone marrow	Induced by IL-1, TNF	Granulocyte-erythrocyte-monocyte-megakaryocyte progenitor cells (CFU-GEMM, CFU-MEG, CFU-Eo, CFU-GM)	Supports the proliferation of macrophage-, eosinophil-, neutrophil-, and monocyte-containing colonies
IFNα, -β, -γ	Epithelial cells, fibroblasts, lymphocytes, macrophages, neutrophils	Induced by viruses (foreign nucleic acids), microbes, microbial foreign antigens, cancer cells	Lymphocytes, macrophages, infected cells, cancer cells	Inhibits viral multiplication. Activates defective phagocytes, direct inhibition of cancer cell multiplication, activation of killer leukocytes, inhibition of collagen synthesis.
IL-1	Endothelial cells, keratinocytes, lymphocytes, macrophages	Induced by TNF-α, IL-1, IL-2, C5a. Suppressed by IL-4, TGF-β	Monocytes, macrophages, T cells, B cells, NK cells, LAK cells	Stimulates T cells, B cells, NK cells, LAK cells. Induces tumoricidal activity and production to other cytokines, endogenous pyrogen (via PGE_2 release). Induces steroidogenesis, acute phase proteins, hypotension; chemotactic neutrophils. Stimulates respiratory burst.
IL-1ra	Monocytes	Induced by GM-CSF, LPS, IgG	Blocks type 1 IL-1 receptors on T cells, fibroblasts, chondrocytes, endothelial cells	Blocks type 1 IL-1 receptors on T cells, chondrocytes, endothelial cells. Ameliorates animal models of arthritis, septic shock, and inflammatory bowel disease.
IL-2	Lymphocytes	induced by IL-1, IL-6	T cells, NK cells, B cells, activated monocytes	Stimulates growth of T cells, NK cells, and B cells
IL-4	T cells, NK cells, mast cells	Induced by cell activation, IL-1	All hematopoietic cells and many others express receptors	Stimulates B cell and T cell growth. Induces HLA class II molecules.
IL-6	Endothelial cells, fibroblasts, lymphocytes, some tumors	Induced by IL-1, TNF-α	T cells, B cells, plasma cells, keratinocytes, hepatocytes, stem cells	B cell differentiation. Induction of acute phase proteins, growth of keratinocytes. Stimulates growth of T cells and hematopoietic stem cells.
IL-8	Endothelial cells, fibroblasts, lymphocytes, monocytes	Induced by TNF, IL-1, LPS, cell adherence (monocytes)	Basophils, neutrophils, T cells	Induces expression of endothelial cell LECAM-1 receptors, β_2 integrins, and neutrophil transmigration. Stimulates respiratory burst.
M-CSF	Endothelial cells, fibroblasts, monocytes	Induced by IL-1, LPS, IFN-α	Committed monocyte progenitors (CFU-M, Mono)	Supports the proliferation of monocyte-forming colonies. Activates macrophages.

(continued)

Table 8–1. Cytokines and growth factors. (continued)

Peptide	Site of Synthesis	Regulation	Target Cells	Effects
MCP-1, MCAF	Monocytes. Some tumors secrete a similar peptide.	Induced by IL1, LPS, PHA	Unstimulated monocytes	Chemoattractant specific for monocytes
TNF-α (LT has almost identical effects)	Macrophages, NK cells, T cells, transformed cell lines, B cells (LT)	Suppressed by PGE_2, TGF-β, IL-4. Induced by LPS.	Endothelial cells, monocytes, neutrophils	Stimulates T cell growth. Direct cytotoxin to some tumor cells. Profound proinflammatory effect via induction of IL-1 and PGE_2. Systemic administration produces many symptoms of sepsis. Stimulates respiratory burst and phagocytosis.

Key:
CFU = Colony-forming unit
G-CSF = Granulocyte colony-stimulating factor
GM-CSF = Granulocyte-macrophage colony-stimulating factor
IFN = Interferon
IL = Interleukin
IL1ra = Interleukin-1receptor antagonist
LPS = Lipopolysaccharide
LT = Lymphotoxin
MCAF = Monocyte chemotactic and activating factor
M-CSF = Macrophage colony-stimulating factor
MCPO-1 = Monocyte chemotactic peptide-1
NK= Natural killer (cell)
PHA= Phytohemagglutinin
TGF-β= Transforming growth factor beta
TNF-α= Tumor necrosis factor alpha

C. Imaging Studies

Radiologic examination is frequently helpful, particularly for the diagnosis of pulmonary infections. Whenever infection is close to bone, radiologic examination is indicated to detect early signs of osteomyelitis, which might require more aggressive surgical or antibiotic therapy. MRI imaging is most useful in detecting bone edema, an early sign of osteomyelitis. For detecting abscesses in solid organs, CT scanning is useful. CT scanning and ultrasonography are particularly useful in localizing occult infection.

Numerous radionuclide scans have been tested, all with fair results. The best radionuclides for labeling leukocytes are gallium (^{67}Ga) and indium (^{111}In). Nuclear imaging modalities are rarely used today for localization of infection.

D. Source of Infection

An early diagnosis of sepsis is usually based on a combination of suspicion and inconclusive evidence, since the results of blood cultures are often unavailable during this stage. An important initial step is to identify the source. Surgical or traumatic wounds, surgical infections in the abdomen or thorax, and clostridial infections are all common, but so are urinary tract infections, pneumonia, and even sinus infections. Once identified, any septic focus amenable to surgical therapy should be excised or drained.

Treatment

A. Incision and Drainage

Abscesses must be opened and bacteria, necrotic tissue, and toxins drained to the outside. The pressure and the number of bacteria in the infected space are lowered; this decreases the spread of toxins and bacteria. An abscess with systemic manifestations is a surgical emergency.

Fluctuation is a reliable but late sign of a subcutaneous abscess. Abscesses in the parotid or perianal area

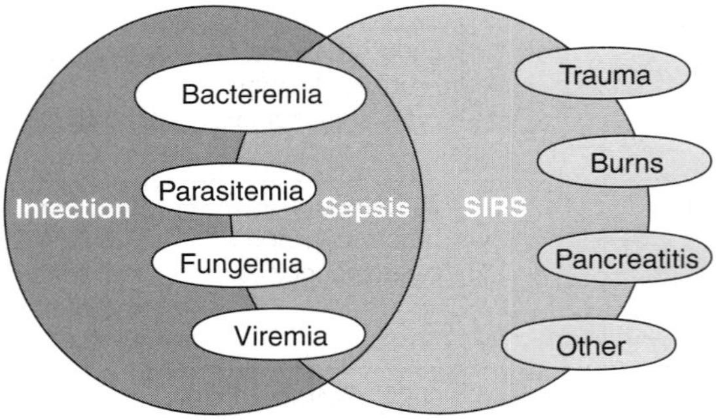

Figure 8–1. Interrelationships among systemic inflammatory response syndrome (SIRS), sepsis, and infection. (Modified, with permission, from Crit Care Med 1992;20:864.)

may never become fluctuant, and if the surgeon waits for this sign, serious sepsis may result. Drainage creates an open wound, but the tissue will heal by second intention with remarkably little scarring. Deep abscesses difficult to drain surgically may be drained by a catheter placed percutaneously under guidance by CT scanning or ultrasonography.

It may appear that a patient with sepsis cannot withstand operation. In fact, operation to drain an abscess may be the most important of all therapeutic measures. One can hardly imagine delaying removal of infarcted bowel because the patient is in shock. There is no substitute for obliteration of the focus of infection when it is surgically accessible.

B. Excision

Some surgical infections may be excised (eg, an infected appendix or gallbladder). In these cases, drainage may not be necessary, and the patient is cured on the operating table. Clostridial myositis may require amputation of the infected limb. The success of such operations is greatly facilitated by intensive specific adjuvant antimicrobial therapy.

C. Circulatory Enhancement

Just as infections due to vascular ischemia are cured by restoring arterial patency, chronic infections in poorly vascularized areas, as in osteoradionecrosis, may be cured by transplanting a functioning vascular bed (eg, a musculocutaneous flap or omental transposition) into the affected area.

D. Antimicrobial Therapy

Antibiotics are not necessary for simple surgical infections that respond to incision and drainage alone—furuncles and uncomplicated wound infections. Infections likely to spread or persist require antibiotic therapy, best chosen on the basis of sensitivity tests. In "toxic" infections, including septic shock, antibiotics must be started promptly and empirically and the regimen modified later from the results of blood cultures. The choice of drugs must take into account the organisms most often cultured from similar infections in previous patients, the results of body fluid gram-stained smears, and specific characteristics of the patient.

E. Nutritional Support

In malnourished, septic, or severely traumatized patients, the ability to ward off or recover from infection is often enhanced by aggressive nutritional therapy. Specific measurable effects include improved immunocompetency and blunting or reversal of catabolism. Protection or restoration of visceral and skeletal muscle allows the patient to cough better and be more mobile.

Prognosis

The mortality rate ranges from 10% in septic patients with manifestations limited to fever, chills, and toxicity, to almost 100% in those who manifest shock and multiple organ failure. Factors that have independent influences on outcome include the causative microorganism, blood pressure, body temperature (inverse relationship), primary site of infection, age, predisposing factors, and place of acquisition of infection (hospital or home). Of patients with low-grade fever and an elevated leukocyte count after antibiotics have been discontinued, 60% will have a relapse. Nevertheless, continuation of antibiotics in questionable cases is often contraindicated because it only delays recognition of infection and may enhance morbidity, as well as increasing antibiotic resistance.

Bone RC: Sir Isaac Newton, sepsis, SIRS, and CARS. Crit Care Med 1996;24:1125.

Bone RC et al: Definitions for sepsis and organ failure and guidelines for the use of innovative therapies in sepsis. The ACCP/SCCM Consensus Conference Committee: American College of Chest Physicians/Society of Critical Care Medicine. Chest 1992;101:1644.

Hoffman JA et al: Phylogenetic perspectives in innate immunity. Science 1999;284:1313.

Lederer JA et al: The effects of injury on the adaptive immune response. Shock 1999;11:153.

O'Grady NP et al: Practice parameters for evaluating new fever in critically ill adult patients. Task Force of the American College of Critical Care Medicine of the Society of Critical Care Medicine in collaboration with the Infectious Disease Society of America. Crit Care Med 1998;26:392.

NOSOCOMIAL INFECTIONS & INFECTION CONTROL

Nosocomial infections affect approximately 2 million patients annually in the United States and add approximately $3.5 billion to the cost of health care. Patients may acquire infection in hospital through contact with personnel or from a nonsterile environment, or infection may develop from bacteria harbored by the patient before operation.

Hospital Personnel as a Source of Infection

Most nosocomially acquired bacteria are transmitted through human contact. In order to minimize transmission in hospital, rules made for behavior, dress, and hygiene should be obeyed.

Unwashed hands are by far the most frequent sources of nosocomial infections such as pneumonia, intravenous catheter-related sepsis, burn wound infections, and even pseudomembranous colitis. Therefore, hand washing is the single most important procedure for preventing nosocomial infections. Routine hand washing should be a matter of reflex conditioning. In today's atmosphere, failure to wash one's hands between patient contacts in a hospital is essentially an unethical act.

The Operating Room as a Source of Infection

Any break in operative technique noted by any member of the operating team should be corrected immediately. Members of the team should not operate if they have cutaneous infections or upper respiratory or viral infections that may cause sneezing or coughing.

Scrub suits should be worn only in the operating room and not in other areas of the hospital. If they must be worn outside the operating room, they should be changed before reentering. Physicians and nurses should always wash their hands between patients. Careful hand washing should follow all contact with infected patients. For preoperative preparation, hands and forearms up to the elbows should be scrubbed for 2–5 minutes with any approved agent if the surgeon has not scrubbed within the past week. Shorter scrubs are allowable between operations. Traffic and talking in the operating room should be minimized.

Though many parts of the operating environment are sterile, the operative field is not—it is merely as sterile as it can be made. Attempts to achieve a level of sterility beyond normal standards have not led to further reductions in wound infection rates. This reflects the fact that bacteria are also present in the patient, and host defense mechanisms are also important determinants of infection not affected by more aggressive attempts to achieve sterility.

Many special and expensive techniques have been devised to minimize bacterial contamination in the operating room. Ultraviolet light, laminar flow ventilation, and elaborate architectural and ventilation schemes have been advocated, but none have been definitively proved more effective than observation of current infection control guidelines and surgical discipline.

The only completely reliable methods for sterilization of surgical instruments and supplies are steam under pressure (autoclaving), dry heat, and ethylene oxide gas. Saturated steam at 2 atm pressure and a temperature of 120 °C destroys all vegetative bacteria and most resistant dry spores in 13 minutes, but exposure of surgical instrument packs should usually be extended to 30 minutes to allow heat and moisture to penetrate to the center of the package. Shorter times are allowable for unwrapped instruments with the vacuum-cycle or high-pressure autoclaves now widely used. Continuous dry heat at 170 °C for 1 hour sterilizes articles that cannot tolerate moist heat. If grease or oil is present on instruments, safe dry-heat sterilization requires 4 hours at 160 °C.

Gaseous ethylene oxide destroys bacteria, viruses, fungi, and various spores. It is used for heat-sensitive materials, including telescopic instruments, plastic and rubber goods, sharp and delicate instruments, electrical cords, and sealed ampules. It damages certain plastics and pharmaceuticals. The technique requires a special pressurized-gas autoclave, with 12% ethylene oxide and 88% Freon-12 at 55 °C, 8 psi pressure above atmospheric pressure. Most items must be aerated in sterile packages on the shelf for 24–48 hours before use in order to rid them of the dissolved gas. Implanted plastics should be stored for 7 days before use. Ethylene oxide is toxic and represents a safety hazard unless it is used according to strict regulations.

Miscellaneous sterilization procedures include soaking in antiseptics such as 2% glutaraldehyde to remove viruses from instruments with lenses. Total sterilization by this method requires 10 hours. Chemical antiseptics are often used to clean operating room surfaces and instruments that need not be totally sterile. Other disinfectant solutions include synthetic phenolics, polybrominated salicylanilides, iodophors, alcohols, other glutaraldehyde preparations, and 6% stabilized hydrogen peroxide. These agents maintain high potency in the presence of organic matter and usually leave effective residual antibacterial activity on surfaces. They are also used to clean anesthetic equipment that cannot be sterilized. Prepackaged instruments and supplies can be sterilized with gamma radiation by manufacturers. Synthetic fabrics have now proved to be superior barriers to bacteria and less costly than the traditional cotton. They can be used in gowns and drapes.

The Patient as a Source of Infection

When possible, preexisting infections should be treated before operation. Secretions from patients with a history of respiratory tract infections should be cultured and appropriate treatment given. The urinary tract should be cultured and specific antibiotics administered before instruments are introduced; this precaution has eliminated septic shock as a complication of urologic surgery. The colon should be prepared as discussed in Chapter 31. Dental extractions for caries are imperative prior to cardiac valve replacement.

Bacteria on the patient's skin are a common cause of infection. Preoperative showers or baths with antiseptic soap reduce the infection rate in clean wounds by 50%. Shaving of the operative field hours prior to incision is associated with a 50% increase in wound infection rates and should not be done. If the patient has a heavy growth of hair, an area just large enough to accommodate the wound and its closure should be clipped rather than shaved immediately before operation. Razor shaving more than a few minutes before operation raises the wound infection rate.

The skin to be included in the operative field should be cleansed with antiseptic. Nonirritating agents such as benzalkonium salts should be used in or around the nose or eyes. For other skin areas, the iodophors (eg, povidone-iodine) and chlorhexidine are used most commonly.

Isolation Procedures: Universal Precautions

Traditionally, patients with infection were individually isolated. Since 1985—partly in response to the HIV epidemic—a more general kind of isolation called "universal precautions" has been substituted. In this system, *any* procedure involving close contact with *any* patient—and especially those involving contact with blood—is performed by hospital personnel wearing gloves and other protective devices. The concept of universal precautions emphasizes (1) prevention of needlestick injuries, (2) the use of traditional barriers such as gloves and gowns, (3) the use of masks and eye coverings to prevent mucous membrane exposure during procedures, and (4) the use of individual ventilation devices when the need for resuscitation is predictable. The CDC recommends that universal precautions apply to blood, semen, and vaginal secretions; to amniotic, cerebrospinal, pericardial, peritoneal, pleural, and synovial fluids; and to other body fluids contaminated with blood. Universal precautions are not recommended for feces, nasal secretions, sputum, sweat, tears, urine, or vomitus unless they contain visible blood. The need for hand washing is not diminished by this system.

http://www.cdc.gov/ncidod/hip/isolat/isolat.htm

Antibiotic Prophylaxis Against Surgical Infections

Prophylactic use of antibiotics can decrease the incidence of infections, especially surgical site infections, but at the risk of toxic and allergic reactions to the drug, drug interactions, bacterial resistance, and superinfection. The principles of antibiotic prophylaxis are simple: (1) Choose antibiotics effective against the expected type of contamination. (2) Use antibiotics only if the risk of infection justifies doing so. (3) Give antibiotics in appropriate doses and at appropriate times. (4) Stop dosing before the risk of side effects outweighs benefits.

Antibiotics for preventive use must not be highly toxic and should not be "first-line" antibiotics for treatment of established infection. Because resistance to antibiotics may develop quickly, agents that have been used frequently for prophylaxis are likely to lose their effectiveness for later treatment. Prophylactic agents should be chosen for cost-effectiveness and safety as well as for efficacy.

Prophylactic antibiotics should be selected to target the organisms most likely to be encountered in the anticipated operative procedure. A first-generation cephalosporin (eg, cefazolin) is preferred for most procedures since it is effective against common gram-positive and gram-negative bacteria and has a moderately long serum half-life. The routine use of vancomycin for prophylaxis is discouraged in light of the emergence of vancomycin-resistant organisms—especially enterococcus and staphylococcus. Agents with better gram-negative and anaerobic bacterial activity (eg, cefoxitin, cefotetan) are preferred for colorectal and gynecologic procedures. A single dose of antibiotic given 30 minutes prior to making the skin incision should provide adequate tissue concentrations for most procedures. Additional doses are advisable for longer procedures (over 4 hours) or those that require large volumes of resuscitative fluids (larger volume of distribution). Postoperative doses of prophylactic antibiotics are usually not necessary; in general, no prophylactic antibiotics should be given after wound closure. The American Heart Association recommends that patients with valvular heart disease or prosthetic heart valves receive antibiotics prior to procedures that result in bacteremia in order to prevent endocarditis. A similar argument has been made for patients with indwelling prosthetic joints.

Antibiotic prophylaxis cannot and is not intended to eliminate bacteria. Use of multiple antibiotics increases the risk of drug reactions, diminishes effectiveness in the long run by promoting the emergence of resistant strains, and increases costs. Antibiotics should be given only when a significant rate of infection is encountered without them or when the consequences of infection would be disastrous, as with placement of vascular, cardiac, or joint prostheses.

The surgeon may be tempted to give every patient antibiotics in order to have an infection-free record, but there are several reasons why this strategy is not appropriate: (1) Clean wounds may become infected with organisms for which prophylactic antibiotics are ineffective. (2) Resistant organisms will eventually develop, creating a higher risk of infection within the hospital. (3) The expense and risks associated with antibiotics (eg, kidney failure, hearing loss, anaphylaxis, skin rashes, fungal infections, enterocolitis) overshadow the minimal beneficial effects of using antibiotics in clean cases. The number of antibiotic-resistant strains has been correlated with the number of kilograms of antibiotics used in any given hospital.

Control of Infection Within the Hospital

Considering the cost of hospital-associated infections, infection control is a very sound investment. Data indicate that infection control programs can prevent approximately one-third of nosocomial infections. Consequently, the Joint Commission on Accreditation of Healthcare Organizations in the USA requires each hospital to have an infection control committee with established infection control procedures. This multidisciplinary committee establishes rules for isolation of infected patients and for protection of hospital personnel exposed to infection, procedures for disposal of materials contaminated by bacteria, and guidelines for limiting the spread of infection. Infection control specialists usually record and analyze patterns of infection. Isolates of bacteria cultured from patients are routinely analyzed for potential significance to the hospital environment. Attempts are made to determine the source of "epidemics." These efforts are coordinated at the national level by the CDC to monitor and report nosocomial infection trends. These data are then used to generate recommendations and guidelines to improve outcomes.

Antimicrobial prophylaxis in surgery. Med Lett Drugs Ther 1999;41:75.

CDC Guidelines on Prevention of Nosocomial Infections, Hospital Infections Program, Centers for Disease Control and Prevention: http://www.cdc.gov/ncidod/hip/

SPECIFIC TYPES OF INFECTIONS

SURGICAL SITE INFECTIONS

Surgical site infections, previously called postoperative wound infections, result from bacterial contamination during or after a surgical procedure. The most recent data from the National Nosocomial Infection Surveillance (NNIS) of the CDC indicate that surgical site infections are the third most frequently reported hospital-associated infection, accounting for 14–16% of all infections in hospitalized patients. Among surgical patients, surgical site infections are the most frequent cause of such infections, accounting for 38% of the total.

Infection usually is confined to the subcutaneous tissues. Despite every effort to maintain asepsis, most surgical wounds are contaminated to some extent. However, infection rarely develops if contamination is minimal, if the wound has been made without undue injury, if the subcutaneous tissue is well perfused and well oxygenated, and if there is no dead space. The criteria used to define surgical site infections have been standardized and describe three different anatomic levels of infection (see Table 8–2).

Table 8–2. Types of surgical site infections (SSIs).

Incisional SSIs
Superficial: Incisional (skin and subcutaneous tissues)
Deep: Incisional (deeper soft deep fascia, muscles, and tissues beneath subcutaneous tissue of the incision)
Organ/space SSIs
Any part of the anatomy other than body wall layers that was manipulated during the procedure

The degree of intraoperative contamination can be divided into four categories: (1) clean (no gross contamination from exogenous or endogenous sources); (2) lightly contaminated (clean-contaminated); (3) heavily contaminated; and (4) infected (in which obvious infection has been encountered during operation). The infection rate is about 1.5% in clean cases. Clean-contaminated wounds (eg, with gastric or biliary surgery) are infected about 2–5% of the time. Heavily contaminated wounds, as in operations on the unprepared colon or emergency operations for intestinal bleeding or perforation, may have an infection risk of 5–30%. Wise use of isolation techniques, preoperative antibiotics, and delayed primary closure will keep rates of surgical site infections within acceptable limits. Since even a minor surgical site infection significantly prolongs hospitalization and increases economic loss, all reasonable efforts must be made to keep the infection rate as low as possible.

The risk of wound infection is influenced but not entirely determined by the degree of contamination. Multiple patient risk factors and perioperative characteristics can increase the likelihood of surgical site infections (Table 8–3).

The susceptibility of the host is usually but not always local. Susceptibility is also proportionate to the oxygen tension in the operative wound. Wound tissue PO_2 in turn is proportionate to arterial PO_2 and the perfusion rate. The perfusion rate is generally determined by the cardiac output and by the tone of the sympathetic nervous system. Sympathetic tone, ie, the degree of peripheral vasoconstriction, is determined by the patient's surface temperature, the degree of pain, the blood volume, and the degree of fear. Therefore, susceptibility to infection can be reduced by such simple methods as rapid infusion of additional fluids, warming, better pain control, and oxygen administration (but only after perfusion has been ensured). Contrary to popular opinion, urinary output correlates poorly with the incidence of wound infection. When the infection risk is high, wound tissue PO_2 can be measured, monitored, and supported. Appropriate technology is available.

Table 8–3. Surgical site infection risk factors.

Host factors
Diabetes mellitus
Hypoxemia
Hypothermia
Leukopenia
Nicotine (tobacco smoking)
Long-term use of steroid or immunosuppressive agents
Malnutrition
Nares colonization with *S aureus*
Poor skin hygiene
Perioperative factors
Operative site shaving
Breaks in operative sterile technique
Early or delayed initiation of antimicrobial prophylaxis
Inadequate intraoperative dosing of antimicrobial prophylaxis
Infected or colonized surgical personnel (skin or surgical attire)
Prolonged hypotension
Poor operating room air quality (contaminated ventilation)
Contaminated operating room instruments or environment
Poor wound care postoperatively

Clinical Findings

Wound infections usually appear between the fifth and tenth days after surgery, but they may appear as early as the first postoperative day or even years later. The first sign is usually fever, and postoperative fever requires inspection of the wound. The patient may complain of pain at the surgical site. The wound rarely appears severely inflamed, but edema may be obvious because the skin sutures appear tight.

Palpation of the wound may disclose an abscess. A good method is to pour surgical soap on the wound and, using it as a lubricant, palpate gently with the gloved hand. Firm or fluctuant areas, crepitus, or tenderness can be detected with minimal pain and contamination. The rare infection deep to the fascia may be difficult to recognize. In doubtful cases, one can carefully open the wound in the suspicious area using meticulous sterile technique. If no pus is present, the wound can be closed immediately with skin tapes. Cultures even of clean wounds that are successfully reclosed are often positive.

Differential Diagnosis

Differential diagnosis includes all other causes of postoperative fever, wound dehiscence, and wound herniation (see Chapter 4).

Prevention

Detailed recommendations for the prevention of surgical site infections (and the relevant supporting data) have been published by the CDC. In general, there are three main aspects to prevention of infection: (1) careful, gentle, clean surgery; (2) reduction of contamination; and (3) support of the patient's defenses, including use of prophylactic antibiotics. The surgeon who traumatizes tissue, leaves foreign bodies or hematomas in wounds, uses too many ligatures, and exposes the wound to drying or pressure from retractors is exposing patients to needless risks of infection.

The purpose of sutures is to approximate tissues and hold them securely, and the right number to use is as few as will accomplish this aim. Since sutures strangulate tissue, they should be tied as loosely as the requirements of approximation permit. Subcutaneous sutures should be used rarely. Using skin tapes instead of skin sutures or staples lowers infection rates, especially in contaminated wounds.

Severely contaminated wounds in which subcutaneous infection is likely to develop are best left open initially and managed by delayed primary closure. This means that the deep layers are closed while skin and subcutaneous tissues are left open, dressed with sterile gauze, inspected on the fourth or fifth day, and then closed (preferably with skin tapes) if no sign of infection is seen. A clean granulating open wound is preferable to a wound infection. Scarring from secondary healing is usually minimal.

Prophylactic antibiotics are indicated whenever wound contamination during the operation can be predicted to be high (eg, operations on the colon). Excessively liberal use of antibiotics is not reasonable. The incidence of postoperative infections in clean operations is not diminished by administration of antimicrobials, and the prophylactic use of these drugs must be reserved for selected cases at high risk for infection.

Treatment

The basic treatment of established wound infection is to open the wound and allow it to drain. Antibiotics are not necessary unless the infection is invasive, manifested by a surrounding zone of soft tissue inflammation (erythema and edema). Culture should be performed to help locate the source and prevent further infection in other patients; to gain a preview of bacterial flora in case other infections develop deep to the wound or in case the existing infection becomes invasive; and to select preoperative antibiotics in case the wound must be entered again.

Prognosis

Most wound infections make illness more severe. Wound infection correlates positively with death rates but is not often the cause of death. It may tip the scales against successful operation.

Bergamini TM et al: The importance of tissue antibiotic activity in the prevention of operative wound infection. J Antimicrob Chemother 1989;23:303.

Culver DH et al: Surgical wound infection rates by wound class, operative procedure, and patient risk index. National Nosocomial Infections Surveillance System. Am J Med 1991;91:152S.

CELLULITIS

Cellulitis is a common invasive nonsuppurative infection of connective tissue. The term is loosely used and often misapplied. The microscopic picture is one of severe inflammation of the dermal and subcutaneous tissues. Although PMNs predominate on Gram stain, there is no gross suppuration except perhaps at the portal of entry.

Clinical Findings

Cellulitis usually appears on an extremity as a brawny red or reddish-brown area of edematous skin. It advances rapidly from its starting point, and the advancing edge may be vague or sharply defined (eg, in erysipelas). A surgical wound, puncture, skin ulcer, or patch of dermatitis is usually identifiable as a portal of entry. The disease often occurs in susceptible patients, eg, alcoholics with postphlebitic leg ulcers. Most cases are caused by streptococci or staphylococci, but other bacteria have been involved. A moderate or high fever is almost always present.

Lymphangitis arising from cellulitis produces red, warm, tender streaks 3–4 mm wide leading from the infection along lymphatic vessels to the regional lymph nodes. There is no suppuration. Bacteria are difficult to obtain for culture, but blood culture is sometimes positive.

Differential Diagnosis

Since the visible features of cellulitis are all due to inflammation, the words inflammation and cellulitis have sometimes been used imprecisely as synonyms. Some forms of inflammation are associated with suppuration requiring incision and drainage, whereas cellulitis as such is not.

Thrombophlebitis is often difficult to differentiate from cellulitis, but phlebitic swelling is usually greater, and tenderness may localize over a vein. Homans' sign does not always make the differentiation—nor does lymphadenopathy. Fever is usually greater with cellulitis, and pulmonary embolization does not occur in cellulitis.

Contact allergy, such as poison oak, may mimic cellulitis in its early phase, but dense nonhemorrhagic vesiculation soon discloses the allergic cause.

Chemical inflammation due to drug injection may also mimic streptococcal cellulitis.

The appearance of hemorrhagic bullae and skin necrosis suggests necrotizing fasciitis.

Treatment

Therapy should consist of rest, elevation, warm packs, and an oral or intravenous antibiotic. Warm packs elevate subcutaneous tissue temperature, and if regional blood supply is normal they can raise local oxygen tension, which should support clearing of infection. Semisynthetic penicillins or first-generation cephalosporins are usually effective. If a clear response has not occurred in 12–24 hours, one should suspect an abscess or consider the possibility that the causative agent is a gram-negative rod or resistant organism. The patient must be examined once daily or more often to detect a hidden abscess masquerading within or under an area of cellulitis.

DIFFUSE NECROTIZING INFECTIONS

These infections are particularly dangerous because they frequently are difficult to diagnose, are extremely toxic, and spread rapidly, often leading to limb amputation. It is for these reasons that the popular press has characterized the causative bacteria as "flesh-eating" or "meat-eating." Although several classification systems for diffuse necrotizing infections have been published, most are not practical since they are based upon historical descriptions and eponyms. The American College of Surgeons recently published a classification system based on clinical presentation, anatomic site of primary tissue involvement, and the microbiology of the causative organisms (Table 8–4). The four known pathogenic factors are the presence of an anaerobic wound, bacterial exotoxins, bacterial synergy, and thrombosis of nutrient bridging vessels.

Classification & Clinical Findings

A. Clostridial Infections

Clostridia are saprophytes. Vegetative and spore forms are widespread in soil, sand, clothing, and feces. They are generally fastidious anaerobes requiring a low redox potential to grow and to initiate conversion of the spores into vegetative, toxin-producing pathogens. Tis-

Table 8–4. Classification of diffuse necrotizing infections.

Clostridial
Necrotizing cellulitis
Myositis
Nonclostridial
Necrotizing fasciitis
Streptococcal gangrene

sue redox potentials in vivo are diminished by impaired blood supply, muscle injury, pressure from casts, severe local edema, foreign bodies, or oxygen-consuming organisms. On Gram stain they appear as relatively large, gram-positive, rod-shaped bacteria. Clostridial infections frequently occur in the presence of other bacteria, especially gram-negative bacilli. A broad spectrum of disease is caused by clostridia, ranging from negligible surface contamination through invasive cellulitis of connective tissue to invasive anaerobic infection of muscle with massive tissue necrosis and profound shock. Six species cause infection in humans; *Clostridium perfringens* (80% of cases), *C novyi,* and *C septicum* are the species most frequently isolated.

Clostridia proliferate and produce toxins that diffuse into the surrounding tissue. *C tetani* and *C botulinum* produce extremely potent biologic toxins. As the pathogens responsible for tetanus and food-borne botulism, respectively, they owe their virulence to toxin production (see below). Other clostridia, however, are highly invasive. For example, *C perfringens* produces a large number of exotoxins that destroy the local microcirculation. This allows further invasion, which can advance at an astonishing rate. The alpha toxin, a necrotizing lecithinase, is thought to be particularly important in this sequence, but other toxins, including collagenase, hyaluronidase, leukocidin, protease, lipase, and hemolysin, also contribute. When the disease has advanced sufficiently, toxins enter the systemic circulation, causing the features of SIRS and, if untreated, ultimately septic shock, multiple organ dysfunction syndrome (MODS), and death. The severity and progress of the local lesion can be judged by the general state of the patient as well as by the local signs of infection. Immunosuppressed patients are particularly susceptible.

Many open wounds are superficially infected or contaminated with clostridia without developing significant infections. The condition is not invasive because the surrounding tissue is basically healthy and the clostridia are confined to necrotic surface tissue. Debridement of dead surface tissue is usually the only treatment necessary. A crepitant abscess or cellulitis has a characteristic brown seropurulent exudate and mousy odor. Invasion is usually superficial to the deep fascia and may spread very quickly, producing discoloration of the skin. Delayed or inadequate debridement of injured tissue after devascularizing injury is the most common setting. Severe pain suggests extension into muscle compartments (myositis). The disease characteristically progresses rapidly, with loss of blood supply to the infected muscle. Profound shock can appear early, rapidly leading to organ dysfunction (MODS). Air bubbles—often visible on plain radiographs (gas gangrene)—and crepitus may be present. However, gas in the tissues is not a good differentiating point, since some clostridial species do not produce gas (eg, *C novyi*); since nonclostridial organisms often produce gas (eg, *E coli*); and since air can enter tissues through a penetrating wound.

B. Nonclostridial Infections

Necrotizing fasciitis is caused by multiple nonclostridial bacterial pathogens. Infection usually involves a mixed microbial flora, often including microaerophilic streptococci, staphylococci, aerobic gram-negative bacteria, and anaerobes, especially peptostreptococci and bacteroides. Fasciitis usually begins in a localized area such as a puncture wound, leg ulcer, or surgical wound. The infection spreads along the relatively ischemic fascial planes, leading to thrombosis of penetrating vessels. Overlying subcutaneous tissue and skin are thus devascularized. Externally, hemorrhagic bullae are usually the first sign of skin death. The skin is usually anesthetic, and crepitus is occasionally present. The fascial necrosis is usually wider than the skin appearance indicates. The patient often seems alert and unconcerned but appears toxic. At operation, the finding of edematous, dull-gray, and necrotic fascia and subcutaneous tissue confirms the diagnosis. Thrombi in penetrating vessels are often visible.

Group A streptococcus (*S pyogenes*) is a bacterium frequently found on the skin and in the throat. Severe invasive infections with group A streptococci associated with shock and organ failure (streptococcal gangrene) are uncommon but have been reported with increasing frequency since the 1980s. This type of infection is also referred to as streptococcal toxic shock syndrome. The incidence of these infections was one to ten cases per 100,000 population in the United States in 1998. Those with chronic immunosuppressive illnesses, such as cancer, diabetes, and end-stage renal disease, and those taking corticosteroids are at increased risk.

Streptococcal organisms release at least five different types of exotoxins. The sudden onset of severe pain is the most common presenting symptom, usually in an extremity associated with a wound. Fever and other signs of systemic infection are frequently present at the time of presentation. Shock and renal dysfunction are usually present within the first 24 hours after admission. Invasion of deeper layers, especially muscle, is uncommon.

Treatment

The major emphasis in treatment is inevitably surgical. Suspicion should be directed toward any wound incurred out of doors and contaminated with a foreign body, soil, or feces and any wound in which tissue (particularly muscle) has been extensively injured. This type of wound should be carefully examined, with the patient under sufficient anesthesia to permit full inspection and debridement of devitalized tissue, including muscle.

It is often difficult to distinguish necrotic from edematous tissue. Careful daily inspections of the wound will determine whether repeated debridement will be necessary. Daily debridement under anesthesia may be required, since these lesions are extensive and the degree of tissue viability is often difficult to assess in the operating room. Tight fascial compartments must be decompressed. Wide-open drainage is essential and may require extensive denudation. A functional extremity can usually be salvaged in fasciitis; if not, amputation can be safely performed later.

It is important to avoid confusing fasciitis with deep gangrene. It is a tragic error to amputate an extremity when removal of dead skin and fascia will suffice. Immediate amputation is necessary when there is diffuse myositis with complete loss of blood supply or when adequate debridement would clearly leave a useless limb. When viability of the remaining tissue is assured and the infection has been controlled, soft tissue deficits can be covered with skin grafts.

Antibiotics are often essential but are ineffective without primary surgical intervention. Given the polymicrobial nature of many necrotizing infections and the difficulty of distinguishing them clinically, broad-spectrum antibiotic therapy is indicated. Broad empiric regimens include intravenous (1) penicillin and an aminoglycoside plus clindamycin; (2) imipenem-cilastatin; or (3) Unasyn plus an aminoglycoside. Some authorities recommend also giving immune globulin (400 mg/kg/d intravenously for 5 days) for documented streptococcal toxic shock syndrome. Gram stain and intraoperative culture of the infected tissue will help to narrow the antibiotic spectrum once bacterial sensitivities are available.

In severe cases of infection, the importance of resuscitative therapy cannot be overemphasized. Debridement often leaves a large raw surface that may bleed extensively and contribute to massive insensible water losses. Intravascular volume must be maintained by infusions of crystalloid; plasma and blood are transfused as needed to correct coagulopathy or anemia. Diabetes mellitus, if present, must be treated aggressively.

Hyperbaric oxygenation has been reported anecdotally to be beneficial adjuvant therapy for clostridial infections, but it cannot replace the primary role of surgical intervention as no amount of increased arterial PO_2 can force oxygen into dead tissue. Hyperbaric oxygen inhibits bacterial invasion but does not eliminate the focus of infection.

Prognosis

Diffuse necrotizing infections are potentially lethal diseases. With adequate treatment, deaths should occur only when treatment is delayed or when patients are already severely ill with other comorbidities (eg, diabetes mellitus) or have advanced bacterial invasion of vital structures. About 20% of patients with necrotizing fasciitis and more than half of patients with streptococcal toxic shock syndrome die. The prognosis for salvage of functioning limbs is not favorable. Limbs affected with myonecrosis often become useless and must be amputated to save life.

Stevens DL: Streptococcal toxic-shock syndrome: spectrum of disease, pathogenesis, and new concepts in treatment. Emerg Infect Dis 1995;1:69.

FURUNCLE, CARBUNCLE, & HIDRADENITIS

Furuncles and carbuncles are cutaneous abscesses (primary pyodermas) that begin in skin glands and hair follicles. Hair follicles normally contain bacteria. Furuncles (boils) usually start in infected hair follicles, though some are caused by retained foreign bodies and other injuries. If the pilosebaceous apparatus becomes obstructed at the skin level, the development of a furuncle can be anticipated. Because the base of the hair follicle may lie in subcutaneous tissue, the infection can spread as cellulitis or it can form a subcutaneous abscess. If a furuncle results from confluent infection of hair follicles, a central core of skin may become necrotic and will slough when the abscess is drained. Furuncles may take a phlegmonous form, ie, extend into the subcutaneous tissue, forming a long, flat abscess. A carbuncle is a deep-seated mass of fistulous tracts between infected hair follicles. Furuncles are the most common surgical infections, but carbuncles are rare.

Furuncles can be multiple and recurrent (furunculosis). Furunculosis usually occurs in young adults and is associated with hormonal changes resulting in impaired skin function. The commonest organisms are staphylococci and anaerobic diphtheroids.

Hidradenitis suppurativa is a serious skin infection of the axillae or groin consisting of multiple abscesses of the apocrine sweat glands. The condition often becomes chronic and disabling. The cause is unknown but may involve a defect of terminal follicular epithelium.

Clinical Findings

Furuncles itch and cause pain. The skin first becomes red and then turns white and necrotic over the top of the abscess. There is usually some surrounding erythema and induration. Regional nodes may become enlarged. Systemic symptoms are rare.

Carbuncles usually start as furuncles, but the infection dissects through the dermis and subcutaneous tissue in a myriad of connecting tunnels. Many of these small extensions open to the surface, giving the appearance of large furuncles with many pustular openings. As carbuncles enlarge, the blood supply to the skin is destroyed and the central tissue becomes necrotic. Carbuncles on the back of the neck are seen almost exclusively in diabetic patients or other relatively immunocompromised patients. The patient is usually febrile and mildly toxic. This is a serious problem that demands immediate surgical attention. Diabetes or some other immunosuppressive condition (eg, HIV disease) must be suspected and treated when a carbuncle is found.

Differential Diagnosis

On occasion, the surgeon may be confronted with a localized area of erythema and induration without obvious suppuration. Many such lesions will go on to central suppuration and become obvious furuncles. On the other hand, when these lesions are located near joints or over the tibia or when they are widely distributed, one must consider such differential diagnoses as rheumatoid nodules, gout, bursitis, synovitis, erythema nodosum, fungal infections, some benign or malignant skin tumors, and inflamed (but not usually infected) sebaceous or epithelial inclusion cysts.

Hidradenitis is differentiated from furunculosis by skin biopsy, which shows typical involvement of the apocrine sweat glands. One suspects hidradenitis when abscesses are concentrated in the apocrine gland areas, ie, the axillae, groin, and perineum. Carbuncles are rarely confused with any other condition.

Complications

Any of these infections may cause suppurative phlebitis when located near major veins. This is particularly important when the infection is located near the nose or eyes. Central venous thrombosis in the brain is a serious complication, and abscesses on the face usually must be treated with antibiotics as well as by prompt incision and drainage.

Hidradenitis may disable the patient but rarely has systemic manifestations. Carbuncles on the back of the neck may in rare cases lead to epidural abscess and meningitis.

Treatment

The classic therapy for furuncle is drainage, not antibiotics. Invasive carbuncles, however, must be treated by excision and adjuvant antibiotic therapy. Between these two extremes, the use of antibiotics depends on the location of the abscess and the extent of infection.

Patients with recurrent furunculosis may be diabetic or immunodeficient. Approximately 50% of patients in a recent study had impaired neutrophil function; treatment with vitamin C appeared to improve neutrophil function and the clinical response. Frequent washing with soaps containing hexachlorophene or other disinfectants is advisable. It may also be necessary to advise extensive laundering of all personal clothing and disinfection of the patient's living quarters in order to reduce the reservoirs of bacteria.

When an abscess fails to resolve after a superficial incision, the surgeon must look for a small opening to a deeper and larger subcutaneous abscess, ie, a **collar-button abscess.**

Carbuncles are often more extensive than the external appearance indicates. Incision alone is almost always inadequate, and excision with electrocautery is required. Excision is continued until the many sinus tracts are removed—usually far beyond the cutaneous evidence of suppuration. It is sometimes necessary to produce a large open wound. This may appear to be drastic treatment, but it achieves rapid cure and prevents further spread. The large wound usually contracts to a small scar and does not usually require skin grafting, because carbuncles tend to occur in loose skin on the back of the neck and on the buttocks, where contraction is the predominant form of repair.

Hidradenitis is usually treated by drainage of the individual abscess followed by careful hygiene. The patient must avoid astringent antiperspirants and deodorants. Painting with mild disinfectants is sometimes helpful. Fungal infections should be searched for if healing after drainage does not occur promptly. If none of these measures is successful, the apocrine sweat-bearing skin must be excised; if the deficit is large, closure with a skin graft may be indicated. The choice of antibiotic must reflect the frequent polymicrobial origin of these infections, including mixed aerobic and anaerobic bacteria. Topical clindamycin was beneficial in a randomized controlled trial. In a separate trial, systemic therapy with tetracycline yielded similar results when compared with topical clindamycin. Isotretinoin may be useful in some cases.

Brook I et al: Aerobic and anaerobic microbiology of axillary hidradenitis suppurativa. J Med Microbiol 1999;48:103.

Brown TJ et al: Hidradenitis suppurativa. South Med J 1998;91:1107.

Jemec GB et al: Topical clindamycin versus systemic tetracycline in the treatment of hidradenitis suppurativa. J Am Acad Dermatol 1998;39:971.

Levy R et al: Vitamin C for the treatment of recurrent furunculosis in patients with impaired neutrophil functions. J Infect Dis 1996;173:1502.

ANTIBIOTIC-ASSOCIATED COLITIS

The incidence of colonic dysfunction secondary to antibiotic use has increased over the past decade. Although all antimicrobial agents are implicated, aminopenicillins, cephalosporins, and clindamycin are commonly used in clinical care and, thus, are most often implicated. Illness results from antibiotic-induced relative changes in normal colonic flora, with resultant overgrowth of some commensals, usually *C difficile.* These bacteria, normally present in the feces of 5% of healthy persons, can be induced to release two types of toxins (cytotoxin A and cytotoxin B) that induce inflammation and mucosal damage. The spectrum of disease ranges from diarrhea to severe, potentially life-threatening colitis associated with mucosal ulceration, bacteremia, and septic shock. The pathognomonic finding on colonoscopy is an elevated, yellow pseudomembrane of necrotic mucosa ("pseudomembranous colitis"). The clinical presentation is characterized by fever, abdominal distention, and usually copious diarrhea in postoperative patients who have recently been exposed to antimicrobial therapy. Although not commonly assessed, stool smear shows numerous fecal leukocytes. *C difficile* toxin A and B can be readily detected by commercially available cytotoxic assays or enzyme immunoassays (EIA). Other organisms that rarely cause colitis include salmonella species, *Clostridium perfringens, Candida albicans,* and *Staphylococcus aureus.*

Treatment includes intravenous fluid resuscitation, correction of electrolyte disorders, and withdrawal of antibiotics if possible. Moderate to severe cases are treated with metronidazole, 250 mg orally three to four times per day, for 14 days. Oral vancomycin is also effective, but current guidelines suggest that use be reserved for those who are critically ill or who have not responded to metronidazole—or in whom this agent is contraindicated because of allergy. Recurrence of symptoms, which occurs in up to 20% of cases, requires repeated antibiotic treatment; many experts also recommend adjunctive attempts to normalize colonic flora with either probiotic therapy or fecal instillations.

Environmental spread of *C difficile* has been reported, poor hand washing has been implicated, and use of hypochlorite solution as an environmental control strategy has been an effective intervention to control high rates of endemicity.

Cleary RK: *Clostridium difficile*-associated diarrhea and colitis: clinical manifestations, diagnosis, and treatment. Dis Colon Rectum 1998;41:1435.

Cunha BA: Nosocomial diarrhea. Crit Care Clin 1998;14:329.

Frost F et al: Increasing hospitalization and death possibly due to *Clostridium difficile* diarrheal disease. Emerg Infect Dis 1998;4:619.

Mayfield JL et al Environmental control to reduce transmission of *Clostridium difficile.* Clin Infect Dis 2000;31:995.

Surawicz CM et al: Pseudomembranous colitis: causes and cures. Digestion 1999;60:91.

TETANUS

Tetanus is a specific anaerobic infection mediated by a neurotoxin that causes nervous irritability and tetanic muscular contractions. The causative organism, *Clostridium tetani,* enters and flourishes in hypoxic wounds contaminated with soil or feces (eg, deep puncture from stepping on a nail). The tetanus-prone wound is usually a puncture wound or one containing devitalized tissue or a foreign body. The occurrence of tetanus in the United States has dropped over the last 5 decades; the lowest annual average ever was reported recently (41 cases, 1995–1997). This improvement is attributed to the increasingly widespread use of tetanus toxoid and improved wound management (see below), including the use of prophylaxis against tetanus in emergency rooms. Tetanus continues to be a severe disease primarily of older adults who are unvaccinated or inadequately vaccinated; during 1995–1997, a disproportionately high number of cases (35%) were reported in persons aged 60 or older.

Tetanus is a clinical diagnosis, as confirmatory laboratory tests are not routinely available. Wound isolation of the organism is neither sensitive nor specific. Symptoms of tetanus may occur as soon as 1 day following exposure or as long as several months later; the median incubation period is 7 days. The first symptoms are usually pain or tingling in the area of injury, limitation of movements of the jaw ("lockjaw"), and spasms of the facial muscles (risus sardonicus). These are followed typically by stiffness of the neck, dysphagia, and laryngospasm. In more severe cases, spasms of the muscles of the back produce opisthotonos. As chest and diaphragm spasms occur, longer and longer periods of apnea follow. The temperature is normal or slightly elevated. The severity of cases varies widely; some are very mild and barely recognizable.

The CDC regularly revises its recommendations for the prevention and treatment of tetanus (www.cdc.gov/nip). Importantly, serosurveys indicate that at least 40% of adults over the age of 60 may lack protective levels of circulating tetanus antitoxin. Because people of all ages are exposed to tetanus, each person should be actively immunized with tetanus toxoid, beginning with routine childhood immunization and continuing with booster injections every 10 years (Table 8–5). It is thus imperative that all patients with traumatic wounds be queried regarding previous tetanus prophylaxis. Tetanus prophylaxis in injured patients depends on the history of immunization and the type of wound. A tetanus-diphtheria (Td) booster (active immunization for clean wounds), tetanus immune globulin (TIG; passive immunization for contaminated wounds), or both may be indicated.

Table 8–5. Tetanus immunization and prophylaxis.

Indication	Immunization or Prophylaxis[1]
Routine adult immunization	Td 0.5 mL every 10 years (or a single booster at age 50)[2]
Clean minor wounds	
Prior immunization unknown or < 3 doses	Td 0.5 mL
Prior immunization > 3 doses	Td 0.5 mL if last dose > 10 years ago
Other wounds	
Prior immunization unknown or < 3 doses	Td 0.5 mL and TIG
Prior immunization > 3 doses	Td 0.5 mL (unless last dose < 5 years ago)

[1]Td = adult tetanus-diphtheria booster; TIG = tetanus immune globulin 250 units IM. If given concurrently with Td, give at separate site.

[2]Patients who have never received an initial vaccination series should receive the complete series.

If established tetanus is suspected, intensive treatment should be started immediately. Mainstays of therapy include neutralization of the toxin with TIG, excision and debridement of the suspected wound, intravenous high-dose penicillin, ventilatory support if indicated, and protection from sudden stimuli. The death rate is approximately 18% in established tetanus. An attack of tetanus does not confer lasting immunity, and patients who have recovered from the disease require active immunization according to the usual recommended schedules.

[CDC National Immunization Program—Epidemiology and Prevention of Vaccine-Preventable Diseases] http://www.cdc.gov/nip/publications/pink/tetanus.pdf

Diphtheria, tetanus, and pertussis: recommendations for vaccine use and other preventive measures: recommendations of the Immunization Practices Advisory Committee (ACIP), Centers for Disease Control and Prevention. MMWR Morb Mortal Wkly Rep 1991;40(RR-10):1.

Tetanus surveillance: United States, 1995–1997. MMWR Morb Mortal Wkly Rep 1998;47(SS-2):1.

Tetanus surveillance: United States, 1991–1994. MMWR Morb Mortal Wkly Rep 1997;46(SS-2):15.

RABIES

Rabies is a preventable viral encephalitis of mammals transmitted through the saliva of an infected animal. Humans are usually inoculated by the bite of a rabid bat, raccoon, skunk, fox, or other wild animal; however, about 30% of victims have no memory or evidence of a bite. Other reported modes of transmission include mucous membranes (eyes, nose, mouth), aerosolization, and corneal transplantation. In 1997, there were 8513 reported cases of rabies (93% in wild animals), but only four were in humans. The number of human deaths due to rabies in the United States decreased dramatically during the 20th century, down to one to four deaths per year in the late 1990s.

Since the established disease is almost invariably fatal, early preventive measures are essential. The wound should be washed thoroughly with soap and water. Information useful in determining the risk of potential rabies infection includes the geographic location of the incident, the type of animal involved, how the exposure occurred, the vaccination status of the animal, and whether it can be safely captured and tested for rabies. Rabies prophylaxis has proved nearly 100% successful, as most human deaths now occur in people who fail to seek medical assistance. Each year, approximately 18,000 people receive rabies vaccine prophylaxis before exposure, and an additional 40,000 receive prophylaxis (vaccine plus immune globin) after exposure. The latest information regarding both pre- and postexposure prophylaxis is available at the CDC's Rabies Section website (http://www.cdc.gov/ncidod/dvrd/rabies).

The rabies virus has a distinctive bullet shape and a nonsegmented, negative-stranded RNA genome. After local (primary) infection, the virus enters peripheral nerves and is transported to the central nervous system, making it difficult to detect (eclipse phase). The subsequent incubation period varies in humans from several days to typically 1–3 months. Clinical symptoms begin with pain and numbness around the site of the wound, followed by nonspecific flu-like symptoms of fever, irritability, malaise, and progressive cerebral dysfunction. Delirium, hallucinations, insomnia, paralysis, and convulsions occur terminally.

The direct fluorescent antibody (DFA) test on brain tissue is used most frequently to diagnose rabies in animals. A complement of tests are used routinely in humans, because no single test can rule out rabies absolutely: serum and cerebrospinal fluid are tested for antibodies, skin biopsy is examined by DFA, and saliva can be tested by nested reverse transcription polymerase chain reaction (RT-PCR).

Rabies Section, Viral and Rickettsial Zoonoses Branch, Division of Viral and Rickettsial Diseases, National Center for Infectious Diseases, Centers for Disease Control and Prevention, Atlanta, Georgia. http://www.cdc.gov/ncidod/dvrd/rabies

ECHINOCOCCOSIS

Echinococcosis (hydatid disease) is caused by the microscopic cestode parasites *Echinococcus granulosus* and *E multilocularis* (1–4 mm tapeworms), which form larval cysts in mammalian tissue. Foxes, coyotes, dogs, and cats are the definitive hosts that harbor the adult tapeworms in their intestines; these animals are not harmed by the worms and have no symptoms. Ova are passed in the feces and are ingested by intermediate hosts such as cattle, humans, rodents, and particularly sheep. The ova penetrate the intestine and pass via the portal vein to the liver (75%) and then to the lung (15%) or other tissues. In the liver, the ovum typically develops into a cyst filled with clear fluid. Brood capsules containing scoleces bud into the cyst lumen. Such "endocysts" may cause secondary intraperitoneal cyst formation if spilled into the peritoneal cavity. Because the cysts grow slowly, patients may be asymptomatic for several years. Pain or discomfort in the upper abdominal region and weight loss may occur as a result of the cyst enlarging. Eosinophilia is present in about 40% of patients. Serologic diagnosis may be substantiated by immunoassays. Ultrasonography and CT scanning readily demonstrate cysts. In some patients, the parasite dies, the cyst wall calcifies, and therapy is not required. However, surgery is most often required, though removal of the cyst is not usually 100% effective for eradication of infection. Excision of the cyst intact, if practical, is preferred. Because of the dangers of anaphylaxis or implantation, care must be taken to avoid rupturing the cyst and spilling its contents into the peritoneal cavity. In some cases, the cyst fluid can be aspirated and replaced by a scolicidal agent (hypertonic sodium chloride solution or sodium hypochlorite solution). After surgery, albendazole or mebendazole may be necessary to keep the cyst from growing back. The overall death rate is about 15%, but it is only 4% in surgically treated cases.

Ammann RW et al: Cestodes. Echinococcus. Gastroenterol Clin North Am 1996;25:655.

Clarkson MJ: Hydatid disease. J Med Microbiol 1997;46:24.

http://www.dpd.cdc.gov/dpdx/HTML/Echinococcosis.htm

Taylor BR et al: Current surgical management of hepatic cyst disease. Adv Surg 1997;31:127.

ACTINOMYCOSIS & NOCARDIOSIS

Actinomycosis and nocardiosis are chronic, slowly progressive infections that may involve many tissues, resulting in the formation of granulomas and abscesses that drain through sinuses and fistulas. Although the causative organisms are true bacteria, the lesions resemble those produced by mycobacteria, fungi, and cancer, making accurate diagnosis difficult.

Actinomyces israelii is a gram-positive, non-acid-fast, filamentous organism that usually shows branching and may break up into short bacterial forms. It is a strict anaerobe and part of the normal flora of the human oropharynx and upper intestinal tract. Inflammatory nodular masses, abscesses, and draining sinuses occur most commonly in the head and neck. One-fifth of patients with actinomycosis have primary lesions in the chest and an equal proportion in the abdomen, most commonly involving the appendix and cecum. Multiple sinuses are commonly formed, and the pus may contain yellow "sulfur granules" of tangled filaments. The inflammatory lesions are often hard and relatively painless and nontender. Systemic symptoms, including fever, are variably present. The discharging sinus tracts or fistulas usually become secondarily infected with other bacteria. Abdominal actinomycosis may produce an abdominal mass mimicking a malignant process or may give rise to appendicitis. If the appendix perforates, multiple lesions and sinuses of the abdominal wall form. Thoracic actinomycosis may give rise to cough, pleural pain, fever, and weight loss, simulating mycobacterial or mycotic infection. Later in the course of the disease, the sinuses perforate the pleural cavity and the chest wall, often involving ribs or vertebrae. CT scanning and needle aspiration may be helpful diagnostically. All forms of actinomycosis are treated with penicillin G for many weeks. Although long-term antibiotic therapy appears to be very successful and can avoid the need for operation, preoperative exclusion of other diagnoses is difficult. Surgical extirpation or drainage of lesions therefore is frequently performed.

Nocardiae are gram-positive, branching, filamentous organisms that may be acid-fast; *Nocardia asteroides* is the most common isolate. The filaments often fragment into bacillary forms. They are aerobes rarely found in the normal flora of the respiratory tract. Nocardiosis may present in two forms. One is localized, chronic granuloma with suppuration, abscess, and sinus tract formation resembling actinomycosis. A specialized disorder occurs in the extremities as Madura foot (mycetoma), with extensive bone destruction but little systemic illness. The second form is a systemic infection, usually beginning as pneumonitis with suppuration and progressing via the bloodstream to involvement of other organs, eg, meninges or brain. Systemic nocardiosis produces fever, cough, and weight loss and resembles mycobacterial or mycotic infections. The mortality rate of nocardial bacteremia is as high as 50%. It is particularly apt to occur as a complication of immunodeficiency in patients with chronic obstructive pulmonary disease, cancer, chronic granulomatous disease, HIV-associated disease, or immunoremittive drug regimens. Nocardiosis is best treated with sulfonamides (eg, sulfadiazine or trimethoprim-sulfamethoxazole) or, when severe, with imipenem and amikacin, for many weeks. Surgical drainage of abscesses, excision of fistulas, and repair of defects are essential features of management.

Cintron JR et al: Abdominal actinomycosis. Dis Colon Rectum 1996;39:105.

Conant EF et al: Actinomycosis and nocardiosis of the lung. J Thorac Imaging 1992;7:75.

Kontoyiannis DP et al: *Nocardia* bacteremia. Report of 4 cases and review of the literature. Medicine 1998;77:255.

Lerner PI: Nocardiosis. Clin Infect Dis 1996;22:891.

Menendez R et al: Pulmonary infection with *Nocardia* species: a report of 10 cases and review. Eur Respir J 1997;10:1542.

Smego R Jr et al: Actinomycosis. Clin Infect Dis 1998;26:1255.

Tarabichi M, Schloss M: Actinomycosis otomastoiditis. Arch Otolaryngol 1993;119:561.

Threlkeld SC et al: Update on management of patients with *Nocardia* infection. Curr Clin Top Infect Dis 1997;17:1.

Warren NG: Actinomycosis, nocardiosis, and actinomycetoma. Dermatol Clin 1996;14:85.

VENOMOUS BITE INJURIES

SNAKEBITE

About 8000 people a year in the United States are bitten by venomous snakes. About one-third of these snakebites do not result in envenomation, as the snake may bite but not inject venom, or may eject it onto the skin in a superficial fashion. Death from serious envenomation occurs in only 9–15 victims per year in the United States. In comparison, there are about 120 United States deaths a year from wasp and bee stings and about 150 deaths per year from lightning.

Identification of Snake

The vast majority of snakebites in the United States are from nonvenomous snakes. Distinguishing whether the patient has been bitten and envenomed by a venomous snake, bitten but not envenomed, or bitten by a nonvenomous snake is critical prior to starting treatments that may not only cause discomfort but may also produce serious side effects. These distinctions require identification of the attacking snake through knowledge of snake taxonomy, anatomy, and geographic distribution. Coloration patterns and fang or tooth marks are deceptive and unreliable identification criteria.

There are about 120 species of snakes in the United States, of which 26 are venomous. The indigenous venomous snakes of North America can be placed in four groups. Three groups are pit vipers of the subfamily Crotalidae: rattlesnakes, with multiple species within the two genera (*Crotalus* and *Sistrurus*); the cottonmouth or water moccasin (*Agkistrodon piscivorus*); and the copperhead (*Agkistrodon contortrix*). Pit vipers can be distinguished from nonvenomous snakes by a round mouth and a pit between the eyes and the nares on each side. They have retractable canaliculated fangs that can rapidly spring into biting position and deliver venom. The large venom glands also give the head a triangular or diamond appearance. North American pit vipers have vertically oriented elliptiform irises. The vast majority of North American pit vipers have a primarily hemotoxic venom, but some, particularly the Mojave rattlesnake, have primarily neurotoxic venom.

The coral snake is in the fourth group of indigenous North American venomous snakes. It is a member of the family Elapidae, which also includes the much more dangerous cobras and kraits. Two different genera of coral snakes (the Western coral snake, *Micruroides euryxanthus,* and the Eastern coral snake, *Micrurus fulvius*) are found chiefly in the western and southern states, respectively, with distinct nonoverlapping geographic distributions. Coral snakes have small mouths, short teeth, and deliver secreted venom into prey through created lacerations. A coral snake bite lacks the characteristic fang marks of bites by pit vipers, sometimes making the bite hard to detect. The degree of envenomation depends upon the size of the snake and the duration of contact; rapid removal of the snake from the victim reduces the risk of significant poisoning. Coral snake venom is primarily neurotoxic and unrelated to that of the pit vipers. Victims may experience respiratory paralysis, one of the hazards of neurotoxic venom.

Some nonpoisonous snakes such as the red milk snake and the scarlet king snake mimic the bright red, yellow, and black coloration of the coral snake. True coral snakes will have red bands immediately adjacent to yellow bands; the nonvenomous mimics will have black bands immediately adjacent to the red bands, thus giving rise to the colloquial mnemonic: "Red on black, venom lack; red on yellow, kill a fellow." This rhyming maxim applies only to North American coral snakes.

The family Elapidae includes the cobras, kraits, and mambas, common in Asia and Africa. Their fangs are at the front of the mouth and are small to moderate in size. Cobra venoms are quite toxic and internationally are a major cause of human snakebite morbidity and mortality.

Sea snakes of the family Hydrophiidae are closely related to the cobras. They are native to the Indian and Pacific Oceans, live primarily in an aquatic—usually marine—environment, and have short fixed fangs and flattened tails. Their venom is quite toxic, and envenomation is a significant risk for fishermen in areas where these snakes are indigenous.

The family Atractaspidae consists of the side-fanged vipers, including the mole vipers and stiletto snakes. They are confined to Africa and the Middle East. Their venom contains sarafotoxins, which are endothelin-like compounds causing potent smooth muscle contraction and vasoconstriction.

Snake Venom

The poison glands of snakes are modified salivary glands that secrete a complex mixture of specialized proteins and enzymes. Snake venom has several functions, including rapid immobilization of prey, predigestion of prey, and defense against predators. Snake venom effects are often broadly and superficially classified as primarily hemotoxic or neurotoxic. Caution should be used, as a combination of multiple effects may present either concurrently or consecutively.

Hemotoxic effects are mediated by proteolytic enzymes, peptides, and metalloproteins that can cause local tissue destruction directly and by intimal injury to blood vessels, followed by thrombosis and necrosis. Activation of the coagulation cascade can occur at multiple points, resulting in net anticoagulation. Direct lysis of red blood cells can cause acute hemolytic anemia and produce acute tubular necrosis. Bites on extremities may cause subcutaneous tissue destruction and loss of digits. Myotoxins can cause compromise of muscle compartments from direct myonecrosis as well as from local pressure effects. Secondary edema can develop rapidly in tissues from both cytokine release and from hemorrhage into local tissues. Systemic effects can include pulmonary edema. Intravascular injection can cause a more severe systemic reaction, with diffuse bleeding from thrombocytopenia and hypofibrinogenemia.

Snake venom neurotoxins often act upon the acetylcholine receptor system, with different components causing postsynaptic antagonism and acetylcholinesterase activity. Other components may cause direct presynaptic nerve cell destruction.

Clinical Findings

Bites by nonvenomous snakes are much more common than bites by venomous snakes. These should be treated as simple puncture wounds, employing an appropriate antitetanus agent.

The excitement and hysteria associated with any snakebite may give rise to symptoms of disorientation, faintness, dizziness, hyperventilation, a rapid pulse, and even primary shock (even with nonvenomous snakebites).

A bite by a venomous snake results in envenomation in only 50–70% of cases. Envenomation may be classified as mild (scratch followed by minimal swelling and not much pain), moderate (fang marks, local swelling, and definite pain), or severe (fang marks, severe and progressive swelling and pain).

Most rattlesnakes, copperheads, water moccasins, and coral snakes tend to bite superficially, but a few bites penetrate muscle. The severity of the poisoning will depend upon the species and size of the snake; the age and size of the victim; the location, depth, nature, and number of bites; the amount of venom injected; the victim's sensitivity to the venom; the microbes present in the snake's mouth; and the availability of appropriate first-aid treatment and subsequent medical care.

Local signs of envenomation include puncture marks, local ecchymosis and discoloration, vesicles and bullae, and rapid appearance of swelling and edema at the injured area, with further progression to adjacent areas. The pain of the bite can be quite severe. Additional signs of hypotension, diaphoresis, nausea, weakness, and faintness are common. Perioral or peripheral paresthesias, taste changes, and fasciculations can be seen. Signs suggestive of neurotoxic envenomation include dysphagia, dysphonia, diplopia, headache, weakness, and respiratory distress. Laboratory findings may include hemoconcentration initially due to fluid shifts, with later decreases in red blood cells and platelets. Urinalysis may show hematuria, glycosuria, and proteinuria. Prothrombin and partial thromboplastin times are often abnormal.

Treatment

The presence and degree of envenomation dictate treatment measures; other factors, such as time elapsed since being bitten, prehospital care, and the age and size of the victim, are also critical.

Wash the bite with soap and water or an antiseptic if available. Apply a broad, firm compressing bandage over the bite which does not restrict arterial and venous blood flow, and immobilize the bitten area at a level below the heart. Remove rings and constrictive devices, and keep the victim at rest and warm. Popular conceptions of first-aid measures including tourniquets, wound incision and suction, application of ice, cryotherapy, electrical shock, and ingestion of alcohol are of no proved value and may be hazardous to both the patient and the caregiver, particularly in the field setting. Transporting the patient to a medical facility is an important field management objective. Identification of the snake is helpful but of lower priority.

Standard evaluation and support of respiratory and cardiovascular function are initial priorities. Laboratory evaluation should include blood typing and crossmatching, coagulation studies, a complete blood count, and urinalysis. Local wound management includes cleansing and disinfection. Systemic measures include administration of antitetanus agent for tetanus prophylaxis and broad-spectrum antibiotic therapy. Fasciotomy should be reserved only for the uncommon compartment syndrome with compartment pressures documented above 30–40 mm Hg. Local bite area excision is not useful and should not be done.

The decision to use antivenin is based upon identification of the offending snake as venomous, discernment of the degree and manifestations of envenomation, time elapsed since the bite, and laboratory abnormalities. Several grading systems have been proposed but are inadequate at present, and the decision to use antivenin must be individualized to each patient and his or her specific reaction to the snakebite.

Effective specific antivenins are available for the bites of both pit vipers and Eastern coral snakes. Crotalidae polyvalent antivenin is effective against all North American pit vipers; North American coral snake antivenin is effective only for the Eastern coral snake. Because these equine antivenins have serious potential side effects, including both allergic reactions and serum sickness, their administration should be reserved for patients with significant bites or after early signs of envenomation have appeared.

Antivenin should ideally be administered early and as a diluted continuous intravenous infusion; local injection in or around the bite is contraindicated. Crotalidae polyvalent antivenin is most effective if given within 4 hours after a bite, of less value after 8 hours, and of questionable value after 30 hours. Severe envenomations may require over 30 vials; antivenin may be appropriate for moderate envenomation, but the risks outweigh the benefits if envenomation is minimal. Coral snake antivenin may be started prior to any neurologic symptoms if the offending snake is suspected or confirmed to be a coral snake.

Chippaux JP et al: Venoms, antivenoms and immunotherapy. Toxicon 1998;36:823.

Holstege CP et al: Crotalid snake envenomation. Crit Care Clin 1997;13:889.

Thwin MM et al: Snake envenomation and protective natural endogenous proteins: a mini review of the recent developments (1991–1997). Toxicon 1998;36:1471.

ARTHROPOD BITES

Stings and bites of arthropods are most often merely a nuisance. Some arthropods, however, can produce death by direct toxicity or by hypersensitivity reactions. Because of their prevalence and numbers, bees and wasps kill more people than any other venomous animal, including snakes.

Bees & Wasps

When a bee stings, it becomes anchored by the two barbed lancets, so that withdrawal is impossible. In the struggle, a bee will usually avulse its stinging apparatus and die. After being stung by a bee, one should scrape the exuded poison sac with a sharp knife. Any attempt to pull the poison apparatus out will simply cause more venom to be squeezed into the tissue. The stinger, once embedded, remains present. If this has occurred in an eyelid, it may irritate the globe of the eye months after the sting.

The stinging lancets of the wasp are not barbed and can easily be withdrawn by the insect to allow it to reinsert or to escape. It is unusual, therefore, to find a stinger left in place after a wasp sting. The females of the variety called yellow jackets are very aggressive. These insects sometimes bite before stinging.

The venom of bees and wasps contains histamine, basic protein components of high molecular weight, free amino acids, hyaluronidase, and acetylcholine. Antigenic proteins are species-specific and may lead to cross-reactivity between insects. Symptoms of arthropod stings may vary from minimal erythema to a marked local reaction of severe systemic toxicity (especially from multiple stings). Infection may occur. A generalized allergic reaction has been described that resembles serum sickness.

Early application of ice packs to reduce swelling is indicated. Elevation of the extremity is also useful. Oral antihistamines may be of some use in reducing urticaria. Parenteral corticosteroids may reduce delayed inflammation. If infection occurs, treatment consists of local debridement and antibiotics. Moderately severe reactions will present as generalized syncope or urticarial reactions. If an anaphylactic reaction or severe reaction is present, aqueous epinephrine, 0.5–1 mL of 1:1000 solution, should be given intramuscularly. A repeat dose may be given in 5–10 minutes, followed by 5–20 mg of diphenhydramine slowly intravenously. Administration of corticosteroids and general supportive measures such as oxygen administration, plasma expanders, and pressor agents may be required in case of shock. Previously sensitized patients should carry identifying tags and a kit for emergency intramuscular injection of epinephrine.

It is possible to immunize persons against bee and wasp stings, but cost-benefit analyses indicate that this is rarely if ever indicated.

Spiders

While all spiders have poison glands and use venom for killing prey, only a few spider venoms are harmful to humans. As with all toxic exposures, the very young, the elderly, and patients with comorbid medical conditions are at greatest risk for adverse outcomes.

A. Lactrodectism

The bite of the Lactrodectus species of spiders (widow and red-back spiders), including the black widow (*Latrodectus mactans*) and the red-backed spider (*L hasseltii*), has primarily systemic neurotoxic effects. The female black widow spider can be identified by its characteristic black body with a red hourglass-like pattern on the abdomen; the male of the species does not bite, and is smaller. The potent venom of this genus acts by destabilization of cell membranes and degranulation at nerve terminals with release of neurotransmitters. Neuromuscular toxic effects of black widow venom occur by presynaptic motor end plate neurotransmitter release, with release of norepinephrine and acetylcholine causing excessive stimulation and eventual fatigue of the motor end plate and muscle.

Symptoms of envenomation begin with pain at the bite location, followed by later development of abdominal wall muscle rigidity, abdominal pain and cramping, respiratory difficulty with potential paralysis, and lower extremity weakness. Massive hemolysis, severe hypotension, and cardiovascular collapse can be seen. Local skin changes are often minimal and can make identification of the bite difficult.

Intravenous administration of calcium gluconate may relieve muscle pain and spasm, but similar relief can be obtained from intravenous opioids and benzodiazepines. Ice packs may improve localized pain from the bite. Most symptoms are self-limited and, with appropriate supportive therapy, resolve within 48 hours, though full recovery may take over a week. A horse antivenin is available but may cause allergic reactions. Antivenin may be indicated in severely symptomatic patients to speed recovery and perhaps to prevent development of long-term symptoms related to neurologic dysfunction.

B. Loxoscelism

The brown recluse spider (*Loxosceles reclusa*) is dark tan and has a violin-shaped mark on the back of the main body. Envenomation can have significant and prolonged local dermonecrotic effects, with development of deep necrotic wounds at the bite site that are very slow to heal. Systemic loxoscelism with intravascular coagulation and renal failure has been seen but is uncommon. The venom appears to cause local tissue necrosis by dissociating normal neutrophil responses of adhesion and degranulation from transmigration and shape changes. Phospholipase D and sphingomyelinase D also contribute to the local necrosis, as well as venom-induced platelet aggregation. Alterations in complement activation and binding of venom to erythrocyte membranes contribute to hemolysis.

The bite may have local signs of erythema and edema but usually minimal associated pain. With serious envenomation, hemorrhagic bullae surrounded by localized ischemia develop over 24–48 hours. The local lesion usually progresses to a very slowly healing ulcer. Systemic effects of fever, urticaria, lymphangitis, nausea, and emesis can develop. Hemolysis and disseminated intravascular coagulation are rare.

Loxoscelism is managed by supportive measures. Cleansing of the bite, rest, and elevation of the affected area are appropriate. While tissue loss is common, early excision of lesions is also associated with poor wound healing. Conflicting data exist regarding systemic treatment with corticosteroids; evidence for efficacy of dapsone (50–100 mg/d) treatment remains anecdotal.

Anderson PC: Spider bites in the United States. Dermatol Clin 1997;15:307.

Bond GR: Snake, spider, and scorpion envenomation in North America. Pediatr Rev 1999;20:147.

Clark RF et al: Clinical presentation and treatment of black widow spider envenomation: a review of 163 cases. Ann Emerg Med 1992;21:782.

Gendron B: *Loxosceles reclusa* envenomation. Am J Emerg Med 1990;8:51.

Gomez HF et al: Loxosceles spider venom induces the production of alpha and beta chemokines: implications for the pathogenesis of dermonecrotic arachnidism. Inflammation 1999;23:207.

Hobbs GD et al: Comparison of hyperbaric oxygen and dapsone therapy for Loxosceles envenomation. Acad Emerg Med 1996;3:758.

Phillips S et al: Therapy of brown spider envenomation: a controlled trial of hyperbaric oxygen, dapsone, and cyproheptadine. Ann Emerg Med 1995;25:363.

Wilson DC et al: Spiders and spider bites. Dermatol Clin 1990;8:277.

Wright SW et al: Clinical presentation and outcome of brown recluse spider bite. Ann Emerg Med 1997;30:28.

ANTIMICROBIAL CHEMOTHERAPY

PRINCIPLES OF SELECTION OF ANTIMICROBIAL DRUGS

Initial & Subsequent Selection of Antimicrobial Agents

The decision to initiate, continue, and stop antimicrobial chemotherapy should be prudently determined. This involves a series of decisions: (1) The judgment, on the basis of clinical impression, that a microbial infection probably exists. (2) Formulation of a differential diagnosis and associated microbial pathogens. (3) Procurement of specimens likely to provide a microbiologic diagnosis. (4) Prompt, initial empiric therapy presumed to be effective against the suspected organisms. (5) Observation of the clinical response to the prescribed antimicrobial and laboratory identification of a putative microbial pathogen. (6) Continuation of the empiric regimen or a switch to pathogen-directed therapy. The clinical status of the patient contributes to the speed with which therapy must be instituted, the route of administration, and the type of therapy. Although laboratory data need not always overrule a decision based on clinical and empiric grounds, judicious targeted use of antimicrobial therapy minimizes drug exposure, adverse events, costs, and the emergence of multidrug-resistant organisms (MDROs).

Selection of an Antimicrobial Drug by Laboratory Tests

When an organism has been identified from a clinical isolate, it is often possible to select the drug of choice on the basis of current clinical experience (see Table 8–6). Given the rising rates of MDROs and geographic differences in antibiogram data (tables of pathogen-specific antibiotic sensitivities), laboratory tests for antimicrobial drug susceptibility are necessary, particularly if the isolated organism is of a type that often exhibits drug resistance, eg, enteric gram-negative rods.

The US National Committee for Clinical Laboratory Standards (NCCLS) has published several consensus recommendations, with updates, for bacterial susceptibility testing. Susceptibility testing methods include disk diffusion and dilution (broth microdilution, plates, and E-tests) procedures. Disk diffusion tests indicate whether a microbial culture is susceptible or resistant to serum-achievable, in vivo drug concentrations with conventional dosage regimens. In contrast, dilution procedures allow reporting of the minimal inhibitory concentration (MIC) and minimal bactericidal concentration (MBC). The MIC is the lowest concentration of a specific antimicrobial agent that inhibits the test organism, while the MBC is the lowest concentration of a specific antimicrobial agent that kills the test organism. The NCCLS prefers reporting of susceptibility via disk diffusion or MIC over MBC. The duration of appropriate therapy depends on the nature of the infection and the severity of the clinical presentation. When clinical improvement does not occur after initiation of putatively appropriate antimicrobial therapy, possible explanations include the following:

(1) The organism isolated from the specimen may not be the one responsible for the infectious process. The usual cause is failure to culture tissue instead of pus.

(2) There may have been failure to drain a collection of pus, debride necrotic tissue, or remove a foreign body. Antimicrobials can never take the place of surgical drainage and removal.

(3) Superinfection may occur in the course of prolonged chemotherapy. New microorganisms may have replaced the original infectious agent. This is particularly common with open wounds or sinus tracts.

(4) The drug may not reach the site of active infection in adequate concentration. The pharmacologic properties of antimicrobials determine their absorption and distribution. Certain drugs penetrate phagocytic cells poorly and thus may not reach intracellular organisms. Some drugs may diffuse poorly into the eye, central nervous system, or pleural space unless injected directly into the area.

(5) At times, two or more microorganisms participate in an infectious process but only one may have been isolated from the specimen. The antimicrobial being used may be effective only against the less virulent organism.

(6) In the course of drug administration, resistant microorganisms may have been selected from a mixed population, and these drug-resistant organisms continue to grow in the presence of the drug.

Assessment of Drug & Dosage

An adequate therapeutic response is an important but not always sufficient indication that the right drug is being given in the right dosage. Proof of drug activity in serum against the original infecting organisms may provide important support for a selected drug regimen even if fever or other signs of infection are continuing. In sepsis, extended-interval administration of aminoglycosides has efficacy and toxicity similar to what is associated with traditional dosing regimens, but costs are less and convenience is increased. This dosing regimen is not recommended for patients with endocarditis, pregnancy, cystic fibrosis, burns covering more than 20% of body surface area, mycobacterial infections, and anasarca. The initial dose is gentamicin or tobramycin, 5 mg/kg intravenously, or amikacin, 15 mg/kg intravenously. A follow-up random serum drug level 6–14 hours later is compared with a nomogram to determine follow-up dosing intervals.

Determining Duration of Therapy

The duration of drug therapy depends on the nature of the infection and the severity of the clinical presentation. Treatment of acute uncomplicated infections should be continued until the patient has been afebrile and clinically well for at least 72 hours. Infections at certain sites (eg, endocarditis, septic arthritis, osteomyelitis) require more prolonged therapy. In evaluating the patient's clinical response, the possibility of adverse reactions to drugs must be considered. Such reactions may mimic continuing activity of the infectious process by causing fever, skin rashes, central nervous system disturbances, and changes in blood and urine. In the case of many drugs, it is desirable to assess hepatic and renal function at intervals. Adverse events may require dose reduction or drug discontinuation.

Oliguria & Renal Failure

Oliguria and renal failure have an important influence on antimicrobial drug dosage, since most of these drugs are excreted—to a greater or lesser extent—by the kidneys. Some drugs require minor adjustments in dosage or frequency of administration. Others, such as aminoglycosides (eg, tobramycin), tetracyclines, and vancomycin, must be reduced in dosage or frequency of administration to avert toxicity in the presence of nitro-

Table 8–6. Antimicrobial drugs of choice for suspected and empiric regimens. Pathogen-directed therapy should utilize antibiogram data from regional clinical microbiology laboratory.*

Suspected or Confirmed Etiologic Agent	Drugs of First Choice	Alternative Drugs
Gram-negative cocci		
Moraxella catarrhalis	Amoxicillin-clavulanic acid or TMP-SMZ[1]	Cephalosporins,[2] erythromycin,[3] tetracycline[4]
Neisseria gonorrhoeae	Ceftriaxone	Cefixime, ciprofloxacin
Meningococcus	Penicillin[5]	Cephalosporins,[2] ampicillin, chloramphenicol
Gram-positive cocci		
Streptococcus pneumoniae (penicillin-susceptible)	Penicillin,[5] ceftriaxone ± vancomycin	Penicillin[5]
S pneumoniae (penicillin-resistant)	macrolide, cephalosporin,[6] vancomycin (combination therapy may be indicated)	
Streptococcus, hemolytic, groups A, B, C, G	Penicillin[5]	Erythromycin,[3] cephalosporin,[6] vancomycin
Viridans streptococci	Penicillin[5] ± aminoglycosides[7]	Cephalosporin,[6] vancomycin
Staphylococcus, methicillin-resistant	Vancomycin + gentamicin or rifampin (or both)	TMP-SMZ, ciprofloxacin
Staphylococcus, non-penicillinase-producing	Penicillin	Cephalosporin, vancomycin
Staphylococcus, penicillinase-producing	Penicillinase-resistant penicillin[8]	Vancomycin, cephalosporin[6]
Enterococci	Ampicillin ± gentamicin	Vancomycin + gentamicin
Gram-negative rods		
Acinetobacter	Aminoglycoside[7] + imipenem	Minocycline, TMP-SMZ[1]
Bacteroides, oropharyngeal strains	Penicillin,[5] clindamycin	Metronidazole, cephalosporin[2,6]
Bacteroides, gastrointestinal strains	Metronidazole	Cefoxitin, chloramphenicol, clindamycin, TMP-SMZ[1]
Brucella	Tetracycline[4] + streptomycin	Tetracycline,[4] ciprofloxacin
Campylobacter	Erythromycin[3]	Imipenem, newer cephalosporins[2]
Enterobacter	TMP-SMZ,[1] aminoglycoside[7]	Ampicillin, TMP-SMZ[1]
Escherichia coli (sepsis)	Aminoglycoside,[7] newer cephalosporins[2]	Ampicillin, cephalosporin[6]
E coli (first urinary infection)	Sulfonamide,[9] TMP-SMZ[1]	Ampicillin and chloramphenicol[1]
Haemophilus (meningitis, respiratory infections)	Cephalosporins[2]	TMP-SMZ,[1] aminoglycoside[7]
Klebsiella	Cephalosporins[2]	TMP-SMZ
Legionella (pneumonia)	Macrolide + rifampin	3rd generation fluoroquinolone Chloramphenicol
Pasteurella (Yersinia) (plague, tularemia)	Streptomycin, tetracycline[4]	Cephalosporins,[2] aminoglycoside[7]
Proteus mirabilis	Ampicillin	Aminoglycoside[7]
Proteus vulgaris and other species	Newer cephalosporins[2]	Ceftazidime or cefoperazone + aminoglycoside; imipenem + aminoglycoside; aztreonam
Pseudomonas aeruginosa	Aminoglycoside[7] + antipseudomonal penicillin[10]	Chloramphenicol, tetracycline,[4] TMP-SMZ
Burkholderia pseudomallei (melioidosis)	Ceftazidime	Chloramphenicol + streptomycin
Burkholderia mallei (glanders)	Streptomycin + tetracycline[4]	TMP-SMZ,[1] ciprofloxacin, ampicillin, chloramphenicol
Salmonella	Ceftriaxone	TMP-SMZ[1]
Serratia, Providencia	Cephalosporins,[2] aminoglycoside[7]	Ampicillin, tetracycline,[4] ciprofloxacin, chloramphenicol
Shigella	TMP-SMZ[1]	

(continued)

Table 8–6. Antimicrobial drugs of choice for suspected and empiric regimens. Pathogen-directed therapy should utilize antibiogram data from regional clinical microbiology laboratory.* (continued)

Suspected or Confirmed Etiologic Agent	Drugs of First Choice	Alternative Drugs
Stenotrophomonas maltophilia	TMP-SMZ[11] Timentum	Clavulanate/ticarcillin
Vibrio (cholera, sepsis)	Tetracycline[4]	TMP-SMZ[1]
Gram-positive rods		
Actinomyces	Penicillin[5]	Tetracycline[4]
Bacillus (eg, anthrax)	Penicillin[5]	Erythromycin[3]
Clostridium (eg, gas gangrene, tetanus)	Penicillin[5]	Metronidazole, chloramphenicol, clindamycin
Corynebacterium diphtheriae	Macrolide	Penicillin[5]
Corynebacterium jeikeium	Vancomycin	Ciprofloxacin
Listeria	Ampicillin + aminoglycoside[7]	TMP-SMZ[1]
Acid-fast rods		
Mycobacterium tuberculosis	INH + rifampin + pyrazinamide + ethambutol	Other antituberculosis drugs
Mycobacterium leprae	Dapsone + rifampin, clofazimine	Ethionamide
Mycobacterium kansasii	INH + rifampin + ethambutol	Other antituberculosis drugs
Mycobacterium avium-intracellulare	Ethambutol + rifampin + clarithromycin	Other antituberculosis drugs
Mycobacterium fortuitum chelonei	Amikacin + doxycycline	Cefoxitin, erythromycin, sulfonamide
Nocardia	Sulfonamide,[9] TMP-SMZ[1]	Minocycline
Spirochetes		
Borrelia (Lyme disease, relapsing fever)	Tetracycline,[4] ceftriaxone	Penicillin,[5] erythromycin[3]
Leptospira	Penicillin[5]	Tetracycline[4]
Treponema (syphilis, yaws, etc)	Penicillin[5]	Ceftriaxone erythromycin,[3] tetracycline[4]
Mycoplasmas	Macrolide or tetracycline[4]	3rd generation fluoroquinolone
Chlamydiae		
C psittaci	Tetracycline[4]	Chloramphenicol
C trachomatis (urethritis or pelvic inflammatory disease)	Doxycycline or erythromycin[3]	Ofloxacin or azithromycin
C pneumoniae	Tetracycline[4]	Erythromycin[3]
Rickettsiae	Tetracycline[4]	Chloramphenicol

*N Engl J Med 1997;336:708. (From the New England Journal of Medicine.)

[1]TMP-SMZ is a mixture of 1 part trimethoprim and 5 parts sulfamethoxazole.

[2]Cephalosporins include cefotaxime, cefuroxime, ceftriaxone, ceftazidime, ceftizoxime, and others.

[3]The oldest macrolide, erythromycin estolate, is best absorbed orally but carries the highest risk of hepatitis; erythromycin stearate and erythromycin ethyl succinate are also available.

[4]All tetracyclines have similar activity against microorganisms. Dosage is determined by rates of absorption and excretion of various preparations.

[5]Penicillin G is preferred for parenteral injection; penicillin V for oral administration—to be used only in treating infections due to highly sensitive organisms.

[6]Older cephalosporins are cephalothin, cefazolin, cephapirin, and cefoxitin for parenteral injection; cephalexin and cephradine can be given orally.

[7]Aminoglycosides—gentamicin, tobramycin, amikacin, netilmicin—should be chosen on the basis of local patterns of susceptibility.

[8]Parenteral nafcillin or oxacillin; oral dicloxacillin, cloxacillin, or oxacillin.

[9]Oral sulfisoxazole and trisulfapyrimidines are highly soluble in urine; parenteral sodium sulfadiazine can be injected intravenously in treating severely ill patients.

[10]Antipseudomonal penicillins: ticarcillin, carbenicillin, mezlocillin, azlocillin, piperacillin.

[11]First choice for previously untreated urinary tract infection is a highly soluble sulfonamide or TMP-SMZ.

gen retention. General guidelines for the administration of such drugs to patients with renal failure are set forth in Table 8–7. The administration of particularly nephrotoxic antimicrobials such as aminoglycosides to patients in renal failure requires guidance by direct assays of serum drug concentrations.

In the newborn or premature infant, excretory mechanisms for some antimicrobials are poorly developed, and for this reason special dosage schedules must be used in order to avoid accumulation of drugs.

Prevention & Control of Spread of Vancomycin Resistance Genes

In an attempt to prevent and control the spread of vancomycin resistance, judicious uses of vancomycin were identified. Vancomycin should not be used routinely in the following circumstances: (1) for surgical prophylaxis in a patient without a severe beta-lactam allergy; (2) for empiric therapy of a febrile neutropenic patient unless initial evidence suggests an infection with gram-positive bacteria; (3) for treatment of a single positive blood culture with a coagulase-negative staphylococcus; (4) for continued empiric administration against presumed infection when cultures do not confirm a beta-lactam-resistant gram-positive organism; (5) as prophylaxis against infection of a central or peripheral intravascular catheter; (6) for first-line treatment of *C difficile* colitis; and (7) for topical application or irrigation.

Distinction should be made between colonization and infection with methicillin-resistant *S aureus* (MRSA) or vancomycin-resistant enterococci (VRE). For MRSA, the majority of bloodstream infections are treated with either vancomycin (dosed to therapeutic trough levels of 15) or linezolid (600 mg IV or orally twice daily). Eradication of MRSA nasal carriage begins with a 5-day course of twice-daily intranasal mupirocin. For VRE, the majority of bloodstream infections are treated with either chloramphenicol or linezolid. No regimen has been effective in eradicating enteric carriage of VRE. Spontaneously clearance of enteric VRE, to vancomycin-susceptible enterococci, has been reported in healthy hosts after discontinuation of selective antimicrobial drug pressure.

ANTIMICROBIAL DRUGS USED IN COMBINATION

Indications

Possible reasons for employing two or more antimicrobials simultaneously instead of a single drug are as follows:

(1) To provide prompt treatment in a severely ill patient suspected of having a serious microbial infection. A good guess about the most probable two or three pathogens is made, and drugs are empirically targeted to those organisms. Before such treatment is started, it is essential that adequate specimens be obtained for identifying the etiologic agent in the laboratory.

(2) To delay the emergence of antimicrobial resistance to one drug in chronic infections by the use of a second or third non-cross-reacting drug. Treatment of active tuberculosis is a good example.

(3) To aid in the presence of mixed infections, particularly those following massive trauma.

(4) To achieve bactericidal synergism (see below). In a few infections, eg, enterococcal sepsis, a combination of drugs is more likely to eradicate the infection than either drug used alone. Unfortunately, such synergism is unpredictable, and a given drug pair may be synergistic for only a single microbial strain.

Disadvantages

The following disadvantages of using antimicrobial drugs in combinations must always be considered:

(1) There is a greater chance of adverse drug reactions or drug hypersensitivity.

(2) Expense is greater.

(3) There is potentially no greater efficacy than an effective single drug.

(4) Empiric, broad-spectrum antimicrobial coverage may compromise the effort to establish a specific etiologic diagnosis.

(5) On rare occasions, drug antagonism with resultant increased rates of illness and death (as noted in bacterial meningitis when a bacteriostatic drug (eg, tetracycline or chloramphenicol) was given with (or prior to) a bactericidal drug (eg, penicillin or ampicillin). Notably, antagonism can usually be overcome by giving a larger dose of one of the drugs in the pair and is therefore an infrequent problem in clinical therapy.

Synergism

Antimicrobial synergism occurs in the situations listed below. Synergistic drug combinations must be selected by specialized laboratory procedures.

(1) One drug inhibits a microbial enzyme that might destroy a second drug. For example, clavulanic acid inhibits bacterial beta-lactamase and protects simultaneously administered amoxicillin from destruction.

(2) Sequential block of a metabolic pathway. Sulfonamides inhibit utilization of extracellular *p*-aminobenzoic acid by susceptible bacteria. Trimethoprim inhibits the reduction of folates, the next metabolic step. Simultaneous use of sulfamethoxazole and trimethoprim can be strikingly more effective in some bacterial infections than use of either drug alone. Similarly, sulfamethoxazole plus pyrimethamine has greatly en-

hanced activity in *Pneumocystis jiroveci* pneumonia and toxoplasma infections.

(3) One drug enhances greatly the uptake of a second drug. Cell-wall inhibitor (beta-lactam) drugs enhance the penetration of various bacteria by aminoglycosides and thus increase the overall bactericidal effect. Eradication of infections by enterococci is enhanced by combinations of a cell wall-active agent and an aminoglycoside. Similarly, the control of sepsis by pseudomonas and other gram-negative rods may be enhanced by combination of a cephalosporin and an aminoglycoside.

Antifungal Therapy

The clinical presentations of yeast and molds are protean and not pathogen specific. Yeastlike fungi are typically round or oval and reproduce by budding; molds are composed of tubular structures called hyphae that grow by branching and longitudinal extension. The selection of an antifungal drug is usually based on the result of a culture obtained for clinical indications or persistent systemic symptoms in a host already receiving broad-spectrum antibacterial therapy. Given the extensive and prolonged use of antibacterial agents, the rising number of immunocompromised hosts, and the availability of antifungal therapeutic options, there has been an increasing need for the judicious use of antifungal therapeutic agents. Recommendations for treatment will depend upon the characterization of the yeast in the mycology laboratory, perhaps supplemented by in vitro testing of fungi. Assessment of drug, dosage, duration of therapy, and evaluation of adverse events is often best done in consultation with an infectious disease specialist. Drug options include the following.

A. Amphotericin B

Amphotericin B is a polyene antimicrobial agent that disrupts the fungal cell by binding to ergosterol in the plasma membrane. Historically, this has been the drug of choice for most systemic mycoses except *Pseudallescheria boydii* and some Fusarium species. Amphotericin B is poorly absorbed and must be administered intravenously except for topical therapy in AIDS patients with azole-resistant oral candidiasis. The initial and total intravenous infusion dose is often determined by the severity of the infection. An initial dose of 0.5–1 mg/kg is usually given over 2–4 hours. In most instances, daily prehydration with 500 mL of normal saline solution will reduce the risk of nephrotoxicity. Recognized adverse events (fever, chills, headache, myalgias, nausea and vomiting) may be reduced by premedicating the patient with acetaminophen, 600 mg orally, and diphenhydramine, 50 mg orally, plus hydrocortisone, 25–100 mg intravenously. Nephrotoxicity may occur over time in the form of distal renal tubular acidosis, hyperkalemia, hypermagnesemia, or impairment of glomerular filtration.

B. Lipid Preparations of Amphotericin B

These formulations include amphotericin B lipid complex, amphotericin B colloidal dispersion, and liposomal amphotericin B. These formulations alter the pharmacokinetics and distribution of the drug and are often substituted for treatment of infections in patients intolerant of or not responding to regular amphotericin B. Lipid formulations of amphotericin B may be indicated for patients who have documented or suspected severe systemic mycoses that are unsuitable for treatment with azoles or who have baseline renal insufficiency or risk factors for development of renal insufficiency, including a (1) Cr greater than 2.5 mg/dL or Cr clearance (Cl_{Cr}) of less than 40 mL/minute, (2) Cr greater than 2 mg/dL or Cl_{Cr} less than 60 mL/minute and receiving one nephrotoxic medication, or (3) Cr greater than 1.5 mg/dL or Cl_{Cr} less than 75 mL/minute and receiving at least two nephrotoxic medications. The nephrotoxic medications of most concern are cisplatin, cyclosporin A, aminoglycosides, foscarnet, pentamidine, cidofovir, and scheduled nonsteroidal anti-inflammatory drugs.

C. Flucytosine

Flucytosine, 25–37.5 mg/kg orally every 6 hours, is an effective agent against some isolates of candida species and *Cryptococcus neoformans.* This drug, when used in combination with amphotericin B, will enhance fungicidal activity. Flucytosine is not recommended as monotherapy and is excreted in the kidney, thus requiring alteration of dosage with renal insufficiency. The primary adverse effect is bone marrow suppression, which is dose-related and occurs with peak serum levels greater than 100 μg/mL.

D. Azoles

There are four fungistatic azoles: ketoconazole, fluconazole, itraconazole, and voriconazole. Ketoconazole is the oldest of these drugs, has the highest frequency of drug interactions, and is markedly hepatotoxic.

Fluconazole is widely distributed in the body and penetrates readily into the cerebrospinal fluid. It has been effective in the treatment of fungal urinary tract infections, oropharyngeal and esophageal candidiasis, and fungal peritonitis. For most indications, one gives 200 mg orally or intravenously as a loading dose followed by a maintenance dose of 100 mg intravenously or orally daily. Adverse events include headache, gastrointestinal side effects, elevated serum aminotransferases, and rashes.

Itraconazole is a triazole with a broad antifungal spectrum. This drug is approved by the Food and Drug Administration (FDA) for the treatment of histoplasmosis and blastomycosis both in immunocompetent and in

Table 8–7. Use of antibiotics in patients with renal failure and hepatic failure.

	Principal Mode of Excretion or Detoxification	Approximate Half-Life in Serum		Proposed Dosage Regimen in Renal Failure		Removal of Drugs by Hemodialysis	Dose After Hemodialysis	Dosage in Hepatic Failure[3]
		Normal	Renal Failure[1]	Initial Dose[2]	Maintenance Dose			
Acyclovir	Renal	2.5–3.5 hours	20 hours	2.5 mg/kg	2.5 mg/kg q24h	Yes	2.5 mg/kg	NC
Ampicillin	Tubular secretion	0.5–1 hour	8–12 hours	1 g	1 g q8–12h	Yes	1 g	NC
Azlo-, mezlo-, piperacillin	Renal 50–70%; biliary 20–30%	1 hour	3–6 hours	3 g	2 g q6–8h	Yes	1 g	1–2 g q8h
Azithromycin	Mainly liver/biliary	> 24 hours	> 24 hours	500 mg	250 mg/d	No	No	NC
Aztreonam	Renal	1.7 hours	6 hours	1–2 g	0.5–1 g q6–8h	Yes	0.5–1 g	NC
Carbenicillin	Tubular secretion	1 hour	16 hours	4 g	2 g q12h	Yes	2 g	NC
Chloramphenicol	Mainly liver	3 hours	4 hours	0.5 g	0.5 g q6h	Yes	0.5 g	0.25–0.5 g q12h
Ciprofloxacin	Renal and liver	4 hours	8.5 hours	0.5 g	0.25–0.75 g q24h	No	None	NC
Clindamycin	Liver	2–4 hours	2.4 hours	0.6 g IV	0.6 g q8h	No	None	0.3–0.6 q8h
Clarithromycin	Mainly biliary/liver	5–7 hours	22 hours	0.5–1.0 g	0.5 g q12h	Limited	Give after dialysis	NC
Erythromycin	Mainly liver	1.5 hours	1.5 hours	0.5–1 g	0.5–1 g q6h	No	None	0.25–0.5 g q6h
Fluconazole	Renal	30 hours	98 hours	0.2 g	0.1 g q24h	Yes	Give q24h dose	NC
Ganciclovir	Renal	3 hours	11–28 hours	1.25 mg/kg	1.25 mg/kg q24h	Yes	Give q24h dose	NC
Imipenem	Glomerular filtration	1 hour	3 hours	0.5 g	0.25–0.5 g q12h	Yes	0.25–0.5 g	NC
Metronidazole	Liver	6–10 hours	6–10 hours	0.5 g IV	0.5 g q8h	Yes	0.25 g	0.25 g q12h
Gatifloxacin	Renal	7–14 hours	36 hours	400 mg po/IV	200 mg q24h	No	None	NC
Levaquin	Renal	4–6 hours	76 hours	500 mg po/IV	250 mg q48h	No	None	NC

Nafcillin	Liver 80%, kidney 20%	0.75 hour	1.5 hours	1.5 g	1.5 g q5h	No	None	2–3 g q12h
Penicillin G	Tubular secretion	0.5 hour	7–10 hours	1–2 million units	1 million units q8h	Yes	500,000 units	NC
Ticarcillin	Tubular secretion	1.1 hour	15–20 hours	3 g	2 g q6–8h	Yes	1 g	NC
Trimethoprim-sulfamethoxazole	Some liver	TMP 10–12 hours; SMZ 8–10 hours	TMP 24–48 hours; SMZ 18–24 hours	320 mg TMP + 1600 mg SMZ	80 mg TMP + 400 mg SMZ q12h	Yes	80 mg TMP + 400 mg SMZ	NC
Vancomycin	Glomerular filtration	6 hours	6–10 days	1 g	1 g q6–10 days based on serum levels	None	None	NC
Cefazolin	Renal	90 min		0.5 g	0.5 g qd	Yes	0.5 g	NC
Cefuroxime	Renal	80 min		1–2 g	1–2 g qd	Yes	0.5 g	NC
Cefotetan	Renal	150 min		0.5–1 g	0.5–1 g qd	Yes	0.5 g	NC
Cefoxitin	Renal	60 min		1–2 g	1–2 g qd	Yes	0.5 g	NC
Ceftriaxone	Renal and liver	480 min		1–2 g	1–2 g qd	No	None	NC
Ceftazidime	Renal	120 min		0.5–1 g	0.5–1 g qd	Yes	0.5 g	NC

[1]Considered here to be marked by creatinine clearance of 10 mL/min or less.
[2]For a 70-kg adult with a serious systemic infection.
[3]NC = No change.

immunocompromised hosts. Formulations exist both as tablets and as an elixir and are best taken on an empty stomach, with absorption improved by increased gastric acidity. Adverse events include nausea, vomiting, rash, and early hepatitis.

Voriconazole is FDA approved for the treatment of invasive aspergillosis, where it demonstrates typical response rates of 40–50% and superiority over conventional amphotericin B.

E. Echinocandin

Caspofungin acetate, the first available drug in this class of antifungal agents, has fungicidal activity against most *Aspergillus* and *Candida* species, including azole-resistant *Candida* strains. It to be at least as effective as, and better tolerated than, amphotericin B for the treatment of esophageal candidiasis, candidemia, and invasive candidiasis.

Antiviral Agents

Eleven drugs have been approved by the FDA for the treatment of viral infections (other than those known for HIV infection). Antiviral drugs can be used for prophylaxis, suppression, preemptive therapy, or treatment of overt disease. The goals of treating acute viral infections in immunocompromised patients are to reduce the severity of illness and potential complications as well as reduction of viral transmission. The goal of antiviral therapy in patients with chronic viral infections is to prevent damage to visceral organs, especially the liver, lungs, gastrointestinal tract, and the central nervous system. The currently most commonly used drugs are acyclovir, valacyclovir, and famciclovir.

A. Acyclovir

Acyclovir is active against herpes simplex virus (HSV) and varicella zoster virus (VZV). This drug is used for the treatment of primary and recurrent genital herpes, severe herpes dermatitis, and herpes simplex encephalitis in normal hosts as well as disseminated VZV and herpes zoster ophthalmicus. For severe systemic infections, the dose is 5 mg/kg intravenously every 8 hours for HSV infections to 10 mg/kg intravenously every 8 hours for HSV encephalitis or VZV infections. The oral dose is 400 mg three times daily for HSV infection and 800 mg five times daily for localized herpes zoster infections. Dosage must be adjusted in renal failure. Side effects are uncommon.

B. Valacyclovir

Valacyclovir is an orally administered prodrug of acyclovir approved for treatment of a first herpes zoster infection or for recurring episodes of genital HSV.

C. Famciclovir

Famciclovir is an oral drug that has activity against VZV, HSV, and Epstein-Barr virus (EBV). It is approved for acute herpes zoster and treatment of recurring episodes of genital HSV at a dosage of 500 mg orally every 8 hours for 7 days or, in recurring HSV episodes, 100 mg orally every 12 hours for 5 days. Headache, nausea, and diarrhea have been reported as adverse events.

Antimycobacterial Therapy

Depending on the location of the surgical practice, empiric or pathogen-directed antituberculous therapy may be a common necessity. Effective treatment of *Mycobacterium tuberculosis* infections requires combination chemotherapy, and initial four-drug regimens are recommended in geographic areas where the prevalence of multidrug-resistant tuberculosis is greater than 4%. Primary treatment regimens include isoniazid, rifampin, ethambutol, and pyrazinamide—with or without streptomycin. Surgical patients suspected of having tuberculosis need to be placed in negative pressure rooms for the protection of health care workers and other patients. Given the public health ramifications, it is often best for the surgical team to include an infectious disease specialist in the initiation and follow-up of patients receiving antituberculous therapy.

Bailey TC et al: A meta-analysis of extended-interval dosing versus multiple daily dosing of aminoglycosides. Clin Infect Dis 1997;24:786.

Balfour HH: Antiviral drugs. N Engl J Med 1999;340:1255.

Bass JB Jr et al: Treatment of tuberculosis and tuberculosis infection in adults and children. Am J Respir Crit Care Med 1994;149:1359.

Herbrecht R et al: Voriconazole versus amphotericin B for primary therapy of invasive aspergillosis. N Engl J Med 2002;347:408.

Mondy KE et al: Evaluation of zinc bacitracin capsules vs. placebo for enteric eradication of vancomycin-resistant *Enterococcus faecium*. Clin Infect Dis 2001;33:473.

Polk R: Optimal use of modern antibiotics: emerging trends. Clin Infect Dis 1999;29:264.

Quagliarello VJ et al: Drug therapy: treatment of bacterial meningitis. N Engl J Med 1997;336:708.

Recommendations for preventing the spread of vancomycin resistance. Hospital Infection Control Practices Advisory Committee (HICPAC). MMWR Morb Mortal Wkly Rep 1995;44(RR-12):1.

Sun KO et al: Management of tetanus: a review of 18 cases. J R Soc Med 1994;87:135.

Walsh TJ et al: Voriconazole compared with liposomal amphotericin b for empirical antifungal therapy in patients with neutropenia and persistent fever. N Engl J Med 2002;346:225.

Fluid & Electrolyte Management 9

Gerard M. Doherty, MD, & Michael H. Humphreys, MD

The surgical patient is at risk for several derangements of body fluid volume and composition, some of which may be iatrogenic. Understanding the physiologic mechanisms that regulate the composition and volume of the body fluids and the principles of fluid and electrolyte therapy is essential for optimal patient management.

BODY WATER & ITS DISTRIBUTION

Total body water comprises 45–60% of body weight; the percentage in any individual is influenced by age and the lean body mass, but in healthy individuals it remains remarkably constant from day to day. Table 9–1 lists the average values of total body water as a percentage of body weight for men and women of different ages. Total body water is divided into intracellular (ICF) and extracellular (ECF) compartments. Intracellular water represents about two-thirds of total body water, or 40% of body weight. The remaining one-third of body water is extracellular. ECF is divided into two compartments: (1) plasma water, comprising approximately 25% of ECF, or 5% of body weight; and (2) interstitial fluid, comprising 75% of ECF, or 15% of body weight.

The solute composition of the intracellular and extracellular fluid compartments differs markedly (Figure 9–1). ECF contains principally sodium, chloride, and bicarbonate, with other ions in much lower concentrations. ICF contains mainly potassium, organic phosphate, sulfate, and various other ions in lower concentrations.

Even though plasma water and interstitial fluid have similar electrolyte compositions, plasma water contains more protein than interstitial fluid. This results in slight differences in electrolyte concentrations, as governed by the Gibbs-Donnan equilibrium. The plasma proteins, chiefly albumin, account for the high colloid osmotic pressure of plasma, which is an important determinant of the distribution of fluid between vascular and interstitial compartments, as defined by the Starling relationships.

The kidneys maintain constant volume and composition of body fluids by two distinct but related mechanisms: (1) filtration and reabsorption of sodium, which adjusts urinary sodium excretion to match changes in dietary intake; and (2) regulation of water excretion in response to changes in secretion of antidiuretic hormone. These two mechanisms allow the kidneys to keep the volume and osmolality of body fluid constant within a few percentage points despite wide variations in intake of salt and water. A corollary is that analysis of the composition and volume of the urine usually provides valuable clues in the diagnosis of disorders of body fluid volume and composition.

Although the movement of certain ions and proteins between the various body fluid compartments is restricted, water is freely diffusible. Consequently, the osmolality (total solute concentration) of all the body compartments is identical—normally, about 290 mosm/kg H_2O. The solutes dissolved in body fluids contribute to total osmolality in proportion to their molar concentration: In ECF, sodium and its salts account for most of the osmolality, whereas in ICF, salts of potassium are chiefly responsible. Control of osmolality occurs through regulation of water intake (thirst) and water excretion (urine volume, insensible loss, and stool water), with the kidneys being the chief regulator. If water intake is low, the kidneys can reduce urine volume and raise urine solute concentration fourfold above plasma (ie, to 1200–1400 mosm/kg H_2O). If water intake is high, the kidneys can excrete a large volume of dilute (50 mosm/kg H_2O) urine.

Concentrations of electrolytes are usually expressed as equivalent weights: A 1-molar (M) solution contains 1 gram molecular weight of a compound dissolved in 1 liter (L) of fluid; 1 equivalent (eq) of an ion is equal to 1 mole (mol) multiplied by the valence of the ion. For example, in the case of the monovalent sodium ion, 1 eq is equal to 1 mol. In the case of calcium, which is divalent, 1 eq is equal to 0.5 mol. In the relatively dilute conditions of body fluids, the sum of the molar concentrations of ions is approximately equal to total fluid osmolality. However, because the chemical activities of these solutes differ, it is usually more accurate to estimate osmolality by multiplying the serum sodium concentration by 2.

The sensitive regulation of salt and water excretion by the kidney produces an intimate relationship

Table 9–1. Total body water (as percentage of body weight) in relation to age and sex.

Age	Male	Female
10–18	59	57
18–40	61	51
40–60	55	47
Over 60	52	46

between body fluid osmolality and volume. Edelman and his coworkers showed that the osmolality of plasma or any other body fluid can be closely approximated by the sum of exchangeable sodium (Na_e^+) and its anions (A^-) plus exchangeable potassium (K_e^+) and its anions divided by total body water (TBW):

$$\text{Osmolality} = \frac{(Na_e^+ + A^-) + (K_e^+ + A^-)}{\text{TBW}} \qquad (1)$$

The plasma sodium concentration (P_{Na}) can be determined by the expression shown in equation 2:

$$P_{Na} = \frac{(Na_e^+ + (K_e^+)}{\text{TBW}} \qquad (2)$$

Although it is neither practical nor necessary to measure exchangeable sodium, exchangeable potassium, or total body water routinely, equation 2 illustrates the major factors that affect the serum sodium concentration and are important to the cause and therapy of many fluid and electrolyte disturbances.

In a steady state, the volume and composition of the urine depend upon the intake of water and dietary solutes. An average North American diet generates about 600 mosm of solute daily that must be excreted by the kidneys. Most people ingest more than 5 g of sodium chloride per day, equivalent to about 85 meq of Na^+ (1 g NaCl = 17 meq Na^+). Potassium excretion averages 40–60 meq/d. Water intake is more variable but usually amounts to about 2 L/d; an additional 400 mL of water per day is generated from cellular metabolism. Extrarenal (insensible) water loss amounts to 10 mL/kg body weight/24 h equally divided among losses from the lungs, from the skin, and in the stool. Losses from the lungs and skin may vary under physiologic conditions, but stool water rarely exceeds 200 mL/d in health. Thus, a typical 24-hour urine volume is 1500 mL and has the approximate solute concentrations shown in Table 9–2.

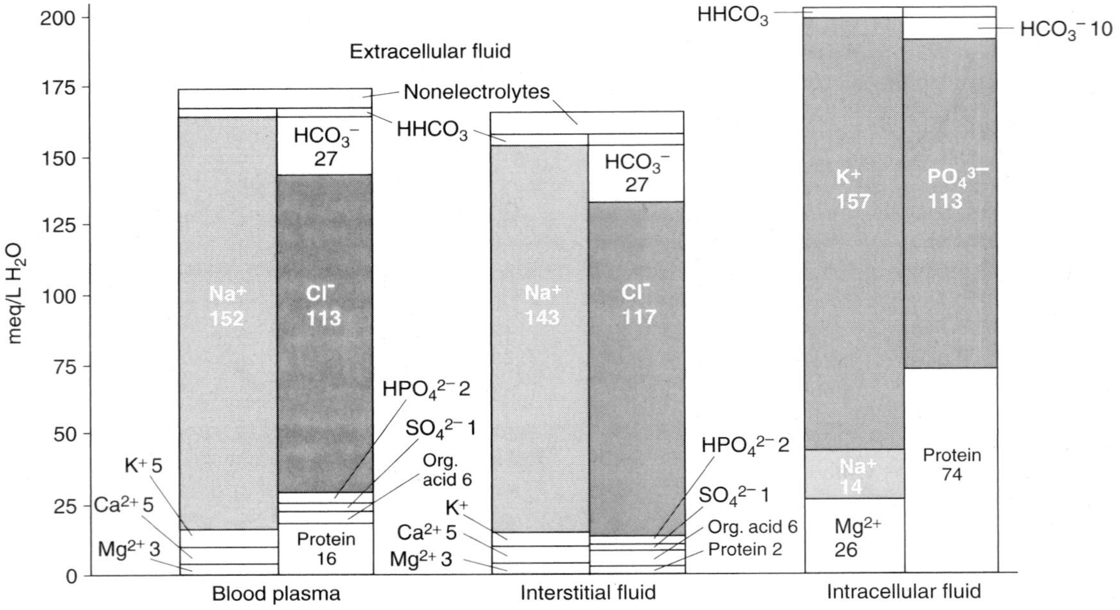

Figure 9–1. Electrolyte composition of human body fluids. Note that the values are in meq/L of water, not of body fluid. (From Leaf A, Newburgh LH: *Significance of the Body Fluids in Clinical Medicine,* 2nd ed. Thomas, 1955. Reproduced by permission from Blackwell Publishing.)

Table 9–2. Typical daily solute balances in normal subjects.

	Concentration	Total Amount
Intake		
Water	...	2 L
Ingested	...	0.4 L
Cell metabolism	...	600 mosm
Total solute	...	100 meq
Sodium	...	60 meq
Potassium		
Urinary excretion		
Water	400 mosm/kg H_2O	1.5 L
Total solute	60 meq/L	600 mosm
Sodium	36 meq/L	90 meq[1]
Potassium		54 meq[1]

[1]Small amounts of sodium and potassium are lost extrarenally (stool, sweat).

VOLUME DISORDERS

RECOGNITION & TREATMENT OF VOLUME DEPLETION

Since volume depletion is common in surgical patients, a general approach to the diagnosis and treatment of volume depletion should be developed and applied to each patient systematically. The clinical manifestations of volume depletion are low blood pressure, narrow pulse pressure, tachycardia, poor skin turgor, and dry mucous membranes. The history may suggest the reason for volume depletion. Records of intake and output, changes in body weight, urine specific gravity, and analysis of the chemical composition of the urine should confirm the clinical impression and be useful when a treatment plan is being devised. Therapy must aim to correct the volume deficit and associated aberrations in electrolyte concentrations.

VOLUME DEPLETION

The simplest form of volume depletion is water deficit without accompanying solute deficit. However, in surgical patients, water and solute deficits more often occur together. Pure water deficits occur in patients who are unable to regulate intake. They may be debilitated or comatose or may have increased insensible water loss from fever. Patients given tube feedings without adequate water supplementation and those with diabetes insipidus may also develop this syndrome. Pure water deficit is reflected biochemically by hypernatremia; the magnitude of the deficit can be estimated from the P_{Na} (equations 2, 3).

Associated findings are an increase in the plasma osmolality, concentrated urine, and a low urine sodium concentration (< 15 meq/L) despite hypernatremia. The clinical manifestations are chiefly caused by hypernatremia, which can depress the central nervous system, resulting in lethargy or coma. Muscle rigidity, tremors, spasticity, and seizures may occur. Since many patients suffering from water deficit have primary neurologic disease, it is often difficult to tell if the symptoms were caused by hypernatremia or by the underlying disease.

Treatment involves replacement of enough water to restore the plasma sodium (P_{Na}) concentration to normal. The excess sodium for which water must be provided can be estimated from equation 3:

$$\Delta Na = (140 - P_{Na}) \times TBW \qquad (3)$$

The ΔNa represents the total milliequivalents of sodium in excess of water. Divide ΔNa by 140 to obtain the amount of water required to return the serum sodium concentration to 140 meq/L. Because of the dehydration, an estimate of total body water (TBW) should be used that is somewhat lower than the normal values listed in Table 9–1. In addition to correction of the existing water deficit, ongoing obligatory water losses (due to diabetes insipidus, fever, etc) must be satisfied. Treat the patient with 5% dextrose in water unless hypotension has developed, in which case hypotonic saline should be used. Rarely, isotonic saline may be indicated to treat shock due to dehydration even though the patient is hypernatremic.

VOLUME & ELECTROLYTE DEPLETION

Combined water and electrolyte depletion may occur from gastrointestinal losses due to nasogastric suction, enteric fistulas, enterostomies, or diarrhea. Other causes are excessive diuretic therapy, adrenal insufficiency, profuse sweating, burns, and body fluid sequestration following trauma or surgery. Diagnosis of combined volume and electrolyte deficiency can be made from the history, physical signs, and records of intake and output. The clinical findings are similar to those of pure volume depletion. However, the urine Na^+ concentration is often less than 10 meq/L, a manifestation of renal sodium conservation resulting from the action of aldosterone on the renal tubule. The urine is usually hypertonic (> 1.020), with an osmolality greater than 450–500 mosm/kg. The decreased blood volume diminishes renal perfusion and often produces prerenal azotemia, reflected by elevated blood urea nitrogen

(BUN) and serum creatinine. Prerenal azotemia is characterized by a disproportionate rise of BUN compared to creatinine; the normal BUN/creatinine ratio of 10:1 is exceeded and may go as high as 20–25:1. This relationship helps differentiate prerenal azotemia from acute tubular necrosis, in which the BUN/creatinine ratio remains close to normal as the serum levels of both substances rise.

Combined water-electrolyte deficits are corrected by restoring volume and the deficient electrolytes. The magnitude of the volume deficit can be estimated by serial measurements of body weight, since acute changes in body weight primarily reflect changes in body fluid. Central venous or pulmonary artery pressure may be low in blood volume deficits and may be useful for monitoring replacement therapy.

The composition of the replacement fluid should take into account the plasma sodium concentration: If the P_{Na} is normal, fluid and electrolyte losses are probably isotonic, and the replacement fluid should be isotonic saline or its equivalent. Hyponatremia may result from salt loss exceeding water loss (ie, the decrease in Na^+_e will be greater than the decrease in TBW; equation 2) or from previous administration of hypotonic solutions. In this situation, the magnitude of the salt deficit can be calculated from equation 3.

Replacement therapy should be planned in two steps: (1) the sodium deficit should be calculated, and (2) the volume deficit should be estimated from clinical signs and changes in body weight. From these calculations, a hypothetical replacement solution can be devised in which the sodium deficit is administered as NaCl and the volume deficit as isotonic NaCl solution. Then administer isotonic NaCl solutions and monitor the patient's response (ie, urine volume and composition, serum electrolytes, and clinical signs). With restoration of ECF volume, renal perfusion improves, and excretion of water will occur while Na^+ continues to be reabsorbed. When replacement is adequate, renal function and serum Na^+ and Cl^- concentrations will return to normal.

VOLUME OVERLOAD

Hormonal and circulatory responses to surgery result in postoperative conservation of sodium and water by the kidneys that is independent of the status of the ECF volume. Antidiuretic hormone, released during anesthesia and surgical stress, promotes water conservation by the kidneys. Renal vasoconstriction and increased aldosterone activity reduce sodium excretion. Consequently, if fluid intake is excessive in the immediate postoperative period, circulatory overload may occur. The tendency for water retention may be exaggerated if heart failure, liver disease, renal disease, or hypoalbuminemia is present. Clinical manifestations of volume overload include edema of the sacrum and extremities, jugular venous distention, tachypnea (if pulmonary edema develops), increased body weight, and elevated pulmonary artery and central venous pressure. A gallop rhythm would indicate cardiac failure.

Volume overload may precipitate prerenal azotemia and oliguria. Examination of the urine usually shows low sodium and high potassium concentrations consistent with enhanced tubular reabsorption of Na^+ and water.

Management of volume overload depends upon its severity. For mild overload, sodium restriction will usually be adequate. If hyponatremia is present, water restriction will also be necessary. Diuretics must be used for severe volume overload. If cardiac failure is present, other measures must be employed, and a cardiology consultation may be necessary.

Inappropriate secretion of antidiuretic hormone (which may occur with head injury, some cancers, and burns) will produce a syndrome characterized by hyponatremia, concentrated urine, elevated urine sodium concentration, and a normal or mildly expanded ECF volume. The serum Na^+ values may drop below 110 meq/L and produce confusion and lethargy. In most cases, restriction of water intake alone will be sufficient to correct the abnormality. Occasionally, a potent diuretic (eg, furosemide) should be given and intravenous isotonic saline infused at a rate equal to the urine output; this will rapidly correct the hyponatremia. Patients with intracranial disease may also develop the syndrome of cerebral salt wasting and present with hyponatremia. However, these patients are volume-depleted, and correct treatment is sodium and volume replacement rather than water restriction.

SPECIFIC ELECTROLYTE DISORDERS

SODIUM

Regulation of the sodium concentration in plasma or urine is intimately associated with regulation of total body water (equation 2) and clinically reflects the balance between total body solute and TBW.

Hypernatremia represents chiefly loss of water; this condition has been discussed above. Current neurosurgical management of traumatic brain injury utilizes controlled hypernatremia by infusion of hypertonic saline to maintain serum Na^+ between 155 and 160 meq/L.

In addition to dilutional hyponatremia and isotonic dehydration, apparent hyponatremia developed in patients with marked hyperlipidemia or hyperproteinemia due to earlier measurement techniques since fat and protein contribute to plasma bulk even though they are not dissolved in plasma water. The sodium concentration of plasma water in this situation is usually normal. Current laboratory techniques use ion-specific electrode measurements of the serum electrolytes, so apparent hyponatremia is no longer a clinical concern.

Hyponatremia in severe hyperglycemia results from the osmotic effects of the elevated glucose concentration, which draws water from the intracellular space to dilute ECF sodium. In hyperglycemia, the magnitude of this effect can be estimated by multiplying the blood glucose concentration in mg/dL by 0.016 and adding the result to the existing serum sodium concentration. The sum represents the predicted serum sodium concentration if the hyperglycemia were corrected. A recent study has suggested that this correction factor may be even higher, particularly at very high (> 400 mg/dL) glucose concentrations.

Acute, severe hyponatremia occasionally develops in patients undergoing elective surgery. In these patients, the hyponatremia results from excessive intravenous sodium-free fluid administration coupled with the post-surgical stimulation of antidiuretic hormone release and causes severe permanent brain damage. Premenopausal women are at greater risk for developing this complication. This outcome underscores the need to limit post-operative free water administration and monitor serum electrolytes.

In most cases, hyponatremia can be successfully treated by administering the calculated sodium needs in isotonic solutions. Infusion of hypertonic saline solutions is rarely indicated and could precipitate circulatory overload. Only when severe hyponatremia (usually with P_{Na} < 120 meq/L) produces mental obtundation and seizures should the patient be treated with hypertonic sodium solutions. The rate of correction of hyponatremia is a major factor in determining outcome. Rapid correction of severe hyponatremia may cause permanent brain damage due to the osmotic demyelination syndrome. For this reason, serum Na^+ should be increased at a rate not to exceed 10–12 meq/L/h. Hyponatremia with volume overload usually indicates impaired renal ability to excrete sodium.

POTASSIUM

The potassium in extracellular fluids constitutes only 2% of total body potassium (Figure 9–1); the remaining 98% is within body cells.

The serum potassium concentration ([K^+]) is thought to be determined primarily by the pH of ECF and the

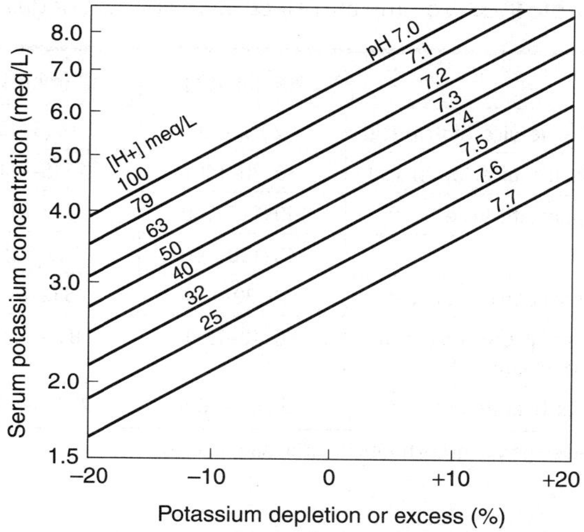

Figure 9–2. **Relationship of serum potassium to total body potassium stores at different blood pH levels.** (Reprinted, with permission, from *University of Washington Teaching Syllabus for the Course on Fluid and Electrolyte Balance.* Edited by Belding Scribner, MD.)

size of the intracellular K^+ pool (Figure 9–2). With extracellular acidosis from administration of inorganic (strong) acids, it has been shown that a large proportion of the excess hydrogen is buffered intracellularly by an exchange of intracellular K^+ for extracellular H^+; this movement of K^+ may produce dangerous hyperkalemia. However, states of clinical metabolic acidosis result from derangements in intracellular metabolism to produce organic acidosis, which may not exert the same effects on the serum K^+. Likewise, simple alkalosis does not regularly result in hypokalemia from movement of K^+ into cells.

In the absence of an acid-base disturbance, serum K^+ reflects the total body pool of potassium (Figure 9–2). With excessive external losses of potassium (eg, from the gastrointestinal tract) (Table 9–3), the serum [K^+] falls: A loss of 10% of total body K^+ drops the serum [K^+] from 4 to 3 meq/L at a normal pH.

Although pH and body composition influence potassium metabolism, measurements of potassium intake and urinary potassium excretion allow the clinician to control potassium balance. Renal excretion of potassium is regulated by mineralocorticoid (aldosterone) levels. Renal failure—particularly acute oliguric renal failure—results in potassium retention and hyperkalemia. Adrenal insufficiency may produce hyperkalemia through impaired renal excretion. Hypokalemia from excessive renal excretion may follow administration of diuretics, adrenal steroid excess, and certain renal tubular disorders associated

Table 9–3. Volume and electrolyte content of gastrointestinal fluid losses.

	Na^+ (meq/L)	K^+ (meq/L)	Cl^- (meq/L)	HCO_3^- (meq/L)	Volume (mL)
Gastric juice, high in acid	20 (20–30)	10 (5–40)	120 (80–150)	0	1000–9000
Gastric juice, low in acid	80 (70–140)	15 (5–40)	90 (40–120)	5–25	1000–2500
Pancreatic juice	140 (115–180)	5 (3–8)	75 (55–95)	80 (60–110)	500–1000
Bile	148 (130–160)	5 (3–12)	100 (90–120)	35 (30–40)	300–1000
Small bowel drainage	110 (80–150)	5 (2–8)	105 (60–125)	30 (20–40)	1000–3000
Distal ileum and cecum drainage	80 (40–135)	8 (5–30)	45 (20–90)	30 (20–40)	1000–3000
Diarrheal stools	120 (20–160)	25 (10–40)	90 (30–120)	45 (30–50)	500–17,000

[1]Average values/24 h with range in parentheses.

with potassium wasting. Rarely, potassium deficiency can arise from deficient dietary potassium intake, as in alcoholic patients or in those receiving total parenteral nutrition with inadequate potassium replacement.

1. Hyperkalemia

Hyperkalemia is a treatable problem that may prove fatal if undiagnosed. Blood potassium levels must be closely monitored in susceptible patients such as those with severe trauma, burns, crush injuries, renal insufficiency, or marked catabolism from other causes. Hyperkalemia may also be due to Addison's disease. Clinical evidence of significant hyperkalemia is usually not present. Nausea and vomiting, colicky abdominal pain, and diarrhea may occur. The electrocardiographic changes are the most helpful indicators of the severity of the disorder: Early changes include peaking of the T waves, widening of the QRS complex, and depression of the ST segment. With further elevation of the blood potassium level, the QRS widens to such a degree that the tracing resembles a sine wave, a finding that portends imminent cardiac standstill.

A number of factors must be rapidly considered in assessing the hyperkalemic patient. First, one should determine whether the serum potassium level is a true metabolic abnormality or has been elevated by hemolysis, marked leukocytosis, or thrombocytosis. Platelet counts greater than 1 million/mL may elevate the serum potassium, since the ion is liberated from platelets as they are consumed during clotting. Second, the acid-base status should be assessed to ascertain its influence (Figure 9–2). Finally, the rapidity with which the elevated serum potassium should be corrected must be determined.

There are five approaches to the emergency treatment of hyperkalemia. Initially, an intravenous infusion of 100 mL of 50% dextrose solution containing 20 units of regular insulin will lower extracellular K^+ by promoting its intracellular transport in association with glucose. Intravenous $NaHCO_3$ solutions may lower serum K^+ as acidosis is corrected, though this point remains controversial. Calcium antagonizes the tissue effects of potassium; an infusion of calcium gluconate will transiently reverse cardiac depression from hyperkalemia without changing the serum potassium concentration. A slower method of controlling hyperkalemia is to administer the cation exchange resin sodium polystyrene sulfonate (Kayexalate) orally or by enema at a rate of 40–80 g/d. This drug binds potassium in the intestine in exchange for sodium. It is often given with sorbitol to induce osmotic diarrhea and enhance the rate of potassium removal. Finally, when hyperkalemia is a manifestation of renal failure, hemodialysis is often necessary; beta-adrenergic stimulation with inhaled albuterol is also helpful in these patients.

2. Hypokalemia

Hypokalemia usually results from renal wasting of potassium; potassium deficiency and hypokalemia from inadequate dietary intake occur only after weeks of a deficient diet. Alcoholics and elderly people with restricted diets are at risk for potassium depletion due to insufficient dietary intake. The clinical manifestations of hypokalemia relate to neuromuscular function: Decreased muscle contractility and muscle cell potential develop, and in extreme cases death may result from paralysis of the muscles of respiration.

When the clinician assesses hypokalemia, the initial goal is to identify the cause. If alkalosis is present, the K^+ needs can be estimated from the nomogram in Figure 9–2. If there is no acid-base imbalance, or if hypokalemia persists after alkalosis is corrected, renal losses are probably excessive. Urine potassium excretion of more than 30 meq/24 h associated with a serum [K^+] under 3.5 meq/L indicates renal potassium wasting. The primary problem in this situation is usually diuretic therapy, alkalosis, or increased aldosterone activity. If renal potassium excretion is less than 30 meq/24 h, the kidneys are conserving potassium appropriately, and hypokalemia reflects a total body deficit.

Treatment consists of correcting the cause of hypokalemia and administering potassium. If the patient is able to eat, potassium should be given orally; otherwise, it should be given intravenously. Usually, potassium concentrations in intravenous solutions should not exceed 40 meq/L. In moderate to severe hypokalemia ([K^+] < 3 meq/L), potassium may be administered at a rate of 20–30 meq/h. With mild hypokalemia ([K^+] 3–3.5 meq/L), potassium should be replaced slowly to avoid hyperkalemia. Potassium should usually be administered intravenously as the chloride salt; in metabolic alkalosis, potassium chloride is specific, since it helps to correct the acid-base abnormality as well as the hypokalemia. Occasional patients may have persistent hypokalemia refractory to replacement therapy because of coexistent magnesium deficiency. Therefore, serum magnesium concentration should be measured in hypokalemic patients, particularly since many of the causes of potassium deficiency will also result in magnesium depletion (see below).

CALCIUM

Calcium is an important mediator of neuromuscular function and cellular enzyme processes even though most of the body calcium is contained in the skeleton. The usual dietary intake of calcium is 1–3 g/d, most of which is excreted unabsorbed in the feces.

The normal serum calcium concentration (8.5–10.3 mg/dL, 4.2–5.2 meq/L) is maintained by humoral factors, mainly vitamin D, parathyroid hormone, and calcitonin. Acidemia increases and alkalemia decreases the serum ionized calcium concentration. Approximately half of the total serum calcium is bound to plasma proteins, chiefly albumin; a small amount is complexed to plasma anions, such as citrate; and the remainder (approximately 40%) of the total serum calcium is free, or ionized, calcium, which is the fraction responsible for the biologic effects. The ionized calcium usually remains constant when the total serum calcium concentration changes with different serum albumin concentrations. Unless the ionized calcium is measured, the serum calcium can only be reliably assessed if accompanied by measurement of the serum albumin concentration.

Severe disturbances of calcium concentration are uncommon in surgical patients, although transient asymptomatic hypocalcemia is common. After operations on the thyroid or parathyroids, the serum calcium concentration should be measured at regular intervals to detect hypocalcemia early if it appears.

1. Hypocalcemia

Hypocalcemia occurs in hypoparathyroidism, hypomagnesemia, severe pancreatitis, chronic or acute renal failure, severe trauma, crush injuries, and necrotizing fasciitis. The clinical manifestations are neuromuscular: hyperactive deep tendon reflexes, a positive Chvostek sign, muscle and abdominal cramps, carpopedal spasm, and, rarely, convulsions. Hypocalcemia is reflected in the ECG by a prolonged QT interval.

The initial step is to check the whole blood pH; if alkalosis is present, it should be treated. Intravenous calcium, as calcium gluconate or calcium chloride, may be needed for the acute problem (eg, after parathyroidectomy). Chronic hypoparathyroidism requires vitamin D, oral calcium supplements, and often aluminum hydroxide gels to bind dietary phosphate in the intestine.

2. Hypercalcemia

Hypercalcemia most frequently is caused by hyperparathyroidism, cancer with bony metastases, ectopic production of parathyroid hormone, vitamin D intoxication, hyperthyroidism, sarcoidosis, milk-alkali syndrome, or prolonged immobilization (especially in young patients or those with Paget's disease). It is also a rare complication of thiazide diuretics.

The symptoms of hypercalcemia are fatigability, muscle weakness, depression, anorexia, nausea, and constipation. Long-standing hypercalcemia may impair renal concentrating mechanisms, resulting in polyuria and polydipsia and in metastatic deposition of calcium. Severe hypercalcemia can cause coma and death. *A serum calcium concentration above 12 mg/dL should be regarded as a medical emergency!*

With severe hypercalcemia (Ca^{2+} > 14.5 mg/dL), intravenous isotonic saline should be given to expand ECF, increase urine flow, enhance calcium excretion, and reduce the serum level.

Furosemide and intravenous sodium sulfate are other methods of increasing renal calcium excretion. Plicamycin is particularly useful for hypercalcemia associated with metastatic cancer. Adrenal corticosteroids are useful for hypercalcemia associated with sarcoidosis, vitamin D intoxication, and Addison's disease. Calcitonin is indicated in patients with impaired renal and cardiovascular function. When renal failure is present, hemodialysis may be required.

MAGNESIUM

Magnesium is largely present in bone and cells, where it serves an important role in cellular energy metabolism.

The normal plasma magnesium concentration is 1.5–2.5 meq/L. Magnesium is excreted primarily by the kidneys. The serum magnesium concentration reflects total body magnesium. Serum magnesium levels may be elevated in hypovolemic shock as magnesium is liberated from cells.

1. Hypomagnesemia

Hypomagnesemia occurs with poor dietary intake, intestinal malabsorption of ingested magnesium, or excessive losses from the gut (eg, severe diarrhea, enteric fistulas, use of purgatives, or nasogastric suction). It may also be caused by excessive urinary losses (eg, from diuretics), chronic alcohol abuse, hyperaldosteronism, and hypercalcemia. Hypomagnesemia occasionally develops in acute pancreatitis, in diabetic acidosis, in burned patients, or after prolonged total parenteral nutrition with insufficient magnesium supplementation. The clinical manifestations resemble those of hypocalcemia: hyperactive tendon reflexes, a positive Chvostek sign, and tremors that may progress to delirium and convulsions.

The diagnosis of hypomagnesemia depends on clinical suspicion with confirmation by measurement of the serum magnesium. Treatment consists of administering magnesium, usually as the sulfate or chloride. In moderate magnesium deficiency, oral replacement is adequate. In more severe deficits, parenteral magnesium must be administered intravenously (40–80 meq of $MgSO_4$ per liter of intravenous fluid). When large doses are infused intravenously, there is a risk of producing hypermagnesemia, with tachycardia and hypotension. The ECG should be inspected for prolongation of the QT interval. Magnesium should be administered cautiously to oliguric patients or those with renal failure and only after magnesium deficiency has been unequivocally documented. Magnesium deficiency may also be accompanied by refractory hypokalemia.

2. Hypermagnesemia

Hypermagnesemia usually occurs in patients with renal disease; it is rare in surgical patients. In patients with renal insufficiency, serum magnesium levels should be monitored closely. Strict attention must be paid to excess magnesium intake, which can occur from a variety of commonly administered antacids and laxatives and which may produce severe and even fatal hypermagnesemia in renal insufficiency.

The initial signs and symptoms of hypermagnesemia are lethargy and weakness. Electrocardiographic changes resemble those in hyperkalemia (widened QRS complex, ST segment depression, and peaked T waves). When the serum level reaches 6 meq/L, deep tendon reflexes are lost; with levels above 10 meq/L, somnolence, coma, and death may ensue.

Treatment of hypermagnesemia consists of giving intravenous isotonic saline to increase the rate of renal magnesium excretion. This may be accompanied by slow intravenous infusion of calcium, since calcium antagonizes some of the neuromuscular actions of magnesium. Patients with hypermagnesemia and severe renal failure may need dialysis.

PHOSPHORUS

Phosphorus is primarily a constituent of bone, but it is also an important intracellular ion with a role in energy metabolism. The serum phosphorus level is only an approximate indicator of total body phosphorus and can be influenced by a number of factors, including the serum calcium concentration and the pH of blood. In urine, phosphorus is an important buffer that facilitates the excretion of acids formed by intermediary metabolism. Urine phosphate buffer is reflected by the excretion of titratable acid.

1. Hypophosphatemia

Clinically important hypophosphatemia may follow poor dietary intake (especially in alcoholics), hyperparathyroidism, and antacid administration (antacids bind phosphate in the intestine). Hypophosphatemia was at one time a frequent complication of total parenteral nutrition until phosphate supplementation became routine. Clinical manifestations appear when the serum phosphorus level falls to 1 mg/dL or less. Neuromuscular manifestations include lassitude, fatigue, weakness, convulsions, and death. Red blood cells hemolyze, oxygen delivery is impaired, and white cell phagocytosis is depressed. Cardiac contractility may be impaired, and rhabdomyolysis can occur. Chronic phosphate depletion has been implicated in the development of osteomalacia.

2. Hyperphosphatemia

Hyperphosphatemia most often develops in severe renal disease, after trauma, or with marked tissue catabolism. It is rarely caused by excessive dietary intake. Hyperphosphatemia is usually asymptomatic. Because it raises the calcium-phosphorus product, the serum calcium concentration is depressed. A high calcium-phosphate product predisposes to metastatic calcification of soft tissues. Treatment of hyperphosphatemia is by diuresis to increase the rate of urinary phosphorus excretion. Administration of phosphate-binding antacids, such as aluminum hydroxide gels, will diminish the gastrointestinal absorption of phosphorus and lower the serum phosphorus concentration. In patients with renal disease, dialysis may be required.

ACID-BASE BALANCE

NORMAL PHYSIOLOGY

During the course of daily metabolism of protein and carbohydrate, approximately 70 meq (or 1 meq/kg of body weight) of hydrogen ion is generated and delivered into the body fluids. In addition, a large amount of carbon dioxide is formed that combines with water to form carbonic acid (H_2CO_3). If efficient mechanisms for buffering and eliminating these acids were not available, the pH of body fluids would fall rapidly. Although mammals have a highly developed system for handling daily acid production, disturbances of acid-base balance are common in disease.

Hydrogen ions generated from metabolism are buffered through two major systems. The first involves intracellular protein, eg, the hemoglobin in red blood cells. More important is the bicarbonate/carbonic acid system, which can be understood from the Henderson-Hasselbalch equation:

$$pH = pK + \log \frac{[HCO_3^-]}{0.03 \times Pco_2} \quad (4)$$

where pK for the $\frac{HCO_3^-}{H_2CO_3}$ system is 6.1.

Hydrogen ion concentration is related to pH in an inverse logarithmic manner. The following transformation of equation 4 is easier to use, because it eliminates the logarithms:

$$[H^+] = \frac{24 \times Pco_2}{[HCO_e^-]} \quad (5)$$

There is an approximately linear inverse relationship between pH and hydrogen ion concentration over the pH range of 7.9–7.50: For each 0.01 decrease in pH, the hydrogen ion concentration increases 1 nmol. Remembering that a normal blood pH of 7.40 is equal to a hydrogen ion concentration of 40 nmol/L, one can calculate the approximate hydrogen ion concentration for any pH between 7.10 and 7.50. For example, a pH of 7.30 is equal to a hydrogen ion concentration of 50 nmol/L. This estimation introduces an error of approximately 10% at the extremes of this pH range. (See also Figure 9–2.)

A consideration of the right-hand side of equation 5 demonstrates that hydrogen ion concentration is determined by the ratio of the $PaCO_2$ to the plasma bicarbonate concentration. In body fluids, CO_2 is dissolved and combines with water to form carbonic acid, the acid part of the acid-base pair. If any two of these three variables are known, the third can be calculated using this expression.

Equation 5 also illustrates how the body excretes acid produced through metabolic processes. Blood PCO_2 is normally controlled within narrow limits by pulmonary ventilation. The plasma bicarbonate concentration is regulated in the renal tubules by three major processes: (1) Filtered bicarbonate is reabsorbed, mostly in the proximal tubule, to prevent excessive bicarbonate loss in the urine; (2) hydrogen ions are secreted as titratable acid to regenerate the bicarbonate that was buffered when these hydrogen ions were initially produced and to provide a vehicle for excretion of about one-third of the daily acid production; and (3) the kidneys also excrete hydrogen ion in the form of ammonium ion by a process that regenerates bicarbonate initially consumed in the production of these hydrogen ions. Volume depletion, increased $PaCO_2$, and hypokalemia all favor enhanced tubular reabsorption of HCO_3^-.

ACID-BASE ABNORMALITIES

The management of clinical acid-base disturbances is facilitated by the use of a nomogram (Figure 9–3) that relates the three variables in equation 5.

Primary respiratory disturbances cause changes in the blood $PaCO_2$ (the numerator in equation 5) and produce corresponding effects on the blood hydrogen ion concentration. Metabolic disturbances primarily affect the plasma bicarbonate concentration (the denominator in equation 5). Whether the disturbance is primarily respiratory or metabolic, some degree of compensatory change occurs in the reciprocal factor in equation 5 to limit or nullify the magnitude of perturbation of acid-base balance. Thus, changes in blood PCO_2 from respiratory disturbances are compensated for by changes in the renal handling of bicarbonate. Conversely, changes in plasma bicarbonate concentration are blunted by appropriate respiratory changes.

Because acute respiratory changes allow insufficient time for compensatory renal mechanisms to respond, the resulting pH disturbances are often great and the abnormalities may be present in pure form. By contrast, chronic respiratory disturbances allow the full range of compensatory mechanisms by the kidneys to come into play, so that blood pH may remain near normal despite wide variations in the blood PCO_2. On the other hand, respiratory compensation for metabolic disturbances occurs almost instantaneously, so that there is little difference in the acid-base variables between acute and chronic disorders.

1. Respiratory Acidosis

Acute respiratory acidosis occurs when respiration suddenly becomes inadequate. CO_2 accumulates in the blood (the numerator in equation 5 increases), and

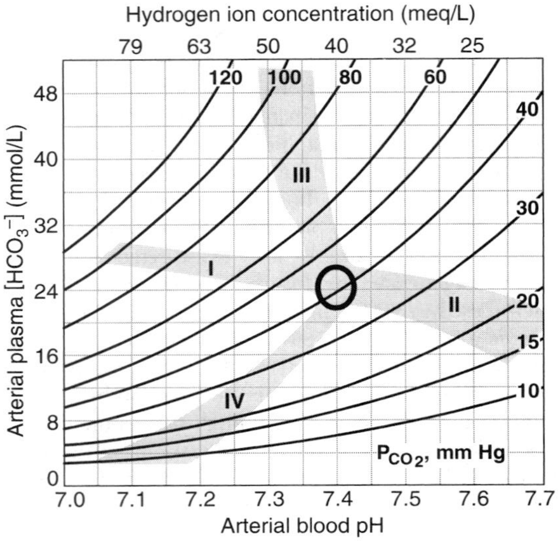

Figure 9–3. Acid-base nomogram for use in evaluation of clinical acid-base disorders. Hydrogen ion concentration (top) or blood pH (bottom) is plotted against plasma HCO_3^- concentration; curved lines are isopleths of CO_2 tension (Pa_{CO_2}, mm Hg). Knowing any two of these variables permits estimation of the third. The circle in the center represents the range of normal values; the shaded bands represent the 95% confidence limits of four common acid-base disturbances: I, acute respiratory acidosis; II, acute respiratory alkalosis; III, chronic respiratory acidosis; IV, sustained metabolic acidosis. Points lying outside these shaded areas are mixed disturbances and indicate two primary acid-base disorders. (Courtesy of Anthony Sebastian, MD, University of California Medical Center, San Francisco.)

hydrogen ion concentration increases. This occurs most often in acute airway obstruction, aspiration, respiratory arrest, certain pulmonary infections, and pulmonary edema with impaired gas exchange. There is acidemia and an elevated blood P_{CO_2} but little change in the plasma bicarbonate concentration. Over 80% of the carbonic acid resulting from the increased Pa_{CO_2} is buffered by intracellular mechanisms—about 50% by intracellular protein and another 30% by hemoglobin. Because relatively little is buffered by bicarbonate ion, the plasma bicarbonate concentration may be normal. An acute increase in the Pa_{CO_2} from 40 to 80 mm Hg will increase the plasma bicarbonate by only 3 meq/L. This is why the 95% confidence band for acute respiratory acidosis (I in Figure 9–3) is nearly horizontal; ie, increases in Pa_{CO_2} directly increase hydrogen ion concentration and decrease pH with little change in plasma bicarbonate concentration. Treatment involves restoration of adequate ventilation. If necessary, tracheal intubation and assisted ventilation or controlled ventilation with sedation should be employed.

Chronic respiratory acidosis arises from chronic respiratory failure in which impaired ventilation gives a sustained elevation of blood P_{CO_2}. Renal compensation raises plasma bicarbonate to the extent illustrated by the 95% confidence limits in Figure 9–3 (the area marked by III). Rather marked elevations of Pa_{CO_2} produce small changes in blood pH, because of the increase in plasma bicarbonate concentration. This is achieved primarily by increased renal excretion of ammonium ion, which enhances acid excretion and regenerates bicarbonate, which is returned to the blood. Chronic respiratory acidosis is generally well tolerated until severe pulmonary insufficiency leads to hypoxia. At this point, the long-term prognosis is very poor. Paradoxically, the patient with chronic respiratory acidosis appears better able to tolerate additional acute increases in blood P_{CO_2}.

Treatment of chronic respiratory acidosis depends largely on attention to pulmonary toilet and ventilatory status. Rapid correction of chronic respiratory acidosis, as may occur if the patient is placed on controlled ventilation, can be dangerous, since the Pa_{CO_2} is lowered rapidly and the compensated respiratory acidosis may be converted to a severe metabolic alkalosis (posthypercapnic metabolic acidosis).

2. Respiratory Alkalosis

Acute hyperventilation lowers the Pa_{CO_2} without concomitant changes in the plasma bicarbonate concentration and thereby lowers the hydrogen ion concentration (II in Figure 9–3). The clinical manifestations are paresthesias in the extremities, carpopedal spasm, and a positive Chvostek sign. Acute hyperventilation with respiratory alkalosis may be an early sign of bacterial sepsis.

Chronic respiratory alkalosis occurs in pulmonary and liver disease. The renal response to chronic hypocapnia is to decrease the tubular reabsorption of filtered bicarbonate, increasing bicarbonate excretion, with a consequent lowering of plasma bicarbonate concentration. As the bicarbonate concentration falls, the chloride concentration rises. This is the same pattern seen in hyperchloremic acidosis, and the two can only be distinguished by blood gas and pH measurements. Generally, chronic respiratory alkalosis does not require treatment; if the Pa_{CO_2} is allowed to return to normal rapidly, posthypocapnic metabolic acidosis with hyperchloremia may occur.

3. Metabolic Acidosis

Metabolic acidosis is caused by increased production of hydrogen ion from metabolic or other causes or from excessive bicarbonate losses. In either case, the plasma bicarbonate concentration is decreased, producing an increase in hydrogen ion concentration (see equation 5). With excessive bicarbonate loss (eg, severe diarrhea, diuretic treatment with acetazolamide or other carbonic anhydrase inhibitors, certain forms of renal tubular disease, and in patients with ureterosigmoidostomies), the decrease in plasma bicarbonate concentration is matched by an increase in the serum chloride, so that the anion gap (the sum of chloride and bicarbonate concentrations subtracted from the serum sodium concentration) remains at the normal level, below 15 meq/L. On the other hand, metabolic acidosis from increased acid production is associated with an anion gap exceeding 15 meq/L. Conditions in which this occurs are renal failure, diabetic ketoacidosis, lactic acidosis, methanol ingestion, salicylate intoxication, and ethylene glycol ingestion. The lungs compensate by hyperventilation, which returns the hydrogen ion concentration toward normal by lowering the blood PCO_2. In long-standing metabolic acidosis, minute ventilation may increase sufficiently to drop the $PaCO_2$ to as low as 10–15 mm Hg. The shaded area marked IV on the nomogram (Figure 9–3) represents the confidence limits for sustained metabolic acidosis.

Treatment of metabolic acidosis depends on identifying the underlying cause and correcting it. Often, this is sufficient. In some conditions, particularly when there is an increased anion gap, alkali administration is required. The amount of sodium bicarbonate required to restore the plasma bicarbonate concentration to normal can be estimated by subtracting the existing plasma bicarbonate concentration from the normal value of 24 meq/L and multiplying the resulting number by half the estimated total body water. This is a useful empiric formula. In practice, it is not usually wise to administer enough bicarbonate to return the plasma bicarbonate completely to normal. It is better to raise the plasma bicarbonate concentration by 5 meq/L initially and then reassess the clinical situation. The administration of sodium bicarbonate may cause fluid overload from the large quantity of sodium and may overcorrect the acidosis. The long-term management of patients with metabolic acidosis entails providing adequate alkali, either as supplemental sodium bicarbonate tablets or by dietary manipulation. In all cases, attempts should be made to minimize the magnitude of bicarbonate loss in patients with chronic metabolic acidosis.

4. Metabolic Alkalosis

Metabolic alkalosis is probably the most common acid-base disturbance in surgical patients. In this condition, the blood hydrogen ion concentration is decreased as a result of accumulation of bicarbonate in plasma. The pathogenesis is complex but involves at least three separate factors: (1) loss of hydrogen ion, usually as a result of loss of gastric secretions rich in hydrochloric acid; (2) volume depletion, which is often severe; and (3) potassium depletion, which almost always is present.

HCl secretion by the gastric mucosa returns bicarbonate ion to the blood. Gastric acid, after mixing with ingested food, is subsequently reabsorbed in the small intestine, so that there is no net gain or loss of hydrogen ion in this process. If secreted hydrogen ion is lost through vomiting or drainage, the result is a net delivery of bicarbonate into the circulation. Normally, the kidneys are easily able to excrete the excess bicarbonate load. However, if volume depletion accompanies the loss of hydrogen ion, the kidneys work to preserve volume by increasing tubular reabsorption of sodium and whatever anions are also filtered. Consequently, because of the increased sodium reabsorption, the excess bicarbonate cannot be completely excreted. This perpetuates the metabolic alkalosis. At first, some of the filtered bicarbonate escapes reabsorption in the proximal tubule and reaches the distal tubule. Here it promotes potassium secretion and enhanced potassium loss in the urine. The urine pH will be either neutral or alkaline, because of the presence of bicarbonate. Later, as volume depletion becomes more severe, the reabsorption of filtered bicarbonate in the proximal tubule becomes virtually complete. Now, only small amounts of sodium, with little bicarbonate, reach the distal tubule. If potassium depletion is severe, sodium is reabsorbed in exchange for hydrogen ion. This results in the paradoxically acid urine sometimes observed in patients with advanced metabolic alkalosis.

Assessment should involve examination of the urine electrolytes and urine pH. In the early stages, bicarbonate excretion will obligate excretion of sodium as well as potassium, so the urine sodium concentration will be relatively high for a volume-depleted patient and the urine pH will be alkaline. In this circumstance, the urine chloride will reveal the extent of the volume depletion: A urine chloride of less than 10 meq/L is diagnostic of volume depletion and chloride deficiency. Later, when bicarbonate reabsorption becomes virtually complete, the urine pH will be acid, and urine sodium, potassium, and chloride concentrations will all be low. The ventilatory compensation in metabolic alkalosis is variable, but the maximal extent of compensation can only raise the blood PCO_2 to about 55 mm Hg. A $PaCO_2$ greater than 60 mm Hg in metabolic alkalosis suggests a mixed disturbance also involving respiratory acidosis.

To treat metabolic alkalosis, fluid must be given, usually as saline solution. With adequate volume repletion, the stimulus to tubular sodium reabsorption is diminished, and the kidneys can then excrete the excess bicarbonate. Most of these patients are also substantially potassium-depleted and will require potassium supplementation. This should be administered as KCl, since chloride depletion is another hallmark of this condition and potassium given as citrate or lactate will not correct the potassium deficit.

5. Mixed Acid-Base Disorders

In many situations, mixed disorders of acid-base balance develop. The most common example in surgical patients is metabolic acidosis superimposed on respiratory alkalosis. This problem can arise in patients with septic shock or hepatorenal syndrome. Since the two acid-base disorders tend to cancel each other, the disturbance in hydrogen ion concentration is usually small. The reverse situation, ie, respiratory acidosis combined with metabolic alkalosis, is less common. Combined metabolic and respiratory acidosis occurs in cardiorespiratory arrest and obviously constitutes a medical emergency. Circumstances involving both metabolic and respiratory alkalosis are rare. The clue to the presence of a mixed acid-base disorder can come from plotting the patient's acid-base data on the nomogram in Figure 9–3. If the set of data falls outside one of the confidence bands, then by definition the patient has a mixed disorder. On the other hand, if the acid-base data fall within one of the confidence bands, it suggests (but does not prove) that the acid-base disturbance is pure or uncomplicated.

PRINCIPLES OF FLUID & ELECTROLYTE THERAPY

The development of a rational plan of fluid and electrolyte therapy requires an understanding of the principles developed earlier in this chapter. First, maintenance fluid requirements must be determined. Second, existing deficits of volume or composition should be calculated. This involves the analysis of four aspects of the patient's fluid and electrolyte status based on weight changes, serum electrolyte concentrations, and blood pH and P_{CO_2}: (1) the magnitude of the volume deficit present, (2) the pathogenesis and treatment of abnormal sodium concentration, (3) assessment of any potassium requirement, and (4) management of any coexistent acid-base disturbance. Finally, therapy must also recognize the presence of ongoing obligatory fluid losses and include these losses in the daily plan of treatment.

Normal maintenance requirements can be determined using the guidelines in Table 9–2. Fever or elevated ambient temperature will increase insensible losses and thereby increase these requirements. The normal response to the stress of surgery is to conserve water and electrolytes, so maintenance requirements are decreased in the immediate postoperative period. In addition, increased catabolism will deliver more potassium to the circulation, so that this ion can be omitted from maintenance solutions for several days postoperatively.

Correction of preexisting deficits must be based on the four factors listed above. Volume deficit is best estimated on the basis of acute changes in weight or from clinical estimates; the clinician should remember that deficits less than 5% of body water will not be detectable and that loss of 15% of body water will be associated with severe circulatory compromise. The relationship of net sodium to net fluid deficit is given by the serum sodium concentration according to equation 3. If the serum sodium concentration is normal, fluid losses have been isotonic; if hyponatremia is present, more sodium than water has been lost. In either case, initial replacement should be with isotonic saline solutions. Any potassium excess or deficit must be assessed in the light of the blood pH according to Figure 9–2. If hypokalemia exists at normal pH, the magnitude of the total body potassium deficit can also be estimated using Figure 9–2. For example, a serum potassium concentration of 2.5 meq/L at pH 7.40 suggests a 20% depletion of total body potassium. A normal human has a potassium capacity of 45 meq/kg body weight; a moderately wasted patient, 35 meq/kg. For a normal 70-kg man, total potassium capacity is 45 × 70, or 3150 meq; the deficit is 20% of this, or 630 meq, and this amount must be considered in therapy calculations. Principles of acid-base therapy have already been outlined.

Two rules of thumb should be applied in prescribing parenteral therapy for fluid and electrolyte deficits. The first is that for most problems, half of the calculated deficits should be replaced in a 24-hour period, with subsequent reassessment of the clinical situation. The second is that a fluid or electrolyte abnormality should take as long to correct as it took to develop. By adherence to these guidelines, overly vigorous replacement will be avoided and, along with it, the production of a different (iatrogenic) electrolyte abnormality.

Ongoing losses must be considered also in the daily fluid therapy plan, with regard to both volume and composition. Characteristic measurements for fluids removed from different segments of the gastrointestinal tract are shown in Table 9–3.

REFERENCES

General

Seldin DW, Giebisch G (editors): *The Kidney: Physiology and Pathophysiology,* 3rd ed. Lippincott Williams & Wilkins, 2000.

Fluid Volume & Sodium Concentration

Adrogue HJ et al: Hypernatremia. N Engl J Med 2000;342:1493.

Adrogue HJ et al: Hyponatremia. N Engl J Med 2000;342:1581.

Anderson RJ: Hospital-associated hyponatremia. Kidney Int 1986; 29:1237.

Arieff AI: Hyponatremia, convulsions, respiratory arrest, and permanent brain damage after elective surgery in healthy women. N Engl J Med 1986;314:1529.

Ayus JC et al: Chronic hyponatremic encephalopathy in postmenopausal women. Association of therapies with morbidity and mortality. JAMA 1999;281:2342.

Ayus JC et al: Postoperative hyponatremic encephalopathy in menstruant women. Ann Intern Med 1992;117:891.

Brater DC: Use of diuretics in cirrhosis and nephrotic syndrome. Semin Nephrol 1999;19:575.

Doyle JA et al: The use of hypertonic saline in the treatment of traumatic brain injury. J Trauma 2001;50:367.

Ellison DH: Diuretic resistance: physiology and therapeutics. Semin Nephrol 1999;19:581.

Fried LF et al: Hyponatremia and hypernatremia. Med Clin North Am 1997;81:585.

Harrigan MR: Cerebral salt wasting syndrome: a review. Neurosurgery 1996;38:152.

Hilliard TA et al: Hyponatremia: evaluating the correction factor for hyperglycemia. Am J Med 1999;106:399.

Hirshberg B et al: The syndrome of inappropriate antidiuretic hormone secretion on the elderly. Am J Med 1997;103:270.

Katz MA: Hyperglycemia-induced hyponatremia—calculation of expected serum sodium depression. N Engl J Med 1973;289:843.

Knochel JP: Hypoxia is the cause of brain damage in hyponatremia. JAMA 1999;281:2342.

Kumar S et al: Sodium. Lancet 1998;352:220.

Palevsky PM: Hypernatremia. Semin Nephrol 1998;18:20.

Palevsky PM et al: Hypernatremia in hospitalized patients. Ann Intern Med 1996;124:197.

Singer I et al: The management of diabetes insipidus in adults. Arch Intern Med 1997;157:1293.

Steele A et al: Postoperative hyponatremia despite near-isotonic saline infusion: a phenomenon of desalination. Ann Intern Med 1997;126:20.

Wilcox CS: Metabolic and adverse effects of diuretics. Semin Nephrol 1999;19:557.

Acid-Base Disturbances & Potassium

Adrogue HJ et al: Management of life-threatening acid-base disorders. (Two parts.) N Engl J Med 1998;338:26, 107.

Greenberg A: Hyperkalemia: treatment options. Semin Nephrol 1998;18:46.

Ishihara K et al: Anion gap acidosis. Semin Nephrol 1998;18:83.

Krapf R et al: Plasma potassium response to acute respiratory alkalosis. Kidney Int 1995;47:217.

Krapf R et al: Chronic respiratory alkalosis. The effect of sustained hyperventilation on renal regulation of acid-base equilibrium. N Engl J Med 1991;324:1394.

Kruse JA et al: Rapid correction of hypokalemia using concentrated intravenous potassium chloride infusions. Arch Intern Med 1990;150:613.

Luft FC: Lactic acidosis update for critical care clinicians. J Am Soc Nephrol 2001;12: S 15.

Potkin RT et al: Resuscitation from severe acute hypercapnia: determinants of tolerance and survival. Chest 1992;102: 1742.

Whang R et al: Refractory potassium repletion: a consequence of magnesium deficiency. Arch Intern Med 1992;152:40.

Calcium, Magnesium, & Phosphorus

Aguilera IM et al: Calcium and the anaesthetist. Anaesthesia 2000;55:779.

Barri YM et al: Hypercalcemia and electrolyte disturbances in malignancy. Hematol Oncol Clin North Am 1996;10:775.

Bilezikian JP: Management of acute hypercalcemia. N Engl J Med 1992;326:1196.

Body JJ: Current and future directions in medical therapy: hypercalcemia. Cancer 2000;88(12 Suppl):3054.

Brooks MJ et al: The refeeding syndrome: an approach to understanding its complications and preventing its occurrence. Pharmacotherapy 1995;15:713.

Brown DL et al: Developments in the therapeutic applications of bisphosphonates. J Clin Pharmacol 1999;39:651.

Bugg NC et al: Hypophosphataemia. Pathophysiology, effects and management on the intensive care unit. Anaesthesia 1998;53: 895.

Kelepouris E et al: Hypomagnesemia: renal magnesium handling. Semin Nephrol 1998;18:58.

Miller DW et al: Hypophosphatemia in the emergency department therapeutics. Am J Emerg Med 2000;18:457.

Subramanian R et al: Severe hypophosphatemia. Pathophysiologic implications, clinical presentations, and treatment. Medicine 2000;79:1

Whang R: Clinical disorders of magnesium metabolism. Compr Ther 1997;23:168.

Ziegler R: Hypercalcemic crisis. J Am Soc Nephrol 2001;12(Suppl 17):S3.

Surgical Metabolism & Nutrition 10

Sean C. Glasgow, MD, & Virginia M. Herrmann, MD

The effects of malnutrition on the surgical patient are well-characterized in the literature but are often overlooked in the clinical arena. Between 30% and 50% of hospitalized patients are malnourished. Protein-calorie malnutrition produces a reduction in lean muscle mass, alterations in respiratory mechanics, impaired immune function, and intestinal atrophy. These changes result in diminished wound healing, predisposition to infection, and increased postoperative morbidity. Although most healthy individuals can tolerate up to 7 days of starvation (with adequate glucose and fluid replacement), those subjected to major trauma, the physiologic stress of surgery, sepsis, or cancer-related cachexia require nutritional intervention much sooner. Methods to identify those at greatest need for supplemental nutrition and to adequately address their needs are discussed in this chapter.

NUTRITIONAL ASSESSMENT

Nutrition screening is the process of identifying patients who are either malnourished or at risk for developing malnutrition. Major trauma and surgical stress alter the intake and absorption of nutrients, as well as their utilization and storage by the body. In select patients (eg, those with severe malnutrition as determined below), preoperative nutritional support has been shown to significantly reduce perioperative morbidity and mortality. Although most patients will not require this level of support, nutrition screening is imperative to identify the patient at high risk for malnutrition or its sequelae. A comprehensive nutritional assessment incorporates the initial history, physical examination, and laboratory testing to provide a snapshot of the patient's recent nutritional health.

History & Physical Examination

The history and physical examination make up the foundation of nutritional assessment. A complete medical history is essential to identify factors that predispose the patient to alterations in nutritional status (Table 10–1). Chronic illnesses such as alcoholism are commonly associated with protein-calorie malnutrition as well as vitamin and mineral deficiencies. Previous operative procedures such as gastrectomy or ileal resection may predispose to generalized malabsorption or isolated deficiency of iron, vitamin B_{12}, or folate. In most cases, the possibility of malnutrition is suggested by the underlying disease or by a history of recent weight loss. Patients with renal failure who require hemodialysis lose amino acids, vitamins, trace elements, and carnitine in the dialysate. Cirrhotics often suffer from whole-body sodium overload despite being hyponatremic, and they are typically protein-deficient. Patients with inflammatory bowel disease, particularly those with ileal involvement, may develop protein deficiency due to a combination of poor intake, chronic diarrhea, and treatment with corticosteroids. Furthermore, alterations in the enterohepatic circulation of bile salts lead to fat, vitamin, calcium, magnesium, and trace element deficiencies. Approximately 30% of patients with cancer have protein, calorie, and vitamin deficiencies due either to the underlying disease or to antimetabolite chemotherapy (eg, methotrexate). Patients infected with HIV are frequently malnourished and have protein, trace metal (selenium and zinc), mineral, and vitamin deficiencies.

A complete history of current medications is essential to alert caregivers to potential underlying deficiencies and drug-nutrient interactions. Although rarely the sole cause of malnutrition, certain over-the-counter herbal preparations can alter nutrient absorption. Agents containing ephedra and caffeine may be abused to induce excessive weight loss. Gingko and other preparations enhance cytochrome p450 metabolism of various drugs. Information about socioeconomic factors and a detailed dietary history may uncover other risk factors.

A careful physical examination begins with an overall assessment of the patient's appearance. Patients with severe malnutrition may appear frankly emaciated, but more subtle signs of malnutrition include temporal muscle wasting, skin pallor, edema, and generalized loss of body fat. Protein status is evaluated from the bulk and strength of the extremity muscles and visible evidence of temporal and thenar muscle wasting. Cardiac flow murmurs may result from anemia. Vitamin deficiencies may be indicated by changes in skin texture, the presence of follicular plugging or a skin rash, corneal vascularization, cracks at the corners of the mouth (cheilosis), hyperemia of the oral mucosa (glossitis), cardiac enlargement, altered sensation in the hands and feet, absence of vibration and position sense (dorsal and lateral column defi-

Table 10–1. Nutritional assessment.

History (Factors Predisposing to Malnutrition)
Absorption disorders (eg, celiac sprue)
AIDS
Alcoholism
Chronic renal insufficiency
Cirrhosis
Diabetes mellitus
Enteric obstruction
Inflammatory bowel disease
Malignancy
Past surgical history, especially involving gastrointestinal tract
Prolonged starvation
Psychiatric disorders (eg, anorexia nervosa)
Recent major surgery, trauma, or burn
Severe cardiopulmonary disease
Physical Examination
Skin: Quality, texture, rash, follicles, hyperkeratosis, nail deformities
Hair: Quality, texture, recent loss
Eyes: Keratoconjunctivitis, night blindness
Mouth: Cheilosis, glossitis, mucosal atrophy (eg, temporal wasting), dentition
Heart: Chamber enlargement, murmurs
Abdomen: Hepatomegaly, abdominal mass, ostomy, fistulas
Rectum: Stool color, perineal fistula, Guaiac test
Neurologic: Peripheral neuropathy, dorsolateral column deficit, mental status
Extremities: Muscle size and strength, pedal edema
Laboratory Tests
CBC: Hemoglobin, hematocrit, mean corpuscular volume (MCV), white blood cell count and differential, total lymphocyte count, platelet count
Electrolytes: Sodium, potassium, chloride, calcium, phosphate, magnesium
Liver function tests: AST (SGOT), ALT (SGPT), alkaline phosphatase, bilirubin, albumin, prealbumin, retinol-binding protein, prothrombin/INR
Miscellaneous: BUN, creatinine, triglycerides, cholesterol, free fatty acids, ketones, uric acid, calcium, copper, zinc, magnesium, transferrin

cits), or abnormal quality and texture of the hair. Trace metal deficiencies produce cutaneous and neurologic abnormalities similar to those associated with vitamin deficiency and may cause changes in the mental status of the patient.

Anthropometric Measurements

Anthropometry is the science of assessing body size, weight, and proportions. Anthropometric measurements gauge body weight and composition with the intent of providing specific information about lean body mass and fat stores. Body composition studies may be used to determine total body water, fat, nitrogen, and potassium. Anthropometric measurements that can be easily performed in the clinic or at the bedside include determination of height and weight, with calculation of body mass index (BMI). More advanced techniques allow the clinician to assess the patient's visceral and somatic protein mass and fat reserve.

Accurate measurement of height, either directly or by alternative means (arm span, body part summation, or knee-height measurement) is essential for nutrition assessment. Accurate weight is similarly important, as is current weight expressed as a percentage of ideal body weight. Ideal body weight can be obtained from life insurance actuarial tables.

The BMI is used to measure protein-calorie malnutrition as well as overnutrition (eg, obesity). A BMI between 18.5 and 24.9 is considered normal in most Western civilizations. Overweight is defined as a BMI from 25 to 29.9, and a BMI greater than 30 defines obesity. BMI is calculated as follows:

$$\text{BMI} = \frac{\text{Weight (kg)}}{\text{Height}^2\text{(m)}} = 703 \times \frac{\text{Weight (lb)}}{\text{Height}^2\text{(in)}}$$

Dual-energy x-ray absorptiometry (DEXA) is increasingly available in hospitals and can be used to assess various body compartments (mineral, fat, lean muscle mass). Most protein resides in skeletal muscle. Somatic (skeletal) protein reserve is estimated by measuring the midhumeral circumference. This measurement is corrected to account for subcutaneous tissue, yielding the midhumeral muscle circumference (MHMC). The result is compared with normal values for the patient's age and gender to determine the extent of protein depletion. Fat reserve is commonly estimated from the thickness of the triceps skin fold (TSF). Reliability of anthropometric measurements is dependent on the skill of the person performing the measurement and is subject to error if performed by different caregivers on the same patient.

Laboratory Data

The visceral protein reserve is estimated from various serum protein levels, total lymphocyte count, and antigen skin testing (Table 10–2). The serum albumin level provides a rough estimate of the patient's nutritional status but is a better prognostic indicator than tool for nutritional assessment. Serum albumin less than 3.5 mg/dL correlates with increased perioperative morbidity and mortality and increased length of hospital stay. Because albumin has a relatively long half-life (20 days), other serum proteins with shorter half-lives have greater utility

Table 10–2. Staging of malnutrition.

Clinical & Laboratory Parameters	Extent of Malnutrition: *Mild*	*Moderate*[1]	*Severe*[1]
Albumin (g/dL)	2.8–3.5	2.1–2.7	< 2.1
Transferrin (mg/dL)	200–250	100–200	< 100
Prealbumin (mg/dL)	10–17	5–10	< 5
Retinol-binding protein (mg/dL)	4.1–6.1 (normal)	< 4.1	
Total lymphocyte count (cells/μL)	1200–2000	800–1200	< 800
Creatinine-height index (%)	60–80	40–60	< 40
Ideal body weight (%)	80–90	70–80	< 70
Weight loss/time	< 5%/month < 7.5%/3 months < 10%/6 months	< 2%/week > 7.5%/3 months > 10%/6 months	> 2%/week
Skin antigen testing (No. reactive/No. placed)	4/4 (normal)	1–2/4 (weak)	0/4 (anergic)

Anthropometric Measurements	Male	Female
Triceps skin fold (mm)	≤12.5	≤16.5
Midhumeral circumference (cm)	> 29	> 28.5

[1]Nutritional supplementation is indicated.

for assessing response to nutritional repletion. Transferrin has a shorter half-life of 8–10 days and is a more sensitive indicator of adequate nutrition repletion than albumin. Prealbumin has a half-life of 2–3 days, and retinol-binding protein has a half-life of 12 hours. Unfortunately, their serum levels are also influenced by other factors, limiting their utility in assessing nutritional status or repletion.

Immune function may be assessed by hypersensitivity skin testing as well as total lymphocytic count, a reflection of T- and B-cell status. Subcutaneous injection of common antigens provides a semi-objective assessment of the antibody-mediated immune response, commonly impaired in malnourished patients. A low total lymphocyte count (TLC) correlates directly with the degree of malnutrition, though the count may be altered by infection, chemotherapy, and other factors, thus limiting its usefulness.

Nutritional Indices

Indices provide a means of risk-stratification and objective comparison among patients (Table 10–3). Additionally, many nutritional indices have been prospectively validated and can provide prognostic information to further guide nutrition support services. Along with the BMI, these indices can assist surgeons in determining the correct timing for intervention and the progress being made toward the goal of adequate nourishment.

A. Creatinine-Height Index (CHI)

CHI may be used to determine the degree of protein malnutrition, although it is less valid in patients who are severely catabolic or have chronic renal disease. A 24-hour urinary creatinine excretion is measured and compared with normal standards. CHI is calculated by the following equation:

$$\text{CHI} = \frac{\text{Actual 24-hour urine creatinine excretion}}{\text{Predicted creatinine excretion}}$$

The urinary excretion of 3-methylhistidine is a more precise measurement of lean body mass and associated protein stores. The amino acid histidine is irreversibly methylated in muscle. During protein turnover, 3-methylhistidine is not reutilized for synthesis, so the urinary excretion of this compound correlates well with muscle protein breakdown. Unfortunately, measurement of 3-methylhistidine is too expensive for use as a routine clinical test.

B. Prognostic Nutrition Index (PNI)

The PNI has been validated in patients undergoing either major cancer or gastrointestinal surgery and found to accurately identify a subset of patients at

Table 10–3. Nutritional indices.

Body Mass Index (BMI)	
BMI = weight (kg)/height^2 (m) = 703 × weight (lb)/height^2 (in)	
Normal	18.5–24.9
Overweight	25–29.9
Obese	30–40
Morbid obesity	> 40
Prognostic Nutritional Index (PNI)	
PNI = 158 – [16.6 × Alb] – [0.78 × TSF] – [0.2 × TFN] – [5.8 × DH]	
Note: for DH, > 5 mm induration = 2; 1–5 mm induration = 1; anergy = 0	
Risk for complications:	
Low	< 40%
Intermediate	40–49%
High	≥50%
Nutrition Risk Index (NRI)	
NRI = [15.19 × Alb] + 41.7 × [actual weight (kg) / ideal weight (kg)]	
Well-nourished	> 100
Mild malnutrition	97.5–100
Moderate malnutrition	83.5–97.5
Severe malnutrition	< 83.5
Catabolic Index (CI)	
CI = [24-hr urine urea nitrogen excretion in g] – [0.5 × (dietary nitrogen intake in g)]	
No physiologic stress	0
Mild stress	0–5
Moderate/severe stress	> 5

Alb, albumin (g/dL).
TSF, triceps skin fold (mm).
TFN, transferrin (mg/dL).
DH, delayed cutaneous hypersensitivity.

increased risk for complications. Furthermore, preoperative nutritional repletion has been shown to reduce postoperative morbidity in this patient group. The PNI has been widely adapted to identify patients at risk in other (nonsurgical) populations, who may benefit from nutritional support.

C. Nutrition Risk Index (NRI)

The NRI was used by the VA TPN Cooperative Study Group for determining preoperative malnutrition, and it has since been prospectively cross-validated against other nutritional indices with good results. The index successfully stratifies perioperative morbidity and mortality using serum albumin and weight loss as predictors of malnutrition. Of note, the NRI is not a tool for tracking the adequacy of nutritional support, since supplemental nutrition often fails to improve serum albumin levels.

D. Subjective Global Assessment (SGA)

Subjective Global Assessment is the only clinical method that has been validated as reproducible and which encompasses the patient's history and physical examination. It is based on five features of the medical history (weight loss in the past 6 months, dietary intake, gastrointestinal symptoms, functional status or energy level, and metabolic demands) along with four features of the physical examination (loss of subcutaneous fat, muscle wasting, edema, and ascites). Limitations of the SGA include its focus on chronic instead of acute nutritional changes and its enhanced specificity at the expense of sensitivity.

Determining Energy Requirements

Adult basal energy expenditure (BEE) is calculated using a modification of the Harris-Benedict equation (Table 10–4). Calculation includes four variables—height (cm), weight (kg), gender, and age (yr). Total energy expenditure (TEE) represents the caloric demands of the body under certain physiologic stresses. TEE is determined by multiplying BEE by a disease-specific stress factor. TEE should be used to guide nutritional supplementation.

Indirect calorimetry is the most accurate method for direct measurement of daily caloric requirements. Using a metabolic cart, oxygen consumption ($\dot{V}O_2$) and carbon dioxide production ($\dot{V}CO_2$) are directly measured from

Table 10–4. Total energy expenditure equation for adults.

Basal energy expenditure (BEE) in kcal/day	
Male:	
66.4 + [13.7 × weight (kg)] + [5.0 × height (cm)] – [6.8 × age (yr)]	
Female:	
655 + [9.6 × weight (kg)] + [1.7 × height (cm)] – [4.7 × age (yr)]	
Stress factors	
Starvation	0.80–1.00
Elective surgery	1.00–1.10
Peritonitis	1.05–1.25
Adult respiratory distress syndrome (ARDS) or sepsis	1.30–1.35
Bone marrow transplant	1.20–1.30
Cardiopulmonary disease (uncomplicated)	0.80–1.00
Cardiopulmonary disease with dialysis or sepsis	1.20–1.30
Cardiopulmonary disease with major surgery	1.30–1.55
Acute renal failure	1.30
Liver failure	1.30–1.55
Liver transplantation	1.20–1.50
Pancreatitis or major burns	1.30–1.80
Total energy expenditure (TEE) in kcal/day	
TEE = BEE × stress factor	

the patient's pulmonary gas flow. Based on these measurements and the amount of nitrogen excreted in the urine, the resting energy expenditure (REE) can be derived using the Weir formula as follows:

$$\text{REE (kcal/min)} = 3.9(\dot{V}O_2) + 1.1(\dot{V}CO_2) - 2.2(\text{urine nitrogen})$$

where $\dot{V}O_2$ and ($\dot{V}CO_2$ are expressed in milliliters per minute and urine nitrogen is in grams per minute. The utility of this technique is limited by the expense and cumbersomeness of the metabolic cart.

The nonprotein respiratory quotient (RQ) is the ratio of carbon dioxide production to oxygen consumption in the metabolism of fuels by the body. When the RQ is 1, pure carbohydrate is being oxidized. Patients metabolizing lipids only will have an RQ of 0.67. Lipogenesis occurs in patients with excess caloric intake (overfeeding). When excessive calories are ingested or administered, the RQ is greater than 1 and can theoretically approach 9. The excess production of CO_2 may impair ventilator weaning in patients with intrinsic lung disease (eg, chronic obstructive pulmonary disease).

NUTRIENT REQUIREMENTS & SUBSTRATES

The body requires an energy source to remain in steady state. About 50% of the basal metabolic rate (BMR) reflects the work of ion pumping, 30% represents protein turnover, and the remainder represents recycling of amino acids, glucose, lactate, and pyruvate. Total energy expenditure is the sum of energy consumed in basal metabolic processes, physical activity, the specific dynamic action of protein, and extra requirements resulting from injury, sepsis, or burns. Energy consumed in physical activity constitutes 10–50% of the total in normal subjects but decreases to 10–20% for hospitalized patients. Energy expenditure and requirements vary, depending on the illness or trauma. The increase in energy expenditure above basal needs is about 10% for elective operations, 10–30% for trauma, 50–80% for sepsis, and 100–200% for burns (depending on the extent of the wound). Metabolic energy can be derived from carbohydrates, proteins, or fats.

Carbohydrate Metabolism

Carbohydrates are the body's primary fuel source under usual conditions, accounting for 30–40% of total caloric intake. Each gram of enteric carbohydrate provides 4 kilocalories (kcal) of energy. Parenterally administered carbohydrates (eg, intravenous dextrose) yield 3.4 kcal per gram.

Carbohydrate digestion is initiated by the action of salivary amylase, and absorption is generally completed within the first 1.0–1.5 m of the small intestine. Salivary and pancreatic amylases cleave starches into oligosaccharides on contact. Surface oligosaccharidases then hydrolyze and transport these molecules across the GI tract mucosa. Deficiencies in carbohydrate digestion and absorption are rare in surgical patients. Pancreatic amylase is abundant, and maldigestion of starch does not usually occur, even in patients with limited pancreatic exocrine function. Patients with diseases such as celiac sprue, Whipple's disease, and hypogammaglobulinemia often have generalized intestinal mucosal flattening and consequent oligosaccharidase deficiency and diminished uptake of carbohydrate.

More than 75% of ingested carbohydrate is broken down and absorbed as glucose. Hyperglycemia stimulates insulin secretion from pancreatic β-cells, which influences protein synthesis. A minimum intake of 400 kcal of carbohydrate per day minimizes protein breakdown, particularly after adaptation to starvation. Cellular uptake of glucose, stimulated by insulin, inhibits lipolysis and promotes glycogen formation. Conversely, the pancreatic hormone glucagon is released in response to starvation or stress; it promotes proteolysis, glycogenolysis, lipolysis, and increased serum glucose. Glucose is essential for wound repair, but excessive carbohydrate intake or repletion with excessive amounts of glucose can cause hepatic steatosis and neutrophil dysfunction.

Protein Metabolism

Proteins are comprised of amino acids and metabolism produces 4 kilocalories per gram of protein. Digestion of proteins yields dipeptides and single amino acids, which are actively absorbed by the gastrointestinal tract. Gastric pepsin initiates the process of digestion. Pancreatic proteases, activated on exposure to enterokinase found throughout the duodenal mucosa, are the principal effectors of protein degradation. Once digested, almost 50% of protein absorption occurs in the duodenum, and complete protein absorption is achieved by the mid-jejunum.

Protein absorption occurs effectively at every level of the small intestine; therefore, clinically significant protein malabsorption is relatively infrequent even after extensive intestinal resection. Protein balance reflects the sum of protein synthesis and degradation. Because protein turnover is in constant flux, the published requirements for protein, amino acids, and nitrogen are only approximations.

Total body protein in a 70-kg person is approximately 10–11 kg, concentrated predominantly in skeletal muscle. Daily protein turnover is 250–300 g, or roughly 3% of total body protein. The daily protein requirement in healthy adults is 0.8 g/kg body weight. In the United States, the typical daily intake averages twice this amount.

Protein synthesis or breakdown can be determined by measuring the nitrogen balance (Table 10–5). Protein intake of 6.25 g is equivalent to 1 g of nitrogen. Nitrogen intake is the sum of nitrogen delivered from enteric and parenteral feeding. Nitrogen output is the sum of nitrogen excreted in the urine and feces, plus losses from any other source of drainage (eg, exudative wounds, gastrocutaneous fistula). Urea nitrogen losses are determined from a 24-hour urine collection. Fecal nitrogen loss can be approximated by 1 g per day, and an additional 2–3 g per day of non-urea nitrogen loss occurs in the urine (eg, ammonia). The accuracy of nitrogen balance calculations can be improved through measurement over several weeks. When losses of nitrogen are large (eg, diarrhea, protein-losing enteropathy, fistula, or burn exudate), measurements of nitrogen balance lose accuracy because of the difficulty in collecting all of the secretions. Despite these shortcomings, 24-hour urine collection for nitrogen balance determination is the best practical means of measuring net protein synthesis and breakdown.

The 20 amino acids are divided into essential amino acids (EAAs) and nonessential amino acids (NEAAs) depending on whether they can be synthesized de novo in the body. They are further divided into aromatic (AAAs), branched chain (BCAAs), and sulfur-containing amino acids. Only the L-isotype of an amino acid is utilized in human protein. Amino acids contain highly reactive thiol, imidazole, aromatic, and dicarboxylic acid groups, which catalyze chemical reactions and determine the tertiary structures of protein molecules via polar, hydrophobic, nonionic, disulfide, and hydrogen bonding. Certain amino acids have unique metabolic functions, particularly during starvation or stress. For example, alanine and glutamine participate in a cycle with glucose that preserves carbon during starvation; leucine stimulates protein synthesis and inhibits catabolism; and BCAAs are the fuels preferred by cardiac and skeletal muscle during starvation. Specific amino acids are addressed below.

A. Glutamine

Although classified as a nonessential amino acid, glutamine plays an important role in the metabolically stressed patient. Glutamine is the crucial respiratory fuel for enterocytes. It is metabolized in the small intestine to ammonia, citrulline,alanine, and proline, and the carbon skeleton serves as an energy precursor for the enterocyte.

Table 10–5. Nitrogen balance.

$\textbf{Nitrogen}_{\textbf{(balance)}} = \textbf{Nitrogen}_{\textbf{(intake)}} - \textbf{Nitrogen}_{\textbf{(output)}}$
$\text{Nitrogen}_{(\text{intake})} = \text{g protein}_{(\text{intake})} / 6.25$
$\text{Nitrogen}_{(\text{output})} = (\text{UUN} \times \text{Vol}) + 3$

UUN is urine urea nitrogen; Vol is the volume of urine produced over the time of measurement.

Following injury and other catabolic events, intracellular glutamine stores may decrease by over 50% and plasma levels by 25%. The decline of glutamine associated with injury or stress exceeds that of any other amino acid and persists during recovery after the concentrations of other amino acid have normalized. Supplementation with glutamine maintains intestinal cell integrity, villous height, and mucosal DNA activity and helps minimize reduction in numbers of T- and B-cells during stress.

Glutamine is avidly consumed by replicating cells, such as fibroblasts, lymphocytes, neoplastic cells, and intestinal epithelium. Catabolic states are characterized by accelerated skeletal muscle proteolysis and translocation of amino acids from the periphery to the visceral organs. Glutamine accounts for a major portion of the amino acids released by muscle in these states. Supplementation with glutamine may improve neutrophil and macrophage function in burn patients and other critically ill patients. Uniquely formulated diets that incorporate glutamine show promise for treating patients with short gut syndrome by accelerating intestinal adaptation.

B. Arginine

Arginine is a substrate for the urea cycle and nitric oxide production and a secretagogue for growth hormone, prolactin, and insulin. Formulas supplemented with arginine have been shown to improve nitrogen balance and wound healing, stimulate T-cell response, and reduce the incidence of infectious complications. T-cell proliferation and function in humans are stimulated in response to arginine supplementation, and albumin synthesis has also been shown to improve with additional amounts of this amino acid. The effects of arginine on T cells may be very important in maintaining the gut barrier. Arginine has been identified as the sole precursor of nitric oxide (endothelial-derived relaxing factor).

C. Taurine

Levels of taurine in the circulation decline markedly in severely catabolic states such as sepsis or major traumatic injury. For this reason, taurine should be considered a "conditionally" essential amino acid. The liver produces organic osmolytes to respond to changes in plasma osmolarity. Taurine is the major osmolyte released in response to hypo-osmotic stress and is the most important osmolyte under normo-osmolar conditions. Additionally, taurine may act to reduce circulating toxins by binding chlorinated oxidants. Taurine release by the liver is increased with glutamine supplementation, demonstrating a complex coregulation between the amino acids.

Lipid Metabolism

Lipids comprise 25–45% of caloric intake in the typical diet. Each gram of lipid provides 9 kcal of energy. Digestion and absorption of lipids is complex and requires coordination between biliary and pancreatic secretions, as well as a functional jejunum and ileum. The introduction of fat to the duodenum results in secretion of cholecystokinin and secretin, leading to gallbladder contraction and pancreatic enzyme release, respectively. Pancreatic secretions contain a combination of lipase, cholesterol esterase, and phospholipase A_2. The alkaline environment of the duodenum facilitates hydrolysis of triglycerides to a monoglyceride and two fatty acids by lipase. Bile salts lead to emulsification. Micelle formation is the most important step in lipid absorption, facilitating absorption of fats across the mucosal barrier. Reabsorption of bile salts (eg, the enterohepatic circulation) is necessary to maintain the bile salt pool. The liver is able to compensate for moderate intestinal bile salt losses by increased synthesis from cholesterol. Major ileal resection may lead to depletion of the bile salt pool and subsequent fat malabsorption. Lipolysis is stimulated by steroids, catecholamines, and glucagon but is inhibited by insulin.

Dietary fats are the sole precursors to eicosanoid production and are potent immunomodulators. Fats or fatty acids are hydrocarbon chains ranging from 2 to 24 carbons in length. The body can synthesize fats from other dietary substrates, but two of the long-chain fatty acids (linoleic and linolenic) are essential. Insufficient intake of these essential fats leads to fatty acid deficiency and can be prevented by supplying a minimum of 3% of the total caloric intake as essential fatty acids.

The polyunsaturated fatty acids (PUFAs) are grouped into two families: ω-6 and ω-3 fatty acids. Linoleic acid is an example of the ω-6 PUFAs; ω-linolenic acid of the ω-3 PUFAs. Vegetable oils such as corn, safflower, sunflower, and soybean oils are good sources of linoleic acid (ω-6 PUFA). Linseed, canola, walnut, and soybean oils are good sources of ω-linolenic acid (ω-3 PUFA). Coldwater fish are a rich source of ω-3 fatty acids, specifically eicosapentaenoic acid (EPA) and docosahexaenoic acid (DHA). Both linoleic and linolenic acid can be processed into arachidonic acid, a precursor in the synthesis of eicosanoids. Eicosanoids are potent biochemical mediators of cell-to-cell communication and are involved in inflammation, infection, tissue injury, and immune system modulation. They also modulate numerous events involving cell-mediated and humoral immunity and can be synthesized in varying amounts by all immune cells, particularly macrophages and monocytes. Diets high in ω-6 fatty acids suppress immune function by inhibiting mitogenesis due to increased prostaglandin E_2 synthesis, which inhibits T-cell proliferation. The administration of additional ω-3 PUFAs has been shown to negate this effect.

Medium-chain fatty acids are generally not components of most oral diets but are widely used in enteral tube feedings. They are easily digested, absorbed, and oxidized and are not precursors to the inflammatory or immunosuppressive eicosanoids. Short-chain fatty acids, such as butyrate and to a lesser extent propionate, are utilized by colonocytes and provide up to 70% of their energy requirements. Since butyrate is not synthesized endogenously, the colonic mucosa relies on intraluminal bacterial fermentation to obtain this fuel.

Nucleotides, Vitamins, & Trace Elements

In addition to the principal sources of metabolic energy (calories), many other substances are necessary to ensure adequate nutrition. Long considered as simple end products of anabolism, nucleotides are now recognized as an important nutritional substrate in critically ill patients. Vitamins are essential for normal metabolism, wound healing, and immune function. They are essential parts of the diet because they cannot be synthesized de novo. The normal requirements for vitamins are shown in Table 10–6. Vitamin requirements may increase in illness. Trace elements are integral cofactors for many enzymatic reactions and are generally not stored by the body in excess of requirements.

A. Nucleotides

Nucleic acids are precursors of DNA and RNA and participate in a number of metabolic reactions fundamental to cellular activity. They have generally not been considered essential for human growth and development. The need for dietary nucleotides increases in severe stress and critical illness. Nucleotides are formed from purines and pyrimidines, and their abundance is especially important for rapidly dividing cells such as enterocytes and immune cells. Immunosuppression has been reported in renal transplant patients being maintained on nucleotide-free diets. Dietary nucleotides are necessary for helper-inducer T-lymphocyte activity. Diets supplemented with RNA or the pyrimidine uracil have been shown to restore delayed hypersensitivity and augment both the lymphoproliferative response and IL-2 receptor expression. Nucleotides may facilitate recovery from infection, as shown in animal studies where increased resistance to *Candida albicans* and *Staphylococcus aureus* infections occurred in groups receiving diets enriched with uracil or RNA. These substrates are incorporated into enteral formulas as potential immunomodulators.

B. Fat-Soluble Vitamins

Vitamins A, D, E, and K are fat soluble and are absorbed in the proximal small bowel in association with bile salt micelles and fatty acids. After absorption, they are delivered to the tissues in chylomicrons and stored in large quantities in the liver (vitamins A and K) or subcutaneous tissue and skin (vitamins D and E). Although rare, there are reports of toxicity from excessive intake of fat-soluble vitamins (eg, hypervitaminosis A from consuming polar bear liver). Fat-soluble vitamins participate in immune function and

Table 10–6. Daily electrolyte, trace element, vitamin, and mineral requirements for adults.

	Enteral	Parenteral
Electrolytes		
Sodium	90–150 meq	90–150 meq
Potassium	60–90 meq	60–90 meq
Trace elements		
Chromium[1]	5–200 μg	10–15 μg
Copper[1]	2–3 mg	0.15–0.5 mg
Manganese[1]	2.5–5 mg	0.15–0.8 mg
Zinc	15 mg	2.5–4 mg
Iron	10 mg	2.5 mg
Iodine	150 μg	...
Fluoride[1]	3 mg	...
Selenium[1]	50–200 μg	20–40 μg
Molybdenum[1]	150–500 μg	20–120 μg
Tin[2]	...	...
Vanadium[2]	...	...
Nickel[2]	...	...
Arsenic[2]	...	...
Silicon[2]	...	...
Vitamins		
Ascorbic acid (C)	60 mg	100 mg
Retinol (A)	1000 μg	3300 IU
Vitamin D	5 μg	200 IU
Thiamin (B_1)	1.4 mg	3 mg
Riboflavin (B_2)	1.7 mg	3.6 mg
Pyridoxine (B_6)	2.2 mg	4 mg
Niacin	19 mg	40 mg
Pantothenic acid	4–7 mg	15 mg
Vitamin E	10 mg	10 IU
Biotin	100–200 μg	60 μg
Folic acid[1]	200 μg	200 μg
Cyanobalamin (B_{12})	2 μg	5.9 μg
Vitamin K[3]	70–149 mg	10 mg
Minerals		
Calcium	1300 mg	0.2–0.3 meq/kg
Phosphorous	800 mg	300–400 meq/kg
Magnesium	350 mg	0.34–0.45 meq/kg
Sulfur	2–3 g	...

[1]Estimated safe and adequate dose.
[2]No available data regarding human requirements.
[3]Weekly requirement.

wound healing. For example, intake of vitamin A 25,000 IU daily counteracts steroid-induced inhibition of wound healing, largely through increases in TBG-β.

C. Water-Soluble Vitamins

Vitamins B_1, B_2, B_6, and B_{12}, vitamin C, and niacin, folate, biotin, and pantothenic acid are absorbed in the duodenum and proximal small bowel, transported in portal vein blood, and utilized in the liver and peripherally. Water-soluble vitamins serve as cofactors to facilitate reactions involved in the generation and transfer of energy and in amino acid and nucleic acid metabolism. Water-soluble vitamins have limited storage in the body. Only vitamin B_{12} is stored to any extent. Because of their limited storage, water-soluble vitamin deficiencies are relatively common.

D. Trace Elements

The daily requirements for the trace elements (Table 10–6) vary geographically depending on differences in soil composition. There are currently nine identified essential trace minerals for humans (Fe, Zn, Cu, Se, Mn, I, Mb, Cr, Co), although others can be found in key enzymatic reactions (eg, boron, fluoride). Trace elements have important functions in metabolism, immunology, and wound healing. Subclinical trace element deficiencies occur commonly in hospitalized patients and various disease states.

Iron serves as the core of the heme prosthetic group in hemoglobin and in the mitochondrial cytochrome respiratory process. Impaired cerebral, muscular, and immunologic function can occur in patients with iron deficiency before anemia becomes clinically evident. Particular attention should be paid to assessing iron stores in pregnant and lactating women.

Zinc is a cofactor for a number of metalloenzymes involved in carbohydrate, fat, amino acid, and nucleic acid metabolism. Deficiency may develop in patients with large fecal losses or after prolonged total parenteral nutrition (TPN) in the absence of zinc supplementation. Clinically, zinc deficiency is characterized by a perioral pustular rash, darkening of skin creases, neuritis, cutaneous anergy, hair loss, and alterations in taste and smell.

Copper is a component of a number of metalloenzymes, including cytochrome oxidase (the terminal enzyme of the electron transport chain), dopamine hydroxylase (a key enzyme in catecholamine metabolism), and lysyl oxidase (which is involved in collagen cross-linkage). Ceruloplasmin is an acute phase reactant that binds the majority of circulating copper and is often used as a surrogate marker for copper stores. This protein stimulates iron release from the liver. Copper deficiency is manifested by microcytic anemia (unresponsive to iron), defective keratinization, or pancytopenia.

Chromium forms a complex with a small peptide containing nicotinic acid to produce glucose tolerance factor (GTF). GTF facilitates the binding of insulin to membrane receptors. Chromium may improve glucose tolerance in patients with adult-onset diabetes mellitus. Chromium deficiency presents as sudden glucose intolerance during prolonged TPN administration without evidence of concomitant sepsis.

Selenium is part of the enzyme glutathione peroxidase. A decrease in the activity of this enzyme leads to peroxidation of membrane lipids, resulting in elevated concentrations of pentane in expired air. Selenium deficiency, which can occur in patients receiving TPN for a prolonged period, is manifested by proximal neuromuscular weakness or cardiac failure with electrocardiographic changes.

Manganese is the cofactor for the metalloenzymes pyruvate carboxylase and manganese-superoxide dismutase, which are involved in the initial step of gluconeogenesis and in cellular antioxidant capability, respectively. Manganese deficiency is associated with weight loss, altered hair pigmentation, nausea, and low plasma levels of phospholipids and triglycerides.

Molybdenum is involved in uric acid, purine, and amino acid metabolism as a cofactor for the metalloenzymes xanthine oxidase and aldehyde oxidase. Molybdenum deficiency results in elevated plasma methionine levels and depressed uric acid concentrations, producing a syndrome consisting of nausea, vomiting, tachycardia, and central nervous system disturbances.

Iodine is a key component of thyroid hormone. Deficiency is rare in the USA because of the widespread use of iodinated salt. Chronically malnourished patients can become iodine-deficient. Since thyroxine participates in the neuroendocrine response to trauma and sepsis, iodine should be included in TPN solutions.

NUTRITIONAL PATHOPHYSIOLOGY

Physiologic processes, immunocompetence, wound healing, and recovery from critical illness all depend upon adequate nutrient intake. A working knowledge of nutritional pathophysiology is essential in planning nutritional regimens.

Starvation

During an overnight fast, liver glycogen is rapidly depleted after a fall in insulin and parallel rise in plasma glucagon levels (Figure 10–1). Carbohydrate stores are depleted after a 24-hour fast. In the first few days of starvation,

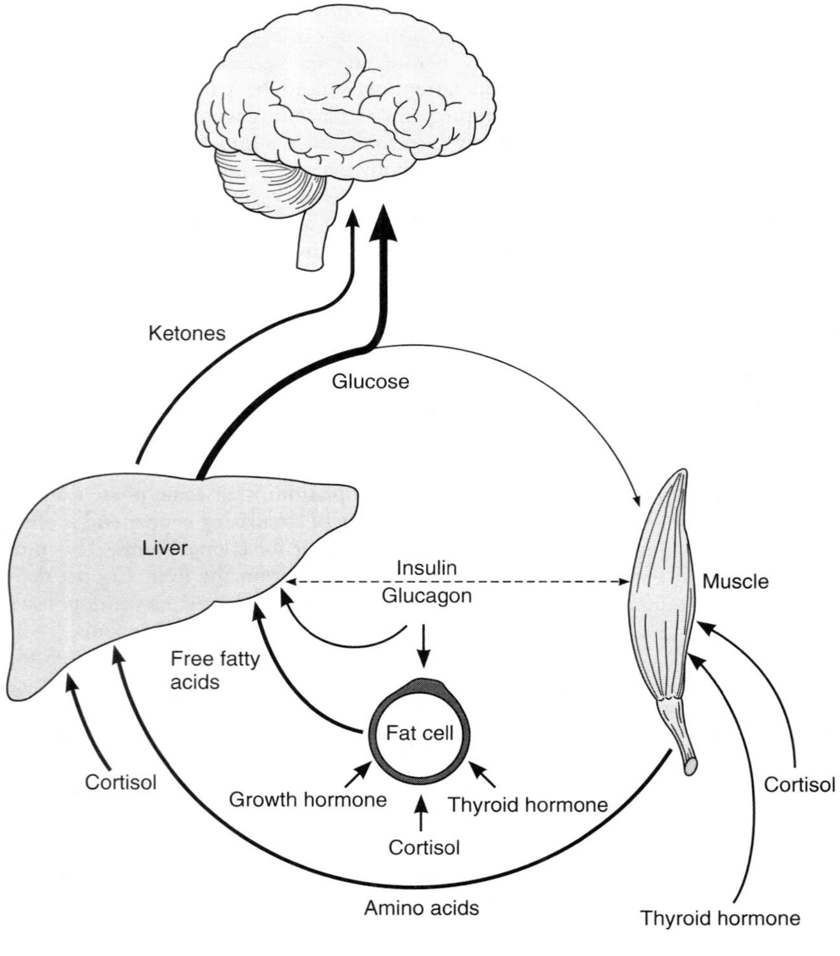

Figure 10–1. The plasma substrate concentrations and hormone levels following an overnight fast. The brain is dependent on glucose, which is supplied predominantly by hepatic glycogenolysis until glycogen supplies are exhausted.

caloric needs are met by fat and protein degradation. There is an increase in hepatic gluconeogenesis from amino acids derived from the breakdown of muscle protein. Hepatic glucose production must satisfy the energy demands of the hematopoietic and the central nervous systems, particularly the brain, which is dependent on glucose oxidation during acute starvation. The release of amino acids from muscle is regulated by insulin, which signals hepatic amino acid uptake, polyribosome formation, and protein synthesis. The periodic rise and fall of insulin associated with ingestion of nutrients stimulates muscle protein synthesis and breakdown. During starvation, chronically depressed insulin levels result in a net loss of amino acids from muscle. Protein synthesis drops while protein catabolism remains unchanged. Hepatic gluconeogenesis requires energy, which is supplied by the oxidation of FFA. The fall in insulin along with a rise in plasma glucagon levels leads to an increase in the concentration of cAMP in adipose tissue, stimulating hormone-sensitive lipase to hydrolyze triglycerides and release FFA. Gluconeogenesis and FFA mobilization require the presence of ambient cortisol and thyroid hormone (a permissive effect).

During starvation, the body attempts to conserve energy substrate by recycling metabolic intermediates. The hematopoietic system utilizes glucose anaerobically, leading to lactate production. Lactate is recycled back to glucose in the liver via the glucogenic (not gluconeogenic) Cori cycle (Figure 10–2). The glycerol released during peripheral triglyceride hydrolysis is converted into glucose via gluconeogenesis. Alanine and glutamine are the preferred substrates for hepatic gluconeogenesis from amino acids and contribute 75% of the amino acid-derived carbon for glucose production.

Branched chain amino acids (BCAAs) are unique because they are secreted rather than taken up by the liver during starvation; they are oxidized by skeletal and cardiac muscle to supply a portion of the energy requirements of these tissues; and they stimulate protein synthesis and inhibit catabolism. The amino groups that are derived from oxidation of BCAAs or transamination of other amino acids are donated to pyruvate or α-ketoglutarate to form alanine and glutamine. Glutamine is taken up by the small bowel, transaminated to form additional alanine, and released into the portal circulation. Along with glucose, these amino acids participate in the glucose-alanine/glutamine-BCAA cycle, which shuttles amino groups and carbon from muscle to liver for conversion into glucose.

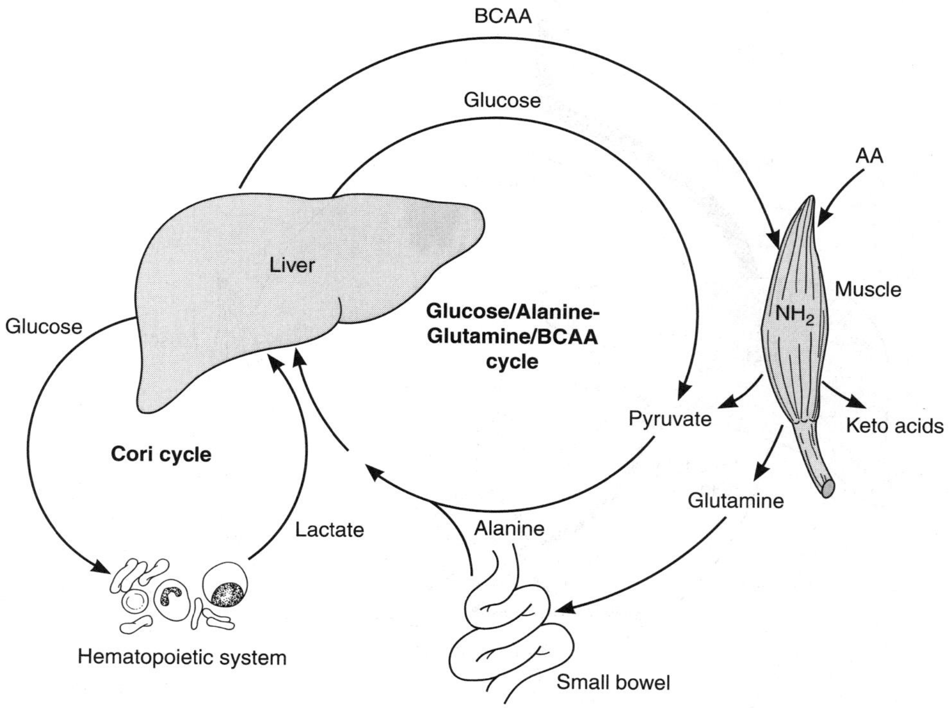

Figure 10–2. The cycles that preserve metabolic intermediates during fasting. Lactate is recycled to glucose via the Cori cycle, while pyruvate is transaminated to alanine in skeletal muscle and converted to glucose by hepatic gluconeogenesis.

Gluconeogenesis from amino acids results in a urinary nitrogen excretion of 8–12 g per day, predominantly as urea, which is equivalent to a loss of 340 g per day of lean tissue. At this rate, 35% of the lean body mass would be lost in 1 month, a uniformly fatal amount. However, starvation can be survived for 2–3 months as long as water is available. The body adapts to prolonged starvation by decreasing energy expenditures and shifting the substrate preference of the brain to ketones (Figure 10–3). After roughly 10 days of starvation, the brain adapts to use lipid as its primary fuel in the form of ketones. The basal metabolic rate decreases by slowing the heart rate and reducing stroke work, while voluntary activity declines owing to weakness and fatigue. The RQ, which in early starvation is 0.85 (reflecting mixed carbohydrate and fat oxidation), falls to 0.70, indicating near-exclusive fatty acid utilization. Blood ketone levels rise sharply, accompanied by increased cerebral ketone oxidation. Brain glucose utilization drops from 140 g to 60–80 g per day, decreasing the demand for gluconeogenesis. Ketones also inhibit hepatic gluconeogenesis, and urinary nitrogen excretion falls to 2–3 g per day. The main component of urine nitrogen is now ammonia (rather than urea), derived from renal transamination and gluconeogenesis from glutamine, and it buffers the acid urine that results from ketonuria. Acute or chronic starvation is characterized by hormone and fuel alterations orchestrated by changing blood substrate levels and can be conceptualized as a "substrate-driven" process. In summary, the adaptive changes in uncomplicated starvation are a decrease in energy expenditure (as much as a 30% reduction), a change in type of fuel

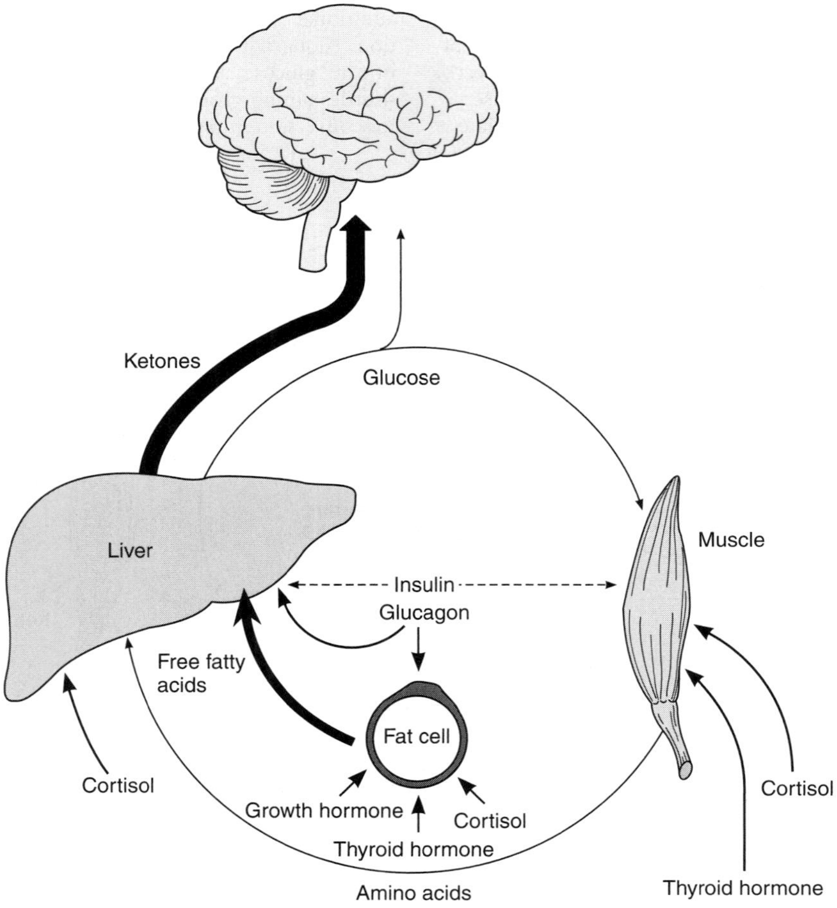

Figure 10–3. The metabolic adaptation to chronic starvation whereby the brain shifts its substrate preference to ketones produced by the liver. Hepatic gluconeogenesis falls and protein breakdown is diminished, thus conserving lean tissue.

consumed to maximize caloric potential, and preservation of protein.

Elective Operation or Trauma

The metabolic effects of elective operations and trauma (Figure 10–4) differ from those of simple starvation due to neurohormonal activation, which accelerates the loss of lean tissue and inhibits the metabolic adaptation characteristic of starvation. Following injury, neural impulses carried via spinothalamic pathways activate the brain stem and thalamic and cortical centers, which stimulate the hypothalamus. Hypothalamic stimulation triggers combined neural and endocrine discharges. Norepinephrine is released from sympathetic nerve endings, epinephrine from the adrenal medulla, aldosterone from the adrenal cortex, ADH from the posterior pituitary, insulin and glucagon from the pancreas, and ACTH, TSH, and growth hormone from the anterior pituitary. These hormones produce secondary elevations of cortisol, thyroid hormone, and somatomedins. The effects of the heightened neuroendocrine secretion include (1) peripheral lipolysis from the synergistic activation of hormone-sensitive lipase by glucagon, epinephrine, cortisol, and thyroid hormone; (2) accelerated catabolism, consisting of a rise in proteolysis stimulated by cortisol; and (3) decreased peripheral glucose uptake due to insulin antagonism by growth hormone and epinephrine. The consequences are a marked rise in plasma concentrations of FFA, glycerol, glucose, lactate, and amino acids. The liver responds with an

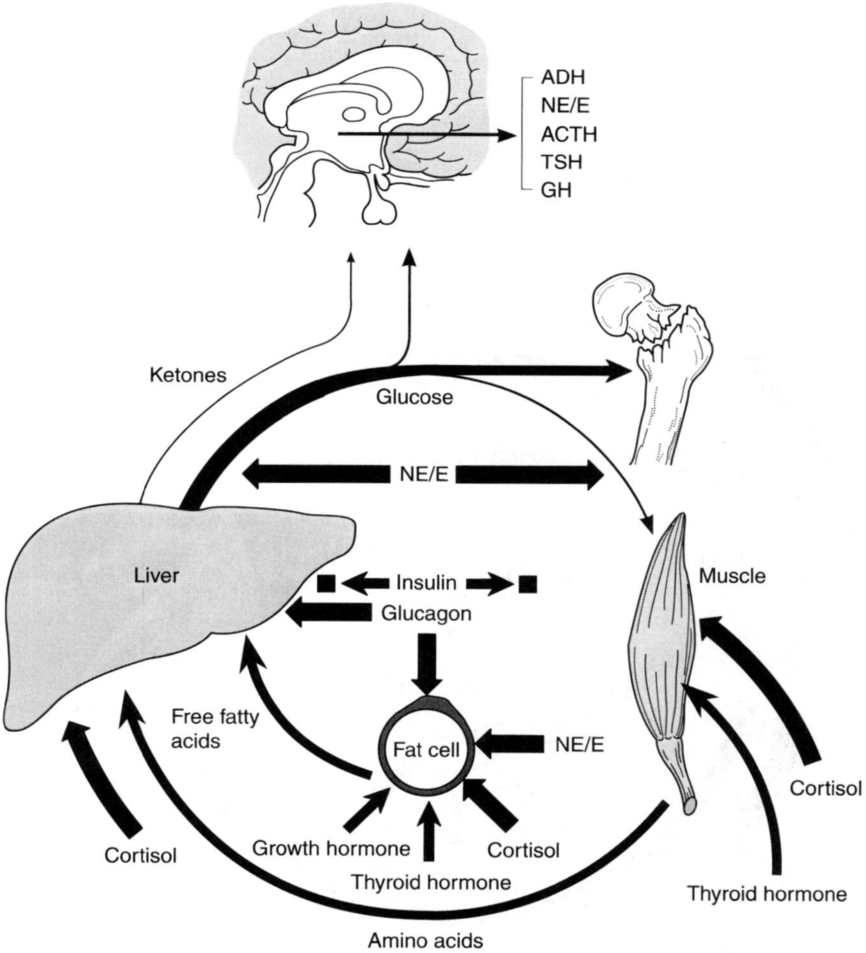

Figure 10–4. The metabolic response to trauma is a result of neuroendocrine stimulation, which accelerates protein breakdown, stimulates gluconeogenesis, and produces glucose intolerance.

increase in substrate uptake and glucose production, as a result of glucagon-stimulated glycogenolysis and enhanced gluconeogenesis induced by cortisol and glucagon.

This accelerated glucose production, along with inhibited peripheral uptake, produces the glucose intolerance commonly observed in traumatized patients. The kidney avidly retains water and sodium because of the effects of ADH and aldosterone. Urinary nitrogen excretion increases to 15–20 g per day in severe trauma, equivalent to a daily lean tissue loss of 750 g. Without exogenous nutrients, the median survival under these circumstances is about 15 days.

There are several reasons for the different metabolic responses observed following elective surgery versus major trauma. The neuroendocrine response is blunted in the operating room through the liberal use of analgesics and immobilization. Sedated patients lack cortical stimulation to the hypothalamus. Atraumatic surgical handling of tissues reduces proinflammatory cytokine release. The net result is that the REE rises only 10% in postoperative patients, compared with 25–30% after severe accidental trauma. In contrast to the substrate dependency of uncomplicated starvation, operation and trauma are "neuroendocrine-driven" processes.

Sepsis

The metabolic changes during sepsis differ from those observed after injury (Figure 10–5). The REE rises 50–

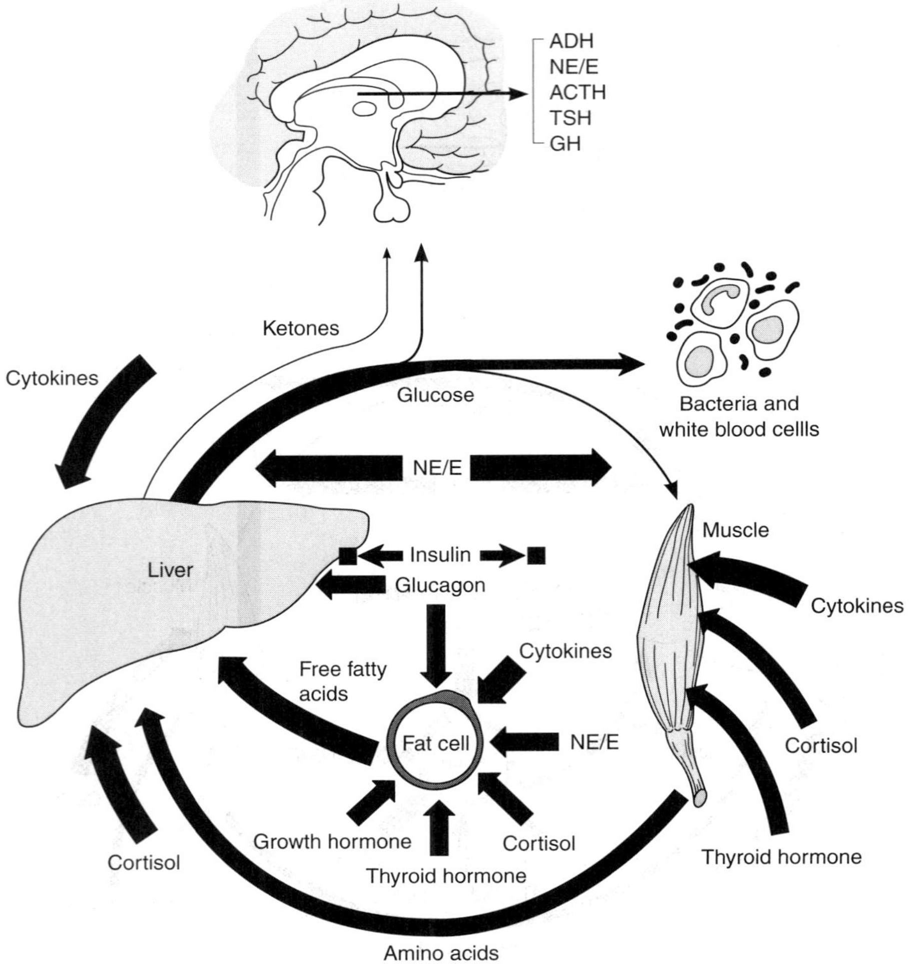

Figure 10–5. During sepsis, cytokines (IL-1, IL-2, TNF) released by lymphocytes and macrophages contribute to catabolism of muscle and adipose tissue and amplify the neurohormonal response to antecedent trauma.

80% above the norm, and urinary nitrogen excretion reaches 20–30 g per day, predominantly due to profound muscle catabolism and impaired synthesis. Catabolism at this rate equates to a median survival of 10 days without nutritional input. The plasma glucose, amino acid, and FFA levels increase more than with trauma. Hepatic protein synthesis is stimulated, with both enhanced secretion of export protein and accumulation of structural protein. The RQ falls to 0.69–0.71, indicative of intense lipid oxidation. This unchecked lipolysis and gluconeogenesis continues despite supplementation with carbohydrate or fat, leading to the hyperglycemia and insulin resistance commonly observed in septic patients.

Sepsis results in elaboration of inflammatory cytokines, most notably TNF-α, IL-1, and IL-6. Alteration in hepatic protein synthesis towards production of acute-phase proteins is triggered by IL-6. Septic patients also develop an abnormal plasma amino acid pattern (increased levels of AAAs and decreased levels of BCAAs) similar to that of patients with liver failure. In contrast to simple starvation, protein conservation does not occur in sepsis. Terminal sepsis results in further increases in plasma amino acids and a fall in glucose concentration, as hepatic amino acid clearance declines and gluconeogenesis ceases.

Boelens PG et al: Plasma taurine concentrations increase after enteral glutamine supplementation in trauma patients and stressed rats. Am J Clin Nutr 2003;77:250.

Braga M et al: Preoperative oral arginine and n-3 fatty acid supplementation improves the immunometabolic host response and outcome after colorectal resection for cancer. Surgery 2002; 132:805.

Gianotti L et al: A prospective, randomized clinical trial on perioperative feeding with an arginine-, omega-3 fatty acid, and RNA-enriched enteral diet: effect on host response and nutritional status. JPEN J Parenter Enteral Nutr 2001; 23:314.

Gibbs J et al: Preoperative serum albumin level as a predictor of operative mortality and morbidity. Arch Surg 1999;134:36.

Hambidge M: Biomarkers of trace mineral intake and status. J Nutr 2003;133:948S.

Nagel M: Nutrition screening: identifying patients at risk for malnutrition. Nutr Clin Pract 1998;8:171.

Nathens AB et al: Randomized, prospective trial of antioxidant supplementation in critically ill surgical patients. Ann Surg 2002;236:814.

Sax HC: Effect of immune enhancing formulas (IEF) in general surgery patients. JPEN J Parenter Enteral Nutr 2001;25: 519.

Schloerb PR: Immune-enhancing diets: products, components, and their rationales. JPEN J Parenter Enteral Nutr 2001;25:53.

Sungurtekin H et al: Comparison of two nutrition assessment techniques in hospitalized patients. Nutr 2004;20:248.

The Veterans Affairs Total Parenteral Nutrition Cooperative Study Group: Perioperative total parenteral nutrition in surgical patients. N Engl J Med 1991;325:527.

ENTERAL NUTRITIONAL THERAPY

Enteral versus Parenteral Nutrition

Postoperative enteral nutritional support is safer and less expensive that parenteral nutrition and has the added benefit of preserving gut functionality. Prospective, randomized trials have demonstrated the superiority of enteral nutrition in reducing postoperative complications and length of hospital stay. "Feeding the gut" also results in fewer all-source infectious complications. Without a doubt, parenteral nutrition has a role in the management of surgical patients, but utilizing the gastrointestinal tract should remain the preferred treatment option. However, enteral supplementation is not risk-free. Physicians must know how to prevent and treat these complications so that enteral feedings can be administered successfully and safely.

Benefits of Enteral Feeding

A. Physiologic and Metabolic Benefits

The gastrointestinal tract can be used for administration of complex nutrients (eg, intact protein, peptides, fiber) that cannot be given intravenously. Gut processing of intact nutrients provides a stimulus for hepatic synthetic function of proteins, whereas administration of nutrients directly into the systemic circulation bypasses the portal circulation. In addition to its systemic benefits, enteral feeding has beneficial local effects on gastrointestinal mucosa. These include trophic stimulation and maintenance of absorptive structures by nourishing the enterocytes directly, thus supporting epithelial cell repair and replication. Luminal nutrients such as glutamine and short-chain fatty acids are used as fuel by the cells of the small bowel and colon, respectively.

B. Immunologic Benefits

The presence of food in the gut, particularly complex proteins and fats, supports the mucosa's critical function as an immunologic barrier by triggering feeding-dependent neuroendocrine activity. This activity stimulates the production of immunoglobulins in the gut, particularly secretory immunoglobulin A, which is important for preventing bacterial adherence to gut mucosa and bacterial translocation. The presence of nutrients in the gut also helps maintain normal gut pH and flora, thus diminishing opportunistic bacterial overgrowth in the small bowel.

C. Safety Benefits

Enteral feeding is generally considered safer than parenteral feeding. Meta-analysis of prospective trials has demonstrated fewer infectious complications with enteral nutrition compared with parenteral nutrition. Subset analysis suggests that enteral nutrition does not result in a lower risk of infection, but rather that parenteral nutrition results in a higher risk. Hyperglycemia, and its resulting inhibition of neutrophil-mediated immunity, also occurs more frequently with parenteral feeding. Enteral nutrition has its own potential complications (discussed below).

D. Cost Benefits

The direct costs of enteral feeding are generally less than those with parenteral nutrition. Direct costs include formula, feeding pumps, and tube placement. The cost advantage for enteral feeding is even greater when indirect costs (eg, central line infection or thrombosis, home health care) are considered.

Indications for Enteral Feeding

Enteral nutrition is the preferred method of nutrition support for malnourished patients (or those who are at risk for developing malnutrition) with an intact gastrointestinal tract. Certain patients are either unable or unwilling to eat in order to meet two-thirds to three-quarters of their daily needs; these patients are also candidates for enteral support. Factors influencing the timing of initiation of enteral nutrition include evidence of preexisting malnutrition, expected degree of catabolic activity, duration of the current illness, and anticipated return to intake by mouth. Patients with partially functioning GI tracts (eg, short bowel syndrome, proximal enterocutaneous fistula) often can tolerate some enteral feeding but may require a combined regimen (both parenteral and enteral) to meet total caloric needs.

Possible Contraindications to Enteral Feeding

Contraindications to enteral feeding are relative or temporary rather than absolute. Patients with short bowel, gastrointestinal obstruction, gastrointestinal bleeding, protracted vomiting and diarrhea, fistulas, ileus, or active gastrointestinal ischemia may require a period of bowel rest. In times of physiologic stress, the body shunts blood away from the splanchnic circulation. Feeding a patient who is hemodynamically unstable or requiring vasopressors may produce bowel ischemia in the setting of preexisting tenuous perfusion. The choice of an appropriate feeding site, administration technique, formula, and equipment may circumvent many of these contraindications.

Implementing Enteral Supplementation

A. Delivery Methods

Prepyloric access via nasogastric tube is beneficial because it is less expensive, easier to secure and maintain, and less labor-intensive than small bowel access. Contraindications to delivery in the stomach are delayed gastric emptying, gastric outlet obstruction, and a history of repeated aspiration of tube feedings due to reflux. Some physicians consider the inability to protect the airway (eg, comatose patients) a relative contraindication to gastric feeding. Diabetics and patients with severe head injuries may have profound gastroparesis. Postpyloric access via a duodenal or jejunal nasoenteric tube is preferred when gastric feedings are not tolerated, when patients are at risk for reflux or aspiration, or when early enteral nutrition is desired. In general, a jejunal tube is preferable since the shorter duodenal tubes have an increased incidence of reflux of feedings or tube migration into the stomach. The literature particularly supports the exclusive use of nasojejunal tubes in patients with severe burns. Patients with nasal obstruction or severe facial fractures should not have these tubes inserted nasally but can have the tube inserted orally once skull base fractures are ruled out. Although a number of bedside methods (eg, auscultation, feeding tube aspirate pH measurements, observation for patient coughing) have been described to check tube placement, these methods can be unreliable. Therefore, tube position below the diaphragm should always be confirmed radiographically before initiating enteral feeding.

Permanent gastrostomy or jejunostomy tubes may be inserted when long-term enteral feeding is indicated. Placement of a feeding tube at the time of the initial operation requires forethought, with consideration given to the patient's expected postoperative course, anticipated ileus, and possible future need for supplementation (eg, during chemoradiation therapy). Surgically placed jejunal feeding tubes are superior to gastrostomy tubes with respect to ease of care, patient tolerance, and need for subsequent manipulation or reintervention.

B. Formulas

Currently available dietary formulations for enteral feedings may be divided into polymeric commercial formulas (blenderized and nutritionally complete), chemically defined formulas (elemental diets), and modular formulas (Table 10–7). Selection of the correct formulation is predicated on patient need, cost, availability and institutional custom.

Blenderized tube feedings may be composed of any food that can be ground in a blender. Caloric distribution of these formulas parallels a normal diet. Nutritionally complete commercial formulas (standard enteral diets) vary in protein, carbohydrate, and fat composition. Most formulas use sucrose or glucose as the carbohydrate source and are suitable for lactose-deficient patients. Commercial formulas are convenient, sterile, and affordable. They are recommended for patients experiencing minimal metabolic stress who have normal gut function.

Chemically defined formulas are commonly called elemental diets. The nutrients are provided in a predigested and readily absorbed form. They contain protein in the form of low-molecular-weight free amino acids or polypeptides. Amino acid (elemental) and polypeptide diets are efficiently absorbed in the presence of compromised gut function. However, they are more expensive than nutritionally complete commercial formulas and are hyperosmolar, which may cause cramping, diarrhea, and fluid losses.

Modular formulations include special formulas used for specific clinical situations (eg, pulmonary, renal, or hepatic failure or immune dysfunction). The available preparations vary in (1) caloric and protein content; (2) protein, carbohydrate, and fat compositions; (3) nonprotein carbohydrate calorie-to-gram nitrogen ratio; (4) osmolality; (5) content of minor trace metals (selenium, chromium, and molybdenum); and (6) content of various amino acids (glutamine, glutamate, BCAAs).

C. Initiating Feedings

In the past, elaborate protocols for initiating tube feedings were used. It is currently recommended that feedings be started with full-strength formula at a slow rate and steadily advanced. This approach reduces the risk of microbial contamination and achieves full nutrient intake earlier. Formulas are often introduced at full strength at 10–40 mL per hour initially and advanced to the goal rate in increments of 10–20 mL per hour every 8 hours as tolerated. Conservative initiation and advancement rates are recommended for patients who are critically ill, those who have not been fed for some time, and those who are receiving high-osmolality or calorie-dense formula. In such patients, starting feeding at 10 mL per hour yields the trophic benefit of enteral feeds without unduly stressing the gut. In patients with active lifestyles, gastric feeds can be provided as boluses of up to 400 mL each, delivered at intervals of 4–6 hours.

D. Monitoring Feedings

Assessing gastrointestinal tolerance to enteral feeding includes monitoring for abdominal discomfort, nausea and vomiting, abdominal distention, and abnormal bowel sounds or stool patterns. Gastric residual volumes are used to evaluate gastric emptying of enteral feedings. High residuals raise concerns about intolerance to gastric feedings and the potential risk for regurgitation and aspiration. When the gastric residual is greater than 200 mL or is associated with signs or symptoms of intolerance, feedings should be held. Further workup with radiographs may be indicated. If the abdominal examination is unremarkable, feedings should be postponed for at least an hour and the residual volume rechecked. If high residuals persist without associated clinical signs and symptoms, a promotility agent (eg, erythromycin, metoclopramide) may be added to the feeding regimen.

Complications of Enteral Feeding

Technical complications occur in about 5% of enterally fed patients and include clogging of the tube; esophageal, tracheal, bronchial, or duodenal perforation; and tracheobronchial intubation with tube feeding aspiration. Patients with decreased consciousness or impaired gag reflexes or those who have undergone endotracheal intubation are at increased risk for technical complications. The tip of the feeding tube must be positioned and verified radiographically. Other methods to evaluate tube placement are not consistently reliable. Generally, the wire stylet used for positioning should not be reinserted once removed. The incidence of tube clogging can be reduced by periodic tap-water flushes and avoiding administration of syrup-based medications through the tube.

Functional complications occur in up to 25% of tube-fed patients and include nausea, vomiting, abdominal distention, constipation, and diarrhea. Feeding the small bowel instead of the stomach can diminish abdominal symptoms. In the critically injured patient, diarrhea is typically multifactorial; it results from polypharmacy (eg, multiple antibiotics), mechanical gut dysfunction (eg, partial small bowel obstruction), intestinal bacterial overgrowth (eg, *Clostridium difficile*), and the protein content or osmolarity of the diet. Treatment consists of stopping any unnecessary medications, correcting gut dysfunction, changing enteral formulation (eg, intact protein versus amino acid or polypeptide formula), or reducing the osmolarity of the formula. In some circumstances, adding pectin or fiber to the diet or administering antidiarrheal agents can be beneficial, but these measures usually are not needed.

In the surgical population, *C difficile* is a common cause of diarrhea due to the routine use of perioperative antibiotics. The diagnosis of pseudomembranous colitis

Table 10–7. Enteral formulas.

	Per 1000 mL											
Product	***Description***	***kcal/mL***	***mosm***	***Protein g (%kcal)***	***Carbohydrate g (%kcal)***	***Fat g (% kcal)***	***H_2O (mL)***	***Na (meq)***	***K (meq)***	***Ca (mg)***	***PO_4 (mg)***	***Vitamin K (mg)***
Standard												
Ensure	Lactose-free, low-residue	1.06	470	37.2 (14)	145 (54.5)	37.2 (31.5)	845	36.8	40	530	530	43
Osmolite	Isotonic, lactose-free, low-residue	1.06	300	37.2 (14)	145 (54.6)	38.5 (31.4)	841	27.6	25.9	530	530	43
Jevity	Isotonic, lactose-free, high dietary fiber (14.4 g/L)	1.06	310	44.4 (16.7)	151.7 (53.3)	36.8 (30)	833	40.4	40	909	756	61
Glucerna	Lactose-free, low-carbohydrate, high-fiber (14.4 g/L)	1	375	41.8 (16.7)	93.7 (33.3)	55.7 (50)	873	40.3	40	703	703	57
Low-volume												
Ensure Plus	Lactose-free, low-residue	1.5	690	54.9 (14.7)	200 (53.3)	53.3 (32)	769	45.9	49.7	704	704	57
Magnacal	Lactose-free, low-residue	2	590	70 (14)	250 (50)	80 (34)	690	43.5	32	1000	1000	300
Low-volume, high-nitrogen												
Ensure Plus HN	Lactose-free, low-residue	1.5	650	62.6 (16.7)	199.9 (53.3)	50 (30)	769	51.5	46.5	1056	1056	85
Perative*	Lactose-free, low-residue	1.3	425	66.6 (20.5)	177 (54.5)	37.3 (25)	789	45.2	44.3	867	867	70

Very high nitrogen												
Replete with fiber	Lactose-free, high-fiber (14 g/L)	1	300	62.5 (25)	113 (45)	34 (30)	840	21.7	40	1000	1000	80
Sustacal	Lactose-free, low-residueZPZP	1.01	650	61 (24)	140 (55)	23 (21)	840	40	54	1010	930	240
Elemental												
Vivonex TEN	Elemental, low-fat, low-residue	1	630	38.2 (15.3)	205.6 (82.2)	2.77 (2.5)	845	20	20	500	500	22.3
Pudding (per 5-oz serving)												
Ensure pudding	Contains lactose	250		6.8	34	9.7		10.4	8.5	200	200	12
Modulars (analysis per tablespoon)												
Polycose Liquid	Glucose polymer	30			7.5							
ProMod	Protein supplement	17		3	0.4	0.4		0	1	15.6	15.6	
Microlipid	Fat supplement	67.5				7.5						
MCT Oil	Medium-chain triglycerides	115.5				14						

*Perative may be contraindicated in transplant patients.

is confirmed by *C difficile* toxin assay or sigmoidoscopy. The primary treatment is stopping unnecessary antibiotics. Additionally, either metronidazole (oral or intravenous) or vancomycin (oral or retention enema) can be started.

Abnormalities in serum electrolytes, calcium, magnesium, and phosphorus can be minimized through vigilant monitoring. Hyperosmolarity (hypernatremia) may lead to mental lethargy or obtundation. The treatment of hypernatremia includes the administration of free water by giving either D_5W intravenously or additional water in the tube feedings. Volume overload and subsequent congestive heart failure may occur as a result of excess sodium administration and is frequently observed in patients with impaired ventricular function or valvular heart disease. Hyperglycemia may occur in any patient but is particularly common in individuals with preexisting diabetes or sepsis. The serum glucose level should be determined frequently and regular insulin administered accordingly.

Alverdy J: Effect of nutrition on gastrointestinal barrier function. Semin Respir Infect 1994;9:248.

Bozetti F et al: Postoperative enteral versus parenteral nutrition in malnourished patients with gastrointestinal cancer: a randomised multicentre trial. Lancet 2001;358:1487.

Braunschweig CL et al: Enteral compared with parenteral nutrition: a meta-analysis. Am J Clin Nutr 2001;74:534.

Cresci GA: The use of probiotics with the treatment of diarrhea. Nutr Clin Pract 2001;16:30.

DeLegge MH: Enteral access—the foundation of feeding. J Parenter Enteral Nutr 2001;25:58.

Heys SD et al: Enteral nutritional supplementation with key nutrients in patients with critical illness and cancer: a meta-analysis of randomized controlled clinical trials. Ann Surg 1999; 229:467.

Ibanez J et al: Incidence of gastroesophageal reflux and aspiration in mechanically ventilated patients using small-bore nasogastric tubes. JPEN J Parenter Enteral Nutr 2000;24: 103.

McClave SA et al: Use of residual volume as a marker for enteral feeding intolerance: prospective blinded comparison with physical examination and radiographic findings. JPEN J Parenter Enteral Nutr 1992; 16:99.

Metheny NA et al: Bedside methods for detecting aspiration in tube-fed patients. Chest 1997;111:724.

Orlando R: Gastrointestinal motility and tube feeding. Crit Care Med 1998;26:1472.

The Veterans Affairs Total Parenteral Nutrition Cooperative Study Group: perioperative total parenteral nutrition in surgical patients. N Engl J Med 1991;325:527.

Williams MS et al: Diarrhea management in enterally fed patients. Nutr Clin Pract 1998; 13:225.

PARENTERAL NUTRITION THERAPY

The development of parenteral nutritional support in the late 1960s revolutionized care of the surgical patient, particularly those with permanent inability to obtain adequate enteral nourishment (eg, short bowel syndrome). Despite its utility in select patients and circumstances, overuse of parenteral nutrition is not only costly but also poses unnecessary risk to patients. In general, parenteral nutrition should be employed only when the gastrointestinal tract cannot be utilized. Parental formulas usually deliver 75–150 nonprotein carbohydrate kcal per gram of nitrogen infused, a ratio that maximizes carbohydrate and protein assimilation and minimizes metabolic complications (aminoaciduria, hyperglycemia, and hepatic glycogenesis). Non-enteral nutrition can be given as peripheral parenteral nutrition (PPN) or total parenteral nutrition (TPN). In addition to route of administration, the two differ in (1) dextrose and amino acid (protein) content of the parenteral solution, (2) primary caloric source (glucose versus fat), (3) frequency of fat administration, (4) infusion schedule, and (5) potential complications.

1. Peripheral Parenteral Nutrition (PPN)

Because PPN avoids the complications associated with central venous access, it is safer to administer than TPN. PPN is indicated for patients with compromised gut function who require supplemental nutrition for less than 14 days. It can be infused via an 18-gauge peripheral IV catheter or via a peripherally inserted central catheter (PICC line). The osmolarity of the solution is limited to 1000 mosm to avoid phlebitis. Consequently, unacceptably large volumes of solution (greater than 2.5 L per day) are needed to fulfill the typical patient's total nutritional requirements. Standard PPN therapy orders should include the administration schedule for the PPN solution and fat supplement, as well as explicit catheter care orders and monitoring guidelines.

PPN Formulation

One liter of standard PPN solution contains $D_{20}W$, 500 mL, and 10% amino acids, 500 mL, plus electrolytes, vitamins, minerals, and trace metals. $D_{20}W$ contains 20 g glucose per 100 mL (100 g per 500 mL). Therefore, 1 L of standard PPN solution yields 340 nonprotein kcal. One gram of nitrogen is equivalent to 6.25 g of protein. One liter of standard PPN provides 50 g of protein, or the equivalent of 8 g of nitrogen. This results in a ratio of nonprotein energy to grams of nitrogen of approximately 43:1. Since 1 L of standard PPN solution contains adequate nitrogen but inadequate calories, the daily PPN regimen must also include 500 mL of 20% fat emulsion (approximately 2 kcal/mL). By infusing PPN solution at 125 mL per hour and supplementing it with 500 mL of 20% fat emulsion daily, the patient receives about 2200 kcal and 150 g protein (24 g nitrogen) daily.

Since the final dextrose concentration of a PPN solution should not exceed 12.5% (due to osmolarity concerns), it is impossible to formulate a concentrated PPN solution for patients with fluid restrictions (eg, cardiac disease, renal failure). Consequently, PPN is contraindicated in the treatment of fluid-restricted patients. Patients with nonoliguric renal failure can receive PPN formulations with none or low amounts of potassium, magnesium, and phosphorus. Likewise, PPN solutions containing primarily BCAAs and low sodium content (40 meq/L) can be provided for patients with hepatic failure.

2. Total Parenteral Nutrition (TPN)

TPN is indicated for patients who cannot obtain adequate nourishment via the GI tract, or rarely as a supplement to oral intake in patients with severe preoperative malnutrition. A minimum duration of treatment of 7–10 days of adequate TPN is needed for preoperative nutritional repletion. Likewise, the use of postoperative TPN for only 2 or 3 days (eg, while awaiting return of bowel function) is discouraged, as the risks outweigh the benefits incurred over this short a period of time.

TPN Formulation

TPN is typically formulated for patients based on their individual nutritional assessment. Most frequently, TPN is prepared in the pharmacy and provided as a 3-in-1 admixture of protein, as amino acids (8.5–10% per volume; 4 kcal/g); carbohydrate, as dextrose (up to 65%; 3.4 kcal/g); and fat, as a lipid emulsion of soybean or safflower oil (20–25%; 9 kcal/g). Alternatively, the lipid emulsion can be administered as a separate intravenous "piggyback" infusion. One liter of TPN solution containing $D_{50}W$, 500 mL, and 8.5% amino acids, 500 mL, provides approximately 1000 kcal and 6.8 g of nitrogen, with the ratio of nonprotein energy to grams of nitrogen being approximately 125:1. Other additives, vitamins, and trace minerals are added to TPN formulations as required (Table 10–8).

Administration

The high osmolarity of TPN solutions necessitates administration via a central vein. The use of multilumen central venous catheters (CVCs) for TPN does not increase the risk of catheter infection; however, a port should be designated for exclusive use for TPN infusion to minimize handling of the line. CVC placement in the subclavian vein is ideal and well tolerated by the patient. Furthermore, the rate of catheter infection is lower for catheters placed in the subclavian compared to catheters placed in either the femoral or internal jugular vein. Femoral vein catheterization has a complication rate over 25% and therefore should be avoided if possible. The CVC should be dressed with a sterile, dry gauze and transparent (nonocclusive) dressing, without antibiotic ointment.

The introduction of TPN should be gradual, with approximately 1000 kcal provided over the first 24 hours. This amount is increased by 500 kcal per day until the patient's goal is reached. Additional maintenance IV fluids should be tapered or discontinued accordingly to maintain an even fluid balance. Standard

Table 10–8. TPN solution formulation.

Components in 1 L of standard TPN:	
Routine additives	
$D_{50}W$[1]	500 mL
8.5% amino acid[1]	500 mL
Sodium chloride[2]	0–140 meq
Sodium phosphate[3]	0–20 mmol
Potassium chloride[4]	0–40 meq
Magnesium sulfate[5]	0–12 meq
Calcium gluconate[5,6]	4.5–9.0 meq
Trace element-5[7]	1 mL
M.V.I.-12[7]	10 mL
Optional additives	
Sodium acetate[2]	0–140 meq
Potassium acetate[4]	0–40 meq
H_2 antagonist[8]	variable
Regular insulin[9]	0–40 units
Vitamin K[10]	10 mg
Heparin[11]	variable
Fat emulsion schedule:	
Infuse 20–25% fat emulsion intravenously via pump at least 3 times per week	

[1]The solution is formulated to deliver 125 nonprotein kcal per gram of nitrogen infused.
[2]Add sodium chloride if the serum CO_2 > 25 meq/L. Add sodium acetate if the serum CO_2 ≤25 meq/L.
[3]The total phosphate dosage should not exceed 20 mmol/L or 60 mmol daily.
[4]Add potassium chloride if the serum CO_2 > 25 meq/L. Add potassium acetate if the serum CO_2 ≤25 meq/L. The potassium dosage should not exceed 40 meq/L.
[5]Added to each liter.
[6]Add calcium gluconate 9 meq to each liter if the serum calcium < 8.5 meq/L. Add 4.5 meq if the serum calcium ≥8.5 meq/L.
[7]Administered in only 1 L per day.
[8]Dosage depends upon the H_2 antagonist selected. Divide the daily dosage equally in all liters of TPN administered.
[9]Total dosage should not exceed 40 units/L.
[10]Administered only once per week.
[11]Heparin administration in TPN is not required, but it may be added in place of subcutaneous dosing.

TPN therapy orders (Figure 10–6) should include the administration schedule for the TPN solution and fat supplement, as well as explicit catheter care orders and monitoring guidelines. For active patients on long-term TPN, cycling the intravenous nutrition therapy over 8–16 hours at night allows freedom from the infusion pump during the remainder of the day.

1. TPN components:

ROUTINE ADDITIVES	Recommended Dosage Ranges per Liter TPN	BAG #___	BAG #___	BAG #___
$D_{50}W$	500 mL	500 mL	500 mL	500 mL
AA 8.5%	500 mL	500 mL	500 mL	500 mL
NaCl	0–140 meq	meq	meq	meq
$NaPO_4$	0–20 mmol	mmol	mmol	mmol
K*Cl	0–40 meq	meq	meq	meq
$MgSO_4$	0–12 meq	meq	meq	meq
Ca gluconate	4.5 or 9 meq	meq	meq	meq
MVI-12®	10 mL/d	10 mL		
Multitrace®	5 mL/d	5mL		
OPTIONAL ADDITIVES				
Na acetate	0–140 meq	meq	meq	meq
K* acetate	0–40 meq	meq	meq	meq
Regular insulin	0–40 units	units	units	units
H_2 antagonist**				
25% albumin***	25 g	g	g	g
NURSE'S SIGNATURE				

* TOTAL POTASSIUM CONTENT PER LITER OF TPN SHOULD NOT EXCEEED 40 meq.
** DIVIDE THE DAILY DOSAGE EQUALLY INTO EACH LITER OF TPN.
*** ONLY IF THE SERUM ALBUMIN < 2.5g/dL AND ENTERAL DIET THERAPY IS ANTICIPATED.

RATE:____40____mL/h via pump.
Final dextrose concentration__25__% Final AA concentration__4.25__%

2. Pharmacy to add vitamin K 10 mg to 1 L of TPN solution every Mon. and Thurs.
3. Fat emulsion 20% 500 mL every Mon., Wed., and Fri. IVPB per pump over 6–8 hours via at least an 18-gauge peripheral IV or via the subclavian catheter.
4. STAT upright and expirational portable chest x-ray to check the position of the subclavian catheter and to rule out a pneumothorax. Notify the physician when the chest x-ray is completed.
5. Heparin lock the TPN catheter with 2 mL of heparin (100 units/mL) until notified by the physician to start the first liter of TPN solution.
6. Strict I/O every shift. Total the I/O every 24 hours.
7. Record the daily weight in kilograms on the vital signs sheet.
8. Check the urine for sugar and acetone every shift and record on the vital signs sheet. If the urine sugar is 4+, request a STAT serum glucose measurement to be drawn by the physician. If the serum glucose is > 160 mg/dL, contact the physician for treatment orders.
9. Notify the physician if the oral temperature is >38C (>100.4F).
10. Routine TPN laboratory tests are to be drawn weekly on the days and times specified below:
    Sun. AM: CBC, SMAC-20
    Tues. AM: Electrolytes, BUN, creatinine, and glucose
    Thurs. AM: CBC, SMAC-20, copper, zinc, magnesium, transferrin, and triglycerides
11. Begin a 24-hour urine collection for urinary urea nitrogen (UUN) at 6:00 AM every Mon. and Thurs. for nitrogen balance determination.
12. TPN catheter dressing and tubing changes per the hospital TPN protocol.
13. Contact the physician for all problems related to TPN.
14. All changes in TPN therapy must be approved by the physician.

Figure 10–6. TPN therapy orders.

Special TPN Solutions

The TPN solution may be concentrated for patients who require fluid restriction (eg, those with pulmonary and cardiac failure). One liter of concentrated TPN solution usually contains a combination of $D_{60}W$ or $D_{70}W$, 500 mL, and 10% or 15% amino acids, 500 mL, plus additives.

Patients in renal failure (serum creatinine greater than 2 mg/dL) who cannot be dialyzed and who require fluid restriction should receive low-nitrogen TPN solution. These solutions contain a combination of $D_{60}W$ or $D_{70}W$ and ideal amino acids (essential amino acids), plus limited amounts of sodium, potassium, magnesium, and phosphate. Patients in renal failure who can undergo dialysis may receive the standard or high-nitrogen TPN formulations, with special attention directed toward minimizing potassium and phosphate intake. Cirrhotic patients with hepatic encephalopathy should receive a TPN solution containing a combination of $D_{30}W$ or $D_{40}W$ and a special hepatic failure amino acid solution (BCAAs) plus additives. Sodium intake in patients with hepatic encephalopathy should be limited to 40 meq/L.

COMPLICATIONS OF PARENTERAL NUTRITION

PPN Therapy

Technical complications of PPN are few. The most common problem is maintaining adequate venous access. Because it causes phlebitis, the PPN infusion catheter must be moved frequently to other sites. Since most patients have few usable peripheral veins, prolonged PPN is rarely possible. The addition of fat, heparin, or corticosteroids to PPN solutions has not decreased the incidence of phlebitis. Infectious complications such as catheter site skin infections and septic phlebitis develop in 5% of patients.

TPN Therapy

Technical, infectious, and metabolic complications each occur in approximately 5% of patients, and the overall mortality rate directly attributable to TPN is 0.2% (Table 10–9). Many of the complications originate from the central venous catheter, with more than 15% of patients developing some line-related complication. Other morbidity is attributable to line infection (typically bacterial) or metabolic abnormalities.

A. Technical Complications

The risks of patient injury while placing a CVC are directly related to surgeon expertise with the procedure, although some risk is present regardless of experience.

Table 10–9. Complications of nutritional therapy.

Enteral Nutrition	Parenteral Nutrition
Technical	***Technical***
Abscess of nasal septum	Air embolus
Acute sinusitis	Arterial laceration
Aspiration pneumonitis	Arteriovenous fistula
Esophagitis (ulceration/stenosis)	Brachial plexus injury
Gastrointestinal perforation	Cardiac perforation
Hemorrhage (local erosion)	Catheter embolism
Hoarseness	Catheter malposition
Intestinal obstruction	Hemothorax
Intracranial passage	Pneumothorax
Knotting/clogging of tube	Subclavian vein thrombosis
Nasal/alar erosions	Thoracic duct injury
Otitis media	Thromboembolism
Pneumatosis intestinalis	Venous laceration
Skin excoriation	
Tracheoesophageal fistula	
Tube dislodgement	
Variceal rupture	
Functional	***Infectious***
Abdominal distention	Catheter-based bacteremia
Constipation	Catheter colonization
Diarrhea	Exit-site infection/cellulites
Nausea/vomiting	
Metabolic	***Metabolic***
Dehydration	Azotemia
Hypercalcemia	Essential fatty acid deficiency
Hyperglycemia	Fluid overload
Hyperkalemia	Hyperchloremic metabolic acidosis
Hypermagnesemia	Hypercalcemia
Hypernatremia	Hyperglycemia
Hyperphosphatemia	Hyperkalemia
Hypocalcemia	Hypermagnesemia
Hypokalemia	Hypernatremia
Hypomagnesemia	Hyperphosphatemia
Hyponatremia	Hypocalcemia
Hypophosphatemia	Hypokalemia
Hypozincemia	Hypomagnesemia
Overhydration	Hyponatremia
Vitamin deficiency	Hypophosphatemia
	Intrinsic liver disease
	Metabolic bone disease
	Trace element deficiency
	Ventilatory failure
	Vitamin deficiency

Arterial puncture (more common in internal jugular or femoral insertion) occurs in up to 15% of patients, while pneumothorax (predominantly from subclavian insertion) develops in up to 3%. The risk for injury increases dramatically after three failed insertions at the same site.

Air embolism occurs when negative intrathoracic pressure draws air into a catheter or needle residing in a central vein. This situation is particularly serious in the presence of pulmonary-systemic shunts (eg, patent foramen ovale). It is characterized by sudden, severe respiratory distress (tachypnea), hypotension, and a cogwheel cardiac murmur. To reduce the risk of air embolism, the patient should be placed in the Trendelenburg position during line insertion to increase central venous pressure. After accurately diagnosing air embolism, treatment involves placing the patient in the Durant position (Trendelenburg and left lateral decubitus) to direct the embolus to the apex of the right ventricle. Catheter-based aspiration can then be attempted.

B. Infectious Complications

Infection of the catheter exit-site is characterized by mild fever (37.5–38 °C), pus around the catheter tract, and erythema and tenderness of the surrounding skin. Late changes include induration of the skin and systemic sepsis. Local wound care and sterile dressing changes every 2–3 days can minimize site infections.

Primary line (catheter) infection may occur in as many as 26% of patients with CVCs. Contrary to conventional wisdom, the number of lumina does not directly affect the rate of catheter-related complications. However, the use of antibiotic-impregnated catheters can reduce colonization rates fourfold. As noted above, insertion in the subclavian vein also reduces the rate of infection. Line infection should be strongly considered in any patient with a CVC who develops fever, new-onset glucose intolerance, leukocytosis (WBC greater than 10,000 cells/μL), or positive blood cultures. The most common offending organisms are skin flora (*S aureus, S epidermidis*), although gram-negative rods from remote sources can also colonize an indwelling catheter. Table 10–10 depicts one treatment algorithm for treating suspected CVC infections. Patients with a suspected line infection who have negative blood cultures and no cardiovascular compromise should have the catheter exchanged over a guidewire and the tip sent for bacterial and fungal cultures. If the fever resolves and subsequent cultures remain negative, no further therapy is necessary. If the patient remains febrile after catheter exchange or continues to have positive blood or catheter cultures, a new central catheter should be inserted at another site. Antibiotics should be started empirically in patients presenting with sepsis.

Table 10–10. Complications of TPN.

Complication	Treatment
Catheter sepsis Incidence: Single-lumen catheter: 3–5% Triple-lumen catheter: 10% Diagnosis: • Unexplained hyperglycemia (> 160 mg/dL) • "Plateau" temperature elevation (> 38 °C) for several hours or days. (***Note:*** *An isolated spike or "picket fence" temperature pattern is usually not indicative of an infected catheter.*) • Leukocytosis (> 10,000/μL) • Exclusion of other potential sources of infection, *or* • A positive blood culture (> 15 colony count) aspirated via the TPN catheter or obtained peripherally, *or* • Catheter site induration, erythema, or purulent drainage.	**Algorithms:** *Negative blood cultures and no cardiovascular signs of sepsis:* (1) Aspirate a blood specimen via the TPN catheter and peripherally for bacterial and fungal culture and then sterilely exchange the preexisting TPN catheter for a new catheter over a guidewire; submit the previous catheter tip for bacterial and fungal culture and colony count; and continue the TPN infusion. *then* (2) Monitor the patient's temperature closely. If the patient defervesces, no further therapy is necessary. If the fever continues or recurs, remove the catheter and insert a new one on the contralateral side and continue the TPN infusion. *Positive blood culture or cardiovascular signs of sepsis:* (1) Aspirate a blood specimen via the TPN catheter and peripherally for bacterial and fungal culture. Then remove the catheter immediately, and submit the catheter tip for bacterial and fungal culture and colony count. *then* (2) Insert a new TPN infusion catheter on the contralateral side and continue the TPN infusion. *then* (3) Initiate appropriate antibiotic therapy.
Hyperglycemia (> 160 mg/dL)	**Algorithms:** (1) Maintain the current TPN infusion rate and begin adding regular insulin to the TPN solution in 10-unit increments until the serum glucose is maintained at ≤160 mg/dL. (***Note:*** *The maximum allowable insulin dosage per liter of TPN is 40 units.*) Until the hyperglycemia is controlled by adding insulin to the TPN solution, simultaneously administer intravenous regular insulin. (***Note:*** *One unit of regular insulin results in an approximately 10 mg/dL increase in the serum glucose. The maximum intravenous dose of regular insulin should not exceed 15 units.*) If the serum glucose remains > 160 mg/dL despite the addition of a total of 40 units of regular insulin per liter of TPN and intravenous regular insulin therapy, *then* (2) Maintain the current TPN infusion rate but begin gradually decreasing the final dextrose concentration of the TPN solution. (***Note:*** *The lower limit for the final dextrose concentration is 15%.*) In addition, begin adding regular insulin to the TPN solution in 10-unit increments until the serum glucose is maintained at ≤160 mg/dL or the maximum allowable insulin dosage (40 units) is reached. Regular insulin should also be simultaneously administered intravenously as in (1) above until the hyperglycemia is controlled by adding insulin to the TPN solution. If the serum glucose remains > 160 mg/dL despite the addition of 40 units of regular insulin per liter of TPN solution, decreasing the final TPN dextrose concentration to 15%, and intravenous regular insulin therapy, *then* (3) Restart the original TPN solution as in (1) above but begin decreasing the TPN infusion rate. Also begin insulin therapy as discussed in (2) above while simultaneously increasing the frequency of fat emulsion therapy from every Monday, Wednesday, and Friday to daily to provide adequate caloric intake.

Table 10–10. Complications of TPN. (continued)

Complication	Treatment
Hypoglycemia (< 65 mg/dL)	May occur with the sudden discontinuance of TPN infusion. If the TPN infusion administered to either an NPO patient or a patient consuming inadequate oral calories is suddenly discontinued, immediately begin an infusion of D_{10} NS at the previous TPN infusion rate via either the TPN catheter or a peripheral IV to prevent rebound hypoglycemia.
Hypernatremia (> 145 meq/L)	Determine the cause. Hypernatremia secondary to dehydration is treated by administering additional "free water" and providing only the daily maintenance sodium requirements (90–150 meq/L) via the TPN infusion. Hypernatremia secondary to increased sodium intake is treated by reducing or deleting sodium from the TPN solution until the serum sodium ≤145 meq/L.
Hyponatremia (< 135 meq/L)	Determine the cause. Hyponatremia secondary to dilution is treated by fluid restriction and by providing only the daily maintenance sodium requirements (90–150 meq/L). Hyponatremia secondary to inadequate sodium intake is treated by increasing the sodium content of the TPN solution until the serum sodium is ≥135 meq/L. (***Note:*** *The maximum sodium content per liter of TPN should not exceed 154 meq.*)
Hyperkalemia (> 5 meq/L)	Immediately discontinue the current TPN infusion containing potassium and begin an infusion of D_{10}NS at the previous TPN infusion rate. Then reorder a new TPN solution without potassium and continue to delete potassium from the TPN solution until the serum potassium ≤ 5 meq/L.
Hypokalemia (< 3.5 meq/L)	A TPN solution should not be utilized for the primary treatment of hypokalemia. The potassium content per liter of TPN solution should not exceed 40 meq. If additional potassium is necessary, it should be administered via another route, eg, IV interrupts.
Hyperphosphatemia (> 4.5 mg/dL)	Immediately discontinue the present phosphate-containing TPN infusion and begin an infusion of D_{10}NS at the previous infusion rate. Then reorder a new TPN solution without phosphate and continue to delete phosphate from the TPN solution until the serum phosphate is ≤4.5 mg/dL.
Hypophosphatemia (< 2.5 mg/dL)	Increase the phosphate content of the TPN solution to a maximum of 20 mmol/L. (***Note:*** *The total daily phosphate dosage should not exceed 60 mmol.*) If severe hypophosphatemia exists, carbohydrate infusion or delivery should be restricted.
Hypermagnesemia (> 3 mg/dL)	Immediately discontinue the present magnesium-containing TPN infusion and begin an infusion of D_{10}NS at the previous infusion rate.
Hypomagnesemia (<1.6 mg/dL)	Increase the magnesium content of the TPN solution to a maximum of 12 meq/L. (***Note:*** *The total daily dosage of magnesium should not exceed 36 meq.*)
Hypercalcemia (> 10.5 mg/dL)	Immediately discontinue the present calcium-containing TPN infusion and begin an infusion of D_{10}NS at the previous TPN infusion rate. Then reorder a new TPN solution without calcium and continue to delete calcium from the TPN dilution until the serum calcium is ≤10.5 mg/dL.
Hypocalcemia (< 8.5 mg/dL)	Increase the calcium content of the TPN solution to a maximum of 9 meq/L. (***Note:*** *The total daily calcium dosage should not exceed 27 meq.*)
High serum zinc (> 150 μg/L)	Discontinue the trace metal supplement (Multitrace 5 mL) in the TPN solution until the serum zinc is ≤150 μg/L.
Low serum zinc (< 55 μg/dL)	Add elemental zinc 2–5 mg daily to 1 L of TPN solution only until the serum zinc is ≥55 μg/dL. (***Note:*** *The elemental zinc is added in addition to the daily supplement.*)

(continued)

Table 10–10. Complications of TPN. (continued)

Complication	Treatment
High serum copper (> 140 μg/dL)	Discontinue the trace metal supplement in the TPN solution until the serum copper is ≤140 μg/dL.
Low serum copper (< 70 μg/dL)	Add elemental copper 2–5 mg daily to 1 L of TPN solution only until the serum copper is ≥70 μg/dL. (***Note:*** *The elemental copper is added in addition to the daily Multiracial 5 mL.*)
Hyperchloremic metabolic acidosis (CO_2 < 22 mmol/L and Cl^- > 110 meq/L)	Reduce the chloride intake by administering the Na^+ and K^+ in the acetate form as either sodium or potassium acetate (or both) until the acidosis resolves (serum CO_2 ≥22 mmol/L) and the serum chloride level returns to normal (< 110 meq/L).

C. Metabolic Complications

The refeeding syndrome was first described in prisoners freed from concentration camps after World War II. Similar pathophysiology may develop when initiating TPN in patients with severe malnutrition and weight loss (greater than 30% of their usual weight). In starvation, energy is derived principally from fat metabolism. TPN results in a shift from fat to glucose as the predominant fuel, and rapid anabolism increases the production of phosphorylated intermediates of glycolysis. These intermediates trap phosphate, producing profound hypophosphatemia. Hypokalemia and hypomagnesemia also occur. The lack of phosphate and potassium lead to a relative ATP deficiency, resulting in the insidious onset of respiratory failure and reduced cardiac stroke volume. Because of these risks, the rate of TPN administration in a severely malnourished patient should be slowly increased over several days. Instead of attempting to meet the patient's nutritional requirements within 72 hours, increases in the infusion rate should be made only while the patient remains nontachycardic. Twice-daily monitoring of electrolytes is also indicated, with repletion as appropriate.

Hepatic dysfunction is a common manifestation of long-term parenteral nutrition support. The exact etiology is unclear; however, in part it is related to the initial bypassing of the portal circulation when providing intravenous nutrition. Severe hepatic steatosis may progress to cirrhosis. Acalculous cholecystitis can also occur in these patients, likely from biliary stasis and lack of gallbladder contraction. Patients on TPN need weekly liver function tests and lipid panels.

Abrupt discontinuation of TPN can produce rebound hypoglycemia in patients with limited oral intake. Infusion of $D_{10}NS$ may be initiated prior to stopping the TPN. The TPN infusion rate does not need to be tapered if the patient can consume 75% or more of daily caloric requirements, or if receiving less than 1000 kcal per day parenterally.

Alverdy JC, Aoys E, Moss GS: Total parenteral nutrition promotes bacterial translocation from the gut. Surgery 1988;104:185.

Dudrick SJ et al: Long-term total parenteral nutrition with growth, development, and positive nitrogen balance. Surgery 1968;64:397.

Fleming CR: Trace element metabolism in adult patients requiring total parenteral nutrition. Am J Clin Nutr 1989;49:573.

Granato D et al: Effects of parenteral lipid emulsions with different fatty acid composition on immune cell functions in vitro. JPEN J Parenter Enteral Nutr 2000;24:113.

McGee DC, Gould MK: Preventing complications of central venous catheterization. N Engl J Med 2003;348:1123.

Seidner DL et al: Parenteral nutrition-associated metabolic bone disease: pathophysiology, evaluation and treatment. Nutr Clin Pract 2000;15:163.

Van Acker BA et al: Response of glutamine metabolism to glutamine-supplemented parenteral nutrition. Am J Clin Nutr 2000;72:79.

Van den Berghe G et al: Intensive insulin therapy in critically ill patients. N Engl J Med 2001;345:1359.

The Veterans Affairs Total Parenteral Nutrition Cooperative Study Group: Perioperative total parenteral nutrition in surgical patients. N Engl J Med 1991;325:527.

DIETS

Optimal Diet

The optimal diet should have the following distribution of energy sources: carbohydrate 55–60%, fat 30%, and protein 10–15%. Refined sugar should constitute less than 15% of dietary energy and saturated fats no more than 10%, the latter balanced by 10% monounsaturated and 10% polyunsaturated fats. Cholesterol intake should be limited to about 300 mg per day (one egg yolk contains 250 mg of cholesterol). The amount of salt in the average American diet, 10–18 g daily, far exceeds the recommended 3 g/day. For Western societies to meet the criteria for an optimal diet, consumption of fat must decrease (from 40%) and consumption of complex carbohydrate should increase.

Meat is presently overemphasized as a protein source, at the expense of grain, legumes, and nuts. Diets that include substantial fish intake have been associated with a decrease in mortality from cardiovascular disease and are attributed to high concentrations of ω-3 fatty acids, principally eicosapentaenoic and docosahexaenoic acids.

Many adults, particularly those who do not drink milk, consume inadequate amounts of calcium. In women this may result in calcium deficiency and skeletal calcium depletion, predisposing women to osteoporosis and axial bony fractures. "Fiber" is the generic term for a chemically complex group of indigestible carbohydrate polymers, including cellulose, hemicellulose, lignins, pectins, gums, and mucilages. The amount of fiber in Western diets averages 25 g per day, but some people ingest as little as 10 g daily. Those who consume low-fiber diets are more likely to develop chronic constipation, appendicitis, diverticular disease, and possibly diabetes mellitus and colonic neoplasms. Bran cereals and bread, fruit, potatoes, rice, and leafy vegetables are rich sources of fiber.

Regular Diets

Many concepts regarding diets are archaic and based on currently unaccepted views of illness. For example, the utility of a low-residue diet in diverticular disease is questionable. The "progressive diet," designed for postoperative feeding and consisting of a clear liquid (high in sodium), then a full liquid (high in sucrose), then a regular diet, is based on outmoded concepts. When peristalsis returns after operation, as evidenced by bowel sounds and ability to tolerate water, most patients are able to ingest a regular diet. Regular diets have an unrestricted spectrum of foods and are most attractive to the patient. An average regular hospital diet for 1 day contains 230–275 g of carbohydrate, 70–75 g of fat, and 95–110 g of protein, with a total caloric content of 2000–2500 kcal. This composition reflects the nutritional needs of healthy persons of average height and weight and will not meet the increased demands imposed by malnutrition or disease.

Lactose Intolerance & Lactose-Free Diets

A lactose-free diet is indicated for patients who have symptoms such as diarrhea, bloating, or flatulence after the ingestion of milk or milk products. Lactose intolerance is genetically determined and occurs in 5–10% of European Caucasians, 60% of Ashkenazi Jews, and 70% of African Americans. Subclinical lactose intolerance may become unmasked following surgery on gastrointestinal tract (eg, gastrectomy). Similarly, avoidance of lactose-containing products is often beneficial advice for patients with Crohn's disease, ulcerative colitis, and AIDS. The efficiency of lactose digestion and absorption can be measured by giving 100 g of oral lactose, then measuring the blood glucose concentration at 30-minute intervals over 2 hours. Patients with lactose intolerance exhibit a rise in blood glucose of 20 mg/dL or less. A lactose-free diet may be deficient in calcium, vitamin D, and riboflavin.

DISEASE-SPECIFIC NUTRITION SUPPORT

Burns

Thermal injury has a tremendous impact on metabolism because of prolonged, intense neuroendocrine stimulation. Extensive burns can double or triple the REE and urinary nitrogen losses, producing a loss of 1500 g per day of lean tissue and a median survival of 7–10 days without nutritional support. The increase in metabolic demands following thermal injury is proportional to the extent of ungrafted body surface. The principal mediators of burn hypermetabolism are catecholamines, which return to baseline only when skin coverage is complete. Decreasing the intensity of neuroendocrine stimulation by providing adequate analgesia and a thermoneutral environment lowers the accelerated metabolic rate and helps to decrease catabolic protein loss until the burned surface can be grafted. Burned patients are prone to infection, and the cytokines activated by sepsis further augment catabolism.

Because infection often complicates the clinical course of patients with burn injury, and infectious complications are more likely with parenteral nutrition, the enteral route of feeding is preferred whenever tolerated. Enteral feeding may be started within the first 6–12 hours postburn to reduce the hypermetabolic response and improve postburn survival. Gastric ileus can be avoided through the use of a nasojejunal tube.

Patients with burns have increased caloric requirements. In addition to estimated maintenance needs (females, 22 kcal/kg/day; males, 25 kcal/kg/day), these patients require an additional 40 kcal per percent of burned total body surface area (TBSA). A 70-kg man with 40% TBSA burns would require 48 kcal/kg/day. Protein requirements are also markedly increased from the normal 0.8 g/kg/day to approximately 2.5 g/kg/day in severely burned patients. Of course, these are initial estimates, and periodic reassessment of nutritional status (eg, prealbumin levels, nitrogen balance) is required in these patients. During the hypermetabolic phase of burn injury (0–14 days), the ability to metabolize fat is restricted, so a diet that derives calories primarily from carbohydrate is preferable. Following the hypermetabolic phase, the metabolism of fat becomes normal. The burn patient should also be given supplemental arginine, nucleotides, and ω-3 polyunsaturated fat to stimulate and maintain immunocompetence.

Diabetes

Glucose intolerance often complicates nutritional supplementation, particularly with parenteral administration. Complications associated with TPN administration (eg, catheter-related sepsis) occur more frequently during prolonged hyperglycemia. Unopposed glycosuria may lead to osmotic diuresis, loss of electrolytes in the urine, and possibly nonketotic coma. Additionally, it is now evident that strict maintenance of serum glucose levels below 110 mg/dL improves mortality and decreases infectious morbidity in critically ill patients. Factors that may aggravate hyperglycemia include the use of corticosteroids, certain vasopressors (eg, epinephrine), preexisting diabetes mellitus, and occult infection.

Maintaining normoglycemia in injured or postoperative patients may be challenging. Whenever feeding (enteral or parenteral) is initiated, serial serum glucose levels should be determined for the first 48 hours. If hyperglycemia does not occur, these measurements can be obtained less frequently once the nutritional goal is reached. Nondiabetic patients may require subcutaneous insulin administered on a sliding scale. Critically ill patients may receive continuous intravenous insulin infusions to control their hyperglycemia. For patients receiving TPN, the previous day's insulin total may be determined and half that amount added to the next TPN order to provide a more uniform administration.

Cancer

Cancer is the second leading cause of death in the United States, and over two-thirds of patients with cancer will develop nutritional depletion and weight loss at some time during the course of the illness. Malnutrition and its sequelae are the direct cause of death in 20–40% of these patients. Weight loss is an ominous presenting sign in many malignancies. Furthermore, antineoplastic treatments, such as chemotherapy, radiation therapy, or operative extirpation, can worsen preexisting malnutrition. Cancer cachexia manifests as progressive involuntary weight loss, fatigue, anemia, wasting, and tissue depletion. It may occur at any stage of the disease. Nutrition support has become an essential adjunct in caring for the cancer patient.

Many studies have evaluated the effectiveness of nutrition support in patients with cancer, with varying results. Klein reported a meta-analysis of 28 prospective, randomized controlled trials evaluating TPN in patients with cancer. Only one of ten surgical trials showed a significant decrease in mortality in the patients receiving TPN, and no other significant benefit was seen in survival, tolerance to treatment, toxicity, or tumor response in patients receiving chemotherapy or radiation therapy. Increasing efforts have been directed toward the use of enteral nutrition because it is simpler, presumably safer, and less costly. Seven prospective, randomized controlled trials of enteral nutrition in patients with cancer who were undergoing surgery showed little if any difference in mortality or morbidity in patients who received enteral feedings. In summary, nutritional supplementation in cancer patients *may* reduce infectious complications or perioperative morbidity, but convincing evidence of improvement in overall survival is lacking.

Patients with cancer may have altered energy expenditure and abnormalities of protein and carbohydrate metabolism. REE increases by 20–30% in certain malignant tumors. The increases in REE can occur even in patients with extreme cachexia in whom a similar degree of uncomplicated starvation would produce profound decreases in REE. Whether the increase in REE correlates with the extent of disease or tumor burden is unknown. Changes in carbohydrate metabolism consist of impaired glucose tolerance, elevated glucose turnover rates, and enhanced Cori cycle activity. Owing to the high rate of anaerobic glucose metabolism in neoplastic tissue, patients with extensive tumors are susceptible to lactic acidosis when given large glucose loads during TPN. These patients also exhibit increased lipolysis, elevated free fatty acid and glycerol turnover, and hyperlipidemia.

Patients with cancer avidly retain nitrogen despite losses in most lean tissue. Animal carcass analysis has shown that the retained nitrogen resides in the tumor, which behaves as a nitrogen trap. Synthesis, catabolism, and turnover of body protein are all increased, but the change in catabolism is greatest.

The utility of enteral supplementation with immune-enhancing agents is unclear. These substances include arginine, glutamine, essential fatty acids, RNA, and branched chain amino acids. Several studies have attempted to examine outcomes in patients with cancer who are fed with enteral formulas supplemented with immune-enhancing agents, compared to routine enteral feeding alone. The findings have been summarized by Heys and coworkers. Meta-analysis of six studies with a total of 487 cancer patients demonstrated a decrease in overall infectious morbidity and hospital stay, but no change in survival, for patients receiving such "targeted therapy." Exactly which elements confer these benefits remains unknown. Megestrol acetate (Megace) stimulates appetite and food intake and improves fat gain and patient mood, but does not alter outcome.

Renal Failure

Whether nutritional support improves the outcome from acute renal failure is difficult to determine due to the metabolic complexities of the disease. Patients with acute renal failure may have normal or increased metabolic rates. Renal failure precipitated by x-ray contrast agents, antibiotics, aortic or cardiac surgery, or periods of hypotension is associated with a normal or slightly elevated REE and a moderately negative nitrogen balance (4–8 g per day). When renal failure follows severe trauma, rhabdomyolysis, or sepsis, the REE may be markedly increased and the nitrogen balance sharply negative (15–25 g per day). When dialysis is frequent, losses into the dialysate of amino acids, vitamins, glucose, trace metals, and lipotrophic factors can be substantial.

The method of measuring nitrogen balance in renal failure is presented in Table 10–11. Nitrogen output is calculated from the urea nitrogen appearance (UNA) and the application of a correction factor for nitrogen loss in stool, skin, and feces. The UNA is the difference in BUN levels between dialysis intervals multiplied by a factor for the volume of distribution of urea in total body water plus the change in weight (assuming weight change is due entirely to water).

Patients in renal failure (serum creatinine over 2 mg/dL) with a normal metabolic rate who cannot undergo dialysis should receive a concentrated (minimal volume) enteral or parenteral diet containing just the essential amino acids, dextrose, and limited amounts of sodium, potassium, magnesium, and phosphate.

Hepatic Failure

Most patients with hepatic failure present with acute decompensation superimposed on chronic hepatic insufficiency. Typically, a history of poor dietary intake contributes to the chronic depletion of protein, vitamins, and trace elements. Water-soluble vitamins, including folate, ascorbic acid, niacin, thiamin, and riboflavin, are especially likely to be deficient. Fat-soluble vitamin deficiency may be a result of malabsorption due to bile acid insufficiency (vitamins A, D, K, and E), deficient storage (vitamin A), inefficient utilization (vitamin K), or failure of conversion to active metabolites (vitamin D). Hepatic iron stores may be depleted either from poor intake or as a result of gastrointestinal blood loss. Total body zinc is decreased owing to the above factors plus increased urinary excretion. The contribution of amino acid abnormalities to hepatic encephalopathy is discussed in Chapter 24.

Table 10–11. Calculation of nitrogen balance in renal failure.

$\text{Nitrogen}_{(\text{balance})} = \text{Nitrogen}_{(\text{intake})} - \text{Nitrogen}_{(\text{output})}$
$\text{Nitrogen}_{(\text{intake})} = \text{g protein}_{(\text{intake})} / 6.25$
$\text{Nitrogen}_{(\text{output})} = 0.97(\text{UNA}) + 1.93$
UNA = UUN + Dialysate urea nitrogen + Change in body urea nitrogen
Change in body urea nitrogen = $(\text{BUN}_f - \text{BUN}_I) \times \text{BW}_I \times 0.6 + (\text{BW}_f - \text{BW}_I)(\text{BUN}_f)$

UUN is urine urea nitrogen (g/L), UNA is urea nitrogen appearance (g/L), BUN is blood urea nitrogen, and BW is body weight. The factor 0.6 represents the volume of distribution of urea. f = final; I = initial.

The use of BCAA-enriched amino acid formulations for TPN in patients with liver disease is controversial because the results of controlled trials are inconclusive. Nonetheless, only BCAAs should be utilized in patients with clinical signs of encephalopathy. In contrast, patients without clinical signs of encephalopathy may receive a concentrated enteral or parenteral diet with reduced carbohydrate content, a combination of EFAs and other lipids, a standard mixture of amino acids, and limited amounts of sodium and potassium.

Cardiopulmonary Disease

Malnutrition is associated with myocardial dysfunction, particularly in the late stages, and fatal cardiac failure can develop in extreme cachexia. Cardiac muscle uses FFAs and BCAAs as preferred metabolic fuels instead of glucose. During starvation, the heart rate slows, cardiac size decreases, and the stroke volume and cardiac output decrease. As starvation progresses, cardiac failure ensues, along with chamber enlargement and anasarca.

The profound nutritional depletion that may accompany chronic heart failure, particularly in valvular disease, results from anorexia of chronic disease, passive congestion of the liver, malabsorption due to venous engorgement of the small bowel mucosa, and enhanced peripheral proteolysis due to chronic neuroendocrine secretion. Attempts at aggressive nutritional repletion in patients with cardiac cachexia have produced inconclusive results. Concentrated dextrose and amino acid preparations should be used to avoid fluid overload. Nitrogen balance should be measured to ensure adequate nitrogen intake. Lipid emulsions must be administered cautiously because they can produce myocardial ischemia and negative inotropy. Feeding these patients with either enteral or parenteral nutrition should be undertaken cautiously to avoid refeeding syndrome and hypophosphatemia.

Patients with severe chronic obstructive pulmonary disease may have difficulty weaning from the ventilator if they are overfed. This relates to the respiratory quotient (RQ), a measure of oxygen consumption and carbon dioxide production by the body in metabolism. An RQ of 1 reflects pure carbohydrate utilization, while an RQ greater than 1 occurs during lipogenesis (energy storage). Although normal lungs can tolerate increased CO_2 production (RQ greater than 1) without adversely affecting respiration, patients with chronic obstructive pulmonary disease may experience CO_2 retention and inability to wean. The treatment is to increase the percentage of calories delivered as lipid and to avoid overfeeding at all costs.

Disease of the Gastrointestinal Tract

Benign gastrointestinal disease (eg, inflammatory bowel disease, fistula, pancreatitis) often leads to nutritional problems due to intestinal obstruction, malabsorption, or anorexia. Chronic involvement of the ileum in inflammatory bowel disease produces malabsorption of fat- and water-soluble vitamins, calcium and magnesium, anions (phosphate), and the trace elements iron, zinc, chromium, and selenium. Protein-losing enteropathy, accentuated by transmural destruction of lymphatics, can add to protein depletion. Treatment with sulfasalazine can produce folate deficiency, and glucocorticoid administration may accelerate breakdown of lean tissue and enhance glucose intolerance owing to stimulation of gluconeogenesis. Patients with inflammatory bowel disease who require elective surgery should be evaluated for malnutrition preoperatively.

Patients with gastrointestinal fistulas can develop electrolyte, protein, fat, vitamin, and trace metal deficiencies; dehydration; and acid-base imbalance. Aggressive fluid replacement is often needed. Patients with fistulas often require nutritional support. The choice of feeding route or formula will depend on the level and length of dysfunctional bowel. Patients with proximal enterocutaneous fistulas (from the stomach to the midileum) should receive TPN with no oral intake. Patients with low fistulas should receive TPN initially, but after infection is brought under control they can often be switched to an enteral formula or even a low-residue diet. The management of enterocutaneous fistulas is discussed further in Chapter 29.

The diagnosis of pancreatitis often mandates strict bowel rest for extended periods of time. Ranson's criteria can serve as a rough estimate of the need for nutritional support (see Chapter 26). Patients with acute pancreatitis who present with three or fewer Ranson criteria should be treated with fluid replacement, nasogastric suction, and bowel rest for at least a week before considering parenteral nutrition. Most of these patients can resume an oral diet and do not benefit from TPN. Those with more than three Ranson criteria should receive TPN. Enteral diets, including elemental and polypeptide formulas, have not been recommended in the past because of concerns these diets may stimulate the pancreas and aggravate the disease. Recent data, however, document the successful use of enteral diets in many patients with pancreatitis.

Short Bowel Syndrome

Inadequate intestinal absorptive surface leads to malabsorption, excessive water loss, electrolyte derangements, and malnutrition. The absorptive capacity of the small intestine is highly redundant, and resection of up to half its functional length is reasonably well tolerated. Short bowel syndrome typically occurs when less than 200 cm of anatomic small bowel remain, although the presence of the ileocecal valve may reduce this length to 150 cm. However, short bowel syndrome also may occur from functional abnormalities of the small bowel resulting from severe inflammation or motility disorder. The optimal nutritional therapy for a patient with short bowel syndrome must be tailored individually and depends upon the underlying disease process and the remaining anatomy. Following resection, the remaining bowel undergoes long-term adaptation, with observed increases in villous height, luminal diameter, and mucosal thickness. The estimated minimum length of small bowel required for adult patients to become independent of TPN is 120 cm.

Adaptation to short gut occurs over time, and initial management should be directed at avoiding electrolyte imbalance and dehydration while providing daily caloric requirements through TPN. Some patients may eventually supplement TPN with oral intake. In these patients, dietary management includes consuming frequent small meals, avoiding hyperosmolar foods, restricting fat intake, and limiting consumption of foods high in oxalate (precipitates nephrolithiasis). Uniquely formulated diets containing glutamine and human growth hormone have shown promise for accelerating intestinal adaptation.

AIDS

Patients with AIDS frequently develop protein-calorie malnutrition and weight loss. Many factors contribute to deficiencies of electrolytes (sodium and potassium), trace metals (copper, zinc, and selenium), and vitamins (A, C, E, pyridoxine, and folate). Enteropathy may impair fluid and nutrient absorption and produce a voluminous life-threatening diarrhea. Standard antidiarrheal agents do not control the diarrhea in AIDS patients, but the synthetic somatostatin analogue octreotide may help. Dehydration occurs as a consequence of refractory diarrhea.

Malnourished AIDS patients require a daily intake of 35–40 kcal and 2.0–2.5 g protein. Those with normal gut function should be given a high-protein, high-calorie, low-fat, lactose-free oral diet. Patients with compromised gut function require an enteral (amino acid or polypeptide) diet or TPN.

Barrera R: Nutritional support in cancer patients. JPEN J Parenter Enteral Nutr 2002;26:S63.

Beale RJ, Bryg DJ, Bihari DJ: Immunonutrition in the critically ill: a systematic review of clinical outcome. Crit Care Med 1999; 27:2799.

Bozzetti F et al: Perioperative total parenteral nutrition in malnourished gastrointestinal cancer patients: a randomized, clinical trial. JPEN J Parenter Enteral Nutr 2000;24:7.

Byrne TA et al: Beyond the prescription: optimizing the diet of patients with short bowel syndrome. Nutr Clin Pract 2000;15:306.

Clark RH et al: Nutritional treatment for acquired immunodeficiency virus-associated wasting using beta-hydroxy beta-methylbutyrate, glutamine, and arginine: a randomized, double-blind, placebo-controlled study. JPEN J Parenter Enteral Nutr 2000;24:133.

Curreri PW et al: Dietary requirements of patients with major burns. Nutr Clin Pract 2001;16:169.

Fischer JE: Branched-chain-enriched amino acid solutions in patients with liver failure. JPEN J Parenter Enteral Nutr 1990; 14(Suppl):226.

Heyland DK et al: Should immunonutrition become routine in critically ill patients? A systematic review of the evidence. JAMA 2001;286:944.

Heys SD et al: Enteral nutritional supplementation with key nutrients in patients with critical illness and cancer: a meta-analysis of randomized controlled clinical trials. Ann Surg 1999; 229:467.

Klein S et al: Nutrition support in patients with cancer: what do the data really show? Nutr Clin Pract 1994;9:91.

MacFie J et al: Oral dietary supplements in pre- and postoperative surgical patients: a prospective and randomized clinical trial. Nutr 2000;16:723.

Moore FA: Effects of immune-enhancing diets on infectious morbidity and multiple organ failure. JPEN J Parenter Enteral Nutr 2001;25:536.

Anesthesia

11

Ronald D. Miller, MD

Anesthesiology is concerned not only with the administration of anesthesia for surgery but also with many other areas of patient care, including critical care medicine, management of chronic pain, and respiratory therapy. In this chapter, the discussion will be limited to anesthesia during surgery and the overall perioperative period, including preoperative evaluation, care in the postanesthetic care unit (PACU), and postoperative pain management.

The development of anesthesia represents one of the most interesting aspects of United States medical history. In 1842, Crawford Long was the first physician to administer diethyl ether by inhalation to produce surgical anesthesia, but his work went largely unrecognized. In 1846, a dentist, William Morton, administered diethyl ether for the removal of a submandibular tumor by surgeon John Warren. This event took place at the Massachusetts General Hospital before an audience of surgeons, medical students, and a newspaper reporter and was therefore well publicized. Another dentist, Horace Wells, allowed nitrous oxide to be administered to him by Gardner Colton, a showman, while a fellow dentist performed a painless tooth extraction. Unfortunately, Wells failed to appreciate the marginal potency of nitrous oxide and was unable to reproduce surgical anesthesia during a demonstration at the Massachusetts General Hospital. Between 1844 and 1886, nitrous oxide continued to be used by showmen who staged public displays of the exhilarating effects of the gas. Diethyl ether was often used for similar purposes. Since then, many techniques for general anesthesia have been developed and improved upon.

In the late 19th century, within a year after Karl Koller, a Viennese surgeon, discovered the topical anesthetic properties of cocaine, William Halsted, of Johns Hopkins University, gave the drug by injection for the production of peripheral nerve block. In 1898, after a trial on himself that led to the first-described lumbar puncture headache, August Bier, in Germany, administered the first spinal anesthetic. In the years that followed, the development of local anesthetics with different durations of action led to the widespread use of regional anesthesia.

Larson MD: History of anesthetic practice. In: *Anesthesia,* 6th ed. Miller RD (editor). Elsevier, 2005.

OVERALL ANESTHETIC RISK

Anecdotal reports of anesthetic mishaps are difficult to evaluate, partly because morbidity and mortality resulting from problems related to the anesthesia itself are difficult to distinguish from those due to the surgical procedure. Yet, in an age of increasing assessment and accountability, databases, including closed claims analysis, are being scrutinized to determine the benefit and hazards of surgery in general and anesthesia specifically. Anesthetic-related deaths have decreased dramatically in the past 2 decades and are now rare. The Institute of Medicine's analysis of medical errors (*To Err Is Human*) has received much national attention and complimented anesthesia for its marked decrease in morbidity and mortality over the past 30 years.

Nevertheless, anesthesiologists worry about issues regarding difficult airway management, neurologic deficits, patients with coronary artery disease, the administration of anesthesia in remote locations (eg, offices and radiology laboratories), and inadequate times for preoperative evaluation. Airway management is still the most frequent concern for anesthetic-induced morbidity, with medication errors and technical central venous access as contributory causes.

Increased use of outpatient and office-based anesthesia requires increased surveillance to ensure that proper safety measures are followed.

Stoelting R: Results of APSF survey regarding anesthesia patient safety issues. Anesthetic Patient Safety Foundation Newsletter 1999;13:6.

Voelker R: Anesthesia-related risks have plummeted. JAMA 1995; 275:445.

PREOPERATIVE PROCEDURES ASSOCIATED WITH ANESTHESIA

Preoperative Evaluation for Anesthetic Risk

Anesthetic risk is difficult to ascertain precisely in most cases. Perioperative complications and deaths are frequently caused by a combination of factors, including concurrent disease, complexity of the operation, and adverse effects of anesthesia. A few complications are due entirely to anesthesia, such as aspiration pneumonitis and hypoxemia due to failure to maintain a patent airway. While many classifications exist, the patient's physical status according to the criteria given in Table 11–1 is the most widely known. This classification system was not specifically designed to estimate anesthetic risk but does provide a "common language" of evaluation for use by different institutions.

A. Method and Site of Evaluations

Historically, patients were evaluated the night before surgery in the hospital. That approach has mostly been abandoned because most patients (even for complicated surgery) enter the hospital the morning of surgery. Although low-risk patients are interviewed by telephone, higher-risk patients should be evaluated in a preoperative evaluation clinic (or its equivalent) one or more days preoperatively. Preoperative clinics not only prepare patients for anesthesia and surgery but also enhance the efficiency and economics of the perioperative experience (eg, decreased surgical cancellations). They also follow protocols, which can ensure that only proper and necessary laboratory and radiologic tests are performed. However, the logistics dictate that the person performing the preoperative evaluation will not be the anesthesiologist who will be delivering the anesthetic. Nevertheless, all the preoperative information will be ready for the anesthesia team actually giving the anesthetic. The team will actually meet the patient in person for the first time 1 hour or less before surgery. This places tremendous emphasis on the adequacy of the telephone and clinic visits to make certain that patients are adequately prepared for anesthesia and surgery.

Table 11–1. Physical status classification of the American Society of Anesthesiologists.

Class	Physical Status
1	Patient has no organic, physiologic, biochemical, or psychiatric disturbance.
2	Patient has mild to moderate systemic disturbances that may or may not be related to the disorder requiring surgery (eg, essential hypertension, diabetes mellitus).
3	Patient has severe systemic disturbances that may or may not be related to the disorder requiring surgery (eg, heart disease that limits activity, poorly controlled essential hypertension).
4	Patient has severe systemic disturbance that is life-threatening with or without surgery (eg, congestive heart failure, persistent angina pectoris).
5	Patient is moribund and has little chance for survival, but surgery is to be performed as a last resort (resuscitative effort) (eg, uncontrolled hemorrhage, as from a ruptured abdominal aneurysm).
E	Patient requires emergency operation.

B. History and Physical Examination

The history should include a review of the patient's previous experiences with anesthesia, and data should be elicited regarding any allergic reactions, delayed awakening, prolonged paralysis from neuromuscular blocking drugs, and jaundice. Knowledge of exercise tolerance, history of the present illness, and the last visit with the patient's primary care doctor is helpful. The presence and severity of any concurrent diseases (eg, hepatitis), coagulopathies, endocrine abnormalities (eg, diabetes mellitus), or cardiorespiratory dysfunction should be noted. The patient's social history (ie, drug, alcohol, and tobacco use, and family history) should be sought.

The physical examination should focus on the cardiovascular system, lungs, and upper airway. It should include measurements of heart rate and of arterial blood pressure obtained in both the supine and standing positions and auscultation for cardiac murmurs, carotid artery bruits, or abnormal breathing. If abnormalities are found, additional tests (electrocardiography, pulmonary function tests, etc) may be indicated. The airway, head, and neck should be examined for factors that could make endotracheal intubation difficult, eg, fat or short neck, limited temporomandibular mobility. Since over 50% of all anesthetic-induced morbidity and mortality is related to inability to maintain the airway, examination of the airway demands special emphasis. The most common scoring of the airway as an assessment of a possible difficult endotracheal intubation is the "Mallampati classification." When the patient's uvula is visible with the mouth open, the score is grade I (easy intubation); in contrast, grade IV exists when the hard palate is visible but not the soft palate. Grade IV suggests a technically difficult endotracheal intubation.

Peripheral venous sites, including the external jugular vein, should also be checked. If regional anesthesia is planned, the proposed site of injection should be examined for abnormalities and signs of infection, and a limited neurologic examination should be performed.

C. Evaluation of Concurrent Drug Therapy

Concurrent drug therapy must be reviewed. Although many drugs can interact with anesthetic drugs (Table 11–2), the influence of concurrent drug therapy on overall or perioperative care is substantial. Smoking and alcohol are well-known factors influencing anesthetic requirement and the postoperative outcome. Tricyclic antidepressants exag-

Table 11–2. Mechanisms by which drugs may influence effects of anesthesia.

Anesthetic requirements may be increased or decreased.
Neuromuscular blockade from muscle relaxants may be enhanced.
Cardiovascular response to sympathomimetics and anesthetics may be exaggerated.
Peripheral sympathetic nervous system activity may be reduced, and cardiovascular depressant reactions to anesthetics may be augmented.
Metabolism may be enhanced or impaired.

gerate the sympathomimetic response of many vasopressors, but antihypertensive and antiarrhythmic drugs can decrease peripheral sympathetic activity and augment the depressant effect of anesthetics. Patients whose hypertension is being treated with angiotensin receptor antagonists seem to have more trouble with hypotension intraoperatively. Certainly, drug therapy associated with concurrent diseases must be individually considered and continued as guided by specific disease-designated protocols (eg, hypertension, diabetes, ischemic heart disease, etc). Lastly, patients are increasingly taking complementing and alternative medications about which little is known but that have the potential for serious interactions with other drugs and anesthesia. Herbal medicines and dietary supplements are of special concern. Increasing amounts of information are becoming available. Obviously, the safety of continuing drug therapy depends on awareness of potential drug interactions.

Certain drugs probably should be started preoperatively, especially for moderately or extensively invasive procedures. These include beta-adrenergic receptor blockade and statins for 2 weeks preoperatively. Small-dose aspirin, unless surgically contraindicated, a physical activity regimen, and smoking cessation are all helpful.

D. Laboratory Tests

In the past, hospital rules mandated that a large battery of screening laboratory tests be given prior to anesthesia; however, many of these tests have been found to be unnecessary, and the advisability of others has been questioned. For example, one common rule is that elective surgery should not be performed if the hemoglobin concentration is less than 10 g/dL. There is no evidence, however, that correction of normovolemic anemia decreases perioperative morbidity and mortality rates. More important is the need to determine why the patient is anemic.

The history and physical examination are the most valuable guides for determining which laboratory tests are necessary (eg, a long history of smoking dictates a thorough examination of pulmonary status by means of pulmonary function tests). Men aged 40 years or younger with no history of problems with anesthesia and normal findings on physical examination usually require no laboratory tests; women of this age and health status usually require only hemoglobin measurements. Recently, the American Society of Anesthesiologists produced a preoperative testing advisory in which it divided surgical procedures into three classes: minimally or moderately invasive procedures and those that disrupt normal physiology.

For the last, most invasive category, a complete blood count, platelet count, and measurement of electrolytes and creatinine are usually recommended. An electrocardiogram is indicated for the last two categories. Other tests are based on comorbid conditions. A creatinine level measurement is usually indicated when the patient is to receive contrast dye.

Questionnaires, some via computers, are a useful means of identifying patients likely to have complications who would therefore benefit from preoperative laboratory testing. This is especially important with increasing emphasis on same-day surgery. Because increasing numbers of medical centers have integrated computerized systems, the results from preoperative and preprocedure assessment clinics will be a prominent part of these systems. Excessive testing can even be hazardous, because borderline abnormalities may lead to additional—sometimes invasive—tests or therapy. An example is potassium treatment for borderline low potassium levels.

E. Summary

The three major goals of preoperative evaluation can be briefly stated as follows: (1) to make certain that the patient is in optimal condition for anesthesia (eg, antibiotic therapy for respiratory infection in a patient with emphysema); (2) to understand the patient's concurrent diseases and drug therapy; and (3) to ensure that all of the patient's questions and concerns are adequately addressed.

Ang-Lee MK, Yuan CS, Moss J: Complementary and alternative Therapies. In: *Anesthesia,* 6th ed, p. 605. Miller RD (editor). Elsevier, 2005.

Pollard JB, Zboray AL, Mazze RI: Economic benefits attributed to opening a preoperative evaluation clinic for outpatients. Anesth Analg 1996;83:407.

Practice Advisory for Preoperative Evaluation & A Report by the American Society of Anesthesiologists Task Force on Preanesthetic Evaluation. Anesthesiology 2000;96:485.

Roizen MF: Preoperative evaluation. In: *Anesthesia,* 6th ed, p. 927. Miller RD (editor). Elsevier, 2005.

Roizen MF: More preoperative assessment by physicians and less by laboratory tests. N Engl J Med 2000;342:204.

Wyatt WJ, Reed DN Jr, Apelgren KN: Pitfalls in the role of standardized pre-admission laboratory screening for ambulatory surgery. Am Surg 1989;55:343.

Informed Consent

Informed consent involves advising the patient of what to expect from administration of anesthesia and of possible adverse effects and risks. Key components of an informed consent include decision-making capacity, patient voluntariness, disclosure, preferences of the reasonable person, legal issues in disclosure, recommendations, the patient's understanding, clinical decisions, and autonomous authorization. Controversial issues include emergency, refusing to provide care, Jehovah's Witnesses beliefs, and confidentiality. In general, the general scenario of the perioperative period should be described, and the patient should be allowed to ask questions. Table 11–3 lists concerns that the anesthesiologist should routinely address. A signed consent form should be obtained, and the physician should make notes and file them in the patient's medical record (see Chapter 6). Many hospitals use a common consent form for both surgery and anesthesia. Although that procedure is acceptable, a separate consent form for anesthesia is increasingly being recommended.

"Informed consent" is a term that is becoming increasingly difficult to define for both surgery and anesthesia. While one might argue that a patient should be informed of every possible complication, in actuality this is not practical and may even be harmful by causing undue worry. In anesthesia, patient autonomy must be balanced with medical needs in deciding what constitutes informed consent. This balance should be based on the anesthesiologist's best judgment. The anesthesiologist's conversation with the patient should be recorded as a separate note in the chart.

Table 11–3. Issues that should be discussed with patients preoperatively.

Risks of anesthesia (dental, heart, vomiting)
Preoperative insomnia and its treatment
Preoperative medication (time, route of administration, and effect)
Anticipated time of transport to the operating room
Sequence of events prior to induction of anesthesia
Anticipated duration of surgery
Description of where awakening from anesthesia will occur
Presence of catheters (eg, epidural, tracheal, bladder, arterial) on awakening
Expected time of return to hospital ward room
Likelihood of postoperative nausea and vomiting
Magnitude of postoperative pain and methods for treatment
Whether they will receive blood transfusions, with associated risks

IMMEDIATE PREOPERATIVE MANAGEMENT

Selection of Preoperative Medication

The principal goals of preoperative medication are (1) to relieve anxiety and provide sedation; (2) to induce amnesia; (3) to decrease secretion of saliva and gastric juices; (4) to increase the gastric pH; (5) to prevent allergic reactions to anesthetic drugs; and (6) to prevent postoperative nausea and vomiting. Medication is usually given 0.5–2 hours before the induction of anesthesia. It is not necessary to give medication specifically to facilitate the induction of anesthesia. The selection of drugs is largely subjective. Sedation can be achieved by benzodiazepines and sometimes opioids (or both), if the patient has acute pain. To avoid an intramuscular injection, diazepam, 0.12 mg/kg, is especially effective for sedation when given orally 1–2 hours preoperatively. Midazolam is a benzodiazepine with powerful amnestic properties and can be given intravenously 10–30 minutes before going into the operating room, usually at a dose of 1.0–2.0 mg/70 kg. Patients should be observed for possible respiratory depression. Also, α_2-adrenergic agonists (eg, clonidine and depomedetomidine) are being used for premedication. Gastric secretion can be decreased both in volume and pH by H_2-receptor antagonists such as cimetidine or ranitidine. These drugs need to be given 2–3 hours preoperatively. Antacids, such as sodium citrate, can be given acutely to decrease gastric fluid pH. Sometimes, drugs that stimulate gastric emptying (eg, metoclopramide) are used. Anticholinergics such as atropine or scopolamine are rarely indicated. The traditional practice of prolonged fasting (eg, NPO after midnight or for 8 hours before induction of anesthesia) in patients without risk factors (eg, obesity, bowel obstruction, severe pain) is being reevaluated. The volume and pH of gastric contents are not affected by fluids ingested more than 2 hours previously. Although it is reasonable to allow clear fluids orally up to 2 hours before induction of anesthesia, this does not apply to patients with known risks for aspiration or those who have ingested solid food.

In the past few years, emphasis has been on pharmacologic approaches to decreasing the incidence of postoperative nausea and vomiting. Certain types of patients, surgical procedures, and anesthetics (eg, opioids) are known to enhance postoperative nausea and vomiting. For moderate- to high-risk patients, ondansetron or dolasetron are effective. Droperidol was commonly used, but was given a "black box" warning by the Food and Drug Administration in 2001 because of QT prolongation.

The anesthesiologist's explanation to the patient of what will occur can substantially alleviate fears about anesthesia and surgery. In fact, it has been shown that a thorough explanation has a calming effect comparable to that of medications given to relieve anxiety.

For some other conditions associated with surgery, it is better to give medication as the need arises. Cardiac vagal activity is best controlled with glycopyrrolate given just before anticipated vagal stimulation. Postoperative analgesia is better achieved by giving opioids intravenously just before they are needed.

Selection of Anesthesia

Many factors influence the choice of anesthesia for a given patient, and it is common practice to discuss the question with the patient preoperatively. The site of surgery and positioning of the patient on the operating table are obviously important factors. Epidural anesthesia and analgesia, along with some peripheral nerve blocks, are increasingly being used not only for sometime superior intraoperative anesthesia but also as options for postoperative analgesia. Yet, a regional nerve block may be contraindicated in a patient with neuropathy due to diabetes mellitus. Spinal anesthesia is inappropriate for thyroidectomy. Different types of anesthesia may be given for elective or emergency surgery, particularly if the patient requiring emergency surgery has a full stomach. Coexisting diseases (eg, hypertension, cardiac disease) must be considered. The age and preferences of the patient must also be taken into account.

The need for pain management and the incidence of nausea and vomiting postoperatively may influence the choice of anesthesia (eg, epidural opioids for pain or propofol for nausea and vomiting).

Preparation for Administration of Anesthesia

Anesthesia usually begins by starting an intravenous infusion and engaging standard monitors, which include noninvasively measured arterial blood pressure, electrocardiography, pulse oximetry, and in some cases peripheral nerve stimulation and body temperature.

The machine for administering anesthesia must be checked for proper functioning, and drugs and other necessary supplies must be at hand (eg, the apparatus needed to suction the pharynx and ventilate the lungs with oxygen via a cuffed endotracheal tube).

National standards are evolving for patient monitoring during anesthesia. In general, minimum monitoring dictates measurement of arterial blood pressure and heart rate every 5 minutes, and the ECG should be displayed continuously.

In addition, standard practice during anesthesia is the use of pulse oximetry, capnography, an oxygen analyzer in the anesthetic circuit, a disconnect alarm, and measurement of body temperature. Other monitors, such as transcutaneous PaO_2, intra-arterial blood pressure, central venous pressure, transesophageal echocardiography, and Bispectral Index, are optimal depending on the anticipated extent of surgery and the anticipated duration and depth of anesthesia. The Bispectral Index is derived from continuous electroencephalographic monitoring and is thought to reflect the hypnotic component of anesthesia. Whether use of this type of monitoring will decrease the incidence of intraoperative "awareness" during general anesthesia is controversial. Even the definition of "intraoperative awareness" during general anesthesia is not well defined. The use of automated anesthetic records, in which all vital sign and other data are downloaded to a common record that can be connected to all activities in the perioperative period (eg, the postanesthetic care unit) is increasingly being recommended by organizations such as the Anesthesia Patient Safety Foundation.

Positioning of the Patient on the Operating Table

The patient must be positioned properly on the operating table to avoid physical or physiologic complications. Immediate complications (eg, decreased cardiac output) or long-term complications (eg, peripheral neuropathy) can result from improper positioning. In fact, nerve damage is the second most common type of anesthetic complication represented in the American Society of Anesthesiologists closed claims database. Nerve damage can be caused by placing the patient in a position that stretches or applies pressure to a nerve. Pressure on a vulnerable area may lead to skin necrosis and ulceration, which in rare cases requires skin grafting. Damage to the toes or fingers may occur when positioning of equipment (eg, Mayo stand) is adjusted. Because anesthesia blunts the normal compensatory mechanisms, a sudden change in the patient's position can cause cardiovascular changes (eg, a shift from the supine to a sitting position may result in hypotension and cerebral hypoperfusion).

Some peripheral nerves are at risk of trauma during anesthesia. Ulnar nerve injury is the most common postoperative peripheral neuropathy (28%). If the elbow is allowed to hang over the edge of the operating table, the ulnar nerve, which runs superficially along the medial aspect of the elbow, may be compressed between the medial epicondyle and the operating table. Injury to the brachial plexus nerves usually results from extension of the arm more than 90 degrees while the patient is supine. The radial nerve may be injured if the patient's arm slips off the operating table or if pressure is applied to the nerve at the point where it traverses the spiral groove of the humerus.

The sciatic nerve may be damaged if the patient is in the lithotomy position with thighs and legs extended outward and rotated or if the knees are extended. The common peroneal nerve is typically damaged by compression between the fibula and the metal brace used in the lithotomy position.

The American Society of Anesthesiologists has specific guidelines that may facilitate prevention of peripheral neuropathies; they include preoperative assessment, upper and lower extremity positioning, protective padding, equipment (eg, shoulder braces), postoperative assessment, and documentation.

Apfel CC et al: A factorial trial of six interventions for the prevention of postoperative nausea and vomiting. N Engl J Med 2004;350:2441.

ASAT Task Force on prevention of perioperative peripheral neuropathies: Practice advisory for the prevention of perioperative neuropathies. Anesthesiology 2000;92:1168.

Particular requirements for anesthesia workstations and their components. American Society for Testing and Materials, 1998.

Warner MA et al: Practice guidelines for preoperative fasting and the use of pharmacologic agents to reduce the risk of pulmonary aspiration: application to healthy patients undergoing elective procedures. Anesthesiology 1999;90:896.

MANAGEMENT OF GENERAL ANESTHESIA DURING OPERATION

Induction of General Anesthesia

General anesthesia can be induced by giving drugs intravenously, by inhalation, or by a combination of both methods.

A. Rapid-Sequence Induction

Anesthesia is probably most commonly induced by the method of rapid-sequence induction, in which rapid administration of thiopental or propofol (possibly in combination with an opioid) is followed by a depolarizing muscle relaxant (eg, succinylcholine) or a nondepolarizing muscle relaxant with a rapid onset time (rocuronium). While other drugs (eg, ketamine, etomidate) can be used for rapid-sequence induction of anesthesia, the combination of thiopental or propofol and succinylcholine is the standard against which others must be compared. This approach allows anesthesia to be induced within 30 seconds and the trachea to be intubated within 60–90 seconds. Oxygen is usually given by mask beforehand to allow maximum time for the tracheal intubation procedure while the patient is apneic.

Rapid-sequence induction of anesthesia minimizes the time during which the trachea is unprotected. Consequently, this method is often used in emergency surgery in patients who have eaten recently. The disadvantage of giving depressant drugs rapidly is that hypotension may occur in patients with questionable cardiovascular status or marginal circulatory volume. Also, this technique should not be used if a difficult endotracheal intubation is anticipated. If the surgery should be performed urgently in a patient with a "full stomach" and a difficult airway, then an awake fiberoptic-facilitated intubation should be considered before induction of anesthesia. Anesthesiologists are now all trained to perform this procedure.

B. Inhalation Induction of Anesthesia

Inhalation of nitrous oxide plus a potent volatile anesthetic (eg, halothane, sevoflurane, desflurane, or isoflurane) can produce anesthesia within 3–5 minutes. After induction, a depolarizing or nondepolarizing neuromuscular blocking drug can be given intravenously to facilitate tracheal intubation. If there is some question about the difficulty of intubation, it can be attempted while the patient is breathing spontaneously, without giving a muscle relaxant. Although conditions for intubation may not be as good with this method, the patient will still be breathing if difficulties with intubation prolong the time before complete airway control is achieved.

The advantage of inhalation induction is that anesthetic drugs can be titrated according to the patient's needs. This allows for administration of more precise doses and minimizes the risk of an accidental overdose with resultant cardiovascular depression. The disadvantages are a slower induction time and lack of protection for the airway for a longer period of time.

C. Combined Intravenous-Inhalation Induction

Short-acting anesthetic drugs such as thiopental, propofol, or midazolam are often administered intravenously before inhalation of a volatile anesthetic. This is done to minimize the discomfort of wearing the anesthetic mask and to facilitate inhalation of the anesthetic, which many people consider to have an offensive odor. This technique combines the advantages of both the intravenous and inhalation approaches. Anesthesia is induced rapidly, and anesthetic drug dosages can be titrated according to the patient's requirements.

Maintaining the Airway

Historically, administering general anesthesia without endotracheal intubation was uncommon. While this approach avoids the complications of intubation, it has many disadvantages. If the patient vomits even a small amount, the airway is unprotected and aspiration will occur. Furthermore, the anesthesiologist must hold the mask with one hand during the entire procedure, and this hinders performance of the many other tasks required (eg, administration of other drugs or blood, record keeping, and monitoring). With the use of the laryngeal mask airway (LMA)(see below), administration of anesthesia via a mask is increasingly rare.

A. Approach to Airway Management Other Than Traditional Endotracheal Intubation

In the last 10 years, many other options have become available for managing the airway in both the awake and the anesthetized patient. The two most important are the LMA and the fiberoptic laryngoscope. The

LMA is an alternative to endotracheal intubation when less invasive approaches are desired or when endotracheal intubation is difficult or impossible; it provides an excellent airway but does not protect against pulmonary aspiration of gastric contents. The fiberoptic laryngoscope represents a major advance in the management of difficult airways in both awake and anesthetized patients. Other valuable but less often used devices include the lighted stylet (lightwand) and the Bullard intubatory laryngoscope as well as many types of endotracheal tests. Since the introduction of the LMA, many derivatives have been developed, including the intubating LMA, the Pro Seal LMA, the Combitube, and many others—all designed to overcome disadvantages of the original LMA or extend its clinical opportunities.

B. Indications for Endotracheal Intubation

Endotracheal intubation is now almost routinely performed during general anesthesia (Table 11–4). Clearly, any patient who has recently eaten or has intestinal obstruction should be managed by rapid intubation. Tracheal intubation is also usually mandatory for patients requiring positive-pressure ventilation (eg, during thoracotomy or when neuromuscular blocking drugs are given). When the patient must be placed in a position other than supine, endotracheal intubation is often required.

C. Complications of Endotracheal Intubation

The most important complication is failure to intubate the trachea, the most common cause of serious anesthesia-induced morbidity. The difficulty of tracheal intubation is related to body weight, head and neck movement, jaw movement, receding mandible, and buck teeth. A variety of techniques are available, including fiberoptic laryngoscopy, to facilitate intubation. Complications occurring during direct laryngoscopy and passage of the tube most often involve injuries to the teeth. The laryngoscope blade should not be used as a lever on the teeth. If a tooth is dislodged, it must be removed. If the tooth cannot be located, radiographs of the chest and abdomen should be obtained to ascertain that the tooth has not passed through the glottic opening.

Hypertension and tachycardia may be associated with endotracheal intubation, but they are usually transient and of no clinical significance. They can be minimized by ensuring that the depth of anesthesia is adequate and by giving lidocaine, 100 mg/70 kg intravenously, to susceptible patients. Administration of small doses of a potent opioid (eg, 150 mg/70 kg of fentanyl) during induction of anesthesia will attenuate the cardiovascular responses to tracheal intubation.

The endotracheal tube can be obstructed or accidentally removed. If it has been incorrectly placed (eg, into the bronchus or esophagus), hypoxemia will result. Auscultation of the lungs and stomach will determine whether the tube is in the esophagus. As well as monitoring the end-tidal CO_2 (ie, the end-tidal CO_2 will dramatically decrease if in the esophagus). If too much pressure is applied by the balloon cuff to the tracheal wall, the tracheal mucosa may become ischemic. Previously, endotracheal tubes had "high-pressure cuffs" that required 80–250 mm Hg of pressure before they expanded enough to seal the tracheal lumen. The currently available "low-pressure cuffs" adapt to irregularities in the tracheal circumference and produce a seal at pressures of 15–30 mm Hg. With these cuffs, the incidence of tracheal ischemia is minimal. However, there is no way to entirely avoid laryngotracheal damage. For example, ciliary denudation can occur over the tracheal rings with only 2 hours of intubation and tracheal pressures of less than 25 mm Hg.

The most common complications following extubation are laryngospasm, aspiration of gastric contents, pharyngitis (sore throat), laryngitis, and laryngeal or subglottic edema. Later complications include laryngeal ulceration with or without granuloma formation, tracheitis, tracheal stenosis, vocal cord paralysis, and arytenoid cartilage dislocation.

The incidence of many of these complications can be reduced by using low-pressure endotracheal tube cuffs to minimize tissue damage and by performing prompt extubation when clinically possible.

Table 11–4. Indications for endotracheal intubation.

To provide a patent airway
To prevent aspiration of gastric contents
To provide tracheal or bronchial suctioning
To facilitate positive-pressure ventilation
To provide adequate ventilation when—
the position of the patient is other than supine,
ventilation provided by mask or laryngeal mask airway is not sufficient, and
disease of the upper airway is present

Maintaining General Anesthesia

The main objectives of general anesthesia are analgesia, unconsciousness, skeletal muscle relaxation, and control of sympathetic nervous system responses to noxious stimulation. Inhaled and intravenous anesthetics, opioids, and muscle relaxants should be selected with specific pharmacologic goals in mind.

A. Nitrous Oxide, Volatile Anesthetics, and Narcotics

Since nitrous oxide does not provide total anesthesia, it is frequently given in combination with a volatile anesthetic, opioid, or both. The main disadvantage of most volatile anesthetics is dose-dependent decrease in arterial blood pressure; when they are used in combination with nitrous oxide, which is relatively free of cardiovascular effects, their total dose can be decreased. Delivery of potent volatile anesthetics is controlled by a machine that allows the anesthesiologist to titrate the dose to the needs of the patient.

Conceptually, most volatile and intravenous anesthetics (eg, propofol, midazolam, etc) are not considered to provide sufficient analgesia for anesthesia. As a result, narcotics or opioids, which generally do not depress the cardiovascular system, are often combined with nitrous oxide. However, in patients with normal ventricular function, the lack of opioid-induced cardiovascular depression in the face of unblocked sympathetic nervous system responses may produce hypertension. If this happens, the addition of low concentrations of a volatile anesthetic will usually control arterial blood pressure. With a combined opioid-nitrous oxide anesthetic, muscle relaxants are more frequently needed to facilitate skeletal muscle relaxation.

B. Total Intravenous Anesthesia (TIVA)

With the introduction of propofol in 1977, the concept of TIVA evolved, which eliminated the need for gaseous (nitrous oxide) or volatile anesthetics. The combination of propofol, other hypnotics, opioids, and muscle relaxants provides all the components of a proper general anesthetic. Delivery systems can deliver precise doses of these drugs.

C. Monitoring the Depth of Anesthesia

Although paralysis by muscle relaxants simplifies exposure of the operative site and decreases the need for volatile or intravenous anesthetics, many signs of anesthesia are absent in the paralyzed patient. It is essential that the anesthesiologist continuously assess the depth of anesthesia. Failure to do so may result in the patient being awake but paralyzed during the procedure.

The Bispectral Index is a monitor that can be used in many cases to assess anesthetic depth. It is measured from superficial scalp electrodes and is a processed electroencephalogram. It is possible that this type of monitoring approach will be increasingly used to assess anesthetic depth.

D. Neuromuscular Blockade

One of the greatest challenges for the anesthesiologist is to administer the proper dosage of muscle relaxant—ie, a dosage large enough to facilitate the surgical procedures but not so large as to cover up inadequate doses of anesthetic drugs and thereby expose the patient to the risk of prolonged postoperative paralysis. A peripheral nerve stimulator is of help in gauging the extent of neuromuscular blockade intraoperatively. Usually, the ulnar nerve is stimulated, and adduction of the thumb is observed. If anesthesia is sufficient, obliteration of 90% of the response will in general result in adequate relaxation. The increasing need or surgical demand for profound muscular relaxation can increase the incidence of weakness causing inadequate ventilation in the recovery room. This can be partly ascribed to difficulties in pharmacologically (ie, neostigmine) reversing profound neuromuscular blockade. Increasing evidence indicates the need to demonstrate, via clinical signs and peripheral nerve stimulation monitoring, objective evidence that neuromuscular blockade (ie, paralysis) has been completely reversed. As a result, the surgical team should also take all other measures to aid in exposure (eg, correct positioning and adequate depth of anesthesia), so that the amount of muscle relaxant can be kept to a minimum. This decreases the incidence of prolonged paralysis and dependence on mechanical ventilation postoperatively.

Benumof JL: Laryngeal mask airway and the ASA difficult airway algorithm. Anesthesiology 1996;84:686.

Viby-Mogensen V: Postoperative residual curarization and evidence-based anesthesia. Br J Anesth 2000;84:301.

REGIONAL ANESTHESIA DURING OPERATION

With the increased use of thoracic (as opposed to lumbar) epidurals and peripheral nerve blocks, regional anesthesia has become a more prominent part of intraoperative anesthesia and especially for postoperative pain relief. A regional anesthetic can be used when it is desirable that the patient remain conscious during the operation. Skeletal muscle relaxation is usually excellent, especially with spinal and epidural anesthesia. Thus, muscle relaxants (eg, vecuronium or rocuronium) are unnecessary. Patients often have misconceptions about regional anesthesia that require detailed explanation of the safety of this technique. One disadvantage of regional anesthesia is the occasional failure to produce adequate anesthesia; another is hypotension due to sympathetic blockade. While regional anesthesia was used most often for surgery of the lower abdomen or lower extremities, upper abdominal, thoracic, and upper extremity surgery is increasingly being conducted under regional anesthesia.

Despite its limitations, regional anesthesia does have many attractive features. Anesthetizing only the part of the body upon which surgery is being performed (eg, spinal anesthesia for lower abdominal surgery or brachial plexus nerve block for arm surgery) may decrease postoperative morbidity. Some examples are as follows:

(1) Blood loss from total hip arthroplasty or prostatectomy is decreased by spinal or epidural anesthesia.

(2) Thromboembolic complications after hip and prostate operations are less.

(3) Lung function may be less affected.

(4) Hospital stay is decreased for colon surgery.

(5) Postoperative impairment of immune function is avoided.

(6) Convalescence may be shorter.

Spinal & Epidural Blocks

Spinal anesthesia is achieved by injecting a local anesthetic into the lumbar intrathecal space. This blocks the spinal nerve roots and dorsal root ganglia and probably also blocks the periphery of the spinal cord. Epidural anesthesia is accomplished by injecting a local anesthetic into the extradural (epidural) space. The epidural space is usually identified via the lumbar approach. The gastrointestinal tract is usually contracted with spinal and epidural anesthesia, facilitating exposure of the surgical site. A limitation not only of spinal and epidural anesthesia but of regional anesthesia generally is the need to provide some sedation. Proper selection will eliminate those patients who need excessive sedation. When enough sedatives are given, the result is a comfortable-appearing, sleep-like state in which there is no spontaneous verbalization. Excess sedation can produce respiratory insufficiency leading to cardiac arrest. Monitoring with a pulse oximeter should allow detection of more subtle degrees of respiratory insufficiency.

There are several complications of spinal anesthesia. Headache is the most common and is seen most frequently in young patients. The incidence is only 1% when a 25-gauge needle is used. For severe headache, a "blood-patch" epidural injection should be performed. This involves injecting 5–10 mL of the patient's blood into the epidural space at the site of the previous lumbar puncture. Pain relief is usually prompt, and headache usually does not recur. This technique is thought to plug the leak of cerebrospinal fluid, restoring pressure in the subarachnoid space to normal.

Because spinal anesthesia blocks innervation of the bladder, administration of large amounts of intravenous fluids may cause bladder distention, and a urethral catheter may be required. This usually occurs with minor operations such as inguinal hernia repairs and can be avoided by keeping fluids to a minimum. Nausea and vomiting may occur when a spinal anesthetic is begun, especially if hypotension is present. If nausea and vomiting persist despite successful treatment of hypotension, diazepam or droperidol may be effective. Peripheral nerve damage is rare.

In the past few years, epidurals have increasingly been used not so much for their intraoperative advantages but for their ability to provide excellent postoperative analgesia via local anesthetics and opioids administered epidurally. For example, patients frequently can ambulate more rapidly following epidural anesthesia versus general anesthesia and still have pain relief. One of the problems with epidurals is the increasing use of low-molecular-weight heparin (eg, enoxaparin) to prevent deep vein thrombosis, especially in hip surgery. If used, the incidence of epidural hematomas may increase.

Recently, the technique of combined spinal-epidural anesthesia has been used. It provides the intense block from spinal anesthesia intraoperatively but also allows the advantages of epidural analgesia to occur postoperatively.

Complications from epidural anesthesia are the same as those for spinal anesthesia, with the exception of headache.

Nerve Blocks

Nerve blocks are most appropriate for surgery of the extremities. Intercostal nerve blocks are useful for postoperative pain relief. In a well-organized anesthesia department, nerve blocks can be performed with a minimum of turnaround time between cases, and patient comfort can be assured with adequate premedication. Several wound infiltration and peripheral nerve techniques (femoral, sciatic-popliteal, brachial plexus) are very effective for postoperative analgesic.

MONITORED ANESTHETIC CARE DURING OPERATION (STANDBY ANESTHESIA)

Monitored (standby) anesthesia is the use of local anesthesia by the surgeon along with administration of sedative-hypnotics (eg, diazepam, midazolam) and opioids (eg, fentanyl) by the anesthesiologist. In elderly or fragile patients—especially those with unprotected airways—these cases can become quite challenging. When unexpectedly large amounts of sedative-hypnotics are required, the decision to interrupt surgery and convert to a general anesthetic with endotracheal intubation is often difficult but obviously crucial.

Brown DL: Spinal, epidural, and caudal anesthesia. In: *Anesthesia,* 6th ed, p. 1653. Miller RD (editor). Elsevier, 2005.

Wedel DJ, Horlocker TT: Nerve blocks. In: *Anesthesia,* 6th ed, p. 1685. Miller RD (editor). Elsevier, 2005.

POSTOPERATIVE PROCEDURES ASSOCIATED WITH ANESTHESIA

Postanesthetic Care Unit (PACU)

The PACU is designed for the monitoring and care of patients during the period immediately following anesthesia and surgery. The PACU must be near the operating room, so that the physician is available for consultation and assistance. The size of the PACU depends on the number and kind of operations performed, with approximately one and one-half beds for each operating room.

Equipment and drugs must be available to provide routine care and advanced organ support. An electrical defibrillator, appropriate airway equipment, and drugs must be available to provide cardiopulmonary resuscitation. In a way, the PACU functions like an intensive care unit with special emphasis on the immediate postoperative period. Of course, appropriate personnel (eg, nurses and an anesthesiologist) must be available to provide care. Standards for PACU care have been formulated by many professional organizations, including the American Society of Anesthesiologists and the American Society of Post Anesthesia Nurses.

Recovery from anesthesia begins in the operating room with the discontinuation of anesthetic drugs and extubation of the trachea. Volatile anesthetics are eliminated by the lungs and intravenous anesthetics by metabolism or renal excretion. Residual activity of muscle relaxants should be assessed with a peripheral nerve stimulator, and any residual blockade should be treated with antagonists. Patients sometimes enter the PACU in a state of hypothermia. Rewarming is important to minimize the adverse effects of shivering on oxygen consumption. Surgeons could help keep their patients from becoming hypothermic by allowing operating room temperatures to be warmer. Postoperative shivering can be treated with body surface warming with devices such as the Bair Huggar system or with meperidine, 10–25 mg/70 kg intravenously.

The most common immediate postoperative complications are upper airway obstruction, arterial hypoxemia, alveolar hypoventilation, hypotension, hypertension, cardiac dysrhythmias, and agitation (delirium tremens).

The physician must make sure that the patient is breathing adequately before initiating the transfer from the PACU to the ward, where monitoring is much less intense. While discharge from the PACU requires clinical judgment, a commonly used scoring system is the Aldrete Score, which quantitates the ability of the patient to move the extremities, the adequacy of breathing and circulation, consciousness, and oxygen saturation as measured by pulse oximetry.

Nausea & Vomiting

Nausea and vomiting is a common problem in the immediate postoperative period. Most pharmacologic medications (eg, small doses of droperidol) are reactive instead of preventive. This problem can be ameliorated by preoperative administration of antiemetics (eg, ondansetron) to high-risk patients (eye surgery, gynecologic surgery). Also, the intraoperative use of opioids augments the incidence of nausea and vomiting. Ketorolac tromethamine, a nonsteroidal, nonopioid anti-inflammatory drug, can produce postoperative analgesia (ie, equivalent to morphine) without respiratory depression and minimal nausea and vomiting. A variety of drugs can be used in the PACU for treatment of nausea and vomiting, including ondansetron, tropisetron, and granisetron.

Postoperative Analgesic

The adequacy of pain management has received national attention, including that of the Joint Commission on the Accreditation of Healthcare Organizations. Most certainly, postoperative pain relief has received prime attention. As a result, many medical centers with high-acuity surgery have a specific Acute Pain Service, which provides postoperative pain relief and the institutional need for education, documentation, and administration regarding all pain relief to patients.

Historically, morphine has been the foundation of postoperative analgesia. Opioids are first given intravenously and later intramuscularly. Regional anesthesia can also be used for postoperative pain relief.

Epidural or occasionally intrathecal administration of opioids is an important advance in pain relief. Complete analgesia can be obtained for 12–24 hours with no interference with autonomic or motor function. If the epidural catheter remains in place postoperatively, the analgesia can be sustained for several days. Several complications can occur from epidural opioids including pruritus and respiratory depression. Now local anesthetics and opioids are given in combination into the epidural space. This combination allows decreases in problems with each drug because of smaller doses of each. Also, inserting the epidural dural catheter at the site of pain (ie, high thoracic to upper lumbar) allows smaller and more precise doses to be given. Lastly, respiratory depression is always to be feared and can be detected by standard nursing care, with specific monitoring orders, on the ward. Even smaller community hospitals that do not have continuous physician coverage are now using this technique. However, epidural catheters should be used cautiously in patients receiving prophylactic small doses or low-molecular-weight heparin against venous thromboembolism.

The addition of clonidine, an α_2-adrenergic agonist, to epidural opioids markedly reduces the required dose of opioid. The ultimate role of clonidine has yet to be determined. Also, a small dose of local anesthetic may be infused that will reduce the dose of opioid and improve the quality of analgesia. The analgesics can be given by intermittent injections or, more commonly, by a continuous infusion.

A technique called patient-controlled analgesia (PCA) can be used for both intravenous and epidurally administered analgesics. With this system a PCA device can be programmed for the bolus dose, lockout interval, and background infusion. Basically this is a negative-feedback loop controlled by the patient. When pain is experienced, the analgesic is given and when pain is reduced, analgesics are not given.

To achieve such profound analgesia postoperatively, the complexity of pain management has markedly increased. This has led to the development of acute pain management teams, usually but not always led by anesthesiologists. As a result, standards for postoperative analgesia have been established, including standard order and evaluation forms.

Aldrete JA: The post anaesthesia recovery score revisited. J Clin Anesth 1995;7:89.

OUTPATIENT SURGERY: HOSPITAL, SURGICENTER, OR OFFICE-BASED

To decrease the cost of hospitalization, outpatient surgery is conducted in a variety of settings, including within a hospital or satellite (surgicenter) unit that is either part of the hospital or free-standing. Physician's offices have increasingly been used for surgery and even general anesthesia. If surgery is performed in an office, the same high standards should be observed as are required in a hospital operating room or surgicenter-based outpatient facility. When this option is used, access to a hospital is needed for the rare unexpected hospitalization that may be required.

Patients who report to the hospital on the day of surgery must be given detailed instructions well in advance (Table 11–5). Local or general anesthesia is usually used in ambulatory surgical procedures. Peripheral nerve blocks are often ideal (especially intravenous Bier block) for superficial surgery of the extremities. Although epidural anesthesia can be used, spinal anesthesia may be followed by postanesthesia headache.

Table 11–5. Written instructions given to patients receiving anesthesia on an outpatient basis.

Complete all laboratory tests requested prior to surgery.
Notify the surgeon if your medical condition changes before surgery.
Do not eat solids for 6 hours or more before surgery.
Clear fluids can be taken up to 2 hours before induction of anesthesia if approved by the anesthesiologist.
Do not wear cosmetics or jewelry.
Report for surgery ___[where and when]___.
The estimated time of discharge will be __[when]__.
You must be accompanied by an adult when you leave the hospital or clinic after surgery.
Following surgery, eat when hungry, starting with fluids and progressing to solid food.
Do not drive or make important decisions during the 24–48 hours following surgery.
Contact the physician in case of complications: _[phone number]_

Recovery from anesthesia is accompanied by return of vital signs to normal, normal level of consciousness, and ability to walk without assistance. After regional anesthesia, it is important to document complete return of sensory and motor function. Nausea, vomiting, and vertigo should be absent, and the patient should not have excessive pain. The patient should be able to drink fluids. Hoarseness or stridor in a patient who was intubated must be watched carefully. Significant laryngeal edema, if present, typically becomes evident within the first hour following extubation of the trachea. Most patients with stridor improve and can be discharged without hospitalization.

The patient should be reminded that mental clarity and dexterity may remain impaired for 24–48 hours, despite an overall feeling of well-being. Driving motor vehicles or operating complex equipment should not be attempted during this period. The use of alcohol or depressant drugs should be avoided, since additive interactions with residual amounts of anesthetic are possible. Oral analgesics should be provided when appropriate. Lastly, the patient should be given the physician's telephone number and instructed to report any new symptoms or other concerns.

Dexter F, Traub RD: The lack of systematic month-to-month variation over one-year periods in ambulatory surgery caseload. Anesth Analg 2000;91:1426.

Marshall SI, Chung F: Discharge criteria and complications after ambulatory surgery. Anesth Analg 1999;88:508.

Pavlin DJ et al: Factors affecting discharge times in outpatients. Anesth Analg 1998;816.

White PE: Criteria for fast-tracking outpatients after ambulatory surgery. J Clin Anesth 1999;11:78.

COMPLICATIONS

Aspiration Pneumonitis

A significant percentage of anesthesia-related deaths are the result of aspiration of food particles, foreign bodies, blood, gastric acid, oropharyngeal secretions, or bile during induction of anesthesia.

Aspiration pneumonitis usually takes one of two forms. Undigested food may be aspirated, producing airway obstruction and respiratory distress. Depending on the amount of material aspirated, respiratory distress can be severe, with cyanosis and cardiac arrest. Other cases may follow a milder, chronic course, leading to lobar pneumonia and lung abscess formation. Treatment involves removal of the particles by suction and bronchoscopy, followed by intensive care support. The second (more common) form of aspiration pneumonitis is caused by aspiration of gastric secretions with a pH less than 2.50, producing sudden bronchospasm, tachypnea, labored respiration, diffuse rales, cyanosis, and hypotension. Cardiac arrest may occur in severe cases.

Prevention is obviously most desirable. Generally, any patient who has eaten solid food within 8 hours should be considered to have a full stomach and therefore at risk of vomiting during induction. However, it should be recognized that 8 hours of fasting does not guarantee a small gastric volume. In traumatized or pregnant patients, gastric emptying may be delayed, and the interval between eating and elective surgery should be lengthened to 12 hours. Premedication with H_2-receptor blockers such as cimetidine and other drugs such as metoclopramide is frequently recommended. Drinking sodium citrate will increase the gastric pH in most patients, but this must be done 45–75 minutes before induction. If time does not permit such a wait, either endotracheal intubation with the patient awake or rapid-sequence induction must be performed.

Warner MA et al: Practice guidelines for preoperative fasting and the use of pharmacologic agents to reduce the risk of pulmonary aspirations. Anesthesiology 1999;90:896.

Malignant Hyperthermia

Malignant hyperthermia associated with anesthesia is an inherited disease manifested by a rapid increase in body temperature, which is often lethal if not promptly treated. The caffeine-halothane contracture test, which measures the concentration of caffeine required to trigger contracture in freshly biopsied skeletal muscle, is the standard test used to establish susceptibility to malignant hyperthermia. A linkage has been established between the human gene for malignant hyperthermia and the ryanodine receptor gene. This receptor is a protein that comprises the calcium release channel of skeletal muscle sarcoplasmic reticulum. Genetic studies suggest that the caffeine-halothane contracture test may yield many false-positive results. In any event, the incidence during anesthesia is approximately 1:15,000 for pediatric patients and 1:50,000 for adult patients. This disease is due to a defect in excitation-contraction coupling in skeletal muscles and high calcium concentrations in the myoplasm. Exposure to a triggering drug such as a volatile anesthetic, succinylcholine, or an amide local anesthetic causes unusually high and sustained levels of calcium in the myoplasm and persistent skeletal muscle contraction. This results in hypermetabolism, including tachycardia, arterial hypoxemia, metabolic and respiratory acidosis, and profound hyperthermia. Dantrolene, up to 10 mg/kg intravenously, is the treatment of choice.

Patients who will require anesthesia and are susceptible to malignant hyperthermia should be pretreated with dantrolene, 5 mg/kg/d orally in four divided doses for 1–3 days; drugs known to trigger the syndrome should be avoided during anesthesia. No anesthetic approach is completely safe in these patients, though the drugs usually used are opioids, barbiturates, nitrous oxide, and local anesthetics.

Fulminant malignant hyperthermia is increasingly rare because of sophisticated monitoring in the operating room and systematic education by groups such as the North American and European Malignant Hyperthermia Group of anesthesiologists and nurse anesthetists. The mortality rate has decreased from about 38% to almost zero with proper management.

Larach MG et al: A clinical grading scale to predict malignant hyperthermia susceptibility. Anesthesiology 1994;80:771.

Ørding HD et al: Between-center variability of results of the in vitro contracture test for malignant hyperthermia susceptibility. Anesth Analg 2000;91:452.

Pessah IN, Lynch C, Gronert GA: Complex pharmacology of malignant hyperthermia. Anesthesiology 1996;84:1275.

Shock & Acute Pulmonary Failure in Surgical Patients

12

James W. Holcroft, MD, & John T. Anderson, MD

I. INITIAL TREATMENT OF SHOCK

Cardiovascular failure, or shock, can be caused by (1) depletion of the vascular volume, (2) compression of the heart or great veins, (3) intrinsic failure of the heart itself, (4) loss of autonomic control of the vasculature, (5) severe untreated systemic inflammation, and (6) severe but partially compensated systemic inflammation. If the shock is decompensated, the blood pressure or the cardiac output will be inadequate for peripheral perfusion; in compensated shock, the perfusion will be adequate but only at the expense of excessive demands on the heart. Depending on the type and severity of cardiovascular failure and on response to treatment, shock can go on to compromise other organ systems. For discussion of gastrointestinal failure, see Chapter 3; for hepatic failure and psychiatric problems, see Chapter 4; for glucose intolerance and kidney failure, see Chapter 5; for complications of wound healing, see Chapter 6; for infectious problems, see Chapter 8; and for problems of catabolism, see Chapter 10. This chapter discusses the cardiovascular and pulmonary disorders associated with shock.

HYPOVOLEMIC SHOCK

Diagnosis

Hypovolemic shock (shock caused by inadequate circulating blood volume) is most often caused by bleeding, but it can also be a consequence of protracted vomiting or diarrhea, sequestration of fluid in the gut lumen (eg, bowel obstruction), or loss of plasma into injured or burned tissues. The body's response to the shock, however, is the same, no matter what the cause. Aldosterone and vasopressin are released; sodium and water are actively reabsorbed from the glomerular filtrate. Adrenergically mediated constriction of the arterioles in the skin, skeletal muscle, gut, pancreas, spleen, and liver (but not the brain or heart) diverts blood flow away from organs that can withstand ischemia for longer periods of time (perhaps hours) to those that cannot. Adrenergically mediated constriction of the venules and small veins in the skin, fat, skeletal muscle, and viscera displaces blood from the peripheral capacitance vessels to the heart, to reestablish ventricular end-diastolic volumes. And adrenergic stimulation of the heart maximizes diastolic and systolic function of the myocardium and adjusts the heart rate to deal with the stresses imposed by the shock state. The result is preservation of organs with high rates of metabolism but at the expense of inefficient use of oxygen by the heart.

The physical findings associated with these compensatory mechanisms can be subtle. In mild hypovolemic shock (a deficit of less than 20% of the blood volume), the only findings will be postural hypotension, cutaneous vasoconstriction, collapse of neck veins, and oliguria. If the shock is caused by blood loss, the hematocrit will decrease with administration of fluids.

Postural hypotension—a fall in the systolic blood pressure of more than 10 mm Hg that persists for more than 1 minute when the patient sits up—is one of the most sensitive signs of hypovolemic shock. It can be elicited by nonphysician personnel, and it can be used in patients who are suspected of being hypovolemic from either dehydration or occult internal blood loss (eg, in a patient who might have gastrointestinal bleeding). This sign cannot be used in the patient with multiple injuries.

Cold skin or difficulty in establishing venous access is sometimes the first manifestation of cutaneous hypoperfusion in a patient in hypovolemic shock, but cutaneous pallor is more sensitive and specific. Pallor, which can be detected in all patients, including those with deeply pigmented skin, is best detected by compressing a toe, to produce blanching on its plantar surface, and then releasing the compression and watching for color return. In a normovolemic patient without peripheral vascular disease, the color should return within 2 seconds; in a hypovolemic patient, the refill takes longer. The test is usually done with the foot at the level of the heart, but if the patient is not badly injured, it is more sensitive if it can be done with the foot raised above the level of the heart, to a height of perhaps 30 cm.

Low filling pressures in the right atrium are always present in hypovolemic shock, even in cases of mild shock, assuming there is no accompanying cardiac compression, and can sometimes be detected by observation of the neck veins. Looking for collapsed neck veins is best done with the patient's head, neck, and torso elevated 30 degrees. A normal right atrial pressure will distend the neck veins to about 2 cm above the manubrium. Failure to see the veins suggests hypovolemia.

Oliguria is another consistent finding in early shock. A Foley catheter should be inserted in any patient suspected of being hypovolemic. Urine output is considered to be potentially inadequate if it is less than 0.5 mL/kg/h in an adult, or less than 1 mL/kg/h in a child, or less than 2 mL/kg/h in an infant.

Administration of asanguinous fluids to a patient who has bled will drop the hematocrit in proportion to the initial degree of blood volume depletion. A fall of 3–4% indicates that the blood volume has been depleted by about 10%; a fall of 6–8% indicates a deficit of about 20% (or 1 L in an average adult). These calculations assume that the patient has been given enough fluid to correct the hypovolemia. (The initial hematocrit in a patient who has recently bled will be normal. Noticeable plasma expansion by compensatory responses, without exogenous administration of fluids, takes at least 30 minutes.)

The shock becomes easier to recognize when it becomes more severe. In moderate hypovolemic shock (a deficit of 20–40% of the blood volume), the patient can be thirsty. Hypotension can be present, even in the supine position. A metabolic acidemia, usually with a compensatory rapid respiratory rate, can develop after initial resuscitation. (The acidemia is usually not present before resuscitation. The products of anaerobic metabolism in the ischemic tissues are only flushed into the circulating blood volume once some degree of reperfusion has been achieved.)

In severe hypovolemic shock (a deficit of more than 40% of blood volume), the blood pressure will always be low, even in the supine position. Cerebral and cardiac perfusion can become inadequate. Signs of the former include changes in mental status, eg, restlessness, agitation, confusion, lethargy, or the appearance of inebriation; signs of the latter include an irregular heartbeat or electrocardiographic evidence of myocardial ischemia, such as ST–T segment depression or the appearance of Q waves.

There are many pitfalls in making the diagnosis of hypovolemic shock, and every clinician will miss the diagnosis on occasion. In some patients, especially young patients, the compensatory mechanisms brought into play against the shock are potent enough to maintain the blood pressure at completely normal levels. In other patients, one might not know if the observed pressure is abnormally low. A young patient might normally have systolic pressures in the low 100's. The same pressure in a chronically hypertensive patient might presage catastrophe.

The heart rate is notoriously unreliable as a sign of hypovolemic shock. Although the heart rate in anesthetized animals increases proportionately in response to graded hemorrhage, the correlation between hypovolemia and heart rate in unanesthetized human beings is poor. Unanesthetized hypovolemic human beings often have normal heart rates, and severe hypovolemia can even produce bradycardia as a preterminal event, as the cardiovascular system makes a last attempt to allow filling of the ventricles during diastole. A normal heart rate provides no assurance that the patient is not in shock.

As last examples of pitfalls, the vasoconstriction of hypovolemic shock can be ablated by the vasodilation of inebriation with alcohol. The oliguria of shock can be overcome by the diuresis induced by the hyperosmolar state of high blood alcohol or glucose levels. And an altered mental status can be a consequence of drug use or alcoholic inebriation, but it can also arise from the most ominous of all of the consequences of shock—inadequate cerebral blood flow.

The physician should consider the diagnosis of shock in any patient who is potentially at risk.

Treatment

A. Airway, Ventilation, Bleeding

Resuscitation of patients in hypovolemic shock, either hemorrhagic or nonhemorrhagic, begins with making sure that the airway is secure, by ensuring that ventilation and oxygenation are adequate, and, in the case of hemorrhagic shock, by controlling bleeding.

With regard to the airway, if there is any question, intubate. The physician cannot let uncertainty about the airway interfere with evaluation and resuscitation of other problems in the often confusing picture of shock. The patient can be extubated later if it turns out that there is no continuing need for the intubation.

If the patient requires mechanical ventilation, and almost all patients intubated for shock do, we prefer volume control ventilation, or some variant thereof. The ventilator is set up to minimize the mean airway pressure. The tidal volume is set at 7 mL/kg ideal body weight; the inspiratory time at 1 s; and the respiratory rate at 15 breaths/min. No end-expiratory pressure is used. To maintain adequate arterial oxygen saturation, the inspired oxygen concentration is set at 1.00.

External bleeding is controlled by application of pressure over the bleeding areas, surgical control, or, in a rare case, by tourniquet. Blood in the pleural cavities is drained, to reestablish ventilation from the compressed lung and to stop further bleeding from the pulmonary parenchyma. Major fractures are immobilized. Preparations are made to operate on patients who are bleeding internally.

B. Initial Fluid Resuscitation

Vascular access is best obtained with percutaneously placed, large-bore (ideally 14-gauge or larger) venous catheters. The catheters can be percutaneously placed in superficial veins in the upper extremities, in central veins at the thoracic outlet, or in the femoral veins; catheters can also by placed in the saphenous veins, by cutdown. Choice of access depends on the severity of the shock, patterns of injury, and experience of the physician gaining the access. Care must be taken to not complicate an already complicated situation. If a central venous catheter is to be placed, the physician placing the catheter has to be confident that the likelihood of injuring a large intrathoracic artery or a lung is low. If veins in the lower extremities are to be used, they must be decannulated within 24 hours, to minimize the risk of phlebitis.

Initial fluid resuscitation begins with a warmed crystalloid solution. Either normal saline or lactated Ringer's solution can be used. Use of lactate in the resuscitative fluid is reasonable if the shock seems to be severe and if the arterial pH is likely to be less than 7.20. The lactate will buffer the hydrogen ions that are released into the central circulation with the initiation of resuscitation, by absorbing hydrogen ion to form lactic acid. The lactic acid is then oxidized in the liver in the Cori cycle to carbon dioxide and water, which are excreted by the lungs and kidneys. This buffering will be effective even in severe shock, when the blood flow to the liver is minimal, assuming that the liver was normal before the shock was induced. There will still be enough flow and enough hepatic reserve for oxidation of the lactic acid. Lactate should not be used, however, if the patient has severe preexisting liver disease.

If the arterial pH is not likely to be excessively low, there is probably no advantage in using lactate or any buffer in the resuscitative fluids. In fact, experiments in animals suggest that there might some advantage in avoiding buffers altogether and using chloride exclusively as the anion in the resuscitative fluid. A modest hyperchloremic acidemia in the immediate postresuscitative state might favorably affect the confirmation of albumen molecules, to decrease some of the permeability produced by the shock, and might favorably affect cardiac function.

The rate at which the initial crystalloid resuscitation should be given depends on the severity of the shock. In an adult patient in severe shock, 2 L is given as fast as possible, followed by a third liter infused over 10 minutes. This amount of fluid will resuscitate most patients in whom hemorrhage has been arrested. Incomplete resuscitation indicates continued bleeding. The patient might need operative control of hemorrhage.

There is no general agreement about how much fluid should be given after the initial 3 L, especially in the patient who might be continuing to bleed. Giving excessive amounts of fluid, in an effort to restore the blood pressure to normal or supranormal levels, can increase the blood loss. It can create edema in wounded tissues, which can hinder wound healing and the ability to fight off infection, by widening the distance between the capillaries in the edematous tissue. Edema in the gut can create an abdominal compartment syndrome, with compression of the inferior vena cava, displacement of the diaphragm into the chest, and compression of the heart and lungs. Edema in the lungs can hinder ventilation and oxygenation. On the other hand, inadequate resuscitation can leave the patient exposed to the many adverse late effects of prolonged shock, such as multiorgan failure.

The primary goal in fluid resuscitation for all forms of shock is the same; namely, restoration of perfusion to the end organs: Circulation to the skin, urine output, acid-base balance, mental status, and myocardial perfusion should all be brought back to the point where there are no observable abnormalities. The blood pressure has to be high enough to ensure a cushion of perfusion for the brain and the heart and any organ that might have obstruction in its nutrient circulation, like kidneys with atherosclerosis in the renal arteries, or the spinal cord in a patient with a thoracoabdominal aneurysm, or the extremities in a patient with peripheral arterial disease. In many patients, however, pressure less that what is usually thought to be normal will be enough to achieve the primary goal of restoration of perfusion to the end organs at risk. Resuscitation does not necessarily have to generate a normal blood pressure in all patients.

Our current goal for fluid therapy in the initial management of shock is to achieve a brachial systolic blood pressure of 90 mm Hg or more, assuming that the causes of the shock, like bleeding, are being rapidly corrected. If the patient can be monitored in an intensive care unit (ICU), the goals for the pressure become more flexible. In most cases, the pressure will usually come up to normal levels on its own accord, assuming that the underlying cause of the shock has been treated. In some cases it will not, especially if the patient begins to develop a systemic inflammatory state. In those cases, a lower pressure can be preferable. See the following sections on inflammatory shock.

C. Blood

Bleeding patients will often need blood, but, if possible, tranfusions should be withheld until the bleeding is controlled. Bank blood administered during continuing hemorrhage can end up in the suction canisters in the operating room, depleting the supply of blood that might be needed later on. If blood has to be given and it there is no time for a full crossmatch, type-specific non-crossmatched cells, which can usually be obtained within 10 minutes, are used. The risk of a transfusion reaction is negligible compared with the risks of inadequate oxygen delivery to the tissues. If type-specific cells are not available, Rh-negative type O cells reconstituted in normal saline are used. Rh-negative universal donor cells are also indicated in treating mass casualties, to minimize the chance of giving the wrong type of blood to a misidentified patient.

The number of red blood cells to be transfused depends primarily on the heart, a working muscle that even under nonstressed conditions uses most of the oxygen delivered to it by the coronary arteries. In shock, the heart will extract even a larger proportion of the delivered oxygen. Wounds will heal with hematocrits as low as 15%, and the other organs of the body can survive with quite low hematocrit levels. The stressed heart cannot.

The decision to transfuse and the magnitude of the transfusion can also depend on the status of the lungs. The level of oxygenation of the systemic arterial blood in a patient with pulmonary dysfunction will fall with a low hematocrit. Markedly desaturated mixed venous blood, which will be a consequence of a low hematocrit, when shunted through lungs with damaged parenchyma will contribute to desaturation of the blood entering the left atrium. At times it is necessary to transfuse in order to treat the arterial desaturation to decrease the inspired oxygen concentration, or to turn down the pressure settings on the ventilator.

At the same time, unnecessary use of bank blood wastes a limited community resource, and excessively high hematocrits, in some patients, can be harmful. The few trials that have randomized patients into a low-hematocrit arm versus a high-hematocrit arm have generally found that the lower hematocrits (with certain limits) have tended to be associated with better survival. Increased viscosity can limit perfusion of the microvasculature of metabolizing tissues, including wounds and areas of infection, especially in the face of low flow rates. Hyperviscosity can limit microvascular flow to the skin, making it difficult for the body to regulate its core temperature. And hyperviscosity could possibly contribute to turbulence at arterial branching points, leading to a loss in energy that could be used for flow in the microvasculature.

The goal for the hematocrit when resuscitating with blood, or the hematocrit value that should trigger transfusion, depends on several factors. A patient with coronary blood flow limited by atherosclerotic plaque needs to have a higher hematocrit than one with normal coronary arteries. A higher hematocrit is safer if the patient cannot be monitored in an ICU. And some patients are more likely to bleed than others. They need to have a cushion.

A hematocrit of 18% might be adequate in a patient in an ICU who is unlikely to bleed and who has no coronary disease. A hematocrit of 39% could conceivably be wise in a patient with active coronary disease who has a condition associated with a high likelihood of bleeding and who is being cared for in a busy emergency room. Table 12–1 lists hematocrit values that can be used as triggers depending on some of these factors. We do not intend that these values be taken literally. They should only be used to initiate thinking about when blood should be given.

D. Modalities to Be Avoided

Albumin-containing solutions should not be used in the initial resuscitation of patients in hypovolemic shock. Shock is associated with a generalized increase in microvascular permeability, which results in extravasation of protein, including administered protein, into the interstitial space. The protein in the interstitium can only be returned to the blood volume via the lym-

Table 12–1. Hemocrit triggers for transfusion: Influence of coronary artery disease (CAD), environment in which the patient is being treated (emergency department versus intensive care unit), and likelihood of bleeding.

Coronary Artery Disease	Environment	Likelihood of Bleeding	Desired Hematocrit
No	ICU	Unlikely	18%
No	ICU	Possible	21%
No	ED	Unlikely	24%
No	ED	Possible	27%
Yes	ICU	Unlikely	30%
Yes	ICU	Possible	33%
Yes	ED	Unlikely	36%

phatics, which have limited flow capabilities. Mobilization of this edema can take hours or even days. The protein-poor edema produced by crystalloid resuscitation does not rely on lymphatic drainage and is much easier to mobilize.

Vasopressors should not be used in resuscitating neurologically intact hypovolemic patients, except in desperate situations, while the vascular volume is being reexpanded. And even under those circumstances, the pressors should only be used for a matter of minutes. The idea that vasopressors divert flow from nonessential organs to essential organs is ill-conceived. Although some organs can withstand ischemia for longer periods of time than others, there are very few parts of the body that are not essential. Use of vasopressors for periods longer than 1 hour in the hypovolemic patient can lead to necrosis of the skin in the extremities (and major amputations), necrosis of the gut, and necrosis of the kidneys. (Vasopressors, however, are often indicated in patients in neurogenic shock, but those patients have lost critical physiological compensatory responses; see below.)

Elevation of the lower extremities above the level of the heart (Trendelenburg's position) in a normovolemic subject shifts blood to the heart and increases ventricular end-diastolic volumes. In the hypovolemic patient, however, adrenergically mediated venoconstriction will already have achieved this shift. Thus the position is of no value in treating hypovolemic shock, and its awkwardness can make evaluation and treatment of other problems more complicated. The position, however, is useful for the treatment of neurogenic shock. See below.

In trauma patients, the pneumatic antishock garment can be useful for temporary compression of bleeding sites that cannot be controlled by other means, for temporary stabilization of pelvic fractures, and as a temporary expedient to increase the blood pressure during transport in patients in neurogenic shock. The garment is of no use for displacing blood from the periphery to the heart in neurologically intact patients. Discharge of the adrenergic system will already have achieved that goal. Furthermore, the garment can be harmful. It can hinder filling of the ventricles by compressing the inferior vena cava and the renal and hepatic veins. It can hinder left ventricular ejection by compressing the arterioles in the lower body. It can push the diaphragm into the chest and interfere with ventilation. It limits the physical examination, and it precludes use of the veins in the lower part of the body as sites for venous access.

CARDIAC COMPRESSIVE SHOCK

Diagnosis

Cardiac compressive shock can arise from any condition that compresses the heart or great veins, including pericardial tamponade; tension pneumothorax; hemothorax; rupture of the diaphragm with encroachment of abdominal viscera into the chest; and distention of the abdomen with compression of the intra-abdominal great veins and elevation of the diaphragm into the chest. All of these conditions are worsened if the patient has to be mechanically ventilated.

The signs of compressive shock are similar to those of hypovolemic shock—postural hypotension, poor cutaneous perfusion, oliguria, hypotension, mental status changes, electrocardiographic signs of myocardial ischemia, metabolic acidemia, and hyperventilation—combined with distended neck veins. The only other type of shock that can produce the combination of poor perfusion associated with distended neck veins is cardiogenic shock, which rarely poses a problem in differential diagnosis. Cardiogenic shock usually develops against a background of evident disease that predisposes to primary myocardial dysfunction (see Cardiogenic Shock, below). Cardiac compression usually follows trauma or occurs in a setting where mechanical compromise of the heart or great veins is a recognized possibility.

The so-called paradoxic pulse is occasionally helpful in diagnosis. A spontaneous breath in a normovolemic subject without cardiac compression produces little effect on systemic blood pressure. If the heart is compressed, the systolic pressure can fall by more than 10 mm Hg. (In contrast, a fall in the blood pressure with positive-pressure ventilation is common and nonspecific, especially in hypovolemic patients; the concept of a paradoxic pulse only applies to patients who are breathing on their own.)

The diagnosis of cardiac compression is facilitated if the patient can be monitored in an ICU with a Swan-Ganz catheter (see Diagnosis of Pulmonary Failure in Surgical Patients), where small stroke volumes in the face of high filling pressures can be documented by direct measurement. In addition, the catheter can be used to compare pressures in the left and right atria. Under normal circumstances, the pressure in the left atrium is about 5 mm Hg higher than in the right. In tamponade, the pressures are identical.

Treatment

Infusion of fluid can transiently overcome some of the ill effects of cardiac compression, but the cause of shock in these patients is mechanical, and definitive treatment must correct the mechanical abnormality. Pericardial tamponade, tension pneumothorax, massive hemothorax, intra-abdominal bleeding, and ruptured diaphragm are discussed in Chapter 13 and bowel obstruction in Chapter 29. Treatment of compressive shock caused by large-volume, high-pressure mechanical ventilation is discussed later in this chapter in the section on mechanical ventilation.

CARDIOGENIC SHOCK

Diagnosis

Cardiogenic shock can arise from several causes including arrhythmias, ischemia-induced myocardial failure, valvular or septal defects, systemic or pulmonary hypertension, myocarditis, and myocardiopathies. Of all the forms of shock, it can be the most resistant to treatment. If the heart cannot pump, there may be nothing that can be done. On the other hand, in less severe cases, it is possible to improve the efficiency of the pumping capability that remains.

The diagnosis of cardiogenic shock usually depends on recognizing an underlying medical condition predisposing the heart to dysfunction in conjunction with an abnormal ECG. The shock is frequently associated with distended neck veins, unless the patient also happens to be hypovolemic, as in a bleeding patient with a recent myocardial infarction. It can also be associated with peripheral edema, an enlarged and tender liver, an enlarged heart on physical examination or x-ray, a third heart sound, rales or x-ray evidence of pulmonary edema, and electrocardiographic signs of ischemia. The diagnosis is usually easy, but two common situations may pose a problem.

The first is a ruptured abdominal aortic aneurysm in a patient with coronary artery disease. The patient might have abdominal pain consistent with a myocardial infarction and electrocardiographic signs of ischemia—the ischemia being caused by hypovolemia and shock. The key is to observe the neck veins.

The second is to ascribe shock to myocardial contusion in a patient who has just suffered a blunt injury to the chest. Although blunt chest trauma can damage the heart, the damage is usually either fatal, with death at the scene of the injury, or, far more often, of no clinical significance. A contusion that produces failure but not death is rare. Shock after blunt trauma in a patient who survives to reach the hospital is almost never caused by contusion—it is far more likely to be caused by hypovolemia or cardiac compression.

Treatment

A. Arrhythmias

In general, hypotension in a patient with a heart rate less than 50 beats/min deserves treatment, even if the ventricular contractions are well coordinated. Treatment begins with the intravenous administration of atropine, at a dose of 0.5 mg, repeated at 2-minute intervals as needed. If the rate remains slow and the patient remains unstable, the heart should be paced, by transvenous or external means.

Too-rapid heart rates also have to be treated, especially if the contractions are dyscoordinated. Short times during diastole limit filling of the ventricles and limit the time for perfusion of the myocardium. The upper limits of the heart rate depend on the patient's age and underlying cardiac status. In a subject with no underlying cardiac disease, the heart rate should not exceed 0.8 multiplied by 220 minus the patient's age in years. In a patient with a compromised heart, a heart rate that exceeds 100 may be too rapid. In some cases the rate might be sinus in origin, but in life-threatening cases, the rapid rates are usually associated with arrhythmias. Treatment of these arrhythmias should follow the guidelines described by Ursic and Harken. The approach depends on the hemodynamic effects of the arrhythmia.

Moribund patients should be cardioverted. The cardioversion takes precedence over securing the airway, and it takes precedence over obtaining vascular access; it even takes precedence over making a precise diagnosis of the arrhythmia. If the patient is near death, the treatment is shock. One hundred joules should be used initially. If unsuccessful, the energy should be rapidly escalated to 360 J.

Cardioversion will be of no value in patients in asystole or with a fine ventricular fibrillation, but successful resuscitation to full neurologic functioning of patients with these arrhythmias is rare. The goal is to get the heart pumping effectively as quickly as possible in those patients who have some hope for recovery, such as those with coarse ventricular fibrillation, ventricular tachycardia, and supraventricular arrhythmias with unsustainably rapid ventricular responses. Cardioversion can be successful in all of these cases.

The nonmoribund patient with a tachyarrhythmia associated with abnormal ventricular conduction should also be cardioverted. If the tachyarrhythmia is associated with normal ventricular conduction—that is, if the patient has a supraventricular tachycardia—the treatment is calcium-channel blockade. Verapamil is a good choice, in an initial dose of 10 mg, followed as needed with a drip at 1 mg/min until the rate slows.

In summary, all critical patients with a tachyarrhythmia should be cardioverted, with the exception of the more stable patient with a supraventricular tachycardia, who should receive a calcium-channel blocker. The simplicity of this approach translates into the possibility of rapid reestablishment of normal blood flow to the brain, which cannot be achieved with chest compressions but which can be achieved with a beating heart. The result of quickly reestablishing a beating heart can be a patient who survives with intact neurologic function.

This approach will suffice as initial treatment for all of the potentially salvageable life-threatening arrhythmias in the surgical patient, but treatment becomes more complicated once the original arrhythmia has been dealt with. This topic—maintenance of an acceptable rhythm after initial resuscitation—has to be left to other textbooks.

B. Opioids

Opioids can be especially effective in treating cardiac failure after myocardial infarction. They relieve pain, provide sedation, block adrenergic discharge to the arterioles, block discharge to the venules and small veins, redistribute the blood from the atria and ventricles to the venous capacitance vessels in the periphery, and decrease myocardial oxygen requirements.

C. Diuretics

Diuretics are the keystone of therapy in congestive heart failure with large ventricular end-diastolic volumes. By decreasing vascular volume, diuretics decrease atrial pressures and mobilize peripheral and pulmonary edema. Pulmonary vascular pressures and volumes decrease; effectiveness of right ventricular contraction increases. Coronary blood flow increases as coronary sinus pressure drops. Decreasing pressures in the ventricles during diastole alleviates compression of the coronary vasculature in the endocardium, when the ventricular muscle receives its nutrient blood flow. And decreasing pressures in the right atrium decreases the stiffness of the coronary vasculature, which decreases the stiffness of the ventricles during diastole (the garden hose effect). The ventricular end-diastolic volumes potentially can increase without much of an associated increase in the end-diastolic pressures.

D. Beta-Blockers

Almost all patients in cardiac failure with ischemia and a rapid heart rate will benefit from a beta-adrenergic blocking agent (eg, esmolol or metoprolol). Decreasing the rate and reducing ventricular stiffness during systole decreases myocardial oxygen requirements. Increasing time in diastole and decreasing ventricular stiffness during diastole augments ventricular filling and increases efficiency of ventricular contraction. All of these effects reduce myocardial oxygen consumption and potentially salvage marginal myocardium. In many patients, the reduced oxygen requirements can be achieved with only minimal loss of energy output from the ventricles. The only contraindication to the use of beta-blockers, beyond the rare development of bronchospasm with administration of the drugs, is hypotension. This latter problem is easily monitored.

E. Vasodilators

Hypertension is unusual but not unheard of in patients with cardiogenic shock. The hypertension is usually associated with inefficient delivery of energy into the aortic root. Treatment should begin with opioids, if the patient is in pain, and then diuresis, if the ventricular end-diastolic volumes are large, and then beta-blockade, if the heart rate is rapid. Vasodilation is the next step. The most useful vasodilators in surgical patients with cardiac failure are morphine, nitroprusside, and nitroglycerin, all of which are either easily reversible or short-acting. All of these agents dilate the systemic arterioles; nitroglycerin and morphine also dilate the systemic venules and small veins.

The drugs can have many beneficial effects. Edema can be mobilized. Atrial and ventricular diastolic volumes and pressures can be decreased. Perfusion of the myocardium can be increased. Myocardial work and oxygen consumption can decrease. Ischemia can be reversed. On the other hand, excessive venous dilation can decrease cardiac filling enough so that stroke volumes and blood pressures fall; excessive arteriolar dilation can make the pressure fall further.

The drugs can be used initially without invasive monitoring. They are usually used in patients with high mean systemic arterial pressures but can occasionally be used (with caution) in patients with normal arterial pressures as long as the blood pressure is adequate for perfusion of the brain and heart and organs with potentially obstructed nutrient arteries. The patient should be monitored for chest pain and electrocardiographic evidence of myocardial ischemia while the drugs are being given. If it seems that the drugs are going to be necessary for more than an hour or two, a Swan-Ganz catheter should be inserted.

F. Inotropic Agents

Administration of inotropic agents, such as dobutamine or milrinone, can increase cardiac output in selected patients in cardiogenic shock, but not all. The agents will usually not increase the pressure. They almost always result in increased myocardial oxygen requirements, and the patients receiving the drugs need to be monitored in an ICU. Development of chest pain or ischemic changes in the electrocardiogram suggests that oxygen demand is exceeding supply. If it is necessary to use inotropic agents for more than 1 hour, a Swan-Ganz catheter should be inserted. Systemic arterial pressures, atrial filling pressures, and cardiac outputs should be determined at different infusion rates. If any question remains about the adequacy of volume resuscitation, cardiovascular parameters should be measured before and after a fluid bolus is given.

Digitalis compounds should not be used in acute cardiac failure except to control ventricular rates in patients with supraventricular tachydysrhythmias. Toxicity may develop, especially when pH and electrolyte changes are unpredictable. The inotropic actions of digitalis are no different from those of dopamine and milrinone.

G. Chronotropic Agents

Patients in cardiac failure with a heart rate in the 60s may on a rare occasion temporarily benefit from administration of a chronotropic agent, such as dopamine. (Isoproterenol is almost never used nowadays.) If dopamine is to be used, the heart rate should only be increased to levels that can be tolerated comfortably. A 60-year-old patient with normal coronary arteries gains little with a heart rate that exceeds 120/min; the limit is about 90/min in the presence of coronary artery disease. In most cases, however, the price to be paid for using a chronotropic agent exceeds the potential benefit. Chronotropic agents increase myocardial work and oxygen requirements and shorten the time during diastole for coronary blood flow and ventricular filling. They should only be used as a temporary expedient. If they are used for more than 30 minutes, a Swan-Ganz catheter should be inserted. The goal of therapy is a normal or slightly supranormal cardiac output. Trying to achieve more than that only increases the risk of myocardial ischemia.

H. Vasoconstrictors

Vasoconstrictors are occasionally useful to increase perfusion pressures for a heart supplied by arteries that are blocked proximally by pathologic processes. On the negative side, the constrictors will increase myocardial oxygen requirements. To be effective, the vasoconstrictors have to increase the aortic pressure enough so that the increased perfusion of the myocardium makes up for the increase in the myocardial oxygen requirements.

Vasoconstrictor use can result in necrosis of organs in the periphery, like the extremities or the gut. They will not increase perfusion to the brain, assuming that the carotid arteries are open and that the patient has a functioning adrenergic nervous system. The endogenous adrenergic nervous system is ideally suited for ensuring adequate blood flow to the brain. The baroreceptors are not placed in the carotid bifurcations by accident. Constrictors should be used only when absolutely necessary and for no more than 60 minutes unless a pulmonary arterial catheter is in place.

I. Transaortic Balloon Pump

The transaortic balloon pump decreases the hindrance that the left ventricle faces when it ejects its blood into the aortic root and can be very effective in resuscitating selected patients with severe reversible left ventricular dysfunction (eg, after cardiopulmonary bypass or acute myocardial infarction). It should only be used if a Swan-Ganz catheter is in place.

J. Extracorporeal Membrane Oxygenation

Extracorporeal membrane oxygenation is most often used in conditions in which one can expect cardiac function to recover within a matter of a few days. Bleeding complications make it impractical for periods exceeding that time.

K. Operative Correction

Although listed last, an operation is sometimes the best early approach. Ruptured valves, occluded arteries, aneurysmal ventricular walls, and certain arrhythmias can potentially be returned to normal with a surgical approach. A surgical solution should not always be the last to be tried. Persisting with a nonsurgical approach can convert a potentially curable problem into one that is hopeless.

NEUROGENIC SHOCK

Diagnosis

Shock caused by failure of the autonomic nervous system can arise from regional or general anesthetics, injuries to the spinal cord, or administration of autonomic blocking agents. The venules and small veins lose tone, worsened by paralysis of surrounding skeletal muscles. Blood pools in the periphery, ventricular end-diastolic volumes decrease, and stroke volumes and blood pressure fall. Loss of arteriolar tone in the denervated areas makes the pressure fall further. If the lesion is below the midthoracic sympathetic outflow, activation of the cardiac adrenergic nerves will increase the heart rate and augment ventricular systolic function; if the lesion is more cephalad, the heart will not be able to compensate. Cardiovascular decompensation in neurogenic shock can be profound.

The diagnosis rests on knowledge of the circumstances preceding the onset of shock and on the physical examination. The patient will always be hypotensive, and the skin will be warm and flushed in the denervated areas. The cause is usually obvious.

Nonfatal head injury—as opposed to spinal cord injury—does not produce neurogenic shock or any other kind of shock. In fact, increased intracranial pressure typically increases blood pressure and slows the heart rate (Cushing reflex). Hypotension and tachycardia should never be attributed to head injury—even severe head injury with cerebral dysfunction—until concomitant hypovolemia has been ruled out. It is a tragedy to ascribe shock to a head injury when the problem is bleeding from a ruptured spleen.

Treatment

Trendelenburg's position, if it does not complicate other aspects of care, is useful. Intravenous fluids, to fill the dilated venules and small veins, should be given. Vasoconstrictors should be used if fluids and Trendelenburg's position are not enough. Norepinephrine and phenylephrine are good choices if the heart rate is rapid; dopamine is a good choice if the heart rate is slow.

The primary purpose of the constrictors is to restore tone in the venules and small veins; a secondary goal is to constrict dilated arterioles. The blood pressure should be increased to the point that coronary perfusion is sustained—as judged by normal ST–T segments on electrocardiography and absence of chest pain—and to the point that perfusion to the brain and spinal cord is supported. The pressure also has to be high enough to perfuse organs with preexisting obstructing proximal arterial lesions. If vasoconstrictors are expected to be needed for more than 1 hour, the patient should be placed in an ICU and monitored with a Swan-Ganz catheter.

LOW-OUTPUT INFLAMMATORY SHOCK

Diagnosis

Bowel perforation, necrotic intestine, abscesses, gangrene, and soft tissue infections can produce low-output inflammatory shock, as can inadequate resuscitation of massive injuries or large burns. The cytokinemia arising from the systemic inflammation can disrupt the microvascular endothelium and prompt the loss of plasma into the interstitium. The shock mimics the clinical picture of severe hypovolemic shock, with signs of adrenergic discharge, oliguria, obtundation, and metabolic academia. The ECG may show signs of ischemia. The patient may, or may not, have a fever. Sometimes, the patient will be hypothermic. The diagnosis is usually clear from the clinical circumstances.

Treatment

Treatment consists of administration of intravenous fluids and antibiotics, correction of gastrointestinal leaks, debridement of dead tissue, and drainage of pus. The patient will probably need to be transferred to an ICU. Vasoconstrictors can be given for very short periods of time if the hypotension is so profound that it is threatening the brain, the heart, or an organ with an obstructed arterial supply. Inotropes can be used more liberally, while the vascular volume is being replenished, but even then they should not be given for more than an hour, unless the patient has a Swan-Ganz catheter in place. The purpose of the volume expansion is to convert the low-output inflammatory shock into a high-output state.

HIGH-OUTPUT INFLAMMATORY SHOCK

Diagnosis

High-output inflammatory shock can precede low-output inflammatory shock or can be the result of successful treatment of low-output shock. The shock usually, but not always, is associated with a fever. The patient is hypotensive with warm, well-perfused extremities, as the body attempts to control its core temperature by offloading heat to the environment. If a pulmonary arterial catheter is placed, the cardiac output will be found to be high, assuming that the ventricular end-diastolic volumes have been brought back to normal levels. The outputs will remain high, occasionally as high as twice normal, as long as the inflammatory state persists. The oxygen consumption may be increased by a factor of 1.5.

Treatment

Treatment consists of control of the underlying cause and fluid administration. Inotropes may be useful. If large amounts of fluids seem to be necessary for the resuscitation and if inotropes are being considered, a Swan-Ganz catheter should be inserted. The goal is to perfuse the inflamed tissues with adequate power so that the product of the cardiac output and the mean arterial pressure is normal. In many patients, the result will be a cardiac output that is increased by a factor of 1.5 with a blood pressure that is decreased to a value that is two-thirds of normal. As in other forms of shock, the pressure has to be high enough to perfuse the heart and brain and organs with potentially obstructed arteries, but it does not have to be normal. Vasoconstrictors can be dangerous, especially if there is any degree of hypovolemia, potentially leading to necrosis of the limbs, the gut, and the kidneys. They should not be used unless the clinician is positive that both the right and left ventricular end-diastolic volumes are normally expanded.

Bernard GR et al: Efficacy and safety of recombinant human activated protein C for severe sepsis. N Engl J Med 2001;344:699.

Carson JL et al: Mortality and morbidity in patients with very low postoperative Hb levels who decline blood transfusion. Transfusion 2002;42:812.

Chang MC et al: Maintaining survivors' values of left ventricular power output during shock resuscitation: a prospective pilot study. J Trauma 2000;49:26; discussion 34.

Chang MC et al: Redefining cardiovascular performance during resuscitation: ventricular stroke work, power, and the pressure-volume diagram. J Trauma 1998;45:470.

Chang MC et al: Effects of abdominal decompression on cardiopulmonary function and visceral perfusion in patients with intra-abdominal hypertension. J Trauma 1998;44:440.

Ciesla DJ et al: Hypertonic saline attenuation of polymorphonuclear neutrophil cytotoxicity: timing is everything. J Trauma 2000;48:388.

Demetriades D et al: Relative bradycardia in patients with traumatic hypotension. J Trauma 1998;45:534.

Diebel LN, Tyburski JG, Dulchavsky SA: Effect of acute hemodilution on intestinal perfusion and intramucosal pH after shock. J Trauma 2000;49:800.

Fleisher LA, Eagle KA: Clinical practice. Lowering cardiac risk in noncardiac surgery. N Engl J Med. 2001;345:1677.

Forsythe SM, Schmidt GA: Sodium bicarbonate for the treatment of lactic acidosis. Chest 2000;117:260.

Gattinoni L et al: A trial of goal-oriented hemodynamic therapy in critically ill patients. SvO_2 Collaborative Group. N Engl J Med 1995;333:1025.

Gore DC et al: Influence of glucose kinetics on plasma lactate concentration and energy expenditure in severely burned patients. J Trauma 2000;49:673; discussion 677.

Hébert PC et al: A multicenter, randomized, controlled clinical trial of transfusion requirements in critical care. Transfusion Requirements in Critical Care Investigators, Canadian Critical Care Trials Group. N Engl J Med 1999;340:409.

Heughan C, Grislis G, Hunt TK: The effect of anemia on wound healing. Ann Surg 1974;179:163.

Ho HS et al: Hypertonic perfusion inhibits intracellular Na and Ca accumulation in hypoxic myocardium. Am J Physiol Cell Physiol 2000;278:C953.

Human albumin administration in critically ill patients: systematic review of randomised controlled trials. Cochrane Injuries Group Albumin Reviewers. BMJ 1998;317:235.

Jonsson K et al: Tissue oxygenation, anemia, and perfusion in relation to wound healing in surgical patients. Ann Surg 1991;214:605.

Kraut EJ et al: Right ventricular volumes overestimate left ventricular preload in critically ill patients. J Trauma 1997;42:839; discussion 845.

Miller PR, Meredith JW, Chang MC: Randomized, prospective comparison of increased preload versus inotropes in the resuscitation of trauma patients: effects on cardiopulmonary function and visceral perfusion. J Trauma 1998;44:107.

Perdue PW et al: "Renal dose" dopamine in surgical patients: dogma or science? Ann Surg 1998;227:470.

Sibbald WJ et al: The Trendelenburg position: hemodynamic effects in hypotensive and normotensive patients. Crit Care Med 1979;7:218.

Ursic C, Harken AH: Critical care: Acute cardiac dysrhythmia. *ACS Surgery: Principles & Practice,* pp. 1052–1065. WebMed Inc., 2004.

Velmahos GC et al: Endpoints of resuscitation of critically injured patients: normal or supranormal? A prospective randomized trial. Ann Surg 2000;232:409.

Victorino GP, Battistella FD, Wisner DH: Does tachycardia correlate with hypotension after trauma? J Am Coll Surg 2003;196:679.

Wade CE et al: Individual patient cohort analysis of the efficacy of hypertonic saline/dextran in patients with traumatic brain injury and hypotension. J Trauma 1997;42(5 Suppl):S61.

II. INITIAL TREATMENT OF ACUTE PULMONARY FAILURE

DIAGNOSIS OF PULMONARY FAILURE IN SURGICAL PATIENTS

Most causes of severe pulmonary failure in the surgical patient can be ascribed to one or more of nine causes: the acute respiratory distress syndrome, inability to effectively expand the lungs because of mechanical abnormalities, atelectasis, aspiration, pulmonary contusion, pneumonia, pulmonary embolus, cardiogenic pulmonary edema, and, rarely, neurogenic pulmonary edema.

The **acute respiratory distress syndrome** (ARDS) typically follows shock and either trauma or sepsis. Activated coagulation and inflammation in the injured or infected tissues release coagulative and inflammatory mediators into the circulation. The lungs bear at least some of the brunt of the activated mediators because they receive all the venous blood that returns to the heart. If the injured or infected tissues are in the nonsplanchnic portions of the body, the lungs are even further at risk because they contain the first microvasculature that the mediators will encounter. (In the case of injury or infection in the splanchnic viscera, the liver bears the initial brunt of the insult.) The mediators disrupt the microvascular endothelium, and plasma extravasates into the interstitium and, in the case of the lungs, into the alveoli. The resultant pulmonary edema impairs both ventilation and oxygenation; the embolization to the lungs impairs perfusion. Arterial oxygen saturation decreases and carbon dioxide content increases—assuming that no compensatory mechanisms come into play.

A number of different mediators of coagulation and inflammation have been implicated as causes of the increased permeability. Proteases, kinins, complement, oxygen radicals, prostaglandins, thromboxanes, leukotrienes, lysosomal enzymes, and other mediators are released from aggregates of platelets and white cells or from the endothelium or plasma as a consequence of the interaction between the aggregates and the vessel wall. Some of these substances are chemoattractants of more platelets and white blood cells, and a vicious cycle of inflammation develops that worsens the disruption of the vascular endothelium. Infection, disease, injury, and ischemia in nonpulmonary tissues thus lead to damage and dysfunction in previously healthy pulmonary tissues.

The diagnosis is made by the development of hypoxemia approximately 24 hours after resuscitation from shock and either trauma or sepsis in the absence of other common causes of hypoxemia under these conditions—mechanical failure, atelectasis, aspiration, and pulmonary contusion. The chest x-ray usually shows a diffuse infiltrate. The lungs develop a nonspecific inflammatory reaction. Monocytes and neutrophils invade the interstitium. Edema appears within a few hours, alveolar flooding is florid within 1 day, and scar tissue begins to form within a week. If the process is unchecked, the lungs become sodden and resemble liver tissue on gross inspection; scar tissue appears within a week and function-limiting fibrosis begins to develop within 2 weeks. If early treatment is effective, the lungs return to normal, both grossly and microscopically. The process of diagnosis and the pathologic features of ARDS are identical to those of the so-called **fat embolism syndrome,** which is, for practical purposes, merely a special case of ARDS in which the release of marrow fat into the blood contributes to the development of pulmonary microvascular damage. Nothing is gained by making a distinction between the two entities.

Mechanical failure can arise from chest wall trauma, pain and weakness after surgery and anesthesia, debility caused by the catabolic metabolism of long-term illness, or bronchopleural fistula. Massive trauma to the chest with multiple fractures of multiple ribs or bilateral disruption of the costochondral junctions can result in a free-floating segment of chest wall known as a **flail chest:** Expansion and relaxation of the rest of the chest wall with spontaneous breathing results in paradoxic motion of the free segment in response to changes in intrathoracic pressure; ventilation becomes compromised; and the arterial P_{CO_2} increases. Lesser degrees of chest wall injury can lead to hypoventilation because of pain associated with breathing. Prolonged mechanical ventilation with loss of muscle mass and power in the diaphragm and the accessory muscles of respiration can require ventilatory support until muscle function returns to normal. A bronchopleural fistula—a communication from the airway to the pleural cavity to the atmosphere, either through a chest tube or through a hole in the chest wall—can develop after pulmonary surgery, trauma, or infection. Large air leaks can compromise ventilation to the uninvolved lung as well as to the diseased side because insufflated air preferentially goes to the side with the fistula.

Atelectasis—localized collapse of alveoli—can develop with prolonged immobilization, as during anesthesia or in association with bed rest. The problem is usually full-blown within a few hours after the initiating event. Only mechanical failure (to which it is related), aspiration, cardiogenic pulmonary edema, and pulmonary embolism can produce equivalent levels of hypoxemia so soon. The diagnosis is supported by auscultation of bronchial breath sounds at dependent portions of the lung and occasionally, if severe enough, by x-ray confirmation of plate-like collapse of pulmonary parenchyma. The most reliable confirmation of the diagnosis, however, comes with response to therapy, which can include encouragement of deep breathing and coughing, ambulation, bronchoscopy, and intubation and mechanical ventilation. Atelectasis should respond within a few hours. No other form of pulmonary insufficiency responds as quickly.

Aspiration of gastric contents or blood can occur in any patient who cannot protect the airway, eg, one who has just been injured or anesthetized or who is debilitated or obtunded for any reason. Gastric acid or particulate matter in the airways leads to disruption of the alveolar and microvascular membranes, causing interstitial and alveolar edema. The resultant hypoxemia is usually evident within a few hours and is associated with a localized infiltrate on x-ray. Recovery of gastric contents by suctioning from the endotracheal tree confirms the diagnosis.

Pulmonary contusion arises from direct trauma to the chest wall and the underlying lung parenchyma. Hypoxemia associated with a localized infiltrate on x-ray develops over 24 hours as the injured lung becomes edematous.

Pneumonia can arise primarily or can be superimposed on aspiration, pulmonary contusion, or ARDS. Generally, the diagnosis is made by recovery of bacteria and purulent material from the endotracheal tree, hypoxemia, signs of systemic sepsis, and a localized infiltrate on x-ray. Recently, there has been interest in a Clinical Pulmonary Infection Score (CPIS) derived from these parameters. The CPIS provides a quantitative value that aids in accurate diagnosis of pneumonia. Diagnosis of the CPIS bronchoscopy, with bronchoalveolar lavage and culture, may be a useful adjunct to distinguish pneumonia from ARDS.

Pulmonary embolism typically presents with sudden deterioration of pulmonary function 3 days or more after an event—such as an operation, injury, or the beginning of immobilization—that can stimulate deposition of clot in a large systemic vein. (See also Chapter 37.) Patients with cancer are at particularly high risk, and in any patient the greater the magnitude of operation or injury, the greater the chance of venous thrombosis and embolization. The chest film is usually nonspecific. A fairly definite diagnosis can often be made by high-definition computed tomograms of the chest. The study requires transfer to the radiology suite and the use of large amounts of radiographic contrast material. Pulmonary arteriography carries the same risks—transfer to the radiology suite and use of contrast—and requires right-heart catheterization, but it does have advantages. It gives a definitive diagnosis with one test. At the end of the diagnostic study, an indwelling catheter can be placed proximal to the clot and used for infusion of lytic agents. And, if needed, a filter can be placed in the inferior vena at the end of the study, before the patient leaves the angiography suite.

Clot emboli must be organized to be clinically significant; embolism to the lung of fresh soft clot rarely causes any difficulty. The pulmonary endothelium contains potent fibrinolysins that can break up any poorly organized embolus. Sudden deterioration in pulmonary function sooner than 3 days after an event that stimulates clot formation is only rarely caused by an embolus; the deterioration is more likely to be caused by mechanical failure, atelectasis, aspiration, or pneumonia.

Cardiogenic pulmonary edema arises from high left atrial and pulmonary microvascular hydrostatic pressures. Patients who have suffered an acute myocardial infarction can present this way, as can patients with underlying myocardial or coronary artery disease when faced with fluid shifts and surgical stress. Occasionally, the rapid administration of intravenous fluid—especially in elderly patients with poor myocardial performance—will outstrip the heart's ability to pump, and pulmonary edema will result. Acute valvular disease, though quite rare after injury or cardiac surgery, is another possible cause of inability of the left heart to pump effectively. The diagnosis is made on the basis of hypoxemia, rales, a third heart sound, perihilar infiltrates, Kerley's lines, and cephalization of blood flow on x-ray along with elevated pulmonary arterial wedge pressures on Swan-Ganz catheterization. A wedge (or left atrial) pressure of 24 mm Hg can produce cardiogenic pulmonary edema even in the presence of an intact endothelium in the pulmonary microvasculature; wedge pressures less than 24 mm Hg will not produce pulmonary edema in and of themselves, but pressures exceeding 16 mm Hg can worsen the edema associated with increased permeability. The goal for the wedge pressure in a patient with uncomplicated cardiogenic pulmonary edema in the absence of an inflammatory process in the lungs should be 20 mm Hg or less; the goal in a patient with an inflammatory process should be 16 or, better, 12 mm Hg.

Neurogenic pulmonary edema is associated both experimentally and clinically with head injury and increased intracranial pressure. The exact mechanism by which this occurs is unknown, but it is probably related to sympathetic discharge with postmicrovascular vasoconstriction in the lungs and a resultant increase in pulmonary microvascular hydrostatic pressure. This form of pulmonary edema and oxygenation defect is rare, and other causes should be considered also in patients with head injury.

INDICATIONS FOR INTUBATION & USE OF MECHANICAL VENTILATION

Intubation of the airway and mechanical ventilation are indicated for treatment of established pulmonary failure, prophylaxis against potential failure, airway protection, and pulmonary toilet. The decision to intubate and initiate mechanical ventilation is usually best made on the basis of clinical criteria. A respiratory rate exceeding 36 breaths/min, labored ventilatory efforts, use of accessory muscles of ventilation, and tachycardia are all indications for intervention, especially if the patient appears to be frightened or anxious. Another indication for intubation and mechanical ventilation is anticipation of treatment that can worsen the pulmonary status, such as fluid resuscitation, manipulation and immobilization of broken bones, or administration of sedatives or narcotics.

Blood gases are not useful in making decisions about intubation and mechanical ventilation in patients in extremis. These patients should be intubated no matter what the gases might show. Blood gases, however, can help in making the decision to intubate and mechanically ventilate in less severely stressed patients. In general, the patient should be intubated if the partial pressure of oxygen, on room air, is less than 60 mm Hg or if the partial pressure of carbon dioxide is greater than 45 mm Hg. But these guidelines should be put in the clinical context. A $PaCO_2$ of 40 mm Hg in a patient breathing 40 times per minute is as alarming as a $PaCO_2$ of 60 mm Hg in a patient with a respiratory rate of 10/min. A PaO_2 of 60 mm Hg on room air in a patient with chronic lung disease may be acceptable; the same value in a patient who is tensing the sternocleidomastoid and intercostal muscles with each breath, making excessive or dyscoordinated use of the abdominal musculature, and who seems to be struggling to draw in enough air, would mandate immediate intubation. A patient with stridor or with maxillofacial trauma or pharyngeal edema may need intubation to maintain the airway. A patient with a severe head injury and depressed mental status may require intubation to protect the airway from aspiration. Intubation may also be indicated for repeated suctioning of the tracheobronchial tree in a patient with a weak gag reflex or inability to cough and clear secretions.

The indications for intubation should be more liberal for a surgical patient than for a medical patient. The medical patient with an exacerbation of chronic obstructive lung disease can be poorly served by placement of a foreign body in his or her trachea. Airway resistance increases, coughing effectiveness decreases, and opportunistic organisms obtain a foothold on and near the tube. Benefit from intubation may be minimal—it is quite possible that the patient may respond to treatment without mechanical ventilation.

Circumstances for the seriously ill surgical patient are usually different. The patient who has multiple injuries, for example, can temporarily tolerate the increased airway resistance, loss of cough, and increased likelihood of tracheobronchial infection. What cannot be tolerated is respiratory arrest during trauma resuscitation. Furthermore, in all likelihood, such patients will eventually require mechanical ventilation anyway. ARDS strikes the lungs 2 days after the injury, not initially. It is safest to secure the airway early; the tube can be removed later if the patient's condition improves faster than expected.

The indications for intubation in the patient with a suspected or known injury to the cervical spine are the same as those in patients with no likelihood of injury. Under no circumstances should concern about the cervical spine lead to procrastination about securing the airway. The consequences of respiratory arrest and anoxic brain damage are as tragic as those of exacerbating a cervical spine injury.

TYPES OF INTUBATION

The trachea can be intubated via the mouth, the nose, the cricothyroid membrane (cricothyroidostomy), or directly (tracheostomy). The tubes used for intubation come with either of two different types of cuffs. Tubes with high-pressure, low-volume cuffs are easy to insert and are useful for short-term intubation and ventilation. The high cuff pressure, however, can interfere with tracheal blood supply and lead to tracheomalacia, erosion into the innominate artery (tracheo-innominate fistula), erosion into the esophagus (tracheoesophageal fistula), or airway stenosis. Tubes with low-pressure, high-volume cuffs are more difficult to insert but should be used for intubation if the intubation is expected to be longer than 24 hours.

Of the four methods available for intubation, the orotracheal route is usually the easiest. Nasotracheal intubation requires the presence of spontaneous ventilation in order to guide tube placement; cricothyroidostomy and tracheostomy require surgical exposure. Orotracheal intubation allows for passage of a larger tube than the nasotracheal route and avoids the problems of sinusitis and necrosis of the nares, which can occur with nasotracheal intubation. On the other hand, nasotracheal intubation can be accomplished in the awake patient without any need for heavy sedation, and some patients seem to find the long-term presence of a nasotracheal tube more comfortable than that of an orotracheal tube. Neither nasotracheal nor orotracheal intubation requires require neck flexion or axial rotation. Either approach can be used in patients with suspected injuries to the cervical spine, assuming that axial traction is maintained during the intubation.

Cricothyroidostomy is indicated when an urgent surgical airway is needed. Extensive maxillofacial trauma can make intubation by the orotracheal or nasotracheal route impossible. Translaryngeal intubation can also be difficult because of poor patient cooperation, altered anatomy, or airway or laryngeal swelling. If the patient is in extremis and respiratory collapse is imminent, attempts at orotracheal or nasotracheal intubation should not be prolonged. As a rule, if transpharyngeal intubation is not successful after one or two attempts, cricothyroidostomy should be done. The cricothyroid membrane in the midline is bounded superiorly by the lower border of the thyroid cartilage. It is located by palpation and is incised by a stab incision. After the hole has been enlarged with the knife handle, a No. 4 or No. 6 tracheostomy tube should be inserted into the trachea. The patient can then be supported with mechanical ventilation and supplemental oxygen as necessary. Cricothyroidostomies maintained for longer than 2 or 3 days may produce glottic and subglottic stenosis; tracheostomies are less likely to do so. Cricothyroidostomies should be converted to tracheostomies as soon as it is safe and practical, assuming that continued intubation is needed.

Tracheostomies have several advantages over translaryngeal intubation: Airway resistance is lower; nursing care is simpler; suctioning is more direct; the tubes do not damage the vocal cords or larynx; and accidental extubation is less serious—a well-established tracheostomy tract can usually be easily reintubated and the patient can usually breathe through the stoma while the tube is being replaced. Tracheostomy is also of benefit when weaning from mechanical ventilation is slow and the patient has been on and off the ventilator a number of times. The presence of a tracheostomy allows for prolonged periods off the ventilator without the requirement for extubation. If the patient develops respiratory distress off the ventilator and a tracheostomy is present, the ventilator can simply be reconnected to the tracheostomy tube.

Translaryngeal intubation, however, has three major advantages over a tracheostomy. First, a tube passed through the larynx can be repositioned, distributing pressure on the tracheal mucosa over a larger area, compared with the balloon on the end of a tracheostomy tube, which is fixed in place. The result is a much lower incidence of late tracheal stenosis and tracheo-innominate artery and tracheoesophageal fistulas, compared with a tracheostomy. Second, because the opening of a translaryngeal tube is well away from the neck and chest, intravenous catheters in these areas can be kept sterile. Third, the cuffs on translaryngeal tubes usually lie in a more axial position in the trachea than those on a tracheostomy tube and are better able to maintain a seal in patients with poor pulmonary compliance and high inspiratory pressures.

The timing of conversion from a translaryngeal intubation to a tracheostomy is controversial. Recommendations as short as 3 days have been made, but large numbers of patients have been intubated for months by the orotracheal or nasotracheal route without serious sequelae. Patients should be converted when airway protection, pulmonary toilet, or any of the other indications outlined above are present. If, in addition, the need for more than 2–3 weeks of intubation is obvious, the threshold for performing tracheostomy should be lowered.

Conversion to tracheostomy should be done as an elective procedure under controlled conditions. A transverse incision overlying the upper trachea is developed by separating the strap muscles of the neck in the midline. Often the thyroid isthmus must be either displaced or divided to allow for adequate exposure of the anterior surface of the trachea. The tracheostomy tube is placed through the second or third tracheal ring.

MODES OF MECHANICAL VENTILATION

Ventilators can be constructed either to deliver a preset volume or a preset pressure during inspiration.

Volume Modes

Volume mode ventilation is most often used today in situations in which the ventilation needs to be kept simple and in which the efforts made by the patient need to be minimized, as in the acutely injured or ill patient. The assist-control mode is the most commonly used mode of volume ventilation. It is designed to assist any ventilatory efforts made by the patient by delivering a machine breath. Whenever the patient begins to inspire, the ventilator is triggered and the preset machine tidal volume is given. A machine backup rate is also set to ensure a minimal number of machine breaths in the absence of spontaneous ventilatory efforts.

The triggers for delivery of an assisted breath can be either pressure-based or flow-based. Most older ventilators use inspiratory pressure as the trigger. The patient initiates a breath, the pressure in the ventilator tubing falls below a preset value, and the ventilator detects this fall in pressure and responds by delivering a breath. The time involved in generating and delivering the breath to the patient, however, can make this form of breathing uncomfortable for the patient. Modern ventilators avoid this problem of triggering by using a "flow-by" circuit. The ventilator delivers a constant flow of air through the ventilator tubing during expiration, usually at a low level of approximately 5 L/min. The ventilator compares the expiratory and inspiratory flow rates. If the patient is making no inspiratory effort, the rates will be the same. If the patient begins to take a breath, the expiratory rate will fall below the inspiratory rate. The ventilator is programmed to trigger a breath when the difference in the flow rates reaches a preset value, usually around 2 L/min, or when the expiratory flow rate falls to 3 L/min. The patient is rewarded with the free flow of at least some air as soon as the effort is initiated. The great majority of patients prefer flow-by over pressure triggering.

Five parameters remain to be determined—the backup ventilatory rate, the tidal volume of the machine-delivered breaths, the time spent in inspiration, the inspired oxygen concentration (FIO_2), and the level of positive end-expiratory pressure (PEEP)—after the decision is made about the type of triggering. The first two of these parameters are the most important in determining ventilation; the latter three are the most important in determining oxygenation.

The minute ventilation—that is, the product of the ventilatory rate and the tidal volume—determines the carbon dioxide levels in the arterial blood, when adjusted for the carbon dioxide production by the body and when adjusted for the amount of dead space ventilation. In most patients, the backup ventilator rate should be set between 12 and 15 breaths per minute. The rate can be increased or decreased as necessary based on the carbon dioxide tension and pH of the arterial blood. The PCO_2 is usually kept close to 40 mm Hg unless hyperventilation is desired, as may be indicated in some in patients with increased intracranial pressure.

Setting the tidal volume dictates how much volume will be delivered with each machine breath. The normal tidal volume during resting spontaneous ventilation is 7 mL/kg ideal body weight. (Fat is metabolically inactive and produces little carbon dioxide; the tidal volume should reflect the mass of actively metabolizing tissues.) Initially, the tidal volume in a ventilated patient should be set at this normal baseline value. Larger tidal volumes associated with higher airway pressures can damage the epithelium lining the small airways and alveoli. If more ventilation is needed, it is preferable to increase the ventilatory rate. If ventilation remains less than normal, as manifested by a persistently elevated $PaCO_2$, it is better to accept the hypercapnia as long as the patient does not have a respiratory acidemia with an arterial pH below 7.20. Hyperexpansion of the alveoli is more damaging to the lungs than hypercapnia is to the body, as long as the pH is acceptable. Either the rate or the tidal volume or both will have to be increased if the patient has a pH less than 7.20. Very high rates or volumes may also be necessary when a bronchopleural fistula is present, to compensate for the volume lost through the fistula.

The time spent in inspiration influences the number of alveoli that become inflated during the breath—the longer the breath, the greater the number of opened alveoli—and thus has a direct influence on the oxygenation. The inspiratory time to expiratory time is usually set in a ratio of 1:2 to 1:3, to give inspiratory times of approximately 1 second. Shorter times during inspiration usually limit filling of the alveoli; longer times can leave too little time for expiration.

The inspired oxygen concentration should be kept high enough so that, in most cases, the oxygen saturation of arterial blood exceeds 92%. Patients with chronic obstructive pulmonary disease and long-standing CO_2 retention are an exception. Such patients have lost the ability to increase their respiratory drive in response to increases in PCO_2 and rely instead on their response to hypoxemia. Increasing the arterial oxygen saturation by adding exogenous oxygen takes away this hypoxic ventilatory stimulus and makes weaning from ventilatory support more difficult. And no patient should have an excessively high inspired oxygen concentration.

All of the nonoxygen volume of ventilator gas is made up of nitrogen, which, unlike oxygen, is not absorbed from alveoli. Nitrogen can be of great value in stenting open the alveoli. When it is replaced by increasing concentrations of oxygen, increased atelectasis caused by oxygen absorption can occur. In addition, high concentrations of oxygen can cause chronic pulmonary fibrosis. Ideally the inspired oxygen concentration should be kept at 50% or less.

Keeping the inspired oxygen levels at acceptably low levels is frequently facilitated by the use of PEEP. The pressure is generated by closure of a valve in the expiratory circuit of the ventilator, to keep the airway pressure above a preset level during expiration and to minimize alveolar collapse. Placement of an endotracheal tube bypasses the normal physiologic PEEP present during spontaneous ventilation from closure of the glottis at the end of expiration. Low levels of "physiologic" PEEP (5 cm H_2O) should probably be used in most intubated patients, and many surgical patients can benefit with higher levels.

Excessively high levels of PEEP, however, can damage the alveolar epithelium, rupture a bronchus with decompression of air under positive pressure into the mediastinum or pleural cavity, and compromise cardiac function. These risks are frequently a problem in medical patients with pulmonary blebs or with preexisting cardiac failure. Surgical patients with the consolidated lungs of ARDS and normal preexisting cardiac function are more protected. At the same time, one has to minimize the risks even in surgical patients.

Damage to the alveolar epithelium and rupture of the bronchi are associated more with peak inspiratory airway pressures than with mean pressures or PEEP and, occasionally, PEEP will decrease the peak inspiratory pressure by expanding atelectatic areas of the lungs. In most cases, however, the PEEP will increase the peak airway pressure by an amount equivalent to the level of the PEEP. As a guideline, the PEEP should never be more than two-thirds of the depth of the chest wall, measured from the spinous processes to the sternum. Levels higher than this are unlikely to be of any benefit in expanding the lungs.

The remaining risk of PEEP, or with any setting on the ventilator that increases the mean airway pressure, is that hyperexpanded lungs can decrease the cardiac output. First, the high pressures can compress the superior and inferior vena cava and the pulmonary veins, compromising diastolic filling of the ventricles (in contrast with a spontaneous inspiration, which augments filling). Second, the high pressures can compress the thin-walled atria and right ventricle, further compromising end-diastolic volumes (again in contrast with a spontaneous inspiration). And third, the high pressures can compress the interalveolar pulmonary microvasculature, making it difficult for the right ventricle to push its blood into and through the pulmonary vasculature. The remedy for the decreased cardiac output, assuming that the mean airway pressures have already been minimized, is usually fluid infusion. The potential problem with this remedy is worsening of the pulmonary failure that prompted the use of the PEEP in the first place. Frequently a balance, or a compromise, has to be struck. Measurements from a Swan-Ganz catheter can be useful in striking this balance.

The main advantage of the volume modes of ventilation is that they are simpler than the pressure modes, which are described below. The main disadvantage is that they limit what the patient can do for himself or herself. In particular, when compared with the pressure support mode, they do not allow for varying times for inspiration and do not allow for sighs.

Pressure Modes

The pressure modes of ventilation are more complicated to use, but they have several advantages over the volume modes, and we preferentially use pressure modes once the patient is in an ICU, where sophisticated monitoring is available.

In **pressure control ventilation,** the medical personnel select the inspiratory pressure and the inspiratory and expiratory times. The inspiratory pressure is kept at a constant level during the entirety of the inspiration by a computer circuit inside the ventilator, which adjusts the inspiratory flow rate to produce the desired pressure. Physiologic inspiratory times and inspiratory/expiratory ratios are usually chosen to make the breaths comfortable for the patient. An inspiratory time of 1 second with an expiratory time of 2 or 3 seconds is typical. Longer inspiratory times with shorter expiratory times (**inverse ratio ventilation**) can be used if the physiologic times prove inadequate to provide enough support. The long inspiratory times, along with the short expiratory times, produce air trapping, which is thought to minimize alveolar collapse and improve the distribution of inspired volume.

If physiologic times are used, the patient can trigger the ventilator to set the ventilatory rate, or a backup rate can be used to ensure adequate minute ventilation. If unphysiologic times are used, the patient will have to be heavily sedated, or even pharmacologically paralyzed. In that case the patient's ventilatory rate will be the same as the machine's rate. In all cases, the tidal volume is determined by the level of the inspired pressure and the inspired time, in conjunction with the resistance of the airways and the compliance of the lungs and chest wall.

Pressure control ventilation can provide adequate ventilation and oxygenation to almost any patient with pulmonary failure, but our preference is to switch the patient over to **pressure support ventilation** as soon as the patient can reliably trigger the ventilator. In this mode, the patient triggers the breath, which is then supported by the ventilator with varying flow rates for as long as the patient makes a substantial inspiratory effort. As in pressure control ventilation, the ventilator adjusts the flow to maintain a constant pressure during the inspiration. The inspiratory time, however, is determined by the interaction of these flows with the patient's own inspiratory efforts. To do this, the ventilator keeps a real-time record of the inspiratory flow rates needed to maintain the pressure during the breath. The flow rate usually reaches a maximum value early in the inspiration and then tapers off as the patient's inspiratory effort decreases. When the flow rate decreases to a predetermined fraction of the maximal flow, the ventilator terminates its support of the breath, and the patient is allowed to exhale. The cutoff value is determined by analog circuits within the ventilator and is usually on the order of 25%, in most ventilators. It cannot be adjusted by the physician, but that is rarely a problem. The great majority of patients are comfortable with a wide range of cutoffs, just as long as they receive the pressure support while they are making their more active inspiratory efforts.

The level of the pressure support is set so that the patient breathes comfortably at a reasonable rate, usually at no more than 24 breaths/min. The goal of the support is to ensure adequate oxygenation and a pH greater than 7.30. The tidal volume generated under these circumstances is usually unimportant. It need only be taken into account if it is thought that the tidal volumes being generated with the pressure support are excessively large or small.

The mode has several advantages. It is usually comfortable for the patient. It overcomes resistance to inspiratory flow in the endotracheal tube and in the ventilatory apparatus and decreases the work of breathing. It makes it impossible for the ventilator to deliver excessively high pressures. The flow is maintained for as long as the patient continues to make an inspiratory effort, so that the mode allows the patient to take sighs at will, minimizing the likelihood of the patient developing atelectasis and achieving this minimization safely, without excessive airway pressure. And it is ideally suited for preparing the patient for weaning and extubation.

The engineering that goes into the pressure modes, however, is more complicated than that which is used for the volume modes, and the engineering of the pressure support mode is more complicated than that for the pressure control mode. The safety of these modes depends on accurate measurements of flow rates, which depend on occasionally erroneous calibration. There is no guarantee that the patient will receive adequate minute ventilation and there is no guarantee that the patient will initiate a breath. To minimize the risk of inadequate ventilation, all ventilators that have pressure mode capabilities have alarms for expired minute ventilation; they also have alarms for apnea. The alarms have to be adjusted properly. These modes of ventilation should not be used unless the personnel taking care of the patient are fully familiar with the equipment and the technique.

Hybrid Modes

For many years, it has been possible with many ventilators to deliver hybrid modes of ventilation, which incorporate features of both volume modes and pressure modes. **Intermittent mandatory ventilation** (IMV) is one such mode. It is designed to overcome the limitations of the assist-control mode. Intermittent machine breaths are delivered at a predetermined rate and—unlike assist-control—are given to the patient regardless of the spontaneous respiratory rate. Between the intermittent mandatory ventilations, however, the patient's spontaneous respiratory efforts are assisted with pressure support breaths. Synchronized intermittent mandatory ventilation (SIMV) is a modification of IMV designed to deliver the preset number of machine breaths in synchrony with some of the patient's own ventilatory efforts, but the principle of spontaneously generated tidal volumes between machine breaths is the same as with IMV.

Intermittent mandatory ventilation requires increased work of breathing by the patient as compared with assist-control, but the rate of machine breaths can be varied to increase or decrease the patient's contribution to ventilation. At very high IMV rates, all ventilation is done by the ventilator, and the patient's contribution is minimal. As the rate is gradually decreased, the patients must increasingly ventilate themselves to maintain minute volume. Incrementally decreasing the IMV rate can be used as a means of weaning from the ventilator. Clinical status, respiratory rate, and the arterial PCO_2 are used to guide the weaning process.

Over the past 5 years, it has become possible to ventilate patients with even more sophisticated hybrid modes. Some ventilators can be set up to deliver constant pressure during the inspiration in such a way that the tidal volume delivered falls in a preset range. Some ventilators can be set up to deliver a preset tidal volume, but without exceeding a preset pressure. Some ventilators can be set up with gradually decreasing ventilatory support, with algorithms built into the system to minimize the need for physician adjustment of the ventilator during weaning. We usually find it unnecessary to use these modes of ventilation, but other clinicians like the added options.

WEANING FROM MECHANICAL VENTILATION

Patients who seem to be doing well and who have required mechanical ventilation for less than 24 hours can frequently be extubated quickly, after undergoing a trial of spontaneous ventilation. Patients must be capable of maintaining their own airway, and their acute illness has to be resolved. They should indicate that they want to be extubated, and should have a twinkle in their eye. Patients should be able to maintain adequate oxygenation with an inspired oxygen concentration of 0.40 or less and with a PEEP of 5 cm water or less.

The majority of ventilated patients are most effectively weaned with daily spontaneous breathing trials. The breathing trial can be given with T-piece ventilation in which the endotracheal tube is attached to a length of tubing connected to a blow-by oxygen source. Alternatively, the trial can be accomplished with a low level (typically 5 cm of water) of pressure support with PEEP, or with continuous positive airway pressure (CPAP). In either case, the patient is asked to support his or her own breathing for 30 minutes. If the patient is breathing comfortably at the end of the trial, the patient can be extubated. If a question arises as to the degree of comfort, blood gases can be obtained, and the patient should be put back on the ventilator, while waiting for the gases to come back from the laboratory. If the patient was reasonably comfortable at the end of the 30-minute trial and if the pH comes back at a normal value, the patient can be extubated. The patient should not be kept on a mode of spontaneous ventilation while waiting for the results from the laboratory. The patient needs to be well rested when the endotracheal tube is removed. If patients do not tolerate the breathing trials, they should be put back on the ventilator and given full support for the rest of the day, allowing them to rest for at least 23.5 hours, to avoid chronic exhaustion.

Weaning from mechanical ventilation can also be achieved with IMV, although we rarely use this technique nowadays. The IMV rate is gradually decreased, requiring the patient to contribute increasingly to the maintenance of adequate minute ventilation. The patient's overall clinical status, respiratory rate, and arterial PCO_2 are used as guidelines to determine the rate of weaning. When an IMV of 4/min or less is well tolerated for long periods, a trial of spontaneous ventilation without any machine support is conducted. The criteria for extubation are the same as when wind-sprints or workouts are used.

Patients who repeatedly fail extubation or are severely deconditioned benefit from a more deliberate and gradual weaning of the ventilator. Frequently, these patients benefit from tracheostomy and optimization of nutritional status as adjuncts to weaning. Mechanical factors increasing work of breathing, ie, reactive airway disease, should be treated and minimized.

EXTUBATION

Both objective and subjective criteria are used to determine if a patient is ready for extubation. Objective measures of pulmonary function include the respiratory rate, the arterial PCO_2, and the patient's ability to oxygenate. The respiratory rate on a T-piece should be less than 24/min if extubation is being considered and in ideal circumstances should be below 20/min. In most instances, the PCO_2 should be 42 mm Hg or less with an acceptably low respiratory rate. In patients with chronic CO_2 retention or metabolic alkalosis with respiratory compensation, higher PCO_2 levels are acceptable as long as the arterial pH is 7.34 or greater. A pH lower than this indicates that the elevation in PCO_2 is acute and poorly tolerated. The patient should have an arterial oxygen saturation of greater than 90% on an FIO_2 of 40% or less and a PEEP of 5 cm H_2O or less.

Subjective criteria for extubation are also important. The patient's underlying disease process will often dictate whether extubation is appropriate. A critically ill patient requiring further operative procedures and with a guarded prognosis may require continued intubation and mechanical ventilatory support in spite of current fairly good pulmonary function. Inability to protect the airway is another indication for continued intubation even when the patient's ability to oxygenate and ventilate are adequate. Finally, there is a gestalt determination of a patient's ability to tolerate extubation and spontaneous ventilation. A patient who can lift his or her head off the pillow, has a sparkle in his or her eye, and obviously wants the endotracheal tube removed is a good candidate for extubation; a lethargic, diaphoretic patient is not.

ADJUVANT TREATMENT

Mechanical ventilation is the mainstay of therapy for treatment of severe pulmonary insufficiency in the surgical patient. Mechanical ventilation, however, introduces problems, such as bacterial colonization of the tracheobronchial tree, which may require adjuvant treatment. The underlying disease process may also require adjuvant treatment.

ANTIBIOTICS

Bacteria can be recovered from tracheal secretions of any patient who has been intubated and on mechanical ventilation for several days. The question is when to treat with antibiotics. Indications include purulent sputum associated with abundant white cells on Gram-stained smears; pathogenic organisms recovered from suctioning; signs of systemic sepsis with increasing fluid requirements and increasing blood glucose concentrations; worsening pulmonary function, as judged by the need to increase inspired oxygen concentrations or end-expiratory pressure; and worsening signs on chest x-ray. If all of these are present, antibiotics should be started. If only one or two are present, antibiotics are probably best withheld to avoid overgrowth of resistant organisms that could later cause fatal pneumonia. Older patients may have only one chance to survive a critical period of illness and should probably be given antibiotics sooner than younger patients, who are better able to recover after prolonged illness. Thus, an 80-year-old patient with flail chest should probably be given antibiotics early; a 20-year-old patient who was hospitalized for a gunshot wound involving the colon and who develops questionable pneumonia 2 weeks later should probably be given antibiotics only when infection is definitely confirmed and the causative organisms are identified. Calculation of a Clinical Pulmonary Infection Score (CPIS) provides a quantitative value to guide diagnosis of pneumonia and avoid overtreatment and antimicrobial resistance or superinfection. Antibiotics can safely be discontinued in patients empirically started on antibiotics for suspected pneumonia who have a CPIS value of < 6 at 72 hours.

CORRECTION OF COAGULATION ABNORMALITIES

After severe trauma or major sepsis, many patients will demonstrate signs of intravascular coagulation, with prolonged clotting times, low platelet counts, decreased fibrinogen levels, and production of fibrin degradation products or fibrin monomers. Nevertheless, if the patient is not bleeding, fresh-frozen plasma and platelets should not be given; they will only add fuel to the fire of systemic inflammation and coagulation. They should, however, be given to patients who are bleeding and to those with severe head injuries who could develop a sudden irretrievable and devastating hemorrhage.

MUSCLE RELAXANTS

Muscle relaxants sometimes greatly simplify ventilatory management in patients with severe pulmonary insufficiency, particularly those with recent injuries or sepsis. Because struggling against the ventilator can compromise ventilatory and cardiovascular function, it may be necessary to paralyze the patient when mechanical ventilation is being instituted. Muscle relaxants are dangerous, however, and should only be used when absolutely necessary and for the shortest possible time. Undetected malfunction of a ventilator may mean death for the paralyzed patient.

CHEST X-RAYS

Chest x-rays should be obtained daily in patients being treated with mechanical ventilation. Films are unreliable in differentiating cardiogenic from noncardiogenic edema, however, and visible changes lag behind clinical changes. Films are helpful in diagnosing contusion, aspiration, and pneumonia and may demonstrate a small pneumothorax or mediastinal emphysema. They show positioning of endotracheal tubes, nasogastric tubes, feeding tubes, central venous catheters, and pulmonary arterial catheters. They may show dilation of the trachea at the site of the balloon on the end of the endotracheal tube.

The Acute Respiratory Distress Syndrome Network: Ventilation with lower tidal volumes as compared with traditional tidal volumes for acute lung injury and the acute respiratory distress syndrome. N Engl J Med 2000;342:1301.

Aldrich TK et al: Weaning from mechanical ventilation: adjunctive use of inspiratory muscle resistive training. Crit Care Med 1989;17:143.

Amato MB et al: Effect of a protective-ventilation strategy on mortality in the acute respiratory distress syndrome. N Engl J Med 1998;338:347.

Bernard GR et al: The American-European Consensus Conference on ARDS. Definitions, mechanisms, relevant outcomes, and clinical trial coordination. Am J Respir Crit Care Med 1994;149(3 Pt 1):818.

Bidani A et al: Permissive hypercapnia in acute respiratory failure. JAMA 1994;272:957.

Blaisdell FW et al: Pulmonary microembolism. A cause of morbidity and death after major vascular surgery. Arch Surg 1966;93:776.

Brochard L et al: Inspiratory pressure support prevents diaphragmatic fatigue during weaning from mechanical ventilation. Am Rev Respir Dis 1989;139:513.

Chastre J et al: Comparison of 8 vs 15 days of antibiotic therapy for ventilator-associated pneumonia in adults: a randomized trial. JAMA 2003;290:2588.

Esteban A et al: Effect of spontaneous breathing trial duration on outcome of attempts to discontinue mechanical ventilation. Spanish Lung Failure Collaborative Group. Am J Respir Crit Care Med 1999;159:512.

Esteban A et al: A comparison of four methods of weaning patients from mechanical ventilation. Spanish Lung Failure Collaborative Group. N Engl J Med 1995;332:345.

Fu Z et al: High lung volume increases stress failure in pulmonary capillaries. J Appl Physiol 1992;73:123.

Gattinoni L et al: Regional effects and mechanism of positive end-expiratory pressure in early adult respiratory distress syndrome. JAMA 1993;269:2122.

Gausche M et al: Effect of out-of-hospital pediatric endotracheal intubation on survival and neurological outcome: a controlled clinical trial. JAMA 2000;283:783.

Heyland DK et al: The attributable morbidity and mortality of ventilator-associated pneumonia in the critically ill patient. The Canadian Critical Trials Group. Am J Respir Crit Care Med 1999;159(4 Pt 1):1249.

Hickling KG, Henderson SJ, Jackson R: Low mortality associated with low volume pressure limited ventilation with permissive hypercapnia in severe adult respiratory distress syndrome. Intensive Care Med 1990;16:372.

Iregui M et al: Clinical importance of delays in the initiation of appropriate antibiotic treatment for ventilator-associated pneumonia. Chest 2002;122:262.

Klocke RA: Carbon dioxide transport. In: *Handbook of Physiology,* Sect 3, vol 4, p. 173. American Physiological Society, 1987.

Kress JP et al: Daily interruption of sedative infusions in critically ill patients undergoing mechanical ventilation. N Engl J Med 2000;342:1471.

MacIntyre NR: Respiratory function during pressure support ventilation. Chest 1986;89:677.

MacIntyre NR et al: Evidence-based guidelines for weaning and discontinuing ventilatory support: a collective task force facilitated by the American College of Chest Physicians; the American Association for Respiratory Care; and the American College of Critical Care Medicine. Chest 2001;120(6 Suppl): 375S.

Marelich GP et al: Protocol weaning of mechanical ventilation in medical and surgical patients by respiratory care practitioners and nurses: effect on weaning time and incidence of ventilator-associated pneumonia. Chest 2000;118:459.

Maziak DE, Meade MO, Todd TR: The timing of tracheotomy: a systematic review. Chest 1998;114:605.

Minei JP et al: Alternative case definitions of ventilator-associated pneumonia identify different patients in a surgical intensive care unit. Shock 2000;14:331; discussion 336.

Pugin J et al: Diagnosis of ventilator-associated pneumonia by bacteriologic analysis of bronchoscopic and nonbronchoscopic "blind" bronchoalveolar lavage fluid. Am Rev Respir Dis 1991;143(5 Pt 1):1121.

Ranieri VM et al: Effect of mechanical ventilation on inflammatory mediators in patients with acute respiratory distress syndrome: a randomized controlled trial. JAMA 1999;282:54.

Saito S, Tokioka H, Kosaka F: Efficacy of flow-by during continuous positive airway pressure ventilation. Crit Care Med. 1990;18:654.

Sassoon CS et al: Inspiratory work of breathing on flow-by and demand-flow continuous positive airway pressure. Crit Care Med 1989;17:1108.

Schweickert WD et al: Daily interruption of sedative infusions and complications of critical illness in mechanically ventilated patients. Crit Care Med 2004;32:1272.

Singh N et al: Short-course empiric antibiotic therapy for patients with pulmonary infiltrates in the intensive care unit. A proposed solution for indiscriminate antibiotic prescription. Am J Respir Crit Care Med 2000;162(2 Pt 1):505.

Stewart TE et al: Evaluation of a ventilation strategy to prevent barotrauma in patients at high risk for acute respiratory distress syndrome. Pressure- and Volume-Limited Ventilation Strategy Group. N Engl J Med 1998;338:355.

III. TREATMENT OF THE MORE CHALLENGING PATIENT

So far, the discussion of shock and pulmonary failure in the surgical patient has concentrated on making a clinical diagnosis and directing treatment on the basis of that diagnosis. This approach works well in many patients, but in some it is not enough. Effective treatment in the more seriously ill patient frequently has to take into account the underlying physiological abnormalities if the treatment is to work. With this approach the clinical diagnosis becomes less important. Dealing with the underlying physiological problem becomes paramount.

COMMON PHYSIOLOGICAL RESPONSES TO SEVERE SHOCK

The body responds to the shock state with compensatory responses. These responses help the patient deal with the initial abnormalities of the shock but can contribute to the later consequences of cardiac and pulmonary failure. Understanding these responses can help the physician in managing the consequences.

Neurohumoral Responses

The neurohumoral responses to shock include discharge of the cardiovascular nerves and release of vasoactive, metabolically active, and volume-conserving hormones. The responses can be lifesaving before therapy begins and serve to maintain homeostasis once therapy has started.

Adrenergic discharge constricts the arterioles, venules, and small veins in all parts of the body except the brain and heart and augments myocardial systolic function. The result is increased cardiac output and blood pressure and diversion of flow to the brain and heart.

The vasoactive hormones angiotensin II and vasopressin act in concert with discharge of the cardiovascular adrenergic nerves. Angiotensin II constricts the vasculature in the skin, kidneys, and splanchnic organs and diverts blood flow to the heart and brain. It also stimulates the adrenal medulla to release aldosterone, resulting in reabsorption of sodium ions from the glomerular filtrate. Vasopressin, like adrenergic discharge and angiotensin II, constricts the vascular sphincters in the skin and splanchnic organs (it does not constrict the renal vasculature) and diverts blood flow to the heart and brain. It also stimulates reabsorption of water from the distal tubules.

Metabolic Responses

In all severe shock states, intracellular hydrogen ion concentrations increase. To compensate, extracellular sodium flows down its electrochemical gradient into the cells, along with chloride and water, in exchange for intracellular hydrogen ion. Intracellular pH increases back toward normal, but the cells swell, with perhaps an increase of 3 L in the intracellular volume.

Hypovolemia, hypotension, pain, and other stresses of critical illness stimulate the release of cortisol, glucagon, and epinephrine—all of which increase extracellular glucose concentrations (see Chapter 11). Thus, glucose should not be used in the initial fluid resuscitation of the patient in shock—it is not necessary and can even induce an osmotic diuresis, worsening hypovolemia and confusing the clinical picture. Glucose-containing solutions should be reserved for those patients who might be in insulin shock.

On the other hand, the endogenously produced glucose generated by the physiological release of the counter-regulatory hormones provides fuel for nervous system function, metabolism of blood cells, and wound healing. The modest increase in extracellular osmolality also helps to replenish vascular volume by drawing water out of the cells and by increasing the interstitial hydrostatic pressure. The increased interstitial pressure drives interstitial protein into the lymphatics and from there into the vascular space. Interstitial oncotic pressure falls, and plasma oncotic pressure rises. The augmented oncotic gradient between the vascular and interstitial spaces draws water, sodium, and chloride into the vascular space, from the interstitial space. This replenishment of vascular volume will continue as long as interstitial hydrostatic pressures are maintained and as long as interstitial protein stores, which constitute more than half of the total extracellular protein content, can be recruited. A certain degree of hyperglycemia might be beneficial in the postresuscitative phase. Once the patient has recovered, however, it appears that it is best to aggressively keep the blood glucose levels low, at 120 mg% or less.

Other hormones with potential metabolic actions, including insulin and growth hormone, are also released during critical illnesses. They have little effect, however, compared with cortisol, glucagon, and epinephrine. Indeed, infusion of cortisol, glucagon, and epinephrine in normal subjects can produce most of the metabolic changes of critical illness.

Microvascular Responses

In severely ill patients, three responses—dilation of systemic arterioles, failure of cell membrane function, and disruption of the vascular endothelium—serve to worsen the patient's condition. In decompensated shock, the systemic arterioles lose their ability to constrict, while the postcapillary sphincters remain constricted. Microvascular hydrostatic pressure rises. Water, sodium, and chloride are driven out of the vascular space and into the interstitium. The process is limited, however, because the oncotic gradient, which increases as fluid is lost from plasma, prevents further fluid losses.

Trauma and sepsis activate coagulation and inflammation, which can disrupt microvascular endothelial integrity in severely ill patients. Platelet and white cell microaggregates that form in injured or infected tissues embolize to the lungs or liver, where they lodge in the capillaries. The microaggregates, endothelium, and plasma in the regions of embolization release kinins, platelet-activating factors, fibrin degradation products, thromboxanes, prostacyclin, prostaglandins, complement, leukotrienes, lysosomal enzymes, oxygen radicals, and other toxic factors, which damage the endothelium and dilate the vasculature in the region of the emboli and distally. Protein, water, sodium, and chloride extravasate into the interstitium. The amount of extravasation is limited only by the increases in interstitial hydrostatic pressure that arise from interstitial flooding. The edema that results can be massive and can involve any tissue in the body.

SWAN-GANZ CATHETER

The Swan-Ganz catheter can be useful in evaluating the cardiovascular consequences associated with the physiological responses described above, and it can be invaluable in directing treatment in selected, seriously ill patients. The modern Swan-Ganz catheter is equipped with a thermistor and an oximeter on its tip. It permits measurement of the cardiac output; right atrial, pulmonary arterial, and pulmonary arterial wedge pressures; and mixed venous oxygen contents. Knowledge of the cardiac output and filling pressures can be used to assess ventricular function as fluid is administered or withheld. The mixed venous oxygen saturation reflects the adequacy of oxygen delivery to the periphery; a value less than 60% indicates inadequate peripheral oxygenation and can be used to evaluate adequacy of the cardiac output and of systemic arterial oxygen content. It can also be used to determine oxygen consumption, which is calculated as the cardiac output multiplied by the difference of the oxygen contents of blood in the systemic and pulmonary arteries. Oxygen consumption can fall in severely ill patients, and measurements of consumption can help assess the patient's response to resuscitation. All of this information can help in dealing with the physiological abnormalities of the shock state and the pulmonary failure that can arise from the shock.

The catheter is particularly useful when treatment of one organ system might harm another. For example, fluid administration might be needed to treat septic shock, but excess fluid might contribute to pulmonary failure; a diuretic might be indicated in an oliguric patient in congestive heart failure, but excessive diuresis might decrease the cardiac output to the point that the kidneys fail; and fluid might be needed for cardiovascular resuscitation in a patient with multiple injuries, but too much fluid might exacerbate cerebral edema. The pulmonary arterial catheter can be extremely helpful in these situations.

Data obtained from the Swan-Ganz catheter can be misleading, however, if mistakes are made in performing the measurements. The cardiac output, as measured by thermodilution, is obtained by injecting a known volume of a solution cooler than blood into the right atrium and measuring the temperature drop in the blood as it flows past a thermistor on the end of the pulmonary arterial catheter or by generating an impulse of heat in the right ventricle and measuring the temperature rise in the pulmonary artery. The greater the area under the temperature curve, the lower the amount of flow through the right heart. Injections should be probably be made at random times during the respiratory cycle, to give the best indication of the output available to the patient, but some prefer to make the injections at a consistent time in the cycle, to minimize variability in the cardiac output–associated heart-lung interactions. Calculations of the cardiac output are made by computer.

When one is obtaining pulmonary arterial or mixed venous blood, the balloon on the end of the catheter should be deflated, and the blood should be withdrawn slowly. If the blood is withdrawn too quickly, the walls of the pulmonary artery will collapse around the end of the catheter, and the specimen will be contaminated by blood that is pulled back, in a retrograde manner, past ventilated and nonperfused alveoli. The oximeter on the tip of the catheter has to be calibrated frequently, by comparing the oxygen saturations of blood obtained from the pulmonary artery with the saturations readout by the oximeter. One has to be sure that the blood that is to be used for calibration is truly representative.

The pressures measured with the pulmonary arterial catheter will be displayed on an oscilloscope and will include a mean pressure that is calculated by computer circuitry in the monitoring equipment. We now use these mean pressures in patient management. They have the advantage that they represent the pressures throughout the respiratory cycle and thus average in the variability associated with heart-lung interactions. Others prefer to read the end-expiratory pressures off of the oscilloscope screen and use those values in patient management. Those pressures are relatively independent of heart-lung interactions but they can be difficult to interpret, even by the most experienced ICU nurse or physician.

Of the five pressures obtained from the catheter, only two—the right atrial and the mean pulmonary arterial pressures—can be taken at face value; the other three—the pulmonary arterial systolic, diastolic, and wedge pressures—are subject to errors of measurement and interpretation. The pulmonary arterial wedge pressure usually is the same as the left atrial pressure. The wedge pressure will not reflect left atrial pressure, however, if the catheter is in a portion of the vasculature occluded by inflated alveoli. If the wedge pressure varies by more than 10 mm Hg with cycles of mechanical ventilation, one should assume that the tip of the catheter is facing the pressure in the alveoli rather than the pressure in the left atrium.

To account for variations in size of the patient, the cardiac output can be indexed to the calculated body surface area. We now prefer, however, to use the patient's desirable body weight, calculated on the assumption that a desirable weight is one that is associated with longevity and freedom from diabetes. A body mass index of 21 is convenient to use, for both men and women. We start with making a rough approximation of the patient's height, to the nearest half-foot. The desirable weights associated with that height, assuming a body mass index of 21, are indicated in Table 12–2. The cardiac outputs associated with that weight are also indicated, assuming that the subjects are supine, nonstressed, resting, fasting, and in a thermoneutral environment. The resting oxygen consumptions under these conditions will be 3.5 mL ×

Table 12–2. Approximate desirable weight, cardiac output, and oxygen consumption in young resting, supine, fasting individuals of varying heights, in a thermoneutral environment.

Height (ft, in)	Desirable Weight[1] (kg)	Cardiac Output[2] (L/min)	Oxygen Consumption[3] (mL/min)
5′0″	49	5	170
5′6″	59	6	205
6′0″	70	7	245
6′6″	83	8	290

[1]Calculated with assumption that the desirable weight is that which gives a body mass index of 21.
[2]Calculated as 100 mL • kg^{-1}• $minutes^{-1}$.
[3]Calculated as 3.5 mL • kg^{-1} • $minutes^{-1}$.

weight^{-1} × minutes^{-1}. We adjust the outputs and the consumptions for patients older than 50 years of age with the assumption that metabolic activity decreases by 10% per decade after the age of 50 years. Thus, for a 70-year-old subject who is 6 feet tall, we assume that a normal cardiac output is 7 L/min multiplied by 0.8 or 5.6 L/min. The oxygen consumption is 245 mL/min multiplied by 0.8 or 195 mL/min.

OXYHEMOGLOBIN DISSOCIATION

The amount of oxygen contained in the blood and the amount of oxygen available to be delivered to the tissues can be expressed as a concentration, a saturation, or as a partial pressure. All three have their value. Understanding their relationships can help in understanding the cardiac and pulmonary pathophysiology of the critically ill surgical patient.

The concentration of oxygen in the blood, or oxygen content (Co_2), is expressed as milliliters of O_2/dL of blood, or vol%. The Co_2 can be measured directly, but the measurement is time-consuming, and the content is usually calculated on the basis of the other two measures of blood oxygenation, the oxygen saturation (So_2) and the Po_2. The Co_2 is related to these other quantities by the following formula:

$$Co_2 = 1.34 \times [Hb] \times So_2 + 0.0031 \times Po_2 \qquad (1)$$

where [Hb] is expressed as g/dL and the Po_2 as mm Hg. Thus, for example, the Co_2 of a blood specimen with a [Hb] of 12 g/dL, an So_2 of 90%, and a Po_2 of 60 mm Hg is 14.7 vol%.

The first term in the equation represents the O_2 carried by the hemoglobin molecule; the second, the O_2 dissolved in the blood water. This second term is small compared with the first as long as the [Hb] is greater than (say) 7 g/dL and the Po_2 is less than (say) 100 mm Hg. Omitting the second term then simplifies the formula to read as follows:

$$Co_2 = 1.34 \times [Hb] \times So_2 \qquad (2)$$

For the previous set of blood gases, this would give a Co_2 of 14.5 vol%.

The formula can be made even simpler by substituting the fraction $^4/_3$ for the decimal 1.34:

$$Co_2 = \frac{4}{3} \times [Hb] \times So_2 \qquad (3)$$

Because [Hb] and the So_2 can usually be approximated by integers with little loss of accuracy, the calculation frequently allows cancellation of the 3 and can be done mentally. For the previous example, the Co_2 would be 14.4 vol%.

Calculation of the Co_2 requires knowledge of the So_2. Many pulmonary arterial catheters are now equipped with sensors mounted on their tips that directly measure the saturation of the blood in the pulmonary artery. Alternatively, blood can be withdrawn from the tip of the catheter and sent to the laboratory, where the So_2 can be easily measured by an instrument known as a co-oximeter. Most laboratories will make this measurement by specific request, but some will calculate the So_2 from the Po_2. This calculation is frequently inaccurate for mixed venous specimens but is usually accurate for arterial blood. The calculation is made from equations that are based on the oxyhemoglobin dissociation curve (Figure 12–1), an empirically derived relationship between the So_2 of human blood and its Po_2. The saturation for a given Po_2 depends on blood temperature, [H^+], and Pco_2 and on the red cell concentration of 2,3-diphosphoglycerate (2,3-DPG). The laboratory should be told the temperature, and it will measure the [H^+] and Pco_2. It will then calculate the So_2 from the Po_2 with the assumption that the 2,3-DPG concentration is normal.

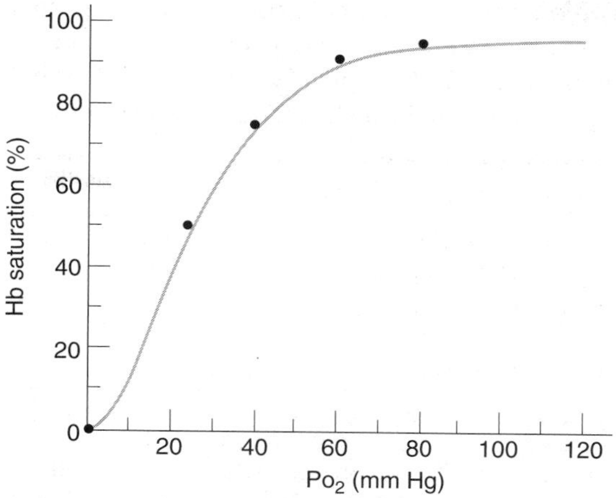

Figure 12–1. Oxyhemoglobin dissociation curve for human blood at 37 °C with a Pco_2 of 40 mm Hg, a pH of 7.40, and a normal 2,3-DPG red cell concentration. Approximate values from Table 12–4 fall close to the idealized curve.

It is helpful, however, to have some guidelines for converting back and forth between So_2 and Po_2. Five approximations for points on the dissociation curve for a patient with normal temperature, [H^+], Pco_2, and 2,3-DPG level are given in Table 12–3. The P_{50} of human hemoglobin—the Po_2 at which the molecule is half-saturated—is 27 mm Hg (approximated as 25 mm Hg in the table). The Po_2 and So_2 for mixed venous blood in a person with a [Hb] of 15 g/dL and a normal O_2 consumption and cardiac output are 40 mm Hg and 75%, respectively. A Po_2 of 60 mm Hg—a value that should be exceeded by most

Table 12–3. Approximate correlations for partial pressures of oxygen and oxygen saturation in blood at 37 °C with a pH of 7.4, a PCO_2 of 40 mm Hg, and a normal 2,3-DPG red cell concentration.

PO_2	SO_2
0 mm Hg	0%
25 mm Hg	50%
40 mm Hg	75%
60 mm Hg	90%
80 mm Hg	95%

patients in an ICU—corresponds to an SO_2 of 90%. A PO_2 of 80 mm Hg corresponds to an SO_2 of 95%. Remembering the values in the table allows construction of a dissociation curve and facilitates conversion from one measure of oxygenation to the other. For example, in a patient with a normal temperature, [H+], PCO_2, and 2,3-DPG and a [Hb] of 10 g/dL, a PO_2 of 60 mm Hg in the systemic arterial blood would create a CO_2 of 12 vol% (from Equation 1), a value that would be adequate if the patient had normal coronary arteries and a good heart. Such a value would be inadequate, however, in the face of underlying heart disease.

CAUSES OF AN ELEVATED $Paco_2$

The patient in pulmonary failure will frequently have an elevated arterial carbon dioxide tension. The arterial PCO_2 is proportionate to CO_2 production divided by alveolar ventilation—defined as the volume of air exchanged per unit time in functioning alveoli. Since CO_2 production is usually fairly constant in adequately perfused patients, the PCO_2 comes to be inversely proportionate to alveolar ventilation. An elevated PCO_2 in the presence of normal CO_2 production means inadequate alveolar ventilation. Ventilation should be assessed with respect to how much work is required to generate the PCO_2. In the case of spontaneous ventilation, this assessment involves the frequency and depth of breathing; in the case of mechanical ventilation, the frequency of the machine-generated breaths and the tidal volume of those breaths.

The PCO_2 also gives an indication of dead space ventilation—the ventilation of nonperfused airways. Since minute or total ventilation is dead space ventilation plus alveolar ventilation, a normal PCO_2 combined with a normal minute ventilation implies a normal dead space ventilation. A normal PCO_2 that must be generated by a supranormal minute ventilation implies increased dead space ventilation. Normal dead space ventilation is one-third of total ventilation, but many critically ill surgical patients will have a dead space ventilation that is up to two-thirds of total ventilation. Increased dead space ventilation can be caused by hypovolemia with poor perfusion of nondependent alveoli, ARDS, pulmonary emboli, pulmonary vasoconstriction, and mechanical ventilation-induced compression of the pulmonary vasculature. Hypovolemia should be treated by expansion of the vascular volume. Emboli should be treated by anticoagulation or by elimination of their source. Dead space generated by mechanical ventilation should be minimized by adjustment of the ventilator, usually by decreasing tidal volumes or end-expiratory pressures, while at the same time maintaining enough mechanical support to generate a normal PCO_2 and alveolar ventilation.

CAUSES OF A LOW Pao_2

Almost all surgical patients with pulmonary failure will have systemic arterial hypoxemia. There are five physiological causes: low inspired O_2 concentration, diffusion block between alveolar gas and capillary blood, subnormal alveolar ventilation, shunting of blood through completely nonventilated portions of the lung or bypassing of blood past the lung, and perfusion of parts of the lung that have low ventilation/perfusion ratios. In addition, any process that decreases the mixed venous CO_2 in the presence of any of the above can lower the arterial PO_2 even further. Low mixed venous CO_2 can be caused by a low arterial CO_2, low cardiac output, or high O_2 consumption.

Arterial hypoxemia in the surgical patient is usually caused by shunting, low ventilation/perfusion ratios, low mixed venous CO_2, or a combination of these factors. Low inspired O_2 concentrations at sea level are impossible so long as the ventilator is functioning properly. (This must be checked, however, as the first step in diagnosing and correcting the cause of a low PO_2.) Diffusion block is exceedingly rare in surgical patients. Subnormal alveolar ventilation can be ruled out with a normal arterial PCO_2 assuming CO_2 production is not depressed. Thus, shunting and areas of low ventilation/perfusion ratios, along with low mixed venous CO_2, remain as causes for almost all cases of hypoxemia in the surgical patient. Shunting and low ventilation/perfusion ratios do not need to be distinguished from each other very often, but the distinction can be made by increasing the inspired O_2 concentration to 100%: Hypoxemia caused by areas of low ventilation/perfusion ratios will be at least partially corrected by 100% O_2; hypoxemia caused by shunting will not. The mixed venous CO_2 can be measured with the Swan-Ganz catheter.

ACID-BASE BALANCE

Acid-base abnormalities can arise from the hypoventilation of pulmonary insufficiency or from the metabolic abnormalities of shock. The former has already been discussed. The latter can become more involved.

The hydrogen ion, carbon dioxide gas, and bicarbonate equilibrate with one another in the plasma water, and if two of the quantities are known, the third can be calculated. In practice, the P_{CO_2} and $[H^+]$, which are measured directly with the blood gas apparatus, will be known. The $[HCO_3^-]$ can then be calculated by the Henderson-Hasselbalch equation, which can be written in the following form (see Chapter 10):

$$[HCO_3^-] = \frac{24 \times P_{CO_2}}{[H^+]} \quad (4)$$

where $[HCO_3^-]$ is expressed as mmol/L, P_{CO_2} as mm Hg, and [H+] as nmol/L. This form of the equation requires conversion of pH, the more common expression of [H+], into nmol/L, the more logical expression, but the conversion is not difficult (Table 12–4). The values in the table are easy to remember if one notes that each value in the column under [H+] is 80% of the value immediately above, with the exception of 80 and 63, which are off by 1. Thus, by Equation 2, if the P_{CO_2} is 60 mm Hg and the pH is 7.30, the $[HCO_3^-]$ is 29 mmol/L.

The $[HCO_3^-]$ calculated by this equation is the amount of bicarbonate ion dissolved in the plasma water and can be obtained only from a specimen of blood that is obtained and processed without exposure to the atmosphere. The "CO_2 combining power," which is typically measured along with electrolyte concentrations in blood that is not processed anaerobically, includes not only the $[HCO_3^-]$ but any CO_2 gas and carbonic acid that is dissolved in the plasma as well. The CO_2 combining power is usually about 2 mmol/L greater than the calculated (and actual) $[HCO_3^-]$.

The base deficit or excess is determined by comparing the calculated $[HCO_3^-]$ with the $[HCO_3^-]$ that might be expected in a patient with a given P_{CO_2} and $[H^+]$. These expected values have been determined by analyzing blood obtained from patients with a wide variety of pulmonary disorders. For example, the kidneys in a patient with chronic respiratory acidemia can usually compensate to the extent that a chronic elevation in P_{CO_2} of 10 mm Hg will generate an increase in $[HCO_3^-]$ of 3 mmol/L. A patient with chronic obstructive lung disease and a chronically elevated P_{CO_2} of 60 mm Hg would be expected to have a $[HCO_3^-]$ of 30 mmol/L—6 mmol/L more than a normal value of 24. If such a patient had a pH of 7.30, the actual $[HCO_3^-]$ would be 29 mmol/L (from Equation 2; see the example in the preceding paragraph). That is, the observed value would be 1 mmol/L less than predicted, and the patient would be said to have a base deficit of 1 mmol/L.

Table 12–4. Conversion of pH to hydrogen ion concentration.

pH	Hydrogen Ion Concentration (mol/L)
7.0	100
7.1	100 × 0.8 = 80
7.2	80 × 0.8 = 63
7.3	63 × 0.8 = 50
7.4	50 × 0.8 = 40
7.5	40 × 0.8 = 32
7.6	32 × 0.8 = 25

Note: Values not indicated in the table can be derived by interpolation. For example, a pH of 7.35 corresponds to a hydrogen ion concentration of approximately 45.

The difficulty with the concept of base deficit and excess is that it rests on historically determined values, which may not be applicable to the patient at hand. For example, if a surgical patient with previously normal lungs lost his or her airway after an operation and began to hypoventilate, one would expect the $[HCO_3^-]$ to be normal—24 mmol/L—because the kidneys would not have had time to compensate for the hypercapnia. If the P_{CO_2} were 60 mm Hg and the pH 7.30, the physician should be concerned because the $[HCO_3^-]$ is 29 mmol/L (these values are the same as in the preceding paragraphs). A value of 29 mmol/L should alert the physician to the fact that the $[HCO_3^-]$ is too high, perhaps because $NaHCO_3$ had been given unnecessarily. The base deficit, however, would be 1 mmol/L, suggesting that the patient's $[HCO_3^-]$ was appropriate. The base deficit would be misleading.

The use of base deficit and excess should probably be abandoned in surgical patients. Errors in patient evaluation are more likely to be minimized if the physician concentrates on the $[HCO_3^-]$ and interprets that value in the light of a particular patient's situation. If a chronically ill patient in the ICU has severe ARDS and a P_{CO_2} of 60 mm Hg with a pH of 7.30, no attempt should be made to change the accompanying $[HCO_3^-]$ of 29 mmol/L—that value represents the expected renal compensation for such a chronic hypercapnia (though the impaired alveolar ventilation should be of concern). On the other hand, if the patient's P_{CO_2} is 60 mm Hg and the pH is 7.45, the patient has an inappropriately high $[HCO_3^-]$ of approximately 40 mmol/L (calculated from Equation 2), perhaps because of unreplaced losses of hydrogen ion from the stomach, chronic use of a loop diuretic, or administration of excessive amounts of acetate in the patient's parenteral nutrition. In this situation, the $[HCO_3^-]$ should be brought down into the low 30s. The excessively high $[HCO_3^-]$ and its resultant alkalemia may be blunting the patient's ventilatory drive.

Thus, in dealing with acid-base disorders, we take the calculation of the bicarbonate concentration in arterial plasma from the blood gas laboratory, or calculate it ourselves. In the case of a metabolic acidemia, we try to correct the underlying abnormality and then, if the pH remains less than 7.20, give sodium bicarbonate, but only after resuscitation has been initiated. The bicarbonate produces carbon dioxide and water locally, in the interstitial fluid at the sites where the hydrogen ions are being produced. In the absence of resuscitation, the locally generated carbon dioxide can cross back into the cell, worsening intracellular acidosis. There is no problem with bicarbonate if it is given after some local flow has been achieved. The generated carbon dioxide will be washed centrally into the pulmonary vasculature, where it will be eliminated by the lungs.

Metabolic alkalemias in the surgical patient are usually easy to recognize and treat. Contraction alkalemias are treated with fluid expansion. Hypokalemic, hypochloremic metabolic alkalemias caused by unreplaced loss of gastric fluids are treated with normal saline supplemented with potassium chloride. Hypokalemic hypochloremic alkalemias caused by use of loop diuretics are treated with the addition of acetazolamide to the diuretic regimen and, if necessary, the administration of 0.1 N hydrochloric acid, given as a slow central intravenous drip, over a period of 48 hours. The amount of acid to be given is calculated on the basis of the presumed extracellular chloride deficit, with the assumption that the interstitial chloride concentration is the same as the plasma concentration, that is, with the assumption that the Donnan factor for chloride is 1.

RISK ASSESSMENT

Predicting the likelihood of survival in critically ill surgical patients is best accomplished by evaluating clinical and laboratory findings. Computation of a severity of illness score is usually unnecessary. Nonetheless, several scoring systems have been developed with the intention of increasing the precision of the estimate. All such systems assign a mathematical probability for survival in groups of patients, and many are useful for research purposes because they allow comparisons of patients between different institutions. None of them, however, are accurate enough to predict survival for an individual patient, though some are still clinically useful for assessing the effects of therapy.

The APACHE II score, in which clinical data and 14 measured variables are entered into a formula to assess the probability of survival, takes about 30 minutes to calculate by hand—less by computer. The score can predict survival in critically ill medical patients; it has not been found to be of value in the usual surgical patient, and in any case it is too cumbersome unless one has a particular interest in this kind of methodology.

Methods for predicting survival in trauma patients are well established, though most trauma systems are designed to evaluate all trauma patients and not the specific subset of critically ill trauma patients. The Injury Severity Score, the Revised Trauma Score, and the ASCOT score have proved to be most reliable. The Glasgow Coma Scale Score is quite accurate for predicting survival in patients with head injuries. Combining the Glasgow Coma Scale Score with a simple measurement of fluid requirement has also proved to be accurate in critically injured trauma patients.

Barie PS et al: Comparison of APACHE II and III scoring systems for mortality prediction in critical surgical illness. Arch Surg 1995;130:77.

Bessey PQ: Critical care: metabolic response to critical illness. In: *ACS Surgery: Principles & Practice,* pp. 1417–1443. WebMed Inc., 2004.

Griffiths RD, Jones C, Palmer TE: Six-month outcome of critically ill patients given glutamine-supplemented parenteral nutrition. Nutrition 1997;13:295.

Horan TC et al: Nosocomial infections in surgical patients in the United States, January 1986–June 1992. National Nosocomial Infections Surveillance (NNIS) System. Infect Control Hosp Epidemiol 1993;14:73.

Houdijk AP et al: Randomised trial of glutamine-enriched enteral nutrition on infectious morbidity in patients with multiple trauma. Lancet 1998;352:772.

O'Quin R, Marini JJ: Pulmonary artery occlusion pressure: clinical physiology, measurement, and interpretation. Am Rev Respir Dis 1983;128:319.

Vassar MJ et al: Prediction of outcome in intensive care unit trauma patients: a multicenter study of Acute Physiology and Chronic Health Evaluation (APACHE), Trauma and Injury Severity Score (TRISS), and a 24-hour intensive care unit (ICU) point system. J Trauma 1999;47:324.

Vassar MJ et al: Comparison of APACHE II, TRISS, and a proposed 24-hour ICU point system for prediction of outcome in ICU trauma patients. J Trauma 1992;32:490; discussion 499.

Wilmore DW: Metabolic response to severe surgical illness: overview. World J Surg 2000;24:705.

Management of the Injured Patient 13

Mark R. Hemmila, MD, & Wendy L. Wahl, MD

EPIDEMIOLOGY OF TRAUMA

Trauma is the medical term that refers to life-threatening or serious injuries that require specialized surgical care if the patient is to survive without disability. As a "disease," trauma is a major public health problem. In the USA, it is the leading cause of death among people from age 1–45 and the fifth leading cause of death for all age groups. For persons under age 30, trauma is responsible for more deaths than all other diseases combined. A total of 150,000 lives are lost per year because of injuries and homicide. Overall, trauma accounts for 6% of all deaths in the country, and an additional 300,000 injured persons suffer some form of permanent disability. Because trauma adversely affects a young population, it results in the loss of more working years than all other causes of death. In 2001 trauma accounted for 2.7 million years of life lost before age 65, with the next closest disease being malignant neoplasms, which was responsible for 1.9 million years of life lost. Presence of alcohol is a significant contributor to trauma fatalities, and 41% of all traffic deaths in 2002 were alcohol related. The financial costs of injury are staggering and exceed $500 billion annually. Regrettably, nearly 40% of all trauma deaths could be avoided by injury prevention measures, alcohol cessation, and the establishment of regional trauma systems that would expedite the evaluation and treatment of seriously injured patients.

Trauma deaths have been classically described as having a trimodal distribution (Figure 13–1), with peaks that correspond to the types of intervention that would be most effective in reducing mortality. The first peak, the **immediate deaths**, represents patients who die of their injuries before reaching the hospital. The injuries accounting for these deaths include major brain or spinal cord trauma and those resulting in rapid exsanguination. Few of these patients would have any chance of survival even with access to immediate care since almost 60% of these deaths occur at the same time as the injury. Prevention remains the major strategy to reduce these deaths.

The second peak, the **early deaths**, are those that occur within the first few hours after injury. Half are caused by internal hemorrhage and the other half are due to central nervous system injuries. Almost all of these injuries are potentially treatable. However, in most cases, salvage requires prompt and definitive care of the sort available at a trauma center, ie, a specialized institution that can provide immediate resuscitation, identification of injuries, and access to a ready operating room 24 hours a day. Development of well-organized trauma systems with rapid transport and protocol-driven care can reduce the mortality in this time period from 30% to less than 10%.

The third peak, the **late deaths**, consists of patients who die days or weeks after injury. Ten percent to 20% of all trauma deaths occur during this period. Mortality for this period has traditionally been attributed to infection and multiple organ failure. However, development of trauma systems has changed the epidemiology of these deaths. During the first week, refractory intracranial hypertension following severe head injury is now responsible for a significant number of these deaths. Improvements in critical care management continue to be essential in reducing deaths during this phase. It is paramount that surgeons caring for trauma patients have genuine expertise in surgical critical care.

TRAUMA SYSTEMS

The purpose of a trauma system is to provide timely, organized care in order to minimize preventable morbidity and mortality following injury. The system includes prehospital care designed to identify, triage, treat, and transport victims with serious injuries. Criteria for staging patients with major trauma consist of standardized scoring systems based on readily discernible anatomic and physiologic variables. The criteria are designed to identify not only the more severe and complex single injuries but also combinations of injuries that require tertiary care. Patients are transported to a trauma center organized to provide the highest possible level of care to patients with major injuries. When a patient arrives in the trauma center, additional triage occurs. The most severely injured patients are identified and receive more intensive care.

The terrorist events of September 11, 2001, have highlighted the need for national and state trauma systems that can handle both routine events and mass casualty situations. Trauma centers that are part of a larger trauma system are already organized to respond

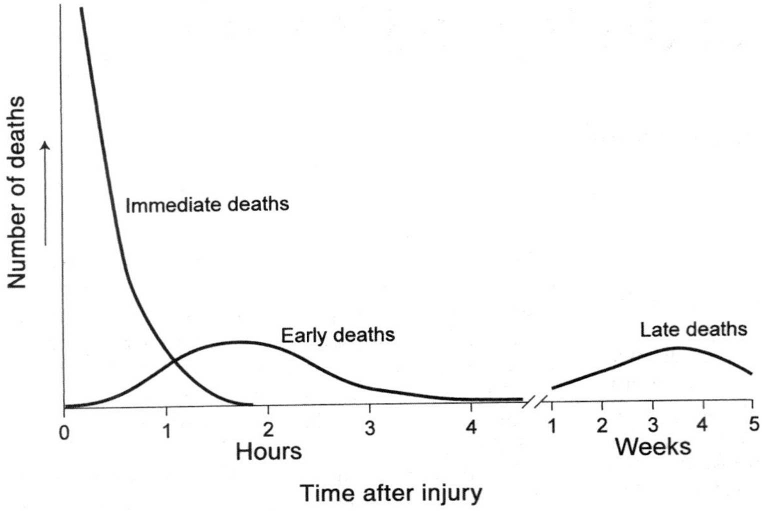

Figure 13–1. Periods of peak mortality after injury. (Modified from Hoyt DB, Coimbra R: Trauma: Introduction. In: Greenfield LJ, Mulholland MW, Oldham KT, et al: *Surgery, Scientific Principles and Practice*, 3rd ed. Lippincott Williams & Wilkins, 2001; p 271.)

to unexpected multiple casualty events. These centers have established linkages with emergency medical service providers and participate in systemwide patient triage and quality improvement. Gaps remain, however, in areas of the country not served by trauma systems, and a wide range in the degree of disaster preparedness exists at all levels of trauma care.

Presently, the majority of the United States population still lives in a geographic area not served by a regional trauma system. Every state in the country has at least one designated trauma center of some level. The total number of trauma centers in the United States has doubled since 1991 to 1154 in 2002; this includes 190 Level I and 263 Level II centers. However, wide variations remain at the state level in the availability and configuration of hospital trauma resources. The issue of need for trauma systems is best highlighted by a study in which it was found that the percentage of preventable deaths in Orange County, California, dropped from 11% to 1% after establishment of a regionalized trauma care facility. Similar data are available for other areas of the country.

The American College of Surgeons (ACS) has defined four levels of institutional trauma care. **Level I** is the highest designation a trauma center can receive. It indicates that the hospital has committed itself to the care of trauma patients and offers the highest level of skill available in trauma care. A level I trauma center is directed by a board-certified surgeon specializing in trauma care and is staffed by a team of board-certified trauma care specialists available 24 hours a day—including emergency room physicians, trauma surgeons, neurosurgeons and neurologists, orthopedic surgeons, plastic surgeons, anesthesiologists, and radiologists. The level I center maintains a quality improvement program including a trauma registry and has an active commitment to research, teaching, and community outreach/injury prevention. **Level II** trauma centers provide 24-hour care by in-hospital and on-call physicians. They are able to deliver the same quality of care as a level I center but without the same teaching and research obligations. Immediate operating room capability must be maintained 24 hours a day in level II centers. The **level III** trauma center provides prompt assessment, resuscitation, and stabilization followed by surgical treatment or inter-hospital transfer as appropriate. Although they may not be able to provide definitive care in all circumstances, level III centers serve a valuable function in less populated areas where resuscitation and stabilization before transport may be lifesaving. **Level IV** centers are designed to provide advanced trauma life support prior to patient transfer in remote areas in which no higher level of care is available.

Only 20% of the hospitals in the United States have sought certification and received a trauma center level I, II, or III designation since the ACS began the program in 1987.

PREHOSPITAL CARE & TRIAGE

The effectiveness of paramedics in the treatment of trauma victims remains controversial due to a lack of data regarding the success of specific prehospital treatments. Evidence of improved survival of cardiac arrest victims treated by well-trained paramedical teams has been inappropriately extrapolated to trauma victims. In the urban setting, where transportation from the scene of an accident to the hospital is typically 5–10 minutes, it is questionable whether any treatment by paramedics other than airway management, simple first aid, and splinting is beneficial. The principal causes of immediate death from trauma are head injury (35%), exsanguination (50%), and airway or pulmonary problems (15%). Only the last of these can be treated in the field. Patients with head injury or airway and pulmonary problems benefit from endotracheal intubation to maintain effective ventilation and prevent aspiration and hypercapnia.

Most life-threatening injuries require hospital facilities and a well-organized team that can provide immediate treatment, including surgery, and any delay in the field usually worsens the outcome. One study showed that trauma victims with cardiac wounds who were treated by paramedics had longer delays in transportation and lower survival rates compared with victims treated by emergency medical technicians (EMTs) or nonmedical personnel. However, recent information shows that well-trained paramedics can prepare patients for transport quickly and then perform life-support procedures en route with a high rate of patient survival. Further studies are required to identify the procedures other than airway intubation that would improve the survival of these patients.

IMMEDIATE MEASURES AT THE SCENE OF AN ACCIDENT

When first seen, the victim of an accident may not appear to be badly injured. There may be little external evidence of injury, so when the mechanism of trauma is sufficient to produce severe injury, the victim must be handled as if a severe injury has occurred. The injured person must be protected from further trauma. First aid at the scene of an accident should be administered by trained personnel whenever possible. The simple act of moving a victim from one position to another, if done improperly, may compress or lacerate the spinal cord, puncture a lung, sever a major blood vessel, or compound a fracture, thereby converting a simple injury into a major one.

Whether the patient is first seen on the battlefield, beside a road, in the emergency ward, or in the hospital, the basic principles of initial management are the same:

(1) Is the victim breathing? If not, provide an airway and establish mouth-to mouth ventilation.

(2) Is there a pulse or heartbeat? If not, begin closed-chest compression.

(3) Is there gross external bleeding? If so, elevate the part if possible and apply enough external pressure to stop the bleeding. A tourniquet is rarely needed.

(4) Is there any question of injury to the spine? If so, protect the neck and spine before moving the patient.

(5) Splint obvious fractures.

As soon as these steps have been taken, the patient can be safely transported.

Specific details of prehospital management are considered in the following paragraphs.

1. Airway Management

The most important therapy that can be provided before the patient gets to the hospital is airway management. If there is any chance of cervical spine injury, inline immobilization of the neck should be maintained as airway maneuvers are done. Simple measures such as clearing the airway of debris, positioning the mandible, and the use of oral airways may be all that is necessary to ensure adequate ventilation. This can often be done by simple manipulation of the mandible or traction on the tongue, particularly in unconscious or semiconscious patients. After the mouth is forced open, the tongue can be grasped between the thumb and forefinger covered with a handkerchief or gauze bandage. The tip of the tongue should be pulled forward beyond the front teeth. The mandible should be manipulated either by pulling forward the angles of the lower jaw or by inserting the thumb between the upper and lower rows of teeth, grasping the mandible in the midline, and drawing it forward until the lower teeth are leading (Figure 13–2).

Suctioning the mouth and pharynx may clear them of blood, mucus, or vomitus so as to permit normal respiration. Repeated suctioning may be required to maintain an adequate airway at the scene of the accident and during transit to a medical facility. Aspiration of vomitus, a frequent cause of sudden death, must be prevented at all costs. A lateral and slightly head-down position is best for patients who are liable to vomit. In respiratory arrest, a clear airway must be provided and mouth-to-mouth breathing instituted if other means of ventilation are not available. In extreme situations, where the upper airway is occluded and the foreign body cannot be removed, it can be lifesaving to insert a large-bore needle or Angiocath (14-gauge) through the cricothyroid membrane (Figure 13–3). Trained personnel can also perform an open cricothyroidotomy if other airway attempts are unsuccessful. Whenever possible, patients who are unconscious or in profound shock should have the airway controlled with an endotracheal tube (Figure 13–4).

Although endotracheal intubation is the only prehospital treatment of proven benefit to trauma victims with potentially lethal injuries, few paramedics are trained or proficient in this skill. Extensive evaluation of the field use of endotracheal intubation by paramedics in emergency care systems has shown that relatively limited training is needed, that intubation is successful in 85–95% of cases, and that paramedics

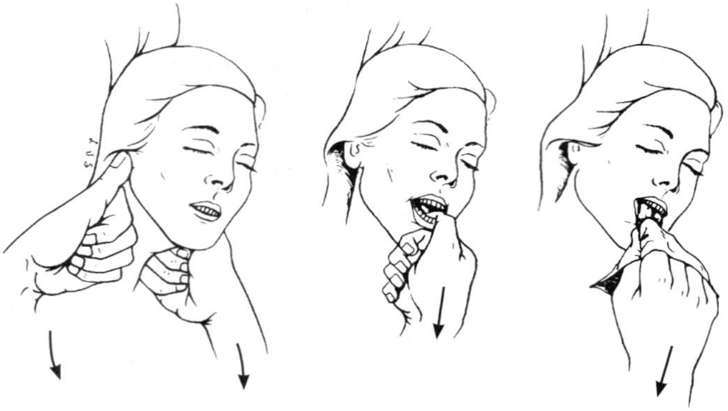

Figure 13–2. Relief of airway obstruction.

retain their skill in this technique even when the frequency of field use is only moderate. For these reasons, endotracheal intubation should be taught to all paramedics.

2. Intravenous Lines

Intravenous lines are critical for intravenous volume resuscitation. However, starting intravenous lines in the field may be counterproductive because the amount of fluid given during a brief trip to the hospital rarely compensates for the loss of blood that occurs during the time it takes to place the line. When extended delays to definitive treatment are inevitable because of long transport distances, intravenous infusions are more apt to be of benefit. Infusion of Ringer's lactate solution is the current recommended crystalloid resuscitation fluid. Two large-bore catheters of 14- to 16- gauge should be placed in the uninjured extremities with 2 L of Ringer's lactate infused for adults. This is the equivalent of 20 mL/kg bolus for a child. The role of other crystalloid or colloid solutions is yet to be clearly defined in the initial resuscitation setting.

3. Prehospital Cardiac Arrest

Cardiac arrest following trauma, when encountered at the scene of an accident, is usually fatal unless a correctable cause such as airway obstruction can be immediately identified. If blunt trauma is the cause

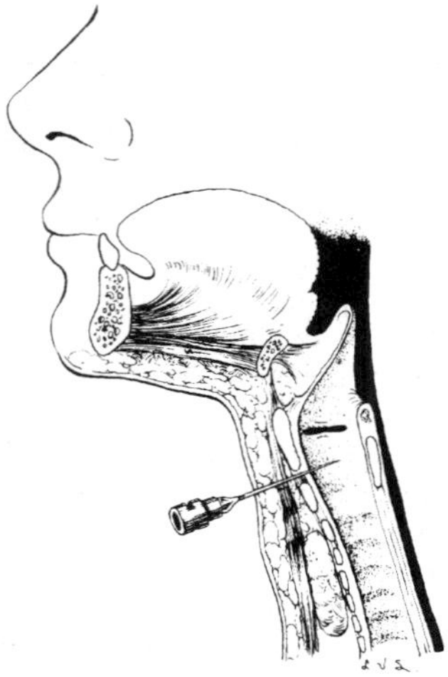

Figure 13–3. Needle in trachea to establish temporary airway.

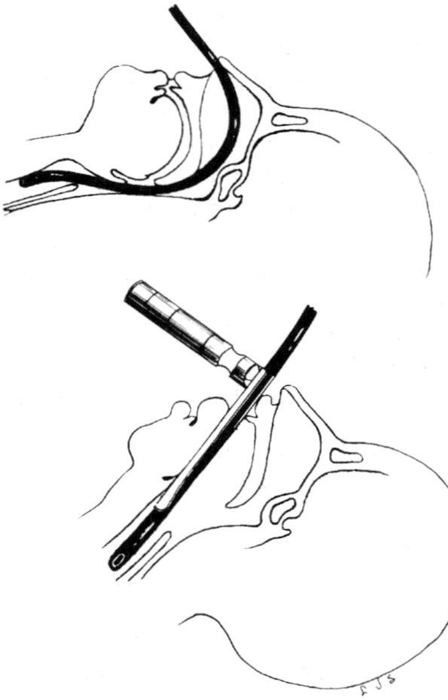

Figure 13–4. *Top:* Nasotracheal intubation. *Bottom*: Orotracheal intubation.

of prehospital arrest, the salvage rate almost is nil. If the cause is penetrating trauma—particularly stab wounds—the salvage rate is highest if the patient can be rapidly delivered to a trauma center. In such cases, ventilation by mouth-to-mouth resuscitation or a manual device should be initiated during transport, and closed-chest cardiac compression should be performed.

4. Neck, Spine, & Fracture Immobilization

All patients with major blunt trauma should be suspected of having spinal injury, and precautions should be taken to immobilize the spine and prevent further injury. Recognition and splinting of major fractures and immobilization of all injured parts before transportation are essential features of early management. Improper handling of the injured patient may worsen or prolong shock and aggravate existing trauma beyond the possibility of definitive repair. "Splint' em where they lie!" is a time-honored rule of emergency care of fractures that has only a few exceptions—when it is necessary to remove an injured patient from imminent danger of fire, explosion, escaping gas, etc. Immobilization should be achieved rapidly and should not delay transfer to the hospital.

5. Triage

Triage at the accident scene seeks to identify the patients who are most at risk of dying from their injuries and thus would benefit most from a trauma center. The ACS has published guidelines for the triage of trauma victims (Figure 13–5). Whenever in doubt, the patient should be transported to a trauma center.

6. Prehospital Transport

Transportation by ground or air ambulance is preferable when feasible. The choice of helicopter or ambulance depends upon time and distance and the level of care that must be provided en route. Ideally, transport should not exceed 15 minutes and the total prehospital time should not exceed 30 minutes. Resuscitation of the seriously injured patient should be continued during transportation, and a constant effort must be made to avoid airway obstruction and aspiration if the patient is vomiting.

If no ambulance is available, a station wagon or truck is preferable to a passenger car. The manipulation necessary to load a seriously injured person into a passenger car may be more harmful than the time lost in waiting for proper transportation. Except in unusual circumstances, injured patients should be transported in the supine position.

EVALUATION OF THE TRAUMA PATIENT

In most cases the history is obtained from prehospital personnel via radio communication or when the patient arrives at the hospital. In the case of motor vehicle accidents, for example, it is important to determine the circumstances of the injury, including the speed of impact, the condition of the vehicle, the position of the patient at the scene, evidence of blood loss, and the condition of other passengers. Record the time the injury occurred and the treatment rendered while en route. Every person who may have information about the circumstances of the injury should be questioned. Knowing the mechanism of the injury often gives a clue to concealed trauma. Information regarding serious underlying medical problems should be sought from Medic Alert bracelets or wallet cards. If the patient is conscious and stable, the examiner should obtain a complete history and use this information to direct the examination in order to avoid unnecessary tests.

Trauma victims require a precise, rapid, systematic approach to initial evaluation in order to ensure their survival. The Advanced Trauma Life Support (ATLS) system developed by the ACS Committee on Trauma represents the best current approach to the severely injured patient. The sequence of evaluation includes primary survey, resuscitation, secondary survey, and definitive management. The primary survey attempts to identify and treat immediate life-threatening conditions. Resuscitation is performed, and the response to therapy is evaluated. The secondary survey includes a comprehensive physical examination designed to detect all injuries and establish a treatment priority for potentially life-threatening ones. During the primary and secondary survey, appropriate laboratory and imaging studies are performed to aid in the identification of injuries and prepare the patient for definitive care.

1. Primary Survey

The Advanced Trauma Life Support manual and provider course published by the ACS Committee on Trauma is the accepted guideline for the primary survey. The primary survey is a rapid assessment to detect life-threatening injuries following the "A, B, Cs..." for Airway, Breathing, Circulation, Disability and Exposure/Environment.

AIRWAY

The establishment of an adequate airway has the highest priority in the primary survey. Oxygen by high flow nasal

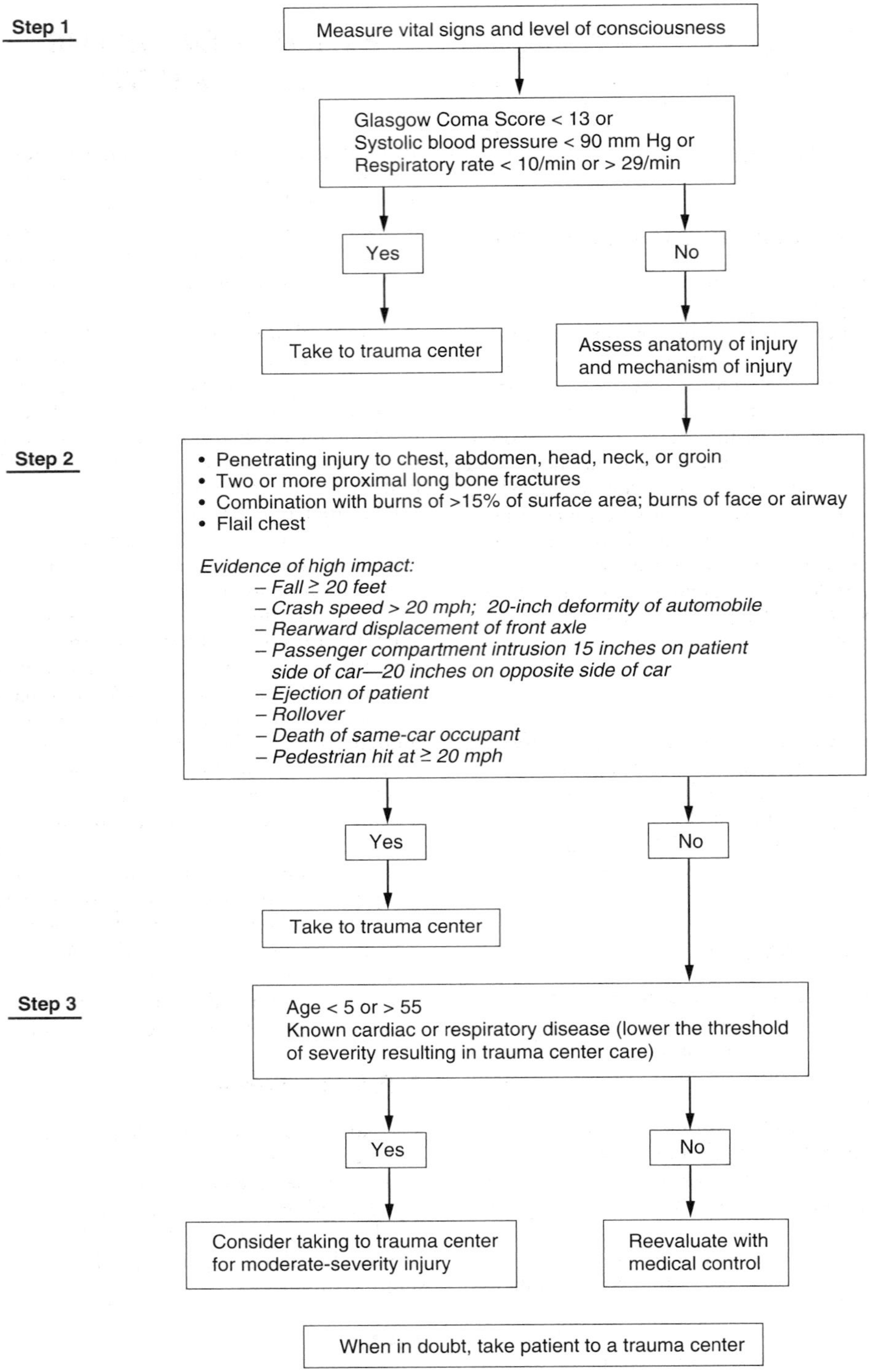

Figure 13–5. Triage scheme for trauma victims as published by the American College of Surgeons Committee on Trauma.

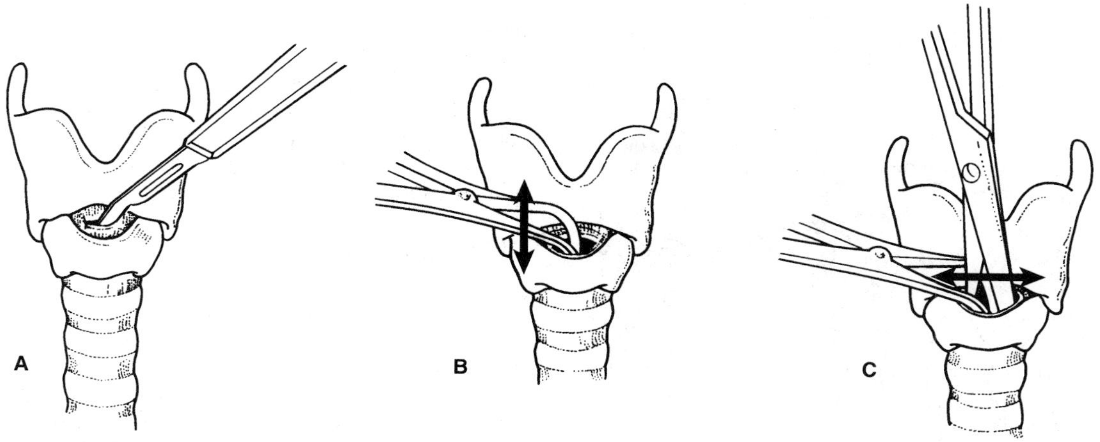

Figure 13–6. Surgical cricothyroidotomy.

cannula (10–12 L/min), 100% non-rebreather mask, or bag-mask ventilation with pulse oximetry should be started if not already in place. Maneuvers used in the trauma patient to establish an airway must consider a possible cervical spine injury. Any patient with multisystem trauma, especially those with an altered level of consciousness or blunt trauma above the clavicles, should be assumed to have a cervical spine injury. The rapid assessment for signs of airway obstruction should include inspection for foreign bodies and facial, jaw, or tracheal/laryngeal fractures that may result in acute loss of airway patency. Techniques that can be used to establish a patent airway while protecting the cervical spine include the chin lift or jaw thrust maneuvers.

Patients who can communicate verbally without difficulty are unlikely to have an impaired airway. Repeated assessment of airway patency is always prudent. Those patients with severe head injury, an altered level of consciousness, or a Glasgow Coma Scale (GCS) score of 8 or less usually require placement of a definitive airway. Orotracheal or nasotracheal intubation can be attempted with cervical spine precautions if a second person maintains axial immobilization of the head to prevent destabilization of the spine. If ventilatory failure occurs and an adequate airway cannot be obtained readily by orotracheal or nasotracheal intubation, surgical cricothyroidotomy should be performed as rapidly as possible (Figure 13–6).

BREATHING

Once the airway has been established, it is necessary to make certain that ventilation is adequate. Examine the patient to determine the degree of chest expansion, breath sounds, tachypnea, crepitus from rib fractures, subcutaneous emphysema, and the presence of penetrating or open wounds. Immediately life-threatening pulmonary injuries that must be detected and treated include presence of a tension pneumothorax, open pneumothorax, flail chest, and massive hemothorax. Chest injury is the second most common cause of asphyxia in the trauma patient. The following are examples of life-threatening pulmonary injuries:

(1) **Tension pneumothorax** occurs when air becomes trapped in the pleural space under pressure. The harmful effects result primarily from shift of the mediastinum, impairment of venous return, and potential occlusion of the airway. Tension pneumothorax is difficult to diagnose even when the patient reaches the hospital. The clinical findings consist of hypotension in the presence of distended neck veins, decreased or absent breath sounds on the affected side, hyperresonance to percussion, and tracheal shift away from the affected side. These signs may be difficult to detect in a hypovolemic patient with a cervical collar in place. Cyanosis may be a late manifestation. Emergency treatment consists of insertion of a large-bore needle or plastic intravenous cannula through the chest wall into the pleural space in the second intercostal space along the mid-clavicular line to relieve the pressure and convert the tension pneumothorax to a simple pneumothorax. The needle or cannula should be left in place while a thoracostomy tube is inserted for definitive management (Figure 13–7).

(2) **Open pneumothorax** results from an open wound of the chest wall with free communication between the pleural space and the atmosphere. The resulting impairment of the thoracic bellows and its ability to expand the lung results in inadequate ventilation. With chest expansion during a breath, air moves in and out

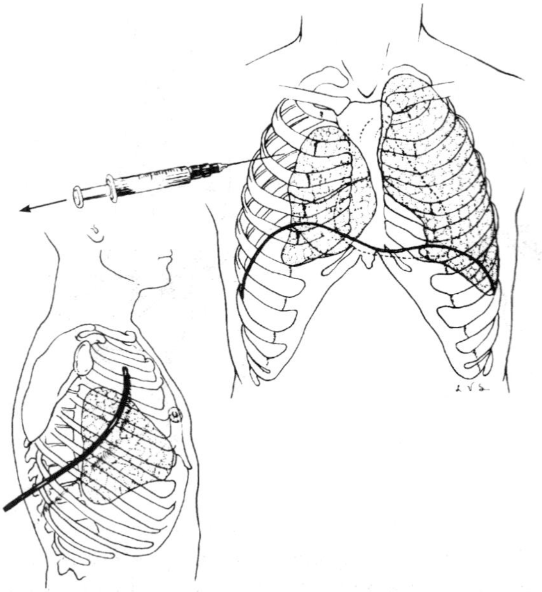

Figure 13–7. Relief of pneumothorax. Tension pneumothorax must be immediately decompressed by a needle introduced through the second anterior intercostal space. A chest tube is usually inserted in the mid-axillary line at the level of the nipple and is directed posteriorly and superiorly toward the apex of the thorax. The tube is attached to a "three-bottle" suction device, and the rate of escape of air is indicated by the appearance of bubbles in the second of the three bottles. Cessation of bubbling suggests that the air leak has become sealed.

of the chest wall opening instead of through the trachea, producing hypoventilation that can be rapidly fatal. Emergency treatment consists of sealing the wound with an occlusive sterile dressing tapped on three sides to act as a flutter-type valve or with any material if nothing sterile is available. Definitive treatment requires placement of a chest tube to reexpand the lung and surgical closure of the defect. Airway intubation with positive-pressure mechanical ventilation can be helpful in massive open pneumothorax.

(3) **Flail chest**: Multiple rib fractures resulting in a free-floating segment of chest wall may produce paradoxic motion that occurs with ventilatory efforts and impairs lung expansion (Figure 13–8). In patients with flail chest, injury-associated pulmonary contusion is common and is often the major cause of respiratory failure. The injury is identified by careful inspection and palpation during physical examination. Patients with large flail segments will almost always require prompt endotracheal intubation and mechanical ventilation, both to stabilize the flail segment and to optimize gas exchange. Smaller flail segments may be well tolerated if supplemental oxygen and adequate analgesia are provided. The work of breathing is increased considerably, and many patients who initially appear to be compensating well may suddenly deteriorate a few hours later. Therefore, most patients with flail chest require monitoring in an intensive care unit.

CIRCULATION

Hemorrhage

Free hemorrhage from accessible surface wounds is usually obvious and can be controlled in most cases by local pressure and elevation of the bleeding point. Firm pressure on the major artery in the axilla, antecubital space, wrist, groin, popliteal space, or at the ankle may suffice for temporary control of arterial hemorrhage distal to these points. When all other measures have failed, a tourniquet may be necessary to control major hemorrhage from extensive wounds or major vessels in an extremity. Failure to release the tourniquet periodically may cause irreparable vascular or neurologic damage. For this reason, the tourniquet should rarely be used and must be kept exposed and loosened at least every 20 minutes for 1 or 2 minutes while the patient is in transit and permanently removed as soon as definitive care is attained. It is wise to write the letters "TK" on the patient's forehead with a skin-marking pen or on adhesive tape.

Vascular Access

All patients with significant trauma should have large-caliber peripheral intravenous catheters inserted imme-

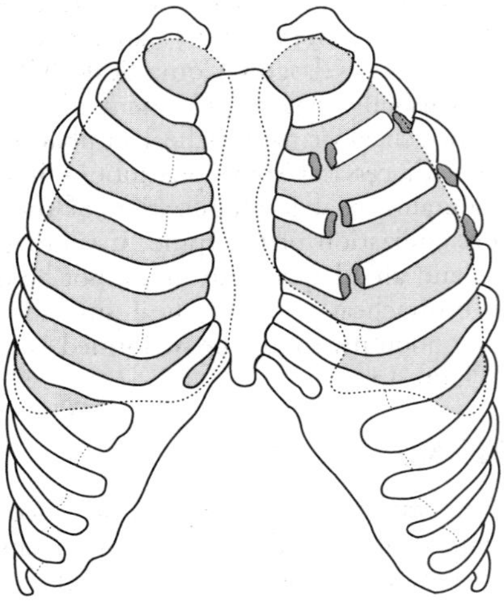

Figure 13–8. Flail chest.

diately for administration of crystalloid fluids as needed. If any degree of shock is present, at least two 14–16 gauge percutaneous intravenous lines should be established, usually in the antecubital fossa. If severe shock, hypovolemic cardiac arrest, or major vascular lesions are present, three intravenous lines are necessary, and one of the venous lines should be placed so that central venous pressure can be monitored as fluids are administered. If venous access cannot be obtained by percutaneous peripheral or central venous cannulation, a venous cutdown of the saphenous vein at the ankle using a sterile 8–10F feeding tube or intravenous extension tubing with the tip cut off can be performed. A blood sample for type and crossmatch should be sent from the venous line, if not already drawn.

As soon as the first intravenous line is inserted, rapid crystalloid infusion should begin. Adult patients should be given 2 L of Ringer's lactate or normal saline. An additional 2 L of crystalloid may be administered if there is no improvement in blood pressure or only a transient response. Beyond this amount, packed red blood cells must also be given in combination with crystalloid solutions to avoid excessive hemodilution. For children, the initial administered volume should be 20 mL/kg. Group O, Rh-negative packed red blood cells should be immediately available for any patient with impending cardiac arrest or massive hemorrhage. Type-specific blood should be available within 15 minutes of patient arrival to the hospital.

Monitoring

As intravenous access is obtained, electrocardiogram leads for continuous cardiac monitoring should be placed. Noninvasive blood pressure measurements of both upper extremities should be obtained with a time-cycled blood pressure cuff. Pulse oximetry is valuable in ensuring that adequate hemoglobin saturation is present in the injured patient.

NEUROLOGIC DISABILITY

A brief neurologic examination should be documented to assess the patient's degree of neurologic impairment, if any. Many factors may contribute to altered levels of consciousness and should be considered in addition to central nervous system injury in all trauma patients. Other than the direct trauma, the most common contributing causes of altered mental status for trauma patients are alcohol intoxication, other central nervous system stimulants or depressants, diabetic ketoacidosis, cerebrovascular accident, and hypovolemic shock. Less common causes are epilepsy, eclampsia, electrolyte imbalances associated with metabolic and systemic diseases, anaphylaxis, heavy metal poisoning, electric shock, tumors, severe systemic infections, hypercalcemia, asphyxia, heat stroke, severe heart failure, and hysteria. These uncommon causes of coma or diminished mental status should be considered if routine testing such as blood alcohol and glucose level, urine toxicology, and head computerized tomography (CT) are unrevealing as to the etiology of mental impairment. In such cases further laboratory and diagnostic testing may be warranted.

The differential diagnosis depends upon a careful history and complete physical examination, with particular attention to the neurologic examination with documentation of the patient's GCS score (Table 13–1), and an urgent head CT scan. The GCS score is useful in monitoring acute changes in neurologic function and is used for prognosticating outcomes after severe head injury. Lateralizing signs may also suggest evidence of an intracranial mass effect or carotid injury, while loss of distal motor or sensory function may help localize potential spinal cord injuries.

EXPOSURE/ENVIRONMENT

All clothing should be removed at once (cut off with trauma shears, usually) from the seriously injured patient, with great care being taken to avoid unnecessary movement. The removal of helmets or other protective clothing may require additional personnel to stabilize the patient and prevent further injury. All skin surfaces should be examined to identify injuries that may not be readily apparent, such as posterior penetrating trauma or open fractures. After inspecting all surfaces, warm blankets or warming devices should be placed to avoid hypothermia in the seriously injured patient.

Table 13–1. Glasgow Coma Scale Score.

Parameter	Score
Best motor response	
Normal	6
Localizes	5
Withdraws	4
Flexion	3
Extension	2
None	1
Best verbal response	
Oriented	5
Confused	4
Verbalizes	3
Vocalizes	2
None	1
Eye opening	
Spontaneous	4
To command	3
To pain	2
None	1

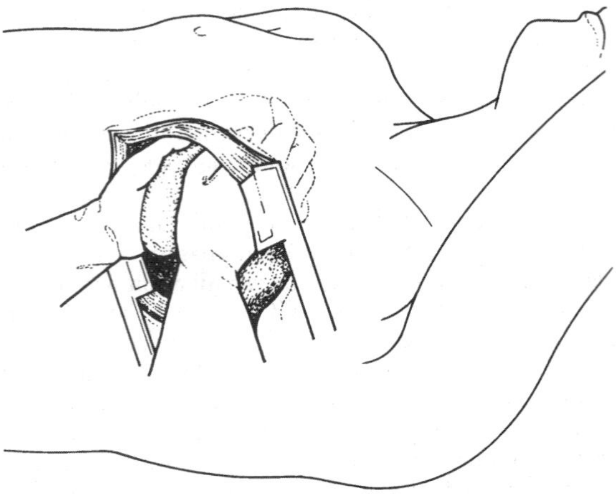

Figure 13–9. Emergency thoracotomy and open cardiac massage.

EMERGENCY ROOM THORACOTOMY

Certain injuries are so critical that operative treatment must be undertaken as soon as the diagnosis is made. In these cases, resuscitation is continued as the patient is being operated on. For cardiopulmonary arrest that occurs in the emergency room as a direct result of trauma, external cardiac compression is rarely successful in maintaining effective perfusion of vital organs. An emergency left anterolateral thoracotomy should be performed in the fourth or fifth intercostal space, and the pericardium should be opened anterior to the phrenic nerve (Figure 13–9). Open cardiac massage, cross-clamping of the descending thoracic aorta, repair of cardiac injuries, and internal defibrillation can be performed as appropriate. Wounds of the lung producing severe hemorrhage or systemic air embolus may require hilar cross-clamping.

Emergency room thoracotomy is most useful for cardiac arrest due to penetrating thoracic trauma, particularly in patients with pericardial tamponade. This extreme procedure is ineffective for most patients with arrest due to blunt trauma and for all patients who have no detectable vital signs in the field (< 1% survival). If vital signs are present in the emergency room but arrest appears imminent, the patient should be transferred rapidly to the operating room, since the conditions there are optimal for operation.

RESUSCITATION PHASE

Shock

Some degree of shock accompanies most severe injuries and is manifested initially by pallor, cold sweat, weakness, lightheadedness, hypotension, tachycardia, thirst, air hunger, and, eventually, loss of consciousness. Patients with any of these signs should be presumed to be in shock and evaluated thoroughly. All patients determined to be in any degree of shock should be reexamined at regular intervals. The degree of shock has been categorized to help guide resuscitation and recognize the severity of symptoms (Table 13–2).

A. Hypovolemic Shock

Hypovolemic shock is due to loss of whole blood or plasma. Blood pressure may be maintained initially by vasoconstriction. Tissue hypoxia increases when hypotension ensues, and shock may become irreversible if irreparable damage occurs to the vital organs. Massive or prolonged hemorrhage, severe crushing injuries, major fractures, and extensive burns are the most common causes. The presence of any of these conditions is an indication for prompt intravenous fluid infusion.

The patient must be kept recumbent and given reassurance and analgesics as necessary. If opioids are necessary for pain, they are best administered intravenously in

Table 13–2. Classification of hypovolemic shock.

	Class I	Class II	Class III	Class IV
Blood loss (mL)	Up to 750	750–1500	1500–2000	> 2000
Blood loss (%BV)	Up to 15%	15–30%	30–40%	> 40%
Pulse rate (beats/min)	< 100	> 100	> 120	> 140
Blood pressure	Normal	Minimal decrease	Decreased	Significantly decreased
Pulse pressure	Normal	Narrowed	Narrowed	Unobtainable or very narrow
Hourly urine output	≥ 0.5 cc/kg	≥ 0.5 cc/kg	< 0.5 cc/kg	Minimal
CNS/mental status	Slightly anxious	Mildly anxious	Anxious & confused	Confused or lethargic

small doses. Subcutaneous injections are poorly absorbed in these circumstances.

The most reliable clinical guide in assessing hypovolemic shock is skin perfusion. In mild or class 1 shock (< 15% blood volume loss), compensatory mechanisms may preserve adequate perfusion and no skin or physiologic changes may be apparent. In moderate or class 2 shock (15–30% blood loss), the skin on the extremities becomes pale, cool, and moist as a result of vasoconstriction and release of epinephrine. Systolic blood pressure is often maintained at near-normal levels, but urine output will usually decrease. With severe or class 3 shock (30–40% blood volume loss), these changes—particularly diaphoresis—become more marked, and urine output decreases significantly. Hypotension ensues. In addition, changes in cerebral function become evident, consisting chiefly of agitation, disorientation, and memory loss. A common error is to attribute uncooperative behavior to intoxication or drug use when in fact it may be due to cerebral ischemia from blood loss. With class 4 shock (> 40% blood volume loss), profound hypotension is typically accompanied by loss of consciousness and anuria. In this situation, rapid resuscitation with crystalloid and blood products is necessary to prevent imminent death.

With any degree of shock, balanced salt solution (eg, lactated Ringer's solution) should be given rapidly intravenously until the signs of shock abate and urine output returns to normal. If shock appears to be due to blood loss, blood transfusion should be given, starting with two units of uncross-matched O– blood if cross-matched blood is unavailable. Two to 4 liters of crystalloid solution can be given rapidly if needed to resuscitate the patient in severe shock. Successful resuscitation is indicated by warm, dry, well-perfused skin, a urine output of 30–60 mL/h, and an alert sensorium.

As a general principle, measurements of blood pressure and pulse are less reliable than changes in urine output in assessing the severity of shock. Young patients and athletic older ones have compensatory mechanisms that often maintain adequate blood pressure even with moderate volume loss. Older patients and those taking cardiac or blood pressure medications often do not exhibit tachycardia even with extreme volume loss. Therefore, a urinary catheter should be inserted for monitoring urine output in any patient with major injuries or shock. Oliguria is the most reliable sign of moderate shock, and successful resuscitation is indicated by a return of urine output to 0.5–1 mL/kg/h. Absence of oliguria is an unreliable index of the absence of shock if the patient has an osmotic diuresis due to alcohol, glucose, mannitol, or intravenous contrast material.

A patient who is receiving intravenous fluids at a high rate may not exhibit signs of shock even in the setting of ongoing hemorrhage. If a patient continues to require high volumes of fluid after initial resuscitation in order to maintain urine output, mental status, and blood pressure, further investigation must be performed to rule out occult hemorrhage.

B. Neurogenic Shock

Neurogenic shock is due to the pooling of blood in autonomically denervated venules and small veins and is usually due to spinal cord injury. Neurogenic shock is not caused by an isolated head injury, and in those patients other causes of shock should be sought. A patient thought to be in neurogenic shock should be given a 2 L crystalloid fluid bolus—followed by an additional bolus if the response is suboptimal. If shock persists with fluid resuscitation, phenylephrine or another vasopressor should be given as a drip with the dosage adjusted until the blood pressure is maintained at a satisfactory level. If the patient does not improve quickly, other kinds of shock must be considered. Patients with neurogenic shock may require central venous pressure monitoring to ensure an optimal volume status.

C. Cardiac Compressive Shock

Cardiac compressive shock is caused by compression of the thin-walled chambers of the heart—the atria and the right ventricle—or by compression or distortion of the great veins entering the heart. The usual causes of this type of shock in the trauma patient are pericardial tamponade, tension pneumothorax, massive hemothorax, diaphragmatic rupture with herniation of abdominal contents into the chest, and an elevated diaphragm from massive abdominal hemorrhage. Treatment consists of urgent decompression depending on the specific cause. In severe cases, emergency thoracotomy may be necessary to restore adequate cardiac function.

D. Cardiogenic Shock

Cardiogenic shock is caused by decreased myocardial contractility and is most commonly caused by myocardial infarction or arrhythmia. Older trauma patients may develop a myocardial infarction as a complication of their injuries. Rarely, a severe myocardial contusion may lead to cardiogenic shock. Treatment is supportive, with volume replacement guided by hemodynamic monitoring and administration of inotropic agents to augment cardiac output as necessary to maintain adequate organ perfusion.

Laboratory Studies

Immediately after intravenous catheters are placed, blood should be drawn for blood typing and cross-matching. If the patient has a history of renal, hepatic or cardiac disease or is taking diuretics or anticoagulants, serum electrolytes and coagulation parameters should be measured.

In most patients with serious injuries an arterial blood gas provides rapid data about acidosis and base deficit, both markers of under-resuscitation in addition to oxygenation (pO_2) and ventilation (pCO_2). Gross blood in the urine indicates the need for further diagnostic testing with abdominal CT scan or in selected cases, a cystogram and urethrogram. Patients with obvious severe head injury, where intracranial pressure monitoring may be indicated, should have coagulation studies and a platelet count performed. Measurement of blood alcohol level and urine toxicology screen may be useful in patients with altered mental status.

Imaging Studies

Radiographic plain films of the chest and pelvis are required in all major injuries. Lateral C-spine films may be helpful in patients with neurologic deficit or unexplained hypotension. Bedside Focused Assessment with Sonography for Trauma (FAST) imaging is now an acceptable triage method for determining the presence of hemoperitoneum in blunt trauma patients or cardiac tamponade in blunt and penetrating trauma patients. The presence of hemoperitoneum in an unstable patient on FAST may be an indication for exploratory laparotomy. Presence of hemoperitoneum in a stable patient or a negative FAST in a patient with abdominal pain is indication for further evaluation with abdominal CT scan. Abnormal chest radiographs with a mechanism for blunt aortic injury should undergo further screening with either helical chest computerized tomography done at the time of abdominal imaging or with aortography, if necessary. Cervical spine imaging should be obtained for patients who are unconscious, have pain in the cervical region, have neurologic deficits, or who have painful or distracting injuries. CT scanning of the head should be performed in all patients with loss of consciousness or more serious neurologic impairment. Radiographs of the long bones and non-cervical spine can usually be deferred until the more critical injuries of the thorax and abdomen have been delineated and stabilized.

2. Secondary Survey & Treatment Priorities

A rapid and complete history and physical examination (with a written record of the findings) are essential for patients with serious or multiple injuries. Progressive changes in clinical findings are often the key to correct diagnosis, and negative findings that change to positive may be of great importance in revising an initial clinical evaluation. This is particularly true in the case of abdominal, thoracic, and intracranial injuries, which frequently do not become manifest until hours after the trauma.

Certain kinds of trauma are apt to cause more than one injury. For example, fractures of the calcaneus resulting from a fall from a great height are often associated with central dislocation of the hip and fractures of the spine and of the skull base. A crushed pelvis is often combined with laceration of the posterior urethra or bladder, vagina, or rectum. Crush injuries of the chest are often associated with lacerations or rupture of the spleen, liver, or diaphragm. Penetrating wounds of the chest may involve not only the thoracic contents but also the abdominal viscera. These combinations occur frequently and should always be suspected.

TREATMENT PRIORITIES

In all cases of patients with multiple injuries, there must be a "captain of the team" who directs the resuscitation, decides which x-rays or special diagnostic tests should be obtained, and establishes priority for care by continuous consultation with other surgical specialists and anesthesiologists. A trauma surgeon or a general surgeon experienced in the care of injured patients usually has this role.

After controlling the airway if necessary, resuscitation and blood volume replacement have first priority. Deepening stupor in patients under observation should arouse suspicion of an expanding intracranial lesion requiring repeated neurologic examination and head computerized tomography. Too often, obvious signs of acute alcohol intoxication have been assumed to be the cause of unconsciousness, and intracranial hemorrhage has been overlooked.

Cerebral injuries take precedence in care only when there is rapidly deepening coma. Extradural bleeding is a critical emergency, requiring operation for control and cerebral decompression. Subdural bleeding may produce a similar emergency. If the patient's condition permits, CT scanning should be performed for localization of the bleeding. In many cases of combined cerebral and abdominal injury with massive bleeding, laparotomy and craniotomy should be performed simultaneously.

In most cases, fractures of the skull have a low priority and can be dealt with after more critical abdominal or thoracic injuries have been treated.

Most urologic injuries are managed at the same time as associated intra-abdominal injuries. Pelvic fractures present special problems and are discussed in Chapters 40 and 42.

Unless there is associated vascular injury with threatened ischemia of the limb, fractures of the long bones can be splinted and treated on an urgent basis. Open contaminated fractures should be cleansed and debrided as soon as possible.

Injuries of the hand run the risk of infection that may result in a lifelong handicap without early effective treatment. Early treatment of the hand at the same time as treatment of any life-threatening injuries avoids infection and preserves the means of livelihood.

Tetanus prophylaxis should be given in all instances of open contaminated wounds, puncture wounds, and burns.

Details of definitive management of injuries are discussed in the sections on trauma that follow and in the various organ system chapters of this book.

NECK INJURIES

All injuries to the neck are potentially life-threatening because of the many vital structures in this area. Injuries to the neck are classified as blunt or penetrating, and the treatment is different for each.

Penetrating injuries of the neck are divided into three anatomic zones (Figure 13–10). Zone I injuries occur at the thoracic outlet, which extends from the level of the cricoid cartilage to the clavicles. Included in this area are the proximal carotid arteries, the subclavian vessels, and the major vessels in the chest. Proximal control of injuries to vascular structures in this zone often requires a thoracotomy or sternotomy. Zone II injuries occur in the area between the cricoid and the angle of the mandible. Injuries here are the easiest to expose and evaluate. Zone III injuries are between the angle of the mandible and the base of the skull. Exposure is much more difficult in this zone and in some cases may require disarticulation of the mandible. High injuries can be inaccessible, and control of hemorrhage may require ligation of major proximal vessels or angiographic embolization.

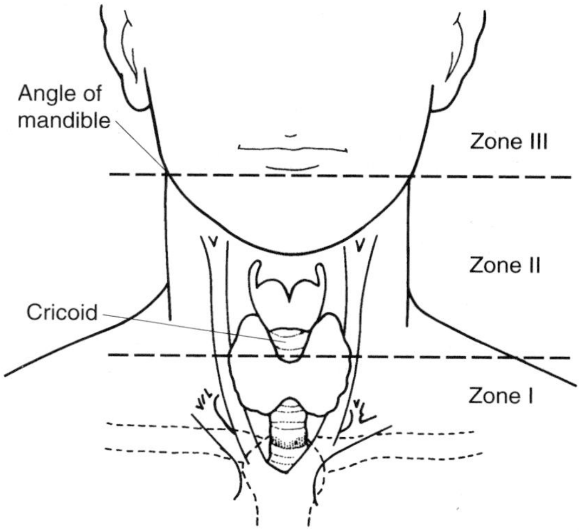

Figure 13–10. Zones of the neck.

Penetrating trauma to the posterior neck may injure the vertebral column, the cervical spinal cord, the interosseous portion of the vertebral artery, and the neck musculature. Penetrating trauma to the anterior and lateral neck may injure the larynx, trachea, esophagus, thyroid, carotid arteries, subclavian arteries, jugular veins, subclavian veins, and thoracic duct.

Blunt cervical trauma may cause fracture or dislocation of the cervical vertebrae (with the risk of spinal cord injury), traumatic occlusion or dissection of the carotid arteries, cerebrospinal fluid cysts, or laryngeal and tracheal injuries complicated by hemorrhage and airway obstruction.

The patient must be examined closely for associated head and chest injuries. The initial level of consciousness is of paramount importance; progressive depression of the sensorium may signify intracranial bleeding or cerebral ischemia and requires neurosurgical evaluation. Trauma to the base of the neck may lacerate major blood vessels. Hemorrhage into the pleural cavity may occur suddenly as contained hematomas rupture.

Clinical Findings

Injuries to the larynx and trachea can be asymptomatic or may cause hoarseness, laryngeal stridor, or dyspnea secondary to airway compression or aspiration of blood. Subcutaneous emphysema in the neck can be present if the wall of the larynx or trachea has been disrupted.

Esophageal injuries are rarely isolated and by themselves may not cause immediate symptoms. Severe chest pain and dysphagia are characteristic of esophageal perforation. Hours later, as mediastinitis develops, progressive sepsis may occur. Mediastinitis results because the deep cervical space is in direct continuity with the mediastinum. Esophageal injuries can be recognized promptly if the surgeon is alert to the possibility and seeks out early diagnosis. Exploration of the neck, radiographic examination of the esophagus with contrast medium, and in selected cases flexible esophagoscopy confirm the diagnosis.

Cervical spine and cord injuries should always be suspected in deceleration injuries or following direct trauma to the neck. If the patient complains of cervical pain or tenderness or if the level of consciousness is depressed, the head and neck should be immobilized (eg, with a rigid cervical collar or sandbags) until cervical radiographs can be taken to rule out cervical fracture or ligamentous injury.

Injury to the great vessels (subclavian, common carotid, internal carotid, and external carotid arteries; subclavian, internal jugular, and external jugular veins) may follow blunt or penetrating trauma. Fractures of the clavicle or first rib may lacerate the subclavian artery and vein. With vascular injuries, the patient typically presents with visible external blood loss, neck hematoma formation, and in varying degrees of shock. Occasionally, bleeding may be contained and the injury may go undetected for a short time. Auscultation may reveal bruits that suggest arterial injury.

Diagnosis

With any penetrating cervical trauma, the likelihood of significant injury is high because there are so many vital structures in such a small space. Any patient with shock, expanding hematoma, or uncontrolled hemorrhage should be taken to the operating room for emergency exploration. The location of the injury suggests which structures may be involved. Vascular injuries at the base of the neck require thoracotomy to obtain proximal control of injured blood vessels before the site of probable injury is exposed. If the patient is stable after resuscitation, additional diagnostic testing may be considered.

Arteriography is usually recommended for patients with injuries in zones I and III because precise identification of the location and extent of injury may alter the operative approach. If possible, arteriography should be performed before exploration of any injury in which blood vessels may be damaged below the level of the cricoid cartilage or above a line connecting the mastoid process with the angle of the jaw. Arterial injuries above this line are practically inaccessible. If injury to the carotid artery at the base of the skull is confirmed by arteriography, repair may not be possible and ligation may be required to control bleeding. Injured carotid arteries that have produced a neurologic deficit should be repaired if possible. The morbidity and mortality of patients undergoing carotid artery repair are significantly lower than those who have ligation of the carotid artery (15% versus 50%). Carotid artery ligation is indicated in the patient who presents with uncontrollable hemorrhage or coma with no prograde flow in the carotid artery.

Since exposure of injuries in zone II is relatively easy to obtain, a policy of mandatory exploration has been the traditional recommendation for all injuries penetrating the platysma in this area. Although this approach is safe, reliable, and time-tested, recent studies have demonstrated that a selective approach is as safe provided that diagnostic testing does not detect a major injury. High-resolution helical CT scanning of the neck has been used recently to guide surgical decision making in zone II penetrating injuries. In the absence of an obvious vascular injury on clinical examination, ultrasound with color flow Doppler has been demonstrated to be reliable in ruling out carotid artery injuries. Arteriography can also be used in this setting and may offer the advantage of identifying an unsuspected vertebral artery injury. Vertebral artery injuries should also be suspected when bleeding from a posterior or lateral neck wound cannot be controlled by pressure on the carotid artery or when there is bleeding from a posterolateral wound associated with fracture of a cervical transverse process. Flexible or rigid endoscopy can be used to evaluate the trachea and esophagus. A contrast study of the upper esophagus should be performed to identify esophageal injuries that might not be readily apparent on endoscopy. These injuries can be difficult to detect and are occasionally missed on surgical exploration. In either case, repeated, careful examinations should be performed.

Fractures of the cervical spine can be confirmed by plain radiographs or CT scan. Radiographic studies of the soft tissues can locate opaque foreign bodies if present and help determine the trajectory and path of the missile in patients with penetrating trauma to the neck.

The most important injuries resulting from blunt cervical trauma are (1) cervical fracture, (2) cervical spinal cord injury, (3) vascular injury, and (4) laryngeal and tracheal injury. Radiographs of the cervical spine and soft tissues are essential. Careful neurologic examination can differentiate between injuries to the spinal cord, brachial plexus, and brain.

Complications

The complications of untreated neck trauma are related to the individual structures injured. Injuries to the larynx and trachea can result in acute airway obstruction, late tracheal stenosis, and sepsis. Cervicomediastinal sepsis can result from esophageal injuries. Carotid artery injuries can produce death from hemorrhage, stroke, or cerebral ischemia, and arteriovenous fistula with cardiac decompensation. Major venous injury can result in exsanguination, air embolism, and arteriovenous fistula formation if there is concomitant arterial injury. Cervical fracture can result in paraplegia, quadriplegia, or death.

Prevention of these complications depends upon immediate resuscitation by intubation of the airway, prompt control of external hemorrhage and blood replacement, protection of the head and neck when cervical fracture is possible, accurate and rapid diagnosis, and prompt operative treatment when indicated.

Treatment

Control of the airway with early intubation is the first key maneuver to successful management of severe neck injuries. Any wound of the neck that penetrates the platysma requires prompt surgical exploration or diagnostic workup to rule out major vascular injury. In patients with zone II injuries, color flow Doppler imaging may provide a reliable way to assess for vascular injury and can be a safe alternative to routine contrast angiography. Arteries damaged by high-velocity missiles require debridement. End-to-end anastomosis of the mobilized vessels is preferred, but if a significant segment is lost, an autogenous vein graft can be used. Vertebral artery injury presents a formidable technical problem because of the interosseous course of the artery shortly after it arises from the subclavian artery. Although unilateral vertebral artery ligation has been followed by fatal midbrain or cerebellar necrosis, because of inadequate communication to the basilar artery, only 3% of patients with left vertebral ligation and 2% of patients with right vertebral ligation develop these complications. Therefore, in the face of massive hemorrhage from a partially severed vertebral artery, ligation with surgical clips applied to the vessel between the transverse processes above and below the laceration is accepted.

Subclavian artery injuries are best approached through a combined cervicothoracic incision. Proper exposure is the key to success in the management of these difficult and too often fatal injuries. Ligation of the subclavian artery is relatively safe, but primary repair is preferable. Care should be taken to avoid phrenic nerve and thoracic duct injury when operating in this region of the neck.

Venous injuries are best managed by ligation. The possibility of air embolism must be kept constantly in mind. A simple means of preventing this complication is to lower the patient's head using the Trendelenburg position until bleeding is controlled.

Esophageal injuries should be sutured closed primarily and drained. Use of muscle flaps to cover the repair can be helpful. Drainage is the mainstay of treatment. Extensive injury to the esophagus is often immediately fatal, because of associated injuries to the spinal cord. Systemic antibiotics should be administered routinely to patients with esophageal injuries.

Minor laryngeal and tracheal injuries do not require treatment, but immediate tracheostomy should be performed when airway obstruction exists. If there has been significant injury to the thyroid cartilage, a temporary laryngeal stent (Silastic) should be employed to provide support. Mucosal lacerations should be approximated before insertion of the stent. Conveniently located small perforations of the trachea can be utilized for tracheostomy. Otherwise, the wounds can be closed after they are debrided and a distal tracheostomy performed. Extensive circumferential tracheal injuries may require resection and anastomosis or reconstruction using synthetic materials.

Primary neurorrhaphy should be attempted for nerve injury. Bilateral vagal nerve injury results in hoarseness and dysphagia. Cervical spinal cord injury should be managed in such a way as to prevent further damage. When there is cervical cord compression from hematoma formation, vertebral fractures, or foreign bodies, decompression laminectomy is necessary.

Blunt trauma to the neck rarely requires direct surgical treatment. More commonly, the soft tissues are contused, but hematomas may develop and cause tracheal compression and respiratory compromise. Tracheostomy is indicated in this instance. Cervical fractures are managed with external immobilization using rigid collars or a halo/vest apparatus. In some selected cases operation to perform reduction and internal fixation with implantable hardware is undertaken. Vascular injuries may occur in cases of severe or localized blunt neck trauma. The common or internal carotid arteries can be torn or can undergo disruption of the intima and require vascular reconstruction. Carotid arteriograms are essential to the diagnosis and should be considered in selected patients. Sometimes blunt carotid injuries are not amenable to operative intervention due to the location or extent of injury. The use of endovascular stent techniques to repair or control blunt carotid artery injuries is feasible, but the indications and determination of outcomes are still in evolution. The value of anticoagulation after blunt injury to the carotid artery continues to be debated, and antiplatelet therapy is a reasonable alternative to full systemic anticoagulation.

Prognosis

Severe laceration of the cervical spinal cord often results in paralysis. Injuries to the soft tissues of the neck, trachea, and esophagus have a good to excellent prognosis if promptly treated. Major vascular injuries have a good prognosis if promptly treated before the onset of irreversible shock or neurologic deficit. The overall death rate for cervical injuries is about 10%.

Barba CA et al: A new cervical spine clearance protocol using computed tomography. J Trauma 2001;51:652.

Cothren CC et al: Anticoagulation is the gold standard therapy for blunt carotid injuries to reduce stroke rate. Arch Surg 2004; 139:540.

Demetriades D et al: Penetrating injuries of the neck in patients in stable condition. Physical examination, angiography, or color flow Doppler imaging. Arch Surg 1995;130:971.

Eddy VA and the Zone 1 Penetrating Neck Injury Study Group: Is routine arteriography mandatory for penetrating injury to zone 1 of the neck? J Trauma 2000;48:208.

Gonzalez RP et al: Penetrating zone II neck injury: does dynamic computed tomographic scan contribute to the diagnostic sensitivity of physical examination for surgically significant injury? A prospective blinded study. J Trauma 2003;54:61.

Gracias VH et al: Computed tomography in the evaluation of penetrating neck trauma. Arch Surg 2001;136:1231.

Grossman MD et al: National survey of the incidence of cervical spine injury and approach to cervical spine clearance in U.S. trauma centers. J Trauma 1999;47:684.

Irish JC et al: Penetrating and blunt neck trauma: 10-year review of a Canadian experience. Can J Surg 1997;40:33.

Liekweg WG, Greenfield LJ: Management of penetrating carotid arterial injury. Ann of Surg 1978;188:587.

Mazolewski PJ et al: Computed tomographic scan can be used for surgical decision making in zone II penetrating neck injuries. J Trauma 2001;51:315.

Schenarts P et al: Prospective comparison of admission CT scan and plain films of the upper cervical spine in trauma patients with altered mental status. J Trauma 2000;49:1163.

Sofianos C et al: Selective surgical management of zone II gunshot injuries of the neck: a prospective study. Surgery 1996;120:785.

Wahl WL et al: Antiplatelet therapy: an alternative to heparin for blunt carotid injury. J Trauma 2002;52:896.

THORACIC INJURIES

Thoracic trauma accounts directly for or is a contributing factor in 50% of deaths due to trauma. Early deaths are commonly due to (1) airway obstruction, (2) flail chest, (3) open pneumothorax, (4) massive hemothorax, (5) tension pneumothorax, and (6) cardiac tamponade. Later deaths are due to respiratory failure, sepsis, and unrecognized injuries. The preponderance of blunt thoracic injuries are the result of automobile accidents. Even what appears as a minor blunt thoracic injury leading to rib fractures and pulmonary contusions can have a profound effect on elderly patients. Near-side collisions are responsible for a higher incidence of blunt aortic injury among older adults and are associated with lower delta V forces compared to those in younger patients. Penetrating chest injuries from knives, bullets, etc, are deadly and can result in complex patterns of injury. The death rate in hospitalized patients with isolated chest injury is 4–8%; it is 10–15% when one other organ system is involved and rises to 35% if multiple additional organs are injured.

Combined injuries of multiple intrathoracic structures are typical. There are often other injuries to the abdomen, head, or skeletal system. Eighty-five percent of chest injuries do not require open thoracotomy, but immediate use of lifesaving measures is often necessary and should be within the competence of all surgeons.

When the physician is confronted with a patient who has sustained thoracic injuries, a rapid estimate of cardiorespiratory status and possible associated injuries gives a valuable overview. For example, patients with upper airway obstruction appear cyanotic, ashen, or gray; examination reveals stridor or gurgling sounds, ineffective respiratory excursion, constriction of cervical muscles, and retraction of the suprasternal, supraclavicular, intercostal, or epigastric regions. The character of chest wall excursions and the presence or absence of penetrating wounds can be observed. If respiratory excursions are not visible, ventilation is probably inadequate. Severe paradoxic chest wall movement in flail chest is usually located anteriorly and can be seen immediately. Sucking wounds of the chest wall should be obvious. A large hemothorax can usually be detected by percussion, and subcutaneous emphysema is easily detected. Both massive hemothorax and tension pneumothorax may produce absent or diminished breath sounds and a shift of the trachea to the opposite side, but in massive hemothorax the neck veins are usually collapsed. If the patient has a thready or absent pulse and distended neck veins, the main differential diagnosis is between cardiac tamponade and tension pneumothorax. In moribund patients, diagnosis must be immediate, and treatment may require chest tube placement, pericardiocentesis, or thoracotomy in the emergency room. The first priority of management should be to provide an airway and restore circulation. One can then reassess the patient and outline definitive measures. A cuffed endotracheal tube and assisted ventilation are required for apnea, ineffectual breathing, severe shock, deep coma, airway obstruction, flail chest, or open sucking chest wounds. Persistent shock or hypoxia may be due to massive hemorrhage, cardiac tamponade, or tension pneumothorax. Shock due to thoracic trauma may be caused by any of the following: massive hemopneumothorax, cardiac tamponade, tension pneumothorax or massive air leak, or air embolism. If hemorrhagic shock is not explained readily by findings on chest x-ray or external losses, it is almost certainly due to intra-abdominal bleeding.

Types of Injuries

A. Chest Wall

Rib fracture, the most common chest injury, varies across a spectrum from simple fracture to fracture with hemopneumothorax to severe multiple fractures with flail chest, pulmonary contusion, and internal injuries. With simple fractures, pain on inspiration is the principal symptom; treatment consists of providing adequate analgesia. In cases of multiple fractures, intercostal nerve blocks or epidural analgesia may be required to ensure adequate ventilation. Measures such as strapping the chest wall with adhesive tape or the placement of elastic binders will interfere with adequate ventilation and lead to the development of atelectasis—and they have no place in the modern management of rib fractures. Multiple fractures may be associated with voluntarily decreased ventilation and subsequent pneumonitis, particularly in the elderly patient.

Flail chest occurs when a portion of the chest wall becomes isolated by multiple fractures and paradoxically moves in and out with inspiration and expiration with a potentially severe reduction in ventilatory efficiency. The magnitude of the effect is determined by the size of the flail segment and the amount of pain with breathing. The rib fractures are usually anterior and there are at least two fractures of the same rib. Bilateral costochondral separation and sternal fractures can also cause a flail segment. An associated lung contusion may produce a decrease in lung compliance not fully manifest until 12–48 hours after injury. Increased negative intrapleural pressure is then required for ventilation, and chest wall instability becomes apparent. If ventilation becomes inadequate, atelectasis, hypercapnia, hypoxia, accumulation of secretions, and ineffective cough occur. Arterial PO_2 is often low before clinical findings appear. Serial blood gas analysis is the best way to determine if a treatment regimen is adequate. For less severe cases, intercostal nerve block or continuous epidural analgesia may be adequate treatment. However, most cases require ventilatory assistance for variable periods of time with a cuffed endotracheal tube and a mechanical ventilator. External fixation of the chest wall is less reliable than positive-pressure ventilation for the average case but may be useful for severe sternal flail or other extensive injuries associated with chest wall instability.

B. Trachea and Bronchus

Blunt tracheobronchial injuries are often due to compression of the airway between the sternum and the vertebral column in decelerating or high-velocity crush accidents. The distal trachea or main stem bronchi are usually involved and 80% of all injuries are located within 2.5 cm from the carina. Penetrating tracheobronchial injuries may occur at any location. Most patients have pneumothorax, subcutaneous emphysema, pneumomediastinum, and hemoptysis. Cervicofacial emphysema may be dramatic. Tracheobronchial injury should be suspected when there is a massive air leak or when the lung does not readily reexpand after chest tube placement. In penetrating injuries of the trachea or main stem bronchi, there is usually massive hemorrhage and hemoptysis. Systemic air embolism resulting in cardiopulmonary arrest may occur if a bronchovenous fistula is present. If air embolism is suspected, emergency thoracotomy should be performed with cross-clamping of the pulmonary hilum on the affected side. The diagnosis is confirmed by aspiration of air from the heart. In blunt injuries, the tracheobronchial injury may not be obvious and may be suspected only after major atelectasis develops several days later. Diagnosis may require flexible or rigid bronchoscopy. Immediate primary repair is indicated for all tracheobronchial lacerations.

C. Pleural Space

Hemothorax (blood within the pleural cavity) is classified according to the amount of blood: minimal, 350 mL; moderate, 350–1500 mL; or massive, 1500 mL or more. The rate of bleeding after evacuation of the hemothorax is clinically even more important. If air is also present, the condition is called hemopneumothorax.

Hemothorax should be suspected with penetrating or severe blunt thoracic injury. There may be decreased breath sounds and dullness to percussion, and a chest x-ray should be promptly obtained (Figure 13–11). In experienced hands ultrasound can diagnose pneumothorax and hemothorax, but this technique is not widely employed at this time. Tube thoracostomy should be performed expeditiously for all hemo- or pneumothoraces. In 85% of cases, tube thoracostomy is the only treatment required. If bleeding is persistent, as noted by continued output from the chest tubes, it is more likely to be from a systemic (eg, intercostal) rather than a pulmonary artery. When the rate of bleeding shows a steady trend of greater than 200 mL/h or the total hemorrhagic output exceeds 1500 mL, thoracoscopy or thoracotomy should usually be performed. The trend and rate of thoracic bleeding is probably more important than the absolute numbers in deciding to perform surgical intervention. Thoracoscopy has been shown to be effective in controlling chest tube bleeding in 82% of cases. This technique has also been shown to be 90% effective in evacuating retained hemothoraces. In most of these cases, the chest wall is the source of hemorrhage. Thoracotomy is required for management of injuries to the lungs, heart, pericardium, and great vessels.

Pneumothorax occurs in lacerations of the lung or chest wall following penetrating or blunt chest trauma. Hyperinflation (eg, blast injuries, diving accidents) can also rupture the lungs. After penetrating injury, 80% of patients with pneumothorax also have blood in the pleural cavity. Most cases of pneumothorax are readily diagnosed on chest x-ray. In some cases, an occult pneumothorax will be identified on an abdominal CT scan that includes sections of the lower chest. Pneumothorax or hemothorax may be identified on the lateral scans that are performed as part of the FAST examination of the abdomen for trauma (see section on abdominal trauma). Most cases of traumatic pneumothorax should be treated with immediate tube thoracostomy.

Tension pneumothorax develops when a flap-valve leak allows air to enter the pleural space but prevents its escape; intrapleural pressure rises, causing total collapse of the lung and a shift of the mediastinal viscera to the

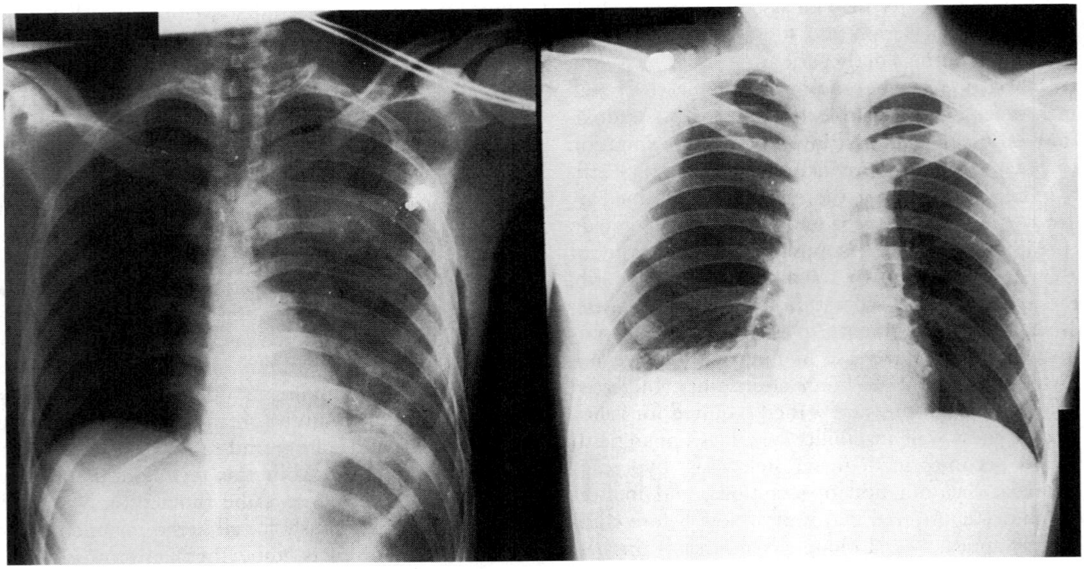

Figure 13–11. Hemopneumothorax. Supine (*left*) and upright films (on different patients).

opposite side, interfering with venous return to the heart. It must be relieved immediately to avoid impairment of cardiac function. Immediate treatment involves placement of a large-bore needle or plastic angiocatheter in the pleural space with care being taken to avoid injury to the intercostal vessels. After this emergency measure has been instituted, tension pneumothorax should be treated definitively by tube thoracostomy.

Sucking chest wounds, which allow air to pass in and out of the pleural cavity, should be promptly treated by an occlusive dressing and tube thoracostomy. The pathologic physiology resembles flail chest except that the extent of associated lung injury is usually less. Definitive management includes surgical closure of the defect in the chest wall.

D. Lung Injury

Pulmonary contusion due to sudden parenchymal concussion occurs after blunt trauma or wounding with a high-velocity missile. Pulmonary contusion occurs in 75% of patients with flail chest but can also occur following blunt trauma without rib fracture. Alveolar rupture with fluid transudation and extravasation of blood are early findings. Fluid and blood from ruptured alveoli enter alveolar spaces and bronchi and produce localized airway obstruction and atelectasis. Increased mucous secretions and overzealous intravenous fluid therapy may combine to produce copious secretions and further atelectasis. The patient's ability to cough and clear secretions effectively is weakened because of chest wall pain or mechanical inefficiency from fractures. Elasticity of the lungs is decreased, resistance to air flow increases, and, as the work of breathing increases, blood oxygenation and pH drop and pCO_2 rises. The cardiac compensatory response may be compromised, because as many as 35% of these patients have an associated myocardial contusion.

Treatment is often delayed because clinical and x-ray findings may not appear until 12–48 hours after injury. The clinical findings are copious thin, blood-tinged secretions, chest pain, restlessness, apprehensiveness, and labored respirations. Eventually, dyspnea, cyanosis, tachypnea, and tachycardia develop. X-ray changes consist of patchy parenchymal opacification or diffuse linear peribronchial densities that may progress to diffuse opacification ("white-out") characteristic for acute respiratory distress syndrome.

Mechanical ventilatory support permits adequate alveolar ventilation and the use of enriched oxygen mixtures and thus reduces the work of breathing. Blood gases should be monitored frequently and arterial saturation adequately maintained. There is some controversy over the best regimen for fluid management, but excessive hydration or blood transfusion should be avoided. Optimal management may require placement of a pulmonary artery catheter, preferably with a thermistor tip for measurement of continuous cardiac output by thermodilution. Serial measurement of central venous pressure, pulmonary arterial pressure, wedge pressures, mixed venous oxygen saturation, and cardiac output helps to avoid either under- or overtransfusion. Despite optimal therapy, about 15% of patients with pulmonary contusion die. Use of protective mechanical ventilator strategies is essential in these patients to avoid progressive ventilator induced lung injury.

Most lung lacerations are caused by penetrating injuries, and hemopneumothorax is usually present. Tube thoracostomy is indicated to evacuate pleural air or blood and to monitor continuing leaks. Since expansion of the lung tamponades the laceration, most lung lacerations do not produce massive hemorrhage or persistent air leaks. Should a pulmonary laceration require operative intervention, lung-sparing techniques should be employed when feasible, rather than formal anatomic lung resection to reduce morbidity and mortality.

Lung hematomas are the result of local parenchymal destruction and hemorrhage. The x-ray appearance is initially a poorly defined density that becomes more circumscribed a few days to 2 weeks after injury. Cystic cavities occasionally develop if damage is extensive. Most hematomas resolve adequately with expectant treatment.

E. Heart and Pericardium

Blunt injury to the heart occurs most often from compression against the steering wheel in auto accidents. This injury is in decline with the increasing prevalence of airbag technology in motor vehicles. The injury varies from localized contusion to cardiac rupture. Autopsy studies of victims of immediately fatal accidents show that as many as 65% have rupture of one or more cardiac chambers and 45% have pericardial lacerations. The incidence of blunt myocardial injury in patients who reach the hospital is unknown but is probably higher than generally suspected. The clinical relevance of this diagnosis is widely debated. Most trauma surgeons advocate the diagnosis and treatment of the actual clinical problem such as acute heart failure, valvular injury, cardiac rupture, or dysrhythmia.

Early clinical findings include friction rubs, chest pain, tachycardia, murmurs, dysrhythmias, or signs of low cardiac output. Patients with risk factors for blunt myocardial injury should undergo evaluation with a 12-lead electrocardiogram (ECG). If the ECG is normal and the patient is asymptomatic, the workup is complete. An abnormal ECG should prompt further evaluation with an echocardiogram. If the patient has proven injury on echocardiogram or hemodynamic instability (or both), the patient should be admitted to the ICU and managed appropriately for the diagnosed injury. An abnormal ECG with a normal echocardiogram merits at least 24 hours of monitoring in a telemetry unit and daily repeat ECGs until stable or the dysrhythmia resolves. Standard measurement of cardiac enzymes is not useful and has no role in the diagnosis of blunt myocardial injury. If the patient is suspected of having a myocardial infarction or acute myocardial ischemia, then cardiac enzymes and cardiology consultation should be obtained.

Management of symptomatic blunt myocardial injury should be the same as for acute myocardial infarction. Hemopericardium may occur without tamponade and can be treated by pericardiocentesis. Tamponade in blunt cardiac trauma is often due to myocardial rupture or coronary artery laceration. Tamponade produces distended neck veins, shock, and cyanosis. Immediate thoracotomy and control of the injury are indicated. If cardiopulmonary arrest occurs before the patient can be transported to the operating room, emergency room thoracotomy with relief of tamponade should be performed. Treatment of injuries to the valves, papillary muscles, and septum must be individualized; and when tolerated, delayed repair is usually recommended.

Pericardial lacerations from stab wounds tend to seal and cause tamponade, whereas gunshot wounds frequently leave a sufficient pericardial opening for drainage. Gunshot wounds produce more extensive myocardial damage, multiple perforations, and massive bleeding into the pleural space. Hemothorax, shock, and exsanguination occur in nearly all cases of cardiac gunshot wounds. The clinical findings are those of tamponade or acute blood loss. Use of ultrasound and the FAST examination technique can reveal the presence of clinically significant blood in the pericardial space.

Treatment of penetrating cardiac injuries requires prompt thoracotomy, pericardial decompression, and control of hemorrhage. Most patients do not require cardiopulmonary bypass. The standard approach has been to repair the laceration using mattress sutures with pledgets while controlling hemorrhage with a finger on the heart. Suture control of cardiac lacerations may be technically difficult when working with a beating heart or in patients with large or multiple lacerations. Several studies have demonstrated that in most cases, emergency temporary control of hemorrhage from cardiac lacerations can be achieved with the use of a skin stapler (Figure 13–12). Following stabilization of the patient, the staples can be removed after definitive suture repair is performed in the operating room. Hemostatic sealants such as FloSeal offer significant promise as additional tools in the surgical armamentarium when dealing with lacerations to the heart or great vessels. Regardless of the approach utilized, care must be taken to avoid injury to the coronary arteries.

Pericardiocentesis or creation of a pericardial window is reserved for selected cases when the diagnosis is uncertain or in preparation for thoracotomy. In approximately 75% of cases of stab wounds and 35% of cases of gunshot cardiac wounds, the patient survives the operation. However, it is estimated that 80–90% of patients with gunshot wounds of the heart do not reach the hospital.

F. Esophagus

Anatomically, the esophagus is well protected, and perforation from external penetrating trauma is relatively

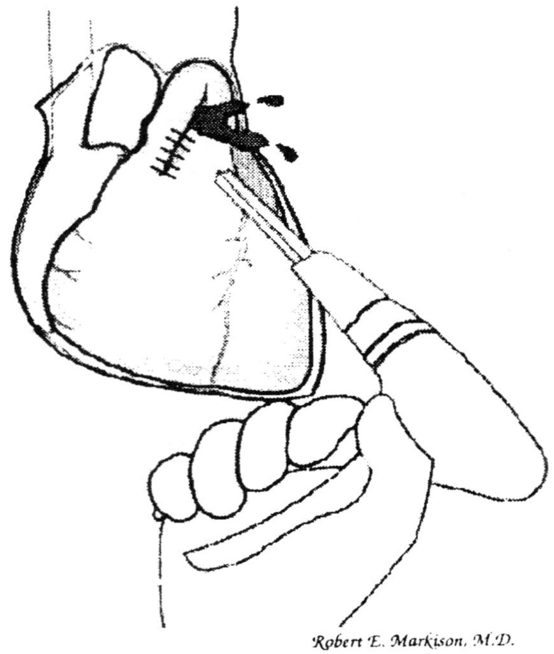

Figure 13–12. **Technique of cardiac stapling. Finger pressure (not shown) is used to maintain hemostasis during stapling.** (Reproduced, with permission, from Macho JR, Markison RE, Schecter WP: Cardiac stapling in the management of penetrating injuries of the heart: rapid control of hemorrhage and decreased risk of personal contamination. J Trauma 1993;34:711.)

infrequent. Blunt injuries are exceedingly rare. The most common symptom of esophageal perforation is pain; fever develops within hours in most patients. Hematemesis, hoarseness, dysphagia, or respiratory distress may also be present. Physical findings include shock, local tenderness, subcutaneous emphysema, or Hamman's sign (pericardial or mediastinal "crunch" synchronous with cardiac sounds). Leukocytosis occurs soon after injury. X-ray findings on plain chest films include evidence of a foreign body or missile and mediastinal air or widening. Pleural effusion or hydropneumothorax is frequently seen, usually on the left side. Contrast x-rays of the esophagus should be performed but are positive in only about 70% of proven perforations.

A nasogastric tube should be passed to evacuate gastric contents. If recognized within 24–48 hours after injury, the esophageal perforation should be closed and pleural drainage instituted with large-bore catheters. Repair of these perforations requires special techniques that include buttressing of the esophageal closure with pleural or pericardial flaps; pedicles of intercostal, diaphragmatic, or cervical strap muscles; and serosal patches from stomach or jejunum. Illness and death are due to mediastinal and pleural infection.

G. Thoracic Duct

Chylothorax and chylopericardium are rare complications of trauma but are difficult to manage when they occur. Penetrating injuries of the neck, thorax, or upper abdomen can injure the thoracic duct or its major tributaries.

Symptoms are due to mechanical effects of the accumulations, eg, shortness of breath from lung collapse or low cardiac output from tamponade. The diagnosis is established when the fluid is shown to have characteristics of chyle.

The patient should be maintained on a fat-free, high-carbohydrate, high-protein diet and the effusion aspirated. Chest tube drainage should be instituted if the effusion recurs. Lipid-free total parenteral nutrition with no oral intake may be effective in treating persistent leaks. Three or 4 weeks of conservative treatment usually are curative. If daily chyle loss exceeds 1500 mL for 5 successive days or persists after 2–3 weeks of conservative treatment, the thoracic duct should be ligated via a right thoracotomy. Intraoperative identification of the leak may be facilitated by preoperative administration of fat containing a lipophilic dye.

H. Diaphragm

Penetrating injuries of the diaphragm outnumber blunt diaphragmatic injuries by a ratio of at least 6:1. Diaphragmatic lacerations occur in 10–15% of cases of penetrating wounds to the chest and in as many as 40% of cases of penetrating trauma to the left chest. Injuries to the right diaphragm are more common than previously thought. The injury is rarely obvious. Wounds of the diaphragm must not be overlooked because they rarely heal spontaneously and because herniation of abdominal viscera into the chest can occur with catastrophic complications either immediately or years after the injuries.

Associated injuries are usually present, and as many as 25% of patients are in shock when first seen. There may be abdominal tenderness, dyspnea, shoulder pain, or unilateral breath sounds. The diagnosis is often missed. Although chest radiography is a sensitive diagnostic tool, it may be entirely normal in 40% of cases. The most common finding is ipsilateral hemothorax, which is present in about 50% of patients. Occasionally, a distended, herniated stomach is confused with a pneumothorax. Passage of a nasogastric tube before x-rays will help to identify an intrathoracic stomach. CT scan or contrast x-rays may be necessary to establish the diagnosis in some cases. Newer-generation helical CT scanners that allow sagittal reformatting can be helpful in definitively diagnosing diaphragmatic injury. Laparoscopy is a useful but invasive technique for detecting occult diaphragmatic injuries in patients who have no other indications for formal laparotomy.

Once the diagnosis is made, a transabdominal surgical approach should be used in cases of acute rupture. Laparoscopic suturing for repair of the injury may be possible in selected cases. The diaphragm should be reapproximated and closed with interrupted or running nonabsorbable sutures. Chronic herniation is associated with adhesions of the affected viscera to the thoracic structures and should be approached via thoracotomy, with the addition of a separate laparotomy when indicated. These cases can be quite challenging and appropriate preoperative planning is recommended.

Asensio JA et al: Penetrating cardiac injuries: a prospective study of variables predicting outcomes. J Am Coll Surg 1998;186:24.

Bergeron E et al: Elderly trauma patients with rib fractures are at greater risk of death and pneumonia. J Trauma 2003;54:478.

Brasel KJ et al: Treatment of occult pneumothoraces from blunt trauma. J Trauma 1999;46:987.

Carrillo EH et al: Video-assisted thoracic surgery in trauma patients. J Am Coll Surg 1997;184:316.

Cothren C et al: Lung-sparing techniques are associated with improved outcome compared with anatomic resection for severe lung injuries. J Trauma 2002;53:483.

Dulchavsky SA et al: Prospective evaluation of thoracic ultrasound in the detection of pneumothorax. J Trauma 2001;50:201.

Feliciano DV, Rozycki GS: Advances in the diagnosis and treatment of thoracic trauma. Surg Clin North Am 1999;79:1417.

Gasparri M et al: Pulmonary tractotomy versus lung resection: viable options in penetrating lung injury. J Trauma 2001;51: 1092.

Karmy-Jones R et al: Timing of urgent thoracotomy for hemorrhage after trauma. Arch Surg 2001;136:513.

Karmy-Jones R et al: Urgent and emergent thoracotomy for penetrating chest trauma. J Trauma 2004;56:664.

Lowdermilk GA, Naunheim KS: Thoracoscopic evaluation and treatment of thoracic trauma. Surg Clin North Am 2000;80: 1535.

Macho JR, Markison RE, Schecter WP: Cardiac stapling in the management of penetrating injuries of the heart: rapid control of hemorrhage and decreased risk of personal contamination. J Trauma 1993;34:711.

Mansour KA: Trauma to the diaphragm. Chest Surg Clin North Am 1997;7:373.

Miller PR et al: ARDS after pulmonary contusion: accurate measurement of contusion volume identifies high-risk patients. J Trauma 2001;51:223.

Rozycki GS et al: The role of ultrasound in patients with possible penetrating cardiac wounds: a prospective multicenter study. J Trauma 1999;46:543.

Schultz JM, Trunkey DD: Blunt cardiac injury. Crit Care Clin 2004;20:57.

Stassen NA et al: Reevaluation of diagnostic procedures for transmediastinal gunshot wounds. J Trauma 2002;53:635.

ABDOMINAL INJURIES

The distribution of blunt and penetrating injury in a given population is highly dependent upon geographic location. Blunt injuries predominate in rural areas, while penetrating injuries are more common in urban areas. The specific type of injury varies according to whether the trauma is penetrating or blunt. The mechanism of injury in blunt trauma is rapid deceleration, and noncompliant organs such as the liver, spleen, pancreas, and kidneys are at greater risk of injury due to parenchymal fracture. Occasionally, hollow organs may be injured, with the duodenum and urinary bladder being particularly susceptible. The small bowel occupies a large portion of the total abdominal volume and is more likely to be injured by penetrating trauma. Most blunt abdominal injuries are related to motor vehicle accidents. Although the use of restraints has been associated with a decrease in the incidence of head, chest, and solid organ injuries, their use may be associated with pancreatic, mesenteric, and intestinal injuries due to compression against the spinal column. These injuries should be considered in the evaluation of patients who have signs of seat belt-related abrasions or hematomas. Internal injury may be present in as many as 30% of these cases. As many as 35% of patents with significant hemoperitoneum may not manifest clinical signs of peritoneal irritation. Retroperitoneal injury may be more subtle and difficult to diagnose during the initial evaluation.

Deaths from abdominal trauma result principally from hemorrhage or sepsis. Most deaths from abdominal trauma are preventable. Patients at risk of abdominal injury should undergo prompt and thorough evaluation. In some cases, dramatic physical findings may be due to abdominal wall injury in the absence of intraperitoneal injury. If the results of diagnostic studies are equivocal, diagnostic laparoscopy or exploratory laparotomy should be considered, since they may be lifesaving if serious injuries are identified early.

Types of Injuries

If the abdomen is the probable source of exsanguinating hemorrhage, the patient should be transferred to the operating room for immediate laparotomy. The hemodynamically stable patent can be more thoroughly assessed within the framework of the secondary survey. Evaluation always includes comprehensive physical examination with pelvic and rectal examinations and may require specific laboratory and radiologic tests. Serially performed examinations may be necessary to detect subtle findings.

A. Penetrating Trauma

Penetrating injuries may cause sepsis if they perforate a hollow viscous. When a full bowel is injured, the contents are evacuated into the peritoneal cavity, and clinical signs of injury are obvious. When an empty bowel is injured or when the retroperitoneal portion of the bowel is penetrated, spillage of bowel contents may be negligible initially, and findings may be minimal. Increasing abdominal tenderness demands surgical exploration. White blood cell count elevations and fever appearing several hours following injury are keys to early diagnosis.

Penetrating injuries can cause severe and early shock if they involve a major vessel or the liver. Penetrating injuries of the spleen, pancreas, or kidneys usually do not bleed massively unless a major vessel to the organ (eg, the renal artery) is damaged. Bleeding must be controlled promptly. A patient in shock with a penetrating injury of the abdomen who does not respond to 2 L of fluid resuscitation should be operated on immediately following chest x-ray.

The treatment of hemodynamically stable patients with penetrating injuries to the lower chest or abdomen varies. All surgeons agree that patients with signs of peritonitis or hypovolemia should undergo surgical exploration, but treatment is less certain for patients with no signs of peritonitis or sepsis who are hemodynamically stable.

Most stab wounds of the lower chest or abdomen should be explored, since a delay in treatment of a hollow viscous perforation can result in severe sepsis. Some surgeons have recommended a selective policy in the management of these patients. When the depth of injury is in doubt, local wound exploration may rule out peritoneal penetration. Laparoscopy may ultimately have a role in the evaluation of penetrating injuries. All gunshot wounds of the lower chest and abdomen should be explored, because the incidence of injury to major intra-abdominal structures exceeds 90% in such cases.

B. Blunt Trauma

A major addition in management of blunt trauma has been the Focused Assessment with Sonography for Trauma (FAST) examination. Ultrasound has proved to be an ideal modality in the immediate evaluation of the trauma patient because it is rapid and accurate for the detection of intra-abdominal fluid or blood and is readily repeatable. It provides valuable information that augments the surgeon's diagnostic capabilities. The use of ultrasonography for the evaluation of trauma patients is not new; it has been used in Europe for the past two decades. Since its introduction in North America in 1989, the technique has been adopted rapidly and a recent survey reports that 78% of United States trauma centers routinely use the FAST examination in the evaluation of patients.

The goal of the FAST examination is the identification of abnormal collections of blood or fluid. In this regard, it obviates the need for diagnostic peritoneal lavage. The primary focus is on the peritoneal cavity, but attention is directed also to the pericardium and to the pleural space. Unclotted blood or fluid allows transmission of ultrasound waves without echoes and thus appears black (Figure 13–13). In the standard FAST examination, four areas are scanned: the right upper quadrant, the subxiphoid area, the left upper quadrant, and the pelvis (Figure 13–14). Most surgeons recommend scanning initially in the right upper quadrant because more than half of the positive tests will reveal blood or fluid in this area. Unstable patients with a pos-

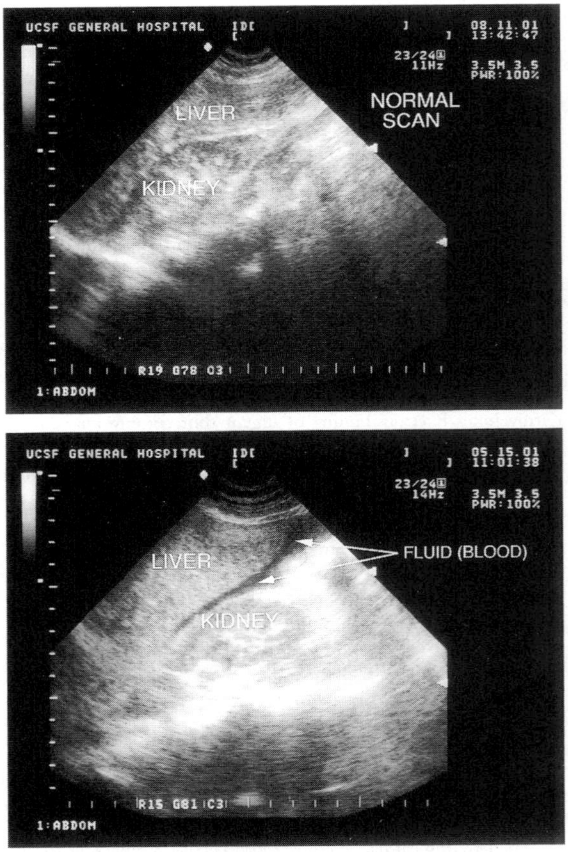

Figure 13–13. *Top:* Normal ultrasound of the right upper quadrant. *Bottom:* Right upper quadrant ultrasound revealing blood between the liver and the kidney and between the liver and the diaphragm. (Courtesy of San Francisco General Hospital.)

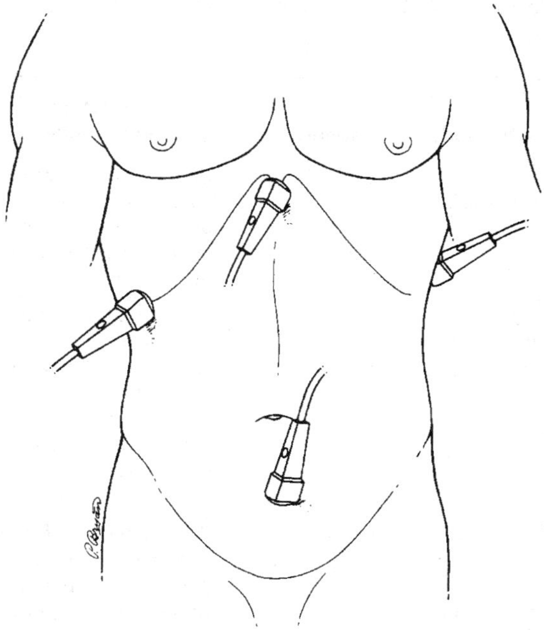

Figure 13–14. Transducer positions for FAST. Pericardial area, right and left upper quadrants, and pelvis. (Reproduced, with permission, from Rozycki GS et al: Surgeon-performed ultrasound for the assessment of truncal injuries: lessons learned from 1540 patients. Ann Surg 1998;228:557.)

itive FAST examination should undergo urgent exploratory laparotomy.

The other diagnostic procedures most commonly used in patients without obvious indications for laparotomy include peritoneal lavage, CT scanning, and diagnostic laparoscopy.

Diagnostic Peritoneal Lavage

Diagnostic peritoneal lavage is designed to detect the presence of intraperitoneal blood. Although its use has decreased significantly at many centers with the use of the FAST examination, it is still considered to be an important test in certain circumstances because of its high sensitivity and specificity. Additional determinations of leukocytes, particulate matter, or amylase in the lavage fluid may indicate the presence of a bowel injury. Drainage of lavage fluid from a chest tube or urinary catheter may indicate a lacerated diaphragm or bladder. Lavage can be performed easily and rapidly, with minimal cost and morbidity. It is an invasive procedure that will affect the findings on physical examination, and it should be performed by a surgeon.

The procedure is neither qualitative nor quantitative. It cannot identify the source of hemorrhage, and relatively small amounts of intraperitoneal bleeding may result in a positive study. It may not detect small and large injuries to the diaphragm and cannot rule out injury to the bowel or retroperitoneal organs. The indications for diagnostic peritoneal lavage include abdominal pain or tenderness, low abdominal rib fractures, unexplained hypotension, spinal or pelvic fractures, paraplegia or quadriplegia, and assessment hampered by altered mental status due to neurologic injury or intoxication. The only contraindication is a need for emergency laparotomy.

The procedure may be performed with careful technique on patients with prior abdominal surgery and in pregnant patients. It should usually be performed through a small infra-umbilical incision with placement of the catheter under direct vision (Figure 13–15). Closed techniques of catheter placement utilizing trocars or guidewires have been shown to be about as safe as the open technique, but the rate of failure with the closed technique is higher, thus eliminating most of the potential advantage. After placement of the catheter, 1 L of normal saline solution is instilled into the peritoneal cavity and then allowed to drain by gravity. At least 200 mL of lavage fluid should be recovered to allow for accurate interpretation. A portion of the recovered fluid is sent for laboratory analysis of cell counts, the presence of particulate matter, and amylase. Criteria for evaluation of results are summarized in Table 13–3.

Computed Tomography

CT is noninvasive, qualitative, sensitive, and accurate for the diagnosis of intra-abdominal injury. Mod-

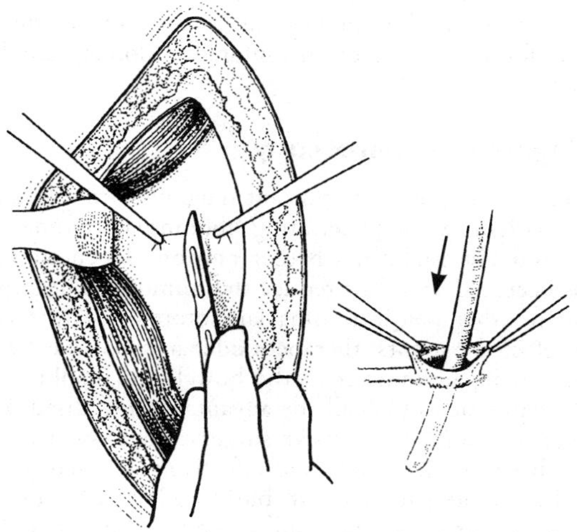

Figure 13–15. Diagnostic pericardial lavage.

Table 13–3. Criteria for evaluation of peritoneal lavage fluid.

Positive
20 mL gross blood on free aspiration (10 mL in children)
≥ 100,000 red cells/μL
≥ 500 white cells/μL (if obtained 3 hours or more after injury)
≥ 175 units amylase/dL
Bacteria on Gram-stained smear
Bile (by inspection or chemical determination of bilirubin content)
Food particles (microscopic analysis of strained or spun specimen)
Intermediate
Pink fluid on free aspiration
50,000–100,000 red cells/μL in blunt trauma
100–500 white cells/μL
75–175 units amylase/dL
Negative
Clear aspirate
≤ 100 white cells/μL
≤ 75 units amylase/dL

ern spiral scanners have greatly decreased the time required for obtaining high-quality images. However, CT scanning remains expensive and the scans require an experienced radiologist for proper interpretation. CT scanning requires transport from the acute care area and should not be attempted in the unstable patient.

CT scanning has a primary role in defining the location and magnitude of intra-abdominal injuries related to blunt trauma. It has the advantage of detecting most retroperitoneal injuries, but it may not identify some gastrointestinal injuries. The information provided on the magnitude of injury allows for nonoperative management of patients with solid organ injuries. Nonsurgical therapy is now used in more than 80% of blunt liver and spleen injuries. A comparison of time, costs, advantages and disadvantages of nonoperative methods used for evaluation of the injured abdomen can be found in Table 13–4.

Diagnostic Laparoscopy

Laparoscopy has an important diagnostic role in stable patients with penetrating abdominal trauma. It can quickly establish whether peritoneal penetration has occurred and thus reduce the number of negative and nontherapeutic trauma laparotomies performed. In selected patients, therapeutic laparoscopy has been used to repair injuries to the bowel and diaphragm. This approach offers all the advantages and disadvantages of minimally invasive surgery. Laparoscopy has also been applied safely and effectively as a screening tool in stable patients with blunt abdominal trauma. However, its use in this context requires further study. Concerns regarding the use of laparoscopy in trauma include the possibility of missed injuries, air embolism, hemodynamic instability related to the pneumoperitoneum, and complications related to trocar placement.

Table 13–4. Comparison of diagnostic methods for abdominal trauma.

Methods	Time/Cost	Advantages/ Disadvantages
Physical examination	Quick/No cost	Useful for serial examinations, very limited by other injuries, coma, drug intoxication, poor sensitivity and specificity.
Diagnostic Peritoneal Lavage (DPL)	Quick/ Inexpensive	Rapid results in unstable patient, but invasive and may be overly sensitive for blood and not specific for site of injury; requires experience and may be limited if previous surgery.
Focused Assessment with Sonography for Trauma (FAST)	Quick/ Inexpensive	Rapid detection of intra-abdominal fluid and pericardial tamponade, may be limited by operator experience, large body habitus, subcutaneous air, poor for detection of bowel injury. Fairly sensitive but not highly specific.
Helical Computerized Abdominal Tomography (CT)	Slower/ Expensive	Most specific for site of injury and can evaluate retroperitoneum, very good sensitivity but may miss bowel injury, risk of reaction to contrast dye.

Exploratory Laparotomy

The three main indications for exploration of the abdomen following blunt trauma are peritonitis, unexplained hypovolemia, and the presence of other injuries known to be frequently associated with intra-abdominal injuries. Peritonitis after blunt abdominal trauma is rare but always requires exploration. Signs of peritonitis can arise from rupture of a hollow organ, such as the duodenum, bladder, intestine, or gallbladder; from pancreatic injury; or occasionally from the presence of retroperitoneal blood.

Emergency abdominal exploration should be considered for patients with profound hypovolemic shock and a normal chest x-ray unless extra-abdominal blood loss is sufficient to account for the hypovolemia. In most cases a rapidly performed FAST examination or peritoneal lavage will confirm the diagnosis of intraperitoneal hemorrhage. Patients with blunt trauma and hypovolemia should be examined first for intra-abdominal bleeding even if there is no overt evidence of abdominal trauma. For example, hypovolemia may be due to loss of blood from a large scalp laceration, but it may also be due to unsuspected rupture of the spleen. Hemoperitoneum may present with no signs except hypovolemia. The abdomen may be flat and nontender. Patients whose extra-abdominal bleeding has been controlled should respond to initial fluid resuscitation with an adequate urine output and stabilization of vital signs. If hypovolemia recurs, intra-abdominal bleeding must be considered to be the cause.

Injuries frequently associated with abdominal injuries are rib fractures, pelvic fractures, abdominal wall injuries, and fractures of the thoracolumbar spine (eg, 20% of patients with fractures of the left lower ribs have a splenic laceration).

Treatment

A. Abdominal Wall Injuries

Abdominal wall injuries from blunt trauma are most often due to shear forces, such as being run over by the wheels of a tractor or bus. The shearing often devitalizes the subcutaneous tissue and skin, and if debridement is delayed, a serious necrotizing anaerobic infection may develop. The management of penetrating abdominal wall injuries is usually straightforward. Debridement and irrigation are appropriate surgical treatment. Every effort must be made to remove foreign material, shreds of clothing, necrotic muscle, and soft tissue. Abdominal wall defects may require insertion of prosthetic material (eg, polypropylene mesh) or coverage with a myocutaneous flap.

B. Liver Injuries

Approximately 85% of all patients with blunt hepatic trauma are stable following resuscitation. In this group, nonoperative management has been shown to be superior to operation in avoiding complications. The primary requirement for nonoperative therapy is continued hemodynamic stability. Patients are monitored in the intensive care unit with frequent assessment of vital signs and serial hematocrits. If transfusion with more than two units of packed red blood cells is required, arteriography with possible embolization of bleeding vessels should be considered. Associated injuries are present in 1–4% of patients in whom nonoperative management is attempted. Many of these injuries—particularly those involving bowel—may not be evident on the initial CT scans. Therefore, patients must be monitored carefully for the development of peritoneal irritation and sepsis.

Nonoperative management of blunt hepatic trauma is successful in more than 90% of cases. With more severe injuries, repeat CT scanning may be necessary to evaluate for possible complications such as parenchymal infarction, hematoma, or biloma. Extrahepatic bile collections should generally be drained percutaneously. Intrahepatic collections of blood and bile usually resolve spontaneously over the course of several months.

Severe liver injury may result in exsanguinating hemorrhage with hypotension that does not respond to fluid resuscitation. For these patients, exploration is warranted. At laparotomy, immediate efforts should be directed to control of hemorrhage. In addition to stopping ongoing blood loss, this will allow for stabilization of the patient by restoration of circulating blood volume. The initial techniques for the control of hepatic hemorrhage include manual compression, perihepatic packing, and the Pringle maneuver. Manual compression or perihepatic packing with laparotomy pads will control hemorrhage in most cases. The Pringle maneuver—clamping of the hepatic pedicle—should be performed when life-threatening hemorrhage is encountered and will control all hepatic bleeding except that from the hepatic veins or the intrahepatic vena cava. In most cases, the Pringle maneuver should not be maintained for more than 1 hour in order to prevent ischemic damage to the liver. Hepatic bleeding can be controlled by suture ligation or application of surgical clips directly to the bleeding vessels. Electrocautery or the argon beam coagulator can be used to control bleeding from raw surfaces of the liver. Microfibrillar collagen or hemostatic gelatin foam sponges soaked in thrombin can be applied to bleeding areas with pressure to control diffuse capillary bleeding. Fibrin glue has been used in treating both superficial and deep lacerations and appears to be the most effective topical agent. Reports of fatal anaphylactic reactions have limited its use. When injury has already resulted in massive blood loss, packing of the abdomen with laparotomy pads and planned reexploration should be considered. At the time of reexploration in 24–48 hours, hemorrhage is usually well controlled and can be managed with individual vessel ligation and debridement. Evidence of persistent hemorrhage should prompt earlier reexploration. Angiographic embolization may be a useful adjunct to surgical packing if arterial hemorrhage is still present or not well controlled. Rarely, selective hepatic artery ligation, resectional debridement, or hepatic lobectomy may be required to control hemorrhage. The raw surface of the liver may then be covered with omentum. Drains should always be used. Decompression of the biliary system is contraindicated, though sutures or clips should be used to control leaking biliary ducts in the hepatic parenchyma.

Hepatic vein injuries frequently bleed massively. Hepatic venous or intrahepatic vena caval injury should be suspected immediately when the Pringle maneuver fails to control bleeding. Several techniques have been described for isolation of the intrahepatic cava prior to attempted repair of these injuries. Unfortunately, even with the use of these techniques, mortality remains very high.

C. Biliary Tract Injuries

Injury to the gallbladder should be treated in most cases by cholecystectomy, but minor lacerations may be closed with absorbable suture material.

Most injuries to the common bile duct can be treated by suture closure and insertion of a T-tube. Avulsion of the common bile duct due to duodenal or ampullary trauma may require choledochojejunostomy in conjunction with total or partial pancreatectomy, duodenectomy, or other diversion procedures. Segmental loss of the common bile duct is best treated by choledochojejunostomy.

D. Splenic Injuries

The spleen is the most commonly injured organ in cases of blunt abdominal trauma. Splenic injuries in children have been managed traditionally without surgery. Until recently, most splenic injuries in adults were managed with splenorrhaphy or splenectomy. Currently, 50–80% of adults with blunt splenic injuries are treated nonoperatively. Patients must be monitored closely in the intensive care unit, and immediate availability of an operating room is essential. Patients should be evaluated frequently for the possibility of other missed injuries or recurrent bleeding. Stable patients who have high-grade splenic injuries on CT or have evidence of ongoing bleeding on CT may be candidates for angiographic embolization. Unstable patients with splenic injuries should undergo splenectomy or attempts at splenic repair if appropriate. Diagnosis and management are covered in detail in Chapter 27.

E. Pancreatic Injuries

Pancreatic injuries may present with few clinical manifestations. Injury should be suspected whenever the upper abdomen has been traumatized, especially when serum amylase levels remain persistently elevated. The best diagnostic study for pancreatic injury (other than exploratory celiotomy) is CT scan of the abdomen. Peritoneal lavage is usually not helpful. Upper gastrointestinal studies with water-soluble contrast material may suggest pancreatic injury by demonstrating widening of the duodenal C-loop. Endoscopic retrograde cholangiopancreatography may be used in selected cases to evaluate for injuries to the major ducts.

The treatment of pancreatic injury depends on its grade and extent. Minor injuries not involving a major duct may be treated nonoperatively. Moderate injuries usually require operative exploration, debridement, and the placement of external drains. More severe injuries, including those with major duct injury or transection of the gland, may require distal resection or external drainage. Traumatic injuries to the head of the pancreas often include associated vascular injuries and carry a high mortality rate. Efforts should be directed at controlling hemorrhage, and drains can be placed in the area of the pancreatic injury. In most cases, pancreaticoduodenectomy should not be attempted in the setting of an unstable patient with multiple injuries.

The late complications of pancreatic injuries include pseudocyst, pancreatic fistula, and pancreatic abscess. Patients treated without resection may require reoperation for resection or Roux-en-Y internal gastrointestinal drainage.

F. Gastrointestinal Tract Injuries

Most injuries of the stomach can be repaired. Large injuries, such as those from shotgun blasts, may require subtotal or total resection.

Duodenal injuries may not be evident from the initial physical examination or x-ray studies. Abdominal films will reveal retroperitoneal gas within 6 hours after injury in most patients. Computed tomography performed with a contrast agent will frequently identify the site of perforation. Most duodenal injuries can be treated with lateral repair, but some may require resection with end-to-end anastomosis. Occasionally, pancreaticoduodenectomy is required to manage a severe injury. A duodenostomy tube is useful in decompressing the duodenum and can be used to control a fistula caused by an injury. Jejunal or omental patches may also aid in preventing a suture line leak.

Duodenal hematomas causing high-grade obstruction usually resolve with nonoperative management. Patients may require total parenteral nutrition. In some cases, a small-bore enteral feeding tube can be passed beyond the area of obstruction utilizing interventional radiology techniques. Large hematomas may require operative evacuation, particularly when the obstruction lasts for more than 10–14 days and a persistent hematoma is seen on CT scan.

Most small bowel injuries can be treated with a two-layer sutured closure, though devascularizing injuries to the mesentery or small bowel will require resection. The underlying principle is to preserve as much small bowel as possible.

For injuries to the colon, the past approach has been to divert the fecal stream or exteriorize the injury. However, more recent studies have shown a higher complication rate with colostomy formation rather than primary repair. Wounds should be considered for primary repair if the blood supply is not compromised. Primary repair is more likely to be associated with complications in patients with ongoing shock, in the patient requiring multiple transfusions, or if there has been a delay of more than 6 hours between injury and operation or if there is gross contamination or peritonitis. Small, clean rectal injuries may be closed primarily if conditions are favorable. The treatment of larger rectal wounds involving pelvic fracture should include proximal diversion with insertion of presacral drains. In this latter case, direct repair of the rectal injury is not mandatory but should be performed if it can be readily exposed. Irrigation of the distal stump should be performed in most cases unless it would further contaminate the pelvic space.

G. Genitourinary Tract Injuries

The most commonly injured genitourinary tract organs are the male genitalia, the uterus, the urethra, the bladder, the ureters, and the kidneys. The workup for these injuries consists primarily of radiologic examinations, which may include abdominal CT scan, intravenous urogram, cystogram, and urethrogram. In unstable patients with associated injuries, it may not be possible to obtain these studies prior to emergency laparotomy. In these patients, an intraoperative single-shot intravenous urogram is safe and of high quality in most cases. This study often provides important information that facilitates rapid and accurate decision making. It can confirm function in the noninjured kidney and help in identifying blunt renal injuries that may be safely observed.

1. Injuries to the male genitalia—Injuries to the male genitalia usually result in skin loss only; the penis, penile urethra, and testes are usually spared. Skin loss from the penis should be treated with a primary skin graft. Scrotal skin loss should be treated by delayed reconstruction; an exposed testis can be temporarily protected by placing it in a subcutaneous tissue pocket in the thigh.

2. Uterine injuries—Injuries of the female reproductive organs are infrequent except in combination with genitourinary or rectal trauma. Injuries to the uterine fundus can usually be repaired with absorbable sutures; drainage is not necessary. In more extensive injuries, hysterectomy may be preferable. The vaginal cuff may be left open for drainage, particularly if there is an associated urinary tract or rectal injury. Injuries involving the uterus in a pregnant woman usually result in death of the fetus. Bleeding may be massive in such patients, particularly in women approaching parturition. Cesarean section plus hysterectomy may be the only alternative.

3. Urethral injuries—Membranous prostatic urethral disruption is often associated with pelvic fracture or deceleration injuries. Blood at the urethral meatus associated with scrotal hematoma and high-riding prostate on digital rectal examination are the classic signs of injury to the male urethra. The prostate may be elevated superiorly by the pelvic hematoma and will be free-riding and high on rectal examination. If these signs are present, urethrography should be performed before attempts at catheter placement, which may convert an incomplete injury to a complete disruption. If an injury is present, urethrography will demonstrate free extravasation of contrast medium from the urethra into the preperitoneal space.

Penetrating injuries are best treated with primary repair. Suprapubic bladder drainage and delayed reconstruction of blunt urethral disruption injuries are safe and effective in the majority of cases. Immediate realignment with cystourethroscopy and placement of a urethral catheter is an attractive minimally invasive alternative. In cases of partial disruption it has been shown to result in stricture-free outcomes.

Major injuries to the bulbous or penile urethra should be managed by suprapubic urinary diversion. A voiding cystourethrogram may later reveal a stricture, but operative correction or dilation is usually not necessary.

4. Bladder injuries—Rupture of the bladder, like urethral disruption, is frequently associated with pelvic fractures. Seventy-five percent of ruptures are extraperitoneal and 25% intraperitoneal. A ruptured bladder should be repaired through a midline abdominal incision. Rupture of the anterior wall of the bladder can be repaired by direct suture; rupture of the posterior wall can be repaired from inside the bladder after an opening has been made in the anterior wall. Care should be taken to avoid entering a pelvic hematoma. Postoperatively, urine should be diverted for at least 7 days.

5. Kidney injuries—Advances in the imaging and staging of renal trauma as well as in treatment strategies have decreased the need for operation and increased renal preservation. More than half of renal injuries can be treated nonoperatively. Management criteria are based on radiographic, laboratory, and clinical findings. Nonoperative treatment of penetrating renal lacerations is appropriate in hemodynamically stable patients without other injuries. Small to moderate injuries can be treated nonoperatively, but severe injuries are associated with a significant risk of delayed bleeding if treated expectantly. Renal exploration should be considered if laparotomy is indicated for associated injuries. A midline transabdominal approach is preferred. The renal artery and vein are secured before Gerota's fascia is opened. The injury should be managed by suture repair, partial nephrectomy, or, rarely, total nephrectomy. Pedicle grafts of omentum or free peritoneal patch grafts can be used to cover defects. Renal vascular injuries require immediate operation to save the kidney. Meticulous attention to reconstructive techniques in renal exploration can ensure an excellent renal salvage rate. Adherence to the principles of early proximal vascular control, debridement of devitalized tissue, hemostasis, closure of the collecting system, and coverage of the defect will maximize the salvage of renal function while minimizing potential complications.

Perirenal hematomas found incidentally at celiotomy should be explored if they are expanding, pulsatile, or not contained by retroperitoneal tissues or if a preexploration urogram shows extensive urinary extravasation.

6. Ureteral injuries—Ureteral injuries are easily missed since urinalysis and imaging studies can be unreliable. Most such injuries can be successfully reconstructed by primary repair, ureteroureterostomy, or ureteral reimplantations.

Armenakas NA, Duckett CP, McAninch JW: Indications for nonoperative management of renal stab wounds. J Urol 1999;161:768.

Asensio JA et al: Operative management and outcomes in 103 AAST-OIS grades IV and V complex hepatic injuries: trauma surgeons still need to operate, but angioembolization helps. J Trauma 2003;54:647.

Asensio JA et al: Approach to the management of complex hepatic injuries. J Trauma 2000;48:66.

Bradley EL 3rd et al: Diagnosis and initial management of blunt pancreatic trauma: guidelines for a multiinstitutional review. Ann Surg 1998;227:861.

Brandes SB, McAninch JW: Reconstructive surgery for trauma of the upper urinary tract. Urol Clin North Am 1999;26:183.

Brasel KJ et al: Trends in the management of hepatic injury. Am J Surg 1997;174:674.

Brown RL et al: Observation of splenic trauma: when is a little too much? J Pediatr Surg 1999;34:1124.

Carrillo EH et al: Evolution in the treatment of complex blunt liver injuries. Curr Probl Surg 2001;38:1.

Cathey KL et al: Blunt splenic trauma: characteristics of patients requiring urgent laparotomy. Am Surg 1998;64:450.

Chappuis CW et al: Management of penetrating colon injuries. A prospective randomized trial. Ann Surg 1991;213:492.

Chen RJ et al: Surgical management of juxtahepatic venous injuries in blunt hepatic trauma. J Trauma 1995;38:886.

Coburn MC, Pfeifer J, DeLuca FG: Nonoperative management of splenic and hepatic trauma in the multiply injured pediatric and adolescent patient. Arch Surg 1995;130:332.

Croce MA et al: Nonoperative management of blunt hepatic trauma is the treatment of choice for hemodynamically stable patients. Results of a prospective trial. Ann Surg 1995;221:744.

Curran TJ, Borzotta AP: Complications of primary repair of colon injury: literature review of 2,964 cases. Am J Surg 1999;177:42.

Fakhry SM et al: Relatively short diagnostic delays (< 8 hours) produce morbidity and mortality in blunt small bowel injury: an analysis of time to operative intervention in 198 patients from a multicenter experience. J Trauma 1999;47:207.

Fulcher AS et al: Magnetic resonance cholangiopancreatography in the assessment of pancreatic duct trauma and its sequelae: preliminary findings. J Trauma 2000;48:1001.

Jacobs IA et al: Nonoperative management of blunt splenic and hepatic trauma in the pediatric population: significant differences between adult and pediatric surgeons? Am Surg 2001;67:149.

Kielb SJ, Voeltz ZL, Wolf JS Jr: Evaluation and management of traumatic posterior urethral disruption with flexible cystourethroscopy. J Trauma 2001;50:36.

Malhotra AK et al: Blunt bowel and mesenteric injuries: the role of screening computed tomography. J Trauma 2000;48:991.

Myers JG et al: Blunt splenic injuries: dedicated trauma surgeons can achieve a high rate of nonoperative success in patients of all ages. J Trauma 2000;48:801.

Nicholas JM et al: Changing patterns in the management of penetrating abdominal trauma: the more things change, the more they stay the same. J Trauma 2003;55:1095.

Pachter HL, Grau J: The current status of splenic preservation. Adv Surg 2000;34:137.

Patton JH et al: Pancreatic trauma: a simplified management guideline. J Trauma 1997;43:234.

Peitzman AB et al: Blunt splenic injury in adults: multi-institutional study of the eastern association for the surgery of trauma. J Trauma 2000;49:177.

Rozycki GS, Newman PG: Surgeon-performed ultrasound for the assessment of abdominal injuries. Adv Surg 1999;33:243.

Sartorelli KH et al: Nonoperative management of hepatic, splenic, and renal injuries in adults with multiple injuries. J Trauma 2000;49:56.

Shapiro MB et al: Damage control: collective review. J Trauma 2000;49:969.

Takishima T et al: Serum amylase level on admission in the diagnosis of blunt injury to the pancreas: its significance and limitations. Ann Surg 1997;226:70.

Uecker J, Pickett C, Dunn E: The role of follow-up radiographic studies in nonoperative management of spleen trauma. Am Surg 2001;67:22.

Udobi KF et al: Role of ultrasonography in penetrating abdominal trauma: a prospective clinical study. J Trauma 2001;50:475.

Wahl WL et al: The need for early angiographic embolization in blunt liver injuries. J Trauma 2002;52:1097.

Zantut LF et al: Diagnostic and therapeutic laparoscopy for penetrating abdominal trauma: a multicenter experience. J Trauma 1997;42:825.

VASCULAR INJURIES

Historical Perspective

Much of our knowledge of blood vessel injuries was developed during the course of military conflicts in the 20th century. Although techniques for the management of vascular injuries were in use prior to World War I, arterial ligation to save a life rather than arterial repair to salvage a limb was generally employed, and amputation frequently resulted after vascular injury.

During World War II, only 33% of arterial injuries were repaired. The amputation rate was 49% following arterial ligation and 36% following arterial repair. In the Korean War, with the advent of antibiotics and advanced vascular surgical techniques, the amputation rate decreased to 13% of cases. The amputation rate associated with arterial injuries during the Vietnam War fell to about 10% due to more rapid evacuation and better resuscitation despite the use of high-velocity weapons.

Amputation rates have dropped to less than 10% for arterial injuries in the extremities in many recent civilian series. This is a result of more rapid transport of injured people, improved blood volume replacement, selective use of arteriography, and better operative techniques.

The Epidemiology of Vascular Trauma

The epidemiology of vascular trauma has been studied in three different settings: military conflicts, large urban locations, and, to a lesser extent, rural areas. The types of injuries seen in civilian vascular trauma, once much different from military varieties, are now more similar to military wounds, and the incidence is increasing as a result of the rise in urban violence, motor vehicle crashes, and iatrogenic injuries owing to more frequent use of minimally invasive diagnostic and therapeutic procedures.

Peripheral vascular trauma typically occurs in young men between the ages of 20 and 40 years. In both urban and rural environments, penetrating mechanisms dominate, accounting for 50–90% of vascular injuries. Because many vascular injuries of the head, neck, and torso are immediately fatal, most patients with vascular injuries surviving transport have extremity trauma. This is especially true in the military experience—eg, in Vietnam, extremity vascular injuries accounted for approximately 90% of all arterial trauma. In the urban civilian experience, extremity vascular injuries comprise about 50% of arterial injuries. In rural vascular trauma, blunt injuries occur more frequently than in urban populations.

Mortality and utilization of medical resources is higher among patients with vascular injuries than among patients who do not have blood vessel injuries. Vascular injuries from automobile accidents or falls from heights and crush injuries account for up to half of all noniatrogenic vascular injuries in United States hospitals. The likelihood of vascular injury after blunt trauma correlates with the overall severity of the injury and the presence of specific orthopedic injuries. For example, up to 30–40% of patients with knee dislocations or severe instability from blunt trauma sustain popliteal artery injury.

The number of iatrogenic vascular injuries has risen dramatically in recent decades. Most involve diagnostic and therapeutic procedures utilizing the femoral (less frequently the brachial or axillary) vessels, which serve as access routes. In order of decreasing frequency, injuries include hemorrhage and hematoma, pseudoaneurysm, arteriovenous fistula formation, vessel thrombosis, and embolization. Rates of injury range from 0.5% for diagnostic procedures to as high as 10% for therapeutic procedures involving large catheters. Increasing age, female gender, use of anticoagulation, and the presence of atherosclerosis increase the risk of these complications. Complications remote from the puncture site include vessel rupture and dissection. Operative procedures (especially hepatic and pancreaticobiliary surgery) are associated with iatrogenic vascular trauma. In addition, anterior and retroperitoneal approaches to the lumbar spine and other orthopedic procedures such as total joint replacement and arthroscopy can produce vascular injuries.

Types of Injuries

A. Penetrating Trauma

The local and regional effects of penetrating wounds are determined by the mechanism of vessel injury. Stab wounds, low-velocity (< 2000 ft/s) bullet wounds, iatrogenic injuries from percutaneous catheterization, and inadvertent intra-arterial injection of drugs produce less soft tissue injury and disrupt collateral circulation less than injuries from sources with greater kinetic energy. The high-velocity missiles responsible for war wounds produce more extensive vascular injuries, which involve massive destruction and contamination of surrounding tissues. The temporary cavitational effect of high-velocity missiles causes additional trauma to the ends of severed arteries and may produce arterial thrombosis due to disrupted intima even when the artery has not been directly hit. This blast effect can also draw material such as clothing, dirt, or pieces of skin along the wound tract, which contributes to the risk of infection. Associated injuries are often major determinants of the eventual outcome.

Shotgun blasts present special problems. Although muzzle velocity is low (about 1200 ft/s), the multiple pellets produce widespread damage, and shotgun wadding entering the wound enhances the likelihood of infection. Similar to high-velocity injuries, the damage is often much greater than might be anticipated from inspection of the entry wound. Moreover, the multiplicity of potential sites of arterial damage often mandates diagnostic arteriography, even in the presence of obvious arterial insufficiency.

B. Blunt Trauma

Motor vehicle accidents are a major cause of blunt vascular trauma. Multiple injuries include fractures and dislocations; and while direct vascular injury may occur, in most instances the damage is indirect due to fractures. This is especially likely to occur with fractures near joints, where vessels are relatively fixed and vulnerable to shear forces. For example, the popliteal artery and vein are frequently injured in association with posterior dislocation of the knee. Fractures of large heavy bones such as the femur or tibia transmit forces that have cavitation effects similar to those caused by high-velocity bullets. There is extensive damage to soft tissues and neurovascular structures, and edema formation interferes with evaluation of pulses. Delay in diagnosis and the presence of associated injuries decrease the chances of limb salvage. Contusions or crush injuries may result in complete or partial disruption of arteries, producing intimal flaps or intramural hematomas that impede blood flow.

Blunt thoracic aortic injury (BTAI) is a serious traumatic injury that continues to have a high initial mortality and is associated with modern high-speed methods of transportation. Autopsy data from cases of fatal BTAI demonstrated that 57% of patients were dead at the scene or on arrival to the hospital, 37% died during the first 4 hours at the hospital, and only 6% died after 4 hours in the hospital. The disruption generally occurs at the aortic isthmus (between the left subclavian artery and the ligamentum arteriosum) due to a deceleration injury in which the heart, the ascending aorta, and the transverse arch continue to move forward while movement of the isthmus and the descending aorta is limited by their posterior attachments. Clinical findings associated with traumatic rupture of the thoracic aorta are listed in Table 13–5 and radiographic findings in Table 13–6. Blunt traumatic injury to the abdominal aorta is uncommon, but this has been reported from lap seat belt trauma.

Almost any vessel can be injured by blunt trauma, including the extracranial cerebral and visceral arteries. Blunt carotid arterial injuries are associated with mortality rates of 20–30%, with over 50% of survivors having permanent severe neurologic deficits. Whereas in the past vertebral artery injuries were considered innocuous, recent studies have reported devastating complications related to these injuries, including a 70% incidence of coexistent cervical spine injuries. Traumatic injury to the superior mesenteric artery is associated with a 50% mortality rate. The brachial and popliteal arteries, which cross joints and are exposed to direct trauma, are particularly susceptible to injury as a result of fractures and dislocations.

Table 13–5. Clinical features of traumatic aortic rupture.

History of high-speed deceleration injury
Flail chest
Fractured sternum
Superior vena cava syndrome
Multiple or first or second rib fractures
Upper extremity hypertension or pulse deficits
Hematoma in the carotid sheaths
Interscapular bruits
Hoarseness with normal larynx

Table 13–6. Radiographic features of traumatic aortic rupture.

Widening of mediastinum
Fractured sternum
Multiple or first rib or second rib fractures
Esophageal deviation to the right
Tracheal deviation to the right
Apical cap
Depression of left main stem bronchus
Obliteration of the aortic knob
Obliteration of the descending aorta
Obliteration of the aortopulmonary window
Obliteration of the medial left upper lobe
Widened paravertebral stripe

Clinical Findings

A. Hemorrhage

When pulsatile external hemorrhage is present, the diagnosis of arterial injury is obvious, but when blood accumulates in deep tissues of the extremity, the thorax, abdomen, or retroperitoneum, the only manifestation may be shock. Peripheral vasoconstriction may make evaluation of peripheral pulses difficult until blood volume is restored. If the artery is completely severed, thrombus may form at the contracted vessel ends and a major vascular injury may not be suspected. The presence of arterial pulses distal to a penetrating wound does not preclude arterial injury; as many as 20% of patients with injuries of major arteries in an extremity have palpable pulses distal to the injury, either because the vessel has not thrombosed or because pulse waves are transmitted through soft clot. Conversely, the absence of a palpable pulse in an adequately resuscitated patient is a sensitive indicator of arterial injury.

B. Ischemia

Acute arterial insufficiency must be diagnosed promptly to prevent tissue loss. Ischemia should be suspected when the patient has one or more of the "five Ps": pain, pallor, paralysis, paresthesia, or pulselessness. The susceptibility of different cells to hypoxia varies (eg, sudden occlusion of the carotid artery results in brain damage within minutes unless collateral circulation can maintain adequate perfusion, but a kidney can survive severe ischemia for up to an hour). Peripheral nerves are quite vulnerable to ischemia because they have a high basal energy requirement to maintain ion gradients over large membrane surfaces and because they have few glycogen stores. Hence, interruption of arterial flow for relatively short periods can result in neural damage due to interrupted substrate delivery. In contrast, skeletal muscle is more tolerant of decreased arterial flow. Muscle can be ischemic for up to 4 hours without developing histologic changes. In general, complete interruption of all arterial inflow (including collateral blood supply) results in neuromuscular ischemic damage after 4–6 hours. Restoration of flow can actually worsen this damage as part of the reperfusion syndrome and can increase the severity of the original ischemic insult.

Prolonged ischemia can produce muscle necrosis and rhabdomyolysis, which releases potassium and myoglobin into the circulation. Myoglobin is an oxygen-transporting protein similar in structure to hemoglobin; it is innocuous unless it dissociates into hematin, which is nephrotoxic in an acidic milieu. Precipitation of hematin pigment also occurs when urine flow is reduced by hypotension or hypovolemia, obstructing renal tubules and worsening nephrotoxicity. Myoglobinemia can lead to acute tubular necrosis and renal failure, hyperkalemia, and a risk of life-threatening arrhythmias. Thus, in addition to limb loss, acute arterial ischemia can produce organ failure and death.

C. False Aneurysm

Disruption of an arterial wall as a result of trauma may lead to formation of a false aneurysm. The wall of a false aneurysm is composed primarily of fibrous tissue derived from nearby tissues, not arterial tissue. Because blood continues to flow past the fistulous opening, the extremity is seldom ischemic. False aneurysms may rupture at any time. They continue to expand because they lack vascular wall integrity. Spontaneous resolution of pseudoaneurysms larger than 3 cm is unlikely, and operative repair becomes increasingly difficult as the aneurysms increase in size and complexity with time. Symptoms gradually appear as a result of compression of adjacent nerves or collateral vessels or from rupture of the aneurysm—or as a result of thrombosis with ischemic symptoms. Iatrogenic false aneurysms after arterial puncture thrombose spontaneously within 4 weeks when they are less than 3 cm in diameter. Simple ultrasound follow-up rather than operative therapy is indicated. Color flow duplex-guided compression of iatrogenic pseudoaneurysms is successful in 70–90% of attempts, but the procedure is uncomfortable and may take hours of probe pressure. Ultrasound-guided thrombin injection has been effective for thrombosing large false aneurysms in a matter of seconds, but distal arterial thrombosis has also been described using this technique.

D. Arteriovenous Fistula

With simultaneous injury of an adjacent artery and vein, a fistula may form that allows blood from the artery to enter the vein. Because venous pressure is lower than arterial pressure, flow through an arteriovenous fistula is continuous; accentuation of the bruit and thrill can be detected over the fistula during systole. Traumatic arteriovenous fistulas may occur as operative complications (eg, aortocaval fistula following removal of a herniated intervertebral disk). Iatrogenic femoral arteriovenous fistulas after arteriograms and cardiac catheterization are seen with increasing frequency. Long-standing large arteriovenous fistulas may result in high-output cardiac failure. Similar to iatrogenic pseudoaneurysms occurring after arteriography, spontaneous resolution of acute arteriovenous fistulas usually occurs.

Diagnosis

Arterial injury must be considered in any injured patient. Patients who present in shock following penetrating injury or blunt trauma should be assumed to have vascular injury until proven otherwise. Any injury near a major artery should arouse suspicion. A plain film may be helpful in demonstrating a fracture whose fragments could jeopardize an adjacent vessel or a bullet fragment that could have passed near to a major vessel. Before the x-ray is taken, entrance and exit wounds should be marked with radiopaque objects such as safety pins or paper clips.

Diagnosis is usually established on the basis of physical examination. In addition to checking for obvious hemorrhage and the "five Ps," the physician should listen for a bruit, palpate for a thrill (eg, of an arteriovenous fistula), and look for an expanding hematoma (eg, of a false aneurysm). Secondary hemorrhage from a wound is an ominous sign that may herald massive hemorrhage. The finding of these "hard" signs reliably reflects the presence of a vascular injury; hard signs mandate immediate exploration in most instances. The presence of "soft" signs (history of bleeding, diminished but palpable pulse, injury in proximity to a major artery, neurapraxia) requires further tests or serial observation.

Doppler flow studies have gained importance in the diagnosis of arterial trauma. An ankle brachial index (ABI), determined by dividing the systolic pressure in the injured limb by the systolic pressure in an uninjured arm, is highly reliable for excluding arterial injury after both blunt and penetrating trauma. An ABI < 0.9 has sensitivity of 95%, specificity of 97%, and negative predictive value of 99% for determining the presence of clinically significant arterial injury. Thus, only patients with "soft" signs and an ABI of < 0.9 require arteriography.

Color flow duplex ultrasonography combines real-time B mode (brightness modulation) ultrasound imaging with a steerable pulsed Doppler flow detector. This technology can provide images of vessels and velocity spectral analysis. Color flow duplex scanning of an area of injury is noninvasive, painless, portable, and easily

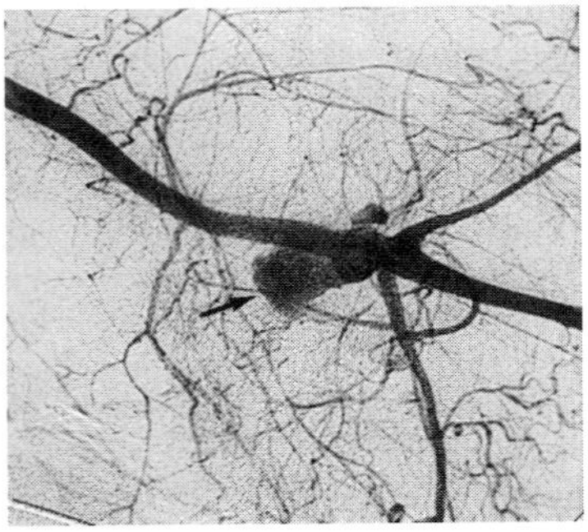

Figure 13–16. Arteriogram showing traumatic pseudoaneurysm of subclavian/axillary artery from penetrating injury.

repeated for follow-up examinations. When compared with arteriography and performed by experienced examiners, duplex ultrasound identifies nearly all major injuries that require treatment, potentially at considerable cost savings. In addition to screening for arterial trauma, duplex scanning has been used to detect pseudoaneurysms, arteriovenous fistulas, and intimal flaps. However, potential logistical and resource problems exist. The technology is sophisticated and requires skill in operation and interpretation, which is not always immediately available.

Arteriography is the most accurate diagnostic procedure for identifying vascular injuries (Figure 13–16). Arteriography to exclude vascular injury for soft signs results in a negative exploration rate of 20–35% and an arteriography-related complication rate of 2–4%. Proximity as the sole indication for arteriography has an extremely low yield, ranging from nil to 10%. Patients with unequivocal signs of arterial injury on physical examination or plain films should have urgent operation. The false-negative rate of arteriography is low, and a normal arteriogram precludes the need for surgical exploration. Virtually all arteriographic errors are due to false-positives, which occur in 2–8% of patients. Technical considerations in performing arteriography include the following: (1) entrance and exit wounds should be marked with a radiopaque marker; (2) the injection site should not be near the suspected injury; (3) an area 10–15 cm proximal and distal to the suspected injury should be included in the arteriographic field; (4) sequential films should be obtained to detect early venous filling; (5) any abnormality should be considered an indication of arterial injury unless it is obviously the result of preexisting disease; and (6) two different projections should be obtained.

Emergency center arteriography not using the Seldinger technique but rather cannulating the artery to be studied with an 18-gauge catheter (antegrade in the lower extremity and prograde in the upper extremity arteries) is quick and surprisingly accurate. The use of fluoroscopy, especially if equipped with subtraction capability, simplifies the timing of contrast injection and x-ray exposure. Fluoroscopy is particularly helpful to visualize distal arteries and minimize the amount of contrast media needed. Arteriography may be particularly useful in differentiating arterial injury from spasm. In general, it is risky to attribute abnormal physical findings in an injured patient to arterial spasm; an arteriogram is indicated in such patients.

Arteriography is also valuable when arterial injuries may have occurred at multiple sites or to localize an injury when a long parallel penetration makes this determination difficult. Complications of arteriography include groin hematomas, iatrogenic pseudoaneurysms, arteriovenous fistulas, embolic occlusions, and delays in diagnosis that may lead to irreversible ischemia in marginally perfused limbs.

For patients suspected of having BTAI based on mechanism of injury, the chest x-ray is a good screening tool to determine the need for further investigation. The most significant radiographic findings for possible BTAI include widened mediastinum, obscured aortic knob, deviation of the left mainstem bronchus or nasogastric tube, and opacification of the aortopulmonary window. Contrast CT scanning of the chest is a useful diagnostic tool for screening and diagnosis of BTAI in selected patients. A negative chest CT can obviate the need for further evaluation with a contrast aortogram. Patients with indeterminate CT scans or positive scans should have confirmation of BTAI with arteriography. In selected instances cardiothoracic or trauma surgeons may consider helical CT scanning alone to be an adequate and complete workup for BTAI. However, in general most surgeons will require the obtaining of an aortic arteriogram prior to performing operative intervention. The use of either transesophageal echocardiography or intraluminal ultrasound in the diagnosis of BTAI continues to evolve, but they are not considered standard diagnostic modalities.

Management

A. Initial Treatment

A rapid but thorough examination should be performed to determine the complete extent of injury. The physician must establish the priority of arterial injury in the overall management of the patient and should remember that delay in arterial repair decreases chances of a favorable outcome. When repair is performed within 12 hours after injury, amputation is rarely necessary; if repair is performed later, the incidence of amputation is about 50%. Depending on the degree of ischemia, delay in arterial repair will lead to lasting neuromuscular damage after as short a period as 4–6 hours.

Restoration of blood volume and control of hemorrhage are done simultaneously. If exsanguinating hemorrhage precludes resuscitation in the emergency room, the patient should be moved directly to the operating room. External bleeding is best controlled by firm direct pressure or packing. Probes or fingers should not be inserted into the wound because a clot may be dislodged, causing profuse bleeding. Tourniquets occlude venous return, disturb collateral flow, and further compromise circulation and should not be employed. Atraumatic vascular clamps may be applied to accessible vessels by trained surgeons, but blind clamping can increase damage and injure adjacent nerves and veins.

After hemorrhage has been controlled and general resuscitation accomplished, further assessment is possible. The extent of associated injuries is determined and a plan of management made. Large-bore intravenous catheters should be placed in extremities with no potential venous injuries. It is prudent to preserve the saphenous or cephalic vein in an uninjured extremity for use as a venous autograft for vascular repair.

B. Nonoperative Treatment

Some arterial injuries remain asymptomatic and heal. Data supporting the practice of observation of small or asymptomatic arterial injuries have emerged from experimental animal studies and clinical reports showing resolution, improvement, or stabilization of arterial injuries. In well-defined settings, this strategy has proved safe in follow-up reports covering periods of up to 10 years. Thus, a nonoperative approach may be appropriate for compliant patients willing to return for follow-up who have (1) no active hemorrhage, (2) low-velocity injuries (particularly stab wounds or iatrogenic punctures), (3) minimal arterial wall disruptions (< 5 mm), (4) small (< 5 mm) intimal defects, and (5) intact distal circulation.

Follow-up must include frequent physical examinations and carefully performed noninvasive studies, and patients should be asymptomatic—and the strategy must be reconsidered if symptoms develop. Adjuvant therapy with antiplatelet agents is usually recommended to improve patency in patients with intimal flaps.

Endovascular management has assumed a greater role in the treatment of arterial trauma in recent years. Transcatheter embolization with coils or balloons has been successful in managing selected arterial injuries such as pseudoaneurysms, arteriovenous fistulas, and active bleeding from nonessential arteries. Coils are made of stainless steel with wool or polyester tufts. They are extruded at the site of vessel injury through 5F or 7F catheters. After deployment, the coils expand and lodge at the extrusion site and the tufts promote thrombosis. Catheter-based intra-arterial infusion of vasodilators has also been used to treat vasospasm in small distal arteries.

The recent popularity of endovascular grafting in elective vascular surgery (see Chapter 34) has been applied to the treatment of arterial trauma. A fixation device such as a stent is attached to a graft, and the stent-graft is inserted endoluminally from a remote site and deployed at the site of injury to repair false aneurysms or arteriovenous fistulas. The indications for endovascular grafting are likely to change as technology advances, but the most frequent application currently is in stable patients with delayed presentations who have complex false aneurysms or arteriovenous fistulas. Use of stent grafts in the acute setting requires the availability of a wide variety of sizes and lengths of grafts and advanced catheter skills. Endovascular repair of BTAI can be performed either electively or even emergently. In small case series this approach has been associated with reduced morbidity. Further study is needed to determine the long-term outcome using endovascular techniques to repair BTAI. Commercial grafts have yielded better results than the noncommercial "homemade" grafts. Thoracic aorta lacerations of more than 1.5 cm resulting in graft apposition length less than 2 cm or those near or in the curvature of the aortic arch are associated with an increased risk of endoleak.

In selected cases of BTAI repair, whether it is operative or endovascular, is delayed because treatment and recovery from other more life-threatening injuries has priority (eg, severe pulmonary contusion, brain injury). This is acceptable and the incidence of aortic rupture after 4 hours in the hospital is low. Systemic blood pressure and heart rate should be controlled with a beta-blocker and other pharmacologic agents as necessary to minimize the risk of rupture while waiting for definitive repair of the injured aorta.

C. Operative Treatment

General anesthesia is preferable to spinal or regional anesthesia. When vascular injuries involve the neck or thoracic outlet, endotracheal intubation must be performed carefully to avoid dislodging a clot and to protect the airway. Moreover, care is necessary to avoid neurologic damage in patients with associated cervical spine injuries. At least one uninjured extremity should also be prepared for surgery, so that saphenous or cephalic vein conduit may be obtained if a vein graft is required. Provision should also be made for operative arteriography.

Incisions should be generous and parallel to the injured vessel. Meticulous care in handling incisions is essential to avoid secondary infections; all undamaged tissue should be conserved for use in covering repaired vessels. Preservation of all arterial branches is important in order to maintain collateral circulation. Atraumatic control of the vessel should be achieved proximal and distal to the injury, so that the injured area may be dissected free of other tissues and inspected without risk of further bleeding. When large hematomas and multiple wounds make exposure and clamping of vessels difficult, it is wise to place a sterile orthopedic tourniquet proximal to the injury that can be inflated temporarily if needed.

The extent of arterial injury must be accurately determined. Arterial spasm generally responds to gentle hydraulic or mechanical dilation. Local application of warm saline or drugs such as papaverine, tolazoline, lidocaine, or nitroglycerin is occasionally effective in relieving spasm. Intra-arterial injection of nitroglycerin or papaverine is also very effective in alleviating spasm. If spasm persists, however, it is best to assume that it is caused by an intramural injury, and the vessel should be opened for direct inspection. An old adage is that spasm is spelled "c-l-o-t."

All devitalized tissue, including damaged portions of the artery, must be debrided. One should resect only the grossly injured portion of the vessel—margins of healthy vessel do not need to be removed. The method of reconstruction depends on the degree of arterial damage. In some instances, the ends of injured vessels can be approximated and an end-to-end anastomosis created. If the vessels cannot be mobilized well enough to provide a tension-free anastomosis, an interposition graft should be used. Early experience with prosthetic interposition grafts was disappointing since postoperative infection, thrombosis, and anastomotic disruption were common. These problems have decreased considerably with the use of grafts made of expanded polytetrafluoroethylene (PTFE). Nevertheless, most surgeons still prefer to use an autogenous graft (ie, vein or artery) in severely contaminated wounds. Saphenous vein grafts should be obtained from the *noninjured* leg to avoid impairment of venous return on the side of the injury. Patch angioplasty using saphenous vein is performed when closure of a partially transected vessel would result in narrowing. Suturing should be done with fine 5-0 or 6-0 monofilament material.

In the unusual circumstance of isolated vascular injury, 5000–10,000 units of intravenous heparin should be given to prevent thrombosis. Otherwise, a small amount of dilute heparin solution (100 units/mL) may be gently injected into the proximal and distal lumen of the injured vessel before clamps are applied. Proximal and distal thrombi are removed with a Fogarty embolectomy catheter. Back-bleeding from the distal artery is not a sure indication that thrombus is absent. A completion operative arteriogram is indicated to determine distal patency and to check on the adequacy of the reconstruction—even when distal pulses are palpable.

It was formerly taught that fractures should be stabilized before vascular injuries were repaired so that manipulation of bones would not jeopardize vascular repair. The disadvantages of this dictum were delay in restoration of flow to ischemic tissue and interference with vascular reconstruction and subsequent arteriographic study of the completed repair by the fixation device. It is currently recommended that vascular repair be performed first, followed by careful application of external traction devices that allow easy access to the wound for observation and dressing changes. Another alternative is to place an intraluminal shunt temporarily across the vascular injury to decrease ischemia while fractures or other injuries are dealt with. There is controversy about the best time to repair injured peripheral nerves; the trend favors concomitant repair except for high-velocity or complicated injuries.

Repaired vessels must be covered with healthy tissue. If left exposed, they invariably desiccate and rupture. Skin alone is inadequate, because subsequent necrosis of the skin would leave the vessels exposed, greatly endangering the reconstruction. Generally, an adjacent muscle (eg, sartorius muscle for coverage of the common femoral artery) can be mobilized and placed over the repair. Musculocutaneous flaps can be constructed by plastic surgeons to cover almost any site. In an extensive or severely contaminated wound, a remote bypass may be routed through clean tissue planes to circumvent difficult soft tissue coverage problems.

D. Venous Injuries

Venous injuries commonly accompany arterial injuries. In order of decreasing frequency, the most common extremity venous injuries are the superficial femoral vein, the popliteal vein, and the common femoral vein. The relative importance and timing of venous repair in an injured extremity is controversial. Advocates of routine venous repair contend that ligation is associated with significant postoperative morbidity, including more frequent failure of arterial repairs due to compromised outflow, venous insufficiency, compartment syndrome, and limb loss. Proponents of venous ligation argue that venous repairs are difficult (requiring interposition, compilation, and spiral grafting), time-consuming (dangerous in the multiply-injured patient), and likely to cause occlusion (patency rates are only about 50%). The presence of postoperative edema after combined arterial and venous injuries is not reliably reduced by attempted venous repair. It seems reasonable to recommend repair of venous injuries when the repair is not too technically difficult (lateral venorrhaphy) and the patient is hemodynamically stable. Thus, the decision to repair the vein depends on the condition of the patient and the condition of the vein. When venous ligation is necessary, postoperative edema can be controlled by elevation of the extremity and use of compression stockings. In patients undergoing venous repair, patency should be monitored using duplex scanning. If thrombosis of the repair is detected and there are no contraindications, anticoagulation should be instituted and maintained for at least 3 months postoperatively.

Fasciotomy is an important adjunctive treatment in many cases of arterial trauma. Indications include the following: (1) combined arterial and venous injury, (2) massive soft tissue damage, (3) delay between injury and repair (4–6 hours), (4) prolonged hypotension, and (5) excessive swelling or high tissue pressure measured by one of several techniques. Whenever compartment pressures (measured with a needle and manometer) approach diastolic pressure, fasciotomy should be performed promptly. Fasciotomies must be performed through adequate skin incisions because when edema is massive the skin envelope itself can compromise neurovascular function.

Fasciotomies are not benign procedures. They create large open wounds, and chronic venous insufficiency is a recognized late complication even in the absence of venous reflux or obstruction. The chronic swelling is thought to be related to loss of integrity of the ensheathing fascia of the calf muscles, reducing the efficiency of the calf muscle pump. Thus, many authorities recommend against routine use of fasciotomies at the initial operation. In the postoperative period, compartmental pressures can be measured using a handheld solid-state transducer as often as clinically indicated. Normal intracompartmental pressure is less than 10 mm Hg. In general, a pressure of 30 mm Hg requires either fasciotomy or continuous monitoring. When the pressure exceeds 45 mm Hg, fasciotomy is mandatory.

E. Immediate Amputation

High-energy or crush injuries of the extremities are associated with high morbidity and a poor prognosis for useful limb function—there is a high late amputation rate despite initial limb salvage. Vascular injuries are now repaired with a high rate of success, but associated orthopedic, soft tissue, and nerve injuries are the critical factors that determine long-term function. A number of scoring systems or indices have been proposed to help determine when to amputate immediately and thus reduce the number of protracted reconstructive procedures that ultimately fail. Management of the mangled extremity is particularly difficult, and none of the scoring systems are universally accepted. Evaluation and management of these patients should be multidisciplinary and the decision to amputate emergently should be made by two independent surgeons whenever possible.

F. Arterial Injuries in Athletes

A number of recent reports have addressed the problem of the increased frequency of arterial injuries in athletes due to certain features of soft tissue hypertrophy and overuse. For example, baseball pitchers frequently develop complications related to thoracic outlet syndrome, producing axillary artery aneurysms and occlusions. Popliteal artery entrapment syndrome, producing popliteal artery aneurysms and occlusions, has been reported in soccer players and long-distance runners. Blunt arterial injuries leading to false aneurysms and occlusions occur in athletes participating in martial arts and other contact sports. Finally, repeated leg motion is thought to be responsible for external iliac artery lesions that have been frequently described in avid cyclists.

Arko FR et al: Vascular complications in high-performance athletes. J Vasc Surg 2001;33:935.

Asensio JA et al: Visceral vascular injuries. Surg Clin North Am 2002;82:1.

Asensio JA et al: Operative management and outcome of 302 abdominal vascular injuries. Am J Surg 2000;180:528.

Biffl WL et al: The devastating potential of blunt vertebral arterial injuries. Ann Surg 2000;231:672.

Biffl WL et al: The unrecognized epidemic of blunt carotid arterial injuries: early diagnosis improves neurologic outcome. Ann Surg 1998;228:462.

Brandt MM, Kazanjian S, Wahl WL: The utility of endovascular stents in the treatment of blunt arterial injuries. J Trauma 2001;51:901.

Brinker MR et al: Tibial shaft fractures with an associated infrapopliteal arterial injury: a survey of vascular surgeons opinions on the need for vascular repair. J Orthop Trauma 2000;14:194.

Brown KR et al: Determinates of functional disability after complex upper extremity trauma. Ann Vasc Surg 2001;15:43.

Buckman RF Jr, Miraliakbari R, Badellino MM: Juxtahepatic venous injuries: a critical review of reported management strategies. J Trauma 2000;48:978.

Caps MT: The epidemiology of vascular trauma. Semin Vasc Surg 1998;11:227.

Carrillo EH et al: Common and external iliac artery injuries associated with pelvic fractures. J Orthop Trauma 1999;13:351.

Cox CS Jr et al: Blunt versus penetrating subclavian artery injury: presentation, injury pattern, and outcome. J Trauma 1999;46:445.

Dennis JW et al: Validation of nonoperative management of occult vascular injuries and accuracy of physical examination alone in penetrating extremity trauma: 5- to 10-year follow-up. J trauma 1998;44:243.

Demetriades D et al: Penetrating injuries to the subclavian and axillary vessels. J Am Coll Surg 1999;188:290.

Fujikawa T et al: Endovascular stent grafting for the treatment of blunt thoracic aortic injury. J Trauma 2001;50:223.

Gasparri MG et al: Physical examination plus chest radiography in penetrating periclavicular trauma: the appropriate trigger for angiography. J Trauma 2000;49:1029.

Granchi T et al: Prolonged use of intraluminal arterial shunts without systemic anticoagulation. Am J Surg 2000;180:493.

Hemmila MR et al: Delayed repair for blunt thoracic aortic injury: is it really equivalent to early repair? J Trauma 2004;56:13.

Kalakuntla V et al: Six-year experience with management of subclavian artery injuries. Am Surg 2000;66:927.

Kang SS et al: Percutaneous ultrasound guided thrombin injections: a new method for treating postcatheterization femoral pseudoaneurysms. J Vasc Surg 1998;27:1032.

Karmy-Jones R et al: Endovascular stent grafts and aortic rupture: a case series. J Trauma 2003;55:805.

Knudson MM et al: Outcome after major renovascular injuries: a Western trauma association multicenter report. J Trauma 2000;49:1116.

Lyden SP et al: Common iliac artery dissection after blunt trauma: case report of endovascular repair and literature review. J Trauma 2001;50:339.

Martinez D et al: Popliteal artery injury associated with knee dislocations. Am Surg 2001;67:165.

McEwan L, Woodruff P, Archibald C: Lap belt abdominal aortic trauma. Australas Radiol 1999;43:369.

McKinley AG, Carrim AT, Robbs JV: Management of proximal axillary and subclavian artery injuries. Br J Surg 2000;87:79.

McQueen MM et al: Acute compartment syndrome. Who is at risk? J Bone Joint Surg Br 2000;82:200.

Nagy K et al: Guidelines for the diagnosis and management of blunt aortic injury: and EAST practice management guidelines work group. J Trauma 2000;48:1128.

Naidoo NM et al: Angiographic embolisation in arterial trauma. Eur J Vasc Endovasc Surg 2000;19:77.

Nair R, Robbs JV, Muckart DJ: Management of penetrating cervicomediastinal venous trauma. Eur J Vasc Endovasc Surg 2000;19:65.

Nehler MR, Taylor LM, Porter JM: Iatrogenic vascular trauma. Semin Vasc Surg 1998;11:283.

Nehler MR et al: Iatrogenic vascular injuries from percutaneous vascular suturing devices. J Vasc Surg 2001;33:943.

Ofer A et al: CT angiography of the carotid arteries in trauma to the neck. Eur J Vasc Endovasc Surg 2001;21:401.

Ott MC et al: Management of blunt thoracic aortic injuries: endovascular stents versus open repair. J Trauma 2004;56:565.

Pagan-Marin H, Bettmann MA, Boxt LM: Blunt abdominal or pelvic trauma—suspected vascular injury. American College of Radiology. ACR Appropriateness Criteria. Radiology 2000;215(Suppl):41.

Rozycki GS et al: Blunt vascular trauma in the extremity: diagnosis, management, and outcome. J Trauma 2003;55:814.

Sparks SR, DeLaRosa J, Bergan JJ: Arterial injury in uncomplicated upper extremity dislocations. Ann Vasc Surg 2000;14:110.

Velmahos GC, Toutouzas KG: Vascular trauma and compartment syndromes. Surg Clin North Am 2002;82:125.

Velmahos GC et al: Angiographic embolization for arrest of bleeding after penetrating trauma to the abdomen. Am J Surg 1999;178:367.

Wahl WL et al: Blunt thoracic aortic injury: delayed or early repair? J Trauma 1999;47:254.

BLAST INJURY

Blast injuries in civilian populations occur as a result of fireworks, household explosions, or industrial accidents. Urban guerrilla warfare or terrorist tactics may take the form of letter bombs, suitcase bombs, car bombs or truck bombs, and suicide bombers. Injuries occur from the effects of the blast itself, propelled foreign bodies, or, in large blasts, from falling objects. Military blast injuries may also involve personnel submerged in water. Water increases energy transmission and the possibility of injury to the viscera of the thorax or abdomen. The pathophysiology of blast injuries involves two mechanisms. **Crush injury** results from rapid displacement of the body wall and may result in laceration and contusion of underlying structures. Minor displacements may produce serious injury if the body wall velocity is high. In addition, the motion of the body wall generates waves that propagate within the body and transfer energy to internal sites.

Clinical Findings

A. Symptoms and Signs

The injury is dependent upon proximity to the blast, space confinement, and detonation size. Large explosions cause multiple foreign body impregnations, bruises, abrasions, and lacerations. Gross soilage of wounds from clothing, flying debris, or explosive powder is usual. About 10% of all casualties have deep injuries to the chest or abdomen. Blast-induced circulatory shock may be caused by immediate myocardial depression without a compensatory vasoconstriction. Lung damage usually involves rupture of the alveolus with hemorrhage. Air embolism from bronchovenous fistula may cause sudden death. The mechanisms of lung injury are thought to be due to spalling effects (splintering forces produced when a pressure wave hits a fluid-air interface), implosion effects, and pressure differentials. Hypoxia may result from a ventilation-perfusion mismatch caused by the pulmonary hemorrhage. Patients with pulmonary blast injury may die despite intensive respiratory support.

Blast injury causing pneumatic disruption of the esophagus or bowel has been reported. Tension pneumoperitoneum is a known although rare complication of barotrauma. Letter bombs cause predominantly hand, face, eye, and ear injuries. Energy transmission within the fluid media of the eye can cause globe rupture, dialysis of the iris, hyphema of the anterior chamber, lens capsule tears, retinal rupture, or macular pucker. Ear injuries may consist of drum rupture or cochlear damage. There may be nerve or conduction hearing deficit or deafness. Tinnitus, vertigo, and anosmia are also seen in letter bomb casualties.

B. Imaging Studies

Chest x-ray may initially be normal or may show pneumothorax, pneumomediastinum, or parenchymal infiltrates. In mass casualty situations it may be necessary to reserve the use of CT scans for those patients with acute changing neurologic examinations during the immediate intake period. Patients with multiple penetrating injuries from shrapnel may benefit from full-body CT scanning following initial stabilization and evaluation. Correlation of radiologic imaging studies with clinical examination is useful in guiding which injuries may need operative intervention when the number of skin surface wounds is high and it is impractical to explore all of these wounds.

Treatment

Severe injuries with shock from blood loss or hypoxia require resuscitative measures to restore perfusion and oxygenation. The usual criteria for exploring penetrating wounds of the thorax or abdomen are employed. Perforation of hollow organs should be suspected in patients with appropriate histories, particularly those that were submerged at the time of injury. Respiratory insufficiency may result from pulmonary injury or may be secondary to shock, fat embolism, or other causes. Tracheal intubation and prolonged respiratory care with mechanical ventilation may be necessary. In cases of tension pneumoperitoneum, surgical decompression may dramatically improve respiratory and hemodynamic functions. Surgical treatment of extremity injuries requires wide debridement of devitalized muscle, thorough cleansing of wounds, and removal of foreign materials. The possibility of gas gangrene in contaminated muscle injuries may warrant open treatment. Eye injuries may require immediate repair. Ear injuries are usually treated expectantly.

Cernak I et al: Blast injury from explosive munitions. J Trauma 1999;47:96.

Coupland RM, Meddings DR: Mortality associated with the use of weapons in armed conflicts, wartime atrocities, and civilian mass shootings: literature review. BMJ 1999;319:407.

Davis TP et al: Distribution and care of shipboard blast injuries (USS Cole DDG-67). J Trauma 2003;55:1022.

Frykberg ER: Medical management of disasters and mass casualties from terrorist bombings: how can we cope? J Trauma 2002; 53:201.

Guy RJ et al: Physiologic responses to primary blast. J Trauma 1998; 45:983.

Irwin RJ et al: Shock after blast wave injury is caused by a vagally mediated reflex. J Trauma 1999;47:105.

Leibovici D, Gofit ON, Shapira SC: Eardrum perforation in explosion survivors: is it a marker of pulmonary blast injury? Ann Emerg Med 1999;34:168.

Mallonee S et al: Physical injuries and fatalities resulting from the Oklahoma City bombing. JAMA 1996;276:382.

Oppenheim A et al: Tension pneumoperitoneum after blast injury: dramatic improvement in ventilatory and hemodynamic parameters after surgical decompression. J Trauma 1998;44:915.

Shaham D et al: The role of radiology in terror injuries. Isr Med Assoc J 2002;4:564.

Stein M, Hirshberg A: Medical consequences of terrorism. The conventional weapon threat. Surg Clin North Am 1999;79:1537.

DROWNING

Drowning is a major cause of accidental death in the United States, particularly in children, and has resulted in 5500 deaths yearly for the last four decades. During summer vacation weekends, the number of deaths may rise to 50 per day. Approximately 25% of drowning victims are teenagers; 20% are less than 10 years of age; and 10% occur in each decade of life from age 20 to age 70. Drowning victims are males in 85% of cases. In the United States, most cases of drowning occur in fresh water, usually lakes, rivers, swimming pools, or spas. Only about one-fourth of drownings occur in seawater. Alcohol ingestion is a factor in as many as 40% of the cases of adult drowning. Inadequate supervision and improperly covered pools or spas are the chief causes of childhood drowning.

The effects of drowning or near-drowning are due principally to hypoxemia and aspiration. The physiologic effects of aspiration differ according to whether the drowning medium is fresh water or salt water, which is hypotonic and hypertonic, respectively, compared with plasma. It is possible for a drowning victim to die of hypoxemia without aspiration, but this occurs rarely. In animal studies, arterial PO_2 falls rapidly after tracheal obstruction, reaching a PO_2 of 10 mm Hg within 3 minutes. In human volunteers who hyperventilated, then held their breath as long as possible, PO_2 declined to 58 mm Hg after 146 seconds of breath holding without exercise but reached 43 mm Hg at 85 seconds if the subject was exercising. Within 3–5 minutes after total immersion in water, this degree of hypoxemia would be enough to cause loss of consciousness in all victims.

If fresh water is aspirated, the fluid is rapidly absorbed from the alveoli, producing intravascular hypervolemia, hypotonicity, dilution of serum electrolytes, and intravascular hemolysis. Animal studies show that the intravascular volume may increase 50% within 3 minutes after fresh water aspiration. In addition, the direct injury to pulmonary surfactant results in increased surface tension and damage to the pulmonary capillary membrane. This can result in a form of noncardiogenic pulmonary edema. Debris and microorganisms are deposited in the alveoli, setting the stage for later infectious complications if the victim survives.

Salt water aspiration produces opposite effects because water is drawn into the alveoli from the vascular space, producing hypovolemia, hemoconcentration, and hypertonicity. Hemolysis is not significant after salt water near-drowning.

Treatment of the near-drowning victim should be directed toward immediate restoration of ventilation, as the degree of hypoxemia and resulting damage increases rapidly. Time should not be wasted in trying to drain the victim's lungs of water, since the actual amount of water aspirated is not large, and in fresh water drowning it is rapidly absorbed from the alveoli in any case.

After restoration of ventilation, the major goals of treatment are to evaluate and correct residual hypoxemia or acidosis and electrolyte abnormalities. If the patient has aspirated significant quantities of fluid, endotracheal intubation and ventilation will usually be necessary. Metabolic acidosis will be self-correcting if the circulation can be restored. In extreme cases, sodium bicarbonate may be given intravenously if the pH is below 7.2. No specific drugs appear to be useful other than those normally used in cardiopulmonary resuscitation. Prophylactic antibiotics and corticosteroids have specifically been shown not to be beneficial.

If immediate resuscitation is successful, the victim is still at high risk of acute respiratory failure if aspiration occurred. This is the major cause of late fatalities. Treatment is identical to that for acute respiratory failure due to any cause—specifically, intubation and the initiation of positive pressure mechanical ventilation with supplemental O_2.

Neurologic damage is the next most common sequela of near-drowning and results from the period of hypoxemia. If the victim never lost consciousness during the drowning episode, the chance of neurologic damage is negligible. In patients who sustain neurologic damage, the neurologic changes and the prognosis are similar to those after cerebral damage from other forms of cardiopulmonary arrest. The kidney may also be affected if significant intravascular hemolysis has occurred. Hemoglobinuria is treated initially by osmotic diuretics and alkalinization of the urine. If acute renal failure occurs, dialysis may be necessary.

Immersion associated with hypothermia may represent a special situation since studies have shown that young, otherwise healthy people can survive accidental deep hypothermia with minimal or no cerebral impairment, even with prolonged circulatory arrest. Rewarming strategies include immersion, body cavity lavage, or, preferably, the use of cardiopulmonary bypass. The latter technique has the advantage of immediately restoring organ perfusion in patients with inadequate circulation.

American Academy of Pediatrics Committee on Injury, Violence, and Poison Prevention: Prevention of Drowning in infants, children, and adolescents. Pediatrics 2003;112:437.

Cummings P, Quan L: Trends in unintentional drowning: the role of alcohol and medical care. JAMA 1999;281:2198.

DeNicola LK et al: Submersion injuries in children and adults. Crit Care Clin 1997;13:477.

Gheen KM: Near-drowning and cold water submersion. Semin Pediatr Surg 2001;10:26.

Giesbrecht GG: Cold stress, near drowning and accidental hypothermia: a review. Aviat Space Environ Med 2000;71:733.

Graf WD, Quan L, Cummings P: Outcome of children after near drowning. Pediatrics 1998;101:160.

Modell JH et al: Survival after prolonged submersion in freshwater in Florida. Chest 2004;125:1948.

Walpoth BH et al: Outcome of survivors of accidental deep hypothermia and circulatory arrest treated with extracorporeal blood warming. N Engl J Med 1997;337:1500.

Burns & Other Thermal Injuries 14

Robert H. Demling, MD

BURNS

A severe thermal injury is one of the most devastating physical and psychological injuries a person can suffer. Over 2 million injuries due to burns require medical attention each year in the USA, with 14,000 deaths resulting. Fires in the home are responsible for only 5% of burn injuries but for 50% of burn deaths—most due to smoke inhalation. About 75,000 patients require hospitalization every year, and 25,000 of those remain hospitalized for over 2 months—evidence of the severity of illness associated with this injury.

ANATOMY & PHYSIOLOGY OF THE SKIN

The skin is the largest organ of the body, ranging in area from 0.25 m^2 in the newborn to 1.8 m^2 in the adult. It consists of two layers: the epidermis and the dermis (corium). The outermost cells of the epidermis are dead cornified cells that act as a tough protective barrier against the environment. The second, thicker layer, the corium (0.06–0.12 mm), is composed chiefly of fibrous connective tissue. The corium contains the blood vessels and nerves to the skin and the epithelial appendages of specialized function. Since the nerve endings that mediate pain are found only in the corium, partial-thickness injuries may be extremely painful, whereas full-thickness burns are usually painless.

The corium is a barrier that prevents loss of body fluids by evaporation and loss of excess body heat. Sweat glands help maintain body temperature by controlling the amount of water that evaporates. They also excrete small amounts of sodium chloride and cholesterol and traces of albumin and urea. The corium is interlaced with sensory nerve endings that mediate the sensations of touch, pressure, pain, heat, and cold. This is a protective mechanism that allows an individual to adapt to changes in the physical environment.

The skin produces vitamin D, which is synthesized by the action of sunlight on certain intradermal cholesterol compounds. The skin also acts as a protective barrier against infection by preventing penetration of the subdermal tissue by microorganisms.

DEPTH OF BURNS

The depth of the burn (Figure 14–1) significantly affects all subsequent clinical events. The depth may be difficult to determine and in some cases is not known until after spontaneous healing has occurred or when the eschar is surgically removed or separates, exposing the wound bed.

Traditionally, burns have been classified as first-, second-, and third-degree, but the current emphasis on burn healing has led to classification as partial-thickness burns, which can heal spontaneously, and full-thickness burns, which require skin grafting, although deep partial-thickness burns are usually excised and grafted as well.

A **first-degree burn** involves only the epidermis and is characterized by erythema and minor microscopic changes; tissue damage is minimal, protective functions of the skin are intact, skin edema is minimal, and systemic effects are rare. Pain, the chief symptom, usually resolves in 48–72 hours, and healing takes place uneventfully. In 5–10 days, the damaged epithelium peels off in small scales, leaving no residual scarring. The most common causes of first-degree burns are overexposure to sunlight and brief scalding.

Second-degree or partial-thickness burns are deeper, involving all of the epidermis and some of the corium or dermis. The systemic severity of the burn and the quality of subsequent healing are directly related to the amount of undamaged dermis. Superficial burns are often characterized by blister formation, while deeper partial-thickness burns have a reddish appearance or a layer of whitish nonviable dermis firmly adherent to the remaining viable tissue. Blisters, when present, continue to increase in size in the postburn period as the osmotically active particles in the blister fluid attract water. Complications are rare from superficial second-degree burns, which usually heal with minimal scarring in 10–14 days unless they become infected.

Deep dermal burns heal over a period of 25–35 days with a fragile epithelial covering that arises from the residual uninjured epithelium of the deep dermal sweat

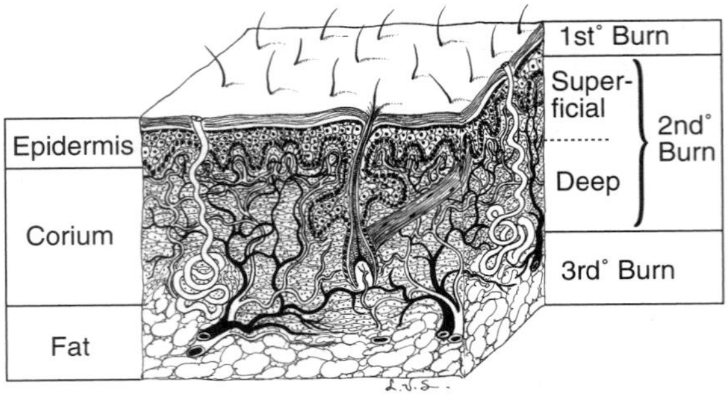

Figure 14–1. Layers of the skin showing depth of first-degree, second-degree, and third-degree burns.

glands and hair follicles. Severe hypertrophic scarring occurs when such an injury heals; the resulting epithelial covering is prone to blistering and breakdown. Evaporative losses after healing remain high compared with losses in normal skin. Conversion to a full-thickness burn by bacteria is common. Skin grafting of deep dermal burns, when feasible, improves the physiologic quality and appearance of the skin cover.

Full-thickness (third-degree) burns have a characteristic white, waxy appearance and may appear to the untrained eye as unburned skin. Burns caused by prolonged exposure, with involvement of fat and underlying tissue, may be brown, dark red, or black. The diagnostic findings of full-thickness burns are lack of sensation in the burned skin, lack of capillary refill, and a leathery texture that is unlike normal skin. All epithelial elements are destroyed, leaving no potential for reepithelialization.

DETERMINATION OF SEVERITY OF INJURY

Illness and death are related to the size (surface area) and depth of the burn, the age and prior state of health of the victim, the location of the burn wound, and the severity of associated injuries, if any—particularly lung injuries.

The total body surface area involved in the burn is most accurately determined by using the age-related charts designed by Lund and Browder (Figure 14–2). A set of these charts should be filled out for every burn patient on admission and when resuscitation is begun.

A careful calculation of the percentage of total body burn is useful for several reasons. First, there is a general clinical tendency to both underestimate and overestimate the size of the burn and thus its severity. The American Burn Association has adopted a severity index for burn injury (Table 14–1). Second, prognosis is directly related to the extent of injury. Third, the decision about who should be treated in a specialized burn facility or managed as an outpatient is based in part on the estimate of burn size.

Patients under age 2 years and over age 60 years have a significantly higher death rate for any given extent of burn. The higher death rate in infants results from a number of factors. First, the body surface area in children relative to body weight is much greater than in adults. Therefore, a burn of comparable surface area has a greater physiologic impact on a child. Second, immature kidneys and liver do not allow for removal of a high solute load from injured tissue or the rapid restoration of adequate nutritional support. Third, the incompletely developed immune system increases susceptibility to infection. Associated conditions such as cardiac disease, diabetes, or chronic obstructive pulmonary disease significantly worsen the prognosis in elderly patients.

Burns involving the hands, face, feet, or perineum will result in permanent disability if not properly treated. Patients with such burns should always be admitted to the hospital, preferably to a burn center. Chemical and electrical burns or those involving the respiratory tract are invariably far more extensive than is evident on initial inspection. Therefore, hospital admission is necessary in these cases also.

PATHOLOGY & PATHOPHYSIOLOGY OF THERMAL INJURIES

The microscopic pathologic feature of the burn wound is principally coagulation necrosis. Beneath any obviously charred tissue there are three distinct zones. The first is the zone of "coagulation," or necrosis with irreversible cell death and no capillary blood flow. The depth of this most severely damaged zone is determined by the temperature and duration of exposure. Surrounding this is a zone of injury or stasis, characterized by sluggish capillary blood flow and injured cells. Although damaged, the tissue is still viable. Further tissue injury is caused by products of inflammation such as oxidants and vasoconstrictor mediators. Environmental insults such as hypoperfusion desiccation or infection can also cause the injured tissue to become necrotic. This process is called **wound conversion.** The third zone is that of "hyperemia," which is the usual inflammatory response of healthy tissue to nonlethal injury. Vasodilatation is typically present.

A rapid loss of intravascular fluid and protein occurs through the heat-injured capillaries. The volume loss is greatest in the first 6–8 hours, with capillary integrity returning toward normal by 36–48 hours. In addition, there is an increase in interstitial osmotic pressure that accentuates the edema. A transient increase in vascular permeability also occurs in nonburned tissues, probably as a result of the initial release of vasoactive mediators. How-

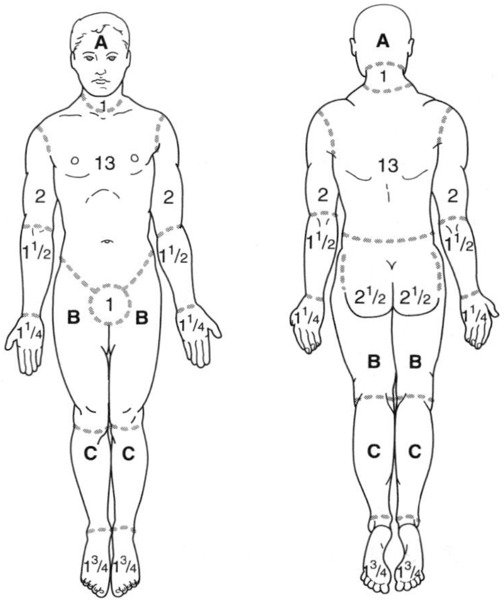

Relative Percentages of Areas Affected by Growth

Area	Age 10	Age 15	Adult
A = half of head	$5\ ^1/_2$	$4\ ^1/_2$	$3\ ^1/_2$
B = half of one thigh	$4\ ^1/_4$	$4\ ^1/_2$	$4\ ^3/_4$
C = half of one leg	3	$3\ ^1/_4$	$3\ ^1/_2$

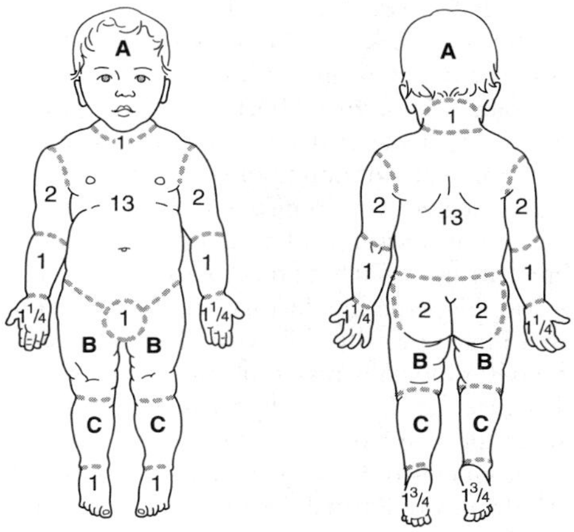

Relative Percentages of Areas Affected by Growth

Area	Age 0	Age 1	Age 5
A = half of head	$9\ ^1/_2$	$8\ ^1/_2$	$6\ ^1/_2$
B = half of one thigh	$2\ ^3/_4$	$3\ ^1/_4$	4
C = half of one leg	$2\ ^1/_2$	$2\ ^1/_2$	$2\ ^3/_4$

Figure 14–2. Table for estimating extent of burns. In adults, a reasonable system for calculating the percentage of body surface burned is the "rule of nines": Each arm equals 9%, the head equals 9%, the anterior and posterior trunk each equal 18%, and each leg equals 18%; the sum of these percentages is 99%.

Table 14–1. Summary of American Burn Association burn severity categorization.

Major burn injury
- Second-degree burn of > 25% body surface area in adults
- Second-degree burn of > 25% body surface area in children
- Third-degree burn of > 10% body surface area
- Most burns involving hands, face, eyes, ears, feet, or perineum
- Most patients with the following:
  - Inhalation injury
  - Electrical injury
  - Burn injury complicated by other major trauma
- Poor-risk patients with burns

Moderate uncomplicated burn injury
- Second-degree burn of 15–25% body surface area in adults
- Second-degree burn of 10–20% body surface area in children
- Third-degree burn of < 10% body surface area

Minor burn injury
- Second-degree burn of < 15% body surface area in adults
- Second-degree burn of < 10% body surface area in children
- Third-degree burn of < 2% body surface area

ever, the edema that develops in nonburned tissues during resuscitation appears to be due in large part to the marked hypoproteinemia caused by protein loss into the burn itself. A systemic inflammatory response occurs in response to a large body burn, resulting in the release of oxidants and other inflammatory mediators into unburned tissues. A generalized decrease in cell energy and membrane potential occurs as a result. This leads to a shift of extracellular sodium and water into the intracellular space. This process is also corrected as hemodynamic stability is restored, but will return if the systemic inflammation is amplified. Smoke inhalation markedly increases the hemodynamic instability, fluid requirements, and mortality rates by adding another source of intense inflammation leading to local lung and systemic tissue damage.

METABOLIC RESPONSE TO BURNS & METABOLIC SUPPORT

The initial metabolic response appears to be activated by proinflammatory cytokines and in turn oxidants.

The secretion of catecholamines, cortisol, glucagon, renin-angiotensin, antidiuretic hormone, and aldosterone is also increased. Early in the response, energy is supplied by the breakdown of stored glycogen and by the process of anaerobic glycolysis.

A profound hypermetabolism occurs in the postburn period, characterized by an increase in metabolic rate that approaches doubling of the basal rate in severe burns. The degree of response is proportionate to the degree of injury, with a plateau occurring when the burn involves about 70% of total body surface. The initiating and perpetuating factors are the mediators of inflammation, especially the cytokines and endotoxin. Added environmental stresses such as pain, cooling, and sepsis increase the obligatory hypermetabolism.

During the first postburn week, the metabolic rate (or heat production) and oxygen consumption rise progressively from the normal level present during resuscitation and remain elevated until the wound is covered and no other sources of inflammation remain. The specific pathophysiologic mechanism remains undefined, but increased and persistent catecholamine secretion and excessive evaporative heat loss from the burn wound are major factors, as is increased circulating endotoxin absorbed from wound or gut.

The evaporative water loss from the wound may reach 300 mL/m^2/h (normal is about 15 mL/m^2/h). This produces a heat loss of about 580 kcal/L of water evaporated. Covering the burn with an impermeable membrane, such as skin substitute, reduces the hypermetabolism. Similarly, placing the burn patient in a warm environment, where convection and radiant loss of heat are minimized, also modestly reduces the metabolic rate. Placing the burn patient in an unwarmed environment (room temperature at or below 27 °C) accentuates heat loss and markedly increases the hypermetabolic state. The persistently elevated circulating levels of catecholamines and cortisol stimulate an exaggerated degree of gluconeogenesis and protein breakdown. Protein catabolism, glucose intolerance, and marked total body weight loss result.

Aggressive nutritional support along with rapid wound closure and control of pain, stress, and sepsis will help control the hypermetabolic state. Recently controlled use of a beta-blocker has been shown to decrease catabolism. In addition, insulin, growth hormones, and testosterone analogues have been shown to both decrease catabolism and increase anabolism.

IMMUNOLOGIC FACTORS IN BURNS

A number of immunologic abnormalities in burn patients predispose to infection. Serum IgA, IgM, and IgG are frequently depressed, reflecting depressed B cell function. Cell-mediated immunity or T cell function is also impaired, as demonstrated by prolonged survival of homografts and xenografts. A decrease in interleukin-2 production due to circulating mediators may be responsible.

PMN chemotactic activity is suppressed. This has been attributed by some to a circulating inhibitory factor released from the burn wound. A decrease in chemotaxis predates evidence of clinical sepsis by several days. Decreased oxygen consumption and impaired bacterial killing have also been demonstrated in PMNs. Depressed killing is probably due to decreased production of hydrogen peroxide and superoxide; this has been demonstrated by decreased PMN chemiluminescent activity in burn patients. An increase in plasma procalcitonin, a metabolite of calcitonin, has recently been reported to be an early marker of sepsis.

BURN MANAGEMENT

ACUTE RESUSCITATION

The burn patient should be assessed and treated like any patient with major trauma. The first priority is to ensure an adequate airway. If there is a possibility that smoke inhalation has occurred—as suggested by exposure to a fire in an enclosed space or burns of the face, nares, or upper torso—arterial blood gases and arterial oxygen saturation of hemoglobin and carboxyhemoglobin CoHgb levels should be measured and 100% oxygen should be administered. If CoHgb is elevated, 100% oxygen should be administered until levels return to normal.

Endotracheal intubation is indicated if the patient is semicomatose, has deep burns to the face and neck, or is otherwise critically injured. Intubation should be done early in all doubtful cases, because delayed intubation will be difficult to achieve in cases associated with facial and pharyngeal edema or upper airway injury, and an emergency tracheostomy may become necessary later under difficult circumstances. If the burn exceeds 20% of body surface area, a urinary catheter should be inserted to monitor urine output. A large-bore intravenous catheter should be inserted, preferably into a large peripheral vein. There is a significant complication rate with the use of central lines in burn patients owing to the increased risk of infection.

Severe burns are characterized by large losses of intravascular fluid, which are greatest during the first 8–12 hours. Fluid loss occurs as a result of the altered capillary permeability, severe hypoproteinemia, and the shift of sodium into the cells. Both fluid shifts diminish significantly by 24 hours postburn. The lung appears to be reasonably well protected from the early edema process, and pulmonary edema is uncommon during the resuscitation period unless there is a superimposed inhalation injury.

Initially, an isotonic crystalloid salt solution is infused to counterbalance the loss of plasma volume into the extravascular space and the further loss of extracellular fluid into the intracellular space. Lactated Ringer's solution is commonly used, the rate being dictated by urine output, pulse (character and rate), state of consciousness, and, to a lesser extent, blood pressure. Urine output should be maintained at 0.5 mL/kg/h and the pulse at 120 beats/min or slower. Base deficit has been shown to be an excellent marker, with an increasing deficit indicating inadequate perfusion.

Swan-Ganz catheters and central venous pressure lines are seldom needed except in the case of severe smoke inhalation injury or unless the patient has sufficient cardiopulmonary disease so that accurate monitoring of volume status would be difficult without measurement of filling pressures or unless a persistent base deficit is present, indicating continued impaired perfusion. It has been estimated that the amount of lactated Ringer's necessary in the first 24 hours for adequate resuscitation is approximately 3–4 mL/kg of body weight per percent of body burn. This is the amount of fluid needed to restore the estimated sodium deficit. At least half of the fluid is given in the first 8 hours because of the greater initial volume loss. Dextrose-containing solutions are not used initially because of early stress-induced glucose intolerance.

Although the importance of restoring colloid osmotic pressure and plasma proteins is well recognized, the timing of colloid infusion remains somewhat varied. Plasma proteins are ordinarily not infused until after the initial plasma leak begins to decrease. This usually occurs about 4–8 hours postburn. The addition of a protein infusion to the treatment regimen after this period will decrease the fluid requirements and—in very young or elderly patients and in patients with massive burns (in excess of 50% of body surface)—will improve hemodynamic stability.

After intravenous fluids are started and vital signs stabilized, the wound should be debrided of all loose skin and dirt. To avoid severe hypothermia, debridement is best done by completing one body area before exposing a second. An alternative is to use an overhead radiant heater, which will decrease net heat loss. Cool water is a very good analgesic on a small superficial burn; however, it should not be used for larger burns because of the risk of hypothermia. Pain is best controlled with the use of intravenous rather than intramuscular narcotics. Tetanus toxoid, 0.5 mL, should be administered to patients with any significant burn injury.

POSTRESUSCITATION PERIOD

Intravenous fluid therapy during the second 24 hours should consist of glucose in hypotonic salt solution to replace evaporative losses and of plasma proteins to maintain adequate circulating volume. Evaporative losses are considerable and will continue until the wound is healed or has been grafted. An estimate of these losses in milliliters per hour is arrived at as follows, where TBS is total body surface:

$$(25 \times \%\ \text{burn}) \times \text{m}^2\ \text{TBS}$$

Treatment should aim to decrease excessive catecholamine stimulation and provide enough calories to offset the effects of the hypermetabolism. Hypothermia, pain, and anxiety all need to be aggressively controlled. Hypovolemia should be prevented by giving enough fluid to make up for the body losses.

Nutritional support should begin as early as possible in the postburn period to maximize wound healing and minimize immune deficiency. Patients with moderate body burns may be able to meet nutritional needs by voluntary oral intake. Patients with large burns invariably require calorie and protein supplementation. This can usually be accomplished by administering a formula diet through a small feeding tube. Parenteral nutrition is also occasionally required, but the intestinal route is preferred if needs can be met this way. Early restoration of gut function will also decrease gut bacterial translocation and endotoxin leak. The reader should consult Chapter 11 for detailed information on nutrition.

The use of penicillin prophylactically in burned patients is controversial. It is probably better to treat streptococcal infections in the few patients who acquire them than to cover all patients. Broad-spectrum antibiotics should never be given for prophylaxis.

Vitamins A, E, and C and zinc should be given until the burn wound is closed. Low-dose heparin therapy may have some benefit, as with other immobilized patients with soft tissue injury.

CARE OF THE BURN WOUND

In the management of superficial partial or second-degree burns, one must provide as aseptic an environment as possible to prevent infection. However, superficial burns generally do not require the use of topical antibiotics. Occlusive dressings are used to minimize exposure to air, increase the rate of reepithelialization, and decrease pain. The exception would be the face, which can be treated open. If there is no infection, burns will heal spontaneously.

The goals in managing deep partial-thickness or full-thickness (third-degree) burns are to prevent invasive infection (ie, burn wound sepsis), to remove dead tissue, and to cover the wound with skin or skin substitutes as soon as possible.

All topical antibiotics retard wound healing to some degree and therefore should be used only on deep second- or third-degree burns or wounds with a high risk of infection.

Topical Antibacterial Agents

Topical agents have definitely advanced the care of burn patients. Although burn wound sepsis is still a major problem, the incidence is lower and the death rate has been reduced, particularly in burns of less than 50% of body surface area. Silver sulfadiazine is now the most widely used preparation. Mafenide, silver nitrate, povidone-iodine, and gentamicin ointments are also used. Silver release dressings are now very popular, silver being a very potent antimicrobial.

Silver sulfadiazine is effective against a wide spectrum of gram-negative organisms and is moderately effective in penetrating the burn eschar. A transient leukopenia secondary to bone marrow suppression often occurs with use of silver sulfadiazine in large burns, but the process is usually self-limiting and the agent does not have to be discontinued.

Mafenide penetrates the burn eschar and is a more potent antibiotic, but there are more complications with its use. Mafenide causes considerable pain upon application in over half of patients. It is also a carbonic anhydrase inhibitor, and metabolic acidosis can result if it is used over a large surface area, particularly in children or the elderly. This agent is used chiefly on burns already infected or when silver sulfadiazine is no longer effective in controlling bacterial growth.

Silver Release Dressings

Several slow-release dressings are now available that release silver ions for several days, decreasing dressing changes and improving patient comfort.

Exposure versus Closed Management

There are two methods of management of the burn wound with topical agents. In **exposure therapy,** no dressings are applied over the wound after application of the agent to the wound twice or three times daily. This approach is typically used on the face and head. Disadvantages are increased pain and heat loss as a result of the exposed wound and an increased risk of cross-contamination.

In the **closed method,** an occlusive dressing is applied over the agent and is usually changed twice daily. The disadvantage of this method is the potential increase in bacterial growth if the dressing is not changed twice daily, particularly when thick eschar is present. The advantages are less pain, less heat loss, and less cross-contamination. The closed method is generally preferred.

Temporary Skin Substitutes

Skin substitutes are another alternative to topical agents for the partial-thickness burn or the clean excised wound. A number of synthetic and biologically active temporary skin substitutes are in use. Reepithelialization is accelerated. Also, pain is better controlled. **Homografts (human skin)** work better for this purpose on large excised wounds but are difficult to obtain. Other alternatives include a number of tissue engineered skin substitutes, which contain bioactive matrix components.

Hydrotherapy

The use of hydrotherapy for wound management remains controversial. A number of studies have shown that the infection rate is actually increased when patients are immersed in a tub because of the generalized inoculation of burn wounds with bacteria from what was previously a localized infection. Hydrotherapy, however, is a very useful form of physical therapy once the wounds are in the process of being debrided and closed. Showering is also effective for wound cleansing in the more stable patient.

Debridement & Grafting

Burn wound inflammation, even in the absence of infection, can result in organ dysfunction and perpetuation of the hypermetabolic state. Early wound closure would be expected to control this process more effectively. Surgical management of burn wounds has now become much more aggressive, with operative debridement beginning within the first several days postburn rather than after eschar has sloughed. More rapid closure of burn wounds clearly decreases the rate of sepsis and, in full-thickness burn injuries in excess of 60% of body surface, significantly decreases the death rate. The approach to operative debridement varies from an extensive burn excision and grafting within several days of injury to a more moderate approach of limiting debridements to less than 15% of the burned area and no more than four units of blood loss per procedure. Excision can be carried down to fascia or to viable remaining dermis or fat. Excision to fascia is more commonly used when the burn extends well into the fat. The mesh can be covered with a biologic dressing to avoid desiccation of the uncovered wound. Excision to viable tissue, referred to as tangential excision, is advantageous because it provides a vascular base for grafting while preserving remaining viable tissue, especially dermis. Blood loss is substantial in view of the vascularity of the dermis. The procedures can be performed on an extremity, using a tourniquet to decrease blood loss.

A number of **permanent skin substitutes** could further facilitate wound closure, particularly in massive burns with insufficient donor sites. Autologous cultures of epithelium have been applied with some success. Permanent skin substitutes composed of both dermis and epidermis have been designed in order to maintain coverage and improve skin function. The efficacy of skin substitutes remains uncertain.

Maintenance of Function

The maintenance of functional motion during evolution of the burn wound is especially desirable to avoid loss of motion at joints. Wound contraction, a normal event during healing, may result in extremity contracture. Immobilization may produce joint stiffness, which at one time was thought to be caused by edema but probably is more due to pain, disuse, or immobilizing dressings. Contracture of the scar, muscles, and tendons across a joint also causes loss of motion and can be diminished by traction, early motion, and pressure distributed directly over the wound to decrease hypertrophic scar formation.

The scar is a metabolically active tissue, continually undergoing reorganization. The extensive scarring that frequently occurs after burns can lead to disfiguring and disabling contractures, but it may be avoided by the use of splints and elevation to maintain a functional position before grafting. Following application of the skin graft, maintenance of proper positioning with splints is indicated. In the convalescent period, application of a pressure dressing and pressure and isoprene splints may result in less hypertrophic scarring and contracture. The pressure should be maintained with elastic garments for at least 6 months and in some cases may be necessary for as long as a year. Early burn contractures can usually be stretched by constant light force.

If reinjury does not occur, the amount of collagen in the scar tends to decrease with time. Stiff collagen becomes softer, and on flat surfaces of the body, where reinjury and inflammation are prevented, remodeling may totally eliminate contracture. However, around joints or the neck, contractures usually persist and surgical reconstruction is often necessary. The sooner the burn wound can be covered with skin grafts, the less likely is contracture.

MANAGEMENT OF COMPLICATIONS

Infection remains a critical problem in burns, though the incidence has been reduced by modern therapy with topical antibacterial agents. A quantitative culture of the burn indicates infection when a concentration of 10^5 organisms—the level defining invasive infection—is present. The cultures also show the sensitivity of the bacteria, and when the bacterial concentration passes 10^5 organisms per gram, systemic administration of specific antibiotics should be instituted (Tables 14–2 and 14–3).

Table 14–2. Diagnosis of burn wound infection.

Systemic Changes	Colonized or Clean	Wound Infection
Body temperature	Increased	Variable
White blood cell count	Increased Mild left shift	High or low Severe left shift
Wound appearance	Variable—may appear purulent or benign	Purulence may be present, or wound surface may appear dry and pale
Bacterial content		
Surface	Scant to large amount	Variable
Quantitative	Usually < 10^5/g	Usually > 10^5/g
Biopsy	No invasion of normal tissue	Invasion of normal tissue by organisms

Sepsis can be difficult to diagnose, since fever and leukocytosis are often present with a burn alone. Hemodynamic instability is a late sign. The temperature may fall below normal, the appearance of the wound may deteriorate, and the white count may fall, ending finally with septic shock. Aggressive antibiotic therapy must be initiated and an attempt made to identify the source of the infection. Pneumonitis, urinary tract infection, and intravenous catheter sepsis should be considered in the differential diagnosis. If other causes are not found, the wound is usually the septic focus and will have to be debrided. Blood volume, nutrition, and oxygenation must be assessed.

Circumferential burns of an extremity or of the trunk pose special problems. Swelling beneath the unyielding eschar may act as a tourniquet to blood and lymph flow, and the distal extremity may become swollen and tense. More extensive swelling may compromise the arterial supply. Escharotomy or excision of the eschar may be required. To avoid permanent damage, escharotomy must be performed before arterial ischemia develops. Constriction involving the chest or abdomen may severely restrict ventilation and may require longitudinal escharotomies. Anesthetics are rarely required, and the procedure can usually be performed in the patient's room.

Acute gastroduodenal (Curling's) ulcers were at one time a frequent complication of severe burns, but the incidence is now extremely low, largely as a result of the

Table 14–3. Most common pathogens in burn infections.

	S aureus	*P aeruginosa*	*C albicans*
Wound appearance	Loss of wound granulation	Surface necrosis; patchy, black	Minimal exudate
Course	Slow onset over 2–5 days	Rapid onset over 12–36 hours	Slow (days)
CNS signs	Disorientation	Modest changes	Often no change
Temperature	Marked increase	High or low	Modest changes
White blood count	Marked increase	High or low	Modest changes
Hypotension	Modest	Often severe	Minimal change
Mortality rate	5%	20–30%	30–50%

early and routine institution of antacid and nutritional therapy and the decrease in the rate of sepsis. Management of Curling's ulcers is discussed in Chapter 23.

A complication unique to children is seizures, which may result from electrolyte imbalance, hypoxemia, infection, or drugs; in one-third of cases, the cause is unknown. Hyponatremia, the most frequent cause, is becoming less common with the diminishing use of topical silver nitrate. Drugs that have been implicated include penicillin, phenothiazine antipsychotic agents, diphenhydramine, and aminophylline.

Acute gastric dilation, which occurs in the first week after injury, should be suspected when the patient repeatedly vomits small quantities of food. Fecal impaction resulting from immobilization, dehydration, and narcotic analgesics is a fairly common occurrence. Systemic hypertension occurs in about 10% of cases in the postresuscitation period.

RESPIRATORY TRACT INJURY IN BURNS

Today the major cause of death after burns is respiratory tract injury or complications in the respiratory tract. The problems include inhalation injury, aspiration in unconscious patients, bacterial pneumonia, pulmonary edema, pulmonary embolism, and posttraumatic pulmonary insufficiency.

Direct inhalation injuries, which predispose to other complications, are divided into three categories: carbon monoxide poisoning (Table 14–4), heat injury to the airway, and inhalation of noxious gases (Table 14–5).

Direct inhalation of dry heat is a rare cause of damage below the vocal cords because in most cases the upper airway effectively cools the inspired gases before they reach the trachea and because reflex closure of the cords and laryngeal spasm halt full inhalation of the hot gas. Direct burns to the upper airway are associated with burns of the face, lips, and nasal hairs and necrosis or swelling of the pharyngeal mucosa. Acute edema of the upper tract may cause airway obstruction and asphyxiation without lung damage. Laryngeal edema must be anticipated in patients with airway burns, and endotracheal intubation should be performed well before manifestations of airway obstruction appear. The endotracheal tube should be large enough to allow removal of thick copious secretions during subsequent care. Tracheostomies performed through burned tissue are associated with a prohibitively high complication rate and should only be done if endotracheal intubation is impossible.

Treatment is primarily supportive, including maintenance of pulmonary toilet, mechanical ventilation (when indicated), and antibiotics.

Table 14–4. Carbon monoxide poisoning.

Carboxyhemoglobin Level	Severity	Symptoms
< 20%	Mild	Headache, mild dyspnea, visual changes, confusion
20–40%	Moderate	Irritability, diminished judgment, dim vision, nausea, easy fatigability
40–60%	Severe	Hallucinations, confusion, ataxia, collapse, coma
> 60%	Fatal	

Table 14–5. Sources of noxious chemicals in smoke.

Polyethylene, polypropylene	Clean burning combustion to CO_2 and H_2O
Polystyrene	Copious black smoke and soot—CO_2, H_2O, some CO
Wood, cotton	Aldehydes (acrolein)
Polyvinylchloride	Hydrochloric acid
Acrylonitrile, polyurethane, nitrogenous compounds	Hydrogen cyanide
Fire retardants may produce toxic fumes	Halogens (F_2, Cl_2, Br_2), ammonia

Carbon monoxide poisoning must be considered in every patient suspected of having inhalation injury on the basis of having been burned in a closed space, physical evidence of inhalation, or dyspnea. Arterial blood gases and carboxyhemoglobin levels must be determined. Levels of carboxyhemoglobin above 5% in nonsmokers and above 10% in smokers indicate carbon monoxide poisoning. Carbon monoxide has an affinity for hemoglobin 200 times that of oxygen, displaces oxygen, and produces a leftward shift in the oxyhemoglobin dissociation curve (P_{50}, the oxygen tension at which half the hemoglobin is saturated with oxygen, is lowered). Measurements of oxyhemoglobin saturation may be misleading because the hemoglobin combined with carbon monoxide is not detected and the percentage saturation of oxyhemoglobin may appear normal.

Mild carbon monoxide poisoning (< 20% carboxyhemoglobin) is manifested by headache, slight dyspnea, mild confusion, and diminished visual acuity. Moderate poisoning (20–40% carboxyhemoglobin) leads to irritability, impairment of judgment, dim vision, nausea, and fatigability. Severe poisoning (40–60% carboxyhemoglobin) produces hallucinations, confusion, ataxia, collapse, and coma. Levels in excess of 60% carboxyhemoglobin are usually fatal.

Various **toxic chemicals** in inspired smoke produce specific respiratory injuries. Inhalation of kerosene smoke, for example, is relatively innocuous. Smoke from a wood fire is extremely irritating because it contains aldehyde gases, particularly acrolein. Direct inhalation of acrolein, even in low concentrations, irritates mucous membranes and produces an outpouring of fluid. A concentration of 10 ppm will cause pulmonary edema. Smoke from some plastic compounds, such as polyurethane, is the most serious kind of toxic irritant. Poisonous gases such as chlorine, sulfuric acid, or cyanides are given off. Cyanide absorption can be lethal. Oxidants are released after all smoke exposures.

Inhalation injury causes severe mucosal edema followed soon by sloughing of the mucosa. The destroyed mucosa in the larger airways is replaced by a mucopurulent membrane. The edema fluid enters the airway and, when mixed with the pus in the lumen, may form casts and plugs in the smaller bronchioles. Terminal bronchioles and alveoli may contain carbonaceous material. Acute bronchiolitis and bronchopneumonia commonly develop within a few days. Sputum smears should be examined daily to detect early bacterial tracheobronchial infection.

When inhalation injury is suspected, early endoscopic examination of the airway with fiberoptic bronchoscopy is helpful in determining the area of injury, ie, whether just the upper airway is involved or the lower airway as well. Unfortunately, the severity of the injury cannot be accurately quantified by bronchoscopy—it can only be shown that an injury is present. Direct laryngoscopy probably gives as much information.

Less common causes of respiratory failure are pulmonary embolus and overload pulmonary edema. Emboli usually occur later in the course of treatment after prolonged bed rest and should be suspected if respiratory function suddenly deteriorates. Heparin anticoagulation is indicated for pulmonary embolism (see Chapter 37). Pulmonary edema from fluid overload during resuscitation usually occurs only in patients with preexisting heart disease. The inhalation-injured lung is very susceptible to edema, which is difficult to manage, since systemic hypoperfusion must be avoided by attempts at diuresis.

Probably the most common cause of respiratory failure is bacterial pneumonia due to either inhalation injury, contamination of the lungs through a tracheostomy or endotracheal tube, airborne infection, or hematogenous spread of bacteria from the burn wound. Alteration of oropharyngeal normal flora with colonization by pathogens and subsequent aspiration of infected secretions is the most common cause of the lung infections.

Pulmonary insufficiency is associated with systemic sepsis. Differentiating acute respiratory distress syndrome (ARDS) from bacterial pneumonia may be difficult. There is damage to the pulmonary capillaries and leakage of fluid and protein into the interstitial spaces of the lung, resulting in loss of compliance and difficulty in oxygenation of the blood. Modern methods of ventilatory support and vigorous pulmonary toilet have significantly reduced the death rate from pulmonary insufficiency.

Treatment

Management of a burn patient should include frequent evaluation of the lungs throughout the hospital course. All patients who initially have evidence of smoke inhalation should receive humidified oxygen in high concentrations. If carbon monoxide poisoning has occurred, 100% oxygen should be given until the carboxyhemoglobin content returns to normal levels and until symptoms of carbon monoxide toxicity resolve. With severe exposures, carbon monoxide may still be bound to the cytochrome enzymes, leading to cell hypoxia even after carboxyhemoglobin levels have returned to near normal. Continued oxygen administration will also reverse this process.

The use of corticosteroids for inhalation injuries is no longer controversial and is clearly contraindicated with the exception of bronchiolitis obliterans. The exception would be the patient with a relative steroid insufficiency.

Bronchodilators by aerosol or aminophylline intravenously may help if wheezing is due to reflex bronchospasm. Chest physical therapy with postural drainage is also required.

When endotracheal intubation is used without mechanical ventilation (eg, for upper airway obstruction), mist and continuous positive pressure ventilatory assistance should be included. The humidity will help loosen the secretions and prevent drying of the airway; the continuous positive pressure will help prevent atelectasis and closure of lung units distal to the swollen airways. Tracheostomy is indicated in the first several days for patients who are expected to require ventilatory support for a few weeks or more. If the neck is burned, excision and grafting followed by tracheostomy is indicated in order to improve pulmonary toilet.

Mechanical ventilation should be instituted early if a significant pulmonary injury is anticipated. A large body burn with chest wall involvement will result in decreased chest wall compliance, increased work of breathing, and subsequent atelectasis. Tracheobronchial injury from inhaled chemicals is accentuated by the presence of a body burn, with a resultant increase in the potential for atelectasis and infection. Controlled ventilation along with sedation will diminish the degree of injury and also conserve energy expenditure. A discussion of ventilatory support is presented in Chapters 3 and 14. Early excision of the deep chest wall burn will help remove the constricting component. Wound closure in turn will decrease the excessive CO_2 production caused by the hypermetabolic state.

REHABILITATION OF THE BURNED PATIENT

Plastic surgical revisions of scars are often necessary after the initial grafting, particularly to release contractures over joints and for cosmetic reasons. The physician must be realistic in defining an acceptable result, and the patient should be told that it may take years to achieve. Burn scars are often unsightly, and—although hope should be extended that improvement can be made—total resolution is not possible in many cases.

Skin expansion techniques utilizing a subdermal Silastic bag that is gradually expanded have greatly improved scar revision management. The ability to enlarge the available skin to be used for replacement of scar improves both cosmetic appearance and function. Advances in microvascular flap surgery have also resulted in substantial improvements in outcome.

The patient must take special care of the skin of the burn scar. Prolonged exposure to sunlight should be avoided, and when the wound involves areas such as the face and hands, which are frequently exposed to the sun, ultraviolet screening agents should be used. Hypertrophic scars and keloids are particularly bothersome and can be diminished with the use of pressure garments, which must be worn until the scar matures—approximately 12 months. Since the skin appendages are often destroyed by full-thickness burns, creams and lotions are required to prevent drying and cracking and to reduce itching. Substances such as lanolin, vitamin A and D ointment, and Eucerin cream are all effective.

Barton R et al: Resuscitation of thermally injured patients with oxygen transport criteria as goals of therapy. J Burn Care Rehabil 1997;18:1.

Boyce S et al: Cultured skin substitutes combined with Integra Artificial Skin to replace native skin autograft and allograft for the closure of excised full thickness burns. J Burn Care Rehabil 1999;20:453.

DeSanti L et al: Development of a burn rehabilitation unit: impact on burn center length of stay and functional outcome. J Burn Care Rehabil 1998;19:414.

Forjuoh SN: The mechanisms, intensity of treatment and outcomes of hospitalized burns: issues for prevention. J Burn Care Rehabil 1998;19:456.

Holm C et al: The relationship between oxygen delivery and oxygen consumption during fluid resuscitation of burn-related shock. J Burn Care Rehabil 2000;21:147.

Kaups KL et al: Base deficit as an indicator of resuscitation needs in patients with burn injuries. J Burn Care Rehabil 1998;19:346.

Mayes T et al: Clinical nutritional protocols for continuous quality improvements in the outcomes of patients with burns. J Burn Care Rehabil 1997;18:365.

Peck MD et al: Surveillance of burn wound infections: a proposal for definitions. J Burn Care Rehabil 1998;19:386.

Schulz JT: A 10-year experience with toxic epidermal necrolysis. J Burn Care Rehabil 2000;21:199.

Smith PD et al: Efficacy of growth factors in the accelerated closure of interstices in explanted meshed human skin grafts. J Burn Care Rehabil 2000;21:5.

ELECTRICAL INJURY

There are three kinds of electrical injuries: electrical current injury, electrothermal burns from arcing current, and flame burns caused by ignition of clothing. Occasionally, all three will be present in the same victim.

Flash or arc burns are thermal injuries to the skin caused by a high-tension electrical current reaching the skin from the conductor. The thermal injury to the skin is intense and deep, because the electrical arc has a temperature of about 2500 °C (high enough to melt bone). Flame burns from ignited clothing are often the most serious part of the injury. Treatment is the same as for any thermal injury.

The damage from electrical current is directly proportionate to its intensity as governed by Ohm's law:

$$\text{Amperage (intensity of current)} = \frac{\text{Voltage (tension or potential)}}{\text{Resistance}}$$

Thus, the amperage depends on the voltage and on the resistance provided by various parts of the body. Voltages above 40 V are considered dangerous.

Once current has entered the body, its pathway depends on the resistances it encounters in the various organs. The following are listed in descending order of resistance: bone, fat, tendon, skin, muscle, blood, and nerve. The pathway of the current determines immediate survival; for example, if the current passes through the heart or the brain stem, death may be immediate from ventricular fibrillation or apnea. Current passing through muscles may cause spasms severe enough to produce long-bone fractures or dislocations.

The type of current is also related to the severity of injury. The usual 60-cycle alternating current that causes most injuries in the home is particularly severe. Alternating current causes tetanic contractions, and the patient may become "locked" to the contact. Cardiac arrest is common from contact with house current.

Electrical current injuries are more than just burns. Focal burns occur at the points of entrance and exit through the skin. Once inside the body, the current travels through muscles, causing an injury more like a crush than a thermal burn. Thrombosis frequently occurs in vessels deep in an extremity, causing a greater depth of tissue necrosis than is evident at the initial examination. The greatest muscle injury is usually closest to the bone, where the highest heat of resistance is generated. The treatment of electrical injuries depends on the extent of deep muscle and nerve destruction more than any other factor.

Myoglobinuria may develop with the risk of acute tubular necrosis. The urine output must be kept two to three times normal with intravenous fluids. Alkalinization of the urine and osmotic diuretics may be indicated if myoglobinuria is present.

A rapid drop in hematocrit sometimes follows sudden destruction of red blood cells by the electrical energy. Bleeding into deep tissues may occur as a result of disruption of blood vessels and tissue planes. In some cases, thrombosed vessels disintegrate later and cause massive interstitial hemorrhage.

The skin burn at the entrance and exit sites is usually a depressed gray or yellow area of full-thickness destruction surrounded by a sharply defined zone of hyperemia. Charring may be present if an arc burn coexists. The lesion should be debrided to underlying healthy tissue. Frequently there is deep destruction not initially evident. This dead and devitalized tissue must also be excised. A second debridement is usually indicated 24–48 hours after the injury, because the necrosis is found to be more extensive than originally thought. The strategy of obtaining skin covering for these burns can tax ingenuity, because of the extent and depth of the wounds. Microvascular flaps are now used routinely to replace large tissue losses.

In general, the treatment of electrical injuries is complex at every step, and after initial resuscitation these patients should be referred to specialized centers.

Haberal M: An eleven year survey of electrical burn injuries. J Burn Care Rehabil 1995;16:43.

Purdue G et al: *Electrical Injuries in Total Burn Care.* Herndon D (editor). Saunders, 2002.

HEAT STROKE

Heat stroke occurs when core body temperature exceeds 40 °C and produces severe central nervous system dysfunction. Two other related syndromes induced by exposure to heat are heat cramps and heat exhaustion.

Heat cramps—muscle pain after exertion in a hot environment—have usually been attributed to salt deficit. It is probable, however, that many cases are really examples of **exertional rhabdomyolysis.** The latter condition, which may also be a complicating factor in heat stroke, involves acute muscle injury due to severe exertional efforts beyond the limits for which the individual has trained. It often produces myoglobinuria, which rarely affects kidney function except when it occurs in patients also suffering from heat stroke. Complete recovery is the rule after uncomplicated heat cramps.

Heat exhaustion consists of fatigue, muscular weakness, tachycardia, postural syncope, nausea, vomiting, and an urge to defecate caused by dehydration and hypovolemia from heat stress. Although body temperature is normal in heat exhaustion, there is a continuum between this syndrome and heat stroke.

Heat stroke, a result of imbalance between heat production and heat dissipation, kills about 4000 persons yearly in the USA. Exercise-induced heat stroke most often affects young people (eg, athletes, military recruits, laborers) who are exercising strenuously in a hot environment, usually without adequate training. Sedentary heat stroke is a disease of elderly or infirm people whose cardiovascular systems are unable to adapt to the stress of a hot environment. Epidemics of heat stroke in elderly people can be predicted when the ambient temperature surpasses 32.2 °C and the relative humidity reaches 50–76%.

In humans, heat is dissipated from the skin by radiation, conduction, convection, and evaporation. When the ambient temperature rises, heat loss by the first three is impaired; loss by evaporation is hindered by a high relative humidity. Predisposing factors to heat accumulation are dermatitis; use of phenothiazines, beta-blockers, diuretics, or anticholinergics; intercurrent fever from other disease; obesity; alcoholism; and heavy clothing. Cocaine and amphetamines may increase metabolic heat production.

The mechanism of injury is direct damage by heat to the parenchyma and vasculature of the organs. The central nervous system is particularly vulnerable, and cellular necrosis is found in the brains of those who die of heat stroke. Hepatocellular and renal tubular damage are apparent in severe cases. Subendocardial damage and occasionally transmural infarcts are discovered in fatal cases even in young persons without previous cardiac disease. Disseminated intravascular coagulation may develop, aggravating injury in all organ systems and predisposing to bleeding complications.

Clinical Findings

A. Symptoms and Signs

Heat stroke should be suspected in anyone who develops sudden coma in a hot environment. If the patient's temperature is above 40 °C (range: 40–43 °C), the diagnosis of heat stroke is definitive. Measurements of body temperature must be made rectally. A prodrome including dizziness, headache, nausea, chills, and gooseflesh of the chest and arms is seen occasionally but is not common. In most cases, the patient recalls having experienced no warning symptoms except weakness, tiredness, or dizziness. Confusion, belligerent behavior, or stupor may precede coma. Convulsions may occur after admission to the hospital.

The skin is pink or ashen and sometimes, paradoxically, dry and hot; dry skin in the presence of hyperpyrexia is virtually pathognomonic of heat stroke. Profuse sweating is usually present in runners and other athletes who have heat stroke. The heart rate ranges from 140/min to 170/min; central venous or pulmonary wedge pressure is high; and in some cases the blood pressure is low. Hyperventilation may reach 60/min and may give rise to respiratory alkalosis. Pulmonary edema and bloody sputum may develop in severe cases. Jaundice is frequent within the first few days after onset of symptoms.

Dehydration, which may produce the same central nervous system symptoms as heat stroke, is an aggravating factor in about 15% of cases.

B. Laboratory Findings

There is no characteristic pattern to the electrolyte changes: The serum sodium concentration may be normal or high, and the potassium concentration is usually low on admission or at some point during resuscitation. Hypocalcemia is common, and hypophosphatemia may occur. In the first few days, the AST, LDH, and CK may be elevated, especially in exertional heat stroke. Alkalosis may follow hyperventilation; acidosis can result from lactic acidosis or acute renal failure. Proteinuria and granular and red cell casts are seen in urine specimens collected immediately after diagnosis. If the urine is dark red or brown, it probably contains myoglobin. The blood urea nitrogen and serum creatinine rise transiently in most patients and continue to climb if renal failure develops. Hematologic findings may be normal or may be typical of disseminated intravascular coagulation (ie, low fibrinogen, increased fibrin split products, slow prothrombin and partial thromboplastin times, and decreased platelet count).

Prevention

For the most part, heat stroke in military recruits and athletes in training is preventable by adhering to a graduated schedule of increasing performance requirements that allows acclimatization over 2–3 weeks. Heat produced by exercise is dissipated by increased cardiac output, vasodilation in the skin, and increased sweating. With acclimatization there is increased efficiency for muscular work, increased myocardial performance, expanded extracellular fluid volume, greater output of sweat for a given amount of work, a lower salt content of sweat, and a lower central temperature for a given amount of work.

Access to drinking water should be unrestricted during vigorous physical activity in a hot environment. Free water is preferable to electrolyte-containing solutions. Most training regimens should not include the use of supplemental salt tablets, since enough salt (10–15 g/d) will be consumed with food to meet the electrolyte losses in sweat and since hypernatremia can develop if ingested salt tablets are not taken with enough water. Clothing and protective gear should be lightened as heat production and air temperature rise, and heavy exercise should not be scheduled at the hottest times of day, especially at the beginning of a training schedule. Long distance runs with open competition, which attract novice runners, should be held in late summer or fall, when heat acclimatization is more apt to have occurred, and should be started before 8 AM or after 6 PM.

Treatment

The patient should be cooled rapidly. The most efficient method is to induce evaporative heat loss by spraying the patient with water at 15 °C and fanning with warm air. Immersion in an ice water bath or use of ice packs is also effective but causes cutaneous vasoconstriction and shivering and makes patient monitoring more difficult. Monitor the rectal temperature frequently. To avoid overshooting the end point, vigorous cooling should be stopped when the temperature reaches 38.9 °C. Shivering should be controlled with parenteral phenothiazines. Oxygen should be administered, and if the PaO_2 drops below 65 mm Hg, tracheal intubation should be performed to control ventilation. Fluid, electrolyte, and acid-base balance must be controlled by frequent monitoring. Intravenous fluid administration should be based on the central venous or pulmonary artery wedge pressure, blood pressure, and urine output; overhydration must be avoided. On average, about 1400 mL of fluid is required in the first 4 hours of resuscitation. Intravenous mannitol (12.5 g) may be given early if myoglobinuria is present. Renal failure may require hemodialysis. Disseminated intravascular coagulation may require treatment with heparin. Digitalis and occasionally inotropic agents (eg, isoproterenol, dopamine) may be indicated for cardiac insufficiency, which should be suspected if hypotension persists after hypovolemia has been corrected.

Prognosis

Bad prognostic signs are temperature of 42.2 °C or more, coma lasting over 2 hours, shock, hyperkalemia, and an AST greater than 1000 units/L during the first 24 hours. The death rate is about 10% in patients who are correctly diagnosed and treated promptly. Deaths in the first few days are usually due to cerebral damage; later deaths may be from bleeding or may be due to cardiac, renal, or hepatic failure.

Bouchama A, DeVol EB: Acid-base alterations in heatstroke. Intensive Care Med 2001;27:680.

Dematte JE et al: Near-fatal heat stroke during the 1995 heat wave in Chicago. Ann Intern Med 1998;129:173.

Khosla R, Guntupalli KK: Heat-related illnesses. Crit Care Clin 1999;15:251.

FROSTBITE

Frostbite involves freezing of tissues. Ice crystals form between the cells and grow at the expense of intracellular water. The resulting cellular dehydration coupled with ischemia due to vasoconstriction and increased blood viscosity are the mechanisms of tissue injury. Skin and muscle are considerably more susceptible to freezing damage than tendons and bones, which explains why the patient may still be able to move severely frostbitten digits.

Frostbite is caused by cold exposure, whose effects can be magnified by moisture or wind. For example, the chilling effects on skin are the same with an air temperature of 6.7 °C) and a 40-mile-per-hour wind as with an air temperature of –40 °C and only a 2-mile-per-hour wind. Contact with metal or gasoline in very cold weather can cause virtually instantaneous freezing; skin will often stick to metal and be lost. The risk of frostbite is increased by generalized hypothermia, which produces peripheral vasoconstriction as part of the mechanism for preservation of core body temperature.

Two related injuries, trench foot and immersion foot, involve prolonged exposure to wet cold above freezing (eg, 10 °C). The resulting tissue damage is produced by ischemia.

Clinical Findings

Frostnip, a minor variant of this syndrome, is a transient blanching and numbness of exposed parts that may progress to frostbite if not immediately detected and treated. It often appears on the tips of fingers, ears, nose, chin, or cheeks and should be managed by rewarming through contact with warm parts of the body or warm air.

Frostbitten parts are numb, painless, and of a white or waxy appearance. With **superficial frostbite,** only the skin and subcutaneous tissues are frozen, so the tissues beneath are still compressible with pressure. **Deep frostbite** involves freezing of underlying tissues, which imparts a wooden consistency to the extremity.

After rewarming, the frostbitten area becomes mottled blue or purple and painful and tender. Blisters appear that may take several weeks to resolve. The part becomes edematous and to a varying degree painful.

Treatment

The frostbitten part should be rewarmed (thawed) in a water bath at 40–42.2 °C for 20–30 minutes. Thawing should not be attempted until the victim can be kept permanently warm and at rest. It is far better to continue walking on frostbitten feet even for many hours than to thaw them in a remote cold area where definitive care cannot be provided. If a thermometer is unavailable, the temperature of the water should be adjusted to be warm but not hot to a normal hand. Never use the frozen part to test the water temperature or expose it to a source of direct heat such as a fire. The risk of seriously compounding the injury is great with any method of thawing other than immersion in warm water.

After thawing has been completed, the patient should be kept recumbent and the injured part left open to the air, protected from direct contact with sheets, clothing, etc. Blisters should be left intact and the skin gently debrided by immersing the part in a whirlpool bath for about 20 minutes twice daily. No scrubbing or massaging of the injured part should be allowed, and topical ointments, antiseptics, etc, are of no value. Vasodilating agents and surgical sympathectomy do not appear to improve healing.

The tissues will heal gradually, and any dead tissue will become demarcated and will usually slough spontaneously. Early in the course, it is nearly impossible, even for someone with considerable experience in the treatment of frostbite, to judge the depth of injury; most early assessments tend to overestimate the extent of permanent damage. Therefore, expectant treatment is the rule, and surgical debridement should be avoided even if evolution of the injury requires many months. Surgery may be indicated to release constricting circumferential eschars, but rarely should the process of spontaneous separation of gangrenous tissue be surgically facilitated. Even in severe injuries, amputation is rarely indicated before 2 months unless invasive infection supervenes. Nuclear scans may be useful to delineate tissue viability.

Concomitant fractures or dislocations create challenging and complex problems. Dislocations should be reduced immediately after thawing. Open fractures require operative reduction, but closed fractures should be managed with a posterior plastic splint. Anterior tibial compartment syndrome, which may develop in patients with associated fractures, may be diagnosed by arteriography and treated by fasciotomy.

After the eschar separates, the skin is noted to be thin, shiny, tender, and sensitive to cold; occasionally it exhibits a tendency to perspire more readily. Gradually it returns toward normal, but pain on exposure to cold may persist indefinitely.

Prognosis

The prognosis for normal function is excellent if appropriate treatment is provided. Individuals who have recovered from frostbite have increased susceptibility to another frostbite injury on exposure to cold.

Affleck DG et al: Assessment of tissue viability in complex extremity injuries: utility of the pyrophosphate nuclear scan. J Trauma 2001;50:263.

Murphy JV et al: Frostbite: pathogenesis and treatment. J Trauma 2000;48:171.

ACCIDENTAL HYPOTHERMIA

Accidental hypothermia consists of the uncontrolled lowering of core body temperature below 35 °C by exposure to cold. The syndrome may be seen in elderly people living alone in inadequately heated homes, in alcoholics exposed to the cold during a binge, in those engaged in winter sports, and in others who become lost in cold weather. Alcohol facilitates the induction of hypothermia by producing sedation (inhibiting shivering) and cutaneous dilation. Other sedatives, tranquilizers, and antidepressants are occasionally implicated. Diseases that predispose to hypothermia include myxedema, hypopituitarism, adrenal insufficiency, cerebral vascular insufficiency, mental impairment, and cardiovascular disorders.

The heart is the organ most sensitive to cooling and is subject to ventricular fibrillation or asystole when the temperature drops to 21–24 °C. Hypothermia affects the oxyhemoglobin dissociation curve, so less oxygen is released to the tissues. Cardiac standstill may cause death in less than 1 hour in shipwreck victims immersed in cold water (6.7 °C). Increased capillary permeability, manifested by generalized edema and pulmonary, hepatic, and renal dysfunction, may develop as the patient is rewarmed. Coagulopathies and disseminated intravascular coagulation are seen occasionally. Pancreatitis and acute renal failure are common in patients whose temperature on admission is below 32 °C.

Clinical Findings

A. Symptoms and Signs

The patient is mentally depressed (somnolent, stuporous, or comatose), cold, and pale to cyanotic. The clinical findings are not always striking and may be mistaken for the effects of alcohol. The core temperature ranges from 21 to 35 °C. Shivering is absent when the temperature is below 32 °C. Respirations are slow and shallow. Many patients have bronchopneumonia. The blood pressure is usually normal and the heart rate slow. When the core temperature drops below 32 °C, the patient may appear to be dead. The extremities may be frostbitten or frozen.

B. Laboratory Findings

Dehydration may increase the concentration of various blood constituents. Severe hypoglycemia is common, and unless detected and treated immediately, it may become dangerously worse as rewarming produces shivering. The serum amylase is elevated in about half of cases, but autopsy studies show that it does not always reflect pancreatitis. Diabetic ketoacidosis becomes a management problem in some patients whose amylase values are elevated on entry. The AST, LDH, and CK enzymes are usually elevated but are of no predictive significance. The ECG shows lengthening of the PR interval, delay in interventricular conduction, and a pathognomonic J wave at the junction of the QRS complex and ST segment.

Treatment

Hypothermic patients should never be considered dead until all measures for resuscitation have failed—prolonged cardiopulmonary arrest in severe hypothermia is compatible with complete recovery.

Mild hypothermia (body temperature 32–35 °C) can be treated in most cases by passive rewarming (heavy clothing and blankets in a warm environment) for a few hours—especially when the patient is shivering. The patient's temperature should be continuously monitored with a rectal or esophageal probe until body temperature reaches normal. Since the volume of intravenous fluids required for resuscitation is often substantial, their temperature can affect the outcome. Consequently, intravenous fluids should be warmed with a heat exchanger during administration.

Active rewarming is indicated for temperature below 32 °C, cardiovascular instability, or failure of passive rewarming. The methods include immersion in a warm water bath, inhalation of heated air, pleural lavage, peritoneal lavage, and blood warming with an extracorporeal bypass machine. Active external rewarming is most often performed by immersion in a warm (40–42 °C) water bath, which will raise body temperature at a rate of 1–2 degrees per hour. A disadvantage of this method is that the core temperature may continue to decline after initiation of the rewarming efforts (known as after-drop), which is associated with worsening cardiovascular function.

Closed pleural irrigation should be performed by flushing the right hemithorax with warm (40–42 °C) saline solution through two large thoracostomy tubes, one anterior and the other posterior. Rewarming by peritoneal lavage involves giving warm (40–45 °C) crystalloid solutions, 6 L/h, which raises core temperature by 2–4 degrees per hour.

Active core rewarming with partial cardiopulmonary bypass, the most efficient technique, is indicated for patients with ventricular fibrillation and severe hypothermia or those with frozen extremities. At a flow rate of 6–7 L/min, core temperature can be raised by 1–2 °C every 3–5 minutes.

In severe cases, endotracheal intubation should be used for better management of ventilation and protection against aspiration, a common lethal complication. Arterial blood gases should be monitored frequently. Bretylium tosylate in an initial dose of 10 mg/kg is the best drug for ventricular fibrillation. Antibiotics are often indicated for coexisting pneumonitis. Serious infections are often unsuspected upon admission, and delay in appropriate therapy may contribute to the severity of the illness. Hypoglycemia calls for intravenous administration of 50% glucose solution. Fluid administration must be gauged by central venous or pulmonary artery wedge pressures, urine output, and other circulatory parameters. Increased capillary permeability following rewarming predisposes to the development of pulmonary edema and compartment syndromes in the extremities. To minimize these complications, the central venous or wedge pressure should be kept below 12–14 cm water. Drugs should not be injected into peripheral tissues, because absorption will not take place while the patient is cold and because drugs may accumulate to produce serious toxicity as rewarming occurs.

As rewarming proceeds, the patient should be continually reassessed for signs of concomitant disease that may have been masked by hypothermia, especially myxedema and hypoglycemia. Any inexplicable failure to respond should suggest adrenal insufficiency.

Prognosis

Survival can be expected in only 50% of patients whose core temperature drops below 32.2 °C. Coexisting diseases (eg, stroke, neoplasm, myocardial infarction) are common and increase the death rate to 75% or more. Survival does not correlate closely with the lowest absolute temperature reached. Death may result from pneumonitis, heart failure, or renal insufficiency.

Brunette DD, McVaney K: Hypothermic cardiac arrest: an 11-year review of ED management and outcome. Am J Emerg Med 2000;18:418.

Demling R: The rate of re-epithelialization across meshed skin grafts is increased with exposure to silver. Burns 2002:28; 264.

Farstad M et al: Recovering from accidental hypothermia by extracorporeal circulation: a retrospective study. Eur J Cardiothorac Surg 2001;20:58.

Light TD: Real time metabolic monitors, ischemia perfusion, titration endpoints and ultraprecise burn resuscitation. J Burn Care Rehab 2004;25:33.

Peng RY, Bongard FS: Hypothermia in trauma patients. J Am Coll Surg 1999;188:685.

Head & Neck Tumors

15

Samuel W. Beenken, MD, & Marshall M. Urist, MD

In 2005, an estimated 39,250 people in the United States will develop squamous cell carcinoma of the upper aerodigestive tract. When detected and treated at an early stage, these cancers are curable in 80% of cases, but many patients present with a locally advanced primary cancer or with regional lymph node metastases. Accurate staging is essential to determine the best therapy and to permit comparison of treatment results. Therapy often involves collaboration between many disciplines such as surgery, radiation oncology, medical oncology, maxillofacial prosthetics, and speech therapy. The priorities of treatment are to eradicate the cancer, then to maintain function, and finally to preserve appearance.

Carvalho AL et al: Trends in incidence and prognosis for head and neck cancer in the United States: A site-specific analysis of the SEER database. Int J Cancer 2005;114:806.

BIOLOGY OF HEAD & NECK TUMORS

The great majority of upper aerodigestive tract cancers are squamous cell carcinomas, and they are the emphasis of this chapter. The most important etiologic agents in the development of these tumors are tobacco and alcohol. The combination of tobacco and alcohol use accounts for the development of 75% of all oral cavity, oropharyngeal, and hypopharyngeal cancers. It is estimated that more than 80% of laryngeal cancers are due to cigarette smoking. Premalignant lesions include leukoplakia and erythroplakia, with the most important risk factor being the presence of cellular dysplasia. Because the entire mucosal surface of the upper aerodigestive tract is exposed to the same carcinogens, multiple anatomic sites are at risk for the simultaneous or sequential development of second primary cancers. Second primary cancers develop in 10–15% of cases.

The development of squamous cell carcinoma is a multistep process. Deletions of chromosomes 3p and 18q, p16 inactivation, amplification of int-2 and bcl-1, mutation of *P53* and overexpression of transforming growth factor-α (TGF-α) and the epidermal growth factor receptor (EGFr) have all been implicated as important components of the carcinogenic process.

Beckhardt RN et al: HER-2/neu oncogene characterization in head and neck squamous cell carcinoma. Arch Otolaryngol Head Neck Surg 1995;121:1265.

Friedlander PL: Genomic instability in head and neck cancer patients. Head Neck 2001;23:683.

Goldenberg D et al: Habitual risk factors for head and neck cancer. Otolaryngol Head Neck Surg 2004;131:986.

Kim MM et al: Molecular pathology of head-and-neck cancer. Int J Cancer 2004;112:545.

DIAGNOSIS OF HEAD & NECK TUMORS

The evaluation of a patient with an abnormality of the upper aerodigestive tract begins with a complete history and physical examination.

History

Common presenting symptoms are pain, bleeding, obstruction, and a mass. Pain is characterized as to frequency, duration, severity, location, and radiation. The amount and types of analgesics used are determined. Several specific clinical patterns are important. Pain around the eyes can be referred from the nasopharynx. Cancers of the base of the tongue, tonsil, or hypopharynx can cause otalgia. Odynophagia can result from deep penetration by cancers of the base of the tongue or hypopharynx or from extensive cervical lymph node metastases. Hemorrhage is usually mild and intermittent and is most commonly associated with cancers of the nasal cavity, nasopharynx, and oral cavity. Obstruction causing alterations of phonation, breathing, swallowing, or hearing can be a manifestation of either early or advanced cancer. Hoarseness is often an early finding in cancers of the glottis, whereas cancers only a few millimeters away on the false vocal cord can grow and metastasize before causing a change in voice. Trismus usually indicates extension of cancer into the pterygoid muscles. Dysphagia is often a late symptom of cancer growth at the base of the tongue, hypopharynx, or cervical esophagus. Loss of hearing can be the first symptom of cancers arising in or invading the auditory tract from the external auditory canal or nasopharynx.

A history of prior squamous cell carcinoma is common, and accurate documentation of its histologic type, stage, and date of occurrence is necessary. One arising more than 3 years after a previous cancer is considered a new primary cancer. The late appearance of cervical lymph node metastases requires a thorough search for a new primary cancer. The appearance of a lung nodule following treatment of squamous cell carcinoma can signify the development of metastases or a primary lung cancer.

Physical Examination

Examination of the upper aerodigestive tract begins with careful inspection of each anatomic site. Dentures are removed and the lips and tongue retracted to obtain a clear view of the oral cavity. The dimensions of a mass or ulcer can be estimated by placing a tongue blade (2 cm wide) over the area. Bimanual palpation is used to examine the floor of the mouth. Palpation is also used to detect cancers in all areas of the oropharynx, especially the base of the tongue and tonsillar fossas. Parapharyngeal tumors arising from a retromandibular extension of the parotid gland—and from nerves, enlarged lymph nodes, or the carotid body—can present as masses in the tonsillar area. Complete examination of the nasopharynx, larynx, and hypopharynx may require use of a topical anesthetic spray. Although most sites are well seen with a headlight and laryngeal mirror, flexible fiberoptic examination can provide additional information.

A detailed neurologic examination can reveal localizing signs when no other findings are present. Hyposmia (decreased sensitivity to odors) can be caused by primary cancers of the olfactory bulb or cancers of the nasal cavity and paranasal sinuses. Sensory loss in the distribution of the infraorbital nerve can be a manifestation of a maxillary sinus cancer. Dysfunction of cranial nerves III–VII and IX–XII can occur with nasopharyngeal cancer. Horner's syndrome suggests extracapsular invasion of cervical lymph node metastases, extralaryngeal spread of a laryngeal cancer, or involvement of the cervical sympathetic chain by a primary lung cancer.

Jugular chain lymph nodes are best examined by feeling the nodes between the thumb and the index finger while grasping around the sternocleidomastoid muscle. Nevertheless, physical examination of the cervical lymph nodes is not very accurate. Thirty percent of patients with clinically negative cervical lymph nodes have metastases on pathologic staging, and 20% of those with clinically suspicious cervical lymph nodes will be histologically free of cancer. Cervical lymph node metastases originate from a primary cancer above the clavicles in 85% of cases (Figure 15–1). Squamous cell carcinoma of the skin and melanoma are important causes of enlarged regional nodes and must not be overlooked.

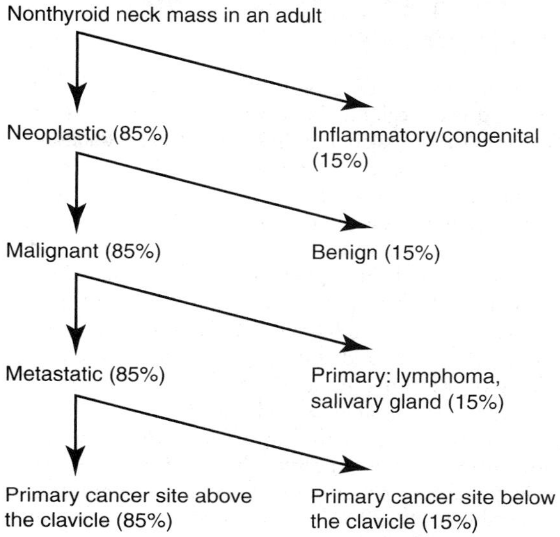

Figure 15–1. Etiology of nonthyroid neck masses in adults.

Biopsy

A biopsy for definitive diagnosis can usually be made at the time of the initial examination. Pinch or punch biopsies of mucosal lesions are generally taken from the margin of the lesion, away from areas of necrosis. Fine-needle aspiration biopsy (FNA) can also be used, particularly for evaluation of palpable cervical lymphadenopathy. If the FNA is reported as showing malignant cells, treatment based on these results can be started. However, if the FNA is read as benign and the cervical lymphadenopathy is clinically suspicious for cancer, repeat FNA or open biopsy is undertaken.

Additional Studies

Examination under anesthesia is often indicated. In addition to palpation of the oral cavity, oropharynx, and neck, direct laryngoscopy, rigid esophagoscopy, nasopharyngoscopy, and bronchoscopy can also be performed. A search can be made for a second cancer. The location and extent of any cancer is described in detail in order to plan appropriate therapy and to assess the results of therapy. A chest x-ray is routine. Barium swallow examination can identify intrinsic or extrinsic compression of the esophagus. Panorex x-rays of the mandible can identify bony invasion from an oral or oropharyngeal cancer. A CT scan of the head and neck is the imaging study of choice for advanced squamous cell carcinoma. Axial and coronal views can demonstrate involvement of the paranasal sinuses, the parapharyngeal and pterygomaxillary spaces, the orbits, and the anterior skull base. MRI is used to determine the extent of cancer involvement at the skull base, in the parapharyngeal space, and in the orbit. PET scans are utilized to detect distant disease.

Weissman JL et al: Current imaging techniques for head and neck tumors. Oncology 1999;13:697.

EXAMINATION OF THE CERVICAL LYMPH NODES

There are three main groups of lymphatic tissue in the head and neck region. The first contains the structures of Waldeyer's ring (palatine tonsils, lingual tonsils, adenoids) and adjacent submucosal lymphatics; the second consists of transitional lymphatics (submental, submandibular, parotid, retroauricular, and occipital nodes); and the third includes the cervical lymph nodes (internal jugular chain, spinal accessory chain, supraclavicular area). Squamous cell carcinoma of the upper aerodigestive tract frequently metastasizes to cervical lymph nodes, as does papillary carcinoma of the thyroid, squamous cell carcinoma of the skin, and melanoma. An accurate prediction of the origin of a metastasis can often be made based on the anatomy of lymphatic drainage in the head and neck. Table 15–1 summarizes the anatomic sites that drain to each lymph node group. The pattern of flow within the lymphatics is predictable unless it has been distorted by a cancer, previous surgery, or radiation therapy.

The cervical lymphatics drain into the thoracic duct on the left side of the neck and into the accessory thoracic duct on the right. The thoracic duct empties into the internal jugular vein near the junction of the internal jugular and subclavian veins. Care must be taken to avoid injury to the duct during neck dissections and supraclavicular lymph node biopsies. Virchow's node, located at the terminus of the thoracic duct in the left supraclavicular region, can sequester metastases from distant primary cancers via the retroperitoneal and posterior mediastinal lymph channels.

Table 15–1. Cervical lymph node metastases by primary cancer site.

Lymph Node Site	Lymph Node Level	Primary Cancer Sites
Submental, submandibular	Level I	Lip, oral cavity, skin, salivary gland
Upper jugular nodes	Level II	Oral cavity, oropharynx, nasopharynx, larynx, salivary gland
Mid-jugular nodes	Level III	Oral cavity, oropharynx, hypopharynx, larynx, thyroid
Lower jugular nodes	Level IV	Oropharynx, hypopharynx, larynx, cervical esophagus, thyroid
Accessory nerve nodes	Level V	Nasopharynx, scalp
Supraclavicular nodes	Level V	Breast, lung, gastrointestinal tract
Suboccipital nodes		Skin
Parotid nodes		Skin, parotid gland

WORKUP OF A NECK MASS

The workup of a patient with a neck mass is an orderly progression of examinations and tests aimed at obtaining information about the mass and possible primary sites of cancer should the mass prove to be metastatic from an unknown primary cancer. The site of a cervical lymph node metastasis often suggests the location of the primary cancer because of specific lymphatic flow patterns in the neck (Table 15–1). Following a thorough history and physical examination, including flexible nasopharyngoscopy for visualization of the nasopharynx, hypopharynx, and larynx, FNA of the neck mass is performed for diagnosis. If the diagnosis is squamous carcinoma from an unknown primary cancer, a CT scan of the head and neck is performed. The patient is subsequently examined under anesthesia. Any abnormal areas are biopsied. The most common sites of occult cancers are the nasopharynx, hypopharynx (piriform sinus), and oropharynx (tonsillar fossa and base of tongue). A neck dissection is performed if the cervical lymph node metastasis is resectable. The neck dissection removes additional ipsilateral cervical lymph nodes that can contain occult metastases. A modified neck dissection may be appropriate, with preservation of the spinal accessory nerve, the sternocleidomastoid muscle, and the internal jugular vein if these structures are not involved with cancer. If more than two cervical lymph nodes contain metastases, if cervical lymph nodes at two or more levels contain metastases, or if there is extracapsular spread of cervical lymph node metastases, then postoperative radiation therapy is recommended. Prophylactic radiation therapy to all potential primary cancer sites is not recommended.

Only 15% of cervical lymph node metastases in the neck come from primaries below the clavicles (Figure 15–1). Metastases in the lower jugular chain and supraclavicular nodes (levels IV and V) can originate from primary cancers below the clavicle. In this case, the most common primary cancer site is the lung; other sites include the pancreas, esophagus, stomach, breast, ovary, testis, and prostate. CT scans of the chest and abdomen, as well as mammography, are performed in the search for a primary cancer, but they reveal the primary cancer in only 25% of cases. PET scan can also be utilized. While many of these cancers cannot be effectively treated, it is important to diagnose lung, breast, prostate, and genital cancers, which often do respond to specific therapy.

Beenken SW et al: Solitary neck mass. In: *Current Surgical Therapy.* Cameron JL (editor). Mosby, 1992.

Califano J et al: Unknown primary head and neck squamous cell carcinoma: molecular identification of the site of origin. J Natl Cancer Inst 1999;91:599.

STAGING OF SQUAMOUS CELL CARCINOMA

Squamous cell carcinoma is staged in order to classify the cancer, to estimate the prognosis, and to plan and assess the results of treatment. This entails an accurate description of the location and size of the primary cancer, the status of the cervical lymph nodes, and the presence or absence of distant metastases. The TNM staging system has done much to standardize the reporting of results of cancer treatment. In the oral cavity, oropharynx, and major salivary glands, T (tumor) stage is defined primarily by cancer size; while in the larynx, hypopharynx, and nasopharynx, T stage depends on the extent of local involvement. The accompanying boxes summarize N (regional lymph nodes) and M (distant metastasis) staging as they apply to squamous cell carcinoma. T stage (primary tumor) is summarized subsequently for the various upper aerodigestive tract anatomic sites. The following definitions are common to all sites: TX: primary tumor cannot be assessed; T0: no evidence of primary tumor; Tis: carcinoma in situ.

N STAGE

NX: Regional lymph nodes cannot be assessed
N0: No regional lymph node metastasis
N1: Metastasis in a single ipsilateral node, 3 cm or less in greatest dimension
N2: metastasis in–
- **N2a:** Single ipsilateral lymph node more than 3 cm but not more than 6 cm in greatest dimension
- **N2b:** Multiple ipsilateral lymph nodes, none more than 6 cm in greatest dimension
- **N2c:** Bilateral or contralateral lymph nodes, none more than 6 cm in greatest dimension

N3: Metastasis in a lymph node more than 6 cm in greatest dimension

M STAGE

MX: Presence of distant metastasis cannot be assessed
M0: No distant metastasis
M1: Distant metastasis

Stage Grouping

Once the TNM classification is established, the cancer stage (Figure 15–2) is defined as follows:

STAGE GROUPING

Stage 0	Tis	N0	M0
Stage I	T1	N0	M0
Stage II	T2	N0	M0
Stage III	T3	N0	M0
	T1	N1	M0
	T2	N1	M0
	T3	N1	M0
Stage IV	T4	N0	M0
	T4	N1	M0
	Any T	N2	M0
	Any T	N3	M0
	Any T	Any N	M1

CANCER OF THE ORAL CAVITY

Anatomy

The vermilion border of the lips is the anterior boundary of the oral cavity, while the anterior tonsillar pillars, the posterior aspect of the hard palate, and the circumvallate papillae of the tongue are the posterior boundary. Subsites are (1) the vermilion surfaces of the lips; (2) the alveolar process of the mandible; (3) the alveolar process of the maxilla; (4) the retromolar trigone, which is the mucosa overlying the ascending ramus of the mandible behind the last lower molar tooth; (5) the hard palate; (6) the buccal

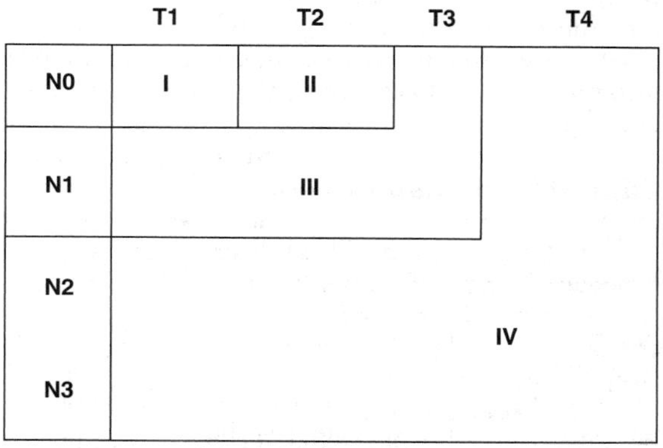

Figure 15–2. Cancer stage groupings for squamous cell carcinoma of the upper aerodigestive tract.

mucosa, which lines the cheeks and inner aspects of the lips and includes the upper and lower buccoalveolar gutters; (7) the floor of the mouth; and (8) the anterior two-thirds of the tongue (oral tongue), which is limited posteriorly by the circumvallate papillae and includes the tip, dorsum, lateral borders, and undersurface of the oral tongue. The mucosa of the oral cavity consists of stratified squamous epithelium.

Pathology

Over 95% of cancers of the oral cavity are squamous cell carcinomas. They are predominantly well and moderately well differentiated and can be preceded by premalignant lesions. Leukoplakia ("white patch") is induced by the same factors (tobacco, alcohol) that cause carcinomas. The malignant potential of leukoplakia corresponds to the degree of cellular dysplasia seen on biopsy. Erythroplakia ("red patch") usually shows severe cellular dysplasia and carries a 50% risk of malignant degeneration. Macroscopically, oral cancers can be exophytic growths, flat cancers with central ulceration and indurated edges, or deeply infiltrating ulcers. Verrucous carcinoma is an exophytic lesion that is histologically well differentiated and has a better prognosis than other oral cancers.

Oral cancers—especially those of the mucosa of the upper and lower alveolar ridges—often invade nearby bone. The mandible is most frequently involved. Minor salivary gland cancers arise in submucosal glands, which are most abundant in the hard palate. Ulceration is a late feature. Melanoma developing in the mucosa of the mouth is rare.

Cancers of the upper lip drain to parotid and submandibular nodes (level I), while those of the lower lip drain to submental and submandibular nodes (level I) and upper and mid jugular nodes (levels II and III). Midline cancers of the lip, the tongue, and the floor of the mouth can drain bilaterally. The incidence of cervical lymph node involvement from cancers of the oral cavity is related to the site and size of the primary cancer. Cancers of the oral tongue and the floor of the mouth have a higher incidence of cervical lymph node involvement than do cancers of the lip, hard palate, or buccal mucosa.

Clinical Findings

Patients with cancer of the oral cavity usually present with ulcerated cancers that have been present for weeks or months. They are typically men aged 50–70 years with a history of heavy tobacco and alcohol use. Dental hygiene is frequently poor, and areas of leukoplakia and erythroplakia can be seen adjacent to the cancer. Submandibular or jugular chain lymph nodes are palpable in 25–35% of patients. Pain is usually not a prominent feature but may become severe with deep infiltration.

T STAGE: ORAL CANCER

T1 Tumor 2 cm or less in greatest dimension
T2 Tumor more than 2 cm but not more than 4 cm in greatest dimension
T3 Tumor more than 4 cm in greatest dimension
T4 Lip: Tumor invades adjacent structures (eg, through cortical bone, tongue, skin)
T4 Oral cavity: Tumor invades adjacent structures (eg, through cortical bone, into deep [extrinsic] muscle of tongue, maxillary sinus, skin)

Treatment

A. Primary Cancer

Surgical excision is the treatment of choice for most oral cancers. Cancers of the vermilion surface of the lip are best treated with full-thickness excision of the lip. Lateral margins of 5 mm of uninvolved lip are taken with the cancer. The defect is closed primarily when one-third or less of the lip is excised. When excision of more than one-third of the lip is required, closure is achieved by transposition of a segment of the opposite lip on a vascular pedicle (Abbe flap). When the entire vermilion of the lip has been damaged, vermilionectomy (lip shave) can be performed along with excision of the cancer and a new vermilion surface created by advancing the labial mucosa.

Within the oral cavity, small cancers can usually be excised through the open mouth taking a margin of 1 cm of normal-appearing tissue. Small defects are closed by direct suture or split-thickness skin grafts. Larger cancers (> 2 cm) require more extensive exposure (ie, cheek flap), resection, and subsequent reconstruction. For cancers involving bone, marginal or segmental resection of the mandible is performed. A **composite resection** involves resection of an oral cancer, resection of a portion of the mandible, and a neck dissection.

Radiation therapy is an alternative to surgery for oral cancers smaller than 4 cm in diameter (T1 and T2 cancers). The side effects of mucositis, xerostomia, and osteoradionecrosis of the mandible must be balanced against potential advantages. T3 and T4 cancers are usually treated with combined surgery and radiation therapy to improve the rate of local control.

B. Management of Neck Metastases

Clinically apparent cervical lymph node metastases can be treated by radical neck dissection, which involves removal of all the lymphatic tissue of the neck along with the sternocleidomastoid muscle, internal jugular vein, and spinal accessory nerve. To save structures not directly involved by cancer, **modified neck dissection** is performed. A **modified radical neck dissection** always preserves the spinal accessory nerve, while a **functional neck dissection** always preserves the sternocleidomastoid muscle, the internal jugular vein, and the spinal accessory nerve. **Selective neck dissections** involve only certain cervical lymph node levels. For example, levels I, II, and III cervical lymph nodes and cervical lymph nodes in the upper portion of level V are removed with a **supraomohyoid neck dissection** while preserving the sternocleidomastoid muscle, the internal jugular vein, and the spinal accessory nerve (Table 15–2).

When modified neck dissections are performed, adjuvant radiation therapy to the neck is frequently required. It is recommended for use when more than two cervical lymph nodes contain metastases, when more than one level of cervical lymph nodes are involved, or when there is extension of metastases through the capsule of a cervical lymph node. Occult cervical lymph node metastases are present in 20–30% of patients with oral cancers (other than lip, buccal mucosa, or hard palate cancers) who present with a clinically negative neck. **Elective neck dissections** have been advocated for these patients to more accurately stage the cancer and to prevent the need for a later and probably more radical neck dissection when the cervical lymph node metastases becomes clinically apparent. A supraomohyoid neck dissection is the dissection of choice in the elective situation.

Prognosis

The five-year survival rates for cancer of the oral cavity with appropriate treatment are as follows: stage I, 72–88%; stage II, 46–80%; stage III, 36–66%; and stage IV, 11–32%. Buccal mucosa cancers have a better prognosis than tongue or hard palate cancers.

Table 15–2. Classification of neck dissections.

Type of Neck Dissection	Node Level of Dissection	Structures Preserved
Radical	I–V	None
Modified radical	I–V	SAN
Functional	II–V (± I)	SCM, IJV, SAN
Anterior	II–IV	SCM, IJV, SAN
Posterior	V	SCM, IJV, SAN
Supraomohyoid	II, III, (± I)	SCM, IJV, SAN

IJV, internal jugular vein; SAN, spinal accessory nerve; SCM, sternocleidomastoid muscle.

Beenken S et al: T1 and T2 squamous cell carcinoma of the oral cavity: prognostic factors and the role of elective lymph node dissection. Head Neck 1999;21:124.

Byers RM et al: Selective neck dissections for squamous carcinoma of the upper aerodigestive tract: patterns of regional failure. Head Neck 1999;21:499.

Ferlito A et al: Changing concepts in the surgical management of the cervical node metastasis. Oral Oncol 2003;39:429.

Matsuo JM et al: Clinical nodal stage is an independently significant predictor of distant failure in patients with squamous cell carcinoma of the larynx. Ann Surg 2003;238:412; discussion 421.

Myers JN et al: Squamous cell carcinoma of the tongue in young adults: increased incidence and factors that predict treatment outcomes. Otolaryngol Head Neck Surg 2000;122:44.

Samant S et al: Evaluation of neck dissection for improved functional outcome. World J Surg 2003;27:805.

CANCER OF THE OROPHARYNX

Anatomy

The oropharynx extends from the hard palate superiorly to the hyoid bone inferiorly. The subsites of the oropharynx are (1) the anterior surface of the soft palate, including the uvula; (2) the posterior pharyngeal wall; (3) the anterior and posterior tonsillar pillars; (4) the tonsils and tonsillar fossas; and (5) the posterior one-third of the tongue, which lies between the circumvallate papillae and the vallecula. The lingual surface of the epiglottis is part of the supraglottic larynx. The mucosa of the oropharynx consists of stratified squamous epithelium.

Pathology

Most oropharyngeal cancers are squamous cell carcinomas, but they tend to be less well differentiated than oral cancers. Deep infiltration is common. Minor salivary gland cancers and lymphomas—particularly non-Hodgkin's lymphoma involving the tonsil and other parts of Waldeyer's ring—also arise in this area. Tumors of the parapharyngeal space may also present as oropharyngeal swellings, causing the mucosa of the lateral pharyngeal wall or soft palate to bulge. These are most often retromandibular parotid tumors or neurogenic tumors (eg, neurilemmoma, neurofibroma, or paraganglioma).

The oropharynx is richly supplied with lymphatics. Posterior pharyngeal wall cancers drain bilaterally to jugular chain nodes (levels II, III, and IV) and the retropharyngeal nodes of Ranvier. Cancers of the tonsillar region drain primarily to the upper and mid jugular chain nodes and to the submandibular nodes (levels I, II, and III). Posterior triangle lymph nodes (level V) become involved following involvement of the jugular chain nodes. The overall incidence of cervical lymph node involvement from cancer of the oropharynx is approximately 70%. Bilateral cervical lymph node metastases are common (50%).

Clinical Findings

Patients with cancer of the oropharynx usually present with ulcerating cancers. Cervical lymph node metastases are a common presenting sign. Approximately 70% of patients with tongue base cancers present with advanced cancer, compared with only 35% of patients with cancer of the oral tongue. Tongue base cancers can spread laterally to involve the mandible, anteriorly to involve the oral tongue, and inferiorly to involve the vallecula and supraglottic larynx. Cancers of the tonsillar region readily extend to the mandible. They can also infiltrate the pterygoid muscles, producing trismus. This is an important presenting symptom, and it may limit access for examination. Referred otalgia is common with deeply infiltrating cancers.

T STAGE: OROPHARYNGEAL CANCER

T1 Tumor 2 cm or less in greatest dimension
T2 Tumor more than 2 cm but not more than 4 cm in greatest dimension
T3 Tumor more than 4 cm in greatest dimension
T4 Tumor invades adjacent structures (eg, through cortical bone, into deep [extrinsic] muscle of tongue, maxillary sinus, skin)

Treatment

A. Primary Cancer

Treatment for cancer of the oropharynx must be individualized. For small cancers (T1 and T2), surgery or radiation therapy gives similar results. For these cancers, surgical access can be achieved through the open mouth or by splitting the lower lip and jaw and retracting the mandible laterally (mandibular swing procedure). Excision of a soft palate cancer is readily accomplished, but when the muscular continuity of the soft palate is completely disrupted, regurgitation of food into the nasal cavity occurs. Therefore, small cancers are usually treated with radiation therapy and surgery is reserved for advanced or recurrent cancer. For more advanced cancers, the choices for therapy are (1) surgery combined with postoperative radiation therapy and (2) initial radiation therapy followed by surgery in the event of recurrence. Combined therapy offers the best chance of local cancer control. Total glossectomy may be necessary to encompass large cancers of the tongue base. Tongue base cancers that extend beyond the vallecula require glossectomy and laryngectomy to remove the cancer completely and to prevent subsequent aspiration pneumonia. Operative defects can be repaired with skin grafts, pedicled myocutaneous flaps (pectoralis major flap), or free flaps (radial forearm and osteomyocutaneous fibular free flaps). Temporary tracheotomy is mandatory in these circumstances.

B. Management of Neck Metastases

Cervical lymph node metastases are treated by radical or modified neck dissection (Table 15–2). If the neck is clinically free of cancer, an elective supraomohyoid neck dissection or radiation therapy is appropriate. If the primary cancer is treated by radiation therapy, the cervical lymph nodes at risk are included in the radiation field. If the primary cancer is treated surgically, an elective neck dissection is appropriate. If postoperative radiation therapy is planned for the primary cancer site, it is reasonable to include the neck in the radiation field instead of performing an elective neck dissection. Initial (induction, neoadjuvant) chemotherapy using cisplatin, fluorouracil, and paclitaxel, singly or in combination, gives response rates of up to 80%, but these responses are rarely of long duration.

Prognosis

The 5-year survival rates for cancer of the oropharynx with appropriate treatment are as follows: stage I, 75%; stage II, 65%; stage III, 45%; and stage IV, less than 30%. Quality of life is a major consideration in the treatment of oropharyngeal cancers, since swallowing and speech are often adversely affected by treatment.

Forastiere AA et al: Radiotherapy and concurrent chemotherapy: a strategy that improves locoregional control and survival in oropharyngeal cancer. J Natl Cancer Inst 1999;91:2065.

Harrison LB et al: Current philosophy on the management of cancer of the base of the tongue. Oral Oncol 2003;39:101.

Parsons JT et al: Squamous cell carcinoma of the oropharynx. Cancer 2002;94:2967.

CANCER OF THE HYPOPHARYNX

Anatomy

The hypopharynx extends from the hyoid bone superiorly to the lower border of the cricoid cartilage inferiorly. It is composed of four subsites: (1) the piriform sinuses, situated lateral to the larynx; (2) the postcricoid area, lying immediately behind the larynx; (3) the posterior pharyngeal wall; and (4) the marginal area where the medial wall of the piriform sinus and the false vocal cord meet superiorly at the aryepiglottic fold. Laterally, the piriform sinuses are bounded by the alae of thyroid cartilage and the thyrohyoid membrane. The hypopharynx, lined by stratified squamous epithelium, has a muscular wall consisting of the middle and inferior constrictor muscles. The retropharyngeal space posterior to the hypopharynx, which contains lymphatics and loose areolar tissue, separates the visceral compartment of the neck from the prevertebral muscles with their overlying prevertebral fascia.

Pathology

Over 95% of hypopharyngeal cancers are squamous carcinomas, which usually present as infiltrating ulcerative lesions. The incidence of poorly differentiated cancer is higher in the hypopharynx than in other regions. The size of these cancers can be deceptive on clinical evaluation because of submucosal lymphatic extension. Minor salivary gland cancers and lymphomas occasionally occur in the hypopharynx, where they usually present as submucosal tumors. Benign hypopharyngeal lesions include webs, strictures, and pharyngoesophageal (Zenker's) diverticula.

Cancer of the hypopharynx has a high propensity for lymphatic invasion, with most patients having cervical lymph node metastases at the time of initial presentation. The hypopharynx—especially the piriform sinus—must always be examined in an adult with cervical lymph node metastases and no obvious primary cancer site. Occult cervical lymph node metastases (ie, clinically negative but histologically positive) are also common, causing the overall incidence of cervical lymph node metastases at presentation to be approximately 75%. The principal cervical lymph node groups involved are the upper, mid, and lower jugular nodes (levels II, III, and IV); the retropharyngeal nodes of Ranvier; and, less frequently, the cervical lymph nodes along the spinal accessory nerve in the posterior triangle (level V).

Clinical Findings

The most common site for hypopharyngeal cancer is the piriform sinus, accounting for 60% of cases. The postcricoid region is affected in 25% of patients and the posterior pharyngeal wall in 15%. Postcricoid lesions are frequently circumferential and cause dysphagia, while piriform sinus lesions tend to remain silent for a long time. Patients with hypopharyngeal cancer are typically men in their fifth to eighth decades with a history of excessive alcohol and tobacco use.

The chief symptoms of hypopharyngeal cancer are pain, dysphagia, and weight loss. Pain can be localized to the site of the cancer or can be referred to the ipsilateral ear. About 25% of patients, especially those with lesions of the piriform sinus, present with palpable cervical lymphadenopathy and no other symptoms. Advanced cancers can invade the larynx and cause vocal cord paralysis and hoarseness. Direct laryngopharyngoscopy and biopsy are necessary to confirm the diagnosis and assess the extent of the cancer.

T STAGE: HYPOPHARYNGEAL CANCER

T1 Tumor limited to one subsite of the hypopharynx and 2 cm or less in size

T2 Tumor invades more than one subsite of the hypopharynx or an adjacent site, or measures more than 2 cm and no more than 4 cm in size, without fixation of the hemilarynx

T3 Tumor invades more than one subsite of the hypopharynx or an adjacent site, with fixation of the hemilarynx

T4 Tumor invades adjacent structures (eg, cartilage or soft tissues of the neck)

Treatment

The goals of treatment are to cure the cancer and maintain functional continuity of the upper aerodigestive tract. Intensive nutritional therapy is necessary if long-standing dysphagia has resulted in cachexia. Patients with cancer of the hypopharynx also commonly have pulmonary disease that must be assessed and managed preoperatively.

A. Primary Cancer

Surgical resection of hypopharyngeal cancers usually requires laryngopharyngectomy. Small (T1, T2) cancers of the piriform sinuses are curable with radiation therapy. Small (T1 and T2) cancers of the posterior pharyngeal wall can be treated with larynx-preserving local excision. Jejunal and tubed radial forearm free flaps permit excellent hypopharyngeal reconstruction. If a cancer extends to or arises in the cervical esophagus, laryngopharyngectomy and esophagectomy may be required. In this circumstance, a gastric pull-up procedure provides for upper aerodigestive tract continuity.

B. Management of Neck Metastases

The incidence of cervical lymph node metastases is so high with hypopharyngeal cancers that some form of neck treatment is appropriate for all patients. Treatment of both sides of the neck is frequently indicated. Radical or modified neck dissection is indicated for clinically evident cervical lymph node metastases. For the clinically negative neck, when the primary cancer is treated with radiation therapy, the neck is also treated with radiation therapy. If the primary cancer is treated surgically, elective neck dissection is performed. If postoperative radiation therapy will be given to the primary cancer site, radiation therapy can also be given to the neck, making an elective neck dissection unnecessary.

Prognosis

In patients with cancer of the hypopharynx, distant metastases appear in 25% of patients—a much higher incidence than with cancers of the oral cavity and oropharynx. The 5-year survival rates for patients with cancer of the hypopharynx receiving appropriate treatment are subsite-specific. Generally, patients with hypopharyngeal cancers do worse than patients with oropharyngeal cancers.

Chu PY et al: Surgical treatment of squamous cell carcinoma of the hypopharynx: analysis of treatment results, failure patterns, and prognostic factors. J Laryngol Otol 2004;118:443.

Urba SG et al: Organ preservation for advanced resectable cancer of the base of tongue and hypopharynx: a Southwest Oncology Group Trial. J Clin Oncol 2005;23:88.

CANCER OF THE LARYNX

Anatomy

The larynx is composed of three anatomic subsites. The supraglottic larynx extends from the epiglottis superiorly to the false cords inferiorly. Sites within the supraglottic larynx include the epiglottis (both lingual and laryngeal surfaces), aryepiglottic folds, arytenoids, and false cords. The glottic larynx consists of the true vocal cords (including the anterior commissure) superiorly and tissues within 5 mm of the inferior surface of the true vocal cords inferiorly. The subglottic larynx extends from the glottis superiorly to the inferior border of the cricoid cartilage inferiorly. Subglottic cancers are uncommon, accounting for less than 1% of all laryngeal cancers. Subglottic extension of a glottic cancer is more common.

Pathology

Squamous cell carcinoma of the supraglottic larynx accounts for 35% of laryngeal cancers. Fifty percent of these patients will present with cervical lymph node metastases. Lymphatic channels drain to the upper, mid, and lower jugular nodes (levels II, III, and IV). Local spread of cancer is usually in a superior or lateral direction. Inferior spread to the anterior commissure is less common.

Cancer of the glottic larynx accounts for nearly 65% of laryngeal cancers. It tends to be well differentiated, to grow slowly, and to metastasize late. Because the true cords have very limited lymphatic drainage, cervical lymph node metastases occur in only 10% of cases. Cervical lymph node metastases usually occur when the cancer infiltrates beyond the limits of the true cord. Submucosal extension occurs early and can lead to involvement of the anterior commissure and the contralateral vocal cord. The cancer can extend laterally, resulting in cartilage destruction, or superiorly, with involvement of the false vocal cords and aryepiglottic folds (transglottic carcinoma). Subglottic extension can also occur.

Subglottic cancers or subglottic extensions of a glottic cancer are associated with a high incidence of cervical lymph node metastases. Lymphatics from the subglottic larynx drain to the mid and lower jugular lymph nodes (levels III and IV) and to the prelaryngeal (cricothyroid or delphian) node. Subsequently, the pretracheal and paratracheal lymph nodes can be involved.

Clinical Findings

The initial presenting symptoms of cancer of the larynx depend upon the site involved. Supraglottic cancers tend to present late with symptoms of dysphagia, odynophagia, hemoptysis, or referred otalgia. Stridor and hoarseness are late findings. Palpable cervical lymphadenopathy is a common presenting sign. Glottic cancers often present early with hoarseness, and palpable lymphadenopathy is uncommon. Late symptoms include dysphagia, odynophagia, stridor, or cough. Subglottic cancer presents with dyspnea, stridor, or palpable cervical lymphadenopathy.

T STAGE: LARYNGEAL CANCER

Supraglottis

T1 Tumor limited to one subsite of the supraglottis with normal vocal cord mobility

T2 Tumor invades more than one subsite of the supraglottis or glottis, with normal vocal cord mobility

T3 Tumor limited to the larynx with vocal cord fixation and/or invades the postcricoid area, medial wall of the piriform sinus, or pre-epiglottic tissues

T4 Tumor invades through the thyroid cartilage and/or extends to other tissues beyond the larynx (eg, to the oropharynx or soft tissues of the neck)

Glottis

T1 Tumor limited to the vocal cord(s) (may involve anterior or posterior commissures) with normal mobility

- **T1a:** Tumor limited to one vocal cord
- **T1b:** Tumor involves both vocal cords

T2 Tumor extends to the supraglottis and/or subglottis, and/or with impaired vocal cord mobility

T3 Tumor limited to the larynx with vocal cord fixation

T4 Tumor invades through the thyroid cartilage and/or extends to other tissues beyond the larynx (eg, to the oropharynx or soft tissues of the neck)

Subglottis

T1 Tumor limited to the subglottis

T2 Tumor extends to the vocal cord(s) with normal or impaired vocal cord mobility

T3 Tumor limited to the larynx with vocal cord fixation

T4 Tumor invades through the thyroid cartilage and/or extends to other tissues beyond the larynx (eg, to the oropharynx or soft tissues of the neck)

Treatment

T1 and T2 cancers of the supraglottic and glottic larynx respond well to radiation therapy. Survival rates are similar to those achieved with surgery, including laser excision, but without the attendant morbidity. Elective radiation therapy to the neck is given to patients with supraglottic carcinomas. T3 and T4 cancers of the supraglottic and glottic larynx are treated with a combination of cisplatin-based chemotherapy and radiation therapy in an effort to avoid the morbidity associated with total laryngectomy. Patients are reevaluated following initial chemotherapy and radiation therapy. If there is complete disappearance of the cancer and biopsies are negative, surgery is avoided. In this way, nearly two-thirds of patients can be spared laryngectomy. Survival rates for patients receiving initial chemotherapy and radiation therapy are the same as those for patients receiving total laryngectomy.

Surgical options for supraglottic and glottic cancer include partial laryngectomy or total laryngectomy. Partial laryngectomy is appropriate for patients with T1 and T2 cancers. Vertical partial laryngectomy removes the ipsilateral vocal cord and overlying laryngeal cartilage. The procedure can be extended superiorly to include the ipsilateral false cord or posteriorly to include the ipsilateral arytenoid cartilage. It is an appropriate procedure for patients with reduced cord mobility due to cancer bulk but not for patients with reduced cord mobility due to invasion of the intrinsic musculature. Horizontal partial laryngectomy is indicated for patients with cancers arising above the level of the true cords. All patients will have some degree of aspiration following this procedure, but careful patient selection can minimize the long-term consequences. Total laryngectomy is appropriate therapy for some patients with T3 laryngeal cancers and for most patients with T4 cancers. In this situation, **wide field laryngectomy** includes removal of the bilateral level II, III, and IV cervical lymph nodes. Ipsilateral thyroid lobectomy is performed to facilitate paratracheal lymph node dissection.

The presence of cervical lymph node metastases is an indication for radical or modified neck dissection. Elective neck dissection or radiation therapy is not indicated for T1 and T2 glottic cancers but is indicated for all supraglottic cancers and for T3 and T4 glottic cancers. If the primary cancer is treated by surgery, an elective neck dissection is appropriate unless adjuvant radiation therapy to the primary cancer site is planned. In that case, elective neck radiation therapy can be given and the neck dissection deferred. If the primary cancer is treated with radiation therapy, elective neck radiation therapy is appropriate and operative dissection can be deferred.

Prognosis

Five-year survival rates for supraglottic cancer with appropriate treatment are as follows: stage I, 90–95%; stage II, 75–80%; stage III, 50%; stage IV, 20–40%.

Five-year survival rates for glottic cancer with appropriate treatment are as follows: stage I, 80–95%; stage II, 70–80%; stage III, 50–70%; stage IV, 20–50%.

Forastiere AA et al: Concurrent chemotherapy and radiotherapy for organ preservation in advanced laryngeal cancer. N Engl J Med 2003;349:2091.

Hinerman RW et al: Carcinoma of the supraglottic larynx: treatment results with radiotherapy alone or with planned neck dissection. Head Neck 2002;24:456.

Hinerman RW et al: Early laryngeal cancer. Curr Treat Options Oncol 2002;3:3.

Mendenhall WM et al: Management of T1-T2 glottic carcinomas. Cancer 2004;100:1786.

CANCER OF THE NASAL CAVITY, NASOPHARYNX, & PARANASAL SINUSES

Anatomy

The nasal cavity is divided into right and left nasal fossae by the nasal septum. Each fossa has an anterior opening (naris or nostril), a posterior opening (choana), and bony projections called turbinates protruding from the lateral walls. Posterior to the nasal cavity is the nasopharynx. Its roof is formed by the skull base, which slopes downward and backward, while the inferior limit is a posterior extension of the plane of the hard palate. The lateral wall is composed of the torus tubularis, the auditory tube orifice, and Rosenmüller's fossa. The paranasal sinuses consist of the maxillary and ethmoid sinuses bilaterally, the frontal sinus, and the sphenoid sinus. Each maxillary sinus shares a common wall with the orbit above, the nasal cavity medially, the oral cavity inferiorly, and the infratemporal fossa posteriorly.

The mucosa of the nasal cavity consists of ciliated pseudostratified columnar epithelium (respiratory mucosa) except in the region of the superior turbinate and the adjacent lateral wall and septum, which is lined by specialized nonciliated epithelium (olfactory mucosa). The sinuses are lined by respiratory epithelium, and melanocytes are scattered throughout the region. The nasopharynx is lined by respiratory epithelium in early life, but squamous metaplasia occurs with aging so that about 60% of the respiratory mucosa is replaced by squamous epithelium in the first decade of life. Initially, this squamous epithelium is nonkeratinizing, but after age 50 more keratinization occurs.

Pathology

The most common cancer of the nasal cavity and paranasal sinuses is squamous cell carcinoma. The maxillary antrum is the most common site, while cancers of the nasal cavity are rare. Adenocarcinoma, sarcoma, melanoma, lymphoma, and minor salivary gland cancers also occur. Esthesioneuroblastoma is an uncommon cancer that arises from olfactory mucosa at the superior aspect of the nasal cavity. It readily invades the ethmoid sinuses and can involve the orbit. In the nasopharynx, squamous carcinomas, 80% of which are nonkeratinizing, also predominate. Lymphoepithelioma, a subgroup of nonkeratinizing squamous carcinoma, is poorly differentiated, lacks squamous or glandular differentiation, and has a lymphocytic component. It is highly radiosensitive.

Cancers of the skin of the vestibule of the nose can drain to parotid, submandibular, or upper jugular nodes (levels I and II). Nasal cavity and maxillary sinus cancers rarely metastasize to the regional lymph nodes unless they are advanced and have invaded adjacent structures. The nasopharynx is richly supplied with lymphatics, and cancers in this region readily drain bilaterally to upper and mid jugular lymph nodes and to posterior triangle lymph nodes (levels II, III, and V). Cervical lymph node metastases occur in 80% of patients with this cancer. Palpable cervical lymphadenopathy is the initial manifestation of 50% of patients with nasopharyngeal cancer. Unlike other squamous cell carcinomas, cancers of the nasopharynx can metastasize to the posterior triangle (level V) in the absence of jugular lymph node involvement.

Clinical Findings

Cancers of the nasal cavity, paranasal sinuses, and nasopharynx are frequently advanced at presentation. Early symptoms such as nasal obstruction, nasal discharge, and sinus congestion are so commonly associated with benign conditions that they are not frequently investigated for the presence of a cancer. Hemorrhage can occur. Bone invasion and involvement of adjacent soft tissue structures are common. Along with the tonsillar fossa, the tongue base, and the piriform sinus, the nasopharynx is an important site of clinically occult primary cancer. Cancers of the maxillary sinus can invade the hard palate and enter the oral cavity. They can also invade the orbital floor, causing visual symptoms and proptosis. Anterior invasion through the skin can occur. In advanced maxillary sinus cancers, cervical lymph node metastases can be the initial manifestation. Cranial nerve symptoms result from invasion of the skull base.

Diagnosis

Diagnosis and assessment of the extent of cancer are more difficult for cancers in this area than for those elsewhere in the upper aerodigestive tract. Histologic examination of an adequate tissue biopsy specimen is always required. CT scanning is performed to delineate the extent of the cancer, though it can be difficult to differentiate between cancer and edematous mucosa. MRI is helpful in making this differentiation.

T STAGE: MAXILLARY SINUS CANCER

T1	Tumor limited to antral mucosa with no erosion or destruction of bone
T2	Tumor with erosion or destruction of the infrastructure, including the hard palate or middle nasal meatus
T3	Tumor invades any of the following: skin of cheek, posterior wall of maxillary sinus, floor or medial wall of orbit, anterior ethmoid sinus
T4	Tumor invades orbital contents and/or any of the following: cribriform plate, posterior ethmoid or sphenoid sinuses, nasopharynx, soft palate, pterygomaxillary or temporal fossas or base of skull

Treatment

Radiation is the principal treatment method for cancer of the nasopharynx. Undifferentiated cancers respond better than well-differentiated ones, and treatment is more successful in younger patients. A dose of 7000 cGy is usually required for the primary cancer. Both sides of the neck are treated because of the high incidence of bilateral cervical lymph node metastases.

Cancers of the maxillary sinus are treated by maxillectomy. For advanced (T3, T4) maxillary sinus cancers, surgery and postoperative radiation therapy provide for the best local control. Orbital exenteration is necessary for maxillary cancers that invade the periorbital tissues. Because the incidence of cervical lymph node metastases is low with cancers of the paranasal sinuses, prophylactic neck dissection or radiation therapy is not necessary. Resectable cancers of the upper nasal cavity and ethmoid sinuses require craniofacial excision, which entails frontal craniotomy to assess the extent of the intracranial extension of the cancer.

Prognosis

Five-year survival rates for nasopharyngeal cancer with appropriate treatment are as follows: stage I, 85%; stage II, 75%; stage III, 45%; stage IV, 10%. One-third of patients die of distant metastases.

Five-year survival rates for maxillary sinus cancer with appropriate treatment are as follows: stage I, 85%; stage II, 65%; stage III, 40%; stage IV, 15–20%.

Oh JL et al: Induction chemotherapy followed by concomitant chemoradiotherapy in the treatment of locoregionally advanced nasopharyngeal cancer. Ann Oncol 2003;14:564.

SALIVARY GLAND TUMORS

Anatomy

The paired major salivary glands consist of the parotid and submandibular glands. Minor salivary glands are widely distributed in the mucosa of the lips, cheeks, hard and soft palate, uvula, floor of mouth, tongue, and peritonsillar region; a few are found in the nasopharynx, paranasal sinuses, larynx, trachea, bronchi, and lacrimal glands.

Pathology

A variety of site-specific and systemic diseases can affect the salivary glands. These are summarized in Table 15–3. Tumors of salivary gland tissue constitute about 5% of head and neck tumors and affect major salivary glands five times more often than minor salivary glands. The incidence of malignancy among salivary gland tumors varies inversely with the size of the gland. About 15% of parotid tumors, 50% of submandibular gland tumors, and 90% of minor salivary gland tumors are malignant.

Table 15–3. Diseases of the salivary glands.

Disease Category	Disease Entity
Inflammatory disease	Actinomycosis
	Acute bacterial sialoadenitis
	Cat scratch disease
	Mumps
	Tuberculosis
Obstructive salivary disease	Kussmaul's disease
	Sialolithiasis
	Sjögren's disease
	Stricture
Neoplasia of the salivary glands	
Benign tumors	Mixed tumor
	Monomorphic adenomas
	Oncocytoma
	Warthin's tumor
Malignant tumors	Acinic cell carcinoma
	Adenocarcinoma
	Adenoidcystic carcinoma
	Malignant mixed tumor
	Mucoepidermoid carcinoma
	Undifferentiated carcinoma

Since 70% of salivary gland tumors occur in the parotid and 85% of these are benign, the majority of salivary gland tumors are benign. These tumors are thought to originate from two cell types: intercalated and excretory duct cells. Myoepithelial cells are present in many salivary gland tumors but rarely present as the principal cell type. The differential diagnosis of a swelling in the parotid region includes parotitis, a primary parotid tumor, upper jugular chain lymph node enlargement, a tumor of the tail of the submandibular gland, an enlarged preauricular or parotid lymph node, a branchial cleft cyst, an epithelial inclusion cyst, or a mesenchymal tumor.

The most common benign salivary gland tumor is the benign mixed tumor or pleomorphic adenoma, which accounts for 70% of parotid tumors and 50% of all salivary gland tumors. Mixed tumors are more common in women than in men, with the peak incidence in the fifth decade. They are slow-growing and lobular and may become very large without interfering with facial nerve function. Although mixed tumors are benign, they will recur after surgery unless they are completely removed. Enucleation is inadequate surgery. When tumor recurs in the parotid region, the facial nerve is at greater risk from damage during reoperation than it was during the initial procedure. Malignant transformation in a benign tumor is uncommon but can occur (malignant mixed carcinoma).

Warthin's tumor (papillary cystadenoma lymphomatosum), the next most common benign tumor, accounts for about 5% of parotid tumors. Warthin's tumors are usually cystic, typically occur in men in the sixth and seventh decades, and are bilateral in about 10% of cases. They occur almost exclusively in the parotid gland and have a typical histologic appearance, consisting of a papillary-cystic pattern with a marked lymphoid component. Oncocytomas are benign tumors composed of large oxyphilic cells called oncocytes. On electron microscopy, the cytoplasm of the oxyphilic cells is packed with mitochondria. Monomorphic tumors are rare benign salivary gland tumors that are usually epithelial but occasionally myoepithelial in origin. They are most commonly seen in the minor salivary glands of the lip.

Mucoepidermoid carcinoma is the most common parotid cancer. These tumors are categorized as high-grade, intermediate-grade, or low-grade cancers. Acinic cell cancers are derived from serous acinar cells and are found almost exclusively in the parotid gland. Adenoid cystic carcinomas, which are uncommon in the parotid, have a great propensity for perineural invasion and local recurrence. Patients with this cancer tend to have protracted illness, with recurrences appearing 15 years or more after treatment. Patients with distant metastases from adenoid cystic carcinoma can survive for 5 or more years. Less common cancers include cancer arising in a mixed tumor and primary squamous cancer, which accounts for approximately 1% of salivary gland cancers and must be differentiated from mucoepidermoid carcinoma and metastatic squamous carcinoma in a parotid lymph node. Among minor salivary gland cancers, adenoid cystic carcinoma is the most common cancer, followed by adenocarcinoma and mucoepidermoid carcinoma. Approximately 70% of all minor salivary gland cancers occur in the oral cavity, principally on the hard palate.

Diagnosis

In most cases, local excision with a margin of normal tissue is the appropriate form of biopsy for a major salivary gland tumor. In the parotid region, this requires identification of the facial nerve. For submandibular tumors, the entire submandibular triangle is cleared. In contrast, minor salivary gland tumors have a higher likelihood of being malignant, and an incisional biopsy is performed initially so that definitive treatment can be planned. In the parotid region, the presence of pain, recent rapid enlargement of a preexisting nodule, skin involvement, or facial nerve paralysis suggests cancer. Enlarged cervical lymph nodes in association with a salivary gland tumor are considered a manifestation of cancer until proved otherwise. Fine-needle aspiration is indicated if accurate diagnosis will allow for better treatment planning.

T STAGE: MAJOR SALIVARY GLAND CANCER

T1 Tumor 2 cm or less in greatest dimension without invasion of surrounding soft tissues

T2 Tumor more than 2 cm but not more than 4 cm in greatest dimension without invasion of surrounding soft tissues

T3 Tumor more than 4 cm in size and/or invading into surrounding soft tissues

T4 Tumor invades skin, mandible, ear canal and/or facial nerve

Treatment

Benign salivary gland tumors are excised. Parotid surgery requires a preauricular incision carried onto the neck to allow adequate exposure of the gland and facial nerve. The aim of the operation is to completely excise the tumor with an adequate margin of normal tissue. Enucleation is avoided because it greatly increases the likelihood of recurrence and nerve damage. When a tumor arises in the parotid gland deep to the facial nerve, the portion of the parotid gland superficial to the facial nerve is removed, the facial nerve is then elevated, and finally the tumor deep to the nerve is removed along with the remaining parotid tissue. Benign tumors of the submandibular gland require total removal of the gland for diagnosis and treatment.

Surgical treatment for parotid cancer depends on the extent of the cancer. Unless the facial nerve is paralyzed or found to be directly invaded by cancer at surgery, it is preserved. When the facial nerve must be divided, it is repaired if it was functioning normally prior to surgery. The facial nerve can be reconstructed using a nerve graft, eg, the greater auricular or sural nerves. Recovery of function can take many months and is often incomplete.

For low-grade salivary gland cancers, complete excision is sufficient treatment. For high-grade cancers, postoperative radiation therapy is indicated for the primary cancer site and regional lymph nodes. Clinically involved lymph nodes are removed by a radical or modified neck dissection. Elective neck dissections are generally not indicated, though removal of level II cervical lymph nodes requires minimal additional surgery after parotidectomy or after removal of the contents of the submandibular triangle.

Prognosis

The prognosis for salivary gland cancer depends on the stage, the histologic grade, the cancer site, the patient's age, and the adequacy of surgical removal. The most important prognostic factor is the cancer stage. The next most important factor is the histologic grade of the cancer. Low-grade cancers such as acinic cell cancers and low-grade mucoepidermoid cancers usually present as stage I or stage II cancers and have an excellent prognosis, with 10-year survival rates of about 80%. On the other hand, the 10-year survival rate after treatment of high-grade stage III and stage IV cancers—such as adenocarcinoma, squamous cell carcinoma, and high-grade mucoepidermoid carcinoma—is about 30%.

Douglas JG et al: Gamma knife stereotactic radiosurgical boost for patients treated primarily with neutron radiotherapy for salivary gland neoplasms. Stereotact Funct Neurosurg 2004;82:84.

Douglas JG et al: Treatment of salivary gland neoplasms with fast neutron radiotherapy. Arch Otolaryngol Head Neck Surg 2003;129:944.

Spiro JF et al: Cancer of the parotid gland: Role of 7th nerve preservation. World J Surg 2003;27:863.

RECONSTRUCTION

The primary aim of head and neck cancer surgery is complete eradication of the cancer. This is most likely to be achieved at the initial attempt, since treatment of recurrences is less successful. Unfortunately, surgery that achieves a good therapeutic result can be cosmetically and functionally unacceptable. Direct wound closure, skin grafting, or tissue transfer can repair surgical defects. Direct wound closure is ideal for small defects of the skin and of the mucosa of the oral cavity and oropharynx. Direct closure of large defects in the oral cavity and oropharynx can create distortion, such as tongue tethering, and is avoided. Skin grafts can be used to close defects of the skin or mucosa of the oral cavity and oropharynx that are not amenable to direct closure.

Tissue to close larger surgical defects can be obtained in several ways, including local rotational cutaneous flaps (forehead and deltopectoral flaps) for closure of defects of the skin of the face, neck, and chest, and rotational flaps of buccal or tongue mucosa for closure of defects in the oral cavity. Tissue can also be transferred from more distant sites using myocutaneous flaps (pectoralis major and latissimus dorsi flaps) and vascularized free flaps (radial forearm and osteomyocutaneous fibular flaps). Each of these techniques has its particular advantages and disadvantages, and the reconstructive procedure must be tailored to the patient and the site and extent of the operative defect.

Jaw reconstruction poses special technical difficulties, but vascularized free flaps such as the osteomyocutaneous fibular free flap appear to be most reliable. If a segment of the horizontal or vertical ramus of the mandible is resected, placement of a mandibular bar with or without transfer of harvested iliac crest bone can provide for a good result. Occasionally in the elderly or debilitated patient, only primary closure of the soft tissues is accomplished. The cosmetic and functional result is usually quite acceptable. Removal of the anterior part of the mandibular arch destroys the contour of the chin and creates the so-called "Andy Gump deformity," which severely affects eating, speech, and cosmetic appearance. Such defects are reconstructed with an osteomyocutaneous fibular free flap when the operative risk is acceptable.

Synthetic prostheses are especially useful following amputation of the nose or ear or after orbital exenteration. Excellent function can be achieved with dental obturators for patients with defects in the hard palate and upper alveolar ridges.

Iizuka T et al: Oral rehabilitation after mandibular reconstruction using an osteocutaneous fibula free flap with endosseous implants. Clin Oral Implants Res 2005;16:69.

Mehta RP et al: Mandibular reconstruction in 2004: an analysis of different techniques. Curr Opin Otolaryngol Head Neck Surg 2004;12:288.

Rashid M et al: Management of oromandibular cancers. J Coll Physicians Surg Pak 2004;14:29.

RADIATION THERAPY

Radiation can be used as definitive treatment with curative intent, as a postoperative adjunct to surgery, or for palliation.

Definitive Radiation Therapy

Squamous cell carcinomas are sensitive to radiation therapy, especially if they are small and only superficially invasive. T1 and T2 cancers of the oral cavity and oropharynx can be treated with surgery or radiation therapy. In some cases, radiation therapy has the advantage of avoiding the disfiguring side effects of surgery. However, mucositis, subsequent xerostomia, and the possibility of osteoradionecrosis of the mandible are disadvantages. Large oral cancers respond poorly to radiation therapy. Surgery with postoperative radiation therapy, if indicated, is the best treatment for these cancers. In the oropharynx, radiation therapy is excellent treatment for small cancers (T1, T2), especially for tonsillar cancers, because the response rate is good and radiation therapy can also treat occult cervical lymph node metastases. Large cancers of the tonsil (T3, T4) require surgery combined with radiation therapy. The surgical treatment of tongue base cancers larger than 3 cm can require total glossectomy and laryngectomy, a procedure with considerable morbidity. Radiation therapy may be the best initial treatment for these cancers, with surgery reserved for persistent cancer.

Nasopharyngeal cancers are responsive to radiation therapy. Surgical resection is usually not possible. A common side effect of radiation therapy in this area is dysfunction of the auditory tube and subsequent otitis media. A myringotomy tube can alleviate this problem. Radiation therapy is excellent treatment for early (T1 or T2) laryngeal cancers and has the advantage of preserving speech. Five-year survival rates range from 70% to 90% depending on the extent of the cancer.

Cervical lymph node metastases can be treated by radiation therapy alone if the lymph nodes measure less than 3 cm in diameter. If lymph nodes remain palpable after treatment, neck dissection is necessary. In general, clinically apparent metastatic cervical lymph nodes are best treated initially by a radical or modified neck dissection.

For most squamous cell carcinomas, radiation therapy is given in fractions of 180–200 cGy 5 days a week for approximately 6 weeks. Doses of 6000–7000 cGy are delivered to the primary cancer. When there is no palpable cervical lymphadenopathy but a high likelihood that the cervical lymph nodes harbor occult metastases, elective radiation therapy to a dose of 5000 cGy to the neck is added. Changes in fraction size and timing have been used to decrease cancer cell regeneration during treatment. Current radiation therapy protocols involve (1) accelerated fractionation, giving two or three fractions per day and shortening the overall duration of treatment; (2) hyperfractionation, giving two or three smaller fractions per day but maintaining the overall treatment duration; (3) accelerated hyperfractionation, reducing overall treatment time through a combination of greater fraction number and smaller fraction size; and (4) concomitant boost, giving a second daily dose radiation to a reduced "field within a field" during the course of conventional radiation therapy.

Adjuvant Radiation Therapy

Radiation therapy is often combined with surgery to improve local and regional control of squamous cell carcinoma. Preoperative radiation therapy (4500–5000 cGy) has been used but has the disadvantage of producing edema and increased vascularity of the operative field, with prolonged wound healing. Postoperative radiation therapy (5000–6000 cGy) is more often employed. Adjuvant radiation therapy is selective, since it is reserved for patients known from surgical or histologic findings to be at high risk of recurrence. Examples of such patients include those with a cancer of high histologic grade or poor differentiation, those with microscopic cancer at the margins of resection or macroscopic residual cancer, and those with perineural extension of cancer. Treatment commences after 4–6 weeks of wound healing.

Palliative Radiation Therapy

In some instances, when primary cancers or cervical lymph node metastases are not resectable, radiation therapy is given in high doses (eg, 6000 cGy or more) with palliation as the goal of treatment.

Adverse Effects of Radiation Therapy

The main acute complications of radiation therapy are skin reaction and mucositis. Long-term complications include fibrosis and vascular sclerosis, xerostomia, and osteoradionecrosis. Patients with carious teeth or advanced periodontal disease must have their teeth extracted before radiation therapy. Those who retain their teeth must maintain excellent dental hygiene. Surgical procedures in a previously irradiated field are technically more difficult. Cancers that have previously been treated by radiation therapy tend to respond poorly to subsequent chemotherapy.

Duan J et al: A dynamic supraclavicular field-matching technique for head-and-neck cancer patients treated with IMRT. Int J Radiation Oncology Biol Phys 2004;60:959.

Mendenhall WM et al: Parameters that predict local control after definitive radiotherapy for squamous cell carcinoma of the head and neck. Head Neck 2003;25:535.

Quon H et al: Brachytherapy in the treatment of head and neck cancer. Oncology (Huntingt) 2002;16:1379.

Robert F et al: Phase I study of anti-epidermal growth factor receptor antibody cetuximab in combination with radiation therapy in patients with advanced head and neck cancer. J Clin Oncol 2001;19:3234.

CHEMOTHERAPY

For patients with advanced squamous cell carcinoma (stage III or IV), surgery and radiation therapy have generally been used sequentially to obtain local and regional control of the cancer. Because many of these patients still develop recurrent cancer, chemotherapy has been used in protocol settings in an effort to improve long-term outcomes.

Induction Chemotherapy

Patients with advanced squamous cell carcinoma who respond to chemotherapy respond better to radiation therapy and live longer. This suggests that if those who respond to initial (induction, neoadjuvant) chemotherapy are subsequently given radiation therapy, surgery might be unnecessary. In a prospective, randomized trial, patients with stage III or stage IV laryngeal cancer were treated with either induction fluorouracil and cisplatin chemotherapy followed by radiation therapy or with surgery followed by radiation therapy. Patients not responding to chemotherapy were treated with surgery plus radiation therapy. The results showed no difference in survival between the two groups, but almost two-thirds of the patients treated with induction chemotherapy and radiation therapy avoided surgery and maintained laryngeal function. Induction chemotherapy followed by radiation therapy for T3 and some T4 laryngeal cancer has become standard therapy at most centers.

Concomitant Chemotherapy

Another strategy under investigation is concomitant chemotherapy and radiation therapy. Chemotherapy is utilized to control microscopic systemic metastases and to enhance the locoregional effects of radiation therapy. When used in this setting, several single agents have been shown to improve cancer-free survival (bleomycin, cisplatin, fluorouracil), though the benefits are small and are offset by the toxicity of the regimen.

Chemotherapy with Reirradiation

Patients with recurrent cancer after primary or adjuvant radiation therapy can benefit from reirradiation combined with fluorouracil and hydroxyurea chemotherapy. Survival is prolonged by 1 or 2 years compared with historical controls.

Adelstein DJ et al: Maximizing local control and organ preservation in stage IV squamous cell head and neck cancer with hyperfractionated radiation and concurrent chemotherapy. J Clin Oncol 2002;20:1405.

Adelstein DJ et al: Mature results of a phase III randomized trial comparing concurrent chemoradiotherapy with radiation therapy alone in patients with stage III and IV squamous cell carcinoma of the head and neck. Cancer 2000; 88:876.

Argiris A et al: Competing causes of death and second primary tumors in patients with locoregionally advanced head and neck cancer treated with chemoradiotherapy. Clin Cancer Res 2004;10:1956.

Brockstein B et al: Patterns of failure, prognostic factors and survival in locoregionally advanced head and neck cancer treated with concomitant chemoradiotherapy: a 9-year, 337-patient, multi-institutional experience. Ann Oncol 2004;15:1179.

Forastiere AA: Is there a new role for induction chemotherapy in the treatment of head and neck cancer? J Natl Cancer Inst 2004;96:1647.

Spencer SA et al: RTOG 96-10: Reirradiation with concurrent hydroxyurea and 5-fluorouracil in patients with squamous cell cancer of the head and neck. Int J Radiat Oncol Biol Phys 2001;51:1299.

CHEMOPREVENTION

Chemoprevention can be defined as the introduction of selected synthetic and natural substances into the diet for the purpose of reducing cancer incidence. Since the early 1960s, vitamin A (retinol) and its derivatives (retinoids) have been used to treat oral leukoplakia, a premalignant lesion of the oral cavity. Several studies have documented resolution of disease. A clinical trial comparing 13-*cis*-retinoic acid (isotretinoin) and placebo in patients with a prior squamous cell carcinoma who had no clinically evident cancer following surgery or radiation therapy was undertaken to investigate isotretinoin's chemopreventive efficacy. After a follow-up of more than 4 years, there was a statistically significant reduction in the rate of development of second primary cancers in the group treated with isotretinoin. Other less toxic compounds such as fenretinide are also being investigated.

Prevention of head and neck cancer: current status and future prospects. Curr Probl Cancer 2004;28:265.

Beenken SW et al: Transforming growth factor-α: A surrogate endpoint biomarker? J Am Coll Surg 2002;195:149.

Lippman SM et al: Oral cancer prevention and the evolution of molecular-targeted drug development. J Clin Oncol 2005;23:346.

Tsao AS et al: Chemoprevention of cancer. CA Cancer J Clin 2004;54:150.

Thyroid & Parathyroid

16

Orlo H. Clark, MD

I. THE THYROID GLAND

EMBRYOLOGY & ANATOMY

See Figure 16–1. The main anlage of the thyroid gland develops as a median entodermal downgrowth from the first and second pharyngeal pouches. During its migration caudally, it contacts the ultimobranchial bodies developing from the fourth pharyngeal pouches. When it reaches the position it occupies in the adult, just below the cricoid cartilage, the thyroid divides into two lobes. The site from which it originated persists as the foramen cecum at the base of the tongue. The path the gland follows may result in thyroglossal remnants (cysts) or ectopic thyroid tissue (lingual thyroid). A pyramidal lobe is frequently present. Agenesis of one thyroid lobe, almost always the left, may occur.

The normal thyroid weighs 15–25 g and is attached to the trachea by loose connective tissue. It is a highly vascularized organ that derives its blood supply principally from the superior and inferior thyroid arteries. A thyroid ima artery may also be present.

PHYSIOLOGY

The function of the thyroid gland is to synthesize, store, and secrete the hormones thyroxine (T_4) and triiodothyronine (T_3). Iodide is absorbed from the gastrointestinal tract and actively trapped by the acinar cells of the thyroid gland. It is then oxidized and combined with tyrosine in thyroglobulin to form monoiodotyrosine (MIT) and diiodotyrosine (DIT). These are coupled to form the active hormones T_4 and T_3, which initially are stored in the colloid of the gland. Following hydrolysis of the thyroglobulin, T_4 and T_3 are secreted into the plasma, becoming almost instantaneously bound to plasma proteins. Most T_3 in euthyroid individuals, however, is produced by extrathyroidal conversion of T_4 to T_3.

The function of the thyroid gland is regulated by a feedback mechanism that involves the hypothalamus and pituitary. Thyrotropin-releasing factor (TRF), a tripeptide amide, is formed in the hypothalamus and stimulates the release of thyrotropin (TSH), a glycoprotein, from the pituitary. Thyrotropin binds to TSH receptors on the thyroid plasma membrane, stimulating increased adenylyl cyclase activity; this increases cAMP production and thyroid cellular function. Thyrotropin also stimulates the phosphoinositide pathway and—along with cAMP—may stimulate thyroid growth.

Cavalieri RR: The effects of nonthyroid disease and drugs on thyroid function tests. Med Clin North Am 1991;75:27.

Sackett WR et al: Thyrothymic thyroid rests: incidence and relationship to the thyroid gland. J Am Coll Surg 2002;195:635.

EVALUATION OF THE THYROID

In a patient with enlargement of the thyroid (goiter), the history (including the family history) and examination of the gland are most important and are complemented by the selective use of thyroid function tests. The surgeon must develop a systematic method of palpating the gland to determine its size, contour, consistency, nodularity, and fixation and to examine for displacement of the trachea and the presence of palpable cervical lymph nodes. The thyroid gland moves cephalad with deglutition, whereas adjacent lymph nodes do not. The isthmus of the thyroid gland is situated immediately caudal to the cricoid cartilage.

Thyroid function is assessed by highly sensitive TSH assays that can differentiate between patients with hypothyroidism (increased TSH levels), euthyroidism, and hyperthyroidism (decreased TSH levels). In most cases, therefore, serum T_3, T_4, and other variables do not need to be measured. A free T_4 level is helpful in some patients with suspected hyper- or hypothyroidism. A serum T_3 level is useful for diagnosing T_3 toxicosis (high T_3 and low TSH), or the euthyroid sick, low T_3 syndrome (low T_3 and normal or slightly increased TSH).

Radioactive iodine (RAI) uptake is useful for differentiating between hyperthyroidism and increased secretion of thyroid hormone (low TSH and increased radioactive iodine uptake) on the one hand and sub-

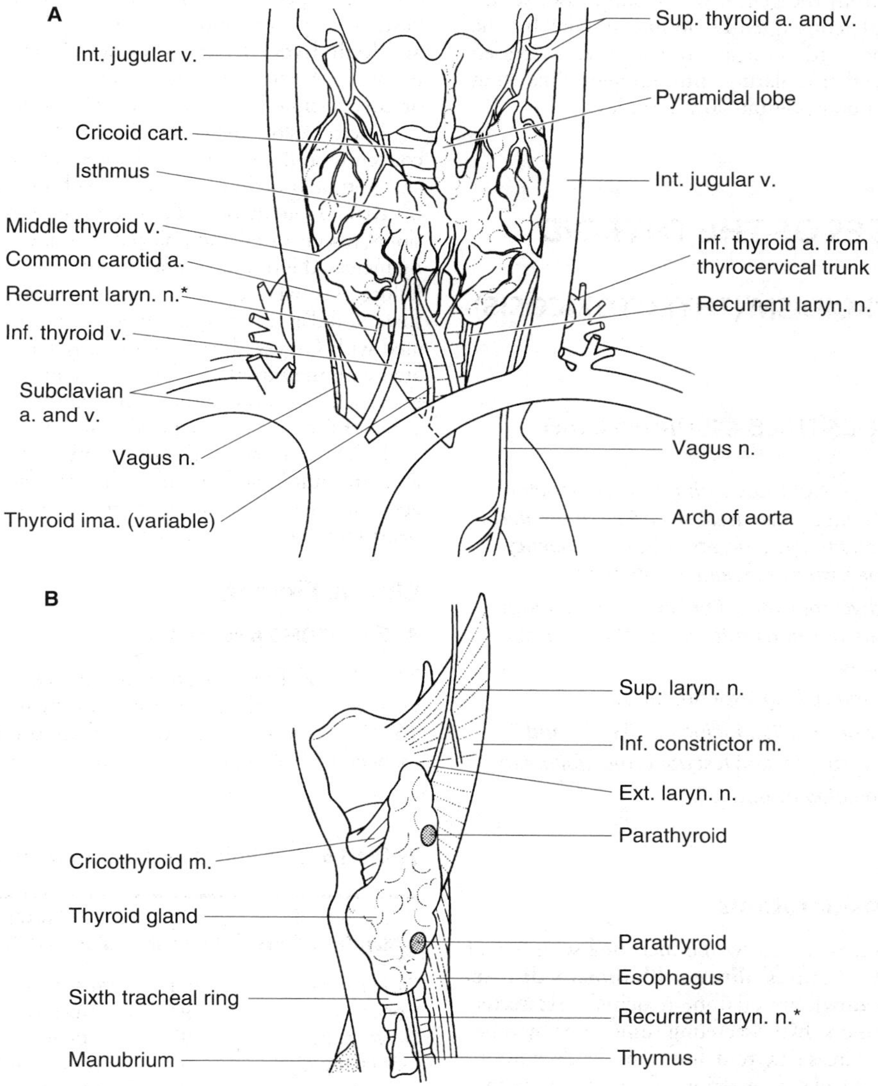

Figure 16–1. Thyroid anatomy.

* The recurrent laryngeal nerve runs in the tracheoesophageal groove on the left and has a slightly more oblique course on the right before it enters the larynx just posterior to the cricothyroid muscle at the level of the cricoid cartilage.

acute thyroiditis (low TSH and low radioactive iodine uptake) on the other. Patients with the latter "leak" thyroid hormone from the gland, which suppresses serum TSH levels and, consequently, iodine uptake by the thyroid. Patients with Graves' disease have increased levels of thyroid-stimulating immunoglobulins that increase iodine uptake despite low TSH levels.

DISEASES OF THE THYROID

HYPERTHYROIDISM (THYROTOXICOSIS)

ESSENTIALS OF DIAGNOSIS

- *Nervousness, weight loss with increased appetite, heat intolerance, increased sweating, muscular weakness and fatigue, increased bowel frequency, polyuria, menstrual irregularities, infertility.*
- *Goiter, tachycardia, atrial fibrillation, warm moist skin, thyroid thrill and bruit, cardiac flow murmur; gynecomastia.*
- *Eye signs: stare, lid lag, exophthalmos.*
- *TSH low or absent; TSI, iodine uptake, T_3, and T_4 increased; T_3 suppression test abnormal (failure to suppress radioiodine uptake).*

General Considerations

Hyperthyroidism is caused by the increased secretion of thyroid hormone (**Graves' disease, Plummer's disease,** iodine **[jodbasedow],** amiodarone toxicity, TSH-secreting pituitary tumors, hCG-secreting tumors) or by other disorders that increase thyroid hormone levels without increasing thyroid gland secretion (factitious hyperthyroidism, subacute thyroiditis, struma ovarii, and, rarely, metastatic thyroid cancers that secrete excess thyroid hormone). The most common causes of hyperthyroidism are diffusely hypersecretory goiter (Graves' disease) and nodular toxic goiter (Plummer's disease).

In all forms, the symptoms of hyperthyroidism are due to increased levels of thyroid hormone in the blood stream. The clinical manifestations of thyrotoxicosis may be subtle or marked and tend to go through periods of exacerbation and remission. Some patients ultimately develop hypothyroidism spontaneously or as a result of treatment. Graves' disease is an autoimmune disease—often with a familial predisposition—whereas the etiology of Plummer's disease is unknown. Most cases of hyperthyroidism are easily diagnosed on the basis of the signs and symptoms; others—eg, mild or **apathetic hyperthyroidism**—which occurs most commonly in the elderly—may be recognized only with laboratory testing for a suppressed TSH level.

Thyrotoxicosis has been described with a normal T_4 concentration, normal or elevated radioiodine uptake, and normal protein binding, but with increased serum T_3 by RIA (**T_3** toxicosis). **T_4** pseudothyrotoxicosis is occasionally seen in critically ill patients and is characterized by increased levels of T_4 and decreased levels of T_3 due to failure to convert T_4 to T_3. Thyrotoxicosis associated with toxic nodular goiter is usually less severe than that associated with Graves' disease and is only rarely if ever associated with the extrathyroidal manifestations of Graves' disease such as exophthalmos, pretibial myxedema, thyroid acropathy, or periodic hypocalcemic paralysis.

If left untreated, thyrotoxicosis causes progressive and profound catabolic disturbances and cardiac damage. Death may occur in thyroid storm or because of heart failure or severe cachexia.

Clinical Findings

A. Symptoms and Signs

The clinical findings are those of hyperthyroidism as well as those related to the underlying cause (Table 16–1). Nervousness, increased diaphoresis, heat intolerance, tachycardia, palpitations, fatigue, and weight

Table 16–1. Clinical findings in thyrotoxicosis.

Clinical Manifestations	Percent	Clinical Manifestations	Percent
Tachycardia	100	Weakness	70
Goiter	98	Increased appetite	65
Nervousness	99	Eye complaints	54
Skin changes	97	Leg swelling	35
Tremor	97	Hyperdefecation (without diarrhea)	33
Increased sweating	91	Diarrhea	23
Hypersensitivity to heat	89	Atrial fibrillation	10
Palpitations	89	Splenomegaly	10
Fatigue	88	Gynecomastia	10
Weight loss	85	Anorexia	9
Bruit over thyroid	77	Liver palms	8
Dyspnea	75	Constipation	4
Eye signs	71	Weight gain	2

*Data from Williams RH: *J Clin Endocrinol Metab* 1946:6:1.

loss in association with a nodular, multinodular, or diffuse goiter are the classic findings in hyperthyroidism. The patient may have a flushed and staring appearance. The skin is warm, thin, and moist, and the hair is fine.

In Graves' disease, there may be exophthalmos, pretibial myxedema, or vitiligo, virtually never seen in single or multinodular toxic goiter. The Achilles reflex time is shortened in hyperthyroidism and prolonged in hypothyroidism. The patient on the verge of thyroid storm has accentuated symptoms and signs of thyrotoxicosis, with hyperpyrexia, tachycardia, cardiac failure, neuromuscular excitation, delirium, or jaundice.

B. Laboratory Findings

Laboratory tests reveal a suppressed TSH and an elevation of T_3, free T_4, and RAI. A history of medications is important, since certain drugs and organic iodinated compounds affect some thyroid function tests, and iodide excess may result in either iodide-induced hypothyroidism or iodine-induced hyperthyroidism (**jodbasedow**). In mild forms of hyperthyroidism, the usual diagnostic laboratory tests are likely to be only slightly abnormal. In these difficult to diagnose cases, two additional tests are helpful: the T_3 suppression test and the thyrotropin-releasing hormone (TRH) test. In the T_3 suppression test, hyperthyroid patients fail to suppress the thyroidal uptake of radioiodine when given exogenous T_3. In the TRH test, serum TSH levels fail to rise in response to administration of TRH in hyperthyroid patients.

Other findings include a high thyroid-stimulating immunoglobulin (TSI) level, low serum cholesterol, lymphocytosis, and occasionally hypercalcemia, hypercalciuria, or glycosuria.

Differential Diagnosis

Anxiety neurosis, heart disease, anemia, gastrointestinal disease, cirrhosis, tuberculosis, myasthenia and other muscular disorders, menopausal syndrome, pheochromocytoma, primary ophthalmopathy, and thyrotoxicosis factitia may be clinically difficult to differentiate from hyperthyroidism. Differentiation is especially difficult when the thyrotoxic patient presents with minimal or no thyroid enlargement. Patients may also have painless or spontaneously resolving thyroiditis and are hyperthyroid because of increased release of thyroid hormone from the thyroid gland. This condition, however, is self-limited, and definitive treatment with antithyroid drugs, radioactive iodine, or surgery is rarely necessary.

Anxiety neurosis is perhaps the condition most frequently confused with hyperthyroidism. Anxiety is characterized by persistent fatigue usually unrelieved by rest, clammy palms, a normal sleeping pulse rate, and normal laboratory tests of thyroid function. The fatigue of hyperthyroidism is often relieved by rest, the palms are warm and moist, tachycardia persists during sleep, and thyroid function tests are abnormal.

Organic disease of nonthyroidal origin that may be confused with hyperthyroidism must be differentiated largely on the basis of evidence of specific organ system involvement and normal thyroid function tests.

Other causes of exophthalmos (eg, orbital tumors) or ophthalmoplegia (eg, myasthenia) must be ruled out by ophthalmologic, ultrasonographic, CT or MRI scans, and neurologic examinations.

Treatment

Hyperthyroidism may be effectively treated by antithyroid drugs, radioactive iodine, or thyroidectomy. Treatment must be individualized and depends on the patient's age and general state of health, the size of the goiter, the underlying pathologic process, and the patient's ability to obtain follow-up care.

A. Antithyroid Drugs

The principal antithyroid drugs used in the USA are propylthiouracil (PTU), 300–1000 mg orally daily, and methimazole, 30–100 mg orally daily. These agents interfere with organic binding of iodine and prevent coupling of iodotyrosines in the thyroid gland. One advantage over thyroidectomy and radioiodine in the treatment of Graves' disease is that drugs inhibit the function of the gland without destroying tissue; therefore, there is a lower incidence of subsequent hypothyroidism. This form of treatment may be used either as definitive treatment or in preparation for surgery or radioactive iodine treatment. When propylthiouracil is given as definitive treatment, the goal is to maintain the patient in a euthyroid state until a natural remission occurs. Reliable patients with small goiters are good candidates for this regimen. A prolonged remission after 18 months of treatment occurs in 30% of patients, some of whom eventually become hypothyroid. Side effects include rashes and fever (3–4%) and agranulocytosis (0.1–0.4%). Patients must be warned to stop the drug and see the physician if sore throat or fever develops.

B. Radioiodine

Radioiodine (^{131}I) may be given safely after the patient has been treated with antithyroid medications and has become euthyroid. Radioiodine is indicated for patients who are over 40 or are poor risks for surgery and for patients with recurrent hyperthyroidism. It is less expensive than operative treatment and is effective. To date, radioiodine treatment at doses necessary to treat hyperthyroidism has not been associated with an increase in leukemia or the induction of congenital anomalies. However, an increased incidence of benign thyroid tumors and rare cases of malignant thyroid tumors has been noted to follow treatment of hyperthyroidism with radioiodine. In young patients, the radiation hazard is certainly increased, and the chance of developing hypothyroidism is virtually 100%. After the first year of treatment with radioiodine, the incidence of hypothyroidism increases about 3% per year. In patients with Graves' ophthalmopathy, steroids should be given when radioiodine therapy is used.

Hyperthyroid children and pregnant women should not be treated with radioiodine.

C. Surgery

1. Indications for subtotal thyroidectomy—The main advantages of subtotal thyroidectomy are rapid control of the disease and a lower incidence of hypothyroidism than can be achieved with radioiodine treatment. Surgery is often the preferred treatment (1) in the presence of a very large goiter or a multinodular goiter with relatively low radioactive iodine uptake; (2) if there is a thyroid nodule that may be malignant; (3) for patients with ophthalmopathy; (4) for the treatment of pregnant patients or children; (5) for the treatment of women who wish to become pregnant within 1 year after treatment; (6) for patients with amiodarone-induced hyperthyroidism; and (7) for the treatment of psychologically or mentally incompetent patients or patients who are for any reason unable to maintain adequate long-term follow-up evaluation.

2. Preparation for surgery—The risk of thyroidectomy for toxic goiter is small since the introduction of the combined preoperative use of iodides and antithyroid drugs. Propylthiouracil or another antithyroid drug is administered until the patient becomes euthyroid and is continued until the time of operation. Two to 5 drops of potassium iodide solution or Lugol's iodine solution are then given for about 10 days before surgery in conjunction with the propylthiouracil to decrease the friability and vascularity of the thyroid, thereby technically facilitating thyroidectomy.

An occasional untreated or inadequately treated hyperthyroid patient may require an emergency operation for some unrelated problem such as acute appendicitis and thus require immediate control of the hyperthyroidism. Such a patient should be treated in a manner similar to one in thyroid storm, since **thyroid storm** or hyperthyroid crises may be precipitated by surgical stress or trauma. Treatment of hyperthyroid patients requiring an emergency operation or those in thyroid storm is as follows: Prevent release of preformed thyroid hormone by administration of Lugol's iodine solution or with ipodate sodium; give the β-adrenergic blocking agent propranolol to antagonize the peripheral manifestations of thyrotoxicosis; and decrease thyroid hormone production and extrathyroidal conversion of T_4 to T_3 by giving propylthiouracil. The combined use of propranolol and iodide has been demonstrated to lower serum thyroid hormone levels. Other important considerations are to treat precipitating causes (eg, infection, drug reactions); to support vital functions by giving oxygen, sedatives, intravenous fluids, and corticosteroids; and to reduce fever. Reserpine may be useful in the patient in whom nervousness is a prominent symptom, and a cooling blanket—not aspirin—should be used in patients requiring an operation.

3. Subtotal thyroidectomy—The treatment of hyperthyroidism by subtotal thyroidectomy eliminates both the hyperthyroidism and the goiter. As a rule, all but about 5 g of thyroid are removed, sparing the parathyroid glands and the recurrent laryngeal nerves.

The death rate associated with the procedure is extremely low—less than 0.1% in a recent collected review. Subtotal thyroidectomy thus provides safe and rapid correction of the thyrotoxic state. The frequency of recurrent hyperthyroidism and hypothyroidism depends on the amount of thyroid remaining and on the natural history of the hyperthyroidism. Given an accomplished surgeon and good preoperative preparation, injuries to the recurrent laryngeal nerves and parathyroid glands occur in less than 2% of cases. Adequate exposure and avoidance of injury to the recurrent laryngeal nerves and parathyroid glands are essential.

Ocular Manifestations of Graves' Disease

The pathogenesis of the ocular problems in Graves' disease remains unclear. Evidence originally supporting the role of either long-acting thyroid stimulator (LATS) or exophthalmos-producing substance (EPS) has not been authenticated.

The eye complications of Graves' disease may begin before there is any evidence of thyroid dysfunction or after the hyperthyroidism has been appropriately treated. Usually, however, the ocular manifestations develop concomitantly with the hyperthyroidism. Relief of the eye problems is often difficult to accomplish until coexisting hyperthyroidism or hypothyroidism is controlled.

The eye changes of Graves' disease vary from no signs or symptoms to loss of sight. Mild cases are characterized by upper lid retraction and stare with or without lid lag or proptosis. These cases present only minor cosmetic problems and require no treatment. When moderate to severe eye changes occur, there is retroorbital soft tissue involvement with proptosis, extraocular muscle involvement, and finally optic nerve involvement. Some cases may have marked chemosis, periorbital edema, conjunctivitis, keratitis, diplopia, ophthalmoplegia, and impaired vision. Ophthalmologic consultation is required.

Treatment of the ocular problems of Graves' disease includes maintaining the patient in a euthyroid state without increase in TSH secretion, protecting the eyes from light and dust with dark glasses and eye shields, elevating the head of the bed, using diuretics to decrease periorbital and retrobulbar edema, and giving methylcellulose or guanethidine eye drops. High doses of glucocorticoids are beneficial in certain patients, but their effectiveness is variable and unpredictable. If exophthalmos progresses despite medical treatment, lateral tarsorrhaphy, retrobulbar irradiation, or surgical decompression of the orbit may be necessary. Total thyroid removal appears to be helpful in some patients. Graves' disease is more likely to worsen after radioiodine treatment than after thyroidectomy. It is important that patients with ophthalmopathy be made aware of the natural history of the disease and also that they be kept euthyroid, since hyper- and hypothyroidism may produce visual deterioration. Operations to correct diplopia should be deferred until after the ophthalmopathy has stabilized.

Franklyn JA et al: Mortality after the treatment of hyperthyroidism with radioactive iodine. N Engl J Med 1998;338:712.

Goldstein R et al: Followup of solitary autonomous thyroid nodules treated with 131 I. N Engl J Med 1983;309:1473.

Ljunggren JG et al: Quality of life aspects and costs in treatment of Graves' hyperthyroidism with antithyroid drugs, surgery, or radioiodine: results from a prospective randomized study. Thyroid 1998;8:653.

McIver B et al: The pathogenesis of Graves' disease. Endocrinol Metab Clin North Am 1998;27:73.

Moleti M et al: Complete thyroid ablation reduces the activity of Graves' ophthalmopathy. Thyroid 2003;13:653.

Nicoloff JT: Thyroid storm and myxedema coma. Med Clin North Am 1985;69:1005.

Park JW et al: Thyroidectomy for Graves' hyperthyroidism. In: *Thyroid Eye Disease.* Dutton JJ, Hark BC (editors). Marcel Dekker, 2002.

Perrier ND et al: Surgery for thyrotoxicosis. In: *Oxford Textbook of Endocrinology and Diabetes.* Wass JAH, Shalet SM (editors.) Oxford University Press, 2002.

EVALUATION OF THYROID NODULES & GOITERS

Thyroid Nodules

The problems facing the clinician when confronted by a patient with a nodular goiter or thyroid nodule are whether the lesion is symptomatic and whether it is benign or malignant. The differential diagnosis includes benign goiter, intrathyroidal cysts, thyroiditis, benign and malignant tumors, and metastatic tumors to the thyroid. The history should specifically emphasize the duration of swelling, recent growth, local symptoms (dysphagia, pain, or voice changes), and systemic symptoms (hyperthyroidism, hypothyroidism, or those from possible tumors metastatic to the thyroid). The patient's age, sex, place of birth, family history, and history of radiation to the neck are most important. Low-dose therapeutic radiation (6.5–2000 cGy) in infancy or childhood is associated with an increased incidence of thyroid cancer (about 10%) in later life. A thyroid nodule is more likely to be a cancer in a man than in a woman and in young (under 20 years) and older (over 60 years) patients rather than in others. In certain geographic areas, endemic goiter is common, making benign nodules more common. Thyroid cancer is familial in about 25% of patients with medullary thyroid cancer (familial medullary thyroid cancer, MEN 2a and 2b) and in about 7% of patients with papillary cancer or Hürthle cell cancer. Papillary thyroid cancer occurs more often in patients with Cowden's syndrome, Gardner's syndrome, or Carney's syndrome.

The clinician must systematically palpate the thyroid to determine whether there is a solitary thyroid nodule or if it is a multinodular gland and whether there are palpable lymph nodes. A solitary hard thyroid nodule is likely to be malignant, whereas most multinodular goiters are benign.

In many patients, the possibility of cancer is difficult to exclude without microscopic examination of the gland itself. Percutaneous needle biopsy is the most cost-effective diagnostic test for most patients and has replaced radioiodine scanning. Cytologic results are classified as malignant, benign, indeterminate or suspicious, and inadequate specimen (Figure 16–2). False-positive diagnoses of cancer are rare, but about 20% of biopsy specimens reported as indeterminate and 5% of those reported as benign are actually malignant. If the specimen is reported as inadequate, biopsy should be repeated. Needle biopsy should in general not be performed in patients with a history of irradiation to the neck or familial thyroid cancer

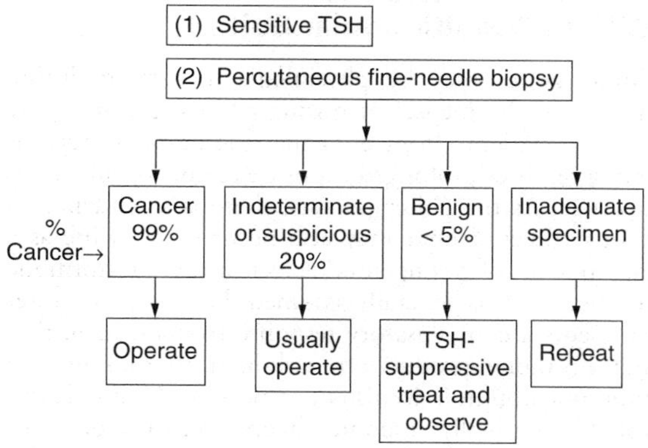

Figure 16–2. Evaluation of thyroid nodule.

because radiation-induced tumors are often multifocal, and a negative biopsy may therefore be unreliable. Radioiodine scanning is used selectively to determine whether a follicular neoplasm by cytologic examination is functioning (warm or hot) or nonfunctioning (cold). Hot solitary thyroid nodules may cause hyperthyroidism but are rarely malignant, whereas cold solitary thyroid nodules have an incidence of cancer of about 20% and should be removed. Thyroid carcinoma is uncommon (1%) in multinodular goiters, but if there is a dominant nodule or one that enlarges, it should be biopsied or removed. Patients with thyroid nodules who received x-ray treatments to the head and neck in infancy and childhood and those with a family history of thyroid cancer have a 40% chance of having thyroid cancer. Thyroid cancer occurs in nearly 50% of the children with solitary cold thyroid nodules; therefore, fine-needle biopsy or thyroidectomy is indicated. Ultrasound differentiates solid and cystic lesions and may detect enlarged lymph nodes. About 15% of cold solitary lesions are cystic. A chest x-ray including the neck is helpful in demonstrating tracheal displacement, calcification of the thyroid nodule, or the presence of pulmonary metastases. CT or MRI scans are usually not necessary but are helpful when the limits of the tumor cannot be defined, such as in patients with large, invasive, or substernal goiters or tumors.

The principal indications for surgical removal of a nodular goiter are (1) suspicion of or documented cancer, (2) symptoms of pressure, (3) hyperthyroidism, (4) substernal extension, and (5) cosmetic deformity. Solitary hard thyroid nodules or nodules that are cold on radioiodine scan and solid by ultrasound or are suspicious for cancer on aspiration biopsy cytology should be removed. Nonoperative treatment is indicated in patients with multinodular goiters and Hashimoto's thyroiditis unless there is a clinically suspicious area that is growing or if the patient was exposed to radiation or has a family history of thyroid carcinoma.

Simple or Nontoxic Goiter (Diffuse & Multinodular Goiter)

Simple goiter may be physiologic, occurring during puberty or the menses or during pregnancy; or it may occur in patients from endemic (iodine-poor) regions or as a result of prolonged exposure to goitrogenic foods or drugs. As the goiter persists, there is a tendency to form nodules. Goiter may also occur early in life as a consequence of a congenital defect in thyroid hormone production. It is generally assumed that nontoxic goiter represents a compensatory response to inadequate thyroid hormone production, although thyroid growth immunoglobulins may also be important. Nontoxic diffuse goiter usually responds favorably to thyroid hormone administration.

Symptoms are usually awareness of a neck mass and dyspnea, dysphagia, or symptoms caused by interference with venous return. In diffuse goiter, the thyroid is symmetrically enlarged and has a smooth surface without areas of encapsulation. However, most patients have multinodular glands by the time they seek medical care. Thyroid function is usually normal, though the sensitive TSH may be suppressed and the radioiodine uptake increased. Surgery is indicated to relieve the pressure symptoms of a large goiter for substernal goiter or to rule out cancer when there are localized areas of hardness or rapid growth. Aspiration biopsy cytology is helpful in these patients.

Alsanea O, Clark OH: Benign disorders of the thyroid gland. In: *Endocrine Tumors,* p. 1. Clark OH, Duh QY, Perrier ND, Jahan TM (editors). BC Decker, 2003.

Bellatone R et al: Management of cystic or predominantly cystic thyroid nodules: the role of ultrasound-guided fine-needle aspiration biopsy. Thyroid 2004;14:43.

Brenta G et al: Comparative efficacy and side effects of the treatment of euthyroid goiter with levo-thyroxine or with triiodothyroacetic. J Clin Endocrinol Metab 2003;88:5287.

Brunaud L et al: Incision length for standard thyroidectomy and parathyroidectomy. Arch Surg 2003;138:1140.

Burguera B et al: Thyroid incidentalomas. Prevalence, diagnosis, significance and management. Endocrinol Metab Clin North Am 2000;29:87.

Cochand-Priollet B et al: The diagnostic value of fine needle aspiration biopsy under ultrasonography in nonfunctioning thyroid nodules: a prospective study comparing cytologic and histologic findings. Am J Med 1994:97:152.

Kang HW et al: Prevalence, clinical, and ultrasonographic characteristics of thyroid incidentalomas. Thyroid 2004;14:29.

Kikuchi S et al: Accuracy of fine needle aspiration cytology in patients with radiation induced thyroid neoplasms. Br J Surg 2003;90:755.

Sadler GP, Clark OH: Total thyroidectomy. In: *Thyroid Cancer,* p. 229. Clark OH, Noguchi S (editors). Quality Medical Publishing, 2000.

Wong CK et al: Thyroid nodules. Rational management. World J Surg 2000;24:934.

Zbar AP, O'Higgins NJ: Use and abuse of thyroid stimulating hormone suppressive therapy in patients with nodular goiter and benign or malignant thyroid neoplasms. In: *Textbook of Endocrine Surgery,* p. 54. Clark OH, Duh QY (editors). Saunders, 1997.

INFLAMMATORY THYROID DISEASE

The inflammatory diseases of the thyroid are termed acute, subacute, or chronic thyroiditis, which can be either suppurative or nonsuppurative.

Acute suppurative thyroiditis is uncommon and is characterized by the sudden onset of severe neck pain accompanied by dysphagia, fever, and chills. It usually follows an acute upper respiratory tract infection; can be diagnosed by percutaneous aspiration, smear, and culture; and is treated by surgical drainage. The organisms are most often streptococci, staphylococci, pneumococci, or coliforms. It may also be associated with a piriform sinus fistula. A barium swallow is therefore recommended in persistent or recurrent cases.

Subacute thyroiditis, a noninfectious disorder, is characterized by thyroid swelling, head and chest pain, fever, weakness, malaise, palpitations, and weight loss. Some patients with subacute thyroiditis have no pain (silent thyroiditis), in which case the condition must be distinguished from Graves' disease. In subacute thyroiditis, the erythrocyte sedimentation rate and serum gamma globulin are almost always elevated, and radioiodine uptake is very low or absent with increased or normal thyroid hormone levels. The illness is usually self-limited, and aspirin and corticosteroids relieve symptoms. These patients eventually become euthyroid.

Hashimoto's thyroiditis, the most common form of thyroiditis, is usually characterized by enlargement of the thyroid with or without pain and tenderness. It is much more common in women (about 15% of women in the USA) and occasionally causes dysphagia or hypothyroidism.

Hashimoto's thyroiditis is an autoimmune disease. Serum titers of antimicrosomal and antithyroglobulin antibodies are elevated. Appropriate treatment for most patients consists of giving small doses of thyroid hormone. Operation is indicated for marked pressure symptoms, for suspected malignant tumor, and for cosmetic reasons. In patients with pressure or choking symptoms, surgical division of the isthmus provides relief. If the thyroid is large or asymmetric and fails to regress after treatment with exogenous thyroid hormone, or if it contains a discrete nodule, percutaneous needle biopsy or thyroidectomy is recommended.

Riedel's thyroiditis is a rare condition that presents as a hard woody mass in the thyroid region with marked fibrosis and chronic inflammation in and around the gland. The inflammatory process infiltrates muscles and causes symptoms of tracheal compression. Hypothyroidism is usually present, and surgical treatment is required to relieve tracheal or esophageal obstruction.

Baker JR: Autoimmune endocrine diseases. JAMA 1997;278:1931.

Hollowell JG et al: Serum TSH, T4, and thyroid antibodies in the United States population (1988–1994): National Health and Nutrition Gramination Survey (NHANES III). J Clin Endocrinol Metab 2002;87:489.

Lal G et al: Thyroiditis. In: *Current Surgical Therapy,* 7th ed. Cameron J (editor). Mosby, 2004.

Moleti M et al: Effects of thyroidectomy alone or followed by radioiodine ablation of thyroid remnants on the outcome of Graves' ophthalmopathy. Thyroid 2003;13:653.

BENIGN TUMORS OF THE THYROID

Benign thyroid tumors are adenomas, involutionary nodules, cysts, or localized thyroiditis. Most adenomas are of the follicular type. Adenomas are usually solitary and encapsulated and compress the adjacent thyroid. The major reasons for removal are a suspicion of cancer, functional overactivity producing hyperthyroidism, and cosmetic disfigurement.

MALIGNANT TUMORS OF THE THYROID

ESSENTIALS OF DIAGNOSIS

- *History of irradiation to the neck in some patients.*
- *Painless or enlarging nodule, dysphagia, or hoarseness.*
- *Firm or hard, fixed thyroid nodule; ipsilateral cervical lymphadenopathy.*
- *Normal thyroid function; nodule stippled with calcium (x-ray), cold (radioiodine scan), solid (ultrasound); positive or suspicious cytology.*
- *Family history of thyroid cancer.*

General Considerations

An appreciation of the classification of malignant tumors of the thyroid is important, because thyroid tumors demonstrate a wide range of growth and malignant behavior. At one end of the spectrum is **papillary adenocarcinoma,** which usually occurs in young adults, grows very slowly, metastasizes through lymphatics, and is compatible with long life even in the presence of metastases (Figure 16–3). At the other extreme is **undifferentiated carcinoma,** which appears late in life and is nonencapsulated and invasive, forming large infiltrating tumors composed of small or large anaplastic cells. Most patients with anaplastic thyroid carcinoma succumb as a consequence of local recurrence, pulmonary metastasis, or both within 6 months. Between these two extremes are follicular, Hürthle cell, and medullary carcinomas, sarcomas, lymphomas, and metastatic tumors. The prognosis depends on the histologic pattern, the age and sex of the patient, the extent of tumor spread at the time of diagnosis, whether the tumor takes up radioiodine, and other factors.

The cause of most cases of thyroid carcinoma is unknown, although persons who received low-dose (6.5–2000 cGy) therapeutic radiation to the thymus, tonsils, scalp, and skin in infancy, childhood, and adolescence

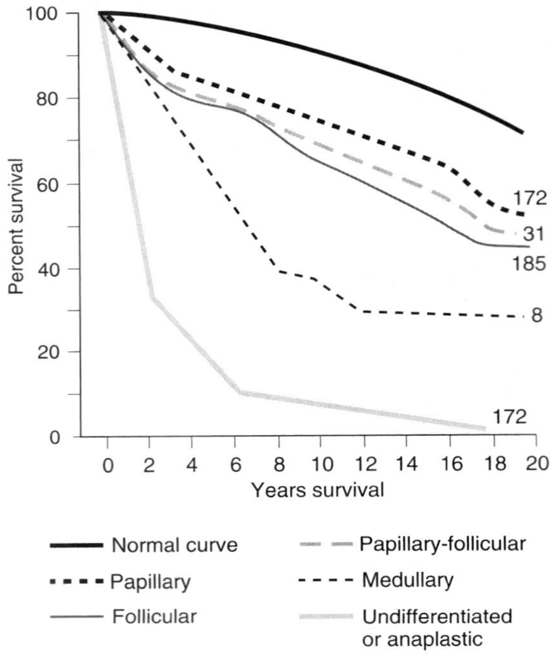

Figure 16–3. Survival rates after thyroidectomy for papillary, mixed papillary-follicular, follicular, medullary, and undifferentiated thyroid cancer.

have an increased risk of developing thyroid tumors. Children are most susceptible to radiation exposure such as occurred with the Chernobyl nuclear accident, but adults up to 50 years of age who were exposed to the atomic blast at Hiroshima had an increased incidence of benign and malignant thyroid tumors. The incidence of thyroid cancer increases for at least 30 years after irradiation.

Types of Thyroid Cancer

A. Papillary Adenocarcinoma

Papillary adenocarcinoma accounts for 85% of cancers of the thyroid gland. The tumor usually appears in early adult life and presents as a solitary nodule. It then spreads via intraglandular lymphatics within the thyroid gland and then to the subcapsular and pericapsular lymph nodes. Fifty percent of children and 20% of adults present with palpable lymph nodes. The tumor may metastasize to lungs or bone. Microscopically, it is composed of papillary projections of columnar epithelium. Psammoma bodies are present in about 60% of cases. Mixed papillary-follicular, follicular variants of papillary carcinoma, and poorly differentiated cancers including tall cell and columnar cell papillary thyroid cancers are sometimes found. The rate of growth may be stimulated by TSH.

B. Follicular Adenocarcinoma

Follicular adenocarcinoma accounts for approximately 10% of malignant thyroid tumors. It appears later in life than the papillary form and may be rubbery or even soft on palpation. Follicular tumors are encapsulated. Microscopically, follicular carcinoma may be difficult to distinguish from normal thyroid tissue. Capsular (invasion through the capsule) and vascular invasion distinguish follicular carcinomas from follicular adenomas. Follicular thyroid cancers only occasionally (7%) metastasize to the regional lymph nodes, but they have a greater tendency to spread by the hematogenous route to the lungs, skeleton, and rarely to the liver. Metastases from this tumor often demonstrate an avidity for radioactive iodine after total thyroidectomy. Skeletal metastases from follicular carcinomas may appear 10 years after resection of the primary lesion. Hürthle cells carcinoma is a variant of follicular carcinoma. It is more likely to be multifocal and involve lymph nodes than follicular carcinoma. Like follicular carcinoma, it makes thyroglobulin, but it does not usually take up radioiodine. The prognosis is not as good for either follicular or Hürthle cell cancers as with the papillary type (Figure 16–3).

C. Medullary Carcinoma

Medullary carcinoma accounts for approximately 7% of malignant tumors of the thyroid and 15% of thyroid cancer deaths. It contains amyloid and is a solid, hard, nodular tumor that does not take up radioiodine and secretes calcitonin. Medullary carcinomas arise from parafollicular cells of the ultimobranchial bodies or C cells. Familial medullary carcinoma occurs in about 25% of patients. It may be isolated or occur with pheochromocytomas—often bilateral—and hyperparathyroidism (MEN 2a). It may also occur with or without pheochromocytomas, marfanoid habitus, multiple neuromas, and ganglioneuromatosis (MEN 2b). Hirschsprung's disease and lichen planus amyloidosis also occur in patients with familial medullary cancer. All patients with medullary thyroid cancer should be screened for an *RET* point mutation on chromosome 10 because 10% of patients without a positive family history have de novo mutations. For patients detected by family genetic screening, most experts recommend prophylactic total thyroidectomy prior to age 6. Isolated familial medullary thyroid cancer is the least aggressive form, whereas this cancer in MEN 2b is the most aggressive form.

D. Undifferentiated Carcinoma

This rapidly growing tumor occurs principally in women beyond middle life and accounts for 1% of all thyroid cancers. This tumor usually evolves from a papillary or follicular neoplasm. It is a solid, quickly enlarging, hard, irregular mass diffusely involving the gland and invading the trachea, muscles, and neurovascular structures early. The tumor may be painful and somewhat tender, may be fixed on swallowing, and may cause laryngeal or esophageal obstructive symptoms. Microscopically, there are three major types: giant cell, spindle cell, and small cell. Mitoses are frequent. Cervical lymphadenopathy and pulmonary metastases are common. Local recurrence after surgical treatment is the rule. Combination treatment with external radiation therapy, chemotherapy, and surgery offers palliation to some patients but is rarely curative (Figure 16–3).

Treatment

The treatment of differentiated thyroid carcinoma is operative removal. For papillary carcinoma, acceptable operations are total lobectomy with isthmectomy, near-total thyroidectomy, and total thyroidectomy—followed by 10-year survival rates of over 80%. Subtotal or partial lobectomy is contraindicated because the incidence of tumor recurrence is greater and survival is shorter. Total thyroidectomy is recommended by the author and many others for papillary (> 1.5 cm), follicular, Hürthle cell, and medullary carcinomas if the operation can be done without producing permanent hypoparathyroidism or injury to the recurrent laryngeal nerves. Total thyroidectomy is preferred over other operations because of the high incidence of multifocal tumor within the gland, a clinical recurrence rate of about 7% in the contralateral lobe if it is spared, and the ease of assessment for recurrence by serum thyroglobulin assay or radioiodine scan during follow-up examinations. It also allows one to treat with radioiodine.

A functional modified radical neck dissection preserving the sternocleidomastoid muscle, spinal accessory nerve, and sensory nerve is performed if lymph nodes in the lateral neck are clinically involved.

Medullary carcinoma is associated with such a high incidence of nodal involvement that a bilateral central neck node cleanout should be done in all patients as well as concomitant ipsilateral and contralateral modified radical neck dissection for primary tumors more than 1.5 cm in diameter and when the central neck nodes are involved. When serum calcitonin or CEA levels remain elevated after thyroidectomy, ultrasound or MRI examination of the neck and MRI of the mediastinum should be done. Laparoscopy should also be done to evaluate for the common miliary metastases on the surface of the liver. If the liver is clear, then central neck dissection and bilateral functional neck dissections should be considered, if not already done, including removal of nodes from the superior mediastinum.

Isolated metastatic deposits of follicular and papillary carcinoma should be removed surgically and treated with ^{131}I after total thyroidectomy or thyroid ablation with radioactive iodine. All patients with thyroid cancer should be maintained indefinitely on suppressive doses of thyroid hormone (mild suppression for low-risk patients). For follow-up, it is helpful to measure serum levels of thyroglobulin (a tumor marker for differentiated thyroid cancer), which are usually increased (> 2 ng/mL) in patients with residual tumor after total thyroidectomy. For **undifferentiated carcinoma, malignant lymphoma,** or **sarcoma,** the tumor should be excised as completely as possible and then treated by radiation and chemotherapy. Doxorubicin (Adriamycin), vincristine, and chlorambucil are the most effective agents. Carcinomas of the kidney, breast, and lung and other tumors sometimes metastasize to the thyroid, but they rarely present as a solitary nodule.

Alsanea O et al: Is familial non-medullary thyroid carcinoma more aggressive than sporadic thyroid cancer? A multicenter series. Surgery 2000;128:1043.

Clark OH: Thyroid cancer: predisposing conditions, growth factors, signal transduction and oncogenes. Aust N Z J Surg 1998;68:469.

Clark OH et al: Management of patients with differentiated thyroid cancer will have positive serum thyroglobulin levels and negative radioiodine. Thyroid 1994;4:501.

Dedivitis RA et al: Thyroglossal duct: a review of 55 cases. J Am Coll Surg 2002;194:274.

Kebebew E et al: Coexisting chronic lymphocytic thyroiditis and papillary thyroid cancer revisited. World J Surg 2001;25:632.

Kebebew E et al: Medullary thyroid cancer: clinical characteristics, treatment, prognostic factors, and comparison of staging systems. Cancer 2000;88:1139.

Kebebew E et al: Differentiated thyroid cancer: "complete" rational approach. World J Surg 2000;24:942.

Latrofe CL et al: Serum antithyroid antibodies disappear after complete thyroid ablation in patients with thyroid cancer. Ann Intern Med 2003;139:346.

Mazzaferri EL et al: Using recombinant human TSH in the management of well-differentiated thyroid cancer: current strategies and future directions. Thyroid 2000;10:767.

Nikioforova MN et al: BRAF mutations in thyroid tumors are restricted to papillary carcinomas and anaplastic or poorly differentiated carcinomas arising from papillary carcinomas. J Clin Endocrinol Metab 2003;88:5399.

Perrier ND et al: Classification and treatment of follicular thyroid neoplasms and discordance between and within medical specialties. Surgery 1999;126:1063.

Pittas AG et al: Bone metastases from thyroid carcinoma: clinical characteristics and prognostic variables in one hundred forty-six patients. Thyroid 2000;10:261.

Yutan E, Clark OH: Hurthle cell carcinoma. Curr Treat Options Oncol 2001 2:337.

II. THE PARATHYROID GLANDS

EMBRYOLOGY & ANATOMY

Phylogenetically, the parathyroids appear rather late, being first seen in amphibia. They arise from pharyngeal pouches III and IV and may be arrested as high as the level of the hyoid bone during their descent to the posterior capsule of the thyroid gland. Four parathyroid glands are present in 85% of the population, and about 15% have more than four glands. Occasionally, one or more may be incorporated into the thyroid gland or thymus and hence are intrathyroidal or mediastinal in location. Parathyroid III, which normally assumes the inferior position, may be found in the anterior mediastinum, usually in the thymus. The upper parathyroids (parathyroid IV) usually remain in close association with the upper portion of the lateral thyroid lobes but may be loosely attached by a long vascular pedicle and migrate caudally along the esophagus into the posterior mediastinum. About 85% of parathyroid glands lie on the posterior capsule of the thyroid gland within 1 cm of where the inferior thyroid artery and recurrent laryngeal nerve cross.

The normal parathyroid gland has a distinct yellowish-brown color, is ovoid, tongue-shaped, polypoid, or spherical, and averages 2 × 3 × 7 mm. The total mean weight of four normal parathyroids is about 150 mg. These encapsulated glands are usually supplied by a branch of the inferior thyroid artery but may be supplied by the superior thyroid or, rarely, the thyroid ima arteries. The vessels can be seen entering a hilum-like structure, a feature that differentiates parathyroid glands from fat.

Mansberger AR Jr et al: Surgical embryology and anatomy of the thyroid and parathyroid glands. Surg Clin North Am 1993;73:727.

PHYSIOLOGY

Parathyroid hormone (PTH), vitamin D, and calcitonin play vital roles in calcium and phosphorus metabolism in bone, kidney, and gut. Specific radioimmunoassays are available to measure PTH, vitamin D, and calcitonin. Ionized calcium, the physiologically important fraction, can now be accurately measured. Total serum calcium concentration is composed of approximately 48% ionized calcium, 46% protein-bound calcium, and 6% calcium complexed to organic anions. Total serum calcium varies directly with plasma protein concentrations, but calcium ion concentrations are unaffected.

PTH and calcitonin work in concert to modulate fluctuations in plasma levels of ionized calcium. When the ionized calcium level falls, the parathyroids secrete more PTH and the parafollicular cells within the thyroid secrete less calcitonin. The rise in PTH and fall in calcitonin produce increased bone resorption and increased resorption of calcium in the renal tubules. More calcium enters the blood, and ionized calcium levels return to normal.

In the circulation, immunoreactive PTH is heterogeneous, consisting of the intact hormone and several hormonal fragments. The amino terminal (N-terminal) fragment is biologically active, whereas the carboxyl terminal (C-terminal) fragment is biologically inert. Measurement of intact PTH by immunoassay is best for screening for hyperparathyroidism and for selective venous catheterization to localize the source of PTH production. PTH-related peptide (PTHrP) that is secreted by nonparathyroid malignant tumors does not cross-react with intact PTH assays.

Because PTH levels rise in normal subjects if ionized calcium levels are low, calcium and PTH must be determined from samples drawn simultaneously to diagnose hyperparathyroidism. The combination of increased PTH levels and hypercalcemia without hypocalciuria is almost always pathognomonic of hyperparathyroidism.

Shattuck TM et al: Somatic and germ-line mutations of the HRPT2 gene in sporadic parathyroid carcinoma. N Engl J Med 2003;349:1722.

Watson PH et al: Parathyroid hormone regulation of syntheses and secretion. Clin Invest Med 1993;16:58.

DISEASES OF THE PARATHYROIDS

PRIMARY HYPERPARATHYROIDISM

ESSENTIALS OF DIAGNOSIS

- *Increased fatigue, weakness, arthralgias, nausea, vomiting, dyspepsia, constipation, polydipsia, polyuria, nocturia, psychiatric disturbances, renal colic, bone, and joint pain. ("Stones, bones, abdominal groans, psychic moans, and fatigue overtones.") Some patients are asymptomatic.*
- *Nephrolithiasis and nephrocalcinosis, osteopenia, osteoporosis, osteitis fibrosa cystica, peptic ulcer disease, renal dysfunction, gout, chondrocalcinosis, pancreatitis.*
- *Hypertension, band keratopathy, neck masses.*
- *Serum calcium, PTH, chloride, usually increased; serum phosphate low or normal; uric acid and alkaline phosphatase sometimes increased; urine calcium increased, normal, or, rarely, decreased; urine phosphate increased; tubular reabsorption of phosphate decreased, osteocalcin and deoxypyridinoline crosslinks increased.*

- *X-rays: subperiosteal resorption of phalanges, demineralization of the skeleton (osteopenia or osteoporosis), bone cysts, and nephrocalcinosis or nephrolithiasis.*

General Considerations

Primary hyperparathyroidism is due to excess PTH secretion from a single parathyroid adenoma (83%), multiple adenomas (6%), hyperplasia (10%), or carcinoma (1%). Fewer abnormal parathyroid glands are identified at focal exploration. Once thought to be rare, primary hyperparathyroidism is now found in 0.1–0.3% of the general population and is the most common cause of hypercalcemia in unselected patients. It is uncommon before puberty; its peak incidence is between the third and fifth decades, and it is two to three times more common in women than in men.

Overproduction of parathyroid hormone results in mobilization of calcium from bone and inhibition of the renal reabsorption of phosphate, thereby producing hypercalcemia and hypophosphatemia. This causes a wasting of calcium and phosphorus, with osseous mineral loss and **osteoporosis.** Other associated or related conditions that offer clues to the diagnosis of hyperparathyroidism are nephrolithiasis, nephrocalcinosis, osteitis fibrosa cystica, peptic ulcer, pancreatitis, hypertension, and gout or pseudogout. Hyperparathyroidism also occurs in both multiple endocrine neoplasia (MEN) type 1, known as **Werner's syndrome,** and MEN type 2, known as **Sipple's syndrome.** The former is characterized by tumors of the parathyroid, pituitary, and pancreas (hyperparathyroidism, pituitary tumors, and functioning or nonfunctioning islet cell pancreatic tumors) that may cause Zollinger-Ellison syndrome (gastrinoma), hypoglycemia (insulinoma), glucagonoma, somatostatinoma, and pancreatic polypeptide tumors (PPomas). Other tumors in MEN 1 syndrome include adrenocortical tumors, carcinoid tumors, multiple lipomas, and cutaneous angiomas. MEN 2a consists of hyperparathyroidism (20%) in association with medullary carcinoma of the thyroid and pheochromocytoma (50%). MEN 2b patients have a marfanoid habitus, multiple neuromas, and pheochromocytomas, but rarely have hyperparathyroidism.

Parathyroid adenomas range in weight from 65 mg to over 35 g, and the size usually parallels the degree of hypercalcemia. Microscopically, these tumors may be of chief cell, water cell, or, rarely, oxyphil cell type.

Primary parathyroid hyperplasia involves all of the parathyroid glands. Microscopically, there are two types: chief cell hyperplasia and water-clear cell (wasserhelle) hyperplasia. Hyperplastic glands vary considerably in size but are usually larger than normal (65 mg).

Parathyroid carcinoma is rare but is more common in patients with profound hypercalcemia and in patients with familial hyperparathyroidism and jaw tumor syndrome. Parathyroid cancers are palpable in half the patients and should be suspected in patients at operation when the parathyroid gland is hard, has a whitish or irregular capsule, or is invasive. Parathyromatosis is a rare condition causing hypercalcemia due to multiple embryologic rests or, more commonly, due to seeding when a parathyroid tumor has ruptured or a tumor capsule has been breached.

Clinical Findings

A. Symptoms and Signs

Historically, the clinical manifestations of hyperparathyroidism have changed. Forty years ago, the diagnosis was based on bone pain and deformity (osteitis fibrosa cystica), and in later years on the renal complications (nephrolithiasis and nephrocalcinosis). At present, over two-thirds of patients are detected by routine screening, and some are asymptomatic. After successful surgical treatment, many patients thought to be asymptomatic become aware of improvement in unrecognized preoperative symptoms such as fatigue, mild depression, weakness, constipation, polydipsia and polyuria, and bone and joint pain. Hyperparathyroidism should be suspected in all patients with hypercalcemia and the above symptoms, especially if associated with nephrolithiasis, nephrocalcinosis, hypertension, peptic ulcer, pancreatitis, or gout. Patients with primary hyperparathyroidism appear to have a shortened life expectancy that improves after successful parathyroidectomy. Younger patients and those with less severe hypercalcemia after parathyroidectomy have the best prognosis.

B. Laboratory Findings, Imaging Studies, and Differential Diagnosis (Approach to the Hypercalcemic Patient)

1. Laboratory findings—See Table 16–2. Hyperparathyroidism and cancer are responsible for about 90% of all cases of hypercalcemia. Hyperparathyroidism is the most common cause of hypercalcemia detected by undirected methods such as routine screening, whereas cancer is the most common cause of hypercalcemia in hospitalized patients. Other causes of hypercalcemia are listed in Table 16–3. In many patients the diagnosis is obvious, while in others it may be difficult. At times, more than one reason for hypercalcemia may exist in the same patient, such as cancer or sarcoidosis plus hyperparathyroidism. A careful history must be obtained documenting (1) the duration of any symptoms possibly related to hypercalcemia; (2) symptoms related to malignant disease; (3) conditions associated with hyperparathyroidism, such as renal colic, peptic ulcer disease, pan-

Table 16–2. Laboratory evaluation of hypercalcemia.

Essential	Selective
Blood Tests	
Calcium Phosphate PTH (intact or two-site assay) Alkaline phosphatase	Creatine and BUN Chloride Uric acid pH Protein electrophoresis or albumin: globulin ratio 25-Dihydroxyvitamin D and 1,25-dihydroxyvitamin D
Radiographic or Nuclear Medicine Procedures	
Chest x-ray Abdominal plain films Ultrasound of kidneys Bone density (hip, lumbar spine, wrist)	Sestamibi scan of neck and ultrasound of neck
Urine tests	
24-hour urinary calcium[1]	Urinalysis Deoxypyridinoline cross-links Osteocalcin

[1]When urine calcium is < 100 mg/24 h, a diagnosis of benign familial hypocalciuric hypercalcemia must be considered.

creatitis, hypertension, or gout; or (4) possible excess use of milk products, antacids, baking soda, or vitamins. In patients with a recent cough, wheeze, or hemoptysis, epidermoid carcinoma of the lung should be considered. Hematuria might suggest hypernephroma, bladder tumor, or renal lithiasis. Chest roentgenograms and intravenous urograms should be performed as appropriate. A long history of renal stones or peptic ulcer disease suggests that hyperparathyroidism is likely.

The most important tests for the evaluation of hypercalcemia are, in order of importance, serum calcium, parathyroid hormone, phosphate, chloride, alkaline phosphatase, creatinine; uric acid, and urea nitrogen; urinary calcium; blood hematocrit and pH; serum magnesium; and erythrocyte sedimentation rate. Measurement of 25-hydroxy and 1,25-hydroxy vitamin D levels, and serum protein electrophoresis are helpful in selected patients when other tests are equivocal.

A high serum calcium and a low serum phosphate suggest hyperparathyroidism, but about half of patients with hyperparathyroidism have normal serum phosphate concentrations. Patients with vitamin D intoxication, sarcoidosis, malignant disease without metastasis, and hyperthyroidism may also be hypophosphatemic, but patients with breast cancer and hypercalcemia are only rarely so. In fact, if hypophosphatemia and hypercalcemia are present in association with breast cancer, concomitant hyperparathyroidism is probable. Measurement of **serum parathyroid hormone** has its greatest value in this situation, since the PTH level is low or nil in patients with hypercalcemia due to *all* causes other than primary or ectopic hyperparathyroidism, or familial hypocalciuric hypercalcemia. In general, serum PTH levels should be measured in all patients with persistent hypercalcemia without an obvious cause and in normocalcemic patients who are suspected of having hyperparathyroidism. Determination of intact serum PTH levels is best since it is sensitive and is not influenced by tumors that secrete parathyroid-related peptide. Nonparathyroid tumors that secrete pure PTH are extremely rare.

An elevated serum chloride concentration is a useful diagnostic clue found in about 40% of hyperparathyroid patients. PTH acts directly on the proximal renal tubule to decrease the resorption of bicarbonate, which leads to increased resorption of chloride and a mild hyperchlo-

Table 16–3. Causes of hypercalcemia

	Approximate Frequency (%)
Cancer Breast cancer Metastatic PTH-related peptide secreting (lung, kidney) Multiple myeloma Leukemias Others	45
Endocrine disorders Hyperparathyroidism Hyperthyroidism Addison's disease, pheochromocytoma Hypothyroidism, VIPoma	46
Increased intake Milk-alkali syndrome Vitamin D and A overdosage Thiazides, lithium, aluminum	4
Granulomatous diseases Sarcoidosis, tuberculosis, etc	3
Benign familial hypocalciuric hypercalcemia and other disorders Paget's disease Immobilization Idiopathic hypercalcemia of infancy Aluminum intoxication Dysproteinemias Rhabdomyolysis	2

remic renal tubular acidosis. Other causes of hypercalcemia do not give increased serum chloride concentrations. Calculation of the **serum chloride to phosphate ratio** takes advantage of slight increases in serum chloride and slight decreases in serum phosphate concentrations. A ratio above 33 suggests hyperparathyroidism.

Serum protein electrophoretic patterns are helpful for excluding multiple myeloma and sarcoidosis. Hypergammaglobulinemia is rare in hyperparathyroidism but is not uncommon in patients with multiple myeloma and sarcoidosis. Roentgenograms of the skull or site of bone pain in patients with elevated alkaline phosphatase levels will often reveal typical "punched-out" bony lesions, and the diagnosis of myeloma can be firmly established by bone marrow examination. Sarcoidosis can be difficult to diagnose, because it may exist for several years with few clinical findings. A chest x-ray revealing a diffuse fibronodular infiltrate and prominent hilar adenopathy is suggestive, and the demonstration of noncaseating granuloma in lymph nodes is diagnostic. The **hydrocortisone suppression test** (150 mg of hydrocortisone per day for 10 days) reduces the serum calcium concentration in most cases of sarcoidosis and vitamin D intoxication and in many patients with carcinoma and multiple myeloma but only rarely in patients with hyperparathyroidism. It is therefore a useful diagnostic maneuver if these conditions are considered. Hydrocortisone suppression is used to treat the hypercalcemic crises that may occur with these disorders.

Serum alkaline phosphate levels are elevated in about 10% of patients with primary hyperparathyroidism and may also be increased in patients with Paget's disease and cancer. When the serum alkaline phosphatase level is elevated, serum 5'-nucleotidase, which parallels liver alkaline phosphatase, should be measured to determine if the increase is from bone, which suggests parathyroid disease, or liver. A 24-hour urine calcium level is helpful for diagnosing hypercalcemic patients who have low urinary calcium levels resulting from benign familial hypocalciuric hypercalcemia and for patients with marked hypercalciuria (> 400 mg/24 h). These patients do not benefit from parathyroidectomy.

2. Bone studies—Bone densitometry and radiographic examination of bone frequently reveals osteopenia (1 standard deviation) or osteoporosis (2 standard deviations from normal), but overt skeletal changes such as subperiosteal resorption or brown tumor are found in only 10% of patients with hyperparathyroidism. Dual photon bone density studies of the femur, lumbar spine, and radius help document osteopenia that occurs in about 70% of female patients with hyperparathyroidism. Bone changes of osteitis fibrosa cystica are rare on x-ray unless the serum alkaline phosphatase concentration is increased. Primary and secondary hyperparathyroidism produce subperiosteal resorption of the phalanges and bone cysts (Figure 16–4). A ground-glass appearance of the skull with loss of definition of the tables and demineralization of the outer aspects of the clavicles are less frequently seen. In patients with markedly elevated serum alkaline phosphatase levels without subperiosteal resorption on x-ray, Paget's disease or cancer must be suspected. A 24-hour urine test for deoxypyridinoline cross-link assay or osteocalcin detects increased bone loss.

3. Differential diagnosis—The differentiation between hyperparathyroidism due to primary parathyroid disease and that due to ectopic hyperparathyroidism or nonparathyroid cancer can now almost always be determined by measuring intact PTH (increase in primary hyperparathyroidism) and PTHrP (increased in nonparathyroid malignant tumors). The most common tumors causing ectopic hyperparathyroidism are squamous cell carcinoma of the lung, renal cell carcinoma, and bladder cancer. Less commonly it is due to hepatoma or to cancer of the ovary, stomach, pancreas, parotid gland, or colon. Recent onset of symptoms, increased sedimentation rate, anemia, serum calcium greater than 14 mg/dL, and increased alkaline phosphatase activity without osteitis fibrosa cystica suggest **malignancy-associated hypercalcemia;** mild hypercalcemia with a long history of nephrolithiasis or peptic ulcer suggests primary hyperthyroidism. Documented hypercalcemia of 6 months or longer essentially rules out malignancy-associated hypercalcemia.

In **milk-alkali syndrome,** a history of excessive ingestion of milk products, calcium-containing antacids, and baking soda is often obtained. These patients become normocalcemic after discontinuing these habits. Patients with milk-alkali syndrome usually have renal insufficiency and low urinary calcium concentrations and are usually alka-

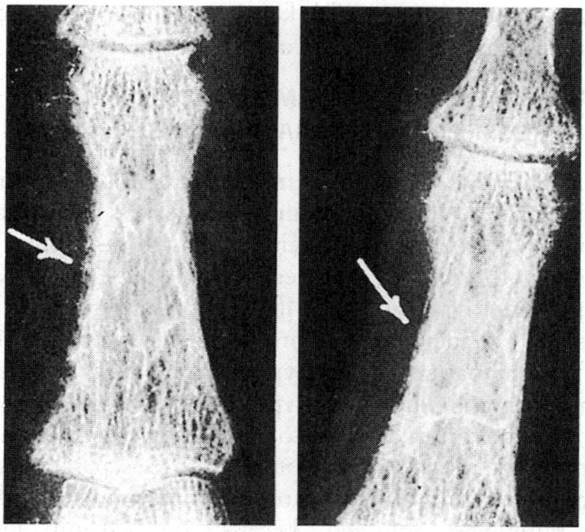

Figure 16–4. Subperiosteal resorption of radial side of second phalanges.

lotic rather than acidotic. Because of the high incidence of ulcer disease in hyperparathyroidism, milk-alkali syndrome may occasionally coexist with that disorder.

Hyperthyroidism, another cause of hypercalcemia and hypercalciuria, can usually be differentiated because manifestations of thyrotoxicosis rather than hypercalcemia bring the patient to the physician. Occasionally, an elderly patient with apathetic hyperthyroidism may be hypercalcemic. A sensitive TSH test should be evaluated in hypercalcemic patients whose PTH levels are not increased. Treatment of hyperthyroidism with antithyroid medications causes serum calcium to return to normal levels within 8 weeks.

Normal subjects taking **thiazide diuretics** may develop a transient increase in serum calcium levels, usually less than 1 mg/dL. Larger rises in serum calcium induced by thiazides have been reported in patients with primary hyperparathyroidism and idiopathic juvenile osteoporosis. Most patients who have hypercalcemia while taking thiazides have another reason for the increase. The best way to evaluate these patients is to switch them to a nonthiazide antihypertensive agent or diuretic and to measure the PTH level. Thiazide-induced hypercalcemia is not associated with increased serum PTH in patients without hyperparathyroidism.

Benign familial hypocalciuric hypercalcemia is one of the few conditions that causes chronic hypercalcemia and mildly elevated PTH levels. It can be difficult to distinguish from primary hyperparathyroidism. The best way to diagnose this disorder is to document a low urinary calcium and a family history of hypercalcemia, especially in children.

Other miscellaneous causes of hypercalcemia are Paget's disease, immobilization (especially in Paget's disease or in young patients), dysproteinemias, idiopathic hypercalcemia of infancy, aluminum intoxication, and rhabdomyolysis (Table 16–3).

C. Approach to the Normocalcemic Patient With Possible Hyperparathyroidism

Renal failure, hypoalbuminemia, pancreatitis, deficiency of vitamin D or magnesium, and excess phosphate intake may cause serum calcium levels to be normal in hyperparathyroidism. Correction of these disorders results in hypercalcemia if hyperparathyroidism is present. The incidence of normocalcemic hyperparathyroidism in patients with hypercalciuria and recurrent nephrolithiasis (idiopathic hypercalciuria) is not known. Because the serum calcium concentration may fluctuate, it should be measured on more than three separate occasions. The serum calcium should be determined the day the sample is obtained, because the calcium level decreases with refrigeration or freezing. Determination of serum ionized calcium is also useful, since it may be increased in patients with normal total serum calcium levels.

If a patient has elevated serum levels of ionized calcium and PTH, the diagnosis of normocalcemic hyperparathyroidism has been confirmed. There are three major causes of hypercalciuria and nephrolithiasis: (1) increased absorption of calcium from the gastrointestinal tract (absorptive hypercalciuria), (2) increased renal leakage of calcium (renal hypercalciuria), and (3) primary hyperparathyroidism. Patients with absorptive hypercalcemia absorb too much calcium from the gastrointestinal tract and therefore have low serum PTH levels. Patients with renal hypercalciuria lose calcium from leaky renal tubules and have increased PTH levels. They can be distinguished from patients with normocalcemic hyperparathyroidism by their response to treatment with thiazides. In renal leak hypercalcemia, serum PTH levels become normal because thiazides correct the excessive loss of calcium, whereas in primary hyperparathyroidism increased serum PTH levels persist and the patient often becomes hypercalcemic.

Natural History of Untreated & Treated Hyperparathyroidism

Patients with untreated hyperparathyroidism have an increased risk of dying prematurely, mainly from cardiovascular and malignant disease. There is decreased respiratory muscular capacity and increased frequency of hypertrophic cardiomyopathy with left ventricular hypertrophy and decreased vascular compliance even in hyperparathyroid patients without hypertension. Hyperparathyroid patients have more hypertension, nephrolithiasis, osteopenia, peptic ulcer disease, gout, renal dysfunction, and pancreatitis. After successful parathyroidectomy, previously hyperparathyroid patients still have an increased risk of premature death. Younger patients and those with less severe disease, however, return to a normal survival curve sooner than do older patients or those with more severe hyperparathyroidism. Most patients with hyperparathyroidism—even those with normocalcemic hyperparathyroidism—have symptoms and associated conditions. In 80% of patients, these clinical manifestations improve or disappear after parathyroidectomy.

Treatment

The only successful treatment of primary hyperparathyroidism is parathyroidectomy. The author feels that virtually all patients with either asymptomatic or symptomatic hyperparathyroidism benefit from the operation both symptomatically and metabolically as well as with improved survival. There are no convincing data to support a plan of medical observation, and considerable data support a surgical approach. Once associated conditions such as hypertension and renal dysfunction become well-established, they seem to progress despite correction of the primary hyperparathyroidism. Thus, it is better to intervene early while it is still possible to correct these problems. In all patients, however, the diagnosis should be established, and short delays to clarify the diagnosis are justified.

A. Marked Hypercalcemia (Hypercalcemic Crisis)

The initial treatment in patients with marked hypercalcemia and acute symptoms is hydration and correction of hypokalemia and hyponatremia. While the patient is being hydrated, assessment of the underlying problem is essential so that more specific therapy may be started. Milk and alkaline products, estrogens, thiazides, and vitamins A and D should be immediately discontinued. Furosemide is useful to increase calcium excretion in the rehydrated patient. Etidronate, plicamycin, and calcitonin are usually effective for short periods in treating hypercalcemia regardless of cause. Glucocorticoids are very effective in vitamin D intoxication and sarcoidosis and in many patients with cancer, including those with peptide-secreting tumors, but are less effective when there is extensive bone disease. As mentioned previously, hyperparathyroid patients only occasionally respond to glucocorticoid administration.

In patients with marked hypercalcemia, once the diagnosis of hyperparathyroidism is established, localization studies, cervical exploration, and parathyroidectomy should be performed in a vigorously hydrated patient, since this is the most rapid and effective method of reducing serum calcium.

B. Localization

Preoperative localization of parathyroid tumors can now be accomplished in about 75% of patients with ultrasonography and 85% with sestamibi scans. These studies, however, are helpful in only about 35% of patients with parathyroid hyperplasia (Figure 16–5). Localization studies are essential in patients with persistent or recurrent hyperparathyroidism and can direct a focused exploration in patients with sporadic primary hyperparathyroidism. An experienced surgeon can find the tumors in about 95% of patients who have not had previous parathyroid or thyroid surgery without preoperative tests. Selective venous catheterization with parathyroid hormone immunoassay is also recommended for patients who have had an unsuccessful previous operation when the noninvasive localization tests are negative or equivocal. This study helps localize the tumor in about 80% of patients. Digital subtraction angiography is useful, while arteriography is now rarely used.

C. Operation

Three approaches are now acceptable for patients with sporadic primary hyperparathyroidism. The bilateral approach is safe and does not require preoperative tests or intraoperative PTH testing. A unilateral approach can be elected when one or more localization tests identify a solitary parathyroid tumor. At operation, a normal and abnormal parathyroid should be identified on the side of the localized tumor. A focal operation can be done in similar patients and the operation completed when the intraoperative PTH level decreases by more than 50% from the highest pre-removed value 10 minutes after the parathyroid tumor is removed. Endoscopic parathyroidectomy is recommended by a minority of surgeons.

In over 80% of cases, the parathyroid tumor is found attached to the posterior capsule of the thyroid gland. The parathyroid glands are usually symmetrically placed, and lower parathyroid glands are situated anterior to the recurrent laryngeal nerve, whereas the upper parathyroid glands lie posterior to the recurrent laryngeal nerve, where it enters the cricothyroid muscle. Parathyroid tumors may also lie cephalad to the superior pole of the thyroid gland, along the great vessels of the neck in the tracheoesophageal area, in thymic tissue, in the substance of the thyroid gland itself, or in the mediastinum. Care must be taken to avoid bleeding and not to traumatize the parathyroid gland or tumors, since color is useful in distinguishing them from surrounding thyroid, thymus, lymph node, and fat. Furthermore, rupture of the parathyroid gland may result in parathyromatosis (seeding of parathyroid tissue) and possible recurrent hyperparathyroidism. Two helpful maneuvers for localizing parathyroid tumors at operation are following the course of a branch of the inferior thyroid artery and gently palpating for the parathyroid tumor. One should attempt to identify four parathyroid glands when a bilateral approach is elected, though there may be more than four or fewer than four.

If a probable parathyroid adenoma is found, it is removed and the diagnosis confirmed by frozen section or by a greater than 50% decrease in PTH. It seems unwise to remove a grossly normal parathyroid gland intentionally, both because this has no beneficial effect and because the gland may be needed to maintain normal function after all the hyperfunctioning tissue is removed. If two adenomas are found, both are removed, and both normal glands are marked and biopsied but not removed.

The presence of a normal parathyroid gland at operation indicates that the tumor removed is an adenoma rather than parathyroid hyperplasia, since in hyperplasia all the parathyroid glands are involved. A compressed rim of normal parathyroid tissue is also suggestive of an adenoma. When all parathyroid glands are hyperplastic, the most normal gland should be subtotally resected, leaving a 50 mg remnant, and confirmed histologically before removal of the remaining glands.

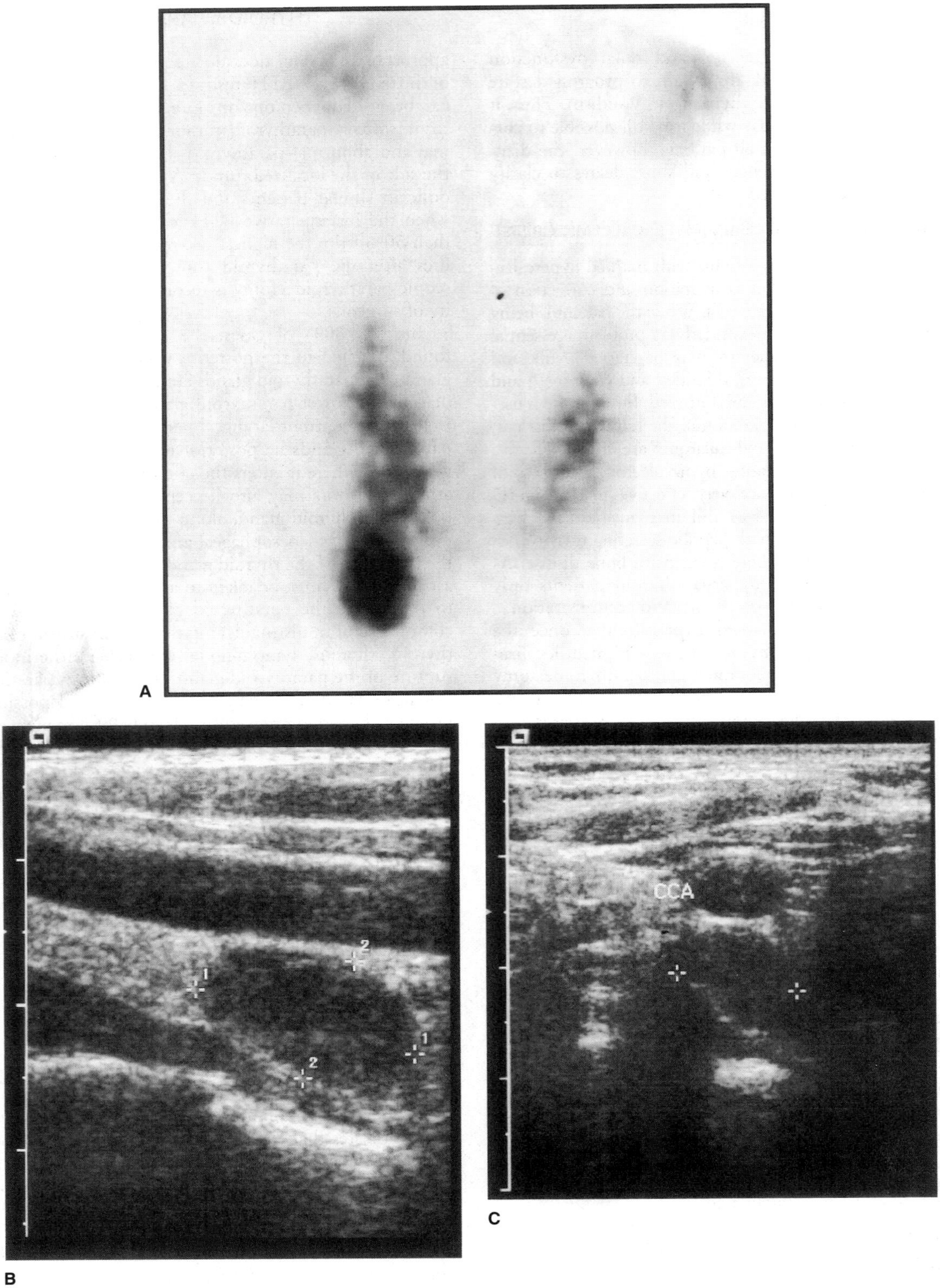

Figure 16–5. Parathyroid adenomas. **A:** Sestamibi scan of right lower parathyroid adenoma. **B:** Longitudinal ultrasound scan of left lower parathyroid adenoma. **C:** Transverse ultrasound scan of left lower parathyroid adenoma.

The upper thymus and perithymic tract should be removed in patients with hyperplasia, because a fifth parathyroid gland is present in 15% of cases.

If exploration fails to reveal a parathyroid tumor, a missing lower gland is often in the thymus (anterior mediastinum), whereas a missing upper gland is usually paraesophageal (or in the posterior mediastinum). One should therefore perform a thymectomy, thyroid lobectomy, or partial thyroidectomy on the side that has only one parathyroid gland, since tumors may be found within the thymus or intrathyroidally. If thyroid nodules are present and clinically a problem, they should be treated as nodular goiter and possible thyroid cancer. Differentiated thyroid carcinoma occurs in 3% of patients with hyperparathyroidism and more frequently in patients with a history of radiation exposure.

The recurrence rate of hyperparathyroidism after the removal of a single adenoma in patients with sporadic hyperparathyroidism is 2% or less. In patients with multiple endocrine neoplasia and familial hyperparathyroidism, recurrent hyperparathyroidism is more common (approximately 33%); therefore, extra care should be taken to remove all abnormal parathyroid tissue and to carefully mark the remaining parathyroid tissue. These hyperparathyroid patients are candidates for possible prophylactic subtotal parathyroidectomy. Total parathyroidectomy with autotransplantation to the forearm is recommended by some surgeons for patients with multiple endocrine neoplasia or familial hyperparathyroidism. The author prefers subtotal parathyroidectomy leaving a well-marked parathyroid remnant because not all parathyroid autografts function effectively.

Exploration of the mediastinum via a sternal split at the initial operation is necessary in only 1–2% of cases and is only recommended in patients with a serum calcium level above 13.5 mg/dL. If cervical exploration was nonproductive or if localization studies suggest a mediastinal tumor, the patient should be allowed to recover from the initial operation and return in 6–8 weeks for mediastinal exploration. Preoperative localization tests are essential before reoperation. Angiographic ablation is possible for poor-risk patients with mediastinal parathyroid adenomas not easily removed via a cervical incision.

D. Postoperative Care

Following removal of a parathyroid adenoma or hyperplastic glands, the serum calcium concentration falls to normal or below normal in 24–48 hours. Patients with severe skeletal depletion ("hungry bones"), long-standing hyperparathyroidism, or high calcium levels may develop profound hypocalcemia with paresthesias, carpopedal spasm, or even seizures. If the symptoms are mild and serum calcium falls slowly, oral supplementation with calcium is all that is required. When marked symptoms develop, it is necessary to give calcium gluconate intravenously. If the response is not rapid, the serum magnesium concentration should be determined and magnesium given if low. Treatment with calcitriol, 1 μg daily, is sometimes required. (See section on Hypoparathyroidism, below.)

E. Reoperation

Reexploration for persistent or recurrent hyperparathyroidism or after a previous thyroidectomy presents formidable problems and an increased risk of complications. First ascertain that the diagnosis is correct and that the patient does not have benign familial hypocalciuric hypercalcemia or hypercalcemia due to another cause such as a malignant tumor. Ultrasound, CT or MRI, and sestamibi scanning should be done first. If these studies are unsuccessful or equivocal, digital subtraction angiography and highly selective venous catheterization with parathyroid hormone immunoassay are recommended. Most such patients have a parathyroid tumor that can be removed through a cervical incision, making mediastinal exploration unnecessary. The success rate of parathyroidectomy performed by experienced surgeons is 95% or better at an initial operation versus a success rate of about 75% with surgeons less experienced at this procedure. The success rate for patients requiring reoperation is about 90%. This success rate is lower in patients with negative or equivocal localization tests and in patients with parathyromatosis and parathyroid cancer.

Al-Fehaily M, Clark OH: Persistent or recurrent hyperparathyroidism. Ann Ital Chir 2003;LXXIV:4:423.

Barney RE et al: Health status improvement after surgical correction of primary hyperparathyroidism in patients with high and low preoperative calcium levels. Surgery 1999;125:608.

Bilezikian J et al: Clinical utility of an immunoradiometric assay for parathyroid hormone (1-84) in primary hyperparathyroidism. JCEM 2003;88:4725.

Brunaud L et al: Incision length for standard thyroidectomy and parathyroidectomy: When is it minimally invasive? Arch Surg 2003;138:1140.

Clark OH: Editorial. How should patients with primary hyperparathyroidism be treated? J Clin Endocrinol Metab 2003;88:3011.

Clark OH: Changing surgical approaches to patients with primary hyperparathyroidism. Curr Surg 2000;57:546.

Clark OH: "Asymptomatic" primary hyperparathyroidism: is parathyroidectomy indicated? Surgery 1994;116:947.

Eng C: Editorial: dissecting the genetics of hyperparathyroidism—new clues from an old friend. J Clin Endocrinol Metab 2000; 85:1752.

Genc H et al: Differing histologic findings after bilateral and focused parathyroidectomy. J Am Coll Surg 2003;196:535.

Haciyanli M et al: Accuracy of preoperative localization studies and intraoperative parathyroid hormone assay in patients with primary hyperparathyroidism and double adenoma. J Am Col Surg 2003;197:739.

Kebebew E et al: Parathyroidectomy for primary hyperparathyroidism in octogenarians and nonagenarians. Arch Surg 2003; 138:867.

Lal G, Clark OH: Primary hyperparathyroidism: controversies in surgical management. Trends Endocrinol Metab 2003;14:417.

Miccoli P et al: Minimally invasive video assisted parathyroidectomy (MIVAP). Eur J Surg Oncol 2003;29:188.

Perrier ND et al: Parathyroid surgery—separating promise from reality. J Clin Endocrinol Metab 2002;87:1024.

Sebag F et al: Reoperative parathyroid operations and intraoperative parathyroid hormone assay. Surgery 2003;134:1049.

Silverberg SJ et al: A 10-year prospective study of primary hyperparathyroidism with or without parathyroid surgery. N Engl J Med 1999;341:1249.

Sokol LJ et al: Intraoperative parathyroid hormone analysis: a study of 200 consecutive cases. Clin Chem 2000;46:1662.

Utiger RD: Treatment of primary hyperparathyroidism (editorial). N Engl J Med 1999;341:1301.

SECONDARY & TERTIARY HYPERPARATHYROIDISM

In secondary hyperparathyroidism, there is an increase in parathyroid hormone secretion in response to low plasma concentrations of ionized calcium, usually owing to renal disease and malabsorption. This results in chief cell hyperplasia. When secondary hyperparathyroidism occurs as a complication of renal disease, the serum phosphorus level is usually high, whereas in malabsorption, osteomalacia, or rickets it is frequently low or normal. Secondary hyperparathyroidism with renal osteodystrophy is a frequent if not universal complication of hemodialysis and peritoneal dialysis. Factors that play a role in renal osteodystrophy are (1) phosphate retention secondary to a decrease in the number of nephrons; (2) failure of the diseased or absent kidneys to hydroxylate 25-dihydroxyvitamin D to the biologically active metabolite 1,25-dihydroxyvitamin D, with decreased intestinal absorption of calcium; (3) resistance of the bone to the action of parathyroid hormone; and (4) increased serum calcitonin concentrations. The resulting skeletal changes are identical with those of primary hyperparathyroidism but are often more severe.

Most patients with secondary hyperparathyroidism may be treated medically. Maintaining relatively normal serum concentrations of calcium and phosphorus during hemodialysis and treatment with calcitriol (orally or intravenously) have decreased the incidence of bone disease.

Occasionally, a patient with secondary hyperparathyroidism develops relatively autonomous hyperplastic parathyroid glands. In most patients after successful renal transplantation, the serum calcium concentration returns to normal, and the hyperplastic parathyroid glands regress. One should, therefore, wait at least 6 months after surgery before considering parathyroidectomy for persistent mild hypercalcemia. In some patients, however, profound hypercalcemia develops (**tertiary hyperparathyroidism**). In general, surgical therapy for so-called tertiary hyperparathyroidism should be delayed until all medical approaches, including treatment with vitamin D, calcium supplementation, and phosphate binders, have been exhausted. Indications for operation in patients with secondary hyperparathyroidism include (1) a calcium × phosphate product > 70, (2) severe bone disease and pain, (3) pruritus, and (4) extensive soft tissue calcification with tumoral calcinosis, and (5) calciphylaxis. Most patients with secondary hyperparathyroidism requiring parathyroidectomy have very high serum PTH levels, whereas patients with aluminum bone disease who do not warrant parathyroidectomy may be hypercalcemic with bone pain, but PTH levels are normal or only slightly increased. In the patient with secondary hyperparathyroidism in whom subtotal parathyroidectomy or total parathyroidectomy with autotransplantation is indicated, all but about 50 mg of the most normal parathyroid gland should be removed, or fifteen 1-mm slices of parathyroid tissue should be transplanted into individual muscle pockets in the forearm. Some parathyroid tissue should also be cryopreserved in case the autotransplanted tissue does not function. These patients usually respond with dramatic relief of bone and joint pain and pruritus. Profound hypocalcemia frequently results following subtotal parathyroidectomy for renal osteodystrophy, both because of "hungry bones" and because of decreased parathyroid hormone secretion. Hypocalcemia due to "hungry bones" can be anticipated in patients with markedly elevated alkaline phosphatase levels.

Clark OH: Secondary hyperparathyroidism. In: *Endocrine Surgery of the Thyroid and Parathyroid Glands.* Clark OH (editor). Mosby, 1985.

Pasieka JL et al: A prospective surgical outcome study assessing the impact of parathyroidectomy on symptoms in patients with secondary and tertiary hyperparathyroidism. Surgery 2000;128: 531.

Sancho JJ, Sitges-Serra A: Surgical approach to secondary hyperparathyroidism. In: *Textbook of Endocrine Surgery,* p. 403. Clark OH, Duh QY (editors). Saunders, 1997.

Savio RM et al: Parathyroidectomy for tertiary hyperparathyroidism associated with X-linked dominant hypophosphatemic rickets. Arch Surg 2004;139:218.

HYPOPARATHYROIDISM

ESSENTIALS OF DIAGNOSIS

- *Paresthesias, muscle cramps, carpopedal spasm, laryngeal stridor, convulsions, malaise, muscle and abdominal cramps, tetany, urinary frequency, lethargy, anxiety, psychoneurosis, depression, and psychosis.*

- *Surgical neck scar. Positive Chvostek and Trousseau signs.*
- *Brittle and atrophied nails, defective teeth, cataracts.*
- *Hypocalcemia and hyperphosphatemia, low or absent urinary calcium, low or absent circulating parathyroid hormone.*
- *Calcification of basal ganglia, cartilage, and arteries as seen on x-ray.*

General Considerations

Hypoparathyroidism, although uncommon, occurs most often as a complication of thyroidectomy, especially when performed for carcinoma or recurrent goiter. Idiopathic hypoparathyroidism, an autoimmune process associated with autoimmune adrenocortical insufficiency, is also unusual, and hypoparathyroidism after ^{131}I therapy for Graves' disease is rare. Neonatal tetany may be associated with maternal hyperparathyroidism. Hypothyroidism as well as hypoparathyroidism may occur in patients with Riedel's struma.

Clinical Findings

A. Symptoms and Signs

The manifestations of acute hypoparathyroidism are due to hypocalcemia. Low serum calcium levels precipitate tetany. Latent tetany may be indicated by mild or moderate paresthesias with a positive Chvostek or Trousseau sign. The initial manifestations are paresthesias, circumoral numbness, muscle cramps, irritability, carpopedal spasm, convulsions, opisthotonos, and marked anxiety. Dry skin, brittleness of the nails, and spotty alopecia including loss of the eyebrows are common. Since primary hypoparathyroidism is rare, a history of thyroidectomy is almost always present. Generally speaking, the sooner the clinical manifestations appear postoperatively, the more serious the prognosis. After many years, some patients become adapted to a low serum calcium concentration, so that tetany is no longer evident.

B. Laboratory Findings

Hypocalcemia and hyperphosphatemia are demonstrable. The urine phosphate is low or absent, tubular resorption of phosphate is high, and the urine calcium is low.

C. Imaging Studies

In chronic hypoparathyroidism, x-rays may show calcification of the basal ganglia, arteries, and external ear.

Differential Diagnosis

A good history is most important in the differential diagnosis of hypocalcemic tetany. Occasionally, tetany occurs with alkalosis and hyperventilation. Symptomatic hypocalcemia occurring after thyroid or parathyroid surgery is due to parathyroid removal or injury by trauma or devascularization or is secondary to "hungry bones." Other major causes of hypocalcemic tetany are intestinal malabsorption and renal insufficiency. These conditions may also be suggested by a history of diarrhea, pancreatitis, steatorrhea, or renal disease. Laboratory abnormalities include decreased concentrations of serum proteins, cholesterol, and carotene and increased concentrations of stool fat in malabsorption and an increased blood urea nitrogen and creatinine in renal failure. Serum parathyroid hormone concentrations are low in hypocalcemia secondary to idiopathic or iatrogenic hypoparathyroidism. Consequently, serum calcium concentrations and urinary calcium, phosphorus, and hydroxyproline levels are decreased, whereas serum phosphate concentrations are increased. In hypocalcemia secondary to malabsorption and renal failure, serum PTH concentrations are elevated and the serum alkaline phosphatase concentration is normal or increased.

Treatment

The aim of treatment is to raise the serum calcium concentration, to bring the patient out of tetany, and to lower the serum phosphate level so as to prevent metastatic calcification. Most postoperative hypocalcemia is transient; if it persists longer than 2–3 weeks or if treatment with calcitriol (1,25-dihydroxyvitamin D) is required, the hypoparathyroidism may be permanent.

A. Acute Hypoparathyroid Tetany

Acute hypoparathyroid tetany requires emergency treatment. Make certain an adequate airway exists. Reassure the anxious patient to avoid hyperventilation and resulting alkalosis. Give calcium gluconate, 10–20 mL of 10% solution slowly intravenously, until tetany disappears. Fifty milliliters of 10% calcium gluconate may then be added to 500 mL of 5% dextrose solution and administered by intravenous drip at a rate of 1 mL/kg/h. Adjust the rate of infusion so that hourly determinations of serum calcium are normal. Calcitriol (1,25-dihydroxyvitamin D)(0.25 to 0.5 μg twice daily) is very helpful for managing acute hypocalcemia because of its rapid onset of action (compared to other vitamin D preparations) and its short duration of action. Hypomagnesemia is present in some cases of tetany not responding to calcium treatment. In such cases, magnesium (as magnesium sulfate) should be given in a dosage of 4–8 g/d intramuscularly or 2–4 g/d intravenously.

B. Chronic Hypoparathyroidism

Once tetany has responded to intravenous calcium, change to oral calcium (gluconate, lactate, or carbonate) three times daily or as necessary. The management of the hypoparathyroid patient is difficult, because the difference between the controlling and intoxicating dose of vitamin D may be quite small. Episodes of hypercalcemia in treated patients are often unpredictable and may occur in the absence of symptoms. Vitamin D intoxication may develop after months or years of good control on a given therapeutic regimen. Dihydrotachysterol is useful in the exceptional case, to supplement treatment with calcium, 1,25-dihydroxyvitamin D, when the usual measures fail to control the hypocalcemia. Frequent serum calcium determinations are necessary to regulate the proper dosage of vitamin D and to avoid vitamin D intoxication. The dose of vitamin D required to correct hypocalcemia may vary from 25,000 to 200,000 IU/d. Phosphorus should also be limited in the diet; in most patients, simple elimination of dairy products is sufficient. In some patients, aluminum hydroxide gel may be necessary to bind phosphorus in the gut to increase fecal losses.

PSEUDOHYPOPARATHYROIDISM & PSEUDOPSEUDO-HYPOPARATHYROIDISM

Pseudohypoparathyroidism is an X-linked autosomal syndrome due to a defective renal adenylyl cyclase system. It is characterized by the clinical and chemical features of hypoparathyroidism associated with a round face; a short, thick body; stubby fingers with short metacarpal and metatarsal bones; mental deficiency; and x-ray evidence of calcification. It is also associated with thyroid and ovarian dysfunction. There is evidence of increased bone resorption and osteitis fibrosa cystica despite the hypocalcemia that accompanies the syndrome. Patients with pseudohypoparathyroidism do not respond to intravenous administration of 200 units of parathyroid hormone with phosphaturia (Ellsworth-Howard test) and have increased serum concentrations of PTH. This condition is usually controlled with smaller amounts of vitamin D than idiopathic hypoparathyroidism, and resistance to therapy is uncommon.

Pseudopseudohypoparathyroidism is also a genetically transmitted disease with the same physical findings of pseudohypoparathyroidism but with normal serum calcium and phosphorus concentrations. Patients with this condition may become hypocalcemic during periods of stress, such as pregnancy and rapid growth; this suggests that a genetic defect is common with pseudohypoparathyroidism.

Abugassa S et al: Bone mineral density in patients with chronic hypoparathyroidism. J Clin Endocrinol Metab 1993;76:1617.

Jan de Beur SM et al: Pseudohypoparathyroidism 1b: exclusion of parathyroid hormone and its receptors as candidate disease genes. J Clin Endocrinol Metab 2000;85:2239.

Juppner H et al: The gene responsible for pseudohypoparathyroidism type 1b is paternally imprinted and maps in four unrelated kindreds to chromosome 20q13.3. Proc Natl Acad Sci U S A 1998;95:1179.

Murray TM et al: Pseudohypoparathyroidism with osteitis fibrosa cystica: direct demonstration of skeletal responsiveness to parathyroid hormone in cells cultured from bone. J Bone Min Res 1993;8:83.

Breast

17

Armando E. Giuliano, MD

BENIGN BREAST DISORDERS

FIBROCYSTIC CONDITION

ESSENTIALS OF DIAGNOSIS

- *Painful, often multiple, usually bilateral masses in the breast.*
- *Rapid fluctuation in the size of the masses is common.*
- *Frequently, pain occurs or increases and size increases during premenstrual phase of cycle.*
- *Most common age is 30–50 years. Rare in postmenopausal women not receiving hormonal replacement.*

General Considerations

Fibrocystic condition is the most frequent lesion of the breast. Although commonly referred to as "fibrocystic disease," it does not, in fact, represent a pathologic or anatomic disorder. It is common in women 30–50 years of age but rare in postmenopausal women who are not taking hormonal replacement medications. Estrogen hormone is considered a causative factor. There may be an increased risk in women who drink alcohol, especially women between 18 and 22 years of age. Fibrocystic condition encompasses a wide variety of histologic changes. These lesions are always associated with benign changes in the breast epithelium, some of which are found so commonly in normal breasts that they are probably variants of normal breast histology but have nonetheless been termed a "condition."

The microscopic findings of fibrocystic condition include cysts (gross and microscopic), papillomatosis, adenosis, fibrosis, and ductal epithelial hyperplasia. Although fibrocystic condition has generally been considered to increase the risk of subsequent breast cancer, only the variants in which proliferation (especially with atypia) of epithelial components is demonstrated represent true risk factors.

Clinical Findings

A. Symptoms and Signs

Fibrocystic condition may produce an asymptomatic lump in the breast that is discovered by accident, but pain or tenderness often calls attention to the mass. There may be discharge from the nipple. In many cases, discomfort occurs or is increased during the premenstrual phase of the cycle, at which time the cysts tend to enlarge. Fluctuation in size and rapid appearance or disappearance of a breast mass are common with this condition. Multiple or bilateral masses are common, and many patients will give a history of a transient lump in the breast or cyclic breast pain.

B. Diagnostic Tests

Because a mass due to fibrocystic condition is frequently indistinguishable from carcinoma on the basis of clinical findings, suspicious lesions should be biopsied. Fine-needle aspiration cytology may be used, but if a suspicious mass that is nonmalignant on cytologic examination does not resolve over several months, it must be excised. Surgery should be conservative, since the primary objective is to exclude cancer. Occasionally, core needle biopsy will suffice. Simple mastectomy or extensive removal of breast tissue is rarely, if ever, indicated for fibrocystic condition.

Differential Diagnosis

Pain, fluctuation in size, and multiplicity of lesions are the features most helpful in differentiating fibrocystic condition from carcinoma. If a dominant mass is present, the diagnosis of cancer should be assumed until disproved by biopsy. Final diagnosis often depends on excisional biopsy. Mammography may be helpful, but the breast tissue in these young women is usually too radiodense to permit a worthwhile study. Sonography is useful in differentiating a cystic from a solid mass.

Treatment

When the diagnosis of fibrocystic condition has been established by previous biopsy or is likely because the history is classic, aspiration of a discrete mass suggestive of a cyst is indicated to alleviate pain and, more importantly, to confirm the cystic nature of the mass. The patient is reexamined at intervals thereafter. If no fluid is obtained or if fluid is bloody, if a mass persists after aspiration, or if at any time during follow-up a persistent lump is noted, biopsy is performed.

Breast pain associated with generalized fibrocystic condition is best treated by avoiding trauma and by wearing (night and day) a brassiere that gives good support and protection. A topical nonsteroidal anti-inflammatory gel may be of value. Hormone therapy is not advisable, because it does not cure the condition and has undesirable side effects. Danazol (100–200 mg twice daily orally), a synthetic androgen, has been used for patients with severe pain. This treatment suppresses pituitary gonadotropins, but androgenic effects (acne, edema, hirsutism) usually make this treatment intolerable; in practice, it is rarely used. Similarly, tamoxifen reduces some symptoms of fibrocystic condition, but because of its side effects it is not useful for young women unless it is given to reduce the risk of cancer. Postmenopausal women receiving hormone replacement therapy may stop hormones to reduce pain.

The role of caffeine consumption in the development and treatment of fibrocystic condition is controversial. Some studies suggest that eliminating caffeine from the diet is associated with improvement. Many patients are aware of these studies and report relief of symptoms after giving up coffee, tea, and chocolate. Similarly, many women find vitamin E (400 international units daily) helpful. However, these observations remain anecdotal.

Prognosis

Exacerbations of pain, tenderness, and cyst formation may occur at any time until the menopause, when symptoms usually subside, except in patients receiving hormonal replacement therapy. The patient should be advised to examine her own breasts each month just after menstruation and to inform her physician if a mass appears. The risk of breast cancer in women with fibrocystic condition showing proliferative or atypical changes in the epithelium is higher than that of women in general. These women should be followed up carefully with physical examinations and mammography.

Byrne C et al: Alcohol consumption and incidence of benign breast disease. Cancer Epidemiol Biomarkers Prev 2002;11:1369.

Lucas JH et al: Breast cyst aspiration. Am Fam Physician 2003; 68:1983.

Marchant DJ: Benign breast disease. Obstet Gynecol Clin North Am 2002;29:1.

Morrow M: The evaluation of common breast problems. Am Fam Physician 2000;61:2371.

Norlock FE: Benign breast pain in women: a practical approach to evaluation and treatment. J Am Med Womens Assoc 2002; 57:85.

FIBROADENOMA OF THE BREAST

This common benign neoplasm occurs most frequently in young women, usually within 20 years after puberty. It is somewhat more frequent and tends to occur at an earlier age in black women. Multiple tumors are found in 10–15% of patients.

The typical fibroadenoma is a round or ovoid, rubbery, discrete, relatively movable, nontender mass 1–5 cm in diameter. It is usually discovered accidentally. Clinical diagnosis in young patients is generally not difficult. In women over 30 years, fibrocystic condition of the breast and carcinoma of the breast must be considered. Cysts can be identified by aspiration or ultrasonography. Fibroadenoma does not normally occur after the menopause, but may occasionally develop after administration of hormones.

No treatment is usually necessary if the diagnosis can be made by needle biopsy or cytologic examination. Excision or vacuum-assisted core needle removal with pathologic examination of the specimen is performed if the diagnosis is uncertain. Cryoablation is being attempted as an alternative to excision. It is usually not possible to distinguish a large fibroadenoma from a phyllodes tumor on the basis of needle biopsy results.

Phyllodes tumor is a fibroadenoma-like tumor with cellular stroma that grows rapidly. It may reach a large size and if inadequately excised will recur locally. The lesion can be benign or malignant. If benign, phyllodes tumor is treated by local excision with a margin of surrounding breast tissue. The treatment of malignant phyllodes tumor is more controversial, but complete removal of the tumor with a rim of normal tissue avoids recurrence. Because these tumors may be large, simple mastectomy is sometimes necessary. Lymph node dissection is not performed, since the sarcomatous portion of the tumor metastasizes to the lungs and not the lymph nodes.

Barbosa ML et al: Cytogenetic findings in phyllodes tumor and fibroadenomas of the breast. Cancer Genet Cytogenet 2004;154:156.

El-Wakeel H et al: Systematic review of fibroadenoma as a risk factor for breast cancer. Breast 2003;12:302.

Fine RE et al: Percutaneous removal of benign breast masses using a vacuum-assisted hand-held device with ultrasound guidance. Am J Surg 2002;184:332.

Kaufman CS et al: Cryoablation treatment of benign breast lesions with 12-month follow-up. Am J Surg 2004;188:340.

NIPPLE DISCHARGE

In order of decreasing frequency, the following are the most common causes of nipple discharge in the nonlactating breast: duct ectasia, intraductal papilloma, and carcinoma. The important characteristics of the discharge and some other factors to be evaluated by history and physical examination are as follows:

(1) Nature of the discharge (serous, bloody, or other).
(2) Association with a mass.
(3) Unilateral or bilateral.
(4) Single or multiple duct discharge.
(5) Discharge is spontaneous (persistent or intermittent) or must be expressed.
(6) Discharge is produced by pressure at a single site or by general pressure on the breast.
(7) Relation to menses.
(8) Premenopausal or postmenopausal.
(9) Patient is taking contraceptive pills or estrogen.

Unilateral, spontaneous serous or serosanguineous discharge from a single duct is usually caused by an intraductal papilloma or, rarely, by an intraductal cancer. A mass may not be palpable. The involved duct may be identified by pressure at different sites around the nipple at the margin of the areola. Bloody discharge is suggestive of cancer but is more often caused by a benign papilloma in the duct. Cytologic examination may identify malignant cells, but negative findings do not rule out cancer, which is more likely in women over age 50 years. In any case, the involved duct—and a mass if present—should be excised. Ductography is of limited value since excision of the bloody duct system is indicated regardless of findings. Ductoscopy is being evaluated as a means of identifying intraductal lesions but is not yet practical.

In premenopausal women, spontaneous multiple duct discharge, unilateral or bilateral, most marked just before menstruation, is often due to mammary dysplasia. Discharge may be green or brownish. Papillomatosis and ductal ectasia are usually seen on biopsy. If a mass is present, it should be removed.

A milky discharge from multiple ducts in the nonlactating breast occurs in certain endocrine syndromes, as a result of hyperprolactinemia. Serum prolactin levels should be obtained to search for a pituitary tumor. Thyroid-stimulating hormone (TSH) helps exclude causative hypothyroidism. Numerous antipsychotic drugs and other drugs may also cause a milky discharge that ceases on discontinuance of the medication.

Oral contraceptive agents or estrogen replacement therapy may cause clear, serous, or milky discharge from a single duct, but multiple duct discharge is more common. The discharge is more evident just before menstruation and disappears on stopping the medication. If it does not stop and is from a single duct, exploration should be considered.

A purulent discharge may originate in a subareolar abscess and require removal of the abscess and the related lactiferous sinus.

When localization is not possible, no mass is palpable, and the discharge is nonbloody, the patient should be reexamined every 2 or 3 months for a year, and mammography should be done. Although most discharge is from a benign process, patients may find it annoying or disconcerting. To eliminate the discharge, proximal duct excision can be considered both for treatment and diagnosis. Cytologic examination of the nipple discharge for exfoliated cancer cells may rarely be helpful in diagnosis. However, the duct may be catheterized and lavage performed to evaluate cells for atypia. Ductoscopy, evaluation of the ductal system with a small scope inserted through the nipple, is also being studied to help identify intraductal lesions that may be causing the discharge.

Dietz JR et al: Directed duct excision by using mammary ductoscopy in patients with pathologic nipple discharge. Surgery 2002;132:582.

Dooley WC et al: Office-based breast ductoscopy for diagnosis. Am J Surg 2004;188:415.

Mokbel K et al: Mammary ductoscopy: current status and future prospects. Eur J Surg Oncol 2005;31:3.

Pritt B et al: Diagnostic value of nipple cytology: study of 466 cases. Cancer 2004;102:233.

Sauter ER et al: Fiberoptic ductoscopy findings in women with and without spontaneous nipple discharge. Cancer 2005;103:914.

Simmons R et al: Nonsurgical evaluation of pathologic nipple discharge. Ann Surg Oncol 2003;10:113.

FAT NECROSIS

Fat necrosis is a rare lesion of the breast but is of clinical importance because it produces a mass, often accompanied by skin or nipple retraction, which is indistinguishable from carcinoma. Trauma is presumed to be the cause, though only about 50% of patients give a history of injury. Ecchymosis is occasionally present. If untreated, the mass effect gradually disappears. The safest course is to obtain a biopsy. Needle biopsy is often adequate, but frequently the entire mass must be excised, primarily to exclude carcinoma. Fat necrosis is common after segmental resection, radiation therapy, or flap reconstruction after mastectomy.

Pui MH et al: Fatty tissue breast lesions. Clin Imaging 2003;27:150.

BREAST ABSCESS

During nursing, an area of redness, tenderness, and induration may develop in the breast. The organism most commonly found in these abscesses is *Staphylococcus aureus.* In the early stages, the infection can often be treated while nursing is continued from that breast by administering an antibiotic such as dicloxacillin or oxacillin, 250 mg four times daily for 7–10 days. If the lesion progresses to form a localized mass with local and systemic signs of infection, surgical drainage is performed and nursing is discontinued.

A subareolar abscess may develop (rarely) in young or middle-aged women who are not lactating. These infections tend to recur after incision and drainage unless the area is explored during a quiescent interval, with excision of the involved lactiferous duct or ducts at the base of the nipple. Otherwise, infection in the breast is very rare unless the patient is lactating. In the nonlactating breast, inflammatory carcinoma is always considered. Thus, findings suggestive of abscess or cellulitis in the nonlactating breast are an indication for incision and biopsy of any indurated tissue. If the abscess can be percutaneously drained and completely resolves, the patient may be followed up conservatively.

Dener C et al: Breast abscesses in lactating women. World J Surg 2003;27:130.

DISORDERS OF THE AUGMENTED BREAST

At least 4 million American women have had breast implants. Breast augmentation is performed by placing implants usually under the pectoralis muscle or, less desirably, in the subcutaneous tissue of the breast. Most implants are made of an outer silicone shell filled with a silicone gel, saline, or some combination of the two. About 15–25% of the patients develop capsule contraction or scarring around the implant, leading to a firmness and distortion of the breast that can be painful. Some require removal of the implant and capsule.

Implant rupture may occur in as many as 5–10% of women, and bleeding of gel through the capsule is noted even more commonly. Although silicone gel may be an immunologic stimulant, there is no increase in autoimmune disorders in patients with such implants. The Food and Drug Administration (FDA) has advised symptomatic women with ruptured implants to discuss possible surgical removal with their physicians. However, women who are asymptomatic and have no evidence of rupture of a silicone gel prosthesis should probably not undergo removal of the implant. Women with symptoms of autoimmune illnesses should address the possibility of removal.

Studies have failed to show any association between implants and an increased incidence of breast cancer. However, breast cancer may develop in a patient with a silicone gel prosthesis, as it does in women without them. Detection in patients with implants is made more difficult since mammography is less able to detect early lesions. However, local recurrence after breast reconstruction for cancer is usually cutaneous or subcutaneous and is easily detected by palpation. If a cancer develops, it should be treated in the same manner as in women without implants. Such women should be offered the option of mastectomy or breast-conserving therapy, which may require removal or replacement of the implant. Radiotherapy of the augmented breast often results in marked capsular contracture. Adjuvant treatments should be given for the same indications as for women who have no implants.

Brinton LA et al: Risk of connective tissue disorders among breast implant patients. Am J Epidemiol 2004;160:619.

Englert H et al: Augmentation mammoplasty and "silicone-osis." Intern Med J 2004;34:668.

Fryzek JP et al: Silicone breast implants. J Rheumatol 2005;32:201.

CARCINOMA OF THE FEMALE BREAST

ESSENTIALS OF DIAGNOSIS

- *Risk factors include delayed childbearing, positive family history of breast cancer or genetic mutations (BRCA1, BRCA2), and personal history of breast cancer or some types of mammary dysplasia.*
- *Most women with breast cancer do not have identifiable risk factors.*
- *Early findings: Single, nontender, firm to hard mass with ill-defined margins; mammographic abnormalities and no palpable mass.*
- *Later findings: Skin or nipple retraction; axillary lymphadenopathy; breast enlargement, redness, edema, pain; fixation of mass to skin or chest wall.*

INCIDENCE & RISK FACTORS

Next to skin cancer, breast cancer is the most common type of cancer in women, second only to lung cancer as a cause of death. The probability of developing breast cancer increases throughout life. The mean and the median age of women with breast cancer is between 60 and 61 years.

There will be about 211,240 new cases of breast cancer and about 40,410 deaths from this disease in women in the United States in the year 2005. An additional 59,000 cases of ductal carcinoma in situ will be detected, principally by screening mammography. One out of every eight or nine American women will develop breast cancer during her lifetime. The incidence of breast cancer continues to increase, but recently mortality has appeared to decrease slightly. This reflects both early detection and increased use of systemic therapy. Women whose mothers or sisters had breast cancer are three to four times more likely to develop the disease. Risk is further increased in patients whose mothers' or sisters' breast cancers occurred before menopause or were bilateral and in those with a family history of breast cancer in two or more first-degree relatives. However, there is no history of breast cancer among female relatives in over 75% of patients. Nulliparous women and women whose first full-term pregnancy was after age 35 have a 1.5 times higher incidence of breast cancer than multiparous women. Late menarche and artificial menopause are associated with a lower incidence, whereas early menarche (under age 12) and late natural menopause (after age 50) are associated with a slight increase in risk. Fibrocystic condition, when accompanied by proliferative changes, papillomatosis, or atypical epithelial hyperplasia, is associated with an increased incidence. A woman who has had cancer in one breast is at increased risk of developing cancer in the other breast. Such women develop a contralateral cancer at the rate of 1% or 2% per year. Women with cancer of the uterine corpus have a risk of breast cancer significantly higher than that of the general population, and women with breast cancer have a comparably increased risk for endometrial cancer. In the United States, breast cancer is more common in whites. The incidence of the disease among nonwhites (mostly blacks) is increasing, especially in younger women. In general, rates reported from developing countries are low, whereas rates are high in developed countries, with the notable exception of Japan. Some of the variability may be due to underreporting in the developing countries, but a real difference probably exists. Dietary factors, particularly increased fat consumption, may account for some differences in incidence. Oral contraceptives do not appear to increase the risk of breast cancer. There is evidence that administration of estrogens to postmenopausal women may result in a slightly increased risk of breast cancer, but only with higher, long-term doses of estrogens. Concomitant administration of progesterone and estrogen may markedly increase the incidence of breast cancer compared with the use of estrogen alone. The Women's Health Initiative prospective randomized study of hormone replacement therapy stopped treatment with estrogen and progesterone early because of an increased risk of breast cancer compared with untreated controls or women treated with estrogen alone. Alcohol consumption increases the risk slightly. Some inherited breast cancers have been found to be associated with a gene on chromosome 17. This gene, *BRCA1,* is mutated in families with early-onset breast cancer and ovarian cancer. As many as 85% of women with *BRCA1* gene mutations will develop breast cancer in their lifetime. Other genes are associated with increased risk of breast and other cancers, such as *BRCA2,* ataxia-telangiectasia mutation, and *p53,* the tumor suppressor gene. *p53* mutations have been found in approximately 1% of breast cancers in women under 40 years of age. Genetic testing is now commercially available for women at high risk of breast cancer. Women with genetic mutations who develop breast cancer may be treated in the same way as women who do not have mutations (ie, lumpectomy), though data are emerging to suggest an increased recurrence rate for these women. Such women with mutations often elect bilateral mastectomy as treatment. Some states have enacted legislation to prevent insurance companies from considering mutations as "preexisting conditions," preventing insurability.

Women at greater than normal risk of developing breast cancer (Table 17–1) should be identified by their physicians, taught the techniques of breast self-examination, and followed up carefully. Those with an exceptional family history should be counseled and given the option of genetic testing. Some of these high-risk women may consider prophylactic mastectomy or tamoxifen.

The National Surgical Adjuvant Breast Project (NSABP) conducted the Breast Cancer Prevention Trial (BCPT), which studied the efficacy of tamoxifen as a preventive agent in women who had never had breast cancer but were at high risk for developing the disease. Women who received tamoxifen for 5 years had about a 50% reduction in noninvasive and invasive cancers compared with women taking placebo. However, women above the age of 50 years who received the drug had an increased incidence of endometrial cancer and deep vein thrombosis. Unfortunately, no survival data will be produced from this trial. The selective estrogen receptor modulator (SERM) raloxifene, effective in preventing osteoporosis, has also shown some promise in preventing breast cancer. This, however, requires further investigation. Several large studies examining this hypothesis are under way. Recently, considerable data have become available regarding the efficacy and success of using aromatase inhibitors to treat breast cancer. Based upon this compelling body of evidence, large multicenter studies (International Breast Cancer Intervention Study II [IBIS-II] and MAP-3) of aromatase inhibitors to prevent breast cancer are currently under way.

Table 17–1. Factors associated with increased risk of breast cancer.[1]

Race	White
Age	Older
Family history	Breast cancer in mother, sister, or daughter (especially bilateral or premenopausal)
Genetics	*BRCA1* or *BRCA2* mutation
Previous medical history	Endometrial cancer Proliferative forms of fibrocystic disease Cancer in other breast
Menstrual history	Early menarche (under age 12) Late menopause (after age 50)
Pregnancy	Nulliparous or late first pregnancy

[1]Normal lifetime risk in white women = 1 in 8 or 9.

Andrews L et al: Psychological impact of genetic testing for breast cancer susceptibility in women of Ashkenazi Jewish background: a prospective study. Genet Test 2004;8:240.

Colditz GA: Estrogen, estrogen plus progestin therapy, and risk of breast cancer. Clin Cancer Res 2005;11(2 Pt 2):909s.

Cuzick J: Aromatase inhibitors for breast cancer prevention. J Clin Oncol 2005;23:1636.

Dite GS et al: Familial risks, early-onset breast cancer, and BRCA1 and BRCA2 germline mutations. J Natl Cancer Inst 2003;95:448.

Ettinger B et al: Reduction of vertebral fracture risk in postmenopausal women with osteoporosis treated with raloxifene: results from a 3-year randomized clinical trial. Multiple Outcomes of Raloxifene Evaluation (MORE) Investigators. JAMA 1999;282:637.

Euhus DM: Understanding mathematical models for breast cancer risk assessment and counseling. Breast J 2001;7:224.

Fabian CJ et al: Selective estrogen-receptor modulators for primary prevention of breast cancer. J Clin Oncol 2005;23:1644.

Freedman AN et al: Estimates of the number of US women who could benefit from tamoxifen for breast cancer chemoprevention. J Natl Cancer Inst 2003;95:526.

Jemal A et al: Cancer Statistics, 2005. CA Cancer J Clin 2005;55:10.

King MC et al: Tamoxifen and breast cancer incidence among women with inherited mutations in BRCA1 and BRCA2: National Surgical Adjuvant Breast and Bowel Project (NSABP-P1) Breast Cancer Prevention Trial. JAMA 2001;286:2251.

Narod SA et al: Prevention and management of hereditary breast cancer. J Clin Oncol 2005;23:1656.

Narod SA et al: Oral contraceptives and the risk of breast cancer in BRCA1 and BRCA2 mutation carriers. J Natl Cancer Inst 2002;94:1773.

Rebbeck TR et al: Bilateral prophylactic mastectomy reduces breast cancer risk in BRCA1 and BRCA2 mutation carriers: the PROSE Study Group. J Clin Oncol 2004;22:1055.

Rossouw JE et al: Risks and benefits of estrogen plus progestin in healthy postmenopausal women: principal results from the Women's Health Initiative randomized controlled trial. JAMA 2002;288:321.

Scott CL et al: Average age-specific cumulative risk of breast cancer according to type and site of germline mutations in BRCA1 and BRCA2 estimated from multiple-case breast cancer families attending Australian family cancer clinics. Hum Genet 2003;112:542.

Wrensch MR et al: Breast cancer risk in women with abnormal cytology in nipple aspirates of breast fluid. J Natl Cancer Inst 2001;93:1791.

EARLY DETECTION OF BREAST CANCER

Screening Programs

A number of mass screening programs consisting of physical and mammographic examination of the breasts of asymptomatic women have been conducted. Such programs frequently identify about 10 cancers per 1000 women older than age 50 years and about 2 cancers per 1000 women younger than age 50 years. About 80% of these women have negative axillary lymph nodes at the time of surgery, whereas only 50% of nonscreened women found in the course of usual medical practice have uninvolved axillary nodes. Detecting breast cancer before it has spread to the axillary nodes greatly increases the chance of survival, and about 85% of such women will survive at least 5 years.

Both physical examination and mammography are necessary for maximum yield in screening programs, since about 35–50% of early breast cancers can be discovered only by mammography and another 40% can be detected only by palpation. About one-third of the abnormalities detected on screening mammograms will be found to be malignant when biopsy is performed. The probability of cancer on a screening mammogram is directly related to the Breast Imaging and Reporting Data System (BIRADS) assessment, and workup should be performed based on this classification. Women 20–40 years of age should have a breast examination as part of routine medical care every 2–3 years. Women over age 40 years should have yearly breast examinations. The sensitivity of mammography varies from approximately 60% to 90%. This sensitivity depends on several factors, including patient age (breast density) and tumor size, location, and mammographic appearance. In young women with dense breasts, mammography is less sensitive than in older woman with fatty breasts, in whom mammography can detect at least 90% of malignancies. Smaller tumors, particularly those without calcifications, are more difficult to detect, especially in dense breasts. The lack of sensitivity and the low incidence of breast cancer in young women have led to questions concerning the value of mammography for screening in women 40–50 years of age. The specificity of mammography in women under 50 years varies from about 30% to 40% for nonpalpable mammographic abnormalities to 85% to 90% for clinically evident malignancies.

Doubt exists about the beneficial effect of screening, especially in women under age 50 years. Questions such as the potential harmful effects of x-rays in a large population of young women and the general value of early detection were raised and largely ignored as various groups supported screening between ages 40 and 50 years. Although the Health Insurance Plan Project study did show a beneficial effect of screening in such women, reducing breast cancer mortality 25% between 10 and 18 years after entry into the study, a Canadian trial demonstrated an unexplained shortening of survival from time of random assignment to death in the screening group. The small number of patients in this study experienced no beneficial effect, but the 95% confidence interval included a potential lifesaving effect as well as a potential harmful effect. A very large number of patients is necessary to show a beneficial effect of screening among patients aged 40–49 years, in whom the incidence of breast cancer is low. In addition, the problems of crossover of patients in the control group with women undergoing physician examination and nonscreening mammograms, problems with mammography quality, and problems in recruitment, randomization, and compliance make the interpretation of such trials difficult. The beneficial effect of screening in women aged 50–69 years is undisputed and has been confirmed by all clinical trials. The efficacy of screening in older women—those older than 70 years—is inconclusive and is difficult to determine because few women were screened.

More recent studies showing a beneficial effect of screening young women and the recommendation of a Swedish consensus panel led the National Cancer Institute (NCI) to reconsider its position on screening mammography for women in their 40s. Two Swedish trials that had shown a 13% decrease in breast cancer mortality (not statistically significant) now showed a statistical advantage for screening women in their 40s, and a meta-analysis similarly revealed a statistical survival advantage for screened women with longer follow-up. In March 1997, the National Cancer Advisory Board recommended that women in their 40s with average risk factors should have screening mammography every 1–2 years and that women at higher risk should seek medical advice on when to begin screening. The American Cancer Society then recommended screening every year for asymptomatic women starting at age 40 years. Studies continue to support the value of screening mammography.

Self-Examination

Breast self-examination (BSE) has not been shown to improve survival. Despite this and despite possible increased biopsy rates, it is a useful technique since many patients do detect their own cancer, and women often feel more in control and proactive by using the procedure. Because of the absence of strong evidence supporting the value of BSE, the American Cancer Society no longer recommends monthly BSE beginning at age 20 years. The recommendation is that patients be made aware of the potential benefits, limitations, and harms (increased biopsies or false-positive results) associated with BSE. Women who chose to perform BSE should be advised regarding the proper technique. Premenopausal women should perform the examination 7–8 days after the menstrual period. The breasts should be inspected initially while standing before a mirror with the hands at the sides, overhead, and pressed firmly on the hips to contract the pectoralis muscles. Masses, asymmetry of breasts, and slight dimpling of the skin may become apparent as a result of these maneuvers. Next, in a supine position, each breast should be carefully palpated with the fingers of the opposite hand. Some women discover small breast lumps more readily when their skin is moist while bathing or showering. Physicians should instruct women in the technique of self-examination and advise them to report a mass or other abnormality.

Imaging

Mammography is the most useful technique for the detection of early breast cancer. Film screen mammography delivers less than 0.4 cGy to the mid breast per view and has largely replaced the older xeromammographic technique, which delivers more radiation.

Mammography is the most reliable means of detecting breast cancer before a mass can be palpated. Slowly growing cancers can be identified by mammography at least 2 years before reaching a size detectable by palpation. Although full-field digital mammography provides an easier method to maintain and review mammograms, it has not been proven that it provides better images or increases detection rates more than film mammography. New computer-assisted detection (CAD) has not shown any increase in detection of cancers and is not routinely performed at centers with experienced mammographers.

Calcifications are the most easily recognized mammographic abnormality. The most common findings associated with carcinoma of the breast are clustered polymorphic microcalcifications. Such calcifications are usually at least five to eight in number, aggregated in one part of the breast and differing from each other in size and shape, often including branched or V- or Y-shaped configurations. There may be an associated mammographic mass density or, at times, only a mass density with no calcifications. Such a density usually has irregular or ill-defined borders and may lead to architectural distortion within the breast. A small mass or architectural distortion, particularly in a dense breast, may be subtle and difficult to detect.

Indications for mammography are as follows: (1) to screen at regular intervals women at high risk for developing breast cancer (see above); (2) to evaluate each breast when a diagnosis of potentially curable breast cancer has been made, and at yearly intervals thereafter; (3) to evaluate a questionable or ill-defined breast mass or other suspicious change in the breast; (4) to search for an occult breast cancer in a woman with metastatic disease in axillary nodes or elsewhere from an unknown primary; (5) to screen women prior to cosmetic operations or prior to biopsy of a mass, to examine for an unsuspected cancer; and (6) to follow those women with breast cancer who have been treated with breast-conserving surgery and radiation.

Patients with a dominant or suspicious mass must undergo biopsy despite mammographic findings. The mammogram should be obtained prior to biopsy so that other suspicious areas can be noted and the contralateral breast can be checked. Mammography is never a substitute for biopsy because it may not reveal clinical cancer in a very dense breast, as may be seen in young women with fibrocystic changes, and may not reveal medullary cancers.

Communication and documentation among the patient, the referring physician, and the interpreting physician are critical for high-quality screening and diagnostic mammography. The patient should be told about *how* she will receive timely results of her mammogram; that mammography does not "rule out" cancer; and that she may receive a correlative examination such as ultrasound at the mammography facility if referred for a suspicious lesion. She should also be aware of the technique and need for breast compression and that this may be uncomfortable. The mammography facility should be informed *in writing* of abnormal physical examination findings. It is strongly recommended in the Agency for Health Care Policy and Research (AHCPR) Clinical Practice Guidelines that all mammography reports be communicated with the patient as well as the health care provider in writing. Additional phone communication about any abnormal findings should take place between the interpreting and referring physicians. Magnetic resonance imaging (MRI) and ultrasound are currently being studied as screening tools for breast cancer. They may be useful modalities in women who are at high risk for breast cancer, but not for the general population. The sensitivity of MRI is much higher than mammography; however, the specificity is significantly lower and this results in multiple unnecessary biopsies. The increased sensitivity despite decreased specificity may be considered a reasonable trade-off for those at increased risk for developing breast cancer, but not for a normal-risk population. Additionally, positron emission tomography (PET) may play a role in imaging atypical lesions, but only after diagnostic mammography has been performed.

Baxter N: Canadian Task Force on Preventive Health Care: Preventive health care, 2001 update: should women be routinely taught breast self-examination to screen for breast cancer? CMAJ 2001;164:1837.

Elmore JG et al: Screening for breast cancer. JAMA 2005;293:1245.

Humphrey LL et al: Breast cancer screening: a summary of the evidence for the U.S. Preventive Services Task Force. Ann Intern Med 2002;137(5 Part 1):347.

Kosters JP et al: Regular self-examination or clinical examination for early detection of breast cancer. Cochrane Database Syst Rev 2003;(2):CD003373.

Kriege M et al: The Magnetic Resonance Imaging Screening Study Group: efficacy of magnetic resonance imaging and mammography for breast cancer screening in women with a familial or genetic predisposition. Obstet Gynecol Surv 2005;60:107.

Nystrom L et al: Long-term effects of mammography screening: updated overview of the Swedish randomised trials. Lancet 2001;359:909.

Reddy DH et al: Incorporating new imaging models in breast cancer management. Curr Treat Options Oncol 2005;6:135.

Smith RA et al: American Cancer Society guidelines for the early detection of cancer, 2005. CA Cancer J Clin 2005;55:31.

Taylor P et al: Impact of computer-aided detection prompts on the sensitivity and specificity of screening mammography. Health Technol Assess 2005;9:1.

Clinical Clues to Early Detection of Breast Cancer

A. Symptoms and Signs

The presenting complaint in about 70% of patients with breast cancer is a lump (usually painless) in the breast. About 90% of breast masses are discovered by the patient herself. Less frequent symptoms are breast pain; nipple discharge; erosion, retraction, enlargement, or itching of the nipple; and redness, generalized hardness, enlargement, or shrinking of the breast. Rarely, an axillary mass or swelling of the arm may be the first symptom. Back or bone pain, jaundice, or weight loss may be the result of systemic metastases, but these symptoms are rarely seen on initial presentation.

The relative frequency of carcinoma in various anatomic sites in the breast is shown in Figure 17–1.

Inspection of the breast is the first step in physical examination and should be carried out with the patient sitting, arms at her sides and then overhead. Abnormal variations in breast size and contour, minimal nipple retraction, and slight edema, redness, or retraction of the skin can be identified. Asymmetry of the breasts and retraction or dimpling of the skin can often be accentu-

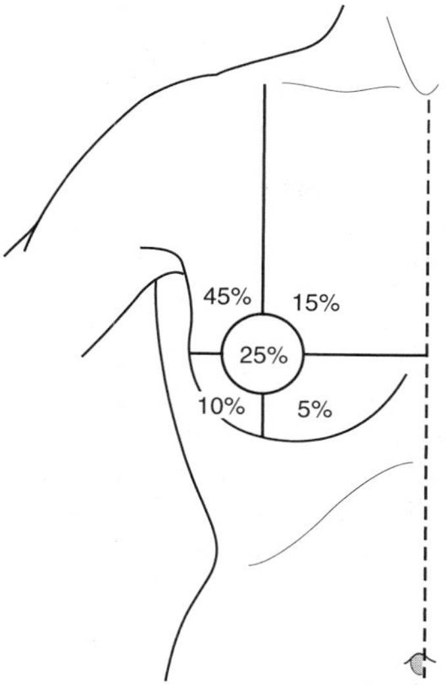

Figure 17–1. Frequency of breast carcinoma at various anatomic sites.

ated by having the patient raise her arms overhead or press her hands on her hips to contract the pectoralis muscles. Axillary and supraclavicular areas should be thoroughly palpated for enlarged nodes with the patient sitting (Figure 17–2). Palpation of the breast for masses or other changes should be performed with the patient both seated and supine with the arm abducted (Figure 17–3). Palpation with a rotary motion of the examiner's fingers as well as a horizontal stripping motion has been recommended.

Breast cancer usually consists of a nontender, firm or hard mass with poorly delineated margins (caused by local infiltration). Slight skin or nipple retraction is an important sign. Minimal asymmetry of the breast may be noted. Very small (1–2 mm) erosions of the nipple epithelium may be the only manifestation of Paget's carcinoma. Watery, serous, or bloody discharge from the nipple is an occasional early sign but is more often associated with benign disease.

A lesion smaller than 1 cm in diameter may be difficult or impossible for the examiner to feel and yet may be discovered by the patient. She should always be asked to demonstrate the location of the mass; if the physician fails to confirm the patient's suspicions, the examination should be repeated in 2–3 months, preferably 1–2 weeks after the onset of menses. During the premenstrual phase of the cycle, increased innocuous nodularity may suggest neoplasm or may obscure an underlying lesion. If there is any question regarding the nature of an abnormality under these circumstances, the patient should be asked to return after her period. Ultrasound is often valuable and mammography essential when an area is felt by the patient to be abnormal but the physician feels no mass.

Metastases tend to involve regional lymph nodes, which may be palpable. One or two movable, nontender, not particularly firm axillary lymph nodes 5 mm or less in diameter are frequently present and are generally of no significance. Firm or hard nodes larger than 1 cm are typical of metastases. Axillary nodes that are matted or fixed to skin or deep structures indicate advanced disease (at least stage III). Microscopic metastases are present in about 30% of patients with clinically negative nodes. On the other hand, if the examiner thinks that the axillary nodes are involved, that impression will be borne out by histologic section in about 85% of cases. The incidence of positive axillary nodes increases with the size of the primary tumor. Noninvasive cancers do not metastasize.

In most cases no nodes are palpable in the supraclavicular fossa. Firm or hard nodes of any size in this location or just beneath the clavicle are suggestive of metastatic cancer and should be biopsied. Ipsilateral supraclavicular or infraclavicular nodes containing cancer indicate that the tumor is in an advanced stage (stage III or IV). Edema of the ipsilateral arm, commonly caused by metastatic infiltration of regional lymphatics, is also a sign of advanced cancer.

B. Laboratory Findings

A consistently elevated sedimentation rate may be the result of disseminated cancer. Liver or bone metastases may be associated with elevation of serum alkaline

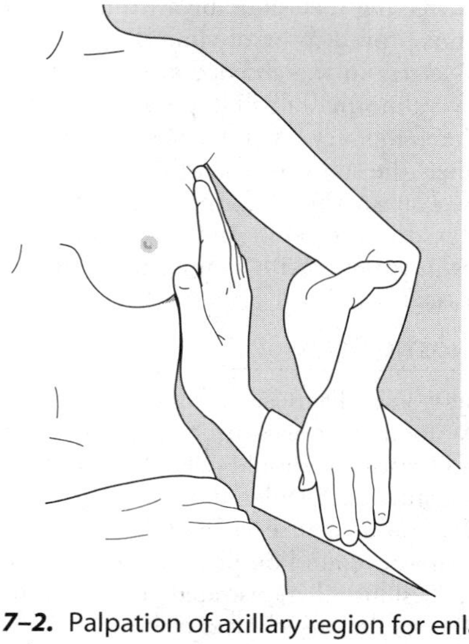

Figure 17–2. Palpation of axillary region for enlarged lymph nodes.

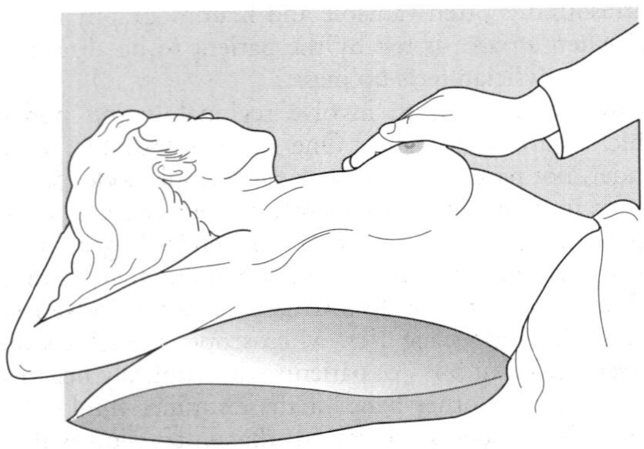

Figure 17–3. Palpation of breasts. Palpation is performed with the patient supine and arm abducted.

phosphatase. Hypercalcemia is an occasional important finding in advanced cancer of the breast. Carcinoembryonic antigen (CEA) and CA 15-3 or CA 27-29 may be used as markers for recurrent breast cancer but are not helpful in diagnosing early lesions. Many scientists are further investigating breast cancer biomarkers through proteomics and hormone assays. These studies are ongoing and may prove to be helpful in early detection or evaluation of prognosis.

C. Imaging for Metastases

Chest x-ray may show pulmonary metastases. Computed tomographic (CT) scanning of the liver and brain is of value only when metastases are suspected in these areas. Bone scans utilizing ^{99m}Tc-labeled phosphates or phosphonates are more sensitive than skeletal x-rays in detecting metastatic breast cancer. Bone scanning has not proved to be of clinical value as a routine preoperative test in the absence of symptoms, physical findings, or abnormal alkaline phosphatase or calcium levels. The frequency of abnormal findings on bone scan parallels the status of the axillary lymph nodes on pathologic examination. PET may prove to be an effective single scan for bone and soft tissue or visceral metastases in patients with symptoms or signs of metastatic disease.

D. Diagnostic Tests

1. Biopsy—The diagnosis of breast cancer depends ultimately upon examination of tissue or cells removed by biopsy. Treatment should never be undertaken without an unequivocal histologic or cytologic diagnosis of cancer. The safest course is biopsy examination of all suspicious masses found on physical examination and of suspicious lesions demonstrated by mammography. About 60% of lesions clinically thought to be cancer prove on biopsy to be benign, and about 30% of lesions believed to be benign are found to be malignant. These findings demonstrate the fallibility of clinical judgment and the necessity for biopsy. A breast mass should not be followed without histologic diagnosis, except perhaps in the premenopausal woman with a nonsuspicious mass presumed to be a fibrocystic condition. A lesion such as this could be observed through one or two menstrual cycles. However, if the mass does not completely resolve during this time, it must be biopsied. Figures 17–4 and 17–5 present algorithms for management of breast masses in premenopausal and postmenopausal patients.

The simplest method is needle biopsy, either by aspiration of tumor cells (fine-needle aspiration cytology) or by obtaining a small core of tissue with a hollow needle.

Fine-needle aspiration cytology is a useful technique whereby cells are aspirated with a small needle and examined by the pathologist. This technique can be performed easily with no morbidity and is much less expensive than excisional or open biopsy. The main disadvantages are that it requires a pathologist skilled in the cytologic diagnosis of breast cancer and that it is subject to sampling problems, particularly because deep lesions may be missed. Furthermore, noninvasive cancers usually cannot be distinguished from invasive cancers. The incidence of false-positive diagnoses is extremely low, perhaps 1–2%. The false-negative rate is as high as 10%. Most experienced clinicians would not leave a suspicious dominant mass in the breast even when fine-needle aspiration cytology is negative unless the clinical diagnosis, breast imaging studies, and cytologic studies were all in agreement.

Large-needle (core needle) biopsy removes a core of tissue with a large cutting needle. Hand-held biopsy devices make large-core needle biopsy of a palpable mass easy and cost-effective in the office with local anesthesia. As in the case of any needle biopsy, the main problem is sampling error due to improper positioning of the needle, giving rise to a false-negative test result.

Open biopsy under local anesthesia as a separate procedure prior to deciding upon definitive treatment is the most reliable means of diagnosis. Needle biopsy or aspiration, when positive, offers a more rapid approach with less expense and morbidity, but when nondiagnostic it must be followed by open biopsy. Open biopsy consists of either an incisional biopsy or an excisional biopsy. An incisional biopsy is one in which an incision is made and a portion of the breast abnormality is removed for histologic evaluation. An excisional biopsy is also done through an incision in the skin, but with the intent to remove the entire abnormality, not simply a sample. Incisional biopsies are rarely performed now.

Additional evaluation for metastatic disease and therapeutic options can be discussed with the patient after the histologic or cytologic diagnosis of cancer has been established. This approach has the advantage of

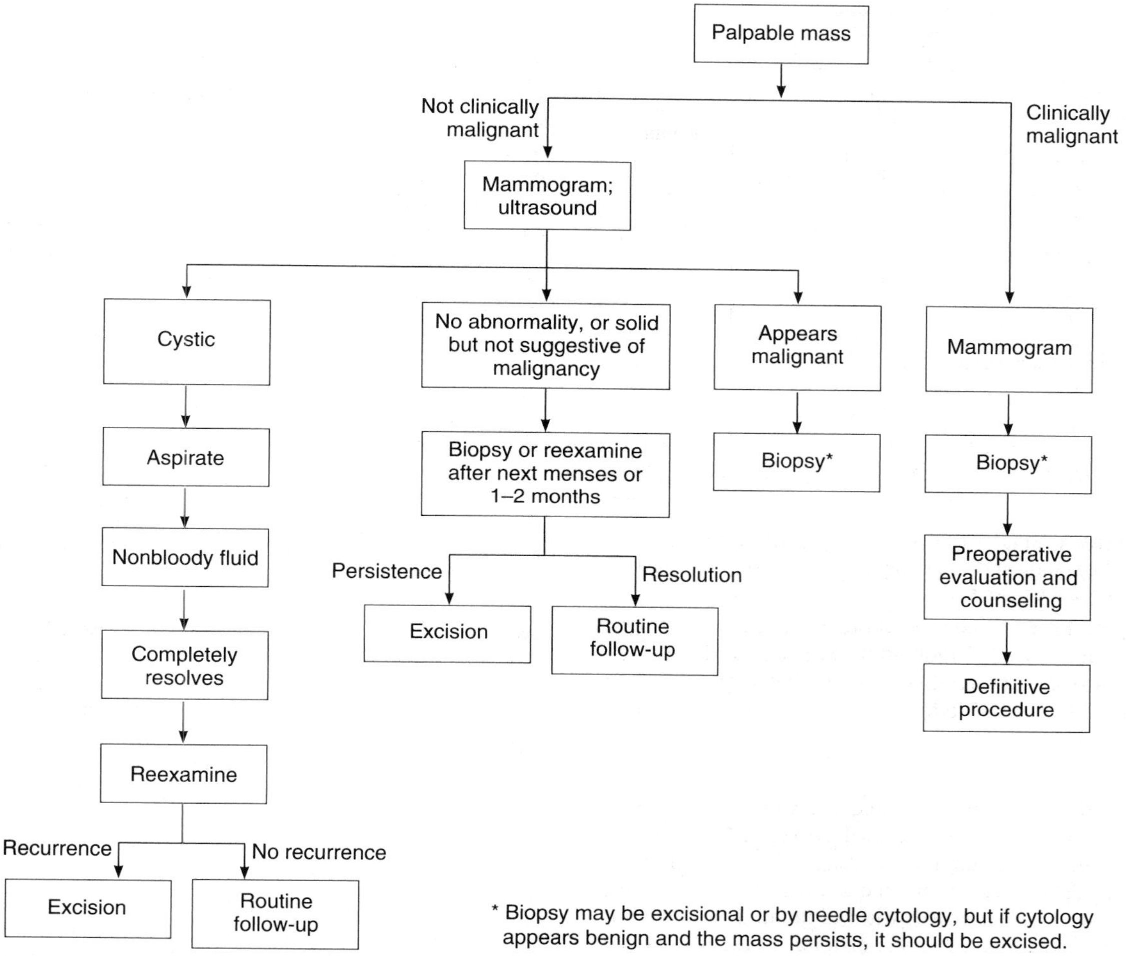

Figure 17–4. Evaluation of breast masses in premenopausal women. (Modified from Giuliano AE: Breast disease. In: *Practical Gynecologic Oncology*, 3rd ed. Berek JS, Hacker NF [editors]. Williams & Wilkins, 2000.)

avoiding unnecessary procedures, since cancer is found in the minority of patients biopsied for a breast lump. In situ cancers are not easily diagnosed cytologically and usually require excisional biopsy.

As an alternative in highly suspicious circumstances, the patient may be admitted to the hospital, where the diagnosis is made on frozen section of tissue obtained by open biopsy under general anesthesia. If the frozen section is positive, the surgeon can proceed immediately with operation. This one-step method is rarely used today except when a cytologic study has suggested cancer but is not diagnostic and there is a high clinical suspicion of malignancy.

In general, the two-step approach—outpatient biopsy followed by definitive operation at a later date—is preferred in the diagnosis and treatment of breast cancer, because patients can be given time to adjust to the diagnosis of cancer, can consider alternative forms of therapy, and can seek a second opinion if they wish. There is no adverse effect from the short (1–2 weeks) delay of the two-step procedure, and this is the current recommendation of the NCI.

2. Ultrasonography—Ultrasonography is performed primarily to differentiate cystic from solid lesions. Though not diagnostic, ultrasound may reveal features highly suggestive of malignancy such as irregular margins on a new solid mass. Ultrasonography may show an irregular mass within a cyst in the rare case of intracystic carcinoma. If a tumor is palpable and feels like a cyst, an 18-gauge needle can be used to aspirate the fluid and make the diagnosis of

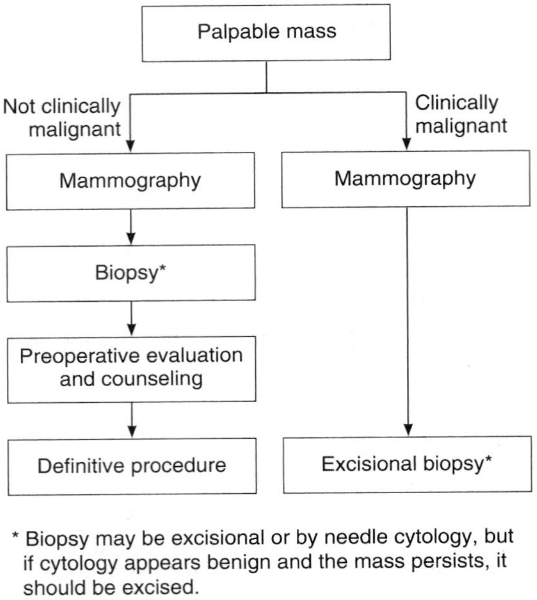

Figure 17–5. Evaluation of breast masses in postmenopausal women. (Modified from Giuliano AE: Breast disease. In: *Practical Gynecologic Oncology*, 3rd ed. Berek JS, Hacker NF [editors]. Williams & Wilkins, 2000.)

cyst. If a cyst is aspirated and the fluid is nonbloody, it does not have to be examined cytologically. If the mass does not recur, no further diagnostic test is necessary. Nonpalpable mammographic densities that appear benign should be investigated with ultrasound to determine whether the lesion is cystic or solid. These may even be needle biopsied with ultrasound guidance.

3. Mammography—When a suspicious abnormality is identified by mammography alone and cannot be palpated by the clinician, the lesion should be biopsied by a **computerized stereotactic guided core needle technique**. These units have been added to mammographic suites to localize abnormalities and perform needle biopsy without surgery. Under mammographic guidance, a biopsy needle can be inserted into the lesion by the mammographer, and a core of tissue for histologic examination or cells for cytology can then be examined. Vacuum assistance increases the amount of tissue obtained and improves diagnosis.

Mammographic localization biopsy is performed by obtaining a mammogram in two perpendicular views and placing a needle or hook-wire near the abnormality so that the surgeon can use the metal needle or wire as a guide during operation to locate the lesion. After mammography confirms the position of the needle in relation to the lesion, an incision is made and the subcutaneous tissue is dissected until the needle is identified. Using the films as a guide, the abnormality can then be localized and excised. It often happens that the abnormality cannot even be palpated through the incision—this is the case with microcalcifications—and thus it is essential to obtain a mammogram of the specimen to document that the lesion was excised. At that time, a second marker needle can further localize the lesion for the pathologist. Stereotactic core needle biopsies have proved equivalent to mammographic localization biopsies. Core biopsy is preferable to mammographic localization for accessible lesions.

4. Other imaging modalities—Other modalities of breast imaging have been investigated. Automated breast ultrasonography is useful in distinguishing cystic from solid lesions but should be used only as a supplement to physical examination and mammography. Ductography may be useful to define the site of a lesion causing a bloody discharge, but since biopsy is always indicated, ductography may be omitted and the blood-filled nipple system excised. Ductosopy has shown some promise in identifying intraductal lesions, especially in the case of pathologic nipple discharge, but the utility of this procedure is still being studied. MRI is highly sensitive but not specific and should not be used for screening, but it may be of value in highly selective cases. It is useful, for example, in differentiating scar from recurrence postlumpectomy and may be valuable to screen high-risk women (eg, women with *BRCA* mutations) and to examine for multicentricity when there is a known primary cancer or to examine the contralateral breast in women with cancer. PET scanning does not appear useful in evaluating the breast but may prove to be of value in examining regional lymphatics.

5. Cytology—Cytologic examination of nipple discharge or cyst fluid may be helpful on rare occasions. As a rule, mammography (or ductography) and breast biopsy are required when nipple discharge or cyst fluid is bloody or cytologically questionable. Ductal lavage, a technique that washes individual duct systems with saline and loosens epithelial cells for cytologic evaluation, is being evaluated as a risk assessment tool but appears to be of little value.

Baker JA et al: Breast US: assessment of technical quality and image interpretation. Radiology 2002;223:229.

Dooley WC: Routine operative breast endoscopy for bloody nipple discharge. Ann Surg Oncol 2002;9:920.

Hollingsworth AB: Perspectives on preoperative staging with breast MRI. J Am Coll Surg 2004;199:173.

Lenahan C et al: The role of tumor markers in breast cancer management. Curr Surg 2004;61:532.

Ljung BM et al: Cytology of ductal lavage fluid of the breast. Diagn Cytopathol 2004;30:143.

van der Hoeven JJ et al: Determinants of diagnostic performance of [F-18] fluorodeoxyglucose positron emission tomography for axillary staging in breast cancer. Ann Surg 2002;236:619.

DIFFERENTIAL DIAGNOSIS

The lesions to be considered most often in the differential diagnosis of breast cancer are the following, in descending order of frequency: mammary dysplasia (fibrocystic condition of the breast), fibroadenoma, intraductal papilloma, lipoma, and fat necrosis.

STAGING

Currently, the American Joint Committee on Cancer and the International Union Against Cancer have agreed on a TNM (tumor, regional lymph nodes, distant metastases) staging system for breast cancer. The use of this uniform TNM staging system enhances communication between investigators and clinicians. Table 17–2 sets forth the TNM classification.

PATHOLOGIC TYPES

Numerous pathologic subtypes of breast cancer can be identified histologically (Table 17–3). These types are distinguished by the histologic appearance and growth pattern of the tumor. In general, breast cancer arises either from the epithelial lining of the large or intermediate-sized ducts (ductal) or from the epithelium of the terminal ducts of the lobules (lobular). The cancer may be invasive or in situ. Most breast cancers arise from the intermediate ducts and are invasive (invasive ductal, infiltrating ductal), and most histologic types are merely subtypes of invasive ductal cancer with unusual growth patterns (colloid, medullary, scirrhous, etc). Ductal carcinoma that has not invaded the extraductal tissue is intraductal or in situ ductal. Lobular carcinoma may be either invasive or in situ.

Except for the in situ cancers, the histologic subtypes have only a slight bearing on prognosis when outcomes are compared after accurate staging. Various histologic parameters, such as invasion of blood vessels, tumor differentiation, invasion of breast lymphatics, and tumor necrosis have been examined, but they too seem to have little prognostic value.

The noninvasive cancers by definition are confined by the basement membrane of the ducts and lack the ability to spread. However, in patients whose biopsies show noninvasive intraductal cancer, associated invasive ductal cancers metastasize to lymph nodes in about 1–3% of cases.

SPECIAL CLINICAL FORMS OF BREAST CANCER

Paget's Carcinoma

The basic lesion is usually an infiltrating ductal carcinoma, usually well differentiated, or a ductal carcinoma in situ (DCIS). The ducts of the nipple epithelium are infiltrated, but gross nipple changes are often minimal, and a tumor mass may not be palpable. The first symptom is often itching or burning of the nipple, with superficial erosion or ulceration. The diagnosis is established by biopsy of the erosion.

Paget's carcinoma is not common (about 1% of all breast cancers), but it is important because the nipple changes appear innocuous. These are frequently diagnosed and treated as dermatitis or bacterial infection, leading to delay in detection. When the lesion consists of nipple changes only, the incidence of axillary metastases is less than 5%, and the prognosis is excellent. When a breast mass is also present, the incidence of axillary metastases rises, with an associated marked decrease in prospects for cure by surgical or other treatment.

Inflammatory Carcinoma

This is the most malignant form of breast cancer and constitutes less than 3% of all cases. The clinical findings consist of a rapidly growing, sometimes painful mass that enlarges the breast. The overlying skin becomes erythematous, edematous, and warm. Often there is no distinct mass, since the tumor infiltrates the involved breast diffusely. The diagnosis should be made when the redness involves more than one-third of the skin over the breast and biopsy shows infiltrating carcinoma with invasion of the subdermal lymphatics. The inflammatory changes, often mistaken for an infection, are caused by carcinomatous invasion of the subdermal lymphatics, with resulting edema and hyperemia. If the physician suspects infection but the lesion does not respond rapidly (1–2 weeks) to antibiotics, biopsy is performed. Metastases tend to occur early and widely, and for this reason inflammatory carcinoma is rarely curable. Mastectomy is seldom indicated unless chemotherapy and radiation have resulted in clinical remission with no evidence of distant metastases. In these cases, residual disease in the breast may be eradicated. Radiation, hormone therapy, and chemotherapy are the measures most likely to be of value, rather than operation.

Breast Cancer Occurring during Pregnancy or Lactation

Breast cancer complicates approximately 1 in 3000 pregnancies. The diagnosis is frequently delayed, because physiologic changes in the breast may obscure the lesion. This results in a tendency of both patients and physicians to misinterpret findings and to delay biopsy. When the cancer is confined to the breast, the 5-year survival rate after mastectomy is about 70%. Axillary metastases are already present in 60–70% of patients, and for them the 5-year survival rate after mastectomy is only 30–40%. Pregnancy (or lactation) is

Table 17–2. TNM staging for breast cancer.

Primary tumor (T)	
Definitions for classifying the primary tumor (T) are the same for clinical and for pathologic classification. If the measurement is made by physical examination, the examiner will use the major headings (T1, T2, or T3). If other measurements, such as mammographic or pathologic measurements, are used, the subsets of T1 can be used. Tumors should be measured to the nearest 0.1 cm increment.	
TX	Primary tumor cannot be assessed
T0	No evidence of primary tumor
Tis	Carcinoma in situ
Tis (DCIS)	Ductal carcinoma in situ
Tis (LCIS)	Lobular carcinoma in situ
Tis (Paget's)	Paget's disease of the nipple with no tumor
Note: Paget's disease associated with a tumor is classified according to the size of the tumor.	
T1	Tumor 2 cm or less in greatest dimension
T1mic	Microinvasion 0.1 cm or less in greatest dimension
T1a	Tumor more than 0.1 cm but not more than 0.5 cm in greatest dimension
T1b	Tumor more than 0.5 cm but not more than 1 cm in greatest dimension
T1c	Tumor more than 1 cm but not more than 2 cm in greatest dimension
T2	Tumor more than 2 cm but not more than 5 cm in greatest dimension
T3	Tumor more than 5 cm in greatest dimension
T4	Tumor of any size with direct extension to (a) chest wall or (b) skin, only as described below
T4a	Extension to chest wall, not including pectoralis muscle
T4b	Edema (including peau d'orange) or ulceration of the skin of the breast, or satellite skin nodules confined to the same breast
T4c	Both T4a and T4b
T4d	Inflammatory carcinoma

N3	Metastasis in ipsilateral infraclavicular lymph node(s) with or without axillary lymph node involvement, or in clinically apparent[1] ipsilateral internal mammary lymph node(s) and in the *presence* of clinically evident axillary lymph node metastasis; or metastasis in ipsilateral supraclavicular lymph node(s) with or without axillary or internal mammary lymph node involvement
N3a	Metastasis in ipsilateral infraclavicular lymph node(s)
N3b	Metastasis in ipsilateral internal mammary lymph node(s) and axillary lymph node(s)
N3c	Metastasis in ipsilateral supraclavicular lymph node(s)
*Pathologic (pN)*2	
pNX	Regional lymph nodes cannot be assessed (eg, previously removed, or not removed for pathologic study)
pN0	No regional lymph node metastasis histologically, no additional examination for isolated tumor cells
Note: Isolated tumor cells (ITC) are defined as single tumor cells or small cell clusters not greater than 0.2 mm, usually detected only by immunohistochemical (IHC) or molecular methods but which may be verified on hematoxylin and eosin stains. ITCs do not usually show evidence of malignant activity, eg, proliferation or stromal reaction.	
pN0(i–)	No regional lymph node metastasis histologically, negative IHC
pN0(i+)	No regional lymph node metastasis histologically, positive IHC, no IHC cluster greater than 0.2 mm
pN0(mol–)	No regional lymph node metastasis histologically, negative molecular findings (RT-PCR)[3]
pN0(mol+)	No regional lymph node metastasis histologically, positive molecular findings (RT-PCR)[3]

(continued)

Table 17–2. TNM staging for breast cancer. (continued)

Regional lymph nodes (N)	
Clinical	
NX	Regional lymph nodes cannot be assessed (eg, previously removed)
N0	No regional lymph node metastasis
N1	Metastasis to movable ipsilateral axillary lymph node(s)
N2	Metastases in ipsilateral axillary lymph nodes fixed or matted, or in clinically apparent ipsilateral internal mammary nodes in the *absence* of clinically evident axillary lymph node metastasis
N2a	Metastasis in ipsilateral axillary lymph nodes fixed to one another (matted) or to other structures
N2b	Metastasis only in clinically apparent[1] ipsilateral internal mammary nodes and in the *absence* of clinically evident axillary lymph node metastasis
pN2	Metastasis in 4–9 axillary lymph nodes, or in clinically apparent4 internal mammary lymph nodes in the *absence* of axillary lymph node metastasis
pN2a	Metastasis in 4–9 axillary lymph nodes (at least one tumor deposit greater than 2.0 mm)
pN2b	Metastasis in clinically apparent[4] internal mammary lymph nodes in the *absence* of axillary lymph node metastasis
pN3	Metastasis in 10 or more axillary lymph nodes, or in infraclavicular lymph nodes, or in clinically apparent[4] ipsilateral internal mammary lymph nodes in the *presence* of 1 or more positive axillary lymph nodes; or in more than 3 axillary lymph nodes with clinically negative microscopic metastasis in internal mammary lymph nodes; or in ipsilateral supraclavicular lymph nodes
pN3a	Metastasis in 10 or more axillary lymph nodes (at least one tumor deposit greater than 2.0 mm), or metastasis to the infraclavicular lymph nodes
pN3b	Metastasis in clinically apparent[4] ipsilateral internal mammary lymph nodes in the *presence* of 1 or more positive axillary lymph nodes; or in more than 3 axillary lymph nodes and in internal mammary lymph nodes with microscopic disease detected by sentinel lymph node dissection but not clinically apparent[4]
pN3c	Metastasis in ipsilateral supraclavicular lymph nodes
pN1	Metastasis in 1–3 axillary lymph nodes, and/or in internal mammary nodes with microscopic disease detected by sentinel lymph node dissection but not clinically apparent[4]
pN1mi	Micrometastasis (greater than 0.2 mm, none greater than 2.0 mm)
pN1a	Metastasis in 1–3 axillary lymph nodes
pN1b	Metastasis in internal mammary nodes with microscopic disease detected by sentinel lymph node dissection but not clinically apparent[4]
pN1c	Metastasis in 1 to 3 axillary lymph nodes and in internal mammary lymph nodes with microscopic disease detected by sentinel lymph node dissection but not clinically apparent.[4] (If associated with greater than 3 positive axillary lymph nodes, the internal mammary nodes are classified as pN3b to reflect increased tumor burden)
Distant metastasis (M)	
MX	Distant metastasis cannot be assessed
M0	No distant metastasis
M1	Distant metastasis

Stage grouping

Stage 0	Tis	N0	M0
Stage I	T1[5]	N0	M0
Stage IIA	T0	N1	M0
	T1[5]	N1	M0
	T2	N0	M0
Stage IIB	T2	N1	M0
	T3	N0	M0
Stage IIIA	T0	N2	M0
	T1[5]	N2	M0
	T2	N2	M0
	T3	N1	M0
	T3	N2	M0
Stage IIIB	T4	N0	M0
	T4	N1	M0
	T4	N2	M0
Stage IIIC	Any T	N3	M0
Stage IV	Any T	Any N	M1

Note: Stage designation may be changed if postsurgical imaging studies reveal the presence of distant metastases, provided that the studies are carried out within 4 months of diagnosis in the absence of disease progression and provided that the patient has not received neoadjuvant therapy.

(continued)

Table 17–2. TNM staging for breast cancer. (continued)

Reproduced from *AJCC Cancer Staging Manual*, 6th ed. Springer, 2002.
[1]*Clinically apparent* is defined as detected by imaging studies (excluding lymphoscintigraphy) or by clinical examination or grossly visible pathologically.
[2]Classification is based on axillary lymph node dissection with or without sentinel lymph node dissection. Classification based solely on sentinel lymph node dissection without subsequent axillary lymph node dissection is designated (sn) for "sentinel node," eg, pN0(i+)(sn).
[3]RT-PCR: reverse transcriptase/polymerase chain reaction.
[4]*Clinically apparent* is defined as detected by imaging studies (excluding lymphoscintigraphy) or by clinical examination. *Not clinically apparent* is defined as not detected by imaging studies (excluding lymphoscintigraphy) or by clinical examination.
[5]T1 includes T1mic.

not a contraindication to operation, and treatment should be based on the stage of the disease as in the nonpregnant (or nonlactating) woman. Overall survival rates have improved, since cancers are now diagnosed in pregnant women earlier than in the past. Breast-conserving surgery may be performed—and radiation and chemotherapy given—even during the pregnancy.

Bilateral Breast Cancer

Clinically evident simultaneous bilateral breast cancer occurs in less than 1% of cases, but there is a 5–8% incidence of later occurrence of cancer in the second breast. Bilaterality occurs more often in familial breast cancer, in women under age 50 years, and when the tumor in the primary breast is lobular. The incidence of second breast cancers increases directly with the length of time the patient is alive after her first cancer—about 1% per year.

In patients with breast cancer, mammography should be performed before primary treatment and at regular intervals thereafter, to search for occult cancer in the opposite breast. Routine biopsy of the opposite breast is usually not warranted even for lobular cancer.

Noninvasive Cancer

Noninvasive cancer can occur within the ducts (ductal carcinoma in situ, DCIS) or lobules (lobular carcinoma in situ, LCIS). LCIS, although thought to be a premalignant lesion or a risk factor for breast cancer, in fact behaves like other carcinomas in situ. In a recent study, patients with LCIS not only went on to develop invasive lobular breast cancer, but also some developed it in the same breast and indexed location of the original LCIS. Although more research needs to be done in this area, the invasive potential of LCIS is being reconsidered. DCIS tends to be unilateral and most often progresses to invasive cancer if untreated. Approximately 40–60% of women who have DCIS treated with biopsy alone develop invasive cancer within the same breast.

The treatment of intraductal lesions is controversial. DCIS can be treated with total mastectomy or by wide excision with or without radiation therapy. Conservative management, excision only, is advised in this patient population until further data are developed. Although research is defining the malignant potential of LCIS, it may be well managed with observation, but patients unwilling to accept the increased risk of breast cancer may be offered surgical excision of the area in question or even bilateral total mastectomy. Currently, accepted standards of care offer the alternative of chemoprevention, using agents such as tamoxifen, which is effective in preventing invasive breast cancer from developing in both LCIS and intraductal carcinoma in situ. Axillary metastases from in situ cancers should not occur unless there is an occult invasive cancer.

Table 17–3. Histologic types of breast cancer.

Type	Frequency of Occurrence
Infiltrating ductal (not otherwise specified)	80–90%
Medullary	5–8%
Colloid (mucinous)	2–4%
Tubular	1–2%
Papillary	1–2%
Invasive lobular	6–8%
Noninvasive	4–6%
Intraductal	2–3%
Lobular in situ	2–3%
Rare cancers	< 1%
Juvenile (secretory)	...
Adenoid cystic	...
Epidermoid	...
Sudoriferous	...

Anderson WF et al: Inflammatory breast carcinoma and noninflammatory locally advanced breast carcinoma: distinct clinicopathologic entities? J Clin Oncol 2003;21:2254.

Fisher ER et al: Pathologic findings from the National Surgical Adjuvant Breast and Bowel Project: twelve-year observations concerning lobular *carcinoma in situ.* Cancer 2004;100:238.

Khan A et al: Diagnosis and management of ductal carcinoma in situ. Curr Treat Options Oncol 2004;5:131.

Marcus E: The management of Paget's disease of the breast. Curr Treat Options Oncol 2004;5:153.

Saunders C et al: Breast cancer during pregnancy. Int J Fertil Womens Med 2004;49:203.

HORMONE RECEPTOR SITES

The presence or absence of estrogen and progesterone receptors in the cytoplasm of tumor cells is of paramount importance in managing patients with breast cancer. Patients whose primary tumors are receptor positive have a more favorable course than those whose tumors are receptor negative. Receptors are of value in determining adjuvant therapy and for treatment of advanced disease. Up to 60% of patients with metastatic breast cancer will respond to hormonal manipulation if their tumors contain estrogen receptors. Fewer than 5% of patients with metastatic, estrogen receptor-negative tumors can be treated successfully in this fashion.

Receptor status is valuable not only in managing metastatic disease but also in helping select patients for adjuvant therapy. Adjuvant hormonal therapy (tamoxifen) with receptor-positive tumors and adjuvant chemotherapy with receptor-negative tumors improve survival rates even in the absence of lymph node metastases (see Adjuvant Systemic Therapy, below).

Progesterone receptors may be a more sensitive indicator than estrogen receptors of patients who may respond to hormonal manipulation. Up to 80% of patients with metastatic progesterone receptor-positive tumors improve with hormonal manipulation. Receptors have no relationship to response to chemotherapy.

The estrogen, progesterone, and HER-2/*neu* receptor status and proliferative indices of the tumor should be determined at the time of initial biopsy. This is performed on paraffin-fixed tissue by immunohistochemistry. HER-2/*neu* assessment in breast cancer by immunohistochemistry is appropriate for patients with tumors that score 3+. Fluorescence in situ hybridization (FISH) is recommended for women with 2+ immunohistochemistry scores to more accurately assess HER-2/*neu* amplification and provide better prognostic information. Receptor status may change after hormonal therapy, radiotherapy, or chemotherapy.

Konecny G et al: Quantitative association between HER-2/*neu* and steroid hormone receptors in hormone receptor-positive primary breast cancer. J Natl Cancer Inst 2003;95:142.

CURATIVE TREATMENT

Treatment may be curative or palliative. Curative treatment is advised for clinical stage I, II, and III disease (Table 17–2). Patients with locally advanced (T3, T4) and even inflammatory tumors may be cured with multimodality therapy, but in most palliation is all that can be expected. Palliative treatment is appropriate for all patients with stage IV disease and for previously treated patients who develop distant metastases or who have unresectable local cancers.

The growth potential of tumors and host resistance factors vary widely from patient to patient and may be altered during the course of the disease. The doubling time of breast cancer cells ranges from several weeks in a rapidly growing lesion to a year in a slowly growing one. Assuming that the rate of doubling is constant and that the neoplasm originates in one cell, a carcinoma with a doubling time of 100 days may not reach clinically detectable size (1 cm) for about 8 years. Rapidly growing cancers have a much shorter preclinical course and a greater tendency to metastasize by the time a breast mass is discovered.

The long preclinical growth phase and the tendency of breast cancers to metastasize have led clinicians to believe that most breast cancer is a systemic disease at the time of diagnosis. Although it may be true that breast cancer cells are released from the tumor prior to diagnosis, variations in the host–tumor relationship prohibit the growth of disseminated disease in many patients. Clearly, not all breast cancer is systemic at the time of diagnosis. For this reason, a pessimistic attitude concerning the management of breast cancer is unwarranted. Most patients can be cured.

Controversy surrounds the timing of surgery with respect to the menstrual cycle. Some suggest that operation during the time of unopposed estrogen adversely affects survival, but most studies support no such effect. Several randomized trials are currently examining this question.

Choice of Primary Therapy

The extent of disease and its biologic aggressiveness are the principal determinants of the outcome of primary therapy. Clinical and pathologic staging help in assessing extent of disease (Table 17–2), but each is to some extent imprecise. Other factors, such as DNA flow cytometry, tumor grade, hormone receptor assays, and oncogene amplification, may be of prognostic value but are not important in determining the type of local therapy.

Controversy surrounds the choice of primary therapy of stage I, II, and III breast carcinoma. A number of states require physicians to inform patients of alternative treatment methods in the management of breast cancer. Currently, the standard of care for stage I, stage II, and most stage III cancer is surgical resection.

Breast-Conserving Therapy

Many nonrandomized trials, the randomized Milan trial, and a large randomized trial conducted by the National Surgical Adjuvant Breast and Bowel Project (NSABP) in the United States show that disease-free survival rates are similar for patients treated by partial mastectomy plus axillary dissection followed by radiation therapy and for those treated by modified radical mastectomy (total mastectomy plus axillary dissection). All patients whose axillary nodes contained tumor received adjuvant chemotherapy.

In the NSABP trial, patients were randomized to three treatment types: (1) "lumpectomy" (removal of the tumor with *confirmed* tumor-free margins) plus whole breast irradiation, (2) lumpectomy alone, and (3) total mastectomy. All patients underwent axillary lymph node dissection, and some had tumors as large as 4 cm with (or without) palpable axillary lymph nodes. With 20 years of follow-up, the lowest local recurrence rate was among patients treated with lumpectomy and postoperative irradiation; the highest—nearly 40% at 20 years of follow-up—was among patients treated with lumpectomy alone. However, no statistically significant differences were observed in overall or disease-free survival among the three treatment groups. This study shows that lumpectomy and axillary dissection with postoperative radiation therapy are as effective as modified radical mastectomy for the management of patients with stage I and stage II breast cancer.

The results of these and other trials have demonstrated that much less aggressive surgical treatment of the primary lesion than has previously been thought necessary gives equivalent therapeutic results and may preserve an acceptable cosmetic appearance.

Tumor size is a major consideration in determining the feasibility of breast conservation. The lumpectomy trial of the NSABP randomized patients with tumors as large as 4 cm. To achieve an acceptable cosmetic result, the patient must have a breast of sufficient size to enable excision of a 4-cm tumor without considerable deformity. Therefore, large size is only a relative contraindication. Subareolar tumors, also difficult to excise without deformity, are not contraindications to breast conservation. Clinically detectable multifocality is a relative contraindication to breast-conserving surgery, as is fixation to the chest wall or skin or involvement of the nipple or overlying skin. The patient—not the surgeon—should be the judge of what is cosmetically acceptable.

Axillary dissection is valuable in preventing axillary recurrences, in staging cancer, and in planning therapy. Intraoperative lymphatic mapping and sentinel node dissection identify lymph nodes most likely to harbor metastases if present in the axillary nodes. Numerous studies have confirmed the validity of this technique. Ongoing trials are examining the replacement of formal axillary dissection with sentinel node dissection. A trial from Milan with very short follow-up showed no difference between axillary dissection and sentinel node biopsy in node-negative women. Results to date suggest that sentinel node biopsy can safely replace axillary dissection for staging and treatment in histopathologically node-negative women at experienced centers. At an international consensus conference in Philadelphia in April 2001, participants recommended sentinel node biopsy as an alternative to axillary dissection in selected patients with invasive cancer. A trial by the American College of Surgeons Oncology Group is examining the role of sentinel node dissection without axillary dissection for node-positive women. Bone marrow biopsy with examination by immunocytochemistry to detect early metastases may be as sensitive a staging procedure as axillary dissection and may identify patients at high risk for disseminating disease.

Recommendations

Earlier consensus held that breast-conserving surgery with radiation was the preferred form of treatment for patients with early-stage breast cancer. Despite the numerous randomized trials showing no survival benefit of mastectomy over breast-conserving partial mastectomy and irradiation, breast-conserving surgery appears underutilized and mastectomy remains the more common treatment. About 25% of patients in the United States with stage I or stage II breast cancer are treated with breast-conserving surgery and radiation therapy, compared with 75% treated with mastectomy. Use of breast-conserving surgery and radiation therapy varies by region of the country, ranging from 15% in the South Central United States to 30% in the Pacific Region.

Modified radical mastectomy (total mastectomy plus axillary lymph node dissection) has been the standard therapy for most patients with breast cancer. This operation removes the entire breast, overlying skin, nipple, and areolar complex as well as the underlying pectoralis fascia with the axillary lymph nodes in continuity. The major advantage of modified radical mastectomy is that radiation therapy may not be necessary. The disadvantage, of course, is the psychological impact associated with breast loss. Radical mastectomy, which removes the underlying pectoralis muscle, should be performed rarely, if at all. Axillary node dissection is not indicated for noninfiltrating cancers, because nodal metastases are rarely present. Skin-sparing mastectomy is currently gaining favor but is appropriate in only a small subgroup of patients. Radiotherapy after partial mastectomy consists of 5–6 weeks of five daily fractions to a total dose of 5000–6000 cGy. Some radiation oncologists use a boost dose. Currently several studies are under way examining the utility and recurrence rates after intraoperative radiation or dose-dense radiation in which the course of radiation is shortened. Current studies suggest that radiotherapy after mastectomy may improve survival, and meta-analyses suggest radiation after lumpectomy may improve survival. The use of radiation in mastectomy patients is being further researched in a large cooperative trial to better identify which subgroups will benefit. Researchers are also examining the utility of axillary irradiation as an alternative to axillary dissection in the clinically node-negative patient with sentinel node metastases.

Preoperatively, full discussion with the patient regarding the rationale for operation and various alternative forms of treatment is essential. Breast-conserving surgery and radiation should be offered whenever possible, since most patients would prefer to save the breast. Breast reconstruction, immediate or delayed, should be discussed with patients who choose or require mastectomy. Patients should have an interview with a reconstructive plastic surgeon to discuss options prior to making a decision regarding reconstruction. Time is well spent preoperatively in educating the patient and family about these matters.

Adjuvant Systemic Therapy

Following surgery and radiation therapy, chemotherapy or hormonal therapy is advocated for most patients with curable breast cancer. The objective of adjuvant systemic therapy is to eliminate the occult metastases responsible for late recurrences while they are microscopic and most vulnerable to anticancer agents. In addition, adjuvant chemotherapy may decrease local recurrence in patients treated with breast conservation, whereas adjuvant hormonal manipulation decreases contralateral breast cancer occurrence.

Even the earliest studies comparing placebo with chemotherapy drugs having minimal activity, such as L-phenylalanine mustard, showed an improvement in both disease-free and overall survival for women who were disease free postoperatively. The landmark study from Milan evaluating the effect of 1 year of adjuvant cyclophosphamide, methotrexate, and fluorouracil (CMF) given on days 1 and 8 of each month for 12 months showed a significant improvement in survival for premenopausal women with node-positive disease. After 20 years of follow-up, significant improvement in survival persisted among those receiving chemotherapy. CMF rapidly became the standard management for premenopausal women with node-positive breast cancer. Subsequently, the use of chemotherapy for postmenopausal women and those at less risk than node-positive women was evaluated. Systemic chemotherapy improved survival in all groups of women treated. The improvement in survival for patients treated appears to be about 30% of the patients' risk of death; that is, a woman with a 30% chance of recurrence and death derives about a 10% overall improvement in survival. This risk-reduction analysis has been confirmed in numerous studies and meta-analyses.

On the basis of the superiority of anthracycline-containing regimens in metastatic breast cancer, both doxorubicin and epirubicin have been studied extensively in the adjuvant setting and have been compared to CMF regimens. Studies comparing Adriamycin (doxorubicin) and cyclophosphamide (AC) or epirubicin and cyclophosphamide (EC) with CMF have shown that treatment with anthracycline-containing regimens are at least as effective, and perhaps more effective, as treatment with CMF. The NSABP B-23 compared four cycles of AC with six cycles of CMF and demonstrated the equivalence of these two regimens in node-negative, estrogen receptor (ER)-negative disease. Whereas four cycles of AC or EC have not demonstrated improved survival compared to CMF, the use of six cycles of fluorouracil plus AC (FAC) or fluorouracil plus EC (FEC) has shown improved survival compared to CMF alone. For node-negative patients, most oncologists offer four cycles of AC or six cycles of CMF in the adjuvant setting.

For node-positive patients, taxanes are now frequently combined with anthracycline-based regimens. The Cancer and Leukemia Group B (CALGB) study comparing four cycles of AC to four cycles of AC followed by four cycles of paclitaxel showed about a 20% proportional reduction in recurrence and a 4% absolute improvement in disease-free survival with the use of paclitaxel. Paclitaxel is now approved for and increasingly employed as adjuvant therapy in node-positive breast cancer.

Unfortunately, a subsequent study by the NSABP failed to show any benefits of the use of paclitaxel except in ER-negative patients with positive nodes. A 2002 National Institutes of Health (NIH) consensus panel felt that firm conclusions about the use of taxanes could not be drawn and recommended that patients receive adjuvant taxanes only in the context of a clinical trial. However, based on trends in improved survival, many oncologists add a taxane to AC for node-positive women. A trial comparing six cycles of FAC to six cycles of docetaxel, doxorubicin, and cyclophosphamide (TAC) showed an improvement in disease-free survival for patients receiving the addition of paclitaxel. This benefit was most marked for patients with positive nodes and was seen in both ER-negative and ER-positive tumors. Until more information is obtained, the role of taxanes in the adjuvant setting remains unclear.

Controversy exists as to whether patients whose tumors overexpress the HER-2/*neu* oncogene benefit more from anthracycline regimens than from CMF regimens. Retrospective analysis of randomized trials suggests that patients with HER-2/*neu* overexpression may benefit more from doxorubicin than patients with

HER-2/*neu*-negative disease. These retrospective studies have numerous problems, including the analysis of HER-2/*neu* on paraffin tissue blocks.

The overall duration of adjuvant chemotherapy still remains uncertain. However, based on the meta-analysis performed in the Oxford Overview (Early Breast Cancer Trialists' Collaborative Group), the current recommendation is for 3–6 months of the commonly used regimens. The addition of taxanes required an additional duration of therapy of up to 6 months. Recently, increasing the frequency of chemotherapy administration (dose-dense chemotherapy) has been shown to be superior to standard dosing.

Adjuvant hormonal therapy is also highly effective in decreasing recurrence and mortality in women with ER-positive tumors. The standard regimen has been tamoxifen for 5 years. Hormonal therapy decreases the risk of mortality by approximately 25%. This appears to be effective regardless of age and may be used in both premenopausal and postmenopausal women. More recently, the aromatase inhibitors have been shown to be effective in the adjuvant setting. The large Arimidex, Tamoxifen, Alone or in Combination (ATAC) trial in postmenopausal women with ER-positive disease showed improved disease-free survival in patients treated with anastrozole compared to those treated with tamoxifen alone or even with the combination of tamoxifen and anastrozole. In addition, anastrozole showed a decrease of over 50% in the recurrence of contralateral breast tumors and fewer side effects such as endometrial cancers, hot flushes, and thromboembolic events. Anastrozole is increasingly being used in the adjuvant setting in postmenopausal women. The American Society of Clinical Oncology, however, has recommended the use of tamoxifen for adjuvant hormonal therapy in the absence of significant contraindications; anastrozole is recommended when there are contraindications to tamoxifen.

Use of high-dose chemotherapy with stem cell support has not demonstrated a consistent, favorable impact on survival and should not be used outside of clinical trials. Although it is clear that dose intensity to a specific threshold is essential, there is no clear benefit to high-dose therapy with stem cell support.

An NIH consensus conference has reexamined the standards for adjuvant therapy of breast cancer. Since the last conference on this topic in 1990, the long-term advantage of systemic therapy has been further established. In the past 10 years, no new prognostic factors have been validated to aid in the selection of patients for adjuvant treatment. Its use should be based on the patient's age; on the size, histopathologic grade, and hormone receptor status of the breast tumor; and on the status of the regional lymph nodes. The value of HER-2/*neu*, *p53*, angiogenesis factors, and vascular invasion is being investigated, but as yet they are not proven prognostic factors. Studies are being conducted evaluating trastuzumab in the adjuvant setting in a group of patients whose tumors overexpress HER-2/*neu*. The panel concluded that regardless of other factors, adjuvant systemic chemotherapy with drug combinations improves survival and should be used for most women who have potentially curable breast cancer. The use of anthracyclines is superior to combinations without anthracyclines. Tamoxifen should be used as a systemic agent in all women whose tumors are hormone receptor positive—regardless of age, menopausal status, or other prognostic factors. HER-2/*neu* status should not affect the choice of agents or the use of hormone therapy. Ovarian ablation in premenopausal patients with estrogen receptor-positive tumors may produce a benefit similar to that of adjuvant systemic chemotherapy. Taxanes have demonstrated benefit in patients with metastatic cancer and are being used in node-negative patients. Adjuvant systemic therapy should not be given to women who have small node-negative breast cancers with favorable histologic subtypes, such as mucinous or tubular carcinoma.

In practice, most medical oncologists are currently using systemic adjuvant therapy for patients with either node-negative or node-positive breast cancer. Prognostic factors other than nodal status being used to determine the patient's risks are tumor size, estrogen and progesterone receptor status, nuclear grade, histologic type, proliferative rate, and oncogene expression (Table 17–4). The assumption is made that all patients with

Table 17–4. Prognostic factors in node-negative breast cancer.

Prognostic Factor	Increased Recurrence	Decreased Recurrence
Size	T3, T2	T1, T0
Hormone receptors	Negative	Positive
DNA flow cytometry	Aneuploid	Diploid
Histologic grade	High	Low
Tumor labeling index	< 3%	> 3%
S phase fraction	> 5%	< 5%
Lymphatic or vascular invasion	Present	Absent
Cathepsin D	High	Low
HER-2/*neu* oncogene	High	Low
Epidermal growth factor receptor	High	Low

node-negative aggressive tumors should receive adjuvant therapy except those who have serious coexistent medical problems. In general, systemic chemotherapy decreases the chance of recurrence by about 30%. Most patients tolerate at least tamoxifen. The use of chemotherapy prior to resection of the primary tumor (neoadjuvant) is gaining popularity. This enables the assessment of in vivo chemosensitivity. A complete tumor response in vivo prior to operation appears to be associated with improvement in survival. Neoadjuvant chemotherapy also permits breast conservation by shrinking the primary tumor in women who would otherwise need mastectomy for local control.

Important questions remaining to be answered are the timing and duration of adjuvant and neoadjuvant chemotherapy, which chemotherapeutic agents should be applied for which subgroups of patients, the use of combinations of hormonal therapy and chemotherapy, and the value of prognostic factors other than hormone receptors in predicting response to adjuvant therapy. Adjuvant systemic therapy is not generally used in patients with small tumors and those with negative lymph nodes who have favorable tumor markers. However, a small disease-free survival benefit, even in patients with small favorable tumors, has been suggested. It appears that adjuvant systemic therapy benefits all breast cancer patients, but the clinician must decide if the benefits outweigh the risks, complications, and expense.

Adjuvant Therapy for Breast Cancer. NIH Consensus Statement 2000. November 1–3;17(4):1–35.

Cady B et al: The surgeon's role in outcome in contemporary breast cancer. Surg Oncol Clin North Am 2000;9:119.

Delaney G: Recent advances in the use of radiotherapy to treat early breast cancer. Curr Opin Obstet Gynecol 2005;17:27.

Early Breast Cancer Trialists' Collaborative Group: Favourable and unfavourable effects on long-term survival of radiotherapy for early breast cancer: an overview of the randomised trials. Lancet 2000;355:1757.

Fisher B et al: Treatment of axillary lymph node-negative, estrogen receptor-negative breast cancer: updated findings from National Surgical Adjuvant Breast and Bowel Project clinical trials. J Natl Cancer Inst 2004;96:1823.

Fisher B et al: Twenty-year follow-up of a randomized trial comparing total mastectomy, lumpectomy, and lumpectomy plus irradiation for the treatment of invasive breast cancer. N Engl J Med 2002;347:1233.

Howell A et al: ATAC Trialists' Group: Results of the ATAC (Arimidex, Tamoxifen, Alone or in Combination) trial after completion of 5 years' adjuvant treatment for breast cancer. Lancet 2005;365:60.

Love RR: Meeting highlights: international consensus panel on the treatment of primary breast cancer. J Clin Oncol 2002;20:1955.

Muller V et al: Bone marrow micrometastases and circulating tumor cells: current aspects and future perspectives. Breast Cancer Res 2004;6:258.

Rouzier R et al: Incidence and prognostic significance of complete axillary downstaging after primary chemotherapy in breast cancer patients with T1 to T3 tumors and cytologically proven axillary metastatic lymph nodes. J Clin Oncol 2002;20:1304.

Veronesi U et al: Full-dose intraoperative radiotherapy with electrons during breast-conserving surgery. Arch Surg 2003;138:1253.

Veronesi U et al: Twenty-year follow-up of randomized study comparing breast-conserving surgery with radical mastectomy for early breast cancer. N Engl J Med 2002;347:1227.

Vinh-Hung V et al: Breast-conserving surgery with or without radiotherapy: pooled-analysis for risks of ipsilateral breast tumor recurrence and mortality. J Natl Cancer Inst 2004;96:115.

Vogel C et al: Efficacy and safety of trastuzumab as a single agent in first-line treatment of HER2-overexpressing metastatic breast cancer. J Clin Oncol 2002;3:719.

Wilke LG et al: Sentinel lymph node biopsy in patients with early-stage breast cancer: status of the National Clinical Trials. Surg Clin North Am 2003;83:901.

PALLIATIVE TREATMENT

This section covers palliative therapy of disseminated disease incurable by surgery (stage IV).

Radiotherapy

Palliative radiotherapy may be advised for primary treatment of locally advanced cancers with distant metastases to control ulceration, pain, and other manifestations in the breast and regional nodes. Irradiation of the breast and chest wall and the axillary, internal mammary, and supraclavicular nodes should be undertaken in an attempt to cure locally advanced and inoperable lesions when there is no evidence of distant metastases. A small number of patients in this group are cured in spite of extensive breast and regional node involvement.

Palliative irradiation is of value also in the treatment of certain bone or soft tissue metastases to control pain or avoid fracture. Radiotherapy is especially useful in the treatment of isolated bony metastasis, chest wall recurrences, brain metastases, and acute spinal cord compression.

Hormone & Targeted Therapy

Disseminated disease may shrink—or grow less rapidly—after endocrine therapy such as administration of hormones (eg, estrogens, androgens, progestins; see Table 17–5); ablation of the ovaries, adrenals, or pituitary; or administration of drugs that block hormone receptor sites (eg, antiestrogens) or drugs that block the synthesis of hormones (eg, aromatase inhibitors). Hormonal manipulation is usually more successful in postmenopausal women even if they have received estrogen replacement therapy. Treatment should be

Table 17–5. Agents commonly used for hormonal management of metastatic breast cancer.

Drug	Action	Dose, Route, Frequency	Major Side Effects
Tamoxifen citrate (Nolvadex)	Selective estrogen receptor modulator	20 mg by mouth daily	Hot flushes, uterine bleeding, thrombophlebitis, rash
Fulvestrant (Faslodex)	Steroidal estrogen receptor (ER) antagonist	250 mg intramuscularly monthly	Gastrointestinal upset, headache, back pain, hot flushes, pharyngitis
Toremifene citrate (Fareston)	Selective estrogen receptor modulator	40 mg by mouth daily	Hot flushes, sweating, nausea, vaginal discharge, dry eyes, dizziness
Diethylstilbestrol (DES)	Estrogen	5 mg by mouth three times daily	Fluid retention, uterine bleeding, thrombophlebitis, nausea
Megestrol acetate (Megace)	Progestin	40 mg by mouth four times daily	Fluid retention
Letrozole (Femara)	Aromatase inhibitor	2.5 mg by mouth daily	Hot flushes, arthralgia/arthritis, myalgia
Anastrozole (Arimidex)	Aromatase inhibitor	1 mg by mouth daily	Hot flushes, skin rashes, nausea and vomiting

based on the presence of estrogen receptor protein in the primary tumor or metastases. The rate of response is nearly equal in premenopausal and postmenopausal women with ER-positive tumors. A favorable response to hormonal manipulation occurs in about one-third of patients with metastatic breast cancer. Of those whose tumors contain estrogen receptors, the response is about 60% and perhaps as high as 80% for patients whose tumors contain progesterone receptors as well. Because only 5–10% of women whose tumors do not contain estrogen receptors respond, they should not receive hormonal therapy except in unusual circumstances, eg, in an older patient who cannot tolerate chemotherapy. Because the quality of life during a remission induced by endocrine manipulation is often superior to a remission following cytotoxic chemotherapy, it is usually best to try endocrine manipulation first in cases in which the estrogen receptor status is unknown. Additionally, women with ER-positive tumors who fail hormone therapy or experience progression should be placed on a different form of hormonal manipulation. Women who have failed tamoxifen and gone on to a third-generation aromatase inhibitor have shown equal if not better response than those who respond to tamoxifen. When receptor status is unknown but the disease is progressing rapidly or involves visceral organs, however, endocrine therapy is rarely successful, and introducing it may waste valuable time.

In addition to radiotherapy, bisphosphonate therapy has shown excellent results in delaying and reducing skeletal events in women with bony metastases. Bisphosphonates are also sometimes used in conjunction with aromatase inhibitors to decrease the potential bony events associated with those drugs. Further research is being conducted examining the utility of bisphosphonates in conjunction with other therapies and in early breast cancer treatment.

In general, only one type of therapy should be given at a time unless it is necessary to irradiate a destructive lesion of weight-bearing bone while the patient is on another regimen. The regimen should be changed only if the disease is clearly progressing. This is especially important for patients with destructive bone metastases, since changes in the status of these lesions are difficult to determine radiographically. A plan of therapy that would simultaneously minimize toxicity and maximize benefits is often best achieved by hormonal manipulation.

The choice of endocrine therapy depends on the menopausal status of the patient. Women within 1 year of their last menstrual period are arbitrarily considered to be premenopausal, whereas women whose menstruation ceased more than a year ago are postmenopausal. If endocrine therapy is the initial choice, it is referred to as primary hormonal manipulation; subsequent endocrine treatment is called secondary or tertiary hormonal manipulation.

Trastuzumab is a monoclonal antibody that binds to HER-2/*neu* receptors on the cancer cell and has been shown to be highly effective in HER-2/*neu*-expressive cancers. In metastatic disease, for patients with HER-2/*neu* oncogene overexpression, trastuzumab has been shown to increase survival when combined with AC or paclitaxel. Ongoing studies are evaluating trastuzumab in combination with others for adjuvant chemotherapy regimens.

A. The Premenopausal Patient

1. Primary hormonal therapy—The potent antiestrogen tamoxifen is the endocrine treatment of choice in the premenopausal patient. Tamoxifen is usually given orally in a dose of 20 mg daily. There is no significant difference in survival or response between tamoxifen therapy and bilateral oophorectomy. Tamoxifen is by far the most common and preferred method of hormonal manipulation for both premenopausal and postmenopausal women. The average remission is about 12 months. Tamoxifen can be given with little morbidity and few side effects. Toremifene, a tamoxifen analogue, is currently available and has similar side effects but is less likely to cause uterine cancer. Controversy continues about whether a response to tamoxifen is predictive of probable success with other forms of endocrine manipulation.

Bilateral oophorectomy is less desirable than primary hormonal manipulation in premenopausal women because tamoxifen is so well tolerated. Oophorectomy can be achieved rapidly and safely by surgery, however, or if the patient is a poor operative risk, by irradiation of the ovaries. Chemical ovarian ablation using a gonadotropin-releasing hormone analogue can also be utilized. Oophorectomy presumably works by eliminating estrogens, progestins, and androgens, which stimulate growth of the tumor.

2. Secondary or tertiary hormonal therapy—Although patients who do not respond to tamoxifen or oophorectomy should be treated with cytotoxic drugs, those who respond and then relapse may subsequently respond to another form of endocrine treatment (Table 17–5). The initial choice for secondary endocrine manipulation has not been clearly defined.

Patients who improve after oophorectomy but subsequently relapse should receive tamoxifen or an aromatase inhibitor. If one fails, the other may be tried but is not likely to succeed. Megestrol acetate may be considered. Megestrol is a progestational agent. Both drugs cause less morbidity and mortality than surgical adrenalectomy, can be discontinued once the patient improves, and are not associated with the many problems of postsurgical hypoadrenalism, so that patients who require chemotherapy are more easily managed. Adrenalectomy or hypophysectomy used in the past induced regression in 30–50% of patients who previously responded to oophorectomy, but these procedures are rarely done today. Pharmacologic hormonal manipulation has in large part replaced these invasive procedures. Toremifene has shown no added value in women whose tumors no longer respond to tamoxifen. Aromatase inhibitors are of value in patients who responded to tamoxifen or oophorectomy but then progress.

B. The Postmenopausal Patient

1. Primary hormonal therapy—Tamoxifen, 20 mg daily, or anastrozole, 1 mg daily, is the initial therapy of choice for postmenopausal women with metastatic breast cancer amenable to endocrine manipulation. Anastrozole (an aromatase inhibitor) has fewer side effects than tamoxifen, the former therapy of choice, and is at least equally as effective. The main side effects of tamoxifen are nausea, vomiting, skin rash, and hot flushes. Rarely, it may induce hypercalcemia in patients with bony metastases. The main side effects of anastrozole are similar but lower in incidence; however, osteoporosis can occur.

2. Secondary or tertiary hormonal therapy—Postmenopausal patients who do not respond to tamoxifen or anastrozole should be given cytotoxic drugs such as CMF or AC. Postmenopausal women who respond initially to tamoxifen or anastrozole but later manifest progressive disease may be crossed over. Aromatase inhibitors have been available for the treatment of advanced breast cancer in postmenopausal women who fail tamoxifen treatment. Recent trials comparing an aromatase inhibitor, anastrozole, with tamoxifen suggest that the former is just as effective and has fewer side effects. Aromatase inhibitors recently have achieved the status of primary hormonal therapy in postmenopausal women. Clinical trials have proved the efficacy of anastrozole and toremifene for such purposes. Androgens have many toxicities and should rarely be used. As in premenopausal patients, neither hypophysectomy nor adrenalectomy is still being performed.

Chemotherapy

Cytotoxic drugs should be considered for the treatment of metastatic breast cancer (1) if visceral metastases are present (especially brain or lymphangitic pulmonary), (2) if hormonal treatment is unsuccessful or the disease has progressed after an initial response to hormonal manipulation, or (3) if the tumor is ER negative. The most useful single chemotherapeutic agent to date is doxorubicin (Adriamycin), with a response rate of 40–50%. Single agents are rarely used but rather are given in combination with other cytotoxic drugs.

Combination chemotherapy using multiple agents has proved to be more effective, with objectively observed favorable responses achieved in 60–80% of patients with stage IV disease. Various combinations of drugs have been used, and clinical trials are continuing in an effort to improve results and reduce undesirable side effects. Nausea and vomiting are well controlled with drugs that directly affect the central nervous system, such as ondansetron and granisetron. These drugs are selective antagonists of serotonin receptors in the central nervous system and block nausea caused by cytotoxic chemotherapy. Doxorubicin (40 mg/m^2 intravenously on day 1) and cyclophosphamide (200 mg/m^2 orally on days 3–6) produce an objective response in about 85% of patients so treated. Other chemotherapeutic regimens have consisted of various combinations of drugs, including cyclophosphamide, vincristine, methotrexate, fluorouracil, and taxanes, with response rates ranging up to 60–70%. Prior adjuvant chemotherapy does not seem to alter response rates in patients who relapse. Growth factors such as erythropoietin (epoetin alfa), which stimulates red blood cell production and mimics the effect of erythropoietin, and filgrastim (granulocyte colony-stimulating factor; G-CSF), which stimulates proliferation and differentiation of hematopoietic cells, prevent life-threatening anemia and neutropenia seen commonly with high doses of chemotherapy. These agents greatly diminish the incidence of infections that may complicate the use of myelosuppressive chemotherapy.

The taxanes (paclitaxel and docetaxel) have been shown to be very effective for patients with metastatic breast cancer. They have usually been given after failure of combination chemotherapy for metastatic disease or relapse shortly after completion of adjuvant chemotherapy. However, they are becoming more important in both the management of metastatic disease and even adjuvant therapy. These drugs have response rates of 30–40% in patients with metastatic disease. They may be especially valuable in treating anthracycline-resistant tumors. Both agents are currently being used after treatment with anthracyclines in patients with advanced disease as well as in adjuvant and neoadjuvant settings. High-dose chemotherapy and autologous bone marrow or stem cell transplantation aroused widespread interest for the treatment of metastatic breast cancer. With this technique, the patient receives high doses of cytotoxic agents, eradicating the marrow, for which the patient subsequently undergoes autologous bone marrow or stem cell transplantation. Complete response rates are as high as 30–35%—considerably better than what can be achieved with conventional chemotherapy. Most randomized trials, however, comparing high-dose chemotherapy with stem cell support show no improvement in survival over conventional chemotherapy. A study purporting to show a survival advantage to high-dose chemotherapy in South Africa was found to be falsified and discredited. Enthusiasm for high-dose chemotherapy with stem cell support has waned, but additional studies continue and recently showed a beneficial effect in some high-risk women. The technique is extremely costly, and the treatment itself is associated with a mortality rate of about 3–7%.

Bernard-Marty C et al: Facts and controversies in systemic treatment of metastatic breast cancer. Oncologist 2004;9:617.

Cristofanilli M et al: New horizons in treating metastatic disease. Clin Breast Cancer 2001;1:276.

Fricker J: Letrozole better than tamoxifen in postmenopausal women. Lancet Oncol 2005;6:137.

Harvey HA: Optimizing bisphosphonate therapy in patients with breast cancer on endocrine therapy. Semin Oncol 2004;31(6 Suppl 12):23.

Hussain SA et al: Endocrine therapy and other targeted therapies for metastatic breast cancer. Expert Rev Anticancer Ther 2004;4:1179.

Mouridsen HT: Aromatase inhibitors in advanced breast cancer. Semin Oncol 2004;31(6 Suppl 12):3.

Pandit-Taskar N et al: Radiopharmaceutical therapy for palliation of bone pain from osseous metastases. J Nucl Med 2004;45:1358.

Slamon DJ et al: Use of chemotherapy plus a monoclonal antibody against HER2 for metastatic breast cancer that overexpresses HER2. N Engl J Med 2001;344:783.

Stadtmauer EA et al: Conventional-dose chemotherapy compared with high-dose chemotherapy plus autologous hematopoietic stem-cell transplantation for metastatic breast cancer. N Engl J Med 2000;342:1069.

PROGNOSIS

Stage of breast cancer is the most reliable indicator of prognosis (Table 17–6). Patients with disease localized to the breast and no evidence of regional spread after microscopic examination of the lymph nodes have by far the most favorable prognosis. Axillary lymph node status is the best-analyzed prognostic factor and correlates with survival at all tumor sizes. In addition, an increased number of axillary nodes involved correlates directly with lower survival rates. Estrogen and progesterone receptors are prognostic variables because patients with hormone receptor-negative tumors and no evidence of metastases to the axillary lymph nodes have a much higher recurrence rate than do patients with hormone

Table 17–6. Approximate survival (%) of patients with breast cancer by TNM stage.

TNM Stage	5 Years	10 Years
0	95	90
I	85	70
IIA	70	50
IIB	60	40
IIIA	55	30
IIIB	30	20
IV	5–10	2
All	65	30

receptor-positive tumors and no regional metastases. The histologic subtype of breast cancer (eg, medullary, lobular, colloid) seems to have little significance in prognosis once these tumors are truly invasive. Flow cytometry of tumor cells to analyze DNA index and S-phase frequency aid in prognosis. Tumors with marked aneuploidy have a poor prognosis (Table 17–4). HER-2/*neu* oncogene amplification, epidermal growth factor receptors, and cathepsin D may have some prognostic value, but no markers are as significant as lymph node metastases in predicting outcome.

The mortality rate of breast cancer patients exceeds that of age-matched normal controls for nearly 20 years. Thereafter, the mortality rates are equal, though deaths that occur among breast cancer patients are often directly the result of tumor. Five-year statistics do not accurately reflect the final outcome of therapy.

When cancer is localized to the breast, with no evidence of regional spread after pathologic examination, the clinical cure rate with most accepted methods of therapy is 75% to greater than 90%. Exceptions to this generalization may be related to the hormonal receptor content of the tumor, tumor size, host resistance, or associated illness. Patients with small mammographically detected estrogen and progesterone receptor-positive tumors and no evidence of axillary spread have a 5-year survival rate greater than 95%. When the axillary lymph nodes are involved with tumor, the survival rate drops to 50–70% at 5 years and probably around 25–40% at 10 years. In general, breast cancer appears to be somewhat more malignant in younger than in older women, and this may be related to the fact that fewer younger women have ER-positive tumors.

For those patients whose disease progresses despite treatment, supportive group therapy may improve survival. As they approach the end of life, such patients will require meticulous efforts at palliative care (see Chapter 5).

Hayes DF: Prognostic and predictive factors for breast cancer: translating technology to oncology. J Clin Oncol 2005;23: 1596.

FOLLOW-UP CARE

After primary therapy, patients with breast cancer should be followed up for life for at least two reasons: to detect recurrences and to observe the opposite breast for a second primary carcinoma. Local and distant recurrences occur most frequently within the first 2 years. During this period, the patient should be examined every 6 months. Thereafter, examination is done annually. Special attention is paid to the contralateral breast, because 10–20% of patients will develop a new primary breast malignancy. The patient should examine her own breast monthly, and a mammogram should be obtained annually. In some cases, metastases are dormant for long periods and may appear 10–15 years or longer after removal of the primary tumor. Estrogen and progestational agents are rarely used for a patient free of disease after treatment of primary breast cancer, particularly if the tumor was hormone receptor positive. Studies nevertheless have failed to show an adverse effect of hormonal agents in patients who are free of disease. Even pregnancy has not been clearly associated with shortened survival of patients rendered disease free—yet most oncologists are reluctant to advise a young patient with breast cancer that she may become pregnant, and most are less than enthusiastic about prescribing hormone replacement therapy for the postmenopausal breast cancer patient. The use of estrogen replacement therapy may be considered for a woman with a history of breast cancer after discussion of the benefits and risks of such therapy for conditions such as osteoporosis and hot flushes, but is not recommended.

Local Recurrence

The incidence of local recurrence correlates with tumor size, the presence and number of involved axillary nodes, the histologic type of tumor, the presence of skin edema or skin and fascia fixation with the primary tumor, and the type of initial local (breast) therapy. As many as 8% of patients develop local recurrence on the chest wall after total mastectomy and axillary dissection. When the axillary nodes are not involved, the local recurrence rate is less than 5%, but the rate is as high as 25% when they are heavily involved. A similar difference in local recurrence rate was noted between small and large tumors. Factors such as multifocal cancer, in situ tumors, positive resection margins, chemotherapy, and radiotherapy have an effect on local recurrence in patients treated with breast-conserving surgery.

Chest wall recurrences usually appear within the first 2 years but may occur as late as 15 or more years after mastectomy. All suspicious nodules and skin lesions should be biopsied. Local excision or localized radiotherapy may be feasible if an isolated nodule is present. If lesions are multiple or accompanied by evidence of regional involvement in the internal mammary or supraclavicular nodes, the disease is best managed by radiation treatment of the entire chest wall including the parasternal, supraclavicular, and axillary areas and usually by systemic therapy.

Local recurrence after mastectomy usually signals the presence of widespread disease and is an indication for studies to search for evidence of metastases. Most patients with locally recurrent tumor will develop distant metastases within 2 years. When there is no evidence of metastases beyond the chest wall and regional nodes, irradiation for cure or complete local excision should be attempted. Patients with local recurrence may be cured with local resection and radiation. After partial mastectomy, local recurrence may not have as serious a prognostic significance as after mastectomy. However, those patients who do develop a breast recurrence have a worse prognosis than those who do not. It is speculated that the ability of a cancer to recur locally after radiotherapy is a sign of aggressiveness and resistance to therapy. Completion of the mastectomy should be done for local recurrence after partial mastectomy; some of these patients will survive for prolonged periods, especially if the breast recurrence is DCIS or more than 5 years after initial treatment. Systemic chemotherapy or hormonal treatment should be used for women who develop disseminated disease or those in whom local recurrence occurs.

Edema of the Arm

Significant edema of the arm occurs in about 10–30% of patients after axillary dissection with or without mastectomy. It occurs more commonly if radiotherapy has been given or if there was postoperative infection. Partial mastectomy with radiation to the axillary lymph nodes is followed by chronic edema of the arm in 10–20% of patients. Because axillary dissection is more accurate for staging operation than axillary sampling, it is recommended that at least level I and II lymph nodes be removed, in combination with partial mastectomy. Sentinel lymph node dissection offers accurate staging without the removal of level I and II nodes and has a much lower risk of lymphedema for node-negative patients. Judicious use of radiotherapy, with treatment fields carefully planned to spare the axilla as much as possible, can greatly diminish the incidence of edema, which will occur in only 5% of patients if no radiotherapy is given to the axilla after a partial mastectomy and lymph node dissection.

Late or secondary edema of the arm may develop years after treatment, as a result of axillary recurrence or of infection in the hand or arm, with obliteration of lymphatic channels. Infection in the arm or hand on the dissected side should be treated with antibiotics, rest, and elevation. When edema develops, careful examination of the axilla for recurrence should be done. If there is no sign of recurrence, the swollen extremity should be treated with rest and elevation. A mild diuretic may be helpful. If there is no improvement, a compressor pump or manual decompression decreases the swelling, and the patient is then fitted with an elastic glove or sleeve. Most patients are not bothered enough by mild edema to wear an uncomfortable glove or sleeve and will treat themselves with elevation or manual decompression alone. Benzopyrones have been reported to decrease lymphedema but are not approved for this use in the United States. Rarely, edema may be severe enough to interfere with use of the limb.

Breast Reconstruction

Breast reconstruction is usually feasible after standard or modified radical mastectomy. Reconstruction should be discussed with patients prior to mastectomy, because it offers an important psychological focal point for recovery. Reconstruction is not an obstacle to the diagnosis of recurrent cancer. The most common breast reconstruction has been implantation of a silicone gel prosthesis in the subpectoral plane between the pectoralis minor and pectoralis major muscles. Although the FDA has placed a moratorium on the purely cosmetic use of silicone gel implants because of possible leakage of silicone and possible associated autoimmune phenomena, they can be used in the reconstructed patient with appropriate prior consent. Most plastic surgeons currently would place a saline-filled prosthesis rather than a silicone gel implant. Alternatively, autologous tissue can be used for reconstruction.

Autologous tissue flaps are aesthetically superior to implant reconstruction in most patients. They also have the advantage of not feeling like a foreign body to the patient. The most popular autologous technique currently is the trans-rectus abdominis muscle flap (TRAM flap), which is done by rotating the rectus abdominis muscle with attached fat and skin cephalad to make a breast mound. The free TRAM flap is done by completely removing the rectus with overlying fat and skin and using microvascular surgical techniques to reconstruct the vascular supply on the chest wall. A latissimus dorsi flap can be swung from the back but offers less fullness than the TRAM flap and is therefore less acceptable cosmetically. Reconstruction may be performed immediately (at the time of initial mastectomy) or may be delayed until later, usually when the patient has completed adjuvant therapy. When considering reconstructive options, concomitant illnesses should be considered, since the ability of an autologous flap to survive depends on medical comorbidities. In addition, the need for radiotherapy may affect the choice of reconstruction.

Risks of Pregnancy

Data are insufficient to determine whether interruption of pregnancy improves the prognosis of patients who are discovered during pregnancy to have potentially curable breast cancer and who receive definitive treatment. Theoretically, the increasingly high levels of estrogen produced by the placenta as the pregnancy progresses could be detrimental to the patient with occult metastases of hormone-sensitive breast cancer. Moreover, occult metastases are present in most patients with positive axillary nodes, and treatment by adjuvant chemotherapy could be potentially harmful to the fetus, although chemotherapy may be given to pregnant women. Under these circumstances, interruption of early pregnancy seems reasonable, with progressively less rationale for the procedure as term approaches. The decision is affected by many factors, including the patient's desire to have the baby and the generally poor prognosis when axillary nodes are involved.

Equally important is the advice regarding future pregnancy (or abortion in case of pregnancy) to be given to women of child-bearing age who have had definitive treatment for breast cancer. Under these circumstances, it must be assumed that pregnancy will be harmful if occult metastases are present, though this has not been demonstrated. Patients whose tumors are ER negative (most younger women) probably would not be affected by pregnancy. To date, no adverse effect of pregnancy on the survival of pregnant women who have had breast cancer has been demonstrated, though most oncologists advise against it.

In patients with inoperable or metastatic cancer (stage IV disease), induced abortion is usually advisable because of the possible adverse effects of hormonal treatment, radiotherapy, or chemotherapy upon the fetus.

Cocquyt VF et al: Better cosmetic results and comparable quality of life after skin-sparing mastectomy and immediate autologous breast reconstruction compared to breast conservative treatment. Br J Plast Surg 2003;56:462.

Langer S et al: Lymphatic mapping improves staging and reduces morbidity in women undergoing total mastectomy for breast carcinoma. Am Surg 2004;70:881.

van der Veen P et al: Lymphedema development following breast cancer surgery with full axillary resection. Lymphology 2004;37:206.

CARCINOMA OF THE MALE BREAST

ESSENTIALS OF DIAGNOSIS

- *A painless lump beneath the areola in a man usually over 50 years of age.*
- *Nipple discharge, retraction, or ulceration may be present.*

General Considerations

Breast cancer in men is a rare disease; the incidence is only about 1% of that in women. The average age at occurrence is about 60—somewhat older than the most common presenting age in women. There may be an increased incidence of breast cancer in men with prostate cancer. The prognosis, even in stage I cases, is worse in men than in women. Blood-borne metastases are commonly present when the male patient appears for initial treatment. These metastases may be latent and may not become manifest for many years. As in women, hormonal influences are probably related to the development of male breast cancer. There is a high incidence of both breast cancer and gynecomastia in Bantu men, theoretically owing to failure of estrogen inactivation by a liver damaged by associated liver disease. It is important to note that first-degree relatives of men with breast cancer are considered to be at high risk. This risk should be taken into account when discussing options with the patient and family. In addition, *BRCA2* mutations are common in men with breast cancer. Men with breast cancer, especially with a history of prostate cancer, should receive genetic counseling.

Clinical Findings

A painless lump, occasionally associated with nipple discharge, retraction, erosion, or ulceration, is the primary complaint. Examination usually shows a hard, ill-defined, nontender mass beneath the nipple or areola. Gynecomastia not uncommonly precedes or accompanies breast cancer in men. Nipple discharge is an uncommon presentation for breast cancer in men, but is an ominous finding associated with carcinoma in nearly 75% of cases.

Breast cancer staging is the same in men as in women. Gynecomastia and metastatic cancer from another site (eg, prostate) must be considered in the differential diagnosis. Benign tumors are rare. Biopsy settles the issue.

Treatment

Treatment consists of modified radical mastectomy in operable patients, who should be chosen by the same criteria as women with the disease. Irradiation is the first step in treating localized metastases in the skin, lymph nodes, or skeleton that are causing symptoms. Examination of the cancer for hormone receptor proteins is of value in predicting response to endocrine ablation. Men commonly have ER-positive tumors. Adjuvant chemotherapy is used for the same indications as in breast cancer in women.

Because breast cancer in men is frequently a disseminated disease, endocrine therapy is of considerable importance in its management. Tamoxifen is the main drug for management of advanced breast cancer in men. Tamoxifen (20 mg daily) should be the initial treatment. There is little experience with aromatase inhibitors, though they should be effective. Castration in advanced breast cancer is a successful measure and more beneficial than the same procedure in women but is rarely used. Objective evidence of regression may be seen in 60–70% of men with hormonal therapy—approximately twice the proportion in women. The average duration of tumor growth remission is about 30 months, and life is prolonged. Bone is the most frequent site of metastases from breast cancer in men (as in women), and hormonal therapy relieves bone pain in most patients so treated. The longer the interval between mastectomy and recurrence, the longer the tumor growth remission following treatment. As in women, there is correlation between estrogen receptors of the tumor and the likelihood of remission following hormonal therapy.

Aromatase inhibitors should replace adrenalectomy in men as it has in women. Corticosteroid therapy alone has been considered to be efficacious but probably has no value when compared with major endocrine ablation. Either tamoxifen or aromatase inhibitors may be primary or secondary hormonal manipulation.

Estrogen therapy—5 mg of diethylstilbestrol three times daily orally—may be effective hormonal manipulation after others have been successful and failed, just as in women. Androgen therapy may exacerbate bone pain. Chemotherapy should be administered for the same indications and using the same dosage schedules as for women with metastatic disease.

Prognosis

The prognosis of breast cancer is poorer in men than in women. The crude 5- and 10-year survival rates for clinical stage I breast cancer in men are about 58% and 38%, respectively. For clinical stage II disease, the 5- and 10-year survival rates are approximately 38% and 10%. The survival rates for all stages at 5 and 10 years are 36% and 17%. For those patients whose disease progresses despite treatment, meticulous efforts at palliative care are essential (see Chapter 5).

Kwiatkowska E et al: Somatic mutations in the BRCA2 gene and high frequency of allelic loss of BRCA2 in sporadic male breast cancer. Int J Cancer 2002;98:943.

Loerzel VW et al: Male breast cancer. Clin J Oncol Nurs 2004;8:191.

Weiss JR et al: Epidemiology of male breast cancer. Cancer Epidemiol Biomarkers Prev 2005;14:20.

Thoracic Wall, Pleura, Mediastinum, & Lung

18

Pierre R. Theodore, MD, & David Jablons, MD

ANATOMY & PHYSIOLOGY

ANATOMY OF THE CHEST WALL & PLEURA

The chest wall is an airtight, expandable, cone-shaped cage. Lung ventilation occurs by generation of negative pressure within the thorax due to simultaneous expansion of the rib cage and downward diaphragmatic excursion.

The ventral wall of the bony thorax is the shortest dimension. It extends from the suprasternal notch to the xiphoid—a distance of approximately 18 cm in the adult. It is formed by the vertically aligned manubrium, sternum, and xiphoid process. The first seven pairs of ribs articulate directly with the sternum, the next three pairs connect to the lower border of the preceding rib, and the last two terminate in the wall of the abdomen. The sides of the chest wall consist of the upper ten ribs, which slope obliquely downward from their posterior attachments. The posterior chest wall is formed by the 12 thoracic vertebrae, their transverse processes, and the 12 ribs (Figure 18–1). The upper ventral portion of the thoracic cage is covered by the clavicle and the subclavian vessels. Laterally, it is covered by the shoulder girdle and axillary nerves and vessels; dorsally, it is covered in part by the scapula.

The superior aperture of the thorax (also called either the thoracic inlet or the thoracic outlet) is a downwardly slanted 5- to 10-cm kidney-shaped opening bounded by the first costal cartilages and ribs laterally, the manubrium anteriorly, and the body of the first thoracic vertebra posteriorly. The inferior aperture of the thorax is bounded by the 12th vertebra and ribs posteriorly and the cartilages of the 7th to 10th ribs and the xiphisternal joint anteriorly. It is much wider than the superior aperture and is occupied by the diaphragm.

The blood supply and innervation of the chest wall are via the intercostal vessels and nerves (Figures 18–2 and 18–3), and the upper thorax also receives vessels and nerves from the cervical and axillary regions. The underside of the sternum's blood supply derives from the internal thoracic artery branches, which anastomose with the intercostal vessels along the lateral aspect of the chest wall.

The parietal pleura is the innermost lining of the chest wall and is divided into four parts: the cervical pleura (cupula), costal pleura, mediastinal pleura, and diaphragmatic pleura. The visceral pleura is a mesodermal layer investing the lungs and is continuous with the parietal pleura, joining it at the hilum of the lung. The potential pleural space is a capillary gap that normally contains only a few drops of serous fluid. However, this space may be enlarged when fluid (hydrothorax), blood (hemothorax), pus (pyothorax or empyema), lymphatic fluid (chylothorax), or air (pneumothorax) is present.

PHYSIOLOGY OF THE CHEST WALL & PLEURA

Mechanics of Respiration

Breathing entails expansion of thoracic volume by elevation of the rib cage and descent of the diaphragm. Infants, in whom the ribs have not yet assumed their oblique contour, are dependent on diaphragmatic breathing. Furthermore, accessory muscles of respiration contribute to the conformational change in the thoracic cage during periods of intense exercise or respiratory distress (Figure 18–4).

Expiration is mainly passive and depends upon elastic recoil of the lungs except with deep breathing, when the abdominal musculature contracts, pulling the rib cage downward and simultaneously elevating the diaphragm by compressing the abdominal viscera against it.

Physiology of the Pleural Space

A. Pressure

The pleural cavity pressure is normally negative, owing to the opposing forces of elastic recoil of the lung and active expansion of the space by the chest wall. During

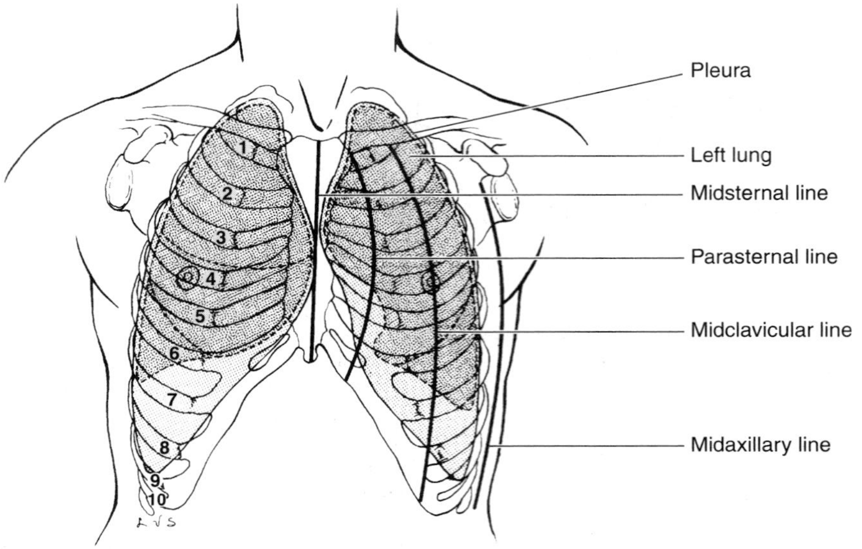

Figure 18–1. The thorax, showing rib cage, pleura, and lung fields.

quiet respiration, it varies from –15 cm H_2O with inspiration to 0–2 cm H_2O during expiration. Deep breathing may cause large pressure changes (eg, –60 cm H_2O during forced inspiration to +30 cm H_2O during vigorous expiration). Because of gravity, pleural pressure at the apex is more negative when the body is erect and changes about 0.2 cm H_2O per centimeter of vertical height.

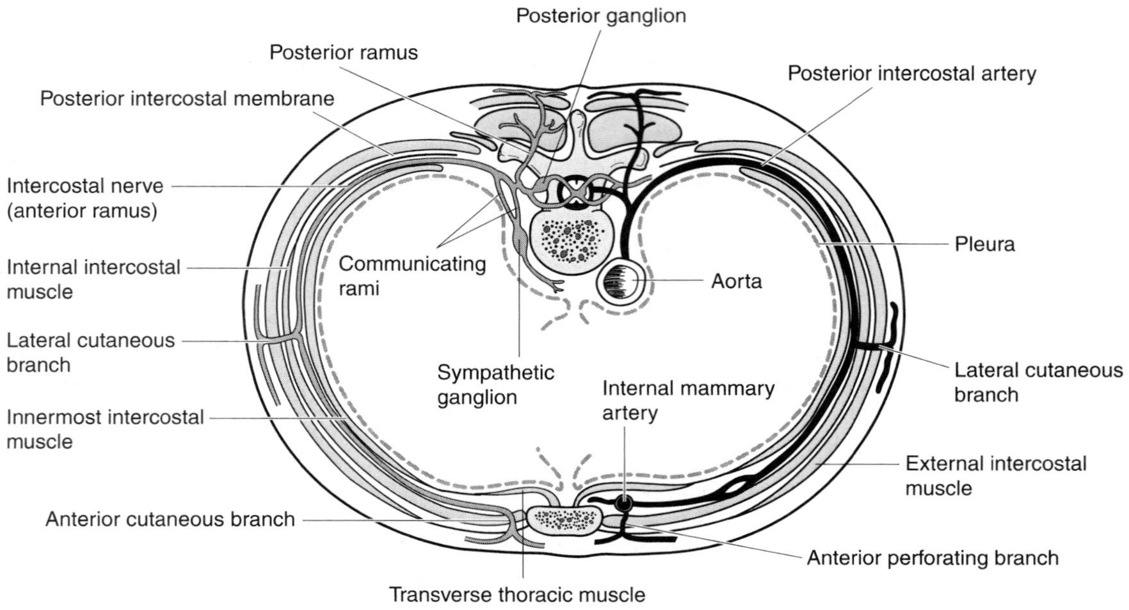

Figure 18–2. Transverse section of thorax.

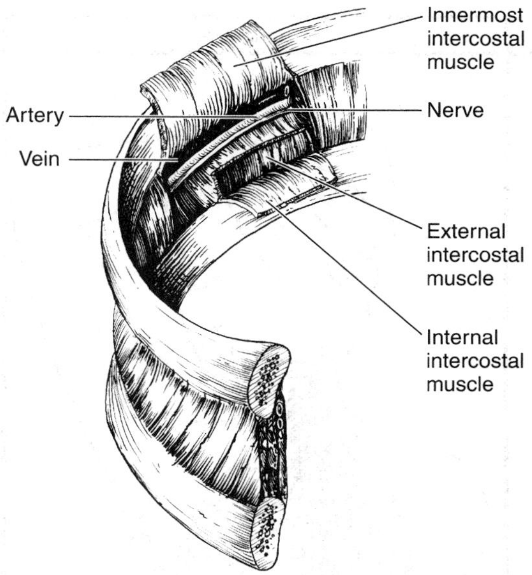

Figure 18–3. Intercostal muscles, vessels, and nerves.

B. Fluid Formation and Reabsorption

Transudation and absorption of fluid within the pleural space normally follow the Starling equation, which depends on hydrostatic, colloid, and tissue pressures in addition to permeability of the pleural membrane. In health, fluid is formed by the parietal pleura and absorbed by the visceral pleura (Figure 18–5). Systemic capillary hydrostatic pressure is 30 cm H_2O, and intrapleural negative pressure averages –5 cm H_2O. Together, these give a net hydrostatic pressure of 35 cm H_2O that causes fluid transudation from the parietal pleura. The colloid osmotic pressure of the systemic capillaries is 34 cm H_2O; this is opposed by 8 cm H_2O of pleural space osmotic pressure. Thus, a net 26 cm H_2O osmotic pressure draws fluid back into systemic capillaries. Systemic hydrostatic pressure (35 cm H_2O) exceeds osmotic capillary pressure (26 cm H_2O) by 9 cm H_2O; thus, there is a 9 cm H_2O net drive of fluid into the pleural space by systemic capillaries in the chest wall. Similar calculations for the visceral pleura involving the low-pressure pulmonary circulation will show that there is a resulting net drive of 10 cm H_2O that attracts pleural fluid into pulmonary capillaries.

In health, pleural fluid is low in protein (<100 mg/dL). When it increases in disease to about 1 g/dL, the net colloid osmotic pressure of the visceral pleural capillaries is equaled and pleural fluid reabsorption becomes dependent on lymphatic drainage. Thus, abnormal amounts of pleural fluid may accumulate (1) when hydrostatic pressure is increased, such as in heart failure; (2) when capillary permeability is increased, as in inflammatory or neoplastic disease; or (3) when colloid osmotic pressure is decreased.

ANATOMY OF THE MEDIASTINUM

The mediastinum is the compartment between the pleural cavities. It extends anteriorly from the suprasternal notch to the xiphoid process and posteriorly from the first to the eleventh thoracic vertebrae. Superiorly, fascial planes in the neck are in direct communication; inferiorly, the mediastinum is limited by the diaphragm. Apertures through the inferior extent of the mediastinum are traversed by the aorta, inferior vena cava, esophagus, and vagus nerve.

In Burkell's classification (Figure 18–6), the **anterior mediastinum** contains the thymus gland, the lymph nodes, the ascending aorta and transverse aorta, the great vessels, and areolar tissue. The **middle mediastinum** contains the heart, the pericardium, the trachea, the hila of the lungs, the phrenic nerves, lymph nodes, and areolar tissue. The **posterior mediastinum** contains the sympathetic chains, the vagus nerves, the esophagus, the thoracic duct, lymph nodes, and the descending aorta.

Congenital abnormalities within the mediastinum are numerous. A defect in the anterior mediastinal pleura with communication of the right and left hemithorax is rare in humans. This retrosternal part of the anterior mediastinum is normally thin, and overexpansion of one pleural space may cause "mediastinal herniation" or a bulge of mediastinal pleura toward the opposite side.

Displacements of the mediastinum occur from masses or from accumulations of air, fluid, blood, or chyle interfering with vital functions. Tracheal compression, vena caval obstruction, and esophageal obstructions cause clinical symptoms. The mediastinum can also be displaced laterally when pathologic processes of one hemithorax cause mediastinal shift. Fibrosis and lung volume loss can shift the mediastinum toward the affected side. Open pneumothorax and massive hemothorax shift the mediastinum away from the affected side. Open pneumothorax produces alternating paradoxic mediastinal shifts with respiration and will adversely affect ventilation. Acute mediastinal displacement may produce hypoxia or reduced venous return and cause dysrhythmias, hypotension, or cardiac arrest.

ANATOMY OF THE LUNG

See Figure 18–7 for lung anatomy.

The lobes of the lung comprise multiple bronchopulmonary segments. The right lung has three lobes: upper, middle, and lower. The left lung consists of two lobes: upper and lower. On the left, the lingular seg-

Anterior view	Posterior view

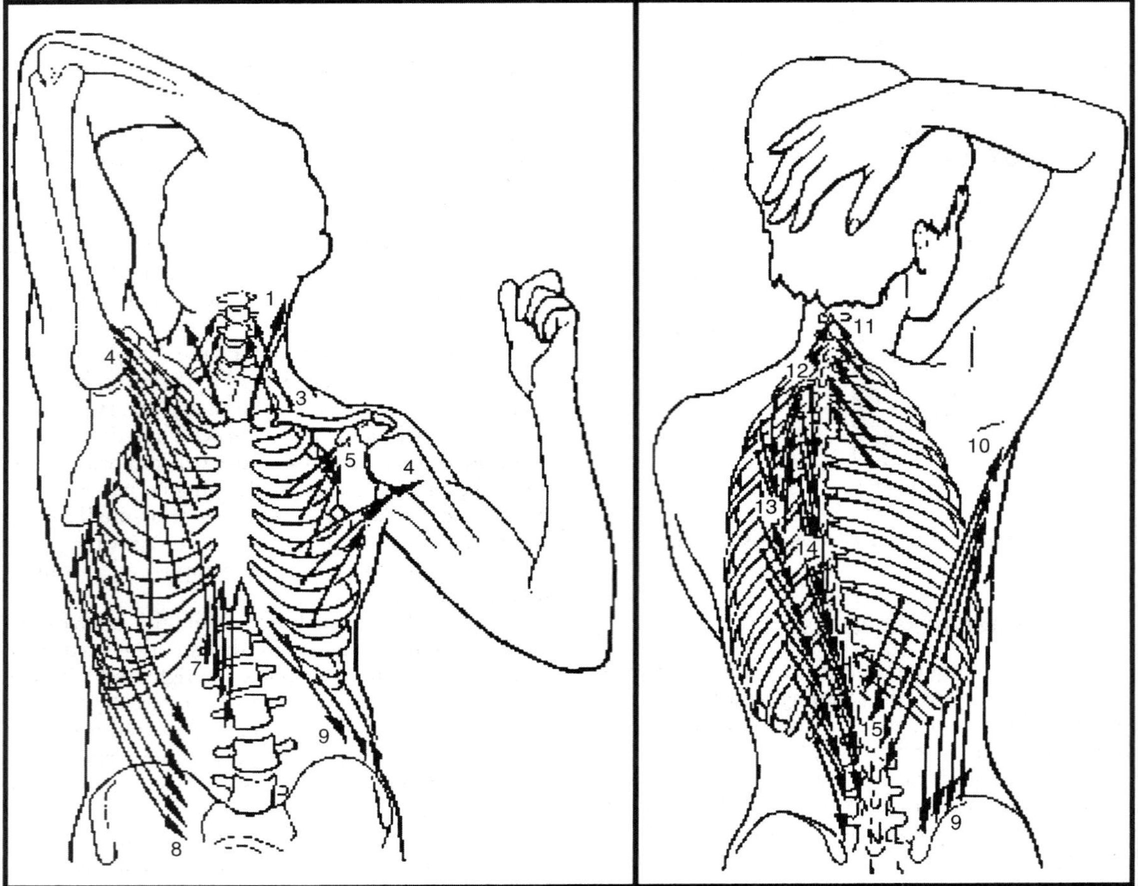

Secondary muscles of inspiration	sternocleidomastoideus (1) scalenes (3) pectoralis major (4) pectoralis minor (5) serratus anterior (10) serratus posterior superior (11) upper iliocostalis (12)
Secondary muscles of expiration	external oblique (8) internal oblique (9) rectus abdominus (7) lower iliocostalis (13) lower longissimus (14) serratus posterior inferior (15)

Figure 18–4. **Accessory muscles of respiration.** (From Kapandji IA: Functional components of the vertebral column. In: IA Kapandji (editor): *The Physiology of the Joints*, Vol. 3: *The Trunk and the Vertebral Column*, Figs. 30 and 29. New York: Churchill Livingstone, 1974.)

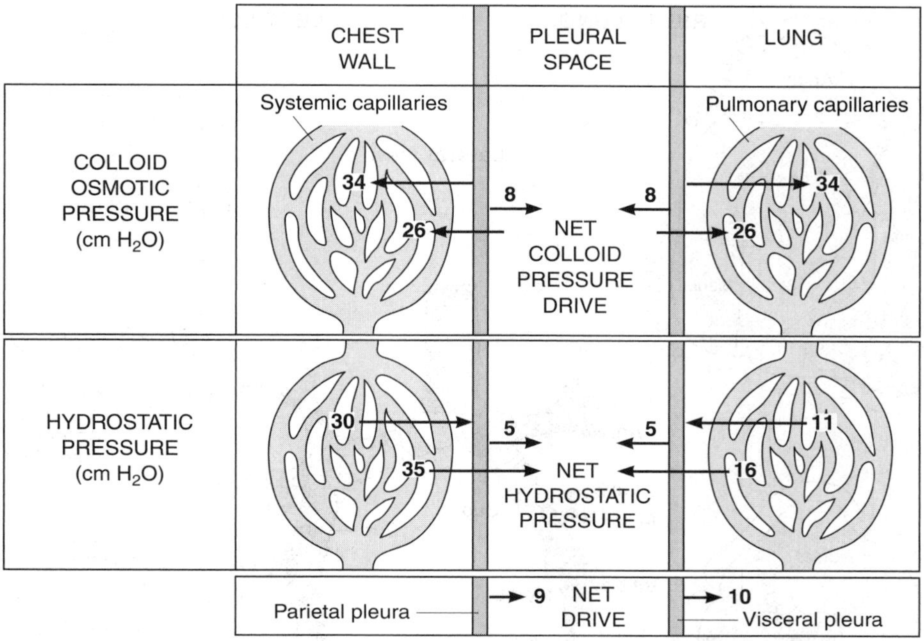

Figure 18–5. Movement of fluid across the pleural space, showing production and absorption of pleural fluid.

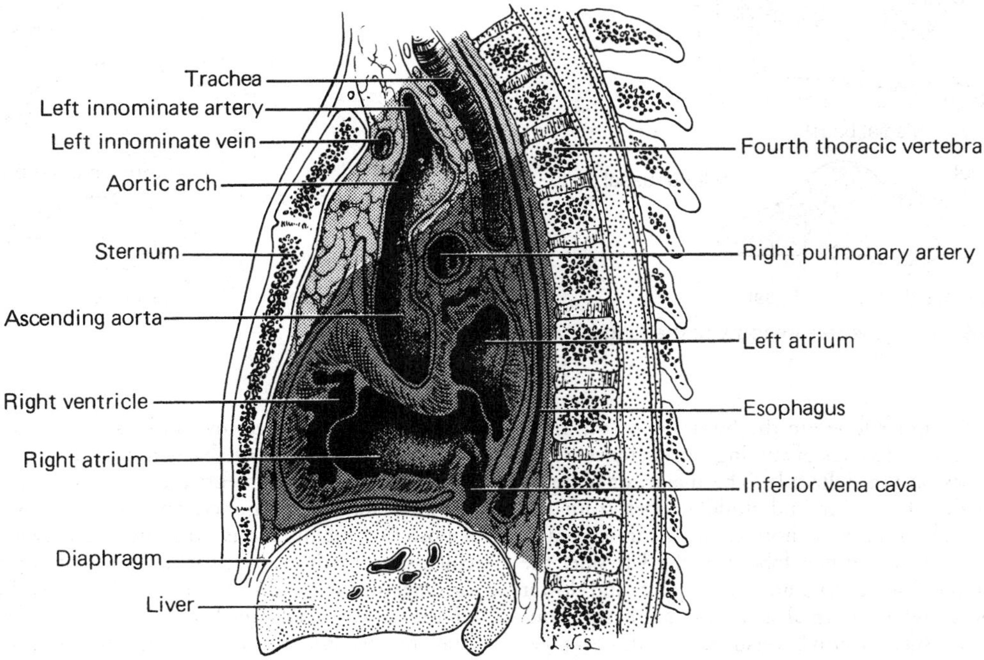

Figure 18–6. Divisions of the mediastinum (Burkell's classification). Light screening: anterior mediastinum; lower dark screening: middle mediastinum; dotted area at right: posterior mediastinum.

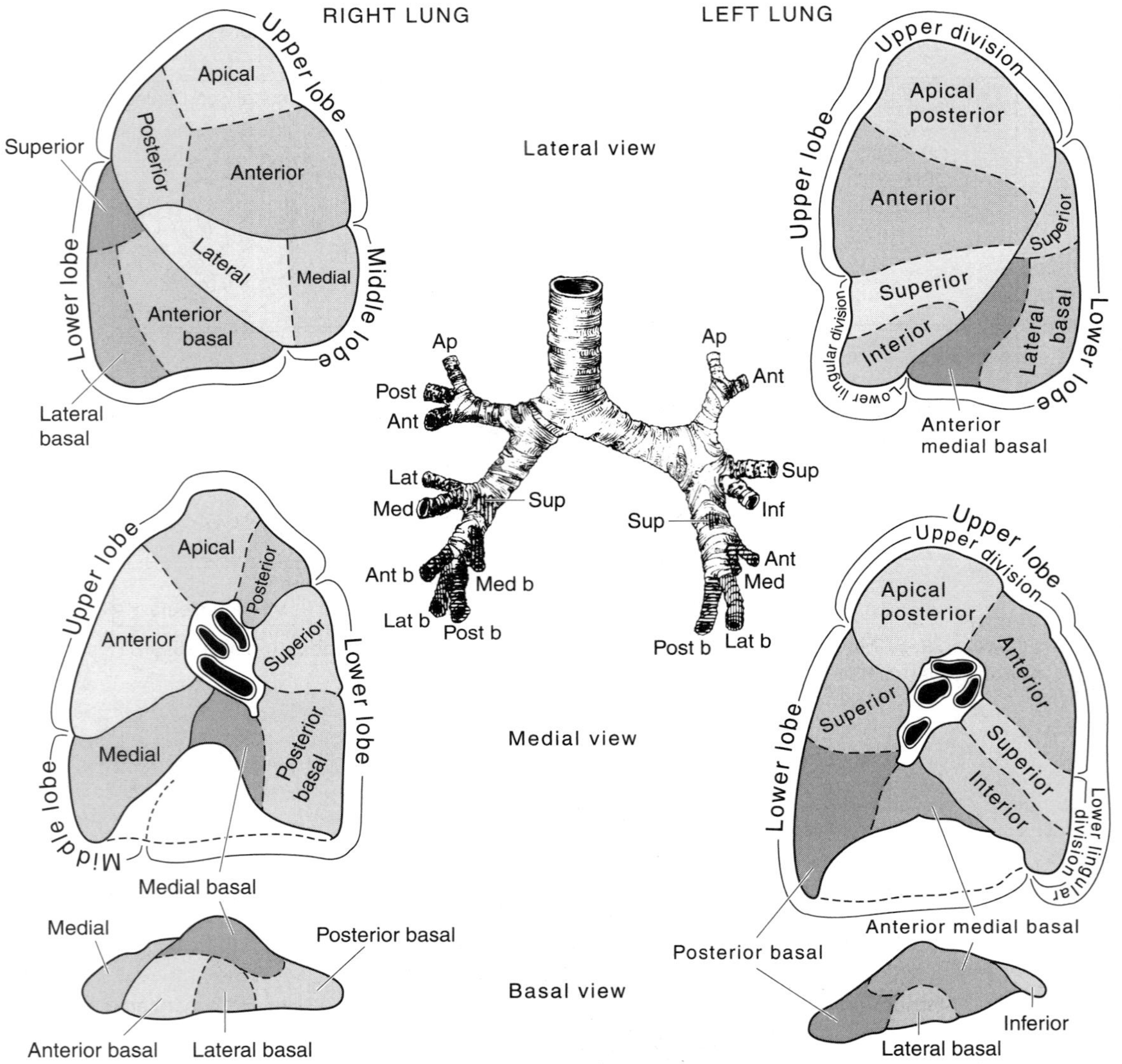

Figure 18–7. Segmental anatomy of the lungs.

ments of the upper lobe are the homolog of the right middle lobe. Two fissures of varying completeness separate the lobes on the right side. The major, or oblique, fissure divides the upper and middle lobes from the lower lobe. The minor, or horizontal, fissure separates the middle from the upper lobe. On the left side, the single oblique fissure separates the upper and lower lobes. These are the normal anatomic segments; congenital defects such as situs inversus reverse this arrangement, and bilateral right-sided anatomy (asplenia) or bilateral left-sided anatomy (polysplenia) can also occur.

The parenchymal anatomy can be seen by studying the sequential division of the bronchopulmonary tree down to the smallest unit of ventilation, the alveolus. The trachea and main stem bronchi and their branches contain a posterior membranous area and are prevented from collapsing by horseshoe-shaped anterior segments of cartilage in their walls. The cartilaginous reinforcement of the airway gradually becomes less complete as the branches become smaller, and reinforcement ceases with bronchi of 1–2 mm. The bronchopulmonary segmental anatomy is designated by numbers (Boyden) or by name (Jackson and Huber). The segmental bronchial anatomy is most constant with the pulmonary vascular structures showing more variability.

The lungs have a dual blood supply: the pulmonary and the bronchial arterial systems. The pulmonary arteries transmit venous blood from the right ventricle for oxygenation. They closely accompany the bronchi. The bronchial arteries usually arise directly from the aorta or nearby intercostal arteries and are variable in number. They transmit oxygenated blood at systemic arterial pressure to the bronchial wall to the level of the terminal bronchioles.

The pulmonary veins travel in the interlobar septa and do not correspond to the distribution of the bronchi or the pulmonary arteries.

THE LYMPHATIC SYSTEM

The lymphatics travel in intersegmental septa centrally as well as to the parenchymal surface to form subpleural networks. Drainage continues toward the hilum in channels that follow the bronchi and pulmonary arteries. The lymphatics eventually enter lymph nodes in the major fissures of the lungs, the hilum, and the paratracheal regions.

The direction of lymphatic drainage—irrespective of the primary site—is cephalad and usually ipsilateral, but contralateral flow may occur from any lobe. The lymphatics from the left lower lobe may be almost equally distributed to the left and right. From the left upper lobe, distribution is often to the anterior mediastinal group (A-P window and para-aortic lymph nodes). Otherwise, the usual sequence of lymphatic spread of pulmonary cancer is first to the regional parabronchial nodes and then to the ipsilateral paratracheal, subcarinal, scalene, or inferior deep cervical nodes.

DIAGNOSTIC STUDIES

Skin Tests

Skin tests are used in the diagnosis of tuberculosis, histoplasmosis, and coccidioidomycosis. Tuberculin testing is usually done with purified protein derivative (PPD) injected intradermally. Intermediate-strength PPD should be used in patients who seem likely to have active disease. Induration of 10 mm or more at the injection site after 48–72 hours is called positive and indicates either active or arrested disease. Because false-negative reactions are rare, a negative test fairly reliably rules out tuberculosis. Mumps antigen is usually placed on the opposite forearm to test for anergy. Skin tests for histoplasmosis and coccidioidomycosis are performed in a similar way, but skin tests for fungal infections are unreliable and serologic tests should be performed instead.

Endoscopy

A. Laryngoscopy

Indirect laryngoscopy is used to assess vocal cord mobility in patients suspected of having lung carcinoma, especially when there has been a voice change. It should be performed also to search for an otherwise occult source for malignant cells in sputum or metastases in cervical lymph nodes.

B. Bronchoscopy

Roentgenographic evidence of bronchial obstruction, unresolved pneumonia, foreign body, suspected carcinoma, hemoptysis, aspiration pneumonia, and lung abscess are only a few of the indications for bronchoscopy. The procedure can be done using either the standard hollow metal (rigid) or the flexible fiber optic bronchoscope under local or general anesthesia. Rigid bronchoscopy must be done under general anesthesia and is most often used for clearing major airways of bulky obstructing lesions such as tumors, foreign bodies, or blood clots. Traditionally the CO_2 laser required use of the rigid bronchoscope, though more recently developed technology (Nd:Yag) can be applied with flexible bronchoscopy.

Flexible bronchoscopy is a highly effective diagnostic and therapeutic tool. It can be performed under local and intravenous sedation. Washings are usually obtained for bacterial or fungal culture and cytologic examination. Visible lesions are biopsied directly, and biopsy specimens are sometimes taken from the carina even though it appears normal. Brush biopsies are obtained from specific bronchopulmonary segments. Occasionally, transcarinal needle biopsy of a subcarinal node is obtained. Thirty to 50 percent of lung tumors are visible bronchoscopically. Brushing, random biopsies, and sputum cytology may still yield a positive diagnosis of cancer or tuberculosis in the absence of a visible lesion. The yield is influenced by size, location, and histologic cell type of the lesion.

Mediastinoscopy

Cervical mediastinoscopy remains a mainstay of evaluation of the mediastinum despite advances in imaging. Properly performed mediastinoscopy samples nodes from at least three stations, including ipsilateral and contralateral paratracheal levels 2, 3, and 4 and subcarinal level 7. Cervical mediastinoscopy is performed through a 3- to 4-cm incision one fingerbreadth above the sternal notch. Dissection proceeds beneath the pretracheal fascia, allowing safe access to mediastinal nodes and avoiding major vascular structures. After palpation, the mediastinoscope can be inserted and nodes biopsied under direct vision. Unclear structures can be aspirated prior to attempted biopsy.

Enlarged lymph nodes in the aorticopulmonary window are technically inaccessible by means of standard cervical mediastinoscopy. Extended cervical mediastinoscopy, however, is a technique that provides access to these aorticopulmonary window nodes. It is performed through the same small neck incision as standard mediastinoscopy except the dissection is carried laterally beside the left carotid artery toward and then over the aorta into the aorticopulmonary space. In older patients with densely calcific aortas, extended mediastinoscopy is contraindicated because of the risk of embolic phenomena and stroke from aortic manipulation.

In experienced hands, the complications of mediastinoscopy are minimal (< 1–2%). Major bleeding complications requiring sternotomy or thoracotomy for repair are infrequent (1–2%). Other possible complications include pneumothorax, recurrent nerve injury, infection, and esophageal injury.

Mediastinoscopy is almost invariably accurate in the diagnosis of sarcoidosis. It is also useful to diagnose tuberculosis, histoplasmosis, Castleman's silicosis, metastatic carcinoma, lymphoma, and carcinoma of the esophagus. It should not be used in the investigation of primary mediastinal tumors, which should be approached by an incision permitting definitive excision.

Chamberlain Procedure

Anterior mediastinotomy (the Chamberlain procedure) is used to sample nodes and biopsy tissue in the anterior mediastinum and most commonly in the aorticopulmonary window. A small (3- to 4-cm) incision is made over the second or third interspace on the appropriate side of the lesion. Alternatively, the procedure can be performed with videoscopic guidance (VATS). The mediastinum is approached through the interspace directly or after excising the costochondral cartilage using either the mediastinoscope or open technique. Careful attention is paid to preserving the mammary vessels encountered in the dissection. The mediastinum is approached extrapleurally unless lesions specifically within the thorax—effusions, tumors invading the hilum or chest wall—need to be investigated. Furthermore, if additional access is required to facilitate the dissection or to treat a complication, the incision can be converted easily to a larger anterior thoracotomy.

Complications resulting from anterior mediastinotomy are similar to those encountered with cervical mediastinoscopy and include bleeding, recurrent nerve injury, and infection. Major morbidity should be less than 1–2%.

Video-Assisted Thoracoscopic Surgery (VATS)

With the advent of sophisticated video technology and optics, video-assisted thoracoscopic surgery (VATS) has evolved as an important tool in thoracic surgery. While thoracoscopic procedures have been used for many years, newer technical advances as well as increasing surgeon familiarity with minimally invasive surgery have made VATS increasingly popular and useful.

VATS plays an important role in the diagnosis and staging of thoracic malignancies (lung cancer, mesothelioma, etc) as well as in the resection of isolated peripheral pulmonary nodules and bullous lung disease. Furthermore, it has been an advance in lung biopsy and pleurodesis procedures.

However, despite gaining popularity, many thoracic surgeons consider the approach suboptimal for lung cancers. Full mediastinal lymph node dissections are not generally obtainable with standard VATS. Even for metastasectomy, concerns over pleural and chest wall seeding with VATS have been documented in the literature, highlighting the need for assiduous attention to detail during these procedures. The improved resolution from new-generation CT scanners have in part supplanted the need for palpation of the entire lung, and increasingly advanced resections are now being performed via VATS approaches. At present VATS is most commonly applied to benign processes, including spontaneous pneumothoraces and pleural effusions, as well as for thoracic sympathectomy and thoracic vertebral discectomy.

As instruments and techniques have evolved, complications from VATS procedures—persistent air leaks, hemorrhage, tumor seeding, etc—have decreased. Overall, major complication rates of 1–2% are reported. Faster patient recovery, shorter hospital stays, decreased pain are major advantages of VATS, although long-term differences between videoscopic and formal thoracotomy using muscle-sparing incisions are yet to be demonstrated.

Scalene Lymph Node Biopsy

Scalene lymph node biopsy has been largely replaced by mediastinoscopy in the evaluation of pulmonary disease since it offers the same information but is less reliable and does not evaluate nodes within the mediastinum. Furthermore, scalene lymph nodes are accessible via cervical mediastinoscopy using the mediastinoscope. In the evaluation of lung cancer, about 15% of scalene node biopsies are positive when the cervical nodes are not palpable compared with 85% when the nodes are palpable. The risk of major complications is about 5%. Deaths are rare.

Pleural Biopsy

A. Needle Biopsy

This procedure is indicated when the cause of a pleural effusion cannot be determined by analysis of the fluid or when tuberculosis is suspected. Any one of three needles can be used: Vim-Silverman, Cope, or Abrams (Harefield). A definitive diagnosis can be obtained in 60–80% of cases of tuberculosis or cancer. The principal complication is pneumothorax. Five to 10 percent of biopsy specimens are inadequate for diagnosis.

B. Surgical Biopsy

Biopsy of the pleura can be performed via videoscopic or open technique with minimal morbidity, providing the pathologist with a specimen superior to that of needle biopsy.

Lung Biopsy

A. Needle Biopsy

The indications for percutaneous needle biopsy are not well established. It may be indicated in diffuse parenchymal disease and in some patients with localized lesions. The diagnosis of interstitial pneumonia, carcinoma, sarcoidosis, hypersensitivity lung disease, lymphoma, pulmonary alveolar proteinosis, and miliary tuberculosis has been established by this method.

Needle biopsies are done by any of three techniques: by aspiration with a cutting needle, by trephine, or by air drill. Needle biopsy of the lung is also possible by a transbronchial technique in which a modified Vim-Silverman or ultrathin needle is used.

There is controversy concerning the risks of spreading the tumor by needle biopsy in localized disease. Complications following percutaneous needle biopsy include pneumothorax (5–30%), hemothorax, hemoptysis, and air embolism. Pulmonary hypertension or cysts and bullae are contraindications. Several deaths have been reported. There is about a 60% chance of obtaining useful information.

B. Surgical Biopsy

Thoracoscopy or VATS has become the procedure of choice for open lung biopsy in patients who can tolerate single lung ventilation. A single anterior axillary line incision can be used for introduction of a stapler and operating thoracoscope. For open biopsies a limited intercostal or anterior parasternal incision is used to remove a 3- to 4-cm wedge of lung tissue in diffuse parenchymal lung disease. The site of incision is selected for accessibility and potential diagnostic value. The incision is generally made at the fifth interspace on the right at the anterior axillary line to allow for access to all three lobes for biopsy—or at the lower lobes bilaterally. The middle lobe and lingula are selected in specific cases when pathology exists only in these areas, as they generally yield results of the poorest quality. Open lung biopsy is associated with a lower death rate, fewer complications, and greater diagnostic yield than needle biopsy. It is especially useful in critically ill, immunosuppressed patients for differentiation of infectious infiltrative lesions from neoplastic infiltrative lesions. Open lung biopsy can be performed in the ICU setting and does not require single lung ventilation. When a focal lesion is biopsied, a larger incision is used. Peripheral lesions are totally excised by wedge or segmental resection, and deeply placed lesions are removed by lobectomy in suitable candidates.

Sputum Analysis

Exfoliative sputum cytology is most valuable for detection of lung cancer. Specimens are obtained by deep coughing or by abrasion with a brush, or bronchial washings are obtained by either bronchoscopic or percutaneous transtracheal washing techniques. Specimens should be collected in the morning and delivered to the laboratory promptly. Centrifugation or filtration can be used to concentrate the cellular elements.

In primary lung cancer, sputum cytology is positive in 30–60% of cases. Repeated sputum examination improves the diagnostic return. Examination of the first bronchoscopic washing material yields a diagnosis in 60% of cases. Postbronchoscopy sputum analysis should always be made at 6–12 and 24 hours, as findings may be positive at these times when previous tests were negative.

Newer technologies, including better sputum-inducing agents, are currently in clinical trials and appear effective. Also, more sophisticated cytologic analysis using immunohistochemistry to molecular markers (cytokeratins, hnRNP, etc) has improved accuracy and sensitivity and the ability to detect premalignant lesions.

Computed Tomography (CT Scan)

Computed tomography is a cornerstone of evaluation of chest pathology. CT scanning is critical in the staging of carcinoma, and has value in defining the extent of metastatic disease. Mediastinoscopy remains the gold standard for evaluation of the mediastinum in lung cancer.

Magnetic Resonance Imaging (MRI)

Although the major value of MRI in the thorax has been in cardiovascular imaging, it has been moderately helpful in showing invasion of lung cancer into the chest wall, vertebrae, and spinal cord as well as mediastinal structures. MRI has a particular niche in the evaluation of superior sulcus (Pancoast) tumors to establish involvement of the brachial plexus, subclavian vessel, or bony chest wall.

Position Emission Tomography (PET)

PET has become an important tool in staging and workup of the cancer patient. PET scanners are more widely available, and current data suggest that PET scanning identifies unsuspected regional or distant disease in 20–30% of patients with lung cancer or esophageal cancer compared with conventional imaging methods (CT, bone scan). PET scanning is more accurate than CT scanning in detection of cancer spread to mediastinal lymph nodes. Because of the high negative predictive value of PET scanning, a negative PET scan in the mediastinum permits direct progression to thoracotomy. The presence of a positive PET scan in the mediastinum mandates either mediastinoscopy or, more recently, endoscopic evaluation of mediastinal lymph nodes because of false-positive PET scan results.

The combined PET/CT is highly accurate (> 90%), but by itself it has a 10–20% false-positive rate in the mediastinum. Therefore, interpretations of PET results must be accepted with caution and must be confirmed by surgical staging when inconsistent with the overall clinical picture.

DISEASES OF THE CHEST WALL

LUNG HERNIA

A lung hernia results from a defect in the chest wall caused by abnormal development, trauma, or surgery. Most lung hernias are thoracic in location, but cervical (defects of Sibson's fascia) or diaphragmatic herniation may occur occasionally. Lung hernias are usually asymptomatic, but some patients experience local tenderness, pain, or mild dyspnea. Operative repair rather than external support produces optimal results if symptoms are present.

CHEST WALL INFECTIONS

Infections that appear to involve only the skin and soft tissues may actually represent outward extensions of deeper infection of the ribs, cartilage, sternum, or even the pleural space (empyema necessitatis). Inadequate drainage of superficial infection can lead to inward extension into the pleural space, causing empyema.

Subpectoral abscess is caused by suppurative adenitis of the axillary lymph nodes, rib or pleural infection, or posterior extension of a breast abscess—or it may occur as a complication of chest wall surgery (eg, mastectomy, pacemaker placement). Symptoms include systemic sepsis, erythema, induration of the pectoral region, and obliteration of the normal infraclavicular depression. Shoulder movement is painful. Organisms most commonly involved include hemolytic streptococci and *Staphylococcus aureus*. Treatment involves incisional drainage along the lateral border of the pectoralis major muscle and administration of systemic antibiotics.

Subscapular abscess may arise from osteomyelitis of the scapula but most commonly follows thoracic operations such as thoracotomy or thoracoplasty. Winging of the scapula or paravertebral induration of the trapezius muscle is usually present. A pleural communication is suggested if a cough impulse is present or if the size of the mass varies with position or direct pressure. The diagnosis is established by needle aspiration. Open drainage is indicated for pyogenic infections not involving the pleural space. Tubercular lesions should be treated by chemotherapy and needle aspiration, if possible.

Osteomyelitis of the Ribs

In the past, osteomyelitis of the ribs was often caused by typhoid fever and tuberculosis. Except in children, hematogenous osteomyelitis is a rare problem today. Thoracotomy incisions may result in osteomyelitis.

Sternal Osteomyelitis

Infection of the sternum most commonly follows median sternotomy incisions, particularly in diabetics. It presents as a postoperative wound infection or mediastinitis with drainage, fever, leukocytosis, and instability of the sternal closure. Treatment consists of open drainage, resection of the involved sternum, and reconstruction of the defect with pectoralis muscle, serratus muscle, or omental coverage. Recently success has been achieved through use of vacuum-assisted closure systems following debridement.

Occasionally, sternal osteomyelitis will be due to tuberculosis.

Infection of the Costal Cartilages & Xiphoid

Costal cartilage infections are relatively unresponsive to antibiotic therapy. Once devascularized, perichondral tissue necroses and remains as a foreign body to perpetuate the infection and sinus tract formation. The infection may be established during the course of septicemia, but the most common cause is direct extension of other surgical infections (eg, wound infection, subphrenic abscess). Surgical division of costal cartilages, as in a thoracoabdominal incision, may predispose to cartilage infection postoperatively if local sepsis develops. A wide variety of organisms have been implicated.

Erythema and induration with fluctuance and often spontaneous drainage can occur. The course can be fulminant or may be indolent over months or years, with periodic exacerbations. Associated osteomyelitis of the sternum, ribs, or clavicle may occur.

The differential diagnosis includes local bone or cartilage tumors, Tietze's syndrome, chest wall metastasis, eroding aortic aneurysm, and bronchocutaneous fistula.

The treatment of choice includes resection of the involved cartilage and adjacent involved bony structures. Recurrence is due to underestimation of the extent of disease and inadequate resection.

Reconstruction of the Chest Wall

Chest wall reconstruction may be necessary following trauma, surgical resection, or infectious processes. Recent advances in the use of musculocutaneous flaps and the supportive use of methyl methacrylate and Marlex mesh to produce solidity below these muscular flaps have facilitated repairs. In massive chest wall defects, vascularization of the area is essential and can be accomplished by use of omental flaps as well as pectoralis, latissimus dorsi, and rectus flaps. Microsurgical techniques for repair of such defects have greatly expanded the ability of plastic surgeons to deal with extensive resectional and infective processes.

Adler BD, Padley SP, Muller NL: Tuberculosis of the chest wall: CT findings. J Comput Assist Tomogr 1993;17:271.

Mansour KA, Anderson TM, Hester TR: Sternal resection and reconstruction. Ann Thorac Surg 1993;55:838.

Pairolero PC, Arnold PG, Harris JB: Long-term results of pectoralis major muscle transposition for infected sternotomy wounds. Ann Surg 1991;213:583.

Siegman-Igra Y et al: Serious infectious complications of midsternotomy: a review of bacteriology and antimicrobial therapy. Scand J Infect Dis 1990;22:633.

Slaughter MS et al: A fifteen-year wound surveillance study after coronary artery bypass. Ann Thorac Surg 1993;56:1063.

TIETZE'S SYNDROME

Tietze's syndrome is a painful nonsuppurative inflammation of the costochondral cartilages and is of unknown cause. Recent evidence suggests that costochondritis may represent a manifestation of seronegative rheumatic disease. Local swelling and tenderness are the only symptoms; they usually disappear without therapy. The syndrome may recur.

Several recent reports have suggested the use of bone scintigraphy and chest CT for diagnosis of infected costochondritis. Bone scanning was effective in localizing and identifying inflamed costochondral junctions. Chest CT was less sensitive in one study. Furthermore, in a small study of patients with Tietze's syndrome, transthoracic echo was able to demonstrate a dishomogeneous increase in echogenicity in the pathologically involved cartilage. Treatment is symptomatic and may include analgesics (NSAIDs) and local or systemic corticosteroids. When symptoms persist longer than 3 weeks and tumefaction suggests neoplasm, excision of the involved cartilage may be indicated and is usually curative.

Aeschlimann A, Kahn MF: Tietze's syndrome: a critical review. Clin Exper Rheumatol 1990;8:407.

MONDOR'S DISEASE (THROMBOPHLEBITIS OF THE THORACOEPIGASTRIC VEIN)

Mondor's disease consists of localized thrombophlebitis of the anterolateral chest wall. It is more prominent in women than in men and occasionally follows radical mastectomy. There are few symptoms other than the presence of a localized tender, cord-like structure in the subcutaneous tissues of the abdomen, thorax, or axilla. The disease is self-limited and devoid of complications such as thromboembolism. The possibility of an infective origin or stasis of the interrupted venous return due to neoplasm must be ruled out.

Bejanga BI: Mondor's disease: analysis of 30 cases. J R Coll Surg Edinb 1992;37:322.

CHEST WALL TUMORS

Chest wall tumors may be simulated by enlarged costal cartilages, chest wall infection, fractures, rickets, scurvy, hyperparathyroidism, and other conditions. Most commonly, chest wall lesions present as a mass with localized or referred pain; less than 25% are asymptomatic. Approximately 60% of all chest wall masses prove to be malignant. Lesions arise from one of the three components of the chest wall, including soft tissues (muscle, nerve, fascia), bone, and cartilage.

The majority of tumors arise from bone or cartilage. Rib involvement is more common than sternal presentation. Chest CT offers the most information for diagnosis and staging. In particular, chest wall sarcomas are associated with pulmonary metastasis. Simple chest x-rays may initially identify a mass, especially if it is calcified. Bone scans should be obtained in all cases.

Initial diagnosis is obtained by limited incisional biopsy (transverse) if the mass is large (> 4 cm). Smaller lesions are excised en bloc, ensuring negative margins, with full knowledge that a malignancy is present in many cases. Classic teaching has been to perform en bloc wide local excisions with immediate reconstruction for all lesions at initial presentations. Progress with adjuvant multimodality therapy, however, for tumors such as rhabdomyosarcomas and Ewing's sarcoma supports the use of initial limited biopsy for tissue diagnosis to guide treatment planning.

Specific Neoplasms

A. Benign Soft Tissue Tumors

1. Lipomas—Lipomas are the most common benign tumors of the chest wall. Occasionally they are very large and lobulated, and they may have dumbbell-shaped extensions that indent the endothoracic fascia beneath the sternum through an intercostal space. They may communicate with a large mediastinal or supraclavicular component.

2. Neurogenic tumors—These may arise from intercostal or superficial nerves. Solitary neurofibromas are most common, followed by neurolemmomas.

3. Cavernous hemangiomas—Hemangiomas of the thoracic wall are usually painful and occur in children. Tumors may be isolated or may involve other tissues (eg, lung), as in Rendu-Osler-Weber syndrome.

4. Lymphangiomas—This rare lesion is seen most often in children. It may have poorly defined borders that make complete excision difficult.

B. Malignant Soft Tissue Tumors

Roughly 50% of all chest wall masses are sarcomas, yet overall they represent only a small percentage (5%) of all malignant soft tissue sarcomas. Survival is determined by the histologic grade, the completeness of resection, and the presence and development of metastases (synchronous or metachronous). Low-grade tumors have 5-year and 10-year survivals approaching 90% and 82%, respectively. With high-grade lesions, however, 5-year survival rates are only 30–50%. The development of metastasis greatly reduces the chances of survival.

Treatment is directed at complete resection with emphasis on achieving negative margins (1–2 cm). En bloc resection techniques include raising skin flaps and reconstruction with soft tissue flaps, Marlex mesh, and methyl methacrylate to correct chest wall deformity and prevent paradoxic chest movement.

Various histologic subtypes of soft tissue sarcoma are encountered. Typically, low-grade sarcomas include desmoids or liposarcomas with low-grade features. Next most frequently seen are malignant fibrosarcoma, rhabdomyosarcoma, and malignant fibrous histiocytoma, which are usually high-grade lesions.

Individual histologic subtype is not by itself a significant prognostic variable, but histologic grade does have that role. Metastases—either synchronous or metachronous—are common to the lungs (75%) and should be resected if negative margins can be achieved and adequate lung function preserved. Therapy for low-grade lesions should consist of complete resection. Incompletely resected lesions can be treated with external beam radiation therapy. High-grade lesions should be resected and patients enrolled into clinical trials evaluating the efficacy of systemic adjuvant chemotherapy. Postoperative radiotherapy is often helpful in the setting of close margins or tumor spillage.

1. Fibrosarcomas—Fibrosarcoma is the most common primary soft tissue cancer of the chest wall. It occurs most frequently in young adults.

2. Liposarcomas—These tumors account for approximately one-third of all primary cancers of the chest wall. They occur more often in men.

3. Neurofibrosarcomas—These uncommon tumors involve the thoracic wall almost twice as often as other parts of the body. They often occur in patients with Recklinghausen's disease and usually originate from intercostal nerves.

C. Benign Skeletal Tumors

1. Chondromas, osteochondromas, and myxochondromas—The combined frequency of these three cartilaginous tumors is about 30–45% of all benign skeletal tumors. Cartilaginous tumors are usually single and occur with equal frequency in males and females between childhood and the fourth decade. The tumors are usually painless and tend to occur anteriorly along the costal margin or in the parasternal area. Wide local excision is curative.

2. Fibrous dysplasia—Fibrous dysplasia (bone cyst, osteofibroma, fibrous osteoma, fibrosis ossificans) accounts for a third or more of benign skeletal tumors of the chest wall. This cystic bone tumor can occur in any portion of the skeletal system, but approximately half involve the ribs. The differential diagnosis includes cystic bone lesions associated with hyperparathyroidism. The tumor is usually single and may be trauma related. Some patients complain of swelling, tenderness, or vague discomfort, but the lesion is usually silent and is detected on routine chest x-ray. Treatment consists of local excision.

3. Eosinophilic granuloma—Eosinophilic granuloma may occur in the clavicle, the scapula, or (rarely) the sternum. Coexisting infiltrates of the lung are often present. This condition often represents a more benign form of Letterer-Siwe disease or Hand-Schüller-Christian disease. Fever, malaise, leukocytosis, eosinophilia, or bone pain may be present. Rib involvement presents as a swelling with cortical bone destruction and periosteal new growth. The clinical picture can resemble osteomyelitis or Ewing's sarcoma. When the disease is localized, excision will result in cure.

4. Hemangioma—Cavernous hemangioma of the ribs presents as a painful mass in infancy or childhood. The tumor appears on chest x-ray either as multiple radiolucent areas or as a single trabeculated cyst.

5. Miscellaneous—Fibromas, lipomas, osteomas, and aneurysmal bone cysts are all relatively rare lesions of the chest wall. The diagnosis is established after excisional biopsy.

D. Malignant Skeletal Tumors

1. Chondrosarcomas—Chondrosarcomas are the most common primary malignant tumor of the chest wall (20–40%). They can involve the sternum but more commonly develop from the costochondral junctions of the first four ribs. About 15–20% of all skeletal chondrosarcomas occur in the ribs or sternum. Most appear in patients 20–40 years of age. Local involvement of pleura, adjacent ribs, muscle, diaphragm, or other soft tissue may develop. Pain is rare, however, and most patients complain only of the mass. Chest x-ray shows destroyed cortical bone, usually with diffuse mottled calcification, and the border of the tumor is indistinct. Successful treatment necessitates wide local excision and en bloc resection to achieve negative margins. Incomplete excision carries a significantly worse prognosis. Overall survival, as in all soft tissue sarcomas, is heavily dependent on the histologic grade. Completely resected low-grade chondrosarcoma has a 60–80% 5-year survival rate. Patients with high-grade lesions who subsequently develop distant metastasis have only 20–30% 5-year survival.

Local recurrence portends future metastatic disease and poor survival. Yet complete resection can often be curative. Therefore, even in the setting of large tumors (> 15–20 cm), resection should be considered even when it necessitates removal of more than six to eight ribs. With advances in epidural pain control and immediate reconstruction techniques, most patients will do surprisingly well. Despite large chest wall resections, most patients can be immediately extubated and will not suffer drastic changes in pulmonary function or chest wall dynamics.

2. Osteogenic sarcoma (osteosarcoma)—Osteosarcoma occurs in the second and third decades, and 60% of cases occur in men. It is more malignant than chondrosarcoma. X-ray findings consist of bone destruction and recalcification at right angles to the bony cortex, which give the characteristic "sunburst" appearance. Osteogenic sarcoma presents commonly as an extremity lesion, with only a small percentage of cases being truncal primaries. Overall, less than 5% of all osteogenic sarcomas arise in the chest wall. Osteogenic sarcoma occurs in the second to fourth decades of life, half-again more commonly in men than in women. Typically, they are more aggressive tumors with a propensity for early metastasis to lung and bone.

Osteogenic sarcoma should be considered a systemic disease upon presentation, and treatment should consist of wide local excision and postoperative chemotherapy. The number of primary osteogenic sarcomas of the chest wall is small, and for that reason it is difficult to draw conclusions about definitive therapy. In the series with the most patients (n = 38), overall 5-year survival after complete resection and postoperative chemotherapy was only 15%.

As in all sarcomas, development of metastasis markedly decreases survival. In osteogenic sarcoma, 60–70% of resected primary cancers will ultimately develop metastasis. While prospective randomized trials of adjuvant chemotherapy are needed, most investigators agree that the current best therapy for osteogenic sarcoma of the chest wall includes resection followed by postoperative chemotherapy.

3. Myeloma (solitary plasmacytoma)—Solitary plasmacytomas of the chest wall are comparatively rare lesions. They constitute 5–20% of all chest wall tumors. Radiologically, they present as classic "punched-out" lytic lesions without evidence of new bone formation. They are more common in men than in women and typically present in the fifth to seventh decades of life.

Over three-fourths of the time, solitary chest wall plasmacytomas are harbingers of diffuse multiple myeloma. Survival is based on the development of systemic disease. Surgery plays a role in diagnosis. Incisional biopsy is performed unless the lesion is small (< 3 cm) and can be full excised. Local control and relief of pain are achieved with radiation therapy (usually 3000–4600 cGy). Once systemic disease is diagnosed, treatment consists of chemotherapy. Overall, 5-year and 10-year survivals for solitary plasmacytomas of the chest wall are 35–40% and 15–20%, respectively. Typical median survivals after treatment with radiation therapy and chemotherapy average 56 months.

4. Ewing's sarcoma (hemangioendothelioma, endothelioma)—Ewing's sarcoma accounts for 10–15% of all primary chest wall tumors. Presentation as a primary chest lesion is not common (< 15%). Typically, Ewing's sarcoma presents as a large, warm, painful soft tissue mass usually associated with pleural effusion. Systemic symptoms such as fever, malaise, and weight loss are common. Radiologic studies demonstrate the classic "onion skin" appearance caused by widening and sclerosis of the cortex as multiple layers of new bone are produced.

Diagnosis can be made usually by fine-needle aspirate or incisional biopsy. Histologically, these tumors are unique and consist of broad sheets of small polyhedral cells with pale cytoplasm and small hyperchromatic nuclei. They stain periodic acid-Schiff-positive.

Ewing's sarcoma is commonly a disease of childhood and adolescence although in several studies, age and gender were not significant prognostic indicators. The most important prognostic indicator for survival was development of distant metastases. Current therapy after diagnosis by needle or incisional biopsy consists of chemotherapy (including cyclophosphamide, dactinomycin, doxorubicin, vincristine) followed by local radiation (5000 cGy) or surgical resection. Some data suggest that better long-term survival may be achieved by resection following chemotherapy. Overall, 5-year survivals range from 15% to 48%. Long-term survivals (10 years) are achievable by patients who do not develop metastases.

E. METASTATIC CHEST WALL TUMORS

Metastases to bones of the thorax are often multiple and are usually from tumors of the kidney, thyroid, lung, breast, prostate, stomach, uterus, or colon. Renal cell and thyroid malignancies have a high propensity for metastasizing to the sternum. Occasionally, they present as a pulsatile mass due to the excessive vascularity of the metastasis. An aneurysm of the ascending thoracic aorta, while rare, must be considered in the differential diagnosis and ruled out prior to attempts at excisional biopsy. Involvement by direct extension occurs in carcinoma of the breast and lung. Primary lung cancer with direct extension to chest wall without nodal involvement (T3 N0) carries a reasonable 5-year survival (40–50%) when treated with radical en bloc resection. Lung metastasis with direct chest wall extension should be treated with radical en bloc resection of the chest wall and underlying lung.

Brodsky JT et al: Desmoid tumors of the chest wall: a locally recurrent problem. J Thorac Cardiovasc Surg 1992;104:900.

Burt M: Primary malignant tumors of the chest wall. The Memorial Sloan-Kettering Cancer Center experience. Chest Surg Clin N Am 1994;4:137.

Burt M et al: Medical tumors of the chest wall. Solitary plasmacytoma and Ewing's sarcoma. J Thorac Cardiovasc Surg 1993;105:89.

Burt M et al: Primary bony and cartilaginous sarcomas of chest wall: results of therapy. Ann Thorac Surg 1992;54:226.

Perry RR et al: Survival after surgical resection for high-grade chest wall sarcomas. Ann Thorac Surg 1990;49:363.

Shamberger RC et al: Malignant small round cell tumor (Ewing) of the chest wall in children. J Pediatr Surg 1989;29:179.

DISEASES OF THE PLEURA

The pleura can be the site of both benign and malignant diseases that may represent primary pleural processes, localized extrapleural diseases, or systemic illnesses. Perhaps the most common pleural problem is the presence of air (pneumothorax) within the pleural space. Pleural effusions—accumulations of fluid—result from benign sterile fluid, malignant fluid, pus, chyle, or blood. Although primary pleural tumors are uncommon, involvement of the pleura with metastatic cancer is common.

Pain and dyspnea are the most common symptoms of pleural disease. The pain most commonly is described as sharp, and it is characteristically worsened by respiratory movements, often inhibiting inspiration. Pleural pain is mediated through somatic intercostal nerves of the chest wall (cervical and costal pleura) and through the phrenic nerve (diaphragmatic and mediastinal pleura), causing chest wall or back pain and pain referred to the shoulder, respectively. The visceral pleura contains only sympathetic and parasympathetic nerve fibers and therefore is insensate; however, extension of visceral processes to involve the parietal pleura can produce typical pleuritic chest pain.

PLEURAL EFFUSION

Pleural effusion is the presence of fluid within the pleural space. More specific terminology may be used when the nature of the fluid is known. **Hydrothorax** is a collection of serous (most often transudative but also exudative) fluid, while pus in the pleural cavity is referred to as a **pyothorax** or **empyema**. Additional terms are used for blood (**hemothorax**) and chyle (**chylothorax**). Abnormal pleural fluid accumulates as a result of one or more of the following mechanisms: (1) increase in the pulmonary vascular hydrostatic pressure (congestive heart failure, mitral stenosis), (2) decrease in the vascular colloidal osmotic pressure (hypoproteinemia), (3) increase in the capillary permeability due to inflammation (pneumonia, pancreatitis, sepsis), (4) decrease in the intrapleural pressure (atelectasis), (5) decrease in the lymphatic drainage (carcinomatosis), (6) transdiaphragmatic movement of abdominal fluid through lymphatics or physical defects (ascites, pancreatic pseudocyst rupture), and (7) rupture of a vascular or lymphatic structure (traumatic injury)

Decreased respiratory excursion, diminished breath sounds (often with a bronchial quality due to compression of underlying lung), dullness to percussion, a pleural friction rub, and local tenderness are signs that indicate the presence of pleural effusion. With longstanding and advanced disease, contraction of the hemithorax with narrowed intercostal spaces and localized bulging, swelling, or redness may occur. Chest radiographs demonstrate varying degrees of opacification of the ipsilateral hemithorax. Accumulation of 300–500 mL fluid causes blunting of the costophrenic angle on x-ray. If the entire hemithorax is opacified, 2000–2500 mL may be present. The mediastinum may be shifted to the contralateral side in the presence of a large effusion or it may remain in the midline—particularly if proximal bronchial obstruction results in lobar or total lung atelectasis, if the mediastinum is fixed from fibrosis or tumor infiltration, if the ipsilateral lung is infiltrated with tumor, or if malignant mesothelioma is present. CT scanning may be required to evaluate complex, loculated, or recurrent pleural fluid collections. Interventional radiology services are useful for loculated pleural effusions that may be managed by percutaneous drain placement under CT guidance

Generally, serous effusions are separated into two broad categories—transudates and exudates—based on the physical and cellular characteristics of the pleural fluid. Identification of the specific type of effusion aids in determination of the cause and most often depends on examination of at least 20 mL of fluid obtained by thoracentesis. Basic tests should include total protein, lactate dehydrogenase (LDH), total and differential cell counts, glucose, pH, cytology, and Gram stain with culture. Furthermore, simultaneous serum total protein, LDH, and glucose should be measured. Effusions with total protein content less than 3 g/dL (or a fluid:serum ratio lower than 0.5), an LDH level < 200 units/dL (or a fluid:serum ratio < 0.6), and a specific gravity below 1.016 represent transudates, while all other effusions are classified as exudates. The results of these basic tests frequently allow the underlying pathologic process to be elucidated (see Table 18–1).

Specific disease processes associated with pleural effusions are described in the following paragraphs.

1. Hydrothorax

Malignancy

More than 25% of all pleural effusions are secondary to cancer, and 35% of patients with lung cancer, 23% of patients with breast cancer (12% of patients with adenocarcinomas of unknown primary site), and 10% of patients with lymphoma develop malignant pleural effusions during the course of their disease. Approximately 10% of malignant effusions are secondary to primary pleural tumors (mostly mesotheliomas). The mechanism (as noted above) is primarily through lymphatic obstruction in either the peripheral lung or central lymph node channels of the mediastinum. Malignant pleural effusions can be serous, serosanguineous, or frankly bloody and are diagnosed primarily by demonstrating malignant cells in the fluid. Cytologic confirmation is successful 50%, 65%, and 70% of the time after one, two, or three thoracenteses, respectively. Closed pleural biopsy alone is successful in only 50% of cases, but coupled with thoracentesis it can increase the diagnostic yield to 80%. Thoracoscopy with direct pleural biopsy, however, is successful in 97% of patients and should be considered in any patient with a suspicious effusion after two negative thoracenteses.

Treatment of malignant effusions is strictly palliative since most patients die within 3–6 months of developing a malignant pleural effusion. Prompt diagnosis and therapy are essential. The goals of treatment are lung reexpansion and pleural symphysis. This is most readily accomplished with placement of a chest tube (20–28F) and closed tube drainage for 24–48 hours (see Figure 18–8). Generally, no more than 1 L is allowed to drain initially. Subsequently, 200–500 mL is allowed to drain every 1–2 hours until the effusion is fully drained. This controlled draining avoids the rare complication of reexpansion pulmonary edema. Once full lung expansion is obtained (regardless of the ongoing drainage), pleurodesis should be performed with an appropriate agent before loculations have formed. Different chemical, radioactive, and infectious agents have been used in the past with varying success rates, including mechlorethamine (success rate 48–57%), thiotepa (nil to 63%), fluorouracil (66%), bleomycin (50–100%), quinacrine (50–83%), tetracycline (83–100%), doxorubicin (80%), mitoxantrone (76%), talc (87–100% insufflation; 83–100% slurry), radioactive colloidal gold and chromium phosphate (50%), and *Corynebacterium parvum* (81%). Finally, mechanical pleurectomy without chemical instillation can control pleural effusions in over 99% of patients, but this requires an operative procedure (although usually only thoracoscopy). Previously, tetracycline was the most popular agent, but this option is no longer available. Doxycycline, bleomycin, and talc are now the most frequently used. Talc is inexpensive, highly effective, and easily administered either as a powder insufflated into the open chest or as a slurry instilled through a chest tube. The other two agents are less successful and are expensive (bleomycin costs $1000 per 30-unit vial). In addition, two randomized trials have proved talc to be superior to both bleomycin and tetracycline. Some hesitancy to use talc has been expressed because of the associated patient discomfort, but there have been no reports of unmanageable pain similar to that seen previously with tetracycline instillation. Furthermore, talc no longer contains asbestos, and the induction of fibrothorax, which is a long-term theoretical concern, is not a problem in these short-lived patients. Talc is a foreign body, however, and use of antibiotics during pleurodesis for empyema prophylaxis may be prudent.

Complications following pleurodesis include pneumothorax, loculated hydrothorax, fever, infection (empyema), acute respiratory distress syndrome (particularly following bilateral simultaneous pleurodeses, which for this reason alone are contraindicated), and recurrence. Fortunately, problems are uncommon, and most patients can have their chest tubes removed within 48–72 hours following talc pleurodesis.

Table 18–1. Differential diagnosis of pleural effusions.[1]

	Tuberculosis	Cancer	Congestive Heart Failure	Pneumonia and Other Nontuberculous Infections	Rheumatoid Arthritis and Collagen Disease	Pulmonary Embolism
Clinical context	Younger patient with history of exposure to tuberculosis.	Older patient in poor general health.	Presence of congestive heart failure.	Presence of respiratory infection.	History of joint involvement; subcutaneous nodules.	Postoperative immobilized, or venous disease.
Gross appearance	Usually serous; often sanguineous.	Often sanguineous.	Serous.	Serous.	Turbid or yellow-green.	Often sanguineous.
Microscopic examination	May be positive for acid-fast bacilli; cholesterol crystals.	Cytology positive in 50%.	. . .	May be positive for bacilli.	. . .	. . .
Cell count	Few have > 10,000 erythrocytes; most have > 1000 leukocytes, mostly lymphocytes.	Two-thirds bloody; 40% >1000 leukocytes, mostly lymphocytes.	Few have > 10,000 erythrocytes or > 1000 leukocytes.	Polymorphonuclears predominate.	Lymphocytes predominate.	Erythrocytes predominate.
Culture	May have positive pleural effusion; few have positive sputum or gastric washings.	. . .	. . .	May be positive.	. . .	. . .
Specific gravity	Most > 1.016.	Most > 1.016.	Most > 1.016.	> 1.016.	> 1.016.	> 1.016.
Protein	90% 3 g/dL or more.	90% 3 g/dL or more.	75% > 3 g/dL.	3 g/dL or more.	3 g/dL or more.	3 g/dL or more.
Sugar	60% < 60 mg/dL.	Rarely < 60 mg/dL.	. . .	Occasionally < 60 mg/dL.	5–17 g/dL (rheumatoid arthritis).	. . .
Other	No mesothelial cells on cytology. Tuberculin test usually positive. pleural biopsy positive.	If hemorrhagic fluid, 65% will be due to tumor; tends to recur after removal.	Right-sided in 55–70%.	Associated with infiltrate on x-ray.	Rapid clotting time; LE cell or rheumatoid factor may be present.	Source of emboli may be noted.

Other exudates: spgr > 1.016. **Fungal infection:** Exposure in endemic area. Source fluid. Microscopy and culture may be positive for fungi. Protein 3 g/dL or more. Skin and serologic tests may be helpful. **Trauma:** Serosanguineous fluid. Protein 3 g/dL or more. **Chylothorax:** History of injury or cancer. Chylous fluid with no protein but with fat droplets.

[1]Modified from: Therapy of pleural effusion: A statement by the Committee on Therapy of the American Thoracic Society. Am Rev Respir Dis 1968;97:479.

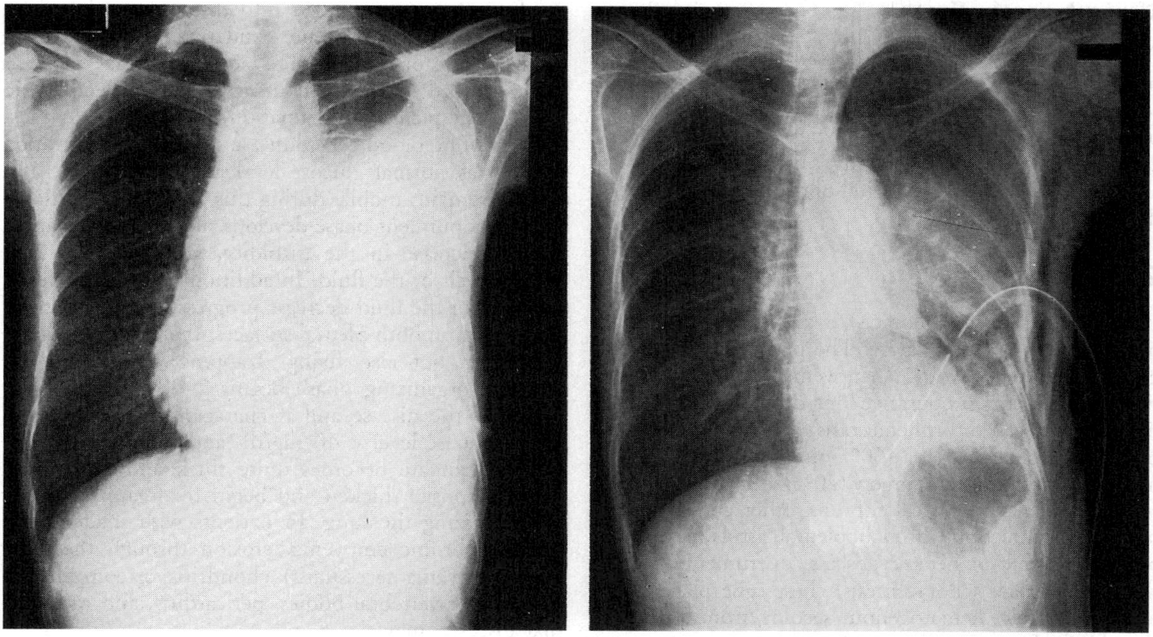

Figure 18–8. Malignant pleural effusion (carcinoma of lung). *Left:* Posteroanterior projection before treatment. *Right:* After chest tube drainage. Note left hilar mass and osteoblastic metastasis to the first lumbar vertebra.

Cardiovascular Disease

Pleural effusions are common findings in patients with moderate to severe congestive heart failure (Figure 18–9). The heart failure may be secondary to ischemia (coronary artery disease), valvular heart disease (mitral stenosis, mitral regurgitation, etc), viral myocarditis, congenital heart disease, and other less common lesions. The effusion may be bilateral or unilateral. When unilateral, the right hemithorax is most often affected. Fluid frequently involves the interlobar fissures (most commonly the minor fissure on the right) and can form localized collections simulating mass lesions known as "pseudotumors." Other cardiovascular causes of pleural effusions include constrictive pericarditis and pulmonary venous obstruction.

Renal Disease

Hydronephrosis, nephrotic syndrome, and acute glomerulonephritis are on occasion associated with pleural effusions. Rupture of the collecting system into the pleural space can also produce a hydrothorax. In this latter case, the pleural fluid creatinine will be elevated (fluid:serum creatinine ratio significantly > 1.0).

Pancreatitis

Moderate to severe pancreatitis is associated with a pleural effusion that characteristically occurs on the left and contains fluid with an amylase concentration substantially higher than that in the serum. Rarely pseudocysts of the capsule of the pancreas may communicate with the pleural space, resulting in high-volume pleural effusions.

Cirrhosis

Approximately 5% of patients with cirrhosis and ascites will develop a pleural effusion. In contrast to pancreatitis, nearly all of these effusions occur on the right side.

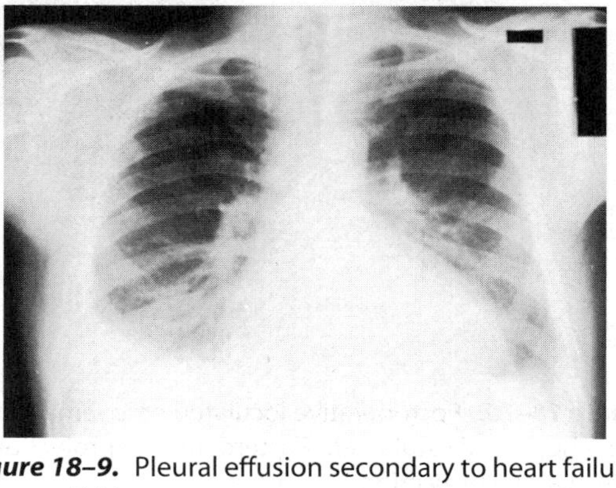

Figure 18–9. Pleural effusion secondary to heart failure (myocarditis).

Thromboembolism

Pulmonary thromboemboli are sometimes accompanied by a pleural effusion. These effusions are typically serosanguineous and small, but they may be frankly bloody and massive. Characteristic x-ray findings are almost always present in the lung. Since the fluid is usually reabsorbed in a short period of time, drainage is seldom necessary.

2. Thoracic Empyema

Pyothorax (empyema thoracis) is the accumulation of pus within the pleural cavity. The pus is usually thick, creamy, and malodorous. If empyema occurs in the setting of underlying suppurative lung disease (ie, pneumonia, lung abscess, or bronchiectasis), it is referred to as a parapneumonic empyema (60% of cases). Other causes of thoracic empyema are surgery (20%; see Figure 18–10), trauma (10%), esophageal rupture, other chest wall or mediastinal infections, bronchopleural fistula, extension of a subphrenic or hepatic abscess, instrumentation of the pleural space (thoracentesis, chest tube placement, etc), and, rarely, hematogenous seeding from a distant site of infection.

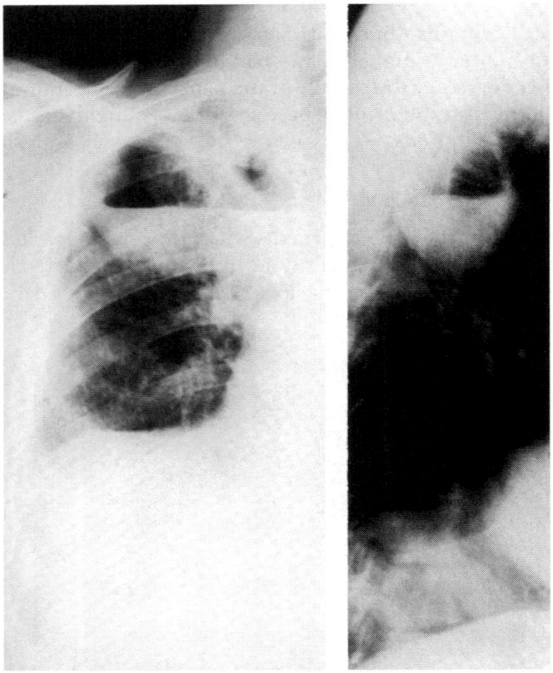

Figure 18–10. Postoperative loculated empyema with bronchopleural fistula. *Left:* Posteroanterior projection. *Right:* Lateral projection.

Empyemas are divided into three phases based on their natural history: acute exudative, fibrinopurulent, and chronic organizing. The acute exudative phase is characterized by the outpouring of sterile pleural fluid (incited by pleural inflammation), which has a low viscosity, white blood cell count, and LDH concentration as well as normal glucose level and normal pH. The pleura remains mobile during this phase. A transitional or fibrinopurulent phase develops subsequently, marked by an increase in the turbidity, white content, and LDH levels of the fluid. In addition, the glucose levels and pH of the fluid decrease progressively and fibrin is deposited on both pleural surfaces, thereby limiting the empyema but also fixing (trapping) the lung. The chronic organizing phase begins 7–28 days after the onset of the disease and is characterized by a pleural fluid glucose level < 40 mg/dL and a pH < 7.0. The pleural exudate becomes quite thick and the pleural fibrin deposits thicken and begin to organize, further immobilizing the lung. In patients with inadequately treated chronic empyema, erosion through the chest wall (empyema necessitatis), chondritis, osteomyelitis of the ribs or vertebral bodies, pericarditis, and mediastinal abscesses may occur.

The bacteriology of thoracic empyema has evolved over the years. Prior to the discovery of penicillin in the 1940s, most empyemas were caused by pneumococci and streptococci (Figure 18–11). With modern antibiotics and improved anaerobic culture techniques, however, the most common isolates from adult empyemas are now anaerobic bacteria, particularly bacteroides species as well as fusobacterium and peptococcus species.

Staphylococcus is the most common organism causing empyema (92% in children under 2 years old), and staphylococcal empyema is one of the most common complications of staphylococcal pneumonias in both adults and children (Table 18–2). Gram-negative bacteria also continue to be significant pathogens, particularly in parapneumonic empyemas. *Escherichia coli* and pseudomonas species account for 66% of aerobic gram-negative empyemas, and other organisms include *Klebsiella pneumoniae,* proteus species, *Enterobacter aerogenes,* and salmonella. Rarely, fungi (aspergillus, *Coccidioides immitis,* blastomyces, and *Histoplasma capsulatum*) and parasites such as *Entamoeba histolytica* can cause empyemas. In a recent review, empyemas were found to contain anaerobic bacteria in only 35% of cases, aerobic bacteria in only 24%, and a combination in 41%. In addition, the average number of bacterial species isolated was 3.2 per patient. Aspiration of oropharygeal flora may represent a source of polymicrobial infection.

Although patients may rarely be completely asymptomatic, most patients with thoracic empyemas present with varying symptoms depending on the underlying disease process, the extent of the pleural involvement,

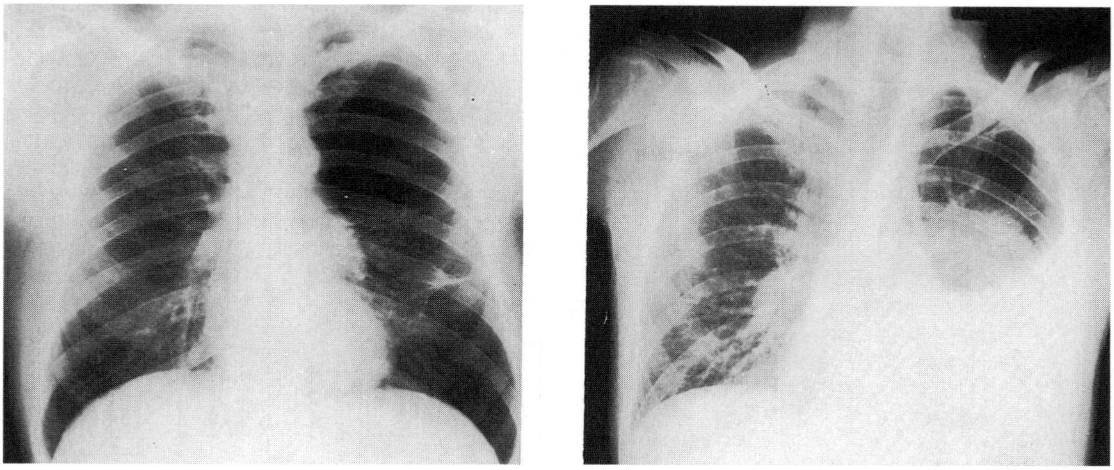

Figure 18–11. Streptococcal empyema. *Left:* Normal x-ray when patient was admitted with high fever. *Right:* Chest x-ray 3 days after admission.

and the immunologic state of the patient. Patients typically complain of fever, pleuritic chest pain or a sense of chest heaviness, dyspnea, hemoptysis, and a cough usually productive of purulent sputum. Signs of thoracic empyema include anemia, tachycardia, tachypnea, diminished breath sounds with dullness to percussion on the involved side, clubbing of fingertips, and occasionally pulmonary osteoarthropathy.

Although the medical history and physical examination often suggest the presence of thoracic empyema, the plain chest radiograph is the most important noninvasive diagnostic test. Empyemas can have almost any appearance and may be associated with an underlying pneumonia, lung abscess, or pleural effusion, but most commonly they appear as posterolateral D-shaped densities on x-ray. In large empyemas the mediastinum may be shifted away from the affected side. Bronchoscopy should be performed on all patients to exclude the presence of endobronchial obstruction. CT scanning provides critical anatomic detail regarding loculations and can assist in differentiation of empyema from lung abscess. Thoracentesis, however, is the procedure of choice for the diagnosis of thoracic empyema. Aspiration of pus establishes the diagnosis, permitting identification of the offending organisms. In early empyemas—particularly those partially treated with antibiotics—the pleural fluid may not be frankly purulent. In these cases, a pleural fluid pH < 7.0, glucose < 40 mg/dL, and an LDH level > 1000 units/L strongly suggests an evolving empyema even if Gram stain and cultures fail to identify organisms.

Goals for the treatment of thoracic empyemas include (1) control of the infection; (2) removal of the purulent material, with obliteration and sterilization of the pleural space and re-expansion of the lung; and (3) elimination of the underlying disease process. Options for treatment include repeated thoracentesis, closed tube thoracostomy, rib resection and open drainage, decortication and empyemectomy, thoracoplasty, and muscle flap closure. Adjunctive maneuvers reported to aid in the disruption and drainage of loculated empyemas include instillation of fibrinolytic enzymes, placement of high (–100 cm H_2O) suction, and video-assisted thoracoscopic debridement. A rational approach to empyema management is outlined in Figure 18–12). Initially, an intercostal catheter of adequate size is carefully inserted into the most dependent portion of the empyema cavity. If after 24–72 hours sepsis persists—or if there is any ques-

Table 18–2. Incidence of various complications of staphylococcal pneumonia in adults and children (in %).

	Adults	Children
Abscess	25	50
Empyema	15	15
Pneumatocele	1	35
Effusion	30	55
Bronchopleural fistula	2	5

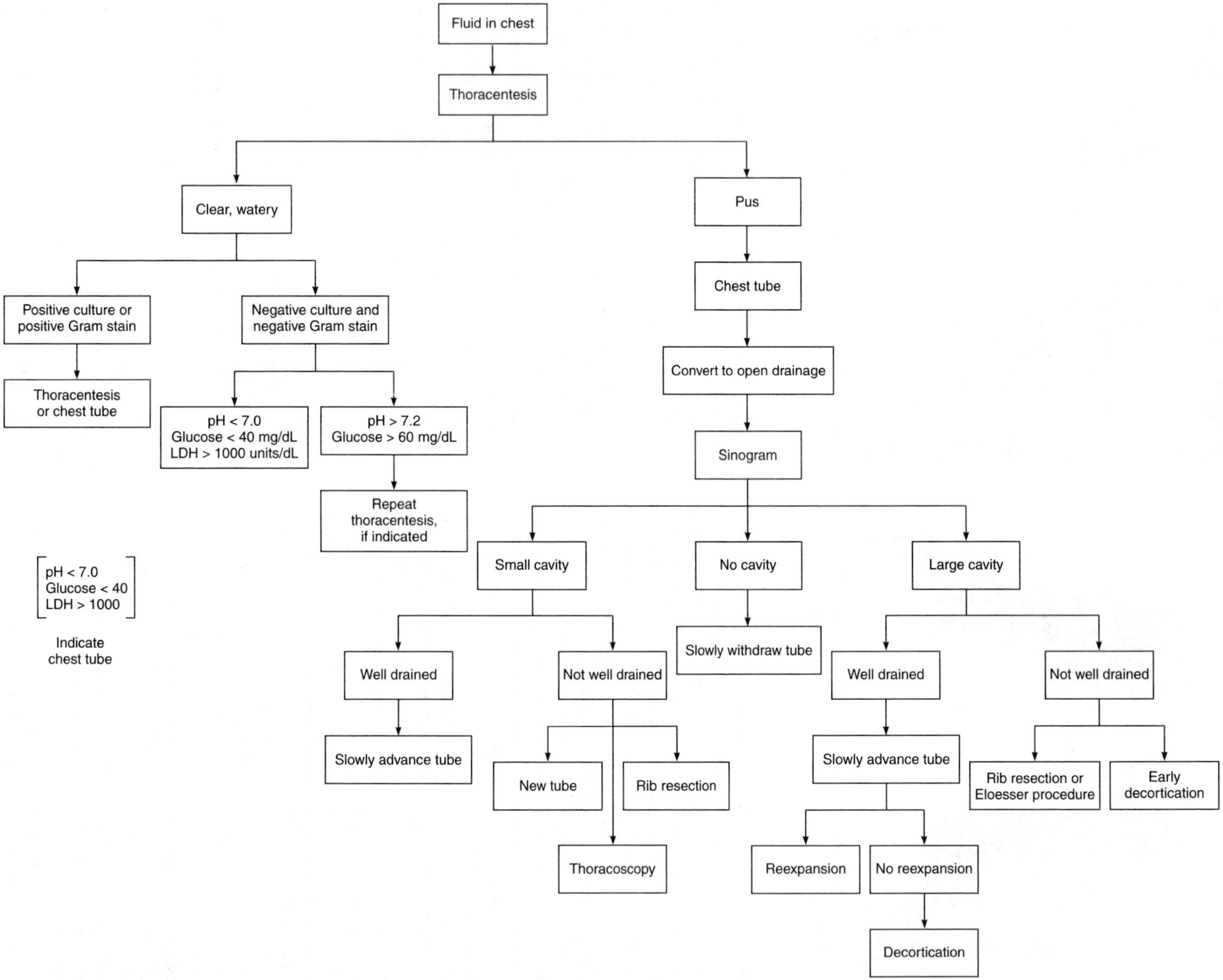

Figure 18–12. Management of empyema. (Modified and reproduced, with permission, from Shields TW: *General Thoracic Surgery,* 3rd ed. Williams & Wilkins, 1989.)

tion as to the adequacy of drainage—a CT scan should be obtained. If, on the other hand, complete drainage and reexpansion of the lung are achieved, no further drainage procedures are necessary.

Patients with residual spaces that are inadequately drained, patients with continued sepsis, and patients thought to require prolonged tube drainage are candidates for open drainage procedures. These can usually be safely performed 10–14 days after closed-tube drainage since the pleurae fuse by that time and the risk of pneumothorax and lung collapse is eliminated. Options for open drainage include simple rib resection and open flap drainage (Eloesser procedure). Simple rib resection involves the removal of short segments (3–6 cm) of one, two, or three ribs at the most dependent portion of the empyema cavity (at or anterior to the posterior axillary line). A tube can be placed through this opening and effective drainage established. A second approach involves the creation of a U-shaped flap of chest wall that is sewn to the parietal pleura after resection of short segments (3–6 cm) of one, two, or three ribs. This creates an epithelialized tract for long-term tubeless drainage of empyema cavities. The flap also acts as a one-way valve allowing fluid and air to escape during exhalation but sealing during inspiration to prevent the ingress of air. Symbas later modified the original Eloesser procedure by changing the flap to an inverted U-shaped flap with the base of the flap placed parallel to and at the level of the inferiormost aspect of the empyema cavity. This type of open drainage allows the empyema cavity to drain reliably and to be easily debrided, irrigated, and cleaned. Ultimately, through lung reexpansion, wound contraction, and granulation, the cavity often completely disappears.

Another option is early decortication and empyemectomy. This has been increasingly advocated in good-risk patients with early loculated empyemas and inadequate tube drainage or lung expansion. Furthermore, if performed early in the course of the process, resection of both parietal and visceral pleural peels (decortication) can be performed via minimally invasive technique without the need for rib spreading. More advanced or chronic disease involves a thoracotomy with decortication with resection of the intact empyema itself (empyemectomy), if possible. The best results with this approach are obtained when the underlying lung is entirely normal and reexpands fully. Posttraumatic empyema, in particular, has been amenable to this treatment.

Empyemas that occur following pulmonary resection often are more difficult to manage. If residual lung is present (resections less than pneumonectomy), the general principles outlined above still apply, although a complicating bronchopleural fistula is often present (Figure 18–13). Simple tube drainage is instituted initially followed by open drainage if necessary. Empyemas following pneumonectomy, however, pose a special problem since there is no longer any lung to obliterate the infected space. In addition, postpneumonectomy empyemas frequently are associated with bronchopleural fistulas. In these patients, specific surgical procedures designed to obliterate residual intrathoracic spaces and in many cases close remaining bronchopleural fistulas may be required (Figure 18–14). In the absence of a bronchopleural fistula, sterilization and closure of a postpneumonectomy space (without obliteration) may be attempted using an irrigation catheter inserted into the apex of the chest cavity. An antibiotic solution specific for the organisms present is then infused into the chest. The solution is allowed to drain through a dependent tube or opening created by simple rib resection. After 2–8 weeks, the catheters are removed and the cavity is closed. The success rate with this technique is quite variable and is reported to be 20–88%. For patients who fail this approach and for those patients with bronchopleural fistulas, the main goal of therapy is to obliterate the residual space and close any bronchopleural fistulas. This is most readily accomplished by the transposition of muscle with or without omentum into the empyema cavity. Multiple muscles may be required, including pectoralis major, latissimus dorsi, serratus anterior, intercostal muscle, and rectus abdominis (Figure 18–15). Use of these muscles is highly successful in closing any remaining bronchopleural fistulas and in completely obliterating the remaining intrathoracic space. The success of muscle flap closure of empyema spaces has made thoracoplasty (once a common procedure for reducing empyema spaces) a rare operation.

Antibiotics are an important adjunct in the treatment of empyemas, but it must be emphasized that drainage is the primary treatment modality. Although antibiotic therapy is always instituted early in the course of therapy when signs of systemic infection generally are present, they need not be continued once effective drainage is established. In fact, overuse of antibiotics may lead to the generation of resistant bacteria and therefore compromise the success of any subsequent procedures designed to obliterate residual intrathoracic space.

Alfageme I et al: Empyema of the thorax in adults: etiology, microbiologic findings, and management. Chest 1993;103:839.

Arnold PG, Pairolero PC: Intrathoracic muscle flaps: an account of their use in the management of 100 consecutive patients. Ann Surg 1990;211:656.

3. Hemothorax

Blood in the pleural space usually occurs secondary to trauma, surgery, diagnostic or therapeutic procedures,

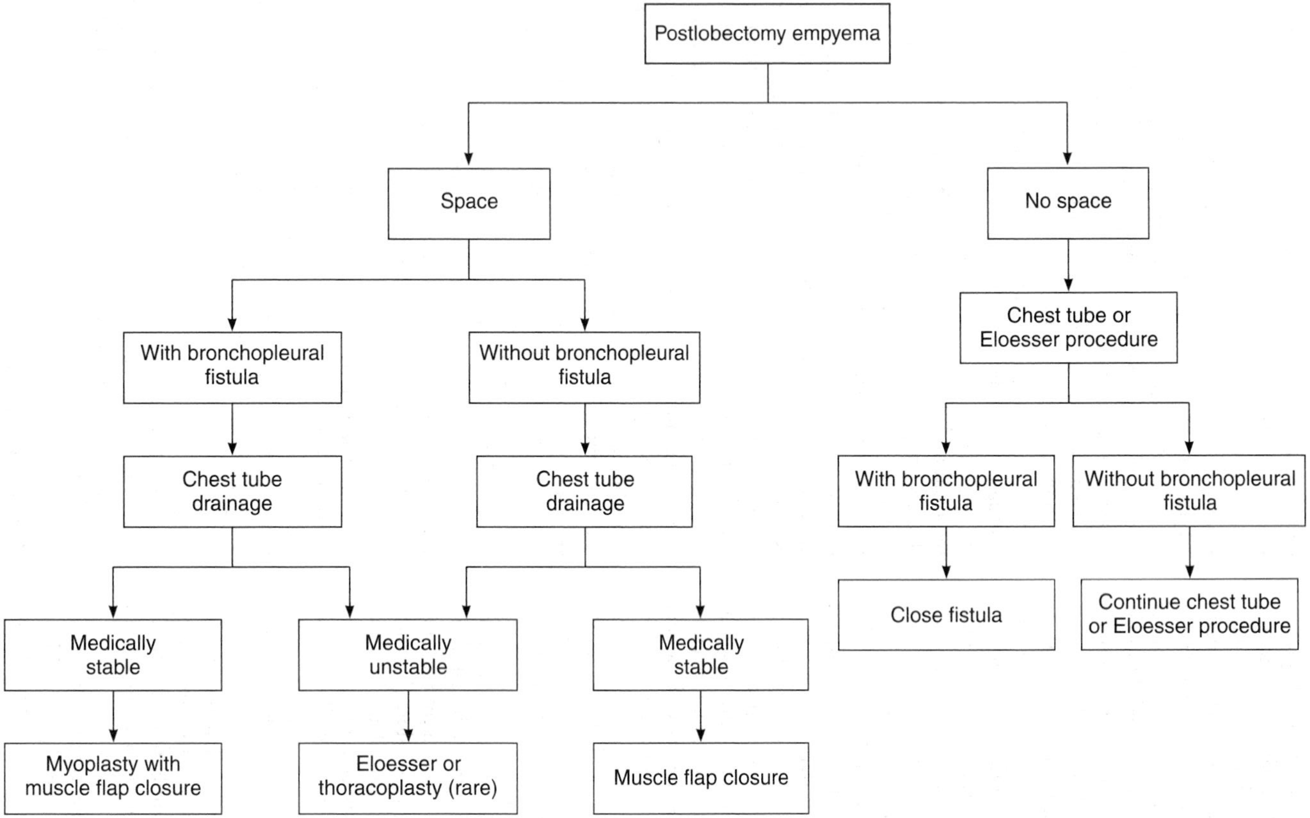

Figure 18–13. Postlobectomy empyema. (Modified and reproduced, with permission, from Shields TW: *General Thoracic Surgery,* 3rd ed. Williams & Wilkins, 1989.)

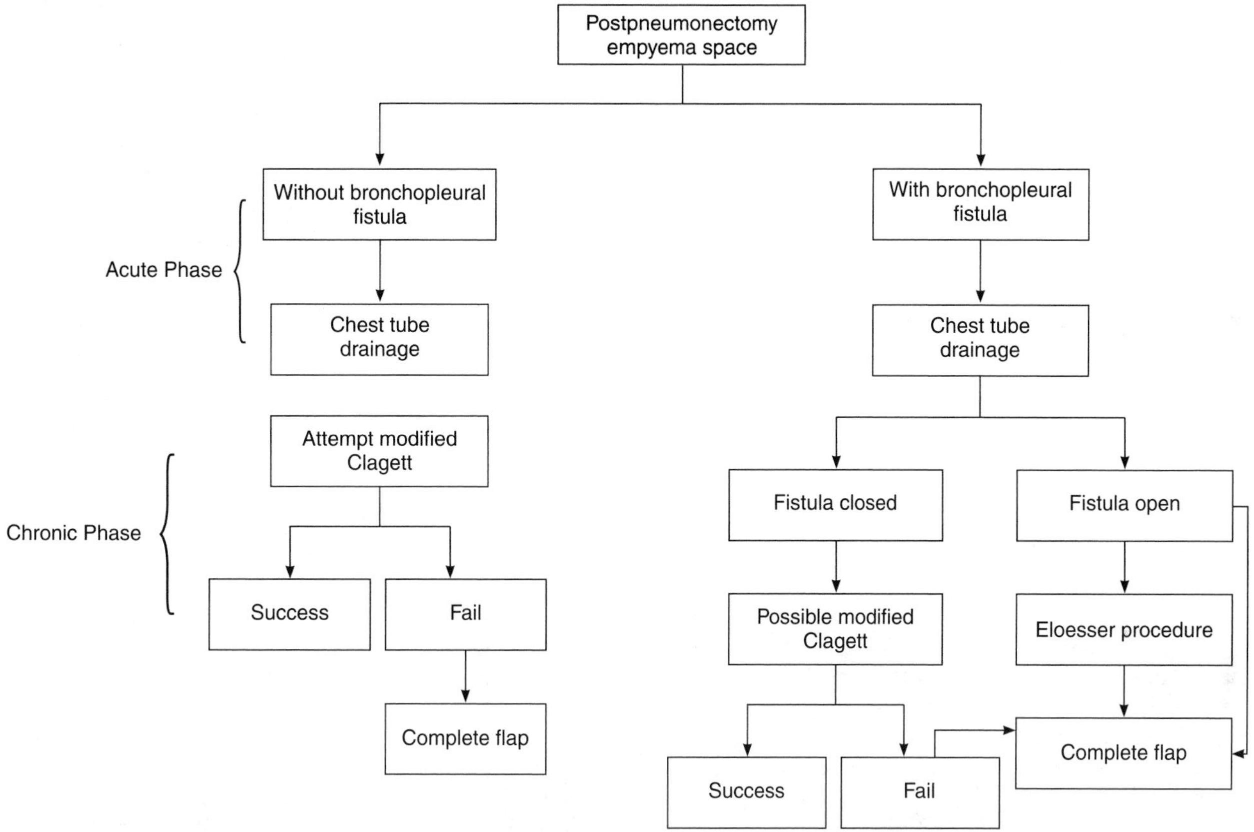

Figure 18–14. Postpneumonectomy empyema. (Modified and reproduced, with permission, from Shields TW: *General Thoracic Surgery,* 3rd ed. Williams & Wilkins, 1989.)

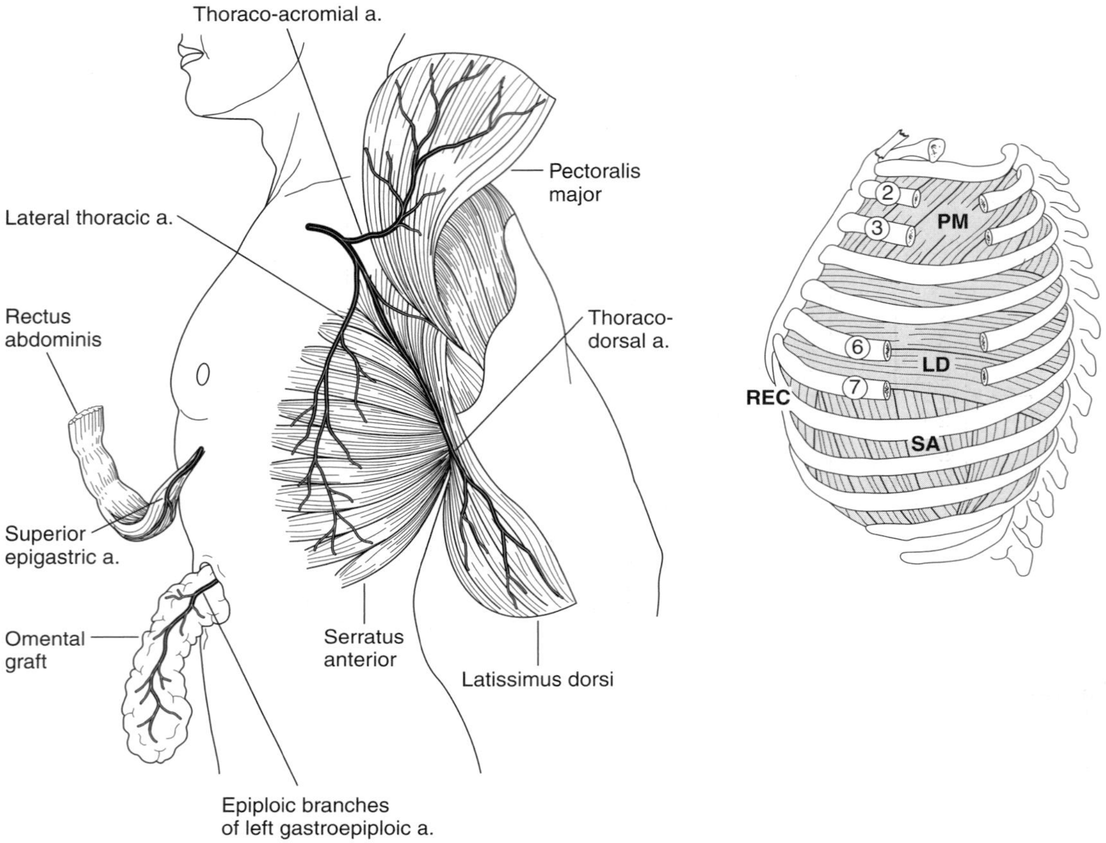

Figure 18–15. Extrathoracic muscle flap closure of a postpneumonectomy empyema cavity. (© 1984 Society for Thoracic Surgery. Reprinted with permission from Society for Thoracic Surgery.)

neoplasms, pulmonary infarction, and infections (tuberculosis). Most hemothoraces can be treated effectively with large-bore (32–36F) closed chest tube drainage, particularly since small amounts of blood (occupying less than one-third of the hemithorax) are readily reabsorbed by the body. However, if significant blood clot has formed (occupying more than one-third of the hemithorax) or if secondary infection occurs, further measures must be taken to avoid the development of an empyema or fibrothorax with pulmonary compromise. Currently, most hemothoraces requiring more than simple tube drainage can be managed with video-assisted thoracic surgical procedures. Rarely, open thoracotomy may be required for complete decortication and evacuation.

4. Chylothorax

Accumulation of chyle within the pleural space is most often due to surgical procedures, particularly cardiothoracic and esophageal operations. Trauma, malignancy, central venous catheterization, congenital lymphatic malformations, thoracic aortic aneurysms, filariasis, and cirrhosis may also rarely cause chylothorax. Penetrating thoracic trauma can lacerate the thoracic duct at any level, but blunt thoracic trauma usually causes a shearing of the duct at the right crus of the diaphragm. This may also occur with violent coughing or hyperextension of the spine. The initial treatment of chylothorax is similar to that of a malignant pleural effusion. Closed chest tube drainage is instituted; the lung is fully reexpanded; and a low-fat diet is started. In some cases, intravenous hyperalimentation (either peripheral or central) may greatly improve the patient's condition. Some evidence supports the use of somatostatin to decrease the output from chylous effusions. The irritating nature of chyle promotes pleurodesis, and in half of patients the leak will stop spontaneously. The instillation of sclerosing agents (see section on pleural effusion, above) has also been advocated to increase the chances of success. If chyle continues to drain for more than 7 days or if significant drainage continues for even a shorter period of time, serious consideration should be given to operation since patients quickly become malnourished from the large associated protein losses. Video-assisted thoracoscopic techniques are usually ideal, making open thoracotomy rarely necessary. The standard approach is via the right chest, where the thoracic duct may be identified as it emerges from beneath the diaphragm between the aorta and the azygos vein. Ligation of the tissues in this area is usually all that is needed.

PNEUMOTHORAX

Air in the pleural space (pneumothorax) can occur as a result of a breach in either the parietal (trauma, esophageal perforation, surgery, etc) or visceral pleura (bulla, fine needle aspirations, etc). Rarely, infections of the pleural space with gas-forming organisms may produce a pneumothorax.. Since a chest radiograph is only a two-dimensional representation of a three-dimensional space, a relatively small separation of the pleural surfaces (eg, 1 cm) on a chest x-ray can translate into a relatively large pneumothorax . A large amount of intrapleural air that causes a shift of the mediastinum toward the contralateral lung is referred to as a tension pneumothorax. A pneumothorax associated with an open chest wound may be termed an open pneumothorax or sometimes a "sucking chest wound." *Tension and open pneumothoraces are surgical emergencies since both ventilation and venous return of blood to the heart are compromised.* Intrapleural air may mix with blood, as frequently occurs after trauma (hemopneumothorax) or esophageal perforation (pyopneumothorax).

Pneumothoraces usually are classified as either spontaneous or acquired (those caused by a specific event such as trauma, invasive procedures, etc). Spontaneous pneumothoraces (Figure 18–16) sometimes are divided into "primary" and "secondary" categories; however, all spontaneous pneumothoraces are secondary to some underlying pathologic process, and such a division is therefore strictly artificial. Most commonly, spontaneous pneumothoraces are caused by rupture of small subpleural blebs due to increased transpulmonary pressure most pronounced at the apex of the lung (apex of the upper lobe and superior segment of the lower lobe). Coughing, rapid falls in atmospheric pressure (> 10 millibars/24 h), rapid decompression (scuba divers), and high altitudes (jet pilots) all are associated with increased transpulmonary pressures and spontaneous pneumothorax. In addition, normal transpulmonary pressures can cause rupture of blebs in patients with connective tissue disorders such as Marfan's syndrome. Other causes of spontaneous pneumothorax include apical bullae (patients with COPD), *Pneumocystis* pneumonia (patients with AIDS), metastatic cancer (particularly sarcomas), lymphangioleiomyomatosis, eosinophilic granuloma, rupture of the esophagus or of a lung abscess, cystic fibrosis, and menstruation (catamenial pneumothorax). Classically, however, spontaneous pneumothoraces occur in asthenic males (male: female ratio 6:1) between the ages of 16 and 24, often with a history of smoking. The true incidence is unknown since up to 20% of patients remain asymptomatic and do not seek medical attention.

Patients with pneumothoraces complain of pleuritic chest pain and dyspnea. If severe underlying cardiopulmonary disease exists or if a tension pneumothorax develops, symptoms become much more dramatic and include diaphoresis, cyanosis, weakness, and symptoms of hypotension and cardiovascular collapse. Physical examination reveals tachypnea, tachycardia, deviation of the trachea away from the involved side (tension pneumothorax), decreased breath sounds, hyperresonance, and diminished vocal fremitus on the involved side. Arterial blood gases may demonstrate hypoxia and occasionally hypocapnia from hyperventilation, and the ECG may show axis deviations, nonspecific ST segment changes, and T wave inversion. The standard test for the diagnosis of pneumothoraces is the posteroanterior (PA) and lateral chest radiograph. Exhalation accentuates the contrast between the collapsed lung and the intrapleural air as well as the magnitude of the collapse. Rarely, a CT scan may be necessary to differentiate a pneumothorax from a large bulla in patients with

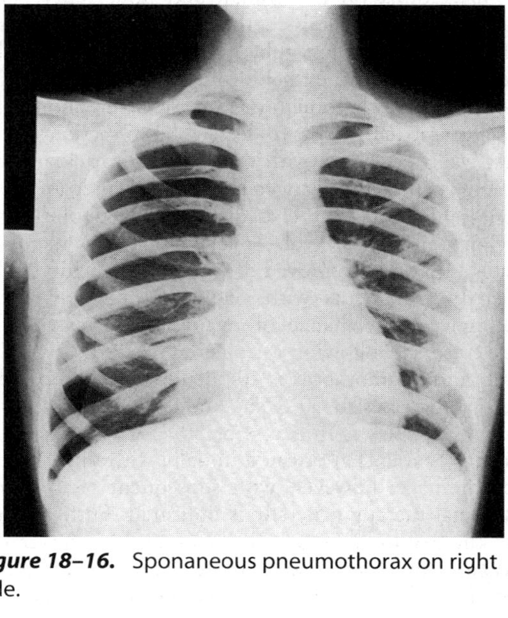

Figure 18–16. Sponaneous pneumothorax on right side.

severe emphysema. In 5–10% of patients, a small pleural effusion may be present and can be hemorrhagic.

The treatment of spontaneous pneumothoraces varies depending on the patient's symptoms and condition, the degree of collapse, the cause, and the estimate of the chance of recurrence. Small (< 20–25%), stable, asymptomatic pneumothoraces in otherwise healthy patients can be followed (often on an outpatient basis) with the expectation of complete resolution within several weeks, since air is normally reabsorbed at a rate of 1–1.25% per day. Larger asymptomatic pneumothoraces taking longer than 2–3 weeks to resolve place the patient at risk for developing trapped lung as a result of deposition of fibrin on the visceral pleura. These patients—as well as patients with symptoms, increasing pneumothoraces, or pneumothoraces associated with pleural effusions—should have them evacuated. In highly selected patients this can be accomplished with simple aspiration as long as the immediate and 2-hour delayed chest radiographs document reexpansion. It should be emphasized, however, that some small breaks in the visceral pleural seal once the lung collapses and can reopen with reexpansion. The chance of recurrence is 20–50% with this method, and follow-up x-ray is therefore mandatory after 24 hours.

Most patients with significant pneumothoraces (> 30%) require placement of a closed-chest catheter (8–20F) for acceptable reexpansion. This catheter then can be placed either to underwater suction drainage or to a Heimlich (one-way) valve. If a Heimlich valve maintains full expansion, the patient may be treated as an outpatient; however, if a Heimlich valve fails to reexpand the lung fully or if the patient's condition is not optimal, admission to hospital and underwater chest tube suction drainage is required. Unless some contraindication exists, chest tubes should be placed in the midaxillary line at the level of the fifth intercostal space (nipple line). In women the breast tissue should be retracted medially and avoided in the dissection to the chest wall. Placement with the use of blunt clamp dissection avoids the dangers of trocar insertion and should almost always be used. Following resolution of any air leakage, the tube may be taken off suction (water seal) and removed if the lung remains fully inflated. In patients with classic spontaneous pneumothoraces, the chance of recurrence increases with each episode. Following a single episode, the risk of a recurrent pneumothorax is 40–50%. After two episodes the risk increases to 50–75%, and with three previous episodes the risk is in excess of 80%. Currently, most first-time patients are treated initially with simple chest tube drainage; however, with subsequent recurrences, additional therapy generally is indicated. Furthermore, with the development of video-assisted thoracic surgery (VATS), some feel that a more aggressive approach should be taken even for first-time pneumothoraces.

Patients with air leaks lasting longer than 7 days, patients who do not fully reexpand their lungs, patients in high-risk occupations (scuba divers, airline pilots, etc), patients with large bullae or poor pulmonary function, and patients with bilateral or recurrent pneumothoraces are candidates for additional medical (pleurodesis) or surgical intervention. Furthermore, patients who frequently travel to places distant from medical care are offered early surgical intervention. Previously, tetracycline pleurodesis was used to decrease the incidence of recurrent pneumothoraces. The use of this substance, however, was associated with significant pain and controversy. It is currently no longer available. The use of talc slurry or powder in this setting is also controversial due to the potential for long-term fibrothorax and restrictive lung disease but has been shown to reduce the recurrence rate to as low as 2%. Many other chemical agents have been used in the past, including mechlorethamine, doxycycline, iodoform, guaiacol, urea, and hypertonic glucose, with varying success rates. Since pleurodesis can make subsequent surgical procedures more difficult, the use of this treatment option continues to generate controversy.

Medically fit patients who are candidates for pleurodesis are also candidates for operation. The procedures used to prevent recurrent pneumothoraces include (1) axillary thoracotomy with apical bullectomy, mechanical pleurodesis, and partial pleurectomy; and (2) complete parietal pleurectomy. Both procedures can be performed with either open or VATS techniques. Complete parietal pleurectomy generally is avoided, since some patients may require future thoracic surgical procedures that are extremely difficult in the face of total parietal pleurectomy. Apical bullectomy, mechanical pleurodesis, and partial apical pleurectomy have been shown to reduce the recurrence rate to near zero. In addition, this procedure is easily accomplished either with VATS techniques or through a small transaxillary thoracotomy, both of which are well tolerated.

Several special situations exist that require particular expertise in treatment decisions. Patients with cystic fibrosis and severe COPD may be candidates for lung transplantation, and both pleurodesis and operation may make subsequent transplantation more dangerous. Therefore, consultation with a transplant surgeon is advisable prior to considering these therapies. AIDS patients with *Pneumocystis* pneumonia and pneumothorax are extremely difficult to manage, having a high rate of persistent bronchopleural fistula, treatment failure, and death. For optimal management, the pulmonary surgeon should have extensive experience in the management of chest catheters.

PRIMARY PLEURAL TUMORS

Primary pleural tumors are uncommon neoplasms of two main types: diffuse malignant pleural mesotheliomas and localized fibrous tumors of the pleura (previously referred to as localized mesotheliomas). Although diffuse malignant pleural mesothelioma is the most common primary pleural tumor, involvement of the pleura with metastatic disease is more frequent and represents the most likely cause of any newly diagnosed pleural malignancy.

1. Localized Fibrous Tumors of the Pleura

Localized fibrous tumors of the pleura arise from subpleural fibroblasts than produce an array of lesions varying from peripheral pulmonary nodules to sessile subpleural masses to the more typical large pedunculated neoplasms. The visceral pleura is involved more often than the parietal pleural, and both benign (70%) and malignant (30%) variations exist. Histologically, benign tumors can exhibit three patterns—fibrous, cellular, and mixed—while malignant ones also have three distinct appearances, ie, tubulopapillary, fibrous, and dimorphic. These tumors behave more like sarcomas of the pleura than diffuse malignant mesotheliomas. Most localized fibrous tumors of the pleura are asymptomatic, discovered only incidentally on chest radiography. Extremely large tumors, however, may produce symptoms of bronchial compression with dyspnea, cough, and chest heaviness—and, rarely, symptoms of hypoglycemia from the production of an insulin-like peptide (4% of patients). On physical examination, signs of clubbing and hypertrophic pulmonary osteoarthropathy (20–35%) may be present. Chest radiography most often demonstrates a well-circumscribed mass that may move with changes in position if the tumor is pedunculated. A pleural effusion is present in 15% of cases and can be bloody, though this does not indicate unresectability. Fine-needle aspiration cytology may be suggestive; however, the diagnosis generally can be established with certainty only at surgery.

The treatment of these lesions is complete resection. Although lobectomy is usually not required for lesions involving the visceral pleura, wedge resection of the pulmonary parenchyma in the area of the tumor is recommended. For neoplasms arising from the parietal pleura, chest wall resection is prudent. Following complete surgical excision, no further therapy is indicated and the prognosis is good, with some patients surviving for over 10 years without recurrence; however, if the resection is incomplete, radiation therapy should be contemplated since the prognosis is poor, with a median survival of only 7 months.

2. Diffuse Malignant Pleural Mesothelioma

Diffuse malignant pleural mesothelioma is the most common primary tumor of the pleura. Since 1960, the disorder has been strongly linked to the use of asbestos. Thick serpentine asbestos fibers (chrysotile) generally are deposited in the proximal airways and are easily cleared with less risk of the development of tumors; however, thin needle-like amphibole fibers (crocidolite, amosite, actinolite, anthrophylite, and tremolite) and the soil silicate zeolite, found in the Anatolia region of Turkey usually lodge in the terminal airways and migrate to the pleura, thereby increasing the risk of diffuse malignant pleural mesothelioma to more than 300 times that of the general population. The increased incidence of mesothelioma in shipbuilders exposed to asbestos-laden insulation from World War II–era ships further implicates asbestosis in the pathophysiology of the disease. The latency period after exposure ranges from 15 years to 50 years. Recent research suggests that the generation of free radicals (including nitric oxide), depression of the immune system (both cellular and humoral), induction of cytokines (TNFα, IL-1α, IL-1β, and IL-6), and the production of genetic defects, eg, abnormalities of chromosomes 1, 3, 4, 6, 7, 9, 11, 17 (p53), and 22 (involves *c-sis,* which encodes for one chain of platelet-derived growth factor) all may play a role in the mechanism of asbestos-related disease.

Histologically, diffuse malignant pleural mesotheliomas are divided into four categories: (1) epithelial or tubopapillary (35–40%), which are associated with pleural effusions and a slightly better prognosis; (2) fibrosarcomatous or mesenchymal (20%), which are often "dry" mesotheliomas; (3) mixed (35–40%); and (4) undifferentiated (5–10%). The right hemithorax (60%) is affected more often than the left (35%), and 5% are bilateral.

Most patients with diffuse malignant pleural mesotheliomas complain of dyspnea on exertion and chest wall discomfort, but other symptoms, such as cough, fever (paraneoplastic), malaise, weight loss, and dysphagia also occur. Complaints of severe chest wall pain, abdominal distention, pericardial tamponade, and superior vena cava syndrome suggest advanced disease. Although most patients develop distant metastases at some time during the course of their disease, these lesions rarely become symptomatic. Chest radiographs are distinctly abnormal, showing pleural thickening, effusion (75%), and narrowing of intercostal spaces. Computed tomography often suggests the diagnosis because of diffuse irregular pleural thickening. The diagnosis generally requires substantial tissue samples and is not generally obtainable from fine-needle aspiration cytology. Tissue can be easily acquired with VATS techniques. Immunohistochemical stains for CEA, LeuM1, B72.3, and BerEP4 are usually negative, while those for vimentin and keratin are generally positive. Calretinin stain, which is specific for cells of mesothelial origin, has recently become available. This immunohistochemical marker can with near certainty determine whether an epithelial malignant tumor is either metastatic to pleura—eg, an adenocarcinoma (calretinin-negative)—or a primary malignant mesothelioma (calretinin-positive). This stain has become an important clinical tool and should be performed on all suspected cases of diffuse malignant pleural mesothelioma. Electron microscopy may also be helpful in distinguishing this disorder from metastatic adenocarcinoma, with which it is often confused. Pathologic staging of diffuse malignant pleural mesothelioma, like its treatment (see below), has been controversial. The original Butchart staging system and a more recently promulgated TNM staging system are set forth in the Table 18–3; however, neither is widely accepted or utilized.

The treatment of diffuse malignant pleural mesothelioma also remains variable. Owing to the low incidence of this disease, its natural history has not been carefully defined with regard to various prognostic factors, and few randomized trials have been conducted to compare treatment strategies. The reported median survival for all patients ranges from 7 months to 16 months. Recent randomized prospective trials have demonstrated benefit of platinum-based chemotherapy in combination with the antifolates pemetrexed or raltitrexed Vogelzang and coworkers randomized 448 patients with unresectable pleural mesothelioma to receive cisplatin versus cisplatin in combination with pemetrexed. Patients treated with pemetrexed in addition to cisplatin demonstrated improved median survival (12.1 versus 9.3 months) and progression-free survival. The improved survival came at a cost of increased bone marrow-related toxicity (neutropenia and leukopenia). van Meerbeeck and coworkers demonstrated similar findings in a randomized sample of patients comparing cisplatin versus combination cisplatin and raltitrexed. Mean survival in the cohort receiving combination cisplatinum and raltitrexed was 11.2 months versus 8.8 months in patients receiving cisplatin alone. Newer chemotherapeutic agents under active investigation include Rampirinase, intrapleural IL-2, and vascular endothelial derived growth factor antagonists (bevacizumab)

Surgery alone has also been used in attempts to improve survival, and two major approaches have been utilized: radical pleuropneumonectomy or parietal pleurectomy with decortication. The initial experience with radical pleuropneumonectomy demonstrated only a higher associated morbidity but not better long-term survival when compared to less radical pleurectomy and decortication. When combined with postoperative chest wall irradiation, the latter procedure results in a median survival of up to 25 months. Other approaches have combined preoperative chemotherapy (MD Anderson), intraoperative and postoperative chemotherapy (Lung Cancer Study Group, Cleveland Clinic), photodynamic therapy (NCI), and immunotherapy with TNFα as well as IFN-α and -γ (NCI, SWOG) with limited success. Currently, the use of intraoperative radiation therapy (UCSF, MSKCC) and gene therapy are also being investigated. Although the gen-

Table 18–3. Staging systems for malignant mesothelioma.

BUTCHART STAGING SYSTEM

Stage I: Tumor is confined within the "capsule" of the parietal pleura—ie, involving the ipsilateral pleura, lung, diaphragm, and external surface of the pericardium within the pleural reflection only.

Stage II: Tumor invades the chest wall or mediastinum (esophagus, trachea, or great vessels). Alternatively, lymph nodes within the chest are involved with metastatic disease.

Stage III: Tumor penetrates the diaphragmatic muscle to involve the peritoneum or retroperitoneum, the pericardium to involve the internal surface or heart, and the mediastinum to involve the contralateral pleura. Alternatively, lymph nodes outside the chest are involved with metastatic disease.

Stage IV: Distant hematogenous metastatic.

TNM STAGING SYSTEM

Tumor Stage

TX: The primary tumor cannot be assessed.
T0: No evidence of primary tumor exists.
T1: The primary tumor is limited to the ipsilateral parietal or visceral pleura.
T2: Tumor invades any of the following: ipsilateral lung, endothoracic fascia, diaphragm, pericardium.
T3: Tumor invades any of the following: ipsilateral chest wall muscles, ribs, mediastinal organs or tissues.
T4: Tumor extends to any of the following: contralateral pleura or lung by direct extension, peritoneum or intra- abdominal organs by direct extension, cervical tissues.

Lymph node stage

NX: Regional lymph nodes cannot be assessed.
N0: No regional lymph node metastases are present.
N1: Metastases are present in ipsilateral bronchopulmonary or hilar lymph nodes.
N2: Metastases are present in ipsilateral mediastinal lymph nodes.
N3: Metastases are present in contralateral mediastinal, internal mammary, supraclavicular, or scalene lymph nodes.

Metastatic stage

MX: The presence of distant metastases cannot be assessed.
M0: No distant metastases exist.
M1: Distant metastases are present.

STAGE GROUPINGS

Stage I: T1–2, N0, M0
Stage II: T1–2, N1, M0
Stage III: T3, N0–1, M0; T1–3, N2, M0
Stage IV: T4, any N, M0; any T, N3, M0; any T, any N, M1

eral impression is that multimodality therapy is superior to any one therapy alone, the exact combination of treatment options for this disease is yet to be defined. It is clear, however, that new therapies are needed.

Antman KH: Natural history and epidemiology of malignant mesothelioma. Chest 1993;103:373S.

Cheng AY: Neoplasms in the mediastinum, chest wall, and pleura. Curr Opin Oncol 1999;6:17.

Patz EF Jr et al: Malignant pleural mesothelioma: value of CT and MR imaging in predicting resectability. AJR Am J Roentgenol 1992;159:961.

Rusch VW, Piantadosi S, Holmes EC: The role of extrapleural pneumonectomy in malignant pleural mesothelioma: a Lung Cancer Study Group trial. J Thorac Cardiovasc Surg 1991; 102:1.

Steele JP, Klabatsa A: Chemotherapy options and new advances in malignant pleural mesothelioma Ann Oncol 2005;16:245.

Sugarbaker DJ et al: Extrapleural pneumonectomy, chemotherapy, and radiotherapy in the treatment of diffuse malignant pleural mesothelioma. J Thorac Cardiovasc Surg 1991;102:10.

van Meerbeeck JP et al: A randomized phase II study of cisplatin with or without raltitrexed in patients (pts) with malignant pleural mesothelioma (MPM): An intergroup study of the EORTC Lung Cancer Group and NCIC. Proc Am Soc Clin Oncol 2004 (Abstr 7021).

Vogelzang NJ, Porta C, Mutti L: Phase III study of pemetrexed in combination with cisplatin versus cisplatin alone in patients with malignant pleural mesothelioma (MPM). J Clin Oncol 2003;21:2696.

DISEASES OF THE MEDIASTINUM

MEDIASTINITIS

Mediastinitis may be acute or chronic. There are four sources of mediastinal infection: direct contamination, hematogenous or lymphatic spread, extension of infection from the neck or retroperitoneum, and extension from the lung or pleura. The most common direct contamination is esophageal perforation. Acute mediastinitis may follow esophageal, cardiac, and other mediastinal operations. Rarely, the mediastinum is directly infected by suppurative conditions involving the ribs or vertebrae. Most direct mediastinal infections are caused by pyogenic organisms. Most mediastinal infections that invade via the hematogenous and lymphatic routes are granulomatous. Contiguous involvement of the mediastinum along fascial planes from cervical infection is frequent; this occurs less commonly from the retroperitoneum because of the influence of the diaphragm. Empyema often loculates to form a paramediastinal abscess, but extension to form a true mediastinal abscess is uncommon. Extension of mediastinal infections to involve the pleura is common.

1. Acute Mediastinitis

Esophageal perforation, the source of 90% of acute mediastinal infections, can be caused by vomiting (Boerhaave's syndrome), iatrogenic trauma (endoscopy, dilation, operation), external trauma (penetrating or blunt), cuffed endotracheal tubes, ingestion of corrosives, carcinoma, or other esophageal disease. Mediastinal infection secondary to cervical disease may follow oral surgery; cellulitis; external trauma involving the pharynx, esophagus, or trachea; and cervical operative procedures such as tracheostomy, mediastinoscopy, and thyroidectomy.

Clinical Findings

Emetogenic esophageal perforation (Boerhaave's syndrome) is usually associated with a history of vomiting but in some cases is insidious in onset. Severe boring pain located in the substernal, left or right chest, or epigastric regions is the chief complaint in over 90% of cases. One-third of patients have radiation to the back, and in some cases pain in the back may predominate. Low thoracic mediastinitis can sometimes be confused with acute abdominal diseases or pericarditis. Acute mediastinitis is often associated with chills, fever, or shock. If pleural extension develops, breathing may aggravate the pain or cause radiation to the shoulder. Swallowing increases the pain, and dysphagia may be present. The patient is febrile, and tachycardia is noted. About 60% of patients have subcutaneous emphysema or pneumomediastinum. A pericardial crunching sound with systole (Hamman's sign) is often a late sign. Fifty percent of patients with esophageal perforation have pleural effusion or hydropneumothorax. Pneumomediastinum or pneumothorax following esophageal endoscopy are sine qua non of esophageal perforation. Neck tenderness and crepitation are more often found in cervical perforations.

The diagnosis may be confirmed by contrast x-ray examination of the esophagus, preferably using water-soluble media. Endoscopic visualization of the perforation is not recommended as an initial diagnostic maneuver as this may inadvertently extend the perforation. Chest CT scan with oral and intravenous contrast is helpful in determining the level of the perforation and the degree of mediastinal soilage as well as possible underlying esophageal or pulmonary pathology. The patient, however, must be clinically stable to be subjected to the rigors of these tests. For more critically ill patients, simple oral administration (or administration through a proximally placed nasogastric tube) of contrast and a simultaneous portable chest x-ray in an ICU setting can often confirm the diagnosis. Myocardial infarction is sometimes mistakenly diagnosed in patients with esophageal perforation when a predisposing cause of pneumomediastinum is not apparent.

Treatment

Surgical management of intrathoracic esophageal perforation depends on the underlying cause (iatrogenic, tumor, stricture, etc) and the amount of elapsed time from leak to diagnosis. All intrathoracic leaks should be surgically explored. Initial management includes immediate drainage of associated pleural contamination by large-bore chest tubes and decompression of the occasional pneumothorax. Broad-spectrum antibiotics, including antifungal therapy, are initiated and vigorous fluid hydration administered.

Typically, a right thoracotomy offers the most access to the intrathoracic esophagus and should be used through the sixth interspace. Even distal left-sided perforations can be managed from the right side. A left thoracotomy, however, is useful when a perforated esophagus from a distal esophageal stricture is encountered.

Treatment of an immediately recognized (< 24 hours) iatrogenic esophageal perforation in an otherwise normal esophagus includes primary two-layer closure with careful attention to complete mucosal closure by interrupted absorbable sutures. Esophageal muscle is then closed over the mucosal injury and buttressed with either a flap of parietal pleura, diaphragm, or intercostal muscle. Copious irrigation and wide drainage is performed. Occasionally, closure over a T-tube drain has been successful.

Esophageal perforations more than 48 hours old are widely drained and the esophagus either defunctionalized or resected. This depends on the degree of mediastinal soilage discovered upon exploration, the extent of sepsis, and the patient's performance status. When perforation occurs secondary to esophageal cancer or manipulation for severe reflux stricture, achalasia, or an otherwise abnormal esophagus, different surgical options exist. If the perforation is recognized immediately and the patient is not floridly septic, esophageal resection is preferred. Reconstruction (usually with a gastric pull-up) can be done at the same setting but only if the patient is stable and the degree of contamination minimal. Otherwise, reconstruction is performed at a later date when the patient has fully recovered from the septic event.

The mortality associated with esophageal perforation remains high (30–60%) despite advances in critical care, nutritional support, and operative management. The specific surgical approach—repair versus diversion or resection—must be tailored to the individual circumstances (mechanism of perforation, underlying pathology, time to diagnosis, and patient performance status) in order to achieve optimal results.

2. Chronic Mediastinitis

Chronic mediastinitis usually involves specific granulomatous processes with associated mediastinal fibrosis and chronic abscesses. Histoplasmosis, tuberculosis, actinomycosis, nocardiosis, blastomycosis, and syphilis have been incriminated. Amebic abscesses and parasitic disease such as echinococcal cysts are rare causes. The infectious process is usually due to histoplasmosis or tuberculosis and involves the mediastinal lymph nodes. Esophageal obstructions may occur. Adjacent mediastinal structures may become secondarily infected. Granulomatous mediastinitis and fibrosing mediastinitis are different manifestations of the same disease. Mediastinal fibrosis is a term used synonymously with idiopathic, fibrous, collagenous, or sclerosing mediastinitis. Eighty or more cases of mediastinal fibrosis have been reported, but the cause has been determined in only 16%, and of these over 90% were due to histoplasmosis. In only 25% of 103 cases of granulomatous mediastinitis has the cause been identified. Histoplasmosis was the most common known cause (60%) and tuberculosis the second most common (25%).

About 85% of patients with mediastinal fibrosis have symptoms from entrapment of mediastinal structures as follows: superior vena caval obstruction in 82%; tracheobronchial obstruction, 9%; pulmonary vein obstruction, 6%; pulmonary artery occlusion, 6%; and esophageal obstruction, 3%. Rarely, inferior vena caval obstruction or involvement of the thoracic duct, atrium, recurrent laryngeal nerve, or stellate ganglion is found. Multiple structures may be simultaneously involved.

Seventy-five percent of patients with granulomatous mediastinitis have no symptoms, and disease is discovered by chest x-ray, which shows a mediastinal mass. The mass is in the right paratracheal region in 75% of cases. In the 25% of patients with symptoms, about half have superior vena caval obstruction and one-third have esophageal obstruction. Occasional patients have bronchial obstruction, bronchoesophageal fistula, or pulmonary venous obstruction.

A mediastinal tuberculous or fungal abscess occasionally dissects long distances to present on the chest wall paravertebrally or parasternally. Secondary rib or costal cartilage infections with multiple draining sinus tracts occur.

Clinical Findings

A. Symptoms and Signs

Granulomatous and fibrosing mediastinitis affects women two to three times more commonly than men. Women aged 20–30 years are most typically affected, though the disorder may present in the fourth to fifth decades. Esophageal involvement results in dysphagia or hematemesis. Tracheobronchial involvement may cause severe cough, hemoptysis, dyspnea, wheezing, and episodes of obstructive pneumonitis. Pulmonary vein obstruction—the most common serious manifestation—produces congestive heart failure resembling advanced mitral stenosis and is usually fatal. Although not diagnostic, the respective skin tests in cases due to histoplasmosis or tuberculosis are strongly positive.

B. Imaging Studies

X-ray findings demonstrate a right paratracheal or anterior mediastinal mass. There may be spotty or subcapsular calcifications. Classically, histoplasmosis presents with hilar node calcification or so-called "popcorn" granuloma appearance. Calcification can also occur in thymoma or teratoma located in the anterior mediastinum. Chest CT (with intravenous and oral contrast) is most effective in defining the extent of mediastinal fibrosis and impingement on vital structures.

Treatment

Specific antimicrobial therapy is indicated when an infecting organism is identified. Patients with symptomatic mediastinal masses and fibrosis can require resection for relief of obstruction.

Prognosis

The prognosis following surgical excision of granulomatous mediastinal masses is good. Operative procedures do not appear to activate fibrosing mediastinitis, but success in treatment has been unpredictable. Most patients with fibrosing mediastinitis—whether treated or not—survive but have persistent symptoms.

Cherveniakov A, Cherveniakov P: Surgical treatment of acute purulent mediastinitis. Eur J Cardiothorac Surg 1992;6:407.

Gottlieb LJ et al: Rigid internal fixation of the sternum in postoperative mediastinitis. Arch Surg 1994;129:489.

Karworde SV et al: Mediastinitis in heart transplantation. Ann Thorac Surg 1992;54:1034.

Marty-Ane CH et al: Descending necrotizing mediastinitis. Advantage of mediastinal drainage with thoracotomy. J Thorac Cardiovasc Surg 1994;57:55.

Ringelman PR et al: Long-term results of flap reconstruction in median sternotomy wound infection. Plast Reconstr Surg 1994;93:1208.

SUPERIOR VENA CAVAL SYNDROME

Superior vena caval obstruction produces a distinctive clinical syndrome. Malignant tumors are the cause in 80–90% of cases; lung cancer accounts for about 90%. The incidence of superior vena caval syndrome in lung cancer patients is 3–5%. The male:female ratio is about 5:1. Other primary mediastinal tumors that may cause superior vena caval obstruction include thymoma, Hodgkin's disease, and lymphosarcoma. Metastatic tumors from the breast or thyroid or from melanoma also occasionally cause superior vena caval obstruction. Benign tumors are an unusual cause, but substernal goiter, any large benign mediastinal masses, and atrial myxoma have been implicated. Thrombotic conditions, either idiopathic or associated with polycythemia, mediastinal infection, or indwelling catheters, are unusual causes. The association of superior vena caval obstruction with chronic mediastinitis is discussed in the preceding section. Trauma may produce acute venous obstruction (eg, traumatic asphyxia, mediastinal hematoma).

The clinical manifestations depend on the abruptness of onset, the location of the obstruction, the completeness of occlusion, and the availability of collateral pathways. Venous pressure measured in the arms or head varies from 200 to 500 mm H_2O, and severity of symptoms is correlated with the pressure. Fatal cerebral edema can occur within minutes of an acute complete obstruction, whereas a slowly evolving one permits development of collaterals and may be only mildly symptomatic. Symptoms are milder when the azygos vein is patent. Azygous blood flow—normally about 11% of the total venous return—can increase to 35% of the venous return from the head, neck, and upper extremities. Thus, the most severe cases occur when occlusion is complete and the azygos vein is involved. The thrombus may propagate proximally to occlude the innominate and axillary veins.

Clinical Findings

Symptoms include puffiness of the face, arms, and shoulders and a blue or purple discoloration of the skin. Central nervous system symptoms include headache, nausea, dizziness, vomiting, distortion of vision, drowsiness, stupor, and convulsions. Respiratory symptoms include cough, hoarseness, and dyspnea, often due to edema of the vocal cords or trachea. Nasal congestion is often an early presenting symptom. These symptoms are made worse when the patient lies flat or bends over. In long-standing cases, esophageal varices may develop and produce gastrointestinal bleeding. The veins of the neck and upper extremities are visibly distended, and in long-standing cases there are marked collateral venous channels over the anterior chest and abdomen. Chronic pleural effusions may develop as a result of impaired lymphatic drainage. Onset of symptoms in fibrosing mediastinitis may be insidious, consisting initially of early morning edema of the face and hands. Occasionally, symptoms and findings are localized to one side when the level of obstruction is above the vena cava and only the innominate vein is blocked. In this situation, symptoms are mild because communicating veins in the neck usually decompress the affected side.

The diagnosis is confirmed by measuring upper extremity venous pressure; in patients with severe symptoms, a pressure of 350 mm H_2O or more is usual. The location and extent of obstruction are best determined by venography. When patients with malignant vena caval obstruction are studied by venography, 35% have thrombosis involving the innominate or axillary veins, 15% have complete caval obstruction without thrombosis, and 50% have partial superior vena caval obstruction. If patency of the azygos vein is in question, interosseous azygography may be useful. Chest x-ray may show a right upper lobe lung lesion or right paratracheal mass. Aortography is occasionally required to exclude aortic aneurysm, though CT scan with contrast enhancement for such lesions is increasingly diagnostic. The differential diagnosis may include angioneurotic edema, congestive heart failure, constrictive pericarditis, and fibrosing mediastinitis. Effort thrombosis of the axillary vein and innominate vein obstruction from elongation and buckling of the innominate artery can be considered in unilateral cases.

Complications

In patients with partial superior vena caval obstruction, thrombosis may suddenly change mild symptoms to marked venous distention, cyanotic swelling, vocal cord edema, and impaired cerebration. Bleeding from esophageal varices is rare except in severe long-standing cases.

Treatment

Superior vena caval obstruction caused by cancer should be treated with diuretics, restriction, avoidance of upper extremity intravenous lines, head elevation, and prompt radiation therapy. Cases of superior vena cava obstruction due to tumor begin to subside by 7–10 days of treatment. Because of the possibility of thrombosis in malignant cases, the use of fibrinolytic agents has been suggested. Caution must be advised in using anticoagulants, however, because many patients have advanced disease and may harbor occult cerebral metastases. Therefore, before starting therapy, patients should undergo CT or MRI brain scanning to prevent the occurrence of intracerebral hemorrhage. Recently, the use of intravascular expansile stents has been pioneered. Limited early experience suggests that the lumen can be reopened and that good venous drainage and decompression can be achieved by minimally invasive interventional radiologic techniques. Long-term results have not been reported, and disadvantages include the need for anticoagulation to prevent recurrent thrombosis. Chemotherapy is sometimes used alone or with radiotherapy. Most cases of malignant superior vena caval obstruction are not remediable by operation. Tissue diagnosis is important for diagnosis and for guiding therapy. Invasive procedures, however, must be tailored to the individual patient and the severity of the caval obstruction. Patients with new, severe, or rapidly progressive symptoms should receive immediate palliative radiation therapy. Patients with subacute presentations can better tolerate the time required to make the diagnosis.

Fine-needle aspiration, bronchoscopy, cervical mediastinoscopy, and anterior mediastinotomy—and even, occasionally, thoracotomy—offer possible approaches for obtaining tissue. Caution must be advised, however, in the setting of acute fulminant superior vena caval obstruction as any invasive procedure will carry a significantly higher morbidity due to bleeding from venous obstruction. In this case, attempts at invasive techniques for tissue diagnosis should be avoided. Most frequently, the disease process has been previously histologically confirmed because superior vena caval obstruction presents typically as a complication of locally advanced disease. In benign incomplete superior vena caval obstruction, surgical excision of the compressing mass can provide an excellent result. In total obstruction, such as occurs in fibrosing mediastinitis, most patients will gradually improve without treatment. There are numerous surgical procedures designed to bypass caval obstruction, replace the superior vena cava, or recanalize the vena caval lumen. These procedures have been dramatically effective in some cases, but only recently have they been sufficiently successful to warrant consideration.

Prognosis

Radiotherapy is most effective when superior vena caval obstruction is incomplete. Mean survival of patients with malignant caval obstruction from lung cancer is 6–8 months. The death rate from causes related to vena caval obstruction itself is only 1–2%.

Doty DB, Doty JR, Jones KW: Bypass of superior vena cava: fifteen years' experience with spiral vein graft for obstruction of superior vena cava caused by benign disease. J Thorac Cardiovasc Surg 1990;99:889.

Kistler AM et al: Superior vena cava obstruction in fibrosing mediastinitis: demonstration of right-to-left shunt and venous collaterals. Nucl Med Commun 1991;12:1067.

Stea B, Kinsella T: Superior vena caval syndrome: clinical features, diagnosis, and treatment. In: *Mediastinal Surgery.* Shields T (editor). Lea & Febiger, 1991.

Urschel HC Jr et al: Sclerosing mediastinitis: improved management with histoplasmosis titer and ketoconazole. Ann Thorac Surg 1990;50:215.

MEDIASTINAL MASS LESIONS

Lesions within the mediastinum represent an interesting variety of masses, both malignant and benign, that arise from the diverse organs and tissues which occupy the central thorax. Overall, the incidence of all mediastinal masses is low, especially compared with the frequency of lesions arising within the lung—bronchogenic cancer, etc. Mediastinal malignancies constitute less than 20% of all thoracic tumors.

Mediastinal masses arise from specific structures that reside in relatively constant anatomic arrangement. The mediastinum itself is defined laterally by the mediastinal pleura of each lung; superiorly and inferiorly by the thoracic inlet and diaphragm, respectively; anteriorly by the sternum; and posteriorly by the vertebral bodies. For purposes of definition, the mediastinum is divided loosely into three main compartments: anterior (or anterosuperior), middle, and posterior. The great vessels and heart, pericardium, trachea, and esophagus define and occupy the middle compartment, which separates anterior from posterior areas. The posterior compartment extends to both sides of the vertebrae to incorporate the paravertebral sulci bilaterally. The distribution and origin of mediastinal masses are summarized in Table 18–4.

The most common mediastinal masses in children are neurogenic tumors (50–60%). In young children (< 4 years of age) they are invariably malignant (neuroblastomas). In adults, neurogenic tumors are the most common mediastinal mass. They arise in the posterior compartment (typically from nerve sheaths) and are usually benign, occasionally calcified, and well circumscribed. Anterior mediastinal masses are more frequently malignant. The most common anterior mediastinal mass is a thymoma, though lymphoma is a close second in prevalence.

Table 18–4. Distribution of tumors and other mass lesions in the mediastinum.

All parts of mediastinum
Lymph node lesions
Middle mediastinum
Aneurysms, vascular lesions
Lipoma
Myxoma
Bronchogenic cysts
Pericardial cysts
Esophageal lesions
Pheochromocytomas
Anterior mediastinum
Thymoma
Lymphoma
Teratoma
Stem cell tumor
Thyroid
Parathyroid
Lipoma

Complete resection is the treatment of choice for all neurogenic tumors. A standard posterolateral thoracotomy offers optimal exposure; however, more limited incisions, including thoracoscopy, can be effective for resection of clinically benign small (< 6 cm) lesions. For lesions that cannot be completely excised, postoperative radiation may decrease local recurrence and symptoms. Incompletely excised or especially large or infiltrative neuroblastomas should receive combination radiation and chemotherapy in conjunction with surgery.

Although classically in adults the majority of mediastinal masses tend to be benign (cysts, neurogenic tumors, etc), recent series have demonstrated a shift toward malignant processes being more prevalent. Whether this represents a true change in tumor incidence or enhanced detection secondary to improved imaging techniques is unclear. Some general rules remain valid, however.

An extensive workup of a mediastinal lesion is usually not required for diagnosis since surgery is usually required both to establish the diagnosis and provide effective treatment. Standard posteroanterior and especially lateral chest films will often provide much useful information; however, contrast CT scanning has become the diagnostic test of choice. MRI, while helpful for assessing vascular or spinal cord extension, has not proved to be more effective than dynamic CT scanning.

Oblique or overpenetrating x-rays are sometimes helpful. Fluoroscopy may show pulsation or variation of shape or location with change of position and respiration. Tomography may reveal calcification or air-fluid levels. Barium swallow is used to evaluate intrinsic esophageal lesions or esophageal displacement by extrinsic masses. Contrast studies of the intestinal tract may reveal the stomach, colon, or small bowel in a hernia. Myelography can be of crucial importance in neurogenic tumors to explain symptoms or plan operative management. Computerized tomographic reconstructed images (virtual bronchography) may be useful to differentiate lung tumors mimicking a mediastinal mass.

CT angiography help to identify aneurysms or displacement. Pulmonary arteriography may be useful to distinguish mediastinal and pulmonary tumors.

Scintiscan is important in evaluating possible substernal goiter in anterior mediastinal lesions, since goiters can generally be removed by the standard cervical approach. Skin tests and serologic studies may be used in suspected granulomatous disease. Bone marrow examination, hormone assays, and serum tumor markers (AFP, β-HCG, LDH) are important adjuncts.

Bronchoscopy and esophagoscopy are occasionally useful to identify primary lung lesions or lesions of the esophagus. Mediastinoscopy and mediastinal biopsy must be used cautiously in mediastinal tumors that are potentially curable. Excisional biopsy is imperative in lesions (eg, thymomas) that are histologically difficult to evaluate since a curable cancer might be dispersed. Mediastinoscopy is useful for the diagnosis of sarcoidosis, Castleman's disease, or disseminated lymphoma.

When substernal goiter is excluded, neurogenic tumors constitute 26% of mediastinal masses, cysts 21%, teratodermoids 16%, thymomas 12%, lymphomas 12%, and all other lesions 12%. About 25% are malignant. In children, the incidence of cancer is about the same, but teratodermoids and vascular tumors are more common.

Clinical Findings

Symptoms are more frequent in malignant than benign lesions. About one-third of patients have no symptoms. Fifty percent of patients have respiratory symptoms such as cough, wheezing, dyspnea, and recurrent pneumonias. Hemoptysis and, rarely, expectoration of cyst contents may occur. Chest pain, weight loss, and dysphagia are found with equal frequency, each in about 10% of patients. Myasthenia (15–20% with thymoma), fever, and superior vena caval obstruction are each found in about 5% of patients.

The following symptoms suggest cancer: hoarseness, Horner's syndrome, severe pain, and superior vena caval obstruction. Malignant tumors, especially lymphomas, may produce chylothorax. Fever may be intermittent in Hodgkin's disease. Thymoma causes myasthenia, hypogammaglobulinemia, Whipple's disease, red blood cell aplasia, and Cushing's disease. Hypoglycemia is a rare complication of mesotheliomas, teratomas, and fibromas. Hypertension and diarrhea occur with pheochromocytoma and ganglioneuroma. Neurogenic tumors may produce specific neurologic findings from cord pressure or may be associated with hypertrophic osteoarthropathy and peptic ulcer disease.

A. Neurogenic Tumors

Neurogenic tumors almost always occur in the posterior mediastinum—often the superior portion—arising from intercostal or sympathetic nerves. Rarely, the vagus or phrenic nerve is involved. The most common variety of tumors (40–65%) arises from the nerve sheath (schwannoma and neurofibroma) and is usually benign. Ten percent of neurogenic tumors are malignant. Malignant tumors occur more frequently in children. Most malignant tumors (neuroblastoma, etc) arise from the nerve cells. Neurogenic tumors may be multiple or dumbbell in type, with widening of the intervertebral foramen. In these cases, MRI is necessary to determine if the mass extends within the spinal canal. Dumbbell tumors have been removed in the past by a two-stage approach, though a single-stage approach is now extensively used.

Pheochromocytomas of the middle mediastinum can be localized using ^{123}I metaiodobenzylguanidine.

B. Mediastinal Cystic Lesions

Cysts of the mediastinum may arise from the pericardium, bronchi, esophagus, or thymus. Pericardial cysts are also called springwater or mesothelial cysts. Seventy-five percent are located near the cardiophrenic angles, and 75% of these are on the right side. Ten percent are actually diverticula of the pericardial sac that communicate with the pericardial space. Bronchogenic cysts arise close to the main stem bronchus or trachea, often just below the carina. Histologically, they contain elements found in bronchi, such as cartilage, and are lined by respiratory epithelium. Enterogenous cysts are known by several names, including esophageal cyst, enteric cyst, or duplication of the alimentary tract. They arise along the surface of the esophagus and may be embedded within its wall. They may be lined by squamous epithelium similar to the esophagus or gastric mucosa. Enterogenous cysts are occasionally associated with congenital abnormalities of the vertebrae. About 10% of cysts in the mediastinum are nonspecific, without a recognizable lining.

C. Germ Cell Tumors

Germ cell tumors are common mass lesions of the anterior mediastinum. Historically, they are both solid and cystic, and the more differentiated ones may contain hair or teeth. Microscopically, ectodermal, endodermal, and mesodermal elements are present. These tumors occasionally rupture into the pleural space, lung, pericardium, or vascular structures.

Most germ cell tumors of the mediastinum are metastatic and present with concomitant retroperitoneal disease. Primary mediastinal extragonadal germ cell malignancies are rare, representing less than 5% of all mediastinal germ cell cancers and less than 5% of all primary mediastinal tumors. Men—in particular white males in their twenties and thirties—are most commonly affected, though extragonadal germ cell tumors can arise in women.

Because germ cells are pluripotent cells, they can give rise to several histologically distinct malignancies, including seminoma (40%), embryonal carcinomas and nongestational choriocarcinomas (20%), and yolk sac tumors (20%). Teratomas (20%) can have both benign and malignant components.

Almost all of these tumors (> 90%) produce tumor markers, including β-hCG and AFP. LDH—a nonspecific tumor marker—is produced by most bulky mediastinal germ cell tumors and is often an effective indicator of tumor burden.

Much progress in treating these tumors has been made with combination therapy (surgery, radiation therapy, and chemotherapy). Currently, over 50% 5-year survival is achievable for nonseminomatous and over 90% 5-year survival is typical for seminomatous mediastinal germ cell cancer. Patients should be screened and followed with AFP, β-hCG, and LDH markers. Surgical resection should be offered after combination chemotherapy has been administered and only after all elevated tumor markers have normalized.

Residual mediastinal masses following chemotherapy and normalization of tumor markers should be resected. At surgery, approximately 40% will be mature teratomas (with the potential for malignant degeneration), 40% necrotic tumors, and 20% residual tumors (requiring postoperative salvage chemotherapy). Rarely is palliative debulking surgery indicated if tumor markers remain elevated after several cycles of chemotherapy. Instead, alternative chemotherapy or investigational therapy should be offered.

D. Lymphoma

Lymphoma is usually associated with disseminated disease metastatic to the mediastinum. It is typically identified in the anterior compartment but can present anywhere through the mediastinum. This is the second most common mass in the anterior mediastinum. Occasionally, lymphosarcoma, Hodgkin's disease, or reticulum cell sarcoma arises as a primary mediastinal lesion.

Treatment

Treatment is tailored to the specific disease process causing the mediastinal mass. In almost all cases, tissue diagnosis is imperative for guiding appropriate therapy. Minimally invasive techniques (FNA or core needle biopsy) or mediastinoscopy and mediastinotomy are appropriate for diagnosis of a mediastinal mass that is secondary to metastatic disease (eg, lymphomas, germ cell tumors). Mediastinal masses, however, that represent primary malignancies (thymoma, neurogenic tumors, etc) are treated usually with initial surgical resection. Surgical approaches include median sternotomy (anterior masses), posterolateral thoracotomy (posterior and middle mediastinal masses) as well as VATS or bilateral anterior thoracotomy (all mediastinal compartments). Adjuvant chemotherapy is important for malignant germ cell lesions, malignant neurogenic tumors, and bulky or advanced thymomas. Postoperative radiation therapy decreases local recurrence in higher-stage thymoma and in other incompletely resected lesions. Radiation and chemotherapy constitutes the principal therapy for primary mediastinal lymphoma.

Prognosis

Overall, the outlook for patients with mediastinal masses has improved, with advances in combined chemotherapy and multimodality therapy. Surgical morbidity and mortality remain low (1–4%). Patients with benign mediastinal lesions do significantly better (> 95% cure rates) compared with those who have malignant mediastinal masses (< 50% overall survival).

Golbey RB: Mediastinal germ cell tumors. A continuing odyssey. Chest Surg Clin N Am 1994;4:195.

Gossot D et al: Thoracoscopy or CT-guided biopsy for residual intrathoracic masses after treatment of lymphoma. Chest 2001; 120:289.

Hagberg H et al: Value of transsternal core biopsy in patients with a newly diagnosed mediastinal mass. Acta Oncol 2000;39:195.

TUMORS OF THE THYMUS & MYASTHENIA GRAVIS

The thymic gland is the site of many neoplasms—thymomas, lymphomas, Hodgkin's granulomas, and other less common tumors. Thymoma, the most common type, may be difficult to differentiate from lymphoma even with an adequate biopsy. About 30% of patients with thymoma have myasthenia gravis, and about 15% of patients with myasthenia develop a thymoma.

Besides myasthenia, thymomas can produce a variety of paraneoplastic syndromes. These include cytopenias, red cell aplasias, and hypogammaglobulinemias as well as autoimmune disorders such as rheumatoid arthritis, lupus erythematosus, and polymyositis.

The relationship of myasthenia gravis to thymoma is interesting and incompletely understood. Myasthenia gravis is a neuromuscular disorder characterized by weakness and fatigability of voluntary muscles owing to decreased numbers of acetylcholine receptors at neuromuscular junctions. Because of the high incidence of thymic abnormalities, improvement after thymectomy, association with other autoimmune disorders, and presence in the serum of 90% of patients of an antibody against acetylcholine receptors, myasthenia gravis is thought to be the result of autoimmune processes. The disease has been induced in several species of laboratory animals by immunization with specific acetylcholine receptors. About 85% of patients with myasthenia gravis have thymic abnormalities consisting of germinal center formation in 70% and thymoma in 15%.

Thymoma may be classified according to predominant cell type into lymphocytic (25%), epithelial (25%), and lymphoepithelial (50%) varieties. Spindle cell tumor, which is sometimes associated with red cell aplasia, is considered among the epithelial tumors. Histologic subtypes, however, classically have not had prognostic significance. Recent reports demonstrate that aneuploidy and the presence of epithelial cells resembling thymic carcinoma have adverse prognostic implications. The histologic classification of thymomas is currently being revised.

Myasthenia gravis may occur in association with tumors of any cell type but is more common with the lymphocytic variety.

Malignant thymoma cannot be determined by the histologic appearance of the tumor alone. Evidence of local invasion grossly or microscopically defines thymoma as malignant. Thymoma is staged according to the Masoaka staging system as set forth in the accompanying box.

THYMOMA STAGING

Stage	Description
I	Macroscopically, completely encapsulated; microscopically, no capsular invasion.
IIa	Macroscopic invasion into surrounding fatty tissues or mediastinal pleura (without microscopic invasion).
IIb	Microscopic evidence of capsular invasion or microscopic invasion of surrounding fatty tissues or mediastinal pleura.
III	Macroscopic invasion into a neighboring organ (pericardium, great vessels, or lung).
IVa	Pleural or pericardial dissemination.
IVb	Lymphatic or hematogenous distant metastases.

Clinical Findings

Fifty percent of thymomas are first identified in an asymptomatic patient on a chest x-ray obtained for another purpose. Symptomatic patients may present with chest pain, dysphagia, myasthenia gravis, dyspnea, or superior vena caval syndrome.

CT scans are useful in making the diagnosis in equivocal cases and in assessing the extent of the lesion. MRI is occasionally helpful to assess vascular invasion.

The diagnosis of myasthenia gravis can be made from the patient's history of easy fatigability and associated decremental response in muscular contraction to repeated stimulation of the motor nerve or from improvement in these abnormalities in response to edrophonium (Tensilon), a short-acting anticholinesterase drug.

Definitive diagnosis of thymoma is based on histologic study of a tissue sample usually after excisional biopsy or complete resection has been performed. Small, well-encapsulated anterior mediastinal masses should not be biopsied, as the procedure penetrates the tumor's capsule and can lead to tumor seeding and recurrence and may jeopardize the chance of cure of an early-stage thymoma.

Treatment

The treatment of choice for thymoma is total thymectomy. The operation is usually performed through a median sternotomy. Posterior lateral thoracotomy as well as "clamshell" (bilateral anterior thoracotomy) or "trapdoor" incisions offers excellent exposure for resection of locally advanced thymomas. Cervical incisions, while useful for thymectomy for benign conditions (myasthenia, etc), have a limited role in the surgical treatment of malignant thymoma. A careful but aggressive resection should be performed for stage III lesions when they can be removed completely without sacrificing vital structures. Postoperative radiotherapy is indicated for invasive thymoma (stage II and stage III).

En bloc resection of the thymoma and associated pericardium, pleura, or lung (including lobectomy or extrapleural pneumonectomy) or great vessel (aorta, superior vena cava) reconstruction is warranted when complete resection is possible. Incomplete resections or debulking procedures do not benefit patients. Administration of neoadjuvant therapy with platinum-based chemotherapy will frequently shrink the tumor and allow subsequent complete resection. Recently, larger thymomas (> 5–6 cm) with evidence of probable invasion are being treated with combined-agent induction chemotherapy. Response rates exceed 70%, and complete resection rates are facilitated.

Large bulky lesions with clinically apparent gross invasion of local structures, pleura, or lung should be biopsied to confirm histologically the diagnosis of thymoma. Neoadjuvant chemotherapy with platinum-based regimens has been effective in shrinking bulky high-grade thymomas, thus allowing for complete resection and greater chances of cure.

Anticholinesterase drugs (eg, neostigmine bromide) are given as initial treatment to patients with myasthenia gravis. Corticosteroids may be given in selected cases, but a high incidence of side effects makes them unsuitable for more liberal use. Early thymectomy is now recommended for all patients with symptomatic myasthenia gravis whether or not a thymoma is suspected. The course of the disease is usually improved, and subsequent development of a malignant thymoma is eliminated. Thymectomy may be postponed in the occasional patient with mild disease well controlled by anticholinesterase therapy.

Following thymectomy, about 75% of patients with myasthenia gravis are improved and 30% achieve complete remission. Younger patients benefit more from thymectomy than do those over age 40 years, but a positive effect also accrues to the latter group. Recently video-assisted thymectomy for myasthenia patients has resulted in reduced length of stay, decreased blood loss and decreased pain in comparison with more traditional partial sternal splitting procedures.

Prognosis

The rates of complication and death with thymectomy are low except when there are extensive tumors. Respiratory care of patients with myasthenia gravis in the immediate postoperative period now presents little difficulty because of the availability of anticholinesterase drugs.

The stage and histologic type of the tumor are the main determinants of survival after thymectomy, though the presence of myasthenia no longer has an adverse effect.

Overall survival rates are extremely good for early-stage thymomas, and 10-year survival rates are excellent. Stage I lesions approach 100% 10-year survival rates. Stage II tumors with resection and postoperative radiation therapy have approximately 75% 10-year survival rates. Patients with locally advanced stage III thymomas, however, have long-term survival rates of less than 25%.Outcomes with multimodality therapy (neoadjuvant chemotherapy, surgery followed by chemotherapy and radiation therapy) are improving, as marked by significant tumor responses and enhanced resectability rates. Long-term survival data with these patients have not yet been reported.

THYMIC CARCINOMA

This tumor is a rare variant (< 15%) of thymic lesions and is histologically and biologically quite different from invasive or malignant thymoma. Thymic carcinomas tend to be very invasive and difficult to resect completely. Unfortunately, even in the setting of complete resection, recurrence is common both locally and at distant sites. Still, when at all possible, an aggressive combined-modality approach (induction chemotherapy, resection, and postoperative chemoradiotherapy) should be employed. Typically, these are young men (< age 50 years) with an otherwise excellent performance status. While a good response to induction therapy and complete resection will provide a significant disease-free interval, long-term survival is still unlikely. Better systemic agents and a molecular understanding of this cancer holds hope for significant improvements in cure rates.

Cooper JD: Current therapy for thymoma. Chest 1993;103(4 Suppl):3345. (Review.)

Maggi G et al: Thymoma: results of 241 operated cases. Ann Thorac Surg 1991;51:152.

Morgenthaler TI et al: Thymoma. Mayo Clin Proc 1993;68:1110. (Review.)

Park HS et al: Thymoma. A retrospective study of 87 cases. Cancer 1994;73:2491.

Rea F et al: Chemotherapy and operation for invasive thymoma. J Thorac Cardiovasc Surg 1993;106:543.

Toker et al: Comparison of early postoperative results of thymectomy: partial sternotomy vs. videothoracoscopy. Thorac Cardiovasc Surg 2005;53:110.

DISEASES OF THE LUNGS

CONGENITAL CYSTIC ANOMALIES OF THE LUNG

Congenital lesions of the lung include primarily tracheobronchial atresia, bronchogenic cysts, pulmonary dysplasia, pulmonary sequestration, congenital cystic adenomatoid malformations, and congenital lobar emphysema. Although many of these lesions present early in life with dramatic symptoms and physical findings, most remain occult until late childhood and even into adult life. These uncommon lesions arise from aberrations in normal aerodigestive tract development, which begins during the fourth week of fetal life when the lung bud forms at the caudal end of a groove in the primordial pharynx. An initial phase of sequential airway branching occurs until as many as 20–25 generations are reached by the 16th week of fetal life. These branches are divided into three zones: a proximal conductive zone (branches 1–16), an intermediate transitional zone (branches 17–19), and a distal respiratory zone (branches 20–25). A second canalicular phase is then entered as capillaries develop in the distal air passages. Finally, the alveolar phase begins at approximately 26 weeks of fetal life as prototype alveolar air sacs appear complete with both type I and type II pneumocytes. The number and size of alveoli continue to increase until the total alveolar surface reaches the adult size of nearly 100 m^2.

1. Tracheobronchial Atresia

Atresia of the tracheobronchial tree can occur at any level and may involve an isolated segment or multiple diffuse areas of the airway. Tracheal atresia is associated with polyhydramnios, prematurity, esophageal atresia, and tracheoesophageal fistula. Typically, neonates present with intractable cyanosis and despite a normal-appearing larynx are unable to be intubated. Emergency tracheostomy can be life-sustaining in babies with isolated subglottic atresia; in other infants with more diffuse disease, mask ventilation can achieve some palliation through anomalous esophagobronchial connections. Diffuse airway involvement, however, is invariably fatal.

Isolated bronchial atresia results in a bronchus that ends in a blind pouch. A mucocele develops distal to the obstruction and, as a result of compression of neighboring normal bronchial structures, causes emphysematous changes in the surrounding lung. Since children frequently develop wheezing, stridor, and pulmonary infections in the involved segments, resection is almost always indicated. Like bronchial atresia, true congenital bronchial stenosis is rare, although right main stem bronchial stenosis occurs not infrequently from iatrogenic airway trauma in chronically ventilated patients.

Related anomalies of the tracheobronchial tree include anomalous tracheal or esophageal bronchi and tracheal diverticula. These rare lesions often present with symptoms of bronchial obstruction and in many cases require resection of involved lung tissue due to chronic infection and the development of bronchiectasis (see below). Similar to pulmonary sequestration, these lesions can have a dominant systemic arterial blood supply that must be kept in mind if operation is contemplated.

2. Bronchogenic Cysts

Abnormal budding of the foregut during development can result in the formation of bronchogenic cysts. These occur most commonly in the pulmonary hilum or mediastinum (primarily in the paratracheal and subcarinal areas) but can also arise in the pulmonary parenchyma. The cysts are usually single, are lined by cuboidal respiratory epithelium, and occur preferentially in the lower lobes. The cyst wall is generally thin, occasionally containing cartilage, and except for mediastinal cysts they frequently communicate with the tracheobronchial tree. Radiographically, these cysts appear as discrete round densities that often are sharply defined and air-filled. They may also present as a solitary pulmonary nodule (if completely fluid-filled) or as a pulmonary abscess with an air-fluid level (see below). In general, mediastinal bronchogenic cysts present with airway compression and parenchymal cysts are manifested by pulmonary infection. Some cysts have been noted to enlarge rapidly and rupture into the pleural space, causing tension pneumothorax. All bronchogenic cysts—regardless of location—are best treated with either simple or segmental resection. Rarely, lobectomy is required.

3. Bronchopulmonary Dysplasia

Bronchopulmonary dysplasia includes pulmonary agenesis and aplasia as well as primary and secondary pulmonary hypoplasia. Unilateral pulmonary agenesis occurs when one lung and the associated vascular structures fail to develop. Neonates with pulmonary agenesis may present with tachypnea and cyanosis, particularly if associated cardiac anomalies exist (50% of cases). Some patients, however, remain asymptomatic until childhood, when they complain of dyspnea and wheezing suggestive of asthma. Physical examination in these patients reveals marked tracheal deviation toward the side of the agenesis, and chest x-ray, barium esophagography, and chest CT may be required to exclude other diagnostic possibilities such as total lung atelectasis from foreign body aspiration, total lung sequestration, and esophageal bronchus. Once bronchopulmonary dysplasia is diagnosed, treatment is limited to supportive care. The prognosis is guarded since only one-half to two-thirds of patients survive for longer than 5 years—succumbing in part from the coexisting cardiac disease. Pulmonary aplasia is essentially identical to pulmonary agenesis except that a blind bronchial tumor stump of varying length exists and can chronically soil the normal lung with infected pooled secretions. This problem necessitates resection of the bronchial stump to prevent this potentially fatal complication.

Pulmonary hypoplasia is defined pathologically as an abnormally low radial alveolus count and low ratio of lung weight to body weight and is considered primary if no inciting cause can be identified. These neonates present with tachypnea and hypoxemia resistant to administration of supplemental oxygen due to abnormal thickening of the pulmonary arteriolar wall. Persistent fetal circulation, hypoxemia, hypercapnia, and acidosis lead to early death in over 75% of patients. Secondary pulmonary hypoplasia results from numerous fetal and maternal abnormalities that physically restrict lung growth and development. The most common of these abnormalities is congenital diaphragmatic hernia (see Chapter 45). Other conditions associated with secondary pulmonary hypoplasia include those that produce oligohydramnios and direct chest compression (eg, bilateral renal agenesis [Potter's syndrome], renal dysplasia, and amniotic fluid leaks); those with abnormal bone development and small rigid chest walls (eg, achondroplasia, chondrodystrophia fetalis calcificans, osteogenesis imperfecta, and spondyloepiphysial dysplasia); those with decreased fetal respiratory movements (eg, phrenic nerve agenesis, abdominal masses or ascites with elevation of the diaphragm, arthrogryposis multiplex congenita, camptodactyly, and congenial myotonic dystrophy); those with intrathoracic mass lesions (eg, congenital cystic adenomatoid malformation, cystic hygroma, and esophageal duplication cysts); and those with pulmonary vascular abnormalities (eg, scimitar syndrome and pulmonary artery agenesis).

dell'Agnola CA et al: Prenatal ultrasonography and early surgery for congenital cystic disease of the lung. J Pediatr Surg 1992;27:1414.

Eber E, Zach MS: Long term sequelae of bronchopulmonary dysplasia (chronic lung disease of infancy). Thorax 2001;56:317.

4. Pulmonary Sequestration

Pulmonary sequestrations are masses of lung parenchyma that arise through abnormal budding of the caudal embryonic foregut and consequently have *no bronchial communication* with the otherwise normal tracheobronchial tree. Sequestrations may occur either within normal lung tissue, termed intralobar sequestrations; or as separate masses with their own visceral pleura, referred to as extralobar sequestrations. The majority (85%) of sequestrations are of the intralobar type. Both types, however, occur in or around the right (42%) or left (58%) lower lobes and have an abnormal systemic blood supply, often from the abdominal aorta. The venous drainage of intralobar sequestrations is through the pulmonary venous system in 96%, and in some cases this may be associated with anomalous venous drainage of the normal lung. The venous drainage of extralobar sequestrations, however, is to the systemic (hemiazygos or azygos) veins. Although some sequestrations (particularly extralobar) present as asymptomatic lower lobe masses, many present with recurrent lower lobe infections due to bacterial seeding that occurs through communications with the remaining normal lung known as the pores of Kohn. In rare instances, patients may present with hemoptysis or congestive heart failure from large left-to-right shunts through the sequestration. The diagnosis is usually suspected on chest x-ray and confirmed with a CT scan of the chest. Although angiography was formerly used to confirm the diagnosis, currently it is indicated only if questions regarding the diagnosis, arterial blood supply, or venous drainage exist despite computed tomography. Treatment consists of segmental resection or, if necessary, lobectomy. Great care must be taken to identify the nature of both the arterial blood supply and the venous drainage to avoid exsanguinating hemorrhage from division of an unrecognized systemic artery or venous infarction of the normal lung from ligation of the common draining vein. Following successful resection, the prognosis is favorable.

Campbell RE et al: Image interpretation session: 1993. Intralobar pulmonary sequestration. Radiographics 1994;14:199.

Dolkart LA et al: Antenatal diagnosis of pulmonary sequestration: a review. Obstet Gynecol Surv 1992;47:515.

Javaid A, Aamir AU: Pulmonary sequestration: a case report and review. Respir Med 1994;88:65.

Louie HW, Martin SM, Mulder DG: Pulmonary sequestration: 17-year experience at UCLA. Am Surg 1993;59:801.

Nicolette LA et al: Intralobar pulmonary sequestration: a clinical and pathological spectrum. J Pediatr Surg 1993;28:802.

5. Congenital Cystic Adenomatoid Malformation

Congenital cystic adenomatoid malformation results from an overgrowth of terminal bronchiolar structures that are lined by typical respiratory epithelium and are associated with disorganized elastic connective tissue and smooth muscle. These "solid" structures are interspersed with cysts that resemble immature alveoli with bronchial-type epithelium, polypoid luminal projections, an absence of mucoserous glands and cartilage, and occasional "intestinal" mucus-secreting cells. These lesions are classified into one of three categories based on their presentation and pathologic features. Some lesions present with a predominantly solid lung mass, occur primarily in stillborn or premature neonates, and are associated with fetal anasarca, ascites, and polyhydramnios. Intermediate lesions with mixed solid and cystic components often present at birth with severe respiratory distress secondary to a large space-occupying mass and the resulting ipsilateral and occasional contralateral pulmonary hypoplasia. Many cystic adenomatoid malformations are detected antenatally, though predominantly cystic lesions frequently escape detection at birth and may present in the older infant, child, or adult with chronic pulmonary infection. The radiographic diagnosis of congenital cystic adenomatoid malformation can be difficult, especially in the newborn, when it can be confused with congenital diaphragmatic hernia and, less frequently, congenital lobar emphysema. A radiograph demonstrating a paucity of intestinal air in the abdomen favors the diagnosis of diaphragmatic hernia, while a chest CT scan may be required in some patients to make a correct diagnosis. The treatment of essentially all lesions is surgical resection, which may be required emergently in neonates who present with severe respiratory distress. The prognosis for the intermediate and predominantly cystic types is good following resection.

6. Congenital Lobar Emphysema

Congenital lobar emphysema is associated with hypoplastic or dysplastic bronchial cartilage in 25–79% of patients and with an increased number of alveoli ("polyalveoli") in up to 37% of affected children. The left upper lobe is most commonly involved, and the right middle lobe is next in frequency. In addition, neonates who require prolonged mechanical ventilation—eg, those with hyaline membrane disease—may develop lobar emphysema from a combination of suction catheter trauma and barotrauma. The right lower lobe is most frequently affected in these patients. Most infants present within the first 6 months of life with respiratory distress. In some patients, severe respiratory distress may occur in the neonatal period, requiring emergent evaluation and treatment. Almost all infants present with tracheal and mediastinal deviation away from the affected side, hyperresonance and decreased breath sounds on the affected side, and a chest x-ray demonstrating hyperlucency in the area of the affected lobe with compression of adjacent lung. A chest x-ray often is all that is necessary prior to operation; however, occasional patients, particularly older children, may require chest CT scans to exclude other pathology, eg, bronchogenic cysts, anomalous pulmonary vessels, and hilar lymphadenopathy. Bronchoscopy also may be necessary to rule out the presence of a foreign body acting as a ball valve. Successful therapy in all patients requires surgical resection, which almost uniformly consists of lobectomy. Great care is necessary with airway management at the time of induction of general anesthesia in these patients as positive-pressure ventilation may result in further shifting of the mediastinum resulting in impaired venous return.

Kennedy CD et al: Lobar emphysema: long-term imaging follow-up. Radiology 1991;180:189.

Stigers KB, Woodring JH, Kanga JF: The clinical and imaging spectrum of findings in patients with congenital lobar emphysema. Pediatr Pulmonol 1992;14:160.

CONGENITAL VASCULAR LESIONS OF THE LUNG

Vascular diseases of the lung include two main processes: arteriovenous malformations and vascular rings. Arteriovenous malformations are uncommon congenital lesions that develop as a result of abnormal capillary formation during the canalicular phase of development. Most arise from the pulmonary artery, but occasionally a systemic arterial source may be involved similar to that in pulmonary sequestration. Rarely, the coronary arteries may be the origin of arteriovenous malformations, with the right coronary artery involved 55% of the time. Coronary arteriovenous fistulas drain into the right ventricle (40%), right atrium (25%), pulmonary artery (20%), coronary sinus (7%), superior vena cava (1%), or left-sided heart chambers (7%). Patients are either asymptomatic or develop signs of congestive heart failure. Myocardial infarction is rare. A continuous murmur and signs reduced left ventricular afterload may be present. Though the diagnosis often can be established with echocardiography and color Doppler imaging, the definitive diagnosis, shunt fraction, and complete preoperative planning requires catheterization and angiography. Operation is indicated for symptomatic patients and for those asymptomatic patients with large shunts.

Vascular rings occur from abnormal development of the aortic arches and major branches, with resulting compression of the trachea and esophagus. In normal fetal development, a dual system of six aortic arches regresses in such a way that the left fourth arch becomes the main left-sided aorta, the left sixth arch develops as the ductus arteriosus, and the right fourth arch persists as the right innominate artery and subclavian artery. Most vascular rings, however, are associated with a right-sided aortic arch and may be classified as complete vascular rings or incomplete rings (arterial slings). Complete vascular rings include a double aortic arch (67%, the most common complete ring), a right aortic arch with a left subclavian and left ductus arteriosus (30%), a right aortic arch with mirror image branching and a left ductus arteriosus (rare), and a left aortic arch with an aberrant right subclavian and right ductus arteriosus (very rare). Incomplete rings consist of an aberrant right subclavian artery that originates on the left side and passes posterior to the esophagus (most common incomplete ring) and an anomalous left pulmonary artery arising from the right pulmonary artery and passing between the trachea and the esophagus (pulmonary artery sling).

Most patients present with symptoms of tracheal or esophageal compression. Patients with an anomalous right subclavian artery may present later in life with swallowing symptoms (dysphagia lusoria) while those with complete vascular rings and pulmonary artery slings typically present early in life (within 6 months) with symptoms of respiratory distress (often frank stridor), particularly with neck flexion and poor feeding. The diagnosis is often suggested by characteristic findings on barium esophagraphy. Bilateral indentations imply double aortic arch. A posterior indentation points to an aberrant right subclavian artery, large right-sided indentations suggest complete rings associated with a right aortic arch, and an anterior impression is typical of a pulmonary artery sling. Often, the diagnosis can be confirmed by echocardiography. MRI/MRA often provides useful anatomic details. Surgical repair of these lesions is indicated once the diagnosis is established and is accomplished by dividing the vascular ring usually through a left thoracotomy. With double aortic arches, the smaller of the two arches is divided distal to the subclavian artery, while other complete rings generally are treated by division of the ligamentum arteriosum. Aberrant right subclavian arteries may be simply divided or, if necessary, reimplanted on the right side. Pulmonary artery slings require reimplantation of the left pulmonary artery and often resection of the compressed trachea which often has severe tracheomalacia and stenosis. Rarely, tracheomalacia secondary to vascular ring compression necessitates suspension of the aortic arch from the sternum.

Anend R et al: Follow-up of surgical correction of vascular anomalies causing tracheobronchial compression. Pediatr Cardiol 1994;51:58.

Lowe GM, Donaldson JS, Backer CL: Vascular rings: 10-year review of imaging. Radiographics 1996,11:637.

van Son JA et al: Surgical treatment of vascular rings: The Mayo Clinic Experience. Mayo Clin Proc 1993;68:1056.

SUPPURATIVE DISEASES OF THE LUNG

1. Lung Abscess

A lung abscess is a localized collection of pus that is contained within a cavity formed by the disintegration of the surrounding tissues. The pus consists of leukocytes and a thin fluid referred to as "liquor puris." Arbitrarily, abscesses are termed acute if the duration is less than 6 weeks and chronic if more than 6 weeks. Although the incidence of lung abscesses fell dramatically following the introduction of effective antibiotics in the 1940s and 1950s, a recent increase in the number of immunocompromised individuals secondary to organ transplantation, chemotherapy, and AIDS has resulted in a resurgence in the numbers of lung abscesses requiring treatment.

Lung abscesses may be divided into two major categories based on etiology: primary and secondary. Primary lung abscesses occur because of aspiration of oropharyngeal contents (most common), acute necrotizing pneumonia (due to *S aureus, K pneumoniae*), chronic pneumonia (due to fungi, tubercle bacilli) and opportunistic infection in an immunodeficient host. Conditions that predispose to aspiration include anesthesia (both general and monitored), neurologic disorders (cerebrovascular accidents, seizures, diabetic coma, head trauma, etc), drug ingestion (alcohol, narcotics, etc), normal sleep, poor oral hygiene (increases bacterial load), and esophageal disease (gastroesophageal reflux, achalasia, cancer, tracheoesophageal fistula). Secondary causes of lung abscesses include bronchial obstruction (cancer, foreign body, hilar lymphadenopathy), cavitating lesions (cancer, pulmonary infarct), direct extension (amebiasis, subphrenic abscess), and hematogenous dissemination (*S aureus, E coli,* etc). It should be noted that secondary infections of congenital or acquired cystic lesions, such as bronchogenic cysts, bullae, tuberculous cavities, and hydatid cysts, are not true pulmonary abscesses because they occur in a preformed spaced. The bacteriologic findings of lung abscesses depend somewhat on the underlying cause and the thoroughness of the laboratory. Classically, aerobic gram-positive cocci *(S aureus, Streptococcus pyogenes)* and facilitative gram-negative bacilli (*K pneumoniae, E coli,* pseudomonas species) have been incriminated: however, with more fastidious culture techniques, anaerobic bacteria (bacteroides species, *Clostridium ramosum,* peptostreptococci, peptococci) are now isolated in over 85% of cultures. In immunocompromised patients, more unusual organisms predominate, eg, *Candida albicans, Legionella micdadei* and *L pneumophila,* and *Pneumocystis carinii.*

Clinical Findings & Diagnosis

Patients with lung abscesses typically complain of cough, fever, dyspnea, and occasionally pleuritic chest pain. The symptoms are often insidious in onset and associated with malaise and weight loss if chronic. Complications include rupture into a bronchus, with initial hemoptysis followed by the production of foul-smelling, purulent sputum (and the potential for life-threatening pneumonia from aspiration of pus into normal lung); rupture into the pleural space with resulting pyopneumothorax, sepsis, and possibly empyema necessitatis; and, rarely, massive hemoptysis requiring emergent pulmonary resection. On physical examination, signs of lobar consolidation predominate; but clubbing, signs of pleural effusion, cachexia, and rarely a draining chest wound (empyema necessitatis) can be present. Laboratory studies should include a differential white blood cell count and sputum culture. Chest radiography may demonstrate an area of intense consolidation or a rounded density with or without an air-fluid level (Figure 18–17). In unusual cases, a CT scan may be required for better radiographic visualization, and in cases of suspected bronchial obstruction or in all patients with unexplained lung abscesses, bronchoscopy is indicated. Fine-needle aspiration of the abscess cavity for diagnostic culture has been shown to isolate the offending pathogens in 94% of patients compared with only 11% and 3% from sputum culture and bronchoalveolar lavage, respectively. In addition, early fine-needle aspiration also has been reported to change the antibiotic regimen in 43% of cases and can be life-saving in immunocompromised patients with unusual organisms.

Treatment

Antibiotic administration has been the mainstay of therapy following general resuscitation measures. The selection of antibiotics varies and depends on the underlying cause, but penicillin and clindamycin are commonly used. In immunocompromised individuals, trimethoprim-sulfamethoxazole, pentamidine, erythromycin, and

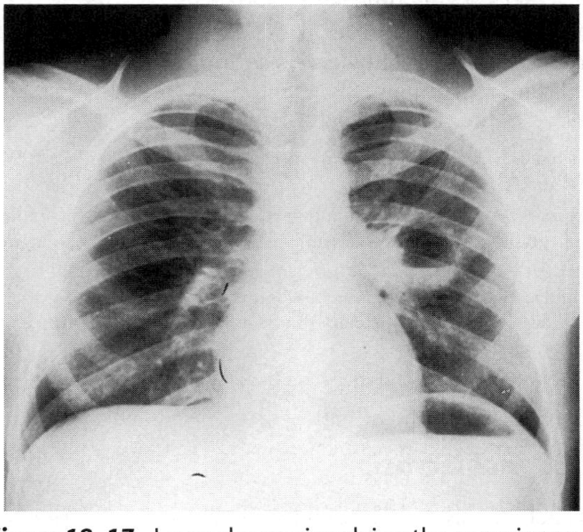

Figure 18–17. Lung abscess involving the superior segment of the left lower lobe.

amphotericin B are often indicated. Once the acute sepsis subsides (after up to 2 weeks), therapy can frequently be changed to an oral outpatient regimen and continued until complete resolution of the abscess occurs (3–5 months). Important adjuncts to antibiotic administration include chest physiotherapy, bronchoscopy (may require repeated examinations to maintain bronchial drainage), and health maintenance measures (general nutrition, dental hygiene, etc). In patients who do not respond to this initial regimen and who do not have surgical indications (see below), early percutaneous drainage has been shown to be a safe and effective procedure (mortality rate 1.5%; morbidity rate 10%). Specific proposed indications for percutaneous drainage include (1) an abscess under tension as evidenced by mediastinal shift, displacement of fissures or downward movement of the diaphragm, (2) radiographic verification of contralateral lung contamination, (3) unremitting signs of sepsis after 72 hours of adequate antibiotic therapy, (4) abscess size > 4 cm or increasing abscess size, (5) rising fluid level, and (6) persistent ventilatory dependency. Thoracotomy today is rarely indicated in the management of lung abscess but continues to be indicated in patients with massive hemoptysis, empyema, bronchial obstruction (particularly if secondary to resectable cancer), and failure of medical therapy. Furthermore, acute rupture into the pleural space (pyopneumothorax) is still a surgical emergency. When surgery is indicated, lobectomy generally is the preferred procedure.

Prognosis

Since the appearance of effective antibiotics, the mortality rate from lung abscesses has declined from 30–50% down to 5–20%. Medical therapy alone is successful in 75–88% of patients, and those requiring operation are cured 90% of the time with a mortality rate of only 1%. In the growing population of ICU and immunocompromised patients, however, the mortality rate remains high (approximately 28%).

Bartlett JG: Antibiotics in lung abscess. Semin Respir Infect 1991; 6:103.

Groskin SA et al: Bacterial lung abscess: a review of the radiographic and clinical features of 50 cases. J Thorac Imaging 1991;6:62.

Lambiase RE et al: Percutaneous drainage of 335 consecutive abscesses: results of primary drainage with 1-year follow-up. Radiology 1992;184:167.

vanSonnenberg E et al: Lung abscess: CT-guided drainage. Radiology 1991;178:347.

2. Bronchiectasis

Bronchiectasis strictly defined is abnormal dilation of the bronchi, but common usage expands the definition to denote the clinical syndrome marked by chronic dilation of bronchi, a paroxysmal cough that produces variable amounts of fetid, mucopurulent sputum, and recurrent pulmonary infections. Bronchiectasis was at one time a common problem frequently complicated by hemoptysis, lung and brain abscesses, empyema, respiratory failure, and death. Since the introduction of vaccination programs, antibiotics, and antituberculous medications, however, it is reported commonly only in isolated geographic locations.

Although congenital diseases (Kartagener's syndrome, cystic fibrosis, Williams-Campbell syndrome, Mounier-Kuhn syndrome, immunoglobulin deficiencies, and α_1-antitrypsin deficiency) can lead to the development of bronchiectasis, most cases are related to acquired disorders and are caused by two factors: infection and bronchial obstruction. Viral and bacterial pneumonias in infancy and childhood—eg, pertussis, measles, influenza, tuberculosis, and bronchopneumonia—were common predisposing conditions that led to bronchiectasis in the past. Either a single severe bout of pneumonia or repeated moderate infections can cause progressive destruction of bronchial cilia, mucosa, musculoelastic tissue, and even cartilage. Healing with fibrosis and contraction of the peribronchial tissues subsequently produces bronchial dilation. Retention of secretions resulting from destruction of normal mucociliary action leads to repeated bouts of infection and progressive scarring and bronchial dilation. Aspirated foreign bodies, endobronchial neoplasms, and hilar lymphadenopathy (see middle lobe syndrome below) also can cause retention of secretions, infections, and progressive bronchiectasis. The presence of true established bronchiectasis, however, must be distinguished from pseudobronchiectasis, which is a cylindric bronchial dilation that is associated with acute bronchopneumonia. When left untreated, true bronchiectasis progresses, while pseudobronchiectasis reverses completely after weeks to months.

Since the original description of bronchiectasis by Laennec in 1826, the disorder has been divided into two main types based on pathologic appearance: saccular and cylindric. Saccular bronchiectasis follows most infections and bronchial obstruction while the cylindric variety is associated with posttuberculosis bronchiectasis. A third type of bronchiectasis is distinguished by alternating saccular and cylindric areas and is referred to as mixed or varicose bronchiectasis. In general, bronchiectasis involves the second-order to fourth-order branches of the segmental bronchi, and its distribution is largely characteristic of the underlying pathology. Congenital disorders, for example, are associated with diffuse bilateral bronchiectasis, while tuberculosis and granulomatous diseases are characterized by unilateral or bilateral disease, most commonly limited to the upper lobes and superior segments of the lower lobes. Furthermore, bronchiectasis following pyogenic and viral pneumonias usually involves only the lower lobes, middle lobe, and lingula, and postobstructive bronchiectasis is generally limited to the obstructed segments (see also middle lobe syndrome, below). Common pathogens in patients with bronchiectasis include *H influenzae, S aureus, K pneumoniae, E coli,* and, in the chronic setting, pseudomonas species. Mycobacteria, fungi, and legionella should also be cultured.

Clinical Findings & Diagnosis

Patients with a history of recurrent febrile episodes often complain of a chronic or intermittent cough that is productive of variable amounts of foul-smelling sputum (up to 500 mL/d). Hemoptysis occurs in 41–66%, but rarely is it massive. Bronchiectasis associated with granulomatous disease may not be associated with a productive cough (so-called "dry" bronchiectasis). Exacerbations and advanced disease are manifested by increased sputum production, fever, dyspnea, anorexia, fatigue, and weight loss. A history of sinus problems, infertility, or a family history of similar problems suggests the presence of an inherited disorder associated with bronchiectasis. Physical examination may reveal cyanosis, clubbing, pulmonary osteoarthropathy, evidence of malnutrition, and, in advanced disease, signs of cor pulmonale. Although bronchiectasis is suspected, an imaging study is usually required for confirmation. Bronchograms were at one time required, but high-resolution, fine-cut (1.5–5 mm) CT scans are now the imaging procedure of choice to document bronchial dilation, particularly with saccular disease. Even with the diagnosis of bronchiectasis, however, endobronchial neoplasm or foreign body must be excluded by flexible fiber optic bronchoscopy.

Treatment

In nearly all patients, conservative medical therapy is indicated and generally is sufficient. This includes broad-spectrum antibiotics, bronchodilators, humidification, expectorants, mucolytics, and effective routine postural drainage. In patients with continued infection, bronchoscopy with bronchoalveolar lavage should be considered to obtain more accurate culture results. Other adjunctive therapies includes influenza and pneumococcal vaccines and, in some patients, chronic "prophylactic" antibiotic administration with trimethoprim-sulfamethoxazole, erythromycin, or ciprofloxacin. A recent advance in controlling underlying bacterial (especially pseudomonas) infection and symptoms associated with bronchiectasis has been the use of inhaled antibiotics. In the cystic fibrosis and chronic bronchiectasis population, nebulized tobramycin or gentamicin has proved effective in controlling infection, sputum production, and symptoms in a significant proportion of patients.

Patients who fail intensive medical therapy may be candidates for surgical resection if the following criteria are met: (1) the disease must be localized and completely resectable; (2) pulmonary reserve must be adequate; (3) the process must be irreversible (ie, not pseudobronchiectasis, bronchial stricture, foreign body, etc); and (4) significant symptoms must persist. Preoperative assessment requires a high-resolution fine-cut CT scan, though some surgeons still prefer a bronchogram as a "road map." Pulmonary function studies generally are not necessary since the involved segments do not function. The goals of surgery are to remove all active disease and to preserve as much functioning lung parenchyma as possible. The surgical approach includes complete segmental resection of the involved areas. Partial resection almost always ends in recurrence. Resection most commonly involves all basal segments (unilaterally or bilaterally) along with the middle lobe or lingula. With tuberculosis, however, removal of the upper lobe or lobes with or without the superior segment of the lower lobes is more likely. During surgery, meticulous maintenance of a clear airway devoid of mucopurulent secretions and blood is essential. Careful dissection of the bronchovascular structures is difficult in patients with chronic inflammation and scarring but is essential to avoid complications.

Prognosis

Although most patients are successfully treated with medical therapy, some require surgery. The results of surgical resection depend on the cause and type of pulmonary involvement. Success with elimination of symptoms occurs in up to 80% of patients with limited localized disease but only 36% of those with diffuse disease. Prognostic factors include (1) unilateral disease restricted to the basal segments, (2) young age, (3) absence of sinusitis and rhinitis, (4) history of pneumonia, and (5) no major airway obstruction. Overall morbidity and mortality rates are surprisingly low at 3–5% and < 1%, respectively.

Ip M et al: Multivariate analysis of factors affecting pulmonary function in bronchiectasis. Respiration 1993;60:45.

McGuinness G et al: Bronchiectasis: CT evaluation. AJR Am J Roentgenol 1993;160:253.

Trucksis M, Swartz MN: Bronchiectasis: a current view. Curr Clin Top Infect Dis 1991;11:170.

3. Middle Lobe Syndrome

Relapsing lateral pneumonia of the middle pulmonary lobe is typically caused by intermittent obstruction, most often extrinsic. In a patient with repeated episodes of right-sided pneumonia, this diagnosis should be entertained, but only after other causes of obstruction (bronchogenic cancer, foreign body, etc), have been ruled out.

Broncholithiasis (see below) and middle lobe syndrome have been considered to be caused by compression or erosion of the bronchus by adjacent diseased lymph nodes. Other factors, such as poor natural drainage and lack of collateral ventilation, probably explain the frequency of middle lobe.

Endobronchial tumors and foreign bodies must be excluded by bronchoscopy.

Most patients respond to intensive medical therapy, and surgery is rarely required. Indications for surgery, which usually involves middle lobectomy, include bronchiectasis, fibrosis (bronchostenosis), abscess, unresolved or intractable recurrent pneumonia, and suspicion of neoplasm.

Ring-Mrozik E et al: Clinical findings in middle lobe syndrome and other processes of pulmonary shrinkage in children (atelectasis syndrome). Eur J Pediatr Surg 1991;1:266.

4. Broncholithiasis

Broncholithiasis is defined as the presence of calculi (broncholiths) within the tracheobronchial tree. In most cases, a calcified parabronchial lymph node erodes through the bronchial wall into the lumen; however, severely inspissated mucus may calcify. Calcified lymph nodes may remain attached to the bronchial wall, lodge in a bronchus, or be expectorated (lithoptysis). The most common cause of broncholithiasis in the United States is histoplasmosis. Tuberculosis is another frequent cause in some parts of the world.

Patients with broncholithiasis often complain of hemoptysis, lithoptysis (30%), cough, sputum production, fever, chills, and pleuritic chest pain. The hemoptysis is characteristically sudden and self-limited, though rarely it may be massive. Symptoms of pneumonia may indicate bronchial obstruction from an impacted broncholith. Signs suggesting broncholithiasis include localized wheezing on physical examination, evidence of hilar calcifications or segmental atelectasis and pneumonia on chest x-ray, and bronchoscopic evidence of peribronchial disease. The diagnosis is confirmed by documentation of lithoptysis or the presence of an endobronchial "lung stone."

The complications of broncholithiasis include hemoptysis, which on occasion can be massive and life-threatening; suppurative lung diseases, eg, pneumonia and bronchiectasis; mid-esophageal traction diverticula; and, rarely, tracheobronchoesophageal fistula. In addition to instituting appropriate therapy for underlying pulmonary diseases, treatment is primarily directed at removal of endobronchial stones. This can be accomplished at the time of bronchoscopy if the broncholith is freely floating within the tracheobronchial tree or if it extends well into the bronchial lumen and can be removed without excessive force or traction (20% of cases). The main danger of transbronchoscopic removal of broncholiths is the real possibility of massive hemorrhage. This results during inappropriate removal of broncholiths that remain substantially attached to the parabronchial tissues. Because of intense peribronchial fibrosis in this situation, the broncholith not infrequently becomes adherent to vascular structures such as the pulmonary artery, which may be torn with vigorous attempts at broncholith removal. Nearly 80% of patients with broncholiths that remain in situ require surgical removal. The goal of surgery in this disease is preservation of lung function. The broncholith may be removed safely with bronchotomy; however, most patients require segmentectomy or lobectomy, particularly if destruction of lung parenchyma has occurred from postobstruction suppurative lung disease. Fistulas between the airway and the esophagus should be repaired with interposition of normal tissue (intercostal muscle flap, etc) between the two structures to prevent recurrence. Following surgery, the prognosis is excellent.

Conces DJ Jr, Tarver RD, Vix VA: Broncholithiasis: CT features in 15 patients. AJR Am J Roentgenol 1991;157:249.

Galdermans D et al: Broncholithiasis: present clinical spectrum. Respir Med 1990;84:155.

Igoe D, Lynch V, McNicholas WT: Broncholithiasis: bronchoscopic vs. surgical management. Respir Med 1990; 84:163.

McLean TR, Beall AC Jr, Jones JW: Massive hemoptysis due to broncholithiasis. Ann Thorac Surg 1991;52:1173.

5. Cystic Fibrosis & Mucoid Impaction of the Bronchi

Cystic fibrosis is a serious congenital disorder that may lead to bronchitis, bronchiectasis, pulmonary fibrosis, emphysema, and lung abscess. Mucoid impaction occurs in patients with asthma and bronchitis. Mucoid plugs are rubbery, semisolid, gray to greenish-yellow in color, and round, oval, or elongated in shape. There is often a history of recurrent upper respiratory infection, fever, and chest pain. Expectoration of hard mucus plugs or hemoptysis may occur.

Bronchogenic carcinoma, fungal infection, tuberculosis, bronchiectasis, abscess, bacterial pneumonia, lipoid pneumonia, pulmonary eosinophilic granuloma, and Löffler's syndrome must be ruled out.

Treatment is with expectorants, detergents, bronchodilators, antibiotics, and aerosol inhalation. The availability of acetylcysteine has largely converted this condition to a purely medical disease. Surgery is indicated when cancer cannot be ruled out, for destroyed lung, or in the treatment of abscess.

Double lung transplantation is a consideration for advanced cystic fibrosis patients with end-stage pulmonary function. Overall, survivals have improved (85% at 1 year, 50% at 5 years) due to improvements in surgical technique (bronchial anastomosis) and immunosuppressive regimens. Still, chronic bronchitis obliterans remains a major obstacle after several years and is the leading cause of eventual transplant failure. Limited donor organ availability prevents the many eligible cystic fibrosis patients from being transplanted.

Fiel SB: Clinical management of pulmonary disease in cystic fibrosis. Lancet 1993;341:1070.

Shennib H et al: Double-lung transplantation for cystic fibrosis. The Cystic Fibrosis Transplant Study Group. Ann Thorac Surg 1992;54:27.

6. Tuberculosis

Tuberculosis markedly declined as a cause of death between 1953 and 1984, but since 1985 this disease has experienced a resurgence due to increased immigration of infected individuals and HIV infection. A reservoir of about 5000–8000 clinical cases exists, and an additional 25,000 new cases occur annually. Less than 20% of the United States population are tuberculin-positive, but tuberculosis remains a common infectious cause of death worldwide.

Several species of the genus mycobacterium may cause lung disease, but 95% of cases of lung disease are due to *Mycobacterium tuberculosis. Mycobacterium bovis* and *Mycobacterium avium* are seldom found in humans. Several "atypical" species of mycobacterium that are chiefly soil-dwellers have become clinically more important in recent years because they are less responsive to preventive and therapeutic measures. Mycobacteria are nonmotile, nonsporulating, weakly gram-positive rods classified in the order Actinomycetales. Dormant organisms remain alive for the life of the host.

The initial infection often involves pulmonary parenchyma in the midzone of the lungs. When hypersensitivity develops after several weeks, the typical caseation appears. Regional hilar lymph nodes become enlarged. Most cases arrest spontaneously at this stage. If the infection progresses, caseation necrosis develops and giant cells produce a typical tubercle. A cause of latent disease in the elderly or debilitated patient is dormant reactivation tubercles. Sites in the apical and posterior segments of the upper lobes and superior segments of the lower lobes are the usual areas of infection.

Clinical Findings

A. Symptoms and Signs

Patients may present with minimal symptoms, including fever, cough, anorexia, weight loss, night sweats, excessive perspiration, chest pain, lethargy, and dyspnea. Extrapulmonary disease may be associated with more severe symptoms, such as involvement of the pericardium, bones, joints, urinary tract, meninges, lymph nodes, or pleural space. Erythema nodosum is seen occasionally in patients with active disease.

B. Laboratory Findings

False-negative tests with intermediate-strength PPD are usually due to anergy, improper testing, or outdated tuberculin. Anergy is sometimes associated with disseminated tuberculosis, measles, sarcoidosis, lymphomas, or recent vaccination with live viruses (eg, poliomyelitis, measles, rubella, mumps, influenza, or yellow fever). Immunosuppressive drugs (eg, corticosteroids, azathioprine) and disease states (eg, AIDS, organ transplantation) may also cause false-negative responses. Mumps skin tests are negative in patients taking immunosuppressive drugs.

Culture of sputum, gastric aspirates, and tracheal washings as well as pleural fluid and pleural and lung biopsies may establish the diagnosis.

C. Imaging Studies

X-ray findings include involvement of the apical and posterior segments of the upper lobes (85%) or the superior segments of the lower lobes (10%). Seldom is the anterior segment of the upper lobe solely involved, as in other granulomatous diseases such as histoplasmosis. Involvement of the basal segments of the lower lobes is uncommon except in women, blacks, and diabetics, but endobronchial disease usually involves the lower lobes, producing atelectasis or consolidation. Differing x-ray patterns correspond to the pathologic variations of the disease: the local exudative lesion, the local productive lesion, cavitation, acute tuberculous pneumonia, miliary tuberculosis, Rasmussen's aneurysm, bronchiectasis, bronchostenosis, and tuberculoma.

Differential Diagnosis

It is critical to distinguish the x-ray findings from bronchogenic carcinoma, particularly when there is tuberculoma without calcification.

Treatment

A. Medical Treatment

Active disease should be treated with one of the chemotherapeutic regimens that have recently been shown to shorten the period of treatment while maintaining their potency. Such drugs include isoniazid, streptomycin, rifampin, and ethambutol (Table 18–5). These multi-

Table 18–5. Antituberculosis drugs and their side effects.

Drug	Dosage (Adult Daily)	Side Effects (Usual)	Monitoring	Remarks
Isoniazid	5–10 mg/kg; 300–600 mg.	Peripheral neuritis, hepatitis, hypersensitivity, convulsions.	SGOT (AST)/SGPT (ALT) (not as routine).	To prevent neuritis, give pyridoxine, 25–50 mg/d orally.
Ethambutol	15–25 mg/kg/d for 60 days, then 15 mg/kg/d.	Optic neuritis (very rare at 15 mg/kg/d).	Visual acuity, red-green color discrimination.	Ocular history and funduscopic examination before use; contraindicated with optic neuritis.
Rifampin	600 mg once daily (children, 10–20 mg/kg to a maximum of 600 mg).	Hepatotoxicity (rare under age 20; 2.5% of cases over age 50). Occasionally, thrombocytopenia, anemia, nephritis.	SGOT (AST)/SGPT (ALT).	Harmless orange staining of urine, sweat, contact lenses, etc. "Flu syndrome" if rifampin given less than twice weekly.
Streptomycin	0.5–1.5 g/d IM (children, 20–40 mg/kg/d IM).	Ototoxicity, nephrotoxicity.	Gross hearing (ticking of watch); if abnormal audiograms, BUN and creatinine.	Used mainly in very ill patients as part of triple-drug regimen.
Aminosalicylic acid	10–12 g/d.	Gastrointestinal intolerance, skin rashes, hypersensitivity.	SGOT (AST)/SGPT (ALT).	Because of poor tolerance, rarely used now.
Pyrazinamide[2]	20–35 mg/kg/d, up to 3 g/d.	Hyperuricemia, hepatotoxicity, arthralgia.	Uric acid, SGOT (AST)/SGPT (ALT).	Sometimes given as first-line drug in short-course regimen (50 mg/kg twice weekly); inexpensive.
Ethionamide[2]	0.5–1 g/d.	Gastrointestinal, hepatotoxicity, hypersensitivity (rash).	SGOT (AST)/SGPT (ALT).	Temporarily stop or reduce dose with gastrointestinal irritation and hepatotoxicity.
Cycloserine[2]	0.5–1 g/d.	Psychosis, personality changes, convulsions, rash.	Drug blood levels if poor renal function.	CNS reactions sometimes controlled by phenytoin.
Capreomycin[2]	20 mg/kg/d IM (up to 1 g/d)	Nephrotoxicity, ototoxicity, hepatotoxicity.	Same as streptomycin with SGOT(AST)/SGPT (ALT) in addition.	Sometimes given as 1 g 2 or 3 times weekly.
Viomycin[2]	1 g twice daily IM 2 or 3 times weekly.	Nephrotoxicity, ototoxicity.	As for streptomycin, plus urinalysis.	As for streptomycin.
Kanamycin[2]	0.5–1 g IM.	See streptomycin.	As for streptomycin, plus urinalysis.	Used mainly for atypical mycobacterial infections.

[1]See also Chambers HF: Antimycobacterial drugs. in: *Basic and Clinical Pharmacology,* 8th ed. Katzung BG (editor). McGraw-Hill, 2001.
[2]Used only as second-line drug in *M tuberculosis* infections, mainly for re-treatment or in drug-resistant cases. Used as first-line drug, in combinations, in atypical mycobacterial infections.

ple-drug regimens are designed to prevent the emergence of resistant strains and minimize toxicity.

B. Surgical Treatment

The role of surgery in treatment of tuberculosis has diminished dramatically since chemotherapy became available. It is now confined to the following indications: (1) failure of chemotherapy, (2) performance of diagnostic procedures, (3) destroyed lung, (4) postsurgical complications, (5) persistent bronchopleural fistula, and (6) intractable hemorrhage.

Surgical resection for diagnosis may be necessary to rule out other diseases, such as cancer, or to obtain material for cultures. Patients with destroyed lobes (Figure 18–18) or

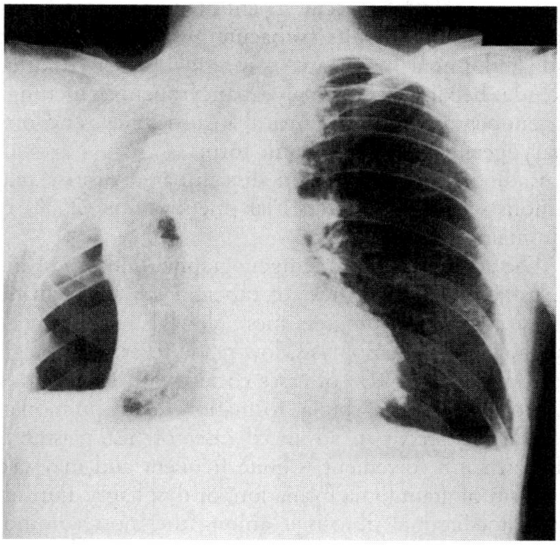

Figure 18–18. Tuberculosis of the right lung with empyema and bronchopleural fistula.

cavitary tuberculosis of the right upper lobe (Figure 18–19) containing large infected foci may sometimes be candidates for resection.

The disease becomes reactivated in some patients who have had thoracoplasty, plombage, or resection, and a few will require reoperation. The most common indications for surgery after plombage therapy are pleural infection (pyogenic or tuberculous) and migration of the plombage material, causing pain or compression of other organs. Following pulmonary resection, tuberculous empyema may develop in the postpneumonectomy space, sometimes associated with a bronchopleural fistula or bony sequestration. Persistent bronchopleural fistula after chemotherapy and closed tube drainage may require direct operative closure. Use of mussel flaps (intercostal, etc.) is highly recommended to cover any bronchial stumps, especially in the setting of pneumonectomy.

Tuberculous empyema poses unique problems of management. Treatment depends upon whether the empyema is (1) associated with parenchymal disease, (2) mixed tuberculous and pyogenic or purely tuberculous, and (3) associated with bronchopleural fistula. The ultimate objective is complete expansion of the lung and obliteration of the empyema space. Pulmonary decortication or resection may be used for tuberculosis, but open or closed drainage is necessary when the process is complicated by pyogenic infection or bronchopleural fistula.

Prognosis

The prognosis is excellent in most cases treated medically; the death rate decreased from 25% in 1945 to less than 10% currently. Perioperative mortality for pulmonary resections for tuberculosis ranges from 10% for pneumonectomy to 3% for lobectomy and 1% for segmentectomy and subsegmental resections.

The relapse rate following modern chemotherapy is about 4%.

Horowitz MD et al: Late complications of plombage. Ann Thorac Surg 1992;53:803.

Langston HT: Thoracoplasty: the how and the why. Ann Thorac Surg 1991;52:1351.

Nolan CM: Failure of therapy for tuberculosis in human immunodeficiency virus infection. Am J Med Sci 1992;304:168.

Pomerantz M et al: Surgical management of resistant mycobacterial tuberculosis and other mycobacterial pulmonary infections. Ann Thorac Surg 1991;52:1108.

Reed CE, Parker EF, Crawford FA Jr: Surgical resection for complications of pulmonary tuberculosis. Ann Thorac Surg 1989;48:165.

FUNGAL INFECTIONS OF THE LUNG

Pulmonary fungal infections are increasing due to the widespread use of broad-spectrum antibiotics, the use of corticosteroids and other immunosuppressive drugs, and the spread of HIV infection. However, infection can occur in immunocompetent hosts. Fungal infections frequently involve the respiratory tract and include histoplasmosis, coccidioidomycosis, blastomycosis, cryptococcosis, aspergillosis, mucormycosis, and candidiasis. Fungal infections, though ubiquitous, are

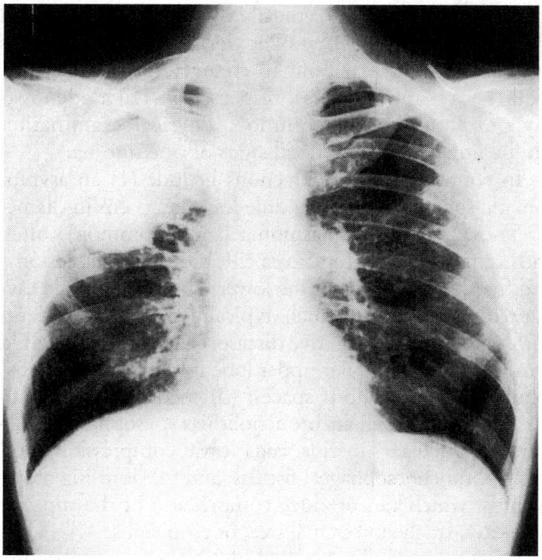

Figure 18–19. Cavitary tuberculosis of the right upper lobe.

notable for several characteristic endemic areas. Candidiasis rarely if ever requires operative treatment and thus will not be discussed here.

1. Histoplasmosis

Histoplasma capsulatum is a dimorphic soil fungus that is frequently found in fowl and bat excreta, pigeon roosts, chicken houses, caves, hollow trees, attics, and lofts. It is endemic in fertile river valleys, such as the Mississippi, Missouri, Ohio, St. Lawrence, and Rio Grande. Infection occurs almost exclusively after inhalation of a large number of spores and occurs with a male:female ratio of 3:1. Once in the lungs, the fungus germinates in yeast form, resulting in caseation, necrosis, fibrosis, and calcification. The diagnosis of histoplasmosis relies on high or rising serum antibody complement fixation titers (> 1:32 or fourfold rise) in the appropriate clinical setting. The histoplasmin skin test, which becomes positive 2–6 weeks following infection, is useful only for epidemiologic studies and not for the diagnosis of acute disease. Sputum culture is positive in less than 10%, but tissue cultures may be more reliable.

Most infections in immunocompetent individuals are asymptomatic. Infections are classified as acute, chronic, or disseminated. Acute infections are manifested either (1) as a flu-like syndrome with fever, chills, dry cough, headache, retrosternal discomfort, arthralgias, and a rash suggesting erythema nodosum; (2) with symptoms similar to a flu-like syndrome but limited to the lungs and occasionally accompanied by a productive cough; or (3) as an acute diffuse nodular disease with mild symptoms. Radiographic findings in these three acute syndromes typically demonstrate ill-defined upper lobe nonsegmental opacities; nonsegmental areas of consolidation that tend to change; and diffuse, discrete 3- to 4-mm nodules, respectively. Hilar adenopathy on chest x-ray is common. Physical examination can be normal or may reveal signs of pneumonia.

In contrast, chronic infections include (1) an asymptomatic solitary, discrete nodule less than 3 cm in diameter known as a histoplasmoma (most common), often with central and concentric calcifications ("target lesion") and frequently located in the lower lobes; (2) chronic cavitary histoplasmosis, which typically occurs in patients with underlying obstructive disease, characteristically mild symptoms, fibronodular upper lobe infiltrates, and centrilobular emphysematous spaces; (3) mediastinal granulomas that may result in broncholithiasis, esophageal traction diverticula, superior vena cava compression, and tracheobronchoesophageal fistulas; and (4) fibrosing mediastinitis, which can produce compression of the superior vena cava, tracheobronchial tree, or esophagus.

Disseminated disease includes an acute, subacute, and chronic form.

These infections occur in children (acute and subacute) as well as adults (subacute and chronic). Fever and abdominal pain are common. Other findings include hepatosplenomegaly, pancytopenia, meningitis, endocarditis, adrenocortical insufficiency, and oropharyngeal ulceration (chronic form).

Radiographic imaging in disseminated disease may demonstrate diffuse interstitial pneumonitis (25%) or minimal findings.

The symptoms and roentgenographic findings of histoplasmosis resemble those of tuberculosis, although the disease appears to progress more slowly. There may be cough, malaise, hemoptysis, low-grade fever, and weight loss. As many as 30% of cases coexist with tuberculosis. Pulmonary fibrosis, bulla formation, and pulmonary insufficiency occur in advanced cases of histoplasmosis. Mediastinal involvement is quite frequent and may take the form of granuloma formation, or dysphagia. Furthermore, mediastinal fibrosis is among the most common benign causes of superior vena caval syndrome (discussed earlier in the chapter). Erosion of inflammatory lymph nodes into bronchi may cause expectoration of broncholiths, hemoptysis, wheezing, or bronchiectasis. Traction diverticula of the esophagus may lead to development of tracheoesophageal fistula. Pericardial involvement may lead to constrictive pericarditis.

In lesions that present as solitary pulmonary nodules, histoplasmosis is diagnosed in about 15–20% of cases. Radiologically, early infections appear as diffuse mottled parenchymal infiltrations surrounding the hila, with enlargement of hilar lymph nodes. Cavitation indicates advanced infection and is the complication about which the surgeon is most often consulted. The diagnosis rests upon finding a positive skin test or complement fixation test and culturing the fungus from sputum or a bronchial aspirate.

Medical therapy of histoplasmosis is indicated only in cavitary and severe disease and for most infections in immunocompromised hosts. Ketoconazole (400 mg/d for 6 months) or itraconazole (200–400 mg/d for 6 months) is useful in cavitary disease, while amphotericin B (1–2 g total dose) is reserved for patients with more serious infections and infections in immunocompromised patients. Surgery is reserved for treatment of complications and to rule out neoplastic disease in the case of suspicious pulmonary nodules. Broncholithectomy with or without pulmonary resection, repair of tracheobronchoesophageal fistulas, decompression of mediastinal granulomas, and spiral saphenous vein bypass of severe symptomatic superior vena cava obstruction are typical examples.

2. Coccidioidomycosis

Coccidioides immitis is a dimorphic soil fungus that is endemic in the Sonoran life zone (Utah, Arizona, California, Nevada, and New Mexico) and is associated with creosote brush. Dry heat with brief intense rain is essential for this fungus, which is spread by strong winds. Infection occurs through inhalation of as few as one to ten arthrospores which then germinate as parasitic spherules. Spherules have a double refractile cell wall and produce endospores that cause the spherule to rupture, spreading the infection into the surrounding tissues. Caseation, suppuration, abscess formation, and fibrosis follow. The diagnosis of coccidioidomycosis relies on the detection of acutely elevated titers of IgM antibodies (by latex agglutination and confirmed by immunodiffusion tube precipitin tests) or rising serum IgG antibody complement fixation titers (seroconversion or fourfold rise) in the appropriate clinical context. The coccidioidin and spherulin skin tests, which become positive 3–21 days following infection, are generally useful only for epidemiologic studies and not for the diagnosis of acute disease. *C immitis* grows well in culture, but it is extremely hazardous to handle and requires a laminar flow hood due to the highly infectious nature of the arthrospores. Identification of the spherules in tissue, lavage samples, and fine-needle aspirates is helpful in making the diagnosis in some patients. Although many stains can be used, including routine fungal (KOH) preparations, Pap staining is most sensitive. Gram stains, however, fail to demonstrate spherules.

Primary infection is asymptomatic in 60% of patients, while most others develop **desert fever**, with fever, productive cough, pleuritic chest pain, pneumonitis, and a rash typical of erythema nodosum or erythema multiforme. Disease that includes arthralgias is known as **desert rheumatism**. Radiographic findings demonstrate segmental or nonsegmental, homogeneous or mottled infiltrates with a predilection for the lower lobes. Physical examination is often unrevealing, but rales and rhonchi may be present. Other findings include eosinophilia (66%), hilar adenopathy (20%), and small exudative pleural effusions (2–20%). Symptomatic persistent infection associated with chest x-ray findings 6–8 weeks after primary infection is classified as one of five types: persistent pneumonia, chronic progressive pneumonia, miliary coccidioidomycosis, coccidioidal nodules, or pulmonary cavities. Persistent pneumonia manifests with symptoms of fever, productive cough, and pleuritic chest pain in association with protracted infiltrates and consolidation on chest x-ray generally resolving within 8 months. Patients with chronic progressive pneumonia complain of fever, cough, dyspnea, hemoptysis, and weight loss, with bilateral apical nodular densities and multiple cavities lasting years. This presentation closely resembles tuberculosis and chronic histoplasmosis. Miliary coccidioidomycosis occurs early and rapidly, associated with bilateral diffuse infiltrates. This form of disease implies the presence of impaired immunity and has an associated mortality rate of 50%. Nearly half of patients with coccidioidal nodules are asymptomatic. These nodular densities (coccidiomas) appear in the middle and upper lung fields, often within 5 cm of the hilum; range from 1 cm to 4 cm in size; and do not calcify, making it hard to distinguish them from malignancy. In endemic areas, 30–50% of all nodules are coccidiomas. Patients develop pulmonary cavities in 10–15% of cases of coccidioidomycosis. Typically, these are solitary (90%), thin-walled, located in the upper lobes (70%), less than 6 cm in size (90%), and close spontaneously within 2 years (50%). Some cavities, however, cross fissures; cause hemoptysis (25– 50%), usually mild; rupture, producing a pyopneumothorax with a bronchopleural fistula; or become infected with aspergillus. Uncommonly, dissemination can occur, particularly in immunocompromised individuals, in pregnancy (third trimester), and in non-Caucasian individuals. Although pulmonary symptoms in disseminated disease are mild, meningeal involvement is common and the mortality rate is high (50%).

Medical therapy is not indicated in asymptomatic, immunocompetent individuals. Patients with persistent or chronic pneumonia, miliary disease, and those at risk for dissemination should be treated with antifungal therapy. Amphotericin B (0.5–2.5 g intravenously as total dose) is the standard treatment, though the newer azole compounds (fluconazole, ketoconazole, and itraconazole) may be used for long-term maintenance therapy since the relapse rate may be as high as 25–50%. Surgery is reserved for patients with coccidiomas when cancer is a concern and in patients with cavities that have an associated radiographic abnormality suggesting carcinoma (ie, thick wall) or that develop a complication, eg, hemoptysis and pyopneumothorax from rupture. Resection should include all diseased tissue and most often requires lobectomy.

3. Blastomycosis

Blastomyces dermatitidis is a dimorphic soil fungus found in warm, wet, nitrogen-rich soil in an endemic area that extends east of a line from the Texas Gulf coast to the border between Minnesota and North Dakota (except Florida and New England). Infection occurs characteristically in males (male:female ratio 6:1–15:1) from 30–60 years of age through inhalation of conidia (asexual spores). At 37 °C the conidia germinate as yeasts, producing caseation in a manner similar to tuberculosis. Rarely, infection may develop through direct skin inoculation. Risk factors include poor hygiene, exposure to dust and wood, manual labor, and poor housing conditions. Since no accurate skin or serologic tests exist, the diagnosis depends on culture or histologic identification of the yeast form. Culture of the mycelial form can be hazardous. *B dermatitidis* grows as white to tan colonies of septate hyphae at room temperature but changes to budding yeast at 37 °C. This temperature-dependent change reflects the uncoupling of oxidative phosphorylation. The yeast form can be found in sputum (33%), bronchoalveolar lavage specimens (38%), lung biopsies (21%), and in fine-needle aspirates (7%) and can be demonstrated with standard KOH preparations or many other histologic stains (but not Gram stain). The yeast, however, does not have a large capsule (distinguishes it from *Cryptococcus neoformans*) and do not grow intracellularly (differentiates it from *Histoplasma capsulatum*).

Manifestations of blastomycosis can occur in many organ systems, including the lungs, skin, bone, genitourinary tract (prostatitis and epididymoorchitis), and central nervous system. Pulmonary infection can be asymptomatic or may present with flu-like symptoms, evidence of pneumonia, or pleurisy. Cough (36%), weight loss (20%), pleuritic pain (26%), fever (23%), hemoptysis (21%), erythema nodosum, and ulcerative bronchitis are common. Radiographic findings include homogeneous or patchy consolidation in a nonsegmental distribution with pleural effusions or thickening or cavitation (15–35%). In some patients, the appearance of pulmonary masses may mimic carcinoma. A predilection for the upper lobes has been noted; however, unlike histoplasmosis and coccidioidomycosis, in blastomycosis hilar and mediastinal adenopathy is unusual.

Limited disease in asymptomatic immunocompetent patients requires no specific therapy. Itraconazole, 100–200 mg/d orally for at least 2–3 months, is now the therapy of choice for nonmeningeal disease, with a response rate of over 80%. Amphotericin B (0.5–2 g), however, is indicated in patients with meningeal disease or failed therapy. Surgical resection is rarely necessary except when the possibility of malignancy cannot be excluded.

4. Cryptococcosis

Cryptococcus neoformans is an encapsulated yeast-like budding fungus. It is a saprophyte existing on the skin, nasopharynx, gastrointestinal tract, and vagina of humans as well as in pigeon excreta, grasses, trees, plants, fruits, bees, wasps, insects (cockroaches), birds, milk products, pickle brine, and soil. Cryptococcal infection generally indicates the presence of an underlying debilitating disease in an immunocompromised host. Infection occurs from inhalation of the yeast form. The diagnosis can be established by the detection of serum antigen (via complement fixation tests) in patients with appropriate clinical and radiographic findings. More commonly, however, histologic identification with India ink stains is used; routine cultures are not performed since they are extremely time-consuming and require multiple biochemical tests for differentiation of cryptococcus from other fungi. No accurate skin test exists for cryptococcosis.

The most common sites of infection are the lungs and central nervous system. Pulmonary infection may remain asymptomatic, or patients may complain of cough, pleuritic chest pain, and fever. Radiographically, cryptococcus can appear as a localized, well-defined 3- to 10-cm pleural-based mass without smooth borders; as single or multiple areas of consolidation, usually within one lobe but in nonsegmental distribution; or as a disseminated miliary nodular infiltrate. A predilection for the lower lobes has been noted. Central nervous system infection usually follows an asymptomatic pulmonary infection. Central nervous system symptoms are highly variable since many patients are severely immunocompromised and do not manifest the usual signs and symptoms of meningitis or cerebritis.

Medical therapy is indicated in most cases of pulmonary infection except for rare cases of limited localized disease. Amphotericin B (0.5–2 g) remains the treatment of choice and is often combined with flucytosine (150/mg/kg per day) for synergy. New azole compounds (eg, fluconazole, itraconazole, and voriconazole) have been used with increasing frequency as first-line therapy both as single agents and in combination. Surgery is rarely indicated and is useful only to exclude the possibility of malignancy or to determine the etiology of an undiagnosed diffuse pulmonary infiltrate by open lung biopsy.

5. Aspergillosis

Aspergillus species are ubiquitous dimorphic soil fungi found in soil and decaying organic matter. The most common pathogenic species include *A fumigatus* (most common), *A niger*, *A flavus*, and *A glaucus*. In culture, these fungi resemble an aspergillum, which is a brush used to sprinkle holy water. Aspergillosis represents the second most common (after candidiasis) opportunistic fungal infection in immunocompromised hosts and the third most common systemic fungal infection requiring hospital care. Infection occurs almost exclusively through inhalation of conidia into areas of lung with impaired mucociliary function (eg, tuberculous cavities). Although the diagnosis is supported by demonstrating immediate and delayed-type hypersensitivity skin reactions, by culturing uniform septate hyphae with dichotomous branching at 45 degrees, and by detecting specific IgG and IgE antibodies, a definitive diagnosis requires demonstration of hyphal tissue invasion or documentation of hyphae on methenamine silver stain in a suspected aspergilloma. Galactomannan enzyme-linked immunosorbent assays have recently become available and serve as a sensitive serum measure of invasive infection.

Infection with aspergillus species usually takes one of three forms: allergic bronchopulmonary aspergillosis, invasive aspergillosis, and aspergilloma. Allergic bronchopulmonary aspergillosis occurs in patients who are atopic (asthmatics) and in patients with cystic fibrosis. Endobronchial fungal growth leads to dilated airways filled with mucus and fungus. Continuous exposure to fungal antigens results in precipitating antibodies, increased IgE levels (which correlate with disease activity), and both immediate and delayed-type hypersensitivity. Patients complain of cough, fever, wheezing, dyspnea, pleuritic pain, and hemoptysis. Chest x-ray shows homogeneous densities in a "gloved-finger," inverted Y, or "cluster of grapes" pattern. Five stages have been defined depending on disease activity and steroid dependency: Stage 1 includes acute infection with characteristic x-ray and laboratory evidence of disease; stage 2 occurs with steroid-induced remission; stage 3 is characterized by asymptomatic exacerbations of laboratory and x-ray findings; steroid-dependent asthma with worsening laboratory tests (total IgE, precipitins, etc) is indicative of stage 4 disease; and end-stage fibrosis, bronchiectasis, and obstruction define stage 5.

Invasive aspergillosis is found exclusively in immunocompromised patients, particularly in patients with leukemia (50–70% of cases). Dissemination occurs frequently, and three types of pulmonary disease have been described: tracheobronchitis (uncommon), necrotizing bronchopneumonia, and hemorrhagic infarction (most common). In tracheobronchitis, disease is usually limited to the larger airways (bronchus more so than trachea) with little parenchymal involvement. Focal or diffuse mucosal ulceration, pseudomembranes, and intraluminal fungal plugs are common. Patients often present with cough, dyspnea, wheezing, and hemoptysis. Occasionally, patchy areas of atelectasis secondary to bronchial obstruction can be seen on chest x-ray. Necrotizing bronchopneumonia should be suspected in patients with unremitting fever, dyspnea, tachypnea, radiologic evidence of bronchopneumonia, and a poor response to standard antibiotic therapy. Finally, hemorrhagic infarction due to vascular permeation with nonthrombotic occlusion of small to medium-sized arteries and necrosis typically results in either a well-defined nodule or a wedge-shaped, pleura-based density. Symptoms are nonspecific and include fever, dyspnea, dry cough, pleuritic chest pain, and hemoptysis. Cavitation is common, and radiologic examination may reveal "round" pneumonia or "air crescents" of a mycotic lung sequestrum.

Aspergillomas ("fungus balls" or mycetomas) are divided into two types: simple, thin-walled cysts lined with ciliated epithelium and surrounded by normal parenchyma; and complex cavities associated with markedly abnormal surrounding lung tissue. Aspergillomas most often occur in the upper lobes and in the superior segments of the lower lobes. Although they may be multiple (22%), calcification and air-fluid levels are rare. Most aspergillomas—particularly complex ones—are associated with cavitary lung disease, ie, tuberculosis (most common), histoplasmosis, sarcoidosis, bronchiectasis, and others. Hemoptysis occurs in 50–80% and can present with frequent minor episodes (30% subsequently have massive bleeding), repeated moderate episodes, or a single episode of massive hemoptysis. Chest x-ray may reveal a 3- to 6-cm round, mobile density with a crescent of air.

Corticosteroids are indicated in patients with allergic bronchopulmonary aspergillosis in addition to measures to relieve bronchospasm (inhaled beta agonists or anticholinergics). In invasive aspergillosis, amphotericin B (0.5–2 g intravenously as total dose) has been standard therapy despite a mortality of 90%. In addition, some patients with complex aspergillomas and severe pulmonary disease are not candidates for surgical resection, and intracavitary amphotericin has been used with modest success. Surgery is indicated for complications of aspergillus infection. Hemoptysis due to aspergillomas is usually best treated by surgical resection. Furthermore, hemoptysis associated with localized invasive aspergillosis (particularly once cavitation has occurred) can be treated by resection and amphotericin B. Generally, wide excision (lobectomy) is required; however, in some high-risk patients with aspergillomas, cavernostomy and muscle flap closure is an alternative.

6. Mucormycosis

Infection with *Rhizopus arrhizus*, absidia species, and rhizomucor species of the class Zygomycetes and the order Mucorales occurs in certain distinct immunosuppressed patient populations: people with poorly controlled diabetes and leukemia patients. These fungi are ubiquitous organisms that are found in decaying fruit, vegetable matter, soil, and manure. Infection occurs following inhalation of sporangiospores, which germinate in a hyphal form. The diagnosis is made by demonstrating the organism in symptomatic patients. No accurate skin or serologic tests exist. Although the fungi do grow in culture as broad irregular nonseptate hyphae that branch at angles up to 90 degrees (occasionally being confused with aspergillus species), most commonly the diagnosis is made on histologic examination. The sine qua non for mucormycosis is hyphal vascular invasion between the internal elastic membrane and the media of blood vessels, causing thrombosis, infarction, and necrosis.

In addition to pulmonary infections, mucormycosis manifests as distinct clinical syndromes such as rhinocerebral infection (direct extension into the central nervous system from paranasal sinus infection), cutaneous infection (burn patients), gastrointestinal infection (children with protein-calorie malnutrition), and disseminated infection (uremic patients receiving deferoxamine therapy). Patients with pulmonary infection complain of fever, cough, pleuritic chest pain, and hemoptysis. Frequently, this type of infection occurs in immunocompromised hosts and follows a fulminant course. Three patterns of infection are noted on chest x-ray: limited disease with involvement of a single lobe or segment, diffuse or disseminated disease with involvement of both lungs and the mediastinum, and endobronchial disease with bronchial obstruction and secondary bacterial infection. Characteristic CT findings include a halo sign (area of low attenuation around a dense infiltrate), ring enhancement, and an air-crescent sign (area of contrast between normal lung and a radiodense cavitating lesion). Amphotericin B is standard treatment. In non-neutropenic patients, the newer azole compounds may be useful; however, infection with these fungi remains highly lethal, with a mortality of 90%. The cause of death in these patients is often fungal sepsis, progressive pulmonary dysfunction, and hemoptysis. In the small group of patients with limited disease, aggressive surgical resection in combination with amphotericin B has lowered the mortality to only 50%. In contrast, the endobronchial form can be effectively treated with transbronchoscopic resection (using the Nd:YAG laser) in a large proportion of patients.

7. Pneumocystosis

Pneumocystis carinii is a fungal organism that has been found in the lungs of a variety of domesticated and wild mammals and is distributed worldwide in humans. Pulmonary involvement leads to progressive pneumonia and respiratory insufficiency. Disease has been seen with increasing frequency in recipients of organ transplants who are undergoing immunosuppressive therapy. Diagnosis is made by open lung biopsy. Without treatment with trimethoprim-sulfamethoxazole, pentamidine, or inhaled antimicrobial therapy, the course is one of relentless progression. With improved antiviral therapy for HIV infections, the incidence of pneumocystosis has been declining.

Benfield TL et al: Prognostic markers of short-term mortality in AIDS-associated *Pneumocystis carinii* pneumonia. Chest 2001;119:844.

Boyars MC, Zwischenberger JB, Cox CS Jr: Clinical manifestations of pulmonary fungal infections. J Thorac Imaging 1992;7:12.

Johnson P, Sarosi G: Current therapy of major fungal diseases of the lung. Infect Dis Clin North Am 1991;5:635.

Ledergerber B et al: Discontinuation of secondary prophylaxis against *Pneumocystis carinii* pneumonia in patients with HIV infection who have a response to antiretroviral therapy. Eight European Study Groups. N Engl J Med 2001;344:168.

Lopez Bernaldo de Quiros JC et al: A randomized trial of the discontinuation of primary and secondary prophylaxis against *Pneumocystis carinii* pneumonia after highly active antiretroviral therapy in patients with HIV infection. Grupo de Estudio del SIDA 04/98. N Engl J Med 2001;344:159.

Russian DA, Levine SJ: *Pneumocystis carinii* pneumonia in patients without HIV infection. Am J Med Sci 2001;321:56.

SARCOIDOSIS (BOECK'S SARCOID, BENIGN LYMPHOGRANULOMATOSIS)

Sarcoidosis is a noncaseating granulomatous disease of unknown cause involving the lungs, liver, spleen, lymph nodes, skin, and bones. The highest incidence is reported in Scandinavia, England, and the United States. The incidence in blacks is 10–17 times that in whites. Half of patients are between ages 20 and 40 years, with women more frequently affected than men.

Clinical Findings

A. Symptoms and Signs

Sarcoidosis may present with symptoms of pulmonary infection, but usually these are insidious and nonspecific. Erythema nodosum may herald the onset, and weight loss, fatigue, weakness, and malaise may appear later. Fever occurs in approximately 15% of cases. Pulmonary symptoms occur in 20–30% and include dry cough and dyspnea. Hemoptysis is rare. One-fifth of patients with sarcoidosis have myocardial involvement, and heart block or failure may occur. Peripheral lymph nodes are enlarged in 75%; scalene lymph nodes are microscopically involved in 80% and mediastinal nodes in 90%; and cutaneous involvement is present in 30%. Hepatic and splenic involvement can be shown by biopsy in 70% of cases. There may be migratory or persistent polyarthritis, and central nervous involvement occurs in a few patients.

B. Imaging Studies

The x-ray findings in sarcoidosis are classified into five descriptive categories or stages (Table 18–6). Pulmonary disease can manifest as a reticulonodular infiltrate, an acinar pattern of opacities, or large nodules with or

Table 18–6. Radiographic stages of sarcoidosis.

Stage 0:	No x-ray abnormality
Stage 1:	Hilar and mediastinal lymph node enlargement without pulmonary abnormalities
Stage 2:	Hilar and mediastinal lymph node enlargement with pulmonary abnormalities
Stage 3:	Diffuse pulmonary disease without adenopathy
Stage 4:	Pulmonary fibrosis

without mediastinal adenopathy. Mediastinal lymph node involvement characteristically includes bilateral symmetric hilar and paratracheal lymphadenopathy. Anterior or posterior mediastinal adenopathy or asymmetric hilar involvement should prompt a suspicion of other diseases, particularly Hodgkin's disease and non-Hodgkin's lymphomas. Pleural effusions and cavitation are rare and, if present, necessitate an evaluation for tuberculosis, congestive heart failure, and coincidental pneumonia.

Diagnosis

Although no single test exists to confirm absolutely the diagnosis of sarcoidosis (the diagnosis remains one of exclusion), it may be suggested by the characteristic radiographic appearance of bilateral hilar and mediastinal lymphadenopathy, by gallium 67 scanning, and by elevated serum and bronchoalveolar fluid levels of angiotensin-converting enzyme and lysozyme. Pathologic documentation of noncaseating granulomas should normally be obtained either via transbronchial biopsy or mediastinoscopy (more reliable, with > 95% success rate). Culture for mycobacteria, fungi, and other atypical infections must also be negative.

Treatment

Asymptomatic patients and those with minimal clinical disease may require no therapy. Corticosteroids have been used in patients with pulmonary impairment and symptomatic disease with good success. Despite the indolent nature of the disease and steroid therapy, long-term mortality is reported as high as 10%. Lung transplantation has been utilized with success in patients refractory to medical management.

NEOPLASMS OF THE LUNG

PRIMARY LUNG CANCER

Lung cancer is the most common cause of cancer-related deaths in both men and women in the United States. In 2004, it is estimated that 165,500 new cases and 155,000 deaths will occur due to pulmonary malignancies. This represents 15% of all new cancer cases and 28% of all cancer-related deaths. In addition, although the incidence in males appears to have stabilized, the incidence continues to rise rapidly in females.

Tobacco smoking accounts for 85% of all lung cancer cases. The effect is greatest for cigarettes and least for pipe smoking and is directly related to the amount of tobacco smoked. Following 5–6 years of smoking cessation, the risk exponentially declines, and after 15 years approaches, but never reaches, that of nonsmokers. "Passive" exposure to cigarette smoke, on the other hand, increases the risk in nonsmokers by two to three times. Exposure to all forms of asbestos (amosite, chrysotile, and crocidolite) has been implicated in as many as 23% of lung cancers, accounting for the high incidence among shipyard workers, insulators, cement makers, truck drivers, and plumbers. The effect is particularly pronounced in smokers and is most commonly associated with squamous cell and small cell carcinoma. Recently, exposure to radon and its alpha-emitting daughter isotopes have been implicated in the increased incidence of lung cancer in both uranium miners and populations living in geographic areas naturally contaminated with high levels of radon gas. Although it has been known for some time that people with high activity of 4-debrisoquine hydroxylase, the so-called debrisoquine metabolic phenotype, have a ten-times increased risk of lung cancer, only recently has the role of genetic factors been appreciated. Chromosome deletions (particularly 11p, 13q, 17p, and 3p), tumor suppressor gene mutations (P53, Hap-1, ErbAb, etc), and constitutive, high-level expression of both growth factor genes (insulin-like and transferrin-like growth factors), epidermal growth factor receptors (HER2/*neu, EGFR1,* etc) and proto-oncogenes (c-, N- and L-*myc;* H-, N-, and K-*ras;* and c-*myb*) have all been implicated in the pathogenesis of lung cancer. Other factors such as vitamin A deficiency, air pollution; exposure to arsenic, cadmium, chromium, ether, and formaldehyde; and employment as bakers, cooks, construction workers, cosmetologists, leather workers, pitchblende miners, printers, rubber workers, and pottery workers have also been incriminated. Finally, certain diseases—eg, progressive systemic sclerosis (scleroderma)—have a defined predisposition for the development of lung cancer. Silencing of genes by aberrant promoter hypermethylation is viewed as a crucial component in lung cancer pathobiology. Newer PCR assays for specific methylation events have permitted identification of genes implicated in the progression of lung cancers.

Pathology

Lung cancer occurs more commonly in the right lung than the left, and the upper lobes are involved more commonly than the lower lobes or the right middle lobe. Synchronous primary lung cancers occur in up to 7% of patients, and 10% of patients will develop a metachronous new tumor (2% per year risk post resection of early stage disease). Furthermore, patients with lung cancer are at higher risk of developing cancers of the upper respiratory tract, oral cavity, esophagus, bladder, and kidney presumably related to the "field effect" of smoking. Lung cancers typically spread by local extension to involve the visceral and parietal pleura, chest wall, great vessels, pericardium, diaphragm, esophagus, and vertebral column. Common sites of metastatic involvement include the ipsilateral pulmonary and hilar lymph nodes, the mediastinal lymph nodes, the lung, liver, bone, brain, adrenal glands, pancreas, kidney, soft tissues, and myocardium. The exact pathologic classification of lung cancer has not been uniform despite attempts at standardization by the World Health Organization. Functionally, however, squamous cell carcinoma, large cell carcinoma, and adenocarcinoma are grouped together under the designation of non-small cell carcinomas and constitute 80% of all lung tumors. Small cell carcinoma represents 15–20%, while bronchial gland adenomas, including carcinoids, comprise the remaining 5%. The differential locations of some of these neoplasms are summarized in Table 18–7.

A. Squamous Cell Carcinoma

The major pathologic features of squamous cell carcinoma are keratinization, cellular stratification, and intercellular bridges. Squamous cell carcinomas account for about 20% of all cases of lung cancer and 70% of non-small cell tumors. Two-thirds are located centrally near the hilum and one-third peripherally. The growth rate and the rate of metastasis tend to be slower than those of other lung tumors.

B. Adenocarcinoma

Adenocarcinomas, which constitute 30% of lung cancers and 60% of non-small cell tumors, are characterized as acinar, papillary, and bronchoalveolar. Acinar adenocarcinoma is composed of glands lined by columnar cells that secrete mucin. Bronchoalveolar carcinoma is characterized by intraluminal papillary fragments that appear in alveoli or small bronchioles. Bronchoalveolar carcinoma may be spread by aerosol transmission. The incidence of adenocarcinoma of the lung is increasing relative to squamous cell carcinoma, perhaps as a consequence of the rise in lung cancer among women, although the exact cause remains unclear.

Table 18–7. Location of lung cancer by histologic type.

Histology	Central (%)	Peripheral (%)
Squamous cell carcinoma	64–81	19–36
Adenocarcinoma	5–29	71–95
Large-cell carcinoma	42–49	51–58
Small-cell carcinoma	74–83	17–26
Overall	63	37

[1]From Cameron RB: Malignancies of the lung. In: *Practical Oncology*. Cameron RB (editor). Originally published by Appleton & Lange. Copyright © 1994 by The McGraw-Hill Companies, Inc.

C. Small Cell Carcinoma

Small cell (oat cell) carcinomas have small, round nuclei with nuclear chromatin and cytoplasm. They are so biologically and clinically distinct from all other cell types that the term non-small cell lung cancer often is applied to all other cell types. Small cell carcinomas comprise 15–20% of all lung cancers. They occur centrally, metastasize early, and are the most resistant to combined-modality treatment.

D. Large Cell Carcinoma

Large cell carcinomas are composed of large polygonal spindle or oval cells arranged in sheets, nests, or clusters. Multinucleated giant cells, intracellular hyalin droplets, glycogen, and acidophilic nuclear inclusions may be present. These tumors are seen peripherally and are less common.

E. Adenosquamous Tumors

Adenosquamous tumors show both cellular features and are more biologically aggressive than other non-small cell lung cancers. Survival percentages of patients with adenosquamous tumors are significantly lower than what is reported for adenocarcinoma or squamous cell cancer.

F. Bronchial Gland Adenomas

Bronchial gland adenoma is a misnomer since the vast majority of these tumors are malignant. Included in this group are carcinoid tumors, adenoid cystic carcinomas, mucoepidermoid carcinoma, mixed tumors of the salivary gland type, and mucous gland adenoma. Carcinoid tumors are derived from Kulchitsky cells, have a vascular stroma, and tend to be located centrally in proximal airways. Although they are slow-growing, they can metastasize widely. Carcinoid syndrome is rarely associated with bronchial carcinoids, as opposed to intestinal carcinoids that metastasize to the liver. Adenoid cystic carcinomas—also referred to as cylindromas—feature groups of epithelial cells that form duct-like structures interspersed with cystic spaces. These neoplasms are locally aggressive and often extend beyond apparent gross pathologic margins. Metastases from adenoid cystic carcinomas often involve the lung, are slow-growing, and are amenable to surgical excision. Mucoepidermoid carcinomas are rare tumors characterized by the presence of squamous cells, mucus-secreting cells, and an intermediate cell type. The cells are bland and less aggressive than those of adenosquamous carcinomas. Mixed tumors of the salivary type are extremely rare infiltrating tumors that are curable with wide local excision. Finally, mucus gland adenomas (papillary or bronchial cyst adenomas) are the only true benign "adenomas" of this group with no metastatic potential. These neoplasms are rare tumors of the major bronchi and consist of numerous mucus-filled cysts lined by a well-differentiated epithelium. Generally, bronchoscopic removal can be accomplished and results in long-term cure.

Clinical Presentation

Nearly 94% of patients present with symptoms from the effects of the primary tumor, regional spread, or metastatic disease. Local effects of the primary tumor account for 27% of presenting symptoms and vary depending on the location of the tumor. Central tumors are associated with cough, hemoptysis, respiratory difficulty (wheezing, stridor, or dyspnea), pain, and pneumonia. Peripheral tumors can cause cough, chest wall pain, pleural effusions, pulmonary abscess, Horner's syndrome (ipsilateral miosis, ptosis, and anhidrosis), and Pancoast's syndrome (ipsilateral shoulder and arm pain in the C8–T1 nerve root distribution, Horner's syndrome, and a superior sulcus—usually squamous—lung cancer). Symptoms due to the effect of regional spread include hoarseness from recurrent nerve paralysis, dyspnea due to phrenic nerve paralysis, dysphagia from compression of the esophagus, superior vena cava syndrome from compression or invasion of the superior vena cava, and pericardial tamponade from invasion of the pericardium. Metastatic disease may present with symptoms of systemic illness (anorexia, weight loss, weakness, and malaise), local manifestations of distant metastases (jaundice, abdominal mass, bony pain or fracture, neurologic deficits, mental status changes, seizures, and soft tissue masses). A number of paraneoplastic syndromes associated with lung cancer have been identified (Table 18–8).

Table 18–8. Paraneoplastic syndromes associated with lung cancer.

Cardiovascular
Thrombophlebitis
Nonbacterial thrombotic endocarditis
Neuromuscular
Subacute cerebellar degeneration
Dementia
Limbic encephalitis
Optic neuritis, retinopathy
Subacute necrotic myelopathy
Autonomic neuropathy (small cell)
Myasthenic (Eaton-Lambert) syndrome (small cell)
Polymyositis
Gastrointestinal
Carcinoid syndrome (carcinoid and small cell)
Anorexia, cachexia
Hematologic
Erythrocytosis
Leukocytosis
Metabolic
Inappropriate ACTH (small cell)
Inappropriate ADH (small cell)
Hypercalcemia (squamous cell carcinoma)
Inappropriate gonadotropins
Dermatologic
Acanthosis nigricans (adenocarcinoma)
Dermatomyositis
Erythema gyratum
Ichthyosis
Other
Hypertrophic pulmonary osteoarthropathy (squamous cell, large cell, and adenocarcinoma)
Nephrotic syndrome
Fever

Diagnosis & Workup

Lung cancer is usually suspected from abnormal findings on a chest x-ray obtained in the course of a routine physical examination or, more commonly, after a complaint of pulmonary symptoms (see above). Findings vary from a small peripheral nodule to an unresolving infiltrate or even total lung atelectasis. Occasionally, the location of the abnormality may suggest certain cell types (Table 18–7; Figure 18–20). Despite the utility of chest x-rays in the diagnosis of lung cancer, prospective randomized trials at three major institutions have failed to demonstrate a survival benefit from mass screening programs incorporating chest x-rays with or without the addition of sputum cytologic examinations. Newer PCR assays of sputum seeking methylation events in expectorated bronchial epithelial cells show promise as a screening tool but are yet to be widely applied or vigorously studied. Once the diagnosis of lung cancer is suspected, a definitive diagnosis can be obtained in over 90% of patients with either bronchoscopy for proximal lesions or fine-needle aspiration cytology for peripheral lesions.

Currently, CT scanning is an integral part of the assessment of patients with lung cancer. Chest CT scans should also include the upper abdomen to assess two of the most common sites of metastases (liver and adrenal glands). Injection of intravenous contrast while the scan is obtained facilitates evaluation of the mediastinum. Additional radiographic workup includes tests to evaluate other common sites of metastases, such as

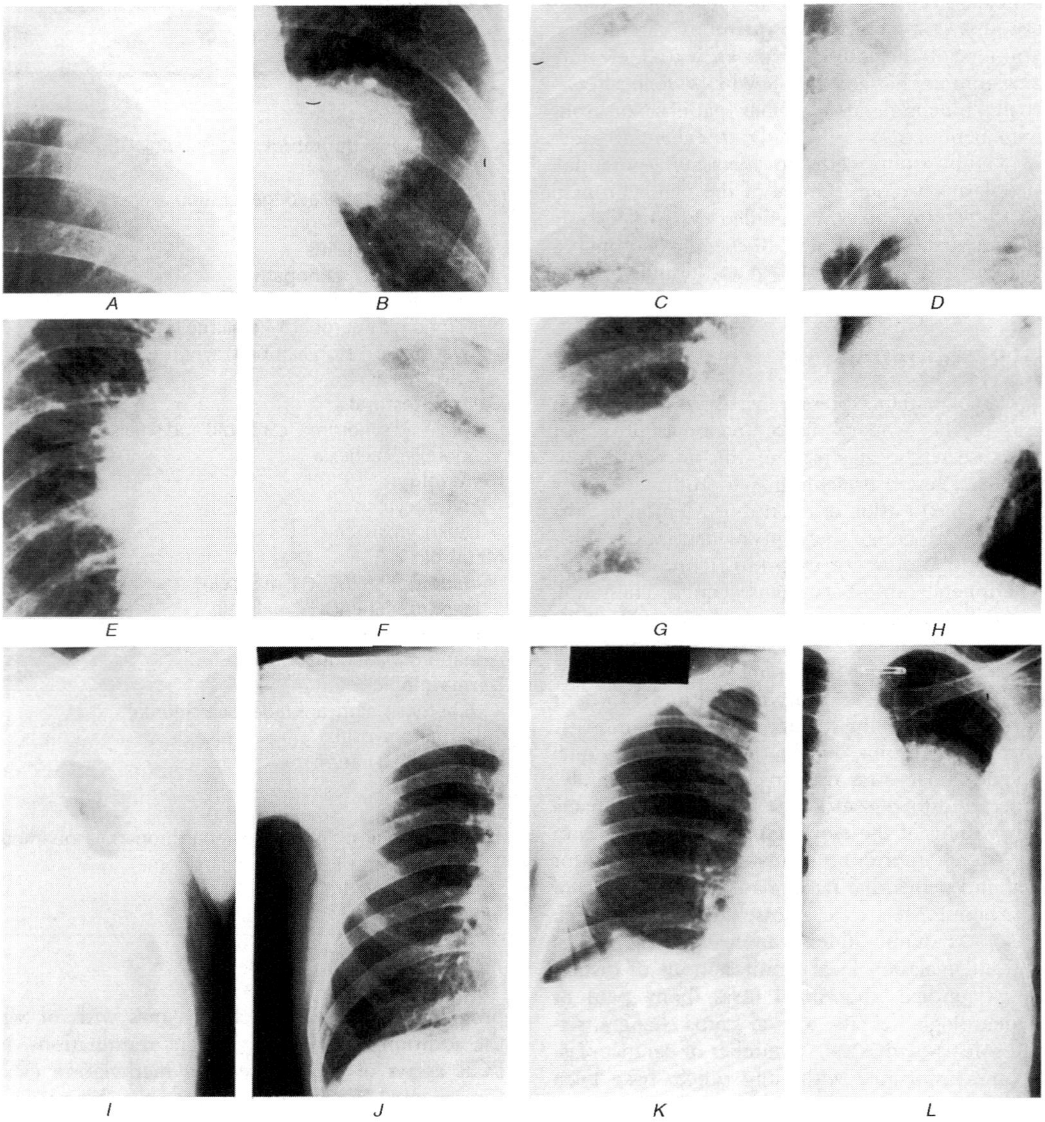

Figure 18–20. X-ray manifestations of lung cancer. ***A:*** Small epidermoid carcinoma in LUL (posteroanterior projection). ***B:*** Large coin lesions; adenocarcinoma in superior segment of LLL (lateral projection). ***C and D:*** Epidermoid carcinoma in RUL. ***E:*** Right hilar mass; small cell carcinoma. ***F:*** Large cavitary epidermoid carcinoma in RUL. ***G*** (posteroanterior projection) and ***H*** (lateral projection): Middle lobe atelectasis from bronchial carcinoid (not visible). ***I:*** Opacification of left hemithorax; large cavitary epidermoid carcinoma. ***J:*** Pancoast's tumor; poorly differentiated epidermoid carcinoma with erosion of third rib and pathologic fracture of fourth rib. ***K:*** Right phrenic nerve paralysis caused by epidermoid carcinoma. ***L:*** Pleural metastasis caused by adenocarcinoma of LLL. (LUL = left upper lobe; LLL = left lower lobe, etc.)

bone and brain. A serum alkaline phosphatase is essential, and a bone scan and brain CT scan (or preferably MRI) should be obtained if indicated by elevated alkaline phosphatase levels, neurologic symptoms, or bone pain or if advanced-stage disease (stage III or beyond) is present. Fluorodeoxyglucose (FDG) positron emission tomography (PET) has evolved into a critical staging test. It is most effective at assay for distant occult disease. It can be helpful for assessing mediastinal node involvement, but it is not definitive. False-positive rates as high as 15–20% have been reported. Furthermore, nodules less than 1 cm in diameter are generally not reliably imaged by PET scanning. Combination high-resolution CT scan and PET scan assessment permits improved correlation of abnormal CT findings with FDG uptake suggestive of tumor. Thoracentesis or thoracoscopy (or both) should be performed in any patient with evidence of a pleural effusion to exclude diffuse involvement of the pleura (T4 or stage IIIB disease), which makes the lesion incurable with surgery. Despite increasing reliance on PET scan to stage the mediastinum, patients with non-small cell lung cancer but without metastatic disease should be evaluated with cervical mediastinoscopy and parasternal mediastinotomy (Chamberlain) if necessary to document the status of the mediastinal nodes in equivocal cases. PET scanning is informative but less accurate than mediastinoscopy. With small cell lung cancer; however, this usually is not necessary. The use of CT scans alone is inaccurate in 40–60% of patients with enlarged lymph nodes over 1 cm (false-positive) and 15% of patients without "significant" lymphadenopathy (false-negative). Once all the information from these staging procedures is in hand, the patient with non-small cell lung cancer can be classified into one of three categories: (1) early lung cancer without mediastinal involvement, or stage I/II (see below); (2) locally advanced lung cancer, or stage IIIA/B, and (3) metastatic lung cancer, or stage IV. Therapy is determined by disease stage. Patients with small cell lung cancer are usually grouped into two categories: disease limited to the ipsilateral hemithorax, including supraclavicular nodes (limited disease); or disease extending beyond the thorax (extensive disease), ie, below the diaphragm or brain metastases.

Staging

By 1987, the American Joint Committee on Cancer (AJCC) and the Union Internationale Contre le Cancer (UICC) had developed a joint staging system for lung carcinoma based on data gathered primarily by Clifford Mountain of the MD Anderson Cancer Center. The lung cancer staging system is based on the tumor (T), the status of regional lymph nodes (N), and the presence or absence of distant metastases (M) as outlined in Table 18–9.

Treatment

Treatment for small cell carcinoma consists primarily of chemotherapy and radiation, though recent data indicate that for early disease (T1–T2 lesions and limited hilar adenopathy) resection may improve local control and result in increased long-term survival (as high as 50%), particularly when combined with postoperative chemotherapy. Treatment for non-small cell lung cancer, however, varies with stage. Early-stage disease (stage I/II) has historically been treated with surgery alone. However, the results of several randomized prospective trials involving adjuvant chemotherapy for early (Ib and higher) non-small cell lung cancer suggest benefit. Locally advanced but surgically resectable disease (stage IIIA) is currently best treated with combined-modality therapy utilizing induction chemotherapy or chemoradiotherapy followed by surgery and, if necessary, postoperative radiotherapy. Locally advanced and surgically unresectable disease (stage IIIB) is best managed with concurrent platinum-based chemotherapy and fractionated radiation therapy. Metastatic disease (stage IV) is only poorly treated with chemotherapy. Radiotherapy in this case is reserved for symptomatic lesions. Combined-agent chemotherapy offers 2–3 months (20%) survival extension to advanced-stage patients. It has been shown to be cost-effective and improve quality of life and is generally well-tolerated by patients with reasonable performance status. New biologic agents—so-called "targeted therapies"—are showing activity in clinical trials and should improve overall survival statistics. It is hoped that with advances in targeted and conventional therapies the current overall survival (< 15% at 5 years) of patients with lung cancer can be improved.

Induction Chemotherapy

Recently completed clinical trials and several ongoing clinical trials suggest survival benefit of treatment with platinum-based chemotherapy prior to definitive resection. Induction chemotherapy has been standard for locally advanced surgically resectable disease, but evidence is accumulating to support induction therapy in early stage non-small cell lung cancer.

A. Surgical Treatment

1. Surgical staging—As noted above, almost all patients with non-small cell lung cancer limited to the thorax should undergo cervical mediastinoscopy to exclude involvement of N2 mediastinal lymph nodes (N2 or N3 disease). A possible exception is a small peripheral (T1) nodule, especially of squamous cell histology without any evidence for mediastinal adenopathy on chest CT scan. PET scan is used with increasing frequency to stage the mediastinum. Surgical staging

Table 18–9. TNM stage groupings.

Primary tumor	
TX	Primary tumor cannot be assessed, or cytologic evidence of malignant cells in sputum or bronchial washings but not visualized by imaging or bronchoscopy
T0	No evidence of primary tumor
Tis	Carcinoma in situ
T1	Tumor 3 cm or less in greatest diameter, completely surrounded by lung or visceral pleura, and without bronchoscopic evidence of involvement of more proximal than a lobar bronchus
T2	Tumor more than 3 cm in greatest diameter, invading the visceral pleura, involving the main stem bronchus but greater than 2 cm distal to the carina, or tumor associated with atelectasis or obstructive pneumonitis extending to the hilum but not involving the entire lung
T3	Tumor of any size invading the chest wall, diaphragm, mediastinal pleura, parietal pericardium, tumor involving the main stem bronchus within 2 cm of but not involving the carina, or tumor associated with atelectasis or obstructive pneumonitis of the entire lung
T4	Tumor of any size invading the mediastinum, heart, great vessels, trachea, esophagus, vertebral body, or carina, or tumor associated with a malignant pleural effusion
Regional lymph nodes (N stage)	
NX	Regional lymph nodes cannot be assessed
N0	No evidence of regional lymph node metastases
N1	Metastases in ipsilateral peribronchial or hilar lymph nodes, including by direct extension
N2	Metastases in ipsilateral mediastinal or subcarinal lymph nodes
N3	Metastases in contralateral mediastinal or hilar lymph nodes or ipsilateral or contralateral scalene or supraclavicular nodes
Distant metastases (M stage)	
MX	Presence of distant metastases cannot be assessed
M0	No evidence of distant metastases
M1	Distant metastases are present
Stage grouping	
Occult disease	TX, N0, M0
Stage 0	Tis, N0, M0
Stage IA	T1, N0, M0
Stage IB	T2 N0 M0
Stage IIA	T1 N1 M0
Stage IIB	T2 N1 M0 T3 N0 M0
Stage IIIA	T1–2, N2, M0, or T3, N0–2, M0
Stage IIIB	T4, Any N, M0, or Any T, N3, M0
Stage IV	Any T, Any N, M1

with cervical mediastinoscopy remains the most accurate staging maneuver. Adenocarcinomas with negative mediastinal nodes by CT have an 18–25% false-negative rate. For left-sided lesions, left parasternal mediastinotomy (Chamberlain) may be required to assess the status of the aorticopulmonary lymph nodes. Without pathologic confirmation of the status of mediastinal lymph nodes, CT scans have been associated with high false-positive and false-negative rates. A surgical assessment of the proximal airways is also required even if this means repeating this invasive procedure, often previously performed by the pulmonologist. Since treatment decisions are based on accurate staging and because treatment of early-stage disease (stage I/II) differs significantly from locally advanced disease (stage IIIA/B), this approach is essential. The importance of accurate staging for patients with non-small cell lung cancer cannot be overstated.

2. Indications and preoperative assessment—Surgical resection is indicated for early-stage lung cancer (stage I/II) and in combination with chemotherapy and radiation in locally advanced resectable disease (stage IIIA or resectable T4, IIIb). In addition, surgery may be indicated for patients with a single site of metastatic disease, such as a solitary brain or adrenal gland metastasis. Both relative and absolute contraindications to surgical resection are listed in Table 18–10.

Preoperative assessment is aimed at evaluating both cardiopulmonary reserve and overall patient fitness. The patient's general performance status or functional classification is probably the most accurate factor in predicting a successful outcome following surgery. Advanced age, by itself, is not a contraindication to surgery. It is the physiologic age—as manifested by functional status—not the chronologic age that is important. A thorough cardiac evaluation is also necessary, since lung cancer and cardiac disease share common risk factors (eg, smoking). Patients with cardiac symptoms, an abnormal ECG, or other findings suggestive of ischemic heart disease should be screened by a stress test (exercise treadmill, dipyridamole- or adenosine-thallium study, dobutamine echocardiogram). Significant left main coronary artery disease should be treated with coronary artery bypass prior to any contemplated pulmonary resection, and other significant disease should be individually assessed for possible bypass or angioplasty. Furthermore, significant pulmonary hypertension and myocardial infarction within 3 months are associated with up to 20% perioperative mortality and constitute absolute contraindications to surgery. Other high-risk findings include myocardial infarction within 6 months, ventricular arrhythmias, and heart block, particularly left posterior fascicular hemiblock. Finally, the patient's pulmonary function and ability to tolerate the required pulmonary resection need to be assessed. This is accomplished with pulmonary function tests (spirometry, diffusing capacity, exercise oximetry) and with differential (quantitative) ventilation-perfusion scanning when appropriate. In a 70 kg patient, the following preoperative studies indicate high morbidity risk and are relative contraindications to resection: FEV_1 < 0.8 L, a predicted postoperative FEV_1 < 0.8, a predicted maximum voluntary ventilation < 50%, a $PaCO_2$ > 45 mm Hg, and a PaO_2 < 50 mm Hg. A diffusion limitation capacity of carbon monoxide (DLCO) < 60% predicted is correlated with an increase in perioperative mortality.

Table 18–10. Medical and surgical contraindications to pulmonary resection.

Absolute	Relative
Myocardial infarction within previous 3 months	Myocardial infarction within previous 6 months
SVC syndrome (due to metastatic tumor)	SVC syndrome (due to primary tumor)
Bilateral endobronchial tumor	Recurrent laryngeal nerve paralysis (due to primary tumor in aorticopulmonary window)
Contralateral lymph node metastases (N3)	Horner's syndrome
Malignant pleural effusion	Small cell histology
Distant metastases (except solitary brain and adrenal metastases)	Metastases higher than the mid-tracheal lymph nodes
	Pericardial involvement
	FEV_1 < 0.8 L (< 50%)
	FEV_1 0.9–2.4 and insufficient pulmonary reserve for planned resection
	Main pulmonary artery involvement

3. Surgical resection

a. Early and locally advanced non-small cell lung cancer—The extent of pulmonary resection is dictated by the location of the primary tumor and the presence or absence of involved hilar (interlobar) lymph nodes. Limited segmental resection for stage I/II non-small cell lung cancer (NSCLC) has been evaluated by the Lung Cancer Study Group and found to result in an increased local recurrence rate (15% versus 3%) and lower overall survival. Segmental resections, therefore, are viewed as compromise procedures only indicated in patients who cannot tolerate lobectomy. Lobectomy continues to be the standard of care for resection for NSCLC. This should include a 1 cm margin of normal proximal bronchus. Samples of interlobar (hilar) lymph nodes are submitted for immediate pathologic examination to exclude involvement that would require pneumonectomy. A "sleeve" resection of main stem bronchus can also be included in the resection, particularly with the right upper lobe. Pneumonectomy is required for proximal lesions involving the main stem bronchus or the interlobar (hilar) lymph nodes. In addition, techniques are available for more extensive resection such as intrapericardial pneumonectomy and tracheal "sleeve" pneumonectomy. The overall mortality rates following segmental resection, lobectomy, and pneumonectomy are 1.4%, 2.9%, and 6.2%, respectively, in centers with large experience. Complications following pulmonary resection include cardiac arrhythmias, hemorrhage, infection (empyema), bronchopleural fistula, respiratory insufficiency, and pulmonary embolism.

b. Advanced (metastatic) non-small cell lung cancer—Patients with solitary brain and adrenal metastases, especially if metachronous, are still candidates for surgical resection and have benefited by prolonged survival in a few small retrospective studies in comparison with historical controls. Systemic preoperative (induction) chemotherapy and radiotherapy, however, should be administered initially. In addition, transbronchial Nd:YAG laser resection of tumors obstructing the proximal airways can significantly palliate selected patients. In addition, improvements in the design and deployment techniques of expansile stents have been a significant advance for palliation of proximal airway obstruction. Finally, photodynamic laser therapy with photosensitizers can alleviate airway obstruction from tumors, albeit not as quickly as Nd:YAG laser ablation.

c. Small cell lung cancer—Resection for small peripheral tumors followed by aggressive postoperative chemotherapy may increase the local control rate and potentially the overall survival rate in the early small cell lung cancer. Survival rates as high as 50% with this approach have been reported.

B. Radiation Therapy

1. Non-small cell lung cancer—Radiation therapy can be administered with curative intent in stage I/II disease in patients who refuse or are not medically suitable candidates for surgery. The 5-year survival rate with this approach, however, is only 22–33%. With locally advanced disease (stage IIIA/B), radiation therapy (5500–6000 cGy) until recently has been the treatment of choice. Although local or nodal recurrence rates are < 30%, long-term survival is < 10% in these patients, and the type of fractionation scheme has not altered the outcome. Adjuvant radiation therapy following surgical resection has been extensively studied by the Lung Cancer Study Group and has been found to decrease local or nodal recurrences but not to prolong overall survival. A much-disputed meta-analysis (the PORT study) showed a decrease in survival for stage II patients treated with postoperative radiation. Differences in radiotherapy techniques within the analysis may account for the worse outcomes. Preoperative radiation has been used with T3 lesions, particularly Pancoast tumors, with improved survival; however, there is no objective evidence that radiation must be given preoperatively. Recently, a multicenter intergroup trial (SWOG) showed a significant survival advantage for combined chemoradiotherapy (etoposide, platinum, and 4500 cGy) prior to resection for Pancoast (superior sulcus) tumors that were N1 or less. Complete resection rates were improved; 20–25% complete pathologic responses were achieved; and survival was significantly improved (45–50% at 3 years) over surgery alone or preoperative radiotherapy and surgery. Intraoperative radiation has been investigated but to date has been associated with unacceptably high morbidity. Finally, in patients with metastatic disease, therapeutic radiation is indicated in patients with symptoms of pain, neurologic symptoms, and symptoms of superior vena cava compression.

2. Small cell lung cancer—Multiple randomized trials comparing the combination of radiation and chemotherapy to chemotherapy alone in limited-stage small cell lung cancer have been conducted. The majority show improved local control and modest (3–4 months) prolonged survival with the combination. This was at the cost of increased morbidity, however. In extensive disease, no benefit has been demonstrated for radiation therapy outside of palliative radiation of symptomatic metastases. Prophylactic cranial irradiation may be beneficial but can cause significant cognitive deficits.

C. Chemotherapy

1. Non-small cell lung cancer—Although chemotherapy alone has not generally been used in the treatment of early or locally advanced NSCLC, combinations of chemotherapy and radiotherapy have been evaluated in locally advanced unresectable disease. In some instances, no benefit to the combination was demonstrated, particularly when only single agents were used; however, improved results with both radiation and combined-agent chemotherapy have recently been documented. In the presence of metastatic disease, multiple trials of combination chemotherapy have demonstrated a modest improvement in overall survival (14 weeks or 25% improved survival) but not without some toxicity. Even so, quality of life assessments and cost analyses support the use of outpatient combined-agent chemotherapy over palliative care alone.

Table 18-11. Adjuvant trials favoring use of chemotherapy in completely resected non-small cell lung cancer.

Study	CT Regimen	Radiation Therapy	Five-Year Survival CT vs. Control
Italian Stage IB Study	Cis/Etoposide × 6	No	63% vs. 45%
IALT LeChevalier	Various platinum	Yes ±	44.5% vs. 40.4%
CALGB 9633 Strauss	Carbo/Taxol × 4	No	69% vs. 54%
NCIC/BR10	Vin/P × 4	No	71% vs. 59%[2]

[1]CT, Carbo/Taxol, carboplatin paclitaxel; Vin/P, vinorelbine cisplatin; Cis, cisplatin.
[2]4-year survival statistics.

a. **Postoperative adjuvant therapy**—A progressive trend in lung cancer therapy has evolved in favor of far more widespread use of adjuvant chemotherapy. Three large multicenter randomized trials in Europe and North America have served as a basis for the increased application of postoperative platinum-based chemotherapy (Italian Stage IB, IALT, CALGB 9633, and NCIC BR10). The benefit of chemotherapy appears to vary based on patient selection but is estimated to be an increase of 5–15% survival measured at 5 years from diagnosis (Table 18–11).

2. Small cell lung cancer—Combination chemotherapy currently produces 85–95% and 75–85% response rates in limited-stage and extensive-stage disease, respectively. Furthermore, median survival is 12–16 months and 7–11 months in each group. Three or four drugs have been shown to be optimal. One of the most effective regimens combines cyclophosphamide, doxorubicin, and vincristine. In addition, a regimen of cisplatin and etoposide has been active in salvage. The optimal duration of therapy has not been defined, but the majority of the effect appears to occur within the first four cycles.

D. Immunotherapy

Immunotherapy using BCG, levamisole, interleukin-2, tumor necrosis factor-α, lymphokine-activated killer (LAK) cells, and tumor-infiltrating lymphocytes has not proved beneficial in any clinical studies to date.

E. Targeted Therapies

Molecular-based therapies targeting overexpressed growth receptors (*EGFR1,* HER2/*neu*) by monoclonal antibody or small molecules are beginning to show clinical effectiveness. Additional agents targeting signal transduction pathways (eg, farnesyl transferase inhibitors) for the *ras* pathway as well as antisense oligonucleotide and gene therapies are all in advanced clinical testing stages and in combination with standard cytotoxic chemotherapy appear to enhance response rates. A current prospective randomized trial from Canada (CAN-NCIC-BR19) is aimed at addressing the effectiveness of EGF inhibition in conjunction with platinum-based chemotherapeutics in the adjuvant setting.

Prognosis

A. Non-Small Cell Lung Cancer

The survival of patients with NSCLC is highly dependent on the pathologic stage. Overall, the 5-year survival of patients with stages I, II, IIIA, IIIB, and IV is 43–64%, 20–40%, 15–25%, 5–7%, and < 2%, respectively. A breakdown of survival by TNM classification is set forth in Table 18–12. Improved survival will likely depend on earlier diagnosis and further coordinated efforts among surgeons, medical oncologists, and radiation oncologists.

B. Small Cell Lung Cancer

Patients with limited-stage disease achieve a median survival of 12–16 months with 5–25% 2-year survival, while those with extensive-stage disease have a median

Table 18–12. Survival in non-small cell lung cancer.

Stage	TNM Description	Five-Year Survival
I		70–76%
a	T1, N0	80–83%
b	T2, N0	60–65%
II		30–40%
a	T1, N1	32–40%
b	T2, N1	28–35%
	T3, N0	
IIIA		10–30%
	T3, N1	30–45%
	T1–2, N2	7–30%
	T3, N2	0–5%
IIIB		<10%
	T4, any N	<10%
	Any T, N3	<10%
IV	M1	<5%
Overall		14.5%

survival of only 7–11 months, with only 1–3% surviving 2 years.

Albain KS et al: Long-term survival after concurrent cisplatin/etoposide (PE) plus chest radiotherapy (RT) followed by surgery in bulky stages IIIA N2 and IIIB non-small cell lung cancer (NSCLC): 6-year outcomes from Southwest Oncology Group study 8805. Proc Am Soc Clin Oncol 1999;18:467a (abst.)

Albain KS et al: Concurrent cisplatin/etoposide plus chest radiotherapy followed by surgery for stages IIIA N2 and IIIB non-small cell lung cancer: mature results of Southwest Oncology Group Phase II study 8805. J Clin Oncol 1995;13:1880.

Friedel G et al: Neoadjuvant chemoradiotherapy of stage III non-small cell lung cancer. Lung Cancer 2000;30:175.

Grunenwald DH et al: Benefit of surgery after chemoradiotherapy in stage IIIB (T4 and/or N3) non-small cell lung cancer. J Thorac Cardiovasc Surg 2001;122:796.

Le Chevalier et al: Should adjuvant chemotherapy become standard treatment in all patients with resected non-small-cell lung cancer? Lancet Oncol 2005;6:182.

Pisters KMW, Le Chevalier T: Adjuvant chemotherapy in completely resected non-small-cell lung cancer. J Clin Oncol 2005;23:3270.

Rosell R et al: A randomized trial comparing preoperative chemotherapy plus surgery with surgery alone in patients with non-small cell lung cancer. N Engl J Med 1994;330:153.

Roth JA et al: A randomized trial comparing perioperative chemotherapy and surgery with surgery alone in resectable stage IIIA non-small cell lung cancer. J Natl Cancer Inst 1994; 86:673.

Schiller JH et al: Comparison of four chemotherapy regimens for advanced non-small cell lung cancer. N Engl J Med 2002; 346:92.

Sugarbaker DJ et al: Results of Cancer and Leukemia Group B protocol 8935: a multiinstitutional phase II trimodality trial for IIIA N2 non-small cell lung cancer. J Thorac Cardiovasc Surg 1995;109:473.

Voltolini L et al: Results of induction chemotherapy followed by surgical resection in patients with stage IIIA (N2) non-small cell lung cancer: the importance of the nodal downstaging after chemotherapy. Eur J Cardiothorac Surg 2001;20:1106.

UNUSUAL PULMONARY NEOPLASMS

Malignant Neoplasms

Bronchial adenomas are a group of low-grade malignancies arising from the bronchial tree. Carcinoid tumors constitute 85–90% of these neoplasms, with adenoid cystic carcinoma (10%) and mucoepidermoid carcinoma (< 5%) accounting for most of the remainder. Carcinoid tumors are classified as either "typical" or "atypical," with markedly different histologic characteristics (Table 18–13). Adenoid cystic carcinomas occur in the lower trachea; infiltrate locally along submucosal and perineural tissue planes, often far beyond the boundaries of gross tumor; and metastasize late. Mucoepidermoid carcinomas resemble salivary tumors, with varying numbers of three distinct cell types: mucous, squamous, and intermediate. Patients with bronchial adenomas complain of cough, recurrent pulmonary infections, hemoptysis, pain, and wheezing. Only 15% of patients are completely asymptomatic. Carcinoid syndrome is rare with pulmonary carcinoid tumors. Most bronchial adenomas are diagnosed with a combination of plain chest radiography, computed tomography, and bronchoscopy. Biopsy at the time of bronchoscopy can be associated with significant bleeding, and measures to control this must be readily available.

Table 18–13. Characteristics of typical and atypical carcinoid tumors.

	Typical	Atypical
Incidence	90%	10%
Central location	80%	50%
Peripheral location	20%	50%
Metastases	10–15%	50–70%

Surgical resection is indicated for these tumors, with lobectomy being the most common procedure. "Sleeve" and bronchoplastic resections are particularly useful to preserve pulmonary function in these patients and make standard pneumonectomy rare. Removal of adenoid cystic carcinomas requires generous margins and frozen section examination of the margins at the time of surgery. Up to 8 cm of trachea can be removed with primary anastomosis. In addition, postoperative radiation may be indicated for close margins. With the possible exception of atypical carcinoid, chemotherapy is generally not indicated in the treatment of these neoplasms.

The long-term outlook is good for patients with metastatic disease. Even patients with adenoid cystic carcinoma and distant metastases may do well for extended periods due to the slow-growing nature of this malignancy; however, lymph node and distant metastases in patients with carcinoid tumors generally carry a poor prognosis.

Benign Neoplasms

Benign neoplasms of the lung are uncommon, accounting for < 1% of all pulmonary tumors. Most are hamartomas, but fibromas, leiomyomas, neurofibromas, myoblastomas, and benign metastasizing leiomyomas also occur. Most lesions are peripheral and asymptomatic; however, central lesions can produce symptoms of cough, wheezing, hemoptysis, and recurrent pneumonia. Typically, the lesions are discovered on routine chest radiographs and appear as a 1- to 2-cm well-circumscribed, bosselated lower lung nodule with calcifications in 10–30%. Central lesions may require bronchoscopy for diagnosis, but a pathologic diagnosis is most often obtained by fine-needle aspiration biopsy or surgery. Surgical resection should be conservative and limited to wedge excision unless the lesion occupies the proximal bronchial airway and is associated with recurrent distal infections or bronchiectasis. In such cases, lobectomy is indicated.

Following resection, the prognosis is excellent.

SPECIAL PROBLEM: THE SOLITARY PULMONARY NODULE

With the frequent use of chest radiography, solitary pulmonary nodules ("coin lesions") are frequently found in patients without pulmonary symptoms. These lesions pose a diagnostic problem for clinicians since they may represent something as benign as a nipple shadow or as malignant as lung cancer (Figure 18–21). The overall incidence of cancer in coin lesions is as low as 10%. Other diagnostic possibilities include (1) infections due to mycobacteria (tuberculosis), fungi (histoplasmosis, coccidioidomycosis), and helminths (echinococcosis); (2) inflammatory nodules from rheumatoid arthritis, focal pneumonitis, and Wegener's granulomatosis; (3) congenital anomalies, such as bronchogenic cysts and arteriovenous malformations; (4) benign neoplasms, eg, hamartomas, hemangiomas, papillary tumors, fibrous tumors of the pleura; (5) malignant neoplasms of the lung; and (6) miscellaneous processes, eg, hematomas, pulmonary infarcts, pleural plaques, loculated effusions, chest wall masses, and mucoid impaction. Although certain radiographic findings may suggest malignancy or benignity, solid pathologic proof that the nodule does not represent a malignancy rests with the clinician. In general, malignant neoplasms are larger and grow rapidly, appear spiculated, often with surface umbilication or notching and eccentric excavation. In addition, cancers often occur in smokers (or former smokers) over the age of 40 with negative skin tests for tuberculosis, histoplasmosis, or coccidioidomycosis (although positive tests do not exclude cancer), and in nodules that lack calcium (CT Hounsfield units < 175). In contrast, benign lesions are small (< 1 cm), stable (> 2 years), and calcified ("target" or "popcorn" distribution; CT Hounsfield units > 175) and are associated with positive skin tests in 70–90% of patients. Evaluation of these patients usually includes chest CT scan, but sputum cytology, cultures, bronchoscopy, and mediastinoscopy are sometimes helpful. FDG-PET scanning plays an important role in

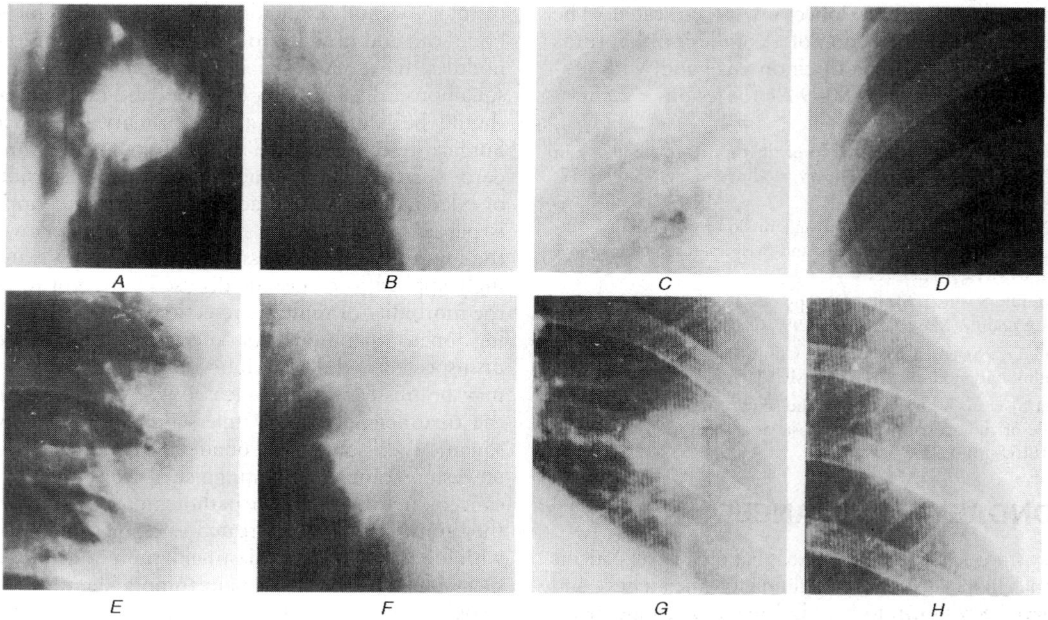

Figure 18–21. Coin lesions. ***A:*** Large-cell undifferentiated carcinoma in RUL (tomogram). ***B:*** Histoplasmosis (tomogram). ***C:*** Hamartoma. ***D:*** Solitary metastasis from epidermoid carcinoma of the cervix. ***E:*** Tuberculoma (tomogram). ***F:*** Foreign body granuloma in heroin addict (tomogram). ***G:*** Adenocarcinoma of LUL (present 6 years). ***H:*** Alveolar cell carcinoma of LUL (present 3 years). (RUL = right upper lobe; LUL = left upper lobe.)

the evaluation of tumors that are suspicious for malignancy. PET scan can often differentiate among lesions suspicious for malignancy.

With the advent of spiral CT scanning, the incidence of asymptomatic pulmonary nodules can vary from 25% to 70%. The vast majority of these lesions now identified are less than 1 cm and often as small as 2–3 mm. In one series, the incidence of lung cancer in the asymptomatic 10 pack-year smoking history population over the age of 50 years was 27% of all lesions identified, followed, and treated. Ongoing trials are assessing the efficacy and cost-effectiveness of CT screening for lung cancer. In the properly selected high-risk patient population (eg, over 60 years of age, moderate COPD, $FEV_1 < 70\%$), and an over 20 pack-year smoking history), spiral CT may prove to be cost-effective and will save lives.

Ultimately, a pathologic diagnosis must be made. In some instances, fine-needle aspiration cytology may be helpful, particularly if a tissue diagnosis of hamartoma can be made or id cultures demonstrating infectious organisms are obtained. The vast majority of solitary pulmonary nodules, however, require surgical excisional biopsy to exclude the possibility of malignancy. Currently, this is accomplished with video-assisted techniques in most patients, particularly if the lesion is in the periphery of the lung. If a benign lesion is encountered, nothing further is warranted; but if a lung cancer is diagnosed, immediate lobectomy is indicated. The prognosis following resection of a coin lesion that turns out to be a bronchogenic carcinoma is good, with a 5-year survival of as high as 80–90% for lesions < 1 cm.

Baaklini WA et al: Diagnostic yield of fiberoptic bronchoscopy in evaluating solitary pulmonary nodules. Chest 2000;117:1049.

Gould MK et al: Accuracy of positron emission tomography for diagnosis of pulmonary nodules and mass lesions: a meta-analysis. JAMA 2001;285:914.

Midthun DE, Swensen SJ, Jett JR: Approach to the solitary pulmonary nodule. Mayo Clin Proc 1993;68:378.

Midthun DE, Swensen SJ, Jett JR: Clinical strategies for solitary pulmonary nodule. Annu Rev Med 1992;43:195.

Swanson SJ et al: Management of the solitary pulmonary nodule: role of thoracoscopy in diagnosis and therapy. Chest 1999; 116(6 Suppl):523S.

SECONDARY LUNG CANCER

Autopsy studies have demonstrated that 30% of all patients with malignancies develop pulmonary metastases, and 12% have been shown to have isolated lung disease that is totally resectable. In addition, 10% of these latter patients (1.2% of all patients) have solitary lung metastases. Most pulmonary metastases occur through hematogenous spread from the primary site; lymphatic or transbronchial spread is extremely rare. Secondary metastatic spread to the pulmonary and mediastinal lymph nodes, however, can also occur. In patients with known extrathoracic primary cancers, multiple pulmonary lesions almost always represent metastatic disease. Solitary lesions, however, may be due to benign disease (18%) or new primary lung cancer (18%) as well as metastatic disease (64%). Most patients with pulmonary metastases are asymptomatic even with extensive disease. If symptoms do develop, cough, hemoptysis, fever, dyspnea, and pain are common. The diagnosis is generally initially suggested by routine chest radiography, and CT of the chest should always be ordered to assess the lungs for other nodules. Although CT scans are more sensitive, detecting nodules as small as 3 mm, they are also less specific (false-positive rate of 55%) than plain x-rays. Pathologic confirmation of the diagnosis is essential and usually is obtained at the time of resection. For patients who are not surgical candidates, fine-needle aspiration cytology is useful for peripheral lesions, while central lesions may require bronchoscopy for tissue diagnosis.

Medically fit patients with resectable disease are surgical candidates as long as the following criteria are fulfilled: (1) the primary tumor must be controlled or imminently controllable; (2) no other sites of disease may exist; (3) no other therapy can offer comparable results; and (4) the operative risk must be low. Since adenocarcinomas (especially breast cancer) commonly involve multiple organs, it is imperative that with this histology a full evaluation be performed, including bone scan and head CT or MRI. Solitary squamous cell nodules, however—even in the presence of a previous squamous cell carcinoma (eg, head and neck tumors)—should be addressed as a new primary (lung) cancer. Surgical resection can be accomplished through a standard posterolateral thoracotomy, median sternotomy, or bilateral anterior thoracotomies. The latter approach is particularly beneficial for bilateral disease involving the lower lobes. Video-assisted thoracoscopy is increasingly applied to metastatic disease in attempt to reduce the morbidity of multiple resections. On occasion, during open operations for metastatic disease, several unsuspected nodules are found by direct palpation that may be missed with thoracoscopy. Wedge resection is the treatment of choice unless the lesion is a solitary squamous cell carcinoma or adenocarcinoma. These latter lesions cannot be distinguished from primary lung cancer on frozen section pathologic examination, and they must therefore be treated as primary lung cancers with lobectomy and mediastinal lymph node dissection. Occasionally, other malignant tumors identified by histologic examination may require lobectomy or rarely even pneumonectomy because of involvement of the proximal pulmonary artery or bronchus.

The success rate with surgical removal of pulmonary metastases has been greatest with testicular (51% 5-year survival) and head-neck cancers (47% 5-year survival). Other types of tumors, such as osteogenic and soft tissue sarcomas, renal cell carcinoma, and colon carcinoma, are all associated with prolonged survival in 20–35% of patients. Results of resection for melanoma are less favorable (10–15% survival benefit). Isolated, resectable pulmonary metastases from rectal cancer can have as high as a 55% 5-year survival with metastasectomy alone.

Furthermore, multiple thoracotomies over periods in excess of 10 years are not unusual with the sarcomas. Numerous studies have been conducted in attempts to identify prognostic factors that could aid in the selection of patients for resection Adverse prognostic factors have included (1) multiple or bilateral lesions, (2) more than four lesions seen on CT scan, (3) tumor doubling time < 40 days, (4) a short disease-free interval, and (5) advanced age.

Although no consensus has developed regarding the selection of candidates for surgical exploration, it is generally agreed that no single criterion should be used to exclude patients from surgical resection. In all series, long-term benefit and survival hinges on complete resection. If complete resection is not deemed possible, resection should not be offered.

LaQuaglia MP: The surgical management of metastases in pediatric cancer. Semin Pediatr Surg 1993;2:75.

Pogrebniak HW, Pass HI: Initial and reoperative pulmonary metastasectomy: indications, technique, and results. Semin Surg Oncol 1993;9:142.

Todd TR: Pulmonary metastectomy: current indications for removing lung metastases. Chest 1993;103(4 Suppl):401S.

The Heart: I. Acquired Diseases 19

Scot H. Merrick, MD

The impact of acquired diseases of the cardiovascular system on the human population is enormous. In the United States alone, cardiovascular disease currently affects over 60 million people and accounts for over 40% of all deaths (Figure 19–1). A subset—coronary artery disease—affects over 12 million people and is responsible for one in every five deaths in the United States.

The spectrum of valvular heart disease is changing as the population ages, increasing the incidence of degenerative valvular disorders and decreasing the incidence of rheumatic valvular diseases. Atherosclerotic disease of the thoracic aorta, more commonly seen in the elderly, is becoming more prevalent as well.

Medical and surgical advances have resulted in a significant decrease in the death rates from cardiovascular diseases over the last decade. Notable exceptions are women and minorities. More importantly, the rate of population expansion is much greater than the development of new therapies, underscoring the need for expanded research in cardiovascular disease prevention.

ISCHEMIC HEART DISEASE

ANGINA PECTORIS

The right and left coronary arteries arise from the sinuses of Valsalva as the first branches of the aorta. The right coronary artery passes deep in the right atrioventricular groove (Figure 19–2) and usually terminates as the posterior descending coronary artery in the posterior interventricular groove. The right coronary artery supplies multiple right ventricular branches and the right marginal artery. In 90% of patients, the right coronary artery gives rise to the posterior descending artery (right coronary dominance) and branches into an atrioventricular nodal artery and several terminal posterolateral left ventricular branches.

The left main coronary artery is usually about 1 cm long and gives rise to the left anterior descending and left circumflex coronary arteries (Figure 19–2). The left anterior descending artery provides several diagonal branches to the anterior wall of the left ventricle and a number of perforating branches to the interventricular septum. In most patients, the left anterior descending artery wraps the apex of the heart, anastomosing with the posterior descending artery. The left anterior descending artery usually is the largest and most important of the coronary arteries. The circumflex coronary artery lies in the left atrioventricular groove (Figure 19–2) and proceeds laterally and posteriorly around the lateral aspect of the left ventricle, usually terminating in several circumflex marginal arteries. In 10% of patients, the circumflex coronary artery provides the posterior descending coronary artery (left coronary dominance).

Coronary blood flow delivers oxygen and metabolic substrates to the myocardium and simultaneously removes carbon dioxide and metabolic by-products via transcapillary exchange. Normal coronary blood flow approximates 1 mL per gram of myocardium per minute and delivers 0.1 mL of oxygen per gram per minute to the heart—a high rate of energy utilization compared with the rest of the body. The extraction of oxygen in the coronary bed averages 75% under normal conditions and increases to nearly 100% during stress. Coronary artery blood flow occurs primarily during diastole because systolic myocardial contraction increases intramyocardial vascular resistance. Normally, mean coronary resistance is three to six times the totally vasodilated value, implying an extreme vasodilator reserve. During stress, oxygen delivery increases as a result of vasodilation in response to the high baseline oxygen extraction. Assuming adequate perfusion pressure, total and regional myocardial blood flow under normal conditions is determined by autoregulation of regional arteriolar resistance modulated by local metabolic demand.

The metabolic activity of heart muscle converts the chemical energy from myocardial oxygen and substrate utilization into mechanical energy in the form of blood pressure and flow. With electrical depolarization of the myocardial cell membrane, chemomechanical alteration of the myosin cross-bridge produces sliding of myosin filaments relative to actin and shortening of the sarcomere. Over the physiologic range of sarcomere lengths (1.6–2 μm), the surface area of available cross-bridge interactions (and therefore the metabolic energy transferred into mechanical work during sarcomere contraction) is directly proportionate to end-diastolic sarco-

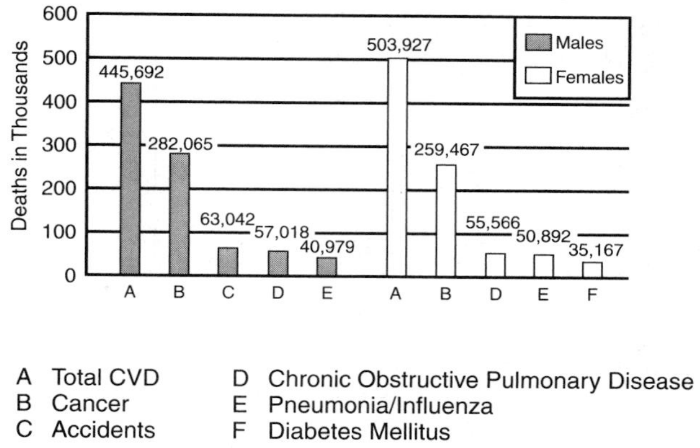

Figure 19–1. Leading causes of death for all males and females in the United States, 1998. (Reprinted with permission of the American Heart Association, 2001 Heart and Stroke Statistical Update. American Heart Association, 2000.)

mere length. The ventricles seem to function as an integrated sum of their component sarcomeres. Mechanical energy production, in the form of pressure and flow (stroke work), is a direct linear function of end-diastolic volume (Figure 19–3) and is not influenced significantly by physiologic changes in afterload. Therefore, short-term alterations in ventricular performance can be assessed by the slope of the stroke work and end-diastolic volume relationship. This basic **Frank-Starling property** of the heart is probably a direct reflection of sarcomere and myosin cross-bridge dynamics. The clinical analog of this principle allows cardiac function to be assessed as the product of cardiac output and mean arterial pressure (circulatory energy) at a given pulmonary capillary wedge pressure. For reference, the normal cardiac hemodynamic values in the adult are presented in Table 19–1.

Pathology

Coronary atherosclerosis is a progressive disease whose earliest microscopic changes have been described in the newborn infant, and advanced lesions are present in half the hearts examined at autopsy during the second decade of life. Early lesions are characterized by intimal incorporation of lipid material, progressing to an expanding plaque surrounded by fibrosis and calcification. In the final stages, rupture of the intimal plaque appears to be a dominant mechanism of worsening symptoms, with deposition of platelets and

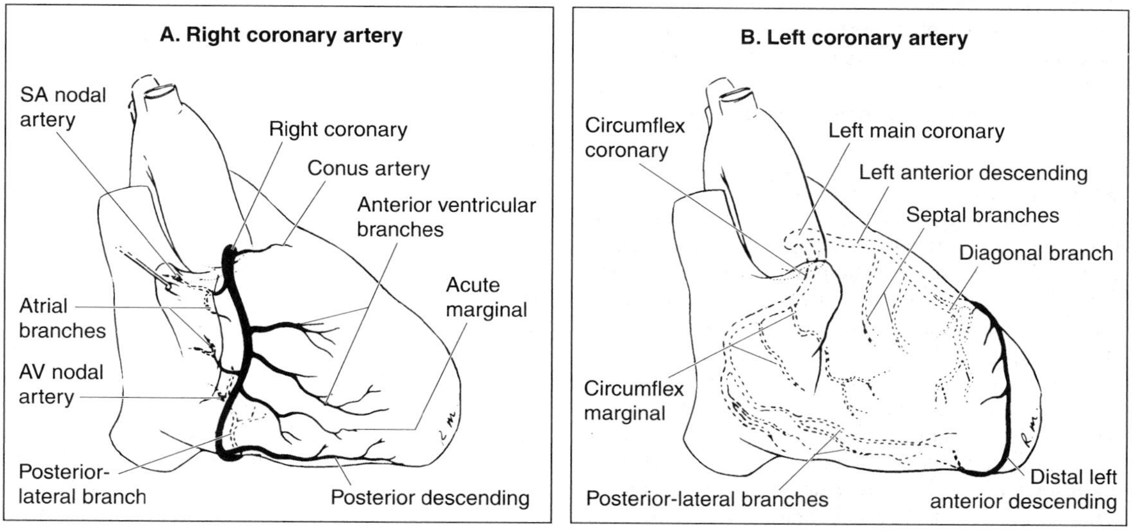

Figure 19–2. Anatomic representation of the right ***(A)*** and left ***(B)*** coronary arteries.

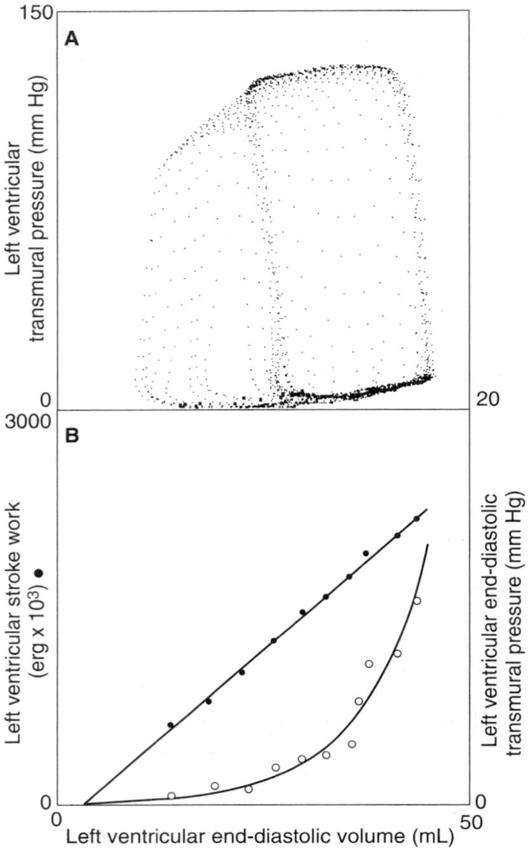

Figure 19–3. A: Left ventricular pressure-volume relationships in a normal conscious dog during a vena caval occlusion. The area of each pressure-volume loop is stroke work. ***B:*** Stroke work versus end-diastolic volume relationships for the pressure-volume loops shown above. The slope is a representation of the inotropic state.

thrombus progressing to thrombotic occlusion and acute myocardial infarction. Subtotal occlusions by "dynamic" thrombotic plaques appear to be of major importance in the pathogenesis of unstable angina. The usual pattern of coronary atherosclerosis is one of multifocal lesions, characteristically involving more than one major trunk in the same heart. The stenoses tend to be short, and lesions in the left anterior descending artery and circumflex system are usually proximal. In the right coronary artery, the disease is more diffuse and involves chiefly the proximal and middle portions of the artery; however, the posterior descending artery and distal branches usually are spared. Type 1 diabetic patients can be an exception, often having diffuse coronary involvement.

When an atherosclerotic plaque decreases the coronary cross-sectional area by 75% (50% reduction in diameter), the resistance to flow becomes significant. The dominant point of coronary vascular resistance becomes the stenosis that limits myocardial perfusion to a fixed value. While flow may be adequate at rest, exercise or other factors that increase myocardial oxygen demand can produce relative ischemia, a fall in coronary pressure distal to the stenosis, and redistribution of blood flow away from the subendocardium. This appears to be the mechanism of exercise-induced angina pectoris. Coronary vasospasm or unstable thrombotic plaques can compound the obstructive physiology. Because of high metabolic demand and tight coupling between energy utilization and expenditure, acute coronary insufficiency—such as occurs with angina pectoris—produces an almost immediate decrement in myocardial segment shortening and work. Even when full reperfusion is accomplished after a 15-minute period of reversible ischemia, dysfunction can be prolonged, requiring 24–48 hours for complete recovery.

Risk Factors

Significant progress has been made in identifying risk factors associated with the development of coronary heart disease (see Table 19–2). Of these, cigarette smoking is the most important. In addition to the adverse effects of carbon monoxide and nicotine on the endothelial cell, cigarette smoke can increase LDL levels, reduce HDL levels, increase fibrinogen levels, and increase platelet aggregation. Exposure to secondhand smoke may increase the death rate from coronary heart disease by 30%. The risk of developing coronary heart disease is reduced 50% after 1 year of smoking abstinence; at 15 years, the risk is no different from that of never-smokers. Niacin, statins, and resins can now modify cholesterol levels effectively.

Clinical Findings

A. Symptoms and Signs

The most common symptom of myocardial ischemia is retrosternal chest pain, or angina pectoris, produced by a reduction in coronary blood flow. The discomfort is often described by the patient as pressure, a choking sensation, or a feeling of tightness. Early in the symptomatic course, a variety of factors such as exercise, cold exposure, eating, and emotional distress can initiate the symptoms. The pain frequently radiates down the left arm and into the left neck and occasionally to the right arm, mandible, or ear. The severity of chest pain can be graded by the New York Heart Association (NYHA) classification, with class I indicating no symptoms; class II, symptoms with severe exertion; class III, chest pain

Table 19–1. Normal cardiac hemodynamic values.

Site	Phasic	Mean	Oxygen Content (vol%)	Oxygen Saturation (%)
Right atrium	7/2	4	16	75
Right ventricle	20/0	5	16	75
Pulmonary artery	20/10	13	16	75
Left atrium	13/3	5–12	20	97
Left ventricle	120/5	12	20	97
Aorta	120/70	85	20	97
Heart rate (HR)		60–90 beats/min		
Forward stroke volume (SV)		73 ± 22 mL/beat		
Cardiac output (CO; HR × SV)		6 L/min		
Cardiac index (CI)		3.5 ± 1.0 L/min/m^2		
End-diastolic volume (EDV)		70 ± 30 mL/m^2		
End systolic volume (ESV)		25 ± 13 mL/m^2		
Ejection fraction (EF)		67 ± 8% (EDV – ESV/EDV)		
Systemic resistance (SVR)		900–1400 dynes•sec•cm^{-2}[(MAP – CVP)/CI)] × 80		
Pulmonary resistance (PVR)		150–250 dynes•sec•cm^{-2}[(PA – CVP)/CI)] × 80		

m^2 = square meter of body surface area
CVP = central venous pressure
MAP = mean arterial pressure
PA = mean pulmonary artery pressure

with mild exertion; and class IV, pain at rest. While minimal anginal symptoms often are easily tolerated and compatible with a normal lifestyle (stable angina), an increasing NYHA class over a short period of time (progressive angina) worsens the prognosis. In the late stages, ischemia occurs at rest and is refractory to medical therapy (unstable angina). Unstable pain patterns imply a very poor outlook, with a high incidence of early infarction and death. Patients who develop pulmonary edema from severe ischemia and those who have angina following a myocardial infarction have a poor prognosis.

A large proportion of patients does not pursue the classic symptomatic progression and present initially with acute myocardial infarction or sudden death. Still others experience *no symptoms at all* during ischemia (silent myocardial ischemia), and coronary artery disease is only discovered in the late stage of congestive heart failure after severe ventricular damage has occurred. The physical examination is frequently unremarkable. Cardiac enlargement may be evident in patients with advanced disease, but the chest radiograph is normal in the majority. While the ECG is normal in at least half of patients, abnormal findings consist of inverted T waves, ST segment abnormalities, or Q waves on the resting ECG. Transient ST segment and T wave changes may occur during an anginal episode or exercise stress test.

B. Imaging Studies

Cardiac catheterization and coronary arteriography are essential for determining the presence and extent of coronary atherosclerosis. In recent years, a trend has favored early angiography in most patients with suspected coronary disease in order to identify individual prognostic characteristics as precisely as possible. This approach has allowed a more objective application of medical therapy to low-risk subsets and selection of patients at high medical risk for elective coronary revascularization. The development of low-cost outpatient catheterization has facilitated this trend. At angiography, the major anatomic predictors of coronary death—such as the number of coronary vessels diseased and the resting left ventricular ejection fraction—are documented. While the extent of obstructive disease can be underestimated in up to 10% of patients, coronary arteriography has the highest sensitivity and specificity of any test available.

Table 19–2. Major risk factors for coronary heart disease.

Cigarette smoking
Serum cholesterol
Total > 240 mg/dL
LDL > 130 mg/dL
HDL < 35 mg/dL
Triglycerides > 200 mg/dL
Male gender
Diabetes mellitus
Hypertension
Family history of early heart disease
Obesity
Inactivity

LDL = low-density lipoprotein
HDL = high-density lipoprotein

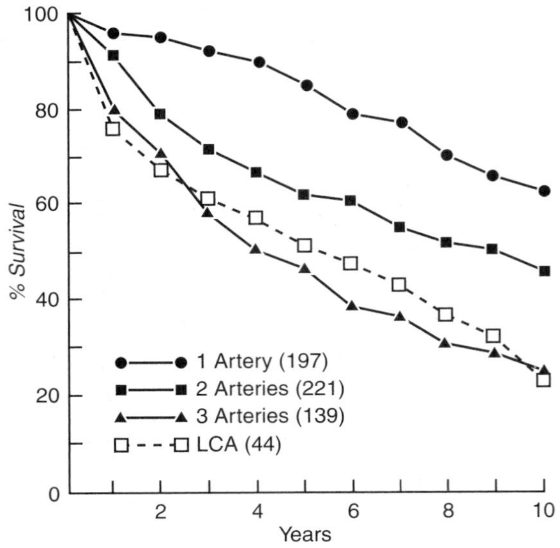

Figure 19–4. Survival in patients with significant lesions of one, two, and three coronary arteries and the left main coronary artery (LCA).

Recently, electron-beam computed tomography has been used to detect and quantify the degree of coronary artery calcification. A coronary calcification scoring system can be correlated with the presence of hemodynamically significant coronary lesions. However, the expense of this study precludes its use as a primary screening tool. In patients with borderline anatomic indications for coronary revascularization, physiologic assessment with radionuclide exercise ventriculography, stress thallium scanning, or exercise echocardiography can be useful in making decisions about operative treatment. In particular, thallium scintigraphy may provide critical information about myocardial viability in patients with poor ventricular function.

Treatment

A. Medical Treatment

Hypertension should be controlled and smoking avoided. Lipid abnormalities should be treated with drugs or diet. After bypass grafting, risk factor modification and continued medical therapy are especially important, since atherosclerotic involvement of saphenous vein grafts is a major long-term risk. When making a choice between medical and surgical therapy, the natural history of angina pectoris should be reviewed. The annual coronary disease mortality rate is directly related to the number of vessels affected and the degree of impairment of left ventricular function (Figures 19–4 and 19–5). In current practice, adverse prognostic factors that might suggest referral for coronary revascularization include severe or progressive angina on medical therapy; refractory unstable angina; significant left main coronary disease; multivessel coronary obstruction (especially with proximal left anterior descending artery involvement); ventricular impairment with a reduced ejection fraction; multivessel coronary disease in diabetics; and ischemic cardiomyopathy. Each of these factors, individually or in combination, significantly reduces survival with medical therapy and predicts an improved longevity after coronary bypass grafting.

In patients with low-risk clinical profiles, medical management is recommended if anginal symptoms and exercise capacity can be maintained satisfactorily. Sublingual nitroglycerin, long-acting nitrate preparations, and nitroglycerin ointment can be useful. Beta-adrenergic blocking agents such as propranolol, atenolol, and timolol are effective and safe. Calcium-channel blocking agents such as nifedipine, diltiazem, and verapamil are also effective. Antiplatelet agents such as aspirin have a definite therapeutic role, and short-term heparinization has been effective in preventing coronary thrombosis and infarction in patients with unstable angina. Patients with unstable syndromes may benefit from glycoprotein IIB/IIIA inhibitors (abciximab, tirofiban), and postinfarction patients are usually prescribed ACE-inhibitors for ventricular remodeling.

B. Surgical Treatment

It is essential that the goals and anticipated results of coronary bypass be explained objectively and in detail to patient and family. Risks and possible complications should be discussed, and all aspects of the history, physical examination, and results of cardiac catheterization should be reviewed, with emphasis on imparting knowl-

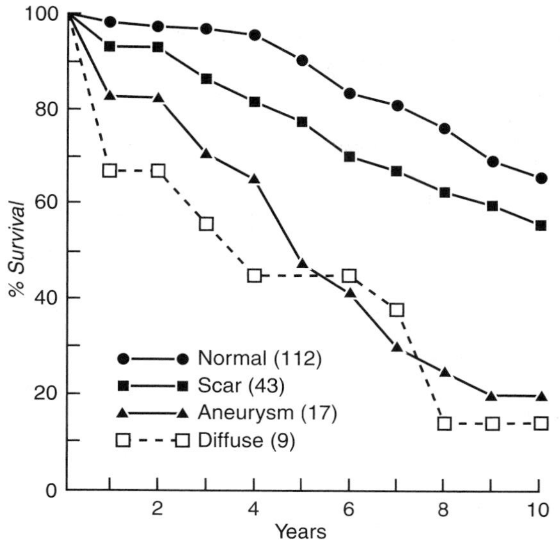

Figure 19–5. Survival according to ventriculographic estimates of resting left ventricular function in patients with ischemic heart disease.

edge about cardiac anatomy and dynamics. Complete revascularization is an important objective and is associated with a better long-term outcome. The presence of carotid bruits should be evaluated, and respiratory status, renal function, and blood coagulation should be assessed. Aspirin should be discontinued, if possible, for 1–2 weeks prior to operation because of an increased risk of postoperative bleeding. Antianginal agents should be continued until the day of operation. If further pharmacologic therapy is required for recurring angina, an intravenous nitroglycerin infusion can be employed. Intra-aortic balloon pumping is also effective for preoperative stabilization of unstable patients in the coronary care unit. Prophylactic broad-spectrum antibiotics are administered intravenously before anesthetic induction and for 24–48 hours postoperatively. Finally, safe and effective cardiac anesthesia is essential for obtaining optimal surgical results.

1. Conventional approach—The vast majority of procedures consist of simple bypass of the obstructed coronary vessels, using either the internal mammary artery or reversed segments of saphenous vein. In most cases, after a median sternotomy incision is made, the left internal mammary artery is dissected from the chest wall. Cardiopulmonary bypass is instituted with or without mild systemic hypothermia, using aortic cannulation for arterial inflow and a single right atrial cannula for venous return to the pump. After clamping of the ascending aorta, cold potassium cardioplegia solution is infused into the aortic root to arrest and protect the heart, reducing myocardial oxygen consumption to minimal levels. The saphenous vein grafts or internal mammary arteries are then sutured to the coronary arteries beyond the stenoses (Figure 19–6), and additional volumes of cardioplegia solution are infused every 20–30 minutes to maintain myocardial temperature below 15 °C. After completion of the distal coronary anastomoses, the aorta is unclamped, proximal aorta–vein graft anastomoses are completed, and cardiopulmonary bypass is discontinued after adequate rewarming.

An average of three or four grafts is inserted. In general, the internal mammary artery is the graft of choice owing to its superior long-term patency. This is in part due to the preservation of a functional endothelium in this graft. At least one internal mammary artery graft is utilized in 95% of procedures, usually to the left anterior descending coronary artery, and adjunctive saphenous vein grafts are used for additional vessels. Multiple internal mammary artery procedures can be performed, using a combination of bilateral mammary artery pedicles, sequential mammary artery anastomoses, and free mammary artery grafts. At present, however, complex internal mammary artery grafting is reserved for patients

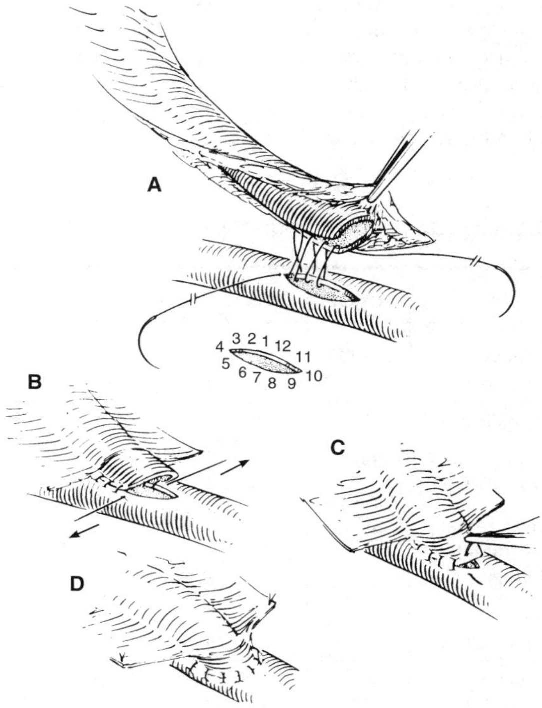

Figure 19–6. Technique of end-to-side internal mammary artery–coronary anastomosis.

with limited saphenous veins, younger patients with longer life expectancies, reoperative cases with previous vein graft failure, and patients with atherosclerotic calcification of the ascending aorta. Other arterial conduits such as the inferior epigastric artery, the gastroepiploic artery, and the radial artery are being used with increasing frequency to improve long-term patency rates. Representative patency rates for these bypass conduits are presented in Table 19–3. Graft closure within the first 30 days after surgery is usually due to technical errors, poor graft quality, or poor target vessel runoff. From 1 month to 3 years, grafts usually occlude from intimal hyperplasia. After 3 years, graft atherosclerosis is the most common reason for closure. Graft patency is adversely affected by persistent cigarette smoking and elevated LDL cholesterol.

2. Minimally invasive approach—Over the past 5 years, a number of alternative surgical methods (minimally invasive direct coronary artery bypass, MIDCAB; off-pump coronary artery bypass, OPCAB; port access) have evolved with the aim of reducing surgical morbidity, mortality, and cost. Of these, the OPCAB approach is the most widely used (approximately 15% of all coronary revascularization procedures) and holds the most promise. With this approach, patients undergo standard median sternotomy and graft harvesting. Cardiopulmonary bypass is eliminated, and grafts are anastomosed to target vessels on the beating heart with the assistance of a stabilizer device designed to keep the target vessel motionless. Although multivessel bypass can be achieved, lesions isolated to the left anterior descending, diagonal, and proximal right coronaries are the most appropriate.

Table 19–3. Long-term graft patency.

Conduit	1 Year	2 Years	5 Years	10 Years
Great saphenous vein	80–90%			50%
Cephalic vein	85%	66%		
Internal mammary artery	98%			90%
Free internal mammary artery	95%		92%	
Gastroepiploic artery	95%		95%	
Radial	94%		83%	
Cryovein[1]		50%		

[1]Cryopreserved cadaver vein.

The primary advantage of the OPCAB approach is elimination of the systemic effects of cardiopulmonary bypass (hypothermia, inflammatory response, micro-emboli, etc). Incomplete revascularization and reduced early graft patency are potential problems. True reductions in morbidity, mortality, and cost await the results of randomized trials.

Transmyocardial laser revascularization has been used in patients with inoperable coronary disease. With this procedure, multiple 1 mm channels are created transmurally to provide access of left ventricular blood into ischemic myocardium. Most channels thrombose quickly; nevertheless, 70% of patients will have symptomatic improvement and better quality of life. Overall survival remains unchanged, and the exact mechanism of improvement from transmyocardial laser revascularization remains unclear.

Prognosis

As a group, patients who are treated by coronary bypass surgery have 5- and 10-year survivals of 92% and 81%, respectively. For the same intervals, freedom from recurrence of angina is 83% and 63%, respectively. The most important predictors of late cardiac mortality after surgery are diabetes, advanced age, reduced ejection fraction, and nonuse of the internal mammary graft. Successful revascularization improves resting left ventricular wall motion in a significant proportion of patients and enhances exercise ventricular performance. Fewer than 1% of patients require repeat revascularization within 4 years of follow-up. Comprehensive morbidity and mortality data are available from the Society of Thoracic Surgeons National Cardiac Surgery Database. For isolated coronary bypass procedures, operative mortality is approximately 2.8%. Univariate predictors of adverse outcome are presented in Table 19–4. In a meta-analysis of the prospective, randomized studies comparing medical to surgical therapy, it is evident that surgery imparts a 39% and 17% reduction in cumulative mortality at 5 and 10 years, respectively (Figure 19–7). This advantage is most evident in patients with multivessel disease, reduced ventricular function, left main coronary involvement, and NYHA class IV symptoms.

THE RELATIVE ROLES OF PTCA, CORONARY STENTS, & CORONARY BYPASS

In 1977, Gruntzig introduced percutaneous transluminal coronary angioplasty (PTCA) for dilating stenotic coronary arterial lesions. Successful dilation rates per stenosis currently exceed 90%; complication rates have fallen below 2%; and procedure-related myocar-

Table 19–4. Preoperative univariate predictors of mortality for coronary bypass procedures.[1]

Variable	Relative Risk
Left main disease	1.58
Female gender	1.69
NYHA class IV	1.74
Previous stroke	1.93
Peripheral vascular disease	2.22
Pulmonary hypertension	2.39
Ejection fraction 25–35%	2.92
Congestive heart failure	2.87
Age > 70	3.13
Prior CABG	3.32
Preop balloon pump	3.43
Renal failure	3.45
Acute myocardial infarction	6.12
Cardiogenic shock	7.89
Emergent operation	12.39

[1]Society of Thoracic Surgeons National Database, 1999.

dial infarction and death remain uncommon. Recent enthusiasm for balloon dilation has been accompanied by its increasing application to more complex forms of coronary disease and a marked increase in the number of procedures performed annually. In many centers, PTCA is now the most commonly used invasive therapy for coronary disease. Comparisons between PTCA and surgery remain controversial. The results of six prospective, randomized studies comparing PTCA and surgery for multi-vessel coronary disease have shown no difference in the overall 5-year survival or nonfatal myocardial infarction rate. However, the risk of repeat revascularization is significantly higher in the PTCA patients. This is particularly evident in patients with diabetes. At 5 years, the cumulative costs for both procedures are similar. Risk-adjusted data from the New York State CABG and PTCA registries show a significant survival advantage for CABG in patients who have single-vessel or double-vessel disease with a proximal ≥ 70% stenosis of the left anterior descending coronary and in any patient with triple-vessel disease. While the addition of coronary stenting to PTCA has reduced the restenosis rate, repeat interventions are still more common when compared with surgical revascularization.

REOPERATION FOR CORONARY ARTERY DISEASE

Since the advent of coronary artery bypass, an increasing number of patients have presented for reoperation. Common reasons for reoperation include progression of atherosclerotic lesions in the native coronary arteries and atherosclerotic involvement of vein bypass grafts. Performing an internal mammary artery graft at the initial operation significantly reduces the need for reoperation. Control of postoperative hyperlipidemia should also reduce the incidence of reoperation.

The technical aspects of the second procedure are more difficult, but the operative mortality rate should be only slightly higher—generally in the range of 3%. Nevertheless, when appropriate clinical indications are present, reoperation should be undertaken with anticipation of excellent long-term results. In patients requiring reoperation for vein graft atherosclerosis and occlusion, arterial grafts offer the potential for a better long-term outcome.

POSTINFARCTION VENTRICULAR SEPTAL DEFECT

Infarction of the interventricular septum with subsequent formation of a ventricular septal defect occurs in less than 1% of patients with acute myocardial infarction. The interval between the acute infarct and septal rupture varies between 1 and 12 days and can be correlated with histologic findings of maximal cardiac mus-

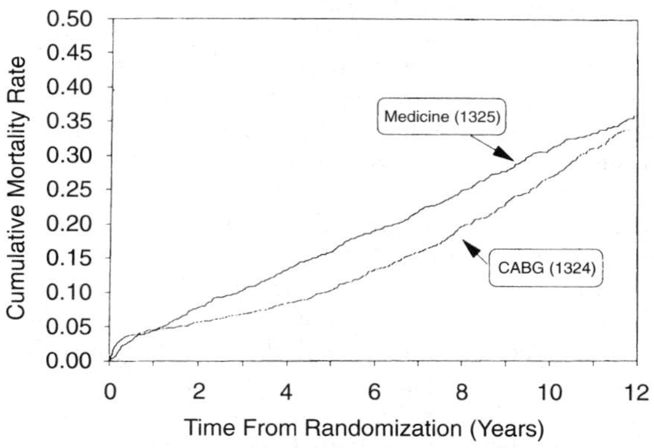

Figure 19–7. Meta-analysis of CABG versus medical survival from 7, prospective, randomized studies. (Reproduced, with permission, from Yusuf S et al: Effect of coronary artery bypass surgery on survival: overview of 10-year results from randomised trials by the Coronary Artery Graft Surgery Trialists. Lancet 1994;344:566. Copyright © 1994. Reprinted with permission from Elsevier.)

cle degeneration and weakening. Once rupture occurs, the prognosis is poor, with 24% of patients dying on the first day after rupture, 65% by the end of 2 weeks, and 81% by 2 months. The syndrome develops classically in a patient with myocardial infarction in whom shock or congestive heart failure suddenly appears.

Clinical Findings

A. Symptoms and Signs

A harsh holosystolic murmur is usually heard along the left sternal border, and two-thirds of patients demonstrate a palpable thrill.

B. Imaging Studies

Although clinical findings may be highly suggestive, the definitive diagnosis is made by Doppler echocardiography and cardiac catheterization. The defects are often irregular, ragged tracts through the anterior apical septum with occlusion of the left anterior descending artery or through the posterior basilar septum in cases of right coronary artery occlusion. In the latter, right ventricular infarction may compound the problem.

Differential Diagnosis

The differential diagnosis includes papillary muscle dysfunction, rupture of a papillary muscle with acute mitral insufficiency, and pericardial friction rub secondary to myocardial infarction.

Treatment

Surgical correction is indicated in nearly all cases, with the possible exception of elderly patients with advanced multiorgan failure. Intervention should not be delayed, and early or even emergency operation should be the rule. A preoperative intra-aortic balloon pump is placed in most patients, and patch closure of the septal defect along with coronary bypass should be performed early to prevent the consequences of acute right ventricular overload or multiorgan failure.

After institution of cardiopulmonary bypass and cardioplegic arrest, an incision is made in the area of infarction, and good exposure of both the left and right ventricles is obtained (Figure 19–8). A portion of the necrotic edge of the defect is resected, and a double patch technique is used for repair (Figure 19–9). Coronary bypass grafts are constructed to all diseased vessels, including the right coronary artery in cases of right ventricular infarction.

Prognosis

Fifty to 80 percent of patients should survive the operative procedure depending on the severity of preoperative shock and multiorgan failure.

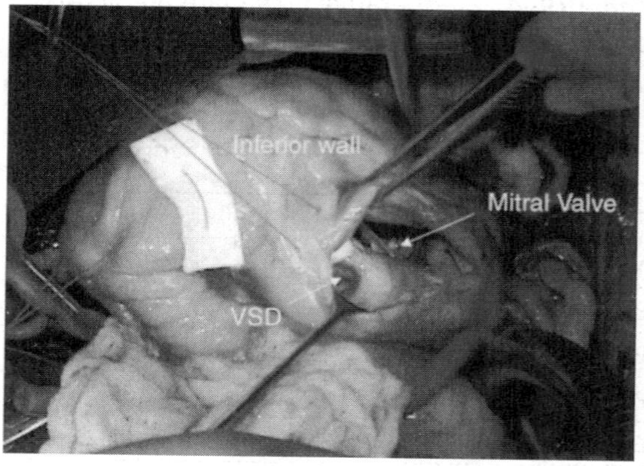

Figure 19–8. Operative photograph of inferior postinfarction ventricular septal defect (VSD). Infarct has been opened to expose fistula into the right ventricle.

LEFT VENTRICULAR ANEURYSM

Left ventricular aneurysm occurs when a large myocardial infarction progresses to a thinned-out transmural scar that bulges paradoxically beyond the normal cavitary contours during systole. While aneurysms have occurred in 2–4% of myocardial infarctions, the incidence is probably decreasing with more aggressive infarct management. Ninety percent of aneurysms involve the anteroseptal left ventricle, and 10% are posterior. Over 50% contain mural thrombus.

Clinical Findings

Patients show signs and symptoms of congestive heart failure, angina, embolization, and ventricular dysrhythmias. Clinical manifestations include a prominent apical impulse, electrocardiographic evidence of an old Q wave myocardial infarction with persistent ST segment elevation, and a localized left ventricular bulge on chest x-ray.

Treatment

Surgical therapy should be considered in most cases, since the prognosis with medical management is poor. Treatment consists of aneurysm resection combined with complete coronary revascularization (Figure 19–10).

Prognosis

The prognosis without surgery is related to the acuity of symptoms, the degree of left ventricular dysfunction, and the extent of associated coronary artery disease.

Significant improvements in symptoms of congestive heart failure and angina are observed in 70–85% of patients surviving after operation, and left ventricular

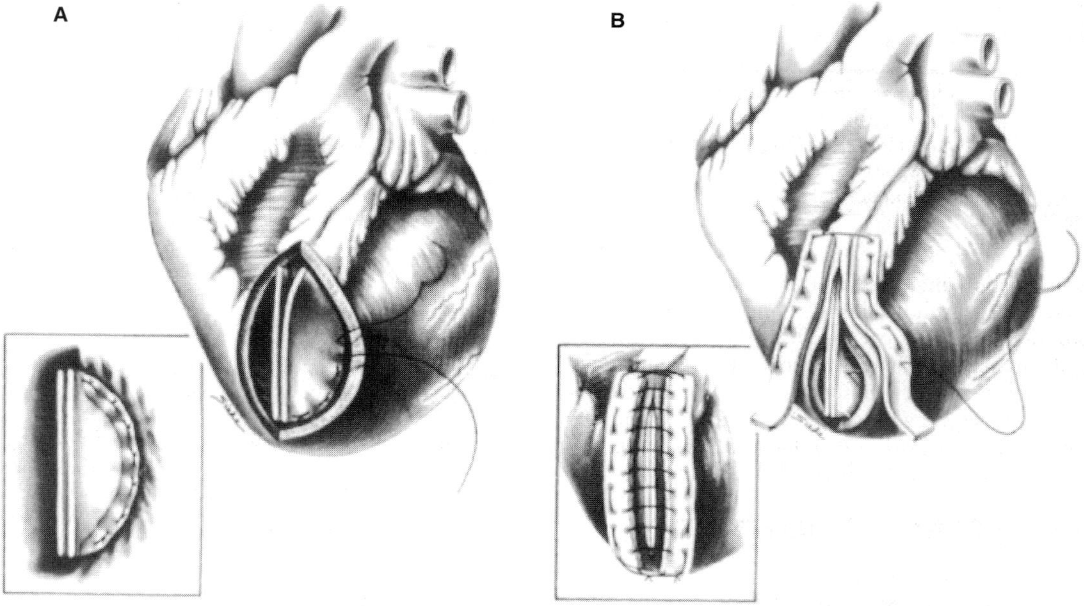

Figure 19–9. Double patch repair technique for anterior postinfarction ventricular septal defect. The ventricular septum is reconstructed by placing sheets of Teflon felt on each side of the septum ***(A)*** and then closing the ventricular walls to the septal patch ***(B)***.

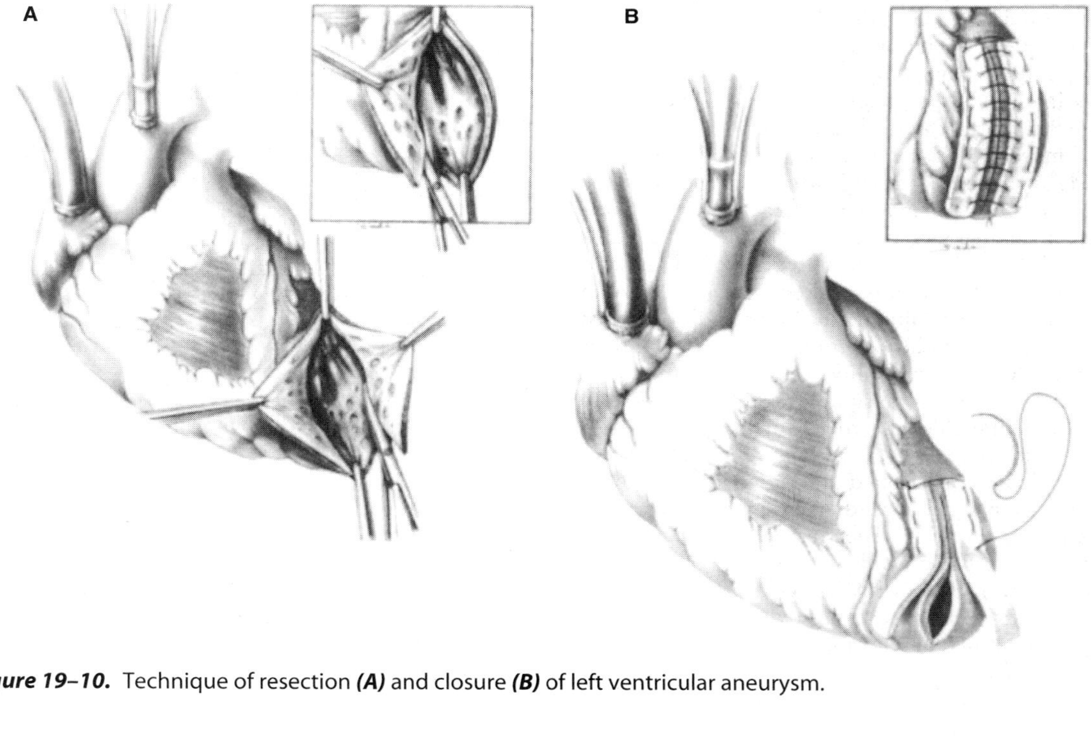

Figure 19–10. Technique of resection ***(A)*** and closure ***(B)*** of left ventricular aneurysm.

Table 19–5. Operations for idiopathic, dilated cardiomyopathy.

Orthotopic heart transplantation
Mitral valve repair
Ventricular reduction surgery
Cardiomyoplasty
Biventricular pacemaker insertion

ejection fraction increases in the majority because of reduced end-diastolic volume. Long-term survival is improved significantly over medical therapy, with 70–80% of patients alive 5 years postoperatively. The operative mortality rate for elective cases is 5% and increases to 20% for emergency procedures. The hospital mortality rate associated with subendocardial resection for ventricular tachycardia has been 11%.

SURGERY FOR CARDIOMYOPATHY

Medical therapy for advanced heart failure carries a dismal prognosis. Approximately 60% of patients with NYHA class IV symptoms will die within 1 year. A small number of these patients may benefit from operative treatment, and the objective is to reduce ventricular chamber size, improve the shape (decrease sphericity), lower filling pressures, and eliminate mitral insufficiency. In so doing, ventricular wall stress and myocardial oxygen demand are reduced.

The type of operation depends on the underlying cause of cardiomyopathy. The two most frequent causes in the United States are ischemic and dilated (idiopathic) cardiomyopathy. The former is not actually a muscle disease but rather severe dysfunction caused by diffuse coronary artery disease. Patients with this condition may be candidates for coronary bypass if suitable target vessels are present and viable myocardium can be demonstrated by thallium scintigraphy or positron emission tomography. Many of these patients have "hibernating" myocardium, which can regain contractile function if blood supply is restored. Operative mortality is acceptable (3–10%), and published 5-year survivals range from 30% to 50%. Idiopathic dilated cardiomyopathy been treated with a number of surgical procedures (Table 19–5). Orthotopic heart transplantation offers the best long-term results in suitable candidates. Mitral valve annuloplasty can be very effective in restoring valve competence in patients with annular stretching from ventricular enlargement. Ventricular reduction surgery (Batista procedure) and dynamic cardiomyoplasty have limited application because of high operative mortality and limited survival. Biventricular pacing is a relatively simple procedure designed to restore the normal depolarization sequence in the ventricular muscle, resulting in significant increases in the ejection fraction.

American Heart Association. 2001 Heart and Stroke Statistical Update.

Bielak LF et al: Probabilistic model for prediction of angiographically defined obstructive coronary artery disease using electron beam computed tomography calcium score strata. Circulation 2000;102:380.

Bishay ES et al: Mitral valve surgery in patients with severe left ventricular dysfunction. Eur J Cardiothorac Surg 2000;17:213.

Braile DM et al: Dynamic cardiomyoplasty: long-term clinical results in patients with dilated cardiomyopathy. Ann Thorac Surg 2000;69:1445.

Chaux AC et al: Postinfarction ventricular septal defect. Semin Thorac Cardiovasc Surg 1998;10:93.

Eagle KA et al: ACC/AHA Guidelines for Coronary Artery Bypass Graft Surgery: a Report of the American College of Cardiology/American Heart Association Task Force on Practice Guidelines (Committee to Revise the 1991 Guidelines for Coronary Artery Bypass Graft Surgery). American College of Cardiology/American Heart Association. J Am Coll Cardiol 1999;34:1262.

Favaloro RG: Landmarks in the development of coronary artery bypass surgery. Circulation 1998;98:466.

Faxon DP: Myocardial revascularization in 1997: angioplasty versus bypass surgery. Am Fam Physician 1997;56:1409.

Frazier OH et al: Transmyocardial revascularization with a carbon dioxide laser in patients with end-stage coronary artery disease. N Engl J Med 1999;341:1021.

Frazier OH et al: Transmyocardial laser revascularization. Does it have a role in the treatment of ischemic heart disease? Tex Heart Inst J 1998;25:24.

Hannan EL et al: A comparison of three-year survival after coronary artery bypass graft surgery and percutaneous transluminal coronary angioplasty. J Am Coll Cardiol 1999;33:63.

He GW: Arterial grafts for coronary artery bypass grafting: biological characteristics, functional classification, and clinical choice. Ann Thorac Surg 1999;67:277.

Kerwin WF et al: Ventricular contraction abnormalities in dilated cardiomyopathy: effect of biventricular pacing to correct interventricular dyssynchrony. J Am Coll Cardiol 2000;35:1221.

Mack MJ: Coronary surgery: off-pump and port access. Surg Clin North Am 2000;80:1575.

Mickleborough LL et al: Results of revascularization in patients with severe left ventricular dysfunction. J Thorac Cardiovasc Surg 2000;119:550.

Motwani JG, Topol EJ: Aortocoronary saphenous vein graft disease: pathogenesis, predisposition, and prevention. Circulation 1998;97:916.

Myers WO et al: CASS Registry long term surgical survival. Coronary Artery Surgery Study. J Am Coll Cardiol 1999;33:488.

Schulze C et al: Reduced expression of systemic proinflammatory cytokines after off-pump versus conventional coronary artery bypass grafting. Thorac Cardiovasc Surg 2000;48:364.

Starling RC, McCarthy PM: Partial left ventriculectomy: sunrise or sunset? Eur J Heart Fail 1999;1:313.

Svennevig JL: Off-pump vs on-pump surgery. A review. Scand Cardiovasc J 2000;34:7.

VALVULAR HEART DISEASE

Developmentally, the fibrous skeleton of the heart, to which the cardiac valves attach, is derived from the endocardial cushions. The fibrous annulus of the mitral valve is a thin, incomplete ring of fibrous tissue, which is most apparent at two points: the right and left fibrous trigones (Figure 19–11). The left fibrous trigone is situated at the left anterior aspect of the mitral ring and consists of fibrous tissue joining the mitral ring to the base of the aorta. The right fibrous trigone, or central fibrous body, lies in the midline of the heart and represents the confluence of fibrous tissue from the mitral valve, the tricuspid valve, the membranous septum, and the posterior aspect of the base of the aorta.

In most patients, two mitral leaflets are evident: the anterior leaflet and the posterior leaflet (Figure 19–11). Both leaflets are approximately the shape of a trapezoid, each attaching by thin fibrous chordae tendineae to both the anterior and the posterior papillary muscles. Stated differently, the chordae from each papillary muscle fan out and attach to nearly half of both cusp margins. The edges of the leaflets have a slightly serrated appearance owing to the insertion of chordae tendineae on the ventricular surface; these serrations mark the line of closure of the normal valve.

The anatomy of the tricuspid valve apparatus is similar, except that three valve leaflets usually are evident: anterior, posterior, and septal (Figure 19–11). The anterior leaflet commonly is the largest of the three and the posterior leaflet the smallest, though many variations occur. The papillary muscles tend to be multiple but can be grouped into three components: anterior (arising from the right ventricular free wall), inferior (arising from the inferior septum), and septal (arising from the high septum in the area of the septal band). As in the mitral valve, papillary muscle groups tend to contribute chordae to multiple leaflets.

The function of the atrioventricular valves is to permit uninhibited flow of blood from the atria to the ventricles during ventricular diastole and to prevent reflux of blood into the atria during ventricular systole. The valves achieve this objective by a coordinated contraction of ventricular myocardium and the papillary muscles during the cardiac cycle. During systole, the valve is closed, and the left atrium serves as a reservoir for blood returning from the lungs. With isovolumic relaxation, left ventricular pressure falls, and when ventricular pressure becomes lower than that of the full atrium, the valve opens and initiates rapid filling of the ventricle.

The aortic valve, located between the outflow tract of the left ventricle and the ascending aorta, is usually tricuspid and is composed of a fibrous skeleton, three cusps, and the sinuses of Valsalva. The fibrous skeleton consists of three U-shaped structures that adjoin one another at the valve commissures as at the points of a crown. Beneath each commissure is the pars membranacea. The skeleton is in fibrous continuity with the anterior leaflet of the mitral valve posterolaterally and with the membranous septum anteriorly. The cusps are delicate fibrous leaflets that insert into the outline of the valve skeleton. The free edge of each cusp is concave, is thicker than the rest of the leaflet, and has at its midpoint a fibrous node. At the beginning of systole, the three cusps rapidly retract to form a triangular orifice. Eddy currents within the sinuses of Valsalva cause a slow wave-like motion of the free edge and billowing of the base of each cusp, thus preventing occlusion of the coronary ostia. During ventricular diastole, the cusps fall passively into the center of the orifice and coapt over a considerable area. The closed valve supports the ejected column of blood and prevents regurgitation into the ventricle. In a healthy valve, approximation of the cusps during diastole is complete, and the three nodes come together near the center of the aortic lumen.

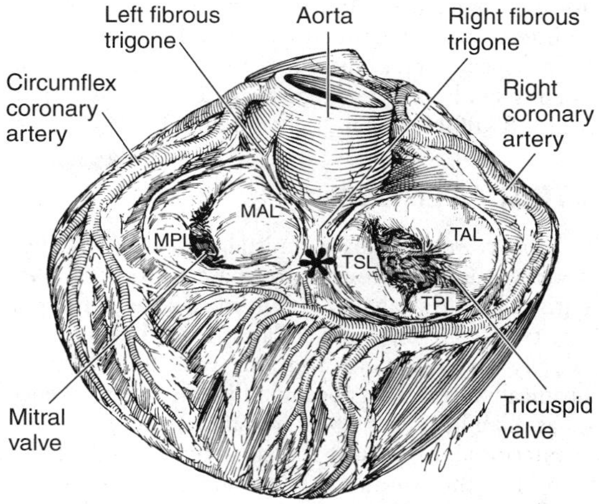

Figure 19–11. Anatomic interrelationships of the atrioventricular valves. (A, anterior leaflet; P, posterior leaflet; S, septal leaflet. The asterisk represents the area of the bundle of His.)

The three sinuses of Valsalva are slightly dilated pockets of the aortic root between the cusps and the aortic wall. The coronary arteries arise from two of the sinuses of Valsalva. Because the aortic valve lies in an oblique plane, the origin of the left coronary artery is posterior and slightly superior to that of the right coronary artery.

A number of disease processes can affect heart valves. By far the most common include rheumatic carditis, degenerative conditions of the valve collagen, and infection. Less frequently, valves may be involved with collagen-vascular disorders, tumors, carcinoid, and Marfan's syndrome. Valvular heart disease was responsible for 89,000 hospital discharges in 1998.

MITRAL STENOSIS

The most common cause of mitral stenosis is still rheumatic fever associated with group A streptococcal pharyngitis. The early valvular lesions of rheumatic fever are characterized by an acute inflammatory infiltrate that gradually heals by organization with fibrous tissue. Chronically, the leaflets become fibrotic and thickened, so that pliability and surface area are reduced. Fusion of the anterior and posterior leaflets may be severe, and in many cases the commissures can no longer be identified. Calcification may occur in the leaflets or the fused commissures, being more common on the posteromedial aspect. The chordae are thickened, shortened, and fused by the same type of fibrosis, and occasionally the subvalvular apparatus may be calcified. The entire process transforms the mitral complex into a rigid funnel-shaped structure with a "fish mouth" opening.

The most significant effects of mitral stenosis occur on the pulmonary vasculature and right ventricle. Congestion of the pulmonary vessels is characteristic, with distention and thickening of pulmonary capillaries. Intimal fibrosis of the pulmonary veins and arterioles also is observed, and in advanced cases medial thickening and fibrosis are common. Pulmonary hypertension progresses with time and may increase to the point of producing systemic levels of systolic blood pressure in the right ventricle and inducing functional tricuspid valve regurgitation.

Clinical Findings

A. Symptoms and Signs

Pulmonary venous hypertension caused by valve obstruction produces the most prominent symptom in mitral stenosis, which is dyspnea. Initially, dyspnea is observed only with effort; but with time and progressive valve obstruction dyspnea begins to occur at rest or at night and is worsened by lying flat (orthopnea). Atrial contraction augments transmitral flow significantly in mitral stenosis, so that development of atrial fibrillation increases mean left atrial pressure and reduces cardiac output by about 20%. In addition, a more rapid ventricular rate decreases diastolic filling time, further exacerbating the problem. Thus, it is common for the clinical status of a patient to deteriorate when atrial fibrillation develops. Death is due to progressive heart failure in 60–70% of patients. Systemic emboli, pulmonary emboli, and infection are the remaining causes.

On physical examination, the patient characteristically appears thin and cachectic, with a washed-out and sallow "mitral facies." Jugular venous pulsations may be prominent with fluid overload or with secondary tricuspid incompetence. If the cardiac rhythm is atrial fibrillation, irregularities in the jugular pulse and prominent v waves are observed. Peripheral edema and hepatic enlargement may be present as well as the classic "hepatojugular reflux." In the presence of pulmonary edema, respirations are rapid and shallow, the work of breathing is increased, and rales are present to varying degrees from the lung bases up the chest. A sternal heave indicates right ventricular enlargement and suggests pulmonary hypertension. In severe cases of pulmonary hypertension, the pulmonary component of the second heart sound is often palpable in the second or third left intercostal space parasternally.

Auscultation of the heart reveals accentuation of the first heart sound (S_1) in the early stages, and with development of pulmonary hypertension the pulmonary component of the second heart sound (S_2) becomes accentuated. An opening snap of the mitral valve is common and appears to be due to sudden tensing of the valve leaflets by chordae after their opening excursion. The opening snap is best heard at the apex and is associated with pliability of the valve leaflets. The mitral opening snap follows S_2 by 40–120 ms, with a shorter interval indicating severe left atrial hypertension. The diastolic murmur of mitral stenosis has a low-pitched rumbling quality, best heard at the apex with the bell of the stethoscope. Because of its low frequency, the murmur can be difficult to detect. The murmur usually commences immediately after the opening snap, and its duration is directly related to the severity of valve obstruction. In sinus rhythm, a presystolic accentuation of the murmur is characteristic, as blood flow is accelerated across the valve by atrial contraction. Presystolic accentuation is lost with development of atrial fibrillation.

B. Electrocardiography

Ninety percent of patients in sinus rhythm exhibit a broad, notched P wave on the ECG, the so-called P mitrale. In later stages, atrial fibrillation and right ventricular hypertrophy are cardinal electrocardiographic signs.

C. Imaging Studies

On x-ray, the overall cardiac silhouette may be normal, with the exception of left atrial enlargement. Pulmonary venous hypertension is accompanied by engorged, transversely oriented superior pulmonary veins. With pulmonary hypertension, the pulmonary arteries and right ventricle become enlarged, displacing the right ventricle toward the sternum on the lateral projection. Severe valvular obstruction is manifested by Kerley B lines and frank pulmonary edema.

Transthoracic echocardiography is the tool of choice in the initial evaluation, providing accurate information on valve anatomy, valve area and gradient, and pulmonary artery pressures. Ventricular function is usually normal in mitral stenosis.

Cardiac catheterization is performed in most patients but can be omitted in young patients with classic clinical and echocardiographic findings. Measurements of transvalvular gradients and calculations of valve area provide useful information about severity of the stenosis. The normal mitral orifice area is 3 cm^2/m^2 BSA, and significant mitral stenosis is suggested when the calculated area approaches 1 cm^2/m^2. Estimation of valve orifice area is subject to some error, however, particularly at low flow rates or in the presence of valvular regurgitation. Moreover, a well-diuresed patient with a contracted blood volume occasionally will exhibit a larger valve area and a lower left atrial pressure than those suggested by the clinical evaluation. Thus, it should be emphasized that catheterization findings are only supplemental, and the entire clinical picture must be considered when making therapeutic decisions.

Treatment

A. Medical Treatment

Most clinicians would agree that asymptomatic patients should be treated medically and carefully observed. Heart rate control is helpful and anticoagulation is recommended for patients in atrial fibrillation. Survival in asymptomatic patients is > 80% at 10 years; however, once limiting symptoms occur, this number drops to 15%.

B. Percutaneous Balloon Valvotomy

Symptomatic patients with moderate to severe mitral stenosis are now being considered for percutaneous valvotomy. The ideal patient has minimal valve calcification and subvalvular scarring, no valve regurgitation, and no atrial thrombus. Successful procedures commonly double the valve area. Mitral regurgitation and persistent atrial septal defect occur in 2–10%. Restenosis-free survival at 10 years is approximately 56%. However, surgical commissurotomy can achieve a larger mitral valve area, better functional recovery, and a lower incidence of late mitral regurgitation.

C. Surgical Treatment

The indications for operative treatment in mitral stenosis are similar to those for the percutaneous balloon approach. All symptomatic patients (NYHA class II or higher) should be considered for operation. Patients with significant pulmonary hypertension, episodic pulmonary edema, new-onset atrial fibrillation, or episodes of thromboembolism are operative candidates as well. Surgical procedures include open commissurotomy and valve replacement. Approximately 50% of stenotic mitral valves treated operatively can be managed with open commissurotomy. Absence of significant leaflet calcification—together with good leaflet mobility and surface area—increases the likelihood of successful repair. Complete incision of fused commissures is performed. The submitral apparatus is inspected, and fused or thickened chordae are resected. The papillary muscle heads can be split to further improve submitral outflow. If significant leaflet calcification or fibrous retraction is evident, a standard prosthetic mitral valve replacement is performed. Whenever possible, the subvalvular attachments to the mitral annulus are preserved to maintain ventricular geometry over time.

Prognosis

The operative mortality rate for isolated primary mitral valve procedures ranges from 1% to 5% depending on the severity of preoperative symptoms, the presence (or not) of severe pulmonary hypertension or right ventricular failure, and the need for mitral valve replacement. Contemporary operations significantly increase long-term survival and patient well-being. After open mitral commissurotomy or valve replacement, most patients experience improvement in symptoms, though repeat operations are necessary at a rate of 2–4% per year after valve repair. The probabilities of systemic embolization and infective endocarditis are lessened significantly by surgical therapy, and patients experiencing atrial fibrillation for less than 1 year have an excellent chance of reverting to sinus rhythm with pharmacologic therapy or cardioversion (or both).

MITRAL REGURGITATION

Competence of the mitral valve depends on an integrated function of the mitral annulus, the valve leaflets, the chordae tendineae, the papillary muscles, and the ventricular wall. Incompetence can be caused by abnormalities of any of these structures.

Rheumatic heart disease accounts for 35–45% of cases of mitral regurgitation. Involvement of the leaflets by the rheumatic process causes shortening, rigidity, and retraction of the cusps. The chordae tendineae also become fibrotic, fused, and shortened.

Idiopathic calcification of the mitral valve and annulus in the elderly can be an important cause of regurgitation and is associated with systemic hypertension, aortic stenosis, diabetes, and chronic renal failure. Calcification may involve the entire annulus and project into adjacent ventricular myocardium. Masses of calcium may protrude into the subvalvular region, immobilizing the valve or preventing leaflet coaptation, and calcium can invade the conduction system or adjacent coronary arteries.

Mitral valve prolapse is present in 3–4% of the general population and can be associated with a midsystolic click and late systolic murmur. Progressive and clinically significant mitral regurgitation develops in approximately 5% of these cases. The primary pathologic process is myxomatous degeneration of the fibrous layer of the valve leaflets and chordae tendineae, producing thinning, elongation, and redundancy. In many patients, rupture of weakened chordae can cause acute mitral regurgitation whose severity depends on the size of chordal rupture and the degree of regurgitation produced. In extreme cases, severe congestive heart failure and acute pulmonary edema may necessitate emergency treatment.

Infective endocarditis is the cause of mitral regurgitation in 5% of cases, and the mitral valve is the most common valve to become infected. Leaflet destruction or chordal rupture can result in sudden, severe incompetence.

The final category of mitral incompetence is **ischemic mitral regurgitation**, defined as moderate to severe valve incompetence precipitated by acute myocardial infarction with no primary leaflet or chordal pathology. This disorder is observed to a significant degree in 3% of patients with coronary artery disease undergoing catheterization and is quite heterogeneous from both the pathophysiologic and the clinical viewpoints. Pathologically, the majority of patients exhibit posterior papillary and annular dysfunction in which regurgitation and congestive heart failure are coincident with the onset of a large posterior wall infarction. Combinations of posterior annular dilation, papillary muscle elongation, loss of papillary muscle shortening, and preexisting congenital leaflet defects produce valve incompetence at the posterior commissural region.

Postinfarction **papillary muscle rupture** occurs more rarely and is observed in only 0.1% of coronary disease patients undergoing catheterization. Congestive heart failure associated with a new murmur usually develops several days after infarction, and the majority have severe regurgitation requiring acute intervention. The infarction usually is posterior and often is small and localized; global ejection fraction is frequently maintained.

Physiologic derangements caused by mitral regurgitation are similar to those associated with mitral stenosis. Left atrial hypertension is transmitted to the pulmonary vasculature, causing dyspnea and pulmonary edema. Pulmonary arterial hypertension, right ventricular failure, and functional tricuspid regurgitation occur by similar mechanisms. However, unlike mitral stenosis, the left ventricle is subjected to a chronic volume overload that ultimately causes myocardial failure.

Clinical Findings

A. Symptoms and Signs

Symptoms produced by mitral regurgitation are related to the level of pulmonary venous hypertension. Exertional dyspnea and orthopnea are common, and chronically reduced cardiac output produces easy fatigability and cardiac cachexia. Moderate to severe regurgitation can be tolerated for many years with relatively minor symptoms until irreversible left ventricular dysfunction develops. Therefore, the severity of symptoms cannot be used as the only criterion for intervention. Hemoptysis is rarely reported, and symptoms occasionally appear with the onset of atrial fibrillation, which complicates 75% of severe cases. Systemic emboli can occur in patients with atrial fibrillation but are not as common as in mitral stenosis. Infective endocarditis should be suspected if there are symptoms of malaise, fever, chills, or a new or worsening murmur or when acute decompensation occurs in a previously stable patient. Angina secondary to mitral regurgitation is rare and should suggest coexisting coronary artery disease. Patients with ischemic mitral regurgitation usually manifest either acute or chronic myocardial ischemic syndromes.

The physical signs of congestive heart failure are similar to those of mitral stenosis. The apical impulse is displaced to the left in proportion to the degree of left ventricular enlargement, and an apical systolic thrill can be palpated. With significant right ventricular enlargement, a sternal heave is evident. On auscultation, the heart sounds usually are normal with the exception of a third heart sound with congestive heart failure or an increased S_2 with pulmonary hypertension. The hallmark of mitral regurgitation is an apical high-pitched, holosystolic murmur that radiates to the axilla and back. On occasion, the murmur will radiate to the base and have a musical quality.

B. Electrocardiography

The ECG may show left ventricular hypertrophy from the chronic volume overload or biventricular hypertrophy with concomitant pulmonary arterial hypertension. In sinus rhythm, P mitrale may be present.

C. Imaging Studies

The chest radiograph illustrates left atrial enlargement in chronic cases, but because of the volume overload the left ventricle also is dilated. Right ventricular enlargement, pulmonary vascular engorgement, and Kerley B lines are common. Transesophageal echocardiography is especially helpful in the evaluation of mitral regurgitation. The site of abnormal mitral valve anatomy can usually be clearly defined along with the degree and location of mitral regurgitation jet (Figure 19–12). Increasing left ventricular end-systolic dimension can be an early sign of impending heart failure even in the absence of symptoms. Cardiac catheterization documents prominent left atrial v waves, elevated left ventricular end-diastolic pressure and increased end-diastolic volume. Pulmonary hypertension in mitral incompetence has the same implications as in mitral stenosis. A reduction in cardiac index below 2 $L/min/m^2$ and a wid-

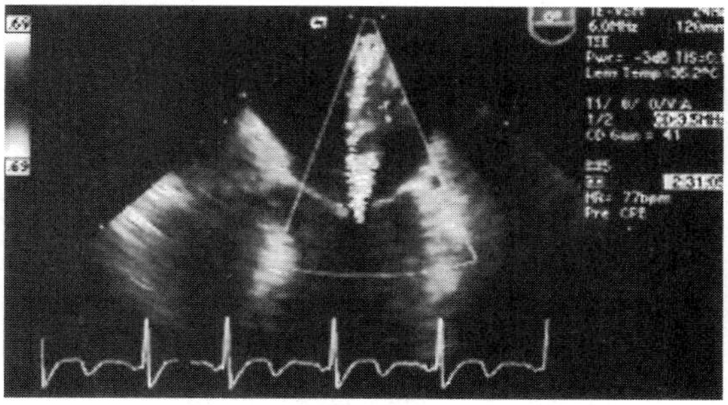

Figure 19–12. Transesophageal echocardiogram showing "central jet" of severe ischemic mitral regurgitation.

ened arteriovenous oxygen difference indicate severe hemodynamic impairment. Regurgitation is graded on the basis of the contrast left ventriculogram as 1–4+.

Treatment

A. Medical Therapy

The typical patient with chronic mitral regurgitation compensates by augmenting preload and reducing afterload (the left ventricle is unloaded by ejecting into the low-pressure left atrium). It is not surprising that patients can be asymptomatic for many years, but the chronic volume overload can result in significant left ventricular dysfunction. The mainstay of medical therapy is preload reduction (diuretics) and afterload reduction (ACE inhibitors). The latter can reduce the regurgitant volume and increase forward output. There are no data to suggest that this approach will benefit the asymptomatic or normotensive patient.

B. Selection of Patients for Operation

The natural history of mitral regurgitation is more variable than that of mitral stenosis because of the greater number of etiologic factors. The clinical course can range from asymptomatic, with moderate mitral regurgitation remaining stable for many years, to a fulminant progression of overwhelming congestive heart failure. There are three determinants of clinical severity: (1) the degree of regurgitation, (2) the status of left ventricular function, and (3) the cause of the valve disease.

Most patients referred for surgery are symptomatic (NYHA class II or greater). Asymptomatic patients should be referred if left ventricular dysfunction is present (ejection fraction < 60%, end-systolic dimension > 45 mm) or if significant pulmonary hypertension or new atrial fibrillation occurs. Exercise echocardiography may be useful in the equivocal patient. Significant left ventricular dysfunction (ejection fraction < 45%) have a higher operative mortality and worse long-term survival.

C. Surgical Treatment

Mitral valve incompetence can be managed by mitral valve repair or replacement. Virtually all myxomatous valves with prolapse can be repaired. Fifty percent have isolated posterior leaflet prolapse or chordal rupture, and posterior leaflet reconstruction along with Carpentier ring annuloplasty (Figure 19–13) is highly effective. Anterior leaflet reconstruction is more difficult and may require chordal transfer (from the posterior leaflet), chordal shortening, or artificial chord insertion to restore competence. In cases of ischemic mitral regurgitation, ring mitral annuloplasty (Figure 19–14) combined with complete coronary revascularization is the procedure of choice. In cases of rheumatic leaflet retraction, valve calcification, or severe endocarditis, prosthetic valve replacement with preservation of the subvalvular apparatus is more appropriate.

Prognosis

Operative mortality rates for elective mitral valve procedures performed under elective conditions approximate 2–5%, and the quality and duration of life are improved. Typical 5- and 10-year survival is 80% and 65%, respectively, and is adversely affected by age and preoperative left ventricular dysfunction (Figure 19–15). Late survival after mitral valve replacement is not as good as after reparative procedures (Figure 19–16).

TRICUSPID VALVE DISEASE

Pathologic disorders of the tricuspid valve can be either functional or organic. Tricuspid regurgitation is usually functional and is secondary to right ventricular dilation and enlargement of the free-wall tricuspid annulus. The annulus in the area of the septal leaflet is spared, and the valve leaflets and chordae generally are normal. Causes of functional tricuspid regurgitation include mitral valve disease, cor pulmonale, primary pulmonary hypertension, right ventricular infarction, and congenital heart disease. In most cases, valve incompetence reflects the presence of—and in turn further aggravates—severe right ventricular failure. The main cause of organic tricuspid regurgitation is infective endocarditis.

Tricuspid stenosis is almost always rheumatic, usually accompanies mitral valve involvement, and is clinically significant in about 5% of patients with rheumatic heart disease. Pathologic changes resemble those in the mitral valve, with thickening and fusion of the leaflets and chordae, producing a stenotic, fixed tricuspid orifice. Carcinoid involvement of the tricuspid valve is characterized by deposition of fibrous carcinoid plaques on the leaflets and ventricular attachments. Rarely, tumors of the right atrium (atrial myxoma) cause secondary obstruction of the tricuspid orifice. Both tricuspid steno-

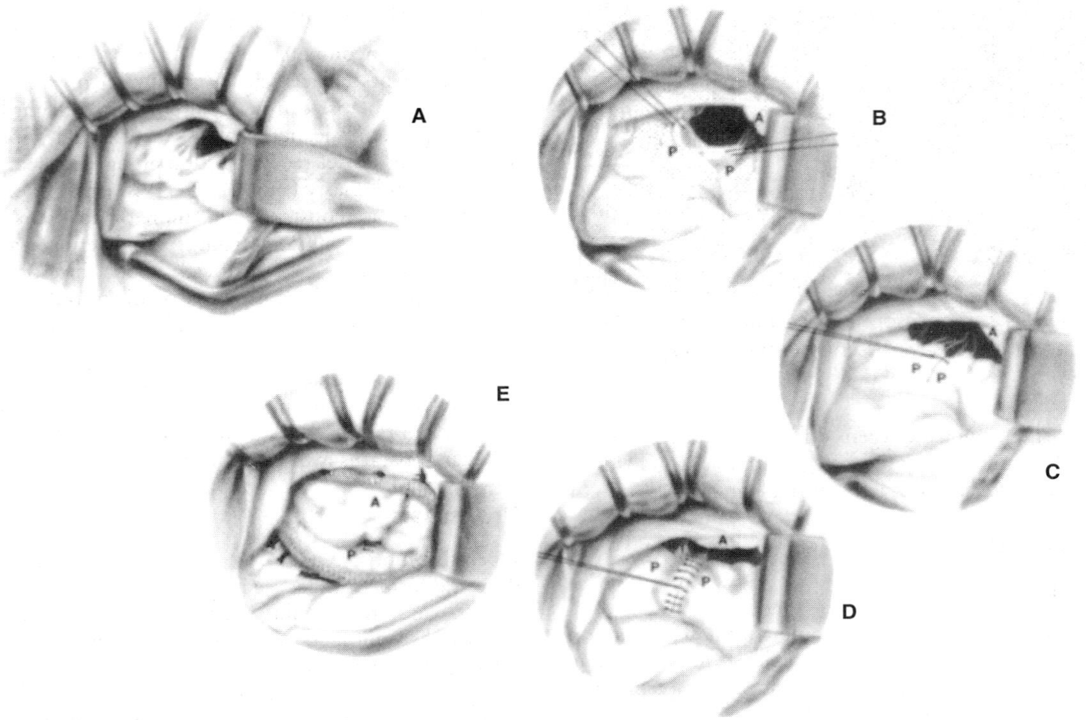

Figure 19–13. Panels ***A–E*** represent atrial views of posterior leaflet reconstruction for isolated posterior leaflet prolapse and insertion of Carpentier annuloplasty ring.

sis and tricuspid regurgitation produce right atrial hypertension, systemic venous engorgement, and hepatic congestion. Severe fluid retention, edema, and debility are characteristic. The process can progress to hepatic failure, cardiac cirrhosis, anasarca, and renal failure.

Clinical Findings

A. Symptoms and Signs

Symptoms in either tricuspid stenosis or regurgitation are related to the degree of systemic venous hypertension. Fatigue and weakness are common, usually without dyspnea or other signs of pulmonary congestion. Isolated tricuspid regurgitation is well tolerated in patients with normal pulmonary artery pressure; but when combined with mitral valve disease, pulmonary hypertension, and right ventricular failure, the clinical status deteriorates rapidly.

Tricuspid valve disease is easily overlooked unless the observer is alert to that diagnostic possibility. In sinus rhythm, contraction of the right atrium against a stenotic valve produces a prominent a wave in the jugular venous pulse; with regurgitant lesions, the jugular v wave is accentuated. The liver is often enlarged and may be pulsatile, but in congestive cirrhosis the liver may be firm and fibrotic. While ascites and edema are common, the lung fields are clear despite engorged

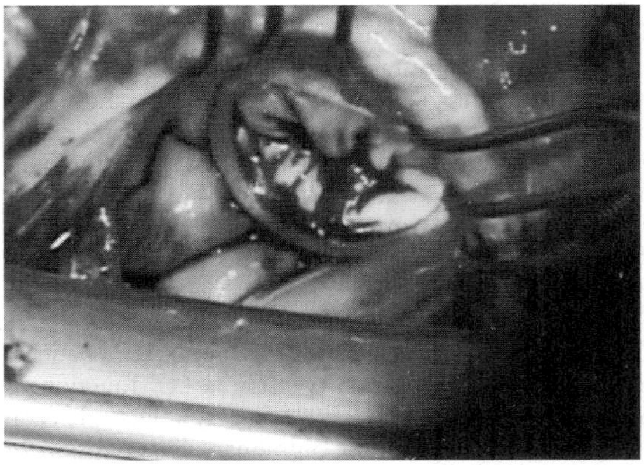

Figure 19–14. Operative photograph of semiflexible mitral ring annuloplasty for ischemic mitral regurgitation. The ring plicates the posterior annulus to restore leaflet coaptation.

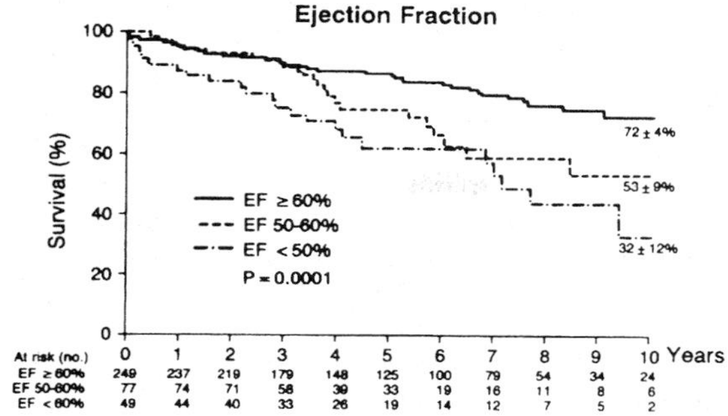

Figure 19–15. Effect of preoperative ventricular function on long-term survival after surgery for mitral regurgitation. (Reproduced with permission, from Enriquez-Sarano M et al: Echocardiographic prediction of survival after surgical correction of organic mitral regurgitation. Circulation 1994;90:830. Copyright © 1994 by American Heart Association.)

neck veins and other signs of congestive heart failure. A tricuspid opening snap may be present. Murmurs with tricuspid valve disease are similar to those observed in mitral disorders, and the two may be difficult to distinguish. Tricuspid murmurs usually are located more toward the left lower sternal border, and both the stenotic and the regurgitant varieties are augmented by inspiration. Both murmurs may be difficult to hear even when the physiologic defects are severe.

B. Electrocardiography

In sinus rhythm, tricuspid valve disease is suggested if the lead II P wave amplitude exceeds 0.25 mV.

C. Imaging Studies

The key radiographic finding is cardiomegaly, with prominence of the right atrial shadow. Echocardiography yields important information on the leaflet anatomy, the location and severity of regurgitation, and right ventricular function. At catheterization, tricuspid stenosis is confirmed by demonstrating a diastolic pressure gradient between the right atrium and right ventricle, utilizing simultaneous pressure measurements. A mean diastolic gradient of 5 mm Hg is significant in tricuspid stenosis, and values as low as 3 mm Hg may produce symptoms; the resting cardiac output is reduced. In tricuspid regurgitation, right atrial pressure is characterized by a prominent v wave, which in severe cases is described as "ventricularization" of atrial pressure. Occasionally, the atrial v wave may be normal despite severe regurgitation because of an enlarged, highly compliant venous system. Pulmonary arterial hypertension favors a functional cause in tricuspid regurgitation, whereas normal pulmonary pressures suggest organic disease.

Treatment

Rheumatic tricuspid stenosis is treated by commissurotomy or valve replacement depending on leaflet mobility, involvement of subvalvular structures, and the presence of regurgitation. Because residual gradients are tolerated poorly, valve replacement should be considered in significantly diseased valves. Because of the high thromboembolic potential of mechanical valves in the low-pressure right atrium, bioprosthetic valves or mitral allografts are preferred for tricuspid valve replacement. Symptomatic cases of carcinoid valve disease require excision of the entire tricuspid apparatus and valve replacement.

Tricuspid endocarditis is a particularly difficult problem. Many patients have septic pulmonary emboli, complicating postoperative recovery. For infections that cannot be eradicated with antibiotics, total excision of the valve has been recommended. Whenever feasible, reparative techniques or tricuspid replacement with a mitral allograft (which is very resistant to reinfection) should be considered.

Moderate to severe functional tricuspid regurgitation secondary to mitral valve disease usually is best managed by correction of the mitral valve disorder followed by tricuspid ring annuloplasty.

AORTIC STENOSIS

Aortic stenosis causes obstruction to left ventricular outflow and can be subvalvular, valvular, or supravalvular. Aortic stenosis in the adult may be due to a congenitally unicuspid or bicuspid valve, congenital subvalvular or supravalvular stenosis, rheumatic heart disease, or, most frequently, degenerative fibrosis and calcification. The cause can often be surmised from the age of

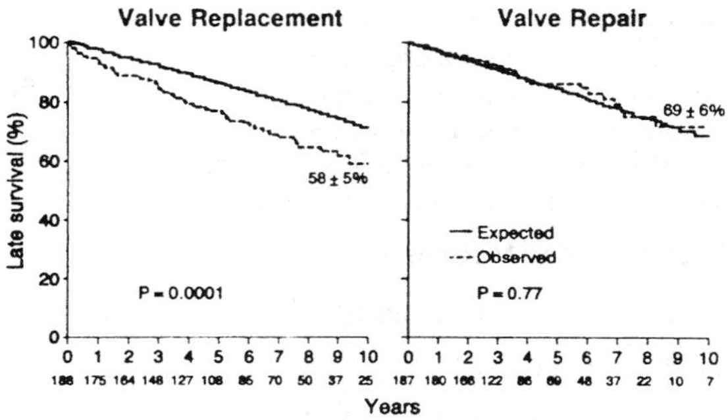

Figure 19–16. Effect of mitral valve replacement versus repair on long-term survival. (Reproduced, with permission, from Enriquez-Sarano M et al: Valve repair improves the outcome of surgery for mitral regurgitation. A multivariate analysis. Circulation 1995;91:1022. Copyright © 1995 by American Heart Association, Inc.)

the patient—congenital lesions accounting for most cases in patients under 30 years of age, rheumatic heart disease or congenital bicuspid valves in patients aged 30–65 years, and degenerative calcific stenosis in patients over 65 years of age.

Resistance to left ventricular outflow produces a pressure overload on the left ventricle that compensates by the development of concentric left ventricular hypertrophy. Hypertrophy is associated with reduced left ventricular diastolic compliance, while systolic function—or ejection fraction—is well maintained. In this setting, atrial systole contributes significantly to left ventricular filling, and the development of atrial fibrillation may precipitate heart failure. Myocardial oxygen consumption is elevated in the hypertrophied ventricle, and the presence of concomitant coronary artery disease may be particularly deleterious by reducing myocardial oxygen delivery.

Clinical Findings

A. Symptoms and Signs

Most patients remain asymptomatic for many years. The classic triad of symptoms includes angina pectoris, syncope, and congestive heart failure and usually denotes an aortic valve gradient greater than 50 mm Hg or a valve area of less than 1 cm^2. Angina pectoris is due to the imbalance between myocardial oxygen demand and delivery caused by increased myocardial oxygen consumption, and in the 25–50% of patients with coronary artery disease it is aggravated by the superimposed reduced oxygen delivery. Syncope is typically exertional and most likely related to inability of the left ventricle to increase cardiac output in the face of a fixed, high-grade obstruction. Congestive heart failure usually occurs late and is an especially ominous sign.

The pulse pressure is often narrowed, with a decreased systolic arterial pressure (parvus et tardus). A harsh midsystolic murmur is heard best at the second intercostal space and along the left sternal border. The murmur may radiate to the carotid arteries, is generally audible at the apex, and typically does not radiate into the axilla. Approximately 25–50% of patients will also have a murmur of aortic regurgitation.

B. Electrocardiography

The ECG demonstrates left ventricular hypertrophy.

C. Imaging Studies

On chest roentgenography, the heart is usually of normal size, though moderate enlargement may exist in the presence of congestive heart failure. Poststenotic dilation of the ascending aorta or calcification in the area of the aortic valve can be observed. Transthoracic echocardiography can evaluate calcification and mobility of aortic valve leaflets, bicuspid aortic leaflet anatomy, left ventricular hypertrophy, left ventricular ejection fraction, transvalvular gradients, and the presence of aortic regurgitation. Cardiac catheterization yields important information on coronary anatomy, cardiac output, transvalvular pressure gradients, overall left ventricular function, and the presence of coexisting valvular lesions. It must be emphasized that because of the compensatory pathologic alterations in preload, left ventricular compliance, and contractility, the measured ejection fraction may underestimate overall myocardial function. Mild aortic stenosis is defined as an aortic valve area of > 1.5 cm^2, moderate as aortic valve area 1–1.5 cm^2, and severe as aortic valve area ≤ 1 cm^2.

Treatment

Symptoms of angina pectoris, congestive heart failure, or syncope in a patient with aortic stenosis are associated with an average life expectancy of 1–3 years if left untreated and constitute the classic indication for aortic valve replacement. In addition, asymptomatic or minimally symptomatic patients in whom the aortic valve gradient is greater than 50 mm Hg or the aortic valve area is less than 1.0 cm^2 are also candidates for valve replacement, especially in the presence of left ventricular dysfunction or coexisting coronary artery disease. Percutaneous balloon valvotomy has a limited role in the treatment of aortic stenosis due to the high rate of restenosis within 6 months. However, patients presenting with severe heart failure may benefit from this approach as a "bridge" procedure for subsequent valve replacement. Every effort should be made to qualify patients for surgery, which offers long-term survival and a better quality of life.

Prognosis

Aortic valve replacement for elective isolated aortic stenosis is associated with a less than 5% operative mortality rate in all categories of patients. Advanced age, left ventricular dysfunction, and acute presentation increase the surgical risk. Regression of ventricular hypertrophy does occur and may continue for 10 years. Long-term survival approximates 85–90% at 5 years, and the outlook is adversely affected by preoperative left ventricular dysfunction, advanced age, and ventricular arrhythmias. Half of all late deaths are from noncardiac causes.

AORTIC INSUFFICIENCY

Aortic insufficiency is caused by abnormal coaptation of the aortic valve leaflets, allowing blood to return to the ventricle from the aorta during diastole. A common cause is rheumatic valvulitis, but varying degrees of annular dilation or annuloaortic ectasia also occur. Cystic medial necrosis, atherosclerosis, syphilitic degeneration, arthritic inflammatory diseases, and congenitally bicuspid valves are among some of the numerous causes of chronic insufficiency, while endocarditis, acute aortic dissection, and trauma account for the majority of cases of acute valve regurgitation.

Clinical Findings

A. Symptoms and Signs

Acute aortic regurgitation is poorly tolerated, and patients commonly present with severe pulmonary edema and failure. Signs of infective endocarditis or trauma may be present. Paradoxically, a diastolic murmur may be absent, indicating complete valve incompetence.

Patients with chronic aortic regurgitation may be asymptomatic for many years but have a reduced life expectancy once symptoms of orthopnea, paroxysmal dyspnea, and congestive failure appear. On physical examination, the pulse pressure is widened and the diastolic pressure is low (Corrigan's pulse). The apical impulse is sustained and laterally and inferiorly displaced. Characteristically, a blowing high-pitched diastolic murmur is heard best along the left lower sternal border with the patient in full expiration. A third heart sound and a diastolic rumble (Austin Flint murmur) may be audible.

B. Electrocardiography

The ECG usually shows left ventricular hypertrophy with left axis deviation.

C. Imaging Studies

Chest roentgenography usually demonstrates normal cardiac size in the acute case. In chronic regurgitation, left ventricular enlargement and pulmonary congestion are typical. Echocardiography permits estimation of left ventricular function and chamber size and the degree of regurgitation. At cardiac catheterization, supravalvular aortography is performed to define the degree of aortic insufficiency. Catheterization also identifies the coronary anatomy along with any associated abnormalities of the aortic root and annulus.

Treatment

For medically treated patients, the 5- and 10-year mortality rates in severe aortic regurgitation are 25% and 50%, respectively. Although vasodilator therapy may be useful in asymptomatic patients, this approach will not reduce the need for subsequent surgery. Aortic valve replacement is the standard operation and should be performed prior to the onset of irreversible left ventricular dilation, which not infrequently occurs prior to the onset of symptoms. The most accurate guide currently available for assessing progression toward irreversibility appears to be echocardiographic measurement of left ventricular dimensions, and significant ventricular dilation (left ventricular end-diastolic dimension > 70 mm or end-systolic dimension > 50 mm) should be used as a guide to recommending valve replacement or repair.

In selected cases of aortic regurgitation due to simple annular dilation, valve repair with subcommissural annuloplasty has been effective.

The prognosis after surgery for severe aortic regurgitation and normal ventricular function is good, with 85% of patients surviving 5 years. Abnormal preoperative ventricular function adversely affects long-term survival.

PROSTHETIC VALVE SELECTION

BIOLOGIC VERSUS MECHANICAL VALVES

Biologic Valves

At the present time, three types of biologic valves are used for replacement of diseased heart valves. The stented porcine bioprosthesis has been used for 25 years. Because of its low incidence of thromboembolic events, postoperative anticoagulation is not necessary for this valve, thereby reducing long-term patient morbidity. However, stented porcine valves are prone to structural failure (from leaflet calcification or leaflet-stent dehiscence), and the incidence of reoperation for this problem is approximately 40% at 10 years. Recently, introduction of the stented pericardial valve (Figure 19–17) has reduced the severity of this problem, and 80% of

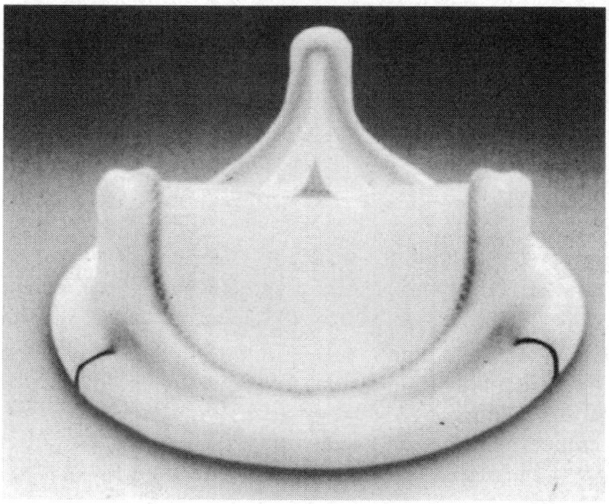

Figure 19–17. Carpentier-Edwards stented pericardial valve.

patients are free from structural failure at 10 years. The is no difference in prosthetic valve endocarditis occurring in porcine, pericardial or mechanical valves (about 2–10% at 10 years), and death rates from this serious complication are similar.

The stentless porcine valve (Figure 19–18) has now been approved for aortic valve replacement. This is a scalloped cylinder of porcine aortic root containing the native valve, with an external Dacron covering. Although somewhat more difficult to implant, this valve has a low transvalvular gradient, and faster regression of ventricular hypertrophy has been observed. Long-term durability will probably be greater than the stented valve, though calcification still remains a problem.

Human allografts have been used for aortic valve replacement for some time, and mitral allografts (Figure 19–19) have been recently introduced. Aortic allografts are virtually free from thromboembolic problems and endocarditis, and the rate of reoperation for structural failure at 10 years is low (8%). Only a handful of centers are implanting the mitral allograft, but the early results are encouraging.

Pulmonary autograft replacement of the aortic valve (Ross procedure) is another biologic option, and the outcomes are similar to those achieved with aortic allografts.

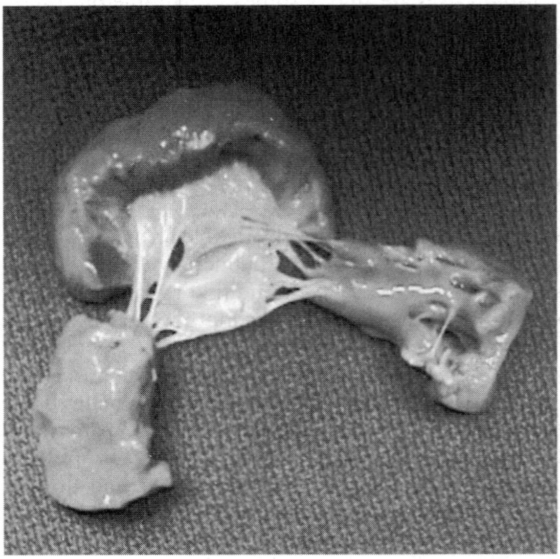

Figure 19–19. Operative photograph of mitral valve allograft.

Mechanical Valves

The most commonly used mechanical valves today include the tilting disk (Medtronic-Hall) and bileaflet (St. Jude) types (Figures 19–20 and 19–21). Both mechanical prostheses offer better predictability of performance and durability than tissue valves and are easier to implant than allografts, stentless valves, or autografts. However, all patients require warfarin therapy, and valve thrombosis or thromboembolism can occur despite adequate anticoagulation. Thromboembolic rates for most mechanical valves with adequate anticoagulation approximate 2–5% per patient year, though thromboembolism is less common with the St. Jude valve. The incidence of minor bleeding episodes is about 2–4% per year, and the incidence of major bleeding is 1–2% per year, with a mortality of 0.5% per year or less. For most mechanical valves, it is recommended that warfarin be given in doses sufficient to achieve an INR of 2.5–3.5. For isolated aortic valve replacement, the INR target can be reduced to 2.0–3.0 if low-dose aspirin is added (81 mg/d).

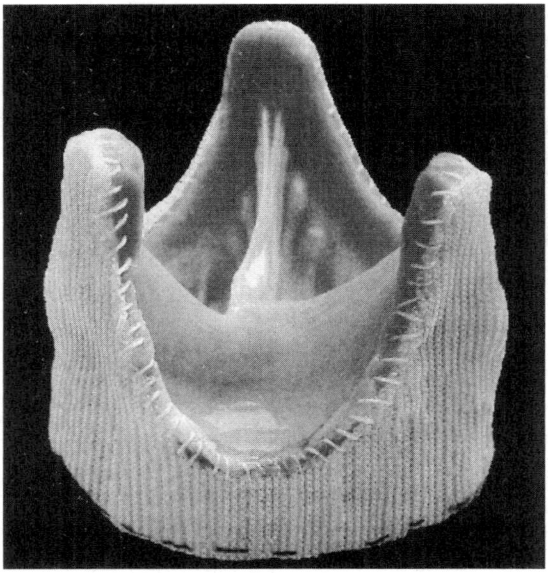

Figure 19–18. St. Jude Medical stentless porcine aortic valve.

Acute thrombosis of mechanical valves can occur if anticoagulation is not monitored carefully, Fortunately, this occurs in less than 2% of patients over 10 years. Structural failures in the currently used valves are rare. For small annuli (< 21 mm), the St. Jude valve offers the lowest transvalvular gradient and the largest effective orifice.

SPECIFIC INDICATIONS FOR VALVE PLACEMENT

Patient age, expected longevity, and ability to take warfarin are the major determinants of prosthetic valve recommendations. For example, young women desiring children

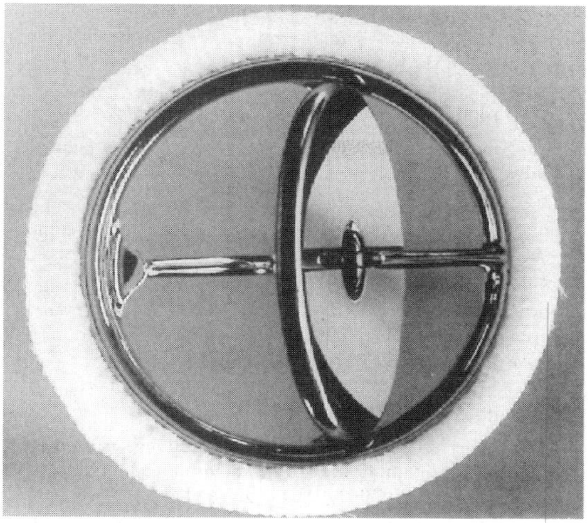

Figure 19–20. Medtronic-Hall tilting disk mechanical valve.

may choose a biologic valve to reduce anticoagulation complications during pregnancy—with the understanding that the prosthesis may eventually require replacement. Young patients or those with chronic renal failure are poor candidates for porcine valves because of the accelerated calcification of these prostheses. Patients with specific contraindications to anticoagulation also are candidates for biologic valves. Many of these patients are elderly and not expected to outlive their prosthetic valves. Patients undergoing complicated valve procedures such as aortic and mitral valve replacement or valve replacement–coronary bypass combinations should receive mechanical valves because of the higher mortality rate associated with reoperation in these groups. Severe infections involving the aortic root are best treated with allograft valves. Tricuspid valve replacement is performed exclusively with porcine valves because of a high incidence of mechanical valve thrombosis even with adequate anticoagulation. With the expanding application of the Maze procedure for correction of atrial fibrillation, younger patients are now being considered for biologic (allograft) valve replacement to avoid long-term anticoagulation.

INFECTIVE ENDOCARDITIS

Endocarditis is infection—usually bacterial—of any part of the cardiac endothelium. The valves are most frequently involved, and the resulting vegetations can cause leaflet destruction or may embolize. Abscess formation can result in heart block or persistent sepsis. Individuals with subacute endocarditis tend to have symptoms for months, and such infections are usually caused by hemolytic streptococci. Acute endocarditis, typically cause by *Staphylococcus aureus,* has a more fulminant course over days to weeks. Patients at risk for endocarditis include those with congenital or preexisting valvular defects, indwelling cardiac catheters, or prosthetic heart valves. Intravenous drug users and patients with prosthetic heart valves have the highest incidence of gram-negative and fungal infections. Infective endocarditis is now the fourth leading cause of life-threatening infection in the United States.

Clinical Findings

A. Symptoms and Signs

Classically, patients present with fever, bacteremia, peripheral emboli, and immunologic vascular phenomena. The latter include glomerulonephritis, Osler's nodes (painful, erythematous nodules usually in the pulp of the fingers), and Roth spots (retinal hemorrhages). Subungual splinter hemorrhages are a sign of peripheral emboli. Less commonly, flat, painless red spots occur on the palms and soles (Janeway lesions). Acute valvular regurgitation and heart failure may dominate the presentation.

B. Laboratory Findings

At least three sets of blood cultures spaced 1 hour apart must be positive. Culture-negative endocarditis occurs in less than 5% of cases and is usually due to prior antibiotic therapy, fastidious organisms, or fungi.

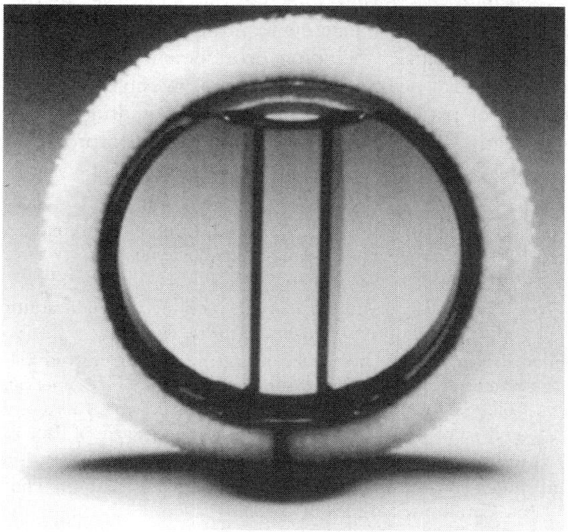

Figure 19–21. St. Jude Medical bileaflet mechanical valve.

C. Electrocardiography

Electrocardiographic findings are not specific. In cases of annular abscess, prolongation of the PR interval may be seen and is an ominous finding.

D. Imaging Studies

The chest x-ray may show signs of heart failure (interstitial pulmonary edema, cardiomegaly). Parenchymal nodules (septic emboli) may be seen in right-sided heart involvement. Echocardiography should be performed in all cases to document the location and degree of valvular involvement, vegetation size, and the presence of annular abscess. Vegetations larger than 1 cm in diameter, especially if located on the mitral valve, are at higher risk for embolization. Cardiac catheterization may be contraindicated in the presence of aortic valve vegetations or abscess of the valve annulus.

Treatment

The mortality of untreated patients with infective endocarditis is virtually 100%. Appropriate parenteral antibiotic therapy for 4–6 weeks has reduced the mortality to 30–50%. Approximately 20–25% of patients will require surgery, further reducing the overall mortality to 10%. Surgery is indicated for the following situations: severe valvular regurgitation with heart failure, abscess of the valve annulus, persistent bacteremia after 7–10 days of adequate antibiotic therapy, fungal or gram-negative infections, recurrent emboli, or mobile vegetations > 1 cm. Acute, severe aortic regurgitation from endocarditis is poorly tolerated because of pulmonary edema and low coronary perfusion pressure. Surgery should be performed promptly. Because of their high resistance to infection, allograft valves are preferred for appropriate patients requiring valve replacement. Mitral valve repair, including debridement of vegetation and pericardial patch reconstruction, is possible in a small number of patients. Success in intravenous drug users is particularly frustrating, since many succumb to prosthetic valve infection or drug overdose.

Acar C et al: Homograft replacement of the mitral valve. Graft selection, technique of implantation, and results in forty-three patients. J Thorac Cardiovasc Surg 1996;111:367.

Bayer AS et al: Diagnosis and management of infective endocarditis and its complications. Circulation 1998;98:2936.

Bonow RO et al: Guidelines for the management of patients with valvular heart disease: executive summary. A report of the American College of Cardiology/American Heart Association Task Force on Practice Guidelines (Committee on Management of Patients with Valvular Heart Disease). Circulation 1998;98:1949.

Carpentier A: Cardiac valve surgery: the French correction. J Thorac Cardiovasc Surg 1983;86:323.

Doty JR et al: Aortic valve replacement with cryopreserved aortic allograft: ten-year experience. J Thorac Cardiovasc Surg 1998;115:371.

Dujardin KS et al: Mortality and morbidity of aortic regurgitation in clinical practice. A long-term follow-up study. Circulation 1999;99:1851.

Elkins RC: The Ross operation: a 12-year experience. Ann Thorac Surg 1999;68(3 Suppl):S14.

Enriquez-Sarano MA et al: Progression of mitral regurgitation: a prospective Doppler echocardiographic study. J Am Coll Cardiol 1999;34:1137.

Enriquez-Sarano M et al: Valve repair improves the outcome of surgery for mitral regurgitation. A multivariate analysis. Circulation 1995;91:1022.

Enriquez-Sarano M et al: Echocardiographic prediction of survival after surgical correction of organic mitral regurgitation. Circulation 1994;90:830.

Ferguson E et al: The surgical management of bacterial valvular endocarditis. Curr Opin Cardiol 2000;15:82.

Grigioni F et al: Ischemic mitral regurgitation: long-term outcome and prognostic implications with quantitative Doppler assessment. Circulation 2001;103:1759.

Kassai B et al: Comparison of bioprosthesis and mechanical valves, a meta-analysis of randomised clinical trials. Cardiovasc Surg 2000;8:477.

Khan JH et al: Maze procedure and homograft replacement of a rheumatic mitral valve. J Heart Valve Dis 1999;8:630.

Khan JH et al: Cardiac valve surgery in octogenarians: improving quality of life and functional status. Arch Surg 1998;133:887.

Knott-Craig CJ et al: Aortic valve replacement: comparison of late survival between autografts and homografts. Ann Thorac Surg 2000;69:1327.

Lambert AS et al: Improved evaluation of the location and mechanism of mitral valve regurgitation with a systematic transesophageal echocardiography examination. Anesth Analg 1999;88:1205.

Ling KH, Enriquez-Sarano M: Long-term outcomes of patients with flail mitral valve leaflets. Coron Artery Dis 2000;11:3.

Maselli D et al: Left ventricular mass reduction after aortic valve replacement: homografts, stentless and stented valves. Ann Thorac Surg 1999;67:966.

Moon MR et al: Treatment of endocarditis with valve replacement: the question of tissue versus mechanical prosthesis. Ann Thorac Surg 2001;71:1164.

Senthilnathan V et al: Heart valves: which is the best choice? Cardiovasc Surg 1999;7:393.

Smedira NG et al: Balloon aortic valvuloplasty as a bridge to aortic valve replacement in critically ill patients. Ann Thorac Surg 1993;55:914.

Westaby S et al: Stentless aortic bioprostheses: compelling data from the Second International Symposium. Ann Thorac Surg 1998;65:235.

THORACIC AORTIC DISEASE

THORACIC AORTIC ANEURYSMS

The most common cause of thoracic aneurysms is arteriosclerosis, which causes a degenerative process in the aortic wall. Atherosclerotic aneurysms can be saccular or fusiform and occur in the ascending or descending thoracic aorta or in the arch. Another common pathophysiologic process is medial degeneration of the aortic wall, characterized by replacement of muscle cells and elastic lamina with mucoid-filled cystic spaces. In Marfan's syndrome, a defect in the fibrillin-1 gene is responsible for abnormal myofibril composition of elastic tissue. The disorder is inherited as an autosomal dominant and has many manifestations. Annuloaortic ectasia can occur in this setting and consists of enlargement of the entire aortic root, including the sinuses of Valsalva. Trauma and infection account for the remaining cases of thoracic aneurysms.

Clinical Findings

A. Symptoms and Signs

Thoracic aneurysms are more common in men, and a history of hypertension is usual. Symptoms, if present, are due to local pressure or obstruction of adjacent thoracic structures. In the ascending aorta, signs may include aortic regurgitation, superior vena cava obstruction, or chest pain with aneurysm expansion. In the arch of the aorta, tracheal compression may occur, while aneurysms of the descending aorta—the most common type—may be associated with recurrent laryngeal nerve compression, phrenic paralysis, dysphagia due to esophageal compression, or stridor due to tracheal compression.

B. Imaging Studies

The chest radiograph may show convexity of the right cardiac border in ascending aneurysms, a prominent aortic knob in transverse aneurysms, and posterior lateral thoracic masses in descending aneurysms. Ultrafast CT scans and MR angiography are now the imaging methods of choice, defining the anatomy and extent of the aneurysm in the majority of cases. Occasionally, aortography may be useful. Because many patients have generalized atherosclerosis, screening for significant coronary artery disease is essential. This is most commonly done with thallium imaging.

Treatment

Symptoms and size are the primary determinants of intervention for thoracic aortic aneurysms. For the asymptomatic patient with an aneurysm ≤ 5.5 cm, aggressive control of blood pressure with drugs (including beta-blockers) is warranted. Any aneurysm > 5.5 cm in diameter should be considered for surgical repair, particularly if symptoms are present. Patients with Marfan's syndrome and a positive family history for rupture or dissection are at higher risk for rupture, and intervention is recommended at 5 cm. Other factors predictive of increased rupture rate include advancing age, COPD, and a growth rate > 0.1 cm per year. Dacron graft replacement is the standard operative procedure and is conducted in different ways depending on the location of the aneurysm.

A. Ascending Aorta and Aortic Arch Aneurysm

Ascending and arch aneurysms require cardiopulmonary bypass for graft replacement, most commonly via right atrial and femoral artery cannulation. The heart is protected during aortic cross-clamping with cold potassium cardioplegia. For aneurysms that extend proximally into the sinuses of Valsalva (annuloaortic ectasia), a composite prosthetic valve–ascending aortic graft conduit is utilized, with reimplantation of the coronary arteries into the graft (as in patients with Marfan's syndrome). More recently, preservation of the aortic valve repair and reconstruction of the aortic root with a Dacron graft (David procedure) has shown promise. For isolated ascending aortic aneurysms, Dacron graft replacement is utilized—again under cardiopulmonary bypass and cardioplegic arrest.

Replacement of a transverse arch aortic aneurysm is made more complex by the need to provide cerebral protection while aortic arch blood flow is interrupted. This may be accomplished by one of several methods. Either standard cardiopulmonary bypass with individual cannulation of arch vessels can be performed, or profound hypothermia can be induced with a period of total circulatory arrest for arch replacement. The latter approach is used most commonly. Core temperatures of 15 °C are required for safe circulatory arrest. Retrograde perfusion via the superior vena cava may be a beneficial adjunct. The brachiocephalic vessels are excised from the native aorta and anastomosed to the Dacron graft as a single button. Great care is taken to remove all air from the grafts before cerebral reperfusion is instituted.

The operative mortality rate for ascending aortic or arch reconstructions has been reduced to about 10% because of advances in myocardial and cerebral protection.

B. Descending Aorta Aneurysm

Descending aorta aneurysms occur distal to the left subclavian artery. Operation is performed through a left thoracotomy incision with one-lung anesthesia. The aorta is clamped above and below the aneurysm, which is replaced with a Dacron tube graft. A major risk in descending thoracic aneurysm repair is spinal cord ischemia with resultant paraplegia. A number of methods have been proposed for protection of the spinal cord. These include cardiopulmonary bypass—with or without deep hypothermia—or left heart bypass. The latter provides distal aortic perfusion by circulating blood from the left atrium to the femoral artery while the aorta is clamped. Heparin-coated circuits available with this method can reduce bleeding. In addition, measured drainage of cerebrospinal fluid may be useful in ischemic cord swelling. For both techniques, reimplantation of large intercostal arteries is recommended because they may provide important collaterals to the cord. Measurement of somatosensory evoked potentials may guide the reimplantation decision.

Prognosis

The operative mortality rate associated with repair of descending aortic aneurysms approximates 5–15%, depending on the age of the patient and coexisting illness. The incidence of paraplegia varies with the extent of the aorta repaired and is now approximately 5–15%. The 10-year survival rate after surgery for ascending aneurysms is 50% and averages 38% for aneurysms of the descending aorta.

THORACIC AORTIC DISSECTION

Acute aortic dissection is the most common cause of aortic rupture and is often a lethal event. Approximately 2000 cases occur each year, and men are affected more commonly than women, usually in the fifth to seventh decades of life. The hallmark of this disease is degeneration of the aortic media. The pathogenesis is controversial. One theory holds that medial degeneration predisposes to rupture of the vasa vasorum, with subsequent intramural hematoma formation as a precursor to the dissection process. Another theory is that the commonly seen intimal tear allows blood to shear the weakened media. The intimal tear is located in the ascending aorta in 62% of cases, in the arch in 10%, and in the isthmus in 16%—and the remainder occur in the distal aorta. Men are more frequently affected, and hypertension is a common predisposing condition. Other causes of aortic dissection include atherosclerosis, iatrogenic injury (catheter, open heart procedures), and closed chest trauma. Patients with Marfan's syndrome and aortic coarctation are more susceptible to aortic dissection.

The DeBakey classification scheme is commonly used to describe the location and extent of aortic dissection. DeBakey type I dissections originate in the ascending aorta and extend into the distal aorta beyond the left subclavian artery; type II dissections involve the ascending aorta only, are frequently chronic, and are associated with aortic valve incompetence; and type III dissections occur distal to the left subclavian artery and commonly extend into the abdominal aorta. The Stanford scheme is simpler and is frequently used to guide therapy: any dissection occurring in the ascending aorta is classified as A; dissections involving only the descending aorta (below the isthmus) are B (Figure 19–22).

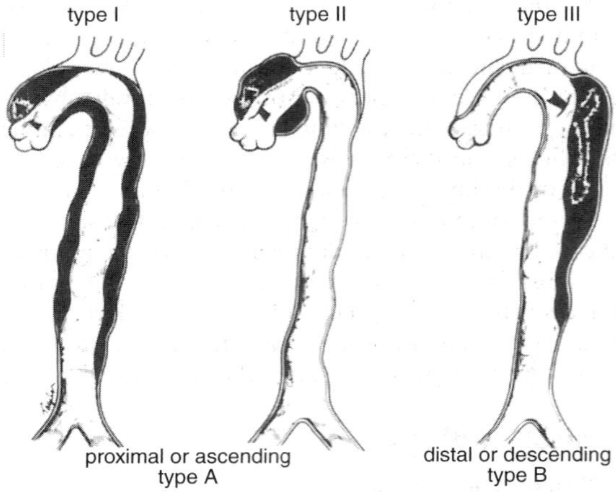

Figure 19–22. DeBakey and Stanford classification schemes for acute aortic dissection. (Reproduced, with permission, from Doroghazi RM, Slater EE [editors]. *Aortic Dissection.* McGraw-Hill, 1983.)

Clinical Findings

A. Symptoms and Signs

The most common symptom is severe chest pain, which often signifies the onset of the intimal tear and formation of the false lumen. The chest pain often is described as a severe tearing sensation that is felt anteriorly in ascending dissections and posteriorly between the scapulas in descending dissections. Hypotension may accompany the pain as a result of loss of blood into the false lumen, free rupture into the mediastinum, or leak into the pericardium. Sudden death may occur from pericardial tamponade or from extension into the aortic root with occlusion of the right or left coronary arteries. Aortic root involvement also is associated with prolapse of the aortic valve commissures and leaflets, causing aortic insufficiency and congestive heart failure.

Other manifestations, occurring as the result of obstruction (by intimal flap or false channel hematoma) of significant aortic branch vessels, include stroke, asymmetric upper extremity pulses and pressures, paraplegia, renal failure, acute mesenteric occlusion, and lower extremity arterial occlusion.

B. Electrocardiography and Laboratory Findings

The ECG and cardiac enzyme determinations are helpful in excluding acute myocardial infarction. This event may mimic many of the signs and symptoms of acute aortic dissection or may be caused by the dissection itself if the false channel occludes one or both coronary ostia. In this situation, administration of thrombolytic therapy or angioplasty would be dangerous.

C. Imaging Studies

The chest radiograph may show a widened mediastinum but is normal in up to half of patients. Cardiomegaly may reflect congestive heart failure or pericardial effusion. With contained rupture, a left pleural effusion may be evident. Ultrafast chest CT is the diagnostic procedure of choice in most centers and is highly sensitive and specific. Transesophageal echocardiography can also be performed rapidly and gives additional information about the myocardial function and aortic valve competence. However, dissections of the aortic arch and branch vessels are not well imaged. MR angiography is being used more frequently but is more time-consuming. Contrast aortography is rarely performed in acute aortic dissection but may be necessary in chronic dissection to determine branch vessel origination from the true or false channel.

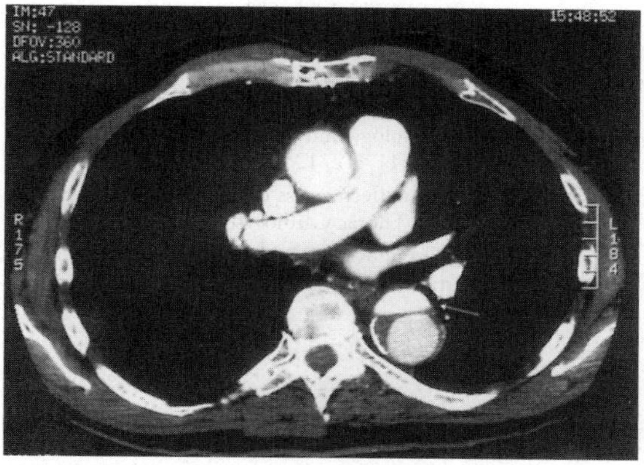

Figure 19–23. CT scan of type B aortic dissection. Arrow points to true lumen of aorta.

Treatment & Prognosis

For the typically hypertensive patient, aggressive control of blood pressure is critical. Intravenous esmolol is commonly used to reduce dP/dT (change in pressure divided by change in time) and the aortic shear forces. Pure vasodilators, if necessary, should be added only after beta-blockade has been achieved.

A. Ascending Dissection

For patients with untreated acute Stanford type A aortic dissection, 3% die suddenly, 27% die within 24 hours, and 70% succumb by 1 week. Rupture with cardiac tamponade, acute coronary occlusion, and acute aortic regurgitation are the major causes of demise. These facts underscore the primary role of urgent surgery for this condition. Replacement of the ascending aorta is required along with resection of the intimal tear. Resuspension of the aortic valve commissures usually restores valve competence. Achieving good hemostasis can be problematic because of the fragile nature of the dissected aorta. Application of new surgical adhesives (BioGlue) may be helpful. Operative mortality for this procedure is about 5%, and the 5-year survival approximates 55%. Since the entire aorta is usually dissected, yearly imaging surveillance is needed to look for aneurysmal changes.

B. Descending Dissection

The majority of patients presenting with acute type B aortic dissection (Figure 19–23) have a benign course. Drug therapy is the treatment of choice. However, approximately 20% of these acute dissection patients require surgery for rupture or significant organ ischemia from branch vessel occlusion. Operative mortality is this situation is at least 15%. Late survival is good, but 20% of patients may develop aneurysmal dilation of the descending aorta requiring operation. Therefore, yearly imaging surveillance is recommended.

Recently, endovascular aortic stent placement, with or without a fenestration procedure, has been applied to descending aortic dissection. However, control of the proximal intimal tear is not always possible, and long-term outcome studies are needed.

Coady MA et al: Natural history, pathogenesis, and etiology of thoracic aortic aneurysms and dissections. Cardiol Clin 1999;17:615.

Coady MA et al: Surgical intervention criteria for thoracic aortic aneurysms: a study of growth rates and complications. Ann Thorac Surg 1999;67:1922.

Coselli JS et al: Cerebrospinal fluid drainage in thoracoabdominal aortic surgery. Semin Vasc Surg 2000;13:308.

Coselli S, LeMaire SA: Left heart bypass reduces paraplegia rates after thoracoabdominal aortic aneurysm repair. Ann Thorac Surg 1999;67:1931.

de Haan P et al: Spinal cord monitoring with myogenic motor evoked potentials: early detection of spinal cord ischemia as an integral part of spinal cord protective strategies during thoracoabdominal aneurysm surgery. Semin Thorac Cardiovasc Surg 1998;10:19.

Elefteriades JA et al: Management of descending aortic dissection. Ann Thorac Surg 1999;67:2002.

Greenberg R, Risher W: Clinical decision making and operative approaches to thoracic aortic aneurysms. Surg Clin North Am 1998;78:805.

Griepp RB et al: Natural history of descending thoracic and thoracoabdominal aneurysms. Ann Thorac Surg 1999;67:1927.

Hartnell GG: Imaging of aortic aneurysms and dissection: CT and MRI. J Thorac Imaging 2001;16:35.

Kouchoukos NT et al: Elective hypothermic cardiopulmonary bypass and circulatory arrest for spinal cord protection during operations on the thoracoabdominal aorta. J Thorac Cardiovasc Surg 1990;99:659.

Leiner T et al: Magnetic resonance angiography of an aortic dissection. Circulation 2001;103:E76.

Meszaros I et al: Epidemiology and clinicopathology of aortic dissection. Chest 2000;117:1271.

Sabik JF et al: Long-term effectiveness of operations for ascending aortic dissections. J Thorac Cardiovasc Surg 2000;119:946.

Umana JP, Mitchell RS: Endovascular treatment of aortic dissections and thoracic aortic aneurysms. Semin Vasc Surg 2000; 13:290.

CARDIAC TUMORS

Primary tumors of the heart are rare, occurring in 0.002–0.3% of autopsy series. They can occur in any age group. Prior to the introduction of echocardiography, most tumors were diagnosed postmortem, since many patients remain asymptomatic until the tumor becomes quite large. Although most primary cardiac tumors are benign, the most common cardiac neoplasm is a metastatic lesion (Table 19–6). Most benign lesions are resectable and potentially curable. With the possible exception of lymphoma, most malignant primary and metastatic lesions are resistant to chemotherapy and radiotherapy and carry a poor prognosis.

Benign myxoma accounts for 75% of all primary benign tumors. Its physical characteristics range from a smooth, round, firm encapsulated mass to a loose conglomeration of gelatinous material, which may be friable (Figure 19–24). Most are attached by a pedicle to the fossa ovalis of the left atrial septum, though some may occur in the right atrium or ventricles. Histologically, myxomas contain various mesenchymal cells; abnormal DNA ploidy may correlate with recurrence after resection. Papillary fibroelastomas typically appear as papillary fronds attached to the aortic valve and are associated with cerebral and coronary embolization.

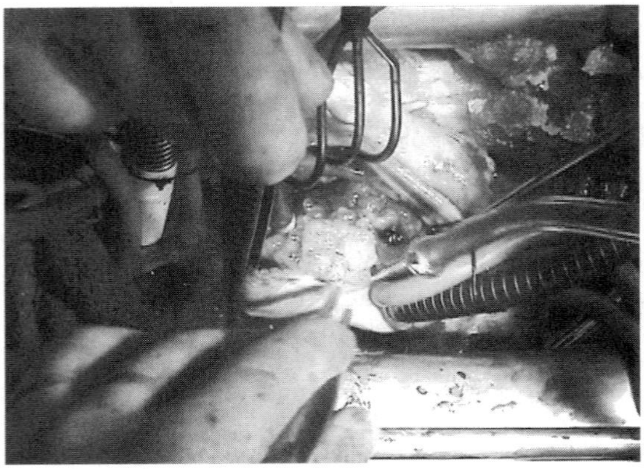

Figure 19–24. Operative photograph of polypoid right atrial myxoma.

Table 19–6. Types of cardiac tumors.

Primary	
Benign (75%)	
	Myxoma
	Rhabdomyoma
	Papillary fibroelastoma
	Fibroma
	Lipoma
	Teratoma
Malignant (25%)	
	Sarcoma (angiosarcoma, rhabdomyosarcoma, fibrosarcoma, osteogenic sarcoma, liposarcoma, lymphoma)
	Teratoma
Metastatic	
Carcinoma (67%) (lung, breast)	
Sarcoma (20%)	
Melanoma (12%)	

Clinical Findings

A. Symptoms and Signs

Clinical findings and presentation are dependent on the type and location of the tumor. As a general rule, malignant lesions usually present with rapidly progressive congestive heart failure from valvular or myocardial infiltration. Patients with myxoma can have protean manifestations. Systemic symptoms and signs include fever, weight loss, and anemia. Patients may also have signs of systemic embolization or mitral valve obstruction (mitral stenosis) from the tumor mass. The latter can produce a characteristic early diastolic sound or "tumor plop." Cardiac fibromas typically occur in the pediatric age group. These tumors grow slowly and tend to invade the conduction system, explaining why patients often die suddenly from arrhythmias.

B. Laboratory and Imaging Studies

Cardiac myxoma may produce abnormalities in the sedimentation rate, gamma globulin, and liver aminotransferases. Anemia and thrombocytopenia are common to many cardiac tumors.

The diagnostic procedure of choice is transesophageal echocardiography. Occasionally, MRI and CT scans are useful for infiltrative lesions.

Treatment

Most benign lesions of the heart are resectable and potentially curable. For cardiac myxomas, it is important to resect a rim of normal tissue around the attachment stalk to reduce future recurrence. The surgeon must be careful not to embolize the tumor during manipulation. Standard cardiopulmonary bypass with cardioplegia arrest is required, and operative mortality should be less than 1%.

Surgery for cardiac sarcomas and metastatic lesions is usually for diagnostic purposes, though palliative resection may occasionally be appropriate. Rarely, orthotopic heart transplantation has been considered in patients with local disease. However, long-term survival for malignant cardiac lesions remains poor.

Araoz PA et al: CT and MR imaging of primary cardiac malignancies. Radiographics 1999;19:1421.

Lobo A et al: Intracardiac masses detected by echocardiography: case presentations and review of the literature. Clin Cardiol 2000;23:702.

Michler RE, Goldstein DJ: Treatment of cardiac tumors by orthotopic cardiac transplantation. Semin Oncol 1997;24:534.

Schaff HV, Mullany CJ: Surgery for cardiac myxomas. Semin Thorac Cardiovasc Surg 2000;12:77.

Shapiro LM: Cardiac tumours: diagnosis and management. Heart 2001;85:218.

Vander Salm TJ: Unusual primary tumors of the heart. Semin Thorac Cardiovasc Surg 2000;12:89.

POSTOPERATIVE CARE

The care of patients after cardiac surgical procedures is assuming a greater role as older and sicker patients are being selected for surgical therapy. While most patients have a smooth and uncomplicated course, 5–10% experience postoperative problems, and a number of parameters are monitored to provide warning of developing complications. The fundamental goal is to provide adequate tissue perfusion. Careful physical examination after surgery is the starting point—to assess mental status, color, jugular venous pressure, pulse strength, and extremity temperature. Standard measurements include radial artery blood pressure, central venous pressure, urinary output, a continuous electrocardiographic tracing, and periodic determinations of arterial blood gases (PO_2, PCO_2) and pH. In complicated cases, cardiac function is assessed with measurements of cardiac output and pulmonary capillary wedge pressure as provided by a thermodilution Swan-Ganz catheter. Bipolar temporary atrial and ventricular pacing wires are left in most patients for control of heart rate or diagnosis of dysrhythmias. Appropriate hematologic and blood chemistry studies as well as chest radiographs are obtained periodically. Body weight is recorded daily to monitor potential fluid retention.

ANTICOAGULATION

Postoperative anticoagulation with aspirin is used routinely for most coronary bypass, valve repair, or bioprosthetic valve replacement procedures. After mechanical valve replacement, all patients should have full warfarin anticoagulation starting with the oral diet and continued indefinitely to maintain the INR at 3.0–3.5.

VENTILATORY SUPPORT

Following uncomplicated elective operations, most patients can be removed from ventilatory support and extubated within a few hours. After anesthetic recovery, criteria for early extubation include good pulmonary gas exchange, adequate ventilatory mechanics, a clear chest radiograph, absence of dysrhythmias and excess bleeding, and stable cardiac and neurologic function. Occasional patients exhibit prolonged pulmonary dysfunction requiring controlled ventilation, positive end-expiratory pressure, diuresis, and transiently increased fractional inspired oxygen. Complicated patients may benefit from prolonged mechanical ventilation by reducing the work of respiration. If pulmonary infection is suggested by radiographic infiltrates, high white blood cell counts, or positive sputum cultures, appropriate antibiotic coverage is added. As the period of required ventilatory support via an endotracheal tube approaches 2 weeks, tracheostomy should be considered. Tracheostomy is especially useful for clearing pulmonary secretions and assisting with ventilatory weaning.

MANAGEMENT OF COMPLICATIONS

Low Cardiac Output

With improving surgical techniques—and especially the introduction of cold potassium cardioplegia—postoperative low cardiac output is now uncommon in most centers. Patients judged by examination or by direct cardiac output determination (eg, cardiac index ≤ 2 L/min/m^2) to have inadequate perfusion must be treated aggressively. Therapeutic options can be categorized as alterations in preload (volume administration), inotropy (dopamine, dobutamine, etc), and afterload (vasoconstrictors, vasodilators). Inadequate heart rate can be treated with epicardial dual-chamber pacing. The most common problem is hypovolemia; volume replacement is usually accomplished with colloid solutions (blood, albumin, hetastarch), and it is not usually necessary to keep the hematocrit over 25%. Central venous pressures or pulmonary capillary wedge pressures of 15 mm Hg usually reflect adequate volume resuscitation.

Additional inotropic agents may be added if low cardiac output persists. These include epinephrine, calcium, and phosphodiesterase inhibitors (milrinone). The latter are particularly useful in situations of high pulmonary artery pressures or systemic vascular resistance. Cases of refractory low output may benefit from intra-aortic balloon counterpulsation. A small catheter is inserted percutaneously into the proximal descending aorta and helium is used to inflate a balloon on the catheter after aortic valve closure, thus augmenting coronary filling. The balloon is deflated with systole, resulting in afterload reduction.

In extreme situations, operative placement of ventricular assist devices may be indicated.

Postoperative Bleeding & Cardiac Tamponade

Cardiopulmonary bypass results in a number of hemostatic perturbations that may affect the clotting process. Residual heparin from the procedure or preoperative anticoagulants, thrombocytopenia, and altered platelet function are the most common problems. Activation of fibrinolysis and dilution of clotting factors also contribute. Most of these problems can be addressed intraoperatively. Administration of antifibrinolytics such as lysine analogs (aminocaproic acid) or serine protease inhibitors (aprotinin) during cardiopulmonary bypass has been shown to reduce postoperative bleeding in complicated patients. Criteria for excessive bleeding after open heart procedures vary widely. However, mediastinal tube outputs greater than 100 mL/h for more than 3 hours postoperatively is of concern. Prompt reexploration of the patient is always preferable to multiple blood transfusions and does not increase wound complication rates.

Cardiac tamponade can be a postoperative surgical emergency. The characteristic hemodynamic finding is elevated and equalized central venous and pulmonary wedge pressures, usually in the setting of excessive mediastinal bleeding. Low cardiac output is a sine qua non of tamponade. The urine output is low, and metabolic acidosis may be present. The chest radiograph may demonstrate mediastinal widening or blood collection. Echocardiography may be helpful in confusing cases, but if a significant question of tamponade exists, reoperation should be considered.

Atrial Dysrhythmias

Atrial dysrhythmias are common following coronary revascularization. Premature atrial contractions, atrial fibrillation, and atrial flutter reflect postoperative atrial irritability and occur in up to 40% of patients. Prophylactic treatment with beta-blocking agents or amiodarone (class III antiarrhythmic) may reduce the incidence of this complication and should be considered in most patients. Other agents that may be effective in controlling the ventricular rate in acute atrial fibrillation include intravenous digoxin, procainamide, and calcium-channel blockers (verapamil). Rapid atrial pacing may be useful in converting atrial flutter. For refractory atrial fibrillation (continuing more than 48 hours after good drug therapy) or in patients with unstable signs (hypotension, ischemia), electrical cardioversion should be performed. Transesophageal echocardiography to rule out atrial thrombus has been recommended prior to cardioversion.

Ventricular Arrhythmias

Ventricular irritability manifested by frequent or multifocal premature ventricular contractions, ventricular tachycardia, or ventricular fibrillation is managed by intravenous lidocaine, procainamide, or amiodarone together with direct-current cardioversion when necessary. Short periods of closed-chest cardiac massage may be necessary, but early cardioversion should be emphasized. Polymorphic ventricular tachycardia and ventricular fibrillation are usually manifestations of significant myocardial ischemia, and problems with the quality of coronary revascularization should be considered. Significant hypokalemia, hypomagnesemia, and hypoxemia should be ruled out. Beta-blocking agents, oral procainamide, or amiodarone can be used for long-term management of persistent ventricular ectopy. Frequent unifocal premature ventricular contractions do not require therapy.

Postoperative conduction disturbances occur frequently. Right bundle branch block is the most common problem and is usually benign. Transient heart block is seen more often after valvular surgery. After 5 days of persistent complete heart block, a permanent pacemaker should be considered.

Renal Dysfunction

Postoperative renal dysfunction after heart surgery occurs in 1–5% of patients and is usually related to preoperative age, diabetic status, and renal insufficiency. The duration of cardiopulmonary bypass may also contribute to this complication. Manifestations may vary from transient oliguric tubular necrosis to permanent renal failure. Proposed mechanisms include perioperative hypotension, atheroembolism, sepsis, or administration of nephrotoxic drugs.

Therapy for renal dysfunction consists of maintaining a higher arterial perfusion pressure (especially in patients with preexisting hypertension), low-dose intravenous dopamine infusion, adequate free water hydration, and general support of cardiac output. Fluid balance and potassium intake are monitored carefully to prevent overhydration or hyperkalemia. Forced diuresis with furosemide or mannitol may reduce the severity of renal failure. Some patients may require temporary venovenous ultrafiltration or hemodialysis. Patients with renal failure are more likely to die during their hospitalization.

Wound Infection

Sternal wound infection should occur in less than 1% of patients after cardiac surgery. Developing sternal instability, fever, leukocytosis, and wound drainage suggest the diagnosis. Severity varies from a superficial subcutaneous infection with a stable sternum to an isolated sternal infection with no mediastinal involvement to full-blown septic mediastinitis. At the first suspicion of a major wound infection, broad-spectrum antibiotics should be instituted and blood cultures obtained. The combination of diabetes and bilateral internal mammary artery harvesting predispose some patients to sternal infection. Infections producing sternal disruption should be treated with early wound debridement and pectoral or omental pedicle flaps. The mortality rate using this approach has been reduced to less than 10%, though morbidity remains high.

Myocardial Infarction

With improvements in myocardial protection and coronary grafting techniques, perioperative myocardial infarction should occur in only 1–2% of patients. Inadequate myocardial protection, incomplete revascularization, and early graft closure are the most common causes. Symptoms are often unreliable, since many patients cannot distinguish incisional pain from angina. Classic electrocardiographic changes and elevated serum troponin or CK are needed for diagnosis. Judicious anti-ischemia therapy is appropriate, and patients with possible vasospasm of arterial grafts should be treated with calcium-channel blockers. Rarely, angioplasty may be used to treat acute graft closure.

Augoustides J et al: Hemodynamic monitoring of the postoperative adult cardiac surgical patient. Semin Thorac Cardiovasc Surg 2000;12:309.

De Feo M et al: Variables predicting adverse outcome in patients with deep sternal wound infection. Ann Thorac Surg 2001; 71:324.

Gorman JH et al: Circulatory management of the unstable cardiac patient. Semin Thorac Cardiovasc Surg 2000;12:316.

Milan BL et al: Management of bleeding and coagulopathy after heart surgery. Semin Thorac Cardiovasc Surg 2000;12:326.

Rho RW et al: Management of postoperative arrhythmias. Semin Thorac Cardiovasc Surg 2000;12:349.

Sirivella S et al: Mannitol, furosemide, and dopamine infusion in postoperative renal failure complicating cardiac surgery. Ann Thorac Surg 2000;69:501.

Suen WS et al: Risk factors for development of acute renal failure (ARF) requiring dialysis in patients undergoing cardiac surgery. Angiology 1998;49:789.

Sural S et al: Etiology, prognosis, and outcome of post-operative acute renal failure. Ren Fail 2000;22:87.

II. Congenital Heart Disease

19

Ronald K. Woods, MD, PhD, & Edward Verrier, MD

DIAGNOSIS

Whereas some newborns may have obvious symptoms and signs of heart disease, others may have complex lesions not detected for days to months. Moreover, the clinical manifestations of a particular anomaly may evolve with age—eg, progressive failure or improvement with ventricular septal defect or increase in pulmonary vasculopathy associated with lesions that cause increased pulmonary blood flow. Although certain anomalies produce certain patterns of symptoms and circulatory dysfunction, specificity is not usually adequate for planning definitive therapy.

An important aspect of postnatal diagnosis is recognition of an abnormal heart sound, murmur, or other symptom referable to the heart. Examples are feeding difficulty, lack of weight gain, frequent respiratory infections, irritability, or cyanosis. Once a clinical abnormality is recognized, an investigation must be pursued until a definitive diagnosis is established. Although most anomalies are diagnosed after birth, prenatal or fetal echocardiography may indicate the presence of an anomaly and in many cases may establish a specific diagnosis.

Chest radiography and electrocardiography should be done in all cases as part of the initial workup. For additional diagnostic screening and anatomic definition, a more specific noninvasive test such as echocardiography is essential. Two-dimensional color flow Doppler echocardiography has eliminated the need to perform cardiac catheterization on every child with suspected congenital heart disease. In most cases, the decision to proceed to operation can be based on echocardiographic findings. However, cardiac catheterization remains relevant to the workup and management of several anomalies because it provides measurements of flow and resistance as well as accurate anatomic detail of the heart, great vessels, and pulmonary vasculature.

A thorough understanding of normal and abnormal anatomy and a consistent systematic means of describing this understanding are vital to the appropriate care of these children. In each case, it is imperative to know the following: (1) the connections of the systemic and pulmonary veins and the location and morphology of the collecting atria; (2) the connections of the atria to the ventricles (concordant, discordant, and biventricular, univentricular, indeterminate) and the mode of connection (one valve, two valves); (3) the ventriculo-arterial connections and the relations and patency of the great vessels; and (4) the origin and course of each coronary artery. The position of the heart in the chest and the direction of the apex may add useful information. While situs and position abnormalities may coexist with serious cardiac malformations, an abnormal heart position (eg, dextrocardia) is not itself diagnostic of a cardiac anomaly.

MANAGEMENT

Management of most congenital cardiac anomalies consists of surgical correction. Medication, diet, and activity regulation are important aspects of management, but the pediatrician or cardiologist should recommend a treatment program leading ultimately to surgical repair at the optimal time to prevent emergence of irreversible complications. The established success of modern care is derived from contributions of several specialties to the multidisciplinary team approach to the care of these children.

In the current era, most surgical procedures for congenital heart anomalies are considered corrective rather than palliative in that abnormal physiology is corrected—and in most cases anatomy is corrected as well. In certain cases in which initial corrective repair is considered too high-risk, it may be preferable to perform a palliative procedure initially and allow the child to grow until a more corrective procedure can be done. Most palliative procedures are designed to increase or decrease pulmonary blood flow. For example, a systemic to pulmonary artery shunt is a common means of increasing pulmonary blood flow in right heart obstructive lesions. At the other extreme, pulmonary artery banding, although used much less frequently in the current era, may be needed to decrease pulmonary blood flow—eg, in a child with a single ventricle and tricuspid atresia.

Most cardiac operations require cardiopulmonary bypass. This is usually accomplished by draining blood through cannulas placed in the right atrium or the venae cavae, through the heart-lung machine, and back to the patient through a small cannula in the aorta. Protection of the heart during the period of aortic cross-clamping or other periods of cardiac ischemia is more commonly done using various cardioplegic techniques quite similar to those described for adult cardiac operations.

Various degrees of hypothermia are employed with cardiopulmonary bypass, depending on the nature of the repair and the anticipated duration of cardiac ischemia. Hypothermia decreases the metabolic rate and oxygen consumption, thereby offering additional protection against ischemia. It also allows lower bypass pump flow rates, which improves visualization of the operative field by decreasing the amount of blood returning to the heart. For certain types of repairs—eg, complex aortic reconstruction in small neonates—deep hypothermic circulatory arrest or regional low-flow hypothermic bypass are considered very useful and in some cases essential options. Cardiopulmonary bypass is used to cool the patient to a core temperature of 15–18 °C (the brain is further cooled by packing the head in ice), at which point the bypass pump is turned off, blood can be drained to the venous reservoir of the pump, and cannulas are removed. With deep hypothermic arrest, most surgeons recommend reestablishing perfusion at low flows for a short time every 20 minutes. Alternatively, with selective arterial cannulation (innominate and possibly descending aorta), flow can be maintained directly to the brain and via collaterals to the lower body at much lower rates without complete circulatory arrest. The incidence of short-term complications secondary to circulatory arrest is considered acceptable; however, the incidence and nature of long-term neurological sequelae are now being more fully appreciated. Because of this, some surgeons advocate avoidance of circulatory arrest if at all possible.

Postoperative Management

After open heart surgery, most patients are maintained with an endotracheal tube in place and controlled mechanical ventilation for 12–24 hours. Drainage catheters in the mediastinum for postoperative bleeding are usually removed 1 or 2 days following surgery. Arterial pressure, blood gas, and oxygen saturation monitoring are routine. For some complex repairs, small venous catheters are left in the major atria or pulmonary artery to accurately measure all major venous and arterial pressure changes. Prophylactic antibiotics are routinely used, usually until lines and drainage tubes are removed.

A relatively common complication after open heart surgery is bleeding, requiring reoperation in 2–5% of patients. Particularly in smaller patients, hemodilution secondary to the prime volume of the bypass pump contributes to a dilutional coagulopathy. Systemic inflammation, factor consumption, and incomplete heparin reversal also contribute to bleeding.

The overall incidence of arrhythmias or significant cardiac dysfunction is low. In most cases, judicious medical management is successful. Nonetheless, mechanical assistance is a recognized utility in this context, most commonly in the form of extracorporeal membrane oxygenator support. Before relying on nonsurgical management or mechanical assist devices, it is imperative to rule out a residual defect, inadequate repair, or mechanical complication of the operation.

Unlike adults, the pulmonary vasculature of newborns and older infants is quite reactive. Postoperative pulmonary artery hypertensive crises are therefore more common in this age group, particularly after repair of certain anomalies such as obstructed pulmonary veins. Measures to reduce pulmonary vascular resistance include controlled mechanical ventilation and administration of bicarbonate to increase pH; high-dose opioid anesthesia to blunt sympathetic responses; increased fraction of inspired oxygen concentration; and, more recently, inhaled nitric oxide.

Castaneda AR et al: *Cardiac Surgery of the Neonate and Infant.* Saunders, 1994.

Fesslova V et al: Evolution and long term outcome in cases with fetal diagnosis of congenital heart disease: Italian multicenter study. Fetal cardiology study group of the Italian Society of Pediatric Cardiology. Heart 1999;82:594.

Kavanaugh-McHugh A et al: Transesophageal echocardiography in pediatric congenital heart disease. Cardiol Rev 2000;8:288.

Limperopoulos OT et al: Neurodevelopmental status of newborns and infants with congenital heart defects before and after open heart surgery. J Pediatr 2000;137:638.

Morris CD et al: 25-year mortality after surgical repair of congenital heart defects in childhood. A population based cohort study. JAMA 1991;266:3447.

Newburger JW et al: A comparison of the perioperative neurologic effects of hypothermic circulatory arrest versus low-flow cardiopulmonary bypass in infant heart surgery. N Engl J Med 1993;329:1057.

Pfammater JP et al: Pediatric open heart operations without diagnostic catheterization. Ann Thorac Surg 1999;68:532.

Wypij D et al: The effect of duration of deep hypothermic circulatory arrest in infant heart surgery on late neurodevelopment: the Boston circulatory arrest trial. J Thorac Cardiovasc Surg 2003;126:1397.

OBSTRUCTIVE CONGENITAL HEART LESIONS

Obstructive lesions impede the forward flow of blood and increase ventricular afterloads. In the absence of a ventricular septal defect, an obstructive lesion in the aortic or pulmonary valve causes the proximal ventricle to become hypertrophied. Sudden death may occur in this context. Ventricular hypertrophy is of concern because of the risk of dysrhythmias, ischemic changes in the myocardium, and potential permanent muscle damage or replacement by fibrosis.

PULMONARY STENOSIS

ESSENTIALS OF DIAGNOSIS

- *No symptoms in patients with mild or moderately severe lesions.*
- *Cyanosis and right-sided heart failure in patients with severe lesions.*
- *High-pitched systolic ejection murmur maximal in the second left interspace. S_2 delayed and soft. Ejection click often present. Increased right ventricular impulse.*
- *No ejection click and inaudible S_2 in severe cases.*

General Considerations

Pulmonary stenosis with intact ventricular septum and a normal aortic root accounts for approximately 5–8% of cardiac anomalies. In most of these patients, the commissures are fused with a flexible tricuspid semilunar valve, producing a domelike structure with a central opening of varying size (Figure 19–25A). Most patients with pulmonary stenosis have a patent foramen ovale; few have true atrial septal defects. In infants, severe valvular stenosis may be associated with a poorly developed right ventricle and can be an extremely serious condition requiring urgent intervention. Less common, isolated infundibular stenosis can produce similar pathophysiology (Figure 19–25B).

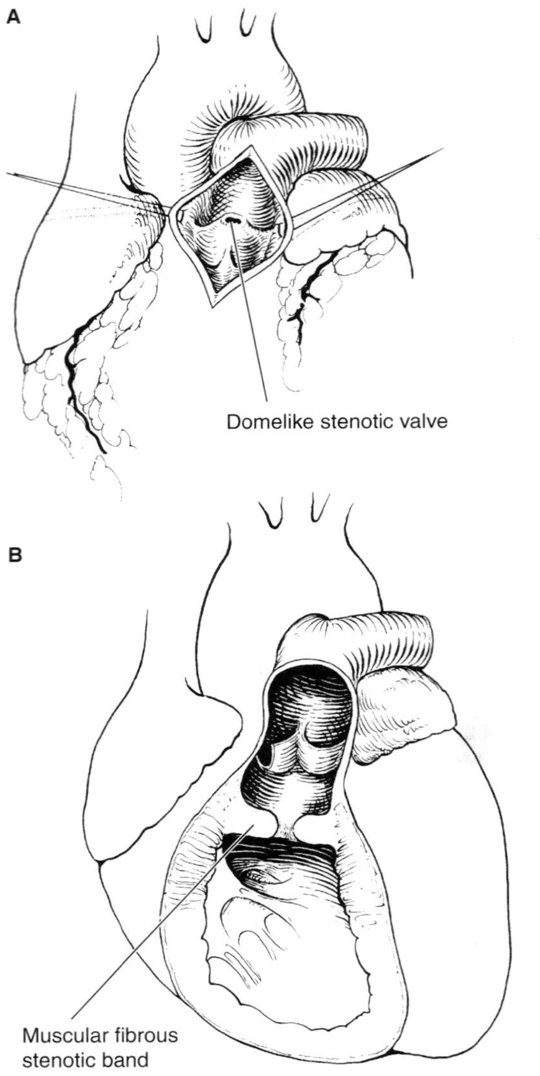

Figure 19–25. Pulmonary stenosis. ***A:*** Valvular pulmonary stenosis. ***B:*** Infundibular pulmonary stenosis.

Clinical Findings

Infants with more severe forms of pulmonary stenosis usually feed poorly and may have hypoxic spells. Sudden death has been reported. Older children usually are asymptomatic and grow normally. A few may complain of fatigue and dyspnea on exertion. When the pulmonary stenosis physiologically worsens as the child grows, shortness of breath, dizziness, and even angina may occur.

Approximately half of the deaths caused by pulmonary stenosis occur in infants. The remainder may be asymptomatic, but the murmurs of pulmonary stenosis are easily heard and usually do not go undetected. Complete evaluation is required. If the gradient between the right ventricle and the pulmonary artery is 50 mm Hg or greater, ventricular hypertrophy is progressive, or tricuspid valve insufficiency develops, repair is usually recommended.

Treatment

Infants with severe right ventricular failure or cyanotic spells require early intervention. In critically ill neonates, prostaglandin E_1 (alprostadil) has proved effective in maintaining pulmonary blood flow through the ductus arteriosus until the pulmonary valve obstruction is relieved. Interventional cardiology and catheter balloon dilation have essentially replaced surgery for most forms of isolated critical pulmonary stenosis. Adequate postdilation gradients with low mortality are attained in over 90% of patients. The procedure is indicated even in the less common scenario of a minimally symptomatic newborn with systemic right ventricular pressure. Surgical valvotomy with cardiopulmonary bypass remains an acceptable approach with equivalent success. It may be necessary for cases in which catheter intervention is not successful or in the context of an extremely small annulus or marked infundibular stenosis, in which case a transannular patch—and perhaps a systemic to pulmonary artery shunt—can be performed.

Prognosis

Posttreatment mortality for critical pulmonary stenosis ranges from 3% to 10%. Restenosis rates are variable and range between 10% and 25%. Right ventricular hypertrophy regresses after relief of the valvular stenosis.

Cheung YF et al: Evolving management for critical pulmonary stenosis in neonates and young infants. Cardiol Young 2000;10:186.

Hanley FL et al: Outcomes in critically ill neonates with pulmonary stenosis and intact ventricular septum: a multiinstitutional study. Congenital Heart Surgeons Society. J Am Coll Cardiol 1993;22:183.

Rao PS: Long-term follow-up results after balloon dilatation of pulmonic stenosis, aortic stenosis, and coarctation of the aorta: a review. Prog Cardiovasc Dis 1999;42:59.

Rao PS: Balloon valvuloplasty in the neonate with critical pulmonary stenosis. J Am Coll Cardiol 1996;27:473.

AORTIC STENOSIS

Four types of congenital aortic stenosis are generally recognized (Figure 19–26). Valvular aortic stenosis is the most common type; subaortic and supravalvular aortic stenosis and asymmetric septal hypertrophy occur infrequently.

1. Valvular Aortic Stenosis

ESSENTIALS OF DIAGNOSIS

- *Usually asymptomatic in children; angina and syncope indicate severe stenosis.*
- *May cause severe heart failure in infants.*
- *Prominent left ventricular impulse; narrow pulse pressure.*
- *Harsh systolic murmur and thrill along left sternal border; systolic ejection click.*

General Considerations

Valvular aortic stenosis accounts for approximately 5% of congenital heart anomalies and is the only type of aortic stenosis that occurs in neonates, accounting for approximately 10% of cases. The clinical characteristics of neonatal critical aortic stenosis differ from those of valvular stenosis in older children in several respects. In neonates, the valve is often unicommissural or bicommissural, and associated anomalies, including other left-sided obstructive lesions, are usually present. Profound clinical deterioration occurs after ductal closure, with severe left ventricular failure, subendocardial ischemia, and endocardial fibroelastosis. In older children, the valve is more frequently tricommissural, and associated anomalies are less common. Most children are asymptomatic, and symptoms, when present—with the exception of sudden death—typically evolve less acutely.

Clinical Findings

Children with severe stenosis develop dyspnea, angina, or syncope with effort. Newborns with aortic stenosis have severe heart failure, variable degrees of cyanosis, metabolic acidosis, and associated respiratory distress. A harsh basilar systolic murmur with thrill along the left sternal border is a common finding. The murmur may at times be inaudible because of heart failure and low cardiac output. In older children, chest radiographs are normal or show only left ventricular hypertrophy. The ascending aorta may be dilated. In the infant, the cardiac silhouette is usually large, and pulmonary venous congestion is present. Echocardiography provides the essential diagnostic information.

Treatment

Valvular stenosis cannot be treated medically. In neonates, clinical presentation alone is the indication to intervene in most cases. In older children, indications include a pressure gradient between the left ventricle and ascending aorta of 50 mm Hg or greater; symptoms of syncope, heart failure, and aborted sudden death; and ischemic electrocardiographic changes. Available interventions include various surgical procedures or balloon dilation. In neonates, suitability for restoration of biventricular physiology can be difficult to ascertain. After initiation of prostaglandin therapy for maintenance or restoration of ductal patency, balloon dilation is typically the initial effort to restore biventricular function in neonates. Other surgeons prefer initial surgical valvotomy with the patient supported on cardiopulmonary bypass. The success of either technique ulti-

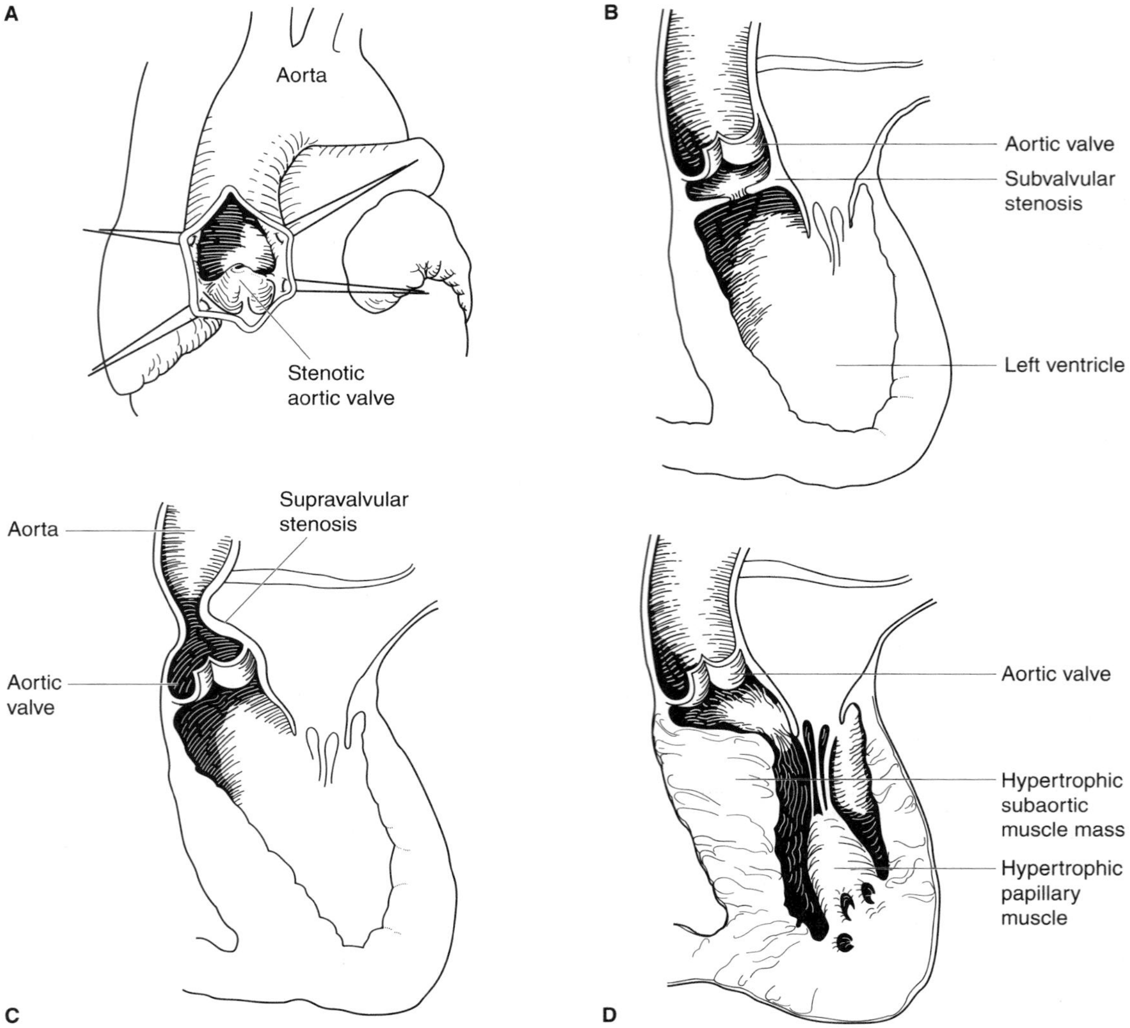

Figure 19–26. Types of congenital aortic stenosis. ***A:*** Valvular aortic stenosis. ***B:*** Subaortic stenosis (discrete fibrous band). ***C:*** Supravalvular aortic stenosis. ***D:*** Hypertrophic obstructive cardiomyopathy.

mately depends on selection of patients appropriate for two-ventricle physiology. For the older child, valve replacement is usually necessary. A variety of replacement options are available, including bioprostheses (stented and unstented porcine and pericardial valves; aortic homografts), pulmonary autografts (Ross procedure), or bileaflet mechanical prostheses.

Prognosis

In general, surgical or balloon valvotomy of a critically stenotic valve in the neonate is not curative. Ultimately, the valve will undergo progressive thickening and stenosis or insufficiency. Mortality ranges between 10% and 40%. Of those surviving, 30–50% will require repeat valvotomy or valve replacement in 5–10 years. Thus, scheduled follow-up is necessary to determine the rate and degree of restenosis or insufficiency. Prognosis after valve repair, a preferred option, is substantially better in the older child, with mortality less than 5%. However, long-term confirmation of durability remains unconfirmed. Results are also good with mechanical replacement, with the acknowledgment that issues of growth of the patient as well as structural deterioration of the valve will necessitate eventual valve replacement. The pulmonary autograft (Ross procedure) is a favored option in children and offers growth potential and freedom from anticoagulation and synthetic surfaces. The pulmonary allograft that is used to replace the harvested autograft remains a source of concern, potentially requiring reintervention when the child is older.

2. Subaortic Stenosis

Subaortic stenosis may exist in two forms: discrete and diffuse subaortic stenosis. The discrete form is more common, consisting of a membranous or fibromuscular ring of tissue located beneath the aortic annulus. Other anomalies may coexist, particularly left-sided obstructive lesions (mitral stenosis, aortic coarctation) associated with the diffuse form. The pathophysiology of left ventricular outflow tract obstruction leads to clinical manifestations similar to those of valvular stenosis. Aortic regurgitation may be seen in 20–30% of patients. The diagnosis is typically confirmed in late childhood and is rare in neonates.

Indications for operative repair include symptoms, a gradient of 50 mm Hg or greater, or evolving aortic regurgitation. Operative repair of the discrete form consists of resection of the membrane and myectomy of the septum. Fifteen-year survival is greater than 95%, with a risk of recurrent obstruction requiring reoperation of 5–20% at 15 years. Repair of the diffuse type requires more extensive modification of the outflow tract, usually with some combination of septal muscle resection, annular and outflow tract enlargement, and in some cases valve replacement, the latter procedures referred to as Konno and Ross-Konno procedures. The operative mortality and the risk of recurrence are greater for the diffuse form of stenosis and depend on the extent of the operation and the severity of associated lesions.

3. Supravalvular Aortic Stenosis

Isolated supravalvular aortic stenosis is typically in the form of an hourglass-shaped constriction of the aorta at the sinotubular junction (top of the commissures). Other forms exist, including a discrete ridge and diffuse narrowing of the entire ascending aorta (20–30% of patients). In fact, obstructive lesions can be found as well in the abdominal aorta (10% of patients) and the pulmonary vasculature or right heart outflow tract (40–70%). This distribution of lesions is due to intrinsically abnormal production of elastin in the media of vessels during development as a consequence of alterations of the elastin gene (7q11.23). It is postulated that decreased elasticity leads to increased shear stresses, leading ultimately to hyperplasia and hypertrophy of smooth muscle in the media, with decreased amounts of broken and disorganized elastin fibers. Therefore, larger arteries, subjected to greater stress, are affected more frequently. Abnormalities of the aortic valve leaflets are present in 20–40% of patients. Less commonly, the left coronary artery may demonstrate various degrees of obstruction.

Supravalvular stenosis is commonly associated with Williams-Beuren syndrome (mental retardation, distinctive facial features, and peripheral pulmonary artery stenosis). It also occurs in autosomal dominant forms and sporadic forms in which the nonvascular aspects of Williams-Beuren syndrome are absent. The various forms depend on the exact abnormality and mode of acquisition of the altered gene. In general, the dominant symptoms relate to the proximal aortic obstruction.

Various types of operative repairs are available. A synthetic or pericardial patch can be inserted to widen the area of narrowing. Another approach consists of limited resection of the stenosis, mobilization of the aorta, and tailoring the proximal and distal ends for primary anastomosis (no synthetic patch). Both techniques are associated with a low operative mortality and excellent relief of obstruction. Subsequent need for aortic valve replacement is a recognized issue. When present, obstruction of the right heart outflow tract or pulmonary vasculature has a tendency to regress with time. For severe lesions, operative repair (patch enlargement) can be conducted at the time of aortic surgery. Balloon angioplasty with or without stenting is a recognized alternative; however, the durability of this approach in this particular patient population is debated.

4. Hypertrophic Obstructive Cardiomyopathy

This genetically transmitted (autosomal dominant) disease of cardiac muscle features a spectrum of ventricular hypertrophy, typically with disproportionate thickening of the septum. The myocardial sarcomeres are hypertrophied and arranged in a bizarre pattern. Stenotic septal coronary arteries are often present. The asymmetric muscle mass may or may not cause obstruction of the left ventricular outflow tract (Figure 19–26D). Mitral regurgitation is a common associated finding. Symptomatic patients nearly always have some degree of obstruction during systole. The severity of this obstruction increases during systole and is related to the force of ventricular contraction and the cross-sectional area of the left ventricular outflow tract during systole. Exercise or various pharmacologic agents may alter these relationships and change the degree of obstruction. The common symptoms in older children are chronic fatigue, episodes of syncope and angina, and dyspnea on exertion. Signs and symptoms of severe congestive heart failure predominate in neonates, and the mortality is extremely high. However, a morphologically similar, nongenetically transmitted form of this disease exists in over 30% of infants of diabetic mothers and typically regresses in the first few months of life.

This disease is quite variable, and the natural history is not entirely predictable. Some patients improve symptomatically with chronic beta-blockade therapy (propranolol). In the pediatric patient in whom a discrete gradient can be demonstrated, operative repair is considered superior to medical therapy. This is accomplished by incising a wide or deep trough of septal muscle under the right coronary leaflet. Extensive resection can cause left bundle branch block or complete heart block. Operative mortality is low, and the need for reoperation for recurrent obstruction is less than 10% at 5 years after repair. Associated mitral regurgitation regresses in the majority of patients after relief of the outflow tract obstruction. Dual-chamber pacing is a more recently advocated alternative but is associated with less reduction in the outflow tract gradient.

Durham LA et al: Ross procedure with aortic root tailoring for aortic valve replacement in the pediatric population. Ann Thorac Surg 1997;64:482.

Gaynor JW et al: Late outcome of survivors of intervention for neonatal aortic valve stenosis. Ann Thorac Surg 1995;60:122.

Gundry SR, Behrendt DM: Prognostic factors in valvotomy for critical aortic stenosis in infancy. J Thorac Cardiovasc Surg 1986;92:747.

Lofland GK et al: Critical aortic stenosis in the neonate: a multi-institutional study of management, outcomes, and risk factors. J Thorac Cardiovasc Surg 2001;121:10.

Lupinetti FM et al: Intermediate-term results in pediatric aortic valve replacement. Ann Thorac Surg 1999;68:521.

Lupinetti FM et al: Optimum treatment of discrete subaortic stenosis. Ann Thorac Surg 1992;54:467.

McElhinney DB et al: Issues and outcomes in the management of supravalvar aortic stenosis. Ann Thorac Surg 2000;69:562.

Mosca RS et al: Critical aortic stenosis in the neonate: a comparison of balloon valvuloplasty and transventricular dilation. J Thorac Cardiovasc Surg 1995;109:147.

Serraf A et al: Surgical treatment of subaortic stenosis: a seventeen-year experience. J Thorac Cardiovasc Surg 1999;117:669.

Stamm C et al: Congenital supravalvar aortic stenosis: a simple lesion? Eur J Cardiothorac Surg 2001;19:195.

Theodoro DA et al: Hypertrophic obstructive cardiomyopathy in pediatric patients: results of surgical treatment. J Thorac Cardiovasc Surg 1996;112:1589.

COARCTATION OF THE AORTA

ESSENTIALS OF DIAGNOSIS

- *Infants may have severe heart failure; children are usually asymptomatic.*
- *Absent or weak femoral pulses.*
- *Systolic pressure higher in upper extremities than in lower extremities; diastolic pressures are similar.*
- *Harsh systolic murmur heard in the back.*

General Considerations

Coarctation of the aorta occurs in 0.2–0.6 per 1000 live births, accounting for 5–8% of congenital cardiovascular anomalies. It occurs two to five times more frequently in males. Fifteen to 30 percent of patients with Turner's syndrome have aortic coarctation. Ninety-eight percent of all aortic coarctations are located at or near the aortic isthmus (the segment of aorta adjacent to the ligamentum arteriosum or ductus arteriosus). Coarctation occurs in three general contexts: as an isolated lesion; with an associated ventricular septal defect; or with associated more severe intracardiac anomalies and more extensive involvement of the aortic arch. Even isolated coarctation has variable morphology and may present as hypoplasia of the isthmus and distal arch. Types of associated anomalies include patent foramen ovale and ductus arteriosus (assumed as part of the anomaly in neonates), ventricular septal defect, bicuspid aortic valve (40% patients), and Shone's syndrome. As a rule, the incidence and severity of associated lesions is inversely proportionate to the age at presentation. Associated anomalies occur in over 70% of neonates and in as few as 10–15% of older children. Theories attempting to explain the embryology and etiology of coarctation describe the effects of decreased flow through the aorta secondary to more proximal left-sided obstruction and the effects of ductal closure and ectopic ductal tissue in the wall of the aorta. No single theory offers an adequate explanation for the spectrum of coarctation morphology.

The general pathophysiology is distal arch–proximal thoracic aortic obstruction. This leads to systolic and diastolic hypertension in the proximal aorta and increased left ventricular afterload. Eventually, collateral vessels develop to maintain distal perfusion. In the neonate, distal flow can be maintained by a patent ductus arteriosus. If left untreated, approximately 50% of patients with isolated coarctation will die by 30 years of age. The common causes of death include congestive heart failure, endocarditis, aortic rupture, and intracranial hemorrhage.

Clinical Findings

The hemodynamic consequences of coarctation of the aorta depend on the rate of closure of the ductus, the severity of obstruction, the development of collaterals, and the presence and severity of associated anomalies. There appear to be two distinct clinical presentations: patients who present in early infancy and those who present in later childhood. Infants with coarctation may have severe congestive heart failure and sudden cardiovascular collapse with ductal closure, necessitating maintenance of ductal patency with prostaglandin E_1.

Many older children with coarctation are asymptomatic and well-developed. Complaints of headache, pains in the calves when running, or frequent nosebleeds are common. Most of these children have hypertension in the upper extremities, and many have electrocardiographic evidence of left ventricular hypertrophy. The classic findings of notched ribs (secondary to enlarged intercostals vessels, seen in children over 4 years of age) or the "reversed 3" sign are seen less frequently in the modern era of earlier diagnosis. When the disorder is suspected, echocardiography is usually sufficient to confirm the diagnosis. Magnetic resonance imaging is another useful modality.

Treatment

With modern surgical techniques and the risk of deleterious consequences of hypertension increasing with age, most surgeons advocate correction soon after confirmation of the diagnosis. In the seriously ill neonate, administration of prostaglandin, mechanical ventilation, administration of bicarbonate and inotropes, and restoration of adequate organ perfusion are critical aspects of management prior to surgical correction. Options for coarctation repair include the following: (1) resection with end-to-end anastomosis; (2) extended resection with primary anastomosis; (3) various versions of subclavian flap aortoplasty with or without concomitant extended resection; (4) patch aortoplasty with polytetrafluoroethylene (Gore-Tex) or Dacron; (5) resection and interposition graft; and (6) percutaneous balloon dilation. Most authors agree that no single technique is optimal for all types of coarctation repair. General principles to consider for first-time repair include resection of the stenotic region and ductal tissue, adequate mobilization to avoid undue tension on suture lines, an attempt to avoid prosthetic material, maintenance of growth potential, and good post-repair patency with no residual pressure gradient across the repair. The timing of repair of associated anomalies is a debated issue. The superiority of staged repair (eg, banding the pulmonary artery for a ventricular septal defect at the time of coarctation repair) versus a single-stage repair via a median sternotomy (bypass, coarctation repair, septal defect closure) continues to be debated; however, there may be a trend toward single-stage repair.

Extended resection via primary repair via a left thoracotomy is a preferred approach in neonates and infants and accommodates various degrees of arch hypoplasia. Extended mobilization of both the descending aorta and the aortic arch proximal to the innominate artery is critical to the success of this technique.

For the young child and a more discrete isolated coarctation, excision with primary repair is a reasonable approach. For the adolescent in whom adequate mobilization may be more difficult, particularly in a reoperative situation, resection with an interposition graft or patch aortoplasty are alternatives.

The experience with balloon angioplasty (with or without stenting in an older child) continues to evolve. With careful patient selection and advanced interventional experience, good results can be obtained. At present, it remains a more selectively applied approach. It continues, however, to be the preferred option for recoarctation (gradient greater than or equal to 20 mm Hg). In most cases, aortography and balloon angioplasty can be performed safely and effectively, thereby eliminating the need for reoperation.

Prognosis

Mortality is variable and depends on the severity of associated anomalies. In general, operative and 2- to 5-year survival is well over 95% but may be as low as 40–50% with an associated severe anomaly. Recurrent coarctation occurs in 5–20% of patients, usually in the first year after repair, and depends on the degree of arch hypoplasia and the technique of repair. Potential complications or morbidity include hemorrhage, damage to the recurrent laryngeal nerve, Horner's syndrome, chylothorax, paraplegia (rare), and various complications related to sacrifice of the subclavian artery (uncommon in young acyanotic patients). Postoperative hypertension is another recognized morbidity. Paradoxic hypertension occurs immediately postoperatively and is often transient. A second phase may evolve days after surgery and may persist. Persistent hypertension is believed to be less common if repair is performed early in life. These forms of postoperative hypertension are believed related to changes in sympathetic tone, baroreceptor sensitivity, and the renin-aldosterone system. Pressure should be carefully monitored, and hypertension should be appropriately treated. There is a recognized risk of postoperative mesenteric vasculitis that may be minimized with good blood pressure control.

Amato JJ et al: Role of extended aortoplasty related to the definition of coarctation of the aorta. Ann Thorac Surg 1991;52:615.

Bacha EA et al: Surgery for coarctation of the aorta in infants weighing less than 2 kg. Ann Thorac Surg 2001;71:1260.

Conte S et al: Surgical management of neonatal coarctation. J Thorac Cardiovasc Surg 1995;109:663.

Dietl CA et al: Risk of recoarctation in neonates and infants after repair with patch aortoplasty, subclavian flap, and combination resection-flap procedure. J Thorac Cardiovasc Surg 1992; 103:724.

Quaegebeur JM et al: Outcomes in seriously ill neonates with coarctation of the aorta: a multiinstitutional study. J Thorac Cardiovasc Surg 1994;108:841.

Rao PS et al: Role of balloon angioplasty in the treatment of aortic coarctation. Ann Thorac Surg 1991;52:621.

Sharma BK et al: Coarctation repair in neonates with subclavian-sparing advancement flap. Ann Thorac Surg 1992;54:137.

INTERRUPTED AORTIC ARCH

Absence of the aortic arch distal to the left subclavian artery (type A, 35%), between the left carotid and left subclavian artery (type B, 60%), or between the innominate and left carotid artery (type C, 5%) is an uncommon but severe form of developmental obstruction within the aorta. The distal aorta receives blood from the patent ductus that may constrict shortly after birth and thus limit flow to the lower extremities. This lesion is almost always accompanied by other intracardiac anomalies such as ventricular septal defect, truncus arteriosus, aortopulmonary window, subaortic stenosis, or transposition of the great vessels. Type B interruption is frequently associated with an aberrant right subclavian artery. Most of these patients are symptomatic in the first few days of life, require prostaglandin E_1 for hemodynamic stabilization, and require early operation for correction. Although staged repair is a reasonable option, the current trend is to repair the arch as well as intracardiac anomalies during the first operation.

Jonas RA et al: Outcomes in patients with interrupted aortic arch and ventricular septal defect: a multiinstitutional study. J Thorac Cardiovasc Surg 1994;107:1099.

Luciani GB et al: One-stage repair of interrupted aortic arch, ventricular septal defect, and subaortic obstruction in the neonate: a novel approach. J Thorac Cardiovasc Surg 1996;111:348.

Serraf A et al: Repair of interrupted aortic arch: a ten-year experience. J Thorac Cardiovasc Surg 1996;112:1150.

HYPOPLASTIC LEFT HEART SYNDROME

ESSENTIALS OF DIAGNOSIS

- *Newborn respiratory distress with varying degrees of cyanosis and hemodynamic failure.*
- *Echocardiographic findings of atretic or stenotic aortic and mitral valves, hypoplastic left ventricle and ascending aorta.*

General Considerations

Hypoplastic left heart syndrome is a spectrum of underdevelopment of left-sided structures, including the mitral and aortic valves, the left ventricle, and the ascending aorta and aortic arch. It accounts for 5–7% of congenital cardiac anomalies and up to 25% of cardiac mortality in the first few days of life. In the more common form of this syndrome, there is atresia of the mitral and aortic valves; the left ventricle is markedly hypoplastic; and the ascending aorta measures 2–3.5 mm. The coronary arteries originate and branch normally but may be stenotic in some cases (aortic atresia, mitral stenosis). The newborn is dependent on a patent interatrial communication and ductus arteriosus. In general, other cardiac anomalies are uncommon. Autopsy data suggest that up to 25% of these children may have developmental abnormalities of the central nervous system as well as various genetically defined disorders. This syndrome is uniformly fatal without intervention. Prenatal diagnosis facilitates counseling and support of parents and is part of a well-prepared multidisciplinary approach to the care of these children.

Clinical Features

The entire cardiac output delivered from the right heart must supply systemic and pulmonary blood flow in a balance that maintains adequate oxygenation of the blood (pulmonary flow) and systemic oxygen delivery. This precarious situation is invariably disrupted by closure of the ductus or an inadequate interatrial communication. The result is respiratory failure, hemodynamic failure, metabolic acidosis, and other organ system failure (gut, kidney). Echocardiography is usually sufficient to confirm the diagnosis. Criteria to reliably distinguish between isolated aortic stenosis and hypoplastic left heart syndrome are under investigation. More so recently, prenatal echocardiographic diagnosis facilitates prenatal counseling and referral to centers with expertise in providing care for these children.

Treatment

Initial management entails resuscitation with mechanical ventilation; judicious use of fluids, pressors, and bicarbonate; and, most importantly, maintenance of ductal patency with prostaglandin infusion. If there is evidence of inadequate mixing, a balloon atrial septostomy can be performed. The fraction of inspired oxygen should be 0.21 or less, and hyperventilation should be avoided. Two types of surgical therapy are currently available for these children—staged reconstruction or transplantation (described elsewhere in this text). Staged reconstruction consists of a Norwood procedure in the neonatal period followed by a Glenn or hemi-Fontan procedure when the child is approximately 6–8 months of age (or 6–8 kg). Staged reconstruction is completed with a Fontan procedure at about 1.5–3 years of age. At the first stage, the pulmonary bifurcation is separated from the main pulmonary artery; the proximal aorta and pulmonary artery are joined; and the remaining aortic arch is reconstructed with pericardium or pulmonary allograft material. An atrial septostomy is also performed. Pulmonary blood flow is provided by a systemic arterial or right ventricular to pulmonary artery shunt. The second stage provides relief of volume overload on the right heart by connecting the superior vena cava to the pulmonary artery and, most commonly, dividing the shunt to the pulmonary artery. Finally, the Fontan procedure directs inferior caval flow to the pulmonary artery, thereby completing the diversion of systemic venous return directly to the pulmonary artery. These children are followed closely, with echocardiographic and angiographic studies being performed prior to each subsequent stage to ensure suitable candidacy for each stage of repair. A more recently described technique for stage 1, stenting the duct and banding the branch pulmonary arteries, offers the advantage of avoiding bypass, but has not yet gained widespread acceptance.

Prognosis

Short-term and intermediate-term outcomes have consistently improved for these children in the past 2 decades. In general, survival at 5 years ranges from 40% to 70%, most deaths occurring soon after the first stage of repair. For those centers with dedicated programs for either staged reconstruction or transplantation, there is no significant difference in 5-year survival rates.

Iannettoni MD et al: Improving results with first-stage palliation for hypoplastic left heart syndrome. J Thorac Cardiovasc Surg 1994;107:934.

Mosca RS et al: Early results of the Fontan procedure in one hundred consecutive patients with hypoplastic left heart syndrome. J Thorac Cardiovasc Surg 2000;119:1110.

Norwood WI: Hypoplastic left heart syndrome. Ann Thorac Surg 1991;52:688.

Norwood WI et al: Fontan procedure for hypoplastic heart syndrome. Ann Thorac Surg 1992;54:1025.

Razzouk AJ et al: Transplantation as a primary treatment for hypoplastic left heart syndrome: intermediate-term results. Ann Thorac Surg 1996;62:1.

Sano S et al: Right ventricle-pulmonary artery shunt in first stage of palliation for hypoplastic left heart syndrome. J Thorac Cardiovasc Surg 2003;126:504.

Starnes VA et al: Current approach to hypoplastic heart syndrome: palliation, transplantation, or both? J Thorac Cardiovasc Surg 1992;104:189.

Tchervenkov CI et al: Congenital Heart Surgery Nomenclature and Database Project: hypoplastic left heart syndrome. Ann Thorac Surg 2000;69:S170.

Weldner PW et al: The Norwood operation and subsequent Fontan operation in infants with complex congenital heart disease. J Thorac Cardiovasc Surg 1995;109:654.

CONGENITAL MITRAL VALVE DISEASE

Congenital mitral valve stenosis or insufficiency is an uncommon form of congenital heart disease with a wide spectrum of abnormalities and continues to be a surgical challenge. Associated anomalies are present in the majority of patients, including ventricular septal defect, atrial septal defect, and coarctation of the aorta. Insufficiency is usually associated with a dilated annulus and restricted leaflet motion due to shortened chordae and leaflet hypoplasia. In mitral stenosis, multiple levels of the valvular apparatus are typically involved, including supravalvular ring, parachute valve, commissural fusion, short chordae, and fused papillary muscles. Shone's anomaly is a recognized syndrome consisting of supravalvar mitral ring, parachute mitral valve, subaortic stenosis, and coarctation of the aorta.

Surgical treatment is indicated for severe symptoms. If feasible, repair—rather than replacement—is a preferred option. Replacement is more likely to be necessary in the case of severe stenosis. Regardless of the type of procedure, careful assessment should be performed to ensure adequate function before leaving the operating room. Valve replacement can provide marked relief of symptoms and, indeed, may be necessary. However, replacement commits the patient to some form of anticoagulation and the need for subsequent repeat replacement when the valve is outgrown. Recent evidence suggests that oversizing the valve to compensate for growth of the child is actually associated with increased mortality. Repair, on the other hand, is associated with a need for reintervention in 25–50% of patients. Balloon valvuloplasty has been described for stenotic lesions; however, the durability of this approach remains to be verified.

Bolling SF et al: Shone's anomaly: operative results and late outcome. Ann Thorac Surg 1990;49:887.

Sousa Uva M et al: Surgery for congenital mitral valve disease in the first year of life. J Thorac Cardiovasc Surg 1995;109:164.

Yoshimura N et al: Surgery for mitral valve disease in the pediatric age group. J Thorac Cardiovasc Surg 1999;118:99.

Zias EA et al: Surgical repair of the congenitally malformed mitral valve in infants and children. Ann Thorac Surg 1998;66:1551.

COR TRIATRIATUM

In this rare anomaly, the pulmonary veins enter an accessory venous chamber demarcated from the true left atrium by a diaphragm. There is typically an obstructive orifice connecting the chamber to the left atrium. Less commonly, the chamber connects to the right atrium. A left-sided superior vena cava is a common finding. The pathophysiology is that of pulmonary venous hypertension, pulmonary congestion, and elevated pulmonary artery pressure. Typically, respiratory compromise occurs early in life. Surgical excision of the membrane corrects the abnormality. With attentive postoperative care and control of pulmonary blood pressure, the prognosis is quite good.

Herlong JR et al: Congenital Heart Surgery Nomenclature and Database Project: pulmonary venous anomalies. Ann Thorac Surg 2000;69:S56.

Salomone G et al: Cor triatriatum: clinical presentation and operative results. J Thorac Cardiovasc Surg 1991;101:1088.

van Son JA et al: Cor triatriatum: diagnosis, operative approach, and late results. Mayo Clin Proc 1993;68:854.

CONGENITAL HEART LESIONS THAT INCREASE PULMONARY ARTERIAL BLOOD FLOW

Approximately 50% of all congenital heart lesions shunt blood from the systemic arterial circulation into the pulmonary circulation (left-to-right shunt). The most common lesions in this group are patent ductus arteriosus, defects of the atrial and ventricular septum, and atrioventricular canal. Rare lesions include ruptured sinus of Valsalva, aortopulmonary window, truncus arteriosus, some types of transposition of the great vessels, double outlet right ventricle, and other more complex lesions.

Differential compliances and pressures between right- and left-sided structures promote shunting of oxygenated blood through abnormal communications to the right heart or pulmonary artery and recirculation through the lungs. The excessive pulmonary circulation causes pulmonary vascular congestion, resulting in frequent respiratory infections, and places an additional volume load on the involved ventricle.

Increased pulmonary blood flow more significantly promotes the development of pulmonary vascular obstructive disease. Elevated flow and pressure lead to endothelial damage or activation—which, in turn, alters smooth muscle cell physiology in the media, leading to hypertrophy of the media of pulmonary arterioles (stage 1), proliferation of intima (stage 2), and, eventually, hyalinization and fibrosis of the intima (stage 3). These morphologic changes, termed pulmonary vascular obstructive disease, are acquired, but they are more likely to occur in congenital lesions producing both high pulmonary arterial pressure and flows (ventricular septal defect, complete atrioventricular canal, truncus arteriosus) than in those producing increased pulmonary blood flow only (atrial septal defect). As the cross-sectional area of the pulmonary vascular bed decreases as a result of the morphologic changes, pulmonary vascular resistance increases and the ratio of pulmonary vascular resistance to systemic vascular resistance also increases. The amount of blood shunted from left to right decreases. When pulmonary vascular resistance equals or exceeds systemic vascular resistance, left-to-right blood flow across the lesion ceases or reverses. In Eisenmenger's syndrome, obstruction of the pulmonary vasculature reduces pulmonary blood flow and causes blood to shunt from right to left. Patients who have advanced pulmonary vascular disease and reversed shunts (Eisenmenger's syndrome) are not candidates for surgery other than lung or heart-lung transplantation.

Pulmonary arterial banding is a palliative operation designed to reduce pulmonary blood flow by placing an anatomically fixed resistance to blood flow across the lungs. The band constricts the main pulmonary artery downstream to the valve and adds a resistance in series to the vascular resistance of the lung. Because of dynamic changes in cardiac output and pressure and resistance within the circulation, addition of a fixed resistance (the band) cannot produce balanced pulmonary and systemic flows under all physiologic conditions. However, a good band can reduce pulmonary arterial blood flow sufficiently to alleviate ventricular failure and prevent rapid progression of pulmonary vascular disease. Unfortunately, preexisting pulmonary vascular disease may not regress after banding. Pulmonary artery banding is only palliative and is used only when other options are not available or are associated with excessive risk.

Horowitz MD et al: Pulmonary arterial banding: analysis of a 25 year experience. Ann Thorac Surg 1989;48:444.

Rabinovitch M: Pathobiology of pulmonary hypertension: impact on clinical management. Pediatr Card Surg Ann Semin Thorac Cardiovasc Surg 2000;3:63.

ATRIAL SEPTAL DEFECT, OSTIUM SECUNDUM TYPE

ESSENTIALS OF DIAGNOSIS

- *Acyanotic, asymptomatic.*
- *Right ventricular lift.*
- *S_2 widely split and fixed.*
- *Grade 1–3/6 pulmonary systolic ejection murmur.*
- *Diastolic flow murmur at the lower left sternal border.*

General Considerations

Ostium secundum defects occur in the region of the fossa ovalis and may be single or multiple. Secundum defects are the most common and, usually, the largest of the atrial septal defects. Defects near the connection to the superior vena cava or inferior vena cava, often associated with partial anomalous pulmonary venous return, are referred to as sinus venosus defects. A patch is used in the repair of many of these atrial defects. For sinus venosus defects, the patch can usually be positioned to baffle the pulmonary venous blood to the left atrium (Figure 19–27).

Heart failure from uncomplicated ostium secundum defects may occur in young children but is less common in adults. Pulmonary vascular disease is also rare, but atrial dysrhythmias are noted with increasing age. The average life expectancy in patients with untreated atrial septal defects is reduced because of right ventricular failure, dysrhythmias, and occasionally pulmonary vascular disease.

Treatment

Most ostium secundum defects should be closed. The optimal time for closure is a debated issue. Paradoxic embolism and endocarditis are small risks associated with delaying repair. Many surgeons advocate proceeding with repair in late infancy or in the second year of life. The issue has changed somewhat more recently with the availability of transluminal percutaneous devices that may be placed in children who have attained an appropriate size (approximately 10 kg or more). In fact, a large percentage of isolated secundum defects are now closed using this technique. For the child in whom device closure is not an option, repair can easily be done on cardiopulmonary bypass using a patch of pericardium, polytetrafluoroethylene (Gore-Tex), or Dacron if primary closure is not feasible. The introduction of minimal access approaches allows surgery to be performed with a much smaller incision and potentially less morbidity. The prognosis after surgical closure is excellent. Although long-term follow-up is not yet available, short-term results of percutaneous device closure are equally promising.

Anderson RH et al: Sinus venosus defect. Am Heart J 1994;128:365.

Berger F et al: Comparison of results and complications of surgical and Amplatzer device closure of atrial septal defects. J Thorac Cardiovasc Surg 1999;118:674.

Jacobs JP et al: Congenital Heart Surgery Nomenclature and Database Project: atrial septal defect. Ann Thorac Surg 2000;69:S18.

Nicholson IA et al: Minimal sternotomy approach for congenital heart operations. Ann Thorac Surg 2001;71:469.

Verrier ED: Secundum atrial defects. In: *Current Therapy in Cardiothoracic Surgery,* vol 1. Grillo HC et al (editors). Bryan Decker, 1989.

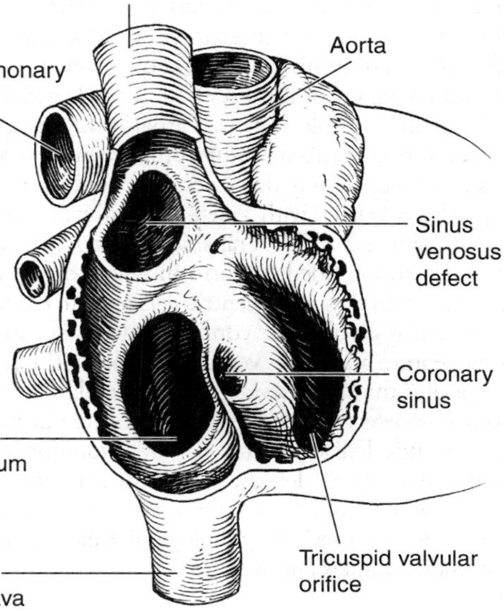

Figure 19–27. Sinus venosus and ostium secundum defects in the atrial septum as viewed from the opened right atrium.

ATRIOVENTRICULAR CANAL DEFECT

ESSENTIALS OF DIAGNOSIS

- *Heart failure common in infancy.*
- *Cardiomegaly, blowing pansystolic murmur, other variable murmurs.*
- *Loud S_2 with fixed splitting.*
- *Electrocardiography shows left axis deviation and a counterclockwise frontal QRS vector loop.*

General Considerations

Atrioventricular canal defect is a deficiency of tissue in the central region of the heart composed of the lower portion of the atrial septum (septum primum), the upper portion of the ventricular septum, and the adjoining components of the left and right atrioventricular valves (LAVV, RAVV: they are not morphologically normal mitral and tricuspid valves). Normal canal development is based on proliferation of endocardial cushion tissue as well as conal tissue, which contributes to formation of the valves. Various aspects of the embryologic process can fail, thereby leading to a spectrum of defects depending on whether one or all three components are affected and to what degree. Anomalies of the atrioventricular valves can range from a cleft in the septal region of the LAVV to a single atrioventricular valve with multiple leaflets. Partial atrioventricular canal defect, formerly called septum primum atrial septal defect, is a deficiency of only the lower aspect of the atrial septum, typically associated with a cleft or commissure in the septal region of the LAVV. Transitional atrioventricular canal defect is an intermediate form in which minor deficiency also occurs in the upper ventricular septum. Complete atrioventricular canal defect consists of deficiency in the lower atrial septum and upper ventricular septum (Figure 19–28). Typically, the more severe valve anomalies are seen with complete defect. Associated anomalies are not uncommon and include left superior vena cava, additional muscular ventricular septal defects, left ventricular outflow tract obstruction, anomalous pulmonary venous connections, patent ductus arteriosus, tetralogy of Fallot, and other less common complex anomalies.

Clinical Findings

The pathophysiology is that of a left-to-right shunt potentially modified by LAVV regurgitation. The severity depends on the degree of abnormality of each structural component of the canal. For partial atrioventricular canal defect, symptoms may be minimal to absent, whereas for an untreated complete defect life expectancy is less than 1 year because of death from congestive heart failure. Pulmonary vascular obstructive disease and progressive LAVV regurgitation are recognized in the natural history of this anomaly. Certain features of this anomaly are modified or exacerbated when it occurs in a child with trisomy 21 (40–60% of surgical cases). Deficiency of valve tissue and obstruction of inflow and outflow of the left ventricle may be less common; however, these children may be more prone to earlier development of pulmonary vascular obstructive disease. Although specific electrocardiographic findings have been described, echocardiography is the best modality for delineating the anatomy. Cardiac catheterization may be needed in infants over 6 months of age in whom pulmonary vascular disease is more of a concern.

Treatment

Surgical correction is indicated, with timing dictated by the degree of the anomaly and symptoms. For complete atrioventricular canal defect, repair is generally performed before 6 months of age. Although repair may be delayed for the asymptomatic child with a partial defect, most surgeons advocate repair by 1 year of age. LAVV regurgitation is also an indication to proceed with repair

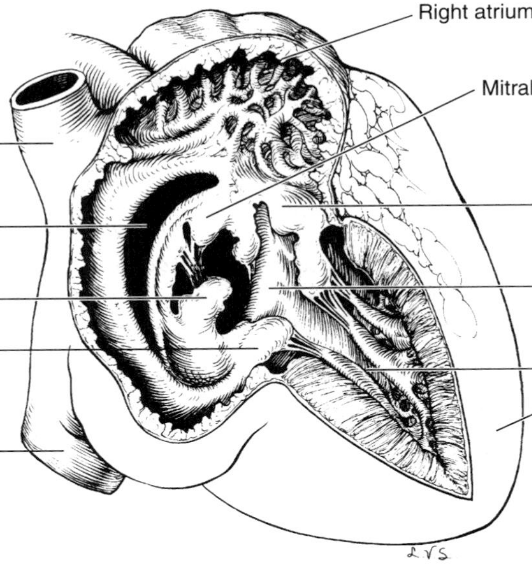

Figure 19–28. Complete atrioventricular canal. The most common type has a divided anterior bridging leaflet. Both the left and right valvular components are attached to the interventricular septum with long, nonfused chordae tendineae. The left and right components of the posterior bridging leaflet are not separated. (Modified from Rastelli GC et al: Surgical repair of the complete form of persistent common atrioventricular canal. J Thorac Cardiovasc Surg 1968;55:299.)

regardless of age. Surgical treatment is directed by the severity of the anomaly. For partial atrioventricular canal defect, repair consists of patch closure, typically using pericardium, and closure of the LAVV cleft, although the merit of the latter if the valve is not insufficient continues to be debated. Transitional or complete atrioventricular canal defect requires patch closure of the septal defects (using single- or double-patch technique) and repair or reconstruction of abnormal valves (suture closure of LAVV cleft with or without annuloplasty).

Prognosis

Mortality varies with the degree of defect, associated cardiac anomalies, age at the time of surgery, and postrepair status of the LAVV. For partial defect, operative mortality is rare, and 10-year survival is greater than 98%. For complete atrioventricular canal defect, operative mortality is approximately 3–5%, with over 90% 10-year survival. An important complication of repair is complete heart block, occurring in 3–5% of patients. The incidence and severity of postoperative LAVV regurgitation is variable (10–40%), with approximately 20% ultimately requiring reoperation. It is expected that many of these children may need additional mitral valve work in adulthood.

Agny M et al: Repair of partial atrioventricular septal defect in children less than five years of age: late results. Ann Thorac Surg 1999;67:1412.

Anderson RH et al: The diagnostic features of atrioventricular septal defect with common atrioventricular junction. Cardiol Young 1998;8:33.

Backer CL et al: Repair of complete atrioventricular canal defects: results with the two-patch technique. Ann Thorac Surg 1995;60:530.

Jacobs JP et al: Congenital Heart Surgery Nomenclature and Database Project: atrioventricular canal defect. Ann Thorac Surg 2000;69:S36.

Najm HK et al: Primum atrial septal defect in children: early results, risk factors, and freedom from reoperation. Ann Thorac Surg 1998;66:829.

Nicholson IA et al: Simplified single patch technique for the repair of atrioventricular septal defect. J Thorac Cardiovasc Surg 1999;118:642.

Reddy VM et al: Atrioventricular valve function after single patch repair of complete atrioventricular septal defect in infancy: how early should repair be attempted? J Thorac Cardiovasc Surg 1998;115:1032.

VENTRICULAR SEPTAL DEFECT

ESSENTIALS OF DIAGNOSIS

- *Asymptomatic if defect is small.*
- *Heart failure with dyspnea, frequent respiratory infections, and poor growth if the defect is large.*
- *Grade 2–6/6 pansystolic murmur maximal at the left sternal border.*
- *S_2 loud with apical diastolic flow murmur and biventricular enlargement if the defect is large.*

General Considerations

Ventricular septal defect is common, accounting for approximately 15–20% of congenital cardiac anomalies. These defects occur in four anatomic positions in the ventricular septum. About 85% occur in the area of the membranous septum (Figure 19–29) (perimembranous). A much smaller percentage of defects occur anterior or distal to the crista supraventricularis (supracristal, conal, or outlet), beneath the septal leaflet of the tricuspid valve (canal or inlet), or in the muscular ventricular septum (muscular).

Ventricular septal defects are often one component of another more complex congenital heart lesion such as truncus arteriosus, atrioventricular canal defect, tetralogy of Fallot, or transposition of the great arteries. Patients with isolated perimembranous defects may have extracardiac lesions such as patent ductus arteriosus or coarctation of the aorta. Patients with outlet defects occasionally have aortic valve regurgitation.

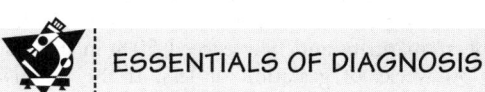

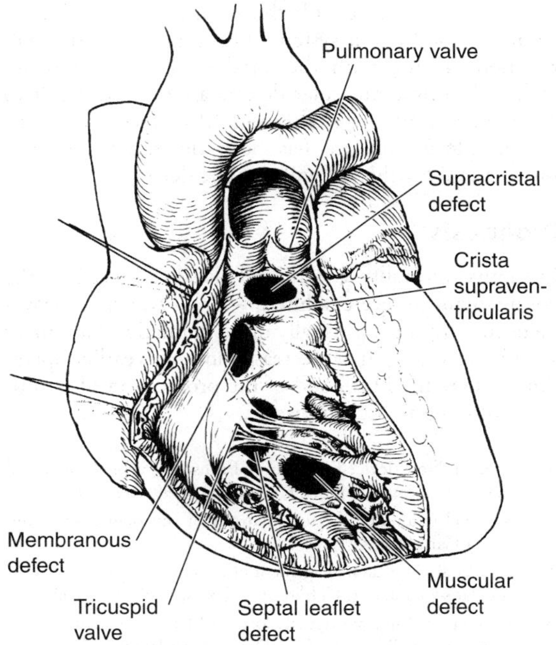

Figure 19–29. Anatomic locations of various ventricular septal defects. The wall of the right ventricle has been excised to expose the ventricular septum.

Clinical Findings

The clinical symptoms relate to pulmonary overcirculation and congestive failure—dyspnea on exertion, poor weight gain, and easy fatigability. Infants with large defects usually fail to grow and have chronic respiratory difficulties and poor feeding habits. In general, the heart is enlarged, and the lung fields are overcirculated. Pulmonary vascular disease may develop as a result of the high pressure and large flow in the lungs. In infants, approximately one-third of defects are small and asymptomatic. Many of these defects will close spontaneously, usually after 7–8 years. About one-third of patients with large or multiple defects are symptomatic in infancy and require aggressive medical management, early diagnosis, and surgical correction. Echocardiography provides sufficient diagnostic information in the majority of cases. In the older asymptomatic child with a persistent defect, consideration may be given to catheterization to assess pulmonary artery pressure and vascular resistance.

Treatment

Indications for surgery include medically refractory symptoms in the infant, elevated pulmonary artery pressure in the asymptomatic infant or older child, the presence of a canal-type defect or a malaligned defect, or the presence of aortic insufficiency with an outlet defect. Optimal treatment consists of synthetic patch closure of the defect with the suture line placed away from the conduction system. The approach is through the right atrium with the child on cardiopulmonary bypass. Multiple muscular defects are often difficult to close due to limited visualization. More recently, percutaneous device closure has been described and may prove useful for this difficult type of defect.

Prognosis

Operative mortality is rare and usually limited to the young infant in severe failure (3–5%). Overall, improvement in symptoms is usually quite dramatic. Pulmonary vascular resistance may decrease; however, earlier operation reduces the likelihood of the progression of significant pulmonary vascular disease.

Amin A et al: New device for closure of muscular ventricular septal defects in a canine model. Circulation 1999;100:320.

Anderson RH et al: The surgical anatomy of ventricular septal defect. J Card Surg 1992;7:17.

Backer CL et al: Surgical management of the conal (supracristal) ventricular septal defect. J Thorac Cardiovasc Surg 1991;102:288.

Hardin JT et al: Primary surgical closure of large ventricular septal defects in small infants. Ann Thorac Surg 1992;53:397.

Jacobs JP et al: Congenital Heart Surgery Nomenclature and Database Project: ventricular septal defect. Ann Thorac Surg 2000;69:S25.

McGrath LB et al: Methods for repair of simple isolated ventricular septal defect. J Card Surg 1991;6:13.

Mehta AVB et al: Ventricular septal defect in the first year of life. Am J Cardiol 1992;70:364.

PATENT DUCTUS ARTERIOSUS

ESSENTIALS OF DIAGNOSIS

- *Older patients with a small or moderately large patent ductus are asymptomatic and have a continuous murmur over the pulmonary area, loud S_2, and bounding peripheral pulses.*
- *Poor feeding, respiratory distress, and frequent respiratory infections in infants with heart failure.*
- *Murmur usually systolic, sometimes continuous.*
- *Widened pulse pressure.*

General Considerations

The ductus arteriosus is a normal component of fetal circulation, connecting the main or proximal left pulmonary artery to the aorta distal to the origin of the left subclavian artery. Elevated pulmonary vascular resistance in utero leads to the majority of flow being directed from the pulmonary artery to the aorta (right-to-left shunt), with the ductus carrying over 60% of the combined ventricular output. In utero, patency is maintained by high flow, prostaglandins (derived from the placenta), and relatively low arterial oxygen tension. In addition to diminished sensitivity to these factors as term approaches, three important events occur at birth: (1) Pulmonary resistance decreases, leading to increased pulmonary flow and decreased ductal flow; (2) the level of prostaglandin decreases as the child is removed from the placenta and increased metabolism occurs with increased flow through the lungs; and (3) the arterial oxygen tension increases. This leads to contraction of smooth muscle in the wall of the ductus with apposition of endothelial cushions (usually within 24 hours) and eventually anatomic closure (3–10 days).

For unknown reasons, closure does not always occur. The incidence of patent ductus is estimated at 2–3% of live births. The incidence increases with the degree of prematurity and may exceed 50% in infants born at 30 weeks of gestation or less. If the ductus remains open and pulmonary vascular resistance decreases, pulmonary blood flow will increase, leading to heart failure and pulmonary congestion. Patent ductus arteriosus also occurs in the context of other cardiac anomalies and may be the critical source of flow from the heart to the lungs or systemic organs.

Clinical Findings

Diagnosis is made by physical examination (wide pulse pressure, to-and-fro murmur) and confirmed by echocardiography. Approximately 5% of full-term infants with untreated patent ductus arteriosus die of heart failure and pulmonary complications in the first year of life. Another 5% have large shunts and ultimately develop pulmonary vascular disease. The remainder are usually asymptomatic, and the ductus is detected during routine examination. In the premature infant, clinical findings of heart failure must be delineated in the context of baseline pulmonary dysfunction of prematurity. Although a murmur is usually present, a widely patent ductus may be associated with minimal turbulence. Inability to wean from mechanical ventilation is a recognized presentation. Echocardiography is diagnostic and has been applied routinely in some centers for the high-risk patient.

Treatment

Optimal treatment depends on the age of the patient. Medical therapy is usually attempted first in the premature infant using indomethacin, a prostaglandin inhibitor, and is successful in over 50% of patients. Effectiveness diminishes with age and gestational maturity. For the term infant or older child or for the premature infant failing medical therapy, optimal treatment consists of surgical obliteration by ligation, clipping, or division through a left thoracotomy or via video thoracoscopic techniques. Transcatheter techniques to place occluding devices are also available for the larger patient. Intermediate-term data have not revealed a significant advantage of catheter-based techniques in terms of cost, effectiveness, or morbidity. More recent data may demonstrate higher success rates and fewer complications.

Prognosis

Operative mortality approaches zero, with recurrence of less than 1% in surgically treated cases. Complications such as injury to the recurrent laryngeal nerve, hemorrhage, and chylothorax are uncommon.

Backer CL et al: Congenital Heart Surgery Nomenclature and Database Project: patent ductus arteriosus, coarctation of the aorta, interrupted aortic arch. Ann Thorac Surg 2000;69:S298.

Hawkins JA et al: Cost and efficacy of surgical ligation versus transcatheter coil occlusion of patent ductus arteriosus. J Thorac Cardiovasc Surg 1996;112:1634.

Laborde F et al: A new video-assisted thoracoscopic surgical technique for interruption of patent ductus arteriosus in infants and children. J Thorac Cardiovasc Surg 1993;105:278.

Mavroudis C et al: Forty-six years of patent ductus arteriosus division at Children's Memorial Hospital of Chicago. Standards for comparison. Ann Surg 1994;220:402.

AORTOPULMONARY WINDOW

Defined as a connection between the ascending aorta and the main pulmonary artery, aortopulmonary window is a rare anomaly, producing a left-to-right shunt and physical findings very similar to those of patent ductus arteriosus. Patients develop heart failure early and are prone to develop pulmonary vascular disease at an early age. Associated anomalies occur in over 50% of patients (atrial and ventricular septal defect, interrupted aortic arch). Once diagnosed, the window should be closed with a patch (synthetic or pericardial) during cardiopulmonary bypass.

Jacobs JP et al: Congenital Heart Surgery Nomenclature and Database Project: aortopulmonary window. Ann Thorac Surg 2000;69:S44.

McElhinney DB et al: Early and late results after repair of aortopulmonary septal defect and associated anomalies in infants < 6 months of age. Am J Cardiol 1998;81:195.

RUPTURED SINUS OF VALSALVA

Rupture of the thin membranous tissue between the aortic sinus of Valsalva and an intracardiac chamber causes an immediate left-to-right shunt. The murmur is usually well localized, parasternal, and continuous, with associated thrill. Most patients rapidly develop heart failure. Rupture is more common in patients with Marfan's syndrome or other autoimmune disorders. Rupture is into the right ventricle in about 70% of cases and into the right atrium in 20%. Precise anatomic diagnosis is by cardiac catheterization and echocardiography. Early operation is indicated.

Barragry TP et al: 15–30 year follow-up of patients undergoing repair of ruptured congenital aneurysms of the sinus of Valsalva. Ann Thorac Surg 1988;46:515.

Mayer ED et al: Ruptured aneurysms of the sinus of Valsalva. Ann Thorac Surg 1986;42:81.

CORONARY ARTERIAL FISTULA

A fistulous communication between the right (60%) or left (40%) coronary artery and the right ventricle (90%), right atrium, or coronary sinus produces a left-to-right shunt and increased pulmonary blood flow. The involved coronary vessels are dilated, and the fistulous openings may be multiple. Many patients are asymptomatic; some develop evidence of myocardial ischemia, and others have some degree of heart failure. A continuous murmur is usually present over the heart. Angiograms are required to determine the number and location of the fistulas. The fistulous connections are ligated at operation without interrupting the coronary artery. Operative mortality is rare.

Mavroudis C et al: Coronary artery fistulas in infants and children: a surgical review and discussion of coil embolization. Ann Thorac Surg 1997;63:1235.

TOTAL ANOMALOUS PULMONARY VENOUS CONNECTION (TAPVC)

ESSENTIALS OF DIAGNOSIS

- *Pulmonary congestion, tachypnea, cardiac failure, and variable cyanosis.*
- *Severe heart failure, cyanosis, poor pulses, acidosis in infants.*
- *Pulmonary midsystolic murmur present, with loud, fixed splitting of S_2 in some patients.*
- *Enlargement of right atrium and ventricle with severe pulmonary vascular congestion.*
- *Blood oxygen saturation similar in aorta and pulmonary artery.*
- *Pulmonary arterial and wedge pressures elevated.*

General Considerations

The term total anomalous pulmonary venous connection (TAPVC) indicates that the pulmonary veins do not make a direct connection with the left atrium. Individual veins usually form a confluence that connects to central systemic veins, thereby draining pulmonary flow to the right atrium. The blood reaches the left atrium only through an atrial septal defect or patent foramen ovale. Mixing of blood in the right atrium leads to similar oxygen saturations in the aorta and pulmonary artery. There are three basic types of total anomalous venous return (Figure 19–30) depending on the site at which the confluence of pulmonary veins connects to the systemic venous system: (1) supracardiac (type 1)—connection to a usually left-sided vertical vein draining to the innominate vein (45%); (2) cardiac (type 2)—connection to the right atrium or coronary sinus (25%); and (3) infracardiac (type 3)—connection to the infradiaphragmatic cava or portal vein (25%). In approximately 5% of cases venous drainage is mixed, with different pulmonary veins draining to different systemic veins. Pulmonary venous obstruction occurs with all types of drainage patterns; however, it may occur more frequently in patients with an infracardiac connection

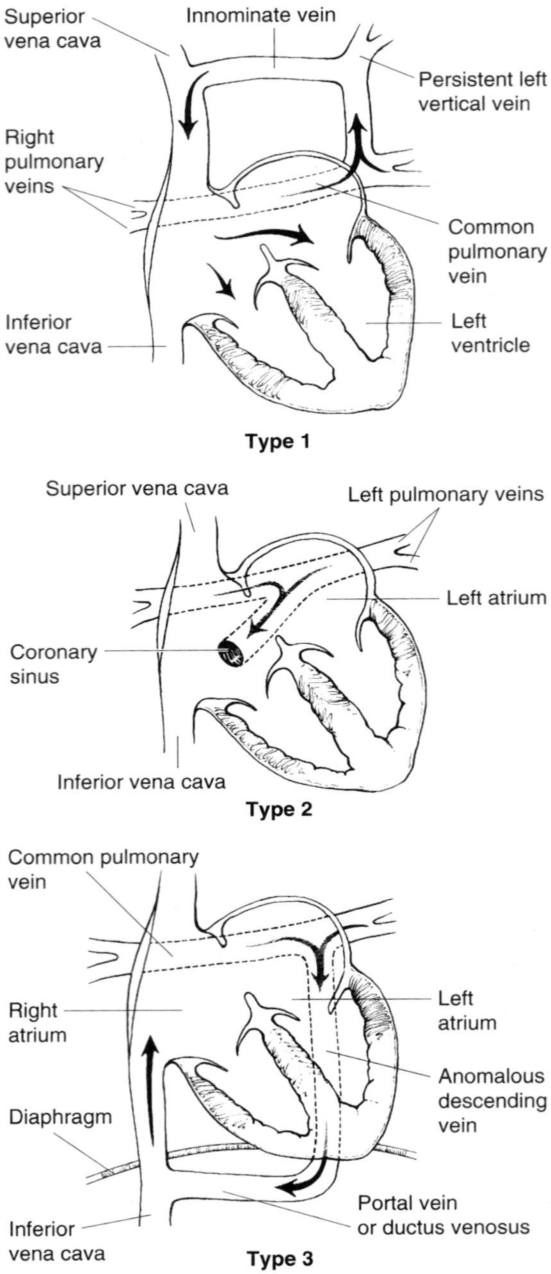

Figure 19–30. Common types of total anomalous pulmonary venous connection. ***Type 1:*** The pulmonary veins connect to a persistent left vertical vein, the innominate vein, and the right superior vena cava. ***Type 2:*** The pulmonary veins connect to the coronary sinus and the right atrium. ***Type 3:*** The pulmonary veins connect to an anomalous descending vein, a portal vein or persistent ductus venosus, and eventually the inferior vena cava.

(more than 50%). The presence of obstruction often leads to elevated pulmonary vascular resistance and is a decisive point in devising a management plan.

Clinical Findings

The presence and degree of obstruction determine the clinical presentation. If obstruction is absent, symptoms relate to the degree of pulmonary overcirculation and hypertension (poor feeding, failure to thrive, tachypnea, diaphoresis). If obstruction is severe, cyanosis, respiratory failure, and hypotension will develop in a few hours after birth. Echocardiography is diagnostic. Catheterization is reserved for cases in which anatomy is unclear after echocardiography or in which balloon septostomy is believed necessary to improve atrial mixing.

Treatment

All forms of TAPVC should be surgically repaired. Timing is dictated by the degree of obstruction. In fact, obstructed TAPVC is one of the few remaining surgical emergencies in pediatric cardiac surgery. Other than intubation and resuscitation, there is no specific medical therapy. Repair of supracardiac and infracardiac drainage is accomplished by anastomosis of the pulmonary venous confluence to the left atrium and ligation of the connection to the systemic vein. Cardiopulmonary bypass or, less frequently, deep hypothermic circulatory arrest is employed for critically ill neonates with obstruction. For TAPVC with cardiac drainage, repair can be accomplished by unroofing the coronary sinus and patch closure of the atrial septum, leaving the coronary sinus to drain to the left atrium. After repair of obstructed TAPVC, measures are employed (alkalosis, increased oxygen tension, sedation, deep analgesia, nitric oxide) to prevent or treat pulmonary artery hypertensive crises.

Prognosis

Hospital mortality is limited primarily to children with severe obstruction (10–15%). Pulmonary hypertension contributes substantially to this mortality. Although very uncommon, children with associated cardiac anomalies experience an exceptionally high mortality (> 30%). Recurrence of pulmonary obstruction occurs in approximately 5–10% of patients. Patients who survive without recurrent obstruction have good cardiac performance, minimal symptoms, and a good long-term prognosis.

Calderone CA et al: Surgical management of total anomalous pulmonary venous drainage: impact of coexisting cardiac anomalies. Ann Thorac Surg 1998;66:1521.

Cobanaglu A et al: Total anomalous pulmonary venous connection in neonates and young infants: repair in the current era. Ann Thorac Surg 1993;55:43.

Lacour-Gayet F et al: Surgical management of progressive pulmonary venous obstruction after repair of total anomalous pulmonary venous connection. J Thorac Cardiovasc Surg 1999;117:679.

COMMON ARTERIAL TRUNK

In common arterial trunk (truncus arteriosus), a single large truncal vessel overrides the ventricular septum and distributes all of the blood ejected from the heart. Although different patterns exist, the truncal root bifurcates, giving rise to a pulmonary trunk or separate pulmonary arteries and the aorta. A ventricular septal defect is present and is usually located directly beneath the truncal valve. Other associated anomalies include atrial septal defect (> 40%), interrupted aortic arch (10%), and abnormal origins of the coronary arteries. In most cases, pulmonary blood flow is increased and signs and symptoms of heart failure are present. Patients develop pulmonary vascular disease at a very early age. Echocardiography is usually sufficient for diagnosis; however, cardiac catheterization is indicated if there are abnormalities of the coronary arteries or if the child is over 3 months of age (to assess pulmonary vasculature).

Surgical correction is indicated once the diagnosis is confirmed. The only contraindication to closure of the septal defect is Eisenmenger's physiology. The principles of repair include closure of the ventricular septal defect, separation of the pulmonary arteries from the truncal root, placing a valved conduit from the right ventricle to the neopulmonary bifurcation, and correction of significant truncal insufficiency (Figure 19–31). Mortality is variable (5–30%), related to truncal valve insufficiency, interrupted arch, coronary anomalies, and pulmonary vascular disease. Survivors remain at risk for the subsequent need for repair or replacement of the truncal valve and replacement of the right ventricle–pulmonary artery conduit.

Bove EL et al: Repair of truncus arteriosus in the neonate and young infant. Ann Thorac Surg 1989;47:499.

Imamura M et al: Improving early and intermediate results of truncus arteriosus repair: a new technique of truncal valve repair. Ann Thorac Surg 1999;67:1142.

Jacobs ML: Congenital Heart Surgery Nomenclature and Database Project: truncus arteriosus. Ann Thorac Surg 2000;69:S50.

Jahangiri M et al: Repair of the truncal valve and associated interrupted arch in neonates with truncus arteriosus. J Thorac Cardiovasc Surg 2000;119:508.

Rajasinghe HA et al: Long-term follow-up of truncus arteriosus repaired in infancy: a twenty-year experience. J Thorac Cardiovasc Surg 1997;113:869.

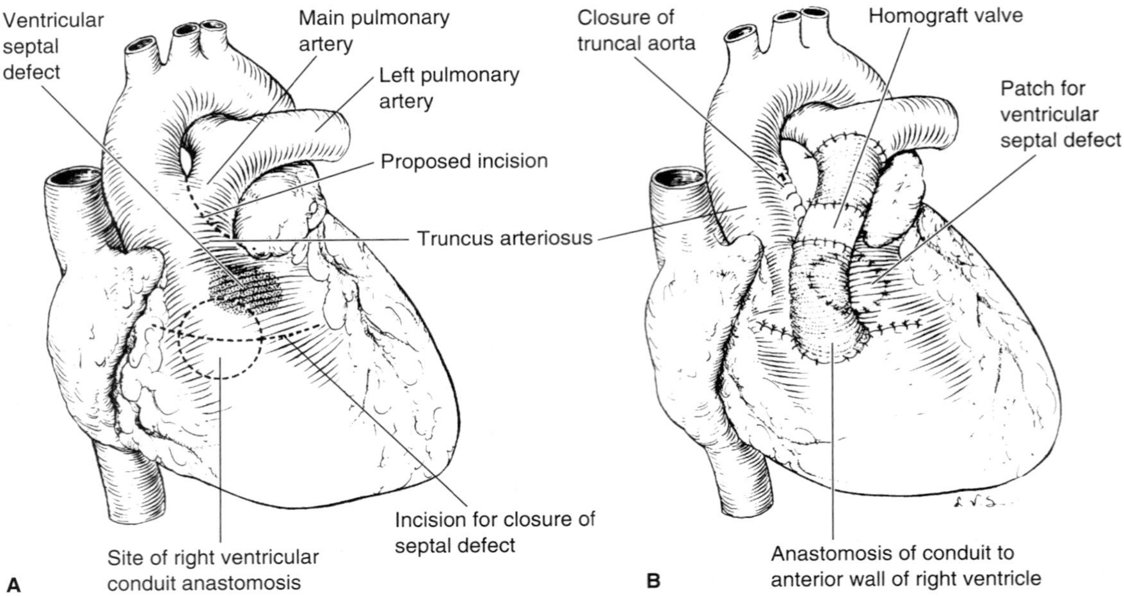

Figure 19–31. Type 1 truncus arteriosus. ***A:*** The main pulmonary artery arises from the truncus arteriosus downstream to the truncal valve. A ventricular septal defect is present. ***B:*** The main pulmonary artery is incised from the truncus. The ventricular septal defect is closed with a patch. A conduit of Dacron that contains a homograft aortic valve is sutured to the anterior wall of the right ventricle and the distal pulmonary artery. A conduit between the right ventricle and pulmonary artery was successfully introduced by J.W. Kirklin in 1964 during correction of severe tetralogy of Fallot.

CONGENITAL HEART LESIONS THAT DECREASE PULMONARY ARTERIAL BLOOD FLOW

Decreased pulmonary blood flow secondary to a primary structural anomaly is more commonly due to obstructive lesions in the right heart or pulmonary artery. A classic example is tetralogy of Fallot, consisting of obstruction in the right ventricular outflow tract (infundibulum), pulmonary valve, or pulmonary artery; a ventricular septal defect; right ventricular hypertrophy; and an overriding aorta. A variety of exceptions exist, however. For example, with transposition of the great arteries, in which the aorta arises from the right ventricle and the pulmonary artery arises from the left ventricle, pulmonary flow can be markedly reduced despite the absence of formal obstruction. Whatever the arrangement, the basic pathophysiology is that of a right-to-left shunt. Systemic return shunted to the systemic output does not circulate through the lungs, resulting in cyanosis and decreased oxygen delivery to the tissues. The degree of cyanosis is inversely proportionate to the amount of effective pulmonary arterial blood flow.

Severe cyanosis stimulates red cell production, which increases the concentration of hemoglobin. This compensatory mechanism increases systemic oxygen delivery simply by increasing the amount of oxygen per unit volume of blood. The hematocrit may increase substantially (to > 70%), in which case the compensatory effects are offset by the risk of decreased flow secondary to increased viscosity and the risk of spontaneous thrombosis.

Variable cyanosis, hypoxic spells, squatting, and clubbing are frequently associated with lesions that reduce pulmonary blood flow. Several factors may alter the degree of cyanosis by altering the ratio of pulmonary and systemic resistances (exercise, acidosis, pain, and the catecholamine response).

Hypoxic spells produce severe cerebral hypoxia and are due to acute reduction of pulmonary blood flow. The classic example is spasm of the infundibular muscle in tetralogy of Fallot, which can occur without warning. Infants and young children become unconscious for varying periods of time and occasionally die. Simple measures such as placing the child in the knee-chest position with the head down (mimics squatting, which increases pulmonary flow by increasing systemic resistance) may help. However, medical therapy may be required to reduce spasm (beta-blockade), increase circulating blood volume and oxygen content (fluid and supplemental oxygen; mechanical ventilation), decrease acidosis (bicarbonate), and increase systemic resistance (norepinephrine). The phenomenon of clubbing of the fingers and toes develops in late infancy and early childhood and is due to proliferation of capillaries and small arteriovenous fistulas in the distal phalanges.

Reduced pulmonary arterial blood flow stimulates enlargement of bronchial and mediastinal arteries. These vessels connect with pulmonary arteries and, in some cases, may provide most of the pulmonary blood flow. At birth, the ductus arteriosus is patent and provides substantial flow to the pulmonary arteries of patients with obstructive right heart lesions. Unfortunately, the ductus nearly always closes during the first few hours or days after birth. The intravenous administration of prostaglandin E_1 will maintain patency of the ductus for hours or days in some infants, thus allowing reversal of acidosis, reduction of cyanosis, and stabilization of the infant prior to definitive therapy.

Several palliative operations that shunt blood from the systemic to the pulmonary arterial circulation have been devised for infants and young children who have insufficient pulmonary arterial blood flow. The Blalock-Taussig shunt operation connects the subclavian artery to the ipsilateral pulmonary artery with an end-to-side anastomosis (Figure 19–32A). The modified Blalock-Taussig shunt interposes a tube graft (3.5–6 mm), usually of polytetrafluoroethylene (Gore-Tex), between the subclavian or innominate artery and the ipsilateral pulmonary artery. The Waterston aortic to right pulmonary arterial anastomosis connects the posterior portion of the ascending aorta to the anterior wall of the right pulmonary artery (Figure 19–32B). The Potts anastomosis joins the left pulmonary artery and the descending thoracic aorta by a side-to-side anastomosis (Figure 19–32C). The Waterston and Potts aortopulmonary shunts are of mostly historical interest because of the difficulty of regulating flow through the shunt and the complexity of shunt take-down at the time of later correction.

Another category of options is to bypass the obstruction in the right heart by diverting part of or all the systemic venous return to the pulmonary circulation. Various connections or procedures have been described. The classic Glenn operation (Figure 19–32D) connects the superior vena cava to the right pulmonary artery in such a way that superior vena caval blood must enter the right pulmonary artery exclusively. The bidirectional Glenn operation connects the superior vena cava end-to-side to the top of the pulmonary artery, allowing flow to both lungs. Complete diversion is provided by the Fontan procedure, in which both superior and inferior caval return are routed to the pulmonary artery. Complete diversion is typically staged—the Fontan procedure is performed several months after the bidirectional Glenn. The modified Fontan procedure employed in recent practice refers to a variety of connections that may be used to divert flow from the inferior vena cava to the pulmonary artery. These include an intra-atrial tunnel (partial tube graft), an extracardiac tube-graft connection between the cava and pulmonary artery (with atrial disconnection oversewn), or an extracardiac pericardial connection.

A final category of surgical therapy includes various procedures that attempt to directly relieve the obstruction and reconstruct the right heart outflow tract. Such procedures include excision of obstructive muscle, patch enlargement of the infundibulum and pulmonary artery, homograft (with valve), replacement of the outflow tract with a valved synthetic conduit, and complex intracardiac baffles.

Castaneda AR et al: *Cardiac Surgery of the Neonate and Infant.* Saunders, 1994.

Gentles TL et al: Fontan operation in 500 consecutive patients: factors influencing early and late outcome. J Thorac Cardiovasc Surg 1997;114:376.

Gold JP et al: A five year clinical experience with 112 Blalock-Taussig shunts. J Card Surg 1993;8:9.

Kopf GS et al: Thirty year follow-up of superior vena cava-pulmonary artery (Glenn) shunts. J Thorac Cardiovasc Surg 1990;100:662.

Reddy V et al: Primary bidirectional superior cavopulmonary shunt in infants between 1 and 4 months of age. Ann Thorac Surg 1995;59:1120.

Watterson KG et al: Very small pulmonary arteries: central end-to-side shunt. Ann Thorac Surg 1991;52:1132.

TETRALOGY OF FALLOT

ESSENTIALS OF DIAGNOSIS

- *History of hypoxic spells and squatting.*
- *Cyanosis and clubbing.*
- *Prominent right ventricular impulse, single S_2.*
- *Grade 1–3/6 ejection murmur in third left intercostal space.*
- *Systolic murmur softens or disappears during cyanotic spell.*
- *Echocardiographic or documentation of stenosis or atresia of the infundibulum or pulmonary valve; ventricular septal defect with overriding aorta; right ventricular hypertrophy.*

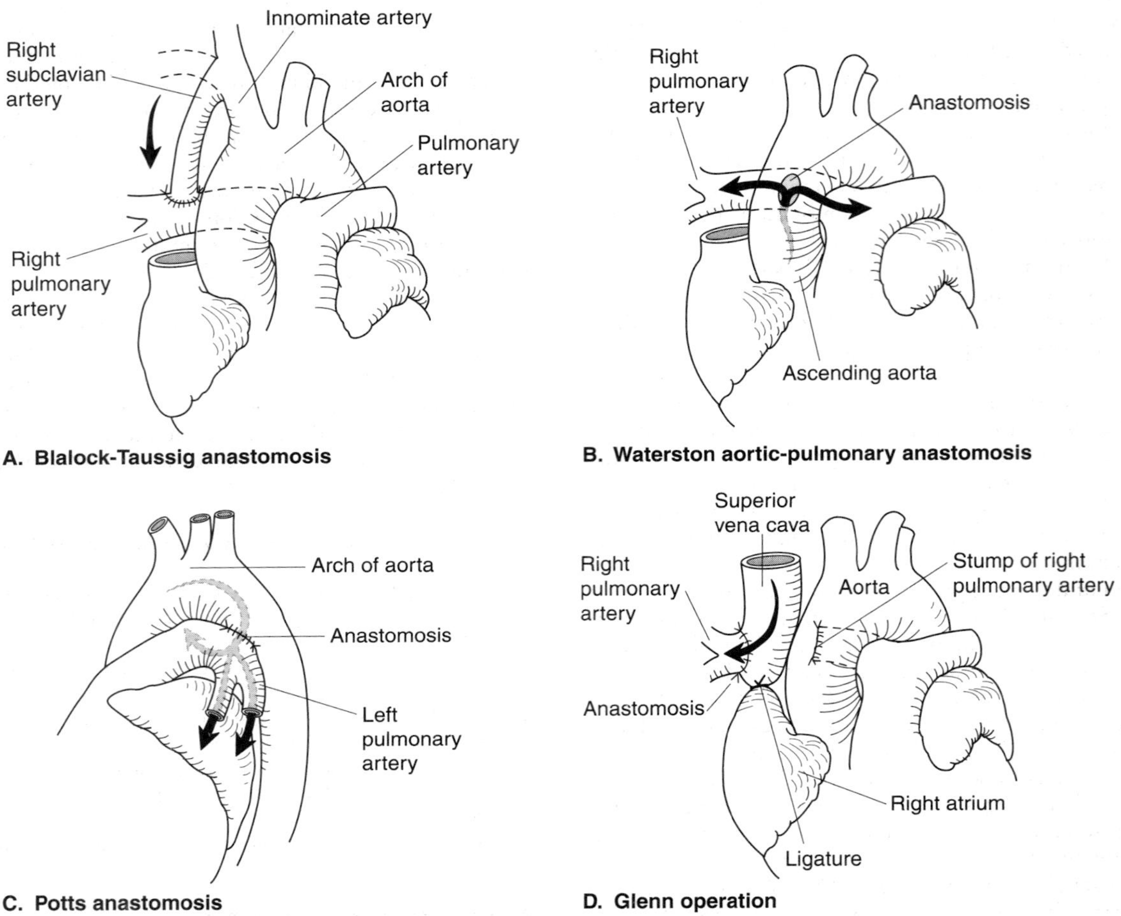

Figure 19–32. Palliative operations to increase pulmonary arterial blood flow. ***A:*** Blalock-Taussig subclavian-pulmonary arterial anastomosis. ***B:*** Waterston aortic to right pulmonary arterial anastomosis. ***C:*** Potts anastomosis between the left pulmonary artery and the descending thoracic aorta. ***D:*** The classic Glenn operation. The end of the right pulmonary artery is connected to the side of the superior vena cava, which is ligated caudad to the anastomosis.

General Considerations

The four basic anatomic abnormalities (Figure 19–33)—ventricular septal defect, infundibular or pulmonary stenosis or atresia, overriding of the aorta (over the ventricular septum), and right ventricular hypertrophy—are believed to result from hypoplasia of the infundibulum (portion of outflow tract just proximal to the pulmonary valve). Pulmonary stenosis may be infundibular, valvular, or may involve the main pulmonary artery. Some degree of hypertrophic muscle mass is present in the pulmonary outflow tract as well. Tetralogy of Fallot may also occur with pulmonary atresia rather than stenosis. As with pulmonary stenosis, the extent of atresia covers a wide spectrum. At the most favorable extreme, atresia is limited to the valve, a large ductus is present, and the size of the pulmonary arteries is normal. At the other extreme (now often regarded as a separate diagnostic entity), central pulmonary arteries and a ductus are absent and aortopulmonary collateral arteries are the sole source of blood flow to the lungs.

The reduction in pulmonary blood flow depends on the degree of outflow tract obstruction and the systemic vascular resistance. In pulmonary atresia, the degree of pulmonary blood flow depends on the presence of normal pulmonary arteries and the extent of aortopulmonary collateral arteries and the degree of stenosis present

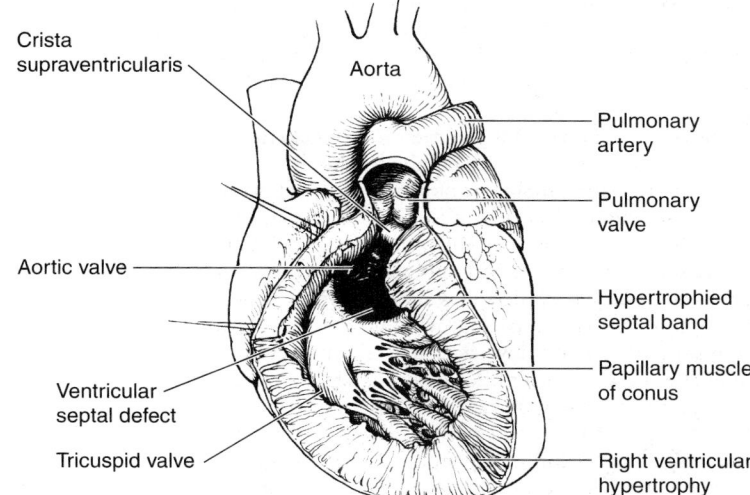

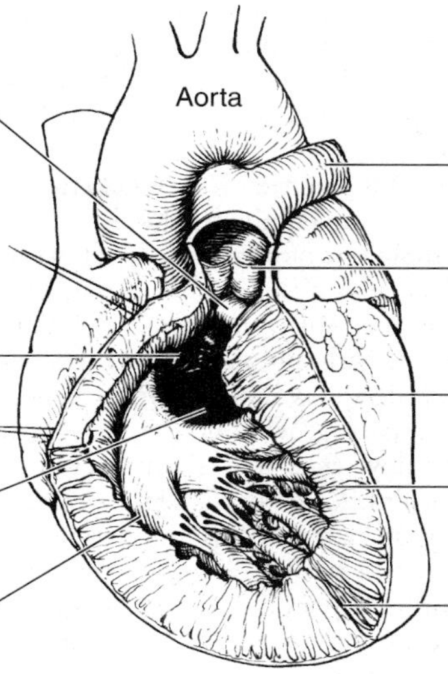

Figure 19–33. Tetralogy of Fallot. The aorta overrides the ventricular septum. A large ventricular septal defect is present, and the hypoplastic infundibulum with hypertrophied muscle bands obstructs blood to the pulmonary arteries.

in those vessels. In fact, extensive unobstructed aortopulmonary collateral arteries may lead to excessive pulmonary blood flow and congestive failure.

Clinical Findings

Symptoms are directly related to the amount of pulmonary blood flow. A patent ductus may mask the lesion and its symptoms in the early days of life. However, with ductal closure, severe pulmonary stenosis in the neonate causes severe cyanosis and acidosis. A systolic murmur is due to the pulmonary stenosis and is heard along the left sternal border. The hypoxic or cyanotic spell is the most serious symptom since it can result in cerebral hypoxia, brain injury, and even death. The diagnosis can usually be made from the cyanosis, small heart size, and diminished pulmonary blood flow seen on the chest radiograph. The ECG shows right ventricular hypertrophy. Echocardiography is usually sufficient to confirm the diagnosis. Cardiac catheterization is necessary in most forms of pulmonary atresia to define the presence and size of central pulmonary arteries (sometimes not possible) and to define the anatomy of aortopulmonary collateral arteries. One aspect of diagnosis is predicting the postrepair capability of the pulmonary vasculature to accommodate the cardiac output. If the vasculature is inadequate and the ventricular septal defect is closed, right heart failure will ensue. Various predictive parameters with variable clinical utility have been described. The McGoon ratio is the combined diameter of pulmonary arteries normalized to the diameter of the descending aorta, an acceptable value being greater than 2.0. The Nakata index is the sum of the cross-sectional areas of the right and left pulmonary arteries normalized to body surface area. Normal values exceed 300 mm_2/m_2; values less than 150 mm_2/m_2 indicate extremely small pulmonary arteries. Another estimate is provided by the normalized pulmonary annulus diameter. Values less than 2 SD below normal warrant concern.

Treatment

In general, most patients are symptomatic at the time of diagnosis, and the diagnosis is therefore an indication for repair. One-stage correction is recommended by many surgeons. This entails cardiopulmonary bypass and patch closure of the ventricular septal defect through the right atrium; a small incision in the infundibulum or proximal main pulmonary artery to resect obstructive muscle (if present); and placement of a patch (pericardium or Gore-Tex) in the infundibulum or artery to widen the outflow tract. In cases in which patch enlargement of the infundibulum is not needed, the repair can be done entirely through the atrium. In other cases it may be necessary to extend the incision and patch insertion across the annulus. The resultant pulmonary insufficiency is usually well tolerated in the child for several years; however, untoward effects of long-standing insufficiency are just beginning to be realized in adult survivors. There are currently no ideal methods to deal with this problem at the time of initial repair. A large ventriculotomy, though, is rarely necessary, can significantly impair ventricular function, and thus should be avoided.

The palliative approach entails initial placement of a systemic to pulmonary artery shunt followed by correction (as described above) at a later age. Proponents acknowledge a lower operative mortality in the sick neonate as well as growth of the pulmonary vasculature induced by the shunt, thereby lowering the risk of post-repair pulmonary hypertension and right ventricular dysfunction.

Initial correction avoids the need for two operations, each with attendant risks, and eliminates the risks associated with the pathophysiology of the anomaly. However, prudent selection of therapy must consider the anatomy of the child and not be based solely on a single technique. For example, the child with pulmonary stenosis and diminutive pulmonary arteries will benefit from a modified approach that induces growth of the vasculature (reconstruction of outflow tract and shunt) yet minimizes relevant risk (such as closure of the septal defect).

Repair of tetralogy of Fallot with pulmonary atresia may also be accomplished with a single procedure or with staged procedures, depending on the degree of development of the central pulmonary vasculature and the complexity of the aortopulmonary collateral artery anatomy. Unifocalization is a term describing the process of disconnecting the collateral arteries from the aorta and joining or focalizing them to a tube of Gore-Tex or one reconstructed from pericardium. This tube (usually one on each side) may then be connected to a reconstructed right heart outflow tract if the pulmonary vasculature is deemed adequate. Alternatively, it may be connected to a systemic shunt to induce growth of the pulmonary vasculature. Closure of the ventricular septal defect is done either at a time when the pulmonary vasculature has undergone enough growth or when enough pulmonary segments have been unifocalized to allow a sufficiently low pulmonary vascular resistance (usually the equivalent of at least one lung). Some surgeons advocate repairing the septal defect with a perforated patch to allow unloading of the right heart and the ability to close the defect percutaneously with a device at a later time. This means that eventual repair of the complex case may require at least three major surgical procedures.

Prognosis

After surgery, patients with tetralogy of Fallot usually have some degree of right ventricular dysfunction due to operative trauma and the newly imposed increased volume work of the ventricle. Judicious medical management is usually successful. In general, mortality is less than 5% in tetralogy with stenosis and may exceed 30–45% in tetralogy with atresia. Subsequent need for reoperation on the outflow tract occurs in approximately 10–15% of patients at 10-year follow-up. Those patients reaching adulthood enjoy normal lives: More than 90% are regularly employed in all types of work; over 50% regularly participate in athletics; and less than 20% require cardiac medications. The incidence of late right ventricular dysfunction and the need for late pulmonary valve replacement is just now being recognized. A definitive statement awaits further studies and follow-up.

Di-Donato RM et al: Neonatal repair of tetralogy of Fallot with and without pulmonary atresia. J Thorac Cardiovasc Surg 1991;101:126.

Discigil B et al: Late pulmonary valve replacement after repair of tetralogy of Fallot. J Thorac Cardiovasc Surg 2001;121:344.

Fraser CD et al: Tetralogy of Fallot: surgical management individualized to the patient. Ann Thorac Surg 2001;71:1556.

Groh MA et al: Repair of tetralogy of Fallot in infancy. Effect of pulmonary artery size on outcome. Circulation 1991;84(5 Suppl):III206.

Karl TR et al: Tetralogy of Fallot: favorable outcome of nonneonatal transatrial, transpulmonary repair. Ann Thorac Surg 1992; 54: 903.

Kirklin JW et al: Morphologic and surgical determinants of outcome events after repair of tetralogy of Fallot and pulmonary stenosis. A two institution study. J Thorac Cardiovasc Surg 1992;103:692.

Knott-Craig CJ et al: A 26-year experience with surgical management of tetralogy of Fallot: risk analysis for mortality or late reintervention. Ann Thorac Surg 1998;66:506.

Lillehei CW et al: The first open heart corrections of tetralogy of Fallot: a 26–31 year follow-up of 106 patients. Ann Surg 1986;204:490.

Norgaard MA et al: Twenty-to-thirty-seven-year follow-up after repair for tetralogy of Fallot. Eur J Cardiothorac Surg 1999;16: 125.

Pagani FD et al: The management of tetralogy of Fallot with pulmonary atresia and diminutive pulmonary arteries. J Thorac Cardiovasc Surg 1995;110:1521.

PULMONARY ATRESIA WITH INTACT VENTRICULAR SEPTUM

In pulmonary atresia with intact ventricular septum, the normally patent pulmonary valve is replaced by a diaphragm or dome of tissue that completely obstructs flow into the pulmonary artery (typically normal size). Since there is no ventricular septal defect, an atrial septal defect and patent ductus arteriosus are necessary for survival beyond the first few hours after birth. The right ventricle may be of normal size but is typically rudimentary, with the cavity obliterated by thickened muscle. Tricuspid annular size is also typically reduced and correlates with the size of the right ventricular cavity. An important associated finding in a significant number of patients is the presence of right ventricular-to-coronary artery fistulas and stenoses of coronary arteries. In fact, the suprasystemic pressure of the right ventricle may be the sole driving force for coronary flow to a major portion of the myocardium.

Cyanosis is usually present at birth. With ductal closure, the child becomes profoundly hypoxic and acidotic and will not survive unless flow is established through the ductus. The ECG shows a relative lack of normal right ventricular dominance. The chest radiograph reveals diminished flow. Diagnosis is confirmed by echocardiography. Cardiac catheterization is usually performed after the child is resuscitated to define the coronary anatomy and assess the probability of a right ventricular dependent coronary circulation.

Optimal surgical therapy depends on the degree of development of the right ventricle. Criteria to guide this decision remain inexact. In general, the procedure entails a systemic-to-pulmonary artery shunt and patch reconstruction of the right heart outflow tract. In cases in which the ventricle is deemed inadequate, a shunt alone is performed. If there is right ventricular dependent coronary circulation, the right ventricle must not be decompressed (only a shunt should be performed), as this would lead to profound myocardial ischemia. Ultimately, if growth of the ventricle and the pulmonary vasculature is adequate, the shunt can be occluded and the atrial septal defect closed, thereby establishing a two-ventricle circulation. If this is not the case, management proceeds along a single-ventricle pathway (eg, Fontan). Although the prognosis for these children is improving, 1-year mortality is in the range of 10–20% in most centers.

Bull C et al: Outcome measures for the neonatal management of pulmonary atresia with intact ventricular septum. J Thorac Cardiovasc Surg 1994;107:359.

Hawkins JA et al: Early and late results in pulmonary atresia, and intact ventricular septum. J Thorac Cardiovasc Surg 1990;100: 492.

Jahangiri M et al: Improved results with selective management in pulmonary atresia with intact ventricular septum. J Thorac Cardiovasc Surg 1999;118:1046.

Rychik J et al: Outcome after operations for pulmonary atresia with intact ventricular septum. J Thorac Cardiovasc Surg 1998;116: 924.

TRICUSPID ATRESIA

Tricuspid atresia is defined by a lack of communication between the right atrium and right ventricle. The ventricular cavity is small. A ventricular septal defect, usually restrictive to flow, connects the ventricles. An interatrial communication is invariably present. The relationship of the great arteries and their connections to the ventricles is abnormal in approximately 30% of patients. This relationship—as well as the degree of obstruction of pulmonary blood flow—provides the basis for classifying subtypes of tricuspid atresia.

A reciprocal relationship exists between the degree of obstruction to systemic and pulmonary blood flow. The clinical presentation can vary depending on the arrangement of the great vessels and the degree of restriction of the atrial and ventricular septal defects. The majority of infants suffer from some degree of reduced pulmonary blood flow and cyanosis and have no obstruction to systemic output. Diagnosis is confirmed by echocardiography; however, cardiac catheterization is often performed to determine the suitability for repair and, in cases with a restrictive atrial septal defect, to perform balloon septoplasty.

In most children, a modified Blalock-Taussig shunt is performed initially to provide adequate balanced pulmonary blood flow. A bidirectional Glenn procedure, followed later by a Fontan (modified) procedure, complete the staged repair. The underlying philosophy is to provide adequate but not excessive pulmonary blood flow and to minimize volume overload of the ventricle and the risk of developing pulmonary vascular disease. This is done by changing the source of pulmonary blood flow from arterial to venous in successive stages (Glenn and subsequent Fontan).

Castaneda AR: From Glenn to Fontan: a continuing evolution. Circulation 1992;86(5 Suppl):II80.

Cleveland DC et al: Surgical treatment of tricuspid atresia. Ann Thorac Surg 1984;38:447.

deLeval MR et al: Total cavopulmonary connection: a logical alternative to atriopulmonary connection for complex Fontan operations. J Thorac Cardiovasc Surg 1988;96:682.

Fontan F et al: Surgical repair of tricuspid atresia. Thorax 1971;26:240.

Franklin RC et al: Tricuspid atresia presenting in infancy: survival and suitability for the Fontan operation. Circulation 1993;87:427.

Jacobs ML et al: Fontan operation: influence of modifications on morbidity and mortality. Ann Thorac Surg 1994;58:945.

EBSTEIN'S ANOMALY

In this malformation, the septal and posterior leaflets of the tricuspid valve are small and deformed and usually displaced toward the right ventricular apex. A large portion of the right ventricle is quite thin and hypoplastic and becomes atrialized. Most patients have an associated atrial septal defect or patent foramen ovale. Cyanosis and arrhythmias in infancy are common. About half of these patients develop right heart failure, some degree of systemic desaturation, hepatomegaly, and dysrhythmias. Operative repair of this lesion without tricuspid valve replacement has been encouraging in approximately half of cases. In these cases, the atrialized portion of the ventricle may be oversewn and the tricuspid valve incompetence corrected. Newer surgical therapies are being developed to provide a functioning right ventricle and tricuspid valve. In others, tricuspid valve replacement is necessary, and in some cases the anatomic deformities are so extensive that effective surgical correction is impossible.

Danielson GK et al: Operative treatment of Ebstein's anomaly. J Thorac Cardiovasc Surg 1992;104:1497.

Dearani JA et al: Congenital Heart Surgery Nomenclature and Database Project: Ebstein's anomaly and tricuspid valve disease. Ann Thorac Surg 2000;69:S106.

Gentles TL et al: Predictors of long term survival with Ebstein's anomaly of the tricuspid valve. Am J Cardiol 1992;69:377.

Knott-Craig CJ et al: Neonatal repair of Ebstein's anomaly: indications, surgical technique, and medium-term follow-up. Ann Thorac Surg 2000;69:1505.

TRANSPOSITION OF THE GREAT ARTERIES—NORMAL VENTRICULAR ARRANGEMENT (D-TRANSPOSITION)

ESSENTIALS OF DIAGNOSIS

- *Situs solitus, levocardia.*
- *Cyanosis from birth; hypoxic spells sometimes present.*
- *Heart failure often present.*
- *Murmurs variable; often absent and not diagnostic.*
- *Echocardiographic confirmation of relationship of great arteries and ventricles.*

General Considerations

Probably nowhere in pediatric cardiac surgery is the terminology potentially more confusing than in descriptions of transposition. This is because carefully developed distinct descriptive systems of embryology and morphology and their respective terminologies have been subsequently incorporated and combined by other authors. The original systems based on concordant or discordant connections, spatial arrangements of the great vessels, or segmental anatomic descriptions remain valid. The segmental description is probably more robust and complete and can be found in standard texts of cardiac embryology. These systems are not defined here. Rather, what follows is a simple explanation to clarify current usage of terms and their relationship to clinical anomalies.

In a general theoretical sense, the great vessels can originate from the ventricles in a number of ways—normal; both great vessels arising from the right or left ventricle; both great vessels arising in an indeterminate fashion from both ventricles in the context of a ventricular septal defect; reversal of the normal arrangement with the aorta arising from the morphologic right ventricle and vice versa; and all variations on this continuum. As a separate issue, the embryologic ventricular looping may occur levo- rather than the normal dextro- (not dextrocardia, which has nothing to do with looping), giving rise to a right-sided morphologic left ventricle and a left-sided morphologic right ventricle. Even with normal ventriculo-arterial connections, the spatial arrangement of the great vessels may differ from the usual rightward posterior aorta and leftward anterior pulmonary artery.

Malposition is the correct general term for implying any abnormal spatial arrangement of the great vessels. Letter designations indicate the position of the aorta relative to the pulmonary artery: D-, to the right; L-, to the left; and A-, anterior. Letter designation does not explicitly define ventriculo-arterial connections. On the other hand, the word "transposition" means the aorta is connected to a morphologic right ventricle regardless of whether it is a right-sided or a left-sided right ventricle. Likewise, the pulmonary artery is connected to a morphologic left ventricle. The spatial relationship of the great vessels can be D-, L-, or A-. Clinically, the more common transposition abnormality consists of normally looped ventricles and a rightward anterior aorta connected to a morphologic right ventricle, hence the term "D transposition" (Figure 19–34). However, other variations of true transposition exist that are treated correctly with an arterial switch yet do not exhibit the "D-" spatial arrangement—side-by-side or anterior-posterior, yet still transposed.

As noted above, the most common spatial arrangement of the great arteries is a rightward anterior aorta. A ventricular septal defect is present in approximately 20–25% of patients, occurring more frequently in the context of unusual great arterial arrangements. Left ventricular outflow tract obstruction may also occur. It is more commonly dynamic in nature owing to leftward septal displacement from higher right ventricular pressures (the systemic ventricle).

The origin and distribution of the coronary arteries are variable. Although the coronary arteries arise from the aortic sinuses facing the pulmonary artery in essentially all patients, the exact origin of the right and left arteries can vary between the two sinuses. The variant that intensifies the difficulty of the arterial switch repair is a left anterior descending artery passing between the great vessels or exhibiting a significant intramural course (passes in the wall of the aorta). In general, coronary arterial variations are more common with the side-by-side great artery arrangement and a ventricular septal defect.

The pathophysiology of transposition is related to the separation and independence of the systemic and pulmonary circulations. Some anatomic communication between the two systems must exist for the patient to survive. The common sites for mixing of blood are a ventricular septal defect, an atrial septal defect, and a patent ductus arteriosus. The degree of cyanosis is proportionate to the relative amount of oxygenated venous blood that reaches the right ventricle and aorta. In the minority of patients who have a

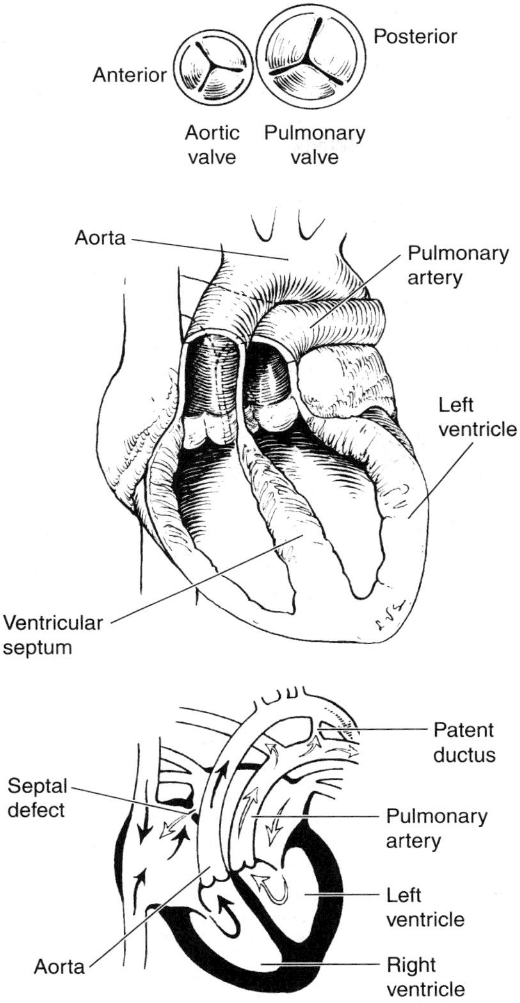

Figure 19–34. Typical transposition of the great arteries. The aorta arises from the morphologic right ventricle and is anterior to and slightly to the right of the pulmonary artery, which originates from the morphologic left ventricle. Inset at bottom illustrates the independent systemic and pulmonary circulations, which may be connected by a patent ductus arteriosus or atrial septal defect. Inset at top illustrates a common relationship of the two great arteries in typical transposition.

ventricular septal defect, mixing is usually adequate; however, increased pulmonary blood flow subjects the child to the risk of rapid development of pulmonary vascular obstructive disease. Residual or induced patency of the ductus also provides good pulmonary blood flow but may lead to excessive pulmonary blood flow, pulmonary edema, and a reduced systemic output, particularly if the foramen ovale or atrial septal defect is restrictive. Balloon atrial septostomy provides adequate mixing and can be performed shortly after the diagnosis is confirmed.

In normal development with normal anatomy, the left ventricle experiences a rapid increase in mass secondary to both volume and pressure workloads. In transposition, physiology promoting this transition is absent or directed to the right ventricle. This has relevance for timing the switch procedure, which restores normal pressure and volume loads to the left ventricle. If performed late (after 3–4 weeks of life), the risk of inadequate left ventricular adaptation may lead to failure and death.

Clinical Findings

Cyanosis is typically present at birth. Clinical deterioration occurs in 24–48 hours as the ductus closes and is manifested as worsening hypoxia and acidosis. In the child with ventricular septal defect or a large persistent ductus arteriosus, symptoms may be minimal during the first few weeks. However, with a progressive decline in pulmonary vascular resistance in the first few days of life, signs of pulmonary overcirculation and heart failure become apparent. The ECG shows right ventricular hypertrophy and the chest radiograph reveals overcirculation and an enlarged heart. Echocardiography is usually sufficient to confirm the diagnosis as well as to demonstrate the branching pattern of the coronary arteries. Cardiac catheterization may be needed to assess coronary anatomy or, in the older infant, to assess pressures and the suitability of the left ventricle for the switch procedure.

Treatment

Without treatment, about half of newborns with transposition of the great arteries die by 1 month of age and 90% die within 1 year. Repair or correction is therefore indicated. Two general types of repairs are possible. The Mustard and Senning operations create intra-atrial baffles and channels to direct the systemic venous return to the left ventricle and the pulmonary venous return to the right ventricle. This restores a series circulation and the capability to oxygenate the blood, albeit leaving the right ventricle as the systemic ventricle. Most surgeons currently advocate switching the circulation at the level of the great arteries rather than the atria. The arterial switch procedure disconnects the pulmonary artery and aorta and reconnects the aorta to the left ventricle and the pulmonary artery to the right ventricle (above the level of the valves). The coronary arteries (buttons) are detached and transferred to the new aortic root. This restores a series circulation and establishes the left ventricle as the systemic ventricle. The current trend is to perform this operation on full flow bypass rather than circulatory arrest.

Timing is important. The optimal sequence is prompt diagnosis, and if necessary, a balloon atrial septostomy. With stabilization of the child, the switch procedure can be performed semi-electively in the first 1–2 weeks of life. If diagnosis has occurred after this time, a two-stage approach to the switch procedure is still possible. A modified Blalock-Taussig shunt is created, and a pulmonary artery band is placed. This provides adequate pulmonary blood flow and a pressure load to acutely condition the left ventricle to function as the systemic ventricle. Approximately 1–2 weeks later, the shunt is taken down, the band removed, and the switch procedure performed. Alternatively, a single stage approach is feasible by rehabilitating the left ventricle after the switch using mechanical support (ECMO or ventricular assist device). If a ventricular septal defect is present, ventricular conditioning is usually not a concern; however, untoward effects of excessive pulmonary blood flow still warrant timely repair. The ventricular and atrial septal defects may be closed at the time of the switch procedure using standard techniques.

The Rastelli procedure is another surgical option, particularly in the context of a ventricular septal defect and left ventricular outflow tract obstruction. This entails enlargement of the ventricular septal defect and placing an intraventricular baffle between the margin of the septal defect and the aortic annulus such that the new left ventricular outflow tract is completely unobstructed. The main pulmonary artery is divided and oversewn, and an infundibulotomy is created. A valved conduit is placed to connect the infundibulotomy to the distal main pulmonary artery or the bifurcation.

Prognosis

The overall results of surgery for transposition of the great arteries are excellent. Mortality in the first year after repair ranges between 2% and 10%. These children are truly corrected and infrequently require reintervention. Mortality and complications occur more frequently in children with left ventricular outflow tract obstruction, complicated coronary artery anatomy, and associated anomalies (eg, interrupted arch). Technical problems with the coronary transfer and coronary artery complications are a recognized contributing factor to postoperative cardiac dysfunction and death. The current experience with atrial level rearrangements is minimal. There are, however, older patients presenting with complications of the Mustard and Senning operations. Tricuspid insufficiency, atrial arrhythmias, and obstruction of the venous pathways are recognized complications. Another issue is the adult with a prior atrial level repair who presents with right ventricular failure. Criteria to direct management toward transplantation versus a double-switch procedure continue to be refined in selected centers.

Alonzo-de-Begona J et al: The Mustard procedure for correction of simple transposition of the great arteries before 1 month of age. J Thorac Cardiovasc Surg 1992;104:1218.

Cochrane AD et al: Staged conversion to arterial switch for late failure of the systemic right ventricle. Ann Thorac Surg 1993;56:854.

Ingram MT et al: Senning repair for transposition of the great arteries without patch augmentation of the septum. J Thorac Cardiovasc Surg 1988;96:485.

Kirklin JW et al: Clinical outcomes after the arterial switch operation for transposition: patient, support, procedural, and institutional risk factors. Circulation 1992;86:1501.

Kreutzer C et al: Twenty-five-year experience with Rastelli repair for transposition of the great arteries. J Thorac Cardiovasc Surg 2000;120:211.

Lupinetti FM et al: Intermediate term survival and functional results after arterial repair for transposition of the great arteries. J Thorac Cardiovasc Surg 1992;103:421.

Mee RBB: Severe right ventricular failure after Mustard or Senning operation. J Thorac Cardiovasc Surg 1986;92:385.

Turley K et al: Intermediate results from the period of the Congenital Heart Surgeons Transposition Study: 1985–1989. Congenital Heart Surgeons Society Database. Ann Thorac Surg 1995;60:505.

Wells WJ et al: Intermediate outcome after the Mustard and Senning procedures: a study by the Congenital Heart Surgeons Society. Pediatr Cardiac Surg Annu of the Semin in Thorac and Cardiovasc Surg 2000;3:186.

Wernovsky G et al: Factors influencing early and late outcome of the arterial switch operation for transposition of the great arteries. J Thorac Cardiovasc Surg 1995;109:289.

CORRECTED TRANSPOSITION OF THE GREAT ARTERIES

As noted in the previous section, commonly used transposition terminology can be confusing at times. Corrected transposition, also referred to as L-transposition, is true transposition, in that the aorta connects to a morphologic right ventricle and the pulmonary artery connects to a morphologic left ventricle. In this case, however, the ventricle has undergone leftward or levo-looping, giving rise to a right-sided morphologic left ventricle and a left-sided morphologic right ventricle. Since the aorta is commonly (though not always) to the left of the pulmonary artery, the "L-" designation is sometimes used (does not refer to the levo-ventricular loop). In this form of transposition, systemic venous blood passes through a morphologic mitral valve into a right-sided morphologic left ventricle, into the pulmonary artery and lungs, through a normal left atrium, and through a morphologic tricuspid valve into a left-sided morphologic right ventricle, to the aorta and systemic circulation. Hence, the transposition is corrected in that a series circulation that oxygenates the blood is maintained.

Associated features include a ventricular septal defect in over 75% of patients and some form of subpulmonary obstruction in less than half of patients. The coronary pattern is relatively invariant but is reversed to correspond to the ventricular arrangement. There is also a corresponding alteration of the conduction system. The conduction bundle passes on the right side of the ventricular septum (morphologically left ventricular). Rather than passing inferior to the septal defect, the conduction bundle passes superior to the defect.

Symptoms are uncommon in infancy. Congestive signs and symptoms eventually develop, however, and are often related to pulmonary stenosis and tricuspid insufficiency, which develop in a significant percentage of patients. First-, second-, or third-degree heart block is another aspect of the natural history of this disease and may be the presenting feature in infancy.

Efforts to design optimal therapy for these children are ongoing. Closure of the ventricular septal defect can be performed through the aorta or left atrium, with sutures placed on the morphologically right ventricular surface. Repair of subpulmonary obstruction remains problematic. Tricuspid insufficiency may be approached surgically through the left or right atrium, with the decision about repair or replacement based on the particular anatomy of the valve and the size of the child. The initiation of pacemaker therapy is based on standard indications. By improving the heart rate and cardiac output and lowering the ventricular volume, tricuspid function may be improved or preserved to some degree. Some surgeons advocate a double-switch procedure (atrial level and arterial level switch), typically in patients without left ventricular (subpulmonary) obstruction. Overall long-term prognosis remains inadequate, with 10-year survivals in the range of 50%.

Alva C et al: The feasibility of complete anatomical correction in the setting of discordant atrioventricular connections. Br Heart J 1999;81:539.

Duncan BW et al: Results of the double switch operation for congenitally corrected transposition of the great arteries. Eur J Cardiothor Surg 2003;24:11.

Hraska V et al: Long-term outcome of surgically treated patients with corrected transposition of the great arteries. J Thorac Cardiovasc Surg 2005;129:182.

Karl TR et al: Senning plus arterial switch operation for discordant (congenitally corrected) transposition. Ann Thorac Surg 1997; 64:495.

Termignon J et al: "Classic" repair of congenitally corrected transposition and ventricular septal defect. Ann Thorac Surg 1996;62:199.

DOUBLE-OUTLET RIGHT VENTRICLE

In double-outlet right ventricle, both great arteries (at least 50% of the annulus of each valve) arise from the right ventricle. This is an uncommon and extremely complex anomaly with a spectrum that anatomically and clinically extends from a tetralogy-like form to a transposition-like form. Because of the rarity and complexity of this anomaly, the discussion here will be limited to brief general comments.

The location of the ventricular septal defect, which is invariably present, determines the classification. It can be subaortic, subpulmonary, noncommitted (quite proximal to the valve annuli), or doubly committed (adjacent to the annuli and flow-directed to both arteries). Subaortic obstruction occurs in approximately one-third of patients with subpulmonary defects, and subpulmonary obstruction occurs in approximately one-third of patients with subaortic defects. Great vessel arrangement and coronary artery branching can also vary. In general, a subaortic ventricular septal defect and a rightward, slightly posterior arrangement are more common. Symptoms vary depending on the location of the septal defect and the degree of outflow tract obstruction. Echocardiography is usually sufficient for diagnosis.

Optimal surgical treatment also depends on the exact anatomy. One option is the creation of an intraventricular baffle to direct left ventricular flow to the aorta in such a way as to close the septal defect and avoid subpulmonary obstruction. An arterial switch is another option if anatomy is not suitable for intraventricular baffling or for baffling combined with some type of rearrangement of the great vessels (but not switch).

Despite the complexity of this anomaly, hospital mortality is acceptably low. Ten-year survival ranges from 60% to 80%. Outflow tract reconstruction and other factors require reintervention in approximately one-third of patients.

Double outlet left ventricle is an even rarer anomaly that will not be discussed in this text.

Aoki M et al: Result of biventricular repair for double-outlet right ventricle. J Thorac Cardiovasc Surg 1994;107:338.

Musumeci F et al: Surgical treatment of double outlet right ventricle at the Brompton Hospital, 1973–1986. J Thorac Cardiovasc Surg 1988;96:278.

Planche C et al: Double-outlet right ventricle with non-committed ventricular septal defect. Eur J Cardiothorac Surg 1999;15:747.

Serraf A et al: Anatomic repair of Taussig-Bing hearts. Circulation 1991;84(5 Suppl):III200.

Takeuchi K et al: Surgical outcome of double-outlet right ventricle with subpulmonary VSD. Ann Thorac Surg 2001;71:49.

SINGLE VENTRICLE

The term "single ventricle" denotes a heart with one ventricular chamber that receives blood from both the tricuspid and mitral valves or a common atrioventricular valve. The anomaly accounts for 3–5% of congenital heart defects. Anomalies such as tricuspid atresia, hypoplastic left heart syndrome, double-inlet ventricles, common ventricle, and various heterotaxy variants (see next section) are often labeled as "single ventricle." The diagnosis of single ventricle and specific associated lesions must be made by echocardiography and often cardiac catheterization.

Clinical findings and prognosis are related to the relative amounts of pulmonary and systemic arterial blood flow. Surgical options include palliation with a shunt or pulmonary arterial band, ventricular partitioning, and staged correction toward a Fontan circulation. The most suitable anatomic types for operation are patients with an anatomic left ventricle and outflow chamber and those with a common ventricle formed from both ventricular sinuses. Prognosis has improved substantially over the past decade. Nonetheless, 1-year survival remains low, ranging between 40% and 80%.

Mayer JE et al: Factors associated with marked reduction in mortality for Fontan operations in patients with single ventricle. J Thorac Cardiovasc Surg 1992;103:444.

Mosca RS et al: Modified Norwood operation for single left ventricle and ventriculoarterial discordance: an improved surgical technique. Ann Thorac Surg 1997;64:1126.

Stein DG et al: Results of total cavopulmonary connection in the treatment of patients with a functional single ventricle. J Thorac Cardiovasc Surg 1991;102:280.

ATRIAL ISOMERISM (HETEROTAXY)

Atrial isomerism refers to the situation of bilaterally similar atria, occurring in approximately 1-2% of liveborn children with congenital heart disease. For right atrial isomerism, both right- and left-sided atria are morphologically right atria—similarly for left atrial isomerism. Serious cardiac anomalies are the norm, particularly with right atrial isomerism. Bilaterality of the bronchial tree and lungs is also present and a reliable indication of the presence of isomerism. The heart resides in the right chest in almost half of cases. Abnormal heart position may indicate isomerism, but location of the heart does not reliably distinguish between right and left isomerism. In most cases, there is also abnormality of visceral situs and splenic status, the latter, either in the form of asplenia or polysplenia, being the original basis for describing these abnormalities as asplenic or polysplenic syndromes. Heterotaxy, referring to the unusual variants of visceral situs (midline liver or mirror image arrangement, bowel rotation, etc) is another term commonly used to refer to these anomalies.

As a general rule, right atrial isomerism is associated with asplenia and bilateral right thoracic organs, whereas left atrial isomerism is associated with polysplenia and bilateral left thoracic organs. Abnormalities of systemic and pulmonary venous connections are common, the latter being to an extracardiac structure more commonly in right atrial isomerism. Most hearts have a common atrioventricular connection guarded by a common valve. Most hearts are also functionally single ventricle, especially with right atrial isomerism. The ventriculo-arterial connections vary considerably; however, pulmonary outflow obstruction is more common with right atrial isomerism, and coarctation or other forms of left heart outflow obstruction are more common with left atrial isomerism. Location of the conduction axis can vary considerably, depending on the morphology of the dominant ventricle. Associated noncardiac abnormalities involve the gastrointestinal, genitourinary, central nervous, and musculoskeletal systems.

Presentation depends on the specific anatomy and associated anomalies for a given child; however, cyanosis with/without obstructed pulmonary venous drainage is more common with right atrial isomerism. Ductal dependent physiology is common. The cardiac workup, based predominantly on echocardiography, must clearly define the anatomy in sequential fashion beginning with the systemic and hepatic venous connections through the cardiac structures to the thoracic aorta. Asplenia (unlike polysplenia) must be detected, using any of a variety of modalities (blood smear and Howell-Jolly or Heinz bodies, ultrasound, computed tomography, radionuclide scanning).

Management will of course depend on the specific pathophysiology; however, in most cases, the strategy will entail resuscitation with prostaglandin (if duct dependent) and palliative rather than corrective surgery. This entails regulation of pulmonary blood flow (shunt or, less commonly, a band) and staged repair to a single ventricle circulation. Obstructed pulmonary venous drainage, which may be masked by proximal obstruction, must be detected and corrected at the time of the initial surgery. Transplantation remains an option for children for whom adequate palliation is deemed improbable.

Prognosis for these children remains poor. Two-year survival is approximately 50%, and may be slightly better with left atrial isomerism. Children surviving to the final stage of palliation also experience higher operative mortality (10%) than that of other Fontan patients, usually due to problems of the atrioventricular valve or the inferior systemic and hepatic venous connections. The available data are insufficient to accurately characterize long-term survival and function.

Anderson RH et al: Defective lateralization in children with congenitally malformed hearts. Cardiol Young 1998;8:512.

Sadiq M et al: Management and outcome of infants and children with right atrial isomerism. Heart 1996;75:314.

MISCELLANEOUS CONGENITAL HEART LESIONS

ANOMALOUS LEFT CORONARY ARTERY

Origin of the left coronary artery from the pulmonary artery causes myocardial ischemia and heart failure in infancy. The right coronary artery is normal and supplies blood to the entire myocardium and intracoronary collaterals, resulting in blood in the anomalous left coronary artery flowing retrograde into the pulmonary artery. This large coronary steal results in myocardial ischemia, dilation of the heart, and, in many cases, fibrosis. Myocardial infarction is not uncommon. The lesion is easily diagnosed by echocardiography and cardiac angiography. The symptoms are usually pallor, sweating, tachycardia, and episodic chest pain that suggests angina pectoris. Repair is indicated at the time of diagnosis and is achieved by direct anastomosis of the left coronary artery to the ascending aorta.

Other surgically relevant coronary anomalies include origin of the left coronary artery from the right sinus and origin of the right coronary artery from the left sinus. Sudden death due to ischemia is a recognized presentation. Potential mechanisms for ischemia include (1) external compression of the artery as it courses between the aorta and pulmonary artery; (2) the slit-like ostium of the anomalous origin; and (3) often an initial intramural course of the anomalous vessel. Interestingly, even for patients presenting with aborted sudden death, an exhaustive workup usually fails to demonstrate ischemia or poor perfusion.

Most surgeons advocate repair once the diagnosis is confirmed in a child or adolescent. This can be accomplished by intraaortic unroofing of the anomalous vessel, thereby translocating the ostium to the correct sinus. Another alternative is detachment and reimplantation to the correct sinus.

Barbero-Marcial M et al: Anomalous origin of the left coronary artery from the pulmonary artery with intramural aortic route: diagnosis and surgical treatment. J Thorac Cardiovasc Surg 1999;117:823.

Cochrane AD et al: Excellent long-term functional outcome after an operation for anomalous left coronary artery from the pulmonary artery. J Thorac Cardiovasc Surg 1999;117:332.

Laks H et al: Aortic implantation of anomalous left coronary artery: an improved surgical approach. J Thorac Cardiovasc Surg 1995;109:519.

Romp RL et al: Outcome of unroofing procedure for repair of anomalous aortic origin of left or right coronary artery. Ann Thorac Surg 2003;76:589.

PERSISTENT LEFT SUPERIOR VENA CAVA

Persistence of a left superior vena cava (left superior cardinal vein) that connects the left jugular and subclavian veins to the coronary sinus is usually asymptomatic. This relatively common anomaly (2–4% of surgical patients) is important to the surgeon in that an otherwise dry operative field remains obscured with venous return. If adequate right-sided venous connections exist or if an innominate vein connects a left cava to the usual right cava, the left cava may be ligated. In other cases, cannulation of the left-sided cava is necessary. Rarely, the right superior vena cava is absent; in 60% cases, an innominate vein and both left and right cavae are present, and each cava is adequate to carry all of the systemic venous return from the upper body.

ENDOCARDIAL FIBROELASTOSIS

This lesion is not operable, but it may occur in association with operable lesions such as coarctation of the aorta, aortic stenosis, anomalous left coronary artery, mitral valvular disease, and hypoplastic left heart syndrome. Hyperplasia of subendocardial elastic and collagenous tissue and proliferation of capillaries cause marked thickening of the ventricular wall and a smooth, glistening lining of the left ventricle. Trabeculae are obliterated, and papillary muscles and chordae tendineae are contracted. The disease affects principally the left ventricle and left atrium; involvement of the right heart chambers is rare. There is some evidence that the disease results from subendocardial ischemia in utero.

Fibroelastosis affects 1–2% of patients with congenital heart disease and may occur primarily without other cardiac lesions. Nearly all infants die of left heart failure within the first year. No specific therapy other than transplantation is available.

CARDIAC TUMORS

Cardiac tumors are uncommon in infancy and childhood, occurring in 0.002–0.08% of patients. In general, primary tumors are more common than tumors metastatic to the heart, though numbers vary depending on the referral patterns for specific institutions. The majority of tumors in children are benign (> 90%). Rhabdomyoma and the somewhat less common fibroma account for the majority of benign tumors. Both tumors are noted more commonly in the ventricle, particularly the septum. Rhabdomyoma appears as pale gray nodules. It may be associated with tuberous sclerosis in over 50% of cases. Fibroma is typically a solid white lesion with distinct borders but no true capsule. In infants, teratoma may be more common than fibroma. Hamartoma is another common tumor in childhood. Myxoma, the most frequently noted cardiac tumor in adults, occurs infrequently in children. Malignant tumors are rare. Malignant teratoma and various types of sarcoma account for most of these tumors.

Symptoms relate to the presence of a space-occupying lesion or to involvement of the conduction system. Therefore, when symptomatic, clinical presentation includes signs and symptoms of failure, outflow tract obstruction, arrhythmias, and embolic events. Echocardiography, cardiac catheterization, computed tomography, and magnetic resonance imaging are all useful diagnostic modalities.

Rhabdomyomas may be observed for spontaneous regression in neonates and young infants. Persistence or enlargement of a tumor in a child of any age, the presence of a tumor in an older child, and symptoms in a child of any age warrant surgical therapy. Complete resection should be the goal; however, excessive myocardial resection resulting in inadequate cardiac function should be avoided.

Chan HS et al: Primary and secondary tumors of childhood involving the heart, pericardium, and great vessels. A report of 75 cases and review of the literature. Cancer 1985;56:825.

Cooley DA et al: Primary cardiac tumors in infants and children: immediate and long-term operative results. Ann Thorac Surg 1996;62:559.

Smythe JF et al: Natural history of cardiac rhabdomyoma in infancy and childhood. Am J Cardiol 1990;66:1247.

PEDIATRIC CARDIAC TRANSPLANTATION

Cardiac transplantation is an established treatment option for infants and children with hypoplastic left heart syndrome, other complex congenital anomalies not amenable to surgical treatment, and various forms of end-stage cardiomyopathy. In certain cases, combined heart-lung transplantation is an option when end-stage cardiac disease is associated with severe pulmonary vascular obstructive disease. In 1998, the International Society for Heart and Lung Transplant recorded over 3000 pediatric cardiac transplants. In contrast to earlier years, congenital heart disease has emerged as the most common diagnosis leading to transplantation, accounting for 50–60% of transplants. Moreover, 20–30% of pediatric cardiac transplants occur in infants. Although similar in several respects to adult cardiac transplantation, there are important differences. The significant number of children with congenital anomalies imposes unique demands on explantation (usually several previous surgeries) and thoughtful preservation of certain structures needed for ultimate reconstruction with the transplanted heart. There is also a greater range of donor-recipient size mismatch and longer ischemic times associated with pediatric cardiac transplantation. Postoperative surveillance may differ as well, particularly in infants, for whom routine transvenous endomyocardial biopsy or intravenous ultrasound may be used less frequently. At its current state of development, ABO-incompatible transplantation is an opportunity uniquely available for infants. This requires use of appropriate type blood products, plasma exchange, and confirmation of absence of antibodies to blood products before reperfusion of the donor heart. Thus far, results appear to be comparable to those in ABO-compatibly transplanted infants.

The decision to transplant occurs in the context of multidisciplinary counseling and consultation and is a decision that obviously cannot be taken lightly by the family or the team. Once a patient is identified as a potential candidate, established protocols guide a thorough evaluation of ultimate suitability for transplantation. Careful analysis of native and palliated or reconstructed anatomy is imperative for successful conduct of the operation.

Immunosuppression is similar to that used in adults and is usually some form of triple therapy consisting of cyclosporine or tacrolimus (FK506), azathioprine, and corticosteroids. Induction therapy with antithymocyte globulin or monoclonal antibodies may be considered in selected cases. Prompt steroid withdrawal or a steroid-free regimen is a recognized practice in children, motivated by the deleterious effects of corticosteroids, particularly growth impairment.

Posttransplantation issues for the child are similar to those for the adult. Bleeding, graft dysfunction, rejection, posttransplant lymphoproliferative disease, and graft vasculopathy (transplant coronary artery disease) are all recognized issues. Transplant coronary artery disease has been a particularly vexing issue that has generated competing explanatory theories. One theory considers vasculopathy a consequence of inadequate immunosuppression and rejection and recommends more intense immunosuppression. At the other extreme is the theory that corticosteroids in some way promote vasculopathy, so that reduced dosage or withdrawal of steroids is recommended. Transplant coronary artery disease occurs in 10–20% of patients, is difficult if not impossible to treat effectively, and typically prompts consideration for retransplantation. Rejection is a common event, occurring with an incidence of approximately 0.5 episodes per patient year, and continues to contribute to mortality. Because of concern for rejection and transplant coronary artery disease, routine surveillance is common practice, using a combination of echocardiography, transvenous endomyocardial biopsy, and intravascular ultrasound. Infection occurs in over 50% of recipients and is another recognized contribution to mortality.

Five-year survival ranges between 60% and 75%. Recent results indicate similar survivals between patients with congenital anomalies and other forms of cardiac disease. Mortality is somewhat higher for infants and may be due to a higher incidence of early graft dysfunction. Outcome analyses do not always include pretransplant mortality. The decision to transplant necessarily invokes a period of waiting for a suitable donor, a period with a mortality that approximates 20%. This is a significant figure that should be acknowledged in the process of choosing between transplantation and another available therapeutic option.

Canter C et al: Survival and risk factors for death after cardiac transplantation in infants: a multi-institutional study. Circulation 1997;96:227.

Hsu DT et al: Heart transplantation in children with congenital heart disease. J Am Coll Cardiol 1995;26:743.

Kanter KR et al: Current results with pediatric heart transplantation. Ann Thorac Surg 1999;68:527.

Pahl E et al: Posttransplant coronary artery disease in children: a multicenter national survey. Circulation 1994;90(part 2):56.

Razzouk AJ et al: Transplantation as a primary treatment for hypoplastic left heart syndrome: Intermediate-term results. Ann Thorac Surg 1996;62:1.

West LJ et al: ABO-incompatible heart transplantation in infants. N Engl J Med 2001;344:793.

DIRECTIONS IN CONGENITAL HEART SURGERY

Creative innovation, multidisciplinary team effort, and advances in hardware development will continue to promote the growth and success of pediatric cardiac surgery. Interventional pediatric cardiology has had a tremendous impact on congenital heart disease. The simultaneous combination of surgical and catheter-based techniques is a newer approach that will continue to receive attention. Cardiopulmonary bypass technology will also continue to improve. Further reduction in oxygenator prime volumes, improvements in biocompatible surfaces, and further modification of ultrafiltration techniques for selective modulation of the inflammatory response will probably occur. Modifications obviating the need for circulatory arrest will be used more frequently in complex neonatal arch surgery. Neuromonitoring, both intraoperatively and postoperatively, will become more commonplace as emphasis on managing the brain and minimizing neuromorbidity evolves. Developments in mechanical assist technology will promote more widespread application to young children. Extracorporeal membrane oxygenation is commonly used in this context at the present time. Miniaturized mobile circuits that can be brought promptly to the bedside for immediate resuscitation are being used more frequently. Prenatal echocardiography, three-dimensional echocardiography, and improvements in transesophageal echocardiography will improve this already extremely versatile diagnostic modality. Prenatal intervention will continue to receive attention in selected centers. Using catheter-based techniques, it may be possible to remove or diminish simple obstructive lesions, thereby eliminating the otherwise inevitable remodeling forces that contribute to abnormal development. Information made available by the genome project will provide some degree of insight into the factors controlling cardiac embryology and development. The clinical transformation and application of this knowledge remain to be seen. Efforts in tissue engineering may ultimately provide more versatile and durable conduits. Although already under way, national and international databases will extend the power of clinical studies and provide answers in a more timely fashion.

However, as is true in other disciplines, the core of future progress is contingent upon the effectiveness and appropriate adaptability of the educational process leading to a career in pediatric cardiac surgery. Recent forces have shaped the environment of clinical surgery in such a way that the traditional sequence of training in general, adult thoracic, and pediatric thoracic (cardiac) surgery is becoming less practical. The consideration of complex issues, difficult decisions, and acceptance of certain tradeoffs will be necessary for the inevitable redesigning of surgical education in the near future.

Esophagus & Diaphragm 20

Marco G. Patti, MD, Pietro Tedesco, MD, & Lawrence W. Way, MD

I. THE ESOPHAGUS

ANATOMY

The esophagus (Figure 20–1) is a muscular tube that serves as a conduit for the passage of food and fluids from the pharynx to the stomach. It originates at the level of the sixth cervical vertebra, posterior to the cricoid cartilage. In the thorax, the esophagus passes behind the aortic arch and the left main stem bronchus, enters the abdomen through the esophageal hiatus of the diaphragm, and terminates in the fundus of the stomach. Its muscle fibers originate from the cricoid cartilage and pharynx above and interdigitate with those of the stomach below. About 2–4 cm of esophagus are normally below the diaphragm. The junction between the esophagus and stomach is maintained in its normal intra-abdominal position by reflections of the peritoneum onto the stomach and of the phrenoesophageal ligament onto the esophagus. The latter is a fibroelastic membrane that lies beneath the peritoneum, on the inferior surface of the diaphragm. When it reaches the esophageal hiatus, the ligament is reflected in an orad direction onto the lower esophagus, where it inserts into the circular muscle layer above the gastroesophageal sphincter, 2–4 cm above the diaphragm.

Three anatomic areas of narrowing occur in the esophagus: (1) at the level of the cricoid cartilage (pharyngoesophageal or upper esophageal sphincter); (2) in the mid thorax, from compression by the aortic arch and the left main stem bronchus; and (3) at the level of the esophageal hiatus of the diaphragm (gastroesophageal or lower esophageal sphincter).

In the adult, the distance as measured from the upper incisor teeth to the cricopharyngeus muscle is 15–20 cm; to the aortic arch, 20–25 cm; to the inferior pulmonary vein, 30–35 cm; and to the gastroesophageal junction, approximately 40–45 cm.

The musculature of the pharynx and upper third of the esophagus is skeletal in type (striated muscle); the remainder is smooth muscle. Physiologically, the entire organ behaves as a single functioning unit, so that no distinction can be made between the upper and lower esophagus from the standpoint of propulsive activity. As in the intestinal tract, the muscle fibers are arranged into inner circular and outer longitudinal layers.

The arterial supply to the esophagus is quite consistent. The upper end is supplied by branches from the inferior thyroid arteries. The thoracic portion receives blood from the bronchial arteries and from esophageal branches originating directly from the aorta. The intercostal arteries may also contribute. The diaphragmatic and abdominal segments are nourished by the left inferior phrenic artery and by the esophageal branches of the left gastric artery.

The venous drainage is more complex and variable. The most important veins are those that drain the lower esophagus. Blood from this region passes into the esophageal branches of the coronary vein, a tributary of the portal vein. This connection constitutes a direct communication between the portal circulation and the venous drainage of the lower esophagus and upper stomach. When the portal system is obstructed, as in cirrhosis of the liver, blood is shunted upward through the coronary vein and the esophageal venous plexus to eventually pass by way of the azygos vein into the superior vena cava. The esophageal veins may eventually form varices as they become distended from the increased blood flow and pressure.

The mucosal lining of the esophagus consists of stratified squamous epithelium that contains scattered mucous glands throughout. The esophagus has no serosal layer and, for this reason, does not heal as readily after injury or surgical anastomosis as other portions of the gastrointestinal tract.

PHYSIOLOGY

The coordinated activity of the upper esophageal sphincter (UES), the esophageal body and the lower esophageal sphincter (LES) is responsible for the motor function of the esophagus.

1. Upper Esophageal Sphincter

The upper esophageal sphincter receives motor innervation directly from the brain (nucleus ambiguous). The sphincter is continuously in a state of tonic contraction,

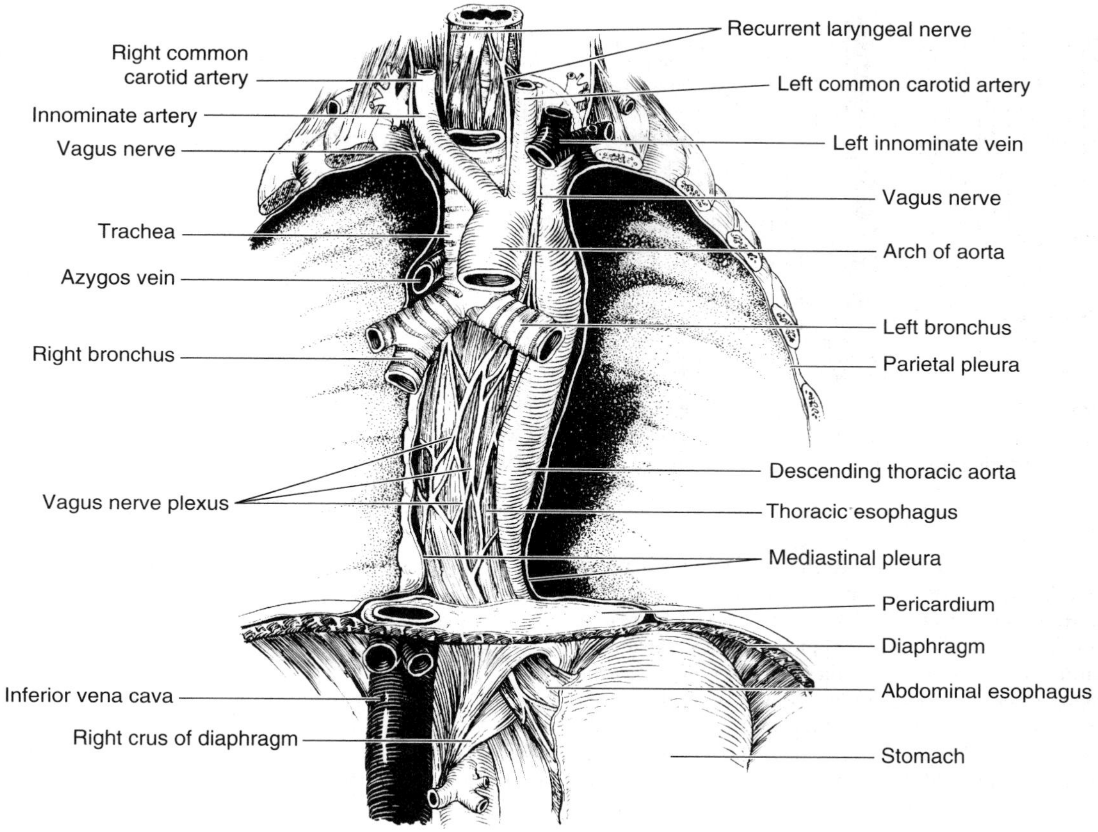

Figure 20–1. Anatomy of the esophagus.

with a resting pressure of about 100 mm Hg (anteroposterior axis). The sphincter prevents passage of air from the pharynx into the esophagus and reflux of esophageal contents into the pharynx. During swallowing, a food bolus is moved by the tongue into the pharynx, which contracts while the UES relaxes. After the food bolus has reached the esophagus, the UES regains its resting tone.

2. Esophageal Body

When food passes through the UES, a contraction is initiated in the upper esophagus, which progresses distally toward the stomach. The wave initiated by swallowing is referred as primary peristalsis (Figure 20–2). It travels at a speed of 3 to 4 cm/s and reaches peak amplitudes of 60–140 mm Hg in the distal esophagus. Local stimulation by distention at any point in the body of the esophagus will elicit a peristaltic wave from the point of stimulus. This is called secondary peristalsis and aids esophageal emptying when the primary wave has failed to clear the lumen of ingested food or when the gastric contents reflux from the stomach. Tertiary waves are considered abnormal, but they are frequently seen in elderly subjects who have no symptoms of esophageal disease.

3. Lower Esophageal Sphincter

The lower esophageal sphincter measures 3–4 cm in length and its resting pressure ranges between 15 and 24 mm Hg. At the time of swallowing, the LES relaxes for 5–10 seconds to allow the food bolus to enter the stomach and then regains its resting tone. The LES relaxation is mediated by vasoactive intestinal polypeptide and nitric oxide, both nonadrenergic, noncholinergic neurotransmitters. The resting tone depends mainly on intrinsic myogenic activity. The LES has a tendency to relax periodically at times independent from swallowing. These periodic relaxations are called **transient lower**

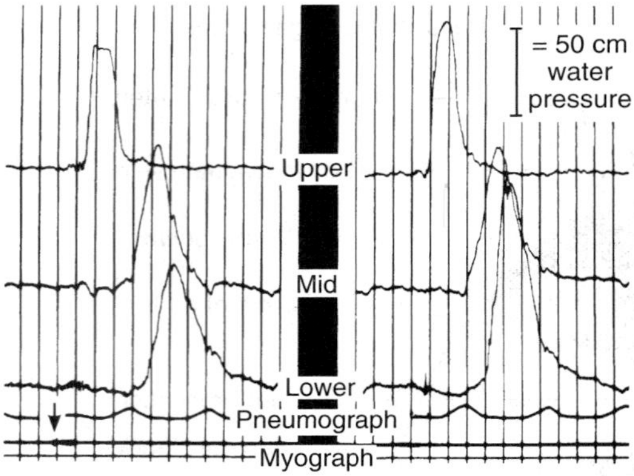

Figure 20–2. Deglutition. Normal esophageal peristaltic waves and pressures during consecutive swallows. Note the orderly downward progression of the waves.

esophageal sphincter relaxations to distinguish them from relaxations triggered by swallows. The cause of these transient relaxations is not known, but gastric distention probably plays a role. Transient LES relaxations account for the small amount of physiologic gastroesophageal reflux present in any individual, and are also the most common cause of reflux in patients with gastroesophageal reflux disease (GERD). Decrease in length or pressure of the LES (or both) is responsible for abnormal reflux in the remaining patients. Overall, it is thought that while transient LES relaxation is the most common mechanism of reflux in volunteers and patients with either absent or mild esophagitis, the prevalence of a mechanically defective sphincter (hypotensive and short) increases in patients with severe esophagitis, particularly when Barrett's metaplasia is present. The crus of the esophageal hiatus of the diaphragm contributes to the resting pressure of the LES. This *pinchcock* action of the diaphragm is particularly important because it protects against reflux caused by sudden increases of intra-abdominal pressure, such as with coughing or bending. This synergistic action of the diaphragm is lost when a sliding hiatal hernia is present, as the gastroesophageal junction is displaced above the diaphragm.

DIAGNOSTIC APPROACH TO ESOPHAGEAL DISEASES

Symptomatic Evaluation

Dysphagia is a unique symptom as it points to an esophageal disorder, either functional (secondary to abnormalities of esophageal peristalsis or lack of coordination between different parts of the esophagus) or mechanical (secondary to a peptic or malignant stricture or an intraluminal mass). Heartburn and regurgitation are considered *typical* of gastroesophageal reflux disease, but they can also be caused by nonesophageal disorders such as biliary disease, irritable bowel syndrome, coronary artery disease, and psychiatric diseases. Gastroesophageal reflux disease can also be responsible for *atypical* symptoms such as cough, hoarseness, and chest pain.

Upper Gastrointestinal Series

The test is performed by giving the patient barium to swallow. Subsequently, multiple images are taken, including the esophagus, the gastroesophageal junction, the stomach, and the duodenum (a barium swallow focuses just on the esophagus and the gastroesophageal junction). This test characterizes a hiatal hernia, an esophageal stricture, an esophageal diverticulum, or an intraluminal mass. A cineesophagram is instead a dynamic evaluation of the swallowing process, and it is particularly useful in patients with functional dysphagia (secondary to a motility disorder, in the absence of a mechanical cause).

Upper Endoscopy

This test allows visualization of the mucosal surface of the esophagus (plus stomach and duodenum). The endoscopist can determine the presence and degree of esophagitis and the presence of an intraluminal mass, and take biopsies.

Endoscopic Ultrasound

An ultrasonographic evaluation can be performed during endoscopy. This test is used in patients with esophageal cancer to define the depth of penetration of the tumor through the esophageal wall (T) and the presence of enlarged periesophageal lymph nodes (N). Fine-needle aspiration of these nodes can be done, and cytologic analysis of the aspirate performed.

Esophageal Manometry

Esophageal manometry allows determination of: (1) lower esophageal sphincter location, length, pressure, and relaxation in response to swallowing; (2) pressure, duration, and velocity of propagation of the peristaltic waves; and (3) location, pressure, relaxation of the upper esophageal sphincter, and coordination with the pharyngeal contraction. The test lasts about 20 minutes, and it is performed by inserting a water-perfused or solid-state catheter through the nostrils (using topical anesthesia) down the esophagus into the stomach, and then withdrawing it gradually while giving the patient sips of water.

Ambulatory 24-hour pH Monitoring

This test measures reflux of acid from the stomach into the esophagus, and it is considered the gold standard for the diagnosis of gastroesophageal reflux disease. By convention, the catheter is placed 5 cm above the upper border of the manometrically determined lower esophageal sphincter and is kept in place for 24 hours, during which the patient does not alter the daily activities and diet. Alternatively, the test can be performed using a wireless capsule implanted in the mucosa of the distal esophagus, avoiding the discomfort of wearing a wire, which comes through the nose for 1 day. In patients in whom cough or hoarseness are thought to be secondary to the upward extent of the gastric refluxate, acid can be measured at different levels in the esophagus. In addition to defining whether a pathologic amount of gastroesophageal reflux is present, the test establishes if there is a temporal correlation between episodes of reflux and symptoms such as heartburn, cough, and chest pain.

Computerized Axial Tomography

A CT scan is used to assess the presence of metastases (lung, liver, adrenals) in patients with esophageal cancer (M).

Positron Emission Tomography

A PET scan is used to assess the metastatic spread of esophageal cancer (M). In addition, it might help predicting the response of esophageal cancer to neoadjuvant therapy.

Laparoscopy/Thoracoscopy

Laparoscopy or thoracoscopy can be used to stage esophageal cancer, particularly when liver metastases or extensive lymphadenopathy are suspected.

Jacobson BC et al: The role of endoscopy in the assessment and treatment of esophageal cancer. Gastrointest Endosc 2003;57:817.

Krasna MJ et al: Thoracoscopy/laparoscopy in the staging of esophageal cancer: Maryland experience. Surg Laparosc Endosc Percut Tech 2002;12:213.

Patti MG et al: Role of esophageal function tests in the diagnosis of gastroesophageal reflux disease. Dig Dis Sci 2001;46:597.

Prakash C, Clouse RE: Value of extended recording time with wireless pH monitoring in evaluating gastroesophageal reflux disease. Clin Gastroenterol and Hepatol 2005;3:329.

Rasanen JV et al: Prospective analysis of accuracy of positron emission tomography, computed tomography, and endoscopic ultrasonography in staging of adenocarcinoma of the esophagus and the esophagogastric junction. Ann Surg Oncol 2003;10:954.

Sampliner RE: Updated guidelines for the diagnosis, surveillance, and therapy of Barrett's esophagus. Am J Gastroenterol 2002;97:1888.

ESOPHAGEAL MOTILITY DISORDERS

The named primary esophageal motility disorders are achalasia, diffuse esophageal spasm, nutcracker esophagus, and the hypertensive lower esophageal sphincter. They occur in the absence of any other esophageal disorder such as reflux, and their cause is unknown. These disorders present with a combination of dysphagia, regurgitation, chest pain, and heartburn. Esophageal manometry is the key test that differentiates these disorders.

ACHALASIA

ESSENTIALS OF DIAGNOSIS

- *Dysphagia.*
- *Regurgitation.*
- *Radiologic evidence of distal esophageal narrowing.*
- *Absence of esophageal peristalsis on esophageal manometry.*

General Considerations

Esophageal achalasia is a primary esophageal motility disorder characterized by the absence of esophageal peristalsis and increased pressure of the lower esophageal sphincter, which fails to relax completely in response to swallowing. These abnormalities lead to impaired propulsion of food with consequent stasis in the esophagus. The incidence of achalasia is about 1/100,000 persons. It affects men more than women, and it can occur at any age.

Pathogenesis

The etiology of esophageal achalasia is still unknown, but two theories exist: (1) a degenerative disease of the neurons; and (2) infections of the neurons by a virus (eg, herpes zoster) or another infectious agent. The latter is supported by the fact that similar findings occur in patients with **Chagas' disease** (American trypanosomiasis), a condition in which the infective organism destroys parasympathetic ganglion cells throughout the body, including the heart and the gastrointestinal, urinary, and respiratory tracts. The degeneration of the myenteric plexus of Auerbach determines loss of the postganglionic inhibitory neurons (which contain nitric oxide and vasoactive intestinal polypeptide), which mediate LES relaxation. Because the postganglionic cholinergic neurons are spared, there is unopposed cholinergic stimulation, which increases LES resting pressure and decreases LES relaxation. There is no propagation of peristaltic waves in response to swallowing, but rather the presence of simultaneous contractions, which are often a mirror image of each other.

Clinical Findings

A. Symptoms and Signs

Dysphagia is the most common symptom, virtually experienced by every patient. It is often for both solids and liquids. Most patients adapt with changes in their diet and are able to maintain a stable weight, while other eventually experience some weight loss. Regurgitation of undigested food is the second most common symptom and is present in about 60% of patients. It occurs more often in the supine position and may lead to aspiration. Heartburn is present in about 40% of patients. It is not due to gastroesophageal reflux, but rather to stasis and fermentation of undigested food in the distal esophagus. Chest pain also occurs in about 40% of patients, and it is usually experienced at the time of a meal.

B. Imaging Studies

A barium swallow should be the first test performed in the evaluation of a patient with dysphagia. It usually shows narrowing at the level of the gastroesophageal junction (Figure 20–3). A dilated, sigmoid esophagus may be present in patients with long-standing achalasia.

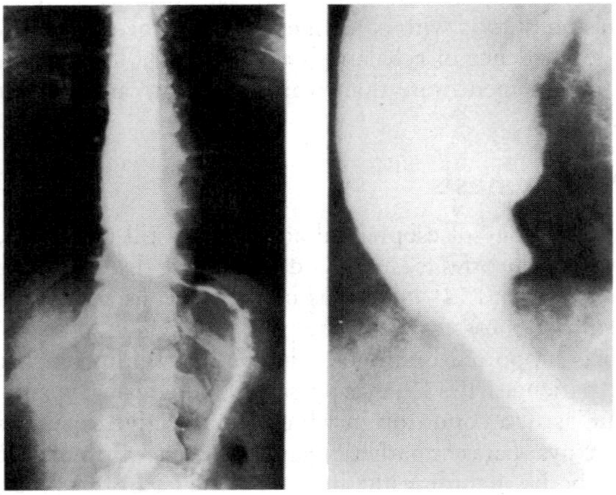

Figure 20–3. Achalasia of the esophagus. *Left:* Moderately advanced achalasia. Note dilated body of esophagus and smoothly tapered lower portion. *Right:* Widely patent cardioesophageal region following cardiomyotomy (Heller procedure).

Endoscopy is performed to rule out a tumor of the gastroesophageal junction.

C. Special Tests

Esophageal manometry is the key test for establishing the diagnosis of esophageal achalasia. The classic manometric findings are: (1) absence of esophageal peristalsis; and (2) hypertensive LES (in about 50% of patients) that relaxes only partially in response to swallowing. When the esophagus is dilated and sigmoid in shape, it may be difficult to pass the catheter through the gastroesophageal junction into the stomach: in these cases the catheter may be placed under fluoroscopic or endoscopic guidance.

Differential Diagnosis

Benign strictures due to gastroesophageal reflux and esophageal carcinoma may mimic the clinical presentation of achalasia. Sometimes an infiltrating tumor of the gastroesophageal junction can mimic not only the clinical and radiological presentation of achalasia but also the manometric profile. This condition is called **secondary or pseudo achalasia**, and should be suspected in patients older than 60 years of age with recent onset of dysphagia (less than 6 months) and excessive weight loss. An endoscopic ultrasound or a CT scan can help establishing the diagnosis.

Complications

Aspiration of retained and undigested food can cause repeated episodes of pneumonia. Achalasia is also a risk factor for esophageal cancer. Squamous cell carcinoma is probably due to the continuous irritation of the mucosa by the retained and fermenting food. Adenocarcinoma can occur in patients who develop gastroesophageal reflux after either pneumatic dilatation or myotomy.

Treatment

Therapy is palliative, and it is directed toward relief of symptoms by decreasing the outflow resistance caused by the dysfunctional LES. Because peristalsis is absent and does not return after any form of treatment, gravity becomes the key factor that allows emptying of food from the esophagus into the stomach. The following treatment modalities are available to achieve this goal:

Medical Therapy

Calcium-channel blockers are used to decrease LES pressure. However, because only 10% of patients benefit from this treatment, it should be used primarily in elderly patients who have contraindications to either pneumatic dilatation or to surgery.

A. Endoscopic Treatment

Intrasphincteric injection of botulinum toxin is used to block the release of acetylcholine at the level of the LES, therefore restoring the balance between excitatory and inhibitory neurotransmitters. This treatment, however, is of limited value as only 60% of treated patients still have relief of dysphagia 6 months after treatment, and this number further decreases to 30% (even after multiple injections) 2.5 years later. In addition, it often causes an inflammatory reaction at the level of the gastroesophageal junction, which makes a subsequent myotomy more difficult. It should be used primarily in elderly patients who are poor candidates for dilatation or surgery.

Pneumatic dilatation has been the main modality of treatment for many years. A balloon is inflated at the level of the gastroesophageal junction to rupture the muscle fibers while trying to leave the mucosa intact. The initial success rate is between 70% and 80% but it decreases to 50% at 10 years, even after multiple dilatations. The perforation rate is around 2–5%. If a perforation occurs, patients are taken emergently to the operating room, where closure of the perforation and a myotomy are performed through a left thoracotomy. The incidence of postdilatation gastroesophageal reflux is about 25–35%. Patients who fail pneumatic dilatation are usually treated by a Heller myotomy.

B. Surgical Treatment

A laparoscopic Heller myotomy and partial fundoplication is the procedure of choice for esophageal achalasia. The operation consists of a controlled division of the muscle fibers (myotomy) of the lower esophagus (6 cm) and proximal stomach (2 cm), followed by an anterior or a posterior partial fundoplication to prevent reflux. Patients remain in the hospital for 24–48 hours and return to regular activities in about 2 weeks. The operation effectively relieves symptoms in about 90% of patients and is effective even in patients who have a low LES pressure after previous dilatation or whose esophagus is dilated. The incidence of postoperative reflux is around 15%. Because of the excellent results, the short hospital stay, and the fast recovery time, a laparoscopic Heller myotomy and partial fundoplication is considered today the primary treatment modality for esophageal achalasia. Persistent or recurrent dysphagia after myotomy can be treated with pneumatic dilatation or a second myotomy. Esophagectomy is reserved for patients with severe dysphagia who have failed both dilatation and myotomy.

Prognosis

A laparoscopic Heller myotomy allows excellent relief of symptoms in the majority of patients and should be preferred to pneumatic dilatation whenever surgical expertise is available. Botulinum toxin and medications should be used only in patients who are not candidates for pneumatic dilatation or laparoscopic Heller myotomy. Periodic follow-up by endoscopy is recommended to rule out the development of esophageal cancer.

DIFFUSE ESOPHAGEAL SPASM

ESSENTIALS OF DIAGNOSIS

- *Dysphagia.*
- *Chest pain.*
- *Intermittent symptoms.*
- *Radiologic evidence of tertiary contractions (corkscrew esophagus).*
- *Intermittent normal and absent peristaltic waves on manometry (> 10%, < 100%).*
- *Normal 24-hour ambulatory pH monitoring.*

General Considerations

The cause of this disorder is not known. Stress might play a role. Progression of diffuse esophageal spasm to achalasia has been documented (complete loss of esophageal peristalsis).

Clinical Findings

A. Symptoms and Signs

The most common symptom is intermittent chest pain, which varies from slight discomfort to severe spasmodic pain that simulates the pain of coronary artery disease. Most patients complain of dysphagia, but weight loss is uncommon.

B. Imaging Studies

The barium swallow is abnormal in 70% of patients. Fluoroscopic studies show segmental spasms, areas of narrowing, and irregular uncoordinated peristalsis *(corkscrew esophagus)* in about 30% of patients. An epiphrenic diverticulum is sometimes present.

C. Manometry

Esophageal manometry is the key test for establishing the diagnosis of diffuse esophageal spasm. The classic manometric findings are: (1) alternation of esophageal peristalsis and simultaneous contractions (> 10% and < 100%). Contrary to old beliefs, the contractions are not hypertensive but of normal or even low amplitude; and (2) normal LES function or abnormalities similar to those seen in achalasia (elevated testing pressure and decreased relaxation in response to swallowing).

D. Ambulatory 24-Hour pH Monitoring

This test is essential as the symptoms and the manometric picture of diffuse esophageal spasm can be caused by gastroesophageal reflux disease. In such cases treatment should be directed toward reflux because the dysmotility is secondary. Therefore, it is crucial to be certain about the diagnosis, as treatment of gastroesophageal reflux disease (acid-reducing medications or a fundoplication) is completely different from that of a primary esophageal motility disorder (pneumatic dilatation or myotomy).

Differential Diagnosis

When chest pain is the predominant symptom, a complete cardiac workup is necessary to exclude a cardiac reason for the pain. Once the heart disease has been excluded, ambulatory pH monitoring must be performed to rule out abnormal gastroesophageal reflux, which is the most common cause of *noncardiac chest pain*. Esophageal manometry is the only test that distinguishes diffuse esophageal spasm from other primary esophageal motor disorders. An endoscopy should be performed to confirm the absence of intraluminal lesions.

Complications

Regurgitation and aspiration may occur, possibly leading to repeated pneumonic infections. An epiphrenic diverticulum may be present, secondary to the motor disorder.

Treatment

The therapeutic approach to diffuse esophageal spasm is similar to that of achalasia. Both disorders can be conceptualized as different points in a spectrum of esophageal motility, where peristalsis is progressively lost and progression from diffuse spasm to achalasia has been documented. In patients with diffuse esophageal spasm, dysphagia is secondary to the abnormal peristalsis and LES, while the chest pain probably results from esophageal distension from poor emptying. Medical therapy (long-acting nitrates, calcium-channel blocking agents) is relatively ineffective. Pneumatic dilatation improves the dysphagia in about 25% of patients. Intra-sphincteric injection of botulinum toxin has also given poor results. In contrast, a laparoscopic Heller myotomy and partial fundoplication (as for patients with achalasia) improves both dysphagia and chest pain in about 80%of patients.

The **hypertensive lower esophageal sphincter** is a rare disorder that manifests with dysphagia and is characterized manometrically by a hypertensive LES (resting pressure > 45 mm Hg), which relaxes in response to swallowing, and normal esophageal peristalsis. Treatment is similar to that of esophageal achalasia.

NUTCRACKER ESOPHAGUS

ESSENTIALS OF DIAGNOSIS

- *Chest pain.*
- *Dysphagia.*
- *Intermittent symptoms.*
- *Peristaltic waves propagate normally but have very high amplitude and long duration.*
- *Normal 24-hour ambulatory pH monitoring.*

General Considerations

The cause of this disorder is not known.

Clinical Findings

A. Symptoms and Signs

Chest pain is the most common symptom. Patients often come to the attention of gastroenterologists only after a thorough cardiac workup has been performed. About half of the patients complain of dysphagia in addition to chest pain.

B. Imaging Studies

The barium swallow is usually normal. An epiphrenic diverticulum is sometimes present.

C. Manometry

Esophageal manometry is the key test for establishing the diagnosis of nutcracker esophagus. The classic manometric findings are as follows: (1) normal propagation of the peristalsis waves (there are no simultaneous contractions). The peristaltic waves in the distal esophagus, however, have very high amplitude (> 180 mm Hg) and duration (> 6 seconds); and (2) normal LES function or abnormalities similar to those seen in achalasia and diffuse esophageal spasm.

D. Ambulatory 24-Hour pH Monitoring

This test is essential because the symptoms and the manometric picture of nutcracker esophagus can be caused by gastroesophageal reflux disease. In such cases treatment should be directed toward reflux because the dysmotility is secondary.

Differential Diagnosis

When chest pain is the predominant symptom, a complete cardiac workup is necessary to exclude a cardiac reason for the pain. Once the heart has been excluded as a cause of the symptom, ambulatory pH monitoring must be performed to rule out abnormal gastroesophageal reflux, which is the most common cause of *noncardiac chest pain*. Esophageal manometry is the only test that distinguishes nutcracker esophagus from other primary esophageal motility disorders.

Complications

Regurgitation and aspiration may occur, possibly leading to repeated pneumonic infections. An epiphrenic diverticulum may be present, secondary to the motor disorder.

Treatment

The nutcracker esophagus is not as well defined as the other primary esophageal motility disorders for both pathophysiology and treatment. Initially it was thought that the high pressures found were the cause of the chest pain, so treatment was aimed at decreasing the high amplitude of the peristaltic waves. However, calcium-channel blockers are unable to improve the chest pain even though they decrease the strength of the contractions. Similarly, the results of surgery have been disappointing, as chest pain persists after myotomy in about 50% of patients. Dysphagia is improved in 80% of patients.

Eckardt VF et al: Pneumatic dilatation for achalasia: late results of a prospective follow-up investigation. Gut 2004;53:629.

Patti MG et al: Spectrum of esophageal motility disorders. Implications for diagnosis and treatment. Arch Surg 2005; 140:442.

Patti MG et al: Impact of minimally invasive surgery on the treatment of esophageal achalasia. A decade of change. J Am Coll Surg 2003;196:698.

Perretta S et al: Achalasia and chest pain. Effect of laparoscopic Heller myotomy. J Gastrointest Surg 2003;7:595.

Richards WO et al: Heller myotomy versus Heller myotomy with Dor fundoplication for achalasia. A prospective double-blind clinical trial. Ann Surg 2004;240:405.

Richter JE: Oesophageal motility disorders. Lancet 2001;358:823.

Rosemurgy A et al: Laparoscopic Heller myotomy provides durable relief from achalasia and salvages failures after botox or dilation. Ann Surg 2005;241:725.

West RL et al: Long-term results of pneumatic dilatation in achalasia followed for more than 5 years. Am J Gastroenterol 2002; 97:1346.

Zaninotto G et al: Randomized controlled trial of botulinum toxin versus laparoscopic Heller myotomy for esophageal achalasia. Ann Surg 2004;239:364.

ESOPHAGEAL DIVERTICULA

Diverticula of the esophagus are mainly located above the upper esophageal sphincter (pharyngoesophageal or Zenker's diverticulum) or the lower esophageal sphincter (epiphrenic diverticulum). They are considered pulsion diverticula and are secondary to abnormalities of the sphincters, in terms of resting pressure, relaxation in response to swallowing, and coordination with the segment above the sphincter. As a consequence, mucosa and submucosa protrude through the muscular layers forming the out-pouching.

1. Pharyngoesophageal Diverticulum (Zenker's Diverticulum)

ESSENTIALS OF DIAGNOSIS

- *Dysphagia.*
- *Regurgitation of undigested food (with risk of aspiration).*
- *Gurgling sounds in the neck.*
- *Halitosis.*

General Considerations

This is the most common of the esophageal diverticula and is three times more frequent in men than in women. Most patients are over age 60. The condition originates from the posterior wall of the esophagus, in a triangular area of weakness (Killian triangle), limited inferiorly by the cricopharyngeus muscle and superiorly by the inferior constrictor muscles. As the diverticulum enlarges, it tends to deviate from the midline, mostly to the left.

Pathogenesis

A Zenker's diverticulum is due to either lack of coordination between the pharyngeal contraction and the opening time of the UES, or to a hypertensive UES. Because of the increased intraluminal pressure, there is progressive herniation of mucosa and submucosa through the Killian triangle. Occasionally, upper esophageal sphincter dysfunction can occur in the absence of a diverticulum (cricopharyngeal achalasia). A hereditary syndrome called oculopharyngeal muscular dystrophy, consisting of ptosis and dysphagia, has been described in patients of French-Canadian ancestry. The dysphagia is the result of weak pharyngeal musculature in the face of normal upper esophageal sphincter function; it is considerably improved by upper esophageal sphincter

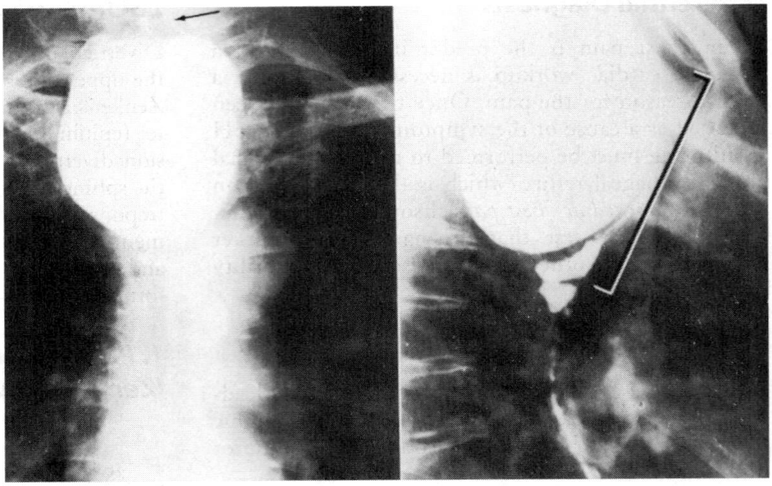

Figure 20–4. Large pharyngoesophageal diverticulum. Note origin in midline *(arrow, left)* and compression of esophagus *(bracket, right)*.

myotomy. This syndrome also manifests with cervical dysphagia. A chronic cough may develop in some patients from aspiration of saliva and ingested food.

Clinical Findings

A. Symptoms

Dysphagia is the most common symptom. Regurgitation of undigested food from the diverticulum often occurs and can lead to aspiration into the tracheobronchial tree and pneumonia. Patients frequently have halitosis and can hear gurgling sounds in the neck. About 30% of patients have associated gastroesophageal reflux disease.

B. Imaging Studies

A barium swallow clearly shows the position and size of the diverticulum, or a prominent cricopharyngeal bar without diverticulum (Figure 20–4). In some patients a hiatal hernia is present.

C. Special Tests

Esophageal manometry shows lack of coordination between the pharynx and the cricopharyngeus muscle and often a hypertensive UES. In addition, it can show a hypotensive LES and abnormal esophageal peristalsis. Ambulatory pH monitoring determines if abnormal esophageal acid exposure is present.

Endoscopy may be dangerous because the instrument can enter the diverticulum rather than the esophageal lumen and cause a perforation.

Differential Diagnosis

Differential diagnosis includes esophageal stricture, achalasia, and esophageal cancer. Pulmonary infection is the most frequent serious complication, and many patients are first seen after experiencing repeated episodes of pneumonia.

Treatment

The standard treatment consists of excision of the diverticulum and myotomy of the cricopharyngeus muscle and the upper 3 cm of the posterior esophageal wall. For small diverticula (< 2 cm), the myotomy alone is sufficient. As an alternative to the conventional treatment, a transoral endoscopic approach (using an endoscopic stapling device that ablates the septum between the diverticulum and the cervical esophagus) can be used for diverticula between 3 and 6 cm in size. If gastroesophageal reflux is present, it should be corrected before dividing the upper esophageal sphincter in order to avoid aspiration.

Prognosis

The prognosis is excellent in about 90% of cases. Complications are rare and the patients are usually able to eat the day after the procedure.

Chang CY et al: Endoscopic staple diverticulostomy for Zenker's diverticulum. Review of the literature and experience in 159 consecutive cases. Laryngoscope 2003;113:957.

Constantini M et al: Oesophageal diverticula. Best Practice & Research Clinical Gastroenterology 2004;18:3.

Counter PR et al: Long-term follow-up of endoscopic stapled diverticulotomy. Ann R Coll Surg Engl 2002;84:89.

Smith SR et al: Endoscopic stapling technique for the treatment of Zenker diverticulum vs standard open-neck technique: a direct comparison and charge analysis. Arch Otolaryngol Head Neck Surg 2002;128:141.

2. *Epiphrenic Diverticulum*

ESSENTIALS OF DIAGNOSIS

- *Dysphagia.*
- *Regurgitation.*
- *Diverticulum evident on barium swallow.*
- *Esophageal motility disorder shown by esophageal manometry.*

General Considerations

Epiphrenic diverticula are located just above the diaphragm. The diverticulum is not a primary anatomic abnormality but rather the consequence of an underlying motility disorder of the esophagus (achalasia is the most common, followed by diffuse esophageal spasm and nutcracker esophagus). The disorder causes an outflow obstruction at the level of the gastroesophageal junction, with consequent increase in intraluminal pressure and progressive herniation of mucosa and submucosa through the esophageal muscle layers.

Clinical Findings

A. Symptoms

The symptoms experienced by the patient are in part due to the underlying motility disorder (dysphagia, chest pain) and in part due to the diverticulum per se (regurgitation with the risk of aspiration). Some diverticula, however, can be asymptomatic.

B. Imaging Studies

A chest radiograph can show an air-fluid level in the posterior mediastinum. A barium swallow clearly shows the position and size of the diverticulum.

C. Special Tests

In the majority of cases esophageal manometry shows the underlying motility disorder. Sometimes it is difficult to position the manometry catheter, and endoscopic or fluoroscopic guidance might be necessary.

Differential Diagnosis

A paraesophageal hernia can be confused with an epiphrenic diverticulum. The barium swallow and the endoscopy help in establishing the diagnosis.

Treatment

The treatment is surgical, and the laparoscopic approach is preferred. It consists of the following:

(1) Resection of the diverticulum.

(2) Long myotomy. This is performed in the side of the esophagus opposite to where the diverticulum is located. It extends proximally to the upper border of the neck of the diverticulum and distally for about 2 cm onto the gastric wall.

(3) A partial fundoplication to prevent gastroesophageal reflux.

Prognosis

A laparoscopic diverticulectomy, with myotomy and fundoplication, is successful in 80–90% of cases.

Fasano NC et al: Epiphrenic diverticulum: clinical and radiographic findings in 27 patients. Dysphagia 2003;18:9.

Nehra D et al: Physiologic basis for the treatment of epiphrenic diverticulum. Ann Surg 2002;235:346.

ESOPHAGEAL MANIFESTATIONS IN SCLERODERMA & OTHER SYSTEMIC DISEASES

Scleroderma and several other systemic diseases may involve the esophagus.

In scleroderma or progressive systemic sclerosis, there is involvement of the gastrointestinal tract in up to 90% of patients. The most common site of gastrointestinal involvement is the smooth muscle portion of the esophagus, where atrophy and fibrosis occur. The upper esophagus (striated muscle) and the upper esophageal sphincter are not involved. As a consequence, the lower esophageal sphincter has a low pressure and the peristalsis is weak (low amplitude or abnormal propagation of the peristaltic waves). These changes can be followed by an increased amount of gastroesophageal reflux with delayed clearance of the refluxed gastric contents. Esophageal symptoms usually appear in patients with the characteristic skin changes and Raynaud's syndrome. In addition to heartburn and regurgitation, patients may have respiratory symptoms due to the upward extent of the gastric refluxate and aspiration. Dysphagia may be due to the abnormal peristalsis or to the presence of a peptic stricture. The diagnostic approach is similar to that of patients with gastroesophageal reflux disease:

- A barium swallow may show a hiatal hernia or a stricture.
- Endoscopy shows esophagitis in 50–60% of patients. Barrett's esophagus is present in about 10% of patients.
- Esophageal manometry usually shows a hypotensive lower esophageal sphincter. Dysmotility is frequent and can progress to complete loss of peristalsis.

- Ambulatory pH monitoring is essential to establish the diagnosis. It can also measure the presence of acid in the proximal esophagus and pharynx in patients with cough or vocal cord problems.
- Gastric scintigraphy is indicated in patient who experience postprandial bloating and fullness to measure the gastric emptying of solids and liquids.

Similar esophageal changes may also occur in rheumatoid arthritis, Sjögren's syndrome, Raynaud's disease, and systemic lupus erythematosus. Similar motor abnormalities are occasionally seen in alcoholism, diabetes mellitus, myxedema, multiple sclerosis, and amyloidosis.

Medical management should always be tried first. A proton pump inhibitor is the drug of choice. If gastroparesis is present, a prokinetic medication such as metoclopramide should be added. A fundoplication should be considered particularly in patients with regurgitation, cough, or vocal cord problems.

Ling TC, Johnston BT: Esophageal investigations in connective tissue disease: which tests are most appropriate? J Clin Gastroenterol 2001;32:33.

Marie I et al: Esophageal involvement and pulmonary manifestations in systemic sclerosis. Arthritis Rheum 2001;45:346.

GASTROESOPHAGEAL REFLUX DISEASE

ESSENTIALS OF DIAGNOSIS

- *Heartburn.*
- *Regurgitation.*
- *Sliding hiatal hernia on barium swallow.*
- *Esophagitis on endoscopy.*
- *Abnormal esophageal motility on manometry.*
- *Abnormal esophageal exposure on ambulatory pH monitoring.*

General Considerations

Gastroesophageal reflux disease (GERD) is the most common upper gastrointestinal disorder of the Western world and accounts for about 75% of esophageal diseases. Heartburn, usually considered synonymous with the presence of abnormal gastroesophageal reflux, is experienced by 20–40% of the adult population of Western countries. However, because many symptomatic patients treat themselves with over-the-counter medications without consulting a physician, the prevalence of the disease is probably higher than reported. The incidence of reflux symptoms increases with age, and both sexes seem to be equally affected. Symptoms are more common during pregnancy, probably due to hormonal effects on the LES and the increased intra-abdominal pressure due to the enlarging uterus.

Pathogenesis

Gastroesophageal reflux disease is caused by the abnormal retrograde flow of gastric contents into the esophagus, resulting in symptoms and mucosal damage. A defective LES is the most common cause of GERD. Transient LES relaxations account for the majority of reflux episodes in patients without mucosal damage or with mild esophagitis, while a short and hypotensive LES is more frequently found in patients with more severe esophagitis. In 40–60% of patients with GERD, abnormalities of esophageal peristalsis are also present. Because esophageal peristalsis is the main determinant of esophageal clearance (the ability of the esophagus to clear gastric contents refluxed through the LES), patients with abnormal esophageal peristalsis have more severe reflux and slower clearance. Therefore, these patients often have more severe mucosal injury and more frequent atypical symptoms such as cough or hoarseness. A hiatal hernia also contributes to the incompetence of the gastroesophageal junction by altering the anatomic relationship between the esophageal crus and the LES. As the gastroesophageal junction is displaced above the diaphragm, the *pinchcock* action of the esophageal crus is lost. In patients with large hiatal hernias, the LES is usually shorter and weaker and the amount of reflux is greater.

Clinical Findings

A. Symptoms

Heartburn, regurgitation, and dysphagia are considered *typical* symptoms of GERD. However, a clinical diagnosis of GERD based on these symptoms is correct in only 70% of patients (when compared with the results of pH monitoring). A good response to therapy with proton pump inhibitors is a good predictor of the presence of abnormal reflux. GERD can also cause *atypical* symptoms such as cough, wheezing, chest pain, hoarseness, and dental erosions. Two mechanisms have been postulated for GERD-induced respiratory symptoms: (1) a vagal reflex arc resulting in bronchoconstriction; and (2) microaspiration into the tracheobronchial tree. ENT symptoms such as hoarseness or dental erosions are instead secondary to the upward extent of the acid with direct damage of the vocal cords or teeth.

B. Barium Swallow

A barium swallow provides information about the presence and size of a hiatal hernia, the presence and length

Table 20–1. Endoscopic grading system for esophagitis.

Grade 1	Reddening of the mucosa without ulceration
Grade 2	Linear ulcerations lined with granulation tissue that bleeds easily when touched
Grade 3	Ulcerations have coalesced to leave islands of epithelium
Grade 4	Stricture

of a stricture, and the length of the esophagus. This test, however, is not diagnostic of GERD, as a hiatal hernia or reflux of barium can be present in the absence of abnormal reflux.

C. Endoscopy

Fifty percent of patients with abnormal reflux do not have esophagitis on endoscopy. Therefore, endoscopy is useful for diagnosing complications of GERD such as esophagitis, Barrett's esophagus, or a stricture. In addition, there is major interobserver variation among endoscopists for the low grades of esophagitis (Table 20–1).

D. Esophageal Manometry

This test provides information about the LES (resting pressure, length, and relaxation) and the quality of esophageal peristalsis. In addition, manometry is essential for proper placement of the pH probe for ambulatory pH monitoring (5 cm above the upper border of the LES).

E. Ambulatory pH Monitoring

This test has a sensitivity and specificity of about 92% and is considered the gold standard for diagnosing GERD (Table 20–2). Medications that affect the production of acid by the parietal cells must be stopped 3 days (H_2 blocking agents) to 14 days (proton pump inhibitors) prior to the study. Diet and exercise are unrestricted during the test in order to mimic a typical day of the patient's life. This test should be performed (1) in patients who do not respond to medical therapy; (2) in patients who relapse after discontinuation of medical therapy; (3) before antireflux surgery; or (4) when evaluating atypical symptoms such as cough and hoarseness. As less than 50% of these patients experience heartburn or have esophagitis on endoscopy, a pH monitoring study becomes the only way to establish a link between reflux and symptoms. A pH probe with 2 sensors, located 5 and 20 cm above the LES, allows determination of the upward extent of the reflux. Tracings are analyzed for a temporal correlation between symptoms and episodes of reflux.

Differential Diagnosis

Heartburn can be the presenting symptom of irritable bowel syndrome, achalasia, cholelithiasis, coronary artery disease, or psychiatric disorders. Esophageal manometry and pH monitoring are essential to determine with certainty if GERD is present and if reflux is the cause of the symptoms.

Complications

Esophagitis is the most common complication. Peptic strictures are uncommon, particularly in the era of proton pump inhibitors. Barrett's esophagus (metaplasia of the esophageal mucosa from squamous to columnar epithelium) is found in about 12% of patients with reflux documented by pH monitoring. Some patients may eventually progress to high-grade dysplasia and adenocarcinoma. Respiratory complications vary from chronic cough to asthma, aspiration pneumonia, and even pulmonary fibrosis. Vocal cord and dental damage can also occur.

Treatment

A. Lifestyle Modifications

Patients should eat frequent small meals during the day (to avoid gastric distention), avoiding fatty foods, spicy foods, and chocolate, as they lower LES pressure. The last meal should be no less than 2 hours before going to bed. In order to increase the effect of gravity, the head of the bed should be elevated over 4- to 6-inch blocks.

B. Medical Therapy

Antacids are useful for patients with mild intermittent heartburn. Acid-suppressing medications are the

Table 20–2. Normal values for ambulatory 24-hour pH monitoring.

Percentage of total time pH < 4.0	4.5%
Percentage of upright time pH < 4.0	8.4%
Percentage of supine time pH < 4.0	3.5%
Number of episodes of reflux < 4.0	47
Number of episodes > 5 minutes	3½
Longest episode (minutes)	20
Composite score[1]	14.7

[1]The composite score indicates the extent to which the patient's values deviate from the normal means of the six variables. It allows one to express in a single figure the degree of the patient's abnormality. Calculation of the composite score is explained in Stein HJ et al: Outpatient physiologic testing and surgical management of foregut motility disorders. Curr Probl Surg 1992;24:495.

mainstay of medical therapy. H_2 blocking agents are usually prescribed for patients with mild symptoms or mild esophagitis. Proton pump inhibitors are superior to H_2 blocking agents, as they determine a more profound control of the acid secretion, with healing of esophagitis in 80–90% of patients. However, symptoms and esophagitis tend to recur in the majority of patients after discontinuation of therapy, so that most patients need chronic maintenance therapy. In addition, about 50% of patients on maintenance proton pump inhibitors require increasing doses to maintain healing of esophagitis. Medical therapy is largely ineffective for the treatment of the extraesophageal manifestations of GERD due to the upward extension of the refluxate. In these patients acid-suppressing medications only alter the pH of the gastric refluxate, but reflux and aspiration can still occur because of an incompetent LES and ineffective esophageal peristalsis.

C. Surgical Therapy

In the past antireflux surgery was considered only for patients who did not respond to medical treatment with antacids or H_2 blocking agents. Today the ideal patient is the one whose heartburn is well controlled by proton pump inhibitors and in whom ambulatory pH monitoring shows abnormal reflux. The operation is indicated in: (1) young patients who require chronic therapy with proton pump inhibitors for control of symptoms; (2) patients in whom regurgitation persists during therapy; (3) patients with respiratory symptoms (cough, asthma, aspiration pneumonia, pulmonary fibrosis); (4) patients with vocal cord damage; or (5) patients with Barrett's esophagus. Recent evidence suggests that an effective antireflux operation may promote regression of the columnar epithelium in up to 50% of patients who have a short segment of Barrett's esophagus (< 3 cm). In addition, it may arrest the progression from metaplasia to dysplasia. However, since the response to therapy is unpredictable, endoscopic surveillance after laparoscopic fundoplication in patients with Barrett's is recommended.

The goal of surgical therapy is to restore the competence of the lower esophageal sphincter. A laparoscopic Nissen fundoplication (360 degrees) is considered today the procedure of choice (Figure 20–5; Figure 20–6), as it increases the resting pressure and length of the LES and decreases the number of transient LES relaxations. The success of the operation is based on the following technical elements:

(1) Dissection of the esophagus in the posterior mediastinum to allow 3–4 cm of esophagus to lie without tension below the diaphragm. By bringing the entire stomach and gastroesophageal junction below the diaphragm, a sliding hiatal hernia is reduced.

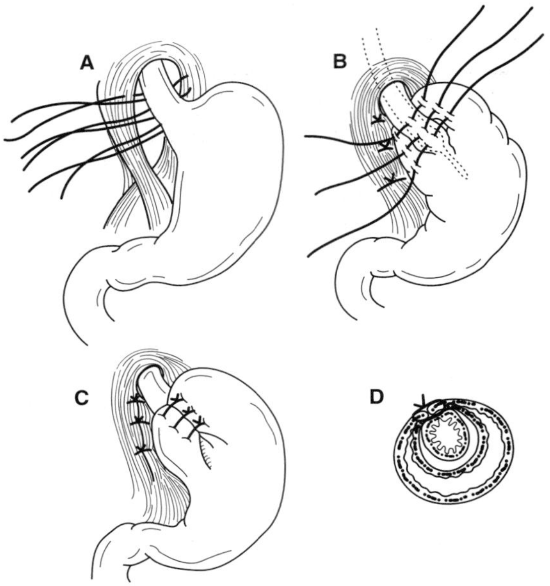

Figure 20–5. ***A:*** Dissection of the hiatus and lower mediastinum to mobilize the distal esophagus and restore about 6 cm to the abdominal position. ***B:*** Closure of the diaphragmatic crura behind the esophagus. ***C:*** Wrapping of the esophagus with the previously dissected fundus of the stomach. ***D:*** The transverse cut shows the gastric wrap around the distal esophagus. Note how increases in intragastric pressure would be transmitted to the esophagus, facilitating closure of the distal esophagus. The radius of this area of the esophagus is reduced, and the sphincter is prevented from dilating further because of the wrap.

(2) Division of the short gastric vessels in order to create a "floppy" fundoplication.

(3) Approximation of the esophageal crus to decrease the size of the esophageal hiatus, therefore avoiding herniation of the wrap.

(4) Construction of a 360-degree fundoplication over a 56–60 French bougie.

The hospital stay is usually 1 day only, and the postoperative discomfort is minimal. Most patients return to work within 2–3 weeks.

Prognosis

Control of *typical* symptoms is obtained in about 90% of patients after a fundoplication. Failures are treated with either medications or a second operation. The success rate is in the 70–90% range for patients with *atypical* symptoms, as it is often more difficult to establish preoperatively a strong correlation between gastroesophageal reflux and symptoms.

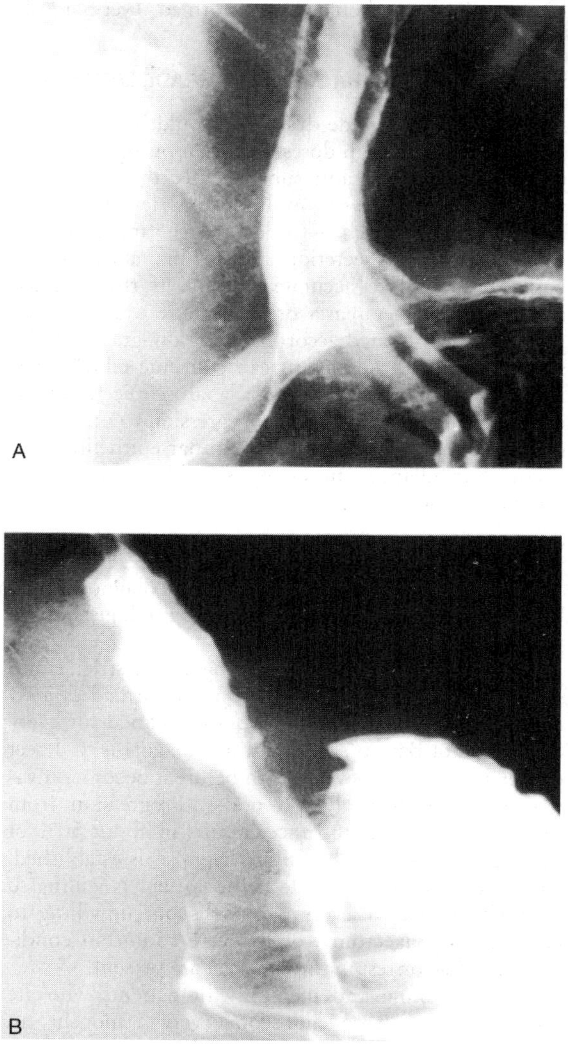

Figure 20–6. Esophagogram before and after Nissen fundoplication in the same patient. A: Wide-open reflux of barium occurs through an incompetent sphincter associated with a sliding hiatal hernia. B: Three months after surgery, the fundic wrap is evident. Note contrast passing through a small channel surrounded by the wrap. The slightly impregnated transverse folds around this channel represent fundal mucosa of the wrap.

Diener U et al: Esophageal dysmotility and gastroesophageal reflux disease. J Gastrointest Surg 2001;5:260.

Halum SL et al: Patients with isolated laryngopharyngeal reflux are not obese. Laryngoscope 2005;115:1042.

Patti MG et al: Total fundoplication is superior to partial fundoplication even when esophageal peristalsis is weak. J Am Coll Surg 2004;198:863.

Patti MG et al: Role of esophageal function tests in the diagnosis of gastroesophageal reflux disease. Dig Dis Sci 2001;46:597.

Patti MG et al: Effect of laparoscopic fundoplication on gastroesophageal reflux disease-induced respiratory symptoms. J Gastrointest Surg 2000;4:143.

Smith CD et al: When fundoplication fails: redo? Ann Surg 2005;241:861.

Triadafilopoulos G: Gastroesophageal reflux. Curr Opin Gastroenterol 2004;20:369.

BARRETT'S ESOPHAGUS

ESSENTIALS OF DIAGNOSIS

- *GERD symptoms (typical and atypical).*
- *Endoscopic evidence of "salmon pink" epithelium above gastroesophageal junction.*
- *Specialized columnar epithelium on esophageal biopsy.*

General Considerations

Barrett's esophagus is a metaplasia of the esophageal mucosa due to replacement of the squamous epithelium by columnar epithelium. About 10–12% of patients undergoing endoscopy for symptoms of GERD are found to have Barrett's epithelium. It occurs more frequently in white men older than 50 years of age. This metaplasia may progress to high-grade dysplasia and eventually adenocarcinoma. Thus, adenocarcinoma represents the final step of a sequence of events in which a benign disease (GERD) evolves into a preneoplastic disease and eventually into cancer.

Pathogenesis

Barrett's esophagus is due to reflux of gastric contents (acid and duodenal juice) into the esophagus. Barrett's metaplasia is considered an advanced stage of GERD characterized by a pan esophageal motor disorder. When compared with patients with GERD with no mucosal injury or less severe esophagitis, patients with Barrett's esophagus have a shorter and weaker LES and decreased amplitude of esophageal peristalsis. As a consequence, the amount of reflux is greater and esophageal clearance is slower. In addition, hiatal hernia is more common in patients with Barrett's metaplasia.

Clinical Findings

A. Symptoms

Patients with Barrett's esophagus typically have a long history of GERD. While most patients experience both typical and atypical symptoms of GERD, others may become asymptomatic over time due to the decreased sensitivity of the metaplastic epithelium.

B. Imaging Studies

Barium swallow may show the presence of ulcerations, a hiatal hernia, or a stricture. Endoscopy shows presence of "salmon pink" epithelium above the gastroesophageal junction, replacing the whitish squamous epithelium. The diagnosis is confirmed by pathologic examination of the esophageal mucosa and requires the identification of intestinal type epithelium, characterized by the presence of goblet cells.

C. Special Tests

Esophageal manometry often shows a short and hypotensive LES and abnormal esophageal peristalsis (decreased amplitude of peristaltic waves, simultaneous waves). Ambulatory pH monitoring usually shows a severe amount of acid reflux. Esophageal exposure to duodenal juice can be quantified by a fiberoptic probe that measures intraluminal bilirubin as a marker for duodenal reflux. In GERD patients, the prevalence of esophageal bilirubin exposure parallels the degree of mucosal injury, being higher in patients with Barrett's esophagus.

Treatment

A. Barrett's Esophagus: Metaplasia

The treatment options are similar to those of patients with GERD without metaplasia and consist of either proton pump inhibitors or a fundoplication. A surgical approach might offer an advantage over medical therapy for the following reasons:

(1) Successful elimination of reflux symptoms with proton pump inhibitors does not guarantee control of acid reflux. When pH monitoring is performed in asymptomatic Barrett's patients treated with these medications, up to 80% of them still have abnormal acid reflux.

(2) Proton pump inhibitors do not eliminate the reflux of bile, a major contributor to the pathogenesis of Barrett's esophagus, while an antireflux operation prevents any of refluxate by restoring the competence of the gastroesophageal junction

(3) A fundoplication may promote regression of the columnar epithelium. Many studies have shown that regression occurs in 15–50% of patients when the length of the Barrett's segment is less than 3 cm. Regardless of the effect of the fundoplication on symptoms, surveillance endoscopy should be performed every 12–24 months.

B. Barrett's Esophagus: Low-Grade Dysplasia

Patients with low-grade dysplasia should be treated for 1–2 months with high doses of proton pump inhibitors (3–4 pills per day) and subsequently the endoscopy should be repeated with multiple biopsies. The rationale for this approach is to decrease the inflammation by blocking acid secretion and reflux, allowing the pathologist a more accurate reading. If the repeated biopsies show metaplasia or high-grade dysplasia, the patient will be treated accordingly. If low-grade dysplasia is confirmed, the patient can continue taking acid-reducing medications or have a laparoscopic fundoplication, as there is evidence that regression to metaplasia or even disappearance of the columnar epithelium can occur. Surveillance endoscopy should be performed every 6–12 months.

C. Barrett's Esophagus: High-Grade Dysplasia

When high-grade dysplasia is found (the diagnosis must be confirmed by two experienced pathologists), two treatment options are available:

(1) Patients can enroll in a program of strict endoscopic surveillance, with endoscopy performed every 3 months and four quadrant biopsies obtained for every centimeter of Barrett's epithelium. The goal is to detect cancer as soon as it develops but before it becomes invasive and spreads to lymph nodes. Progression from high-grade dysplasia to cancer occurs in about 50% of patients 5 years after the initial diagnosis is established. This approach is reasonable if the patient is willing to undergo endoscopy every 3 months but unwilling to have an esophagectomy, or if severe comorbid conditions (cardiac or respiratory disease) are present.

(2) For young and medically fit patients who are unwilling to undergo endoscopy every 3 months, an esophagectomy should be considered. Invasive cancer is already present in about 30% of patients thought to have high-grade dysplasia at the time of the operation. The prognosis depends on the pathologic staging.

New treatment modalities have been devised for endoscopic ablation of the columnar epithelium. The rationale for these new treatment modalities is to ablate the segment of columnar epithelium, allowing regeneration of the squamous mucosa. Different techniques can be used, such as photodynamic therapy, thermal ablation, mucosal resection, radiofrequency application, or argon beam plasma coagulation. These therapies are still considered experimental.

Castell DO: Medical, surgical and endoscopic treatment of gastroesophageal reflux disease and Barrett's esophagus. J Clin Gastroenterol 2001;33:262.

Corley DA et al: Surveillance and survival in Barrett's adenocarcinomas: a population-based study. Gastroenterology 2002;122:633.

Fisher D et al: Quality of life in patients with Barrett's esophagus undergoing surveillance. Am J Gastroenterol 2002;97:2193.

Gerson LB et al: Prevalence of Barrett's esophagus in asymptomatic individuals. Gastroenterology 2002;123:461.

Pagani M et al: Barrett's esophagus: combined treatment using argon beam plasma coagulation and laparoscopic antireflux surgery. Dis Esophagus 2003;16:279.

Rex DK et al: Screening for Barrett's esophagus in colonoscopy patients with and without heartburn. Gastroenterol 2003;125:1670.

Schnell T et al: Long term non surgical management of Barrett's esophagus with high-grade dysplasia. Gastroenterology 2001;120:1607.

Shaheen NJ: Advances in Barrett's esophagus and esophageal adenocarcinoma. Gastroenterology 2005;128:1554.

HIATAL HERNIA

PARAESOPHAGEAL HIATAL HERNIA

ESSENTIALS OF DIAGNOSIS

- *May be asymptomatic.*
- *Symptoms secondary to mechanical obstruction: dysphagia, epigastric discomfort, bleeding.*
- *Symptoms secondary to gastroesophageal reflux.*

General Considerations

There are two types of esophageal hiatal hernia: paraesophageal and sliding (the sliding type has been discussed under gastroesophageal reflux disease; see Figures 20–7 and 20–8). Obesity, aging, and general weakening of the musculofascial structures set the stage for enlargement of the esophageal hiatus and herniation of the stomach into the posterior mediastinum.

There are two types of paraesophageal hernia. In one type, the less common, part of the stomach herniates into the thorax immediately adjacent and to the left of an undisplaced gastroesophageal junction (Figures 20–9 and 20–10). Since the gastroesophageal sphincteric mechanism functions normally in most of these cases, reflux of gastric contents is uncommon. More commonly, however, the paraesophageal herniation occurs in association with the sliding type, and symptoms due to gastroesophageal reflux may occur along symptoms secondary to the mechanical obstruction.

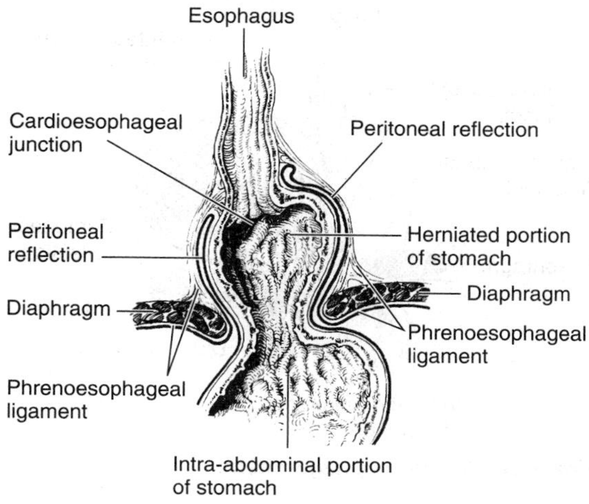

Figure 20–7. Sliding esophageal hernia.

Clinical Findings

Symptoms usually develop in adult life. Patients can experience epigastric discomfort, postprandial bloating, or dysphagia or have anemia secondary to gastric erosions. In addition, they may experience symptoms due to gastroesophageal reflux.

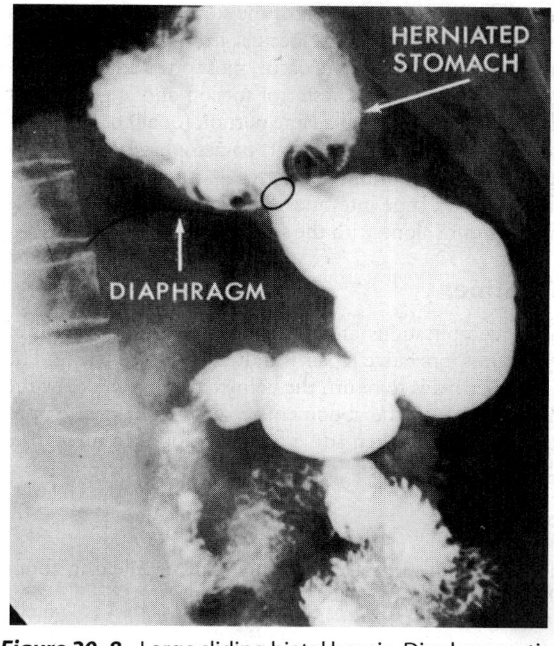

Figure 20–8. Large sliding hiatal hernia. Diaphragmatic hiatus is circled.

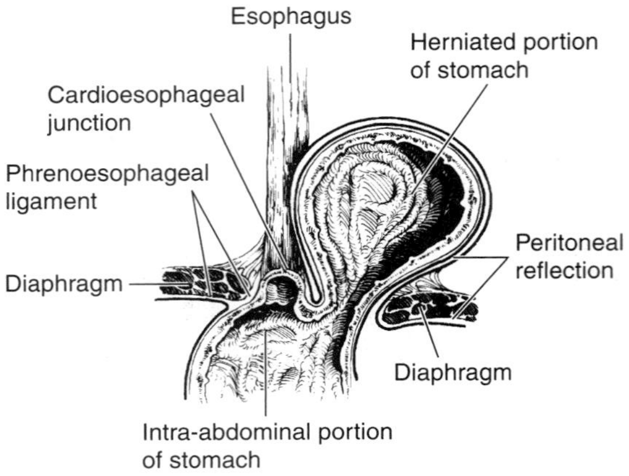

Figure 20–9. Paraesophageal hernia.

Diagnosis

A barium swallow will delineate the anatomy and the type of hiatal hernia. Endoscopy is important to determine if gastric or esophageal inflammation is present and to rule out cancer. If reflux symptoms are present, manometry and pH monitoring should be performed.

Complications

The most frequent complications of paraesophageal hernia are hemorrhage, incarceration, obstruction, and strangulation. The herniated portion of the stomach often becomes congested, and bleeding occurs from erosions of the mucosa. Obstruction may occur, most often at the esophagogastric junction as a result of torsion and angulation at this point—especially if a large portion (or all) of the stomach herniates into the chest. In paraesophageal hiatal hernia—in contrast to the sliding type—other viscera such as the small and large intestine and spleen may also enter the mediastinum along with the stomach.

Treatment

Since complications are frequent even in the absence of symptoms, operative repair is indicated in most cases. The usual method is to return the herniated stomach below the diaphragm into the abdomen, repair the enlarged esophageal hiatus, and then add a fundoplication. In most cases the operation can be performed laparoscopically.

Prognosis

The results of surgical management are excellent in about 90% of patients.

Aly A et al: Laparoscopic repair of larger hiatal hernias. Br J Surg 2005;92:648.

Diaz S et al: Laparoscopic paraesophageal hernia repair, a challenging operation: medium-term outcome of 116 patients. J Gastrointest Surg 2003;7:59.

Luketich JD et al: Laparoscopic repair of giant paraesophageal hernia: 100 consecutive cases. Ann Surg 2000;232:608.

TUMORS OF THE ESOPHAGUS

1. Benign Tumors of the Esophagus

ESSENTIALS OF DIAGNOSIS

- *Dysphagia, epigastric discomfort, heartburn.*
- *Radiographic demonstration of a smooth filling defect within the esophageal lumen.*

General Considerations

Esophageal leiomyomas are the most common benign tumors of the esophagus. They represent 10% of all gas-

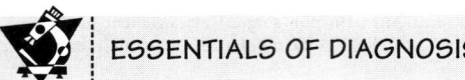

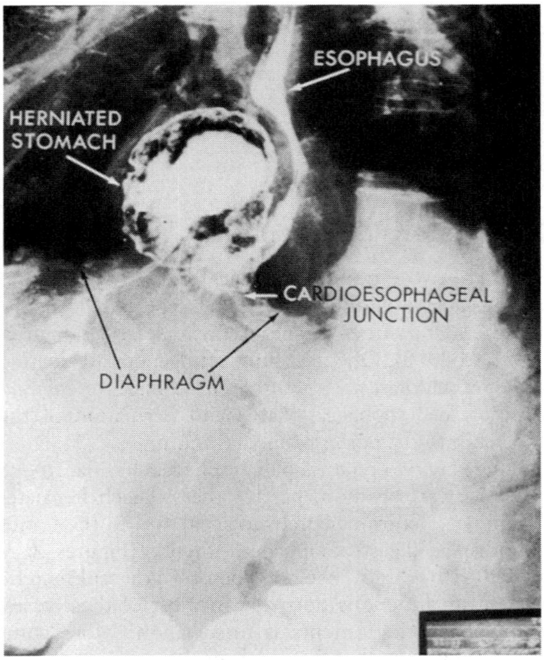

Figure 20–10. Paraesophageal hernia. Note that the cardioesophageal junction remains in its normal anatomic position below the diaphragm.

trointestinal leiomyomas. They originate in the smooth muscle layers, mostly in the lower two-thirds of the esophagus, and narrow the esophageal lumen. These tumors consist of muscle cells surrounded by a capsule of fibrous tissue. The mucosa overlying the tumor is generally intact, but occasionally it may become ulcerated as a result of pressure necrosis by an enlarging lesion. Leiomyomas are not associated with the development of cancer. Other tumors such as fibromas, lipomas, fibromyomas, and myxomas are rare. Congenital cysts or reduplications of the esophagus (the second most common benign lesion after leiomyomas) may occur at any level, although they are most common in the lower esophagus.

Clinical Findings

Many benign lesions are asymptomatic and are discovered incidentally during upper gastrointestinal fluoroscopic examination. Benign tumors or cysts grow slowly and become symptomatic only after reaching a size of 5 cm or more. On barium swallow leiomyomas appear as a smooth filling defect within the esophageal lumen (Figure 20–11). An intraluminal mass covered by normal mucosa can be easily recognized during endoscopy, but biopsies should not be taken, as they may make subsequent enucleation of the tumor more difficult. Endoscopic ultrasound and chest CT help in the characterization of the tumor and in the differential diagnosis.

Differential Diagnosis

Leiomyomas, cysts, and duplications can be distinguished from cancer by their classic radiographic appearance.

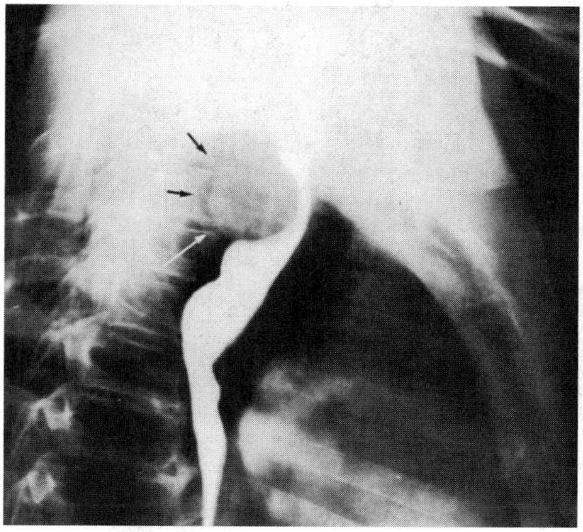

Figure 20–11. Leiomyoma of esophagus. Note smooth, rounded density causing extrinsic compression of esophageal lumen.

Intraluminal papillomas, polyps, or granulomas may be indistinguishable radiographically from early carcinoma, so their exact nature must be confirmed histologically.

Treatment

Small polypoid intraluminal lesions may be removed endoscopically. The treatment of choice for symptomatic leiomyomas is enucleation. While in the past a thoracotomy or a laparotomy was used to expose the esophagus and remove the tumor, today enucleation can be accomplished by either a thoracoscopic or a laparoscopic approach.

Koide N et al: Thoracoscopic enucleation of esophageal stromal tumor. Dis Esophagus 2004;17:104.

Mutrie CJ et al: Esophageal leiomyomas: A 40-year experience. Ann Thorac Surg 2005;79:1122.

2. Carcinoma of the Esophagus

ESSENTIALS OF DIAGNOSIS

- *Progressive dysphagia, initially for solids and later for liquids.*
- *Progressive weight loss.*
- *Diagnosis established by endoscopy and biopsies.*
- *Staging established by endoscopic ultrasound, computed tomography of chest and abdomen, positron emission tomography. Bronchoscopy indicated for cancer of the mid thoracic esophagus.*

General Considerations

In the United States esophageal carcinoma accounts for 10,000 to 11,000 deaths per year. The epidemiology of esophageal cancer in the United States has changed considerably during the last 30 years. In the 1970s, squamous cell carcinoma was the most common type of esophageal cancer, as it accounted for about 90% of the total cases. It was located in the thoracic esophagus and affected mostly black men. Over the past three decades there has been a progressive increase in the incidence of adenocarcinoma of the distal esophagus and gastroesophageal junction, so that today it accounts for more than 50% of all new cases of esophageal cancer. Adenocarcinoma is more frequent in white men with gastroesophageal reflux disease. Squamous cell cancer is still the most common type worldwide. Esophageal cancer occurs mostly during the fifth to seventh decades of life and is more common in men than women.

Pathogenesis

The most common contributing factors for squamous cell carcinoma are cigarette smoking and chronic alcohol exposure. Chronic ingestion of hot liquids or foods, poor oral hygiene, and nutritional deficiencies may play a role. Certain medical conditions such as achalasia, caustic injuries of the esophagus, and Plummer-Vinson syndrome are associated with an increased incidence of squamous cell cancer. Gastroesophageal reflux disease is the most common predisposing factor for adenocarcinoma of the esophagus, where adenocarcinoma represents the last event of a sequence that starts with GERD and progresses to metaplasia, high-grade dysplasia, and cancer. Esophageal cancer arises in the mucosa and subsequently tends to invade the submucosa and the muscle layers. Ultimately, structures located next to the esophagus may be infiltrated (tracheobronchial tree, aorta, recurrent laryngeal nerve). At the same time the tumor tends to metastasize to the lymph nodes (celiac, mediastinal, cervical) and to the liver and lungs.

Clinical Findings

A. Symptoms

Dysphagia is the most common presenting symptom. Dysphagia is initially for solids but eventually it progresses to liquids. Weight loss occurs in more than 50% of patients. Patients can have pain when swallowing. Pain over bony structures may be due to metastases. Hoarseness is usually due to invasion of the right or left recurrent laryngeal nerves with paralysis of the ipsilateral vocal cord. Respiratory symptoms may be due to regurgitation and aspiration of undigested food or to invasion of the tracheobronchial tree, with development of a tracheo-esophageal fistula.

B. Imaging Studies

Barium swallow shows the location and the extent of the tumor. Esophageal cancer usually presents as an irregular intraluminal mass or a stricture (Figure 20–12). Endoscopy allows direct visualization and biopsies of the tumor. For tumors of the upper and mid esophagus, bronchoscopy is indicated to rule out invasion of the tracheobronchial tree.

C. Special Tests

After the diagnosis is established, it is important to determine the staging of the cancer. Abdominal and chest CT scans are useful to detect distant organ metastases (M, metastases) and invasion of structures next to the esophagus. Alternatively, positron emission tomography can be used. Endoscopic ultrasound is the most sensitive test to determine the penetration of the

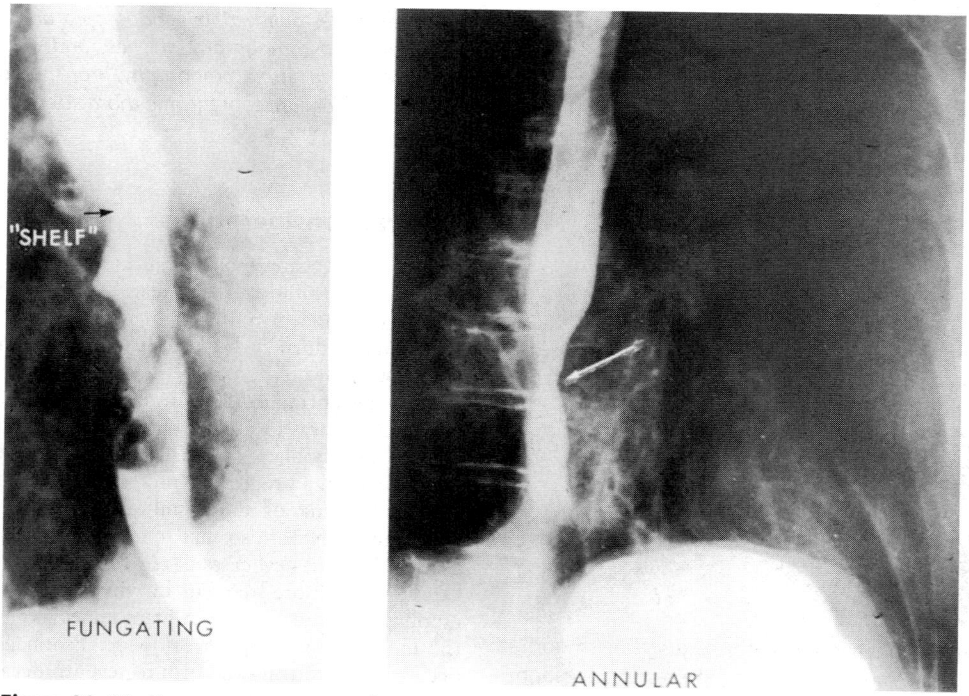

Figure 20–12. Two common types of esophageal carcinoma.

tumor (T, tumor), the presence of enlarged periesophageal lymph nodes (N, nodes) and invasion of structures next to the esophagus. Fine-needle aspiration of enlarged periesophageal lymph nodes can be done under ultrasound guidance. A bone scan is indicated in patients with new onset of bone pain.

Differential Diagnosis

The differential diagnosis includes peptic strictures due to reflux, achalasia, and benign esophageal tumors.

Treatment

Patients with esophageal cancer are considered candidates for esophageal resection if the following criteria are met: (1) there is no evidence of spread of the tumor to structures next to the esophagus such as the tracheobronchial tree, the aorta, or the recurrent laryngeal nerve; (2) there is no evidence of distant metastases; (3) the patient is fit from a cardiac and respiratory point of view. An esophagectomy can be performed by using an abdominal and a cervical incision (with blunt dissection of the thoracic esophagus through the esophageal hiatus; transhiatal esophagectomy), or by using an abdominal and a right chest incision (transthoracic esophagectomy). After removal of the esophagus, continuity of the gastrointestinal tract is reestablished by using either the stomach or the colon. The transhiatal esophagectomy offers the advantage of avoiding the chest incision, with decreased compromise of lung function and decreased postoperative discomfort. The validity of the transhiatal esophagectomy as a cancer operation was initially questioned because part of the operation is not done under direct vision and because of the small number of resected lymph nodes. However, many retrospective studies and prospective randomized trials have shown no difference in survival between the two operations, suggesting that it is not the type of operation that influences survival but rather the stage of the disease at the time the operation is performed. The morbidity rate of the operation is around 30%, and it is mostly due to cardiac (arrhythmias), respiratory (atelectasis, pleural effusion), and septic complications (anastomotic leak, pneumonia). The mortality rate in specialized centers is less than 5%. As with other complex operations (cardiac surgery, liver and pancreatic resections), a lower mortality rate is obtained in "high-volume centers" and is due to the presence of an experienced team composed of surgeons, anesthesiologists, intensivists, cardiologists, radiologists, and nurses.

Because most patients have already lymph node metastases at the time of surgery, the 5-year survival for this disease remains poor. Neoadjuvant therapy based on a combination of radiotherapy and chemotherapy has been tried in the past in order to improve local (radiotherapy) and distant control of the disease (chemotherapy). Unfortunately, most prospective randomized trials have failed to show a survival benefit in patients treated by neoadjuvant therapy followed by surgery as compared to patients undergoing surgery alone. Most studies, however, have shown that there is a subgroup of patients (about 15%) who have a "complete pathologic response" (no tumor found in the specimen) with better 5-year survival. It is unclear if this survival benefit is due to the therapy per se or to more favorable tumor biology. Today is not possible to identify the patients who are likely to benefit from neoadjuvant therapy. No survival benefit is achieved when radiation therapy or chemotherapy or both are administered postoperatively (adjuvant therapy).

Nonoperative therapy is reserved for patients who are not candidates for surgery because of local invasion of the tumor, metastases, or a poor functional status. The goal of therapy in these patients is palliation of the dysphagia, allowing them to eat. The following treatment modalities are available to achieve this goal:

(1) Expandable, coated, metallic stents can be deployed by endoscopy under fluoroscopic guidance in order to keep the esophageal lumen open. They are particularly useful when a tracheo-esophageal fistula is present.

(2) Laser therapy (Nd:YAG laser) relieves dysphagia in up to 70% of patients. However, multiple sessions are usually required to keep the esophageal lumen open;

(3) Radiation therapy is successful in relieving dysphagia in about 50% of patients.

Prognosis

The stage of the disease is the most important prognostic factor. Overall 5-year survival for esophageal cancer remains around 25%.

Kwon RS et al: Gastrointestinal cancer imaging: deeper than the eye can see. Gastroenterology 2005;128:1538.

Ferguson MK, Durkin A: Long-term survival after esophagectomy for Barrett's adenocarcinoma in endoscopically surveyed and non surveyed patients. J Gastrointest Surg 2002;6:29.

Nguyen NT et al: Thoracoscopic and laparoscopic esophagectomy for benign and malignant disease. Lessons learned form 46 consecutive procedures. J Am Coll Surg 2003;197:902.

Rasanen JV et al: Prospective analysis of accuracy of positron emission tomography, computed tomography, and endoscopic ultrasonography in staging of adenocarcinoma of the esophagus and esophagogastric junction. Ann Surg Oncol 2003;10:954.

Urba SG et al: Randomized trial of preoperative chemoradiation versus surgery alone in patients with locoregional esophageal carcinoma. J Clin Oncol 2001;19:305.

Wang KK et al: American Gastroenterological Association technical review on the role of the gastroenterologists in the management of esophageal carcinoma. Gastroenterology 2005;128:1471.

Weber WA et al: Imaging of esophageal and gastric cancer. Semin Oncol 2004;31:530.

OTHER SURGICAL DISORDERS OF THE ESOPHAGUS

PERFORATION OF THE ESOPHAGUS

ESSENTIALS OF DIAGNOSIS

- *History of recent instrumentation of the esophagus or severe vomiting.*
- *Pain in the neck, chest, or upper abdomen.*
- *Signs of mediastinal or thoracic sepsis within 24 hours.*
- *Contrast radiographic evidence of an esophageal leak.*

General Considerations

Esophageal perforations can result from iatrogenic instrumentation (eg, endoscopy, balloon dilation), severe vomiting, external trauma, and other rare causes. The subsequent clinical manifestations are influenced by the site of the perforation (ie, cervical or thoracic) and, in the case of thoracic perforations, whether or not the mediastinal pleura has been ruptured. Morbidity resulting from esophageal perforation is principally due to infection. Immediately after injury, the tissues are contaminated by esophageal contents, but infection has not become established; surgical closure of the defect will usually prevent the development of serious infection. If more than 24 hours have elapsed since the time of injury, severe contamination has occurred. At this time, the esophageal defect usually breaks down if it is surgically closed, and measures to treat mediastinitis and empyema may not be adequate to avoid a fatal outcome. Although serious infection usually occurs if surgical repair is delayed, a few cases of minor instrumental perforations can be managed by antibiotics without operation.

A. Instrumental Perforations

Medical instrumentation is the most common cause of esophageal perforation (diagnostic or therapeutic endoscopy). Instrumental perforations are most likely to occur in the cervical esophagus. The esophagoscope may press the posterior wall of the esophagus against osteoarthritic spurs of the cervical vertebrae, causing contusion or laceration. The cricopharyngeal area is the most common site of injury. Perforations of the thoracic esophagus may occur at any level but are most common at the natural sites of narrowing, at the level of the left main stem bronchus and at the diaphragmatic hiatus. Perforations during pneumatic dilatation for achalasia (2–6%) occur proximal to the gastroesophageal junction.

B. Spontaneous (Postemetic) Perforation (Boerhaave's Syndrome)

Spontaneous perforation usually occurs in the absence of preexisting esophageal disease, but 10% of patients have reflux esophagitis, esophageal diverticulum, carcinoma, etc. Most cases follow a bout of heavy eating and drinking. The rupture usually involves all layers of the esophageal wall and most frequently occurs in the left posterolateral aspect 3–5 cm above the gastroesophageal junction. The tear results from excessive intraluminal pressure, usually caused by violent retching and vomiting. Some cases have also been associated with childbirth, defecation, convulsions, heavy lifting, and forceful swallowing. The overlying pleura are also torn, so that both the mediastinum and the pleural cavity are contaminated with esophageal contents. The second most common site of perforation is at the mid thoracic esophagus, on the right side at the level of the azygous vein.

Clinical Findings

A. Signs and Symptoms

The principal early manifestation is pain, which is felt in the neck with cervical perforations and in the chest or upper abdomen with perforations of the thoracic esophagus. The pain may radiate to the back. With cervical perforations, pain is followed by crepitus in the neck, dysphagia, and signs of infection. Perforations of the thoracic esophagus, which communicate with the pleural cavity in about 75% of cases, are usually accompanied by tachycardia, tachypnea, dyspnea, and the early development of hypotension. With perforation into the chest, pneumothorax is produced followed by hydrothorax and, if not promptly treated, empyema. The left chest is involved in 70% and the right chest in 20%; involvement is bilateral in 10%. The rate of fluid accumulation in the chest may be as high a 1 L/h, which results in hypovolemia and a mediastinal shift. Escape of air into the mediastinum may result in a "mediastinal crunch," which is produced by the heart beating against air-filled tissues (Hamman's sign). If the pleura remain intact, mediastinal emphysema appears more rapidly, and pleural effusion is slow to develop.

B. Imaging Studies

X-ray studies are important to demonstrate that perforation has occurred and to locate the site of the injury. In perforations of the cervical esophagus, x-rays show air in the soft tissues, especially along the cervical spine. The trachea may be displaced anteriorly by air and fluid.

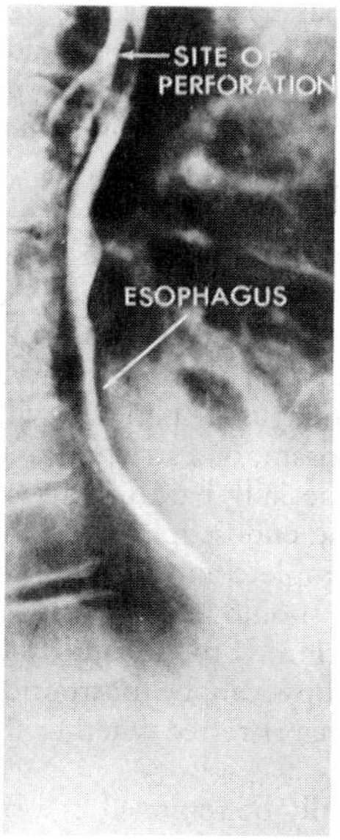

Figure 20–13. Extravasation of contrast material through instrumental perforation of upper thoracic esophagus. Note loculi of air and fluid anterior to esophagus, indicating that mediastinitis has already developed.

Later, widening of the superior mediastinum may be seen. With thoracic perforations, mediastinal widening and pleural effusion with or without pneumothorax are the usual findings. An esophagogram using water-soluble contrast medium should be performed promptly in every patient suspected of having an esophageal perforation (Figure 20–13). If a leak is not seen, the examination should be repeated using barium. A CT scan of the chest is also useful to localize the perforation and eventually to drain mediastinal fluid collections.

C. Special Studies

Thoracentesis will reveal cloudy or purulent fluid, depending on how much time has passed since the time of perforation. The amylase content of the fluid is elevated, and serum amylase levels may also be high as a result of absorption of amylase from the pleural cavity.

Treatment

Antibiotics should be given immediately. The infection is usually polymicrobial with *Staphylococcus, Streptococcus, Pseudomonas,* and *Bacteroides.* Early surgery is appropriate for all but a few cases, and every effort should be made to operate before the perforation is 24 hours old. For lesions treated within this time limit, the operation should consist of closure of the perforation and external drainage. External drainage alone may suffice for small cervical perforations, which may be difficult to find. Patients with achalasia in whom perforation has resulted from balloon dilation of the lower esophageal sphincter should have the tear in the esophagus repaired and a Heller myotomy performed on the opposite side of the esophagus. Definitive therapy (eg, resection) should also be performed in patients with other surgical conditions, such as esophageal carcinoma.

Primary repair has a high failure rate if the perforation is older than 24 hours. The classic recommendation in this situation has been to isolate the perforation (ie, to minimize further contamination) by performing a temporary cervical esophagostomy, ligating the esophagus just proximal to the gastroesophageal junction, and placing a feeding jejunostomy for enteral nutrition. Alternatively, the segment of esophagus where the perforation is located can be resected, bringing the proximal end of esophagus out through the neck and closing the distal end. The mediastinum is drained and a feeding jejunostomy is created. Later, the esophagostomy is taken down and stomach or the colon interposed to bridge the gap at the site of resection. Blunt esophagectomy may be feasible as emergency treatment of instrumental perforation in a patient with lye stricture.

Spontaneous incomplete rupture of the esophagus is seen occasionally. This lesion may be the result of increased intraluminal pressure or may be idiopathic, but the tear is usually located in the mid esophagus. In incomplete rupture, the tear is confined to the mucosal layer; it dissects distally in the submucosal plane, often as far as the gastroesophageal junction. The manifestations consist of chest pain, dyspnea, odynophagia, and, sometimes, bleeding. An esophagogram demonstrates an intramural tract of barium (which may give a double-lumen appearance) and sometimes encroachment on the esophageal lumen by an intramural hematoma. Treatment is with antibiotics and total parenteral nutrition.

Nonoperative management consisting of antibiotics alone may be all that is necessary in a few selected cases of instrumental perforation. This approach should be confined to patients without thoracic involvement (eg, pneumothorax or hydrothorax) whose esophagogram demonstrates just a short extraluminal sinus tract without wide mediastinal spread (ie, the contamination is limited) and who have no systemic signs of sepsis (eg, hypotension and tachypnea).

Prognosis

The survival rate is 90% when surgical treatment is accomplished within 24 hours. The rate drops to about 50% when treatment is delayed.

Dresner SM et al: Spontaneous oesophageal perforation during vaginal delivery. J R Soc Med 2001;94:90.

Vogel SB et al: Esophageal perforation in adults: aggressive, conservative treatment lowers morbidity and mortality. Ann Surg 2005;241:1016.

INGESTED FOREIGN OBJECTS

Most cases of ingested foreign objects occur in children who swallow coins or other small objects. In adults, the problem most often consists of esophageal meat impaction or, less commonly, lodged bones or toothpicks. Dentures and esophageal disease, such as a benign stricture, are the principal predisposing factors in adults. Prisoners and mentally ill persons occasionally swallow foreign objects intentionally.

About 90% of swallowed foreign objects pass into the stomach and from there into the intestine and are eventually passed without problems. Ten percent hang up in the esophagus. If they traverse the esophagus, objects whose dimensions exceed 2–5 cm tend to remain in the stomach. Ten percent of ingested foreign objects require endoscopic removal, and 1% require surgery. About 10% of ingested foreign objects enter the tracheobronchial tree.

The patient's history usually defines the problem adequately. The patient with a foreign object in the esophagus may or may not experience dysphagia or chest pain.

Specific Kinds of Ingested Foreign Objects

A. Coins

Pennies and dimes usually pass into the stomach, but larger coins will lodge in the esophagus at or just beyond the cricopharyngeus. It is important to know if a swallowed coin has remained in the esophagus, and whether or not the patient has symptoms is an unreliable basis for making the determination. Therefore, anteroposterior and lateral chest x-rays should be obtained to determine whether the coin is in the esophagus or trachea. Small children should be x-rayed from the base of the skull to the anus in order to find any additional coins in the gut.

Coins in the esophagus should be removed promptly, since complications may occur if treatment delay exceeds 24 hours. The procedure is best accomplished with a grasping forceps passed through a flexible endoscope. Sedation is adequate for older children or adults, but general endotracheal anesthesia is required in order to protect the airway of infants and young children. A smooth foreign body too large to grasp with a forceps can be removed by passing a dilating balloon beyond it and then withdrawing the endoscope and balloon as a unit. If the object is small enough (< 20 mm), it may be pushed into the stomach.

Once a coin has passed into the stomach, it can be observed by periodic x-rays for as long as a month before the conclusion is reached that spontaneous elimination is unlikely and endoscopic removal is indicated.

B. Meat Impaction

Meat is the most common foreign object that lodges in the esophagus of adults, and many affected patients have underlying esophageal disease. The site of meat impaction is usually at the cricopharyngeus muscle or in the distal esophagus in patients with achalasia, diffuse esophageal spasm, or a stricture.

No x-rays (especially barium studies) are indicated, for they make the endoscopist's task more difficult. If obstruction is complete and the patient cannot handle saliva, endoscopy should be performed as an emergency to prevent aspiration. If the clinical findings are minor, however, endoscopy can be postponed for up to 12 hours (but no longer) to see whether the food will pass spontaneously.

Meat can usually be removed as a single piece using a polypectomy snare passed through a flexible endoscope. In some cases, a meat bolus can be pushed into the stomach, which is safe so long as it passes with minimal pressure. After the esophagus has been cleared, it should be checked endoscopically for underlying disease. An esophageal stricture should be dilated if the esophageal wall is not acutely inflamed as a result of the meat impaction.

C. Sharp and Pointed Objects

Bones, safety pins, hat pins, razor blades, toothpicks, nails, and many others constitute this group of foreign objects. The general principles of management are (1) to remove these objects endoscopically by grasping and pulling a blunt side (eg, the hinge of an open safety pin) with forceps; (2) to remove a piece of glass or a razor blade by pulling it into the lumen of a rigid esophagoscope; or (3) to operate if neither of these methods appears to be safe. Sharp or pointed objects in the stomach should be removed surgically, since 25% of them will perforate the intestine, usually near the ileocecal valve, if they exit the pylorus.

D. Button Batteries

These small batteries are swallowed by children, just like coins, but unlike coins they are highly corrosive and should be removed urgently before a serious complication such as an esophagotracheal or esophagoaortic fistula develops.

E. Cocaine Packets

Cocaine smugglers may swallow small packets of cocaine in balloons or condoms. Rupture of just one of these packets can be fatal, so attempts at endoscopic removal are unsafe. If it appears that the packets will pass spontaneously, the patient may be watched; otherwise, surgical removal is indicated.

Arana A et al: Management of ingested foreign bodies in childhood and review of the literature. Eur J Pediatr 2001;160:468.

Younger RM, Darrow DH: Handheld metal detector confirmation of radiopaque foreign bodies in the esophagus. Arch Otolaryngol Head Neck Surg 2001;127:1371.

CAUSTIC INJURIES OF THE ESOPHAGUS

ESSENTIALS OF DIAGNOSIS

- *History of ingestion of caustic liquids or solids.*
- *Burns of the lips, mouth, tongue, and oropharynx.*
- *Chest pain and dysphagia.*

General Considerations

Ingestion of strong solutions of acid or alkali or of solid substances of similar nature produces extensive chemical burns. The injury usually represents a suicide attempt in adults and accidental ingestion in children. Strong alkali produces "liquefaction necrosis," which involves dissolution of protein and collagen, saponification of fats, dehydration of tissues, thrombosis of blood vessels, and deep penetrating injuries. Acids produce a "coagulation necrosis" involving eschar formation, which tends to shield the deeper tissues from injury. Depending upon the concentration and the length of time the irritant remains in contact with the mucosa, sloughing of the mucous membrane, edema and inflammation of the submucosa, infection, perforation, and mediastinitis may develop.

Ingested lye in solid form tends to adhere to the mucosa of the pharynx and proximal esophagus. Severe acute esophageal necrosis is rare, and the main clinical problems are early edema and late stricture formation, principally of the proximal esophagus. Liquid caustics commonly produce much more extensive esophageal necrosis, and occasionally even tracheo-esophageal and esophago-aortic fistulas. If the patient survives the acute phase, a lengthy nondilatable stricture often develops.

Ingestion of strong acid characteristically produces greatest injury to the stomach, with the esophagus remaining intact in over 80% of cases. The result may be immediate gastric necrosis or late antral stenosis.

Nearly all severe injuries are caused by strong alkali. Weak alkali and acid are associated with less extensive lesions.

Clinical Findings

A. Symptoms and Signs

Systemic symptoms roughly parallel the severity of the caustic burn. The most common finding is inflammatory edema of the lips, mouth, tongue, and oropharynx; in the absence of visible injury in this area, severe esophageal damage is rare. Patients with serious esophageal burns often experience chest pain and dysphagia and drooling of large amounts of saliva. Pain on swallowing may be intense. If the damage is severe, the patient often appears toxic, with high fever, prostration, and shock. The absence of toxicity does not rule out severe injury, however. Tracheobronchitis accompanied by coughing and increased bronchial secretions is frequently noted. Stridor may be present, and in a few patients respiratory obstruction progresses rapidly and requires tracheostomy for relief. Complete esophageal obstruction due to edema, inflammation, and mucosal sloughing may develop within the first few days.

B. Esophagoscopy

Endoscopy is the key test in the evaluation of caustic trauma to the esophagus. Determination of the extent of injury by esophagoscopy contributes substantially to therapeutic decisions. Endoscopy should be performed after the initial resuscitation, usually within 24 hours of admission. The scope is inserted far enough to gauge the most serious degree of burn, which is classified as first-, second-, or third-degree as defined in (Table 20–3).

C. Radiology

A chest x-ray should be taken in all patients. It may show signs of esophageal perforation (subcutaneous emphysema, pneumomediastinum, pneumothorax), or aspiration (pulmonary infiltrates).

A esophagogram is indicated in the initial evaluation if perforation is suspected and in later stages to detect the presence of a stricture.

Treatment

Patients should be hospitalized and intravenous fluids started. Intravenous antibiotics should be given to patients treated for caustic injuries. The use of steroids is still controversial. A nasogastric tube placed under fluoroscopic or endoscopic guidance allows stenting of the esophagus, preventing complete obstruction of the lumen.

Patients with first-degree burns do not require aggressive therapy and may be discharged from the hospital after a short period of observation. Second-degree and minor spotty third-degree injuries are treated by inserting a nasogastric tube. Nutrition can be given through the tube or parenterally using total parenteral

Table 20–3. Endoscopic grading of corrosive burns of esophagus and stomach.[1]

Grade	Definition	Endoscopic Findings
First-degree	Superficial mucosal injury	Mucosal hyperemia and edema; superficial mucosal desquamation.
Second-degree	Full-thickness mucosal involvement. No or partial-thickness muscular injury.	Sloughing of mucosa. Hemorrhage, exudate, ulceration, pseudomembrane formation, and granulation tissue when examined late.
Third-degree	Full-thickness esophageal or gastric injury with extension into adjacent tissues.	Sloughing of tissues with deep ulceration. Complete obliteration of esophageal lumen by edema; charring and eschar formation; full-thickness necrosis; perforation.

[1]Reproduced, with permission, from Estrera A et al: Corrosive burns of the esophagus and stomach: a recommendation for an aggressive surgical approach. Ann Thorac Surg 1986;41:276.

nutrition. Periodic esophagograms are obtained in late follow-up to look for stricture formation, which is treated early in its development by dilations and eventually resection.

Third-degree burns involving extensive esophagogastric necrosis require emergency esophagogastrectomy, esophagostomy, and feeding jejunostomy. Esophagectomy is best performed by the blunt technique using a laparotomy and cervical incision. It is sometimes necessary to resect adjacent organs (eg, transverse colon) that have also been damaged. Reconstruction by substernal colon interposition is performed 6–8 weeks later.

Prognosis

Early and proper management of caustic burns provides satisfactory results in most cases. The ingestion of strong acid or alkaline solutions with extensive immediate destruction of the mucosa produces profound pathologic changes that may result in fibrous strictures that require dilations and, in some cases, esophagectomy and colon interposition.

de Jong AL et al: Corrosive esophagitis in children: a 30-year review. Int J Pediatr Otorhinolaryngol 2001;57:203.

Ertekin C et al: The results of caustic ingestions. Hepatogastroenterology 2004;51:1397.

Huang YC et al: Balloon dilation of double strictures after corrosive esophagitis. J Pediatr Gastroenterol Nutr 2001;32:496.

Kim YT et al: Is it necessary to resect the diseased esophagus in performing reconstruction for corrosive esophageal stricture? Eur J Cardiothorac Surg 2001;20:1.

ESOPHAGEAL BANDS, WEBS, OR RINGS

A narrow mucosal ring (**Schatzki's ring**) may develop at the lower end of the esophagus. Most patients are relatively free from symptoms unless the ring is less than 12 mm in diameter. Dysphagia may be severe, however. In most cases, the ring is located at the squamocolumnar junction and occurs in a patient with gastroesophageal reflux disease. Being confined to the mucosa, it differs from an inflammatory (peptic) stricture, which involves all layers of the esophagus. A barium swallow clearly identifies the problem. Treatment consists of endoscopic dilatation of the ring and treatment of the associated reflux (acid-reducing medications or fundoplication).

Jalil S, Castell DO: Schatzski's ring: a benign cause of dysphagia in adults. J Clin Gastroenterol 2002;35:295.

Winters GR et al: Schatzski's rings do not protect against acid reflux and may decrease esophageal acid clearance. Dig Dis Sci 2003;48:299.

II. THE DIAPHRAGM

The diaphragm (Figure 20–14) is a musculotendinous dome-shaped structure attached posteriorly to the first, second, and third lumbar vertebrae, anteriorly to the lower sternum, and laterally to the costal arches. It separates the abdominal and the thoracic cavities. The diaphragm allows the passage of various normal structures through anatomic foramina. The aortic hiatus lies posteriorly at the level of the 12th thoracic vertebra, and through it pass the aorta, the thoracic duct, and the azygos venous system. The esophageal hiatus lies immediately anteriorly and slightly to the left at the level of the tenth thoracic vertebra and is separated from the aortic hiatus by the decussation of the right crus of the diaphragm. Through this hiatus pass the esophagus and the vagus nerves. At the level of the ninth thoracic ver-

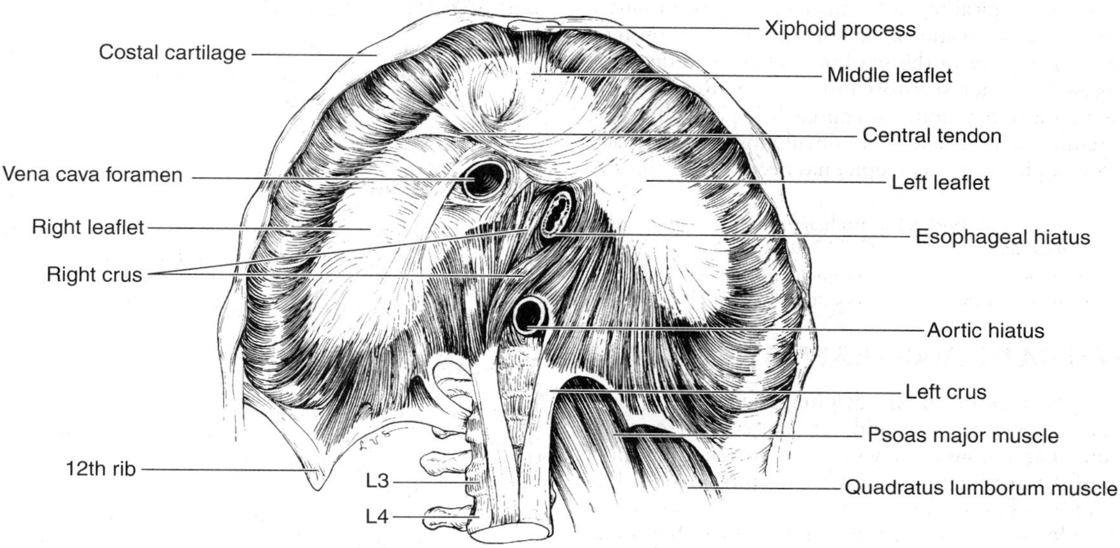

Figure 20–14. Inferior surface of diaphragm.

tebra and slightly to the right of the esophageal hiatus is the vena caval foramen, which allows passage of the inferior vena cava and small branches of the phrenic nerve. The phrenic arteries arising directly from the aorta supply the diaphragm along with the lower intercostal arteries and the terminal branches of the internal mammary arteries.

PARASTERNAL OR RETROSTERNAL (FORAMEN OF MORGAGNI) HERNIA & PLEUROPERITONEAL (FORAMEN OF BOCHDALEK) HERNIA

Failure of fusion of the sternal and costal portions of the diaphragm anteriorly in the midline creates a defect (foramen of Morgagni) through which hernias can occur. Normally, the diaphragm becomes fused, allowing only the internal mammary arteries and their superior epigastric branches, along with lymphatics, to pass through this area. Posterolaterally, failure of fusion of the pleuroperitoneal canal creates a defect though which viscera may herniate to produce a foramen of Bochdalek hernia (Figure 20–15).

Although both types of hernia are congenital, symptoms in the Morgagni hernia usually do not develop until middle life or later. This type of hernia is more frequent in women. These hernias are mostly right-sided and have a hernia sac. The most common contents are the omentum, the colon, and the stomach. On the other hand, the Bochdalek hernia occurs more frequently on the left side and may cause severe respiratory distress at birth, requiring an emergency operation. Routine chest films show a retrosternal solid mass, a retrosternal air-filled viscus, or similar findings in the posterolateral thorax if a Bochdalek hernia is present. Chest CT confirms the diagnosis and identifies the contents of the hernia.

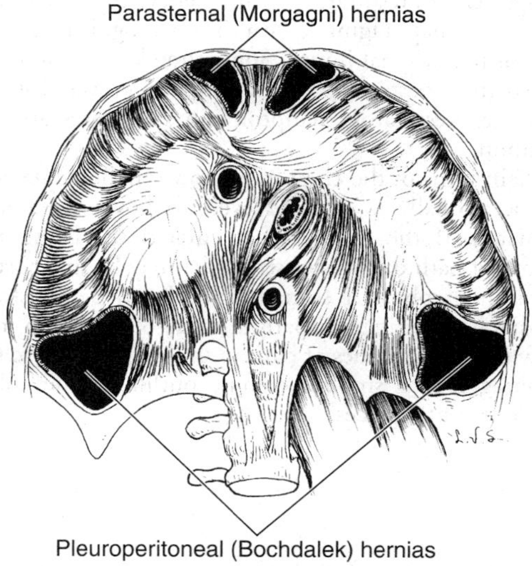

Figure 20–15. Sites of congenital diaphragmatic herniation.

Elective surgical repair is indicated in most instances to prevent complications. An emergency operation may become necessary in the newborn infant who develops progressive cardiorespiratory insufficiency. Repair of the defect by a transabdominal approach is preferable, and the results are excellent. A minimally invasive approach (laparoscopic or thoracoscopic) has been recently used.

Mei-Zahav M et al: Bochdalek diaphragmatic hernia: not only a neonatal disease. Arch Dis Child 2003;88:532.

Minneci PC et al: Foramen of Morgagni hernia: changes in diagnosis and treatment. Ann Thorac Surg 2004;77:1956.

TRAUMATIC DIAPHRAGMATIC HERNIA

Traumatic rupture of the diaphragm may occur as a result of penetrating wounds or severe blunt external trauma. Lacerations usually occur in the tendinous portion of the diaphragm, most often on the left side. The liver provides protection to diaphragmatic injury on the right side except from penetrating wounds. Abdominal viscera may immediately herniate through the defect in the diaphragm into the pleural cavity or may gradually insinuate themselves into the thorax over a period of months or years.

Clinical Findings

Diaphragmatic ruptures present in two ways. In the acute form, the patient has recently experienced blunt trauma or a penetrating wound to the chest, abdomen, or back. The clinical manifestations are essentially those of the associated injuries, but occasionally, massive herniation of abdominal viscera through the diaphragm causes respiratory insufficiency. In the chronic form, the diaphragmatic tear is unrecognized at the time of the original injury. Some time later, symptoms appear from herniation of viscera: pain, bowel obstruction, etc. Respiratory symptoms in such cases are less common.

Plain films of the chest may show a radiopaque area and occasionally an air-fluid level if hollow viscera have herniated. If the stomach has entered the chest, the abnormal path of a nasogastric tube may be diagnostic. Ultrasonography, CT scan, and MRI may demonstrate the diaphragmatic rent. Barium study of the colon may show irregular patches of barium in the colon above the diaphragm or a smooth colonic outline if the colon does not contain feces.

Differential Diagnosis

Traumatic rupture of the diaphragm must be differentiated from atelectasis, space-consuming tumors of the lower pleural space, pleural effusion, and intestinal obstruction due to other causes.

Complications

Hemorrhage and obstruction may occur. If herniation is massive, progressive cardiorespiratory insufficiency may threaten life. The most severe complication is strangulating obstruction of the herniated viscera.

Treatment

For acute ruptures, a transabdominal (most commonly) or transthoracic route is used depending on the procedure required to treat ancillary injuries. When the diaphragmatic tear is the only injury, it is usually fixed by laparotomy. Chronic injuries can be repaired by either approach. Asymptomatic tears of the diaphragm with herniated viscera should be repaired, because the risk of strangulating obstruction is high.

Prognosis

Surgical repair of the rent in the diaphragm is curative, and the prognosis is excellent. The diaphragm supports sutures well, so that recurrence is practically unknown.

Grover SB et al: Simultaneous dual posttraumatic diaphragmatic and abdominal wall hernias. J Trauma 2001;51:583.

Matthews BD et al: Laparoscopic repair of traumatic diaphragmatic injuries. Surg Endosc 2003;17:254.

Reina A et al: Traumatic intrapericardial diaphragmatic hernia: case report and literature review. Injury 2001;32:153.

TUMORS OF THE DIAPHRAGM

Primary tumors of the diaphragm are not common. The majority are benign lipomas. Pericardial cysts develop in the interval between the heart and the diaphragm and are usually unilocular and on the right side. Fibrosarcoma, the most common primary malignant diaphragmatic tumor, is extremely rare.

Benign tumors are usually asymptomatic. Since their benign nature cannot be established except by histology, all lesions of this type should be excised through an appropriate thoracotomy or thoracoabdominal approach.

The Acute Abdomen

21

Gerard M. Doherty, MD

The term "an acute abdomen" denotes any sudden spontaneous nontraumatic disorder whose chief manifestation is in the abdominal area and for which urgent operation may be necessary. Because there is frequently a progressive underlying intra-abdominal disorder, undue delay in diagnosis and treatment adversely affects outcome.

The approach to a patient with an acute abdomen must be orderly and thorough. An acute abdomen must be suspected even if the patient has only mild or atypical complaints. The history and physical examination should suggest the probable causes and guide the choice of initial diagnostic studies. The clinician must then decide if in-hospital observation is warranted; if additional tests are needed; if early operation is indicated; or if nonoperative treatment would be more suitable.

All clinicians should be thoroughly familiar with the presenting pattern of the most common causes of an acute abdomen (Table 21–1). Moreover, they should be familiar with the disease patterns specific to the region and locality where they practice. Other chapters in this book provide detailed descriptions of specific diseases and their management.

HISTORY

Abdominal Pain

History taking by an experienced physician is an active process whereby a cluster of diagnostic possibilities is considered in order to systematically eliminate less likely conditions. Pain is the most common and predominant presenting feature of an acute abdomen. Careful consideration of the location, the mode of onset and progression, and the character of the pain will suggest a preliminary list of differential diagnoses.

A. Location of Pain

Because of the complex dual visceral and parietal sensory network innervating the abdominal area, pain is not as precisely localized as in the extremities. Fortunately, some general patterns do emerge that provide clues to diagnosis. Visceral sensation is mediated primarily by afferent C fibers located in the walls of hollow viscera and in the capsules of solid organs. Unlike cutaneous pain, **visceral pain** is elicited either by distention, by inflammation or ischemia stimulating the receptor neurons, or by direct involvement (eg, malignant infiltration) of sensory nerves. The centrally perceived sensation is generally slow in onset, dull, poorly localized, and protracted. Different visceral structures are associated with different sensory levels in the spine (Table 21–2). Because of this, increased wall tension due to luminal distention or forceful smooth muscle contraction (colic) produces diffuse deep-seated pain felt in the mid epigastrium, periumbilical area, lower abdomen, or flank areas (Figure 21–1). Visceral pain is most often felt in the midline because of the bilateral sensory supply to the spinal cord.

By contrast, **parietal pain** is mediated by both C and A delta nerve fibers, the latter being responsible for the transmission of more acute, sharper, better-localized pain sensation. Direct irritation of the somatically innervated parietal peritoneum (especially the anterior and upper parts) by pus, bile, urine, or gastrointestinal secretions leads to more precisely localized pain. The cutaneous distribution of parietal pain corresponds to the T6–L1 areas. Parietal pain is more easily localized than visceral pain because the somatic afferent fibers are directed to only one side of the nervous system. Abdominal parietal pain is conventionally described as occurring in one of the four abdominal quadrants or in the epigastric or central abdominal area.

Abdominal pain may be referred or may shift to sites far removed from the primarily affected organs (Figure 21–2). The term **referred pain** denotes noxious (usually cutaneous) sensations perceived at a site distant from that of a strong primary stimulus. Distorted central perception of the site of pain is due to the confluence of afferent nerve fibers from widely disparate areas within the posterior horn of the spinal cord. For example, pain due to subdiaphragmatic irritation by air, peritoneal fluid, blood, or a mass lesion is referred to the shoulder via the C4-mediated (phrenic) nerve. Pain may also be referred to the shoulder from supradiaphragmatic lesions such as pleurisy or lower lobe pneumonia, especially in young patients. Although more often perceived in the right scapular region, referred biliary pain may mimic angina pectoris if it is perceived in the anterior chest or left shoulder areas. Posterolateral right flank pain may be seen in retrocecal appendicitis.

Table 21–1. Common causes of the acute abdomen.

Gastrointestinal tract disorders
- *Nonspecific abdominal pain
- **Appendicitis*
- **Small and large bowel obstruction*
- **Perforated peptic ulcer*
- *Incarcerated hernia*
- *Bowel perforation*
- *Meckel's diverticulitis*
- *Boerhaave's syndrome*
- *Diverticulitis
- Inflammatory bowel disorders
- Mallory-Weiss syndrome
- Gastroenteritis
- Acute gastritis
- Mesenteric adenitis
- Parasitic infections

Liver, spleen, and biliary tract disorders
- **Acute cholecystitis*
- *Acute cholangitis*
- *Hepatic abscess*
- *Ruptured hepatic tumor*
- *Spontaneous rupture of the spleen*
- Splenic infarct
- Biliary colic
- Acute hepatitis

Pancreatic disorders
- *Acute pancreatitis

Urinary tract disorders
- *Ureteral or renal colic
- Acute pyelonephritis
- Acute cystitis
- Renal infarct

Gynecologic disorders
- *Ruptured ectopic pregnancy*
- *Twisted ovarian tumor*
- *Ruptured ovarian follicle cyst*
- *Acute salpingitis
- Dysmenorrhea
- Endometriosis

Vascular disorders
- *Ruptured aortic and visceral aneurysms*
- *Acute ischemic colitis*
- *Mesenteric thrombosis*

Peritoneal disorders
- *Intra-abdominal abscesses*
- Primary peritonitis
- Tuberculous peritonitis

Retroperitoneal disorders
- Retroperitoneal hemorrhage

[1]The most common causes are marked with an asterisk. Conditions in italic type often require urgent operation.

Table 21–2. Sensory levels associated with visceral structures.

Structures	Nervous System Pathways	Sensory Level
Liver, spleen, and central part of diaphragm	Phrenic nerve	C3–5
Peripheral diaphragm, stomach, pancreas, gallbladder, and small bowel	Celiac plexus and greater splanchnic nerve	T6–9
Appendix, colon, and pelvic viscera	Mesenteric plexus and lesser splanchnic nerve	T10–11
Sigmoid colon, rectum, kidney, ureters, and testes	Lowest splanchnic nerve	T11–L1
Bladder and rectosigmoid	Hypogastric plexus	S2–4

Spreading or shifting pain parallels the course of the underlying condition. The site of pain at onset should be distinguished from the site at presentation. Beginning classically in the epigastric or periumbilical region, the incipient visceral pain of acute appendicitis (due to distention of the appendix) later shifts to become sharper parietal pain localized in the right lower quadrant when the overlying peritoneum becomes directly inflamed (Figure 21–2). In perforated peptic ulcer, pain almost always begins in the epigastrium, but as the leaked gastric contents track down the right paracolic gutter, pain may descend to the right lower quadrant with even diminution of the epigastric pain.

The location of pain serves only as a rough guide to the diagnosis—"typical" descriptions are reported in only two-thirds of cases. This great variability is due to atypical pain patterns, a shift of maximum intensity away from the primary site, or advanced or severe disease. In cases presenting late with diffuse peritonitis, generalized pain may completely obscure the precipitating event. Pain confined to either upper quadrant may be evaluated by anatomic consideration of acute conditions that affect the underlying organs.

B. Mode of Onset and Progression of Pain

The mode of onset of pain reflects the nature and severity of the inciting process. Onset may be explosive (within seconds), rapidly progressive (within 1–2 hours), or gradual (over several hours). Unheralded, excruciating generalized pain suggests an intra-abdominal catastrophe such as a perforated viscus or rupture of an aneurysm, ectopic pregnancy, or abscess. Accompanying systemic signs

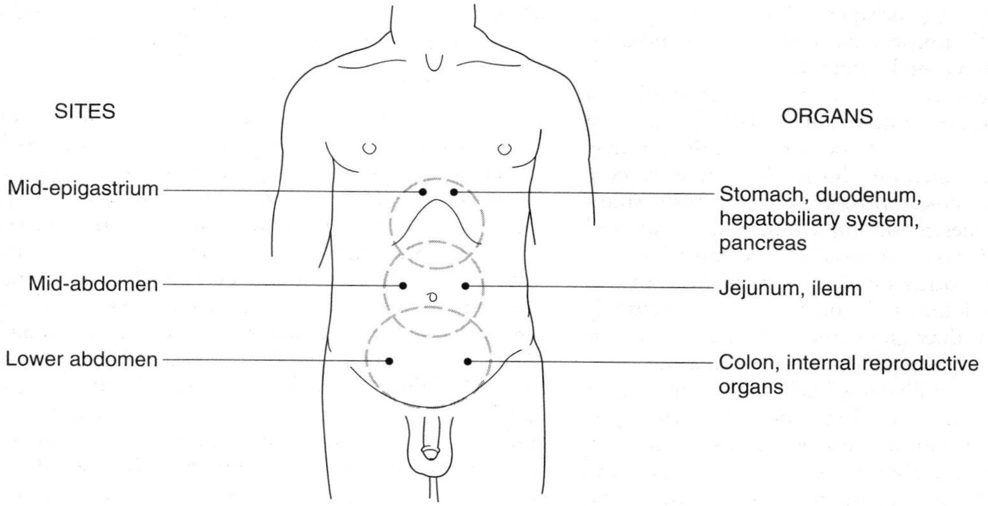

Figure 21–1. Visceral pain sites.

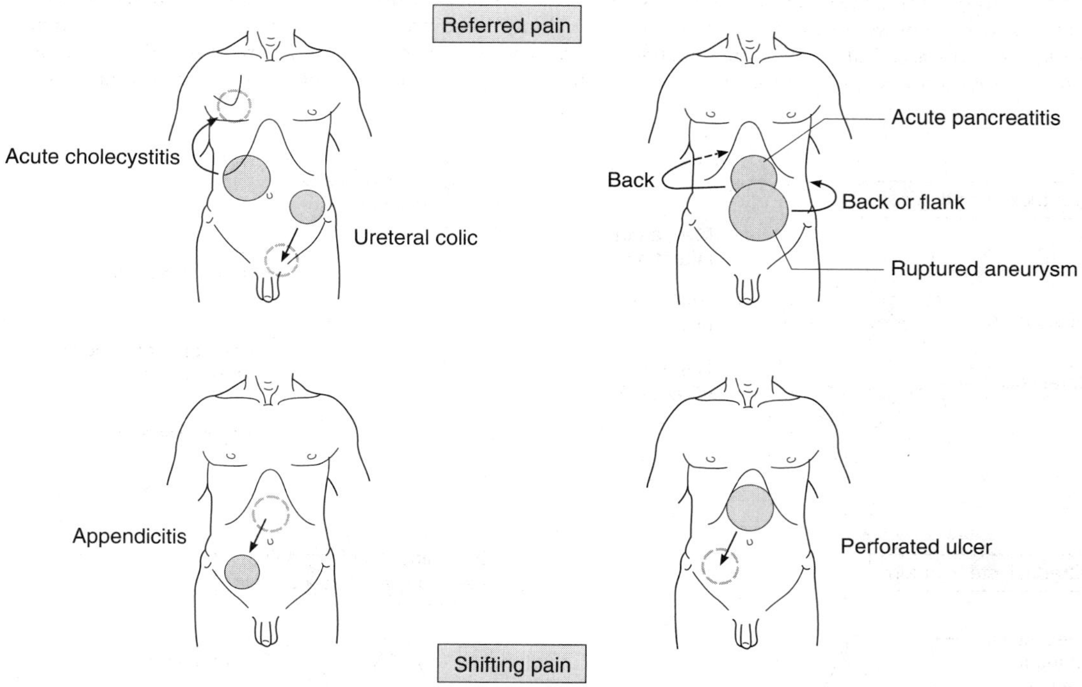

Figure 21–2. Referred pain and shifting pain in the acute abdomen. Solid circles indicate the site of maximum pain; dashed circles indicate sites of lesser pain.

(tachycardia, sweating, tachypnea, shock) soon supersede the abdominal disturbances and underscore the need for prompt resuscitation and laparotomy.

A less dramatic clinical picture is steady mild pain becoming intensely centered in a well-defined area within 1–2 hours. Any of the above conditions may present in this manner, but this mode of onset is more typical of acute cholecystitis, acute pancreatitis, strangulated bowel, mesenteric infarction, renal or ureteral colic, and high (proximal) small bowel obstruction.

Finally, some patients initially have slight—at times only vague—abdominal discomfort that is fleetingly present diffusely throughout the abdomen. It may be unclear whether these patients even have an acute abdomen or whether the illness is likely to be a matter for medical rather than surgical attention. Associated gastrointestinal symptoms are infrequent at first, and systemic symptoms are absent. Eventually, the pain and abdominal findings become more pronounced and steady and are localized to a smaller area. This pattern may reflect a slowly developing condition or the body's defensive efforts to cordon off an acute process. This broad category includes acute appendicitis (especially retrocecal or retroileal), incarcerated hernias, low (distal) small bowel and large bowel obstructions, uncomplicated peptic ulcer disease, walled-off (often malignant) visceral perforations, some genitourinary and gynecologic conditions, and milder forms of the rapid-onset group mentioned in the first paragraph.

C. Character of Pain

The nature, severity, and periodicity of pain provide useful clues to the underlying cause (Figure 21–3). Steady pain is most common. Sharp superficial constant pain due to severe peritoneal irritation is typical of perforated ulcer or a ruptured appendix, ovarian cyst, or ectopic pregnancy. The gripping, mounting pain of small bowel obstruction (and occasionally early pancreatitis) is usually intermittent, vague, deep-seated, and crescendo at first but soon becomes sharper, unremitting, and better localized. Unlike the disquieting but bearable pain associated with bowel obstruction, pain caused by lesions occluding smaller conduits (bile ducts, uterine tubes, and ureters) rapidly becomes unbearably intense. Pain is appropriately referred to as **colic** if there are pain-free intervals that reflect intermittent smooth muscle contractions, as in ureteral colic. In the strict sense, the term "biliary colic" is a misnomer because biliary pain does not remit. The reason is that the gallbladder and bile duct, in contrast to the ureters and intestine, do not have peristaltic movements. The "aching discomfort" of ulcer pain, the "stabbing, breathtaking" pain of acute pancreatitis and mesenteric infarction, and the "searing" pain of ruptured aortic

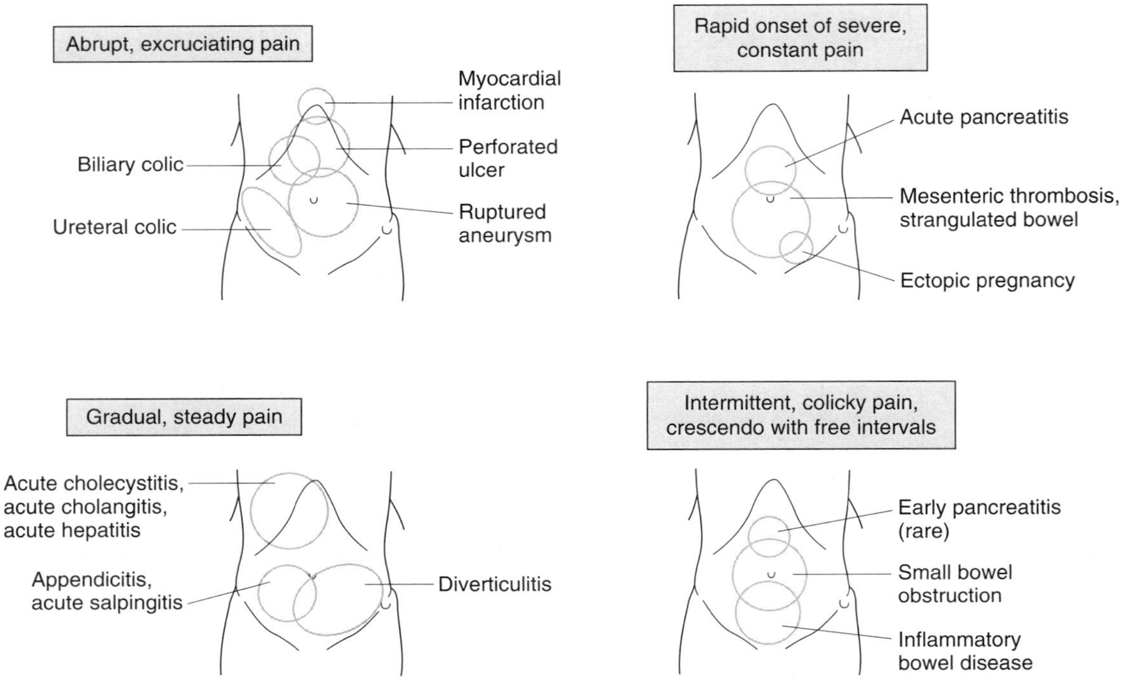

Figure 21–3. The location and character of pain are helpful in the differential diagnosis of the acute abdomen.

aneurysm remain apt descriptions. Despite the use of such descriptive terms, the quality of visceral pain is not a reliable clue to its cause.

Agonizing pain denotes serious or advanced disease. Colicky pain is usually promptly alleviated by analgesics. Ischemic pain due to strangulated bowel or mesenteric thrombosis is only slightly assuaged even by narcotics. Nonspecific abdominal pain is usually mild, but mild pain may also be found with perforated ulcers that have become localized and in mild acute pancreatitis. An occasional patient will deny pain but complain of a vague feeling of abdominal fullness that feels as though it might be relieved by a bowel movement. This visceral sensation **(gas stoppage sign)** is due to reflex ileus induced by an inflammatory lesion walled off from the free peritoneal cavity, as in retrocecal or retroileal appendicitis.

Past episodes of pain and factors that aggravate or relieve pain should be noted. Pain caused by localized peritonitis, especially when it affects upper abdominal organs, tends to be exacerbated by movement or deep breathing.

The clinician should be familiar with the pathophysiology and salient features of the common causes of acute abdomen. The location, character, and severity of the pain in relation to its duration of onset along with the presence or absence of systemic symptoms help to differentiate rapidly progressive (and usually more serious) surgical conditions (eg, intestinal ischemia) from more indolent or medical causes (eg, ruptured ovarian cysts).

Other Symptoms Associated with Abdominal Pain

Anorexia, nausea and vomiting, constipation, or diarrhea often accompanies abdominal pain, but since these are nonspecific symptoms, they do not have much diagnostic value.

A. Vomiting

When sufficiently stimulated by secondary visceral afferent fibers, the medullary vomiting centers activate efferent fibers to induce reflex vomiting. Hence, pain in the acute surgical abdomen usually precedes vomiting, whereas the reverse holds true in medical conditions. Vomiting is a prominent symptom in upper gastrointestinal diseases such as Boerhaave's syndrome, Mallory-Weiss syndrome, acute gastritis, and acute pancreatitis. Severe uncontrollable retching provides temporary pain relief in moderate attacks of pancreatitis. The absence of bile in the vomitus is a feature of pyloric stenosis. Where associated findings suggest bowel obstruction, the onset and character of vomiting may indicate the level of the lesion. Recurrent vomiting of bile-stained fluid is a typical early sign of proximal small bowel obstruction. In distal small or large bowel obstruction, prolonged nausea precedes vomiting, which may become feculent in late cases. Disorders that induce vomiting in younger patients may give rise only to anorexia or nausea in older patients. Although vomiting may present in either acute appendicitis or nonspecific abdominal pain, coexisting nausea and anorexia are more suggestive of the former condition.

B. Constipation

Reflex ileus is often induced by visceral afferent fibers stimulating efferent fibers of the sympathetic autonomic nervous system (splanchnic nerves) to reduce intestinal peristalsis. Hence, paralytic ileus undermines the value of constipation in the differential diagnosis of an acute abdomen. Constipation itself is hardly an absolute indicator of intestinal obstruction. However, **obstipation** (the absence of passage of both stool and flatus) strongly suggests mechanical bowel obstruction if there is progressive painful abdominal distention or repeated vomiting.

C. Diarrhea

Copious watery diarrhea is characteristic of gastroenteritis and other medical causes of an acute abdomen. Blood-stained diarrhea suggests ulcerative colitis, Crohn's disease, or bacillary or amebic dysentery. It is also common with ischemic colitis but often absent in intestinal infarction due to superior mesenteric artery occlusion.

D. Other Specific Symptoms

These are extremely helpful if present. **Jaundice** suggests hepatobiliary disorders; **hematochezia** or **hematemesis**, a gastroduodenal lesion or Mallory-Weiss syndrome; **hematuria**, ureteral colic or cystitis. The passage of blood clots or necrotic mucosal debris may be the sole evidence of advanced intestinal ischemia.

Other Relevant Aspects of the History

A. Gynecologic History

The menstrual history is crucial to the diagnosis of ectopic pregnancy, mittelschmerz (due to a ruptured ovarian follicle), and endometriosis. A history of vaginal discharge or dysmenorrhea may denote pelvic inflammatory disease.

B. Drug History

Anticoagulants have been implicated in retroperitoneal and intramural duodenal and jejunal hematomas; oral contraceptives in the formation of benign hepatic adenomas and in mesenteric venous infarction. Corticosteroids, in particular, may mask the clinical signs of even advanced peritonitis. Pyloric perforation has been caused by "crack" smoking.

C. Family History

This often provides the best information about medical causes of an acute abdomen (see below).

D. Travel History

This may raise the possibility of amebic liver abscess or hydatid cyst, malarial spleen, tuberculosis, *Salmonella typhi* infection of the ileocecal area, or dysentery.

E. Operation History

Any history of a previous abdominal, groin, vascular, or thoracic operation may be relevant to the current illness. Particular attention to the mode of operation (laparoscopic, open, endovascular) and any anatomic reconstructions may clarify aspects of the current complaint. If possible within the time constraints imposed by the urgency of the current problem, operative notes and pathology reports should be obtained and reviewed.

PHYSICAL EXAMINATION

The tendency to concentrate on the abdomen should be resisted in favor of a methodical and complete general physical examination. A systematic approach to the abdominal examination is outlined in Table 21–3. One should search for specific signs that confirm or rule out differential diagnostic possibilities (Table 21–4).

(1) General observation: General observation affords a fairly reliable indication of the severity of the clinical situation. Most patients, although uncomfortable, remain calm. The writhing of patients with visceral pain (eg, intestinal or ureteral colic) contrasts with the rigidly motionless bearing of those with parietal pain (eg, acute appendicitis, generalized peritonitis). Diminished responsiveness or an altered sensorium often precedes imminent cardiopulmonary collapse.

(2) Systemic signs: Systemic signs usually accompany rapidly progressive or advanced disorders associated with an acute abdomen. Extreme pallor, hypothermia, tachycardia, tachypnea, and sweating suggest major intra-abdominal hemorrhage (eg, ruptured aortic aneurysm or tubal pregnancy). Given such findings, one must proceed rapidly with the subsequent examination and tests in order to exclude extra-abdominal causes and to institute treatment.

(3) Fever: Constant low-grade fever is common in inflammatory conditions such as diverticulitis, acute cholecystitis, and appendicitis. High fever with lower abdominal tenderness in a young woman without signs of systemic illness suggests acute salpingitis. Disorientation or extreme lethargy combined with a very high fever (> 39 °C) or swinging fever or with chills and rigors signifies impending septic shock. This is most often due to advanced peritonitis, acute cholangitis, or pyelonephritis. However, fever is often mild or absent in elderly, chronically ill, or immunosuppressed patients with a serious acute abdomen.

(4) Examination of the acute abdomen

(a) Inspection: The abdomen should be thoughtfully inspected before palpation. A tensely distended abdomen with an old surgical scar suggests both the presence and the cause (adhesions) of small bowel obstruction. A scaphoid contracted abdomen is seen

Table 21–3. Steps in physical examination of the acute abdomen.

1. Inspection	7. Punch tenderness
2. Auscultation	Costal area
3. Cough tenderness	Costovertebral area
4. Percussion	8. Special signs
5. Guarding or rigidity	9. External hernias and male genitalia
6. Palpation	10. Rectal and pelvic examination
One-finger	
Rebound tenderness	
Deep	

Table 21–4. Physical findings in various causes of acute abdomen.

Condition	Helpful Signs
Perforated viscus	Scaphoid, tense abdomen; diminished bowel sounds (late); loss of liver dullness; guarding or rigidity.
Peritonitis	Motionless; absent bowel sounds (late); cough and rebound tenderness; guarding or rigidity.
Inflamed mass or abscess	Tender mass (abdominal, rectal, or pelvic); punch tenderness; special signs (Murphy's, psoas, or obturator).
Intestinal obstruction	Distention; visible peristalsis (late); hyperperistalsis (early) or quiet abdomen (late); diffuse pain without rebound tenderness; hernia or rectal mass (some).
Paralytic ileus	Distention; minimal bowel sounds; no localized tenderness.
Ischemic or strangulated bowel	Not distended (until late); bowel sounds variable; severe pain but little tenderness; rectal bleeding (some).
Bleeding	Pallor, shock; distention; pulsatile (aneurysm) or tender (eg, ectopic pregnancy) mass; rectal bleeding (some).

with perforated ulcer; visible peristalsis occurs in thin patients with advanced bowel obstruction; and soft doughy fullness is seen in early paralytic ileus or mesenteric thrombosis.

(b) Auscultation: Auscultation of the abdomen should also precede palpation. Peristaltic rushes synchronous with colic are heard in mid small bowel obstruction and in early acute pancreatitis. These tend to last longer but occur less frequently than in normal patients or in those with acute cholecystitis. They differ from the high-pitched hyperperistaltic sounds unrelated to the crampy pain of gastroenteritis, dysentery, and fulminant ulcerative colitis. An abdomen that is silent except for infrequent tinkly or squeaky sounds characterizes late bowel obstruction or diffuse peritonitis. Except for these more extreme patterns, the many auscultatory variants heard in paralytic ileus and other conditions render them largely useless for specific diagnosis.

(c) Coughing to elicit pain: The patient should be asked to cough and point to the area of maximal pain. Peritoneal irritation so demonstrated may be confirmed afterward without causing unnecessary pain by rigorous testing for rebound tenderness. Unlike the parietal pain of peritonitis, colic is visceral pain and is seldom aggravated by deep inspiration or coughing.

(d) Percussion: Percussion serves several purposes. Tenderness on percussion is akin to eliciting rebound tenderness; both reflect peritoneal irritation and parietal pain. With a perforated viscus, free air accumulating under the diaphragm may efface normal liver dullness. Tympany near the midline in a distended abdomen denotes air trapped within distended bowel loops. Free peritoneal fluid may be detected by demonstrating shifting dullness.

(e) Palpation: Palpation is performed with the patient resting in a comfortable supine position. Incisional and periumbilical hernias are noted. **Guarding** is assessed by placing both hands over the abdominal muscles and depressing the fingers gently. Properly performed, this maneuver is comforting to the patient. If there is voluntary spasm, the muscle will be felt to relax when the patient inhales deeply through the mouth. With true involuntary spasm, however, the muscle will remain taut and rigid ("board-like") throughout respiration. Except for rare neurologic disorders—and, for unknown reasons, renal colic—only peritoneal inflammation (by reflex afferent stimulation of efferent motor fibers) produces rectus muscle rigidity. Unlike peritonitis, renal colic induces spasm confined to the ipsilateral rectus muscle.

Tenderness that connotes localized peritoneal inflammation is the most important finding in patients with an acute abdomen. Its extent and severity are determined first by one- or two-finger palpation, beginning away from the area of cough tenderness and gradually advancing toward it. Tenderness is usually well demarcated in acute cholecystitis, appendicitis, diverticulitis, and acute salpingitis. If there is poorly localized tenderness unaccompanied by guarding, one should suspect gastroenteritis or some other inflammatory intestinal process without peritonitis. Compared with the degree of pain, unexpectedly little and only vague tenderness is elicited in uncomplicated hollow viscus obstruction, walled-off or deep-seated perforations (eg, retrocecal or retroileal appendicitis or diverticular phlegmons), and in very obese patients.

When the patient raises his or her head from the bed or examination table, the abdominal muscles will be tensed. Tenderness persists in abdominal wall conditions (eg, rectus hematoma), whereas deeper peritoneal pain due to intraperitoneal disease is lessened (Carnett's test). Hyperesthesia may be demonstrable in abdominal wall disorders or localized peritonitis, but it is more prominent in herpes zoster, spinal root compression, and other neuromuscular problems. Trigger point sensitivity, lateral costal rib tip tenderness, and pain exacerbated by spinal motion reflect parietal abdominal wall conditions that subside dramatically after infiltration with local anesthetic agents.

Abdominal masses are usually detected by deep palpation. Superficial lesions such as a distended gallbladder or appendiceal abscess are often tender and have discrete borders. If one suspects that abdominal guarding is masking an acutely inflamed gallbladder, the right subcostal area should be palpated while the patient inhales deeply. Inspiration will be arrested abruptly by pain **(Murphy's sign)**, or the gallbladder fundus may be felt as it strikes the examining fingers during descent of the diaphragm.

Deeper masses may be adherent to the posterior or lateral abdominal wall and are often partially walled off by overlying omentum and small bowel. As a result, their borders are ill-defined, and only dull pain may be elicited by palpation. Examples include pancreatic phlegmon and ruptured aortic aneurysm.

Even if a mass cannot be directly felt, its presence may be inferred by other maneuvers. A large psoas abscess arising from a perinephric abscess or perforated Crohn's enteritis may cause pain when the hip is passively extended or actively flexed against resistance **(iliopsoas sign)**. Similarly, internal and external rotation of the flexed thigh may exert painful pressure **(obturator sign)** on a loop of the small bowel entrapped within the obturator canal (obturator hernia). **Punch tenderness** over the lower costal ribs indicates an inflammatory condition affecting the diaphragm, liver, or spleen or its adjacent structures. While this may suggest a hepatic, splenic, or subphrenic abscess, it is also common in acute cholecystitis, acute hepatitis, or splenic infarct. **Costovertebral angle tenderness** is common in acute pyelonephritis. Since they are not invariably present, these special signs are helpful only in conjunction with a compatible history and related physical findings.

(f) Inguinal and femoral rings; male genitalia: The inguinal and femoral rings in both sexes and the genitalia in male patients should be examined next.

(g) Rectal examination: A rectal examination should be performed in most patients with an acute abdomen. Diffuse tenderness is nonspecific, but right-sided rectal tenderness accompanied by lower abdominal rebound tenderness is indicative of peritoneal irritation due to pelvic appendicitis or abscess. Other useful findings include a rectal tumor, blood-stained stool, or occult blood (detected by guaiac testing). Rectal examination may be dispensed with in children diagnosed as having appendicitis because of marked right lower quadrant tenderness, guarding, or rigidity.

(h) Pelvic examination: An acute abdomen is incorrectly diagnosed more often in women than in men, particularly in younger age groups. A pelvic examination is vital in women with a vaginal discharge, dysmenorrhea, menorrhagia, or left lower quadrant pain. A properly performed pelvic examination is invaluable in differentiating among acute pelvic inflammatory diseases that do not require operation and acute appendicitis, twisted ovarian cyst, or tubo-ovarian abscess (see Chapter 41).

INVESTIGATIVE STUDIES

The history and physical examination by themselves provide the diagnosis in two-thirds of cases of an acute abdomen. Supplementary laboratory and radiologic examinations are indispensable for diagnosis of many surgical conditions, for exclusion of medical causes ordinarily not treated by operation, and for assistance in preoperative preparation. Even in the absence of a specific diagnosis, there may already be enough information on which to base a rational decision about management. Additional studies are worthwhile only if they are likely to significantly alter or improve therapeutic decisions. A more liberal use of diagnostic studies is justified in elderly or seriously ill patients, in whom the history and physical findings may be less reliable and an early diagnosis vital to ensure a successful outcome.

The availability and reliability of certain studies vary in different hospitals. The invasiveness, risks, and cost-effectiveness of a test should be weighed when the physician selects diagnostic studies. Test results must always be interpreted within the clinical context of each case. Basic studies should be obtained in all but the most desperately ill patients. Other less vital tests may be requested later as indicated (Table 21–5).

Laboratory Investigations

A. Blood Studies

Hemoglobin, hematocrit, and white blood cell and differential counts taken on admission are highly informative. Only a rising or marked leukocytosis (> 13,000/μL), especially in the presence of a shift to the left on the blood smear, is indicative of serious infection. Moderate leukocytosis, commonly encountered in medical as well

Table 21–5. General principles of timing of diagnostic studies in an acute abdomen.

	Immediate	Same Day[1]	Next Day[1]
Blood	Hematocrit, white blood cell count, urea, creatinine, cross-matching,[1] arterial gases.[1]	Clotting studies, amylase, liver function tests.	Specific tests.
Urine	Microscopy, dipstick testing, culture.[1]		Specific tests.
Stool	Occult blood.	Warm smear, culture.	
Radiography and ultrasound	Chest, abdomen.	Ultrasonography or CT scan, angiography, water-soluble upper gastrointestinal series, HIDA scan (see Chapter 26).	Repeat abdominal films; barium enema or small bowel follow-through, intravenous urogram, and PTC (see Chapter 26); liver-spleen, gallium, and technetium scans.
Endoscopy		Proctosigmoidoscopy, upper endoscopy.	ERCP (see Chapter 26), colonoscopy, laparoscopy.
Other		Paracentesis, culdocentesis.	

[1]When indicated.

as surgical inflammatory conditions, is nonspecific and may be even absent in elderly or debilitated patients with infections. A low white blood cell count (< 8000/μL) is a feature of viral infections such as mesenteric adenitis or gastroenteritis and nonspecific abdominal pain.

A specimen of clotted blood for cross-matching should be sent whenever urgent surgery is anticipated. An additional tube of clotted blood may be reserved in case of such need.

Serum electrolytes, urea nitrogen, and creatinine are important, especially if hypovolemia is expected (ie, due to shock, copious vomiting or diarrhea, tense abdominal distention, or delay of several days after onset of symptoms). Arterial blood gas determinations should be obtained in patients with hypotension, generalized peritonitis, pancreatitis, possible ischemic bowel, and septicemia. Unsuspected metabolic acidosis may be the first clue to serious disease.

A raised serum amylase level corroborates a clinical diagnosis of acute pancreatitis. Moderately elevated values must be interpreted with caution, since abnormal levels frequently accompany strangulated or ischemic bowel, twisted ovarian cyst, or perforated ulcer. Moreover, a normal or even low amylase value may be seen in hemorrhagic pancreatitis or pseudocyst. Cloudy (lactescent) serum in a patient with abdominal pain suggests pancreatitis even though the serum amylase is normal.

In patients with suspected hepatobiliary disease, liver function tests (serum bilirubin, alkaline phosphatase, AST, ALT, albumin, and globulin) are useful to differentiate medical from surgical hepatic disorders and to gauge the severity of underlying parenchymal disease.

Clotting studies (platelet counts; prothrombin time and partial thromboplastin time) and a peripheral blood smear should be requested if the history hints at a possible hematologic abnormality (cirrhosis, petechiae, etc). The erythrocyte sedimentation rate, often nonspecifically raised in the acute abdomen, is of dubious diagnostic value; a normal value does not exclude serious surgical illness.

Antibody titers for amebic, typhoid, or viral disease and other special blood tests may pinpoint a specific disease, but therapeutic decisions often cannot await their results.

B. Urine Tests

Urinalysis is easily performed and may reveal useful information. Dark urine or a raised specific gravity reflects mild dehydration in patients with normal renal function. Hyperbilirubinemia may give rise to tea-colored urine that froths when shaken. Microscopic hematuria or pyuria can confirm ureteral colic or urinary tract infection and obviate a needless operation. Initial antibiotic treatment should be adjusted after culture and sensitivity reports are available. Dipstick testing (for albumin, bilirubin, glucose, and ketones) may reveal a medical cause of an acute abdomen. Pregnancy tests should be ordered if there is a history of a missed period.

C. Stool Tests

Gastrointestinal bleeding is not a common feature of the acute abdomen. Nonetheless, testing for occult fecal blood should be routinely performed. A positive test points to a mucosal lesion that may be responsible for large bowel obstruction or chronic anemia, or it may reflect an unsuspected carcinoma.

Warm stool smears for bacteria, ova, and animal parasites may demonstrate amebic trophozoites in patients with bloody or mucous diarrhea. Stool samples for culture should be taken in patients with suspected gastroenteritis, dysentery, or cholera.

Imaging Studies

A. Plain Chest X-Ray Studies

An erect chest x-ray is essential in all cases of an acute abdomen. Not only is it vital for preoperative assessment, but it may also demonstrate supradiaphragmatic conditions that simulate an acute abdomen (eg, lower lobe pneumonia or ruptured esophagus). An elevated hemidiaphragm or pleural effusion may direct attention to subphrenic inflammatory lesions.

B. Plain Abdominal X-Ray Studies

Plain supine films of the abdomen should be obtained only selectively. In general, erect (or lateral decubitus) views contribute little additional information except in suspected intestinal obstruction. Even though radiologic abnormalities are present in up to 40% of patients, these are diagnostic only half the time. Plain films are indicated in patients who have appreciable abdominal tenderness or distention, abnormal bowel sounds, a history of abdominal surgery, suspected foreign body ingestion, or who have a depressed sensorium or who are in a high-risk category. They are helpful in patients with possible intestinal obstruction or ischemia, perforated viscus, renal or ureteral calculi, or acute cholecystitis. They are seldom of value in patients suspected to have appendicitis or urinary tract infection. They are inappropriate in pregnant patients, unstable individuals in whom clear-cut physical signs mandating laparotomy already exist, or patients with only mild, resolving nonspecific pain. Maximal information is obtained by an experienced radiologist apprised of the clinical situation. However, the surgeon who is familiar with the clinical details should review all x-rays.

One should observe the gas pattern of the hollow viscera; free or abnormal air patterns under the diaphragm, within the biliary radicles, or outside the bowel wall; the outline of solid organs and the peritoneal fat lines; and radiopaque densities.

An abnormal bowel gas pattern suggests paralytic ileus, mechanical bowel obstruction, or pseudo-obstruction. A diffuse gas pattern with air outlining the rectal ampulla suggests paralytic ileus, especially if bowel sounds are absent. Gaseous distention is the rule in bowel obstruction. Air-fluid levels are usually seen in distal small bowel obstruction and a distended cecum with small bowel dilation in large bowel obstruction. Along with the clinical findings, the distinctive radiologic appearances of colonic dilation in toxic megacolon or volvulus establish the diagnosis (see Figure 30–15). Adynamic ileus associated with long-standing acute appendicitis or with an atypical appendix location often produces a pattern that suggests localized right lower quadrant ileus. This radiologic picture in a patient without previous abdominal surgery should influence the diagnostic decision toward appendicitis or other ileocecal disease (tumor, inflammatory disorders). "Thumbprint" impressions on the colonic wall are noted in about half of patients with ischemic colitis. A displaced gastric or colonic air shadow may be the only sign of subcapsular splenic hematoma.

Free gas under the hemidiaphragm must be looked for specifically. Its presence in approximately 80% of perforated ulcers corroborates the clinical diagnosis. Massive pneumoperitoneum is observed in free colonic perforations.

Biliary tree air designates a biliary-enteric communication, such as a spontaneous or surgically created choledochoduodenal fistula or gallstone ileus. Air delineating the portal venous system characterizes pylephlebitis. Air between loops of small bowel may arise from a small localized perforation.

Obliteration of the psoas muscle margins or enlargement of the kidney shadows indicates retroperitoneal disease.

Radiopaque densities of characteristic appearance and location may confirm a clinical suspicion of biliary, renal staghorn, or ureteral calculi; appendicitis; or aortic aneurysm. Whereas pelvic phleboliths are readily distinguishable, a migrant gallstone may be mistaken for a calcified mesenteric lymph node if the accompanying small bowel distention or biliary tree air is overlooked in gallstone ileus.

C. Angiography

Percutaneous invasive angiographic studies, or magnetic resonance angiography (MRA), are indicated if intra-abdominal intestinal ischemia or ongoing hemorrhage is suspected. They should precede any gastrointestinal contrast study that might obscure film interpretation. Selective visceral angiography is a reliable method of diagnosing mesenteric infarction. Emergency angiography may confirm a ruptured liver adenoma or carcinoma or an aneurysm of the splenic artery or other visceral artery. In patients with massive lower gastrointestinal bleeding, angiography may identify the bleeding site, may suggest the likely diagnosis (eg, vascular ectasia, polyarteritis nodosa), and may even be therapeutic if embolization can be performed. Angiography is of little value in ruptured aortic aneurysm or if frank peritoneal findings (peritonitis) are present. It is contraindicated in unstable patients with severe shock or sepsis and seldom warranted if other findings or tests already dictate the need for laparotomy or laparoscopy. Magnetic resonance angiography is most useful to evaluate the aortic, celiac, and mesenteric vasculature in the setting of possible subacute or chronic mesenteric ischemia.

D. Gastrointestinal Contrast X-Ray Studies

Gastrointestinal contrast studies should not be requested routinely or be regarded as screening studies. They are helpful only if a specific condition being considered can be verified or treated by a contrast x-ray examination. For suspected perforations of the esophagus or gastroduodenal area without pneumoperitoneum, a water-soluble contrast medium (eg, meglumine diatrizoate [Gastrografin]) is preferred. If there is no clinical evidence of bowel perforation, a barium enema may identify the level of a large bowel obstruction or even reduce a sigmoid volvulus or intussusception. Only if there is no likelihood of large bowel obstruction should a barium small bowel follow-through study be used to study a partial small bowel obstruction or to look for an intramural duodenal (or jejunal) hematoma that is best managed conservatively.

An emergency intravenous urogram is seldom necessary to evaluate nontraumatic causes of hematuria. It should be performed electively after microscopic examination of a stained and centrifuged urine specimen and cystoscopic examination. Ultrasonography and HIDA scans have replaced intravenous cholangiography in the evaluation of jaundiced patients and those suspected of having acute cholecystitis.

E. Ultrasonography

Ultrasonography is useful in evaluating upper abdominal pain that does not resemble ulcer pain or bowel obstruction and in investigating abdominal masses. Ultrasonography has a diagnostic sensitivity of about 80% for acute appendicitis and is most useful in pregnant patients and those presenting with features suggestive of atypical appendicitis or in young women with mid or lower abdominal pain. Color Doppler studies can distinguish avascular cysts and twisted masses from inflammatory and infectious processes. CT scanning may be more useful if excessive bowel gas, so common in elderly and ill patients, precludes satisfactory ultrasound examination. It is particularly helpful in pancreatic and retroperitoneal lesions and any severe localized infections (eg, acute diverticulitis).

F. CT Scan

Urgent or emergent CT scan of the abdomen is now generally routinely and rapidly available. This has proved extremely useful in the evaluation of abdominal complaints for patients who do not already have clear indications for laparotomy or laparoscopy. CT is helpful in identifying small amounts of free intraperitoneal gas and sites of inflammatory diseases that may prompt (appendicitis, tubo-ovarian abscess) or postpone (diverticulitis, pancreatitis, hepatic abscess) operation. It should not replace or delay operation in a patient for whom the scan will not change the decision to operate.

G. Radionuclide Scans

Liver-spleen scans, HIDA scans, and gallium scans may be useful for localizing intra-abdominal abscesses. However, their utility has been greatly decreased by the routine availability of urgent CT scans. Radionuclide blood pool or Tc-sulfur colloid scans may identify sources of slow or intermittent intestinal bleeding. Technetium pertechnetate scans may reveal ectopic gastric mucosa in Meckel's diverticulum. Tc-99m hexamethylpropyleneamineoxide (HMPAO) scanning may help in patients with vague signs of appendicitis. It has a sensitivity rate of 85%, specificity of 93%, and accuracy rate of 89%. It may also suggest other causes of intra-abdominal inflammation.

Endoscopy

Proctosigmoidoscopy is indicated in any patient with suspected large bowel obstruction, grossly bloody stools, or a rectal mass. Minimal air should be used for bowel insufflation. Besides reducing a sigmoid volvulus, colonoscopy may also locate the source of bleeding in cases of lower gastrointestinal hemorrhage that has subsided. Gastroduodenoscopy and ERCP are usually done electively to evaluate less urgent inflammatory conditions (eg, gastritis, peptic disease) in patients without alarming abdominal signs.

Paracentesis

In patients with free peritoneal fluid, aspiration of blood, bile, or bowel contents is a strong indication for urgent laparotomy. On the other hand, infected ascitic fluid may establish a diagnosis in spontaneous bacterial peritonitis, tuberculous peritonitis, or chylous ascites (see Chapter 22), which rarely require surgery. Culdocentesis may be useful for suspected ruptured corpus luteum cyst.

Peritoneal cytology (obtained by direct aspiration through a fine catheter) or diagnostic peritoneal lavage may disclose tumor or an acute intra-abdominal inflammatory problem. These investigations should be used selectively after imaging studies in patients with equivocal findings and in those who would poorly tolerate a negative laparotomy.

Laparoscopy

Laparoscopy is now a therapeutic as well as a diagnostic modality. In young women, it may distinguish a nonsurgical problem (ruptured graafian follicle, pelvic inflammatory disease, tubo-ovarian disease) from appendicitis. In obtunded, elderly, or critically ill patients, who often have deceptive manifestations of an acute abdomen, it may facilitate earlier treatment in those with positive findings while eliminating the added morbidity of a laparotomy in negative cases. Where appendicitis is confirmed, laparoscopic appendectomy may be performed. Increasingly, surgeons must acquire new laparoscopic skills in order to deal with other acute intra-abdominal conditions (eg, adhesive bowel obstruction) that previously demanded a formal laparotomy.

DIFFERENTIAL DIAGNOSIS

The age and gender of the patient help in the differential diagnosis: Mesenteric adenitis mimics acute appendicitis in the young; gynecologic disorders complicate the evaluation of lower abdominal pain in women of childbearing age; and malignant and vascular diseases are more common in the elderly. Causes of an acute abdomen reflect the disease patterns of the indigenous population, and an awareness of common causes within the physician's locale will improve diagnostic accuracy. The clinical picture in early cases is often unclear. The following observations should be borne in mind:

(1) Any patient with acute abdominal pain persisting for over 6 hours should be regarded as having a surgical problem requiring in-hospital evaluation. Well-localized pain and tenderness usually indicate a surgical condition. Systemic hypoperfusion in conjunction with generalized abdominal pain is seldom due to a medical problem.

(2) Acute cholecystitis, appendicitis, bowel obstruction, cancer, and acute vascular conditions are the most common causes of the surgical acute abdomen in older patients. In children, appendicitis accounts for one-third of all cases and nonspecific abdominal pain for nearly all the remainder.

(3) Acute appendicitis and intestinal obstruction are the most frequent final diagnoses in cases erroneously believed at first to be nonsurgical. Appendicitis should always remain a foremost concern if sepsis or an inflammatory lesion is suspected. It is the commonest cause of

bizarre peritoneal findings that produce ileus or intestinal obstruction. Half of children with appendicitis present with a marked facial flush (due to high serotonin levels). The presence of the gas stoppage sign or x-ray findings of right lower quadrant ileus should raise the possibility of retrocecal or retroileal appendicitis. Appendicitis is less likely in previously healthy individuals if the history exceeds 3 days' duration and the patient has no fever, appreciable tenderness, ileus, or leukocytosis.

Pelvic appendicitis, with mild abdominal pain, vomiting, and frequent loose stools, simulates gastroenteritis. The initial abdominal signs may be mild and the rectal and pelvic examinations unremarkable. A low white blood cell count or lymphocytosis favors gastroenteritis.

Atypical presentations of appendicitis are encountered during pregnancy. Maternal illness and fetal death in such cases are caused mainly by complications following delayed diagnosis. Appendectomy is well tolerated during pregnancy, and removal of a normal appendix is more frequently tolerated than observation of the perforation.

(4) Salpingitis, dysmenorrhea, ovarian lesions, and urinary tract infections complicate the evaluation of the acute abdomen in young women. Many diagnostic errors can be avoided by taking a careful menstrual history and performing a pelvic examination and urinalysis. Ultrasound study and pregnancy tests are helpful in appropriate cases. Compared with patients with appendicitis, patients with acute salpingitis tend to present with a longer history of pain, often related to the menstrual cycle, and to have higher fever, bilateral pelvic signs, and a markedly elevated white blood cell count.

(5) Unusual types or atypical manifestations of intestinal obstruction, especially early cases, are easily missed. Emesis, abdominal distention, and air-fluid levels on x-ray may be negligible in Richter's hernia, proximal or closed-loop small bowel obstructions, and early cecal volvulus.

Intestinal obstruction in an elderly woman who has not had a previous operation suggests an incarcerated femoral hernia or, rarely, an obturator hernia or gallstone ileus. There may be no pain or tenderness in the area of the hernia. Carefully examine the inguinofemoral region; repeat the rectal and pelvic examinations; and check for an obturator sign. Transient mild upper abdominal pain followed several days later by signs of intestinal obstruction is typical of gallstone ileus. Look for a radiopaque stone and air outlining the biliary tree on the plain abdominal x-ray.

(6) Elderly or cardiac patients with severe unrelenting diffuse abdominal pain but without commensurate peritoneal signs or abnormalities on plain abdominal films may have intestinal ischemia. Arterial blood pH should be measured and visceral angiography performed early.

Table 21–6. Medical causes of an acute abdomen for which surgery is not indicated.

Endocrine and metabolic disorders	**Infections and inflammatory disorders**
Uremia	Tabes dorsalis
Diabetic crisis	Herpes zoster
Addisonian crisis	Acute rheumatic fever
Acute intermittent porphyria	Henoch-Schönlein purpura
Acute hyperlipoproteinemia	Systemic lupus erythematosus
Hereditary Mediterranean fever	Polyarteritis nodosa
Hematologic disorders	**Referred pain**
Sickle cell crisis	Thoracic region
Acute leukemia	Myocardial infarction
Other dyscrasias	Acute pericarditis
Toxins and drugs	Pneumonia
Lead and other heavy metal poisoning	Pleurisy
Narcotic withdrawal	Pulmonary embolus
Black widow spider poisoning	Pneumothorax
	Empyema
	Hip and back

(7) Medical causes of the acute abdomen should be excluded before exploratory laparotomy is considered (Table 21–6). Upper abdominal pain may be encountered in myocardial infarction, acute pulmonary conditions (pneumothorax, lower lobe pneumonia, pleurisy, empyema, infarction), and acute hepatitis. Generalized or migratory abdominal discomfort may be felt in acute rheumatic fever, polyarteritis nodosa and other types of diffuse vasculitis, acute intermittent porphyria, and acute pleurodynia. Sharp flank pain, often accompanied by rectus spasm and cutaneous hyperesthesia, may be caused by osteoarthritis with thoracic or spinal nerve compression. Likewise, acute bursitis and hip joint disorders may produce pain radiating into the lower quadrants. Exquisite tingling or pinpricking sensations along a flank dermatome are characteristic of preeruptive herpes zoster.

Medical conditions usually can be distinguished from surgical ones by a careful assessment of the history and physical examination. The family history may furnish the first clue. The history is usually atypical in some aspects, and thoughtful scrutiny will disclose details such as unusual or exaggerated symptoms—or concomitant extra-abdominal complaints—that point to the true cause. Despite the apparent severity of pain, localized abdominal tenderness with involuntary guarding is seldom present. Fever and associated systemic signs may be disproportionate to the degree of pain.

Laboratory and x-ray studies will verify the diagnosis and avoid an operation.

(8) Beware of acute cholecystitis, acute appendicitis, and perforated peptic ulcer in patients already hospitalized for an illness affecting another organ system. Their presentation is often atypical, leading to delayed diagnosis and complications.

(9) Exploration is most often undertaken without benefit for salpingitis, mesenteric adenitis, gastroenteritis, pyelonephritis, and acute viral hepatitis.

(10) Nonspecific abdominal pain, comprising one-third of all cases, is the most common cause of the acute abdomen, especially in children. Generally mild, short-lived, and seldom associated with other serious symptoms, it resolves without specific treatment. Most cases represent undiagnosed viral and mild bacterial infections, irritable bowel syndrome, gynecologic problems, abdominal wall pain, psychosomatic pain, or worm infection.

INDICATIONS FOR SURGICAL EXPLORATION

The need for operation is apparent when the diagnosis is certain, but surgery sometimes must be undertaken before a precise diagnosis is reached. Table 21–7 lists some indications for urgent laparotomy or laparoscopy. Among patients with acute abdominal pain, those over age 65 more often require operation (33%) than do younger patients (15%).

A liberal policy of exploration is advisable in patients with inconclusive but persistent right lower quadrant tenderness. Pain in the left upper quadrant infrequently requires urgent laparotomy, and its cause can usually await elective confirmatory studies.

Table 21–7. Indications for urgent operation in patients with an acute abdomen.

Physical findings
- Involuntary guarding or rigidity, especially if spreading
- Increasing or severe localized tenderness
- Tense or progressive distention
- Tender abdominal or rectal mass with high fever or hypotension
- Rectal bleeding with shock or acidosis
- Equivocal abdominal findings along with—
  - Septicemia (high fever, marked or rising leukocytosis, mental changes, or increasing glucose intolerance in a diabetic patient)
  - Bleeding (unexplained shock or acidosis, falling hematocrit)
  - Suspected ischemia (acidosis, fever, tachycardia)
  - Deterioration on conservative treatment

Radiologic findings
- Pneumoperitoneum
- Gross or progressive bowel distention
- Free extravasation of contrast material
- Space-occupying lesion on scan, with fever
- Mesenteric occlusion on angiography

Endoscopic findings
- Perforated or uncontrollably bleeding lesion

Paracentesis findings
- Blood, bile, pus, bowel contents, or urine

PREOPERATIVE MANAGEMENT

After initial assessment, parenteral analgesics for pain relief should not be withheld. In moderate doses, analgesics neither obscure useful physical findings nor mask their subsequent development. Indeed, abdominal masses may become obvious once rectus spasm is relieved. Pain that persists in spite of adequate doses of narcotics suggests a serious condition often requiring operative correction.

Resuscitation of acutely ill patients is outlined in Chapter 2. Medications should be restricted to only essential requirements. Particular care should be given to use of cardiac drugs and corticosteroids and to control of diabetes. Antibiotics are indicated for some infectious conditions or as prophylaxis during the perioperative period (see Chapter 8).

A nasogastric tube should be inserted in patients likely to undergo surgery and for those with hematemesis or copious vomiting, suspected bowel obstruction, or severe paralytic ileus. This precaution may prevent aspiration in patients suffering from drug overdose or alcohol intoxication, patients who are comatose or debilitated, or elderly patients with impaired cough reflexes. However, since the tube interferes with coughing and is uncomfortable, it should be removed once it is safe to do so.

A urinary catheter should be placed in patients with systemic hypoperfusion. In some elderly patients, it eliminates the cause of pain (acute bladder distention) or unmasks relevant abdominal signs.

Informed consent for surgery may be difficult to obtain when the diagnosis is uncertain. It is prudent to discuss with the patient and family the possibility of multiple staged operations; temporary or permanent stomal openings; impotence or sterility; and postoperative intubation for mechanical ventilation. Whenever the exact diagnosis is uncertain—especially in young or frail or severely ill patients—a frank preoperative discussion of the diagnostic dilemma and reasons for laparotomy or laparoscopy will reduce postoperative anxieties and misunderstanding.

Eskelinen M et al: Contributions of history-taking, physical examination, and computer assistance to diagnosis of acute small-bowel obstruction. A prospective study of 1333 patients with acute abdominal pain. Scand J Gastroenterol 1994;29:715.

Hoekstra HJ et al: Gastrointestinal complications in lung transplant survivors that require surgical intervention. Br J Surg 2001;88:433.

Kraemer M et al: Acute appendicitis in late adulthood: incidence, presentation, and outcome. Results of a prospective multicenter acute abdominal pain study and a review of the literature. Langenbecks Arch Surg 2000;385:470.

Mindelzun RE et al: The acute abdomen: current CT imaging techniques. Semin Ultrasound CT MR 1999;20:63.

Rao PM et al: Effect of computed tomography of the appendix on treatment of patients and use of hospital resources. N Engl J Med 1998;338:141.

Siewert B et al: CT of the acute abdomen: findings and impact on diagnosis and treatment. AJR Am J Roentgenol 1994;163:1317.

Silliman CC et al: Indications for surgical intervention for gastrointestinal emergencies in children receiving chemotherapy. Cancer 1994;74:203.

Simic O et al: Incidence and prognosis of abdominal complications after cardiopulmonary bypass. Cardiovasc Surg 1999;7:419.

Urban BA et al: Targeted helical CT of the acute abdomen: appendicitis, diverticulitis, and small bowel obstruction. Semin Ultrasound CT MR 2000;21:20.

Vander Velpen GC et al: Diagnostic yield and management benefit of laparoscopy: a prospective audit. Gut 1994;35:1617.

Whitney TM et al: Emergent abdominal surgery in AIDS: experience in San Francisco. Am J Surg 1994;168:239.

Peritoneal Cavity

22

Gerard M. Doherty, MD

THE PERITONEUM & ITS FUNCTIONS

The peritoneal cavity is lined by the **parietal peritoneum**, a mesothelial lining. This lining is called the **visceral peritoneum** where it is reflected onto the enclosed abdominal organs. Its relationship to intraperitoneal structures defines discrete compartments within which abscesses may form (see Intra-abdominal Abscesses). The peritoneal surface area is a semipermeable membrane with an area comparable to that of the cutaneous body surface. Nearly 1 m^2 of the total 1.7 m^2 area participates in fluid exchange with the extracellular fluid space at rates of 500 mL or more per hour. Normally, there is less than 50 mL of free peritoneal fluid, a transudate with the following characteristics: specific gravity below 1.016; protein concentration less than 3 g/dL; white blood cell count less than 3000/μL; complement-mediated antibacterial activity; and lack of fibrinogen-related clot formation. The circulation of peritoneal fluid is directed toward lymphatics in the undersurface of the diaphragm. There, particulate matter—including bacteria up to 20 μm in size—is cleared via stomas in the diaphragmatic mesothelium and lymphatics and discharged mainly into the right thoracic duct.

The peritoneal cavity is normally sterile. Small numbers of bacteria can be efficiently disposed of, but peritonitis ensues if the defense mechanisms are overwhelmed by massive or continued contamination. In response to tissue damage, mast cells in the delicate mesothelial lining discharge histamine and other vasoactive substances that enhance vascular permeability. The resulting fibrinogen-rich plasma exudate supplies complement and opsonic proteins that promote bacterial destruction. Tissue thromboplastin released by injured mesothelial cells converts fibrinogen into fibrin, which may in turn lead to collagen deposition and formation of fibrous adhesions. In health, this reaction is limited by a plasminogen activator in the cell lining, but the plasminogen activator is inactivated by injury or infection. Bacterial lipopolysaccharide (endotoxin) and cytokines can stimulate production of tumor necrosis factor (TNF). TNF, in turn, mediates the release of plasminogen activator inhibitor produced by inflamed peritoneal mesothelial cells, which can lead to persistence of fibrin. Fibrin clots segregate bacterial deposits, a source of endotoxins that contribute to sepsis, but segregation may also inadvertently shield bacteria from bacteria-clearing mechanisms.

The **omentum** is a well-vascularized pliable, mobile double fold of peritoneum and fat that participates actively in the control of peritoneal inflammation and infection. Its composition is well suited to sealing off a leaking viscus (eg, perforated ulcer) or area of infection (eg, resulting from a ruptured appendix) and for carrying a collateral blood supply to ischemic viscera. Its bacteria scavenger functions include absorption of small particles and delivery of phagocytes that destroy unopsonized bacteria.

DISEASES & DISORDERS OF THE PERITONEUM

ACUTE SECONDARY BACTERIAL PERITONITIS

Pathophysiology

Peritonitis is an inflammatory or suppurative response of the peritoneal lining to direct irritation. Peritonitis can occur after perforating, inflammatory, infectious, or ischemic injuries of the gastrointestinal or genitourinary system. Common examples are listed in Table 22–1. **Secondary peritonitis** results from bacterial contamination originating from within viscera or from external sources (eg, penetrating injury). It most often follows disruption of a hollow viscus. Extravasated bile and urine, although only mildly irritating when sterile, are markedly toxic if infected and provoke a vigorous peritoneal reaction. Gastric juice from a perforated duodenal ulcer remains mostly sterile for several hours, during which time it produces a chemical peritonitis with large fluid losses; but if left untreated, it evolves within 6–12

Table 22–1. Common causes of peritonitis.

	Cause	Mortality Rate
Mild	Appendicitis Perforated gastroduodenal ulcers Acute salpingitis	< 10%
Moderate	Diverticulitis (localized perforations) Nonvascular small bowel perforation Gangrenous cholecystitis Multiple trauma	< 20%
Severe	Large bowel perforations Ischemic small bowel injuries Acute necrotizing pancreatitis Postoperative complications	20–80%

hours into bacterial peritonitis. Intraperitoneal fluid dilutes opsonic proteins and impairs phagocytosis. Furthermore, when hemoglobin is present in the peritoneal cavity, *Escherichia coli* growing within the cavity can elaborate leukotoxins that reduce bactericidal activity. Limited, localized infection can be eradicated by host defenses, but continued contamination invariably leads to generalized peritonitis and eventually to septicemia with multiple organ failure.

Factors that influence the severity of peritonitis include the type of bacterial or fungal contamination, the nature and duration of the injury, and the host's nutritional and immune status. The grade of peritonitis varies with the cause. Clean (eg, proximal gut perforations) or well-localized (eg, ruptured appendix) contaminations progress to fulminant peritonitis relatively slowly (eg, 12–24 hours). In contrast, bacteria associated with distal gut or infected biliary tract perforations quickly overwhelm host peritoneal defenses. This degree of toxicity is also characteristic of postoperative peritonitis due to anastomotic leakage or contamination. Conditions that ordinarily cause mild peritonitis may produce life-threatening sepsis in an immunocompromised host.

Causative Organisms

Systemic sepsis due to peritonitis occurs in varying degrees depending on the virulence of the pathogens, the bacterial load, and the duration of bacterial proliferation and synergistic interaction. Except for spontaneous bacterial peritonitis, peritonitis is almost invariably polymicrobial; cultures usually contain more than one aerobic and more than two anaerobic species. The microbial picture reflects the bacterial flora of the involved organ. As long as gastric acid secretion and gastric emptying are normal, perforations of the proximal bowel (stomach or duodenum) are generally sterile or associated with relatively small numbers of gram-positive organisms. Perforations or ischemic injuries of the distal small bowel (eg, strangulated hernia) lead to infection with aerobic bacteria in about 30% of cases and anaerobic organisms in about 10% of cases. Fecal spillage, with a bacterial load of 10^{12} or more organisms per gram, is extremely toxic. Positive cultures with gram-negative and anaerobic bacteria are characteristic of infections originating from the appendix, colon, and rectum. The predominant aerobic pathogens include the gram-negative bacteria *E coli,* streptococci, proteus, and the Enterobacter-Klebsiella groups. Besides *Bacteroides fragilis,* anaerobic cocci and clostridia are the prevalent anaerobic organisms. Synergism between fecal anaerobic and aerobic bacteria increases the severity of infections.

Clinical Findings

By estimating the severity of peritonitis from clinical and laboratory findings, the need for specific organ-supportive care and surgery can be determined.

See Chapter 21 for details of radiologic and other investigations.

A. Symptoms and Signs

The clinical manifestations of peritonitis reflect the severity and duration of infection and the age and general health of the patient. Physical findings can be divided into (1) abdominal signs arising from the initial injury and (2) manifestations of systemic infection. Acute peritonitis frequently presents as an acute abdomen. **Local findings** include abdominal pain, tenderness, guarding or rigidity, distention, free peritoneal air, and diminished bowel sounds—signs that reflect parietal peritoneal irritation and resulting ileus. **Systemic findings** include fever, chills or rigors, tachycardia, sweating, tachypnea, restlessness, dehydration, oliguria, disorientation, and, ultimately, refractory shock. Shock is due to the combined effects of hypovolemia and septicemia with multiple organ dysfunction. *Recurrent unexplained shock is highly predictive of serious intraperitoneal sepsis.*

The findings in abdominal sepsis are modified by the patient's age and general health. Physical signs of peritonitis are subtle or difficult to interpret in both very young and very old patients as well as in those who are chronically debilitated, immunosuppressed, or receiving corticosteroids and in postoperative patients. Paracentesis or diagnostic peritoneal lavage may be occasionally useful in equivocal cases and in senile or confused patients. A white blood cell count of greater than 200 cells/μL is indicative of peritonitis, with virtually no false-positive and minimal false-negative errors. Delayed recognition is a major cause of the high mortality rate of peritonitis.

B. Laboratory Findings

Laboratory studies gauge the severity of peritonitis and guide therapy. Blood studies should include a complete blood cell count, cross-matching, arterial blood gases, electrolytes, a blood clotting profile, and liver and renal function tests. Samples for culture of blood, urine, sputum, and peritoneal fluid should be taken before antibiotics are started. A positive blood culture is usually present in toxic patients.

Differential Diagnosis

Specific kinds of infective (eg, gonococcal, amebic, candidal) and noninfective peritonitis may be seen. In the elderly, systemic diseases (eg, pneumonia, uremia) may produce intestinal ileus so striking that it resembles bowel obstruction or peritonitis.

Familial Mediterranean fever (periodic peritonitis, familial paroxysmal polyserositis) is a rare genetic condition that affects individuals of Mediterranean genetic background. Its exact cause is unknown. Patients present with recurrent bouts of abdominal pain and tenderness along with pleuritic or joint pain. Fever and leukocytosis are common. Colchicine prevents but does not treat acute attacks. Provocative testing by infusion of metaraminol (10 mg) induces abdominal pain within 2 days.

Laparoscopy has superseded laparotomy in suspect individuals. Free fluid and inflamed peritoneal surfaces are found, but smears and cultures are negative. The appendix should be removed to simplify diagnosis in subsequent episodes. Amyloidosis with renal failure is a late complication that is preventable by long-term colchicine therapy.

Treatment

Fluid and electrolyte replacement, operative control of sepsis, and systemic antibiotics are the mainstays of treatment of peritonitis.

A. Preoperative Care

1. Intravenous fluids—The massive transfer of fluid into the peritoneal cavity must be replaced by an appropriate amount of intravenous fluid. If systemic toxicity is evident or if the patient is old or in fragile health, a central venous pressure (or pulmonary artery wedge pressure) line and bladder catheter should be inserted; a fluid balance chart should be kept; and serial body weight measurements should be taken to monitor fluid requirements. Sufficient balanced or lactated Ringer's solution must be infused rapidly enough to correct intravascular hypovolemia promptly and to restore blood pressure and urine output to satisfactory levels. Potassium supplements are withheld until tissue and renal perfusion are adequate and urine is produced. Blood is reserved for anemic patients or those with concomitant bleeding.

2. Care for advanced septicemia—Cardiovascular agents and mechanical ventilation in an intensive care unit are essential in patients with advanced septicemia. An arterial line for continuous blood pressure recording and blood sampling is helpful. Cardiac monitoring with a Swan-Ganz catheter is essential if inotropic drugs are used. (See Chapters 9, 10, and 13 for details of fluid resuscitation and the management of septic shock.)

3. Antibiotics—Loading doses of intravenous antibiotics directed against the anticipated bacterial pathogens should be given after fluid samples have been obtained for culture. Initial antibiotics employed include third-generation cephalosporins, ampicillin-sulbactam, ticarcillin-clavulanic acid, aztreonam or imipenem-cilastatin for gram-negative coliforms, and metronidazole or clindamycin for anaerobic organisms. The choice of single-, double- or triple-drug therapy is of less importance than adequate coverage of both anticipated aerobic and anaerobic organisms. Inadequate initial drug dosing and scheduling contribute to treatment failures. Aminoglycosides should be used judiciously because renal impairment is often a feature of peritonitis and because lowered intraperitoneal pH may impair their in vivo activity.

Empirically chosen antibiotics should be modified postoperatively by culture and sensitivity results if there is persistent or subsequent infection (seen in 15–20% of patients). Antibiotics are continued until the patient has remained afebrile with a normal white count and a differential count of less than 3% bands.

B. Operative Management

1. Control of sepsis—The objectives of surgery for peritonitis are to remove all infected material, correct the underlying cause, and prevent late complications. Except in early, localized peritonitis, a midline incision offers the best surgical exposure. Materials for aerobic and anaerobic cultures of fluid and infected tissue are obtained immediately after the peritoneal cavity is entered. Occult pockets of infection are located by thorough exploration, and contaminated or necrotic material is removed. Routine radical debridement of all peritoneal and serosal surfaces does not increase survival rates. The primary disease is then treated. This may require resection (eg, ruptured appendix or gallbladder), repair (eg, perforated ulcer), or drainage (eg, acute pancreatitis). Attempts to reanastomose resected bowel in the presence of extensive sepsis or intestinal ischemia often lead to leakage. Temporary stomas are safer, and these can be taken down several weeks later after the patient has recovered from the acute illness. Surgical wounds should seldom be closed primarily. They should be left open in grossly soiled cases or delayed primary closure employed in those with less contamination.

2. Peritoneal lavage—In diffuse peritonitis, lavage with copious amounts (> 3 L) of warm isotonic crystalloid solution removes gross particulate matter as well as blood and fibrin clots and dilutes residual bacteria. The addition of antiseptics or antibiotics to the irrigating solution is generally useless or even harmful because of induced adhesions (eg, tetracycline, povidone-iodine). Antibiotics given parenterally will reach bactericidal levels in peritoneal fluid and may afford no additional benefit when given by lavage. Furthermore, lavage with aminoglycosides can produce respiratory depression and complicate anesthesia because of the neuromuscular blocking action of this group of drugs. After lavage is completed, all fluid in the peritoneal cavity must be aspirated because it may hamper local defense mechanisms by diluting opsonins and removing surfaces upon which phagocytes destroy bacteria.

3. Peritoneal drainage—Drainage of the free peritoneal cavity is ineffective and often undesirable. Not only are drains quickly isolated from the rest of the peritoneal cavity, but they also still act as a channel for exogenous contamination. Prophylactic drainage in diffuse peritonitis does not prevent abscess formation and may even predispose to abscesses or fistulas. Drainage is useful for residual focal infection or when continued contamination is present or likely to occur (eg, fistula). It is indicated for localized inflammatory masses that cannot be resected or for cavities that cannot be obliterated. Soft sump drains with continuous suction through multiple side perforations are effective for large volumes of fluid. Smaller volumes of fluid are best handled with closed drainage systems (eg, Jackson-Pratt drains). Large cavities with thick walls may be drained by several large Penrose drains placed in a dependent position.

To achieve more effective peritoneal drainage in severe peritonitis, some surgeons have previously left the entire abdominal wound open to widely expose the peritoneal cavity. Besides requiring intensive nursing and medical support to cope with massive protein and fluid losses (averaging 9 L the first day), there are serious complications such as spontaneous fistulization, wound sepsis, segmental colonic necrosis, and large incisional hernias. Consequently, this method is seldom employed now.

An alternative method is to re-explore the abdomen every 1–3 days until all loculations have been adequately drained. The wound may be closed temporarily with a sheet of polypropylene (Marlex) mesh that contains a nylon zipper or Velcro to avoid a tight abdominal closure and to facilitate repeated opening and closing. Other options include the use of a plastic sheet (Bogota bag) or a wound vacuum device bridging over the open fascia. Exploration may even be performed in the intensive care unit with heavy sedation. Available data suggest that this method should be restricted to selected patients with long-standing (more than 48 hours) extensive intraperitoneal sepsis associated with multiple organ failure (high sepsis scores). One prospective study failed to demonstrate a significant difference in mortality rates between the conventional closed (31%) and open (44%) techniques.

4. Management of abdominal distention—Abdominal distention caused by ileus frequently accompanies peritonitis, and decompression of the intestine is often ineffective in reliably decreasing the distention. An alternative approach is to close the abdomen temporarily with a sheet of plastic (Bogota bag) to avoid further distention, increased intra-abdominal pressure, and respiratory or renal problems (abdominal compartment syndrome). A **gastrostomy** may be advantageous if prolonged nasogastric decompression is expected, especially in elderly patients or those with chronic respiratory disease. A central TPN line or needle jejunostomy catheter (for proximal gut lesions) is placed when prolonged nutritional support is anticipated.

C. Postoperative Care

Intensive care monitoring, often with ventilatory support, is mandatory in unstable and frail patients. Achieving hemodynamic stability to perfuse major organs is the immediate objective, and this may entail the use of cardiac inotropic agents besides fluid and blood product supportive measures. Antibiotics are given for 10–14 days, depending on the severity of peritonitis. A favorable clinical response is evidenced by well-sustained perfusion with good urine output, reduction in fever and leukocytosis, resolution of ileus, and a returning sense of well-being. The rate of recovery varies with the duration and degree of peritonitis.

The early removal of all nonessential catheters (arterial, central venous, urinary, and nasogastric) reduces the risk of secondary infected foci. Drains should be removed or advanced once drainage diminishes and becomes more serous in nature. Excessive or prolonged suction may produce fistulas or bleeding even within a few days.

Growing awareness of the association between proximal gut colonization with candida, *Streptococcus faecalis,* pseudomonas, and coagulase-negative staphylococci and secondary nosocomial infections and subsequent multiple organ failure has encouraged early gut feeding and discontinuation of unnecessary antibiotics whenever feasible.

Complications

Postoperative complications are frequent and may be divided into local and systemic problems. Deep wound infections, residual abscesses and intraperitoneal sepsis, anastomotic breakdown, and fistula formation usually become manifest toward the end of the first postoperative week. Persistent high or swinging fever, inability to wean off cardiac inotropes, generalized edema with unexplained continued high fluid requirements, increased abdominal distention, prolonged mental apathy and weakness, or general failure to improve despite intensive treatment may be the sole indicators of residual intra-abdominal infection. This should prompt a thorough examination of the patient for infected catheters and an abdominal CT scan. Percutaneous catheter drainage of localized abscesses or open reexploration is undertaken as needed (see next section).

Uncontrolled sepsis leads inexorably to sequential multiple organ failure affecting the respiratory, renal, hepatic, clotting, and immune systems. Supportive measures, including mechanical ventilation, transfusions, total parenteral nutrition, and hemodialysis, are ineffectual unless primary septic foci are eliminated by combined surgical and antibiotic therapy.

Prognosis

The overall mortality rate of generalized peritonitis is about 40% (Table 22–1). Factors contributing to a high mortality rate include the type of primary disease and its duration, associated multiple organ failure before treatment, and the age and general health of the patient. Mortality rates are consistently below 10% in patients with perforated ulcers or appendicitis; in young patients; in those having less extensive bacterial contamination; and in those diagnosed and operated upon early. Patients with distal small bowel or colonic perforations or postoperative sepsis tend to be older, to have concurrent medical illnesses and greater bacterial contamination, and to have a greater propensity to renal and respiratory failure; their mortality rates are about 50%. Markedly poor physiologic indices (eg, APACHE II or Mannheim Peritonitis Index), reduced cardiac status, and low preoperative albumin levels identify high-risk patients who require intensive treatment to reduce a daunting mortality rate.

INTRA-ABDOMINAL ABSCESSES

1. Intraperitoneal Abscesses

Pathophysiology

An intra-abdominal abscess is a collection of infected fluid within the abdominal cavity. Gastrointestinal perforations, postoperative complications, penetrating trauma, and genitourinary infections are the most common causes. An abscess forms by one of two modes: It may develop (1) adjacent to a diseased viscus (eg, with perforated appendix, Crohn's enterocolitis, or diverticulitis) or (2) as a result of external contamination (eg, postoperative subphrenic abscesses). In one-third of cases, the abscess occurs as a sequela of generalized peritonitis. Interloop and pelvic abscesses form if extravasated fluid gravitating into a dependent or localized area becomes secondarily infected (Figure 22–1).

Bacteria-laden fibrin and blood clots and neutrophils contribute to the formation of an abscess. The pathogenic organisms are similar to those responsible for peritonitis, but anaerobic organisms occupy an important role. Experimentally, mixed aerobic (*E coli*) and anaerobic (*B fragilis*) infections, especially in conjunction with adjuvants (eg, feces or barium), reduce intraperitoneal O_2 and pH, thereby fostering anaerobic proliferation and abscess formation.

Sites of Abscesses

The areas in which abscesses commonly occur are defined by the configuration of the peritoneal cavity with its dependent lateral and pelvic basins (Figure 22–1), together with the natural divisions created by the transverse mesocolon and the small bowel mesentery. The supracolic compartment, located above the transverse mesocolon, broadly defines the subphrenic spaces (Figure 22–2A). Within this area, the subdiaphragmatic (suprahepatic) and subhepatic areas of the subphrenic space may be distinguished. The **subdiaphragmatic space** on each side occupies the concavity between the hemidiaphragms and the domes of the hepatic lobes. The inferior limits of its posterior recess are the attachments of the coronary and triangular ligaments on the dorsal—not superior—aspect of the diaphragm. Anteriorly, the lower limits are defined on the right by the transverse colon and on the left by the anterior stomach surface, omentum, transverse colon, spleen, and phrenicocolic ligament. Although each subdiaphragmatic space is continuous over the convex liver surface, inflammatory adhesions may delimit an abscess in an anterior or posterior position (Figure 22–2B). The falciform ligament separates the right and left subdiaphragmatic divisions.

The **right subhepatic division** (Figure 22–2B) of the subphrenic space is located between the undersurfaces of the liver and gallbladder superiorly and the right kidney and mesocolon inferiorly. The anterior bulge of the kidney partitions this space into an anterior (gallbladder fossa) and posterior (Morison's pouch) section.

The **left subhepatic space** also has an anterior and posterior part (Figure 22–2C). The smaller anterior subhepatic space lies between the undersurface of the left lobe and the anterior surface of the stomach. Left subdiaphragmatic collections often extend into this anterior subhepatic area. The posterior subhepatic space is the lesser sac, which is situated behind the lesser omentum and stomach and lies anterior to the pancreas, duodenum, transverse mesocolon, and left kidney. It extends posteriorly to the attach-

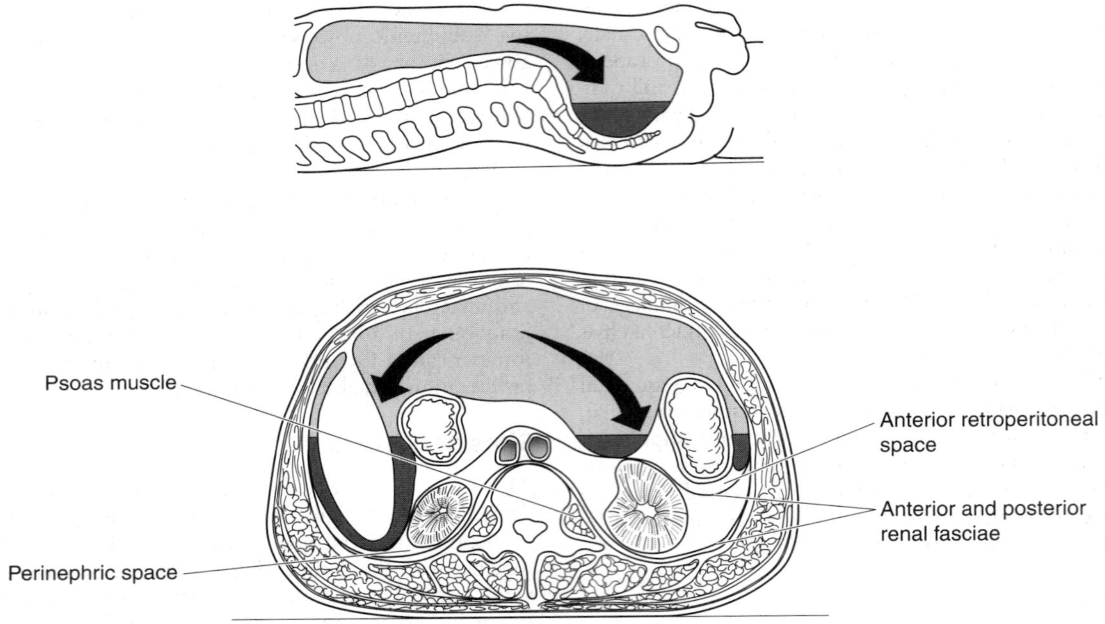

Figure 22–1. Lateral (*top*) and cross-sectional (*bottom*) views of the abdomen, showing fluid gravitating to the dependent areas of the peritoneal cavity. The retroperitoneal compartments are also outlined.

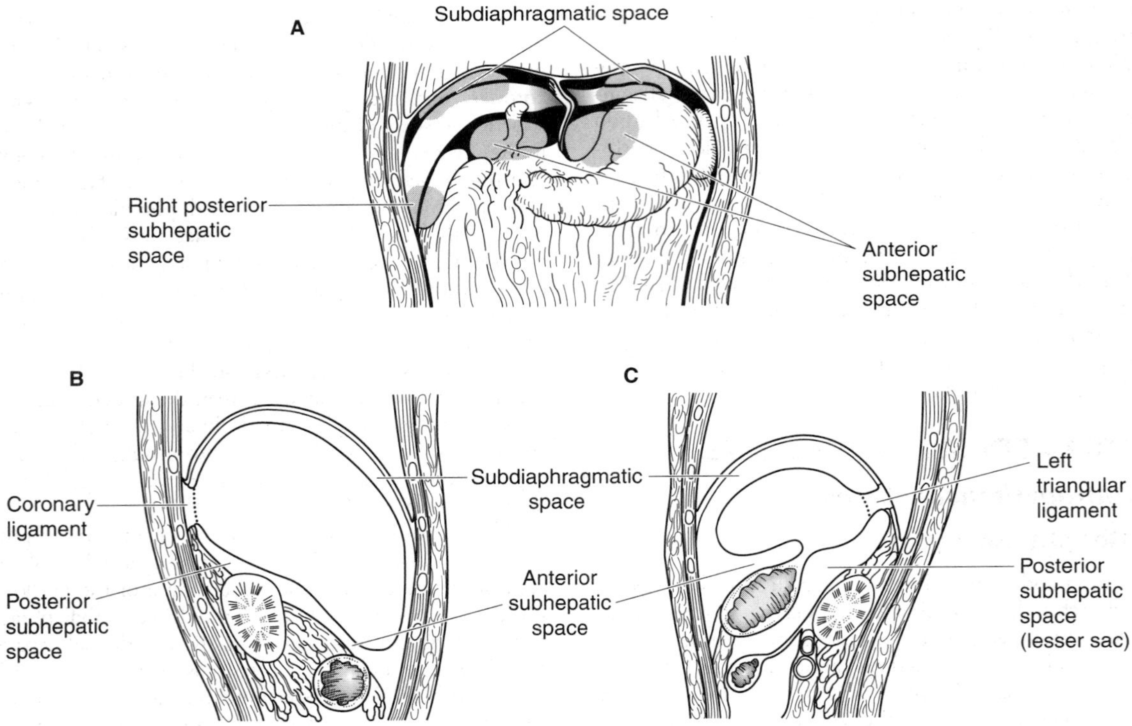

Figure 22–2. Subphrenic spaces. ***A:*** Anterior view. ***B:*** Right lateral view. ***C:*** Left lateral view.

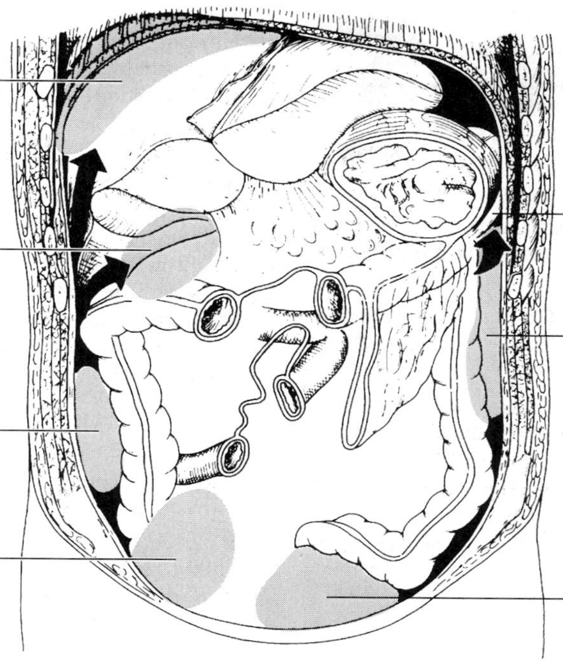

Figure 22–3. The infracolic peritoneal compartment and common abscess sites. Note how paracolic fluid on the right side can migrate up into the subphrenic spaces, whereas collections on the left side are prevented from doing so by the phrenicocolic ligament.

ment of the left triangular ligament superiorly on to the hemidiaphragm. The lesser sac communicates with both the right subhepatic and right paracolic spaces through the narrow foramen of Winslow.

The **infracolic compartment**, below the transverse mesocolon, includes the pericolic and pelvic areas (Figure 22–3). The diagonally aligned root of the small bowel mesentery divides the midabdominal area between the fixed right and left colons into right and left infracolic spaces. Each lateral paracolic gutter and lower quadrant area communicates freely with the pelvic cavity. However, while right paracolic collections may track upward into the subhepatic and subdiaphragmatic spaces, the phrenicocolic ligament hinders fluid migration along the left paracolic gutter into the left subdiaphragmatic area.

The most common abscess sites are in the lower quadrants, followed by the pelvic, subhepatic, and subdiaphragmatic spaces (Table 22–2).

Clinical Findings

A. Symptoms and Signs

An intraperitoneal abscess should be suspected in any patient with a predisposing condition. Fever, tachycardia, and pain may be mild or absent, especially in patients receiving antibiotics. A deep-seated or posteriorly situated abscess may exist in seemingly well individuals whose only symptom is persistent fever. Not infrequently, prolonged ileus or a sluggish recovery in a patient who has had recent abdominal surgery or peritoneal sepsis, rising leukocytosis, or nonspecific radiologic abnormality provides the initial clue. A mass is seldom felt except late in patients with lower quadrant or pelvic lesions. Irritation of contiguous structures may produce lower chest pain, dyspnea, referred shoulder pain or hiccup, or basilar atelectasis or effusion in subphrenic abscesses; or diarrhea or urinary frequency in pelvic abscesses. The diagnosis is more difficult in postoperative, chronically ill, confused, or diabetic patients and in those receiving immunosuppressive drugs, a group particularly susceptible to septic complications.

Sequential multiple organ failure—principally respiratory, renal, or hepatic failure—or stress gastrointestinal bleeding with disseminated intravascular coagulopathy is highly suggestive of intra-abdominal infection.

B. Laboratory Findings

A raised leukocyte count, abnormal liver or renal function test results, hyperglycemia, and abnormal arterial blood gases are nonspecific signs of infection. Serial

Table 22–2. Common sites and causes of intraperitoneal abscesses.

Site	Cause
Right lower quadrant	Appendicitis, perforated ulcer, regional enteritis
Left lower quadrant	Colorectal perforation (diverticulitis, carcinoma, inflammatory bowel diseases)
Pelvis	Appendicitis, colorectal perforation, gynecologic sepsis, postoperative complications
Subphrenic region	Postoperative complications following gastric or hepatobiliary surgery or splenectomy, perforated ulcer, acute cholecystitis, appendicitis, pancreatitis (lesser sac)
Interloop	Postoperative bowel perforation

postoperative measurement of serum lysozyme (derived from phagocytic cells) is a promising but not widely available test that appears to be highly specific for intra-abdominal pus. Persistently positive blood cultures point strongly to an intra-abdominal focus. A cervical smear demonstrating gonococcal infection is of specific value in diagnosing tubo-ovarian abscess.

C. Imaging Studies

1. X-ray studies—Plain x-rays may suggest an abscess in up to one-half of cases. In subphrenic abscesses, the chest x-ray may show pleural effusion, a raised hemidiaphragm, basilar infiltrates, or atelectasis. Abnormalities on plain abdominal films include an ileus pattern, soft tissue mass, air-fluid levels, free or mottled gas pockets, effacement of properitoneal or psoas outlines, and displacement of viscera. Many of these findings are vague or nonspecific, but they may suggest the need for a CT scan. Barium contrast studies interfere with and have been largely superseded by other imaging techniques. A water-soluble upper gastrointestinal series may reveal an unsuspected perforated viscus or outline perigastric and lesser sac abscesses.

2. Ultrasonography—Real-time ultrasonography is sensitive (about 80% of cases) in diagnosing intra-abdominal abscesses. The findings consist of a sonolucent area with well-defined walls containing fluid or debris of variable density. Bowel gas, intervening viscera, skin incisions, and stomas interfere with ultrasound examinations, limiting their efficacy in postoperative patients. Nevertheless, the procedure is readily available, portable, and inexpensive, and the findings are specific when correlated with the clinical picture. Ultrasonography is most useful when an abscess is clinically suspected, especially for lesions in the right upper quadrant and the paracolic and pelvic areas.

3. CT scan—CT scan of the abdomen, the best diagnostic study, is highly sensitive (over 95% of cases) and specific. Neither gas shadows nor exposed wounds interfere with CT scanning in postoperative patients, and the procedure is reliable even in areas poorly seen on ultrasonography. Abscesses appear as cystic collections with density measurements of between 0 and 15 attenuation units. Resolution is increased by contrast media (eg, sodium diatrizoate) injected intravenously or instilled into hollow viscera adjacent to the abscess. One drawback of CT scan is that diagnosis may be difficult in areas with multiple thick-walled bowel loops or if a pleural effusion overlies a subphrenic abscess, so that occasionally a very large abscess is missed. CT- or ultrasonography-guided needle aspiration can distinguish between sterile and infected collections in uncertain cases.

4. Radionuclide scan—Gallium-67 citrate and indium 111-labeled autologous leukocyte scans are rarely indicated because, compared to other modalities, they do not provide a timely answer, have high false-positive and false-negative rates, and provide less anatomic localization.

5. Magnetic resonance imaging—The scanning time, patient inaccessibility during scan acquisition, and upper respiratory motion have limited the usefulness of MRI in the investigation of upper abdominal abscesses. CT scan is generally preferable.

Treatment

Treatment consists of prompt and complete drainage of the abscess, control of the primary cause, and adjunctive use of effective antibiotics. Depending upon the abscess site and the condition of the patient, drainage may be achieved by operative or nonoperative methods. **Percutaneous drainage** is the preferred method for single, well-localized, superficial bacterial abscesses that do not have fistulous communications or contain solid debris. Following CT scan or ultrasonographic delineation, a needle is guided into the abscess cavity; infected material is aspirated for culture; and a suitably large drainage catheter is inserted.

Postoperative irrigation is vital to remove debris and ensure catheter patency. This technique is not appropriate for multiple or deep (especially pancreatic) abscesses or for patients with ongoing contamination, fungal infections, or thick purulent or necrotic material. Percutaneous drainage can be performed in about 75% of cases. The success rate exceeds 80% in simple abscesses but is often less than 50% in more complex ones. It is heavily influenced by the availability of appropriate equipment and the experience of the radiologist performing the drainage. Complications include septicemia, fistula formation, bleeding, and peritoneal contamination.

Open drainage is reserved for abscesses for which percutaneous drainage is inappropriate or unsuccessful. These include many cases where there is a persistent focus of infection (eg, diverticulitis or anastomotic dehiscence) that needs to be controlled. In cases without evidence of continued soiling, the direct extraserous route has the advantage of establishing dependent drainage without contaminating the rest of the peritoneal cavity. Only light general anesthesia or even local anesthesia is necessary, and surgical trauma is minimized. Right anterior subphrenic abscesses can be drained by a subcostal incision (Figure 22–4). Posterior subdiaphragmatic and subhepatic lesions can be decompressed posteriorly through the bed of the resected twelfth rib (Nather-Ochsner incision, Figure 22–4) or by a lateral extraserous method (DeCosse incision). Most lower quadrant and flank abscesses can be drained through a lateral extraperitoneal approach. Pelvic abscesses can often be detected on pelvic or rectal examination as a fluctuant mass distorting the contour of the vagina or rectum. If needle aspiration directly through the vaginal or rectal wall returns pus, the abscess is best drained by making an incision in that area. In all cases, digital or direct exploration must ensure that all loculations are broken down. Penrose and sump drains are used to allow continued drainage postoperatively until the infection has resolved. Serial sonograms or imaging studies help document obliteration of the abscess cavity.

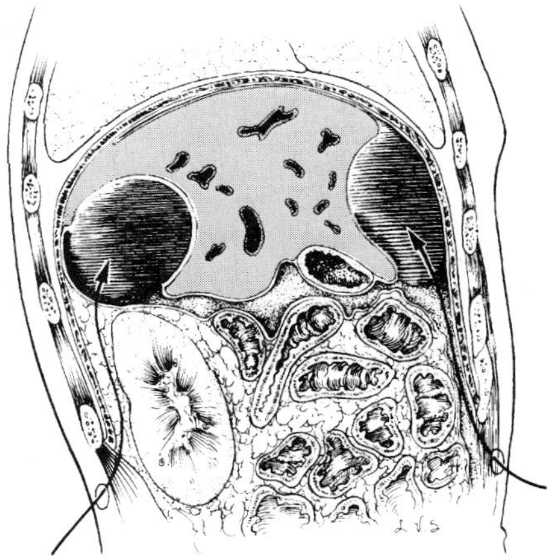

Figure 22–4. Extraperitoneal approaches to the right subphrenic spaces. An abscess in the anterior subhepatic space usually requires transperitoneal drainage. Posterior abscesses may also be drained laterally.

Transperitoneal exploration is indicated if the abscess cannot be localized preoperatively, if there are several or deep-lying lesions, if an enterocutaneous fistula or bowel obstruction exists, or if previous drainage attempts have been unsuccessful. This is especially likely in postoperative patients with multiple abscesses and persistent peritoneal soiling. The need to achieve complete drainage fully justifies the greater stress of laparotomy and the small possibility that infection might be spread to other uninvolved areas. Laparoscopy alone is often inadequate, especially in critically toxic patients without a localized focus.

Satisfactory drainage is usually evidenced by improving clinical findings within 3 days after starting treatment. Failure to improve indicates inadequate drainage, another source of (or ongoing) sepsis, or organ dysfunction. Additional localizing studies and repeated percutaneous or operative drainage should be undertaken urgently (ie, within 24–48 hours, depending on the seriousness of the case). Failure to acknowledge adequate progress delays essential studies and incurs higher mortality.

Prognosis

The mortality rate of serious intra-abdominal abscesses is about 30%. Deaths are related to the severity of the underlying cause, delay in diagnosis, multiple organ failure, and incomplete drainage. Right lower quadrant and pelvic abscesses are usually caused by perforated ulcers and appendicitis in younger individuals. They are readily diagnosed and treated, and the mortality rate is less than 5%. Diagnosis is often delayed in older patients; this increases the likelihood of multiple organ failure. Decompensation of two major organ systems is associated with a mortality rate of over 50%. Shock is an especially ominous sign. Subphrenic, deep, and multiple abscesses frequently require operative drainage and are associated with a mortality rate of over 40%. An untreated residual abscess is nearly always fatal.

Barkhausen J et al: Impact of CT in patients with sepsis of unknown origin. Acta Radiol 1999;40:552.

Farthmann EH et al: Epidemiology and pathophysiology of intraabdominal infections (IA). Infection 1998;25:329.

Kaplan M: Negative pressure wound therapy in the management of abdominal compartment syndrome. Ostomy Wound Management 2004;50:20S.

Schimp VL et al: Vacuum-assisted closure in the treatment of gynecologic oncology wound failures. Gynecol Oncol 2004;92:586.

2. Retroperitoneal & Retrofascial Abscesses

Pathophysiology

The large retroperitoneal space, extending from the diaphragm to the pelvis, is divided into anterior and posterior compartments (Figure 22–1). The **anterior portion** includes structures between the posterior peritoneum and the perinephric fascia (pancreas; parts of the duodenum and the ascending and descending colon). The **posterior portion** contains the adrenals, kidneys, and perinephric spaces. The compartment posterior to the transversalis fascia is involved in retrofascial abscesses.

Abscesses occur less commonly in the retroperitoneum than in the peritoneal cavity. Retroperitoneal abscesses arise chiefly from injuries or infections in adjacent structures: gastrointestinal tract abscesses due to appendicitis, pancreatitis, penetrating posterior ulcers, regional enteritis, diverticulitis, or trauma; genitourinary tract abscesses due to pyelonephritis; and spinal column abscesses due to osteomyelitis or disk space infections.

Psoas abscesses may be primary or secondary. Primary psoas abscesses, which occur without associated disease of other organs, are caused by hematogenous spread of *Staphylococcus aureus* from an occult source and are predominantly seen in children and young adults. They are more common in underdeveloped countries. Secondary psoas abscesses result from spread of infection from adjacent organs, principally from the intestine, and are therefore most often polymicrobial. The most common cause is Crohn's disease.

The pyogenic bacteria (*E coli,* bacteroides, proteus, klebsiella) have replaced *Mycobacterium tuberculosis* as the major causative organism. Surprisingly, only a single causative organism is involved in over one-half of cases. A positive blood culture—especially with *Bacteroides*—is an ominous finding.

Clinical Findings

Although they may be symptomless, retroperitoneal abscesses tend to develop in patients with obvious acute illnesses. Fever and abdominal or flank pain are prominent features, sometimes accompanied by anorexia, weight loss, and nausea and vomiting. The clinical findings in patients with psoas abscess consist of hip pain, flexion of the hip with pain on extension, and a positive iliopsoas sign. Abdominal, thigh, and back pain may also occur. The diagnosis is apt to be overlooked when pain in the hip aggravated by walking is the major complaint. The differential diagnosis includes retroperitoneal tumors and hematomas. Radionuclide scanning, bowel contrast studies, and urograms are the common preliminary investigations, but CT scanning most accurately delineates these lesions. Gas bubbles are diagnostic of an abscess. Awareness of the overall clinical picture is essential for CT scanning to differentiate retroperitoneal abscesses from neoplasms or hematomas. Abscesses are confined to specific compartments, whereas malignant lesions, by contrast, frequently violate peritoneal and fascial barriers and can invade bone.

Treatment

Failure to institute prompt and adequate drainage in addition to systemic antibiotics leads to a fatal outcome. Apart from multiloculated pancreatic abscesses, many retroperitoneal abscesses are amenable to percutaneous CT scan-guided needle aspiration and catheter drainage. Drainage by catheter, however, has a lower success rate for retroperitoneal than intraperitoneal abscesses for the following reasons: (1) Retroperitoneal abscesses often dissect along planes, giving a stellate instead of globular shape; (2) they often contain necrotic debris that will not pass through catheters; and (3) they often invade adjacent muscle (eg, psoas abscess). Operation is indicated if there is no clinical improvement after 2 days of percutaneous drainage. An extraperitoneal approach via the flank is preferred for upper retroperitoneal and perirenal abscesses—and one via the perineum presacrally between the anus and the coccyx for pelvic lesions. Transperitoneal exploration may be unavoidable for deep anterior retroperitoneal abscesses. Resection of necrotic or diseased organs, debridement of the affected compartment, and thorough drainage should be accomplished. In general, retroperitoneal abscesses are difficult to drain completely, and residual or recurrent abscesses are common (especially with regional enteritis). Psoas abscesses may invade the spine or ipsilateral hip to cause osteomyelitis or may track across the midline to cause a contralateral psoas abscess.

The surgical mortality rate is about 25%. Failure of the fever to subside within 3 days indicates inadequate drainage and persistent sepsis that will prove fatal if not corrected promptly.

PRIMARY PERITONITIS

Primary ("spontaneous") peritonitis occurring in the absence of gastrointestinal perforation is caused mainly by hematogenous spread but occasionally by transluminal or direct bacterial invasion of the peritoneal cavity. Impairment of the hepatic reticuloendothelial system and compromised peripheral destruction of bacteria by neutrophils promotes bacteremia, which readily infects ascitic fluid that has reduced bacterium-killing capacity. Primary peritonitis is most closely associated with cirrhosis and advanced liver disease with a low ascitic fluid protein concentration. It is also seen in patients with the nephrotic syndrome or systemic lupus erythematosus, or after splenectomy during childhood. Recurrence is common in cirrhosis and often proves fatal.

Clinical Findings

The clinical presentation simulates secondary bacterial peritonitis, with abrupt onset of fever, abdominal pain, distention, and rebound tenderness. However, one-fourth of patients have minimal or no peritoneal symptoms. Most have clinical and biochemical manifestations of advanced cirrhosis or nephrosis. Leukocytosis, hypoalbuminemia, and a prolonged prothrombin time are characteristic findings. The diagnosis hinges upon examination of the ascitic fluid, which reveals a white blood cell count greater than 500/μL and more than 25% polymorphonuclear leukocytes. A blood-ascitic fluid albumin gradient greater than 1.1 g/dL, a raised serum lactic acid level (> 33 mg/dL), or a reduced ascitic fluid pH (< 7.31) supports the diagnosis. Bacteria are seen on Gram-stained smears in only 25% of cases. Culture of ascitic fluid inoculated immediately into blood culture media at the bedside usually reveals a single enteric organism, most commonly *E coli,* klebsiella, or streptococci, but *Listeria monocytogenes* has been reported in immunocompromised hosts.

Treatment

Antibiotic prophylaxis is of no proven value. Systemic antibiotics with third-generation cephalosporins (eg, cefotaxime) or a beta-lactam-clavulanic acid combination along with supportive treatment are begun once the diagnosis has been established. The 50% average mortality rate is due to peritonitis in only about a third of cases. Multiple organ failure as indicated by gastrointestinal bleeding, hepatic encephalopathy, and renal failure are ominous signs.

Troidle L et al: Differing outcomes of gram-positive and gram-negative peritonitis. Am J Kidney Dis 1998;32:623.

TUBERCULOUS PERITONITIS

Pathophysiology

Tuberculosis peritonitis is encountered in 0.5% of new cases of tuberculosis. It presents as a primary infection without active pulmonary, intestinal, renal, or uterine tube involvement. Its cause is reactivation of a dormant peritoneal focus derived from hematogenous dissemination from a distant nidus or breakdown of mesenteric lymph nodes. Some cases occur as a systemic manifestation of extra-abdominal infection. Multiple small, hard, raised, whitish tubercles studding the peritoneum, omentum, and mesentery are the distinctive finding. A cecal tuberculoma, matted lymph nodes, or omental involvement may form a palpable mass.

The disease affects young persons, particularly women, and is more prevalent in countries where tuberculosis is still endemic. AIDS patients are especially susceptible to development of extrapulmonary tuberculosis.

Clinical Findings

Chronic symptoms (lasting more than a week) include abdominal pain and distention, fever, night sweats, weight loss, and altered bowel habits. Ascites is present in about half of cases, especially if the disease is of long standing, and may be the primary manifestation. A mass may be felt in a third of cases. The differential diagnosis includes Crohn's disease, carcinoma, hepatic cirrhosis, and intestinal lymphoma. One-fourth of patients have acute symptoms suggestive of acute bowel obstruction or peritonitis that mimics appendicitis, cholecystitis, or a perforated ulcer.

Detection of an extra-abdominal site of tuberculosis, evident in half of cases, is the single most useful diagnostic clue. Pleural effusion is present in up to 50% of patients. Paracentesis, laparoscopy, or peritoneal biopsy is applicable only in patients with ascites. The peritoneal fluid is characterized by a protein concentration above 3 g/dL with less than 1.1 g/dL serum-ascitic fluid albumin difference and lymphocyte predominance among white blood cells. Definitive diagnosis is possible in 80% of cases by culture (often taking several weeks) and direct smear. A PPD skin test is useful only when positive (about 80% of cases). Hematologic and biochemical studies are seldom helpful, and leukocytosis is uncommon. The sedimentation rate is elevated in many cases. The presence of high-density ascites or soft tissue masses on ultrasonography or CT scan supports the diagnosis. Young patients from endemic areas who present with classic symptoms or who have suggestive imaging findings should undergo diagnostic laparoscopy, which may obviate laparotomy.

Treatment

In chronic cases, nonoperative therapy is preferable if the diagnosis can be established. Most patients presenting with acute symptoms are diagnosed only by laparotomy. In the absence of intestinal obstruction or perforation, only a biopsy of a peritoneal or omental nodule should be taken. Obstruction due to constriction by a tuberculous lesion usually develops in the distal ileum and cecum, although multiple skip areas along the small bowel may exist. Localized short segments of diseased bowel are best treated by resection with primary anastomosis. Multiple strictured areas may be managed either by side-to-side bypass or a stricturoplasty of partially narrowed segments.

Combination antituberculosis chemotherapy should be started once the diagnosis is confirmed or considered likely. A favorable response is the rule, but isoniazid and rifampin must be continued for 18 months postoperatively.

GRANULOMATOUS PERITONITIS

Pathophysiology

Talc (magnesium silicate), cornstarch glove lubricants, gauze fluffs, and cellulose fibers from disposable surgical fabrics may elicit a vigorous granulomatous (probably a delayed hypersensitivity) response in some patients 2–6 weeks after laparotomy. The condition is uncommon now that surgeons wipe clean their gloves before handling abdominal viscera. Less rarely, granulomatous peritonitis may develop as a hypersensitivity reaction to other foreign material (eg, intestinal ascariasis or food particles from a perforated ulcer). This process should be distinguished from congenital peritoneal encapsulation or abdominal cocoon.

Clinical Findings

Besides abdominal pain, which is often out of proportion to the low-grade fever, there may be nausea and vomiting, ileus, and other systemic complaints. Abdominal tenderness is usually diffuse but mild. Free abdominal fluid, if detectable, should be tapped and inspected for the diagnostic Maltese cross pattern of starch particles.

Treatment

Reoperation achieves little and should be avoided if the diagnosis can be made. Most patients undergo reexploration because they present an erroneous impression of postoperative bowel obstruction or peritoneal sepsis. The diffuse hard, white granulomatous masses studding the peritoneum and omentum are easily mistaken for cancer or tuberculosis unless a biopsy specimen is taken to demonstrate foreign body granulomas.

If granulomatous peritonitis is suspected, the response to treatment with corticosteroids or other anti-inflammatory agents is often so dramatic as to be diagnostic in itself. After clinical improvement, intravenous methylprednisolone can be replaced by oral prednisone for 2–3 weeks. The disease is self-limited and does not predispose to late intestinal obstruction.

ASCITES

1. Chylous Ascites

The accumulation of free chyle in the peritoneal cavity is a rare form of ascites. Most patients are adults—many of them elderly women—with occult cancer, often a lymphoma or adenocarcinoma (of the pancreas or stomach), causing lymphatic obstruction. Chylous ascites resulting from external trauma or operative mishap (portosystemic decompression, abdominal aneurysmectomy and retroperitoneal lymphadenectomy procedures) has a more favorable prognosis. About 15% of cases occur in young children (usually < 1 year old) with congenital lymphatic anomalies.

Clinical Findings

The typical presentation is of abdominal distention and pain along with vague constitutional symptoms. Physical findings—besides ascites—include concomitant pleural effusion and peripheral edema. The combination of fever, night sweats, and lymphadenopathy should arouse suspicion of a lymphoma. The discovery of milky ascitic fluid on paracentesis suggests the correct diagnosis. Only a rough correlation exists between the gross appearance of the fluid and its triglyceride content (> 200 mg/dL, with a mean level of 1500 mg/dL). The fluid leukocyte count (mostly lymphocytes) averages 1000/μL. Hypoalbuminemia, lymphocytopenia, and anemia are frequently present.

Conventional radiologic investigations, particularly CT scan of the abdomen, may be helpful. Lymph node biopsy, where applicable, and laparotomy have the highest diagnostic value.

Treatment

Treatment of spontaneous chylous ascites is largely supportive rather than operative. Symptomatic relief can be obtained by intermittent abdominal and pleural tapping. Repeated punctures seldom arrest the chylous leakage and are not without hazard. Dietary measures should begin with a low-fat diet supplemented by medium-chain triglycerides, the latter being transported via the portal rather than the lymphatic circulation. Two-thirds of pediatric cases resolve spontaneously on expectant management within a month or so as collaterals develop. If dietary measures fail, oral findings should be halted and total parenteral nutrition instituted. In adults, the most hopeful situation is if an underlying cancer (which is rarely amenable to curative resection) producing the chylous ascites regresses with chemotherapy or irradiation. Spontaneous improvement is the rule in posttraumatic cases.

Except for resectable congenital chylous cysts, surgery has little to offer. In refractory traumatic cases, intraoperative lymphangiography or perioperative injection of lipophilic dyes at times identifies a leaking site that can be plicated. At operation, the root of the small bowel mesentery around the superior mesenteric vessels should be carefully examined, as a discrete tear is more common at this site. Peritoneovenous shunting has been successful in some postoperative cases. Other surgical endeavors such as bowel resection and retroperitoneal dissection are uniformly futile.

2. Malignant Ascites

Ascites due to advanced cancer is a distressing complication that often necessitates in-hospital care. Peritoneal implants stimulate production of ascitic fluid while impeding its resorption by diaphragmatic lymphatics. Malignant ascites also occurs in the absence of free peritoneal tumor cells if there is advanced venous or lymphatic obstruction. A positive cytologic diagnosis is obtained in 60–90% of cases and supported by a high LDH (> 500 IU/L) or CEA content. DNA aneuploidy on flow cytometry analysis is confirmatory in cytology-negative cases.

Since this is often a preterminal condition, conservative management is preferred, with diuretics (especially spironolactone), paracentesis if warranted by the symptoms, and chemotherapy.

Peritoneovenous shunting (preferably with the Denver shunt) should be considered in symptomatic patients who have ascites refractory to conservative methods and an expected survival time of at least 2 months. Shunting is not effective for viscous or loculated ascites, heavily blood-stained ascites, or ascites with an unusually high cell count. The procedure is most suitable in patients with breast, gastric, or ovarian adenocarcinoma or cytology-negative ascites. Complications include shunt obstruction, disseminated intravascular coagulation, fluid overload, and sepsis. Surprisingly, dissemination of the tumor is rare. About half of the patients derive substantial benefits but few survive beyond 6 months.

Arroyo V et al: Complications of cirrhosis. II. Renal and circulatory dysfunction. Lights and shadows in an important clinical problem. J Hepatol 2000;32(1 Suppl):157.

Dugernier T et al: Ascites fluid in severe acute pancreatitis: from pathophysiology to therapy. Acta Gastroenterol Belg 2000;63:264.

Heneghan MA et al: Pathogenesis of ascites in cirrhosis and portal hypertension. Med Sci Monit 2000;6:807.

Uriz J et al: Pathophysiology, diagnosis and treatment of ascites in cirrhosis. Baillieres Best Pract Res Clin Gastroenterol 2000;14:927.

PERITONEAL ADHESIONS

Tissue ischemia, mechanical or thermal trauma, infection, radiation injury, and foreign body reaction predispose to adhesion formation. The peritoneal injury underlying these noxious stimuli evokes a serosanguineous inflammatory reaction that leads to fibrin deposition. Ordinarily, local plasminogen activators initiate lysis of the fibrin strands within 3 days of their formation. Metamorphosis of mesodermal cells regenerates a single layer of new mesothelium as early as 5 days after injury. Inadequate fibrinolysis due to reduced mesothelial plasminogen activator activity allows fibroblastic proliferation to produce fibrous adhesions. Adhesions are now the most prevalent cause of acute and recurrent small bowel obstruction (see Chapter 29) and a persistent bane of abdominal and especially pelvic surgery. However, adhesions may also provide useful vascular bridges that promote tissue healing, such as in ischemic areas of a bowel anastomosis.

Adhesions develop in two-thirds of patients after laparotomy, especially after extensive procedures, pelvic operations, or multiple abdominal operations. Spontaneous adhesions, presumably related to subclinical inflammation, are also found in one-quarter of patients on postmortem examination. Postoperative adhesions are most heavily distributed near the operative site. The omentum, small bowel, colon, and rectum (in descending order of frequency) are involved most often. Short obese female patients seem to have a greater tendency to form adhesions.

Prevention & Treatment

Precise operative technique with avoidance of serosal trauma will reduce but not eliminate adhesion formation. Ischemic tissue trauma caused by crushing, cautery, and mass ligation should be minimized. Reperitonealization of the pelvic floor under tension has been shown to promote rather than hinder adhesion formation. Indeed, well-vascularized peritoneal edges will resurface adjacent denuded areas with epithelium within 2 weeks. The use of an omental flap or synthetic absorbable or nonabsorbable material (eg, Gore-Tex) appears useful after extensive pelvic dissections. Abdominal packs, moist or dry, should be used sparingly, because they produce abrasive serosal tears. Blood and foreign bodies alone induce only a slight peritoneal reaction, but this becomes extensive when there are accompanying serosal injuries. Precise hemostasis is vital, because unclotted blood in the peritoneal cavity acts as an additional source of fibrin, and platelets themselves stimulate serosal inflammation. Starch glove powder, lint gauze fluffs, and cellulose fibers from disposable drapes provoke a rigorous foreign body reaction, and care should be taken to prevent such contamination. The differences between similar types of nonreactive suture material are less critical than the manner in which they are employed: A large number of coarse sutures creates more adhesions than well-placed finer sutures. Laparoscopic procedures tend to produce fewer adhesions than laparotomy.

Hyaluronic acid-carboxymethylcellulose film (Sepra film) placed during laparotomy decreases the formation of intraperitoneal adhesions. It is particularly useful in patients likely to need early reoperation, such as those with a temporary bowel diversion.

Beck DE et al: A prospective, randomized, multicenter, controlled study of the safety of Seprafilm adhesion barrier in abdominopelvic surgery of the intestine. Dis Col Rectum 2003;46:1310.

TUMORS OF THE PERITONEUM & RETROPERITONEUM

Most tumors affecting the peritoneum are secondary implants from primary intraperitoneal cancers. Some unusual peritoneal and retroperitoneal lesions present with abdominal masses or ascites that may be confused with carcinomatosis or chronic inflammatory peritonitis.

Peritoneal Mesothelioma

These rare primary neoplasms are derived from the mesodermal lining of the peritoneum. The malignant variety develops most commonly in men, with a long latent period (averaging 40 years) after prolonged asbestos exposure. Pleural malignant mesotheliomas outnumber peritoneal ones by a ratio of 3 to 1. Patients present typically with weight loss, crampy abdominal pain, a large mass or distention due to ascites, and a history of asbestos contact. Fewer than half of these patients have asbestosis demonstrated on plain chest films. In contrast to peritoneal carcinomatosis, mesotheliomas are associated with less ascites than the degree of abdominal distention would suggest, and cytologic studies of ascitic fluid are rarely positive. CT scan of the lower thorax and abdomen will demonstrate ascites, peritoneal and mesenteric thickening, pleural plaques, and soft tissue masses involving the omentum and peritoneum. Multiple fine-needle aspiration biopsies guided by ultrasonography, CT scan, or laparoscopy can establish the diagnosis. Electron microscopy is confirmatory in equivocal cases.

Patients usually undergo laparotomy either for diagnosis or because of bowel obstruction. Localized masses should be resected to avoid subsequent obstruction. Metastases to the liver and lung occur late. Encouraging results have been reported with long-term survival following cytoreductive surgery and intraperitoneal cisplatin-based combination chemotherapy. Long-term survivors (beyond 1 year) have been reported with combined treatment by surgical debulking, intraperitoneal cisplatin-doxorubicin, and whole-abdomen irradiation. One should differentiate malignant mesotheliomas from cystic mesotheliomas and well-differentiated papillary mesotheliomas in women, which are less malignant and carry a better prognosis even though they tend to recur locally.

Pseudomyxoma Peritonei

This unusual disease is caused by a low-grade mucinous cystadenocarcinoma of the appendix or ovary that secretes large amounts of mucus-containing epithelial cells. It should be distinguished from benign appendiceal mucocele, which may also have local mucinous deposits but carries a favorable outlook. Patients seldom complain until advanced stages of disease, at which time they have abdominal distention and pain and, in many instances, intermittent or chronic partial small bowel obstruction. Weight loss and other features of cancer are uncommon. The shed neoplastic cells spread freely to two main areas: the upper abdominal sites of peritoneal fluid resorption (undersurface of diaphragm and omentum) and the dependent peritoneal areas (pelvis and lateral abdominal gutters). Distant metastases and visceral involvement are rare. Ultrasonography and CT scans show a distinctive peritoneal scalloping of the liver margin, calcified plaques, ascites, and low-density masses.

At laparotomy, the surgeon should remove as much of the primary lesion and gelatinous material as possible. The omentum also should be resected and existing or impending bowel obstruction relieved. This often necessitates right hemicolectomy. If there is no apparent primary tumor, the appendix and, in women, both ovaries should be removed. Some surgeons advocate radical peritonectomy (including splenectomy, cholecystectomy, appendectomy, sigmoid colectomy, and hysterectomy) to eliminate potential areas of microscopic spread. Whether the higher morbidity incurred is justified remains debated.

Current therapy favors very early intraperitoneal fluorouracil-based adjuvant chemotherapy. Systemic chemotherapy is generally useless. Adjuvant intracavitary radiotherapy has also been advocated, especially for patients with residual disease. Reexploration should be undertaken either as a planned second-look laparotomy or to debulk residual tumor responsible for recurrent obstruction or debilitating mucous ascites. Two-thirds of patients eventually succumb to local or regional disease. The survival rate is about 50% at 5 years and 30% at 10 years.

Sebbag G et al: Results of treatment of 33 patients with peritoneal mesothelioma. Br J Surg 2000;87:1587.

Sugarbaker PH: Management of peritoneal-surface malignancy: the surgeon's role. Langenbecks Arch Surg 1999;384:576.

Cysts of the Mesentery & Retroperitoneum

These rare developmental lesions are usually ectopic pockets of lymphatic tissue or, more rarely, mucinous ovarian cystadenomas. Patients—one-third of whom are children—present with an asymptomatic abdominal mass, chronic pain, or an acute abdomen. The mass is often large, smooth, round, compressible, and more mobile transversely than longitudinally. CT or ultrasonographic scans along with contrast studies of the gastrointestinal and urinary tracts reveal the cystic nature and location of the mass. The differential diagnosis includes pancreatic pseudocysts, enteric duplication (in children), inflammatory cysts, and retroperitoneal tumors. Laparotomy or laparoscopy reveals the cyst, which contains serous fluid if it is in the mesocolon; chylous fluid if it is in the small bowel mesentery; or blood-stained fluid. Most lesions are benign, and enucleation suffices. Segmental resection may be necessary for cysts that impinge upon the bowel wall or its blood supply. Recurrences are more frequent with retroperitoneal cysts, because they may not be amenable to complete excision, and marsupialization may be required instead.

Mesenteric Lipodystrophy (Mesenteric Panniculitis)

There are fewer than 200 reported cases of mesenteric lipodystrophy, in which chronic fat degeneration and fibrosis affecting the root of the mesentery produce diffuse mesenteric thickening or masses. Its cause is unknown, but it may be a localized form of Weber-Christian disease.

The patient, often an elderly man, has recurrent abdominal pain, weight loss, or symptoms of partial intestinal obstruction. A hard, irregular abdominal mass, usually in the left upper quadrant, is felt in over half of patients. CT or ultrasound examination and barium follow-up studies can outline the lesion. CT scanning shows the characteristic features of nonhomogeneous masses of fat and soft tissue density. MRI may suggest the fibrous nature of the lesion and delineates vascular involvement. The diagnosis is usually made only by biopsy at laparotomy, but resection is neither feasible nor indicated. An occasional patient will require a side-to-side intestinal bypass to relieve obstruction.

The process subsides spontaneously in most cases. A more serious variant **(retractile mesenteritis)** associated with obstruction of the mesenteric lymphatics and veins often proves fatal. Corticosteroids, cyclophosphamide, and azathioprine should be reserved for such cases and for patients with clinical deterioration. Lymphoma occurs in 15% of cases on follow-up.

RETROPERITONEAL FIBROSIS

This uncommon entity is characterized by extensive fibrotic encasement of retroperitoneal tissues. Over two-thirds of cases are idiopathic and the rest secondary to drugs (eg, methysergide, beta-adrenergic blocking agents), retroperitoneal hemorrhage, perianeurysmal inflammation, irradiation, urinary extravasation, or cancer. The fibrosis represents an allergic reaction to insoluble lipid (ceroid) that has leaked from atheromatous plaques, especially those within the aorta. The urinary tract may be involved with a diagnostic triad of hydronephrosis and hydroureter (usually bilateral), medial deviation of the ureters, and extrinsic ureteric compression near the L4–5 level. Desmoplastic involvement of the small and large bowel may give rise to obstructive symptoms. Most patients are men over age 50 who present with renal failure or obstructive uropathy. Pain in the low back or flank is common. Pyuria is present in most patients. The diagnosis is suggested by a CT scan that shows the fibrotic process and any coexisting aneurysmal changes in the aorta. MRI may distinguish fibrosis from lymphoma or metastatic carcinoma. Withdrawal of suspect drugs is usually followed by gradual improvement.

Severe urinary obstruction should be decompressed by ureteric stents or nephrostomy. Prednisone (30–60 mg daily) and immunosuppression have been tried but with inconclusive benefits. These agents should be started early postoperatively before marked fibrosis develops. Tamoxifen has produced regression of desmoid tumors. If surgery becomes necessary, a thick rubbery or fibrotic plaque containing chronic inflammatory cells is found at exploration. Multiple biopsy specimens should be taken to exclude cancer. Ureterolysis should be attempted, and there may be some advantage to wrapping omentum around the freed ureters to reduce the risk of subsequent entrapment. Laparoscopic ureterolysis may occasionally be feasible. The outlook is good as long as there is no underlying cancer.

Amis ES Jr: Retroperitoneal fibrosis. AJR Am J Roentgenol 1991;157:321.

Marcolongo R et al: Immunosuppressive therapy for idiopathic retroperitoneal fibrosis: a retrospective analysis of 26 cases. Am J Med 2004;116:194.

Marzano A et al: Treatment of idiopathic retroperitoneal fibrosis using cyclosporin. Ann Rheum Dis 2001;60:427.

DISORDERS INVOLVING THE OMENTUM

Infection

The omentum plays an important role in protecting against spreading peritonitis. In chronic infections such as tuberculosis, it may become infected and appear as a rolled-up thickened, inflamed mass. Nonspecific inflammation of the omentum, often a sequela of previous torsion, causes vague abdominal pain.

Torsion & Infarction

Primary (spontaneous) torsion of the omentum may develop if a free portion is fixed by an adhesion or trapped within a hernia. Rotation around the pedicle occludes the blood supply and leads to ischemic necrosis. Infarction may also be secondary to abdominal trauma or vascular conditions such as polyarteritis nodosa. Paraesophageal omental herniation may predispose to a hiatal hernia and may mimic a mediastinal lipoma.

Clinically, torsion presents as acute abdominal pain with nausea and vomiting. Tenderness is confined to the involved area, usually on the right side but away from McBurney's point. A mobile, tender mass is noted in one-third of cases. These features may suggest acute appendicitis or cholecystitis but are not typical of those diseases. The clinical findings usually mandate surgical exploration, which reveals serosanguineous fluid, a normal appendix, and the hemorrhagic necrotic segment of omentum. Resection of the affected portion is curative.

Tumors & Cysts of the Omentum

The omentum is frequently involved secondarily by intra-abdominal malignant tumors, especially gastrointestinal and ovarian adenocarcinomas. Primary cysts or vascular anomalies, usually incidentally discovered at laparotomy, are readily resected.

Stomach & Duodenum

23

Gerard M. Doherty, MD, & Lawrence W. Way, MD

I. STOMACH

The stomach receives food from the esophagus and has four functions: (1) It acts as a reservoir that permits eating reasonably large quantities of food at intervals of several hours. (2) Food contained in the stomach is mixed, triturated, and delivered into the duodenum in amounts regulated by its chemical nature and texture. (3) The first stages of protein and carbohydrate digestion are carried out in the stomach. (4) A few substances are absorbed across the gastric mucosa.

ANATOMY

The anatomy of the stomach may be seen in Figures 23–1 to 23–3.

The **cardia** is located at the gastroesophageal junction. The **fundus** is the portion of the stomach that lies cephalad to the gastroesophageal junction. The **corpus** is the capacious central part; division of the corpus from the pyloric antrum is marked approximately by the angular incisure, a crease on the lesser curvature just proximal to the "crow's-foot" terminations of the nerves of Latarjet (Figure 23–3). The **pylorus** is the boundary between the stomach and the duodenum.

The **cardiac gland area** is the small segment located at the gastroesophageal junction. Histologically, it contains principally mucus-secreting cells, though a few parietal cells are sometimes present. The **oxyntic gland area** is the portion containing parietal (oxyntic) cells and chief cells (Figure 23–2). The boundary between this region and the adjacent pyloric gland area is reasonably sharp, since the zone of transition spans a segment of only 1–1.5 cm. The **pyloric gland** area constitutes the distal 30% of the stomach and contains the G cells that manufacture gastrin. Mucous cells are common in the oxyntic and pyloric gland areas.

As in the rest of the gastrointestinal tract, the muscular wall of the stomach is composed of an outer longitudinal and an inner circular layer. An additional incomplete inner layer of obliquely situated fibers is most prominent near the lesser curvature but is of less substance than the other two layers.

Blood Supply

The blood supply of the stomach and duodenum is illustrated in Figure 23–3. The left gastric artery supplies the lesser curvature and connects with the right gastric artery, a branch of the common hepatic artery. In 60% of persons, a posterior gastric artery arises off the middle third of the splenic artery and terminates in branches on the posterior surface of the body and the fundus. The greater curvature is supplied by the right gastroepiploic artery (a branch of the gastroduodenal artery) and the left gastroepiploic artery (a branch of the splenic artery). The mid portion of the greater curvature corresponds to a point at which the gastric branches of this vascular arcade change direction. The fundus of the stomach along the greater curvature is supplied by the vasa brevia, branches of the splenic and left gastroepiploic arteries.

The blood supply to the duodenum is from the superior and inferior pancreaticoduodenal arteries, which are branches of the gastroduodenal artery and the superior mesenteric artery, respectively. The stomach contains a rich submucosal vascular plexus. Venous blood from the stomach drains into the coronary, gastroepiploic, and splenic veins before entering the portal vein. The lymphatic drainage of the stomach, which largely parallels the arteries, partially determines the direction of spread of gastric neoplasms.

Nerve Supply

The parasympathetic nerves to the stomach are shown in Figure 23–3. As a rule, two major vagal trunks pass through the esophageal hiatus in close approximation to the esophageal muscle. The nerves are originally located to the right and left of the esophagus and stomach during embryonic development. When the foregut rotates, the lesser curvature turns to the right and the greater curvature to the left, and corresponding shifts in location of the vagal trunks follow. Hence, the right vagus supplies the posterior and the left the anterior gastric surface. About 90% of the vagal fibers are sensory afferent; the remaining 10% are efferent.

In the region of the gastroesophageal junction, each trunk bifurcates. The anterior trunk sends to the liver a

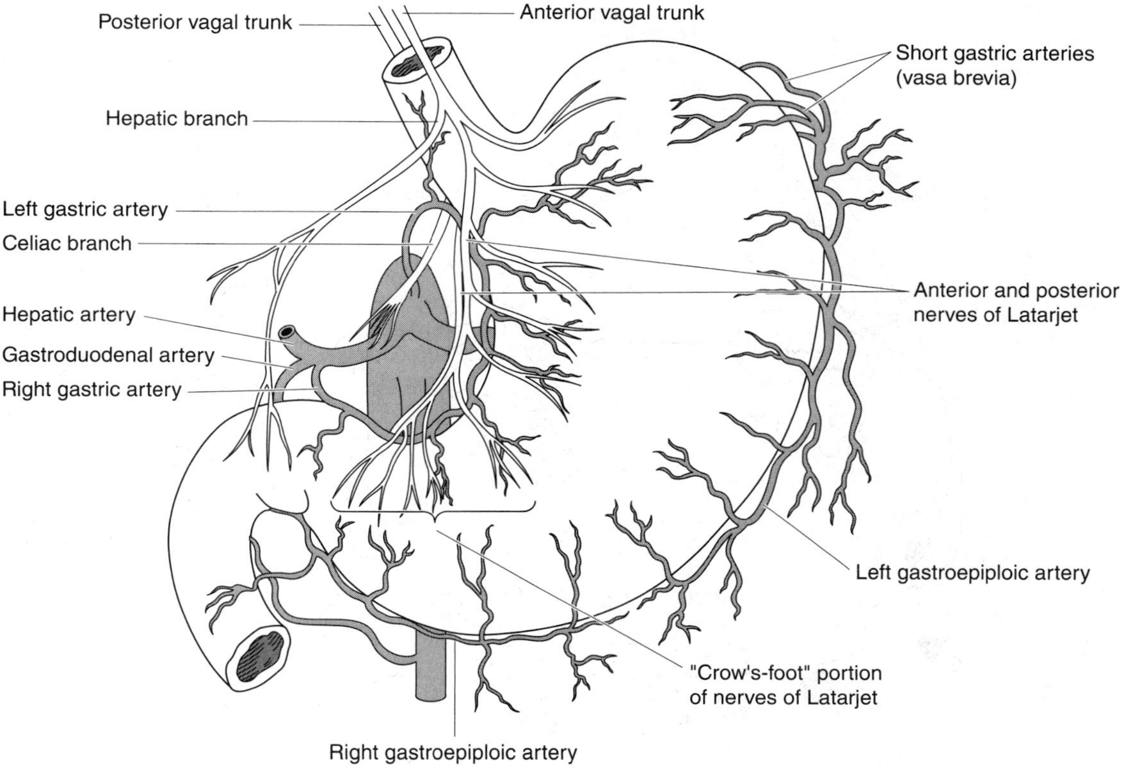

Figure 23–3. Blood supply and parasympathetic innervation of the stomach and duodenum.

D. Blood Group Substances

Seventy-five percent of people secrete blood group antigens into gastric juice. The trait is genetically determined and is associated with a lower incidence of duodenal ulcer than in nonsecretors.

E. Electrolytes

The unique characteristic of gastric secretion is its high concentration of hydrochloric acid, a product of the parietal cells. As the concentration of H^+ rises during secretion, that of Na^+ drops in a reciprocal fashion. K^+ remains relatively constant at 5–10 meq/L. Chloride concentration remains near 150 meq/L, and gastric juice maintains its isotonicity at varying secretory rates.

The Parietal Cell & Acid Secretion

Many of the key events in acid secretion by gastric parietal cells are illustrated in Figure 23–4. The onset of secretion is accompanied by striking morphologic changes in the apical membranes. Resting parietal cells are characterized by an infolding of the apical membrane, called the secretory canaliculus, which is lined by short microvilli. Multiple membrane-bound tubulovesicles and mitochondria are present in the cytoplasm. With stimulation, the secretory canaliculus expands, the microvilli become long and narrow and filled with microfilaments, and the cytoplasmic tubulovesicles disappear. The proton pump mechanism for acid secretion is located in the tubulovesicles in the resting state and in the secretory canaliculus in the stimulated state.

The basal lateral membrane contains the receptors for secretory stimulants and transfers HCO_3^- out of the cell to balance the H^+ output at the apical membrane. Active uptake of Cl^- and K^+ conduction also occur at the basal lateral membrane. Separate membrane-bound receptors exist for histamine (H_2 receptor), gastrin, and acetylcholine. The intracellular second messengers are thought to be cAMP for histamine and Ca^{2+} for gastrin and acetylcholine.

Acid secretion at the apical membrane is accomplished by a membrane-bound H^+/K^+-ATPase (the proton pump); H^+ is secreted into the lumen in exchange for K^+.

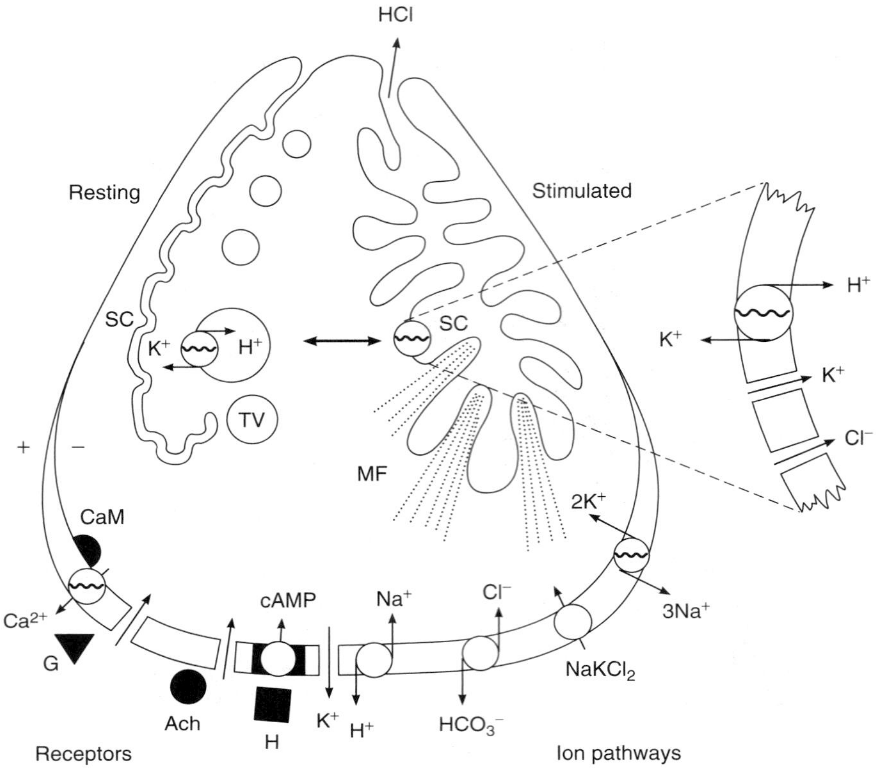

Figure 23–4. Diagram of a parietal cell, showing the receptor systems and ion pathways in the basal lateral membrane and the apical membrane transition from a resting to a stimulated state. Ach, acetylcholine; CaM, calmodulin; G, gastrin; H, histamine; MF, microfilaments; SC, secretory canaliculus; TV, tubulovesicles. (© 1984 Elsevier Inc. Reprinted with permission from Elsevier.)

Mucosal Resistance in the Stomach & Duodenum

The healthy mucosa of the stomach and duodenum is provided with mechanisms that allow it to withstand the potentially injurious effects of high concentrations of luminal acid. Disruption of these mechanisms may contribute to acute or chronic ulceration.

The surface of the gastric mucosa is coated with mucus and secretes HCO_3^- in addition to H^+. Protected by the blanket of mucus, the surface pH is much higher than the luminal pH. HCO_3^- secretion is stimulated by cAMP, prostaglandins, cholinomimetics, glucagon, CCK, and by as yet unidentified paracrine hormones. Inhibitors of HCO_3^- secretion include nonsteroidal anti-inflammatory agents, alpha-adrenergic agonists, bile acids, ethanol, and acetazolamide. Increases in luminal H^+ result in increased HCO_3^- secretion, probably mediated by tissue prostaglandins.

Gastric mucus is a gel composed of high-molecular-weight glycoproteins and 95% water. Since it forms an unstirred layer, it helps the underlying mucosa to maintain a higher pH than that of gastric juice, and it also acts as a barrier to the diffusion of pepsin. At the surface of the layer of mucus, peptic digestion continuously degrades mucus, while below it is continuously being replenished by mucous cells. Gastric acid is thought to enter the lumen through thin spots in the mucus overlying the gastric glands. Secretion of mucus is stimulated by luminal acid and perhaps by cholinergic stimuli. The layer of mucus is damaged by exposure to nonsteroidal anti-inflammatory agents and is enhanced by topical prostaglandin E_2.

Mucosal defects produced by mechanical or chemical trauma are rapidly repaired by adjacent normal cells that spread to cover the defect, a process that can be enhanced experimentally by adding HCO_3^- to the nutrient side of the mucosa. This important phenomenon has not yet been thoroughly studied.

The duodenal mucosa possesses defenses similar to those in the stomach: the ability to secrete HCO_3^- and mucus and rapid repair of mucosal injuries.

Regulation of Acid Secretion

The regulation of acid secretion can best be described by considering separately those factors that enhance gastric acid production and those that depress it. The interaction of these forces is what determines the levels of secretion observed during fasting and after meals.

A. Stimulation of Acid Secretion

Acid production is usually described as the result of three phases that are excited simultaneously after a meal. The separation into phases is of value principally for descriptive purposes.

1. Cephalic phase—Stimuli that act upon the brain lead to increased vagal efferent activity and acid secretion. The sight, smell, taste, or even thought of appetizing food may elicit this response. The effect is entirely vagally mediated and is abolished by vagotomy. The vagal stimuli have a direct effect on the parietal cells to increase acid output.

2. Gastric phase—Food in the stomach (principally protein hydrolysates and hydrophobic amino acids) stimulates gastrin release from the antrum. Gastric distention has a similar but less intense effect.

The presence of food in the stomach excites long vagal reflexes, impulses that pass to the central nervous system via vagal afferents and return to stimulate the parietal cells.

A third aspect of the gastric phase involves the sensitizing effect of distention of the parietal cell area to gastrin that is probably mediated through local intramural cholinergic reflexes.

3. Intestinal phase—The role of the intestinal phase in the stimulation of gastric secretion has been incompletely investigated. Various experiments have shown that the presence of food in the small bowel releases a humoral factor, named entero-oxyntin, that evokes acid secretion from the stomach.

B. Inhibition of Acid Secretion

Without systems to limit secretion, unchecked acid production could become a serious clinical problem. Examples can be found (eg, Billroth II gastrectomy with retained antrum) where acid production rose after surgical procedures that interfered with these inhibitory mechanisms.

1. Antral inhibition—pH below 2.50 in the antrum inhibits the release of gastrin regardless of the stimulus. When the pH reaches 1.20, gastrin release is almost completely blocked. If the normal relationship of parietal cell mucosa to antral mucosa is changed so that acid does not flow past the site of gastrin production, serum gastrin may increase to high levels, with marked acid stimulation. Somatostatin in gastric antral cells serves a physiologic role as an inhibitor of gastrin release (a paracrine function).

2. Intestinal inhibition—The intestine participates in controlling acid secretion by liberating hormones that inhibit both the release of gastrin and its effects on the parietal cells. Secretin blocks acid secretion under experimental conditions but not as a physiologic action. Fat in the intestine is the most potent method of inhibition, affecting gastrin release and acid secretion. Neither somatostatin nor GIP, both released by food in the intestine, seems able to account for the inhibition, and the term enterogastrone is used to denote the still unidentified hormone presumably responsible.

Integration of Gastric Physiologic Function

Ingested food is mixed with salivary amylase before it reaches the stomach. The mechanisms stimulating gastric secretion are activated. Serum gastrin levels increase from a mean fasting concentration of about 50 pg/mL to 200 pg/mL, the peak occurring about 30 minutes after the meal. Food in the lumen of the stomach is exposed to high concentrations of acid and pepsin at the mucosal surface. Food settles in layers determined by sequence of arrival, but fat tends to float to the top. The greatest mixing occurs in the antrum. Antral contents therefore become more uniformly acidic than those in the body of the organ, where the central portion of the meal tends to remain alkaline for a considerable time, allowing continued activity of the amylase.

Peptic digestion of protein in the stomach is only about 5–10% complete. Carbohydrate digestion may reach 30–40%. A lipase originating from the tongue initiates the first stages of lipolysis in the stomach.

The gastric contents are delivered to the duodenum at a rate determined by the volume and texture of the meal, its osmolality and acidity, and its content of fat. A meal of lean meat, potatoes, and vegetables leaves the stomach within 3 hours. A meal with a very high fat content may remain in the stomach for 6–12 hours.

Calam J, Baron JH: ABC of the upper gastrointestinal tract: pathophysiology of duodenal and gastric ulcer and gastric cancer. BMJ 2001;323:980.

PEPTIC ULCER

Peptic ulcers result from the corrosive action of acid gastric juice on a vulnerable epithelium. Depending on circumstances, they may occur in the esophagus, the duodenum, the stomach itself, the jejunum after surgical construction of a gastrojejunostomy, or the ileum in relation to ectopic gastric mucosa in Meckel's diverticulum. When the term peptic ulcer was first used, it was thought that the most important factor was the peptic activity in gastric juice. Since then, evidence has implicated acid as the chief injurious agent; in fact, it is axiomatic that if gastric juice contains no acid, a (benign) peptic ulcer cannot be present. Appreciation of the role of acid has led to the emphasis on therapy with antacids and H_2 blocking agents for the medical therapy of ulcers and to operations that reduce acid secretion as the major surgical approach. In the case of duodenal and gastric ulcers, *Helicobacter pylori* must colonize and weaken the mucosa before acid is able to do the damage, and therapy directed against this organism has a more definitive effect on the disease.

It has been estimated that about 2% of the adult population in the USA suffers from active peptic ulcer disease, and about 10% of the population will have the disease during their lifetime. Men are affected three times as often as women. Duodenal ulcers are ten times more common than gastric ulcers in young patients, but in the older age groups the frequency is about equal. Probably as a result of a declining prevalence of *H pylori* infection, the incidence has declined to less than half what it was 25 years ago.

In general terms, the ulcerative process can lead to four types of disability: (1) **Pain** is the most common. (2) **Bleeding** may occur as a result of erosion of submucosal or extraintestinal vessels as the ulcer becomes deeper. (3) Penetration of the ulcer through all layers of the affected gut results in **perforation** if other viscera do not seal the ulcer. (4) **Obstruction** may result from inflammatory swelling and scarring and is most likely to occur with ulcers located at the pylorus or gastroesophageal junction, where the lumen is narrowest.

The clinical features and prognosis of duodenal ulcer and gastric ulcer are sufficiently different to be dealt with separately here.

DUODENAL ULCER

ESSENTIALS OF DIAGNOSIS

- *Epigastric pain relieved by food or antacids.*
- *Epigastric tenderness.*
- *Normal or increased gastric acid secretion.*
- *Signs of ulcer disease on upper gastrointestinal x-rays or endoscopy.*
- *Evidence of Helicobacter pylori infection.*

General Considerations

Duodenal ulcers may occur in any age group but are most common in the young and middle-aged (20–45 years). They appear in men more often than women. About 95% of duodenal ulcers are situated within 2 cm of the pylorus, in the duodenal bulb.

Considerable evidence implicates *H pylori* as the principal cause of duodenal ulcer disease. This microaerophilic gram-negative curved bacillus can be found colonizing patches of gastric metaplasia within the duodenum in 90% of patients with this disease. The bacilli remain on the surface of the mucosa rather than invading it. They are thought to render the duodenum more vulnerable to the injurious effects of acid and pepsin by releasing urease or other toxins.

The epidemiology of peptic ulcer disease reflects the prevalence of *H pylori* infection in different populations. In areas of the world where peptic ulcer is uncommon (eg, rural Africa), human infection is rare. Duodenal ulcer disease has emerged as a major clinical entity in Western society only since the latter part of the 19th century. The incidence reached a peak about 30 years ago and then declined to reach a lower plateau a few years ago. These changes are thought to be explained by variations in *H pylori* infection resulting from public health factors. Within countries like the USA, the distribution of *H pylori* is explainable by a fecal-oral theory of transmission. The prevalence of infection is higher among lower socioeconomic groups. Interestingly, only a minority of infected persons develop ulcers. *H pylori* also has an important role in the etiology of gastric ulcer, gastric cancer, and gastritis. The 10% of duodenal ulcers that are not associated with helicobacter infection are caused by nonsteroidal anti-inflammatory drugs and other agents.

Gastric acid secretion is characteristically higher than normal in patients with duodenal ulcer compared with normal subjects, but only one-sixth of the duodenal ulcer population have secretory levels that exceed the normal range (ie, acid secretion in normal subjects and those with duodenal ulcer overlap considerably), so the disease cannot be explained simply as a manifestation of increased acid production. Whether acid secretion increases in response to helicobacter infection is doubted. One possibility is that the patches of metaplastic gastric epithelium in the duodenum on which helicobacter take up residence result from the action of acid. Then the colonized patches undergo ulceration.

Chronic liver disease, chronic lung disease, and chronic pancreatitis have all been implicated as increasing the possibility of duodenal ulceration.

Clinical Findings

A. Symptoms and Signs

Pain, the presenting symptom in most patients, is usually located in the epigastrium and is variably described as aching, burning, or gnawing. Radiologic survey studies indicate, however, that some patients with active duodenal ulcer have no gastrointestinal complaints.

The daily cycle of the pain is often characteristic. The patient usually has no pain in the morning until an hour or more after breakfast. The pain is relieved by the noon meal, only to recur in the later afternoon. Pain may appear again in the evening, and in about half of cases it arouses the patient during the night. Food, milk, or antacid preparations give temporary relief.

When the ulcer penetrates the head of the pancreas posteriorly, back pain is noted; concomitantly, the cyclic pattern of pain may change to a more steady discomfort, with less relief from food and antacids.

Varying degrees of nausea and vomiting are common. Vomiting may be a major feature even in the absence of obstruction.

The abdominal examination may reveal localized epigastric tenderness to the right of the midline, but in many instances no tenderness can be elicited.

B. Endoscopy

Gastroduodenoscopy is useful in evaluating patients with an uncertain diagnosis, those with bleeding from the upper intestine, and those who have obstruction of the gastroduodenal segment and for assessing response to therapy.

C. Diagnostic Tests

1. Gastric analysis—A gastric analysis may be indicated in certain cases. The standard gastric analysis consists of the following: (1) Measurement of acid production by the unstimulated stomach under basal fasting conditions; the result is expressed as H^+ secretion in meq/h and is termed the **basal acid output (BAO)**. (2) Measurement of acid production during stimulation by histamine or pentagastrin given in a dose maximal for this effect. The result is expressed as H^+ secretion in meq/h and is termed the **maximal acid output (MAO)**.

Interpretation of the results is outlined in Table 23–1.

Table 23–1. Mean values for acid output during gastric analysis for normals and patients with duodenal ulcer.

		Mean Acid Output (meq/h)	
	Sex	***Normal***	***Duodenal Ulcer***
Basal[1]	Male	2.5	5.5
	Female	1.5	3
Maximal[1] (pentagastrin)	Male	30	40
	Female	20	30

[1]The upper limits of normal are: Basal, 5 meq/h; maximal, 30 meq/h.

2. Serum gastrin—Depending on the laboratory, normal basal gastrin levels average 50–100 pg/mL, and levels over 200 pg/mL can almost always be considered high.

Gastrin concentrations may rise in hyposecretory and hypersecretory states. In the former conditions (eg, atrophic gastritis, pernicious anemia, acid-suppressant medications), the cause is higher antral pH with loss of antral inhibition for gastrin release. More important clinically is elevated gastrin levels with concomitant hypersecretion, where the high gastrin level is responsible for the increased acid and resulting peptic ulceration. The best-defined clinical condition in this category is Zollinger-Ellison syndrome (gastrinoma).

A fasting serum gastrin determination should be obtained in patients with peptic ulcer disease that is unusually severe or refractory to therapy.

D. Radiographic Studies

On an upper gastrointestinal series, the changes induced by duodenal ulcer consist of duodenal deformities and an ulcer niche. Inflammatory swelling and scarring may lead to distortion of the duodenal bulb, eccentricity of the pyloric channel, or pseudodiverticulum formation. The ulcer itself may be seen either in profile or, more commonly, en face.

Differential Diagnosis

The most common diseases simulating peptic ulcer are (1) chronic cholecystitis, in which cholecystograms show either nonfunctioning of the gallbladder or stones in a functioning gallbladder; (2) acute pancreatitis, in which the serum amylase is elevated; (3) chronic pancreatitis, in which ERCP shows an abnormal pancreatic duct; (4) functional indigestion, in which x-rays are normal; and (5) reflux esophagitis.

Complications

The common complications of duodenal ulcer are hemorrhage, perforation, and duodenal obstruction. Each of these is discussed in a separate section. Less common complications are pancreatitis and biliary obstruction.

Prevention

Prevention of ulcer disease entails avoidance of *H pylori* infection.

Treatment

Acute duodenal ulcer can be controlled by suppressing acid secretion in most patients, but the long-term course of the disease (ie, frequency of relapses and of complications) is unaffected unless *H pylori* infection is eradicated. Surgical therapy is recommended principally for the treatment of complications: bleeding, perforation, or obstruction.

A. Medical Treatment

The goals of medical therapy are (1) to heal the ulcer and (2) to cure the disease. Treatment in the first category is aimed at decreasing acid secretion or neutralizing acid. The principal drugs consist of H_2 receptor antagonists (eg, cimetidine, ranitidine) and proton pump blockers (eg, omeprazole). One of the H_2 receptor antagonists is usually the first choice, and when given in therapeutic doses, it will bring about healing of the ulcer in 80% of patients within 6 weeks. Omeprazole is reserved for patients whose ulcers are refractory to H_2 antagonists or for those with Zollinger-Ellison syndrome. Antacids may be used alternatively as primary therapy or on an as-needed basis to treat ulcer pain. Antacids are just as effective as H_2 receptor antagonists but slightly more difficult to administer.

After the ulcer has healed, discontinuation of therapy results in an 80% recurrence rate within 1 year, which may be avoided by chronic nighttime administration of a single dose of H_2 receptor antagonists. A better approach is to treat the *H pylori* infection along with the ulcer, since eradication of *H pylori* eliminates recurrent ulceration unless the infection recurs—an uncommon event. At present, the optimal daily regimen consists of the following combination of drugs: lansoprazole, 30 mg twice daily for 14 days; amoxicillin, 1 g twice daily for 14 days; and clarithromycin, 500 mg twice daily for 14 days.

B. Surgical Treatment

If medical treatment has been optimal, a persistent ulcer may be judged intractable, and surgical treatment is indicated. This is now uncommon.

The surgical procedures that can cure peptic ulcer are aimed at reduction of gastric acid secretion. Excision of the ulcer itself is not sufficient for either duodenal or gastric ulcer; recurrence is nearly inevitable with such procedures.

The surgical methods of treating duodenal ulcer are vagotomy (several varieties) and antrectomy plus vagotomy. All of these procedures can be performed laparoscopically. With rare exceptions, one of the vagotomy operations is sufficient (Figure 23–5).

1. Vagotomy—Truncal vagotomy consists of resection of a 1- or 2-cm segment of each vagal trunk as it enters the abdomen on the distal esophagus. The resulting vagal denervation of the gastric musculature produces delayed emptying of the stomach in many patients unless a drainage procedure is performed. The method of drainage most often selected is **pyloroplasty (Heineke-Mikulicz procedure**; Figure 23–6); **gastrojejunostomy** is used less often. Neither procedure gives a superior functional result, and pyloroplasty is less time-consuming.

Vagal denervation of just the parietal cell area of the stomach is called **parietal cell vagotomy** or **proximal gastric vagotomy**. The technique spares the main nerves of Latarjet (Figures 23–3 and 23–5) but divides all vagal branches that terminate on the proximal two-thirds of the stomach. Since antral innervation is preserved, gastric emptying is relatively normal, and a drainage procedure is unnecessary. Nevertheless, parietal cell vagotomy plus pyloroplasty give better results (ie, fewer recurrent ulcers) than parietal cell vagotomy alone. Parietal cell vagotomy appears to have about the same effectiveness as truncal or selective vagotomy for curing the ulcer disease, but dumping and diarrhea are much less frequent. It is probably the procedure of choice for intractable and perforated duodenal ulcers and is relatively less useful for obstructing and bleeding ulcers.

The vagotomy procedures have the advantages of technical simplicity and preservation of the entire gastric reservoir capacity. The principal disadvantage is recurrent ulceration in about 10% of patients. The recurrence rate after parietal cell vagotomy is about twice as high in patients with prepyloric ulcer, and most surgeons use a different operation for an ulcer in this location.

2. Antrectomy and vagotomy—This operation entails a distal gastrectomy of 50% of the stomach, with the line of gastric transection carried high on the lesser curvature to conform with the boundary of the gastrin-producing mucosa.

The terms antrectomy and hemigastrectomy are loosely synonymous. The proximal remnant may be reanastomosed to the duodenum **(Billroth I resection)** or to the side of the proximal jejunum **(Billroth II resection)**. The Billroth I technique is most popular, but there is no conclusive evidence that the results are superior. When creating a Billroth II (gastrojejunostomy) reconstruction, the surgeon may bring the jejunal loop up to the gastric remnant either anterior to the transverse colon or posteriorly through a hole in the transverse mesocolon. Since either method is satisfactory, an antecolic anastomosis is elected in most cases because it is simpler. Truncal vagotomy is performed as described in the preceding section; antrectomy by itself will not prevent a high recurrence rate. In most instances, the surgeon will be able to remove the ulcerated portion of duodenum in the course of resection.

Vagotomy and antrectomy is associated with a low incidence of marginal ulceration (2%) and a generally good overall outcome, but the risk of complications is higher than after vagotomy without resection.

3. Subtotal gastrectomy—This operation consists of resection of two-thirds to three-fourths of the distal

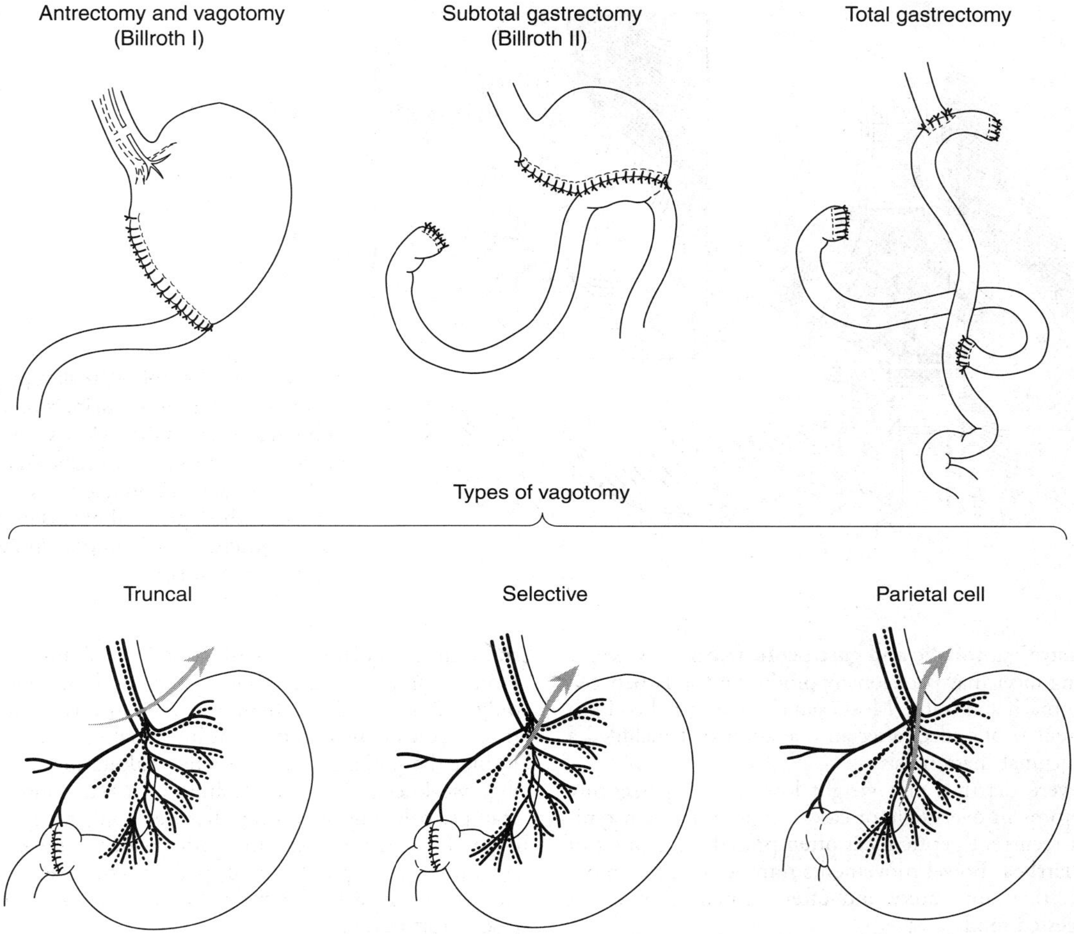

Figure 23–5. Various types of operations currently popular for treating duodenal ulcer disease. Total gastrectomy is reserved for Zollinger-Ellison syndrome. The choice among the other procedures should be individualized according to principles discussed in the text.

stomach. After subtotal gastrectomy for duodenal ulcer, a Billroth II reconstruction is preferable. Subtotal gastrectomy is largely of historical interest.

Complications of Surgery for Peptic Ulcer

A. Early Complications

Duodenal stump leakage, gastric retention, and hemorrhage may develop in the immediate postoperative period.

B. Late Complications

1. Recurrent ulcer (marginal ulcer, stomal ulcer, anastomotic ulcer)—Recurrent ulcers form in about 10% of duodenal ulcer patients treated by vagotomy and pyloroplasty or parietal cell vagotomy; and in 2–3% after vagotomy and antrectomy or subtotal gastrectomy. These figures were accumulated before the emergence of effective treatment against *H pylori,* however, and are likely to be lower with current management. Recurrent ulcers nearly always develop immediately adjacent to the anastomosis on the intestinal side.

The usual complaint is upper abdominal pain, which is often aggravated by eating and improved by antacids. In some patients, the pain is felt more to the left in the epigastrium, and left axillary or shoulder pain is occasionally reported. About a third of patients with stomal ulcer will experience major gastrointestinal hemorrhage. Free perforation is less common (5%).

Diagnosis and treatment are essentially the same as for the original ulcer.

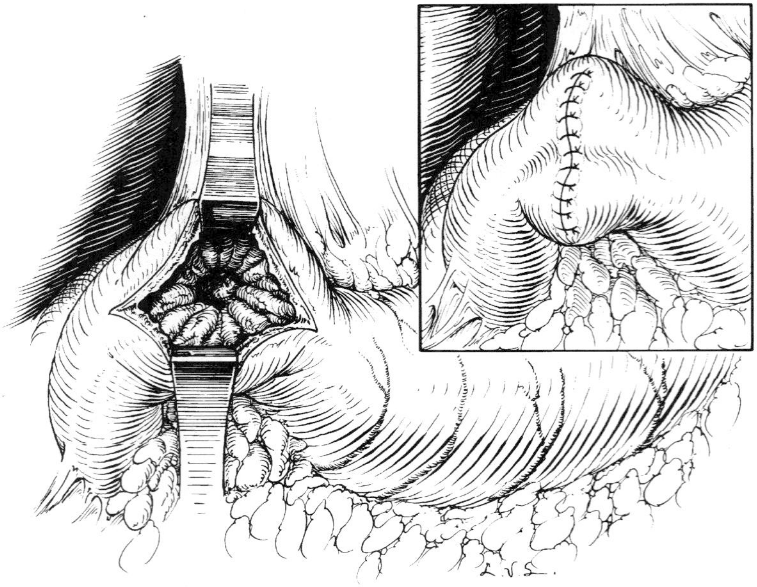

Figure 23–6. Heineke-Mikulicz pyloroplasty. A longitudinal incision has been made across the pylorus, revealing an active ulcer in the duodenal bulb. The insert shows the transverse closure of the incision that widens the gastric outlet. The accompanying vagotomy is not shown.

2. Gastrojejunocolic and gastrocolic fistula—A deeply eroding ulcer may occasionally produce a fistula between the stomach and colon. Most examples have resulted from recurrent peptic ulcer after an operation that included a gastrojejunal anastomosis.

Severe diarrhea and weight loss are the presenting symptoms in over 90% of cases. Abdominal pain typical of recurrent peptic ulcer often precedes the onset of the diarrhea. Bowel movements number 8–12 or more a day; they are watery and often contain particles of undigested food.

The degree of malnutrition ranges from mild to very severe. Laboratory studies reveal low serum proteins and manifestations of fluid and electrolyte depletion. Appropriate tests may reflect deficiencies in both water-soluble and fat-soluble vitamins.

An upper gastrointestinal series reveals the marginal ulcer in only 50% of patients and the fistula in only 15%. Barium enema unfailingly demonstrates the fistulous tract.

Initial treatment should replenish fluid and electrolyte deficits. The involved colon and ulcerated gastrojejunal segment should be excised and colonic continuity reestablished. Vagotomy, partial gastrectomy, or both are required to treat the ulcer diathesis and prevent another recurrent ulcer. Results are excellent in benign disease. In general, the outlook for patients with a malignant fistula is poor.

3. Dumping syndrome—Symptoms of the dumping syndrome are noted to some extent by most patients who have an operation that impairs the ability of the stomach to regulate its rate of emptying. Within several months, however, dumping is a clinical problem in only 1–2% of patients. Symptoms fall into two categories: cardiovascular and gastrointestinal. Shortly after eating, the patient may experience palpitations, sweating, weakness, dyspnea, flushing, nausea, abdominal cramps, belching, vomiting, diarrhea, and, rarely, syncope. The degree of severity varies widely, and not all symptoms are reported by all patients. In severe cases, the patient must lie down for 30–40 minutes until the discomfort passes.

Diet therapy to reduce jejunal osmolality is successful in all but a few cases. The diet should be low in carbohydrate and high in fat and protein content. Sugars and carbohydrates are least well tolerated; some patients are especially sensitive to milk. Meals should be taken dry, with fluids restricted to between meals. This dietary regimen ordinarily suffices, but anticholinergic drugs may be of help in some patients; others have reported improvement with supplemental pectin in the diet, and the use of somatostatin analogues offers some promise.

4. Alkaline gastritis—Reflux of duodenal juices into the stomach is an invariable and usually innocuous situation after operations that interfere with pyloric function, but in some patients, it may cause marked gastritis. The principal symptom is postprandial pain, and the diagnosis rests on endoscopic and biopsy demonstration of an edematous inflamed gastric mucosa. Since a minor degree of gastritis is found in most patients after Billroth II gastrectomy, the endoscopic findings are to some degree nonspecific. Persistent severe pain is an indication for surgical reconstruction. Roux-en-Y gastrojejunostomy with a 40-cm efferent jejunal limb is the treatment of choice.

5. Anemia—Iron deficiency anemia develops in about 30% of patients within 5 years after partial gastrectomy. It is caused by failure to absorb food iron bound in an organic molecule. Before this diagnosis is accepted, the patient should be checked for blood loss, marginal ulcer, or an unsuspected tumor. Inorganic iron—ferrous sulfate or ferrous gluconate—is indicated for treatment and is absorbed normally after gastrectomy.

Vitamin B_{12} deficiency and megaloblastic anemia appear in a few cases after gastrectomy.

6. Postvagotomy diarrhea—About 5–10% of patients who have had truncal vagotomy require treatment with antidiarrheal agents at some time, and perhaps 1% are seriously troubled by this complication. The diarrhea may be episodic, in which case the onset is unpredictable after symptom-free intervals of weeks to months. An attack may consist of only one or two watery movements or, in severe cases, may last for a few days. Other patients may continually produce 3–5 loose stools per day.

Most cases of postvagotomy diarrhea can be treated satisfactorily with constipating agents.

7. Chronic gastroparesis—Chronic delayed gastric emptying is seen occasionally after gastric surgery. Prokinetic agents (eg, metoclopramide) are often helpful, but some cases are refractory to any therapy except a completion gastrectomy and Roux-en-Y esophagojejunostomy (ie, total gastrectomy).

Donahue PE: Parietal cell vagotomy versus vagotomy-antrectomy: ulcer surgery in the modern era. World J Surg 2000;24:264.

Erstad BL: Proton-pump inhibitors for acute peptic ulcer bleeding. Ann Pharmacother 2001;35:730.

Jamieson GG: Current status of indications for surgery in peptic ulcer disease. World J Surg 2000;24:256.

Logan RP, Walker MM: ABC of the upper gastrointestinal tract: epidemiology and diagnosis of *Helicobacter pylori* infection. BMJ 2001;323:920.

Macintyre IM: Peptic ulcer surgery—an obituary. Proc R Coll Physicians Edinb 2000;30:158.

Macintyre IM: Peptic ulcer surgery—an obituary. (Part 2.) Proc R Coll Physicians Edinb 2000;30:245.

Peterson WL, Cook DJ: Antisecretory therapy for bleeding peptic ulcer. JAMA 1998;280:877.

Peura D: *Helicobacter pylori*: rational management options. Am J Med 1998;105:424.

Zittel TT, Jehle EC, Becker HD: Surgical management of peptic ulcer disease today—indication, technique and outcome. Langenbecks Arch Surg 2000;385:84.

ZOLLINGER-ELLISON SYNDROME (GASTRINOMA)

ESSENTIALS OF DIAGNOSIS

- *Peptic ulcer disease (often severe) in 95%.*
- *Gastric hypersecretion.*
- *Elevated serum gastrin.*
- *Non-B islet cell tumor of the pancreas or duodenum.*

General Considerations

Zollinger-Ellison syndrome is manifested by gastric acid hypersecretion caused by a gastrin-producing tumor (gastrinoma). Although the normal pancreas does not contain appreciable amounts of gastrin, most gastrinomas occur in the pancreas; others are found submucosally in the duodenum and rarely in the antrum or ovary. The gastrin-producing lesions (called **apudomas** from the theory of their histogenesis) in the pancreas are non-B islet cell carcinomas (60%), solitary adenomas (25%), and hyperplasia or microadenomas (10%); the remaining cases (5%) are due to solitary submucosal gastrinomas in the first or second portion of the duodenum. About one-third of patients have the multiple endocrine neoplasia type I syndrome (MEN 1), which is characterized by a family history of endocrinopathy and the presence of tumors in other glands, especially the parathyroids and pituitary. Patients with MEN 1 usually have multiple benign gastrinomas. Those without MEN 1 usually have solitary gastrinomas that are often malignant. The tumors may be as small as 2–3 mm and are often difficult to find. In about one-third of cases, the tumor cannot be located at laparotomy.

The diagnosis of cancer can be made only with findings of metastases or blood vessel invasion, because the histologic pattern is similar for benign and malignant tumors. In most patients with malignant gastrinomas, the illness caused by hypergastrinemia (ie, severe peptic ulcer disease) is a greater threat to health than the illness caused by malignant growth and spread.

Clinical Findings

A. Symptoms and Signs

Symptoms associated with gastrinoma are principally a result of acid hypersecretion—usually from peptic ulcer disease. Some patients with gastrinoma have severe diarrhea from the large amounts of acid entering the duodenum, which can destroy pancreatic lipase and produce steatorrhea, damage the small bowel mucosa, and overload the intestine with gastric and pancreatic secretions. About 5% of patients present with diarrhea only.

Ulcer symptoms are often refractory to large doses of antacids or standard doses of H_2 blocking agents. Hemorrhage, perforation, and obstruction are common complications. Marginal ulcers appear after surgical procedures that would cure the ordinary ulcer diathesis.

B. Laboratory Findings

Hypergastrinemia in the presence of acid hypersecretion is almost diagnostic of gastrinoma. Gastrin levels are normally inversely proportionate to gastric acid output; therefore, diseases that result in increased gastric pH may cause a rise in serum gastrin concentration (eg, pernicious anemia, atrophic gastritis, gastric ulcer, postvagotomy state, acid-suppressing medications). Serum gastrin levels should be measured in any patient with suspected gastrinoma or ulcer disease severe enough to warrant consideration of surgical treatment. H_2 receptor blocking agents, omeprazole, or antacids frequently increase serum gastrin concentrations and should be avoided for several days before gastrin measurements are made. It is often helpful to measure gastric acid secretion to rule out H^+ hyposecretion as a cause of hypergastrinemia.

The normal gastrin value is less than 200 pg/mL. Patients with gastrinoma usually have levels exceeding 500 pg/mL and sometimes 10,000 pg/mL or higher. Very high gastrin levels (eg, > 5000 pg/mL) or the presence of alpha chains of hCG in the serum usually indicates cancer. Patients with borderline gastrin values (eg, 200–500 pg/mL) and acid secretion in the range associated with ordinary duodenal ulcer disease should have a secretin provocative test. Following intravenous administration of secretin (2 units/kg as a bolus), a rise in the gastrin level of > 150 pg/mL within 15 minutes is diagnostic.

Marked basal acid hypersecretion (> 15 meq H^+ per hour) occurs in most Zollinger-Ellison patients who have an intact stomach. In a patient who has previously undergone gastrectomy, a basal acid output of 5 meq/h or more is highly suggestive. Since the parietal cells are already under near maximal stimulation from hypergastrinemia, there is little increase in acid secretion following an injection of pentagastrin, and the ratio of basal to maximal acid output (BAO/MAO) characteristically exceeds 0.6.

Hypergastrinemia and gastric acid hypersecretion may be seen in gastric outlet obstruction, retained antrum after a Billroth II gastrojejunostomy, and in antral gastrin cell hyperactivity (hyperplasia). These conditions may be differentiated from gastrinoma by use of the secretin test. Because associated hyperparathyroidism is so common, serum calcium concentrations should be measured in all patients with gastrinoma.

Serum levels of neuron-specific enolase, β-hCG, and chromogranin-A are often elevated in patients with functioning apudomas. Although they are probably of no physiologic importance, the high levels of these peptides may be useful in diagnosing apudomas and following the results of therapy.

C. Imaging Studies

An upper gastrointestinal series usually shows ulceration in the duodenal bulb, though ulcers sometimes appear in the distal duodenum or proximal jejunum. The presence of ulcers in these distal ("ectopic") locations is nearly diagnostic of gastrinoma. The stomach contains prominent rugal folds, and secretions are present in the lumen despite overnight fasting. The duodenum may be dilated and exhibit hyperactive peristalsis. Edema may be detected in the small bowel mucosa. The barium flocculates in the intestine, and transit time is accelerated. A CT or MR scan will often demonstrate the pancreatic tumors. Somatostatin-receptor scintigraphy is extremely sensitive for detection of gastrinoma primary and metastatic sites. Transhepatic portal vein blood sampling to find gradients of gastrin production has been supplanted by the intra-arterial secretin test. Infusion of secretin into the artery supplying a functional gastrinoma causes an increase in hepatic vein gastrin levels. This invasive test is usually reserved for difficult situations.

Treatment

A. Medical Treatment

Initial treatment should consist of H_2 blocking agents (eg, cimetidine, 300–600 mg, four times daily; ranitidine, 300–450 mg, four times daily). The dose should be adjusted to keep gastric H^+ output below 5 meq in the hour preceding the next dose. Although the response to H_2 blocking agents is usually excellent at first, with time, the dose must be increased in order to maintain the same level of control. Omeprazole, a proton pump blocker, is indicated sooner or later in nearly all patients.

A combination of streptozocin, fluorouracil, and doxorubicin is the most effective chemotherapeutic regimen for advanced cancer.

B. Surgical Treatment

Resection is the ideal treatment for gastrinoma and is appropriate in all patients with apparently localized disease and no other significant limitations to their survival. Surgical cure may be possible when there are resectable metastases in peripancreatic lymph nodes or the liver. Overall, about 70% of patients have immediate biochemical cure, and about 30% of patients remain disease-free after 5 years.

Every patient with sporadic Zollinger-Ellison syndrome should be considered a candidate for tumor resection. The preoperative workup should include a CT or MR scan of the pancreas and somatostatin-receptor scintigraphy. Regardless of other findings, exploratory laparotomy is then recommended in the absence of evidence of unresectable metastatic disease. If the tumor is found in the pancreas, it is enucleated if possible. Operative ultrasound may help in the examination of the pancreas. Most lesions will be found either in the head of the pancreas or in the duodenum. All patients should have longitudinal duodenotomy and palpation of the duodenal mucosa to identify the frequent primary tumors in this site.

Prognosis

Since H_2 blocking agents become less effective with time, omeprazole is eventually required in medically treated patients. Because it is usually multifocal, the disease can rarely be cured surgically in patients with MEN 1. Malignant gastrinomas cause death from growth of metastases.

Alexander HR et al: Prospective study of somatostatin receptor scintigraphy and its effect on operative outcome in patients with Zollinger-Ellison syndrome. Ann Surg 1998;228:228.

Brentjens R, Saltz L: Islet cell tumors of the pancreas: the medical oncologist's perspective. Surg Clin North Am 2001;81:527.

Doherty GM et al: Lethality of multiple endocrine neoplasia type I. World J Surg 1998;22:581.

Lairmore TC et al: Duodenopancreatic resections in patients with multiple endocrine neoplasia type 1. Ann Surg 2000;231:909.

Lim JH et al: Prospective study of the utility of somatostatin-receptor scintigraphy in the evaluation of patients with multiple endocrine neoplasia type 1. Surgery 1998;124:1037.

Lowney JK et al: Pancreatic islet cell tumor metastasis in multiple endocrine neoplasia type 1: correlation with primary tumor size. Surgery 1998;124:1043.

Norton JA et al: Surgery to cure the Zollinger-Ellison syndrome. N Engl J Med 1999;341:635.

Norton JA: Intraoperative methods to stage and localize pancreatic and duodenal tumors. Ann Oncol 1999;10(Suppl 4):182.

Norton JA et al: Surgical treatment of localized gastrinoma within the liver: a prospective study. Surgery 1998;124:1145.

Pisegna JR: The effect of Zollinger-Ellison syndrome and neuropeptide-secreting tumors on the stomach. Curr Gastroenterol Rep 1999;1:511.

GASTRIC ULCER

ESSENTIALS OF DIAGNOSIS

- *Epigastric pain.*
- *Ulcer demonstrated by x-ray.*
- *Acid present on gastric analysis.*

General Considerations

The peak incidence of gastric ulcer is in patients aged 40–60 years, or about 10 years older than the average for those with duodenal ulcer. Ninety-five percent of gastric ulcers are located on the lesser curvature, and 60% of these are within 6 cm of the pylorus. The symptoms and complications of gastric ulcer closely resemble those of duodenal ulcer.

Gastric ulcers may be separated into three types with different causes and different treatments. **Type I ulcers**, the most common variety, are found in patients who on the average are 10 years older than patients with duodenal ulcers and who have no clinical or radiographic evidence of previous duodenal ulcer disease; gastric acid output is normal or low. The ulcers are usually located within 2 cm of the boundary between parietal cell and pyloric mucosa, but always in the latter. As noted above, 95% are on the lesser curvature, usually near the incisura angularis.

Antral gastritis is universally present, being most severe near the pylorus and gradually diminishing. This is associated in most cases with the presence of *H pylori* beneath the mucus layer, on the luminal surface of epithelial cells, and gastric ulcer disease is probably the result of infection with this organism.

Type II ulcers are located close to the pylorus (prepyloric ulcers) and occur in association with (most often following) duodenal ulcers. The risk of cancer is very low in these gastric ulcers. Acid secretion measured by gastric analysis is in the range associated with duodenal ulcer.

Type III ulcers occur in the antrum as a result of chronic use of nonsteroidal anti-inflammatory agents.

One must always consider whether the ulcer seen on x-ray or by endoscopy represents an ulcerated malignant tumor rather than a simple benign ulcer. Efforts must be expended during the *initial* stage of the workup to establish this distinction. Despite the generally discouraging results of surgery for gastric adenocarcinoma, those whose tumors are difficult to distinguish from benign ulcer have a 50–75% chance of cure after gastrectomy.

Clinical Findings

A. Symptoms and Signs

The principal symptom is epigastric pain relieved by food or antacids, as in duodenal ulcer. Epigastric tenderness is a variable finding. Compared with duodenal ulcer, the pain in gastric ulcer tends to appear earlier after eating, often within 30 minutes. Vomiting, anorexia, and aggravation of pain by eating are also more common with gastric ulcer.

Achlorhydria is defined as no acid (pH > 6.00) after pentagastrin stimulation. Achlorhydria is incompatible with the diagnosis of benign peptic ulcer and suggests a malignant gastric ulcer. About 5% of malignant gastric ulcers will be associated with this finding.

B. Gastroscopy and Biopsy

Gastroscopy should be performed as part of the initial workup to attempt to find malignant lesions. The rolled-up margins of the ulcer that produce the meniscus sign on x-ray can often be distinguished from the flat edges characteristic of a benign ulcer. Multiple (preferably six) biopsy specimens and brush biopsy should be obtained from the edge of the lesion. False-positives are rare; false-negatives occur in 5–10% of malignant ulcers.

C. Imaging Studies

Upper gastrointestinal x-rays will show an ulcer, usually on the lesser curvature in the pyloric area. In the absence of a tumor mass, the following suggest that the ulcer is malignant: (1) the deepest penetration of the ulcer is not beyond the expected border of the gastric wall; (2) the meniscus sign is present, ie, a prominent rim of radiolucency surrounding the ulcer, caused by heaped-up edges of tumor; and (3) cancer is more common (10%) in ulcers greater than 2 cm in diameter. Coexistence of duodenal deformity or ulcer favors a diagnosis of benign ulcer in the stomach.

Differential Diagnosis

The characteristic symptoms of gastric ulcer are often clouded by numerous nonspecific complaints. Uncomplicated hiatal hernia, atrophic gastritis, chronic cholecystitis, irritable colon syndrome, and undifferentiated functional problems are distinguishable from peptic ulcer only after appropriate radiologic studies and sometimes not even then.

Gastroscopy and biopsy of the ulcer should be performed to rule out malignant gastric ulcer.

Complications

Bleeding, obstruction, and perforation are the principal complications of gastric ulcer. They are discussed separately elsewhere in this chapter.

Treatment

A. Medical Treatment

Medical management of gastric ulcer is the same as for duodenal ulcer. The patient should be questioned regarding the use of ulcerogenic agents, which should be eliminated as far as possible.

Repeat endoscopy should be obtained to document the rate of healing. After 4–16 weeks (depending on the initial size of the lesion and other factors), healing usually has reached a plateau. In order to cure the disease and avoid recurrent ulcers, *H pylori* must be eradicated. The success of therapy in this regard can be checked by serologic testing for *H pylori* antibodies.

B. Surgical Treatment

Before the significance of *H pylori* in the etiology of gastric ulcer was appreciated, the most effective surgical treatment was distal hemigastrectomy (including the ulcer); somewhat less effective but still useful in high-risk patients was vagotomy and pyloroplasty. Parietal cell vagotomy for prepyloric ulcers was followed by a high (eg, 30%) recurrence rate, but parietal cell vagotomy plus pyloroplasty worked well.

Intractability to medical therapy has now become a rare indication for surgery in gastric ulcer disease, since H_2 receptor antagonists or omeprazole can bring the condition under control, and treatment of *H pylori* infection can almost eliminate the problem of recurrence. Consequently, surgery is needed principally for complications of the disease: bleeding, perforation, or obstruction.

Calam J, Baron JH: ABC of the upper gastrointestinal tract: pathophysiology of duodenal and gastric ulcer and gastric cancer. BMJ 2001;323:980.

Miller JS, Hendren SK, Liscum KR: Giant gastric ulcer in a body packer. J Trauma 1998;45:617.

Pai R, Tarnawski A: Signal transduction cascades triggered by EGF receptor activation: relevance to gastric injury repair and ulcer healing. Dig Dis Sci 1998;43(9 Suppl):14S.

Peskar BM, Maricic N: Role of prostaglandins in gastroprotection. Dig Dis Sci 1998;43(9 Suppl):23S.

UPPER GASTROINTESTINAL HEMORRHAGE

Upper gastrointestinal hemorrhage may be mild or severe but should always be considered an ominous manifestation that deserves thorough evaluation. Bleeding is the most common serious complication of peptic ulcer, portal hypertension, and gastritis, and these conditions taken together account for most episodes of upper gastrointestinal bleeding in the average hospital population.

The major factors that determine the diagnostic and therapeutic approach are the amount and rate of bleeding. Estimates of both should be made promptly and monitored and revised continuously until the episode has been resolved. It is important to know at the outset that bleeding stops spontaneously in 75% of cases; the remainder includes those who will require surgery, experience complications, or die.

Hematemesis or melena is present except when the rate of blood loss is minimal. **Hematemesis** of either bright-red or dark blood indicates that the source is proximal to the ligament of Treitz. It is more common from bleeding that originates in the stomach or esophagus. In general, hematemesis denotes a more rapidly bleeding lesion, and a high percentage of patients who vomit blood require surgery. Coffee-ground vomitus is due to vomiting of blood that has been in the stomach long enough for gastric acid to convert hemoglobin to methemoglobin.

Most patients with **melena** (passage of black or tarry stools) are bleeding from the upper gastrointestinal tract, but melena can be produced by blood entering the bowel at any point from mouth to cecum. The conversion of red blood to dark depends more on the time it resides in the intestine than on the site of origin. The black color of melenic stools is probably caused by hematin, the product of oxidation of heme by intestinal and bacterial enzymes. Melena can be produced by as little as 50–100 mL of blood in the stomach. When 1 L of blood was instilled into the upper intestine of experimental subjects, melena persisted for 3–5 days, which shows that the rate of change in character of the stool is a poor guide to the time bleeding stops after an episode of hemorrhage.

Hematochezia is defined as the passage of bright-red blood from the rectum. Bright-red rectal blood can be produced by bleeding from the colon, rectum, or anus. However, if intestinal transit is rapid during brisk bleeding in the upper intestine, bright-red blood may be passed unchanged in the stool.

Tests for Occult Blood

Normal subjects lose about 2.5 mL of blood per day in their stools, presumably from minor mechanical abrasions of the intestinal epithelium. Between 50 and 100 mL of blood per day will produce melena. Tests for occult blood in the stool should be able to detect amounts between 10 and 50 mL/d. False-positive results may be due to dietary hemoglobin, myoglobin, or peroxidases of plant origin. Iron ingestion does not give positive reactions. The various tests using guaiac, benzidine, phenolphthalein, or orthotoluidine have similar specificities. The sensitivity of the guaiac slide test (Hemoccult) is in the desired range, and this is the best test available at present.

Initial Management

In an apparently healthy patient, melena of a week or more suggests that the bleeding is slow. In this type of patient, admission to the hospital should be followed by a deliberate but nonemergency workup. However, patients who present with hematemesis or melena of less than 12 hours' duration should be handled as if exsanguination were imminent. The approach entails a simultaneous series of diagnostic and therapeutic steps with the following initial goals: (1) Assess the status of the circulatory system and replace blood loss as necessary. (2) Determine the amount and rate of bleeding. (3) Slow or stop the bleeding by ice-water lavage. (4) Discover the lesion responsible for the episode. The last step may lead to more specific treatment appropriate to the underlying condition.

The patient should be admitted to the hospital and a history and physical examination performed. Experienced clinicians are able to make a correct diagnosis of the cause of bleeding from clinical findings in only 60% of patients. Peptic ulcer, acute gastritis, esophageal varices, esophagitis, and Mallory-Weiss tear account for over 90% of cases (see Table 23–2). Questions concerning the symptoms and predisposing factors should be asked. The patient should be questioned about salicylate intake and any history of a bleeding tendency.

Of the diseases commonly responsible for acute upper gastrointestinal bleeding, only portal hypertension is associated with diagnostic clues on physical examination. However, gastrointestinal bleeding should not be automatically attributed to esophageal varices in a patient with jaundice, ascites, splenomegaly, spider angiomas, or hepatomegaly; over half of cirrhotic patients who present with acute hemorrhage are bleeding from gastritis or peptic ulcer.

Blood should be drawn for crossmatching, hematocrit, hemoglobin, creatinine, and tests of liver function. An intravenous infusion should be started and, in the massive bleeder, a large-bore nasogastric tube inserted. In cases of melena, the gastric aspirate should be examined to verify the gastroduodenal source of the hemorrhage, but about 25% of patients with bleeding duodenal ulcers have gas-

Table 23–2. Causes of massive upper gastrointestinal hemorrhage.

	Relative Incidence	
Common causes		
Peptic ulcer		45%
Duodenal ulcer	25%	
Gastric ulcer	20%	
Esophageal varices		20%
Gastritis		20%
Mallory-Weiss syndrome		10%
Uncommon causes[1]		5%
Gastric carcinoma		
Esophagitis		
Pancreatitis		
Hemobilia		
Duodenal diverticulum		

[1]Note that cancer is rarely the cause.

tric aspirates that test negatively for blood. The tube must be larger than the standard nasogastric tube (16F) so the stomach can be lavaged free of liquid blood and clots. After its contents have been removed, the stomach should be irrigated with copious amounts of ice water or saline solution until blood no longer returns. If the patient was bleeding at the time the nasogastric tube was inserted, iced saline irrigation usually stops it. The large tube can then be exchanged for a standard nasogastric tube attached to continuous suction so further blood loss can be measured.

It is common to give H_2 receptor antagonists or omeprazole, though controlled trials have shown no benefit. If bleeding continues or if tachycardia or hypotension is present, the patient should be monitored and treated as for hemorrhagic shock.

In acute rapid hemorrhage, the hematocrit may be normal or only slightly low. A very low hematocrit without obvious signs of shock indicates more gradual blood loss.

All of the above tests and procedures can be performed within 1 or 2 hours after admission. By this time, in most instances, bleeding is under control, blood volume has been restored to normal, and the patient is being adequately monitored so that recurrent bleeding can be detected promptly. When this stage is reached, additional diagnostic tests should be performed.

Diagnosis of Cause of Bleeding

Once the patient is stabilized, endoscopy should be the first study. In general, endoscopy should be performed within 24 hours after admission, and under these circumstances the source of bleeding can be demonstrated in about 80% of cases. Longer delays have a lower diagnostic yield. Two lesions are seen in about 15% of patients. An upper gastrointestinal series should be performed if endoscopy is equivocal or unavailable. Although the diagnostic information provided by endoscopy does not appear to have resulted in decreased blood loss or improved outcome, endoscopic therapy, in the form of sclerosis of varices or injection of a bleeding ulcer, may do so. Having the diagnosis will also help in planning subsequent treatment, including the surgical approach if operation becomes necessary.

Rarely, selective angiography will have diagnostic or therapeutic usefulness. For diagnosis, it is most helpful when other studies fail to demonstrate the cause of bleeding. Infusion through the angiographic catheter of vasoconstrictors (eg, vasopressin) and embolization of the bleeding vessel with Gelfoam may be able to halt the bleeding in special cases.

Later Management

Although a precise diagnosis of the cause of the bleeding may be valuable in later management, the patient must not be allowed to slip out of clinical control during the search for definitive diagnostic information. *The decision for emergency surgery depends more on the rate and duration of bleeding than on its specific cause.*

The need for transfusion should be determined on a continuing basis, and blood volume must be maintained. Blood pressure, pulse, central venous pressure, hematocrit, hourly urinary volume, and amount of blood obtained from the gastric tube or from the rectum all enter into this assessment. Many studies have shown the tendency to underestimate blood loss and inadequately transfuse massively bleeding patients who truly need aggressive therapy. Continued slow bleeding is best monitored by serial determinations of the hematocrit.

The following criteria define patients with a very low risk of serious bleeding: age less than 75 years, no unstable comorbid illness, no ascites evident on physical examination, normal prothrombin time, and, within 1 hour after admission, a systolic blood pressure above 100 mm Hg and nasogastric aspirate free of fresh blood. Patients with all six of these findings may be spared emergency endoscopy and discharged from the hospital early to undergo outpatient workup.

Several factors are associated with a worse prognosis with continued medical management of the bleeding episode. These are not absolute indications for laparotomy, but they should alert the clinician that emergency surgery may be required.

High rates of bleeding or amounts of blood loss predict high failure rates with medical treatment. Hematemesis is usually associated with more rapid bleeding and a greater blood volume deficit than melena. The presence of hypotension on admission to the hospital or the need for more than four units of blood to achieve circulatory stability implies a worse prognosis; if bleeding continues and subsequent transfusion requirements exceed 1 unit every 8 hours, continued medical management is usually unwise. The level of serum fibrin degradation products, indicating endogenous fibrinolysis, correlates with the severity of hemorrhage and the death rate. This may be a useful prognostic test, and the results could be used as a guide for the administration of fibrinolytic inhibitors in therapy. Evidence for or against this view is not yet available.

Total transfusion requirements also correlate with death rates. Death is uncommon when fewer than seven units of blood have been used, and the death rate rises progressively thereafter.

In general, bleeding from a gastric ulcer is more dangerous than bleeding from gastritis or duodenal ulcer, and patients with gastric ulcer should always be considered for early surgery. Regardless of the cause, if bleeding recurs after it has once stopped, the chances of success without operation are low. Most patients who rebleed in the hospital should have surgery.

Patients over age 60 tolerate continued blood loss less well than younger patients, and their bleeding should be stopped before secondary cardiovascular, pulmonary, or renal complications arise.

In 85% of patients, bleeding stops within a few hours of admission. About 25% of patients rebleed once bleeding has stopped. Rebleeding episodes are concentrated within the first 2 days of hospitalization, and if the patient has had no further bleeding for a period of 5 days, the chance of rebleeding is only 2%. Rebleeding is most common in patients with varices, peptic ulcer, anemia, or shock. About 10% of patients require surgery to control bleeding, and most of these patients have bleeding ulcers or, less commonly, esophageal varices. The death rate is 30% among patients who rebleed and 3% among those who do not. The mortality rate is also high in the elderly and in patients who are already hospitalized at the onset of bleeding. Analyses of large series of patients suggest that a number of those who died would not have done so if operations had been performed earlier and more often.

Dallal HJ, Palmer KR: ABC of the upper gastrointestinal tract: upper gastrointestinal haemorrhage. BMJ 2001;323:1115.

Palmer KR: Intravenous omeprazole after endoscopic treatment of bleeding peptic ulcers. Gut 2001;49:610.

Peterson WL, Cook DJ: Antisecretory therapy for bleeding peptic ulcer. JAMA 1998;280:877.

Spiegel BM, Vakil NB, Ofman JJ: Endoscopy for acute nonvariceal upper gastrointestinal tract hemorrhage: is sooner better? A systematic review. Arch Intern Med 2001;161:1393.

Van Dam J, Brugge KR: Endoscopy of the upper gastrointestinal tract. N Engl J Med 1999;341:1738.

HEMORRHAGE FROM PEPTIC ULCER

Approximately 20% of patients with peptic ulcer will experience a bleeding episode, and this complication is responsible for about 40% of the deaths from peptic ulcer. Peptic ulcer is the most common cause of massive upper gastrointestinal hemorrhage, accounting for over half of all cases. Chronic gastric and duodenal ulcers have about the same tendency to bleed, but the former produce more severe episodes. Bleeding ulcers are more common in persons with blood group O, though the reason for this association is not known.

Bleeding ulcers in the duodenum are usually located on the posterior surface of the duodenal bulb. As the ulcer penetrates, the gastroduodenal artery is exposed and may become eroded. Since no major blood vessels lie on the anterior surface of the duodenal bulb, ulcerations at this point are not as prone to bleed. Patients with concomitant bleeding and perforation usually have two ulcers, a bleeding posterior ulcer and a perforated anterior one. Postbulbar ulcers (those in the second portion of the duodenum) bleed frequently, though ulcers are much less common in this site than near the pylorus.

In some patients, the bleeding is sudden and massive, manifested by hematemesis and shock. In others, chronic anemia and weakness due to slow blood loss are the only findings. The diagnosis is unreliable when based on clinical findings, so endoscopy should be performed early (ie, within 24 hours) in most cases.

In the preceding section, the management of acute upper gastrointestinal hemorrhage, the selection of diagnostic tests, and the factors suggesting the need for operation were discussed. Most patients (75%) with bleeding peptic ulcer can be successfully managed by medical means alone. Initial therapeutic efforts usually halt the bleeding. H_2 blockers and proton pump inhibitors decrease the risk of bleeding but have no effect on active bleeding.

After 12–24 hours have passed and the bleeding has clearly stopped, a patient who feels hungry should be fed. Twice-daily hematocrit readings should be ordered as a check on slow continued blood loss. Stools should be tested daily for the presence of blood; they will usually remain guaiac-positive for several days after bleeding stops.

Rebleeding in the hospital has been attended by a death rate of about 30%. A policy of early surgery for those who rebleed would improve this figure. Patients who are over age 60, present with hematemesis, are actively bleeding at the time of endoscopy, or whose admission hemoglobin is below 8 g/dL have a higher risk of rebleeding. About three times as many patients with gastric ulcer (30%) rebleed compared with those with duodenal ulcer. Most instances of rebleeding occur within 2 days from the time the first episode has stopped. In one study, only 3% of patients who stopped bleeding for this long bled again.

Endoscopic Therapy

Treatments administered through the endoscope may stop active bleeding or prevent rebleeding. Effective methods include injection into the ulcer of epinephrine, epinephrine plus 1% polidocanol (a sclerosing agent), or ethanol; or cautery using the heater probe, monopolar electrocautery, or the Nd:YAG laser. At least two modalities should be available to the endoscopist in the event one is unsuitable for a specific case or fails to work. Except for the laser, all are inexpensive. The indications for treatment are (1) active bleeding at the time of endoscopy and (2) the presence of a visible vessel in the base of the ulcer. Endoscopic therapy decreases transfusion requirements (by about half) and the rate of rebleeding (by about three-quarters) compared with sham-treated controls. When treatment fails the first time, it may often be repeated with a good chance of success. It is important, however, not to allow the patient to deteriorate during nonoperative attempts at halting the bleeding.

Emergency Surgery

Less than 10% of patients bleeding from a peptic ulcer require emergency surgery. Selection of those most likely to survive with surgical compared with medical treatment rests on the rate of blood loss and the other factors associated with a poor prognosis.

The overall death rate is significantly less after vagotomy and pyloroplasty than after gastrectomy for bleeding ulcer, and rebleeding occurs with about equal frequency after either procedure.

During laparotomy, the first step is to make a pyloroplasty incision if the endoscopic diagnosis is a bleeding duodenal ulcer. If a duodenal ulcer is found, the bleeding vessel should be suture-ligated and the duodenum and antrum inspected for additional ulcers. The pyloroplasty incision should then be closed and a truncal vagotomy performed. If the posterior wall of the duodenal bulb has been destroyed by a giant duodenal ulcer, a gastrectomy and Billroth II gastrojejunostomy may be preferable, since this somewhat uncommon ulcer is especially prone to bleed again if left in continuity with the stomach. Gastric ulcers can be handled by either gastrectomy or vagotomy and pyloroplasty. A thorough search should always be made for second ulcers or other causes of bleeding.

Prognosis

The death rate for an acute massive hemorrhage is about 15%. Careful study of the causes of death suggests that this figure could be improved by (1) more precise blood replacement–since undertransfusion is the cause of some complications and deaths; and (2) earlier surgery in selected patients who fall into serious-risk categories–since the tendency has been to perform surgery on too few patients too late in the illness. Patients who stop bleeding should be treated as outlined in the section on duodenal ulcer.

Rockall TA: Management and outcome of patients undergoing surgery after acute upper gastrointestinal haemorrhage. Steering Group for the National Audit of Acute Upper Gastrointestinal Haemorrhage. J R Soc Med 1998;91:518.

MALLORY-WEISS SYNDROME

Mallory-Weiss syndrome is responsible for about 10% of cases of acute upper gastrointestinal hemorrhage. The lesion consists of a 1- to 4-cm longitudinal tear in the gastric mucosa near the esophagogastric junction; it usually follows a bout of forceful retching. The disruption extends through the mucosa and submucosa but not usually into the muscularis mucosae. About 75% of these lesions are confined to the stomach; 20% straddle the esophagogastric junction; and 5% are entirely within the distal esophagus. Two-thirds of patients have a hiatal hernia.

The majority of patients are alcoholics, but the tear may appear after severe retching for any reason. Several cases have been reported following closed chest cardiac compression.

Clinical Findings

Typically, the patient first vomits food and gastric contents. This is followed by forceful retching and then bloody vomitus. Rapid increases in gastric pressure, sometimes aggravated by hiatal hernia, cause the tear. Actual rupture of the distal esophagus can also be produced by vomiting (Boerhaave's syndrome), but the difference seems to depend on vomiting of food in rupture and nonproductive retching in gastric mucosal tear.

Esophagogastroscopy is the most practical means of making the diagnosis.

Treatment & Prognosis

Initially, the patient is handled according to the general measures prescribed for upper gastrointestinal hemorrhage. In about 90% of patients, the bleeding stops spontaneously after ice-water lavage of the stomach. Patients who are still bleeding vigorously by the time endoscopy is performed are likely to require surgery. The bleeding can sometimes be controlled by endoscopic therapy (eg, electrocautery). If bleeding persists, surgical repair of the tear will be required.

If the diagnosis has been made before laparotomy, the surgeon should make a long, high gastrotomy after the abdomen is opened. The tear may be difficult to expose adequately. The search must be thorough, since in about 25% of patients there are two tears. A running polyglycolic acid (not catgut) suture should be used to oversew the lesion. Postoperative recurrence is rare.

Kortas DY: Mallory-Weiss tear: predisposing factors and predictors of a complicated course. Am J Gastroenterol 2001;96:2863.

Younes Z, Johnson DA: The spectrum of spontaneous and iatrogenic esophageal injury: perforations, Mallory-Weiss tears, and hematomas. J Clin Gastroenterol 1999;29:306.

PYLORIC OBSTRUCTION DUE TO PEPTIC ULCER

The cycles of inflammation and repair in peptic ulcer disease may cause obstruction of the gastroduodenal junction as a result of edema, muscular spasm, and scarring. To the extent that the first two factors are involved, the obstruction may be reversible with medical treatment.

Obstruction is usually due to duodenal ulcer and is less common than either bleeding or perforation. The few gastric ulcers that obstruct are close to the pylorus. Obstruction due to peptic ulcer must be differentiated from that caused by a malignant tumor of the antrum or of the pancreas. Malignancy is becoming the more common cause, and it may be difficult to identify.

Clinical Findings

A. Symptoms and Signs

Most patients with obstruction have a long history of symptomatic peptic ulcer, and as many as 30% have been treated for perforation or obstruction in the past. The patient often notes gradually increasing ulcer pains over weeks or months, with the eventual development of anorexia, vomiting, and failure to gain relief from antacids. The vomitus often contains food ingested several hours previously, and absence of bile staining reflects the site of blockage. Weight loss may be marked if the patient has delayed seeking medical care.

Dehydration and malnutrition may be obvious on physical examination but are not always present. A succussion splash can often be elicited from the retained gastric contents. Peristalsis of the distended stomach may be visible on gross inspection of the abdomen, but this sign is relatively rare. Most patients have upper abdominal tenderness. Tetany may appear with advanced alkalosis.

B. Laboratory Findings

Anemia is found in about 25% of patients. Prolonged vomiting leads to a unique form of metabolic alkalosis with dehydration. Measurement of serum electrolytes shows hypochloremia, hypokalemia, hyponatremia, and increased bicarbonate. Vomiting depletes the patient of Na^+, K^+, and Cl^-; the latter is lost in excess of Na^+ and K^+ as HCl. Gastric HCl loss causes extracellular HCO_3^- to rise, and renal excretion of HCO_3^- increases in an attempt to maintain pH. Large amounts of Na^+ are excreted in the urine with the HCO_3^-. Increasing Na^+ deficit evokes aldosterone secretion, which in turn brings about renal Na^+ conservation at the expense of more renal loss of K^+ and H^+. GFR may drop and produce a prerenal azotemia. The eventual result of the process is a marked deficit of Na^+, Cl^-, K^+, and H_2O. Treatment involves replacement of water and NaCl until a satisfactory urine flow has been established. KCl replacement should then be started. Details of management are found in Chapter 8.

C. Saline Load Test

This is a simple means of assessing the degree of pyloric obstruction and is useful in following the patient's progress during the first few days of nasogastric suction.

Through the nasogastric tube, 700 mL of normal saline (at room temperature) is infused over 3–5 minutes, and the tube is clamped. Thirty minutes later, the stomach is aspirated and the residual volume of saline recorded. Recovery of more than 350 mL indicates obstruction. It must be recognized that the results of a saline load test do not predict how well the stomach will handle solid food. Solid emptying can be measured with technetium Tc 99m-labeled chicken liver.

D. Imaging Studies

Plain abdominal x-rays may show a large gastric fluid level. An upper gastrointestinal series should not be performed until the stomach has been emptied, because dilution of the barium in the retained secretions makes a worthwhile study impossible.

E. Endoscopy

Gastroscopy is usually indicated to rule out the presence of an obstructing neoplasm.

Treatment

A. Medical Treatment

A large (32F) Ewald tube should be passed and the stomach emptied of its contents and lavaged until clean. After the stomach has been completely decompressed, a smaller tube should be inserted and placed on suction for several days to allow pyloric edema and spasm to subside and to permit the gastric musculature to regain its tone. A saline load test may be performed at this point to provide a baseline for later comparison. If chronic obstruction has produced severe malnutrition, total parenteral nutrition should be instituted.

After decompression of the stomach for 48–72 hours, the saline load test should be repeated. If this indicates sufficient improvement, the tube should be withdrawn and a liquid diet may be started. Gradual resumption of solid foods is permitted as tolerated.

B. Surgical Treatment

If 5–7 days of gastric aspiration do not result in relief of the obstruction, the patient should be treated surgically. Persistence of nonoperative effort beyond this point in the absence of progress rarely achieves the result hoped for. Failure of the obstruction to resolve completely (eg, if the patient can take only liquids) and recurrent obstruction of any degree are indications for surgery.

Surgical treatment may consist of a truncal or parietal cell vagotomy and drainage procedure (Figure 23–5). Truncal vagotomy and gastrojejunostomy is the easiest to perform laparoscopically.

Prognosis

About two-thirds of patients with acute obstruction fail to improve sufficiently on medical therapy and require operation to relieve the blockage. Patients who respond to medical treatment should be treated as outlined in the section on duodenal ulcer.

Jamieson GG: Current status of indications for surgery in peptic ulcer disease. World J Surg 2000;24:256.

PERFORATED PEPTIC ULCER

Perforation complicates peptic ulcer about half as often as hemorrhage. Most perforated ulcers are located anteriorly, though occasionally gastric ulcers perforate into the lesser sac. The 15% death rate correlates with increased age, female sex, and gastric perforations. The diagnosis is overlooked in about 5% of patients, most of whom do not survive.

Anterior ulcers tend to perforate instead of bleed because of the absence of protective viscera and major blood vessels on this surface. In less than 10% of cases, acute bleeding from a posterior "kissing" ulcer complicates the anterior perforation, an association that carries a high death rate. Immediately after perforation, the peritoneal cavity is flooded with gastroduodenal secretions that elicit a chemical peritonitis. Early cultures show either no growth or a light growth of streptococci or enteric bacilli. Gradually, over 12–24 hours, the process evolves into bacterial peritonitis. Severity of illness and occurrence of death are directly related to the interval between perforation and surgical closure.

In an unknown percentage of cases, the perforation becomes sealed by adherence to the undersurface of the liver. In such patients, the process may be self-limited, but a subphrenic abscess will develop in many.

Clinical Findings

A. Symptoms and Signs

The perforation usually elicits a sudden, severe upper abdominal pain whose onset can be recalled precisely. The patient may or may not have had preceding chronic symptoms of peptic ulcer disease. Perforation rarely is heralded by nausea or vomiting, and it typically occurs several hours after the last meal. Shoulder pain, if present, reflects diaphragmatic irritation. Back pain is uncommon.

The initial reaction consists of a chemical peritonitis caused by gastric acid or bile and pancreatic enzymes. The peritoneal reaction dilutes these irritants with a thin exudate, and as a result the patient's symptoms may temporarily improve before bacterial peritonitis occurs. The physician who sees the patient for the first time during this symptomatic lull must not be misled into interpreting it as representing bona fide improvement.

The patient appears severely distressed, lying quietly with the knees drawn up and breathing shallowly to minimize abdominal motion. Fever is absent at the start. The abdominal muscles are rigid owing to severe involuntary spasm. Epigastric tenderness may not be as marked as expected because the board-like rigidity protects the abdominal viscera from the palpating hand. Escaped air from the stomach may enter the space between the liver and abdominal wall, and upon percussion the normal dullness over the liver will be tympanitic. Peristaltic sounds are reduced or absent. If delay in treatment allows continued escape of air into the peritoneal cavity, abdominal distention and diffuse tympany may result.

The above description applies to the typical case of perforation with classic findings. In as many as one-third of patients, the presentation is not as dramatic, diagnosis is less obvious, and serious delays in treatment may result from failure to consider this condition and to obtain the appropriate abdominal x-rays. Many of these atypical perforations occur in patients already hospitalized for some unrelated illness, and the significance of the new symptom of abdominal pain is not appreciated. The only way to improve this record is to routinely obtain abdominal films on patients with abdominal pain of recent onset.

Lesser degrees of shock with minimal abdominal findings occur if the leak is small or rapidly sealed. A small duodenal perforation may slowly leak fluid that runs down the lateral peritoneal gutter, producing pain and muscular rigidity in the right lower quadrant and thus raising a problem of confusion with acute appendicitis.

Perforations may be sealed by omentum or by the liver, with the later development of a subhepatic or subdiaphragmatic abscess.

B. Laboratory Findings

A mild leukocytosis in the range of 12,000/μL is common in the early stages. After 12–24 hours, this may rise to 20,000/μL or more if treatment has been inadequate. The mild rise in the serum amylase value that occurs in many patients is probably caused by absorption of the enzyme from duodenal secretions within the peritoneal cavity. Direct measurement of fluid obtained by paracentesis may show very high levels of amylase.

C. Imaging Studies

Plain x-rays of the abdomen reveal free subdiaphragmatic air in 85% of patients. Films should be taken with the patient both supine and upright. A film in the left lateral decubitus position may be a more practical way to demonstrate free air in the uncomfortable patient. If the findings are questionable, 400 mL of air can be insufflated into the stomach through a nasogastric tube and the films repeated. Free air in the abdomen in a patient with sudden upper abdominal pain should clinch the diagnosis.

If no free air is demonstrated and the clinical picture suggests perforated ulcer, an emergency upper gastrointestinal series should be performed. If the perforation has not sealed, the diagnosis is established by noting escape of the contrast material from the lumen. Barium is more reliable than water-soluble contrast media, and, contrary to previous views, does not appear to aggravate infection or to be difficult to remove.

Differential Diagnosis

The differential diagnosis includes acute pancreatitis and acute cholecystitis. The former does not have as explosive an onset as perforated ulcer and is usually accompanied by a high serum amylase level. Acute cholecystitis with perforated gallbladder could mimic perforated ulcer closely but free air would not be present with ruptured gallbladder. Intestinal obstruction has a more gradual onset and is characterized by less sever pain that is crampy and accompanied by vomiting.

The simultaneous onset of pain and free air in the abdomen in the absence of trauma usually means perforated peptic ulcer. Free perforation of colonic diverticulitis and acute appendicitis are other rare causes.

Treatment

The diagnosis is often suspected before the patient is sent for confirmatory x-rays. Whenever a perforated ulcer is considered, the first step should be to pass a nasogastric tube and empty the stomach to reduce further contamination of the peritoneal cavity. Blood should be drawn for laboratory studies, and intravenous antibiotics (eg, cefazolin, cefoxitin) should be started. If the patient's overall condition is precarious owing to delay in treatment, fluid resuscitation should precede diagnostic measures. X-rays should be obtained as soon as the clinical status will permit.

The simplest surgical treatment, laparoscopy (or laparotomy) and suture closure of the perforation solves the immediate problem. The closure most often consists of securely plugging the hole with omentum (Graham-Steele closure) sutured into place rather than bringing together the two edges with sutures. All fluid should be aspirated from the peritoneal cavity, but drainage is not indicated. Reperforation is rare in the immediate postoperative period.

About three-fourths of patients whose perforation is the culmination of a history of chronic symptoms continue to have clinically severe ulcer disease after simple closure. This has gradually led to a more aggressive treatment policy involving a definitive ulcer operation for most patients with acute perforation, eg, parietal cell vagotomy plus closure of the perforation or truncal vagotomy and pyloroplasty. Now that ulcer disease can be cured by eradicating *H pylori,* the value of anything more than simple closure will have to be reexamined.

Concomitant hemorrhage and perforation are most often due to two ulcers, an anterior perforated one and a posterior one that is bleeding. Perforated ulcers that also obstruct obviously cannot be treated by suture closure of the perforation alone. Vagotomy plus gastroenterostomy or pyloroplasty should be performed. Perforated anastomotic ulcers require a vagotomy or gastrectomy, since in the long run, closure alone is nearly always inadequate.

Nonoperative treatment of perforated ulcer consists of continuous gastric suction and the administration of antibiotics in high doses. Although this has been shown to be effective therapy, with a low death rate, it is occasionally accompanied by a peritoneal and subphrenic abscess, and side effects are greater than with laparoscopic closure.

Prognosis

About 15% of patients with perforated ulcer die, and about a third of these are undiagnosed before surgery. The death rate of perforated ulcer seen early is low. Delay in treatment, advanced age, and associated systemic diseases account for most deaths.

Donovan AJ, Berne TV, Donovan JA: Perforated duodenal ulcer: an alternative therapeutic plan. Arch Surg 1998;133:1166.

Hernandez-Diaz S, Rodriguez LA: Association between nonsteroidal anti-inflammatory drugs and upper gastrointestinal tract bleeding/perforation: an overview of epidemiologic studies published in the 1990s. Arch Intern Med 2000;160:2093.

Memon MA, Fitzgibbons RJ Jr: The role of minimal access surgery in the acute abdomen. Surg Clin North Am 1997;77:1333.

Millat B, Fingerhut A, Borie F: Surgical treatment of complicated duodenal ulcers: controlled trials. World J Surg 2000;24:299.

Svanes C: Trends in perforated peptic ulcer: incidence, etiology, treatment, and prognosis. World J Surg 2000;24:277.

STRESS GASTRODUODENITIS, STRESS ULCER & ACUTE HEMORRHAGIC GASTRITIS

The term stress ulcer has been used to refer to a heterogeneous group of acute gastric or duodenal ulcers that develop following physiologically stressful illnesses. There are four major etiologic factors associated with such lesions: (1) shock, (2) sepsis, (3) burns, and (4) central nervous system tumors or trauma.

Etiology

A. Stress Ulcer

Acute ulcers following major surgery, mechanical ventilation, shock, sepsis, and burns (Curling's ulcers) have

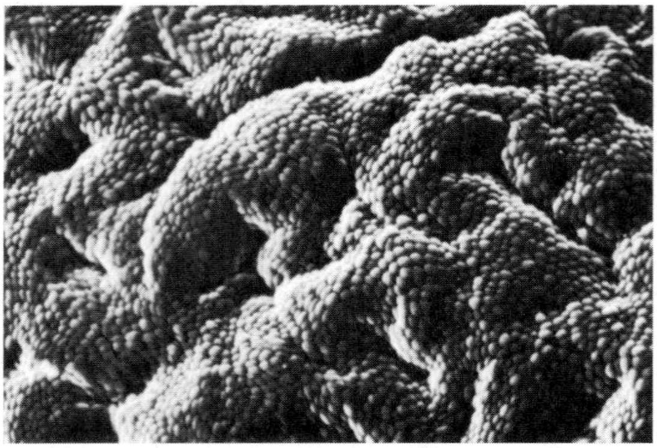

Figure 23–7. Scanning electron photomicrograph of the surface epithelium of a normal subject showing individual cells and numerous gastric pits. (Reduced from × 350.) (Courtesy of Jeanne M. Riddle.)

enough common features to suggest they evolve by a similar pathogenetic mechanism

Hemorrhage is the major clinical problem, though perforation occurs in about 10% of cases. Despite the predilection of stress ulcers to develop in the parietal cell mucosa, in about 30% of patients the duodenum is affected, and sometimes both stomach and duodenum are involved. Morphologically, the ulcers are shallow, discrete lesions with congestion and edema but little inflammatory reaction at their margins. Gastroduodenal endoscopy performed early in traumatized or burned patients has shown acute gastric erosions in the majority of patients within 72 hours after the injury (Figures 23–7 and 23–8). Such studies illustrate how frequently the disease process remains subclinical; clinically apparent ulcers develop in about 20% of susceptible patients. Clinically evident bleeding is usually seen 3–5 days after the injury, and massive bleeding generally does not appear until 4–5 days later.

Decreased mucosal resistance is the first step, which may involve the effects of ischemia (with production of toxic superoxide and hydroxyl radicals) and circulating toxins, followed by decreased mucosal renewal, decreased production of endogenous prostanoids, and thinning of the surface mucus layer. Decreased gastric mucosal blood flow also plays a role by decreasing the supply of blood buffers available to neutralize hydrogen ions that are diffusing into the weakened mucosa. Experimental evidence has implicated platelet-activating factor, released by endotoxin, as a possible mediator of gut ulceration in sepsis. The mucosa is thus rendered more vulnerable to acid-pepsin ulceration and lysosomal enzymes. Acid hypersecretion may be involved to some extent, since burn patients who manifest serious bleeding have higher gastric acid output than patients with a more benign course. Disruption of the gastric mucosal barrier to back diffusion of acid has been found in less than half of patients and is now thought to be a manifestation of the disease rather than a cause.

B. Cushing's Ulcers

Acute ulcers associated with central nervous system tumors or injuries differ from stress ulcers because they are associated with elevated levels of serum gastrin and increased gastric acid secretion. Morphologically, they are similar to ordinary gastroduodenal peptic ulcers. Cushing's ulcers are more prone to perforate than other kinds of stress ulcers.

C. Acute Hemorrhagic Gastritis

This disorder may share some causative factors with the above conditions, but the natural history is different and the response to treatment considerably better. Most of these patients can be controlled medically. When surgery is required for alcoholic gastritis, a high proportion of patients are cured by pyloroplasty and vagotomy.

Clinical Findings

Hemorrhage is nearly always the first manifestation. Pain rarely occurs. Physical examination is not contributory except to reveal gross or occult fecal blood or signs of shock.

Prevention

H_2 receptor antagonists given prophylactically to critically ill patients decrease the incidence of stress erosions

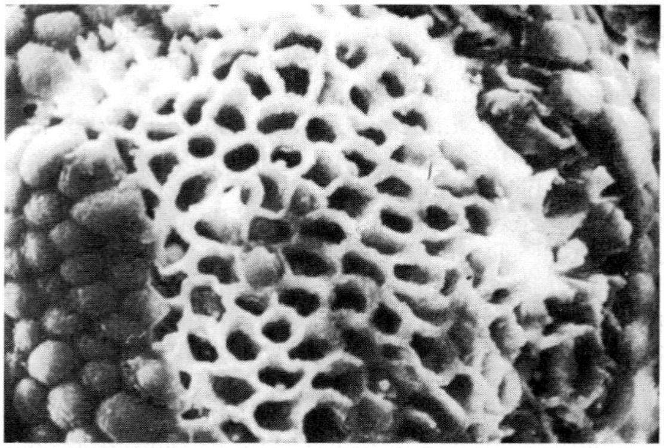

Figure 23–8. Scanning electron photomicrograph of the surface epithelium of a patient with acute gastric mucosal erosions, showing a patch of cellular defoliation. Lesions such as this may account for back diffusion of H^+. (Reduced from × 1145.) (Courtesy of Jeanne M. Riddle.)

and overt bleeding. The drug may be given orally (eg, ranitidine, 150 mg through a nasogastric tube every 12 hours) or intravenously (eg, cimetidine, 50–100 mg/h). Sucralfate is also effective. Patients receiving total parenteral nutrition appear to be protected by this therapy and experience no increased benefit from H_2 antagonists. A concern that decreasing gastric acidity with H_2 blocking agents would increase the rate and severity of nosocomial pneumonia (from gastric bacterial overgrowth) has not been justified by experience.

Treatment

Initial management should consist of gastric lavage with chilled solutions and measures to combat sepsis if present. H_2 receptor blockers are of no value in the actively bleeding patient, but they probably decrease the rate of rebleeding once bleeding has stopped.

Some success has been reported with the selective infusion of vasoconstricting agents (eg, vasopressin) into the left gastric artery through a percutaneously placed catheter. In the sickest patients, if facilities and trained personnel are available, this technique should probably be attempted before operation is considered.

Perform laparotomy if the nonoperative regimen fails to halt the bleeding. Surgical treatment should consist of vagotomy and pyloroplasty, with suture of the bleeding points, or vagotomy and subtotal gastrectomy. There is a trend toward the first of these options, particularly in the sickest patients. When it occurs, rebleeding is nearly always from an ulcer left behind at the initial procedure. Rarely, total gastrectomy has had to be used because of the extent of ulceration and severity of bleeding or because of rebleeding after a lesser operation.

Felig DM, Carafa CJ: Stress ulcers of the stomach. Gastrointest Endosc 2000;51:596.

Phillips JO et al: A randomized, pharmacokinetic and pharmacodynamic, cross-over study of duodenal or jejunal administration compared to nasogastric administration of omeprazole suspension in patients at risk for stress ulcers. Am J Gastroenterol 2001;96:367.

GASTRIC CARCINOMA

There are about 20,000 new cases of carcinoma of the stomach in the USA annually. The incidence has dropped to one-third of what it was 35 years ago. This may reflect changes in the prevalence of *H pylori* infection, which has a role in the etiology of this disease. *H pylori* is known to be a cause of chronic atrophic gastritis, which in turn is a recognized precursor of gastric adenocarcinoma. Epidemiologic studies have linked gastric *H pylori* infection with a 3.6- to 18-fold (all patients versus women) increase in the risk of developing carcinoma of the body or antrum (not the cardia), and the risk is proportionate to serum levels of *H pylori* antibodies.

The present incidence in American males is ten new cases per 100,000 population per year. The highest rate, 63 per 100,000 males, is seen in Costa Rica; in eastern and central European countries, it is about 35 per 100,000 per year. Epidemiologic studies suggest that the incidence of gastric carcinoma is related to low dietary intake of vegetables and fruits and high intake of starches. Carcinoma of the stomach is rare under age 40, from which point the risk gradually climbs. The mean age at discovery is 63. It is about twice as common in men as in women.

Gastric epithelial cancers are nearly always adenocarcinomas. Squamous cell tumors of the proximal stomach involve the stomach secondarily from the esophagus. Five morphologic subdivisions correlate loosely with the natural history and outcome.

1. Ulcerating carcinoma (25%)—This consists of a deep, penetrating ulcer-tumor that extends through all layers of the stomach. It may involve adjacent organs in the process. The edges are shallow by contrast with overhanging edges noted in benign ulcers.

2. Polypoid carcinomas (25%)—These are large, bulky intraluminal growths that tend to metastasize late.

3. Superficial spreading carcinoma (15%)—Also known as early gastric cancer, superficial spreading carcinoma is confined to the mucosa and submucosa. Metastases are present in only 30% of cases. Even when metastases are present, the prognosis after gastrectomy is much better than for the more deeply invading lesions of advanced gastric cancer. In Japan, screening programs have been so successful that early gastric cancer now constitutes 30% of surgical cases, and survival rates have improved accordingly.

4. Linitis plastica (10%)—This variety of spreading tumor involves all layers with a marked desmoplastic reaction in which it may be difficult to identify the malignant cells. The stomach loses its pliability. Cure is rare because of early spread.

5. Advanced carcinoma (35%)—This largest category contains the big tumors that are found partly within and partly outside the stomach. They may originally have qualified for inclusion in the preceding groups but have outgrown that early stage.

Gastric adenocarcinomas can also be classified by degree of differentiation of their cells. In general, rate and extent of spread correlate with lack of differentiation. Some tumors are found histologically to excite an inflammatory cell reaction at their borders, and this feature indicates a relatively good prognosis. Tumors whose cells form glandular structures (intestinal type)

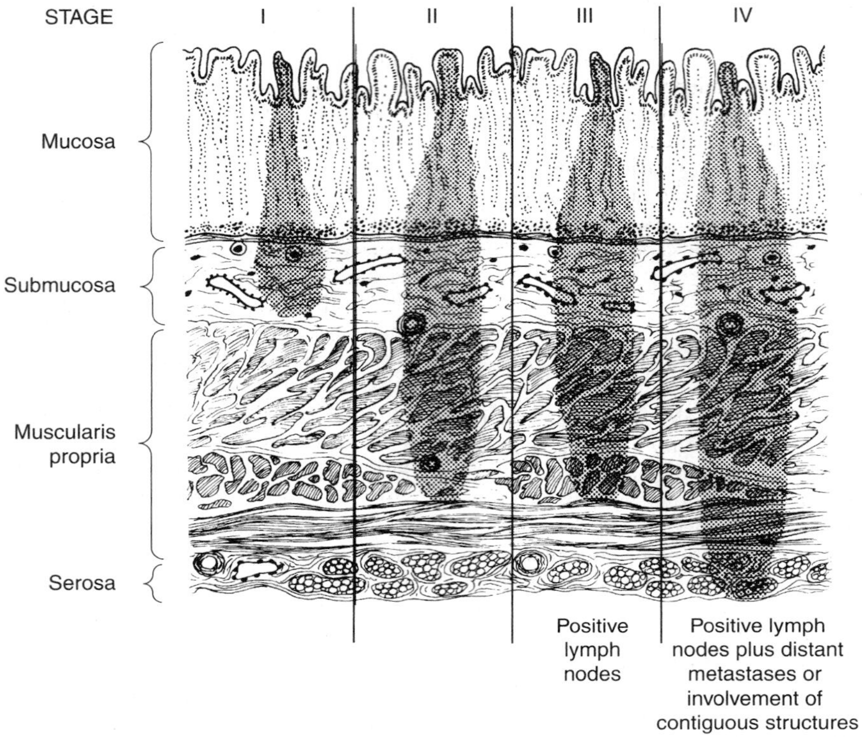

Figure 23–9. Staging system for gastric carcinoma. The darkly shadowed areas represent cancers with different depths of mucosal penetration.

have a somewhat better prognosis than tumors whose cells do not (diffuse type); the diffuse type is often associated with a substantial stromal component. The intestinal type of tumor accounts for a much larger proportion of cases in countries such as Japan and Finland where gastric cancer is especially common. The gradual decline in incidence in these areas is due principally to decreased occurrence of the intestinal type of tumor. Signet ring carcinomas, which contain more than 50% signet ring cells, have become increasingly more common and now constitute one-third of all cases. They behave as the diffuse type of cancer and occur more frequently in women, in younger patients, and in the distal part of the stomach. Previous *H pylori* infection is not associated with the development of any specific histologic type of gastric cancer.

Extension occurs by intramural spread, direct extraluminal growth, and lymphatic metastases. Pathologic staging, which correlates closely with survival, is illustrated in Figure 23–9. Three-fourths of patients have metastases when first seen. Within the stomach, proximal spread exceeds distal spread. The pylorus acts as a partial barrier, but tumor is found in 25% of cases in the first few centimeters of the bulb.

Early gastric cancer, defined as a primary lesion confined to the mucosa and submucosa with or without lymph node metastases, is associated with an excellent prognosis (5-year survival rate of 90%) after resection. In Japan, mass screening programs detect about 30% of patients with this lesion, whereas in the USA, only 10% of patients have early gastric cancer.

Forty percent of tumors are in the antrum, predominantly on the lesser curvature; 30% arise in the body and fundus, 25% at the cardia, and 5% involve the entire organ. Frequency of location has gradually changed, so that proximal lesions are more common now than 10–20 years ago. Benign ulcers develop at the greater curvature and cardia less commonly than malignant ones. Ulcers at these points are particularly suspect for neoplasm.

Clinical Findings

A. Symptoms and Signs

The earliest symptom is usually vague postprandial abdominal heaviness that the patient does not identify as a pain. Sometimes the discomfort is no different from other vague dyspeptic symptoms that have been intermittently present for years, but the frequency and persistence are new.

Anorexia develops early and may be most pronounced for meat. Weight loss, the most common symptom, averages about 6 kg. True postprandial pain suggesting a benign gastric ulcer is relatively uncommon, but if it is present one may be misled if subsequent x-rays show an ulcer. Vomiting may be present and becomes a major feature if pyloric obstruction occurs. It may have a coffee-ground appearance owing to bleeding by the tumor. Dysphagia may be the presenting symptom of lesions at the cardia.

An epigastric mass can be felt on examination in about one-fourth of cases. Hepatomegaly is present in 10% of cases. The stool will be positive for occult blood in half of patients, and melena is seen in a few. Otherwise, abnormal physical findings are confined to signs of distant spread of the tumor. Metastases to the neck along the thoracic duct may produce a Virchow node. Rectal examination may reveal a Blumer shelf, a solid peritoneal deposit anterior to the rectum. Enlarged ovaries (Krukenberg tumors) may be caused by intraperitoneal metastases. Further dissemination may involve the liver, lungs, brain, or bone.

B. Laboratory Findings

Anemia is present in 40% of patients. Carcinoembryonic antigen (CEA) levels are elevated in 65%, usually indicating extensive spread of the tumor.

C. Imaging Studies

An upper gastrointestinal series is diagnostic for many tumors, but the overall false-negative rate is about 20%. Major diagnostic problems are posed by ulcerating tumors, a few of which may not be distinguishable radiologically from benign peptic ulcers. The differential features are listed in the section on gastric ulcer, but x-rays alone will not establish a diagnosis of benign ulcer. All patients with a newly discovered gastric ulcer should undergo gastroscopy and gastric biopsy.

D. Gastroscopy and Biopsy

Large gastric carcinomas can usually be identified as such by their gross appearance at endoscopy. All gastric lesions, whether polypoid or ulcerating, should be examined by taking multiple biopsy and brush cytology specimens during endoscopy. False results are seen occasionally as a result of sampling error, and a minimum of six biopsies is necessary for greatest accuracy.

Treatment

Surgical resection is the only curative treatment. About 85% of patients are operable, and in 50% the lesions are amenable to resection; of the resectable lesions, half are potentially curable (ie, no signs of spread beyond the limits of resection).

The surgical objective should be to remove the tumor, an adjacent uninvolved margin of stomach and duodenum, the regional lymph nodes, and, if necessary, portions of involved adjacent organs. The proximal margin should be a minimum of 6 cm from the gross tumor. If the tumor is located in the antrum, a curative resection would entail distal gastrectomy with en bloc removal of the omentum, a 3- to 4-cm cuff of duodenum and the subpyloric lymph nodes, and, in some instances, excision of the left gastric artery and nearby lymph nodes. Reconstruction after gastrectomy may be by either a Billroth I or II procedure, but the latter is preferable because postoperative growth of residual tumor near the pylorus may obstruct a gastroduodenal anastomosis early.

Total gastrectomy with splenectomy is required for tumors of the proximal half of the stomach and for extensive tumors (eg, linitis plastica). Whether or not the spleen should be removed in such cases is a subject of debate. Alimentary continuity is most often reestablished by a Roux-en-Y esophagojejunostomy. Construction of an intestinal pouch as a substitute food reservoir (eg, Hunt-Lawrence pouch) is of no nutritional value, and it increases the risks of immediate complications.

Esophagogastrectomy plus splenectomy with intrathoracic esophagogastrostomy is the operation usually performed for tumors of the cardia. The procedure is usually done through two separate incisions: first, a laparotomy for the gastric part, and then a right posterolateral thoracotomy for the anastomosis.

Japanese surgeons have devised a more detailed staging system than the one used in most other countries and have also recommended more aggressive lymphadenectomy as a matter of routine in the resection of gastric cancers. The results of resections as reported from Japan are better than those obtained by the standard operations described above, so attempts are being made to determine whether the difference is due to the more radical operations. Most Western surgeons are skeptical, and radical lymphadenectomy (eg, clearing all nodal levels up to and including the para-aortic nodes) is not recommended at present.

The propensity for proximal submucosal spread must be appreciated at surgery. It is often advisable to perform a frozen section at the proximal margin before constructing the anastomosis. If tumor is found, the gastrectomy should be extended.

Palliative resection is usually indicated if the stomach is still movable and life expectancy is estimated to be more than 1–2 months. Palliative gastrectomy is usually performed to remove an antral lesion and prevent obstruction, but in selected cases, total gastrectomy is appropriate palliative treatment if the operation can be done safely and the amount of extragastric tumor is minimal. Whenever technically feasible, palliative gastrectomy is preferable to palliative gastrojejunostomy.

Adjuvant chemotherapy after curative surgery has not been of value with the regimens tested to date. For advanced disease, doxorubicin or fluorouracil alone, each of which results in a 20% response rate, is as good as a combination of chemotherapeutic agents.

Prognosis

In the USA, the overall 5-year survival rate is about 12%. The 5-year survival rate for patients with early gastric cancer is about 90%. The 5-year survival rates in relation to the extent of spread are stage I, 70%; stage II, 30%; stage III, 10%; and stage IV, 0%.

Death from tumor may follow dissemination to other organs or may be the result of progressive gastric obstruction and malnutrition.

Ceelen WP et al: Hyperthermic intraperitoneal chemoperfusion in the treatment of locally advanced intra-abdominal cancer. Br J Surg 2000;87:1006.

De Vivo R et al: The role of chemotherapy in the management of gastric cancer. J Clin Gastroenterol 2000;30:364.

Gastric cancer and *Helicobacter pylori:* a combined analysis of 12 case control studies nested within prospective cohorts. Gut 2001;49:347.

Hardman MJ et al: Barrier formation in the human fetus is patterned. J Invest Dermatol 1999;113:1106.

Hulscher JB et al: Prospective analysis of the diagnostic yield of extended en bloc resection for adenocarcinoma of the oesophagus or gastric cardia. Br J Surg 2001;88:715.

Huntsman DG et al: Early gastric cancer in young, asymptomatic carriers of germ-line E-cadherin mutations. N Engl J Med 2001;344:1904.

Kalmar K et al: Comparison of quality of life and nutritional parameters after total gastrectomy and a new type of pouch construction with simple Roux-en-Y reconstruction: preliminary results of a prospective, randomized, controlled study. Dig Dis Sci 2001;46:1791.

Kelly S et al: A systematic review of the staging performance of endoscopic ultrasound in gastro-oesophageal carcinoma. Gut 2001;49:534.

Lee HK et al: Influence of the number of lymph nodes examined on staging of gastric cancer. Br J Surg 2001;88:1408.

Macdonald JS et al: Chemoradiotherapy after surgery compared with surgery alone for adenocarcinoma of the stomach or gastroesophageal junction. N Engl J Med 2001;345:725.

Yasuda K et al: Risk factors for complications following resection of large gastric cancer. Br J Surg 2001;88:873.

GASTRIC POLYPS

Gastric polyps are single or multiple benign tumors that occur predominantly in the elderly. Those located in the distal stomach are more apt to cause symptoms. Whenever gastric polyps are discovered, gastric cancer must be ruled out.

Gastric polyps can be classified histologically as hyperplastic, adenomatous, or inflammatory. Other polypoid lesions, such as leiomyomas and carcinoid tumors, are discussed elsewhere. Hyperplastic polyps, which constitute 80% of cases, consist of an overgrowth of normal epithelium; they are not true neoplasms and have no relationship to gastric cancer. About 30% of adenomatous polyps contain a focus of adenocarcinoma, and adenocarcinoma can be found elsewhere in the stomach in 20% of patients with a benign adenomatous polyp. The incidence of cancer in an adenomatous polyp rises with increasing size. Lesions with a stalk and those less than 2 cm in diameter are usually not malignant. About 10% of benign adenomatous polyps undergo malignant change during prolonged follow-up.

Anemia may develop from chronic blood loss or deficient iron absorption. Over 90% of patients are achlorhydric after maximal stimulation. Vitamin B_{12} absorption is deficient in 25%, although megaloblastic anemia is present in only a few. Exfoliative cytologic examination of specimens obtained by endoscopy and brush biopsy should be performed in all patients.

Excision with a snare through the endoscope can be performed safely for most polyps. Otherwise, laparotomy is indicated for polyps greater than 1 cm in diameter or when cancer is suspected. Single polyps may be excised through a gastrotomy and a frozen section performed. If the polyp is found to be carcinoma, an appropriate type of gastrectomy is indicated. Partial gastrectomy should be performed for multiple polyps in the distal stomach. If 10–20 polyps are distributed throughout the stomach, the antrum should be removed and the fundic polyps excised. Total gastrectomy may be required for symptomatic diffuse multiple polyposis.

These patients should be followed because they have an increased risk of late development of pernicious anemia or gastric cancer. Recurrent polyps are uncommon.

Abraham SC et al: Hyperplastic polyps of the stomach: associations with histologic patterns of gastritis and gastric atrophy. Am J Surg Pathol 2001;25:500.

Karheuser A et al: Familial adenomatous polyposis associated with multiple adrenal adenomas in a patient with a rare 3' APC mutation. J Med Genet 1999;36:65.

Ohkusa T et al: Disappearance of hyperplastic polyps in the stomach after eradication of *Helicobacter pylori.* A randomized, clinical trial. Ann Intern Med 1998;129:712.

GASTRIC LYMPHOMA & PSEUDOLYMPHOMA

Lymphoma is the second most common primary cancer of the stomach but constitutes only 2% of the total number, 95% being adenocarcinomas. Almost all are non-

Hodgkin's lymphomas and are generally classified as B cell mucosa-associated lymphoid tissue (MALT) lymphomas. They are further subclassified as low-grade or high-grade based on nuclear pattern. About 20% of patients manifest a second primary cancer in another organ.

The principal symptoms are epigastric pain and weight loss, similar to those of carcinoma. Characteristically, the tumor has attained bulky proportions by the time it is discovered; by comparison with adenocarcinoma of the stomach, the symptoms from a gastric lymphoma are usually mild in relation to the size of the lesion. A palpable epigastric mass is present in 50% of patients. Barium x-ray studies will demonstrate the lesion, although it usually is mistaken for adenocarcinoma or, in 10% of cases, for benign gastric ulcer. Gastroscopy with biopsy and brush cytology provides the correct diagnosis preoperatively in about 75% of cases. If a pathologic diagnosis has not been made, the surgeon may incorrectly judge the lesion to be inoperable carcinoma because of its large size. Preoperative staging should include a CT scan and bone marrow biopsy.

Treatment of low-grade gastric lymphoma consists of long-term chemotherapy with cyclophosphamide. Surgical resection followed by total abdominal radiotherapy may be the treatment of choice for high-grade lymphomas, but the subject is debated. Intraoperative staging should consist of needle biopsies of both lobes of the liver and biopsies of celiac and para-aortic lymph nodes. Splenectomy should be performed only if the spleen is directly invaded. Extension into the duodenum or esophagus should not lead to resection of these organs but to postoperative adjunctive therapy. The 5-year disease-free survival rate is 50%. Survival correlates with stage of disease, extent of penetration of the gastric wall, and histologic grade of the tumor. Most recurrences appear within 2 years of surgery. Because two-thirds of recurrences are outside the abdomen, patients at high risk of recurrence should receive postoperative chemotherapy also.

Gastric pseudolymphoma consists of a mass of lymphoid tissue in the gastric wall, often associated with an overlying mucosal ulcer. It is thought to represent a response to chronic inflammation. The lesion is not malignant, though the presentation, which includes pain, weight loss, and a mass on barium studies, cannot be distinguished from that of a malignant lesion.

Treatment of gastric pseudolymphoma consists of resection. The distinction from lymphoma is made on histologic examination of the specimen, which shows mature germinal centers in pseudolymphoma. No additional therapy is indicated postoperatively.

Crump M, Gospodarowicz M, Shepherd FA: Lymphoma of the gastrointestinal tract. Semin Oncol 1999;26:324.

Kolve ME, Fischbach W, Wilhelm M: Primary gastric non-Hodgkin's lymphoma: requirements for diagnosis and staging. Recent Results Cancer Res 2000;156:63.

Steinbach G et al: Antibiotic treatment of gastric lymphoma of mucosa-associated lymphoid tissue. An uncontrolled trial. Ann Intern Med 1999;131:88.

Yamashita H et al: When can complete regression of low-grade gastric lymphoma of mucosa-associated lymphoid tissue be predicted after *Helicobacter pylori* eradication? Histopathology 2000;37:131.

GASTRIC LEIOMYOMAS & GASTROINTESTINAL STROMAL TUMOR (GIST)

Leiomyomas are common submucosal growths that are usually asymptomatic but may cause intestinal bleeding. GIST (previously called leiomyosarcomas) may grow to a large size and most often present with bleeding. Radiologically, the tumor usually contains a central ulceration caused by necrosis from outgrowth of its blood supply. In most cases the tumor arises from the proximal stomach. It may grow into the gastric lumen, remain entirely on the serosal surface, or even become pedunculated within the abdominal cavity. Spread is by direct invasion or blood-borne metastases. CT scans provide useful information on the amount of extragastric extension. Leiomyomas should be removed by enucleation or wedge resection. After the more radical resections required for leiomyosarcomas, the 5-year survival rate is 20%. If technically possible, complete resection of metastases (eg, peritoneal, hepatic) in addition to the primary may improve the outcome. The results are affected by tumor size, DNA ploidy pattern, and tumor grade. Lesions that exhibit ten or more mitoses in a high-powered field rarely can be cured. The tumor is resistant to radiotherapy. Imatinib mesylate (Gleevec) is an effective systemic agent. It is used for disseminated disease and is in trials for adjuvant use.

MÉNÉTRIER'S DISEASE

Ménétrier's disease, a form of hypertrophic gastritis, consists of giant hypertrophy of the gastric rugae; high, normal, or low acid secretion; and excessive loss of protein from the thickened mucosa into the gut, with resulting hypoproteinemia. The etiology may involve altered expression of TGFα. Clinical manifestations include edema, diarrhea, anorexia, weight loss, and skin rash. Chronic blood loss may also be a problem. Indigestion may respond to antacids, but this treatment does not improve the gastric pathologic process or secondary hypoproteinemia. The hypertrophic rugae present as enormous filling defects on upper gastrointestinal series and are frequently misinterpreted as carcinoma. The protein leak from the gastric mucosa may respond to atropine (and other anticholinergic drugs), hexamethonium bromide, eradication of *H pylori,* or H_2 blocking agents or omeprazole. Rarely, total gastrectomy is indicated for severe intractable hypoproteinemia, anemia, or inability to exclude cancer. Medical management is best for most patients, though the gastric abnormalities and hypoproteinemia may persist. Some cases gradually evolve into atrophic gastritis. In children the disease characteristically is self-limited and benign. There is an increased risk of adenocarcinoma of the stomach in adults with Ménétrier's disease.

Badov D et al: *Helicobacter pylori* as a pathogenic factor in Menetrier's disease. Am J Gastroenterol 1998;93:1976.

Burdick JS et al: Treatment of Menetrier's disease with a monoclonal antibody against the epidermal growth factor receptor. N Engl J Med 2000;343:1697.

Madsen LG et al: Menetrier's disease and *Helicobacter pylori:* normalization of gastrointestinal protein loss after eradication therapy. Dig Dis Sci 1999;44:2307.

PROLAPSE OF THE GASTRIC MUCOSA

This uncommon lesion occasionally accompanies small prepyloric gastric ulcers. Episodes of vomiting and abdominal pain simulate peptic ulcer disease. X-ray shows prolapse of antral folds into the duodenum. One must be alert to the presence of gastric or duodenal ulcer as the underlying cause.

Antrectomy with a Billroth I anastomosis is occasionally required. Generally, conservative treatment suffices.

GASTRIC VOLVULUS

The stomach may rotate about its longitudinal axis (organo-axial volvulus) or a line drawn from the mid lesser to the mid greater curvature (mesenterioaxial volvulus). The former is more common and is often associated with a paraesophageal hiatal hernia. In other patients, eventration of the left diaphragm allows the colon to rise and twist the stomach by pulling on the gastrocolic ligament.

Acute gastric volvulus produces severe abdominal pain accompanied by a diagnostic triad (Borchardt's triad): (1) vomiting followed by retching and then inability to vomit, (2) epigastric distention, and (3) inability to pass a nasogastric tube. The situation calls for immediate laparotomy to prevent death from acute gastric necrosis and shock. An emergency upper gastrointestinal series will show a block at the point of the volvulus. The death rate is high.

Chronic volvulus is more common than acute. It may be asymptomatic or may cause crampy intermittent pain. Cases associated with paraesophageal hiatal hernia should be treated by repair of the hernia and anterior gastropexy. When cases are due to eventration of the diaphragm, the gastrocolic ligament should be divided the entire length of the greater curvature. The colon rises to fill the space caused by the eventration, and the stomach will resume its normal position, to be fastened by a gastropexy.

GASTRIC DIVERTICULA

Gastric diverticula are uncommon and usually asymptomatic. Most are pulsion diverticula consisting of mucosa and submucosa only, located on the lesser curvature within a few centimeters of the esophagogastric junction. Those in the prepyloric region generally possess all layers and are more likely to be symptomatic. A few patients have symptoms from hemorrhage of inflammation within a gastric diverticulum, but for the most part these lesions are incidental findings on upper gastrointestinal series. Radiologically, they can be confused with a gastric ulcer.

BEZOAR

Bezoars are concretions formed in the stomach. Trichobezoars are composed of hair and are usually found in young girls who pick at their hair and swallow it. Phytobezoars consist of agglomerated vegetable fibers. Pressure by the mass can create a gastric ulcer that is prone to bleed or perforate.

The postgastrectomy state predisposes to bezoar formation because pepsin and acid secretion are reduced and the triturating function of the antrum is gone. Orange segments or other fruits that contain a large amount of cellulose have been implicated in most cases. Improper mastication of food is a contributing factor that can sometimes be obviated by providing the patient with properly fitted dentures. The fruit may remain in the stomach or pass into the small intestine and cause obstruction. Some surgeons routinely warn postgastrectomy patients to avoid citrus fruits.

Large semisolid bezoars of *Candida albicans* have also been found in postgastrectomy patients. Some can be fragmented with the gastroscope. The patient should also be treated with oral nystatin.

Patients with symptomatic gastric bezoars may complain of abdominal pain. Ulceration and bleeding are associated with a death rate of 20%.

Nearly all gastric bezoars can be broken up and dispersed by endoscopy. Neglected lesions with complications (ie, bleeding or perforation) require gastrectomy.

II. DUODENUM

DUODENAL DIVERTICULA

Diverticula of the duodenum are found in 20% of autopsies and 5–10% of upper gastrointestinal series. Symptoms are uncommon, and only 1% of those found by x-ray warrant surgery.

Duodenal pulsion diverticula are acquired outpouchings of the mucosa and submucosa, 90% of which are on the medial aspect of the duodenum. They are rare before age 40. Most are solitary and within 2.5 cm of the ampulla of Vater. There is a high incidence of gallstone disease of the gallbladder in patients with juxtapapillary diverticula. Diverticula are not seen in the first portion of the duodenum, where diverticular configurations are due to scarring by peptic ulceration or cholecystitis.

A few patients have chronic postprandial abdominal pain or dyspepsia caused by a duodenal diverticulum. Treatment is with antacids and anticholinergics.

Serious complications are hemorrhage or perforation from inflammation, pancreatitis, and biliary obstruction. Bile acid-bilirubinate enteroliths are occasionally formed by bile stasis in a diverticulum. Enteroliths can precipitate diverticular inflammation or biliary obstruction and, rarely, have caused bowel obstruction after entering the intestinal lumen.

Surgical treatment is required for complications and, rarely, for persistent symptoms. Excision and a two-layer closure are usually possible after mobilization of the duodenum and dissection of the diverticulum from the pancreas. Removal of the diverticulum and closure of the defect are superior to simple drainage in the case of perforation. If biliary obstruction appears in a patient whose bile duct empties into a diverticulum, excision might be more hazardous than a side-to-side choledochoduodenostomy.

The rare wind sock type of intraluminal diverticulum usually presents with vague epigastric pain and postprandial fullness, though intestinal bleeding or pancreatitis is occasionally seen. The diagnosis can be made by barium x-ray studies. The diverticulum can be excised through a nearby duodenotomy. In some cases, the narrow diverticular outlet can be enlarged endoscopically.

Lobo DN et al: Periampullary diverticula and pancreaticobiliary disease. Br J Surg 1999;86:588.

DUODENAL TUMORS

Tumors of the duodenum are rare. Carcinoma of the ampulla of Vater is discussed in Chapter 26.

1. Malignant Duodenal Tumors

Most malignant duodenal tumors are adenocarcinomas, leiomyosarcomas, or lymphomas. They appear in the descending duodenum more often than elsewhere. Pain, obstruction, bleeding, obstructive jaundice, and an abdominal mass are the modes of presentation. Duodenal carcinomas, particularly those in the third and fourth portions of the duodenum, are often missed on barium x-ray studies. Endoscopy and biopsy will usually be diagnostic if the examiner is suspicious enough and can reach the lesion.

If possible, adenocarcinomas and leiomyosarcomas should be resected. Pancreaticoduodenectomy is usually necessary if the tumor is localized. Unresectable lesions should be treated by radiotherapy. Biopsy and radiotherapy are recommended for lymphoma.

After curative resections, the 5-year survival rate is 30%. The overall 5-year survival rate is 18%.

2. Benign Duodenal Tumors

Brunner's gland adenomas are small submucosal nodules that have a predilection for the posterior duodenal wall at the junction of the first and second portions. Sessile and pedunculated variants are seen. Symptoms are due to bleeding or obstruction. Leiomyomas may also be found in the duodenum and ordinarily are asymptomatic.

Carcinoid tumors of the duodenum are often endocrinologically active, producing gastrin, somatostatin, or serotonin. Simple excision is the treatment of choice.

Heterotopic gastric mucosa, presenting as multiple small mucosal nodules, is an occasional endoscopic finding of no clinical significance.

Villous adenomas of the duodenum may give rise to intestinal bleeding or may obstruct the papilla of Vater and cause jaundice. As in the colon, the risk of malignant change is high—about 50%. Small pedunculated villous adenomas may be snared during endoscopy, but sessile tumors must be locally excised via laparotomy. Tumors that contain malignant tissue should be treated by a Whipple procedure.

Alarcon FJ et al: Familial adenomatous polyposis: efficacy of endoscopic and surgical treatment for advanced duodenal adenomas. Dis Colon Rectum 1999;42:1533.

Bakaeen FG et al: What prognostic factors are important in duodenal adenocarcinoma? Arch Surg 2000;135:635.

Bouvet M et al: Factors influencing survival after resection for periampullary neoplasms. Am J Surg 2000;180:13.

Isomoto H et al: Clinical and endoscopic features of adult T-cell leukemia/lymphoma with duodenal involvement. J Clin Gastroenterol 2001;33:241.

Kaklamanos IG et al: Extent of resection in the management of duodenal adenocarcinoma. Am J Surg 2000;179:37.

Ryder NM et al: Primary duodenal adenocarcinoma: a 40-year experience. Arch Surg 2000;135:1070.

Wallace MH et al: Randomized, placebo-controlled trial of gastric acid-lowering therapy on duodenal polyposis and relative adduct labeling in familial adenomatous polyposis. Dis Colon Rectum 2001;44:1585.

SUPERIOR MESENTERIC ARTERY OBSTRUCTION OF THE DUODENUM

Rarely, obstruction of the third portion of the duodenum is produced by compression between the superior mesenteric vessels and the aorta. It most commonly appears after rapid weight loss following injury, including burns. Patients in body casts are particularly susceptible.

The superior mesenteric artery normally leaves the aorta at an angle of 50–60 degrees, and the distance between the two vessels where the duodenum passes between them is 10–20 mm. These measurements in patients with superior mesenteric artery syndrome average 18 degrees and 2.5 mm. Acute loss of mesenteric fat is thought to permit the artery to drop posteriorly, trapping the bowel like a scissors.

Skepticism exists regarding the frequency of this condition in adults who have not experienced acute loss of weight. Most often the patient in question is a thin, nervous woman whose complaints of dyspepsia and occasional emesis are more properly explained on a functional basis. When a clear-cut example is encountered, it may actually represent a form of intestinal malrotation with duodenal bands.

The patient complains of epigastric bloating and crampy pain relieved by vomiting. The symptoms may remit in the prone position. Anorexia and postprandial pain lead to additional malnutrition and weight loss.

Upper gastrointestinal x-rays demonstrate a widened duodenum proximal to a sharp obstruction at the point where the artery crosses the third portion of the duodenum. When the patient moves to the knee-chest position, the passage of barium is suddenly unimpeded. Further verification can be provided if angiography shows an angle of 25 degrees or less between the superior mesenteric artery and the aorta. However, this procedure is not recommended for routine evaluation of obvious cases.

Many patients whose superior mesenteric artery makes a prominent impression on the duodenum are asymptomatic, and in ambulatory patients one should hesitate to attribute vague chronic complaints to this finding.

Involvement of the duodenum by scleroderma leads to duodenal dilatation and hypomotility and an x-ray and clinical picture highly suggestive of superior mesenteric artery syndrome. In the latter, increased duodenal peristalsis should be demonstrable proximal to the arterial blockage, whereas diminished peristalsis characterizes scleroderma. Patients with duodenal scleroderma usually have dysphagia from concomitant esophageal involvement.

Malrotation with duodenal obstruction by congenital bands can mimic this syndrome.

Postural therapy may suffice. The patient should be placed prone when symptomatic or in anticipation of postprandial difficulties. Ambulatory patients should be instructed to assume the knee-chest position, which allows the viscera and the artery to rotate forward off the duodenum.

Chronic obstruction may require section of the suspensory ligament and mobilization of the duodenum, or a duodenojejunostomy to bypass the obstruction. Patients with various forms of malrotation should be treated by mobilizing the duodenojejunal flexure, which releases the duodenum from entrapment by congenital bands.

Diwakaran HH, Stolar CG, Prather CM: Superior mesenteric artery syndrome. Gastroenterology 2001;121:516, 746.

Richardson WS, Surowiec WJ: Laparoscopic repair of superior mesenteric artery syndrome. Am J Surg 2001;181:377.

REGIONAL ENTERITIS OF THE STOMACH & DUODENUM

The proximal intestine and stomach are rarely involved in regional enteritis, though this disease has now been reported in every part of the gastrointestinal tract from the lips to the anus. Most patients with Crohn's disease in the stomach or duodenum have ileal involvement as well.

Pain can in many instances be relieved by antacids. Intermittent vomiting from duodenal stenosis or pyloric obstruction is frequent. The x-ray finding of a cobblestone mucosa or stenosis would be suggestive when associated with typical changes in the ileum. The endoscopic appearance is fairly characteristic, and biopsy with the peroral suction device usually gives an adequate specimen for histologic confirmation of the diagnosis.

Medical treatment is nonspecific and consists principally of corticosteroids during exacerbations. Surgery may be indicated for disabling pain or obstruction. If the disease is localized to the stomach, a partial gastrectomy can be performed. Duodenal involvement most often requires a gastrojejunostomy to bypass the obstruction. Vagotomy should also be performed to prevent development of a marginal ulcer. Recurrent Crohn's disease involving the anastomosis is an occasional late complication, but it can usually be managed successfully by reoperation.

Internal fistulas involving the stomach or duodenum usually represent extensions from primary disease in the ileum or colon. Surgical treatment consists of resection of the diseased ileum or colon and closure of the fistulous opening in the upper gut.

Mansari OE et al: Adenocarcinoma complicating Crohn's disease of the duodenum. Eur J Gastroenterol Hepatol 2001;13:1259.

Reynolds HL Jr, Stellato TA: Crohn's disease of the foregut. Surg Clin North Am 2001;81:117.

Worsey MJ et al: Strictureplasty is an effective option in the operative management of duodenal Crohn's disease. Dis Colon Rectum 1999;42:596.

Yamamoto T et al: Gastroduodenal fistulas in Crohn's disease: clinical features and management. Dis Colon Rectum 1998;41:1287.

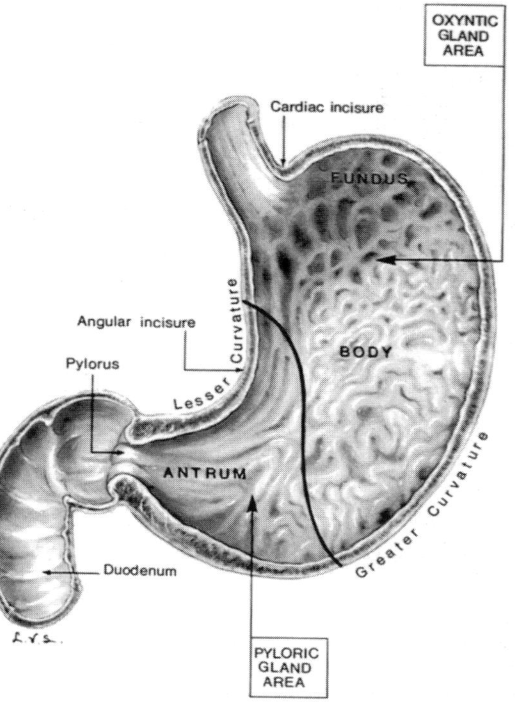

Figure 23–1. Names of the parts of the stomach. The line drawn from the lesser to the greater curvature depicts the approximate boundary between the oxyntic gland area and the pyloric gland area. No prominent landmark exists to distinguish between antrum and body (corpus). The fundus is the portion craniad to the esophagogastric junction.

division that travels in the lesser omentum. The bifurcation of the posterior trunk gives rise to fibers that enter the celiac plexus and supply the parasympathetic innervation to the remainder of the gastrointestinal tract as far as the mid transverse colon. Both trunks, after giving rise to their extragastric divisions, send some fibers directly onto the surface of the stomach and others along the lesser curvature (anterior and posterior nerves of Latarjet) to supply the distal part of the organ. As shown in Figure 23–3, a variable number of vagal fibers ascend with the left gastric artery after having passed through the celiac plexus.

The preganglionic motor fibers of the vagal trunks synapse with ganglion cells in Auerbach's plexus (plexus myentericus) between the longitudinal and circular muscle layers. Postganglionic cholinergic fibers are distributed to the cells of the smooth muscle layers and the mucosa.

The adrenergic innervation to the stomach consists of postganglionic fibers that pass along the arterial vessels from the celiac plexus.

PHYSIOLOGY

Motility

Storage, mixing, trituration, and regulated emptying are accomplished by the muscular apparatus of the stomach. Peristaltic waves originate in the body and pass toward the pylorus. The thickness of the smooth muscle increases in the antrum and corresponds to the stronger contractions that can be measured in the distal stomach. The pylorus behaves as a sphincter, though it normally allows a little to-and-fro movement of chyme across the junction.

An electrical pacemaker situated in the fundal musculature near the greater curvature gives rise to regular (3/min) electrical impulses (pacesetter potential, basic electrical rhythm) that pass toward the pylorus in the outer longitudinal layer. Every impulse is not always followed by a peristaltic muscular contraction, but the impulses determine the maximal peristaltic rate. The frequency of peristalsis is governed by a variety of stimuli mentioned below. Each contraction follows sequential depolarization of the underlying circular muscle resulting from arrival of the pacesetter potential.

Peristaltic contractions are more forceful in the antrum than the body and travel faster as they progress distally. Gastric chyme is forced into the funnel-shaped antral chamber by peristalsis; the volume of contents delivered into the duodenum by each peristaltic wave depends on the strength of the advancing wave and the extent to which the pylorus closes. Most of the gastric contents that are pushed into the antral funnel are propelled backward as the pylorus closes and pressure within the antral lumen rises. Five to 15 mL enter the duodenum with each gastric peristaltic wave.

The volume of the empty gastric lumen is only 50 mL. By a process called receptive relaxation, the stomach can accommodate about 1000 mL before intraluminal pressure begins to rise. Receptive relaxation is an active process mediated by vagal reflexes and abolished by vagotomy. Peristalsis is initiated by the stimulus of distention after eating. Various other factors have positive or negative influences on the rate and strength of contractions and the rate of gastric emptying. Vagal reflexes from the stomach have a facilitating influence on peristalsis. The texture and volume of the meal both play a role in the regulation of emptying; small particles are emptied more rapidly than large ones, which the organ attempts to reduce in size (trituration). The osmolality of gastric chyme and its chemical makeup are monitored by duodenal receptors. If osmolality is greater than 200 mosm/L, a long vagal reflex (the enter-

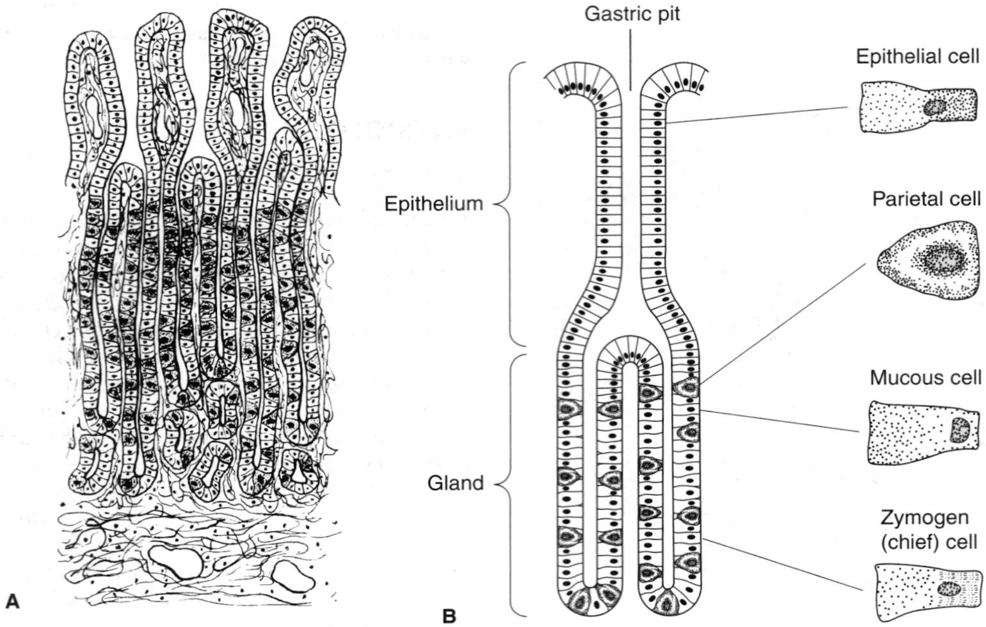

Figure 23–2. Histologic features of the mucosa in the oxyntic gland area. Each gastric pit drains three to seven tubular gastric glands. ***A:*** The neck of the gland contains many mucous cells. Oxyntic (parietal) cells are most numerous in the mid portion of the glands; peptic (chief) cells predominate in the basal portion. ***B:*** Drawing from photomicrograph of the gastric mucosa.

ogastric reflex) is activated, delaying emptying. Gastrin causes delay in emptying. Gastrin is the only circulating gastrointestinal hormone to have a physiologic effect on emptying.

Gastric Juice

The output of gastric juice in a fasting subject varies between 500 and 1500 mL/d. After each meal, about 1000 mL are secreted by the stomach.

The components of gastric juice are as follows:

A. Mucus

Mucus is a heterogeneous mixture of glycoproteins manufactured in the mucous cells of the oxyntic and pyloric gland areas. Mucus provides a weak barrier to the diffusion of H^+ and probably protects the mucosa. It also acts as a lubricant and impedes diffusion of pepsin.

B. Pepsinogen

Pepsinogens are synthesized in the chief cells of the oxyntic gland area (and to a lesser extent in the pyloric area) and are stored as visible granules. Cholinergic stimuli, either vagal or intramural, are the most potent pepsigogues, though gastrin and secretin are also effective. The precursor zymogen is activated when pH falls below 5.00, a process that entails severance of a polypeptide fragment from the larger molecule. Pepsin cleaves peptide bonds, especially those containing phenylalanine, tyrosine, or leucine. Its optimal pH is about 2.00. Pepsin activity is abolished at pH greater than 5.00, and the molecule is irreversibly denatured at pH greater than 8.00.

C. Intrinsic Factor

Intrinsic factor, a mucoprotein secreted by the parietal cells, binds with vitamin B_{12} of dietary origin and greatly enhances absorption of the vitamin. Absorption occurs by an active process in the terminal ileum.

Intrinsic factor secretion is enhanced by stimuli that evoke H^+ output from parietal cells. Pernicious anemia is characterized by atrophy of the parietal cell mucosa, deficiency in intrinsic factor, and anemia. Subclinical deficiencies in vitamin B_{12} have been described after operations that reduce gastric acid secretion, and abnormal Schilling tests in these patients can be corrected by the administration of intrinsic factor. Total gastrectomy creates a dependence on parenteral administration of vitamin B_{12}.

Liver & Portal Venous System

24

William R. Jarnagin, MD

SURGICAL ANATOMY

Segments

The liver develops as an embryologic outpouching from the duodenum by a process described in Chapter 25. The liver is one of the largest organs in the body, representing 2% of the total body weight. In classic descriptions, the liver was characterized as having four lobes: right, left, caudate, and quadrate; however, this is an overly simplistic view that fails to consider the much more complex segmental anatomy, which is depicted in Figure 24–1.

The liver is divided into eight segments based on the branching of the portal triads and hepatic veins. The structures of the portal triad (hepatic artery, portal vein, and biliary duct) are separate extrahepatically but enter the hepatic hilus ensheathed within a thickened layer of Glisson's capsule. The three main hepatic veins divide the liver into four sectors, each of which is supplied by a **portal pedicle**. The caudate lobe is an exception since its venous drainage is directly into the vena cava and therefore independent of the major hepatic veins. The four sectors delimited by the hepatic veins are called the **portal sectors**, and these portions of the parenchyma are supplied by independent portal pedicles arising from the right or left main pedicles. The divisions separating the sectors are called **portal scissurae**, within each of which runs a hepatic vein. Further branching of the pedicles subdivides the sectors into segments. The liver is thus subdivided into segments, numbered one through eight, with the caudate lobe designated as segment I. Segments I–IV comprise the left liver and segments V–VIII the right. Each segment is supplied by an independent portal pedicle, which forms the basis of sub-lobar segmental resections (see below).

The anatomical right and left hemi-livers are separated by an imaginary line running from the medial aspect of the gallbladder fossa to the inferior vena cava, running parallel with the fissure of the round ligament. This division is known as Cantlie's line or the principal plane and marks the course of the middle hepatic vein. The right hepatic vein further subdivides the right liver into anterior (segments V and VIII) and posterior (segments VI and VII) sectors, while the umbilical fissure subdivides the left liver into the medial sector (segment IV) and left lateral segment (segments II and III).

The relationship of the liver to the other abdominal organs is shown in Figure 24–2.

Portal Circulation

The portal vein is formed by the confluence of the splenic and superior mesenteric veins at the level of the second lumbar vertebra behind the head of the pancreas (Figure 24–3). It runs for approximately 6–9 cm to the hilum of the liver, where it divides into the main right and left branches. The left gastric vein usually enters the portal vein on its anteromedial aspect just cephalad to the margin of the pancreas, in which case it must be ligated during the surgical construction of a portacaval shunt; in 25% of cases, the left gastric vein joins the splenic vein. Other small venous tributaries from the pancreas and duodenum are less constant but must be anticipated during surgical mobilization of the portal vein.

The inferior mesenteric vein often drains into the splenic vein to the left of its junction with the superior mesenteric vein; alternatively, it may empty directly into the superior mesenteric vein.

In the hepatoduodenal ligament, the portal vein lies dorsal and slightly medial to the common bile duct. Portocaval lymph nodes are encountered along the right lateral aspect of the portal vein, running from the level of the duodenum to the liver and extending posteriorly. These lymph nodes are routinely removed during resections for certain malignancies and must be dissected before a portocaval shunt can be created.

Venous Blood Supply

The anatomy of venous blood supply is shown in Figure 24–4. Both the portal and hepatic venous systems lack valves. The main portal vein terminates in the porta hepatis by dividing into right and left branches. The right branch typically has a short extrahepatic course before subsequently dividing into anterior and posterior sectoral divisions, usually within the hepatic parenchyma. The left branch has a longer extrahepatic course, running first along the base of segment IV and

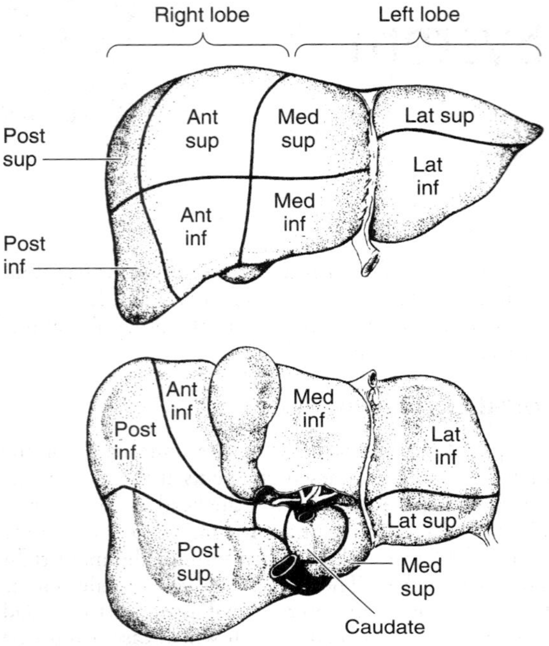

Figure 24–1. Segmental anatomy of the liver. The major lobar fissure, separating the right and left lobes, passes from the inferior vena cava through the gallbladder bed.

then entering the umbilical fissure, where it gives rise to branches to segments II, III, and IV; a large branch to the caudate lobe generally arises from the left portal vein prior to its entry into the umbilical fissure. Variations in the normal portal vein anatomy occur but are less common than aberrancies in the arterial supply or biliary drainage (see below). The most common anomaly of the portal venous system is separate origins of the right anterior and posterior sectoral branches.

The hepatic veins represent the final common pathway for the central veins of the lobules of the liver. There are three major hepatic veins: left, right, and middle. The right hepatic vein drains into the vena cava independently, while the middle and left hepatic veins typically join just outside of the liver, forming a common trunk. The middle hepatic vein runs in the principal plane (Cantlie's line) and provides drainage for segment IV and the anterior sector of the right liver (segments V and VIII). The left hepatic vein drains segments II and III while the right hepatic vein drains the posterior sector (segments VI and VII) and provides additional drainage to the anterior sector. A small umbilical vein runs within the umbilical fissure, providing accessory drainage of segments III and IV and emptying into the left hepatic vein. Several small accessory veins enter the inferior vena cava directly from the posterior aspect of the right lobe and must be carefully ligated during a right mobilization and resection of the right liver.

Arterial Blood Supply

The common hepatic artery arises from the celiac axis, ascends in the hepatoduodenal ligament, and gives rise to the right gastric, gastroduodenal, and proper hepatic arteries; the proper hepatic artery then divides into the right and left hepatic arterial branches in the liver hilum. The hepatic artery supplies approximately 25% of the 1500 mL of blood that enters the liver each minute; the remaining 75% is supplied by the portal vein.

Variations of the standard arterial anatomy of the liver are relatively common, seen in up to 40% of patients. The most common variants involve different origins of the right or left hepatic artery. A replaced right hepatic artery arises entirely from the superior mesenteric artery and courses to the right of the common bile duct within the porta hepatis, which is in contrast to its normal position to the left of the duct. Recognition of this

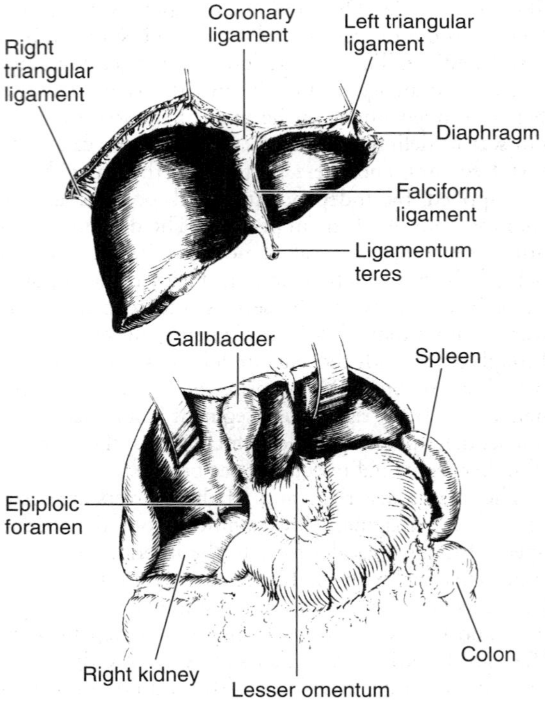

Figure 24–2. Relationships of the liver to adjacent abdominal organs.

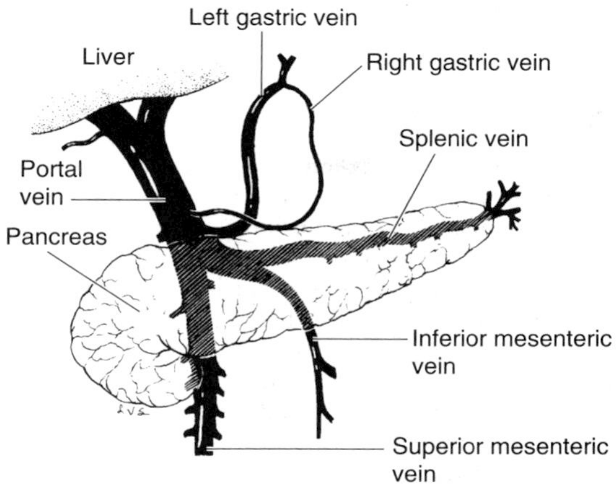

Figure 24–3. Anatomic relationships of portal vein and branches.

anatomical variant is critical during operations on the extrahepatic biliary tree. An accessory right hepatic artery also arises from the superior mesenteric artery and is found in the same location within the porta hepatis but supplies only a portion of the right liver; in this situation, a separate right branch arising from its normal position off the proper hepatic artery is typically present. An accessory or replaced left hepatic artery arises from the left gastric artery and enters the liver through the gastrohepatic ligament. Up to 25% of patients have a replaced or accessory right hepatic artery, and a similar proportion have a replaced or accessory left hepatic artery. Within the liver, the hepatic arterial branches travel with segmental bile ducts and portal vein branches.

Biliary Drainage

The biliary tree arises within the liver from bile canaliculi, formed from specialized segments of the hepatocyte membrane. Bile canaliculi join to form progressively larger biliary ducts, resulting in segmental bile ducts that drain each segment. The right anterior and right posterior sectoral ducts unite to form the main right hepatic duct, while the union of ducts draining segments II, III, and IV forms the left hepatic duct. The left hepatic duct typically is longer and has a longer extrahepatic course than the right hepatic duct. Drainage of segment I (caudate lobe) is principally into the left hepatic duct, but additional smaller ducts enter the right hepatic duct or drain directly into the hepatic duct confluence, which is formed by the union of the major lobar ducts to form the common hepatic duct. The common hepatic duct descends within the hepatoduodenal ligament for a variable distance to the point of insertion of the cystic duct of the gallbladder to give rise to the common bile duct.

Anatomic variations in the biliary ductal anatomy are seen in approximately 30% of patients and most often involve the right hepatic duct. In approximately 25% of patients, the duct from the right posterior sector joins the common hepatic duct or the left hepatic duct independently. Variations are far less common on the left side.

Lymphatics

Lymphatics draining superficial lobules of the liver follow a subcapsular course to the diaphragm, to the suspensory ligaments of the liver, or to the posterior mediastinum, while others enter the porta hepatis. Lymphatics arising from lobules deep within the liver travel either with the hepatic veins along the vena cava or with the portal veins into the porta hepatis. The majority of the lymphatic drainage of the liver is to the hepatoduodenal ligament.

NERVES

The liver and biliary tree are innervated by sympathetic fibers arising from T7 to T10 and by parasympathetic fibers from the right and left vagus nerves. The postganglionic sympathetic nerves arise from the celiac ganglia. Fibers derived from the celiac ganglia and vagus nerves form a plexus of nerves that run along the anterior and posterior aspects of the hepatic artery.

PHYSIOLOGY

Total hepatic blood flow (about 1500 mL/min; 30 mL/min per kg body weight) constitutes 25% of the cardiac

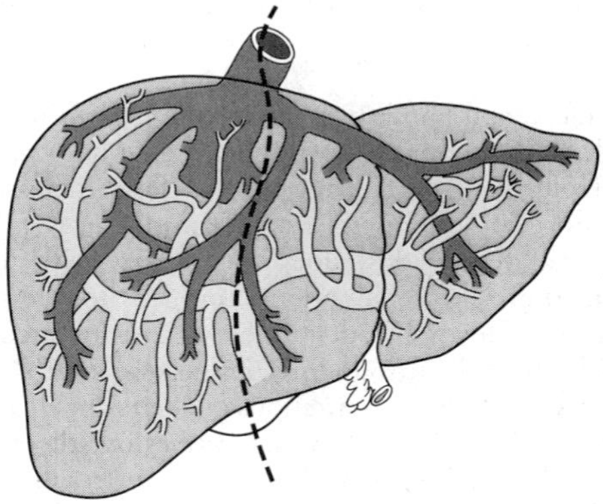

Figure 24–4. Anatomy of the veins of the liver. The major lobar fissure is represented by the dashed line. Branches of the hepatic artery and biliary ducts follow those of the portal vein. The darker vessels represent the hepatic veins and vena cava; the lighter system represents the portal vein and its branches.

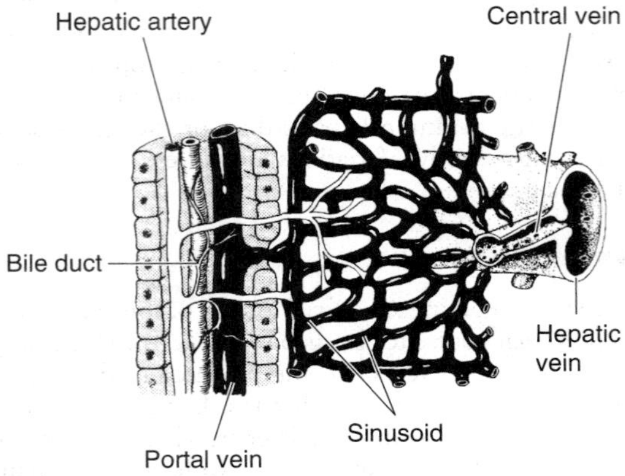

Figure 24–5. Vascular anatomy of the liver lobule.

output, though the liver accounts for only 2.5% of body weight. About 30% of the hepatic volume is blood (12% of total blood volume). Two-thirds of the flow enters through the portal vein and one-third through the hepatic artery. Pressure in the portal vein is normally low (10–15 cm H_2O [7–11 mm Hg]). The liver derives half of its oxygen from hepatic arterial blood and half from portal venous blood.

Blood flow within the liver is uniform, as demonstrated by an even distribution of microspheres injected into the hepatic artery or portal vein. Hepatic blood flow to the liver is regulated by a number of factors. Muscular sphincters at the inlet and outlet of sinusoids represent a major control point and respond to a number of different stimuli, including the autonomic nervous system, circulating hormones, bile salts, and metabolites. The cells lining the hepatic sinusoids (endothelial cells, Kupffer cells, and stellate cells) can also regulate flow to some extent.

Portal venous and hepatic arterial blood becomes pooled after entering the periphery of the hepatic sinusoid (Figure 24–5). Hepatic arterial flow increases or decreases reciprocally with changes in portal flow; however, portal venous flow does not increase with reductions in arterial flow. This arterial compensatory response is controlled largely by adenosine, which is released into the space of Mall surrounding the hepatic arterial resistance vessels. High concentrations of adenosine dilate the vessels, which increases flow and washes out the adenosine. Sudden occlusion of the portal vein results in an immediate 60% rise in hepatic arterial flow. The total flow then gradually returns toward normal. On the other hand, sudden reductions in hepatic arterial supply are not immediately met by significant increases in portal vein flow. In both normal subjects and cirrhotics, total hepatic flow and portal pressure drop following hepatic arterial occlusion. Arterial collaterals develop over the ensuing months, and arterial perfusion is ultimately restored.

HEPATIC RESECTION

Liver resection is most commonly indicated for primary and secondary malignant tumors and symptomatic benign tumors; less common indications include traumatic injury, infection/abscesses, and living donor transplantation. Removal of as much as 80–85% of the normal liver can be performed with the expectation that the liver remnant will regenerate sufficiently for the patient to survive. It must be emphasized, however, that such extensive resections should be considered only in patients with normal hepatic function; those with cirrhosis or significant fibrosis or steatosis (fatty infiltration of the liver) tolerate major hepatic resections poorly. Liver function may be decreased for several weeks after extensive resection, but the extraordinary regenerative capacity of the liver rapidly provides new functioning hepatocytes. Within 24 hours after partial hepatectomy, cell replication becomes active and continues until the original volume of hepatic tissue is restored. Considerable regeneration occurs within 10 days, and the process is essentially complete by 4–5 weeks. Excised portions of liver are not re-formed; rather, the growth consists of formation of new lobules and expansion of residual lobules. The stimuli for hepatic regeneration are thought to include the following: hepatocyte growth factor, TGFα, heparin binding growth factor, hepatopoietin B, and disinhibition by TGFβ_1 (ie, decreased levels of this inhibitor of hepatic growth).

Preoperative Evaluation

Several different disease- and patient-related factors must be assessed before deciding to proceed with hepatic resection. Among the most important of these is the preoperative functional status of the liver. Cirrhosis is a relative contraindication for partial hepatectomy because the limited reserve of the residual cirrhotic liver may be insufficient to meet essential metabolic demands and the cirrhotic liver has a reduced capacity for regeneration. Cirrhosis is a particular concern in patients with hepatocellular carcinoma, which frequently arises in the setting of chronic hepatic parenchymal disease.

Several tests are available to assess hepatic function prior to operation, none of which is perfect. The Child-Pugh classification is the oldest and most widely employed and remains the most useful assessment. The Child-Pugh system classifies hepatic function based on several measures of hepatic function (see below and Table 24–1). Originally used to assess mortality related to porto-systemic shunts, the Child's score also predicts

Table 24–1. Child-Pugh classification of functional status in liver diseases.

	Class: A Risk: Low	B Moderate	C High
Ascites	Absent	Slight to moderate	Tense
Encephalopathy	None	Grades I–II	Grades III–IV
Serum albumin (g/dL)	> 3.5	3.0–3.5	< 3.0
Serum bilirubin (mg/dL)	< 2.0	2.0–3.0	> 3.0
Prothrombin time (seconds above control)	< 4.0	4.0–6.0	> 6.0

mortality in patients with cirrhosis after hepatic resection. In general, only Child's A and highly selected Child's B cirrhotics would be candidates for resection. The indocyanine green clearance (IGC) test is commonly used in centers outside of North America but has not been proven superior to the Child-Pugh scoring system.

Extent of Hepatic Resection

Hepatic resections are classified as anatomical (based on the segmental liver anatomy) or nonanatomical. Wedge resections, enucleations, and resectional debridement of devitalized tissue are examples of the latter. In general, anatomical resections are preferred, since they are associated with lower blood loss and, when performed for malignancy, a lower incidence of positive resection margins.

Major resections must be performed in accordance with the segmental anatomy. Major resections (right or left hepatectomy or extended hepatectomy) are commonly performed; however, the segmental anatomy of the liver allows smaller resections or bilateral resections to be performed when necessary and appropriate. For example, in selected situations, a resection of the anterior (segments V and VIII) or posterior (segments VI and VII) sectors may be performed rather than sacrificing the entire right liver. Such parenchymal-sparing resections on one side would then allow a resection of part of the contralateral lobe, if necessary.

The terminology and extent of the common types of resections are depicted in Figure 24–6. The operation entails removal of a lobe or segment with its afferent and efferent vessels while avoiding injury to vessels and bile ducts supplying the residual tissue.

Most elective hepatic resections can be performed through an abdominal incision, although selected situations (very large right lobe tumors) are probably best performed with a thoracoabdominal approach. The best perioperative results are obtained by minimizing blood, which is accomplished by (1) achieving vascular inflow and outflow control prior to parenchymal transaction; (2) performing careful division of the liver with precise control of intrahepatic vascular structures; (3) using low central venous pressure anesthesia, which reduces hepatic venous blood loss.

Postoperative Course

Patients submitted to major resections require close monitoring for the first several postoperative days; however, a prolonged stay in the intensive care unit is unnecessary in most cases. The major concern in the immediate postoperative period is hemorrhage, although in practice, reoperation for bleeding is rarely necessary. Patients without cirrhosis usually exhibit some metabolic changes consistent with mild liver insufficiency but these quickly normalize, and they are often ready for discharge on the seventh or eighth postoperative day. In the presence of significant hepatic parenchymal disease (ie, cir-

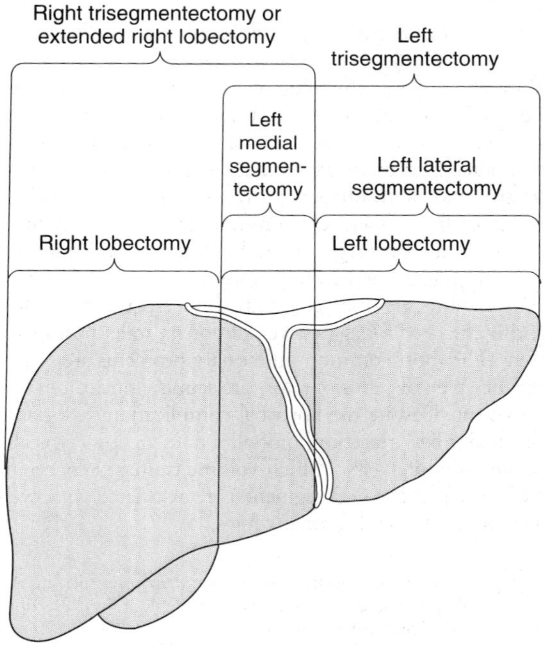

Figure 24–6. Terminology of various segmental resections of the liver. Lobectomy is sometimes referred to as hemihepatectomy.

rhosis, fibrosis, steatosis) or septic complications, postoperative liver function may be significantly impaired.

Many of the postoperative abnormalities can be predicted based on the liver's normal function. The serum bilirubin often increases after major resections but returns to normal as regeneration progresses. A persistent or rising serum bilirubin level should raise concern for a perihepatic fluid collection (biloma) or hepatic failure (especially if other measures of hepatic function are also deteriorating). The serum albumin level usually falls and the prothrombin time often increases; treatment of the latter with fresh frozen plasma is generally needed only when the INR is markedly elevated (> 2). Some patients may develop ascites, which can be treated with diuresis. Although the liver's glycogen stores are necessarily reduced after a major partial hepatectomy, hypoglycemia is almost never a problem postoperatively; normoglycemia can be easily maintained with 5% dextrose solutions, and profound hypoglycemia should raise concern for pending liver failure. Serum levels of phosphate, magnesium, and potassium often decrease during the first several postoperative days and require replacement. The liver enzymes (AST, ALT) are usually increased in the first few days after operation and then normalize. By contrast, the alkaline phosphatase is often initially normal and then increases and can remain elevated for several days to weeks after surgery.

Complications

Complications occur in up to 40% of patients after major liver resection (≥ 3 segments), but many are relatively minor and the overwhelming majority are readily managed and resolve without sequelae. Liver-related complications are the most frequent; perihepatic fluid collections requiring drainage occur in approximately 10–15% of patients. Relative hepatic insufficiency (hyperbilirubinemia, ascites, coagulopathy) is relatively common but resolves in most patients as the liver regenerates; however, hepatic failure is distinctly uncommon in high-volume centers. Pulmonary complications are also seen with some frequency, underscoring the need for aggressive pulmonary toilet postoperatively. The most common pulmonary problems are symptomatic pleural effusions or atelectasis; pneumonia is infrequent. Despite the potential complications associated with major liver resection, mortality rates are low, typically on the order of 1–3% in high-volume centers. Less extensive liver resections (< 3 segments) are associated with even lower morbidity and mortality rates.

Belghiti et al: Seven hundred forty-seven hepatectomies in the 1990's: an update to evaluate the actual risk of liver resection. J Am Coll Surg 2000;191:38.

Ettorre GM et al: Postoperative liver function after elective right hepatectomy in elderly patients. Br J Surg 2001;88:73.

Jackson PG et al: Predictors of outcome in 100 consecutive laparoscopic antireflux procedures. Am J Surg 2001;181:231.

Jarnagin et al: Improvement in perioperative outcome after hepatic resection: analysis of 1803 cases over the past decade. Ann Surg 2002;236:397.

Nagino M et al: Liver regeneration after major hepatectomy for biliary cancer. Br J Surg 2001;88:1084.

Nuzzo G et al: Liver resections with or without pedicle clamping. Am J Surg 2001;181:238.

Papadimitriou JD et al: The impact of new technology on hepatic resection for malignancy. Arch Surg 2001;136:1307.

Strasberg SM: Terminology of liver anatomy and liver resections: coming to grips with hepatic Babel. J Am Coll Surg 1997;184:413.

Takayama T et al: Randomized comparison of ultrasonic vs clamp transection of the liver. Arch Surg 2001;136:922.

Yamashita Y et al: Bile leakage after hepatic resection. Ann Surg 2001;233:45.

DISEASES & DISORDERS OF THE LIVER

HEPATIC TRAUMA

Based on the mechanism of injury, liver trauma is classified as penetrating or blunt. Penetrating wounds, constituting more than half of cases, are typically due to projectiles (such as bullets or shrapnel) or knives. In civilian practice, most of these tend to be clean wounds that are dangerous because of intra-abdominal bleeding but do not result in much devitalization of liver tissue. In contrast, high-velocity projectiles are associated with greater energy that is transferred to the abdominal viscera and can shatter the parenchyma, even if the projectile does not enter the liver directly.

Blunt trauma can be inflicted by a direct blow to the upper abdomen or lower right rib cage or can follow sudden deceleration, as occurs with a fall from a great height. Most often a consequence of automobile accidents, direct blunt trauma tends to produce explosive bursting wounds or linear lacerations of the hepatic surface, often with considerable parenchymal destruction. The stellate, bursting type of injury tends to affect the posterior and superior aspect of the right liver (segments VI, VII, and VIII) because of its relatively vulnerable location, convex surface, fixed position, and concentration of hepatic mass. Damage to the left lobe is much less common than damage to the right. Injuries that involve shearing forces can tear the hepatic veins where they enter the liver substance, producing an exsanguinating retrohepatic injury in an area difficult to surgically expose and repair. The staging system described in Table 24–2 is used to categorize liver injuries and provide a common language in order to allow comparisons of results of treatment between institutions.

The principal surgical goals are to stop bleeding and debride devitalized liver. Because some degree of liver failure is common postoperatively, efforts should be made during each step to maintain adequate oxygenation

Table 24–2. Liver Injury Scale.

Grade	Type	Description
I	Hematoma	Subcapsular, nonexpanding, < 10% surface area.
	Laceration	Capsular tear, nonbleeding; < 1 cm deep in parenchyma.
II	Hematoma	Subcapsular, on expanding, 10–50% surface area; intraparenchymal, non-expanding, < 2 cm in diameter.
	Laceration	Capsular tear, active bleeding; 1–3 cm deep into the parenchyma, < 10 cm long.
III	Hematoma	Subcapsular, > 50% surface area or expanding or ruptured subcapsular hematoma with active bleeding; intraparenchymal hematoma > 2 cm or expanding.
	Laceration	> 3 cm deep into the parenchyma.
IV	Hematoma	Ruptured intraparenchymal hematoma with active bleeding.
	Laceration	Parenchymal disruption involving > 50% of hepatic lobe.
V	Laceration	Parenchymal disruption involving > 50% of hepatic lobe.
	Vascular	Juxtahepatic venous injuries; ie, retro-hepatic vena cava or major hepatic veins.
VI	Vascular	Hepatic avulsion.

[1]Increase by one grade when there are two or more injuries to the liver. Grading applied based on best available evidence, whether from x-rays, operative findings, or autopsy findings.

and perfusion of the liver. Also, when one is debriding liver tissue, care should be taken to avoid injury to the vascular supply of adjacent viable parenchyma.

Clinical Findings

A. Symptoms and Signs

The clinical manifestations of liver injury are those of hypovolemic shock, ie, hypotension, decreased urinary output, low central venous pressure, and, in some cases, abdominal distention.

B. Laboratory Findings

With major injuries, particularly those associated with disruption of hepatic veins, the rate of blood loss is usually so rapid that anemia does not develop. Leukocytosis greater than 15,000/μL is common following rupture of the liver from blunt trauma.

C. Imaging Techniques

CT scans should be obtained in most stable patients suspected of having a hepatic injury. The scans demonstrate the extent of the injury and provide a rough estimate of the amount of blood loss. The findings are useful for triaging, since minor injuries rarely require surgical treatment whereas extensive ones usually do. One must exercise caution, however, in using CT estimates of injury grade, since they correlate poorly (ie, they both understage and overstage) with what is found at surgery.

Sonography has not been helpful other than as the rapid abdominal abdominal sonogram to identify fluid in the abdomen. It does not help to define the injury. Angiography is generally not helpful in the acute setting but may be used to diagnose and treat specific postinjury problems, such as hemobilia.

Treatment

Patients with stable minor liver injuries (and no associated injuries requiring exploration) may be managed expectantly unless symptoms or signs of bleeding appear. The CT findings in patients who may be considered for nonoperative management include contained subcapsular or intrahepatic hematoma, unilobar fracture, absence of devitalized liver, minimal intraperitoneal blood, and absence of injuries to other intra-abdominal organs. Serial CT scans should be obtained to verify that the lesion is stable rather than expanding.

Most patients have CT or clinical evidence of active bleeding or a major injury, however, and require prompt exploration.

Most lacerations have stopped bleeding by the time operation is performed. In the absence of active hemorrhage, these wounds need not be sutured. Active bleeding should be managed by clipping or direct suture of identifiable vessels, if possible, rather than by mass ligatures. Subcapsular hematomas often overlie an active bleeding site or parenchyma in need of debridement and should be explored even though the injury appears to be tamponaded and of limited severity. Blunt injuries associated with substantial amounts of parenchymal destruction may be particularly difficult to manage. Rarely, a very severe pulverizing injury requires formal lobectomy.

Temporary occlusion of the hepatic artery and portal vein can be done quickly by placing a vascular clamp around the entire hepato-duodenal ligament (Pringle's maneuver). This can be done for periods of 15–20 minutes and reduce the hemorrhage sufficiently to permit more accurate ligation of bleeding vessels. With major hepatic venous injuries, however, a Pringle maneuver has little effect, and precise repair of the injury may not be possible. Absorbable gauze mesh (eg, polyglycolic acid) can sometimes be wrapped around an injured lobe and sutured in a way that maintains pressure and tamponades the bleeding; this is difficult to accomplish without rendering the involved liver ischemic, however, and such an approach is rarely applicable. In some cases, control of arterial hemorrhage requires ligation of the hepatic artery or one of the accessible lobar branches in the hilum.

The most difficult problems involve lacerations of the major hepatic veins behind the liver. With such injuries, temporary clamping of the inflow vessels will not slow the bleeding to allow inspection and repair of the injured vessels. For persistent bleeding, the abdominal incision can be extended into a median sternotomy to improve exposure. An ancillary technique, which is used only rarely, is to place a tube through the atrial appendage into the inferior vena cava past the origin of the hepatic veins. Appropriately placed ligatures around the vena cava permit total isolation of the liver circulation without interrupting venous return from the lower extremities to the heart. Resection of the right liver improves exposure of the retrohepatic vena cava but is a difficult to perform in the face of overwhelming hemorrhage.

In many cases, when bleeding is difficult to control and especially when other injuries must be addressed, the best strategy is to pack the liver to achieve hemostasis. The packs are generally left in place for 48–72 hours, during which time the patient remains sedated and intubated in the intensive care unit where adequate resuscitative measures are undertaken. The packs are removed in the operating room; if persistent bleeding is noted, definitive repair of the injury can then be performed.

The majority of patients who come to operation require little in the way of surgical intervention to control bleeding; drainage of substantial liver lacerations and other injuries is reasonable since bile leakage can occur. Suture ligation of bleeding hepatic vessels and debridement of devitalized tissue are indicated in about 30% and 10% of cases, respectively. More extensive procedures are indicated even less often.

Penetrating injuries that also involve the small bowel or colon may result in contamination of perihepatic fluid or devitalized liver tissue, leading to a subhepatic abscess. Placement of drains may help prevent this problem, but a high index of suspicion should be maintained.

Postoperative Complications

With present techniques, hemorrhage at laparotomy is rarely uncontrollable except with retrohepatic venous injuries. Patients who rebleed from the liver wound after initial suture ligation should be treated by reexploration or packing; rarely is a major resection required. Angiography and CT scanning may provide useful diagnostic information preoperatively in such patients. Subhepatic sepsis develops in about 20% of cases; it is more frequent if lobectomy has been done.

Hemobilia may be responsible for gastrointestinal bleeding in the postoperative period and can be diagnosed by selective angiography. Treatment consists of embolization through the arteriography catheter.

Prognosis

The death rate of 10–15% following hepatic trauma depends largely on the type of injury and the extent of associated injury to other organs. About one-third of patients admitted to the emergency department in shock cannot be saved. Only 1% of penetrating civilian wounds are lethal, whereas a 20% death rate attends blunt trauma. The death rate in blunt hepatic injury is 10% when only the liver is injured. If three major organs are damaged, the death rate is close to 70%. Bleeding causes more than half of deaths associated with liver trauma.

Carrillo EH et al: Non-operative management of blunt hepatic trauma. Br J Surg 1998;85:461.

Chen RJ et al: Factors determining operative mortality of grade V blunt hepatic trauma. J Trauma 2000;49:886.

David Richardson J et al: Evolution in the management of hepatic trauma: a 25-year perspective. Ann Surg 2000;232:324.

Leone RJ Jr, Hammond JS: Nonoperative management of pediatric blunt hepatic trauma. Am Surg 2001;67:138.

Pryor JP, Stafford PW, Nance ML: Severe blunt hepatic trauma in children. J Pediatr Surg 2001;36:974.

SPONTANEOUS HEPATIC RUPTURE

Spontaneous rupture of the liver is not common. Most cases of ruptured normal liver are due to preeclampsia-eclampsia, and most cases of ruptured diseased liver are due to hepatic tumors (hepatocellular carcinoma or hepatic adenoma). Hepatic rupture should be suspected in any pregnant or postpartum patient (especially if hypertensive) who complains of acute discomfort in the upper abdomen. Spontaneous rupture has also been reported in association with a number of other conditions, including hepatic hemangioma, typhoid fever, malaria, tuberculosis, syphilis, polyarteritis nodosa, and diabetes mellitus. The diagnosis is best made by CT scanning. Rupture of the liver in the newborn is related to birth trauma in larger infants after difficult deliveries. The typical progression is intrahepatic hemorrhage expanding to subcapsular hematoma and eventually capsular rupture and free intra-abdominal hemorrhage.

Angiography and hepatic artery embolization can be quite effective for controlling hemorrhage in the setting of spontaneous rupture. Emergency laparotomy and intraoperative management (as one would for a traumatic liver injury) are reserved for those who fail hepatic artery embolization or are unsuitable for the procedure.

Chiappa A et al: Emergency liver resection for ruptured hepatocellular carcinoma complicating cirrhosis. Hepatogastroenterology 1999;46:1145.

Risseeuw JJ et al: Liver rupture postpartum associated with preeclampsia and HELLP syndrome. J Matern Fetal Med 1999;8:32.

PRIMARY LIVER CANCER

Liver malignancy may arise from hepatocytes (hepatocellular carcinoma, the most common) or biliary epithelial cells (intrahepatic cholangiocarcinoma). Tumors arising from both cell types (mixed hepatocellular carcinoma/cholangiocarcinoma) have also been described. Neonates may also develop a variant of hepatocellular carcinoma called hepatoblastoma because it is morphologically similar to fetal liver and the occasional presence of hematopoieis. Primary malignancy arising from other liver cell types (endothelial cells, stellate cells, neuroendocrine cells, or lymphocytes) is exceedingly rare.

Primary hepatic cancer is relatively uncommon in the USA, but its incidence is increasing. In Asia and Africa, however, primary liver cancer is extremely common and in some areas represents the single most frequent abdominal tumor and the most common cause of cancer-related death. The etiologic factors in these high-risk areas are environmental or cultural, since persons of similar racial background in the USA are at only slightly greater risk than Caucasians. About 9000 cases—distributed equally between men and women—occur in the USA each year. Most arise in persons over age 50, but a few are found in children, mainly under 2 years of age.

Chronic hepatitis B and C virus (HBV and HCV) infection is the principal etiologic factor worldwide for hepatocellular carcinoma. Patients chronically seropositive for HBsAg constitute a high-risk group for development of hepatocellular carcinoma, which in some cases may be detected early by screening for serum alpha-fetoprotein levels. Hepatitis B virus DNA has been detected integrated into the genome of host hepatocytes and hepatoma cells and has a direct oncogenic effect. Patients with chronic hepatitis B infection may therefore develop hepatocellular carcinoma in the absence of cirrhosis; by contrast, hepatocellular carcinoma arising in the setting of chronic hepatitis C infection is typically associated with cirrhotic change. Cirrhosis from almost any cause (eg, alcoholism, hemochromatosis, α_1-antitrypsin deficiency, or primary biliary cirrhosis) is associated with an increased risk of hepatocellular carcinoma, and the great majority of these tumors arise in the setting of chronic underlying liver disease. Certain fungal metabolites called aflatoxins have been shown experimentally to be capable of producing liver tumors. These substances are present in staple foods (eg, ground nuts and grain) in some parts of Africa where hepatomas are common.

Unlike hepatocellular carcinoma, intrahepatic cholangiocarcinoma is infrequently associated with cirrhosis. Primary sclerosing cholangitis is a predisposing condition in a small minority of patients. Widespread infection with liver flukes *(Clonorchis sinensis)* is at least partly responsible for the higher incidence of these tumors in some parts of Asia. There is some evidence to suggest that chronic hepatitis C infection is associated with the rising worldwide incidence of intrahepatic cholangiocarcinoma, although this relationship remains mechanistically ill-defined. In Western centers, the vast majority of intrahepatic cholangiocarcinomas are sporadic. Intrahepatic cholangiocarcinoma generally presents as a large mass within the liver and is therefore clinically distinct from cholangiocarcinoma arising from the extrahepatic biliary tree.

Hepatomas constitute about 85% of primary hepatic cancers. Previously, differences in morphology were used to separate tumors into three types: **mass-forming** type, characterized by a single predominant mass clearly demarcated from the surrounding liver, occasionally with small satellite nodules; **nodular** type, composed of multiple nodules, often distributed throughout the liver; and a **diffuse** type, characterized by infiltration of tumor throughout the remaining parenchyma. A number of staging systems for HCC are in current use (American Joint Commission on Cancer (TNM), Okuda, Cancer of the Liver Italian Program (CLIP); none fully accounts for extent of disease and underlying hepatic parenchymal function, which is an important predictor of outcome.

About 50% of resectable tumors are surrounded by a fibrous capsule, a structure that develops as a result of compression of adjacent liver stroma. Encapsulated tumors exhibit a lower incidence of tumor microsatellites and venous permeation compared with nonencapsulated tumors, and the finding is a favorable sign. An uncommon variety of the massive type, **fibrolamellar hepatocellular carcinoma**, contains numerous fibrous septa and may resemble focal nodular hyperplasia. Fibrolamellar hepatoma occurs in a younger age group (average 25 years) and is not associated with cirrhosis or hepatitis B virus infection.

A large proportion of patients will have intra- or extrahepatic metastases at presentation. Multiple intrahepatic tumors can arise as a result of infiltration of the portal venous system with subsequent dissemination of tumor cells. Vascular invasion is more common with larger tumors (> 5 cm). The extrahepatic sites most commonly involved with metastatic disease include the hilar and celiac lymph nodes and the lungs; metastases to bone and brain are less common and peritoneal disease (ie, carcinomatosis) is distinctly unusual. Major portal or hepatic veins are often invaded by tumor, and venous occlusion may occur as a result.

Microscopically, there is usually little stroma between the malignant cells, and the tumor has a soft consistency. The tumor may be highly vascularized, a feature that rarely can result in massive intraperitoneal hemorrhage following spontaneous rupture.

Cholangiocarcinoma makes up about 15% of primary liver cancers. They are usually well-differentiated adenocarcinomas that spread invasively in the liver substance.

Intra- or extrahepatic spread of disease is not uncommon by the time the tumor is detected. These tumors infrequently cause symptoms at early stages and therefore often grow to a large size before they become apparent, not infrequently because of pain. The mixed tumors are similar to intrahepatic cholangiocarcinoma in that they are infrequently associated with chronic liver disease.

Angiosarcoma of the liver, a rare fatal tumor, has been seen in workers intensively exposed to vinyl chloride for prolonged periods in polymerization plants.

Clinical Findings

A. Symptoms and Signs

The diagnosis at early and more treatable stages is often difficult, since symptoms are often absent. Screening and surveillance of high-risk patients (with cirrhosis, chronic hepatitis, etc) is helpful in this regard. Patients with more advanced tumors may have epigastric or right upper quadrant pain, which may be associated with referred pain in the right shoulder. Weight loss may be present. Jaundice is rare in patients with small tumors and good liver function; the presence of jaundice suggests either very advanced cancer or deteriorating liver function or both.

Hepatomegaly or a mass is palpable in many patients. An arterial bruit or a friction rub may be audible over the liver. Intermittent fever may be a presenting feature. Ascites or gastrointestinal bleeding from varices indicates advanced disease, and ascites fluid with blood should always suggest hepatoma. An acute deterioration in a previously well-compensated cirrhotic patient should also raise the suspicion of HCC.

The patterns of presentation can thus be extremely variable and may include (1) pain with or without hepatomegaly; (2) sudden deterioration of the condition of a cirrhotic patient owing to the appearance of hepatic failure, bleeding varices, or ascites; (3) sudden, massive intraperitoneal hemorrhage; (4) acute illness with fever and abdominal pain; (5) symptoms related to distant metastases; and (6) no clinical findings or symptoms.

B. Laboratory Findings

Depending on the disease extent and underlying hepatic function, laboratory values may range from entirely normal to suggestive of impending liver failure. Serum transaminase levels (AST and ALT) and alkaline phosphatase may be increased, although this is nonspecific and is often seen in patients with chronic liver disease without HCC. The presence of a moderate to large liver tumor may bring about an increase in the serum alkaline phosphatase in the absence of underlying liver disease. An elevated serum bilirubin is a more ominous finding and reflects some degree of liver dysfunction, either from the underlying chronic liver disease or a large volume of cancer within the liver. Less often, jaundice is the result of tumor involvement of the biliary confluence by direct compression or by intrabiliary tumor extension. Other signs of compromised hepatic function include hypoalbuminemia, coagulopathy, and thrombocytopenia. A large number of patients will be positive for HBsAg or HCV antibody; the proportions of each will vary somewhat by geography.

C. Liver Scan

CT scans, ultrasound scans, and MRI scans demonstrate the principal lesion in nearly all patients. MRI scans with MR angiography or CT angiography may provide more detail regarding vascular involvement. A triple-phase, contrast-enhanced helical CT scan generally provides the best images of disease extent within the liver and will assess for extrahepatic spread.

D. Angiography

Diagnostic angiography was previously used often to assess liver tumors but is now rarely needed for this purpose and is used primarily for treatment (ie, chemoembolization). Hepatomas are supplied primarily by the hepatic artery, and the vast majority are more vascular than adjacent parenchyma (hypervascular). In some cases, the center of the tumor has become necrotic, and only the peripheral areas are hypervascular. Arterial branches supplying the tumor have an irregular appearance compared to the native hepatic artery, and arterial-venous shunting may be seen. By contrast, cholangiocarcinomas usually appear less vascular than adjacent tissue. Hemangiomas have a distinctive pattern of peripheral nodular enhancement and patchy vascular pooling. Other benign tumors, particularly adenomas and focal nodular hyperplasia, are more difficult to diagnose based on angiographic features alone.

The venous phase of a superior mesenteric arterial injection may show invasion or occlusion of the portal vein by tumor.

Angiography may be equivocal in small tumors, which may be demonstrated with greater certainty by a selective injection of iodized oil (Lipiodol) followed 1–2 weeks later by CT scans. Normal liver clears the contrast medium, but hepatomas cannot do so and remain opacified.

E. Liver Biopsy

The diagnosis can be established by percutaneous core biopsy or aspiration biopsy. Fine-needle aspiration biopsy is associated with an approximately 30% false-negative rate. A negative result therefore does not rule out malignant disease, and a core biopsy should be pursued if the index of suspicion is high. Percutaneous biopsy carries some risk of bleeding, although this is rare in experienced hands; tumor dissemination resulting from a biopsy has been reported but is rare. In patients with cirrhosis, the presence of a hypervascular mass > 2 cm on two different imaging studies (ultrasound, CT, MRI, or angiography) or a hypervascular mass > 2 cm on one imaging study combined with a serum alpha-fetoprotein level > 400 ng/mL (see below) is diagnostic of HCC, and a biopsy is therefore not required.

F. Surveillance

In high-risk patients, surveillance with periodic imaging studies is recommended in order to detect early HCC, which is more amenable to treatment. The optimal type and timing of imaging studies is the subject of some debate, but such programs have proved useful in areas with a high incidence of chronic hepatitis, such as Asia, where a large proportion of patients are now identified with a mass 2 cm in diameter or smaller; other studies in high-risk patients have also proved valuable.

G. Tumor Markers

Alpha-fetoprotein (AFP), a glycoprotein normally present only in the fetal circulation, is present in high concentrations in the serum of many patients with primary hepatomas and testicular tumors. Increased levels are rarely seen as a product of other tumor types, such as the lung, stomach, pancreas, and biliary tree.

The upper limit of normal in the serum is 20 ng/mL; values above 200 ng/mL are suggestive of hepatoma, while levels above 400 ng/mL in a cirrhotic patients with a hypervascular liver mass > 2 cm in diameter are diagnostic. Levels in the intermediate range are nonspecific and may occur with benign liver diseases, such as cirrhosis and chronic hepatitis, where they represent a manifestation of liver cell proliferation. As imaging methods have improved, the diagnosis of liver cancer is being made earlier, when AFP levels may be normal or only minimally elevated. Additionally, some patients may have normal AFP levels, despite the presence of advanced disease. In general, AFP levels correlate with tumor size and vascular invasion, and a number of studies have shown a correlation between high AFP levels and recurrent cancer after resection.

Differential Diagnosis

The clinical picture is often nonspecific, and the presenting symptoms may provide little in the way of diagnostic clues. Primary liver cancer is often confused with metastatic cancer arising from other abdominal sites. The presence of cirrhosis and findings consistent with chronic liver disease clearly make hepatocellular carcinoma the leading diagnosis, and this is often confirmed with further testing. In patients without cirrhosis or normal AFP levels (or both), a hypervascular mass in the liver should raise other diagnostic considerations, such as hepatic adenoma, which can be difficult to distinguish from HCC based on imaging alone. In addition, certain types of cancer may give rise to hypervascular liver metastases, including melanoma, neuroendocrine carcinoma, and renal cell carcinoma.

When complications develop suddenly in a cirrhotic patient, the possibility of hepatoma must always be considered. In rare instances, primary hepatocellular cancer is associated with metabolic or endocrine abnormalities such as erythrocytosis, hypercalcemia, hypoglycemic attacks, Cushing's syndrome, or virilization.

Complications

Sudden intra-abdominal hemorrhage may occur from spontaneous bleeding. Obstruction of the portal vein may produce portal hypertension, and obstruction of the hepatic veins may produce the Budd-Chiari syndrome. Liver failure is a common cause of death.

Treatment

A. Partial Hepatectomy

Resection is the most effective therapy and is the treatment of choice in selected patients without cirrhosis or in cirrhotics with well-preserved hepatic function. Initial diagnostic laparoscopy, immediately prior to planned laparotomy, may identify previously undetected spread of tumor within the liver or abdominal cavity that would preclude resection; however, with better imaging, the yield of laparoscopy has decreased. The minimal criteria of resectability that must be met are (1) disease confined to the liver and (2) disease amenable to a complete resection. Multiple tumors in the liver and tumor invasion into major portal or hepatic veins are bad prognostic findings, even if resection is technically feasible; such patients generally not good candidates for resection. For small and peripherally placed lesions, particularly in cirrhotics, sublobar, segmental resections are preferred if technically feasible. Anatomical segmentectomies are preferred to non-anatomical resections. Larger or more central tumors will require more extensive resections. In Western centers, about 25–30% of patients with HCC prove to be candidates for resection; this proportion is over 60% in Japan, due largely to widespread surveillance programs.

If gross tumor is left behind or if the margins of resection are involved microscopically, progressive disease is the rule. After a complete resection, the prognosis is best for patients with a solitary, small, and asymptomatic tumor and well-preserved hepatic function. Several adverse predictors of outcome have been identified, which vary somewhat among studies. However, the presence of vascular invasion (even if microscopic) has been identified in nearly all studies to predict recurrent cancer and poor outcome. Large tumor size (> 5 cm), the presence of satellite tumors, and markedly elevated AFP (> 2000 ng/mL) are also associated with a worse outcome, in part because of their correlation with vascular invasion. Additionally, patients with coexistent hepatocellular disease (ie, cirrhosis) tend to do worse, and this is especially true in the face of significant hepatocellular dysfunction or portal hypertension.

In general, cirrhosis constitutes the major obstacle to resection in patients with HCC. Careful patient selection (Child's A, no portal hypertension) is critical in order to avoid acute liver failure. In addition to this immediate perioperative concern, cirrhotic patients have a late risk of death from progression of the underlying liver disease (bleeding esophageal varices or liver failure) and a high rate (> 75%) of new tumors developing in the residual liver. For these reasons, highly selected patients may be better treated with liver transplantation rather than resection.

Overall, the rate of tumor recurrence is approximately 70% at 5 years (although it is higher, as mentioned above, in patients with cirrhosis). Some patients may be candidates for repeat resection or ablative procedures. The 5-year survival rate is approximately 40% but is lower for patients with cirrhosis. Patients may have a somewhat more favorable outcome, although this may simply reflect the lack of underlying liver disease and younger age.

After surgery, the patient should be followed by periodic physical examinations and blood work to assess liver function. Imaging studies and AFP measurements (if elevated before resection) at regular intervals may help identify early, localized recurrences that may be amenable to repeat resection or palliative therapy.

B. Liver Transplantation

Hepatocellular carcinoma is the only solid neoplasm for which transplantation plays a significant role. Liver transplantation has the advantage of treating not only the malignant disease but also the underlying cirrhosis. Previously, the selection criteria for transplanting hepatoma patients were broad and included patients with very advanced disease. Consequently, 5-year survival rates were < 40%, too low to justify use of a scarce resource. The lessons learned from this early experience have allowed identification of patients most likely to benefit, specifically those with a single tumor = 5 cm in diameter or up to three tumors with none exceeding 3 cm in diameter. Using these strict criteria, 5-year survival rates of 70% can be achieved. It should be emphasized that the benefit of transplantation is realized only when the waiting time for a new graft is < 6 months. Since waiting times can exceed 12 months in many centers, up to 50% of patients will develop cancer progression or otherwise become ineligible. This problem has led to a number of centers to adopt living donor transplantation as a means of increasing the donor pool, an approach that remains controversial because of donor-related morbidity and mortality.

A major concern of transplantation in cancer patients has been that the immunosuppressive therapy required to support the graft would remove an important defense mechanism against progression of residual microscopic disease. Indeed, calculated tumor doubling times for lesions in transplanted patients have been shown to be greater compared to patients not on immunosuppressive agents. Despite this possibility and although the logistical problems and expense are enormous, transplantation is a reasonable option in patients with cirrhosis who are not candidates for resection and have limited malignant disease, as specified in the selection criteria.

At present, transplantation has no role in patients with cholangiocarcinoma outside of controlled clinical trials, since the results to date have been poor.

C. Ethanol Injection

Percutaneous ablative techniques are a reasonable option in patients with small unresectable HCC, of which ethanol injection is the cheapest, easiest, and least morbid. Using ultrasound or CT guidance, 95% ethanol (5–20 mL) is injected through a 22-gauge needle directly into the tumor. This approach can achieve complete necrosis in 90–100% of tumors < 2 cm, but its efficacy declines rapidly as the tumor size increases. The patient is followed up and retreatment given for residual or new primary tumors. In one multi-institutional series from Italy, survival 1, 2, and 3 years after treatment for patients with solitary, small tumors was 90%, 80%, and 63%, respectively.

D. Radiofrequency Ablation

Radiofrequency ablation (RFA) is another percutaneous ablative approach, useful for treating selected patients with unresectable, small tumors. Under ultrasound or CT guidance, a needle is used to access the lesion; the needle is attached to a radiofrequency generator that generates thermal energy to bring about tumor destruction. RFA can be used percutaneously, laparoscopically, or at laparotomy.

The goal of RFA is the same at that of ethanol injection; namely, to achieve complete tumor necrosis. The efficacy of RFA is limited by tumor size but may be somewhat greater than ethanol injection in this regard; RFA is less effective for tumors adjacent to major vascular structures. A randomized study comparing the two techniques found no differences in survival, although RFA may offer better local tumor control rates. In carefully selected patients, 5-year survival rates of 30–40% have been reported.

E. Arterial Embolization

Hepatic artery embolization is another ablative technique that is more broadly applicable than RFA or ethanol injection. This approach takes advantage of the fact that primary liver cancers derive disproportionately greater blood supply from the hepatic arterial circulation compared to the surrounding liver. The strategy is to combine selective hepatic arterial injection of cancer chemotherapeutic agents with arterial embolization, the latter to produce tumor necrosis and slow the washout of the drugs. Embolization can be used in patients with much larger tumors than can be effectively treated with percutaneous procedures, and the procedure can be staged to treat bilobar disease. Patients must have adequate liver function; those with Child class C cirrhosis or thrombosis of the portal vein are not suitable candidates.

A variety of techniques have been used. Embolization is often performed with Gelfoam, which dissolves after a few weeks, but other inert agents are also used. Doxorubicin, mitomycin, and cisplatin in various combinations are the drugs most often given. Lipiodol, which lodges in the tumor, has occasionally been used as a carrier for the drugs. It remains unclear if the addition of chemotherapeutic agents provides much benefit beyond the necrosis produced by occlusion of the hepatic arterial supply. Many patients require multiple treatments, although the optimal schedule is ill-defined. Embolization achieves partial responses in up to 55% of patients. The best 3-year survival rates are approximately 50%. Histologic studies of tumors resected shortly after treatment reveal viable neoplastic cells in the tumor capsule, which receives blood from the portal vein as well as the hepatic artery.

Akriviadis EA et al: Hepatocellular carcinoma. Br J Surg 1998;85:1319.

Baffis V et al: Use of interferon for prevention of hepatocellular carcinoma in cirrhotic patients with hepatitis B or hepatitis C virus infection. Ann Intern Med 1999;131:696.

Bergsland EK, Venook AP: Hepatocellular carcinoma. Curr Opin Oncol 2000;12:357.

Fong Y et al: Hepatocellular Carcinoma: An analysis of 412 HCC at a Western center. Ann Surg 1999;229:790-800.

Grasso A et al: Radiofrequency ablation in the treatment of hepatocellular carcinoma—a clinical viewpoint. J Hepatol 2000;33:667.

Krinsky GA, Lee VS, Theise ND: Focal lesions in the cirrhotic liver: high resolution ex vivo MRI with pathologic correlation. J Comput Assist Tomogr 2000;24:189.

Llovet JM et al: Hepatocellular carcinoma. Lancet 2003;362:1907.

Mor E et al: Treatment of hepatocellular carcinoma associated with cirrhosis in the era of liver transplantation. Ann Intern Med 1998;129:643.

Trevisani F et al: Randomized control trials on chemoembolization for hepatocellular carcinoma: is there room for new studies? J Clin Gastroenterol 2001;32:383.

Tung-Ping Poon R, Fan ST, Wong J: Risk factors, prevention, and management of postoperative recurrence after resection of hepatocellular carcinoma. Ann Surg 2000;232:10.

Weber SM et al: Intrahepatic cholangiocarcinoma: resectability, recurrence pattern and outcome. J Am Coll Surg 2001:193;384.

METASTATIC NEOPLASMS OF THE LIVER

Metastatic cancer is 20 times more common than primary tumors in the liver. Nearly all solid tumors can potentially give rise to liver metastases; primary cancers of the gastrointestinal tract (colon, pancreas, esophagus, stomach, neuroendocrine), breast, lung, genitourinary system (kidney, adrenal), ovary and uterus, melanoma, and sarcomas account for the overwhelming majority of cases. Spread to the liver may be via the systemic or portal venous circulation. The cirrhotic liver, which often gives rise to primary hepatic tumors, seems to be less susceptible than normal liver to implantation of metastases.

Individual tumor types have characteristic patterns of spread. For example, colorectal cancer spreads to the liver as the first site of metastatic disease in a very high proportion of patients; the lung is the next most common site but bone, brain, or adrenal metastases are distinctly unusual. By contrast, metastatic lung cancer to the liver typically occurs concomitantly with spread to other sites, with brain, bone, and adrenal among the most common. In general, the vast majority of patients with metastases to the liver also have disease at other sites. A notable exception is colorectal cancer, which in many cases involves the liver only for a prolonged period. In the past, approximately 20% of patients with hepatic metastases had additional tumor deposits in the liver not seen on preoperative imaging studies. As imaging technology has improved, however, this proportion has become increasingly smaller.

Clinical Findings

A. Symptoms and Signs

The signs and symptoms will vary with the clinical scenario, the disease extent within the liver, and the presence or absence of metastatic disease to other sites. Patients with an undiagnosed primary tumor may come to attention because of symptoms caused by the metastatic disease. Weight loss, fatigue, pain, and anorexia are the presenting general complaints in many such patients. Signs of liver failure, such as ascites and jaundice, are uncommon and suggestive of very advanced cancer. Fever without demonstrable infection is present in 15% of cases. By contrast, patients with a known history of cancer undergoing routine surveillance often develop liver metastases that cause no symptoms; in a small proportion of cases, liver metastases are found on studies done for unrelated reasons.

Physical examination is not infrequently unrevealing. Hepatomegaly or a palpable tumor in the upper abdomen may be present, and either may be tender. Portal hypertension may be manifested by abdominal venous collaterals or splenomegaly. A friction rub is sometimes heard over the liver.

B. Laboratory Findings

Laboratory values may be entirely normal or at most reflect only minor nonspecific changes. Patients with advanced cancer will have anemia and hypoalbuminemia. The alkaline phosphatase is increased in most patients. More significant derangements in liver function will occur in patients with a large volume of liver disease, although this is uncommon at initial presentation. Tumor marker levels (CEA, CA 19-9, CA-125) are often elevated, depending on the tumor type, and may be helpful for monitoring treatment.

The diagnosis can be established in most cases by CT or ultrasound-guided percutaneous liver biopsy or fine-needle aspiration for malignant cells.

C. Imaging Studies

The detection of liver metastases usually relies on CT or ultrasound scans. MRI provides useful additional information and may help distinguish benign from malignant disease. However, a high-quality helical CT scan with IV and oral contrast medium provides excellent assessment of disease extent in the liver and elsewhere in the abdomen. In the past, CT portography was superior to ordinary contrast-enhanced CT and was obtained routinely in patients being considered for hepatic resection, but this is no longer the case. During surgery, intraoperative ultrasound is used to assess the liver for disease not appreciated on imaging studies.

Treatment

For most patients with metastatic liver disease, chemotherapy is the only treatment option, particularly with coexisting metastases outside the liver. Such therapy is generally not curative but rather palliative in most cases. A notable exception is metastatic colorectal cancer, for which resection or other treatments aimed at the liver disease are effective and potentially curative; the recent advent of several active chemotherapeutic agents has further improved the results of treatment. Carefully selected patients with metastases from other primary tumors (sarcoma, breast, ovary, lung, neuroendocrine) may also benefit from resection but represent a small minority of cases.

A. Hepatic Resection

Hepatic resection is most commonly indicated in patients with metastatic colorectal cancer. Of the approximately 130,000 patients diagnosed with colorectal cancer annually in the United States, approximately 50% either have liver metastases at diagnosis or develop liver metastases at some point. In 40% of the latter group, the liver is the only demonstrable site of disease. Hepatic metastases from colorectal cancer thus affect approximately 20,000 patients per year, which is comparable to the annual incidence of pancreatic or esophageal carcinoma.

If a complete resection can be achieved, the 5-year survival rate is 25–40%; systemic or regional chemotherapy or both is frequently given after resection. The presence of extrahepatic metastases and inability to achieve a complete resection are contraindications to resection in most cases. However, the indications for resection continue to evolve as more effective chemotherapeutic agents have emerged. The following are associated with a worse prognosis after resection: (1) original tumor with involved lymph nodes (stage III or Dukes C); (2) multiple liver lesions; (3) less than 1 year since resection of the colon primary (disease-free interval); and (4) CEA level > ng/mL. Variables that do not influence the outcome include (1) histologic grade of the tumor; (2) bilateral rather than unilateral disease; (3) site of the primary tumor within the large intestine; and (4) the gender of the patient. The mortality rate for resection of hepatic metastases is 1–2% in hospitals where this operation is performed frequently.

The liver is the most common site of cancer recurrence after a complete resection. A small proportion of patients may be amenable to a second resection.

The efficacy of liver resection for colorectal cancer has been clearly established and is the most common indication for this procedure. By contrast, for most other tumor types, the benefit of liver resection is much more limited. Rare patients with metastases from renal cell carcinoma, ovarian cancer, adrenocortical carcinoma, or sarcomas appear to derive the most benefit; liver resection for metastatic gastrointestinal cancers other than colorectal is almost never warranted. In selecting patients with noncolorectal liver metastases for resection, the most important factors are: (1) long disease-free interval; (2) solitary resectable liver tumor; and (3) absence of extrahepatic metastases.

Neuroendocrine carcinomas (pancreatic islet cell tumors, carcinoids) represent a unique class of tumors that often give rise to liver metastases. Unlike other metastatic tumor types, patients with neuroendocrine tumors often survive for many years. Multiple liver metastases are the rule with this disease, so complete resection is usually not possible. However, debulking liver resections are sometimes indicated to palliate tumor-related pain or hormonal symptoms. Partial hepatectomy is also sometimes worthwhile to extirpate a tumor invading directly from a contiguous organ.

B. Radiofrequency Ablation

Radiofrequency ablation has been used to treat metastases to the liver from a variety of tumor types. The indications for this procedure remain ill-defined. The best candidates are those with a limited number of small liver lesions with no evidence of extrahepatic cancer.

C. Chemotherapy

In a large proportion of patients with metastatic colorectal cancer, the liver is the only evident site of disease. If the lesions cannot be resected, regional intrahepatic chemotherapy can be given by placing a catheter in the gastroduodenal artery (at its origin with the common hepatic artery) connected to an implantable, subcutaneous infusion pump, which allows the delivery of much higher concentrations of drug to the tumor than is possible with systemic administration. This regimen is generally not used for metastases from other kinds of tumors. The pump is primed with floxuridine, which is delivered by continuous infusion (0.1–0.2 mg/kg/d) for 14-day periods alternating with 14-day rests. Systemic chemotherapy is usually given concomitantly. The discovery of extrahepatic lesions at laparotomy for pump placement is a relative contraindication to proceeding with this approach. Treatment is continued until disease progression or excessive toxicity is seen, or rarely until the response is complete. Toxicity consists mainly of gastroduodenal erosions (caused by unintentional perfusion of these areas), chemical hepatitis, or chemical sclerosing cholangitis. Survival is related principally to the initial amount of liver involvement by tumor, objective response to treatment (which is seen in about 60% of patients), and extent of prior chemotherapy. The median survival of patients with less than 30% of liver replaced by tumor is 24 months, compared with 10 months if the extent of replacement exceeds 30%. There is a general perception that hepatic artery infusion therapy improves survival, but the objective evidence is inconclusive. Cure is not a realistic objective.

Hepatic artery infusion chemotherapy may be a useful adjunctive therapy after complete tumor resection or radiofrequency ablation. Studies of this option are under way.

Systemic chemotherapy (eg, with fluorouracil, irinotecan, or oxaliplatin) after liver resection has not been proved to improve survival, although it is often prescribed.

D. Miscellaneous

Hepatic artery ligation or angiographic embolization of the tumor has been of benefit in a few patients with hepatic metastases from specific tumor types, particularly neuroendocrine tumors.

Prognosis

Survival varies with the site of origin of the primary tumor and the extent of metastatic disease. Patients with extensive hepatic replacement by multiple lesions have a dismal outlook, with a survival measured in months, compared to perhaps 2–3 years for patients with small solitary lesions. The range of treatment options and effective chemotherapeutic agents is greatest for metastatic colorectal cancer compared to most other tumor types, and survival is generally better in this group.

Cady B et al: Surgical margin in hepatic resection for colorectal metastasis: a critical and improvable determinant of outcome. Ann Surg 1998;227:566.

DeMatteo RP et al: Results of hepatic resection for sarcoma metastatic to liver. Ann Surg 2001;234:540.

Fong et al: Clinical score for predicting recurrence after hepatic resection for metastatic colorectal cancer: analysis of 1001 consecutive cases. Ann Surg 1999;230:309.

Gruenberger T et al: Reduction in recurrence risk for involved or inadequate margins with edge cryotherapy after liver resection for colorectal metastases. Arch Surg 2001;136:1154.

Harmon KE et al: Benefits and safety of hepatic resection for colorectal metastases. Am J Surg 1999;177:402.

Heslin MJ et al: Colorectal hepatic metastases: resection, local ablation, and hepatic artery infusion pump are associated with prolonged survival. Arch Surg 2001;136:318.

Kokudo N et al: Anatomical major resection versus nonanatomical limited resection for liver metastases from colorectal carcinoma. Am J Surg 2001;181:153.

Lambert LA, Colacchio TA, Barth RJ Jr: Interval hepatic resection of colorectal metastases improves patient selection. Arch Surg 2000;135:473.

Nagakura S, Shirai Y, Hatakeyama K: Computed tomographic features of colorectal carcinoma liver metastases predict posthepatectomy patient survival. Dis Colon Rectum 2001;44:1148.

Primrose JN: Treatment of colorectal metastases: surgery, cryotherapy, or radiofrequency ablation. Gut 2002;50:1.

Scudamore CH et al: Radiofrequency ablation followed by resection of malignant liver tumors. Am J Surg 1999;177:411.

Strasberg SM et al: Survival of patients evaluated by FDG-PET before hepatic resection for metastatic colorectal carcinoma: a prospective database study. Ann Surg 2001;233:293.

Taylor I, Gillams AR: Colorectal liver metastases: alternatives to resection. J R Soc Med 2000;93:576.

BENIGN TUMORS & CYSTS OF THE LIVER*

Hemangiomas

Hemangioma is the most common benign hepatic tumor, and except for the skin and mucous membranes, the liver is the most common site of origin. Women are affected more often than men—in some series, up to 75% of patients are female. Histologically, hepatic hemangiomata are of the cavernous type rather than the capillary type. Most are small solitary subcapsular growths that are found incidentally during laparotomy or autopsy or on imaging studies. Rarely, hemangiomata grow to very large dimensions (giant hemangiomata) and cause abdominal pain or a palpable mass. Most are small to moderate-sized lesions, however; pain is uncommon in tumors < 8–10 cm in diameter.

Rare complications of liver hemangiomata include hemorrhagic shock resulting from spontaneous rupture and the Kasabach-Merritt syndrome, which is usually seen in children and is associated with thrombocytopenia and a consumptive coagulopathy; both of these complications are exceedingly uncommon. Large congenital hemangiomas of the liver may be associated with others in the skin. Large hemangiomata may also

*Echinococcal cysts are discussed in Chapter 8.

give rise to large-volume arteriovenous shunting, resulting in cardiac hypertrophy and congestive heart failure.

Large-bore needle biopsy is hazardous due to bleeding risks; aspiration biopsy with a fine needle is safe but rarely helpful. Fortunately, biopsy is very rarely indicated, since the diagnosis can be made with certainty in most cases by contrast-enhanced CT or MRI scans. The hallmark features of hemangiomata are nodular peripheral enhancement of the lesion, with slow enhancement of the entire lesion on the more delayed images. MRI is particularly good for hemangiomata, which appear very bright on the T2-weighted images. Angiography is unnecessary and nuclear scans lack sufficient sensitivity and specificity.

The only reasons to resect hemangiomata are for symptoms, most commonly pain, or diagnostic uncertainty. Symptomatic hemangiomas should be excised by lobectomy or enucleation. Even large lesions can be safely removed. Radiotherapy or embolization via a catheter in the hepatic artery may be tried in patients who are poor candidates for surgery, but the efficacy of these approaches is limited. The natural history of asymptomatic hemangiomas, whether large or small, is benign. The vast majority of incidentally discovered hemangiomata remain stable in follow-up, do not give rise to symptoms, and therefore do not require resection. Progressive growth of asymptomatic hemangiomata over a relatively short time interval, particularly in young patients, is considered a relative indication for resection.

Bykov S et al: The role of hepatobiliary scintigraphy in the follow-up of benign liver tumors secondary to oral contraceptive use. Clin Nucl Med 2001;26:946.

Charny CK et al: The management of 155 patients with benign liver tumours. Br J Surg 2001;88:1.

Cherqui D et al: Laparoscopic liver resections: a feasibility study in 30 patients. Ann Surg 2000;232:753.

Popescu I et al: Liver hemangioma revisited: current surgical indications, technical aspects, results. Hepatogastroenterology 2001;48:770.

Terkivatan T et al: Indications and long-term outcome of treatment for benign hepatic tumors: a critical appraisal. Arch Surg 2001;136:1033.

Cysts

A number of different cystic lesions may affect the liver. Simple hepatic cysts, the most common, are unilocular fluid-filled lesions that generally produce no symptoms. The occasional large cyst may present as an upper abdominal mass or discomfort. Small simple cysts may be difficult to diagnose on CT and may be confused for metastatic disease; ultrasound and MRI are better modalities to assess the character of cystic lesions. Many patients have multiple simple cysts, which should not be confused with polycystic liver disease, a progressive condition characterized by cystic replacement of virtually the entire liver. Polycystic liver disease is associated in about half of cases with polycystic renal disease. The possibility of echinococcosis (see Chapter 8) should be considered in patients with cystic liver lesions and the appropriate exposure history, although their radiographic appearance is usually quite distinctive.

Most simple cysts have a serous lining and a smooth, thin wall. Intracystic hemorrhage can occur, which can confuse the radiographic appearance. Solitary cysts lined with cuboidal epithelium are classified as cystadenomas and should be resected, since they are premalignant. Cystadenomas are characterized radiographically as complex, with internal septae, an irregular lining, and papillary projections. Complex, multilocular (septated) cysts (if not echinococcal) are usually neoplastic and should be resected; the possibility of a simple cyst with internal hemorrhage should be kept in mind. There are few indications for aspirating hepatic cysts—simple cysts reaccumulate fluid quickly, neoplastic cysts must be excised, and parasitic cysts might rupture and the parasite thus allowed to spread. It is possible to eliminate small cysts by aspiration of the contents followed by an injection into the lumen of 20–100 mL of absolute alcohol; however, small cysts almost never cause symptoms and generally require no treatment.

Large symptomatic cysts are difficult to eradicate with alcohol injections, and serious superinfection of the cyst cavity may occur. The simplest method of treatment consists of laparoscopic cyst fenestration (wide excision of the cyst wall). A tongue of omentum is fixed so it lies in the residual cyst cavity as an ancillary measure to prevent the edges from coapting. The operation is curative in nearly all patients.

Multiple, small simple cysts do not usually require treatment, but large polycystic livers that cause discomfort or are associated with obstructive jaundice can be managed by partial resection or surgically unroofing the cysts on the surface of the liver and creating windows between superficial cysts and adjacent deep cysts. The opened cysts are allowed to drain into the abdominal cavity. The results of surgery for polycystic liver disease are often disappointing, with quick return of symptoms in many patients.

Cowles RA, Mulholland MW: Solitary hepatic cysts. J Am Coll Surg 2000;191:311.

Hansen P, Ludemann R, Swanstrom LL: Minimally invasive approaches to hepatic surgery. Hepatogastroenterology 2001; 48:37.

Inaba Y et al: Focal attenuation differences in pericystic liver tissue as seen on CT hepatic arteriography and CT arterial portography: observation using a unified helical CT and angiography system. Abdom Imaging 1999;24:360.

Hepatic Adenoma

Hepatic adenomas occur predominantly in women and appear to be related to the widespread use of oral contraceptives. Mestranol-containing compounds have been associated with a disproportionate number of cases, but mestranol has been in use longer than the other agents.

The tumors are soft, yellow-tan, well-circumscribed masses that are usually of moderate size (range of 2–15 cm in diameter). Most of those that cause symptoms are in the 8- to 15-cm range. Two-thirds of hepatic adenomas are solitary; other benign tumors (such as focal nodular hyperplasia, see below) are present in some cases. Transition from benign hepatic adenoma to hepatocellular carcinoma may occur, with liver cell dysplasia as an intermediate step. Histologically, hepatic adenomas consist of an encapsulated homogeneous mass of normal-appearing hepatocytes without bile ducts or central veins. Intra-tumoral hemorrhage or central necrosis may be present.

About half of patients are asymptomatic. Most of those with symptoms present with right upper quadrant pain. Spontaneous hemorrhage into the substance of the tumor with subsequent rupture and intraperitoneal bleeding is a well-known potential complication of adenomas; patients with this life-threatening problem present with acute pain or even hemorrhagic shock. There is a strong association of acute bleeding episodes with pregnancy.

Liver function tests and AFP levels are usually normal or minimally deranged. Adenomas are typically hypervascular compared to the surrounding liver parenchyma, a feature that is apparent on contrast-enhanced CT or MRI scans or angiography. Adenomas can be difficult to distinguish from focal nodular hyperplasia, another benign tumor often found in young women. Differences in tumor vascularity may be demonstrated on angiography; however, MRI is probably the best study for differentiating these lesions. Adenomas often cannot be distinguished from well-differentiated hepatocellular carcinoma on imaging studies and even on biopsy specimens. Needle biopsy is generally safe but often inconclusive and is associated with a small risk of bleeding.

The general consensus is that adenomas should be resected because of the risks of malignant change and spontaneous hemorrhage. Unfortunately, the true likelihood of these events is difficult to estimate, since most series include only treated patients. Symptomatic and large asymptomatic adenomas clearly should be resected. Emergent resection or hepatic artery embolization should be undertaken in patients with evidence of hemorrhage. Small peripheral lesions may be removed with wedge excisions but larger tumors require more extensive resections. Small adenomas may regress when oral contraceptive agents are discontinued, and close follow-up with imaging studies is not unreasonable in such cases; however, any change in symptoms or imaging characteristics (growth, hemorrhage) should prompt resection. The possibility that a presumed adenoma is actually a well-differentiated HCC or contains a focus of malignancy must always be kept in mind; there is no completely reliable means of making the differentiation other than pathologic analysis of the resected specimen.

Most patients recover without sequelae after surgical removal; recurrence is rare. Oral contraceptives should be proscribed permanently in all cases. Radiotherapy and chemotherapy are of no value, but elective hepatic artery embolization may be helpful in patients who are not surgical candidates.

Focal Nodular Hyperplasia

Focal nodular hyperplasia (FNH) is a benign lesion with no malignant potential. Like hepatic adenoma, FNH is much more common in young women. The average age is about 40 years, but the tumor can occur at any age. Unlike hepatic adenoma, however, the use of oral contraceptive agents does not appear to predispose to the development of FNH, although it has been suggested that these agents can stimulate growth.

Grossly, the tumor is a well-circumscribed, firm, tan, usually subcapsular mass measuring 2–3 cm in diameter. In patients with symptoms, the lesions are much larger, usually around 10 cm. Multiple tumors can occur; 80% are solitary. The gross appearance on cut section is quite characteristic, consisting of a central stellate scar (which is actually an aggregation of blood vessels) with radiating fibrous septa that compartmentalize the lesion into lobules. Histologically, there are nodular aggregations of normal-appearing hepatocytes without central veins or portal triads. Bile duct proliferation is present in the nodules.

Most patients with FNH are asymptomatic. The few with symptoms present with a right upper quadrant discomfort. Unlike hepatic adenomas, these lesions rarely, if ever, bleed, and the natural history of asymptomatic lesions is benign. Very rare patients with diffuse FNH develop portal hypertension.

Hepatic function tests and AFP levels are usually normal. Hepatic scintiscans usually do not show a filling defect but are of little practical value. CT scans demonstrate the tumor and may also show the central stellate scar. The arteriographic pattern is one of hypervascularity. In most cases, the diagnosis of FNH can be made with noninvasive studies, although distinguishing FNH from hepatic adenomas can be difficult, even for experienced radiologists. MRI scanning is the best modality, but the imaging features of both tumors overlap somewhat and they occur in similar patient populations. Fine-needle aspiration biopsies are generally not helpful.

Symptomatic lesions should be removed, while asymptomatic tumors (the majority) should be left undisturbed, provided that the diagnosis has been made confidently. In the latter circumstance, a period of observation with imaging studies is recommended to ensure stability. Inability to distinguish FNH from adenoma or malignant disease is an indication for resection in some patients. Discontinuation of oral contraceptives probably has no impact. Focal nodular hyperplasia can be reliably identified on examination of frozen sections.

Bioulac-Sage P, Balabaud C, Wanless IR: Diagnosis of focal nodular hyperplasia: not so easy. Am J Surg Pathol 2001;25:1322.

Leconte I et al: Focal nodular hyperplasia: natural course observed with CT and MRI. J Comput Assist Tomogr 2000;24:61.

Terkivatan T et al: Indications and long-term outcome of treatment for benign hepatic tumors: a critical appraisal. Arch Surg 2001;136:1033.

Terkivatan T et al: Treatment of ruptured hepatocellular adenoma. Br J Surg 2001;88:207.

PORTAL HYPERTENSION

Etiology

The major causes of portal hypertension are listed in Table 24–3. In all but a few instances, the basic lesion is increased resistance to portal flow. Those associated with increased resistance can be subclassified according to the site of the block as prehepatic, hepatic, and posthepatic; hepatic causes of portal hypertension are further classified as presinusoidal, sinusoidal, and postsinusoidal. Cirrhosis accounts for about 85% of cases of portal hypertension in the USA, most commonly from heavy alcohol use. Postnecrotic cirrhosis is next in frequency, followed by biliary cirrhosis. The other intrahepatic causes of portal hypertension are relatively rare in Western countries, although in some parts of the world hepatic schistosomiasis constitutes the largest single group. Idiopathic portal hypertension occurs with greater frequency in southern Asia.

After cirrhosis, extrahepatic portal venous thrombosis or occlusion is the most common cause of portal hypertension in the USA. Patients with this condition are generally younger than cirrhotics, and many are children. Posthepatic obstruction due to Budd-Chiari syndrome or constrictive pericarditis is rare.

Table 24–3. Causes of portal hypertension.

I. Increased resistance to flow
- **A. Prehepatic (portal vein obstruction)**
  1. Congenital atresia or stenosis
  2. Thrombosis of portal vein
  3. Thrombosis of splenic vein
  4. Extrinsic compression (eg, tumors)
- **B. Hepatic**
  1. Cirrhosis
     - a. Portal cirrhosis (nutritional, alcoholic, Laënnec's)
     - b. Postnecrotic cirrhosis
     - c. Biliary cirrhosis
     - d. Others (Wilson's disease, hemochromatosis)
  2. Acute alcoholic liver disease
  3. Chronic active hepatitis
  4. Congenital hepatic fibrosis
  5. Idiopathic portal hypertension (hepatoportal sclerosis)
  6. Schistosomiasis
  7. Sarcoidosis
- **C. Posthepatic**
  1. Budd-Chiari syndrome (hepatic vein thrombosis)
  2. Veno-occlusive disease
  3. Cardiac Disease
     - a. Constrictive pericarditis
     - b. Valvular heart disease
     - c. Right heart failure

II. Increased portal blood flow
- **A. Arterial-portal venous fistula**
- **B. Increased splenic flow**
  1. Banti's syndrome
  2. Splenomegaly (eg, tropical splenomegaly, myeloid metaplasia)

Pathophysiology

Since pressure in the portal venous system is determined by the relationship $P = F \times R$, portal hypertension could result either from increased volume of portal blood flow or increased resistance to flow. In practice, however, the liver has tremendous reserve capacity to accommodate increased blood flow, and portal hypertension due to this mechanism is extremely uncommon. Nearly all clinically relevant cases result from increased resistance, although the site of the resistance varies in different diseases. A pathophysiologic classification of the causes of portal hypertension is given in Table 24–3.

Portal venous pressure normally ranges from 7 to 10 mm Hg. In portal hypertension, portal pressure exceeds 10 mm Hg, averaging around 20 mm Hg and occasionally rising as high as 50–60 mm Hg.

In alcoholic liver disease, the abnormal resistance is predominantly postsinusoidal, as indicated by the results of wedged hepatic vein pressure studies.*

The causes of increased resistance in this disease are thought to be (1) distortion of the hepatic veins by regenerative nodules and (2) fibrosis of perivascular tissue around the hepatic veins and the sinusoids.

Even in the absence of cirrhosis, acute alcoholic hepatitis can raise portal pressure by producing centrilobular swelling and fibrosis. Sinusoidal resistance to flow is also increased by engorgement of adjacent hepatocytes with fat and resultant distortion and narrowing of vascular channels. Documented cases of normalization or

*A catheter wedged in a tributary of the hepatic vein permits estimation of the pressure in the afferent veins to the sinusoid. The gradient between the wedged pressure and that in the hepatic vein reflects resistance at any point between the wedged position and the periphery of the sinusoid. The current view holds that the site of principal resistance in normal persons is in reasonably large hepatic veins. In cirrhosis, it is probably in the sinusoids as well as the hepatic veins.

reduction in portal pressure have occurred with resolution of the pathologic changes.

Schistosomiasis can produce a unique form of presinusoidal obstruction to blood flow from deposition of parasite ova in small portal venules. The subsequent chronic inflammatory reaction leads to fibrosis and cirrhosis. Many patients with schistosomiasis are also at risk for chronic hepatitis, which can exacerbate the liver damage.

Fluctuations in the level of portal hypertension may occur in conjunction with changes in blood volume. This is almost never a problem in patients with a normal liver. However, administration of colloid solutions to a patient with underlying liver disease and a normal or expanded blood volume could theoretically aggravate the clinical manifestations of portal hypertension.

Budd-Chiari syndrome (hepatic vein thrombosis) results from obstruction of flow through the hepatic veins. The resulting sinusoidal hypertension produces prominent ascites and hepatomegaly. Conditions (veno-occlusive disease, inferior vena cava obstruction by tumor or congenital webs, right-sided heart failure) that reduce flow through the hepatic veins will result in a similar clinical picture.

Banti's syndrome was defined as liver disease secondary to primary splenic disease and was incorrectly considered as the cause of portal hypertension now known to result from cirrhosis and other hepatic disorders rather than a consequence of such conditions. Portal hypertension from splenomegaly and increased splenic vein flow has been described in patients with hematologic diseases or tropical splenomegaly and apparently normal liver function. This is uncommon, however, and given the great reserve of the liver to handle increases in portal flow, many such patients probably have some component of liver disease. In cirrhosis, the increased splenic blood flow accompanying "congestive" splenomegaly may occasionally be great enough to warrant splenic artery ligation or splenectomy to decrease portal pressure and improve symptoms, but this situation is rare.

Increased flow may contribute to portal hypertension in patients with traumatic arterial-portal venous fistulas (traumatic, congenital). When an arteriovenous fistula occurs, portal hypertension and its clinical manifestations usually do not appear for several months, because sinusoidal capacity is so great that the immediate rise in portal pressure is only moderate. With time, however, sinusoidal sclerosis develops, resistance increases, and portal pressure gradually reaches high levels, leading to the formation of varices.

The average portal flow in cirrhotic patients with complications of portal hypertension is about 30% of normal, ranging from 0 to 700 mL/min. Hepatic arterial flow is usually reduced by a similar proportion. The range of portal flow rates in different patients may vary greatly; in some, blood in the portal vein moves sluggishly or the direction of flow may even be reversed (hepatofugal) so that the portal vein functions as an outflow tract from the liver. These states of low flow predispose to spontaneous thrombosis of the portal vein, a complication of cirrhosis that usually is associated with acute clinical deterioration and renders the portal vein unsuitable for a shunt.

The obstacle to flow through the liver promotes expansion of collateral channels between the portal and systemic venous systems. As the pathologic process develops, portal pressure increases until a level of about 40 cm H_2O (30 mm Hg) is reached. At this point, increasing hepatic resistance, even to the point of occlusion of the portal vein, diverts a greater fraction of portal flow through collaterals without significant increments in portal pressure.

The type of collateral that develops depends partly on the cause of the portal hypertension. In extrahepatic portal vein thrombosis (without liver disease), collaterals in the diaphragm and in the hepatocolic, hepatoduodenal, and gastrohepatic ligaments transport blood into the liver around the occluded vein (hepatopetal). In cirrhosis, collateral vessels circumvent the liver and deliver portal blood directly into the systemic circulation (hepatofugal); these collaterals give rise to esophageal and gastric varices. Other common spontaneous collaterals are through a recanalized umbilical vein to the abdominal wall, from the superior hemorrhoidal vein into the middle and inferior hemorrhoidal veins, and through numerous small veins (of Retzius) connecting the retroperitoneal viscera with the posterior abdominal wall.

Isolated thrombosis of the splenic vein causes localized splenic venous hypertension and gives rise to large collaterals from spleen to gastric fundus. From there, the blood returns to the main portal system through the coronary vein. In this condition, gastric varices are often present without esophageal varices.

Of the many large collaterals that form as a result of portal hypertension, spontaneous bleeding is relatively uncommon except from those at the gastroesophageal junction; spontaneous bleeding from gastric varices can sometimes occur. Compared with adjacent areas of the esophagus and stomach, the gastroesophageal junction is especially rich in submucosal veins, which expand disproportionately in patients with portal hypertension. The cause of variceal bleeding is most probably rupture due to sudden increases in hydrostatic pressure. Esophagitis is usually mild or absent.

Debernardi-Venon W et al: CO_2 wedged hepatic venography in the evaluation of portal hypertension. Gut 2000;46:856.

Krige JE, Beckingham IJ: ABC of diseases of liver, pancreas, and biliary system. Portal hypertension—1: varices. BMJ 2001;322:348.

Krige JE, Beckingham IJ: ABC of diseases of liver, pancreas, and biliary system: portal hypertension—2. Ascites, encephalopathy, and other conditions. BMJ 2001;322:416.

CIRRHOSIS

Hepatic cirrhosis remains a major public health problem worldwide, with and annual mortality of approximately 23,000 per year in the USA alone. The incidence of the cirrhosis is increasing, due in large measure to hepatitis C, and at present is the third most common cause of death in men in the fifth decade of life.

Alcohol abuse remains the leading cause of cirrhosis in most Western countries. Alcohol exerts direct toxic effects on the liver that are magnified in the presence of protein and other dietary deficiencies that are often present. Even still, cirrhosis develops in a small minority of patients who abuse alcohol. Alcohol induces a specific cytochrome P450 in the liver (ie, P450 2E1) that participates in its metabolism to acetaldehyde, which has a number of deleterious effects, including antibody formation, decreased DNA repair, enzyme inactivation, and alterations in microtubules, mitochondria, and plasma membranes. Acetaldehyde also promotes glutathione depletion, free radical-mediated toxicity, lipid peroxidation, and hepatic collagen synthesis. Hepatic steatosis and alcoholic hepatitis are stages of alcoholic liver injury that may precede cirrhosis. Alcoholic hyalin, a glycoprotein, accumulates in centrilobular hepatocytes of patients with alcoholic hepatitis. There is some evidence that immunologic responses to alcoholic hyalin may be important in the pathogenesis of cirrhosis.

Collagen deposition in cirrhosis results from increased fibroblastic activity as well as from repair following hepatocellular injury and necrosis. The ultimate result is a liver containing regenerative nodules and connective tissue septa linking portal fields with central canals.

The natural history of cirrhosis is difficult to predict. Once the diagnosis has been established, up to 30% of patients die within a year from hepatic failure or complications of portal hypertension, of which bleeding esophageal varices is the most feared. In newly diagnosed cirrhotics, the chances of dying within the subsequent 2–3 years are influenced by the status of liver function (as reflected by the Child-Pugh classification), the presence of varices, and the portal pressure. A group of cirrhotics with varices followed by the Boston Interhospital Liver Group experienced a 1-year death rate of 66%. Cirrhotics without varices may benefit substantially by abstaining from alcohol. Bleeding episodes occur in up to 40% of all patients with cirrhosis, and the initial episode of variceal hemorrhage is fatal in 50% or more. At least two-thirds of those who survive their initial hemorrhage will bleed again, and the risk of dying from the second is similarly high. It is principally for such patients that portal decompressive procedures are recommended.

Menon KV, Kamath PS: Managing the complications of cirrhosis. Mayo Clin Proc 2000;75:501.

Menon KV, Gores GJ, Shah VH: Pathogenesis, diagnosis, and treatment of alcoholic liver disease. Mayo Clin Proc 2001; 76:1021.

ACUTELY BLEEDING VARICES

About half of patients with massive bleeding from varices die as a result of the acute event. This high death rate reflects not only the massive hemorrhage but also the frequent presence of severely compromised liver function and other systemic disease that may or may not be related to alcohol abuse. Malnutrition, pulmonary aspiration and infection, and coronary artery disease are frequent coexisting conditions. Additional complicating factors in this patient population include lack of cooperation with treatment and acute alcohol withdrawal, which in its worst manifestation (delirium tremens) adds greatly to the already high mortality rate.

Clinical Findings

A. Symptoms and Signs

The initial management of the patient with massive gastrointestinal hemorrhage is discussed in Chapter 23. It must be emphasized that bleeding from varices cannot be accurately diagnosed on clinical grounds alone even though the history or the appearance of the patient may strongly suggest the presence of cirrhosis or portal hypertension. Most patients with bleeding varices have alcoholic cirrhosis, and the diagnosis may seem obvious in a patient with hepatomegaly, jaundice, and vascular spiders who admits to recent binge drinking. Splenomegaly, the most constant physical finding, is present in 80% of patients with portal hypertension regardless of the cause. Ascites is frequently present. Massive ascites and hepatosplenomegaly in a nonalcoholic would suggest the much less common Budd-Chiari syndrome. If cirrhosis or varices have been documented on previous examinations, hematemesis would strongly suggest bleeding varices as the cause.

B. Laboratory Findings

Most patients with alcoholic liver disease and acute upper gastrointestinal bleeding have compromised liver function. The bilirubin is usually elevated, and the serum albumin is often below 3 g/dL. The leukocyte count may be elevated. Anemia may be a reflection of chronic alcoholic liver disease or hypersplenism as well as acute hemorrhage. The development of a hepatoma by a cirrhotic may first manifested by hemorrhage from varices; CT scan and determination of serum alpha-fetoprotein will make the diagnosis. Thrombocytopenia and coagulopathy are common.

C. Special Examinations

1. Esophagogastroscopy—Emergency esophagogastroscopy is the most useful procedure for diagnosing bleeding varices and should be scheduled as soon as the patient's general condition is stabilized by blood transfusion and other supportive measures. Endotracheal intubation may be necessary for airway control. Varices appear as three or four large, tortuous submucosal bluish vessels running longitudinally in the distal esophagus. The bleeding site may be identified, but in some cases the lumen fills with blood so rapidly that the lesion is obscured.

2. Upper gastrointestinal series—A barium swallow outlines the varices in about 90% of affected patients, but barium studies are neither as sensitive nor as specific as endoscopy, and they are difficult and dangerous in the bleeding patient.

Treatment of Acute Bleeding

The general goal of treatment is to control the bleeding as quickly and reliably as possible using methods with the fewest possible side effects. The methods currently in use for acute variceal bleeding are listed in Table 24–4.

The patient's condition is stabilized to the extent possible by following the general guidelines for treating major upper gastrointestinal bleeding described in Chapter 23. Other therapy should include measures to treat or prevent encephalopathy, parenteral vitamin K to correct a prolonged prothrombin time, and electrolyte replacement (especially potassium) as required to restore electrolyte balance.

Endoscopic sclerotherapy or banding is the initial therapy of choice. Vasopressin or propranolol may or may not be included in the initial resuscitative regimen. Balloon tamponade is no longer used routinely but is rather reserved for special situations when other methods fail.

These measures are successful in approximately 90% of cases, but the early rebleeding rate is about 30%. When bleeding continues after initial treatment and if the patient is a good operative risk, an emergency shunt procedure should be considered.

Death rates rise rapidly in patients requiring more than ten units of blood, and in general, patients still bleeding after six units—or those whose bleeding is still unchecked 24 hours after admission—should be considered for portal decompression procedures. Even when the bleeding is brought under control by the initial intervention, the mortality rate remains high (about 35%) as a result of liver failure and other complications.

Table 24–4. Measures to control acute bleeding from esophageal varices.

Medical
1. Vasopressin, terlipressin
2. Somatostatin analogues

Mechanical
3. Balloon tamponade

Interventional, nonsurgical
4. Endoscopic sclerotherapy
5. Transphepatic embolization and sclerotherapy

Surgical
6. Emergency portasystemic shunts
7. Esophageal transection and reanastomosis
8. Esophagogastric devascularization
9. Suture ligation of varices

Specific Measures

1. Acute endoscopic sclerotherapy or ligation—Via fiberoptic endoscopy, 1–3 mL of sclerosant solution is injected into the lumen of each varix, causing it to become thrombosed. Variations in the type of endoscope or sclerosant solution or whether or not the varices are physically compressed, etc, appear to have little influence on the outcome. Endoscopy is usually repeated within 48 hours and then once or twice again at weekly intervals, at which time any residual varices are injected.

Sclerotherapy controls acute bleeding in 80–95% of patients, and rebleeding during the same hospitalization is about half (25% versus 50%) the rebleeding rate of patients treated with a combination of vasopressin and balloon tamponade. Even though controlled trials show improvement in the control of bleeding with sclerotherapy, the evidence for increased patient survival is conflicting.

A similar effect can be achieved by endoscopic ligation of the varices. The varix is lifted with a suction tip, and a small rubber band is slipped around the base. The varix necroses to leave a superficial ulcer. A controlled trial has reported rubber band ligation to be more effective in controlling bleeding (eg, fewer episodes of rebleeding; lower mortality rate) than sclerotherapy.

2. Vasopressin and terlipressin (triglycyl lysine vasopressin)—Vasopressin and terlipressin lower portal blood flow and portal pressure by directly constricting splanchnic arterioles, thereby reducing inflow. Vasopressin alone controls acute bleeding in about 80% of patients, and this increases to 95% when used in conjunction with balloon tamponade. Cardiac output, oxygen delivery to the tissues, hepatic blood flow, and renal blood flow are also decreased—effects that occasionally produce complications such as myocardial infarction, cardiac arrhythmias, and intestinal necrosis. These unwanted side effects may sometimes be prevented without interfering with the decrease in portal pressure by simultaneous administration of nitroglycerin or isoproterenol.

Although the results are somewhat contradictory, controlled trials generally indicate that vasopressin plus nitroglycerin is superior to vasopressin alone and that vasopressin alone is superior to placebo in controlling active variceal bleeding. Survival is not increased, however. Vasopressin is given as a peripheral intravenous infusion (at about 0.4 units/min), which is safer than bolus injections. Nitroglycerin can be given intravenously or sublingually. Terlipressin, a synthetic vasopressin analogue, undergoes gradual conversion to vasopressin in the body and is safe to give by intravenous bolus injection (2 mg intravenously every 6 hours). It may cause fewer cardiac side effects than vasopressin.

3. Octreotide acetate—Somatostatin and the synthetic longer-lasting analogue octreotide have the same effect on the splanchnic circulation as vasopressin but without significant side effects. These drugs are as effective as vasopressin in controlling acute variceal bleeding and are now the first choice for the pharmacologic control of acutely bleeding varices. Octreotide is given as an initial bolus of 100 μg followed by a continuous infusion of 25 μ/h for 24 hours.

4. Balloon tamponade—(Figure 24–7) Tubes designed for tamponade have two balloons that can be inflated in the lumen of the gut to compress bleeding varices. There are three or four lumens in the tube, depending on the type: two are for filling balloons within the stomach and the esophagus and the third permits aspiration of gastric contents. A fourth lumen in the Minnesota tube is used to aspirate the esophagus orad to the esophageal balloon. The main effect results from traction applied to the tube, which forces the gastric balloon to compress the collateral veins at the cardia of the stomach. Inflating the esophageal balloon probably contributes little, since barium x-rays suggest that it does not actually compress the varices.

The most common serious complication is aspiration of pharyngeal secretions and pneumonitis.

Another serious hazard is the occasional instance of esophageal rupture caused by inflation of the esophageal balloon. The esophageal balloon is therefore infrequently used.

About 75% of actively bleeding patients can be controlled by balloon tamponade. When bleeding has stopped, the balloons are left inflated for another 24 hours. They are then decompressed, leaving the tube in place. If bleeding does not recur, the tube should be withdrawn.

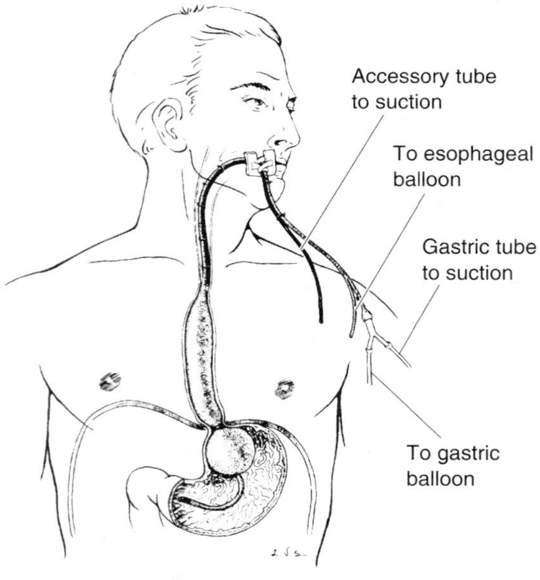

Figure 24–7. Sengstaken-Blakemore tube with both gastric and esophageal balloons inflated.

5. Transjugular intrahepatic portasystemic shunt (TIPS)—TIPS is a minimally invasive means of creating a portasystemic shunt by creating a direct communication between the portal and hepatic venous systems within the liver. A catheter is introduced through the jugular vein and, under radiologic control, positioned in the hepatic vein. From this point, the portal vein is accessed through the liver, the tract is dilated, and the channel is kept open by inserting an expandable metal stent, which is left in place. This technique is of great value in controlling portal hypertension and variceal bleeding and can be used to stop acute bleeding or to prevent rebleeding in a patient who has recovered from an acute episode. The shunts remain open in most patients for up to a year, at which point intimal overgrowth and thrombosis occlude a gradually increasing number.

TIPS has proved most useful as a bridge to transplantation. With current materials, it should not be regarded as definitive therapy, though the shunt will usually remain patent for many months. Thus, patients with advanced liver disease are the principal candidates for TIPS, whereas those with less severe cirrhosis should be considered for beta-blocker therapy or surgery (shunt or devascularization procedure).

6. Surgery—The operative procedures to control active bleeding are emergency portasystemic shunt and variceal ligation or esophageal transection.

a. Emergency portacaval shunt—An emergency portasystemic shunt has a 95% rate of success in stopping variceal bleeding. The death rate of the operation is related to the status of the patient's liver function (eg, Child-Pugh classification) (Table 24–1) as well as the rate and amount of bleeding and its effects on cardiac, renal, and pulmonary function. Some patients with advanced liver disease, especially those with severe encephalopathy and ascites, have an extraordinarily poor survival regardless of the treatment. In such patients, surgery is usually not warranted, even in the face of continued bleeding. On the other hand, patients with good liver function usually recover after an emergency shunt. A controlled trial showed that the death rate in acutely bleeding Child's C patients was insignificantly lower after endoscopic sclerotherapy (44%) than after emergency portacaval shunt (50%).

For active bleeding, an end-to-side portacaval shunt or H-mesocaval shunt is most commonly performed.

The distal splenorenal (Warren) shunt is usually too time-consuming for use in emergency operations. The central splenorenal shunt is more complicated than an end-to-side portacaval shunt and has no specific advantages. A side-to-side portacaval shunt might be preferable in an acutely bleeding patient with severe ascites, and this approach (or a variant such as an H-mesocaval shunt) would be required for someone with Budd-Chiari syndrome.

Hepatic failure is the cause of death in about two-thirds of those who die after an emergency portacaval shunt. Renal failure, which is often accompanied by ascites, is another potentially lethal problem. Metabolic alkalosis and delirium tremens are not uncommon postoperatively in alcoholics.

b. Esophageal transection—Varices may be obliterated by firing the end-to-end stapler in the distal esophagus after tucking a full-thickness ring of tissue into the cartridge with a circumferential tie. This procedure has gained popularity in the past decade, and in many surgical units it is the first choice for therapy when nonsurgical methods fail. If transection is performed, it must be done as soon as it is recognized that a second attempt at sclerotherapy or band ligation has failed. As a last-ditch effort—after many units of blood have been transfused—death from liver failure is all but certain. The results (eg, survival) are better in patients with nonalcoholic cirrhosis. Stapled transection has replaced the older technique of direct suture ligation of the varices. Transection must be viewed as an emergency measure to stop persistent bleeding—not as definitive treatment—since the underlying portal hypertension is not corrected and varices recur months later in many patients.

Cales P et al: Early administration of vapreotide for variceal bleeding in patients with cirrhosis. French Club for the Study of Portal Hypertension. N Engl J Med 2001;344:23.

Gerbes AL et al: Transjugular intrahepatic portosystemic shunt (TIPS) for variceal bleeding in portal hypertension: comparison of emergency and elective interventions. Dig Dis Sci 1998;43:2463.

Mercado MA et al: Comparative study of 2 variants of a modified esophageal transection in the Sugiura-Futagawa operation. Arch Surg 1998;133:1046.

Orozco H et al: A comparative study of the elective treatment of variceal hemorrhage with beta-blockers, transendoscopic sclerotherapy, and surgery: a prospective, controlled, and randomized trial during 10 years. Ann Surg 2000;232:216.

Shibata D et al: Transjugular intrahepatic portosystemic shunt for treatment of bleeding ectopic varices with portal hypertension. Dis Colon Rectum 1999;42:1581.

Woods JE, Kiely JM: Short-term international medical service. Mayo Clin Proc 2000;75:311.

NONBLEEDING VARICES

Patients with varices that have never bled have a 30% chance of bleeding at some point; and of those who bleed, 50% die. For patients who do not bleed during the first year after diagnosis of varices, the risk of bleeding subsequently decreases by half and continues to drop thereafter. Patients who have bled once from esophageal varices have a 70% chance of bleeding again, and about two-thirds of repeat bleeding episodes are fatal.

Evaluation

A. Severity of Hepatic Disease and Operative Risk

The immediate death rate of an elective shunt procedure can be predicted from the patient's hepatic function as reflected by the Child-Pugh classification (Table 24–1). In addition to operative death rate, the figures also correlate with the death rate in the first postshunt year. Thereafter, survival curves of the different risk classes become reasonably parallel.

The severity of histopathologic changes in liver biopsies correlates with the immediate surgical death rate, the most ominous findings being hepatocellular necrosis, polymorphonuclear leukocyte infiltration, and the presence of Mallory bodies. The extent of histologic change also correlates with the more easily obtained data in the Child-Pugh classification (ie, severe changes occur in class C patients), so results of biopsies have no independent predictive value.

B. Portal Flow and Pressure Measurements

Measurements of pressure and flow in the splanchnic vasculature have been used for diagnosis and as a guide to therapy and prognosis in portal hypertension. Portal pressure can be measured directly at surgery or preoperatively by any of the following techniques: (1) Wedged hepatic venous pressure (WHVP), which accurately reflects free portal pressure when portal hypertension is caused by a postsinusoidal (or sinusoidal) resistance, as in cirrhosis. The measurement obtained with the catheter in the wedged position should be corrected by subtracting the free hepatic venous pressure (FHVP). This is the most commonly used technique. (2) Direct measurement of splenic pulp pressure by a percutaneously placed needle. (3) Percutaneous transhepatic catheterization of the intrahepatic branches of the portal vein.

This is the method of choice in patients thought to have presinusoidal block or Budd-Chiari syndrome. (4) Catheterization of the umbilical vein through a small incision, the catheter being threaded into the portal system. With each of these methods, one may also obtain anatomic information by performing angiography through the catheter.

It is not customary to measure portal pressure preoperatively, however, since the information obtained does not influence management in most patients. Duplex ultrasonography is an accurate noninvasive means of assessing the amount and direction of flow in the portal vein. Preoperatively, duplex ultrasonography is useful to determine patency of the portal vein and direction of flow. Because of spontaneous thrombosis, about 10% of patients with cirrhosis have a portal vein unsuitable for a portacaval shunt. If flow in the portal vein is reversed (hepatofugal), a selective shunt is not recommended, because it compromises the ability of portal tributaries to serve as an outflow tract for liver blood. Duplex ultrasonography can also be used to follow changes in portal perfusion after shunt operations.

C. Portal Angiography

The portal venous anatomy is often studied preoperatively by angiographic techniques. The objectives are to determine the patency, location, and size of the veins tentatively chosen for a shunt, to demonstrate the presence of varices, and to estimate the degree of prograde portal flow. Some of this information can now be obtained less invasively by duplex ultrasonography. When a splenorenal shunt is contemplated, the left renal vein should be opacified, either by injection of the renal artery or renal vein.

Treatment

The treatment options consist of expectant management, endoscopic sclerotherapy, beta-blocker (propranolol), portasystemic shunts, devascularization of the esophagogastric junction, and miscellaneous rarely used operations. The treatment of patients with varices that have never bled is usually referred to as prophylactic therapy (eg, prophylactic sclerotherapy or prophylactic propranolol). By convention, procedures performed on patients who have bled previously are referred to as therapeutic (eg, therapeutic shunts).

A. Prophylactic Therapy

Prophylactic therapy could theoretically be of value since the mortality rate of variceal bleeding is high (50%), the risk of bleeding in patients with varices is relatively high (30%), and varices can often be diagnosed before the initial episode of bleeding. In patients who have never had a bleeding episode, the following have been shown to be related to the risk of hemorrhage: Child-Pugh classification, the size of the varices, and the presence of red wale markings (longitudinal dilated venules resembling whip marks) on the varices. This information can be used to select high-risk patients (up to 65% risk of bleeding within a year) for prophylactic propranolol.

B. Therapy of Patients Who Have Bled Previously

As noted earlier, patients who recover from an episode of variceal bleeding have about a 70% chance of bleeding again. Much effort has been expended to ascertain the best treatment for these patients. The methods of greatest interest include endoscopic sclerotherapy, propranolol, and portasystemic shunts.

1. Endoscopic sclerotherapy—The technique of endoscopic sclerotherapy was described earlier in this chapter. Chronic sclerotherapy has been disappointing as a method of preventing future bleeding, and most have come to think of it principally as a way to stop acute bleeding when bleeding recurs.

2. Propranolol—Propranolol, a beta-adrenergic blocking agent, decreases cardiac output and splanchnic blood flow and consequently portal blood pressure. Chronic propranolol therapy, 20–160 mg twice daily (a dose that reduces resting pulse rate by 25%), decreases by about 40% the frequency of rebleeding from esophageal or gastric varices, deaths from rebleeding, and overall mortality. The benefits are greater in Child's A and B than in Child's C cirrhotics. The addition of chronic sclerotherapy to the propranolol regimen does not improve the outcome. Abstinence from alcohol may not necessarily decrease the mortality related specifically to variceal hemorrhage, as was initially thought.

C. Surgery

The objective of surgical procedures used to treat portal hypertension is either to obliterate the varices or to reduce blood flow and pressure within the varices (Table 24–5). A third option, particularly in patients with advanced cirrhosis, is liver transplantation.

1. Liver transplantation—Any relatively young patient with cirrhosis who has survived an episode of variceal hemorrhage should be considered a candidate for liver transplantation, since any other form of therapy carries a much higher (about 80%) mortality rate within the subsequent 1–2 years as a result of repeat bleeding or complications of hepatic failure. Obviously, continued alcohol use is a contraindication to transplantation in most patients. The good transplantation candidates, however, should not be subjected to portasystemic shunts or other procedures if it appears that they will come to transplantation in the near future. In general,

Table 24–5. Surgical procedures for esophageal varices.

A. Direct variceal obliteration
1. Variceal suture ligation
a. Transthoracic
b. Transabdominal
2. Esophageal transection and reanastomosis
a. Suture technique
b. Staple technique
3. Variceal sclerosis
a. Esophagoscopic
b. Transhepatic
4. Variceal resection
a. Esophagogastrectomy
b. Subtotal esophagectomy
B. Reduction of variceal blood flow and pressure
1. Portasystemic shunts
a. End-to-side
b. Side-to-side
1. Side-to-side portacaval
2. Mesocaval
3. Central splenorenal
4. Renosplenic
2. Selective shunts
a. Distal splenorenal (Warren)
b. Left gastric vena caval (Inokuchi)
3. Reduction of portal blood flow
a. Splenectomy
b. Splenic artery ligation
4. Reduction of proximal gastric blood flow
a. Esphagogastric devascularization
b. Gastric transection and reanastomosis (Tanner)
5. Stimulation of additional portasystemic venous collaterals
a. Omentopexy
b. Splenic transposition
C. Measures to preserve hepatic blood flow after portacaval shunt
1. Arterialization of portal vein stump

Child's class A patients are candidates for portal decompression; Child's class C patients are candidates for a transplant. A transjugular intrahepatic shunt (see previous section) is an excellent way to control bleeding while the patient is being prepared for a transplant.

2. Portasystemic shunts—Portasystemic shunts can be grouped into those that shunt the entire portal system (total shunts) and those that selectively shunt blood from the gastrosplenic region while preserving the pressure-flow relationships in the rest of the portal bed (selective shunts). All of the shunt operations commonly used today reduce the incidence of rebleeding to less than 10%, compared with about 75% in unshunted patients. Unfortunately, the price of this achievement is an operative mortality rate of 5–20% (depending on the Child-Pugh classification [Table 24–1]), further impairment of liver function, and an increase in encephalopathy (at least with total shunts). Therefore, since shunts have these potential drawbacks, clinical trials are needed to pinpoint their place within an overall treatment strategy.

In one well-designed trial, patients who had bled previously were randomized to chronic sclerotherapy or a distal splenorenal shunt (Warren shunt). Patients randomized to chronic sclerotherapy who had recurrent episodes of bleeding during treatment (ie, treatment failures, which amounted to 30% of the sclerotherapy group) were then treated surgically (ie, shunted). The results showed that 2-year survival was better among those originally randomized to sclerotherapy (90%) than among those originally assigned to the shunt group (60%). This trial supports a general treatment plan consisting initially of sclerotherapy and reserving portasystemic shunts for the patients in whom sclerotherapy fails to control bleeding adequately.

The choice of shunt has been the subject of much debate and several randomized trials. The principal question in recent years has been whether encephalopathy and survival are better with a selective shunt (eg, a distal splenorenal shunt) than with a total shunt (eg, a mesocaval or an end-to-side portacaval shunt). The results are conflicting, but in general they support the contention that there is about half as much severe encephalopathy following selective shunts. None of the trials have shown any particular shunt to be associated with longer survival.

a. Types of portasystemic shunts—Figure 24–8 depicts the various shunts in use currently. Although they differ technically, physiologically there are only three different types: end-to-side, side-to-side, and selective.

(1) Total shunts— The end-to-side shunt completely disconnects the liver from the portal system. The portal vein is transected near its bifurcation in the liver hilum and anastomosed to the side of the inferior vena cava. The hepatic stump of the vein is oversewn. Postoperatively, the wedged hepatic venous pressure (sinusoidal pressure) drops slightly, reflecting the inability of the hepatic artery to compensate fully for the loss of portal inflow. The side-to-side portacaval, mesocaval, mesorenal, and central splenorenal shunts are all physiologically similar, since the shunt preserves continuity between the hepatic limb of the portal vein, the portal system, and the anastomosis. Flow through the hepatic limb of the standard side-to-side shunt is nearly always away from the liver and toward the anastomosis. The extent to which hepatofugal flow is produced by the other types of "side-to-side" shunts listed above is not known.

The end-to-side portacaval shunt gives immediate and permanent protection from variceal bleeding and is

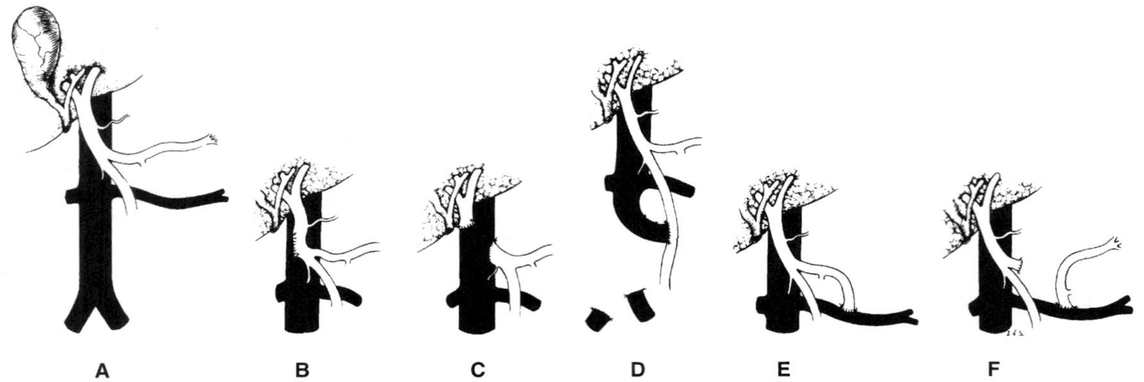

Figure 24–8. Types of portacaval anastomoses: ***A:*** Normal. ***B:*** Side-to-side. ***C:*** End-to-side. ***D:*** Mesocaval. ***E:*** Central splenorenal. ***F:*** Distal splenorenal (Warren). The H-mesocaval shunt is not illustrated.

somewhat easier to perform than a side-to-side portacaval or central splenorenal shunt. Encephalopathy may be slightly more common after side-to-side than end-to-side portacaval shunts. Side-to-side shunts are required in patients with Budd-Chiari syndrome or refractory ascites (when the latter is treated by a portasystemic shunt).

The mesocaval shunt interposes a segment of prosthetic graft or internal jugular vein between the inferior vena cava and the superior mesenteric vein where the latter passes in front of the uncinate process of the pancreas. The mesocaval shunt is particularly useful in the presence of severe scarring in the right upper quadrant or portal vein thrombosis, and in some cases it may be technically easier than a conventional side-to-side portacaval shunt if a side-to-side type of shunt is necessary. In most cases, portal flow to the liver is lost after this shunt. Evidence has been presented, however, that by limiting the diameter of the prosthetic graft to 8 mm (compared with 12- to 20-mm grafts), prograde flow is preserved in the portal vein, which decreases the incidence of postoperative encephalopathy while still preventing variceal hemorrhage.

(2) Selective shunts— Selective shunts lower pressure in the gastroesophageal venous plexus while preserving blood flow through the liver via the portal vein.

The distal splenorenal (Warren) shunt involves anastomosing the distal (splenic) end of the transected splenic vein to the side of the left renal vein, plus ligation of the major collaterals between the remaining portal and isolated gastrosplenic venous system. The latter step involves division of the gastric vein, the right gastroepiploic vein, and the vessels in the splenocolic ligament. The operation is more difficult and time-consuming than conventional shunts and except for the experienced operator is probably too complex for emergency portal decompression. If mobilization of the splenic vein is hazardous, the renal vein may be transected and its caval end joined to the side of the undisturbed splenic vein. The segment of splenic vein between the anastomosis and the portal vein is then ligated. Surprisingly, this seems to have little permanent effect on renal function as long as the remaining tributaries are preserved on the oversewn renal vein stump.

In contrast to total shunts, the Warren shunt does not improve ascites and should not be performed in patients whose ascites has been difficult to control. Preoperative angiography should be performed to determine if the splenic vein and left renal vein are large enough and close enough together for performance of this shunt. Recent pancreatitis may preclude safe dissection of the splenic vein from the undersurface of the pancreas.

Another type of selective shunt (Inokuchi shunt) consists of joining the left gastric vein to the inferior vena cava by a short segment of autogenous saphenous vein. The procedure has not become popular, perhaps because of its technical complexity.

Selective shunts tend to become less selective over several years as new collaterals develop between the high- and low-pressure regions of the portal system. This is accompanied by a gradual decrease in portal pressure (measured by WHVP) and evolution of the procedure into a version of side-to-side total shunt. The enlargement postoperatively of small venous tributaries entering the distal splenic vein from the pancreas suggests that this is the path by which nonselectivity develops. It is possible that this can be avoided by mobilizing the splenic vein all the way to the hilum (dividing these small vessels) before performing the splenorenal anastomosis.

b. Choice of shunt—A reasonable approach to shunt selection is as follows: The distal splenorenal shunt is the first choice for elective portal decompression. If ascites is present or the anatomy is unfavorable, an end-to-side portacaval shunt is preferred. Side-to-side shunts would be done for patients with severe ascites or Budd-Chiari syndrome. The H-mesocaval and central splenorenal shunts are reserved for special anatomic situations in which the above operations are unsuitable. An end-to-side shunt or H-mesocaval shunt is performed for emergency decompression.

Portacaval and distal splenorenal shunts are often followed by a rise in platelet count in patients with secondary hypersplenism. The response is unpredictable, however, and hypersplenism need not necessarily dictate the type of shunt since it rarely produces clinical manifestations. A central splenorenal shunt, in which splenectomy is performed, should not be considered preferable to other kinds of shunt just because the patient has a low platelet count.

c. Results of portasystemic shunts—Over 90% of portasystemic shunts remain patent, and the incidence of recurrent variceal bleeding is less than 10%. The 5-year survival rate after a portacaval shunt for alcoholic liver disease averages 45%. Some degree of encephalopathy develops in 15–25% of patients. Severe encephalopathy is seen in about 20% of alcoholics following a total shunt; its occurrence is not related to the severity of preshunt encephalopathy.

D. Devascularization Operations

The objective of devascularization is to destroy the venous collaterals that transport blood from the high-pressure portal system into the veins in the submucosa of the esophagus.

The Sugiura procedure is done in two stages. In the first stage, performed through a thoracotomy, the dilated venous collaterals between esophagus and adjacent structures are divided, and the esophagus at the level of the diaphragm is transected and reanastomosed. The second stage, a laparotomy, is performed immediately after the thoracotomy if the patient is actively bleeding but is deferred 4–6 weeks in elective cases. In the second stage of the operation, the upper two-thirds of the stomach is devascularized and selective vagotomy, pyloroplasty, and splenectomy are performed. It is possible in some cases to perform the entire operation through the left chest. An analogous operation has been described that consists of splenectomy, gastroesophageal devascularization, and resection of a 5-cm segment of the gastroesophageal junction. Continuity of the gut is restored by esophagogastrostomy with pyloroplasty.

In studies from Japan, where these operations originated, operative mortality is around 5%, variceal rebleeding is 2–4%, and 5-year survival is approximately 80%. Operations of this type performed in patients with alcoholic cirrhosis in North America have had poor results, owing to a high rate (40%) of late rebleeding.

E. Miscellaneous Operations

Attempts have also been made to decrease portal pressure by decreasing splanchnic inflow through splenectomy or splenic artery ligation. Diseases characterized by marked splenomegaly may rarely be associated with portal hypertension as a consequence of increased splenic blood flow, which has been known to reach levels as high as 1000 mL/min. Splenic blood flow may occasionally be increased enough in patients with cirrhosis to contribute significantly to the portal hypertension. However, splenectomy or splenic artery ligation in cirrhosis most often gives only a transient decrease in portal pressure, and over half of patients having these operations bleed again. Some workers have suggested that the absolute size of the splenic artery (a crude index of splenic flow) correlates with the clinical effectiveness of splenic artery ligation, a good result being predictable if the diameter of the artery is 1 cm or greater.

de Franchis R: Updating consensus in portal hypertension: report of the Baveno III Consensus Workshop on definitions, methodology and therapeutic strategies in portal hypertension. J Hepatol 2000;33:846.

Gentilini P et al: Ascites and hepatorenal syndrome during cirrhosis: two entities or the continuation of the same complication? J Hepatol 1999;31:1088.

Krige JE, Beckingham IJ: ABC of diseases of liver, pancreas, and biliary system. Portal hypertension—1: varices. BMJ 2001;322:348.

Lebrec D: Drug therapy for portal hypertension. Gut 2001;49:441.

Sarin SK et al: Comparison of endoscopic ligation and propranolol for the primary prevention of variceal bleeding. N Engl J Med 1999;340:988.

Suzuki H, Stanley AJ: Current management and novel therapeutic strategies for refractory ascites and hepatorenal syndrome. QJM 2001;94:293.

Vlachogiannakos J et al: Angiotensin converting enzyme inhibitors and angiotensin II antagonists as therapy in chronic liver disease. Gut 2001;49:303.

EXTRAHEPATIC PORTAL VENOUS OCCLUSION

Idiopathic portal vein thrombosis (in the absence of liver disease) accounts for most cases of portal hypertension in childhood and for a few cases in adults. Neonatal septicemia, omphalitis, umbilical vein catheterization for exchange transfusion, and dehydration have all been incriminated as possible causes, but collectively they can be implicated in less than half of cases. The causes of portal vein thrombosis in adults include hepatic tumors, cirrhosis, trauma, pancreatitis, pancreatic pseudocyst, myelofibrosis, thrombotic states (eg, protein C deficiency), and sepsis.

Although clinical manifestations may be delayed until adulthood, 80% of patients present between 1 and 6 years of age with variceal bleeding. About 70% of hemorrhages are preceded by a recent upper respiratory tract infection. Some of these children first come to medical attention because of splenomegaly and pancytopenia. Failure to recognize the underlying problem has occasionally led to splenectomy, with the result that portal decompression using the splenic vein is precluded. Ascites is uncommon except transiently after bleeding. Liver function is either normal or only slightly impaired, which probably accounts for the low incidence of overt encephalopathy. There is an increased frequency of neuropsychiatric problems, which may be a subtle form of encephalopathy.

Because the patient's general condition and liver function are good, the death rate for sudden massive bleeding is about 20%, much below the rate in other types of portal hypertension. The diagnosis can be confirmed with cross-sectional imaging or direct mesenteric angiography. Wedged hepatic venous pressure is normal.

Bleeding episodes in children under age 8 are usually self-limited and often do not require endoscopic sclerotherapy, administration of vasopressin, or balloon tamponade. Even if such interventions are necessary, however, the bleeding episodes are self-limited and uncommonly fatal, so emergency operations are rarely necessary.

Thrombosed portal veins are unsuitable for shunt procedures. Cavomesenteric shunts are best for young children, whose vessels are small. In older individuals, treatment should be started with sclerotherapy; if that fails to control the bleeding, a distal splenorenal shunt is preferred. Splenectomy alone has no permanent effect and sacrifices the splenic vein, which might be needed later for a shunt operation. Shunts in small children have a high rate of spontaneous thrombosis and should be avoided, if possible, until approximately 8–10 years of age, when the vessels are of larger caliber. Even still, using precise technique, some surgeons have obtained a high rate of anastomotic patency in the very young. Encephalopathy and hepatic dysfunction many years after a total shunt may be improved if converted to a selective shunt.

Splenectomy alone is never indicated in this disease, either for hypersplenism or in an attempt to reduce portal pressure, because the rebleeding rate is 90% and fatal postsplenectomy sepsis is not uncommon. If it is not possible to construct an adequate shunt, expectant management is the best strategy. Repeated severe bleeding episodes should be treated by transendoscopic sclerosis. Esophagogastrectomy with colonic interposition may be effective but should be considered a last resort.

Janssen HL et al: Extrahepatic portal vein thrombosis: aetiology and determinants of survival. Gut 2001;49:720.

Sheen CL et al: Clinical features, diagnosis and outcome of acute portal vein thrombosis. QJM 2000;93:531.

Valla DC, Condat B: Portal vein thrombosis in adults: pathophysiology, pathogenesis and management. J Hepatol 2000;32:865.

van't Riet M et al: Diagnosis and treatment of portal vein thrombosis following splenectomy. Br J Surg 2000;87:1229.

SPLENIC VEIN THROMBOSIS

Isolated thrombosis of the splenic vein is a rare cause of variceal bleeding that can be cured by splenectomy. The splenic venous blood, blocked from its normal route, flows through the short gastric vessels to the gastric fundus and then into the left gastric vein, continuing toward the liver. As the blood traverses the stomach, large gastric varices are produced that may rupture and bleed. Characteristically, the collateral pattern does not involve the esophagus, so esophageal varices are uncommon.

The principal causes of this syndrome are pancreatitis, pancreatic pseudocyst, neoplasm, and trauma. Splenomegaly is present in two-thirds of patients. Diagnosis can be made by selective splenic arteriography that opacifies the venous phase. Splenectomy is curative. Many cases of splenic vein thrombosis are unaccompanied by bleeding varices, and in such cases, no therapy is required.

de Franchis R: Updating consensus in portal hypertension: report of the Baveno III Consensus Workshop on definitions, methodology and therapeutic strategies in portal hypertension. J Hepatol 2000;33:846.

Gentilini P et al: Ascites and hepatorenal syndrome during cirrhosis: two entities or the continuation of the same complication? J Hepatol 1999;31:1088.

Krige JE, Beckingham IJ: ABC of diseases of liver, pancreas, and biliary system. Portal hypertension—1: varices. BMJ 2001;322:348.

Lebrec D: Drug therapy for portal hypertension. Gut 2001;49:441.

Mercado MA et al: Results of surgical treatment (modified Sugiura-Futagawa operation) of portal hypertension associated to complete splenomesoportal thrombosis and cirrhosis. HPB Surg 1999;11:157.

Sarin SK et al: Comparison of endoscopic ligation and propranolol for the primary prevention of variceal bleeding. N Engl J Med 1999;340:988.

Sakorafas GH, Tsiotou AG: Splenic-vein thrombosis complicating chronic pancreatitis. Scand J Gastroenterol 1999;34:1171.

Sakorafas GH et al: The significance of sinistral portal hypertension complicating chronic pancreatitis. Am J Surg 2000;179:129.

Stein M, Link DP: Symptomatic spleno-mesenteric-portal venous thrombosis: recanalization and reconstruction with endovascular stents. J Vasc Interv Radiol 1999;10:363.

Suzuki H, Stanley AJ: Current management and novel therapeutic strategies for refractory ascites and hepatorenal syndrome. QJM 2001;94:293.

Vlachogiannakos J et al: Angiotensin converting enzyme inhibitors and angiotensin II antagonists as therapy in chronic liver disease. Gut 2001;49:303.

BUDD-CHIARI SYNDROME

Budd-Chiari syndrome is a rare disorder resulting from obstruction of hepatic venous outflow. Most cases are caused by spontaneous thrombosis of the hepatic veins, often associated with polycythemia vera or the use of birth control pills. Some patients present with idiopathic membranous stenosis of the inferior vena cava located between the hepatic veins and right atrium, which is usually associated with secondary thrombosis of the hepatic veins. Many patients with Budd-Chiari syndrome are HBsAg-positive, and others have malignancies (eg, hepatocellular carcinoma). It was originally thought that this condition was congenital, but it is now known to arise secondarily from other conditions.

Posthepatic (postsinusoidal) obstruction raises sinusoidal pressure, which is transmitted proximally to cause portal hypertension. Because the parenchyma is relatively free of fibrosis, filtration across the sinusoids and hepatic lymph formation increase greatly, producing marked ascites.

Symptoms usually begin with a mild prodrome consisting of vague right upper quadrant abdominal pain, postprandial bloating, and anorexia. After weeks or months, a more florid picture develops consisting of gross ascites, hepatomegaly, and hepatic failure. At this stage the AST is usually markedly increased, the serum bilirubin is slightly elevated, and the alkaline phosphatase is inconsistently abnormal.

Except in patients with membranous obstruction of the vena cava, liver scans (CT or MRI) usually demonstrate marked perfusion abnormality throughout most of the liver except for a small central area representing the caudate lobe, whose venous outflow is spared (it goes directly to the vena cava through multiple small tributaries). CT scans show pooling of intravenous contrast media in the periphery of the liver; patent hepatic veins cannot be seen on ultrasound scans. An enlarged azygos vein may be seen on chest x-rays of patients with caval obstruction. Liver biopsy reveals grossly dilated central veins and sinusoids, pericentral necrosis, and replacement of hepatocytes by red blood cells. Centrilobular fibrosis develops late. The clinical diagnosis should be confirmed by venography, which shows the hepatic veins to be obstructed, usually with a beak-like deformity at their orifice. The inferior vena cava should be opacified to verify its patency, which is a requirement for a successful portacaval shunt. Previously direct venography was used, but the required information may now be obtained using noninvasive methods, such as CT or MR angiography. The x-rays may show compression of the intrahepatic cava by the congested liver.

In patients without cancer and in whom the obstruction is confined to the hepatic veins, a side-to-side portacaval or mesocaval shunt can be considered; TIPS is not an option in this situation since the hepatic veins are not patent. Focal membranous obstruction of the suprahepatic cava may be treated by excision of the lesion with or without the addition of a patch angioplasty. Some cases may be managed nonsurgically by percutaneous transluminal balloon dilation of the stenosis.

Occlusion of the inferior vena cava by thrombosis or compression from the liver requires a mesoatrial shunt using a prosthetic vascular graft. Because the incidence of graft thrombosis is relatively high, it may be advisable to perform a second-stage side-to-side portacaval shunt a few months after mesoatrial shunt decompression of the liver in patients with hepatic vein thrombosis whose vena cava was originally blocked by a congested liver. Development of hepatocellular carcinoma is common in patients with membranous obstruction of the vena cava. The postoperative results are excellent in patients without malignant neoplasms.

Liver transplantation is indicated in patients with advanced hepatic decompensation either from cirrhosis or as part of the acute syndrome. The results are excellent, and the risk of later hepatocellular carcinoma is eliminated.

Michl P et al: Successful treatment of chronic Budd-Chiari syndrome with a transjugular intrahepatic portosystemic shunt. J Hepatol 2000;32:516.

Olzinski AT, Sanyal AJ: Treating Budd-Chiari Syndrome: making rational choices from a myriad of options. J Clin Gastroenterol 2000;30:155.

Orloff MJ et al: A 27-year experience with surgical treatment of Budd-Chiari syndrome. Ann Surg 2000;232:340.

ASCITES

Ascites in hepatic disease results from (1) increased formation of hepatic lymph (from sinusoidal hypertension), (2) increased formation of splanchnic lymph, (3) hypoalbuminemia, and (4) salt and water retention by the kidneys. Before therapy is started, paracentesis should be performed and the following examinations made on a sample of ascitic fluid: (1) Culture and leukocyte count: Spontaneous bacterial peritonitis is common and may be clinically silent. A white count above 250/μL is highly suggestive of infection. (2) LDH levels: A ratio of LDH in ascites to serum that exceeds 0.6 suggests the presence of cancer or infection. (3) Serum amylase: A high level suggests pancreatic disease. (4) Albumin: The ratio of serum to ascites albumin concentrations is above 1.1 in liver disease and below 1.1 in malignant ascites. (5) Cytology: This is pertinent only in patients with a cancer diagnosis or a suspicion of cancer.

Medical Treatment

In general, the intensity of medical therapy required to control ascites can be predicted from the pretreatment 24-hour urine Na^+ output as follows: A Na^+ output below 5 meq/24 h will require strong diuretics; 5–25 meq/24 h, mild diuretics; and above 25 meq/24 h, no diuretics. Initial treatment is usually with spironolactone, 200 mg/d. The objective is to stimulate a weight loss of 0.5–0.75 kg/d, except in patients with peripheral edema who can mobilize fluid faster. If spironolactone alone is insufficient, another drug such as furosemide should be added. A loop diuretic (eg, furosemide, ethacrynic acid) should be given only in combination with a distally acting diuretic (eg, spironolactone, triamterene). Alternatively, massive ascites may be treated by one or more large volume (eg, 5-L) paracenteses; this is often accompanied by an intravenous infusion of albumin, although the benefits of albumin are unclear. Close monitoring of serum electrolytes should be done. Salt or water restriction is recommended in refractory cases. Caution is required in patients with evidence of renal dysfunction, since aggressive fluid removal can result in renal failure.

Surgical Treatment

A. Portacaval Shunt

A history of ascites that has been easy to control need not influence the choice of shunt operation intended to treat variceal bleeding. When ascites has been severe, however, a side-to-side shunt (eg, side-to-side portacaval, H-mesocaval, central splenorenal) may be considered, because it reduces sinusoidal as well as splanchnic venous pressure. A side-to-side portacaval shunt is rarely indicated just to treat ascites—eg, in patients in whom several LeVeen shunts have thrombosed—although the incidence of severe postoperative encephalopathy is high under these circumstances.

B. Peritoneal-Jugular Shunt (LeVeen Shunt, Denver Shunt)

Refractory ascites can be treated with a LeVeen shunt—a subcutaneous Silastic catheter that transports ascitic fluid from the peritoneal cavity to the jugular vein. A small unidirectional valve sensitive to a pressure gradient of 3–5 cm H_2O prevents backflow of blood. A modification called the Denver shunt contains a small chamber that can be used as a pump to clear the line by external pressure. In practice, Denver shunts become blocked more often than LeVeen shunts.

In patients with ascites due to cirrhosis, use of a LeVeen shunt should be confined to those who fail to respond to high doses of diuretics (eg, 400 mg of spironolactone and 400 mg of furosemide daily) or who repeatedly develop encephalopathy or azotemia during diuretic therapy.

Peritoneovenous shunts may also be used for ascites associated with cancer. The best results occur in patients whose ascitic fluid contains no malignant cells. A LeVeen shunt is of benefit in Budd-Chiari syndrome but is ineffective for chylous ascites. Because the incidence of complications and early shunt thrombosis is high, a LeVeen shunt is relatively contraindicated if the ascitic fluid is grossly bloody, contains many malignant cells, or has a high protein concentration (> 4.5 g/dL). The incidence of tumor embolization is low (5%).

The ascitic fluid should be cultured a few days before the shunt is inserted. Antibiotics are given pre- and postoperatively. The operation can be done with local anesthesia.

Postoperatively, the patient is outfitted with an abdominal binder and instructed to perform respiratory exercises against mild pressure to increase abdominal pressure and flow through the shunt. Dietary salt should not be restricted. A functioning LeVeen shunt alone is unable to fully eliminate the ascites, but it improves symptoms related to distention and renders the patient much more responsive to diuretics. Therefore, furosemide should be administered postoperatively.

An average of 10 kg of weight is lost during the first 10 days after the operation, and eventually the abdomen assumes a normal configuration. Nutrition and serum albumin levels often improve postoperatively. Urinary sodium excretion increases promptly, and renal function may improve in patients with the hepatorenal syndrome. Serious complications and deaths are most common in patients with advanced hepatorenal syndrome or a serum bilirubin level greater than 4 mg/dL. Although some patients eventually bleed from varices following insertion of a LeVeen shunt, the shunt itself does not increase the risk of bleeding and actually decreases portal pressure. Thus, a previous episode of variceal bleeding is not a contraindication for this procedure. Disseminated intravascular coagulation (DIC), manifested by increased fibrin split products, decreased platelet count, etc, occurs in more than half of cases but is clinically relevant in only a few. The frequency and severity of DIC may be minimized by emptying most of the ascitic fluid from the abdomen during operation and partially replacing it with Ringer's lactate solution. Lethal septicemia may occur if the ascitic fluid is infected at the time the shunt is inserted.

In about 10% of cases, the valve becomes thrombosed and must be replaced.

Hydrothorax, usually on the right side, may develop in patients with cirrhosis and ascites. The fluid reaches the chest through a pinhole opening in the membranous portion of the diaphragm, a pathway that can be demonstrated by aspirating the thoracic fluid, injecting technetium Tc 99m colloid into the ascites fluid, and observing rapid accumulation of the label in the chest. Treatment consists of a peritoneovenous shunt and injection of a sclerosing agent into the pleural cavity after it has been tapped dry. If a leak persists, it may be closed surgically by thoracotomy.

Aslam N, Marino CR: Malignant ascites: new concepts in pathophysiology, diagnosis, and management. Arch Intern Med 2001;161:2733.

Ben-Ami H et al: Acute transient chylous ascites associated with acute biliary pancreatitis. Am J Med Sci 1999;318:122.

Helton WS et al: Transjugular intrahepatic portasystemic shunt vs surgical shunt in good-risk cirrhotic patients: a case-control comparison. Arch Surg 2001;136:17.

Kaser S et al: Transjugular intrahepatic portosystemic shunt (TIPS) augments hyperinsulinemia in patients with cirrhosis. J Hepatol 2000;33:902.

Krige JE, Beckingham IJ: ABC of diseases of liver, pancreas, and biliary system: portal hypertension-2. Ascites, encephalopathy, and other conditions. BMJ 2001;322:416.

Rossle M et al: A comparison of paracentesis and transjugular intrahepatic portosystemic shunting in patients with ascites. N Engl J Med 2000;342:1701.

Suzuki H, Stanley AJ: Current management and novel therapeutic strategies for refractory ascites and hepatorenal syndrome. QJM 2001;94:293.

Zervos EE, Rosemurgy AS: Management of medically refractory ascites. Am J Surg 2001;181:256.

HEPATIC ENCEPHALOPATHY

Central nervous system abnormalities may be seen in patients with chronic liver disease and are especially likely after portocaval shunts. Porta-systemic encephalopathy, ammonia intoxication, hepatic coma, and meat intoxication are terms used to refer to this condition. The manifestations range from lethargy to coma—from minor personality changes to psychosis—from asterixis to paraplegia. Hypothermia and hyperventilation may precede coma.

Pathogenesis

Hepatic encephalopathy is a reversible metabolic neuropathy that results from the action of chemicals absorbed from the gut on the brain. Increased exposure of the brain to these agents is the result of impaired hepatic metabolism due to cirrhosis or spontaneous or surgically created shunts of portal venous blood around the liver and increased permeability of the blood-brain barrier. The chemical agents responsible for encephalopathy form from the action of colonic bacteria on protein within the gut. Potential aggravating factors include gastrointestinal hemorrhage, constipation, azotemia, hypokalemic alkalosis, infection, excessive dietary protein, and sedatives (Table 24–6). Four main theories concerning mediation of this syndrome currently attract the most attention.

Table 24–6. Factors contributing to encephalopathy.

A. Increased systemic toxin levels
1. Extent of portal-systemic venous shunt
2. Depressed liver function
3. Intestinal protein load
4. Intestinal flora
5. Azotemia
6. Constipation

B. Increased sensitivity of central nervous system
1. Age of patient
2. Hypokalemia
3. Alkalosis
4. Diuretics
5. Sedatives, narcotics, tranquilizers
6. Infection
7. Hypoxia, hypoglycemia, myxedema

A. Amino Acid Neurotransmitters

Gamma-aminobutyric acid (GABA), the principal inhibitory neurotransmitter in the brain, produces a state similar to hepatic encephalopathy when given experimentally. It is normally synthesized in the brain and by bacteria within the colon; GABA in the GI tract is normally degraded by the liver and is found in increased levels in the serum of patients with hepatic encephalopathy. The passage of GABA across the blood-brain barrier is increased in hepatic encephalopathy. Experiments also indicate the presence of increased numbers of GABA receptors in encephalopathy and increased GABA-ergic tone, perhaps due to a benzodiazepine receptor agonist ligand on the receptor complex (GABA/benzodiazepine receptor). This has raised the possibility of treating encephalopathy with benzodiazepine antagonists, and the drug flumazenil has shown promise in preliminary trials.

B. Ammonia

Ammonia is produced in the colon by bacteria and is absorbed and transported in portal venous blood to the liver, where it is extracted and converted to glutamine. Ammonia concentrations are elevated in the arterial blood and cerebrospinal fluid of patients with encephalopathy, and experimental administration of ammonia produces central nervous system symptoms.

C. False Neurotransmitters

According to this theory, cerebral neurons become depleted of normal neurotransmitters (norepinephrine and dopamine), which are partially replaced by false neurotransmitters (octopamine and phenylethanolamine). The result is inhibition of neural function. Serum levels of branched-chain amino acids (leucine, isoleucine, valine) are decreased and levels of aromatic amino acids (tryptophan, phenylalanine, tyrosine) are elevated in patients with encephalopathy. Because these two classes of amino acids compete for transport across the blood-brain barrier, the aromatic amino acids have increased access to the central nervous system, where they serve as precursors for false neurotransmitters. Trials of therapy with supplements of branched-chain amino acids have given conflicting results.

D. Synergistic Neurotoxins

This theory postulates that ammonia, mercaptans, and fatty acids, none of which accumulate in the brain in amounts capable of producing encephalopathy, have synergistic effects that produce the full-blown syndrome in patients with liver disease.

Prevention

Encephalopathy is a major side effect of portacaval shunt and is to some extent predictable. Elderly patients are considerably more susceptible. Patients with alcoholic liver disease fare better than those with postnecrotic or cryptogenic cirrhosis, apparently owing to the invariable progression of liver dysfunction in the latter. Good liver function partially protects against encephalopathy. If the liver has adapted to complete or nearly complete diversion of portal blood before operation, a surgical shunt is less apt to depress liver function further. For example, patients with thrombosis of the portal vein (complete diversion and normal liver function) rarely experience encephalopathy after portal-systemic shunt. Encephalopathy is less common after a distal splenorenal (Warren) shunt than after other kinds of shunts.

Increased intestinal protein, whether of dietary origin or from intestinal bleeding, aggravates encephalopathy by providing more substrate for intestinal bacteria. Constipation allows more time for bacterial action on colonic contents. Azotemia results in higher concentration of blood urea, which diffuses into the intestine, is converted to ammonia, and is then reabsorbed. Hypokalemia and metabolic alkalosis aggravate encephalopathy by shifting ammonia from extracellular to intracellular sites where the toxic action occurs.

Laboratory Findings

Arterial ammonia levels are usually high. The presence of high levels of glutamine in the cerebrospinal fluid may help distinguish hepatic encephalopathy from other causes of coma. Electroencephalography is more sensitive than clinical evaluation in detecting minor involvement. The changes are nonspecific and consist of slower mean frequencies. Studies performed at different times can be compared to assess the effects of therapy.

Treatment

Acute encephalopathy is treated by controlling precipitating factors, halting all dietary protein intake, cleansing the bowel with purgatives and enemas, and administering antibiotics (neomycin or ampicillin) or lactulose. Neomycin may be given orally or by gastric tube (two to four times daily) or rectally as an enema (1% solution one or two times daily). At least 1600 kcal of carbohydrate should be provided daily, along with therapeutic amounts of vitamins. Blood volume must be maintained to avoid prerenal azotemia. After the patient responds to initial therapy, dietary protein may be started at 20 g/d and increased by increments of 10–20 g every 2–5 days as tolerated.

Chronic encephalopathy is treated by restriction of dietary protein, avoidance of constipation, and elimination of sedatives, diuretics, and tranquilizers. To avoid protein depletion, protein intake must not be chronically reduced below 50 g/d. Vegetable protein in the diet is tolerated better than animal protein. Lactulose, a disaccharide unaffected by intestinal enzymes, is the drug of choice for long-term control. When given orally (20–30 g three or four times daily), it reaches the colon, where it stimulates bacterial anabolism (which increases ammonia uptake) and inhibits bacterial enzymes (which decreases the generation of nitrogenous toxins). Its effect is independent of colonic pH. A related compound outside the United States, lactitol (β-galactoside sorbitol), is also effective and appears to work faster. As a powder, it is easier to use than liquid lactulose. Intermittent courses of oral neomycin or metronidazole may be given if lactulose therapy and preventive measures are inadequate.

Butterworth RF: Hepatic encephalopathy: a neuropsychiatric disorder involving multiple neurotransmitter systems. Curr Opin Neurol 2000;13:727.

Gill RQ, Sterling RK: Acute liver failure. J Clin Gastroenterol 2001;33:191.

Lockwood AH: Early detection and treatment of hepatic encephalopathy. Curr Opin Neurol 1998;11:663.

Menon KV, Kamath PS: Managing the complications of cirrhosis. Mayo Clin Proc 2000;75:501.

HEPATIC ABSCESS

Hepatic abscesses may be bacterial, parasitic, or fungal in origin. In the USA, pyogenic abscesses are the most common, followed by amebic abscesses (see Chapter 8). Unless otherwise indicated, the remarks in this section refer to bacterial abscesses.

Cases are about evenly divided between those with a single abscess and those with multiple abscesses. About 90% of right lobe abscesses are solitary, while only 10% of left lobe abscesses are solitary.

In most cases, the development of a hepatic abscess follows a suppurative process elsewhere in the body. Many abscesses are due to direct spread from biliary infections such as empyema of the gallbladder or protracted cholangitis. Abdominal infections such as appendicitis or diverticulitis may spread through the portal vein to involve the liver with abscess formation. About 40% of patients have an underlying malignancy. Other cases develop after generalized sepsis from bacterial endocarditis, renal infection, or pneumonitis. In 25% of cases, no antecedent infection can be documented ("cryptogenic" abscesses). Rare causes include secondary bacterial infection of an amebic abscess, hydatid cyst, or congenital hepatic cyst.

In most cases, the organism is of enteric origin. *Escherichia coli, Klebsiella pneumoniae,* bacteroides, enterococci (eg, *Streptococcus faecalis*), anaerobic streptococci (eg, Peptostreptococcus), and microaerophilic streptococci are most common. Staphylococci, hemolytic streptococci, or other gram-positive organisms are usually found if the primary infection is bacterial endocarditis or pneumonitis.

Clinical Findings

A. Symptoms and Signs

When liver abscess develops in the course of another intra-abdominal infection such as diverticulitis, it is accompanied by increasing toxicity, higher fever, jaundice, and a generally deteriorating clinical picture. Right upper quadrant pain and chills may appear.

In other cases, the diagnosis is much less obvious, since the illness develops insidiously in a previously healthy person. In these, the first symptoms are usually malaise and fatigue, followed after several weeks by fever. Epigastric or right upper quadrant pain is present in about half of cases. The pain may be aggravated by motion or may be referred to the right shoulder.

The course of fever is often erratic, and spikes to 40–41 °C are common. Chills are present in about 25% of cases. The liver is usually enlarged and may be tender to palpation. If tenderness is severe, the condition may be confused with cholecystitis.

Jaundice is unusual in solitary abscesses unless the patient's condition is worsening. Jaundice is often present in patients with multiple abscesses and primary disease in the biliary tree and in general is a bad prognostic sign.

B. Laboratory Findings

Leukocytosis is present in most cases and is usually over 15,000/μL. A small group of patients, usually the most seriously ill, may fail to develop leukocytosis. Anemia is present in most. The average hematocrit is 33%.

Serum bilirubin is usually normal except in patients with multiple abscesses or biliary obstruction or when hepatic failure has supervened. Alkaline phosphatase is often elevated even in the presence of a normal bilirubin.

C. Imaging Studies

X-ray changes present in the right lung in about one-third of cases consist of basilar atelectasis or pleural effusion. The right diaphragm may be elevated and less mobile than the left.

Plain films of the abdomen are usually normal or show only hepatomegaly. In a few patients, an air-fluid level in the region of the liver reveals the presence and location of the abscess. Distortion of the contour of the stomach on upper gastrointestinal series may be seen with large abscesses involving the left lobe.

Ultrasound and CT scans are the most useful diagnostic tests, providing accurate information regarding the presence, size, number, and location of abscesses within the liver. CT scans have the added advantage of being able to demonstrate abscesses or neoplasms elsewhere in the abdomen. The radioisotope liver scintiscan is able to demonstrate most liver abscesses but is nonspecific, gives little other useful information, and is therefore not helpful.

Differential Diagnosis

In many cases, early findings may be so vague that hepatic abscess is not even considered. The multiple other causes of malaise, weight loss, and anemia would enter into the differential diagnosis. With spiking fevers, one must consider all the causes of fever of unknown origin. Failure to entertain the idea of hepatic abscess and to obtain the necessary scans leads to most errors in diagnosis.

Once imaging tests have demonstrated the abscess, the responsible organisms must be identified. Amebiasis should be considered in cases of a solitary abscess. Compared with amebic abscesses, pyogenic liver abscesses are seen more often in patients older than 50 years and are associated with jaundice, pruritus, sepsis, a palpable mass, and elevated bilirubin and alkaline phosphatase levels. Patients with amebic abscesses more often have been to an endemic area and have abdominal pain and tenderness, diarrhea, hepatomegaly, and positive serologic tests for amebiasis.

Complications

Intrahepatic spread of infection may create multiple additional abscesses and is responsible for some failures after treatment of an apparently solitary abscess. As the untreated abscess expands, rupture may occur into the pleural or peritoneal cavity, usually with catastrophic results. Septicemia and septic shock are common terminal complications of diffuse hepatic infection. Hepatic failure may develop in addition to uncontrolled sepsis, or it may predominate over signs of infection.

Hemobilia may follow bleeding from the vascular wall into the abscess cavity. In this case, hepatic artery embolization or ligation may be required to control bleeding.

Treatment

Antibiotics should be started promptly. Initial coverage, before culture results are available, should be adequate for *E coli, K pneumoniae,* bacteroides, enterococci, and anaerobic streptococci and consequently would usually include an aminoglycoside, clindamycin or metronidazole, and ampicillin. The regimen may be modified later according to the results of cultures.

About 80% or more of patients with liver abscesses are adequately treated by drainage catheters inserted percutaneously under ultrasound or CT guidance. Whether the patient has a single abscess or multiple abscesses, this is usually the most appropriate initial therapy. The catheters can be removed in 1–2 weeks after output becomes nonpurulent and scant.

In about 40% of patients, the catheters do not drain well following initial placement and must be repositioned. The principal advantage of percutaneous drainage is lower morbidity (not lower mortality). It is easier to provide thorough drainage surgically, so when difficulties are encountered with percutaneous drainage, laparotomy should be performed promptly. Surgical intervention is more often necessary in cases of multiple, loculated collections or when the abscess cavity contains a large amount of necrotic debris. In such cases, open debridement should be considered. Rarely, multiple abscesses are confined to a single lobe and can be cured by lobectomy. Biliary obstruction or other causes of sepsis must also be corrected.

Prognosis

The overall mortality rate of 15% is more closely related to the underlying disease than to any other factor. The mortality rate is about 40% in patients with malignant disease. Pleural effusion, leukocytosis over 20,000/μL, hypoalbuminemia, and polymicrobial infection correlate with a poor outcome. In the USA, whether the abscess is solitary or multiple no longer has a major influence on survival, but where benign biliary disease remains a major cause of this disease, multiple hepatic abscesses are associated with a worse prognosis. Death is rare in patients with a cryptogenic liver abscess.

Dharmarajan TS et al: Pyogenic liver abscess: a geriatric problem. J Am Geriatr Soc 2000;48:1022.

Johannsen EC, Sifri CD, Madoff LC: Pyogenic liver abscesses. Infect Dis Clin North Am 2000;14:547.

Molle I et al: Increased risk and case fatality rate of pyogenic liver abscess in patients with liver cirrhosis: a nationwide study in Denmark. Gut 2001;48:260.

Narayanan S et al: Crohn's disease presenting as pyogenic liver abscess with review of previous case reports. Am J Gastroenterol 1998;93:2607.

Biliary Tract

25

Gerard M. Doherty, MD, & Lawrence W. Way, MD

EMBRYOLOGY & ANATOMY

The anlage of the biliary ducts and liver consists of a diverticulum that appears on the ventral aspect of the foregut in 3 mm embryos. The cranial portion becomes the liver; a caudal bud forms the ventral pancreas; and an intermediate bud develops into the gallbladder. Originally hollow, the hepatic diverticulum becomes a solid mass of cells that later recanalizes to form the ducts. The smallest ducts—the bile canaliculi—are first seen as a basal network between the primitive hepatocytes that eventually expands throughout the liver (Figure 25–1). Numerous microvilli increase the canalicular surface area. Bile secreted here passes through the interlobular ductules (canals of Hering) and the lobar ducts and then into the hepatic duct in the hilum. In most cases, the common hepatic duct is formed by the union of a single right and left duct, but in 25% of individuals, the anterior and posterior divisions of the right duct join the left duct separately. The origin of the common hepatic duct is close to the liver but always outside its substance. It runs about 4 cm before joining the cystic duct to form the common bile duct. The common duct begins in the hepatoduodenal ligament, passes behind the first portion of the duodenum, and runs in a groove on the posterior surface of the pancreas before entering the duodenum. Its terminal 1 cm is intimately adherent to the duodenal wall. The total length of the common duct is about 9 cm.

In 80–90% of individuals, the main pancreatic duct joins the common duct to form a common channel about 1 cm long. The intraduodenal segment of the duct is called the hepatopancreatic ampulla, or ampulla of Vater.

The gallbladder is a pear-shaped organ adherent to the undersurface of the liver in a groove separating the right and left lobes. The fundus projects 1–2 cm below the hepatic edge and can often be felt when the cystic or common duct is obstructed. It rarely has a complete peritoneal covering, but when this variation does occur, it predisposes to infarction by torsion. The gallbladder holds about 50 mL of bile when fully distended. The neck of the gallbladder tapers into the narrow cystic duct, which connects with the common duct. The lumen of the cystic duct contains a thin mucosal septum, the spiral valve of Heister, which offers mild resistance to bile flow. In 75% of persons, the cystic duct enters the common duct at an angle. In the remainder, it runs parallel to the hepatic duct or winds around it before joining the common duct (Figure 25–2).

In the hepatoduodenal ligament, the hepatic artery is to the left of the common duct and the portal vein is posterior and medial. The right hepatic artery usually passes behind the hepatic duct and then gives off the cystic artery before entering the right lobe of the liver, but variations are common.

The mucosal epithelium of the bile ducts varies from cuboidal in the ductules to columnar in the main ducts. The gallbladder mucosa is thrown into prominent ridges when the organ is collapsed, and these flatten during distention. The tall columnar cells of the gallbladder mucosa are covered by microvilli on their luminal surface. Wide channels, which play an important role in water and electrolyte absorption, separate the individual cells.

The walls of the bile ducts contain only small amounts of smooth muscle, but the termination of the common duct is enveloped by a complex sphincteric muscle. The gallbladder musculature is composed of interdigitated bundles of longitudinal and spirally arranged fibers.

The biliary tree receives parasympathetic and sympathetic innervation. The former contains motor fibers to the gallbladder and secretory fibers to the ductal epithelium. The afferent fibers in the sympathetic nerves mediate the pain of biliary colic.

PHYSIOLOGY

Bile Flow

Bile is produced at a rate of 500–1500 mL/d by the hepatocytes and the cells of the ducts. Active secretion of bile salts into the biliary canaliculus is responsible for most of the volume of bile and its fluctuations. Na^+ and water follow passively to establish isosmolality and electrical neutrality. Lecithin and cholesterol enter the canaliculus at rates that correlate with variations in bile salt output. Bilirubin and a number of other organic anions—estrogens, sulfobromophthalein, etc—are actively secreted by the hepatocyte by a different transport system from that which handles bile salts.

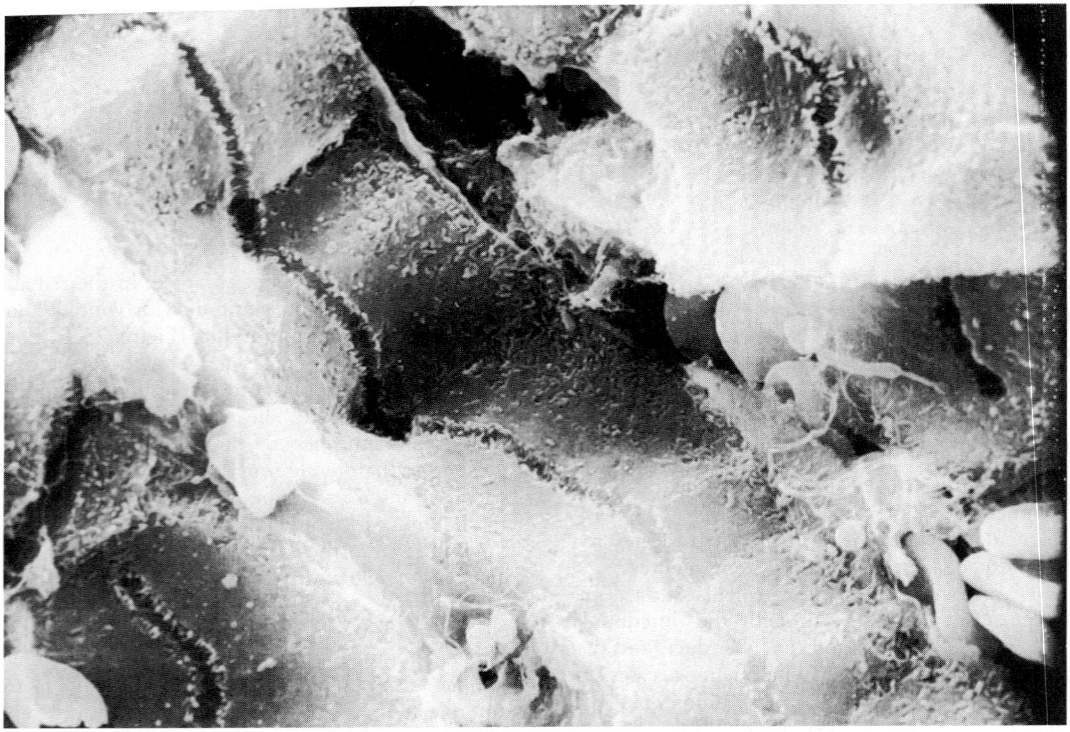

Figure 25–1. Scanning electron photomicrograph of a hepatic plate with adjacent sinusoids and sinusoidal microvilli and a bile canaliculus running in the center of the liver cells. Although their boundaries are indistinct, about four hepatocytes constitute the section of the plate in the middle of the photograph. Occasional red cells are present within the sinusoids. (Reduced from × 2000.) (Courtesy of Dr James Boyer.)

The columnar cells of the ducts add a fluid rich in HCO_3^- to that produced in the canaliculus. This involves active secretion of Na^+ and HCO_3^- by a cellular pump stimulated by secretin, VIP, and cholecystokinin. K^+ and water are distributed passively across the ducts (Figure 25–3).

Between meals, bile is stored in the gallbladder, where it is concentrated at rates of up to 20% per hour. Na^+ and either HCO_3^- or Cl^- are actively transported from its lumen during absorption. The changes in composition brought about by concentration are shown in Figure 25–4.

Three factors regulate bile flow: hepatic secretion, gallbladder contraction, and choledochal sphincteric resistance. In the fasting state, pressure in the common bile duct is 5–10 cm H_2O, and bile produced in the liver is diverted into the gallbladder. After a meal, the gallbladder contracts, the sphincter relaxes, and bile is forced into the duodenum in squirts as ductal pressure intermittently exceeds sphincteric resistance. During contraction, pressure within the gallbladder reaches 25 cm H_2O and that in the common bile duct 15–20 cm H_2O.

Cholecystokinin (CCK) is the major physiologic stimulus for postprandial gallbladder contraction and relaxation of the sphincter, but vagal impulses facilitate its action. CCK is released into the bloodstream from the mucosa of the small bowel by fat or lipolytic products in the lumen. Amino acids and small polypeptides are weaker stimuli, and carbohydrates are ineffective. Bile flow during a meal is augmented by turnover of bile salts in the enterohepatic circulation and stimulation of ductal secretion by secretin, VIP, and CCK. Motilin stimulates episodic partial gallbladder emptying in the interdigestive phase.

Bile Salts & the Enterohepatic Circulation

Bile salts, lecithin, and cholesterol comprise about 90% of the solids in bile, the remainder consisting of bilirubin, fatty acids, and inorganic salts. Gallbladder bile contains about 10% solids and has a bile salt concentration between 200 and 300 mmol/L (Figure 25–4).

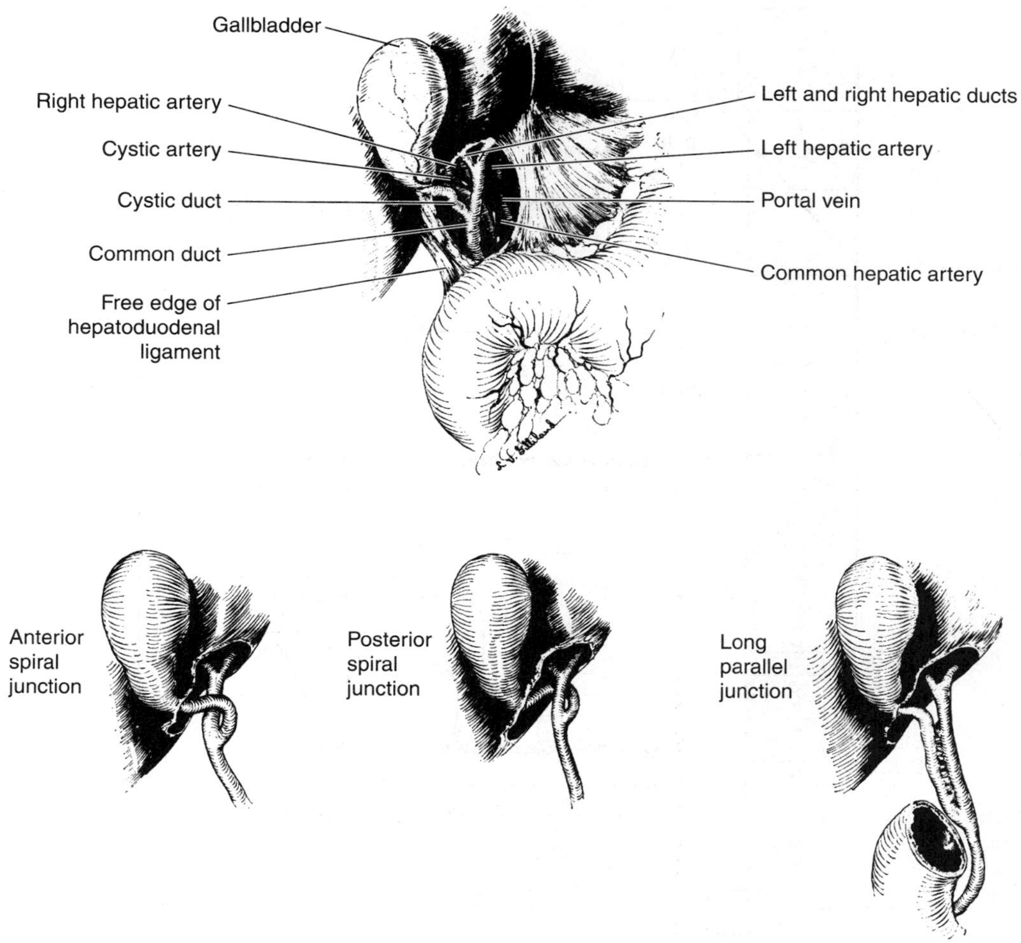

Figure 25–2. Anatomy of the gallbladder and variations in anatomy of the cystic duct.

Bile salts are steroid molecules formed from cholesterol by hepatocytes. The rate of synthesis is under feedback control and can be increased a maximum of about 20-fold. Two **primary** bile salts—cholate and chenodeoxycholate—are produced by the liver. Before excretion into bile, they are conjugated with either glycine or taurine, which enhances water solubility. Intestinal bacteria alter these compounds to produce the **secondary** bile salts, deoxycholate and lithocholate. The former is reabsorbed and enters bile, but lithocholate is insoluble and is excreted in the stool. Bile is composed of 40% cholate, 40% chenodeoxycholate, and 20% deoxycholate, conjugated with glycine or taurine in a ratio of 3:1.

The functions of bile salts are (1) to induce the flow of bile, (2) to transport lipids, and (3) to bind calcium ions in bile. The importance of the last of these is unknown. Bile acid molecules are amphipathic—ie, they have hydrophilic and hydrophobic poles. In bile, they form multimolecular aggregates called micelles in which the hydrophilic poles become aligned to face the aqueous medium. Water-insoluble lipids, such as cholesterol, can be dissolved within the hydrophobic centers of bile salt micelles. Molecules of lecithin, a water-insoluble but polar lipid, aggregate into hydrated bilayers that form vesicles in bile, and they also become incorporated into bile acid micelles to form mixed micelles. Mixed micelles have an increased lipid-carrying capacity compared with pure bile acid micelles. Cholesterol in bile is transported within the phospholipid vesicles and the bile salt micelles.

Bile salts remain in the intestinal lumen throughout the jejunum, where they participate in fat digestion and

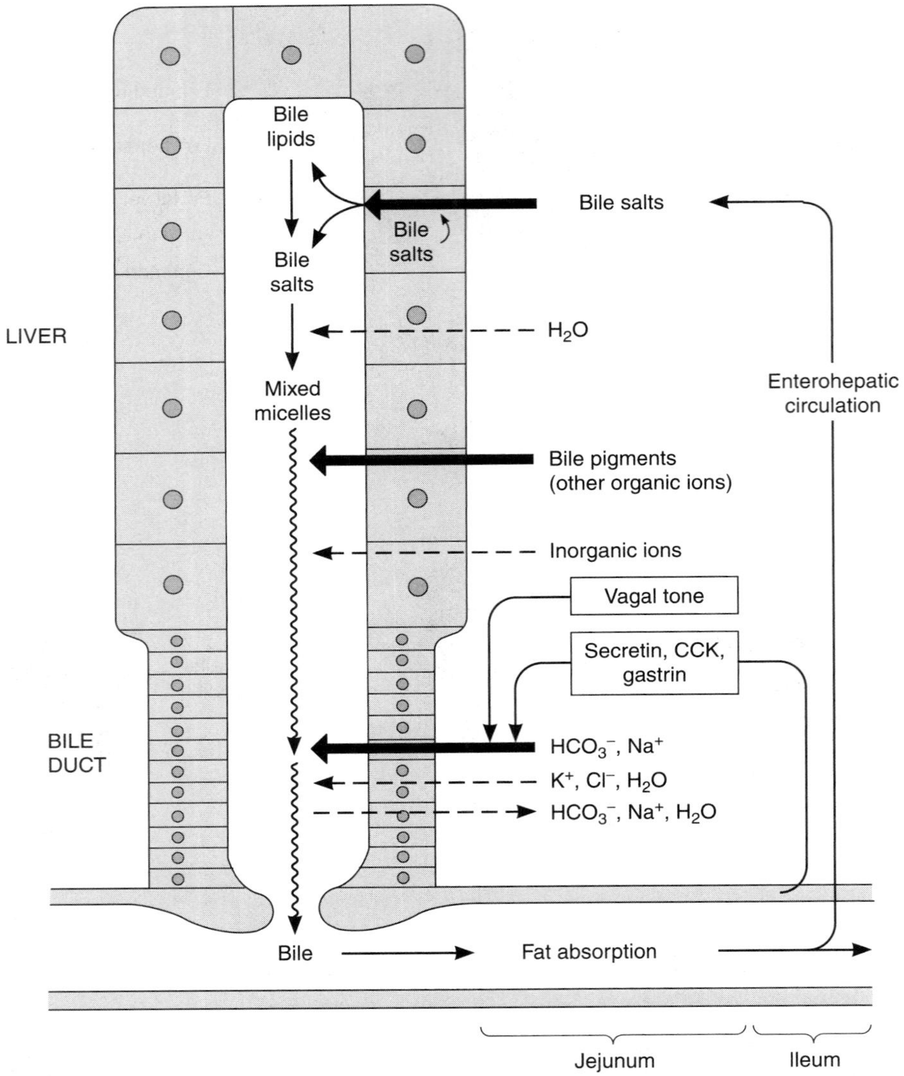

Figure 25–3. Bile formation. Solid lines into the ductular lumen indicate active transport; dotted lines represent passive diffusion.

absorption (Figure 25–5). Upon reaching the distal small bowel, they are reabsorbed by an active transport system located in the terminal 200 cm of ileum. Over 95% of bile salts arriving from the jejunum are transferred by this process into portal vein blood; the remainder enter the colon, where they are converted to secondary bile salts. The entire bile salt pool of 2.5–4 g circulates twice through the enterohepatic circulation during each meal, and six to eight cycles are made each day. The normal daily loss of bile salts in the stool amounts to 10–20% of the pool and is restored by hepatic synthesis.

Arias IM et al: The biology of the bile canaliculus. Hepatology 1993;17:318.

Gustafsson U, Sahlin S, Einarsson C: Biliary lipid composition in patients with cholesterol and pigment gallstones and gallstone-free subjects: deoxycholic acid does not contribute to formation of cholesterol gallstones. Eur J Clin Invest 2000;30:1099.

Hofmann AF: The continuing importance of bile acids in liver and intestinal disease. Arch Intern Med 1999;159:2647.

Kullak-Ublick GA: Regulation of organic anion and drug transporters of the sinusoidal membrane. J Hepatol 1999;31:563.

Sahin M et al: Effect of octreotide (Sandostatin 201-995) on bile flow and bile components. Dig Dis Sci 1999;44:181.

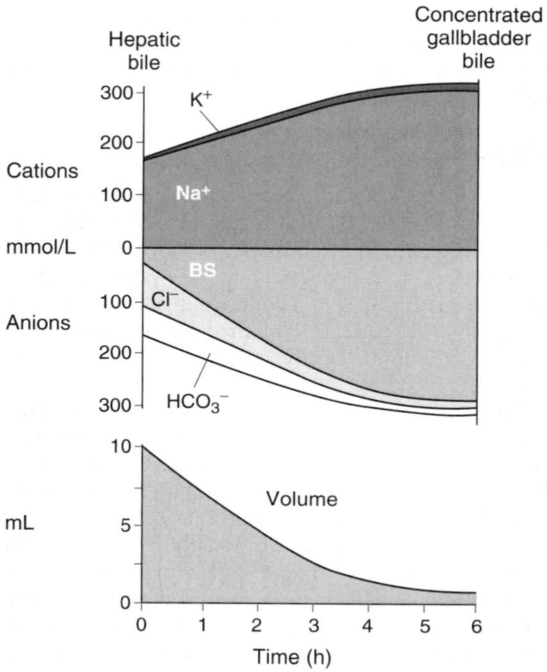

Figure 25–4. Changes in gallbladder bile composition with time. (Courtesy of J Dietschy.)

Bilirubin

About 250–300 mg of bilirubin is excreted each day in the bile, 75% of it from breakdown of red cells in the reticuloendothelial system and 25% from turnover of hepatic heme and hemoproteins. First, heme is liberated from hemoglobin, and the iron and globin are removed for reuse by the organism. Biliverdin, the first pigment formed from heme, is reduced to unconjugated bilirubin, the indirect-reacting bilirubin of the van den Bergh test. Unconjugated bilirubin is insoluble in water and is transported in plasma bound to albumin.

Unconjugated bilirubin is extracted from blood by hepatocytes, where it is conjugated with glucuronic acid to form bilirubin diglucuronide, the water-soluble direct bilirubin. Conjugation is catalyzed by glucuronyl transferase, an enzyme on the endoplasmic reticulum. Bilirubin is transported within the hepatocyte by cytosolic binding proteins, which rapidly deliver the molecule to the canalicular membrane for active secretion into bile. Within bile, conjugated bilirubin is largely transported in association with mixed lipid micelles.

After entering the intestine, bilirubin is reduced by intestinal bacteria to several compounds known as urobilinogens, which are subsequently oxidized and converted to pigmented urobilins. The term urobilinogen is often used to refer to both urobilins and urobilinogens.

DIAGNOSTIC EXAMINATION OF THE BILIARY TREE

Plain Abdominal Film

The posteroanterior supine view of the abdomen will show gallstones in the 10–15% of cases where they are radiopaque. The bile itself sometimes contains sufficient calcium (milk of calcium bile) to be seen. An enlarged gallbladder can occasionally be identified as a soft tissue mass in the right upper quadrant indenting an air-filled hepatic flexure.

In several types of biliary disease, the diagnosis may be suggested by air seen in the bile ducts on a plain film. This usually signifies the presence of a biliary-intestinal fistula (from disease or surgery) but also occurs rarely in severe cholangitis, emphysematous cholecystitis, and biliary ascariasis.

Oral Cholecystography

Tyropanoate sodium or iopanoic acid is taken orally the night before the examination, along with a light meal. The drug is absorbed, bound to albumin in portal blood, extracted by hepatocytes, and secreted in bile. Opacification occurs only with concentration in the gallbladder and on the average is optimal 10 hours after tyropanoate

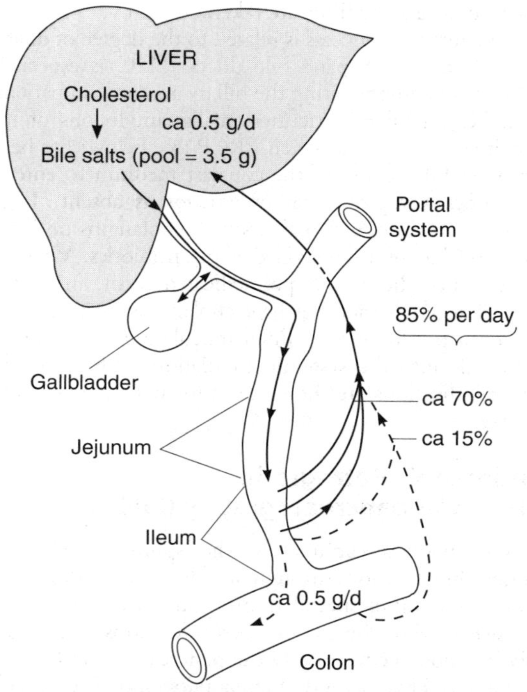

Figure 25–5. Enterohepatic circulation of bile salts. (Courtesy of M. Tyor.)

ingestion. Posteroanterior and oblique supine views and an upright or lateral decubitus film are obtained.

Oral cholecystograms are unsatisfactory if the contrast agent is inefficiently absorbed from the intestine or poorly excreted by the liver. Absorption is often impaired in acute abdominal illnesses with ileus, vomiting, or diarrhea. If the bilirubin level is over 3 mg/dL, hepatic excretion will probably be inadequate. False-negative results are obtained in 5% of tests. A normal gallbladder may not opacify for several weeks after severe trauma or a major illness.

Nonopacification occurs in 20% of patients after the usual single-dose regimen. When a second dose is given and x-rays repeated the following day, opacification is obtained in 25% of these patients. Persistent nonopacification is a highly reliable (> 95% true positive) indication of gallbladder disease. Instead of performing a double-dose oral cholecystogram as the next step when a single dose fails to opacify, it is simpler to obtain an ultrasound scan.

Percutaneous Transhepatic Cholangiography (THC, PTC)

Percutaneous transhepatic cholangiography is performed by passing a fine needle through the right lower rib cage and the hepatic parenchyma and into the lumen of a bile duct. Water-soluble contrast material is injected, and x-ray films are taken.

The technical success is related to the degree of dilatation of the intrahepatic bile ducts. THC is especially valuable in demonstrating the biliary anatomy in patients with benign biliary strictures, malignant lesions of the proximal bile duct, or when ERCP (see below) has been unsuccessful. Failure of the contrast medium to enter a duct does not prove that obstruction is absent. THC should not be done in patients with cholangitis until the infection has been controlled with antibiotics. Virtually all patients should be premedicated with antibiotics regardless of whether they have cholangitis—septic shock has been produced by sudden inoculation of organisms from bile into the systemic circulation. Otherwise, the contraindications are the same as for percutaneous liver biopsy.

Endoscopic Retrograde Cholangiopancreatography (ERCP)

ERCP involves cannulating the sphincter of Oddi under direct vision through a side-viewing duodenoscope. It requires special training involving more than familiarity with the use of fiberoptic endoscopes. Usually it is possible to opacify the pancreatic as well as the bile ducts. This method of cholangiography is especially applicable to patients with an abnormal clotting mechanism who would not be candidates for transhepatic puncture of the ducts. It is usually the preferred method of examining the biliary tree in patients with presumed choledocholithiasis or obstructing lesions in the periampullary region.

Ultrasound

Ultrasonography is both sensitive and specific in detecting gallbladder stones and dilatation of bile ducts. In the investigation of gallbladder disease, false-positive diagnoses for stones are rare, and false-negative reports owing to small stones or a contracted gallbladder occur in only 5% of patients examined by real time ultrasound. Ultrasound usually misses stones in the common duct.

Dilatation of bile ducts in a jaundiced patient indicates bile duct obstruction, but it is fairly common for the ducts to be normal in the presence of obstruction. When ultrasound shows dilated ducts, THC will nearly always be technically successful.

The ultrasonographer occasionally reports that the gallbladder contains "sludge." This material is sonographically opaque, does not cast an acoustic shadow, and forms a dependent layer in the gallbladder. On clinical analysis, it is a fine precipitate of calcium bilirubinate. Sludge may accompany gallstone disease or may be a solitary finding. It is seen in a variety of clinical settings, many of which are characterized by gallbladder stasis (eg, prolonged fasting). By itself, sludge is not an indication for cholecystectomy.

Radionuclide Scan (HIDA Scan)

Technetium 99m-labeled derivatives of iminodiacetic acid (IDA) are excreted in high concentration in bile and produce excellent gamma camera images. Following intravenous injection of the radionuclide, imaging of the bile ducts and gallbladder normally appears within 15–30 minutes and of the intestine within 60 minutes. In patients with acute right upper quadrant pain and tenderness, a good image of the bile duct accompanied by no image of the gallbladder indicates cystic duct obstruction and strongly supports a diagnosis of acute cholecystitis. The test is easy to perform and is occasionally a useful method of confirming this diagnosis.

JAUNDICE

Jaundice is categorized as prehepatic, hepatic, or posthepatic, depending upon the site of the underlying disease. Hemolysis, the most common cause of prehepatic jaundice, involves increased production of bilirubin. Less common causes of prehepatic jaundice are Gilbert's disease and the Crigler-Najjar syndrome.

Hepatic parenchymal jaundice is subdivided into hepatocellular and cholestatic types. The former includes acute viral hepatitis and chronic alcoholic cirrhosis. Some cases of intrahepatic cholestasis may be indistinguishable clinically and biochemically from cholestasis due to bile duct obstruction. Primary biliary cirrhosis, toxic drug jaundice, cholestatic jaundice of pregnancy, and postoperative cholestatic jaundice are the most common forms.

Extrahepatic jaundice most often results from biliary obstruction by a malignant tumor, choledocholithiasis, or biliary stricture. Pancreatic pseudocyst, chronic pancreatitis, sclerosing cholangitis, metastatic cancer, and duodenal diverticulitis are less common causes.

The cause of jaundice can be ascertained in the majority of patients from clinical and laboratory findings alone. In the remainder, THC or ERCP and ultrasound or CT scans will be necessary. The indications for these tests are discussed in later sections.

History

The age, sex, and parity of the patient and possible deleterious habits should be noted. Most cases of infectious hepatitis occur in patients under age 30. A history of drug addiction may suggest serum hepatitis transmitted by shared hypodermic equipment. Chronic alcoholism can usually be documented in patients with cirrhosis, and acute jaundice in alcoholics usually follows a recent binge. Obstructing gallstones or tumors are more common in older people.

Patients with jaundice due to choledocholithiasis may have associated biliary colic, fever, and chills and may report previous similar attacks. The pain in malignant obstruction is deep-seated and dull and may be affected by changes in position. Pain in the region of the liver is frequently experienced in the early stages of viral hepatitis and acute alcoholic liver injury. The patient with extrahepatic obstruction may report that stools have become lighter in color and the urine dark.

Cholestatic diseases are often accompanied by pruritus—a source of severe discomfort in some cases. Pruritus may precede jaundice, but usually it appears at about the same time. The itching is most severe on the extremities and is aggravated by warm, humid weather. The cause remains obscure; itching does not correlate with bile salt levels in the skin, as was once believed. Cholestyramine, an anion exchange resin, usually provides relief by binding bile salts in the intestinal lumen and preventing their reabsorption.

Physical Examination

Hepatomegaly is common in both hepatic and posthepatic jaundice. In some cases, palpation of the liver may suggest cirrhosis or metastatic cancer, but impressions of this kind are unreliable. Secondary stigmas of cirrhosis usually accompany acute alcoholic jaundice; liver palms, spider angiomas, ascites, collateral veins on the abdominal walls, and splenomegaly suggest cirrhosis. A nontender, palpable gallbladder in a jaundiced patient suggests malignant obstruction of the common duct (Courvoisier's law), but absence of a palpable gallbladder is of little significance in ruling out cancer.

Laboratory Tests

In hemolytic disease, the increased bilirubin is principally in the unconjugated indirect fraction. Since unconjugated bilirubin is insoluble in water, the jaundice in hemolysis is acholuric. The total bilirubin in hemolysis rarely exceeds 4–5 mg/dL, because the rate of excretion increases as the bilirubin concentration rises, and a plateau is quickly reached. Greater values suggest concomitant hepatic parenchymal disease.

Jaundice due to hepatic parenchymal disease is characterized by elevations of both conjugated and unconjugated serum bilirubin. An increase in the conjugated fraction always signifies disease within the hepatobiliary system. The direct bilirubin predominates in about half of cases of hepatic parenchymal disease.

Both intrahepatic cholestasis and extrahepatic obstruction raise the direct bilirubin fraction, though the indirect fraction also increases somewhat. Since direct bilirubin is water-soluble, bilirubinuria develops. With complete extrahepatic obstruction, the total bilirubin rises to a plateau of 25–30 mg/dL, at which point loss in the urine equals the additional daily production. Higher values suggest concomitant hemolysis or decreased renal function. Obstruction of a single hepatic duct does not usually cause jaundice.

In extrahepatic obstruction caused by neoplasms, the serum bilirubin usually exceeds 10 mg/dL, and the average concentration is about 18 mg/dL. Obstructive jaundice due to common duct stones often produces transient bilirubin increases in the range of 2–4 mg/dL, and the level rarely exceeds 15 mg/dL. Serum bilirubin values in patients with alcoholic cirrhosis and acute viral hepatitis vary widely in relation to the severity of the parenchymal damage.

In extrahepatic obstruction, modest rises of AST levels are common, but levels as high as 1000 units/L are seen (though rarely) in patients with common duct stones and cholangitis. In the latter patients, the high values last for only a few days and are associated with increases in LDH concentrations. In general, AST levels above 1000 units/L suggest viral hepatitis.

Serum alkaline phosphatase comes from three sites: liver, bone, and intestine. In normal subjects, liver and bone contribute about equally, and the intestinal contribution is small. Hepatic alkaline phosphatase is a product of the epithelial cells of the cholangioles, and increased alkaline phosphatase levels associated with liver disease are the result of increased enzyme production. Alkaline phosphatase levels go up with intrahepatic cholestasis, cholangitis, or extrahepatic obstruction. Since the elevation is from overproduction, it may occur with focal hepatic lesions in the absence of jaundice. For example, a solitary hepatic metastasis or pyogenic abscess in one lobe or a tumor obstructing only one hepatic duct may fail to obstruct enough hepatic parenchyma to cause jaundice but usually is associated with increased alkaline phosphatase. In cholangitis with incomplete extrahepatic obstruction, serum bilirubin levels may be normal or mildly elevated, but serum alkaline phosphatase may be very high.

Bone disease may complicate the interpretation of abnormal alkaline phosphatase levels (Figure 25–6). If one suspects that the increased serum enzyme may be from bone, serum calcium, phosphorus, and 5′-nucleotidase or leucine aminopeptidase levels should be determined. These last two enzymes are also produced by cholangioles and are elevated in cholestasis, but their serum concentrations remain unchanged with bone disease.

Changes in serum protein levels may reflect hepatic parenchymal dysfunction. In cirrhosis, the serum albumin falls and the globulins increase. Serum globulins reach high values in some patients with primary biliary cirrhosis. Biliary obstruction generally produces no changes unless secondary biliary cirrhosis has developed.

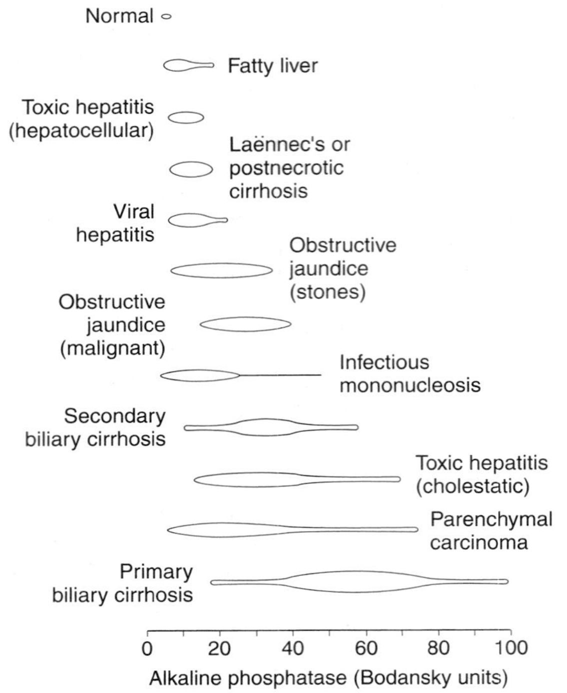

Figure 25–6. Range of alkaline phosphatase values in various hepatobiliary disorders.

Diagnosis

The principal diagnostic objective is to distinguish surgical (obstructive) from nonsurgical jaundice. The history, physical examination, and basic laboratory data allow an accurate diagnosis to be made in most cases without invasive tests (eg, liver biopsy, cholangiograms).

Since most jaundiced patients are not critically ill when first seen, diagnosis and therapy may be conducted in a stepwise fashion, with each test selected according to the information available at that point. Only severe or worsening cholangitis requires urgent intervention. If the jaundice is mild and recent, it often passes within 24–48 hours, at which time an oral cholecystogram or ultrasound scan can be ordered to verify gallstone disease.

In patients with persistent jaundice, the first test will usually be an ultrasound scan, which may show dilated intrahepatic bile ducts (indicating ductal obstruction) or gallbladder stones. The lesion may be further delineated by ERCP or THC. ERCP is preferable when the lower end of the duct is thought to be obstructed (eg, suspected carcinoma of the pancreas or other periampullary tumors). THC is usually preferred for proximal lesions (eg, biliary stricture, neoplasm of the bifurcation of the hepatic ducts), because it gives better opacification of the ducts proximal to the obstruction and therefore provides more information that can be used in planning surgery. If the clinical presentation suggests neoplastic obstruction, a CT scan could be selected in preference to an ultrasound scan, because CT gives better definition of mass lesions while also demonstrating the presence and general location of bile duct obstruction.

If ultrasound or CT scans suggest biliary obstruction, a decision must be made about whether cholangiograms are indicated. In general, patients with gallstone disease do not require preoperative cholangiograms, whereas cholangiograms would be routine in patients with neoplastic obstruction, benign biliary stricture, or rare or unknown causes of obstructive jaundice.

PATHOGENESIS OF GALLSTONES

More than 20 million people in the USA have gallstones in their gallbladders; about 300,000 operations are performed annually for this disease, and at least 6000 deaths result from its complications or treatment. The incidence of gallstones rises with age, so that between 50 and 65 years of age about 20% of women and 5% of men are affected (Figure 25–7).

The gallstones in 75% of patients are composed predominantly (70–95%) of cholesterol and are called cholesterol stones. The remaining 25% are pigment

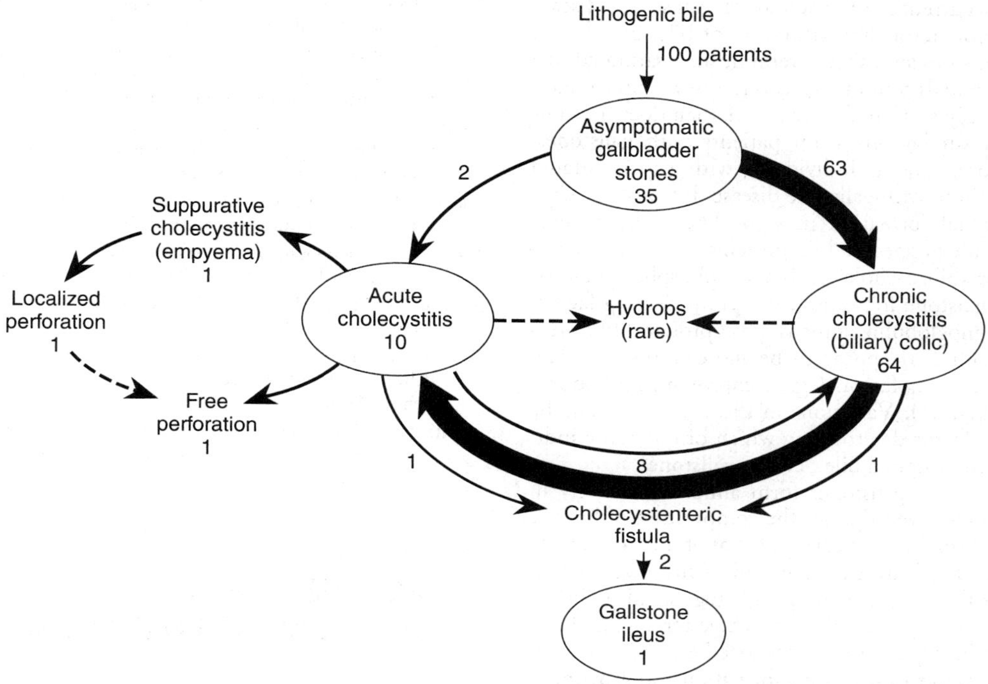

Figure 25–7. The natural history of gallbladder stones. The numbers approximate the percentage of patients in each category. Note that most patients with acute cholecystitis have previously had biliary colic.

stones. Regardless of composition, all gallstones give rise to similar clinical sequelae.

Cholesterol Gallstones

Cholesterol gallstones result from secretion by the liver of bile supersaturated with cholesterol. Influenced by various factors present in bile, the cholesterol precipitates from solution and the newly formed crystals grow to macroscopic stones. Except when the common bile duct is dilated or partially obstructed, the stones in this disease form almost exclusively within the gallbladder. Those found in the ducts usually reach that location after passing through the cystic duct.

The incidence of cholesterol gallstone disease is highest in American Indians, lower in Caucasians, and lowest in blacks, with a twofold gradient from one group to the next. More than 75% of American Indian women over age 40 are affected. Before puberty, the disease is rare but of equal frequency in both sexes. Thereafter, women are more commonly affected than men until after menopause, when the discrepancy lessens. Hormonal effects are also reflected in the increased incidence of gallstones with multiparity and the increased cholesterol saturation of bile and greater incidence of gallstones following ingestion of oral contraceptives. Obesity is the other major risk factor. The relative risk rises proportionately to the extent of overweight due to a progressively increasing output of cholesterol in bile.

As noted previously, cholesterol is insoluble and in bile must be transported within bile salt micelles and phospholipid (lecithin) vesicles. When the amount of cholesterol in bile exceeds the cholesterol holding capacity, cholesterol crystals begin to precipitate from the phospholipid vesicles.

The secretion of bile salt and cholesterol into bile is linked. Bile salt elutes cholesterol from the hepatocyte membrane during passage into the bile canaliculus. At higher bile salt output levels, the amount of cholesterol relative to bile salt entering bile decreases. This means that during low bile flow (eg, during fasting), bile holding capacity for cholesterol is more saturated than during high bile flow. In fact, almost half of persons in Western cultures have bile supersaturated with cholesterol in the morning after an overnight fast. The bile salt pool in patients with cholesterol gallstone disease is about half the size of that of normal subjects, but this is a result of the gallstone disease (eg, gallstones displace bile in the gallbladder) and not a cause.

The occurrence of cholesterol gallstone disease requires cholesterol supersaturation of bile, but that in itself is not sufficient. Cholesterol in supersaturated bile from individuals without gallstone disease precipitates spontaneously at a much slower rate than does the cholesterol in similar bile from patients with gallstones. Furthermore, among individuals with supersaturated bile, only those with gallstone disease demonstrate cholesterol crystal formation in vivo. These observations are the result of specific bile proteins that either stabilize or destabilize cholesterol-laden phospholipid vesicles. For gallstone formation, the pronucleating factors (eg, immunoglobulin, mucus glycoprotein, fibronectin, orosomucoid) appear to be more important than the antinucleating factors (eg, glycoprotein, apolipoprotein, cytokeratin). Variations in these proteins may be the critical factor determining which of the many individuals with saturated bile develop gallstones.

The fact that gallstones form almost exclusively in the gallbladder even though the composition of hepatic bile is abnormal underscores the important role of the gallbladder in gallstone pathogenesis. This includes concentrating the bile, providing nidi (eg, small grains of pigment) for crystallization of cholesterol, supplying mucoprotein to paste the stones together, and serving as an area of stasis to allow stone formation and growth.

Pigment Stones

Pigment stones account for 25% of gallstones in the USA and 60% of those in Japan. Pigment stones are black to dark brown, 2–5 mm in diameter, and amorphous. They are composed of a mixture of calcium bilirubinate, complex bilirubin polymers, bile acids, and other unidentified substances. About 50% are radiopaque, and in the USA they constitute two-thirds of all radiopaque gallstones. The incidence is similar in men and women and in blacks and whites. Pigment stones are rare in American Indians.

Predisposing factors are cirrhosis, bile stasis (eg, a strictured or markedly dilated common duct), and chronic hemolysis. Some patients with pigment stones have increased concentrations of unconjugated bilirubin in their bile. Scanning electron microscopy demonstrates that about 90% of pigment stones are composed of dense mixtures of bacteria and bacterial glycocalix along with pigment solids. This suggests that bacteria have a primary role in pigment gallstone formation, and it also helps to explain why patients with pigment gallstone disease have sepsis more often than do those with cholesterol gallstone disease. It seems likely that bacterial β-glucuronidase is responsible for deconjugating the soluble bilirubin-diglucuronide to insoluble unconjugated bilirubin, which subsequently becomes agglomerated by glycocalix into macroscopic stones.

Beckingham IJ: ABC of diseases of liver, pancreas, and biliary system. Gallstone disease. BMJ 2001;322:91.

Caroli-Bosc FX et al: Cholelithiasis and dietary risk factors: an epidemiologic investigation in Vidauban, Southeast France. General Practitioner's Group of Vidauban. Dig Dis Sci 1998;43:2131.

Cicala M et al: Increased sphincter of Oddi basal pressure in patients affected by gall stone disease: a role for biliary stasis and colicky pain? Gut 2001;48:414.

Glasgow RE et al: The spectrum and cost of complicated gallstone disease in California. Arch Surg 2000;135:1021.

Han T et al: Apolipoprotein B-100 gene Xba I polymorphism and cholesterol gallstone disease. Clin Genet 2000;57:304.

Ko CW, Sekijima JH, Lee SP: Biliary sludge. Ann Intern Med 1999;130(4 Part 1):301.

Wells JE et al: Isolation and characterization of cholic acid 7alpha-dehydroxylating fecal bacteria from cholesterol gallstone patients. J Hepatol 2000;32:4.

Zapata R et al: Gallbladder motility and lithogenesis in obese patients during diet-induced weight loss. Dig Dis Sci 2000;45:421.

DISEASES OF THE GALLBLADDER & BILE DUCTS

ASYMPTOMATIC GALLSTONES

Data on the prevalence of gallstones in the USA indicate that only about 30% of people with cholelithiasis come to surgery. Symptoms of gallstone disease generally do not change in severity. Each year, about 2% of patients with asymptomatic gallstones develop symptoms, usually biliary colic rather than one of the complications of gallstone disease. Patients with chronic colic tend to have symptoms of the same level of severity and frequency. The present practice of operating only on symptomatic patients, leaving the millions without symptoms alone, seems appropriate. A question is often raised about what to advise the asymptomatic patient found to have gallstones during the course of unrelated studies. The presence of either of the following portends a more serious course and should probably serve as a reason for prophylactic cholecystectomy: (1) large stones (> 2 cm in diameter), because they produce acute cholecystitis more often than small stones; and (2) a calcified gallbladder, because it so often is associated with carcinoma. However, most asymptomatic patients have no special features. If coexistent cardiopulmonary or other problems increase the risk of surgery, operation should not be considered. For the average asymptomatic patient, it is not reasonable to make a strong recommendation for cholecystectomy. The tendency, however, is to operate on younger patients and temporize in the elderly.

Beckingham IJ: ABC of diseases of liver, pancreas, and biliary system. Gallstone disease. BMJ 2001;322:91.

GALLSTONES & CHRONIC CHOLECYSTITIS (BILIARY COLIC)

ESSENTIALS OF DIAGNOSIS

- *Episodic abdominal pain.*
- *Dyspepsia.*
- *Gallstones on cholecystography or ultrasound scan.*

General Considerations

Chronic cholecystitis is the most common form of symptomatic gallbladder disease and is associated with gallstones in nearly every case. In general, the term cholecystitis is applied whenever gallstones are present regardless of the histologic appearance of the gallbladder. Repeated minor episodes of obstruction of the cystic duct cause intermittent biliary colic and contribute to inflammation and subsequent scar formation. Gallbladders from symptomatic patients with gallstones who have never had an attack of acute cholecystitis are of two types: (1) In some, the mucosa may be slightly flattened, but the wall is thin and unscarred and, except for the stones, appears normal. (2) Others exhibit obvious signs of chronic inflammation, with thickening, cellular infiltration, loss of elasticity, and fibrosis. The clinical history in these two groups cannot always be distinguished, and inflammatory changes may also be found in patients with asymptomatic gallstones.

Clinical Findings

A. Symptoms and Signs

Biliary colic, the most characteristic symptom, is caused by transient gallstone obstruction of the cystic duct. The pain usually begins abruptly and subsides gradually, lasting for a few minutes to several hours. The pain of biliary colic is usually steady—not intermittent, like that of intestinal colic. In some patients, attacks occur postprandially; in others, there is no relationship to meals. The frequency of attacks is quite variable, ranging from nearly continuous trouble to episodes many years apart. Nausea and vomiting may accompany the pain.

Biliary colic is usually felt in the right upper quadrant, but epigastric and left abdominal pain are common, and some patients experience precordial pain. The pain may radiate around the costal margin into the back or may be referred to the region of the scapula. Pain on top of the shoulder is unusual and suggests direct diaphragmatic irritation. In a severe attack, the patient usually curls up in bed, changing position frequently in order to be more comfortable.

During an attack, there may be tenderness in the right upper quadrant, and, rarely, the gallbladder is palpable.

Fatty food intolerance, dyspepsia, indigestion, heartburn, flatulence, nausea, and eructations are other symptoms associated with gallstone disease. Because they are also frequent in the general population, their presence in any given patient may only be incidental to the gallstones.

B. Laboratory Findings

An ultrasound scan of the gallbladder should usually be the first test. Gallstones can be demonstrated in about 95% of cases, and a positive reading for gallstones is almost never in error. An oral cholecystogram should be obtained if the ultrasound study is equivocal, if the patient is a candidate for lithotripsy or ursodiol therapy, or if symptoms are highly suggestive and an ultrasound study has been read as normal.

About 2% of patients with gallstone disease have normal ultrasound studies and oral cholecystograms. Therefore, if the clinical suspicion of gallbladder disease is high and these two tests are negative, the patient should be studied by ERCP (to opacify the gallbladder in the search for stones) or duodenal intubation and examination of duodenal bile for cholesterol crystals or bilirubinate granules.

Differential Diagnosis

Gallbladder colic may be strongly suggested by the history, but the clinical impression should always be verified by an ultrasound study. Biliary colic may simulate the pain of duodenal ulcer, hiatal hernia, pancreatitis, and myocardial infarction.

An ECG and a chest x-ray should be obtained to investigate cardiopulmonary disease. It has been suggested that biliary colic may sometimes aggravate cardiac disease, but angina pectoris or an abnormal ECG should rarely be indications for cholecystectomy.

Right-sided radicular pain in the T6–T10 dermatomes may be confused with biliary colic. Osteoarthritic spurs, vertebral lesions, or tumors may be shown on x-rays of the spine or may be suggested by hyperesthesia of the abdominal skin.

An upper gastrointestinal series may be indicated to search for esophageal spasm, hiatal hernia, peptic ulcer, or gastric tumors. In some patients, the irritable colon syndrome may be mistaken for gallbladder discomfort. Carcinoma of the cecum or ascending colon may be overlooked on the assumption that postprandial pain in these conditions is due to gallstones.

Complications

Chronic cholecystitis predisposes to acute cholecystitis, common duct stones, and adenocarcinoma of the gallbladder. The longer the stones have been present, the higher the incidence of all of these complications. Complications are infrequent, however, and the presence of gallstones is not reason enough for prophylactic cholecystectomy in a person with asymptomatic or mildly symptomatic disease.

Treatment

A. Medical Treatment

Avoidance of offending foods may be helpful.

1. Dissolution—Cholesterol gallstones in the gallbladder can be dissolved in some cases by chronic treatment with ursodiol, which reduces the cholesterol saturation of bile by inhibiting cholesterol secretion. The resulting undersaturated bile slowly dissolves the solid cholesterol in the gallstones.

Unfortunately, bile salt therapy has marginal efficacy. The gallstones must be small (eg, < 5 mm) and devoid of calcium (ie, nonopaque on CT scans), and the gallbladder must opacify on oral cholecystography (an indication of unobstructed flow of bile between bile duct and gallbladder). About 15% of patients with gallstones are candidates for treatment. Dissolution is achieved within 2 years in about 50% of highly selected patients. Stones recur, however, in 50% of cases within 5 years. In general, dissolution therapy—alone or in conjunction with lithotripsy—is used only rarely.

2. Lithotripsy and dissolution—Extracorporeal shock wave lithotripsy (ESWL) involves focusing shock waves, which pass through tissue and fluids, upon the gallstones. The stones are fragmented by explosion of small air bubbles within interstices of the solid material.

Lithotripsy is of little therapeutic value because the fragments remain in the gallbladder unless they can be dissolved. Consequently, candidates for lithotripsy must also use ursodiol therapy. Complete elimination of gallbladder stones is attained within 9 months in about 25% of appropriately selected patients. Because of the many drawbacks of this form of treatment, it has not been approved by the FDA in the United States.

B. Surgical Treatment

Cholecystectomy is indicated in most patients with symptoms. The procedure can be scheduled at the patient's convenience, within weeks or months after diagnosis. Active concurrent disease that increases the risk of surgery should be treated before operation. In some chronically ill patients, surgery should be deferred indefinitely.

Cholecystectomy is most often performed laparoscopically, but when the laparoscopic approach is contraindicated (eg, too many adhesions) or unsuccessful, it may be performed through a laparotomy. The difference consists of 4 fewer days in the hospital and several fewer weeks off work when done laparoscopically. Regardless of how it is done, operative cholangiography is usually included to look for common duct stones. If stones are found, common duct exploration is performed (see under choledocholithiasis).

Prognosis

Serious complications and deaths related to the operation itself are rare. The operative death rate is about 0.1% in patients under age 50 and about 0.5% in patients over age 50. Most deaths occur in patients recognized preoperatively to have increased risks. The operation relieves symptoms in 95% of cases.

Beyer AJ 3rd, Delcore R, Cheung LY: Nonoperative treatment of biliary tract disease. Arch Surg 1998;133:1172.

Binmoeller KF, Schafer TW: Endoscopic management of bile duct stones. J Clin Gastroenterol 2001;32:106.

Calland JF et al: Outpatient laparoscopic cholecystectomy: patient outcomes after implementation of a clinical pathway. Ann Surg 2001;233:704.

Fletcher DR et al: Complications of cholecystectomy: risks of the laparoscopic approach and protective effects of operative cholangiography: a population-based study. Ann Surg 1999;229:449.

Gadacz TR: Update on laparoscopic cholecystectomy, including a clinical pathway. Surg Clin North Am 2000;80:1127.

Maxwell JG et al: Cholecystectomy in patients aged 80 and older. Am J Surg 1998;176:627.

Montori A et al: Endoscopic and surgical integration in the approach to biliary tract disease. J Clin Gastroenterol 1999;28:198.

Moonka R et al: The presentation of gallstones and results of biliary surgery in a spinal cord injured population. Am J Surg 1999; 178:246.

Sakuramoto S et al: Preoperative evaluation to predict technical difficulties of laparoscopic cholecystectomy on the basis of histological inflammation findings on resected gallbladder. Am J Surg 2000;179:114.

Stuart SA et al: Routine intraoperative laparoscopic cholangiography. Am J Surg 1998;176:632.

Tocchi A et al: The need for antibiotic prophylaxis in elective laparoscopic cholecystectomy: a prospective randomized study. Arch Surg 2000;135:67.

Traverso LW: Risk factors for intraoperative injury during cholecystectomy: an ounce of prevention is worth a pound of cure. Ann Surg 1999;229:458.

Yerdel MA et al: Direct trocar insertion versus Veress needle insertion in laparoscopic cholecystectomy. Am J Surg 1999;177:247.

ACUTE CHOLECYSTITIS

ESSENTIALS OF DIAGNOSIS

- *Acute right upper quadrant pain and tenderness.*

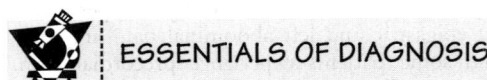

- *Fever and leukocytosis.*
- *Palpable gallbladder in one-third of cases.*
- *Nonopacified gallbladder on radionuclide excretion scan.*
- *Sonographic Murphy sign.*

General Considerations

In 80% of cases, acute cholecystitis results from obstruction of the cystic duct by a gallstone impacted in Hartmann's pouch. The gallbladder becomes inflamed and distended, creating abdominal pain and tenderness. The natural history of acute cholecystitis varies, depending on whether the obstruction becomes relieved, the extent of secondary bacterial invasion, the age of the patient, and the presence of other aggravating factors such as diabetes mellitus. Most attacks resolve spontaneously without surgery or other specific therapy, but some progress to abscess formation or free perforation with generalized peritonitis.

The pathologic changes in the gallbladder evolve in a typical pattern. Subserosal edema and hemorrhage and patchy mucosal necrosis are the first changes. Later, PMNs appear. The final stage involves development of fibrosis. Gangrene and perforation may occur as early as 3 days after onset, but most perforations occur during the second week. In cases that resolve spontaneously, acute inflammation has largely cleared by 4 weeks, but some residual evidence of inflammation may last for several months. About 90% of gallbladders removed during an acute attack show chronic scarring, although many of these patients deny having had any previous symptoms.

The cause of acute cholecystitis is still partially conjectural. Obstruction of the cystic duct is present in most cases, but in experimental animals, cystic duct obstruction does not result in acute cholecystitis unless the gallbladder is filled with concentrated bile or bile saturated with cholesterol. There is also evidence that trauma from gallstones releases phospholipase from the mucosal cells of the gallbladder. This is followed by conversion of lecithin in bile to lysolecithin, which is a toxic compound that may cause more inflammation. Bacteria appear to have a minor role in the early stages of acute cholecystitis, even though most complications of the disease involve suppuration.

About 20% of cases of acute cholecystitis occur in the absence of cholelithiasis (acalculous cholecystitis). Some of these are due to cystic duct obstruction by another process such as a malignant tumor. Rarely, acute acalculous cholecystitis results from cystic artery occlusion or primary bacterial infection by *E coli,* clostridia, or, occasionally, *Salmonella typhi.* Most cases occur in patients hospitalized with some other illness; acute acalculous cholecystitis is particularly common in trauma victims (civilian or military) and in patients receiving total parenteral nutrition. Small-vessel occlusion occurs early, and unless treatment is given promptly, the disease progresses rapidly to gangrenous cholecystitis and septic complications, at which point the death rate is high.

Clinical Findings

A. Symptoms and Signs

The first symptom is abdominal pain in the right upper quadrant, sometimes associated with referred pain in the region of the right scapula. In 75% of cases, the patient will have had previous attacks of biliary colic, at first indistinguishable from the present illness. However, in acute cholecystitis, the pain persists and becomes associated with abdominal tenderness. Nausea and vomiting are present in about half of patients, but the vomiting is rarely severe. Mild icterus occurs in 10% of cases. The temperature usually ranges from 38 to 38.5 °C. High fever and chills are uncommon and should suggest the possibility of complications or an incorrect diagnosis.

Right upper quadrant tenderness is present, and in about a third of patients the gallbladder is palpable (often in a position lateral to its normal one). Voluntary guarding during examination may prevent detection of an enlarged gallbladder. In others, the gallbladder is not enlarged because scarring of the wall restricts distention. If instructed to breathe deeply during palpation in the right subcostal region, the patient experiences accentuated tenderness and sudden inspiratory arrest (Murphy's sign).

B. Laboratory Findings

The leukocyte count is usually elevated to 12,000–15,000/μL. Normal counts are common, but if the count goes much above 15,000, one should suspect complications. A mild elevation of the serum bilirubin (in the range of 2–4 mg/dL) is common, presumably owing to secondary inflammation of the common duct by the contiguous gallbladder. Bilirubin values above this range would most likely indicate the associated presence of common duct stones. A mild increase in alkaline phosphatase may accompany the attack. Occasionally, the serum amylase concentration transiently reaches 1000 units/dL or more.

C. Imaging Studies

A plain x-ray of the abdomen may occasionally show an enlarged gallbladder shadow. In 15% of patients, the gallstones contain enough calcium to be seen on the plain film.

Ultrasound scans show gallstones, sludge, and thickening of the gallbladder wall, and the ultrasonographer can determine even better than the clinician whether the point of maximum tenderness is over the gallbladder (ultrasonographic Murphy's sign). This last finding is often absent, however, when the gallbladder is gangrenous. Usually, ultrasound is the only test needed to make the diagnosis of acute cholecystitis.

If additional diagnostic information is desirable (eg, if ultrasound is equivocal or negative), a radionuclide excretion scan (eg, HIDA scan) should be performed. This test cannot demonstrate gallstones, but if the gallbladder is imaged, acute cholecystitis is ruled out except in rare cases of acalculous cholecystitis (the test is positive in most cases of acute acalculous cholecystitis). Imaging of the duct but not the gallbladder supports the diagnosis of acute cholecystitis. A few false positives are seen in advanced gallstone disease without acute inflammation and in acute biliary pancreatitis.

Differential Diagnosis

The differential diagnosis includes other common causes of acute upper abdominal pain and tenderness. An acute peptic ulcer with or without perforation might be suggested by a history of epigastric pain relieved by food or antacids. Most cases of perforated ulcer demonstrate free air under the diaphragm on x-ray. An emergency upper gastrointestinal series may help.

Acute pancreatitis can be confused with acute cholecystitis, especially if cholecystitis is accompanied by an elevated amylase level. Furthermore, HIDA scans fail to outline the gallbladder in most cases of acute biliary pancreatitis. Sometimes the two diseases coexist, but pancreatitis should not be accepted as a second diagnosis without specific findings.

Acute appendicitis in patients with a high cecum may closely simulate acute cholecystitis.

Severe right upper quadrant pain with high fever and local tenderness may develop in acute gonococcal perihepatitis (Fitz-Hugh-Curtis syndrome). Clues to the proper diagnosis may be found in tenderness in the adnexa, vaginal discharge that shows gonococci on a Gram-stained smear, and a disparity between the patient's high fever and her general lack of toxicity.

Complications

The major complications of acute cholecystitis are empyema, gangrene, and perforation.

A. Empyema

In empyema (suppurative cholecystitis), the gallbladder contains frank pus, and the patient becomes more toxic, with high spiking fever (39–40 °C), chills, and leukocytosis greater than 15,000/μL. Parenteral antibiotics should be given, and percutaneous cholecystostomy or cholecystectomy should be performed.

B. Perforation

Perforation may take any of three forms: (1) localized perforation with pericholecystic abscess; (2) free perforation with generalized peritonitis; and (3) perforation into an adjacent hollow viscus, with the formation of a fistula. Perforation may occur as early as 3 days after the onset of acute cholecystitis or not until late in the second week. The total incidence of perforation is about 10%.

1. Pericholecystic abscess—Pericholecystic abscess, the most common form of perforation, should be suspected when the signs and symptoms progress, especially when accompanied by the appearance of a palpable mass. The patient often becomes toxic, with fever to 39 °C and a leukocyte count above 15,000/μL, but sometimes there is no correlation between the clinical signs and the development of local abscess. Cholecystectomy and drainage of the abscess can be performed safely in many of these patients, but if the patient's condition is unstable, percutaneous cholecystostomy is preferable.

2. Free perforation—Free perforation occurs in only 1–2% of patients, most often early in the disease when gangrene develops before adhesions wall off the gallbladder. The diagnosis is made preoperatively in less than half of cases. In some patients with localized pain, sudden spread of pain and tenderness to other parts of the abdomen suggests the diagnosis. Whenever it is suspected, free perforation must be treated by emergency laparotomy. Abdominal paracentesis may be misleading and has proved to be of little diagnostic usefulness. Cholecystectomy should be performed if the patient's condition will permit; otherwise, cholecystostomy is done. The death rate depends partly on whether the cystic duct remains obstructed or the stone becomes dislodged after perforation. The former leads to a purulent peritonitis that is lethal in 20% of cases. In the latter, a true bile peritonitis ensues and over 50% of patients die. The earlier operation is performed, the better the prognosis.

3. Cholecystenteric fistula—If the acutely inflamed gallbladder becomes adherent to adjacent stomach, duodenum, or colon and necrosis develops at the site of one of these adhesions, perforation may occur into the lumen of the gut. The resulting decompression often allows the acute disease to resolve. If the gallbladder stones discharge through the fistula and if they are large enough, they may obstruct the small intestine (gallstone ileus; see below). Rarely, patients vomit gallstones that have entered the stomach through a cholecystogastric fistula. In most patients, the acute attack subsides and the cholecystenteric fistula is clinically unsuspected.

Cholecystenteric fistulas do not usually cause symptoms unless the gallbladder is still partially obstructed by stones or scarring. Neither oral nor intravenous cholangiograms will opacify the gallbladder or the fistula, but the latter may be shown on upper gastrointestinal series, where it must be differentiated from a fistula due to perforated peptic ulcer. Malabsorption and steatorrhea have been reported in isolated cases of cholecystocolonic fistulas. Steatorrhea in this situation could be due either to absence of bile in the proximal bowel following diversion into the colon or, more rarely, to excess bacteria in the upper intestine.

Symptomatic cholecystenteric fistulas should be treated by cholecystectomy and closure of the fistula. The majority are discovered incidentally during cholecystectomy for symptomatic gallbladder disease.

Treatment

Intravenous fluids should be given to correct dehydration and electrolyte imbalance, and a nasogastric tube should be inserted. For acute cholecystitis of average severity, parenteral cefazolin (2–4 g daily) should be given. Parenteral penicillin (20 million units daily), clindamycin, and an aminoglycoside should be given for severe disease. Single-drug therapy using imipenem is a good alternative.

There are two schools of thought about the treatment of acute cholecystitis. Since the disease resolves with antibiotics and supportive care in about 60% of cases, one approach is to manage the patient expectantly, with a plan to perform elective cholecystectomy after recovery, reserving surgery during the acute attack for those with severe or worsening disease. (This approach is untenable in acute acalculous cholecystitis.)

The preferred plan is to perform cholecystectomy in all patients unless there are specific contraindications to operation (eg, serious concomitant disease). Four controlled trials have supported this approach with the following data: (1) the incidence of technical complications is no greater with early surgery; (2) early surgery reduces the total duration of illness by approximately 30 days, length of hospitalization by 5–7 days, and direct medical costs by several thousand dollars; and (3) the death rate is slightly lower with early surgery because of earlier treatment for some patients whose condition would have worsened during expectant management. Since these trials were completed, the average case appears to have become more severe, and the arguments against expectant management are now even more compelling.

The following are the major factors that affect the decision (Figure 25–8): (1) whether the diagnosis is established; (2) the general health of the patient as modified by coexistent disease or the present illness; and (3) signs of local complications of acute cholecystitis. The diagnosis should be clear-cut and the patient optimally prepared; if perforation or empyema is suspected, emergency surgery is indicated.

In about 30% of cases, the diagnosis of acute cholecystitis is established but the general condition of the patient is unsatisfactory. If possible, surgery should be postponed in these cases until the ancillary disease is controlled.

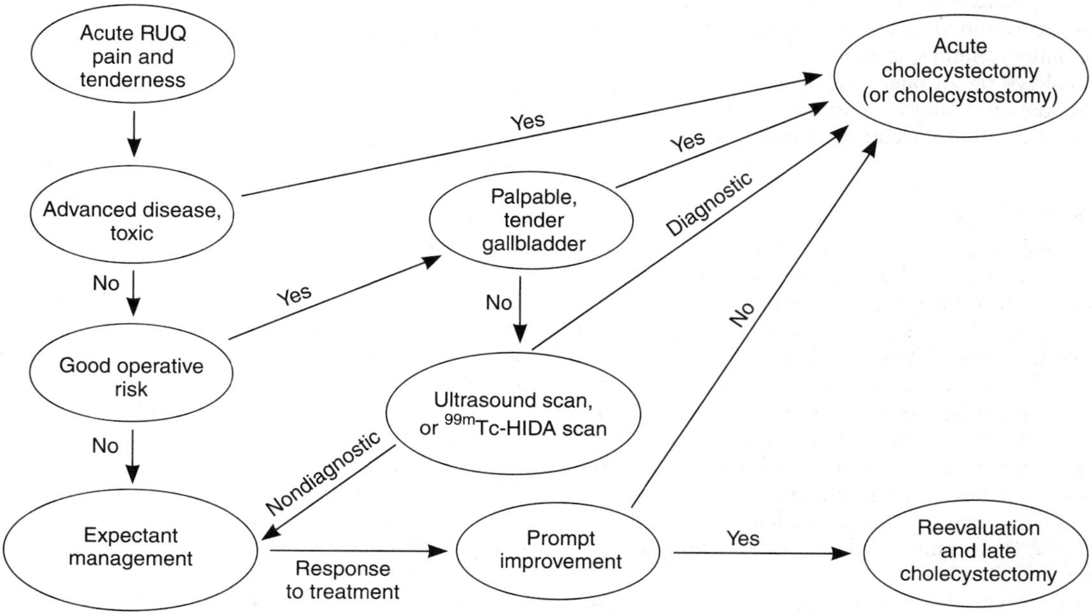

Figure 25–8. Scheme for the management of acute cholecystitis.

Expectant management cannot be rigidly adhered to, however, if the manifestations of cholecystitis worsen.

About 10% of patients require emergency treatment. These are generally clinical situations in which the disease appears to have become complicated or is about to. High fever (39 °C), marked leukocytosis (> 15,000/μL), or chills suggest suppurative progression. Acalculous acute cholecystitis should automatically be placed in this category. When the patient's general condition is poor, percutaneous catheter cholecystostomy is the preferable treatment. Patients in better overall health should be treated by cholecystectomy.

The sudden appearance of generalized abdominal pain may indicate free perforation. Appearance of a mass while the patient is under observation may be a sign of local perforation and abscess formation. Changes of this sort are indications for emergency surgery.

Cholecystectomy is the preferable operation in acute cholecystitis, and it can be performed laparoscopically in about 50% of patients. Operative cholangiography should be performed in most cases, and the common bile duct explored if appropriate indications are present (see section on choledocholithiasis). Patients with severe acute cholecystitis who are in poor condition for emergency cholecystectomy should be treated by percutaneous cholecystostomy. Percutaneous cholecystostomy may also be the preferred therapy for acute acalculous cholecystitis. A catheter inserted under ultrasound or CT guidance is allowed to drain the gallbladder of its bile or pus. The resulting decompression controls the acute disease, including any local infection, but the gallstones cannot be removed. Therefore, cholecystectomy should be performed after the patient recovers in order to avoid recurrent attacks. Cholecystectomy is definitive therapy in the patient with acalculous cholecystitis. At one time, cholecystostomy was performed surgically, but most hospitals now have radiologists skilled in the simpler percutaneous method.

Prognosis

The overall death rate of acute cholecystitis is about 5%. Nearly all of the deaths are in patients over age 60 or those with diabetes mellitus. In the older age group, secondary cardiovascular or pulmonary complications contribute substantially to the death rate. Uncontrolled sepsis with peritonitis and intrahepatic abscesses are the most important local conditions responsible for death.

Common duct stones are present in about 15% of patients with acute cholecystitis, and some of the more seriously ill patients have simultaneous cholangitis from biliary obstruction. Acute pancreatitis may also complicate acute cholecystitis, and the combination carries a greater risk.

Patients who develop the suppurative forms of gallbladder disease such as empyema or perforation are less likely to recover. Earlier admission to the hospital and early cholecystectomy reduce the chances of these complications.

Berber E et al: Selective use of tube cholecystostomy with interval laparoscopic cholecystectomy in acute cholecystitis. Arch Surg 2000;135:341.

Borzellino G et al: Emergency cholecystostomy and subsequent cholecystectomy for acute gallstone cholecystitis in the elderly. Br J Surg 1999;86:1521.

Davis CA et al: Effective use of percutaneous cholecystostomy in high-risk surgical patients: techniques, tube management, and results. Arch Surg 1999;134:727.

Eldar S et al: The impact of patient delay and physician delay on the outcome of laparoscopic cholecystectomy for acute cholecystitis. Am J Surg 1999;178:303.

Geoghegan JG, Keane FB: Laparoscopic management of complicated gallstone disease. Br J Surg 1999;86:145.

Greenwald JA et al: Standardization of surgeon-controlled variables: impact on outcome in patients with acute cholecystitis. Ann Surg 2000;231:339.

Kim KH et al: Percutaneous gallbladder drainage for delayed laparoscopic cholecystectomy in patients with acute cholecystitis. Am J Surg 2000;179:111.

Laycock WS et al: Variation in the use of laparoscopic cholecystectomy for elderly patients with acute cholecystitis. Arch Surg 2000;135:457.

Lillemoe KD: Surgical treatment of biliary tract infections. Am Surg 2000;66:138.

Lobe TE: Cholelithiasis and cholecystitis in children. Semin Pediatr Surg 2000;9:170.

Svanvik J: Laparoscopic cholecystectomy for acute cholecystitis. Eur J Surg 2000;(Suppl 585):16.

EMPHYSEMATOUS CHOLECYSTITIS

Emphysematous cholecystitis is a rare condition in which bubbles of gas from anaerobic infection appear in the lumen of the gallbladder, its wall, the pericholecystic space, and, on occasion, the bile ducts. Clostridia species are the most commonly implicated organisms, but other gas-forming anaerobes such as *E coli* or anaerobic streptococci may be found. Three times as many men as women are affected, and 20% of patients have diabetes mellitus. In contrast to the usual form of acute cholecystitis, the disease probably is a bacterial infection from the earliest moment. In many cases, the gallbladder contains no stones.

The disease begins with sudden and rapidly progressive right upper quadrant pain. Fever and leukocytosis reach high levels quickly, and the patient is considerably more toxic than is usually the case in acute cholecystitis. On examination, a mass can usually be found in the right upper quadrant.

Plain films of the abdomen show tissue emphysema outlining the gallbladder and, in some cases, an air-fluid level in the lumen. The clinical and x-ray pictures are characteristic enough so that the diagnosis is usually obvious. If the changes on plain films are equivocal, a CT scan may bring them out.

The patient should be treated with high doses of antibiotics effective against clostridia and the other species mentioned above. Emergency surgical treatment should follow the initial resuscitative measures. Cholecystectomy can be safely performed in most cases, but the most critically ill might fare better with cholecystostomy. The types of complications are the same as in other forms of acute cholecystitis, but illness is more severe and death rates are higher.

Danse EM, Laterre PF: Images in clinical medicine. Emphysematous cholecystitis. N Engl J Med 1999;341:1126.

Garcia-Sancho Tellez L et al: Acute emphysematous cholecystitis. Report of twenty cases. Hepatogastroenterology 1999;46:2144.

Zeebregts CJ et al: Percutaneous drainage of emphysematous cholecystitis associated with pneumoperitoneum. Hepatogastroenterology 1999;46:771.

GALLSTONE ILEUS

Gallstone ileus is mechanical intestinal obstruction caused by a large gallstone lodged in the lumen. It is seen most often in women, and the average age is about 70.

Clinical Findings

A. Symptoms

The patient usually presents with obvious small bowel obstruction, either partial or complete. The obstructing gallstone enters the intestine through a cholecystenteric fistula located in the duodenum, colon, or, rarely, the stomach or jejunum. The gallbladder may contain one or several stones, but stones that cause gallstone ileus are almost always 2.5 cm or more in diameter. The lumen in the proximal bowel will allow most of these large calculi to pass caudally until the ileum is reached. Obstruction of the large intestine may follow passage of a gallstone through a fistula at the hepatic flexure or may occur even after the stone has traversed the entire small bowel.

B. Signs

In most patients, the findings on physical examination are typical of distal small bowel obstruction. Obstruction of the duodenum or jejunum may give a perplexing clinical picture because of the lack of distention. Right upper quadrant tenderness and a mass may be present in some cases, but the distended abdomen may be difficult to examine accurately.

C. Imaging Studies

In addition to dilated small intestine, plain films of the abdomen may show a radiopaque gallstone, and unless one is alert to the possibility of gallstone ileus, the ectopic stone can be a puzzling finding. In about 40% of cases, careful examination of the film will reveal gas in the biliary tree, a manifestation of the cholecystenteric fistula. When the clinical picture is unclear, an upper gastrointestinal series should be obtained, which will demonstrate the cholecystoduodenal fistula and verify intestinal obstruction.

Treatment

The proper treatment is emergency laparotomy and removal of the obstructing stone through a small enterotomy. The proximal intestine must be carefully inspected for the presence of a second calculus that might cause a postoperative recurrence. The gallbladder should be left undisturbed at the original operation.

Once the patient has recovered, an elective cholecystectomy should be scheduled if the patient complains of chronic gallbladder symptoms. On this basis, interval cholecystectomy will be required in about 30% of patients. The fistula itself is rarely the source of trouble and closes spontaneously in most patients.

Prognosis

The death rate of gallstone ileus remains about 20%, largely because of the poor general condition of elderly patients at the time of laparotomy. In many cases, the patient has developed cardiac or pulmonary complications during a preoperative delay when the diagnosis was unclear.

Lobo DN, Jobling JC, Balfour TW: Gallstone ileus: diagnostic pitfalls and therapeutic successes. J Clin Gastroenterol 2000;30:72.

Scarpa FJ, Borges J, Mullen D: et al: Gallstone ileus. Am J Sug. 2000; 180:99.

CHOLANGITIS (BACTERIAL CHOLANGITIS)

Bacterial infection of the biliary ducts always signifies biliary obstruction, since in the absence of obstruction even heavy bacterial contamination of the ducts fails to produce symptoms or pathologic changes. The block to flow may be partial or, less commonly, complete. The principal causes are choledocholithiasis, biliary stricture, and neoplasm. Less common causes are chronic pancreatitis, ampullary stenosis, pancreatic pseudocyst, duodenal diverticulum, congenital cyst, and parasitic invasion. Iatrogenic cholangitis may complicate transhepatic or T tube cholangiography. Not all obstructing lesions are followed by cholangitis, however. For example, biliary infection develops in only 15% of patients with neoplastic obstruction. The likelihood of cholangitis is greatest when the obstruction occurs after the duct has acquired a resident bacterial population.

With obstruction, ductal pressure rises, and bacteria proliferate and escape into the systemic circulation via the hepatic sinusoids. Experimentally, the incidence of positive blood cultures with ductal infection is directly proportionate to the absolute height of the pressure in the duct.

The symptoms of cholangitis (sometimes referred to as Charcot's triad) are biliary colic, jaundice, and chills and fever, though a complete triad is present in only 70% of cases. Laboratory findings include leukocytosis and elevated serum bilirubin and alkaline phosphatase levels. The predominant organisms in bile (in approximately decreasing frequency) are *E coli,* klebsiella, pseudomonas, enterococci, and proteus. *Bacteroides fragilis* and other anaerobes (eg, *Clostridium perfringens*) can be detected in about 25% of cases, and their presence correlates with multiple previous biliary operations (often including a biliary enteric anastomosis), severe symptoms, and a high incidence of postoperative suppurative complications. Anaerobes are nearly always seen in the company of aerobes. Two species of bacteria can be cultured in about 50% of cases. Bacteremia probably occurs in most cases, and blood cultures obtained at the appropriate time contain the same organisms as the bile. Early in an attack, an ultrasound scan will often give useful diagnostic information. Further workup (THC, ERCP, etc) can proceed later after the acute manifestations are brought under control. Cholangiography is dangerous during active cholangitis.

The term **suppurative cholangitis** has been used for the most severe form of this disease, when manifestations of sepsis overshadow those of hepatobiliary disease. The diagnostic pentad of suppurative cholangitis consists of abdominal pain, jaundice, fever and chills, mental confusion or lethargy, and shock. The diagnosis is often missed because the signs of biliary disease are overlooked.

Most cases of cholangitis can be controlled with intravenous antibiotics. A cephalosporin antibiotic (eg, cefazolin, cefoxitin) is the drug of choice in the average mild to moderately severe case. If disease is severe or progressively worsens, an aminoglycoside plus clindamycin or metronidazole should be added to the regimen.

For patients with severe cholangitis or unremitting cholangitis despite antibiotic therapy, the bile duct must be promptly decompressed. Most cases of severe acute cholangitis are associated with choledocholithiasis, where the best treatment consists of emergency endoscopic sphincterotomy. In the uncommon case where this is unsuccessful, laparotomy is indicated in order to decompress the bile duct. Cholangitis accompanying neoplastic obstruction may be managed by insertion of a transhepatic drainage catheter into the bile duct. A cholangiogram should not be obtained because the procedure could worsen sepsis.

Urgent intervention (eg, endoscopic sphincterotomy, percutaneous transhepatic drainage, or operative decompression) is required in about 10% of patients with acute cholangitis. The remaining 90% are eventually treated by elective surgery or endoscopic sphincterotomy following antibiotic therapy and a thorough diagnostic evaluation.

Elsakr R et al: Antimicrobial treatment of intra-abdominal infections. Dig Dis 1998;16:47.

Hanau LH, Steigbigel NH: Acute (ascending) cholangitis. Infect Dis Clin North Am 2000;14:521.

Poon RT et al: Management of gallstone cholangitis in the era of laparoscopic cholecystectomy. Arch Surg 2001;136:11.

Raraty MG, Finch M, Neoptolemos JP: Acute cholangitis and pancreatitis secondary to common duct stones: management update. World J Surg 1998;22:1155.

CHOLEDOCHOLITHIASIS

ESSENTIALS OF DIAGNOSIS

- *Biliary pain.*
- *Jaundice.*
- *Episodic cholangitis.*
- *Gallstones in gallbladder or previous cholecystectomy.*

General Considerations

Approximately 15% of patients with stones in the gallbladder are found to harbor calculi within the bile ducts. Common duct stones are usually accompanied by others in the gallbladder, but in 5% of cases, the gallbladder is empty. The number of duct stones may vary from one to more than 100.

There are two possible origins for common duct stones. The evidence suggests that most cholesterol stones develop within the gallbladder and reach the duct after traversing the cystic duct. These are called secondary stones. Pigment stones may have a similar pedigree or, more often, develop de novo within the common duct. These are called primary common duct stones. About 60% of common duct stones are cholesterol stones and 40% are pigment stones. The latter are, on the average, associated with more severe clinical manifestations.

Patients may have one or more of the following principal clinical findings, all of which are caused by obstruction to the flow of bile or pancreatic juice: biliary colic, cholangitis, jaundice, and pancreatitis (Figure 25–9). It seems likely, however, that as many as 50% of patients with choledocholithiasis remain asymptomatic.

The common duct may dilate to 2–3 cm proximal to an obstructing lesion, and truly huge ducts develop in patients with biliary tumors. In choledocholithiasis or biliary stricture, the inflammatory reaction restricts dilation, so the dilatation is less marked. Dilation of the ductal system within the liver can also be limited by cirrhosis.

Biliary colic is the result of rapid rises in biliary pressure whether the block is in the common duct or neck of the gallbladder. Gradual occlusion of the duct—as in cancer—rarely produces the same kind of pain as gallstone disease.

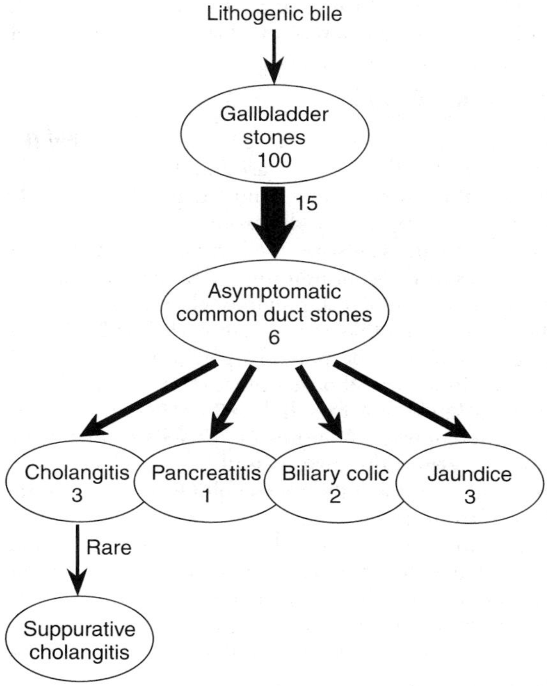

Figure 25–9. The natural history of common duct stones. Of every 100 patients with gallbladder stones, 15 will have common duct stones, which will produce the spectrum of syndromes illustrated. Note that the individual syndromes overlap, indicating that they may appear together in various combinations.

Clinical Findings

A. Symptoms

Choledocholithiasis may be asymptomatic or may produce sudden toxic cholangitis, leading to a rapid demise. The seriousness of the disease parallels the degree of obstruction, the length of time it has been present, and the extent of secondary bacterial infection (see Cholangitis, above). Biliary colic, jaundice, or pancreatitis may be isolated findings or may occur in any combination along with signs of infection (cholangitis).

Biliary colic from common duct obstruction cannot be distinguished from that caused by stones in the gallbladder. The pain is felt in the right subcostal region, epigastrium, or even the substernal area. Referred pain to the region of the right scapula is common.

Choledocholithiasis should be strongly suspected if intermittent chills, fever, or jaundice accompanies biliary colic. Some patients notice transient darkening of their urine during an attack even though jaundice is not evident.

Pruritus is usually the result of persistent long-standing obstruction. The itching is more intense in warm weather when the patient perspires and is usually worse on the extremities than on the trunk. It is much more common with neoplastic obstruction than with gallstone obstruction.

B. Signs

The patient may be icteric and toxic, with high fever and chills, or may appear to be perfectly healthy. A palpable gallbladder is unusual in patients with obstructive jaundice from common duct stone because the obstruction is transient and partial, and scarring of the gallbladder renders it inelastic and nondistensible. Tenderness may be present in the right upper quadrant but is not often as marked as in acute cholecystitis, perforated peptic ulcer, or acute pancreatitis. Tender hepatic enlargement may occur.

C. Laboratory Findings

In cholangitis, leukocytosis of 15,000/μL is usual, and values above 20,000/μL are common. A rise in serum bilirubin often appears within 24 hours after the onset of symptoms. The absolute level usually remains under 10 mg/dL, and most are in the range of 2–4 mg/dL. The direct fraction exceeds the indirect, but the latter becomes elevated in most cases. Bilirubin levels do not ordinarily reach the high values seen in malignant tumors because the obstruction is usually incomplete and transient. In fact, fluctuating jaundice is so characteristic of choledocholithiasis that it fairly reliably differentiates between benign and malignant obstruction.

The serum alkaline phosphatase level usually rises and may be the only chemical abnormality in patients without jaundice. When the obstruction is relieved, the alkaline phosphatase and bilirubin levels should return to normal within 1–2 weeks, with the exception that the former may remain elevated longer if the obstruction was prolonged.

Mild increases in AST and ALT are often seen with extrahepatic obstruction of the ducts; rarely, AST levels transiently reach 1000 units.

D. Imaging Studies

Radiopaque gallstones may be seen on plain abdominal films or CT scans. Ultrasound scans will usually show gallbladder stones and, depending on the degree of obstruction, dilatation of the bile duct. Ultrasound and CT scans are insensitive in the search for stones in the common duct. ERCP is indicated if the patient has had a previous cholecystectomy. If cholecystectomy has not been performed, cholangiography should be part of operative management. Some clinicians choose preoperative ERCP for patients scheduled for cholecystectomy in order to clear the common bile duct. If ERCP is not technically successful, the surgeon will be forced to convert to open common bile duct exploration to clear the duct of stones.

Bilirubin values above 10 mg/dL are so uncommon in choledocholithiasis that when this finding is present, cholangiography should be performed to rule out the possibility of neoplastic obstruction.

Differential Diagnosis

The workup should consider the same possibilities in differential diagnosis as for cholecystitis.

Serum amylase levels above 500 units/dL can result from acute pancreatitis, acute cholecystitis, or choledocholithiasis. Other manifestations of pancreatic disease should be documented before an unqualified diagnosis of pancreatitis is accepted.

Alcoholic cirrhosis or acute alcoholic hepatitis may present with jaundice, right upper quadrant tenderness, and leukocytosis. The differentiation from cholangitis may be impossible from clinical data. A history of a recent binge suggests acute liver disease. A percutaneous liver biopsy may be specific.

Intrahepatic cholestasis from drugs, pregnancy, chronic active hepatitis, or primary biliary cirrhosis may be difficult to distinguish from extrahepatic obstruction. ERCP would be appropriate to make the distinction, particularly if other studies (eg, ultrasound scan) failed to provide evidence of gallstone disease. If jaundice has persisted for 4–6 weeks, a mechanical cause is probable. Since most patients improve during this interval, persistent jaundice should never be assumed to be the result of parenchymal disease unless a normal cholangiogram rules out obstruction of the major ducts.

Intermittent jaundice and cholangitis after cholecystectomy are compatible with biliary stricture, and the distinction requires ERCP.

Biliary tumors usually produce intense jaundice without biliary colic or fever, and once it begins, the jaundice rarely remits.

Complications

Long-standing ductal infection can produce intrahepatic abscesses. Hepatic failure or secondary biliary cirrhosis may develop in unrelieved obstruction of long duration. Since the obstruction is usually incomplete and intermittent, cirrhosis develops only after several years in untreated disease. Acute pancreatitis, a fairly common complication of calculous biliary disease, is discussed in Chapter 26. Rarely, a stone in the common duct may erode through the ampulla, resulting in gallstone ileus. Hemorrhage (hemobilia) is also a rare complication.

Treatment

Patients with acute cholangitis should be treated with systemic antibiotics and other measures as described in the preceding section; this usually controls the attack within 24–48 hours. If the patient's condition worsens or if marked improvement is not observed within 2–4 days, endoscopic sphincterotomy or surgery and common bile duct exploration should be performed.

The typical patient presents with mild cholangitis and evidence on ultrasound scans of gallbladder stones. Laparoscopic cholecystectomy is indicated and, depending on the experience of the surgeon, laparoscopic exploration of the common duct if an operative cholangiogram or laparoscopic ultrasound demonstrates the expected common duct stones. Laparoscopic common duct exploration is usually accomplished through the cystic duct (which may have to be dilated), but when the common duct is enlarged (> 1.5 cm), it may be accomplished through a choledochotomy incision, just as in open surgery. Eventually, nearly all cases of common duct stones should be manageable by laparoscopic techniques, but at this stage the requisite laparoscopic skills are not available in most hospitals. If the surgeon thinks the common duct stones cannot be removed laparoscopically, it is probably best to remove the gallbladder laparoscopically and the common duct stones by endoscopic sphincterotomy. If the stones cannot be removed by sphincterotomy, a second (open) operation may be necessary.

There is also a lack of consensus regarding the importance of operative cholangiography or ultrasound during cholecystectomy when there are no clues suggesting stones in the duct. In such cases the chances of finding a stone are only 3–5%, and some consider the effort unwarranted. On the other hand, operative cholangiograms also provide confirmation of the biliary anatomy, which contributes to avoidance of bile duct injuries, and the natural history of the few overlooked stones is worrisome. Therefore, we side with those who perform operative cholangiography liberally in such cases.

When the common duct is explored through the cystic duct and gallstones are removed, the cystic duct must be ligated, but a drainage catheter is not usually left within the common duct. When the common duct is explored through a choledochotomy (either during a laparoscopic or open operation), a T tube is usually left in the duct, and cholangiograms are taken a week or so postoperatively. Any residual stones discovered on these postoperative x-rays can be extracted 4–6 weeks later through the T tube tract.

Patients with common duct stones who have had a previous cholecystectomy are best treated by **endoscopic sphincterotomy**. Using a side-viewing duodenoscope, the ampulla is cannulated, and a 1-cm incision is made in the sphincter with an electrocautery wire. The opening created in the sphincter permits stones to pass from the duct into the duodenum. Endoscopic sphincterotomy is unlikely to be successful in patients with large stones (eg, > 2 cm), and it is contraindicated in the presence of stenosis of the bile duct proximal to the sphincter. Laparotomy and common duct exploration are required in a few cases.

Stones in the intrahepatic branches of the bile duct can usually be removed without difficulty during common duct exploration. In some cases, however, one or more of the intrahepatic ducts have become packed with stones, and the associated chronic inflammation has produced stenosis of the duct near its junction with the common hepatic duct. It is often impossible in these cases to clear the duct of stones, and if the disease involves only one lobe (usually the left lobe), hepatic lobectomy is indicated.

Binmoeller KF, Schafer TW: Endoscopic management of bile duct stones. J Clin Gastroenterol 2001;32:106.

Lauter DM, Froines EJ: Laparoscopic common duct exploration in the management of choledocholithiasis. Am J Surg 2000; 179:372.

Prat F et al: Prediction of common bile duct stones by noninvasive tests. Ann Surg 1999;229:362.

Rosenthal RJ, Rossi RL, Martin RF: Options and strategies for the management of choledocholithiasis. World J Surg 1998;22: 1125.

Soetikno RM, Montes H, Carr-Locke DL: Endoscopic management of choledocholithiasis. J Clin Gastroenterol 1998;27: 296.

Soper NJ: Intraoperative detection: intraoperative cholangiography vs. intraoperative ultrasonography. J Gastrointest Surg 2000;4: 334.

Suc B et al: Surgery vs endoscopy as primary treatment in symptomatic patients with suspected common bile duct stones: a multicenter randomized trial. French Associations for Surgical Research. Arch Surg 1998;133:702.

Tranter SE, Thompson MH: Potential of laparoscopic ultrasonography as an alternative to operative cholangiography in the detection of bile duct stones. Br J Surg 2001;88:65.

Wu JS, Dunnegan DL, Soper NJ: The utility of intracorporeal ultrasonography for screening of the bile duct during laparoscopic cholecystectomy. J Gastrointest Surg 1998;2:50.

POSTCHOLECYSTECTOMY SYNDROME

This term has been used to signify the heterogeneous group of disorders affecting patients who continue to complain of symptoms after cholecystectomy. It is not really a syndrome, and the term is confusing.

The usual reason for incomplete relief after cholecystectomy is that the preoperative diagnosis of chronic cholecystitis was incorrect. The only symptom entirely characteristic of chronic cholecystitis is biliary colic. When a calculous gallbladder is removed in the hope that the patient will gain relief from dyspepsia, fatty food intolerance, belching, etc, the operation may leave the symptoms unchanged.

The presenting symptom may be dyspepsia or pain. An organic cause for the symptoms is more likely to be discovered in patients with severe episodic pain than in those with other complaints. Abnormal liver function studies, jaundice, and cholangitis are other manifestations that indicate residual biliary disease. Patients with suspicious findings should be studied by ERCP or THC. Choledocholithiasis, biliary stricture, and chronic pancreatitis are the most common causes of symptoms. Evidence is accumulating to implicate sphincter of Oddi dysmotility as a cause of pain in some patients. The diagnosis may be possible by biliary manometry, but experience is still too meager to justify acceptance of this entity without question. Relief of pain may follow endoscopic sphincterotomy. Stenosis of the hepatobiliary ampulla, a long cystic duct remnant, and neuromas have been blamed for continued symptoms, but well-verified cases are uncommon.

CARCINOMA OF THE GALLBLADDER

Carcinoma of the gallbladder is an uncommon neoplasm that occurs in elderly patients. It is associated with gallstones in 70% of cases, and the risk of malignant degeneration correlates with the length of time gallstones have been present. The tumor is twice as common in women as in men, as one would expect from the association with gallstones.

Most primary tumors of the gallbladder are adenocarcinomas that appear histologically to be scirrhous (60%), papillary (25%), or mucoid (15%). Dissemination of the tumor occurs early by direct invasion of the liver and hilar structures and by metastases to the common duct lymph nodes, liver, and lungs. In an occasional case, where carcinoma is an incidental finding after cholecystectomy for gallstone disease, the tumor is confined to the gallbladder as a carcinoma in situ or an early invasive lesion. Most invasive carcinomas, however, have spread by the time of surgery, and spread is virtually certain if the tumor has progressed to the point where it causes symptoms.

Clinical Findings

A. Symptoms and Signs

The most common presenting complaint is of right upper quadrant pain similar to previous episodes of biliary colic but more persistent. Obstruction of the cystic duct by tumor sometimes initiates an attack of acute cholecystitis. Other cases present with obstructive jaundice and, occasionally, cholangitis due to secondary involvement of the common duct.

Examination usually reveals a mass in the region of the gallbladder, which may not be recognized as a neoplasm if the patient has acute cholecystitis. If cholangitis is the principal symptom, a palpable gallbladder would be an unusual finding with choledocholithiasis alone and should suggest gallbladder carcinoma.

B. Imaging Studies

Oral cholecystograms almost never opacify except in patients with small incidental cancers. CT and ultrasound scans may demonstrate the extent of disease, but more often they show only gallstones.

The correct diagnosis is made preoperatively in only 10% of cases.

Complications

Obstruction of the common duct may produce multiple intrahepatic abscesses. Abscesses in or next to the tumor-laden gallbladder are frequent.

Prevention

The incidence of gallbladder cancer has decreased in recent years as the frequency of cholecystectomy has increased. It has been estimated that one case of gallbladder cancer is prevented for every 100 cholecystectomies performed for gallstone disease.

Treatment

If a localized carcinoma of the gallbladder is recognized at laparotomy, cholecystectomy should be performed along with en bloc wedge resection of an adjacent 3–5 cm of normal liver and dissection of the lymph nodes in the hepatoduodenal ligament. If a small invasive carcinoma overlooked during cholecystectomy for gallstone disease is later discovered by the pathologist, reoperation is indicated to perform a wedge resection of the liver bed plus regional lymphadenectomy. Some surgeons also recommend that the common duct be included routinely (ie, even in the absence of gross invasion) in the lymph node dissection for any lesion that involves the full thickness of the gallbladder wall. In the few cases where cancer has not penetrated the muscularis mucosae, cholecystectomy alone should suffice. More extensive hepatectomies (eg, right lobectomy) are not worthwhile. Lesions that invade the bile duct and produce jaundice should be resected if possible. When not, a stent should be inserted endoscopically or percutaneously. There is little that surgery can offer in cases with hepatic metastases or more distant spread.

Prognosis

Radiotherapy and chemotherapy are not effective palliative measures. About 85% of patients are dead within a year after diagnosis.

The 10% of patients who presently survive more than 5 years consist of those whose carcinoma was an incidental finding during cholecystectomy for symptomatic gallstone disease and those in whom an aggressive resection has removed all gross tumor.

Baillie J: Tumors of the gallbladder and bile ducts. J Clin Gastroenterol 1999;29:14.

Bismuth H, Majno PE: Hepatobiliary surgery. J Hepatol 2000; 32(1 Suppl):208.

Kondo S et al: Regional and para-aortic lymphadenectomy in radical surgery for advanced gallbladder carcinoma. Br J Surg 2000;87:418.

Mainprize KS, Gould SW, Gilbert JM: Surgical management of polypoid lesions of the gallbladder. Br J Surg 2000;87:414.

Scott TE et al: A case-control assessment of risk factors for gallbladder carcinoma. Dig Dis Sci 1999;44:1619.

Sugiyama M, Atomi Y, Yamato T: Endoscopic ultrasonography for differential diagnosis of polypoid gall bladder lesions: analysis in surgical and follow up series. Gut 2000;46:250.

MALIGNANT TUMORS OF THE BILE DUCT

ESSENTIALS OF DIAGNOSIS

- *Intense cholestatic jaundice and pruritus.*
- *Anorexia and dull right upper quadrant pain.*
- *Dilated intrahepatic bile ducts on ultrasound or CT scan.*
- *Focal stricture on transhepatic or retrograde endoscopic cholangiogram.*

General Considerations

Primary bile duct tumors are not more common in patients with cholelithiasis, and men and women are affected with equal frequency. Tumors appear at an average age of 60 years but may appear at any time between 20 and 80 years of age. More young people have been seen with this disease in recent years. Ulcerative colitis is a common associated condition, and in occasional cases bile duct cancer develops in a patient with ulcerative colitis who has been known to have sclerosing cholangitis for several years. Chronic parasitic infestation of the bile ducts in the Orient may be responsible for the greater incidence of bile duct tumors in that area.

Most malignant biliary tumors are adenocarcinomas located in the hepatic or common bile duct. The histologic pattern varies from typical adenocarcinoma to tumors composed principally of fibrous stroma and few cells. The acellular tumors may be mistaken for benign strictures or sclerosing cholangitis if adequate biopsies are not obtained. About 10% are bulky papillary tumors, which tend to be less invasive and less apt to metastasize.

At presentation, metastases are uncommon, but the tumor has often grown into the portal vein or hepatic artery.

Clinical Findings

A. Symptoms and Signs

The illness presents with gradual onset of jaundice or pruritus. Chills, fever, and biliary colic are usually absent, and except for a deep discomfort in the right upper quadrant the patient feels well. Bilirubinuria is present from the start, and light-colored stools are usual. Anorexia and weight loss develop insidiously with time.

Icterus is the most obvious physical finding. If the tumor is located in the common duct, the gallbladder may distend and become palpable in the right upper quadrant. The tumor itself is never palpable. Patients with tumors of the hepatic duct do not develop palpable gallbladders. Hepatomegaly is common. If obstruction is unrelieved, the liver may eventually become cirrhotic, and splenomegaly, ascites, or bleeding varices become secondary manifestations.

B. Laboratory Findings

Since the duct is often completely obstructed, the serum bilirubin is usually over 15 mg/dL. Serum alkaline phosphatase is also increased. Fever and leukocytosis are not common, since the bile is sterile in most cases. The stool may contain occult blood, but this is more common with tumors of the pancreas or hepatopancreatic ampulla than those of the bile ducts.

C. Imaging Studies

Ultrasound or CT scans usually detect dilated intrahepatic bile ducts. THC or ERCP clearly depicts the lesion, and both are indicated in most cases. THC is of greater value, since it better demonstrates the ductal anatomy on the hepatic side of the lesion. With tumors involving the bifurcation of the common hepatic duct (Klatskin tumors), it is important to determine the proximal extent of the lesion (ie, whether the first branches of the lobar ducts are also involved). ERCP is of value with proximal tumors because if it shows concomitant obstruction of the cystic duct, the diagnosis will most often prove to be gallbladder cancer invading the common duct (not a primary common duct neoplasm). The typical pattern with distal bile duct cancers consists of stenosis of the bile duct with sparing of the pancreatic duct. Adjacent stenoses of both ducts (the double-duct sign) indicate primary cancer of the pancreas. MR cholangiopancreatography may be useful if high-quality studies are available.

Occasionally, bile samples obtained at the time of THC will show malignant cells on cytologic study, but this is not a particularly useful test since the diagnosis of cancer must be presumed from the cholangiographic findings and a negative cytologic study is unreliable. Angiography may suggest invasion of the portal vein or encasement of the hepatic artery. False positives may occur, however.

Differential Diagnosis

The differential diagnosis must consider other causes of extrahepatic and intrahepatic cholestatic jaundice. Choledocholithiasis is characterized by episodes of partial obstruction, pain, and cholangitis, which contrast with the unremitting jaundice of malignant obstruction. Bilirubin concentrations rarely surpass 15 mg/dL and are usually below 10 mg/dL in gallstone obstruction, whereas bilirubin levels almost always exceed 10 mg/dL and are usually above 15 mg/dL in neoplastic obstruction. A rapid rise of the bilirubin level to above 15 mg/dL in a patient with sclerosing cholangitis should suggest superimposed neoplasm. Dilatation of the gallbladder may occur with tumors of the distal common duct but is rare with calculous obstruction.

The combination of an enlarged gallbladder with obstructive jaundice is usually recognized as being due to tumor. If the gallbladder cannot be felt, primary biliary cirrhosis, drug-induced jaundice, chronic active hepatitis, metastatic hepatic cancer, and common duct stone must be ruled out. In general, any patient with cholestatic jaundice of more than 2 weeks' duration whose diagnosis is uncertain should be studied by THC or ERCP. The finding of focal bile duct stenosis in the absence of previous biliary surgery is almost pathognomonic of neoplasm.

Treatment

Patients without evidence of metastases or other signs of advanced cancer (eg, ascites) are candidates for laparotomy. The 30% of patients who do not qualify may be treated by insertion of a tube stent into the bile duct transhepatically under radiologic control or from the duodenum under endoscopic control. The tube is positioned so that holes above and below the tumor reestablish flow of bile into the duodenum. If both lobar ducts are blocked by a tumor at the bifurcation of the common hepatic duct, it is usually necessary to place a transhepatic tube into only one lobar duct. If the lesion blocks the takeoff of the segmental ducts, stents are rarely beneficial.

Laparotomy is indicated in most cases, however, with the objective of removing the tumor. Preoperative decompression of the bile duct with a percutaneous catheter to relieve jaundice does not lower the incidence of postoperative complications. At operation, which may be immediately preceded by diagnostic laparoscopy, the extent of the tumor should be determined by external examination of the bile duct and the adjacent portal vein and hepatic artery.

Tumors of the distal common duct should be treated by radical pancreaticoduodenectomy (Whipple procedure) if it appears that all tumor would be removed. Secondary involvement of the portal vein is the usual reason for unresectability of tumors in this location. Mid common duct or low hepatic duct tumors should also be removed if possible. If the tumor cannot be excised, bile flow should be reestablished into the intestine by a cholecystojejunostomy or Roux-en-Y choledochojejunostomy. The choice is based on technical considerations.

Tumors at the hilum of the liver should be resected if possible and a Roux-en-Y hepaticojejunostomy performed. The anastomosis is usually between hilum and bowel rather than between individual bile ducts and bowel. A curative operation nearly always requires resection of either the right or the left lobe of the liver and, in all cases, the caudate lobe. Extension into the lobar and segmental ducts and secondary involvement of the hepatic artery and portal vein are the most common reasons for inability to resect the tumor. Subtotal resections offer little in the way of palliation.

Postoperative radiotherapy is commonly recommended.

Prognosis

The average patient with adenocarcinoma of the bile duct survives less than a year. The overall 5-year survival rate is 15%. Following a thorough radical operation, 5-year survival is about 40%. Biliary cirrhosis, intrahepatic infection, and general debility with terminal pneumonitis are the usual causes of death. Palliative resections and stents may improve the length and quality of survival in this disease even though surgical cure is uncommon. Limited experience with liver transplantation for this disease has been discouraging: tumor has recurred postoperatively in most patients.

Ahrendt SA, Nakeeb A, Pitt HA: Cholangiocarcinoma. Clin Liver Dis 2001;5:191.

Burke EC et al: Hilar cholangiocarcinoma: patterns of spread, the importance of hepatic resection for curative operation, and a presurgical clinical staging system. Ann Surg 1998;228:385.

Chamberlain RS, Blumgart LH: Hilar cholangiocarcinoma: a review and commentary. Ann Surg Oncol 2000;7:55.

Jarnagin WR: Cholangiocarcinoma of the extrahepatic bile ducts. Semin Surg Oncol 2000;19:156.

Kosuge T et al: Improved surgical results for hilar cholangiocarcinoma with procedures including major hepatic resection. Ann Surg 1999;230:663.

Lillemoe KD, Cameron JL: Surgery for hilar cholangiocarcinoma: the Johns Hopkins approach. J Hepatobiliary Pancreat Surg 2000;7:115.

Molmenti EP et al: Hepatobiliary malignancies. Primary hepatic malignant neoplasms. Surg Clin North Am 1999;79:43.

BENIGN TUMORS & PSEUDOTUMORS OF THE GALLBLADDER

Various unrelated lesions appear on the cholecystogram as projections from the gallbladder wall. The differentiation from gallstones is based upon observing whether a shift in position of the projections follows changes in posture of the patient, since stones are not fixed. Cancer should be suspected in any polypoid lesion that exceeds 1 cm in diameter.

Polyps

Most of these are not true neoplasms but cholesterol polyps, a local form of cholesterosis. Histologically, they consist of a cluster of lipid-filled macrophages in the submucosa. They easily become detached from the wall when the gallbladder is handled at surgery. It is not known whether cholesterol polyps are important in the genesis of gallstones. Some patients experience gallbladder pain, but whether this is related to the presence of the polyps per se or is a manifestation of functional gallbladder disease has not been established.

Inflammatory polyps have also been reported, but they are quite rare.

Adenomyomatosis

On cholecystography, this entity presents as a slight intraluminal convexity that is often marked by central umbilication. It is usually found in the fundus but may occur elsewhere. It is unclear whether adenomyomatosis is an acquired degenerative lesion or a developmental abnormality (ie, hamartoma). The following synonyms for this lesion appear in the literature: adenomatous hyperplasia, cholecystitis glandularis proliferans, and diverticulosis of the gallbladder. Although the condition is probably asymptomatic in many cases, adenomyomatosis can cause abdominal pain. Cholecystectomy should be performed in such patients.

Adenomas

These appear as pedunculated adenomatous polyps, true neoplasms that may be papillary or nonpapillary histologically. In a few cases they have been found in association with carcinoma in situ of the gallbladder.

BENIGN TUMORS OF THE BILE DUCTS

Benign papillomas and adenomas may arise from the ductal epithelium. Only 90 cases have been reported to date. The neoplastic propensity of the ductal epithelium is widespread, so the tumors are often multiple, and recurrence is common after excision. The affected duct must be radically excised for permanent cure to result.

BILE DUCT INJURIES & STRICTURES

ESSENTIALS OF DIAGNOSIS

- *Episodic cholangitis.*
- *Previous biliary surgery.*
- *Transhepatic cholangiogram often diagnostic.*

General Considerations

Benign biliary injuries and strictures are caused by surgical trauma in about 95% of cases. The remainder result from external abdominal trauma or, rarely, from erosion of the duct by a gallstone. Prevention of injury to the duct depends on a combination of technical skill, experience, and a thorough knowledge of the normal anatomy and its variations in the hilum of the liver. The number of bile duct injuries has risen sharply in the past few years along with the shift from open to laparoscopic cholecystectomy.

The most common lesion consists of excision of a segment of the common duct as a result of mistaking it for the cystic duct. Partial transection, occlusion with metal clips, injury to the right hepatic duct, and leakage from the cystic duct are other examples. A full discussion of how these injuries occur and how they can be prevented is beyond the scope of this text.

A clean incision of the duct without additional damage is best managed by opening the abdomen and suturing the incision with fine absorbable suture material.

Clinical Findings

A. Symptoms

Manifestations of injury to the duct may or may not be evident in the postoperative period. Following laparoscopic surgery, bile ascites, manifested by abdominal distention, bloating, and pain plus mild jaundice, is the usual presentation, since the duct is usually open to the abdomen. The symptoms are relatively mild and may for a time be thought to represent only ileus until a worsening picture requires further investigation.

Injuries following open cholecystectomy more often present with intermittent cholangitis or jaundice as a consequence of a biliary stricture. The first clear-cut symptoms may not be evident for weeks or months after surgery.

B. Signs

Findings are not distinctive. Bile ascites produces abdominal distention and ileus and, rarely, true bile peritonitis with toxicity. The right upper quadrant may be tender but usually is not. Jaundice is usually present during an attack of cholangitis.

C. Laboratory Findings

The serum alkaline phosphatase concentration is elevated in cases of stricture. The serum bilirubin fluctuates in relation to symptoms but usually remains well below 10 mg/dL.

Blood cultures are usually positive during acute cholangitis.

D. Imaging Studies

Bile ascites can be suspected on ultrasound or CT scan. Fluid should be aspirated, and if it is bile, the diagnosis is clear. THC and ERCP are necessary to depict the anatomy. After laparoscopic cholecystectomy, the most common pattern is a blocked (by a metal clip) lower duct and an upper duct draining freely into the abdomen. With a stricture, the findings most often consist of focal narrowing of the common hepatic duct within 2 cm of the bifurcation and mild to moderate dilatation of the intrahepatic ducts.

Differential Diagnosis

Choledocholithiasis is the condition that most often must be differentiated from biliary stricture because the clinical and laboratory findings can be identical. A history of trauma to the duct would point toward stricture as the more likely diagnosis. The final distinction must often await radiologic or surgical findings. THC or ERCP should be definitive.

Other causes of cholestatic jaundice may have to be ruled out in some cases.

Complications

Complications develop quickly if the leak is not controlled. Bile peritonitis and abscesses may form. With stricture, persistent cholangitis may progress to multiple intrahepatic abscesses and a septic death.

Treatment

Bile duct injuries should be surgically repaired in all but a few patients who are likely to improve with a nonoperative approach. Excision of the damaged duct and Roux-en-Y hepaticojejunostomy is indicated for most acute and chronic injuries. The entire biliary tree must be outlined by cholangiograms preoperatively. The key to success is the thoroughness of the dissection and the ability ultimately to suture healthy duct to healthy bowel. This, in turn, depends on the experience of the surgeon with this particular operation.

When a definitive repair is technically impossible, the stricture may be dilated with a transhepatic balloon-tipped catheter. This is particularly applicable to patients with portal hypertension, whose hepatic hilum contains numerous venous collaterals that make operation hazardous.

Prognosis

The death rate from biliary injuries is about 5%, and severe illness is frequent. If the stricture is not repaired, episodic cholangitis and secondary liver disease are inevitable.

Surgical correction of the stricture should be successful in about 90% of cases. Experience at centers with a special interest in this problem indicates that good results can be obtained even if several previous attempts did not relieve the obstruction. There is essentially no place for liver transplantation in this disease.

Nealon WH, Urrutia F: Long-term follow-up after bilioenteric anastomosis for benign bile duct stricture. Ann Surg 1996;223:639.

Savader SJ et al: Laparoscopic cholecystectomy-related bile duct injuries: a health and financial disaster. Ann Surg 1997;225:268.

Strasberg SM, Eagon CJ, Drebin JA: The "hidden cystic duct" syndrome and the infundibular technique of laparoscopic cholecystectomy—the danger of the false infundibulum. J Am Coll Surg 2000;191:661.

Strasberg SM, Hertl M, Soper NJ: An analysis of the problem of biliary injury during laparoscopic cholecystectomy. J Am Coll Surg 1995;180:101.

Strasberg SM, Picus DD, Drebin JA: Results of a new strategy for reconstruction of biliary injuries having an isolated right-sided component. J Gastrointest Surg 2001;5:266.

Yeh TS et al: Value of magnetic resonance cholangiopancreatography in demonstrating major bile duct injuries following laparoscopic cholecystectomy. Br J Surg 1999;86:181.

UNCOMMON CAUSES OF BILE DUCT OBSTRUCTION

Congenital Choledochal Cysts

About 30% of congenital choledochal cysts produce their first symptoms in adults, usually presenting with jaundice, cholangitis, and a right upper quadrant mass. Diagnosis can be made by THC or ERCP. The optimal surgical procedure is excision of the cyst and construction of a Roux-en-Y hepaticojejunostomy. If this is not technically possible or if the patient's condition will not permit a prolonged operation, the cyst should be emptied of precipitated biliary sludge and a cystenteric anastomosis constructed. Congenital cysts of the biliary tree have a high incidence of malignant degeneration, which is another argument for excision rather than drainage.

Vercruysse R, Van den Bossche MR: Choledochal cyst in adults. Acta Chir Belg 1998;98:220.

Watanatittan S, Niramis R: Choledochal cyst: review of 74 pediatric cases. J Med Assoc Thai 1998;81:586.

Caroli's Disease

Caroli's disease, another form of congenital cystic disease, consists of saccular intrahepatic dilatation of the ducts. In some cases, the biliary abnormality is an isolated finding, but more often it is associated with congenital hepatic fibrosis and medullary sponge kidney. The latter patients often present in childhood or as young adults with complications of portal hypertension. Others have cholangitis and obstructive jaundice as initial manifestations. There is no definitive surgical solution to the problem except in rare cases with isolated involvement of one hepatic lobe, where lobectomy is curative. Intermittent antibiotic therapy for cholangitis is the usual regimen.

Hara H et al: Surgical treatment for congenital biliary dilatation, with or without intrahepatic bile duct dilatation. Hepatogastroenterology 2001;48:638.

Parada LA et al: Clonal chromosomal abnormalities in congenital bile duct dilatation (Caroli's disease). Gut 1999;45:780.

Waechter FL et al: The role of liver transplantation in patients with Caroli's disease. Hepatogastroenterology 2001;48:672.

Hemobilia

Hemobilia presents with the triad of biliary colic, obstructive jaundice, and occult or gross intestinal bleeding. Most cases in Western cultures follow several weeks after hepatic trauma with bleeding from an intrahepatic branch of the hepatic artery into a duct. It is seen with less frequency now, because the general principles of management of hepatic trauma are better understood. In the Orient, hemobilia usually follows ductal parasitism *(Ascaris lumbricoides)* or Oriental cholangiohepatitis. Other causes are hepatic neoplasms, rupture of a hepatic artery aneurysm, hepatic abscess, and choledocholithiasis. The diagnosis may be suspected from a technetium 99m-labeled red blood cell scan, but an arteriogram is usually required for diagnosis and planning of therapy. Sometimes the bleeding can be stopped by embolizing the lesion with stainless steel coils, Gelfoam, or autologous blood clot infused through a catheter selectively positioned in the hepatic artery. If this is unsuccessful, either direct ligation of the bleeding point in the liver or proximal ligation of an upstream branch of the hepatic artery in the hilum is required.

Green MH et al: Haemobilia. Br J Surg 2001;88:773.

Pancreatitis

Pancreatitis can cause obstruction of the intrapancreatic portion of the bile duct by inflammatory swelling, encasement with scar, or compression by a pseudocyst. The patient may present with painless jaundice or cholangitis. Occasionally, a distended gallbladder can be felt on abdominal examination. Differentiation from choledocholithiasis and secondary acute pancreatitis depends on biliary x-rays or surgical exploration if the jaundice persists. Jaundice due to inflammation alone rarely lasts more than 2 weeks; persistent jaundice following an attack of acute pancreatitis suggests the development of a pseudocyst, underlying chronic pancreatitis with obstruction by fibrosis, or even an obstructing neoplasm.

Biliary obstruction from chronic pancreatitis may have few or no clinical manifestations. Jaundice is usually present, but the average peak bilirubin level is only 4–5 mg/dL. Some patients with functionally significant stenosis have persistently elevated alkaline phosphatase levels as the only abnormality; when surgical decompression of the bile duct is not performed, these patients often develop secondary biliary cirrhosis within a year or so. Diagnosis of stricture is made by ERCP, which shows a long stenosis of the intrapancreatic portion of the duct, proximal dilatation, and either a gradual or abrupt tapering of the lumen at the pancreatic border, occasionally accompanied by ductal angulation. If cholangiograms show stenosis and if alkaline phosphatase or bilirubin levels remain more than twice normal for longer than 2 months, the stenosis is functionally significant and unlikely to resolve and requires surgical correction. Choledochoduodenostomy is done in most cases. Cholecystoduodenostomy is unreliable because the cystic duct is often too narrow to provide continued biliary decompression.

Patients with obstructive jaundice and pseudocyst usually respond to surgical drainage of the pseudocyst. However, occasionally they do not respond, because chronic scarring—not the cyst—is the cause of obstruction. Procedures to drain both the bile duct and the pseudocyst are indicated if operative cholangiograms demonstrate persistent bile duct obstruction after the cyst has been decompressed.

Ampullary Dysfunction & Stenosis

Stenosis of the hepatopancreatic ampulla (ampullary stenosis) has been implicated as a cause of pain and other manifestations of ampullary obstruction and is often considered as a cause of postcholecystectomy complaints. Some cases are idiopathic, whereas others may be the result of trauma from gallstones. If the patient has secondary manifestations of biliary obstruction (eg, jaundice, increased alkaline phosphatase concentration, cholangitis) in the absence of gallstones or some other obstructing lesion, and cholangiography shows dilatation of the common duct, ampullary stenosis is a plausible explanation. However, the diagnosis is more often proposed as a reason for upper abdominal pain without these more objective findings. Ampullary dysfunction is postulated in these cases.

Sphincter of Oddi dysfunction may be the cause of biliary-like pain and is often considered in patients who remain uncomfortable after cholecystectomy. The pathogenesis of the symptoms is thought to be similar to that of esophageal dysmotility and the irritable bowel syndrome. The patients typically experience severe, intermittent upper abdominal pain that lasts for 1–3 hours, sometimes following a meal.

Residual gallstone and pancreatic disease must first be ruled out. Ampullary dysfunction can then be diagnosed by sphincter of Oddi manometry. Patients are placed in one of three groups depending on the presence of three objective manifestations of biliary obstruction: abnormal liver function tests, prolonged (> 45 minutes) common bile duct emptying of contrast media after ERCP; and a common duct greater than 12 mm in diameter. Patients in group I have all three findings; patients in group II have one or two findings; and patients in group III have none of the findings. Group I patients are thought to have enough evidence of disease that sphincterotomy should be performed without manometry. Group I patients have abnormal motility so rarely that they should not be considered further for sphincterotomy. Thus, motility studies are most often of value in determining which of the group II patients will improve after sphincterotomy.

The abnormalities sought on the motility studies include an elevated (> 40 mm Hg) basal sphincter pressure and a paradoxic rise in sphincter pressure in response to CCK. The former is most reliable. About 50% of group II patients have elevated sphincter pressures, and these are the ones who benefit from sphincterotomy.

A scintigraphic test may be just as accurate. The patient is given a bolus of CCK followed by ^{99m}Tc-DISIDA. Gamma camera images of the liver and bile duct are obtained for 60 minutes. A scoring system (score: 0–12) is based on the rate of passage of the imaging agent past various relevant points (eg, appearance and clearance through the liver, bile duct, and bowel). The normal range is 0–5; abnormal is 6–12.

Sphincter of Oddi dysfunction is an uncommon explanation for abdominal pain, and it is appropriate to remain skeptical unless the objective findings of biliary obstruction are clear-cut. In well-selected cases, however, endoscopic sphincterotomy is truly beneficial.

Chen JW, Saccone GT, Toouli J: Sphincter of Oddi dysfunction and acute pancreatitis. Gut 1998;43:305.

Rosenblatt ML et al: Comparison of sphincter of Oddi manometry, fatty meal sonography, and hepatobiliary scintigraphy in the diagnosis of sphincter of Oddi dysfunction. Gastrointest Endosc 2001;54:697.

Silverman WB et al: Hybrid classification of sphincter of Oddi dysfunction based on simplified Milwaukee criteria: effect of marginal serum liver and pancreas test elevations. Dig Dis Sci 2001;46:278.

Thomas PD et al: Use of (99m)Tc-DISIDA biliary scanning with morphine provocation for the detection of elevated sphincter of Oddi basal pressure. Gut 2000;46:838.

Toouli J et al: Manometry based randomised trial of endoscopic sphincterotomy for sphincter of Oddi dysfunction. Gut 2000;46:98.

Duodenal Diverticula

Duodenal diverticula usually arise on the medial aspect of the duodenum within 2 cm of the orifice of the bile duct, and in some individuals the duct empties directly into a diverticulum. Even in the latter circumstance, duodenal diverticula are usually innocuous. Occasionally, distortion of the duct entrance or obstruction by enterolith formation in the diverticulum produces symptoms. Either choledochoduodenostomy or Roux-en-Y choledochojejunostomy is usually a safer method of reestablishing biliary drainage than attempts to excise the diverticulum and reimplant the duct.

Ascariasis

When the worms invade the duct from the duodenum, ascariasis can produce symptoms of ductal obstruction. Air may sometimes be seen within the ducts on plain films. Antibiotics should be used until cholangitis is controlled, and anthelmintic therapy (mebendazole, albendazole, or pyrantel pamoate) should then be given. The acute symptoms usually subside with antibiotics, but if they do not, endoscopic sphincterotomy should be performed and attempts made to extricate the worms. If this is unsuccessful and the patient remains acutely ill, the duct should be emptied surgically.

Recurrent Pyogenic Cholangitis (Oriental Cholangiohepatitis)

Oriental cholangiohepatitis is a type of chronic recurrent cholangitis prevalent in coastal areas from Japan to Southeast Asia. In Hong Kong it is the third most common indication for emergency laparotomy and the most frequent type of biliary disease. The disease is currently thought to result from chronic portal bacteremia, with portal phlebitis antedating the biliary disease. *E coli* causes secondary infection of the bile ducts, which initiates pigment stone formation within the ducts.

Biliary obstruction from the stones gives rise to recurrent cholangitis, which, unlike gallstone disease in Western countries, may be unaccompanied by gallbladder stones. The gallbladder is usually distended during an attack and may contain pus.

Chronic recurrent infection often leads to biliary strictures and hepatic abscess formation. The strictures are usually located in the intrahepatic bile ducts, and for some unknown reason the left lobe of the liver is more severely involved. Intrahepatic gallstones are common, and their surgical removal may be difficult or impossible. Acute abdominal pain, chills, and high fever are usually present, and jaundice develops in about half of cases. Right upper quadrant tenderness is usually marked, and in about 80% of cases the gallbladder is palpable. ERCP or THC is the best way to study the biliary tree and can help in determining the need for surgery and the type of procedure.

Systemic antibiotics should be given for acute cholangitis. Surgical treatment consists of cholecystectomy, common duct exploration, and removal of stones. Sphincteroplasty should also be performed to allow any residual or recurrent stones to escape from the duct. A Roux-en-Y choledochojejunostomy is indicated for patients with strictures, markedly dilated ducts (eg, > 3 cm), or recurrent disease after a previous sphincteroplasty. The results of surgery are good in 80% of patients. Chronic intrahepatic stones and infection, which often involve only one lobe, may require hepatic lobectomy.

Although many patients are cured, prolonged illness from repeated infection is almost unavoidable once strictures have appeared or the intrahepatic ducts have become packed with stones.

Cosenza CA et al: Current management of recurrent pyogenic cholangitis. Am Surg 1999;65:939.

Harris HW et al: Recurrent pyogenic cholangitis. Am J Surg 1998;176:34.

Kim M et al: MR imaging findings in recurrent pyogenic cholangitis. AJR Am J Roentgenol 1999;173:1545.

Park MS et al: Recurrent pyogenic cholangitis: comparison between MR cholangiography and direct cholangiography. Radiology 2001;220:677.

Sclerosing Cholangitis

Sclerosing cholangitis is a rare chronic disease of unknown cause characterized by nonbacterial inflammatory narrowing of the bile ducts. About 60% of cases occur in patients with ulcerative colitis, and sclerosing cholangitis develops in about 5% of patients with that disorder. Other less commonly associated conditions are thyroiditis, retroperitoneal fibrosis, and mediastinal fibrosis. The disease chiefly affects men 20–50 years of age. In most cases, the entire biliary tree is affected by the inflammatory process, which causes irregular partial obliteration of the lumen of the ducts. The narrowing may be confined, however, to the intrahepatic or extrahepatic ducts, though it is almost never so short as to resemble a post-traumatic or focal malignant stricture. The woody-hard duct walls contain increased collagen and lymphoid elements and are thickened at the expense of the lumen.

The clinical onset usually consists of the gradual appearance of mild jaundice and pruritus. Symptoms of bacterial cholangitis (eg, fever and chills) are uncommon in the absence of previous biliary surgery. Laboratory findings are typical of cholestasis. The total serum bilirubin averages about 4 mg/dL and rarely exceeds 10 mg/dL. ERCP is usually diagnostic, demonstrating ductal stenoses and irregularity, which often gives a beaded appearance. Liver biopsy may show pericholangitis and bile stasis, but the changes are nonspecific.

The complications of sclerosing cholangitis include gallstone disease and adenocarcinoma of the bile duct. The latter is most common in patients with ulcerative colitis. Furthermore, patients with ulcerative colitis and sclerosing cholangitis appear to be at greater risk for colonic mucosal dysplasia and colon cancer than those with ulcerative colitis not associated with sclerosing cholangitis.

Ursodiol (ursodeoxycholic acid), 10 mg/kg/d, improves liver function tests and symptoms. Cholestyramine will give relief from pruritus. Percutaneous transhepatic balloon dilatation can be of value to treat dominant strictures. In cases where the disease is largely confined to the distal extrahepatic duct and the proximal ducts are dilated, a Roux-en-Y hepaticojejunostomy may be indicated. For patients with severe intrahepatic involvement, hepatic transplantation should be considered.

The natural history of sclerosing cholangitis is one of chronicity and unpredictable severity. Some patients seem to obtain nearly complete remission after treatment, but this is not common. Bacterial cholangitis may develop after operation if adequate drainage has not been established. In these cases, antibiotics will be required at intervals. Most patients experience the gradual evolution of secondary biliary cirrhosis after many years of mild to moderate jaundice and pruritus. Liver transplantation is indicated when the disease becomes advanced. The results are good.

Ghosh S, Shand A, Ferguson A: Ulcerative colitis. BMJ 2000;320:1119.

Kim WR et al: A revised natural history model for primary sclerosing cholangitis. Mayo Clin Proc 2000;75:688.

Kubicka S et al: K-ras mutations in the bile of patients with primary sclerosing cholangitis. Gut 2001;48:403.

Ryder SD, Beckingham IJ: ABC of diseases of liver, pancreas, and biliary system. Other causes of parenchymal liver disease. BMJ 2001;322:290.

van Hoogstraten HJ et al: Ursodeoxycholic acid therapy for primary sclerosing cholangitis: results of a 2-year randomized controlled trial to evaluate single versus multiple daily doses. J Hepatol 1998;29:417.

Pancreas

26

Gerard M. Doherty, MD, & Lawrence W. Way, MD

EMBRYOLOGY

The pancreas arises in the fourth week of fetal life from the caudal part of the foregut as dorsal and ventral pancreatic buds. Both anlagen rotate to the right and fuse near the point of origin of the ventral pancreas. Later, as the duodenum rotates, the pancreas shifts to the left. In the adult, only the caudal portion of the head and the uncinate process are derived from the ventral pancreas. The cranial part of the head and all of the body and tail are derived from the dorsal pancreas. Most of the dorsal pancreatic duct joins with the duct of the ventral pancreas to form the main pancreatic duct **(duct of Wirsung)**; a small part persists as the accessory duct **(duct of Santorini)**. In 5–10% of people, the ventral and dorsal pancreatic ducts do not fuse, and most regions of the pancreas drain through the duct of Santorini and the orifice of the minor papilla. In this case, only the small ventral pancreas drains with the common bile duct through the papilla of Vater.

ANATOMY

The pancreas is a thin elliptic organ that lies within the retroperitoneum in the upper abdomen (Figures 26–1 and 26–2). In the adult, it is 12–15 cm long and weighs 70–100 g. The gland can be divided into three portions—head, body, and tail. The head of the pancreas is intimately adherent to the medial portion of the duodenum and lies in front of the inferior vena cava and superior mesenteric vessels. A small tongue of tissue called the uncinate process lies behind the superior mesenteric vessels as they emerge from the retroperitoneum. Anteriorly, the stomach and the first portion of the duodenum lie partly in front of the pancreas. The common bile duct passes through a posterior groove in the head of the pancreas adjacent to the duodenum. The body of the pancreas is in contact posteriorly with the aorta, the left crus of the diaphragm, the left adrenal gland, and the left kidney. The tail of the pancreas lies in the hilum of the spleen. The main pancreatic duct (the duct of Wirsung) courses along the gland from the tail to the head and joins the common bile duct just before entering the duodenum at the ampulla of Vater. The accessory pancreatic duct (the duct of Santorini) enters the duodenum 2–2.5 cm proximal to the ampulla of Vater (Figure 26–1).

The blood supply of the pancreas is derived from branches of the celiac and superior mesenteric arteries (Figure 26–2). The superior pancreaticoduodenal artery arises from the gastroduodenal artery, runs parallel to the duodenum, and eventually meets the inferior pancreaticoduodenal artery, a branch of the superior mesenteric artery, to form an arcade. The splenic artery provides tributaries that supply the body and tail of the pancreas. The main branches are termed the dorsal pancreatic, pancreatica magna, and caudal pancreatic arteries. The venous supply of the gland parallels the arterial supply. Lymphatic drainage is into the peripancreatic nodes located along the veins.

The innervation of the pancreas is derived from the vagal and splanchnic nerves. The efferent fibers pass through the celiac plexus from the celiac branch of the right vagal nerve to terminate in ganglia located in the interlobular septa of the pancreas. Postganglionic fibers from these synapses innervate the acini, the islets, and the ducts. The visceral afferent fibers from the pancreas also travel in the vagal and splanchnic nerves, but those that mediate pain are confined to the latter. Sympathetic fibers to the pancreas pass from the splanchnic nerves through the celiac plexus and innervate the pancreatic vasculature.

PHYSIOLOGY

Exocrine Function

The external secretion of the pancreas consists of a clear, alkaline (pH 7.0–8.3) solution of 1–2 L/d containing digestive enzymes. Secretion is stimulated by the hormones secretin and cholecystokinin (CCK) and by parasympathetic vagal discharge. Secretin and cholecystokinin are synthesized, stored, and released from duodenal mucosal cells in response to specific stimuli. Acid in the lumen of the duodenum causes the release of secretin, and luminal digestion products of fat and protein cause the release of cholecystokinin.

The water and electrolyte secretion is formed by the centroacinar and intercalated duct cells principally in response to secretin stimulation. The secretion is modified by exchange processes and active secretion in the ductal collecting system. The cations sodium and potassium are present in the same concentrations as in

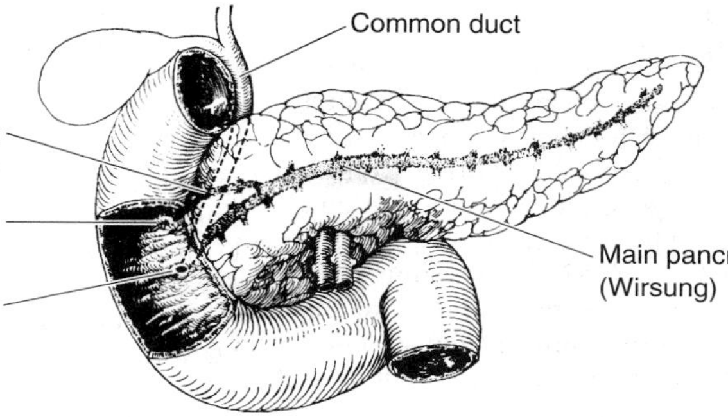

Figure 26–1. Anatomic configuration of pancreatic ductal system. (Courtesy of W Silen.)

plasma. The anions bicarbonate and chloride vary in concentration according to the rate of secretion: with increasing rate of secretion, the bicarbonate concentration increases and chloride concentration falls, so that the sum of the two is the same throughout the secretory range. Pancreatic juice helps neutralize gastric acid in the duodenum and adjusts luminal pH to the level that gives optimal activity of pancreatic enzymes.

Pancreatic enzymes are synthesized, stored (as zymogen granules), and released by the acinar cells of the gland, principally in response to cholecystokinin and vagal stimulation. Pancreatic enzymes are proteolytic, lipolytic, and amylolytic. Lipase and amylase are stored and secreted in active forms. The proteolytic enzymes are secreted as inactive precursors and are activated by the duodenal enzyme enterokinase. Other enzymes secreted by the pancreas include ribonucleases and phospholipase A. Phospholipase A is secreted as an inactive proenzyme activated in the duodenum by trypsin. It catalyzes the conversion of biliary lecithin to lysolecithin.

Turnover of protein in the pancreas exceeds that of any other organ in the body. Intravenously injected amino acids are incorporated into enzyme protein and may appear in the pancreatic juice within 1 hour. Three mechanisms prevent autodigestion of the pancreas by its proteolytic enzymes: (1) The enzymes are stored in acinar cells as zymogen granules, where they are separated from other cell proteins. (2) The enzymes are secreted in an inactive form. (3) Inhibitors of proteolytic enzymes are present in pancreatic juice and pancreatic tissue.

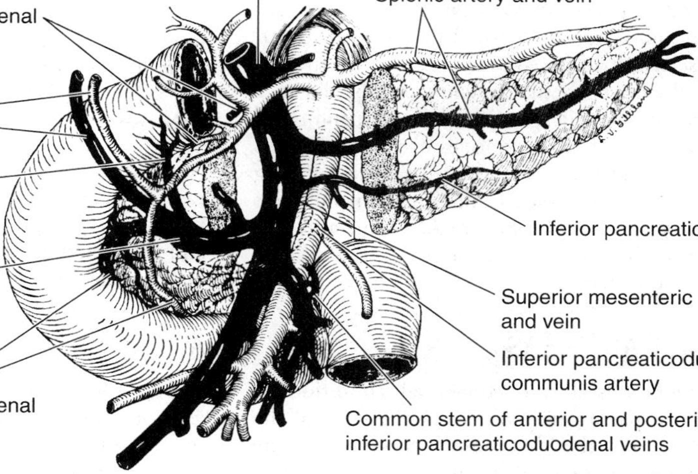

Figure 26–2. Arterial supply and venous drainage of the pancreas. (Courtesy of W Silen.)

Endocrine Function

The function of the endocrine pancreas is to facilitate storage of foodstuffs by release of insulin after a meal and to provide a mechanism for their mobilization by release of glucagon during periods of fasting. Insulin and glucagon, as well as pancreatic polypeptide and somatostatin, are produced by the islets of Langerhans.

Insulin, a polypeptide (MW 5734) consisting of 51 amino acid residues, is formed in the beta cells of the pancreas via the precursor proinsulin. Insulin secretion is stimulated by rising or high serum concentrations of metabolic substrates such as glucose, amino acids, and perhaps short-chain fatty acids. The major normal stimulus for insulin release appears to be glucose. The release and synthesis of insulin are stimulated by activation of specific glucoreceptors located on the surface membrane of the beta cell. Insulin release is also stimulated by calcium, glucagon, secretin, cholecystokinin, vasoactive intestinal polypeptide (VIP), and gastrin, all of which sensitize the receptors on the beta cell to glucose. Epinephrine, tolbutamide, and chlorpropamide release insulin by acting on the adenylyl cyclase system.

Glucagon, a polypeptide (MW 3485) consisting of 29 amino acid residues, is formed in the α cells of the pancreas. The release of glucagon is stimulated by a low blood glucose concentration, amino acids, catecholamines, sympathetic nervous discharge, and cholecystokinin. It is suppressed by hyperglycemia and insulin.

The principal functions of insulin are to stimulate anabolic reactions involving carbohydrates, fats, proteins, and nucleic acids. Insulin decreases glycogenolysis, lipolysis, proteolysis, gluconeogenesis, ureagenesis, and ketogenesis. Glucagon stimulates glycogenolysis from the liver and proteolysis and lipolysis in adipose tissue as well as in the liver. With the increase in lipolysis, there is an increase in ketogenesis and gluconeogenesis. Glucagon increases cAMP in the liver, heart, skeletal muscle, and adipose tissue. The short-term regulation of gluconeogenesis depends on the balance between insulin and glucagon. Studies on insulin and glucagon suggest that the hormones exert their effects via receptors on the cell membrane. Before entering the systemic circulation, blood draining from the islets of Langerhans perfuses the pancreatic acini, and this exposure to high levels of hormones is thought to influence acinar function.

ANNULAR PANCREAS

Annular pancreas is a rare congenital condition in which a ring of pancreatic tissue from the head of the pancreas surrounds the descending duodenum. The abnormality usually presents in infancy as duodenal obstruction with postprandial vomiting. There is bile in the vomitus if the constriction is distal to the entrance of the common bile duct. X-rays show a dilated stomach and proximal duodenum (double bubble sign) and little or no air in the rest of the small bowel.

After correction of fluid and electrolyte imbalance, the obstructed segment should be bypassed by a duodenojejunostomy or other similar procedure. No attempt should be made to resect the obstructing pancreas, because a pancreatic fistula or acute pancreatitis often develops postoperatively.

Occasionally, annular pancreas will present in adult life with similar symptoms.

PANCREATITIS

Pancreatitis is a common nonbacterial inflammatory disease caused by activation, interstitial liberation, and autodigestion of the pancreas by its own enzymes. The process may or may not be accompanied by permanent morphologic and functional changes in the gland. Much is known about the causes of pancreatitis, but despite the accumulation of much experimental data, understanding of the pathogenesis of this disorder is still incomplete.

In **acute pancreatitis**, there is sudden upper abdominal pain, nausea and vomiting, and elevated serum amylase. **Chronic pancreatitis** is characterized by chronic pain, pancreatic calcification on x-ray, and exocrine (steatorrhea) or endocrine (diabetes mellitus) insufficiency. Attacks of acute pancreatitis often occur in patients with chronic pancreatitis. **Acute relapsing pancreatitis** is defined as multiple attacks of pancreatitis without permanent pancreatic scarring, a picture most often associated with biliary pancreatitis. The unsatisfactory term **chronic relapsing pancreatitis**, denoting recurrent acute attacks superimposed on chronic pancreatitis, will not be used in this chapter. Alcoholic pancreatitis often behaves in this way. The term **subacute pancreatitis** has also been used by some to denote the minor acute attacks that typically appear late in alcoholic pancreatitis.

Etiology

Most cases of pancreatitis are caused by gallstone disease or alcoholism; a few result from hypercalcemia, trauma, hyperlipidemia, and genetic predisposition; and the remainder are idiopathic. Important differences exist in the manifestations and natural history of the disease as produced by these various factors.

A. Biliary Pancreatitis

About 40% of cases of pancreatitis are associated with gallstone disease, which, if untreated, usually gives rise to additional acute attacks. For unknown reasons, even repeated attacks of acute biliary pancreatitis seldom produce chronic pancreatitis. Eradication of the biliary disease nearly always prevents recurrent pancreatitis.

The etiologic mechanism most likely consists of transient obstruction of the ampulla of Vater and pancreatic duct by a gallstone. Choledocholithiasis is found in only 25% of cases, but because over 90% of patients excrete a gallstone in feces passed within 10 days after an acute attack, it is assumed that most attacks are caused by a gallstone or biliary sludge traversing the common duct and ampulla of Vater. Other possible steps in pathogenesis initiated by passage of the gallstone are discussed below.

B. Alcoholic Pancreatitis

In the USA, alcoholism accounts for about 40% of cases of pancreatitis. Characteristically, the patients have been heavy users of hard liquor or wine; the condition is relatively infrequent in countries where beer is the most popular alcoholic beverage. Most commonly, 6 years or more of alcoholic excess precede the initial attack of pancreatitis, and even with the first clinical manifestations, signs of chronic pancreatitis can be detected if the gland is examined microscopically. Thus, alcoholic pancreatitis is often considered to be synonymous with chronic pancreatitis no matter what the clinical findings.

Acetaldehyde, an ethanol metabolite, has been implicated as a mediator, since it can generate toxic oxygen metabolites under the influence of xanthine oxidase. In experimental studies, alcohol decreases incorporation of phosphate into parenchymal phospholipids, decreases zymogen synthesis, and produces ultrastructural changes in acinar cells. Acute administration of alcohol stimulates pancreatic secretion and induces spasm in the sphincter of Oddi. This has been compared to experiments that produce acute pancreatitis by combining partial ductal obstruction and secretory stimulation. If the patient can be persuaded to stop drinking, acute attacks may be prevented, but parenchymal damage continues to occur owing to persistent ductal obstruction and fibrosis.

C. Hypercalcemia

Hyperparathyroidism and other disorders accompanied by hypercalcemia are occasionally complicated by acute pancreatitis. With time, chronic pancreatitis and ductal calculi appear. It is thought that the increased calcium concentrations in pancreatic juice that result from hypercalcemia may prematurely activate proteases. They may also facilitate precipitation of calculi in the ducts.

D. Hyperlipidemia

In some patients—especially alcoholics—hyperlipidemia appears transiently during an acute attack of pancreatitis; in others with primary hyperlipidemia (especially those associated with elevated chylomicrons and very low density lipoproteins), pancreatitis seems to be a direct consequence of the metabolic abnormality. Hyperlipidemia during an acute attack of pancreatitis is usually associated with normal serum amylase levels, because the lipid interferes with the chemical determination for amylase; urinary output of amylase may still be high. One should inspect the serum of every patient with acute abdominal pain, because if it is lactescent, pancreatitis will almost always be the correct diagnosis. If a primary lipid abnormality is present, dietary control reduces the chances of additional attacks of pancreatitis as well as other complications.

E. Familial Pancreatitis

In this condition, attacks of abdominal pain usually begin in childhood. The genetic defect appears to be transmitted as a non-X-linked dominant with variable penetrance. Some affected families also have aminoaciduria, but this is not a universal finding. Diabetes mellitus and steatorrhea are uncommon. Chronic calcific pancreatitis develops eventually in most patients, and many patients become candidates for operation for chronic pain. Pancreatic carcinoma is more frequent in patients with familial pancreatitis.

F. Protein Deficiency

In certain populations where dietary protein intake is markedly deficient, the incidence of chronic pancreatitis is high. The reason for this association is obscure, especially in view of the observation that pancreatitis afflicts alcoholics with higher dietary protein and fat intake than those who consume less protein and fat.

G. Postoperative (Iatrogenic) Pancreatitis

Most cases of postoperative pancreatitis follow common bile duct exploration, especially if sphincterotomy was performed. Two practices, now largely abandoned, were often responsible: (1) use of a common duct T tube with a long arm passing through the sphincter of Oddi, and (2) dilation of the sphincter to 5–7 mm during common duct exploration. Operations on the pancreas, including pancreatic biopsy, are another cause. A few cases follow gastric surgery or even operations remote from the pancreas. Pancreatitis is particularly common after cardiac surgery with cardiopulmonary bypass, where the risk factors are preoperative renal failure, valve surgery, postoperative hypotension, and (particularly) the perioperative administration of calcium chloride (> 800 mg calcium chloride per square meter of body surface area). Pancreatitis may also complicate endoscopic retrograde pancreatography or endoscopic sphincterotomy.

Rarely, pancreatitis follows Billroth II gastrectomy, owing to acute obstruction of the afferent loop and reflux of duodenal secretions under high pressure into the pancreatic ducts. The condition has been recreated experimentally in dogs (Pfeffer loop preparation).

H. Drug-Induced Pancreatitis

Drugs are probably responsible for more cases of acute pancreatitis than is generally suspected. The most commonly incriminated drugs are corticosteroids, estrogen-containing contraceptives, azathioprine, thiazide diuretics, and tetracyclines. Pancreatitis associated with use of estrogens is usually the result of drug-induced hypertriglyceridemia. The mechanisms involved in the case of other drugs are unknown.

I. Obstructive Pancreatitis

Chronic partial obstruction of the pancreatic duct may be congenital or may follow healing after injury or inflammation. Over time, the parenchyma drained by the obstructed duct is replaced by fibrous tissue, and chronic pancreatitis develops. Sometimes there are episodes of acute pancreatitis as well.

Pancreas divisum may predispose to a kind of obstructive pancreatitis. If this anomaly is present and further narrowing of the opening of the minor papilla occurs (eg, by an inflammatory process), the orifice may be inadequate to handle the flow of pancreatic juice. The diagnosis of pancreas divisum may be made by ERCP. If a patient with the anomaly is found to have documented episodes of acute pancreatitis and no other cause is found, it is reasonable to assume that the anomaly is the cause.

Surgical sphincteroplasty of the minor papilla or the insertion of a stent has been proposed as treatment, but results have been suboptimal. This may be due to the presence of irreversible parenchymal changes and the persistence of chronic inflammation. In patients with obvious changes of chronic pancreatitis, surgical treatment should consist of pancreatic resection or drainage.

J. Idiopathic Pancreatitis and Miscellaneous Causes

In about 15% of patients, representing the third largest group after biliary and alcoholic pancreatitis, there is no identifiable cause of the condition. If investigated in greater than usual detail (eg, duodenal drainage examination for cholesterol crystals), many of these patients will be found to have gallstones or biliary sludge undetectable by ultrasound scans. Recent data have linked mutations of the cystic fibrosis gene to idiopathic pancreatitis.

Viral infections and scorpion stings may cause pancreatitis.

Pathogenesis

The concept that pancreatitis is due to enzymatic digestion of the gland is supported by the finding of proteolytic enzymes in ascitic fluid and increased amounts of phospholipase A and lysolecithins in pancreatic tissue from patients with acute pancreatitis. Experimentally, pancreatitis can be created readily if activated enzymes are injected into the pancreatic ducts under pressure. Trypsin has not been found in excessive amounts in pancreatic tissue from affected humans, possibly because of inactivation by trypsin inhibitors. Nevertheless, although the available evidence is inconclusive, the autodigestion theory is almost universally accepted. Other proposed factors are vascular insufficiency, lymphatic congestion, and activation of the kallikrein-kinin system.

For many years, trypsin and other proteases were held to be the principal injurious agents, but recent evidence has emphasized phospholipase A, lipase, and elastase as perhaps of greater importance. Trypsin ordinarily does not attack living cells, and even when trypsin is forced into the interstitial spaces, the resulting pancreatitis does not include coagulation necrosis, which is so prominent in human pancreatitis.

Phospholipase A, in the presence of small amounts of bile salts, attacks free phospholipids (eg, lecithin) and those bound in cellular membranes to produce extremely potent lyso-compounds. Lysolecithin, which would result from the action of phospholipase A on biliary lecithin, or phospholipase A itself, plus bile salts, is capable of producing severe necrotizing pancreatitis. Trypsin is important in this scheme, because small amounts are needed to activate phospholipase A from its inactive precursor.

Elastase, which is both elastolytic and proteolytic, is secreted in an inactive form. Because it can digest the walls of blood vessels, elastase has been thought to be important in the pathogenesis of hemorrhagic pancreatitis.

If autodigestion is the final common pathway in pancreatitis, earlier steps must account for the presence of active enzymes and their reaction products in the ducts and their escape into the interstitium. The following are the most popular theories that attempt to link the known etiologic factors with autodigestion:

A. Obstruction-Secretion

In animals, ligation of the pancreatic duct generally produces mild edema of the pancreas that resolves within a week. Thereafter, atrophy of the secretory apparatus occurs. On the other hand, partial or intermittent ductal obstruction, which more closely mimics what seems to happen in humans, can produce frank pancreatitis if the gland is simultaneously stimulated to secrete. The major shortcoming of these experiments has been the difficulty encountered in attempting to cause severe pancreatitis in this way. However, since the human pancreas manufactures ten times as much phospholipase A as does the dog or rat pancreas, the consequences of obstruction in humans conceivably could be more serious.

B. Common Channel Theory

Opie, having observed pancreatitis in a patient with a gallstone impacted in the ampulla of Vater, speculated that reflux of bile into the pancreatic ducts might have initiated the process. Flow between the biliary and pancreatic ducts requires a common channel connecting these two systems with the duodenum. Although these ducts converge in 90% of humans, only 10% have a common channel long enough to permit biliary-pancreatic reflux if the ampulla contained a gallstone. Experimentally, pancreatitis produced by pancreatic duct obstruction alone is similar in severity to pancreatitis following obstruction of a common channel, so biliary reflux is discounted as an etiologic factor in this disease.

C. Duodenal Reflux

The above theories do not explain activation of pancreatic enzymes, a process that normally takes place through the action of enterokinase in the duodenum. In experimental animals, if the segment of duodenum into which the pancreatic duct empties is surgically converted to a closed loop, reflux of duodenal juice initiates severe pancreatitis (Pfeffer loop). Pancreatitis associated with acute afferent loop obstruction after Billroth II gastrectomy is probably the result of similar factors. Other than in this specific example, there is no direct evidence for duodenal reflux in the pathogenesis of pancreatitis in humans.

D. Back Diffusion Across the Pancreatic Duct

Just as the gastric mucosa must serve as a barrier to maintain high concentrations of acid, so must the epithelium of the pancreatic duct prevent diffusion of luminal enzymes into the pancreatic parenchyma. Experiments in cats have shown that the barrier function of the pancreatic duct is vulnerable to several injurious agents, including alcohol and bile acids. Furthermore, the effects of alcohol can occur even after oral ingestion, because alcohol is secreted in the pancreatic juice. Injury to the barrier renders the duct permeable to molecules as large as MW 20,000, and enzymes from the lumen may be able to enter the gland and produce pancreatitis.

The studies by Steer and his coworkers have shown that a very early event in several forms of experimental pancreatitis, including that due to pancreatic duct obstruction, consists of zymogen activation within acinar cells by lysosomal hydrolases (eg, cathepsin B). This may represent the long-sought unifying explanation. Other factors must be postulated, however, to account for the variations in severity of the disease. In biliary pancreatitis, transient obstruction of the ampulla of Vater by a gallstone is most likely the first event. Alcoholic pancreatitis probably has several causes, including partial ductal obstruction, secretory stimulation, acute effects on the ductal barrier, and toxic actions of alcohol on parenchymal cells.

E. Systemic Manifestations

Severe acute pancreatitis may be complicated by multiple organ failure, principally respiratory insufficiency (acute respiratory distress syndrome [ARDS]), myocardial depression, renal insufficiency, and gastric stress ulceration. The pathogenesis of these complications is similar in many respects to that of multiple organ failure in sepsis, and in fact, sepsis due to pancreatic abscess formation is a contributing factor in some of the most severe cases of acute pancreatitis. During acute pancreatitis, pancreatic proteases, bacterial endotoxins, and other active agents are liberated into the systemic circulation. The concentrations of serum factors able to complex with the proteases (eg, α_2-macroglobulin) decrease in proportion to the severity of the illness, and complexed α_2-macroglobulin, which normally is cleared rapidly by macrophages, accumulates. These circulating complexes, which retain proteolytic activity, are thought to contribute to systemic toxicity. The endotoxin probably originates from bacteria that translocate through an abnormally permeable intestinal mucosa. Within the circulation, the proteases and the endotoxin activate the complement system (especially C5) and kinins. Complement activation leads to granulocyte aggregation and accumulation of aggregates in the pulmonary capillaries. The granulocytes release neutrophil elastase, superoxide anion, hydrogen peroxide, and hydroxide radicals, which in concert with bradykinin exert local toxic effects on the pulmonary epithelium that result in increased permeability. Arachidonate metabolites (eg, PGE_2, PGI_2, leukotriene B_4) may also be involved in some way. Analogous events are thought to occur in other organs.

Brady M et al: Cytokines and acute pancreatitis. Baillieres Best Pract Res Clin Gastroenterol 1999;13:265.

Chen JW, Saccone GT, Toouli J: Sphincter of Oddi dysfunction and acute pancreatitis. Gut 1998;43:305.

Cohn JA et al: Relation between mutations of the cystic fibrosis gene and idiopathic pancreatitis. N Engl J Med 1998;339:653.

Cushman R: Apples, oranges, forests, and trees. J Health Polit Policy Law 1999;24:763.

Eckerwall G, Andersson R: Early enteral nutrition in severe acute pancreatitis: a way of providing nutrients, gut barrier protection, immunomodulation, or all of them? Scand J Gastroenterol 2001;36:449.

Etemad B, Whitcomb DC: Chronic pancreatitis: diagnosis, classification, and new genetic developments. Gastroenterology 2001;120:682.

Halangk W et al: Role of cathepsin B in intracellular trypsinogen activation and the onset of acute pancreatitis. J Clin Invest 2000;106:773.

Layer P, Keller J: Pancreatic enzymes: secretion and luminal nutrient digestion in health and disease. J Clin Gastroenterol 1999;28:3.

Miskovitz P: Role of selectins in acute pancreatitis. Crit Care Med 2001;29:686.

Okazaki K et al: Recent concept of autoimmune-related pancreatitis. J Gastroenterol 2001;36:293.

Opie EL: The theory of retrojection of bile into the pancreas. Rev Surg 1970;27:1.

Saluja AK, Steer MLP6: Pathophysiology of pancreatitis. Role of cytokines and other mediators of inflammation. Digestion 1999;60(Suppl 1):27.

Sharer N et al: Mutations of the cystic fibrosis gene in patients with chronic pancreatitis. N Engl J Med 1998;339:645.

Steer ML: How and where does acute pancreatitis begin? Arch Surg 1992;127:1350.

Vaccaro MI et al: Lipopolysaccharide directly affects pancreatic acinar cells: implications on acute pancreatitis pathophysiology. Dig Dis Sci 2000;45:915.

Whitcomb DC, Ulrich CD 2nd: Hereditary pancreatitis: new insights, new directions. Baillieres Best Pract Res Clin Gastroenterol 1999;13:253.

1. Acute Pancreatitis

ESSENTIALS OF DIAGNOSIS

- *Abrupt onset of epigastric pain, frequently with back pain.*
- *Nausea and vomiting.*
- *Elevated serum or urinary amylase.*
- *Cholelithiasis or alcoholism (many patients).*

General Considerations

While edematous and hemorrhagic pancreatitis are manifestations of the same pathologic processes and the general principles of treatment are the same, hemorrhagic pancreatitis has more complications and a higher death rate. In edematous pancreatitis, the glandular tissue and surrounding retroperitoneal structures are engorged with interstitial fluid, and the pancreas is infiltrated with inflammatory cells that surround small foci of parenchymal necrosis. Hemorrhagic pancreatitis is characterized by bleeding into the parenchyma and surrounding retroperitoneal structures and extensive pancreatic necrosis. In both forms, the peritoneal surfaces may be studded with small calcifications representing areas of fat necrosis.

Clinical Findings

A. Symptoms and Signs

The acute attack frequently begins following a large meal and consists of severe epigastric pain that radiates through to the back. The pain is unrelenting and usually associated with vomiting and retching. In severe cases, the patient may collapse from shock.

Depending on the severity of the disease, there may be profound dehydration, tachycardia, and postural hypotension. Myocardial function is depressed in severe pancreatitis, presumably because of circulating factors that affect cardiac performance. Examination of the abdomen reveals decreased or absent bowel sounds and tenderness that may be generalized but more often is localized to the epigastrium. Temperature is usually normal or slightly elevated in uncomplicated pancreatitis. Clinical evidence of pleural effusion may be present, especially on the left. If an abdominal mass is found, it probably represents a swollen pancreas (phlegmon) or, later in the illness, a pseudocyst or abscess. In 1–2% of patients, bluish discoloration is present in the flank **(Grey Turner's sign)** or periumbilical area **(Cullen's sign)**, indicating hemorrhagic pancreatitis with dissection of blood retroperitoneally into these areas.

B. Laboratory Findings

The hematocrit may be elevated as a consequence of dehydration or low as a result of abdominal blood loss in hemorrhagic pancreatitis. There is usually a moderate leukocytosis, but total white blood cell counts over 12,000/μL are unusual in the absence of suppurative complications. Liver function studies are usually normal, but there may be a mild elevation of the serum bilirubin concentration (usually < 2 mg/dL).

The serum amylase concentration rises to more than $2\frac{1}{2}$ times normal within 6 hours after the onset of an acute episode and generally remains elevated for several days. Values in excess of 1000 IU/dL occur early in the attack in 95% of patients with biliary pancreatitis and 85% of patients with acute alcoholic pancreatitis. Those with the most severe disease are more apt to have amylase levels below 1000 IU/dL.

Elevated serum lipase is detectable early and for several days after the acute attack. Since the lipase level tends to be higher in alcoholic pancreatitis and the amylase level higher in gallstone pancreatitis, the lipase/amylase ratio has been suggested as a means to help distinguishing the two.

Elevated amylase levels may occur in other acute abdominal conditions, such as gangrenous cholecystitis, small bowel obstruction, mesenteric infarction, and perforated ulcer, though levels rarely exceed 500 IU/dL. Episodes of acute pancreatitis may occur without rises in serum amylase; this is the rule if hyperlipidemia is present. Furthermore, high levels may return to normal before blood is drawn.

The methods most commonly used for measuring amylase in the serum detect pancreatic amylase, salivary amylase, and macroamylase. However, hyperamylasemia is sometimes present in patients with abdominal pain when the elevated amylase levels consist entirely of salivary amylase or macroamylase and the pancreas is not inflamed.

Urine amylase excretion is also increased and is of diagnostic value. Excretion of more than 5000 units/24 h is abnormal. The urinary clearance of amylase increases during acute pancreatitis owing to a decrease in tubular reabsorption of amylase (normally 75% of filtered amylase). This was once thought to be specific, and the amylase-to-creatinine clearance ratio was used as a diagnostic test for acute pancreatitis. However, the increased amylase clearance results from overload of the tubular reabsorptive pathway with various urine proteins and is a nonspecific effect of tissue damage seen in many acute illnesses or following trauma.

In severe pancreatitis, the serum calcium concentration may fall as a result of calcium being complexed with fatty acids (liberated from retroperitoneal fat by lipase) and impaired reabsorption from bone owing to the action of calcitonin (liberated by high levels of glucagon). Relative hypoparathyroidism and hypoalbuminemia have also been implicated.

C. Imaging Studies

In about two-thirds of cases, a plain abdominal film is abnormal. The most frequent finding is isolated dilation of a segment of gut **(sentinel loop)** consisting of jejunum, transverse colon, or duodenum adjacent to the pancreas. Gas distending the right colon that abruptly stops in the mid or left transverse colon **(colon cutoff sign)** is due to colonic spasm adjacent to the pancreatic inflammation. Both of these findings are relatively nonspecific. Glandular calcification may be evident, signifying chronic pancreatitis. An upper gastrointestinal series may show a widened duodenal loop, swollen ampulla of Vater, and, occasionally, evidence of gastric irritability. Chest films may reveal pleural effusion on the left side.

A CT scan of the pancreas using intravenous contrast media should be obtained in any patient with acute pancreatitis whose illness is not resolving after 48–72 hours. The radiologic findings may be consistent with any of the following: relatively normal appearing pancreas, pancreatic **phlegmon**, pancreatic phlegmon with extension of the inflammatory process to adjacent extrapancreatic spaces, pancreatic **necrosis**, or pancreatic pseudocyst or **abscess** formation.

Occasionally, radiopaque gallstones will be apparent on plain x-rays. Ultrasound study may demonstrate gallstones early in the attack and may be used as a baseline for sequential examinations of the pancreas.

Several weeks after the pancreatitis has subsided, ERCP may be of value in patients with a tentative diagnosis of idiopathic pancreatitis (ie, those who have no history of alcoholism and no evidence of gallstones on ultrasound and oral cholecystogram). This examination demonstrates gallstones or changes of chronic pancreatitis in about 40% of such patients.

Differential Diagnosis

To some extent, acute pancreatitis is a diagnosis of exclusion, for other acute upper abdominal conditions such as acute cholecystitis, penetrating or perforated duodenal ulcer, high small bowel obstruction, acute appendicitis, and mesenteric infarction must always be seriously considered. In most cases, the distinction is possible on the basis of the clinical picture, laboratory findings, and CT scans. The critical point is that the diseases with which acute pancreatitis is most likely to be confused are often lethal if not treated surgically. Therefore, diagnostic laparotomy is indicated if they cannot be ruled out on clinical grounds.

Chronic hyperamylasemia occurs rarely without any relation to pancreatic disease. Some cases are associated with renal failure, chronic sialadenitis, salivary tumors, ovarian tumors, or liver disease, but often there is no explanation. Analysis of serum amylase isoenzymes is the only way to determine whether the amylase originates from salivary glands or pancreas. **Macroamylasemia** is a chronic hyperamylasemia in which normal amylase (usually salivary) is bound to a large serum glycoprotein or immunoglobulin molecule and is therefore not excreted into urine. The diagnosis rests on the combination of hyperamylasemia and low urinary amylase. Macroamylasemia has been found in patients with other diseases such as malabsorption, alcoholism, and cancer. Many patients have abdominal pain, but the relationship of the pain and the macroamylasemia is uncertain.

Complications

The principal complications of acute pancreatitis are abscess and pseudocyst formation. These are discussed in separate sections. Gastrointestinal bleeding may occur from adjacent inflamed stomach or duodenum, ruptured pseudocyst, or peptic ulcer. Intraperitoneal bleeding may occur spontaneously from the celiac or splenic artery or from the spleen following acute splenic vein thrombosis. Involvement of the transverse colon or duodenum by the inflammatory process may result in partial obstruction, hemorrhage, necrosis, or fistula formation.

Early identification of patients at greatest risk of complications allows them to be managed more aggressively, which appears to decrease the mortality rate. The criteria of severity that have been found to be reliable are based either on the systemic manifestations of the disease as reflected in the clinical and laboratory findings or on the local changes in the pancreas as reflected by the findings on CT scan. Ranson used the former approach to develop the staging criteria listed in Table 26–1. Just the single finding of fluid sequestration (ie, fluid admin-

Table 26–1. Ranson's criteria of severity of acute pancreatitis.[1]

Criteria present initially	
	Age > 55 years
	White blood cell count > 16,000/μL
	Blood glucose > 200 mg/dL
	Serum LDH > 350 IU/L
	AST (SGOT) > 250 IU/dL
Criteria developing during first 24 hours	
	Hematocrit fall > 10%
	BUN rise > 8 mg/dL
	Serum Ca^{2+} < 8 mg/dL
	Arterial Po_2 < 60 mm Hg
	Base deficit > 4 meq/L
	Estimated fluid sequestration > 600 mL

[1]Morbidity and mortality rates correlate with the number of criteria present. Mortality rates correlate as follows: 0–2 criteria present = 2%; 3 or 4 = 15%; 5 or 6 = 40%; 7 or 8 = 100%.

istered minus urine output) exceeding 2 L/d for more than 2 days is a reasonably accurate dividing line between severe (life-threatening) and mild-to-moderate disease. The local changes in the pancreas as shown on CT scans may be even more revealing. The presence of any of the following indicates a high risk of local infection in the pancreatic bed: involvement of extrapancreatic spaces in the inflammatory process, pancreatic necrosis (areas in the pancreas that do not enhance with intravenous contrast media), and early signs of abscess formation (eg, gas bubbles in the tissue).

Treatment

A. Medical Treatment

The goals of medical therapy are reduction of pancreatic secretory stimuli and correction of fluid and electrolyte derangements.

1. Gastric suction—Oral intake is withheld, and a nasogastric tube is inserted to aspirate gastric secretions, although the latter has no specific therapeutic effect. Oral feeding should be resumed only after the patient appears much improved, appetite has returned, and serum amylase levels have dropped to normal. Premature resumption of eating may result in exacerbation of disease.

2. Fluid replacement—Patients with acute pancreatitis sequester fluid in the retroperitoneum, and large volumes of intravenous fluids are necessary to maintain circulating blood volume and renal function. Patients with severe pancreatitis should receive albumin to combat the capillary leak that contributes to the pathophysiology. In severe hemorrhagic pancreatitis, blood transfusions may also be required. The adequacy of fluid replacement is the single most important aspect of medical therapy. In fact, undertreatment with fluids may actually contribute to the progression of pancreatitis. Fluid replacement may be judged most accurately by monitoring the volume and specific gravity of urine.

3. Antibiotics—Antibiotics are not useful in mild cases of acute pancreatitis. However, recent studies have shown benefit of antibiotics that penetrate pancreatic tissue for patients with severe pancreatitis. Imipenem is the most commonly used antibiotic. Antibiotics should also be used for treatment of specific operative complications.

4. Calcium and magnesium—In severe attacks of acute pancreatitis, hypocalcemia may require parenteral calcium replacement in amounts determined by serial calcium measurements. Recognition of hypocalcemia is important because it may produce cardiac dysrhythmias. Hypomagnesemia is also common, especially in alcoholics, and magnesium should also be replaced as indicated by serum levels.

5. Oxygen—Hypoxemia severe enough to require therapy develops in about 30% of patients with acute pancreatitis. It is often insidious, without clinical or x-ray signs, and out of proportion to the severity of the pancreatitis. The most pronounced examples accompany severe pancreatitis, often in association with hypocalcemia. The basic lesion, a form of adult respiratory distress syndrome, is poorly understood. Pulmonary changes include decreased vital capacity and an oxygen diffusion defect.

Hypoxemia must be suspected in every patient, and arterial blood gases should be measured every 12 hours for the first few hospital days. Supplemental oxygen therapy is indicated for PaO_2 levels below 70 mm Hg. An occasional patient requires endotracheal intubation and mechanical ventilation. Diuretics may be useful in decreasing lung water and improving arterial oxygen saturation.

6. Peritoneal lavage—Peritoneal lavage has been employed in severe refractory cases to remove toxins in the peritoneal fluid that would otherwise have been absorbed into the systemic circulation. Some patients appear to improve in response to this therapy although controlled trials have not substantiated its efficacy. Severe pancreatitis that fails to show clinical improvement after 24–48 hours of standard inpatient treatment is the usual indication for peritoneal lavage. The technique involves infusing and withdrawing 1–2 L of lactated Ringer's solution through a peritoneal dialysis catheter every hour for 1–3 days. Meta-analysis of the existing data shows no benefit; this treatment is not recommended outside of a clinical trial.

7. Nutrition—Total parenteral nutrition avoids pancreatic stimulation and should be used for nutritional support in any severely ill patient who will be unable to eat for more than 1 week. Elemental diets ingested orally or given by tube into the small intestine do not avoid secretory stimulation. Neither form of nutrition directly affects recovery of the pancreas.

8. Other drugs—Octreotide, H_2 receptor blockers, anticholinergic drugs, glucagon, and aprotinin have shown no beneficial effects in controlled trials.

B. Endoscopic Sphincterotomy

Biliary pancreatitis is caused by a gallstone becoming lodged in the ampulla of Vater. In most cases, the stone passes into the intestine but occasionally it becomes impacted in the ampulla, which results in more severe disease. Less than 10% of cases of biliary pancreatitis are severe (ie, three or more three Ranson criteria), but in severe cases, endoscopic sphincterotomy performed within 72 hours of the onset of the disease has been shown to decrease the incidence of concomitant biliary sepsis and lower the mortality rate from the pancreatitis.

C. Surgical Treatment

Surgery is generally contraindicated in uncomplicated acute pancreatitis. However, when the diagnosis is uncertain in a patient with severe abdominal pain, diagnostic laparotomy is not thought to aggravate pancreatitis.

When laparotomy has been performed for diagnosis and mild to moderate pancreatitis is found, cholecystectomy and operative cholangiography should be performed if gallstones are present, but the pancreas should be left undisturbed. For *severe* edematous pancreatitis, the gastrocolic omentum should be divided and the pancreas inspected. Although some surgeons place drains and irrigating catheters in the region of the pancreas, we prefer to keep foreign bodies out of this area.

The diagnosis of biliary pancreatitis can usually be suspected on the basis of ultrasound studies of the gallbladder early in the acute attack. Cholecystectomy should be performed on these patients during hospitalization for the acute attack soon after the attack resolves. A longer delay (even a few weeks) is associated with a high incidence (80%) of recurrent pancreatitis. Since life-threatening attacks are uncommon in gallstone pancreatitis, operation (common duct exploration; sphincteroplasty) or endoscopic therapy (sphincterotomy) early in an attack is rarely justified. However, when the attack is especially severe, elective cholecystectomy should be deferred up to several months to allow complete recovery from pancreatitis.

It is currently thought that debridement of dead peripancreatic tissue, which is often (40% of cases) colonized by bacteria, reduces the mortality rate of acute severe necrotizing pancreatitis. Historical controls place the mortality rate at 50–80% in the absence of operative treatment and 10–40% among patients subjected to necrosectomy. The diagnosis of necrotizing pancreatitis is suspected from the clinical findings; patients treated surgically have three or more Ranson criteria and average about $4^1/_2$ criteria. Contrast-enhanced CT scans obtained early in the course of the disease are studied for the presence of nonenhancing areas, which indicate lack of vascular perfusion and reflect the presence of necrotic peripancreatic fat or pancreatic parenchyma. Percutaneous needle aspiration of these areas is used to detect the presence of bacterial colonization. A distinction is made between these cases of "infected necrotizing pancreatitis" and "pancreatic abscess," which may appear later in the course of the disease. Patients with infected necrotizing pancreatitis and severe clinical findings benefit most from surgical therapy, but laparotomy may be undertaken just because of a deteriorating condition in patients with necrotizing pancreatitis in the absence of bacterial colonization. At surgery, all peripancreatic spaces are opened and any necrotic tissue is removed by gentle blunt dissection. A T-tube is inserted if there is bile duct obstruction, and cholecystectomy is performed for gallstone disease. Two large drains are placed within the debrided spaces and are used postoperatively for sterile lavage. About 8 L of fluid are infused through this system daily for an average of 2 weeks. Other than CT evidence of necrotic tissue with or without infection, there are presently no other criteria in general use that call for pancreatic surgery in patients with severe pancreatitis.

Surgery for complications of acute pancreatitis, such as abscess, pseudocyst, and pancreatic ascites, is discussed below.

Prognosis

The death rate associated with acute pancreatitis is about 10%, and nearly all deaths occur in a first attack and among patients with three or more Ranson criteria of severity. Respiratory insufficiency and hypocalcemia indicate a poor prognosis. The death rate associated with severe necrotizing pancreatitis is 50% or more, but surgical therapy lowers the figure to about 20%. Persistent fever or hyperamylasemia 3 weeks or longer after an attack of pancreatitis usually indicates the presence of a pancreatic abscess or pseudocyst.

Abu-Zidan FM, Bonham MJ, Windsor JA: Severity of acute pancreatitis: a multivariate analysis of oxidative stress markers and modified Glasgow criteria. Br J Surg 2000;87:1019.

Beckingham IJ, Bornman PC: ABC of diseases of liver, pancreas, and biliary system. Acute pancreatitis. BMJ 2001;322:595.

Bornman PC, Beckingham IJ: ABC of diseases of liver, pancreas, and biliary system. Chronic pancreatitis. BMJ 2001;322:660.

Brivet FG, Emilie D, Galanaud P: Pro- and anti-inflammatory cytokines during acute severe pancreatitis: an early and sustained response, although unpredictable of death. Parisian Study Group on Acute Pancreatitis. Crit Care Med 1999;27:749.

Chang L et al: Preoperative versus postoperative endoscopic retrograde cholangiopancreatography in mild to moderate gallstone pancreatitis: a prospective randomized trial. Ann Surg 2000;231:82.

Dervenis C, Bassi C: Evidence-based assessment of severity and management of acute pancreatitis. Br J Surg 2000;87:257.

Frakes JT: Biliary pancreatitis: a review. Emphasizing appropriate endoscopic intervention. J Clin Gastroenterol 1999;28:97.

Gumaste V: Prophylactic antibiotic therapy in the management of acute pancreatitis. J Clin Gastroenterol 2000;31:6.

Hamano H et al: High serum IgG4 concentrations in patients with sclerosing pancreatitis. N Engl J Med 2001;344:732.

Nealon WH, Matin S: Analysis of surgical success in preventing recurrent acute exacerbations in chronic pancreatitis. Ann Surg 2001;233:793.

Platell C, Cooper D, Hall JC: A meta-analysis of peritoneal lavage for acute pancreatitis. J Gastroenterol Hepatol 2001;16:689.

Schmid SW et al: The role of infection in acute pancreatitis. Gut 1999;45:311.

Toh SK, Phillips S, Johnson CD: A prospective audit against national standards of the presentation and management of acute pancreatitis in the South of England. Gut 2000;46:239.

Uhl W et al: Acute gallstone pancreatitis: timing of laparoscopic cholecystectomy in mild and severe disease. Surg Endosc 1999;13:1070.

Williams M, Simms HH: Prognostic usefulness of scoring systems in critically ill patients with severe acute pancreatitis. Crit Care Med 1999;27:901.

Windsor JA, Hammodat H: Metabolic management of severe acute pancreatitis. World J Surg 2000;24:664.

2. Pancreatic Pseudocyst

ESSENTIALS OF DIAGNOSIS

- *Epigastric mass and pain.*
- *Mild fever and leukocytosis.*
- *Persistent serum amylase elevation.*
- *Pancreatic cyst demonstrated by ultrasound or CT scan.*

General Considerations

Pancreatic pseudocysts are encapsulated collections of fluid with high enzyme concentrations that arise from the pancreas. They are usually located either within or adjacent to the pancreas in the lesser sac, but pancreatic pseudocysts have also been found in the neck, mediastinum, and pelvis. The walls of a pseudocyst are formed by inflammatory fibrosis of the peritoneal, mesenteric, and serosal membranes, which limits spread of the pancreatic juice as the lesion develops. The term pseudocyst denotes absence of an epithelial lining, whereas true cysts are lined by epithelium.

Two different processes are involved in the pathogenesis of pancreatic pseudocysts. Many occur as complications of severe acute pancreatitis, where extravasation of pancreatic juice and glandular necrosis form a sterile pocket of fluid that is not reabsorbed as inflammation subsides. Superinfection of such collections leads to pancreatic abscess instead of pseudocyst. In other patients, usually alcoholics or trauma victims, pseudocysts appear without preceding acute pancreatitis. The mechanism in these cases consists of ductal obstruction and formation of a retention cyst that loses its epithelial lining as it grows beyond the confines of the gland. In posttraumatic pseudocyst, symptoms usually do not appear until several weeks after the injury. Some are iatrogenic, eg, occurring during splenectomy; others follow an external blow to the abdomen.

Pseudocysts develop in about 2% of cases of acute pancreatitis. The cysts are single in 85% of cases and multiple in the remainder.

Clinical Findings

A. Symptoms and Signs

A pseudocyst should be suspected when a patient with acute pancreatitis fails to recover after a week of treatment or when, after improving for a time, symptoms return. Since it is now fairly routine to obtain a CT scan early in an attack of severe acute pancreatitis, the early stages of pseudocyst formation are often demonstrated radiographically before specific clinical findings appear. The first clinical manifestation is usually a palpable tender mass in the epigastrium, consisting of a swollen pancreas and contiguous viscera (a phlegmon). With time, the mass may subside, but if it persists it most likely represents a pseudocyst.

In other cases, the pseudocyst develops insidiously without an obvious attack of acute pancreatitis.

Regardless of the type of prodromal phase, pain is the most common finding. Fever, weight loss, tenderness, and a palpable mass are present in about half of patients. A few have jaundice, a manifestation of obstruction of the intrapancreatic segment of the bile duct.

B. Laboratory Findings

An elevated serum amylase and leukocytosis are present in about half of patients. When present, elevated bilirubin levels reflect biliary obstruction. Of those patients with acute pancreatitis whose serum amylase remains elevated for as long as 3 weeks, about half will have a pseudocyst.

C. Imaging Studies

CT scan (Figure 26–3) is the diagnostic study of choice. The size and shape of the cyst and its relation-

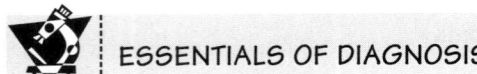

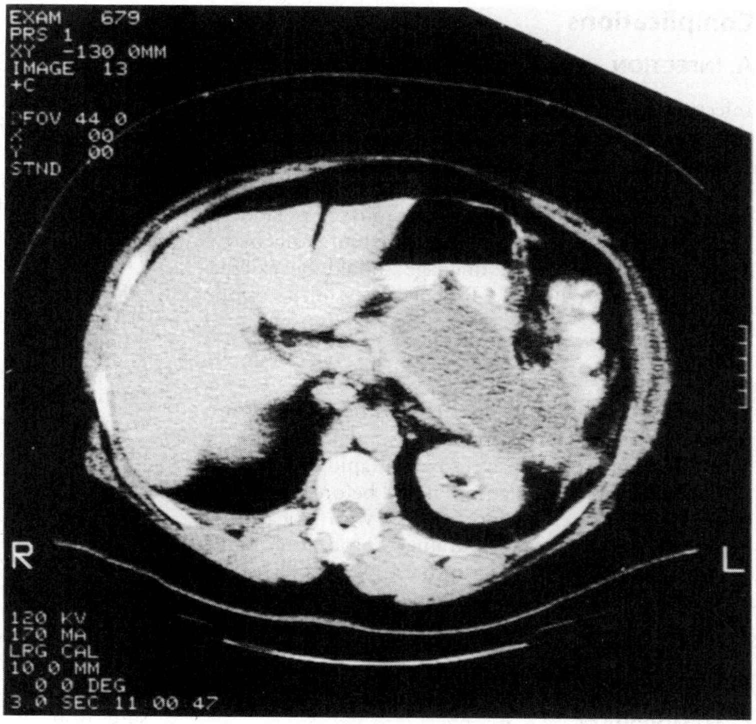

Figure 26–3. CT scan of a large unilocular pseudocyst impinging on the posterior wall of the stomach (which contains contrast media). A cyst in this location is usually best drained into the stomach.

ship to other viscera can be seen. Acute pseudocysts are often irregular in shape; chronic pseudocysts are most often circular or nearly so. An enlarged pancreatic duct may be demonstrated in patients with chronic pancreatitis. A dilated common bile duct would suggest biliary obstruction, either from the cyst or from underlying chronic pancreatitis.

The gallbladder should be studied by ultrasound to look for gallstones, especially in patients with acute pancreatitis. Although ultrasound can also demonstrate pseudocysts, the amount of important detail obtained is less than that from CT scans, and consequently the role of ultrasound is mainly to follow changes in size of an acute pseudocyst already imaged by CT scans, so the amount of x-ray exposure can be kept to a minimum.

ERCP should be performed if there are thought to be significant abnormalities of the bile or pancreatic duct as suggested by CT scans or the results of liver function tests. Either duct may be dilated and in need of surgical drainage in conjunction with drainage of the pseudocyst. ERCP usually opacifies the pseudocyst as well, but the information is not usually of major value in planning treatment, so ERCP is not obtained routinely.

An upper gastrointestinal series will often reveal a mass in the lesser sac that distorts the stomach or duodenum, but this is not particularly useful information. The principal indication for an upper gastrointestinal series is to search for a site of gastric or duodenal obstruction in patients who are vomiting.

With wide use of sensitive imaging studies in the diagnosis of pancreatic disease, small asymptomatic pseudocysts are often demonstrated. The natural history of these subclinical lesions is benign, and there is no indication for prophylactic surgical treatment.

Differential Diagnosis

Pancreatic pseudocysts must be distinguished from pancreatic abscess and acute pancreatic phlegmon. Patients with an abscess exhibit signs of infection.

Rarely, patients with pseudocyst present with weight loss, jaundice, and a nontender palpable gallbladder and are first thought to have pancreatic carcinoma. CT scans show that the lesion is fluid-filled, which suggests the correct diagnosis.

Neoplastic cysts—either cystadenoma or cystadenocarcinoma—account for about 5% of all cases of cystic pancreatic masses and may be indistinguishable preoperatively from pseudocyst. The correct diagnosis can be made from the gross appearance supplemented by a biopsy obtained at operation.

Complications

A. Infection

Infection is a rare complication resulting in high fever, chills, and leukocytosis. Drainage is required as soon as the diagnosis is suspected. Some lesions can be drained externally via a catheter placed percutaneously using ultrasound guidance. Internal drainage of infected pseudocysts adherent to the stomach can be achieved surgically by cystogastrostomy; otherwise, drainage should be external, because the suture line of a Roux-en-Y cystojejunostomy may not heal.

B. Rupture

Sudden perforation into the free peritoneal cavity produces severe chemical peritonitis, with board-like abdominal rigidity and severe pain. Rapid enlargement of the pseudocyst is sometimes noted before it ruptures. The treatment is emergency surgery with irrigation of the peritoneal cavity and a drainage procedure for the pseudocyst. The wall of a ruptured pseudocyst is usually too flimsy to hold sutures securely, so most ruptured cysts must be drained externally. Rupture of a pseudocyst occurs in less than 5% of cases, but even with prompt treatment it may be fatal.

C. Hemorrhage

Bleeding may occur into the cyst cavity or an adjacent viscus into which the cyst has eroded. Intracystic bleeding may present as an enlarging abdominal mass with anemia resulting from blood loss. If the cyst has eroded into the stomach, there may be hematemesis, melena, and blood in the nasogastric aspirate. The rapidity of the blood loss often produces hemorrhagic shock, which may preclude arteriography. If time permits, however, emergency arteriography should be performed to delineate the site of bleeding, which is usually a false aneurysm of an artery in the cyst wall, and to embolize it if possible. If embolization successfully occludes the bleeding vessel, several weeks should elapse to ensure that bleeding will not recur, and at that point the pseudocyst should be drained surgically in the same fashion as a nonbleeding pseudocyst. If the bleeding cannot be stopped by embolization, emergency surgery should be performed. Usually all that can be done is to open the cyst and suture ligate the bleeding vessel in the cyst wall, followed by external or internal drainage of the cyst. Sometimes it is possible to excise the cyst, which is desirable because doing so more certainly avoids the risk of recurrent hemorrhage.

Treatment

The principal indications for treating pancreatic pseudocysts are to improve symptoms and to prevent complications. Recent data indicate that the natural history of these lesions is more benign than previously thought—that in the absence of symptoms or radiographic evidence of enlargement (and irrespective of cyst size), expectant management is not unreasonable, and that a few untreated cysts resolve spontaneously even after being stable for months. Expectant management is especially important in the first 6–12 weeks of existence of cysts that have arisen during an attack of acute pancreatitis. The chances of spontaneous resolution are about 40%; catheter drainage at this stage is meddlesome; and internal drainage of the cyst by surgery may be difficult or even impossible. Thereafter, for cysts greater than 5 cm, treatment is usually recommended over expectant management (in the absence of contraindications, such as serious concomitant disease), because most cysts can be promptly eliminated by percutaneous catheter drainage or surgical drainage into the stomach or intestine. This obviates the need for prolonged follow-up with repeated ultrasound or CT scans and avoids the risks, albeit low, of complications. Patients who present with a symptomatic pseudocyst and no history of recent acute pancreatitis may be treated without the 6- to 12-week delay, because their cyst wall is tough (mature) enough to hold sutures and allow an anastomosis with the gut. Jaundice in a patient with a pseudocyst is usually caused by pressure from the cyst on the bile duct. Draining the pseudocyst usually relieves the obstruction, but an operative cholangiogram should be obtained to make sure.

A. Excision

Excision is the most definitive treatment but is usually confined to chronic pseudocysts in the tail of the gland. This approach is recommended especially for cysts that follow trauma, where the head and body of the gland are normal. Most cysts should be drained either externally or internally into the gut.

B. External Drainage

External drainage is best for critically ill patients or when the cyst wall has not matured sufficiently for anastomosis to other organs. A large tube is sewn into the cyst lumen, and its end is brought out through the abdominal wall. External drainage is complicated in a third of patients by a pancreatic fistula that sometimes requires surgical drainage but on the average closes spontaneously in several months. The incidence of recurrent pseudocyst is about four times greater after external drainage than after drainage into the gut.

C. Internal Drainage

The preferred method of treatment is internal drainage, where the cyst is anastomosed to a Roux-en-Y limb of jejunum (cystojejunostomy), to the posterior wall of the stomach (cystogastrostomy), or to the duodenum (cystoduodenostomy). The interior of the cyst should be inspected for evidence of a tumor and biopsy performed as appropriate. Cystogastrostomy is preferable for cysts behind and densely adherent to the stomach. This may well be done laparoscopically in the future. To accomplish free, dependent drainage, Roux-en-Y cystojejunostomy provides better drainage of cysts in various other locations. Cystoduodenostomy is indicated for cysts deep within the head of the gland and adjacent to the medial wall of the duodenum—lesions that would be difficult to drain by any other technique. The procedure consists of making a lateral duodenotomy, opening into the cyst through the medial wall of the duodenum, and then closing the lateral duodenotomy. Following internal drainage, the cyst cavity becomes obliterated within a few weeks. Even after cystogastrostomy, an unrestricted diet can be allowed within a week after surgery, and x-rays taken at this time usually show only a small residual cyst cavity.

D. Nonsurgical Drainage

External drainage can be established by a percutaneous catheter placed into the cyst under radiographic or ultrasound control. This is the preferred method for infected pseudocysts. In some centers, it is also used for the majority of uncomplicated pseudocysts as the primary mode of therapy. About two-thirds of cysts so treated are permanently eradicated. It may also be useful to shrink a truly huge pseudocyst (eg, one that occupies half of the abdominal cavity), because it is technically difficult to obtain adequate internal drainage of these lesions into the gut. Occasionally, a sterile cyst may become infected when a narrow catheter is inserted into it. This is more likely when the cyst lumen contains debris that is not drained effectively by this technique. Chronic external pancreatic fistula is a potential complication of this method.

Two other drainage techniques have been tried: (1) Passing a catheter percutaneously through the anterior abdominal wall, the anterior wall of the stomach, and through the posterior stomach into the cyst. After several weeks, the catheter is removed, and a chronic tract remains from cyst to gastric lumen. (2) Using a fiberoptic gastroscope to make a small incision through the back wall of the stomach into the cyst. Because of questions about efficacy and safety, neither method is widely used.

Prognosis

The recurrence rate for pancreatic pseudocyst is about 10%, and recurrence is more frequent after treatment by external drainage. Serious postoperative hemorrhage from the cyst occurs rarely—most often after cystogastrostomy. In most cases, however, surgical treatment of pseudocysts is uncomplicated and definitively solves the immediate problem. Many patients later experience chronic pain as a manifestation of underlying chronic pancreatitis.

Cooperman AM: Surgical treatment of pancreatic pseudocysts. Surg Clin North Am 2001;81:411.

Heider R et al: Percutaneous drainage of pancreatic pseudocysts is associated with a higher failure rate than surgical treatment in unselected patients. Ann Surg 1999;229:781.

Heider R, Behrns KE: Pancreatic pseudocysts complicated by splenic parenchymal involvement: results of operative and percutaneous management. Pancreas 2001;23:20.

Mori T et al: Laparoscopic pancreatic cystgastrostomy. J Hepatobiliary Pancreat Surg 2000;7:28.

Neff R: Pancreatic pseudocysts and fluid collections: percutaneous approaches. Surg Clin North Am 2001;81:399.

Vidyarthi G, Steinberg SE: Endoscopic management of pancreatic pseudocysts. Surg Clin North Am 2001;81:405.

3. Pancreatic Abscess

Pancreatic abscess, which complicates about 5% of cases of acute pancreatitis, is invariably fatal if it is not treated surgically. It tends to develop in severe cases accompanied by hypovolemic shock and pancreatic necrosis and is an especially frequent complication of postoperative pancreatitis. Abscess formation follows secondary bacterial contamination of necrotic pancreatic debris and hemorrhagic exudate. The organisms may spread to the pancreas hematogenously as well as directly through the wall of the transverse colon. It is unknown whether prophylactic antibiotics given early in the course of severe acute pancreatitis decrease the incidence of abscess.

Clinical Findings

An abscess should be suspected when a patient with severe acute pancreatitis fails to improve and develops rising fever or when symptoms return after a period of recovery. In most cases, there is improvement for a while before signs of infection appear 2–4 weeks after the attack began. Epigastric pain and tenderness and a palpable tender mass are clues to diagnosis. In many cases, the findings are not especially striking—ie, the temperature is only modestly elevated and the patient does not appear septic. Vomiting or jaundice may be present, but in some cases fever and leukocytosis are the only findings. The serum amylase may be elevated but usually is normal. Characteristically, the serum albumin is below 2.5 g/dL and the alkaline phosphatase is elevated. Pleural fluid and diaphragmatic paralysis may be evident on chest x-rays. An upper gastrointestinal series may show deformity of the stomach or duodenum by a mass, but it usually does not, and the changes are nonspecific in any case. Diagnostic CT scans will usually indicate the presence of a fluid collection in the area of the pancreas. Gas in the collection on plain films or CT scans is virtually diagnostic. Percutaneous CT scan-guided aspiration may be used to aid in diagnosis and obtain a specimen for Gram stain and culture.

In general, the diagnosis is difficult, treatment is often instituted late, illness is severe, and death rates are high.

Treatment

The collection of pus must be drained. Percutaneous catheter drainage may be helpful as a first step in order to decrease toxicity or to obtain a specimen for culture. In some cases, catheter drainage will prove to be definitive, but most often the infected retroperitoneal space is honeycombed and contains necrotic debris that cannot pass through the catheter, so surgical debridement is necessary. It is best to consider catheter drainage as a preparatory step for surgery rather than a curative treatment, for that is the usual relationship. Otherwise, there may be a tendency to delay surgery for too long as futile efforts are repeatedly made to manipulate the catheters into better positions. In fact, the two measures—surgical debridement and catheter drainage—are complementary.

Preoperatively, the patient should be given broad-spectrum antibiotics, since the organisms are usually a mixed flora, most often *Escherichia coli, Bacteroides, Staphylococcus, Klebsiella, Proteus, Candida albicans,* etc. Necrotic debris should be removed and external drainage instituted.

Postoperative hemorrhage (immediate or delayed) from the abscess cavity occurs occasionally.

Prognosis

The death rate is about 20%, a consequence of the severity of the condition, incomplete surgical drainage, and the inability in some cases to make the diagnosis.

Baril NB et al: Does an infected peripancreatic fluid collection or abscess mandate operation? Ann Surg 2000;231:361.

Beger HG, Rau B, Isenmann R: Prevention of severe change in acute pancreatitis: prediction and prevention. J Hepatobiliary Pancreat Surg 2001;8:140.

Kang CY et al: Development of HIV/AIDS vaccine using chimeric gag-env virus-like particles. Biol Chem 1999;380:353.

Tsiotos GG, Sarr MG: Management of fluid collections and necrosis in acute pancreatitis. Curr Gastroenterol Rep 1999;1:139.

Venu RP et al: Endoscopic transpapillary drainage of pancreatic abscess: technique and results. Gastrointest Endosc 2000;51(4 Part 1):391.

4. Pancreatic Ascites & Pancreatic Pleural Effusion

Pancreatic ascites consists of accumulated pancreatic fluid in the abdomen without peritonitis or severe pain. Since many of these patients are alcoholic, they are often thought at first to have cirrhotic ascites. The syndrome is most often due to chronic leakage of a pseudocyst, but a few cases are due to disruption of a pancreatic duct. The principal causative factors are alcoholic pancreatitis in adults and traumatic pancreatitis in children. Marked recent weight loss is a major clinical manifestation, and unresponsiveness of the ascites to diuretics is an additional diagnostic clue. The ascitic fluid, which ranges in appearance from straw-colored to blood-tinged, contains elevated protein (> 2.9 g/dL) and amylase levels. Once this condition is suspected, definitive diagnosis is based on chemical analysis of the ascitic fluid and endoscopic retrograde pancreatography. The latter procedure frequently demonstrates the point of fluid leak and allows a rational surgical approach if operation is required.

Initial therapy should consist of a period of intravenous hyperalimentation and somatostatin. This often cures the problem. If considerable improvement has not occurred within 2–3 weeks, surgery should be performed. A preoperative ERCP is essential to demonstrate the site of the leak. If it is not entirely obvious from the films taken during ERCP, a CT scan should be performed immediately afterward, while contrast media is still in the pancreatic duct. The greater sensitivity of the CT scan will be enough to reveal the tiny trickle from the pancreatic duct into the abdomen. The operation involves suturing a Roux-en-Y limb of jejunum to the site of the leak on the surface of the pancreas or a pancreatic pseudocyst. With appropriate therapy, the outlook is excellent. The death rate is low in patients treated before debilitation becomes severe.

Chronic pleural effusions of pancreatic origin represent a variant in which the pancreatic fistula drains into the chest. The diagnosis is made by measuring high concentrations of amylase (usually > 3000 IU/dL) in the fluid. A CT scan of the pancreas and retrograde pancreatogram should be obtained. Medical therapy consists of draining the fluid with a chest tube, somatostatin, and total parenteral nutrition. If after several weeks the fistula persists or if it recurs after the tube has been removed, the source of the leak on the pancreas should either be drained into a Roux-en-Y limb of jejunum or excised as part of a distal pancreatectomy.

Dugernier T, Laterre PF, Reynaert MS: Ascites fluid in severe acute pancreatitis: from pathophysiology to therapy. Acta Gastroenterol Belg 2000;63:264.

Kaman L et al: Internal pancreatic fistulas with pancreatic ascites and pancreatic pleural effusions: recognition and management. Aust N Z J Surg 2001;71:221.

Takeo C, Myojo S: Marked effect of octreotide acetate in a case of pancreatic pleural effusion. Curr Med Res Opin 2000;16:171.

5. *Chronic Pancreatitis*

ESSENTIALS OF DIAGNOSIS

- *Persistent or recurrent abdominal pain.*
- *Pancreatic calcification on x-ray in 50%.*
- *Pancreatic insufficiency in 30%; malabsorption and diabetes mellitus.*
- *Most often due to alcoholism.*

General Considerations

Chronic alcoholism causes most cases of chronic pancreatitis, but a few are due to gallstones, hypercalcemia, hyperlipidemia, duct obstruction from any cause, or inherited predisposition (familial pancreatitis). Direct trauma to the gland, either from an external blow or from surgical injury, can produce chronic pancreatitis if a ductal stricture develops during the healing process. In such cases, disease is often localized to the segment of gland drained by the obstructed duct. Although gallstone disease may cause repeated attacks of acute pancreatitis, this uncommonly leads to chronic pancreatitis.

There is evidence that pancreatic juice normally contains a specific protein responsible for maintaining calcium carbonate in solution. Levels of this protein are decreased in patients with chronic pancreatitis, a situation that allows calcium carbonate to precipitate and form calculi. Pressure within the duct is increased in patients with chronic pancreatitis (about 40 cm H_2O) compared with normal subjects (about 15 cm H_2O). This is a result of increased viscosity of pancreatic juice, partial obstruction by calculi, and impaired distensibility of the gland because of diffuse fibrosis (eg, a compartment syndrome). Sphincteric pressure remains in the normal range. The increased pressure causes dilation of the duct in the patient whose pancreas has not yet become fixed by scarring. It may also impair nutrient blood flow, causing further functional damage. Pathologic changes in the gland include destruction of parenchyma, fibrosis, dedifferentiation of acini, calculi, and ductal dilation.

Clinical Findings

A. Symptoms and Signs

Chronic pancreatitis may be asymptomatic, or it may produce abdominal pain, malabsorption, diabetes mellitus, or (usually) all three manifestations. The pain is typically felt deep in the upper abdomen and radiating through to the back, and it waxes and wanes from day to day. Early in the course of the disease, the pain may be episodic, lasting for days to weeks and then vanishing for several months before returning again. Attacks of acute pancreatitis may occur, superimposed on the pattern of chronic pain. Many patients become addicted to the narcotics prescribed for pain.

B. Laboratory Findings

Abnormal laboratory findings may result from (1) pancreatic inflammation, (2) pancreatic exocrine insufficiency, (3) diabetes mellitus, (4) bile duct obstruction, or (5) other complications such as pseudocyst formation or splenic vein thrombosis.

1. Amylase—In acute exacerbations, serum and urinary amylase levels may be elevated, but most often they are not, perhaps because pancreatic fibrosis has destroyed so much of the enzyme-forming capacity of the parenchyma.

2. Tests of exocrine pancreatic function—The secretin and cholecystokinin stimulation tests are the most sensitive tests to detect exocrine malfunction but are difficult to perform.

3. Diabetes mellitus—About 75% of patients with calcific pancreatitis and 30% of those with noncalcific pancreatitis have insulin-dependent diabetes. Most of the rest have either abnormal glucose tolerance curves or abnormally low serum insulin levels after a test meal. The margin of reserve is such that partial pancreatectomy is quite likely to convert a patient who does not require insulin into one who does require it postoperatively.

4. Biliary obstruction—Elevated bilirubin or alkaline phosphatase levels may result from fibrotic entrapment of the lower end of the bile duct. The differential diagnosis of biliary obstruction in these patients must consider acute pancreatic inflammation, pseudocyst, or pancreatic neoplasm.

5. Miscellaneous—Splenic vein thrombosis may produce secondary hypersplenism or gastric varices.

C. Imaging Studies

Endoscopic retrograde pancreatography is helpful in establishing the diagnosis of chronic pancreatitis, in ruling out pancreatic pseudocyst and neoplasm, and in preoperative planning for patients thought to be candidates for surgery. The typical findings are ductal stones and irregularity, with dilation and stenoses and, occasionally, ductal occlusion. The discovery of small unsuspected pseudocysts is common. Retrograde cholangiography should be performed simultaneously to determine whether the common bile duct is narrowed by the pancreatitis, to determine whether biliary calculi are present, and to aid the surgeon in avoiding injury to the bile duct during operation.

Complications

The principal complications of chronic pancreatitis are pancreatic pseudocyst, biliary obstruction, duodenal obstruction, malnutrition, and diabetes mellitus. Adenocarcinoma of the pancreas occurs with greater frequency in patients with familial chronic pancreatitis than in the general population.

Treatment

A. Medical Treatment

Malabsorption and steatorrhea are managed with support and measures. Controlled trials have shown that administering pancreatic enzymes has little effect on the pain.

Patients with chronic pancreatitis should be urged to discontinue the use of alcohol. Abstention from alcohol will reduce chronic or episodic pain in more than half of cases even though damage to the pancreas is irreversible. Psychiatric treatment may be beneficial. Diabetes in these patients usually requires insulin.

B. Surgical Treatment

Surgical therapy is principally of value to relieve chronic intractable pain. It is essential that every effort be made to eliminate alcohol abuse. The best surgical candidates are those whose pain persists after alcohol has been abandoned.

Surgical treatment in most cases involves a procedure that facilitates drainage of the pancreatic duct or resects diseased pancreas—or that serves both purposes. The choice of operation can usually be made preoperatively based on the findings of a retrograde pancreatogram and CT scans. Coincidental bile duct obstruction is common and should be treated by simultaneous choledochoduodenostomy.

1. Drainage procedures—A dilated ductal system reflects obstruction, and when dilation is present, procedures to improve ductal drainage usually relieve pain. Calcific alcoholic pancreatitis most often falls into this category.

The usual finding is an irregular, widely dilated duct (1–2 cm in diameter) with points of stenosis ("chain of lakes" appearance) and ductal calculi. For such patients, a longitudinal pancreaticojejunostomy **(Puestow procedure)** is appropriate (Figure 26–4). The duct is opened anteriorly from the tail into the head of the gland and anastomosed side-to-side to a Roux-en-Y segment of proximal jejunum. Pain improves postoperatively in about 80% of patients, but improvement of pancreatic insufficiency is uncommon. This procedure, however, has a low rate of success when the pancreatic duct is narrow (ie, < 8 mm).

Sphincteroplasty and distal (caudal) pancreaticojejunostomy **(Du Val procedure)** are other drainage techniques that were used more often in the past. The latter is only of historical interest, but surgical sphincteroplasty plus extraction of pancreatic ductal calculi continuous in use. Attempts are currently being made to accomplish something similar by subjecting pancreatic calculi to external shock wave lithotripsy, followed by endoscopic sphincterotomy and stone extraction. Another experimental method involves decompression of the duct by an endoscopically placed stent. Questions of safety and efficacy have tempered the early enthusiasm for these procedures.

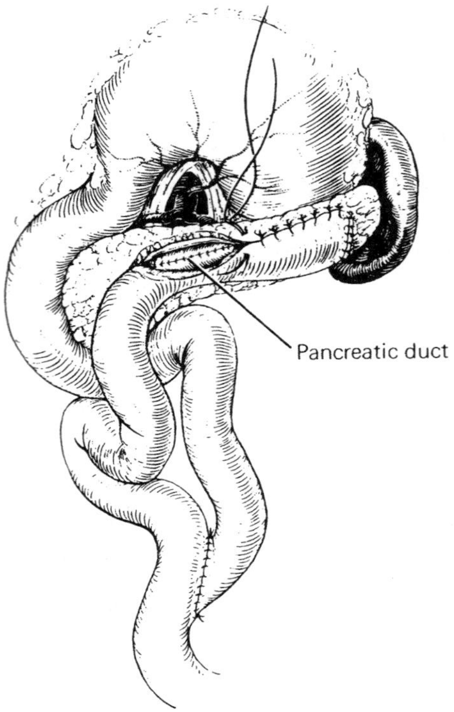

Figure 26–4. Longitudinal pancreaticojejunostomy (Puestow) for chronic pancreatitis.

2. Pancreatectomy—In the absence of a dilated duct, pancreatectomy is the best procedure, and the extent of resection can often be determined from a CT scan and pancreatogram. In patients with small ducts, the most severe disease is usually located in the head of the gland, and **pancreaticoduodenectomy** (Whipple procedure) is the operation of choice. A variant of this procedure involves resection of the head of the gland while preserving the duodenum. A Roux-en-Y limb of jejunum is anastomosed to both cut surfaces of the pancreas. If the duct is also dilated in the body and tail, resection of the head can also be combined with longitudinal pancreaticojejunostomy in that part of the gland. Pain relief is satisfactory in about 80% of patients treated by these operations. **Total pancreatectomy** is indicated when a previous pancreaticoduodenectomy or distal pancreatectomy has failed to give satisfactory pain relief. The reported results are contradictory; pain relief has been excellent in reports from the UK but less than excellent in reports from the USA. Difficulties in controlling diabetes mellitus occur in 30–40% of patients who have had total pancreatectomy and are responsible for occasional deaths. For this reason, total pancreatectomy is contraindicated in active alcoholics. For chronic alcoholic pancreatitis, resections from the left of the gland—eg, **distal subtotal pancreatectomy**—are much less successful than resections of the head and are rarely performed nowadays. The most common indication is chronic focal posttraumatic pancreatitis, in which the head may be normal.

3. Celiac plexus block—Celiac plexus block may be used in an attempts to obtain pain relief before proceeding with a major pancreatic resection in small duct pancreatitis. A newer and more effective variant of this approach consists of **thoracoscopic splanchnicectomy**—resection of segments of the greater and lesser splanchnic nerves as they enter the thorax from the abdomen. When performed thoracoscopically, the procedure is relatively minor, and it interrupts the pain afferents with greater certainty.

Prognosis

Longitudinal pancreaticojejunostomy relieves pain in about 80% of patients with a dilated duct. Weight gain is common but less predictable. The results of pancreaticoduodenectomy are good in 80% of patients, but removal of the distal pancreas is less successful. Total pancreatectomy, which is principally reserved for failures of other operations, gives satisfying relief in 30–90% of patients depending on the series. The reasons for these widely differing results are not known. Celiac plexus block is of lasting benefit to no more than 30% of patients. In some patients, pain subsides with advancing pancreatic insufficiency.

Except in advanced cases with continuous pain, alcoholics who can be persuaded to stop drinking often experience relief from pain and recurrent attacks of pancreatitis. In familial pancreatitis, the progress of the disease is inexorable, and many of these patients require surgery. The results of longitudinal pancreaticojejunostomy are excellent in familial pancreatitis. Narcotic addiction, diabetes, and malnutrition are serious problems in many patients.

Adamek HE et al: Long term follow up of patients with chronic pancreatitis and pancreatic stones treated with extracorporeal shock wave lithotripsy. Gut 1999;45:402.

Apte MV, Keogh GW, Wilson JS: Chronic pancreatitis: complications and management. J Clin Gastroenterol 1999;29:225.

Berney T et al: Long-term metabolic results after pancreatic resection for severe chronic pancreatitis. Arch Surg 2000;135:1106.

Bornman PC, Beckingham IJ: ABC of diseases of liver, pancreas, and biliary system. Chronic pancreatitis. BMJ 2001;322:660.

Izbicki JR et al: Extended drainage versus resection in surgery for chronic pancreatitis: a prospective randomized trial comparing the longitudinal pancreaticojejunostomy combined with local pancreatic head excision with the pylorus-preserving pancreatoduodenectomy. Ann Surg 1998;228:771.

Jimenez RE et al: Outcome of pancreaticoduodenectomy with pylorus preservation or with antrectomy in the treatment of chronic pancreatitis. Ann Surg 2000;231:293.

McCutcheon AD: Neurological damage and duodenopancreatic reflux in the pathogenesis of alcoholic pancreatitis. Arch Surg 2000;135:278.

Pitchumoni CS: Chronic pancreatitis: pathogenesis and management of pain. J Clin Gastroenterol 1998;27:101.

Sakorafas GH et al: Pancreatoduodenectomy for chronic pancreatitis: long-term results in 105 patients. Arch Surg 2000;135:517.

Whitcomb DC: Hereditary pancreatitis: new insights into acute and chronic pancreatitis. Gut 1999;45:317.

PANCREATIC INSUFFICIENCY (Steatorrhea; Malabsorption)

Pancreatic exocrine insufficiency may follow pancreatectomy or pancreatic disease, especially chronic pancreatitis. Many patients with varying degrees of pancreatic insufficiency have no symptoms and require no treatment, whereas others may benefit greatly from a rational medical regimen.

Malabsorption and steatorrhea do not appear until more than 90% of pancreatic exocrine function is lost; with 2–10% of normal function, steatorrhea is mild to moderate; with less than 2% of normal function, steatorrhea is severe. On a diet containing 100 g of fat per day, normal subjects excrete 5–7 g/d, and the efficiency of assimilation is similar over a wide range of fat intake. Total pancreatectomy causes about 70% fat malabsorption. If the pancreatic remnant is normal, subtotal resections may have little effect on absorption.

Pancreatic insufficiency affects fat absorption more than that of protein or carbohydrate, because protein digestion is aided by gastric pepsin and carbohydrate digestion by salivary and intestinal amylase. Malabsorption of vitamins is rarely a significant problem. Water-soluble B vitamins are absorbed throughout the small intestine, and fat-soluble vitamins, although dependent on micellar solubilization by bile salts, do not require pancreatic enzymes for absorption. Vitamin B_{12} malabsorption has been detected in some patients with pancreatic insufficiency, but it is rarely a clinical problem, and vitamin B_{12} replacement is unnecessary.

Thus, the principal problem in otherwise uncomplicated pancreatic insufficiency is fat malabsorption and accompanying caloric malnutrition.

Tests of Pancreatic Exocrine Function

A. Secretin or Cholecystokinin Test

Pancreatic juice is obtained by peroral duodenal intubation, and the response to an intravenous injection of secretin or cholecystokinin is measured. The results vary, depending on the dose and preparation of hormone used. Both tests (using purified hormones or the synthetic octapeptide of cholecystokinin) seem to be reliable. Pancreatic fluid should normally have a bicarbonate concentration greater than 80 meq/L and bicarbonate output above 15 meq/30 min.

B. Pancreolauryl Test

Fluorescein dilaurate is given orally with breakfast, and urinary fluorescein excretion is measured. Release and absorption of fluorescein depend on the action of pancreatic esterase. The test is relatively specific, but considerable exocrine insufficiency is required for a positive result. It is currently the most widely used test of exocrine function because it is inexpensive and easy to do.

C. PABA Excretion (Bentiromide) Test

The patient ingests 1 g of the synthetic peptide bentiromide (Bz-Ty-PABA), and urinary excretion of aromatic amines (PABA) is measured. Cleavage of the peptide to liberate PABA depends on intraluminal chymotrypsin activity. Patients with chronic pancreatitis excrete about 50% of the normal amount of PABA.

D. Fecal Fat Balance Test

The patient ingests a diet containing 75–100 g fat each day for 5 days. The amounts of dietary fat should be measured and should be the same each day. Excretion of less than 7% of ingested fat is normal. Clinically significant steatorrhea is present when fat malabsorption exceeds about 25%. Total pancreatectomy results in about 70% fat malabsorption.

Examination of a stool specimen for fat globules (obviously much simpler than the fat balance test) is specific and relatively sensitive for fat malabsorption.

Treatment

The diet should aim for 3000–6000 kcal/d, emphasizing carbohydrate (400 g or more) and protein (100–150 g). Patients with steatorrhea may or may not have diarrhea, and dietary restriction of fat is important mainly to control diarrhea. Patients with diarrhea may be restricted to 50 g of fat and the amount increased until diarrhea appears. Permissible fat intake averages 100 g/d distributed equally among four meals.

Pancrelipase replacement may be accomplished with pancreatic extracts containing 30,000–50,000 units of lipase distributed throughout each of four daily meals. Lesser amounts are much less effective; an hourly dosage regimen probably has no advantages.

If enzymes alone do not improve the malabsorption enough, the problem is probably due to destruction of lipase by gastric acid. This can be largely alleviated by adding an H_2 receptor blocking agent to the enzyme regimen. A preparation of enzymes as enteric-coated microspheres (Pancrease) is less vulnerable to low pH and may be more effective in refractory cases.

Medium-chain triglycerides (MCT), which can be obtained as a powder or an oil, may be used as a caloric supplement. This product is more rapidly hydrolyzed and the fatty acids more readily absorbed than are long-chain triglycerides, which make up 98% of the fat in a normal diet. Unfortunately, MCT oil is relatively unpalatable and is frequently associated with nausea and vomiting, bloating, and diarrhea, which limit patient acceptance.

DiMagno EP: Gastric acid suppression and treatment of severe exocrine pancreatic insufficiency. Best Pract Res Clin Gastroenterol 2001;15:477.

Durie PR: Pancreatic aspects of cystic fibrosis and other inherited causes of pancreatic dysfunction. Med Clin North Am 2000;84:609.

Layer P, Keller J: Pancreatic enzymes: secretion and luminal nutrient digestion in health and disease. J Clin Gastroenterol 1999;28:3.

Tsiotos GG et al: Long-term outcome of necrotizing pancreatitis treated by necrosectomy. Br J Surg 1998;85:1650.

ADENOCARCINOMA OF THE PANCREAS

An estimated 29,200 patients will develop pancreatic cancer in the United States in 2001, and 28,900 will die of the disease. These nearly equal numbers illustrate the dismal prognosis generally associated with pancreatic carcinoma. The death rate per 100,000 people has been basically unchanged since the mid 1960s at about 10/100,000 for men and 27/100,000 for women. After tumors of the lung and colon, pancreatic carcinoma is the third leading cause of death due to cancer in men between ages 35 and 54. Factors associated with an increased risk of pancreatic cancer are cigarette smoking, dietary consumption of meat (especially fried meat) and fat, previous gastrectomy (> 20 years earlier), and race (in the USA but not Africa, blacks are more susceptible than whites).

The peak incidence is in the fifth and sixth decades. In two-thirds of cases, the tumor is located in the head of the gland; the remainder occur in the body or tail. Ductal adenocarcinoma, mainly of a poorly differentiated cell pattern, accounts for 80% of the cancers; the remainder are islet cell tumors and cystadenocarcinomas, tumors that are discussed later in this chapter. Pancreatic adenocarcinoma is characterized by early local extension to contiguous structures and metastases to regional lymph nodes and the liver. Pulmonary, peritoneal, and distant nodal metastases occur later.

Clinical Findings

A. Symptoms and Signs

1. Carcinoma of the head of the pancreas—About 75% of patients with carcinoma of the head of the pancreas present with weight loss, obstructive jaundice, and deep-seated abdominal pain. Back pain occurs in 25% of patients and is associated with a worse prognosis. In general, smaller tumors confined to the pancreas are associated with less pain. Weight loss averages about 20 lb (44 kg). Hepatomegaly is present in half of patients but does not necessarily indicate spread to the liver. A palpable mass, which is found in 20%, nearly always signifies surgical incurability. Jaundice is unrelenting in most patients but fluctuates in about 10%. Cholangitis occurs in only 10% of patients with bile duct obstruction. A palpable nontender gallbladder in a jaundiced patient suggests neoplastic obstruction of the common duct **(Courvoisier's sign)**, most often due to pancreatic cancer; this finding is present in about half of cases. Jaundice is often accompanied by pruritus, especially of the hands and feet.

2. Carcinoma of the body and tail of the pancreas—Since carcinomas of the body and tail of the pancreas are remote from the bile duct, less than 10% of patients are jaundiced. The presenting complaints are weight loss and pain, which sometimes occurs in excruciating paroxysms. In the few patients with jaundice or hepatomegaly, metastatic involvement has usually occurred. Migratory thrombophlebitis develops in 10% of cases. Once considered relatively specific as a clue to pancreatic cancer, this complication is now known to affect patients with other types of malignant disease.

The diagnosis of pancreatic carcinoma may be extremely difficult. The typical patient who presents with abdominal pain, weight loss, and obstructive jaundice rarely presents a problem, but those with just weight loss, vague abdominal pain, and nondiagnostic x-rays are occasionally labeled psychoneurotics until the existence of cancer becomes obvious. If back pain predominates, orthopedic or neurosurgical causes may be sought at first. One characteristic feature is the tendency for the patient to seek relief of pain by assuming a sitting position with the spine flexed. Recumbency, on the other hand, aggravates the discomfort and sometimes makes sleeping in bed impossible. Sudden onset of diabetes mellitus is an early manifestation in 25% of patients.

B. Laboratory Findings

Elevated alkaline phosphatase and bilirubin levels reflect either common duct obstruction or hepatic metastases. The bilirubin level with neoplastic obstruction averages 18 mg/dL, much higher than that generally seen with benign disease of the bile ducts. Only rarely are serum aminotransferase levels markedly elevated. Repeated examination of stool specimens for occult blood gives a positive reaction in many cases.

Serum levels of the tumor marker CA 19-9 are elevated in most patients with pancreatic cancer, but the sensitivity in resectable (< 4 cm) lesions is probably too low (50%) for this to serve as a screening tool. Elevated levels also occur with other gastrointestinal cancers. The greatest usefulness of CA 19-9 measurements may be in following the results of treatments. After complete resection of a tumor, elevated levels drop to normal, but they rise again with recurrence.

C. Imaging Studies

Nearly all patients should have a CT scan.

1. CT scan—CT scans show a pancreatic mass in 95% of cases, usually with a central zone of diminished attenuation, and in over 90% of patients with a mass there are signs of extension beyond the boundaries of the pancreas. The upstream pancreatic duct is noted to be dilated in 70% of patients, and the bile duct is dilated in 60% (principally in those with jaundice). The presence of both bile duct and pancreatic duct dilation is strong evidence for pancreatic cancer even in the absence of a mass. Findings suggesting unresectability include local tumor extension (eg, behind the pancreas; into the liver hilum), contiguous organ invasion (eg, duodenum, stomach), distant metastases, involvement of the superior mesenteric or portal vessels, or ascites. In general, size of the mass is only loosely related to resectability. CT scans using modern dynamic scanning techniques are as accurate as angiography in assessing vascular involvement.

2. ERCP—In patients with a typical clinical history and a pancreatic mass on CT, ERCP is unnecessary. In the absence of a mass, an ERCP is indicated. It is the most sensitive test (95%) for detecting pancreatic cancer, though specificity in differentiating between cancer and pancreatitis is low. Consequently, a pancreatogram should be obtained early in cases where the existence of a pancreatic lesion is suspected but unproved. The findings consist of stenosis or obstruction of the pancreatic duct. Adjacent lesions of the bile duct and pancreatic duct ("double-duct sign") are highly suggestive of neoplastic disease, especially if the biliary involvement is focal. Although ERCP is useful to distinguish between the various kinds of periampullary tumors, that information rarely alters management.

3. Upper gastrointestinal series—An upper gastrointestinal series is not sensitive in detecting pancreatic cancer, but it provides information about patency of the duodenum that may be useful in deciding whether a gastrojejunostomy will have to be performed. The classic findings consist of widening of the duodenal sweep, narrowing of the lumen, and the "reversed-3 sign," named for the duodenal configuration.

4. Other studies—Angiography has not proved reliable in detecting or staging pancreatic neoplasms, and ultrasound is a poor second to CT scans for imaging.

D. Aspiration Biopsy

Percutaneous aspiration biopsy of pancreatic mass lesions is positive in 85% of malignant tumors. The procedure is relatively safe, but there is a risk of spreading a localized (resectable) tumor, so it is contraindicated in patients who are candidates for surgery. Aspiration biopsy in them should be performed, if desired, during laparotomy. Percutaneous aspiration biopsy is principally of value to verify a presumptive diagnosis of adenocarcinoma of the pancreas in patients with radiographic evidence of unresectability. In these cases, cytologic proof is important, for treatment decisions should not be made solely on the basis of the indirect evidence provided by CT scans and other imaging tests. There is too great a risk of misdiagnosing something unusual, such as a retroperitoneal lymphoma or sarcoma, and administering inappropriate treatment.

Differential Diagnosis

The other periampullary neoplasms—carcinoma of the ampulla of Vater, distal common bile duct, or duodenum—may also present with pain, weight loss, obstructive jaundice, and a palpable gallbladder. Preoperative cholangiography and gastrointestinal x-rays may suggest the correct diagnosis, but laparotomy is sometimes required.

Complications

Obstruction of the splenic vein by tumor may cause splenomegaly and segmental portal hypertension with bleeding gastric or esophageal varices.

Treatment

Pancreatic resection for pancreatic cancer is appropriate only if all gross tumor can be removed with a standard resection. The lesion is considered resectable if the following areas are free of tumor: (1) the hepatic artery near the origin of the gastroduodenal artery; (2) the superior mesenteric artery where it courses under the body of the pancreas; and (3) the liver and regional lymph nodes. Since the pancreas is so close to the portal vein and the superior mesenteric vessels, these structures may be involved early. About 20% of cancers of the head of the pancreas can be resected, but because of local and distant spread, this is rarely possible for lesions of the body and tail.

A histologic diagnosis can usually be made at operation by aspiration biopsy. With small lesions of the head of the gland, it may be difficult to obtain a specimen for histologic diagnosis because much of the palpable mass may consist of inflamed pancreatic tissue. Occasionally, histologic diagnosis is impossible, and clinical decisions must rest on indirect evidence.

For curable lesions of the head, pancreaticoduodenectomy **(Whipple operation)** is required (Figure 26–5). This involves resection of the common bile duct, the gallbladder, the duodenum, and the pancreas to the mid body. There is an increasing tendency to preserve the antrum and pylorus. Involvement of a short (< 1.5 cm) segment of the portal vein is not a contraindication to a curative resection. This is managed by a partial or circumferential resection of the affected area.

When the procedure is performed by surgeons who do it frequently, the operative mortality rate is less than 5%. When it is performed by less experienced surgeons, the mortality rate is 20–30%. Postoperative deaths are due to complications such as pancreatic and biliary fistulas, hemorrhage, and infection.

In an attempt to increase the cure rate, total pancreatectomy has been given a trial on the theory that many pancreatic cancers are multicentric. However, total pancreatectomy produces a brittle type of diabetes mellitus that compromises the quality of life, and cure rates were not higher.

For unresectable lesions, cholecystojejunostomy or choledochojejunostomy provides relief of jaundice and pruritus. A cholangiogram should be obtained to verify patency between the cystic and common bile ducts unless it is grossly obvious. Percutaneous or endoscopically placed biliary stents may also provide effective palliation and are preferable to surgical biliary decompression if the lesion is known to be unresectable. Gastrojejunostomy is required if the tumor blocks the duodenum. If laparotomy has been performed, gastrojejunostomy should be considered regardless of the presence of duodenal obstruction, because with time this often develops before other life-threatening complications.

Laparoscopy is a useful first step in patients scheduled for a possible Whipple procedure. If metastases are seen that militate against a curative resection, laparoscopic gastrojejunostomy or cholecystojejunostomy (or both) can be performed. If not, one should proceed with the laparotomy. About 15% of patients thought to have localized disease from preoperative studies are found to be unresectable at laparoscopy.

Gemcitabine-based chemotherapy has clear benefits in patients with metastatic disease. Its utility in combination with radiation therapy and as adjuvant therapy is being defined.

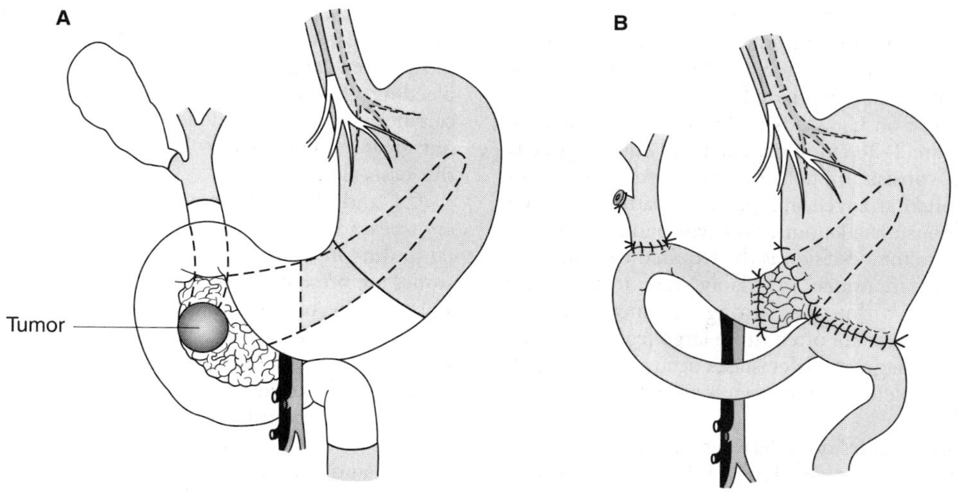

Figure 26–5. Pancreaticoduodenectomy (Whipple procedure). ***A:*** Preoperative anatomic relationships showing a tumor in the head of the pancreas. ***B:*** Postoperative reconstruction showing pancreatic, biliary, and gastric anastomoses. A cholecystectomy and bilateral truncal vagotomy are also part of the procedure. In many cases, the distal stomach and pylorus can be preserved, and vagotomy is then unnecessary.

Prognosis

The mean survival following palliative therapy is 7 months. Following a Whipple procedure, survival averages about 18 months. Factors associated with tumor recurrence and shorter survival include lymph node involvement, tumor size over 2.5 cm, blood vessel invasion, and amount of blood transfused. If tumor cells extend to the margins of the resected specimen, long-term survival is rare. If the margins are clear, about 20% of patients live more than 5 years. Overall 5-year survival is about 10%, but only 60% of these patients are actually free of tumor.

Balci NC, Semelka RC: Radiologic diagnosis and staging of pancreatic ductal adenocarcinoma. Eur J Radiol 2001;38:105.

Bodner WR, Hilaris BS, Mastoras DA: Radiation therapy in pancreatic cancer: current practice and future trends. J Clin Gastroenterol 2000;30:230.

Bornman PC, Beckingham IJ: ABC of diseases of liver, pancreas, and biliary system. Pancreatic tumours. BMJ 2001;322:721.

Crane CH et al: Combining gemcitabine with radiation in pancreatic cancer: understanding important variables influencing the therapeutic index. Semin Oncol 2001;28(3 Suppl 10):25.

Farnell MB, Nagorney DM, Sarr MG: The Mayo clinic approach to the surgical treatment of adenocarcinoma of the pancreas. Surg Clin North Am 2001;81:611.

Kozuch P et al: Treatment of metastatic pancreatic adenocarcinoma: a comprehensive review. Surg Clin North Am 2001;81: 683.

Madura JA et al: Adenosquamous carcinoma of the pancreas. Arch Surg 1999;134:599.

Mangray S, King TC: Molecular pathobiology of pancreatic adenocarcinoma. Front Biosci 1998;3:D1148.

Molinari M, Helton WS, Espat NJ: Palliative strategies for locally advanced unresectable and metastatic pancreatic cancer. Surg Clin North Am 2001;81:651.

Rose DM et al: ^{18}Fluorodeoxyglucose-positron emission tomography in the management of patients with suspected pancreatic cancer. Ann Surg 1999;229:729.

Sohn TA, Yeo CJ: The molecular genetics of pancreatic ductal carcinoma: a review. Surg Oncol 2000;9:95.

CYSTIC NEOPLASMS

Cystic neoplasms of the pancreas usually present with abdominal pain, a mass, or jaundice and are diagnosed from the findings on CT scans.

Cystadenomas can be classified as serous or mucinous. Serous cystadenomas, which are usually microcystic adenomas, are well-circumscribed lesions consisting of multiple small cysts ranging in size from microscopic to about 2 cm. The cut surface has the appearance of a sponge. The multicystic nature of the lesion is usually—but not always—evident on CT scans, which may also show a few calcifications. The epithelium, which is flat to cuboidal, has no malignant potential. Treatment usually entails excision, but in the rare case where this is too hazardous, the lesion may be left in place with the knowledge that complications are rare. An occasional serous cystadenoma will consist of one or more large cysts (ie, macrocystic).

Mucinous cystadenomas (macrocystic adenomas), which are much more common in women than in men, are unilocular or, more often, multilocular lesions that have a smooth lining with papillary projections. The septate appearance on CT scans is characteristic. The cystic spaces measure 2–20 cm in diameter and contain mucus. The lining consists of tall columnar and goblet cells, which are often arranged in a papillary pattern. In time, most mucinous cystadenomas will evolve into cystadenocarcinomas, so total excision is the required treatment.

Cystadenocarcinomas invariably present as a focus of malignancy within an existing mucinous cystadenoma. The tumors are often quite large (eg, 10–20 cm) at the time of diagnosis. Metastases occur in about 25% of cases. Complete excision results in a 5-year survival rate of 70%.

An uncommon lesion, referred to as solid-and-papillary or papillary-cystic neoplasm of the pancreas, occurs almost exclusively in young women (under age 25 years). The tumor is usually large. It may be locally invasive, but metastases are uncommon, and cure is to be expected after resection.

Balci NC, Semelka RC: Radiologic features of cystic, endocrine and other pancreatic neoplasms. Eur J Radiol 2001;38:113.

Balcom JH 4th et al: Cystic lesions in the pancreas: when to watch, when to resect. Curr Gastroenterol Rep 2000;2:152.

Le Borgne J, de Calan L, Partensky C: Cystadenomas and cystadenocarcinomas of the pancreas: a multiinstitutional retrospective study of 398 cases. French Surgical Association. Ann Surg 1999;230:152.

Sarr MG et al: Cystic neoplasms of the pancreas: benign to malignant epithelial neoplasms. Surg Clin North Am 2001;81:497.

Sarr MG et al: Clinical and pathologic correlation of 84 mucinous cystic neoplasms of the pancreas: can one reliably differentiate benign from malignant (or premalignant) neoplasms? Ann Surg 2000;231:205.

Shima Y et al: Diagnosis and management of cystic pancreatic tumours with mucin production. Br J Surg 2000;87:1041.

Verdolini K et al: Laryngeal adduction in resonant voice. J Voice 1998;12:315.

Vihtelic TS, Doro CJ, Hyde DR: Cloning and characterization of six zebrafish photoreceptor opsin cDNAs and immunolocalization of their corresponding proteins. Vis Neurosci 1999; 16:571.

Wilentz RE et al: Pathologic examination accurately predicts prognosis in mucinous cystic neoplasms of the pancreas. Am J Surg Pathol 1999;23:1320.

ADENOMA & ADENOCARCINOMA OF THE AMPULLA OF VATER

Adenoma and adenocarcinoma of the ampulla of Vater account for about 10% of neoplasms that obstruct the distal bile duct. One-third are adenomas and two-thirds adenocarcinomas. Since a remnant of benign adenoma can be found in a majority of adenocarcinomas, it is suspected that malignant change in an adenoma gives rise to most carcinomas. The presenting symptom is most often jaundice or occasionally gastrointestinal bleeding. Weight loss and pain are more common with carcinoma than with adenoma, but the differences are not great enough to allow a distinction to be made on this basis alone.

CT and ultrasound scans reveal dilation of the biliary tree and pancreatic duct. Gallstones are an incidental finding in 20% of patients, and when common duct stones are present, they may incorrectly be held responsible for the biliary obstruction. The most important diagnostic study is ERCP. In 75% of cases, tumor is visible on duodenoscopy as an exophytic papillary lesion, an ulcerated tumor, or an infiltrating mass. An adequate biopsy usually can be obtained from these lesions. In 25% of cases, there is no intraduodenal growth, and endoscopic sphincterotomy is necessary to display the tumor. It is best to wait 10–14 days to biopsy these tumors because of transient artifacts that result from the sphincterotomy. ERCP also demonstrates dilation of the biliary and pancreatic ducts. It has become common to perform a sphincterotomy whenever possible, not only to facilitate performance of a biopsy but also to decompress the biliary tree and allow jaundice to subside in anticipation of subsequent surgical therapy. The value of this step has not been established.

Although some adenomas have been successfully treated by snare excision or, preferably, by neodymium:YAG laser destruction, local resection or pancreaticoduodenectomy is preferable because of the significant chance that an invasive carcinoma will be undertreated at a time that it is curable. These nonsurgical methods should be reserved for patients who are poor candidates for resection.

Treatment of adenocarcinoma consists of pancreaticoduodenectomy as for pancreatic carcinoma. The operative mortality rate is less than 5%, and the 5-year survival rate is about 50%. The presence of metastases in resectable peripancreatic lymph nodes is not a contraindication to pancreaticoduodenectomy, for the 5-year survival rate under these circumstances is still a respectable 25%. Local excision is an alternative for noninfiltrating papillary adenocarcinomas in patients who are too poor a risk for pancreaticoduodenectomy, but this operation is not as successful as pancreaticoduodenectomy. Endoscopic sphincterotomy alone or with retrograde stent placement (the combination is usually required) is indicated when there is definite evidence (eg, hepatic metastases) that the tumor is incurable. Survival averages less than a year with this approach, however.

Bakaeen FG et al: What prognostic factors are important in duodenal adenocarcinoma? Arch Surg 2000;135:635.

Crucitti A et al: Ampullary carcinoma: prognostic significance of ploidy, cell-cycle analysis and proliferating cell nuclear antigen (PCNA). Hepatogastroenterology 1999;46:1187.

Howe JR et al: Factors predictive of survival in ampullary carcinoma. Ann Surg 1998;228:87.

Lee JH et al: Outcome of pancreaticoduodenectomy and impact of adjuvant therapy for ampullary carcinomas. Int J Radiat Oncol Biol Phys 2000;47:945.

Roberts RH et al: Pancreaticoduodenectomy of ampullary carcinoma. Am Surg 1999;65:1043.

PANCREATIC ISLET CELL TUMORS

Islet cell tumors may be functioning (ie, hormone-producing) or nonfunctioning, malignant or nonmalignant. More than half are functioning; less than half are malignant. Insulinoma, the most common functioning islet cell neoplasm, arises from beta cells and produces insulin and symptoms of hypoglycemia. Tumors of the δ or α_1 cells produce gastrin and the Zollinger-Ellison syndrome. Alpha_2 cell neoplasms may produce excess glucagon and hyperglycemia. Non-beta islet cell tumors may secrete serotonin, ACTH, MSH, and kinins (and evoke the carcinoid syndrome). Some produce pancreatic cholera, a severe diarrheal illness.

1. Nonfunctioning Islet Cell Tumors

Most of these lesions are malignant tumors of the head of the gland, which present with abdominal and back pain, weight loss, and, in many cases, a palpable abdominal mass. Jaundice is seen occasionally. CT scans reveal a pancreatic mass, and angiography typically shows it to be hypervascular. The histologic pattern on biopsy specimens is diagnostic of islet cell tumor, but whether or not the lesion is malignant rests on evidence of invasiveness or metastases, not the appearance of the cells. Immunohistochemical staining of the tissue is positive for chromogranin and neuron-specific enolase (markers of APUD tumors). Metastases are present at the time of diagnosis in 80% of patients. Resection of all gross tumor (eg, by a Whipple procedure), the preferred treatment, is possible in less than half of patients because of local extension or distant metastases. A combination of streptozocin and doxorubicin is the most effective chemotherapeutic regimen. The 5-year disease-free survival rate is about 15%.

Bartsch DK et al: Management of nonfunctioning islet cell carcinomas. World J Surg 2000;24:1418.

Jensen RT: Carcinoid and pancreatic endocrine tumors: recent advances in molecular pathogenesis, localization, and treatment. Curr Opin Oncol 2000;12:368.

Somogyi L, Mishra G: Diagnosis and staging of islet cell tumors of the pancreas. Curr Gastroenterol Rep 2000;2:159.

2. Insulinoma

Insulinomas have been reported in all age groups. About 75% are solitary and benign. About 10% are malignant, and metastases are usually evident at the time of diagnosis. The remaining 15% are manifestations of multifocal pancreatic disease—either adenomatosis, nesidioblastosis, or islet cell hyperplasia.

The symptoms (related to cerebral glucose deprivation) are bizarre behavior, memory lapse, or unconsciousness. Patients may be mistakenly treated for psychiatric illness. There may be profuse sympathetic discharge, with palpitations, sweating, and tremulousness. Hypoglycemic episodes are usually precipitated by fasting and are relieved by food, so weight gain is common. The classic diagnostic criteria **(Whipple's triad)** are present in most cases: (1) hypoglycemic symptoms produced by fasting, (2) blood glucose below 50 mg/dL during symptomatic episodes, and (3) relief of symptoms by intravenous administration of glucose.

The most useful diagnostic test and the only one indicated in all but a few patients is demonstration of fasting hypoglycemia in the presence of inappropriately high levels of insulin. The patient is fasted, and blood samples are obtained every 6 hours for glucose and insulin measurements. The fast is continued until hypoglycemia or symptoms appear or for a maximum of 72 hours. If hypoglycemia has not developed after 70 hours, the patient should be exercised for the final 2 hours. Although insulin levels are not always elevated in patients with insulinoma, they will be high relative to the blood glucose concentration. A ratio of plasma insulin to glucose greater than 0.3 is diagnostic. Ratios should be calculated before and during the fast. Proinsulin, which constitutes more than 25% of total insulin (the upper limit of normal) in about 85% of patients with insulinomas, should also be measured. Proinsulin levels greater than 40% suggest a malignant islet cell tumor.

Drugs that release insulin (tolbutamide, glucagon, leucine, arginine, calcium) were used in the past as provocative tests. No provocative tests are currently used.

Localization of the tumor is important but may be difficult. In about 10% of cases, the tumor is so small or located so deeply that it is difficult or impossible to find at laparotomy. High-resolution CT and MR scans are successful in demonstrating about 40% of tumors. Endoscopic (gastroscopic) ultrasound examination of the pancreas may be able to show a much higher percentage. The most important examination is intraoperative ultrasound, which can identify a pancreatic tumor in nearly all cases. It is more sensitive than any preoperative test.

In patients who have had previous resection or significant upper abdominal surgery, exploration with intraoperative ultrasound may be difficult. Invasive preoperative testing may then be useful. Angiography gives a yield of about 50%. Transhepatic portal venous sampling has proved an accurate preoperative localizing method, demonstrating the position in the pancreas in about 95% of lesions. However, this test is time-consuming and somewhat invasive, involving entering the portal vein with a catheter passed percutaneously through the liver and testing blood at various sites within the portal, superior mesenteric, and splenic veins for insulin levels. The point where insulin concentrations rise sharply indicates the site of the tumor. An alternative invasive localizing test uses arteriography with selective calcium infusion into arteries supplying the pancreas. Blood samples from the hepatic veins reveal an increase in insulin level when calcium is infused into an artery supplying the tumor.

Differential Diagnosis

Fasting hypoglycemia may be a manifestation of some nonpancreatic, non-islet cell tumors. Clinically, the condition is identical to that resulting from insulinoma, but the cause is rarely secretion of insulin by the tumors, as serum insulin levels are normal. Most non-islet cell tumors associated with hypoglycemia are large and readily detected on physical examination. The majority are of mesenchymal origin (eg, hemangiopericytoma, fibrosarcoma, leiomyosarcoma) and are located in the abdomen or thorax, but hepatoma, adrenocortical carcinoma, and a variety of other lesions may also produce hypoglycemia. The principal means by which these tumors produce hypoglycemia are the following: (1) secretion by the tumor of insulin-like growth factor II (IGF-II), an insulin-like peptide that normally mediates the effects of growth hormone; and (2) inhibition of glycogenolysis or gluconeogenesis. Rapid utilization of glucose by the tumor, replacement of liver tissue by metastases, and secretion of insulin are other postulated mechanisms that are probably uncommon.

Surreptitious self-administration of insulin is seen occasionally, most often in an individual with access to insulin on the job. If insulin injections have been given for as long as 2 months, insulin antibodies will be detectable in the patient's serum. Circulating C peptide levels are normal in these patients but elevated in most patients with insulinoma. Sulfonylurea ingestion can be detected by measuring the drug in plasma.

Treatment

Surgery should be done promptly, because with repeated hypoglycemic attacks, permanent cerebral damage occurs and the patient becomes progressively more obese. Moreover, the tumor may be malignant. Medical treatment is reserved for surgically incurable lesions.

A. Medical Treatment

Diazoxide is administered to suppress insulin release. For incurable islet cell carcinomas, streptozocin is the best chemotherapeutic agent. Sixty percent of patients live up to 2 additional years. Toxicity is considerable; streptozocin is not recommended as a routine adjunct to surgical therapy.

B. Surgical Treatment

At surgery, the entire pancreas must be palpated carefully because the tumors are usually small and difficult to find. The gland should also be examined intraoperatively with ultrasound, which may be able to locate a tumor that cannot be felt, or to demonstrate signs of invasion (ie, irregular borders) that indicate malignancy—something that cannot be detected by palpation. When the tumor is found, it may be enucleated if it is superficial or resected as part of a partial pancreatectomy if it is deep-seated or invasive. Insulinomas in the head of the gland can nearly always be enucleated.

Tumors that can be localized preoperatively, and that are placed in favorable anatomic locations, can sometimes be resected using a laparoscopic approach. The same principles of local, complete resection should be followed. Laparoscopic ultrasound is often useful to guide this exploration.

In the past, the tumor could not be detected in about 5% of cases by these methods. The traditional recommendation was to resect the distal half of the pancreas and have the pathologist slice the specimen into thin sections and look for the tumor. If the tumor was found, the operation was concluded; if it was not found, additional pancreas would be resected until an 80% distal pancreatectomy had been performed. Since the tumors are evenly distributed, this strategy is 80% successful in removing the tumor. Intraoperative monitoring of blood glucose is often done as a means of determining if the tumor has been excised, but it is unreliable. With the use of operative ultrasound scanning, however, no more than 1–2% of insulinomas remain occult, and blind distal pancreatectomy is rarely even considered.

Patients with insulinoma associated with MEN-1 usually have multiple (average of three) lesions. Because persistence of the disease is much more likely in this condition following the standard surgical approach, the operation recommended here is distal pancreatectomy plus enucleation of any lesions found in the head of the gland.

For islet cell hyperplasia, nesidioblastosis, or multiple benign adenomas, distal subtotal pancreatectomy usually decreases insulin levels enough that medical management is simplified. For islet cell carcinomas, resection of both primary and metastatic lesions is warranted if technically feasible.

Patients with sporadic insulinomas lead a normal life after the tumor has been removed. The outcome is less predictable in patients with MEN-1, who may have several insulin-producing tumors.

Dolan JP, Norton JA: Occult insulinoma. Br J Surg 2000;87:385.

Grant CS: Surgical aspects of hyperinsulinemic hypoglycemia. Endocrinol Metab Clin North Am 1999;28:533.

Grant CS: Insulinoma. Surg Oncol Clin N Am 1998;7:819.

Service FJ: Classification of hypoglycemic disorders. Endocrinol Metab Clin North Am 1999;28:501.

3. Pancreatic Cholera (WDHA Syndrome: Watery Diarrhea, Hypokalemia, & Achlorhydria)

Most cases of pancreatic cholera are caused by a nonbeta islet cell tumor of the pancreas that secretes VIP (vasoactive intestinal polypeptide) and peptide histidine isoleucine. The syndrome is characterized by profuse watery diarrhea, massive fecal loss of potassium, low serum potassium, and extreme weakness. Gastric acid secretion is usually low or absent even after stimulation with betazole or pentagastrin. Stool volume averages about 5 L/d during acute episodes and contains over 300 meq of potassium (20 times normal). Severe metabolic acidosis frequently results from loss of bicarbonate in the stool. Many patients are hypercalcemic, possibly from secretion by the tumor of a parathyroid hormone-like substance. Abnormal glucose tolerance may result from hypokalemia and altered sensitivity to insulin. Patients who complain of severe diarrhea must be studied carefully for other causes before the diagnosis of WDHA syndrome is entertained seriously. Chronic laxative abuse is a frequent explanation.

CT scan is the best initial imaging test; somatostatin receptor scintigraphy is also very useful for localization. Approximately 80% of the tumors are solitary, located in the body or tail, and can be removed easily. About half of the lesions are malignant, and three-fourths of those have metastasized by the time of exploration. Even if all of the tumor cannot be removed, resection of most of it alleviates symptoms in about 40% of patients even though the average survival is only 1 year. Streptozocin has produced remissions in several cases, but nephrotoxicity may limit its effectiveness. Treatment with long-acting somatostatin analogues decreases VIP levels, controls diarrhea, and may even reduce tumor size. The effect persists indefinitely in most patients, but in a few it is transient.

Jensen RT: Overview of chronic diarrhea caused by functional neuroendocrine neoplasms. Semin Gastrointest Dis 1999;10:156.

Soga J, Yakuwa Y: Vipoma/diarrheogenic syndrome: a statistical evaluation of 241 reported cases. J Exp Clin Cancer Res 1998;17:389.

4. Glucagonoma

Glucagonoma syndrome is characterized by migratory necrolytic dermatitis (usually involving the legs and perineum), weight loss, stomatitis, hypoaminoacidemia, anemia, and mild to moderate diabetes mellitus. Scotomas and changes in visual acuity have been reported in some cases. The age range is 20–70 years, and the condition is more common in women. The diagnosis may be suspected from the distinctive skin lesion; in fact, the presence of a prominent rash in a patient with diabetes mellitus should be enough to raise suspicions. Glucagonoma should also be suspected in any patient with new onset of diabetes after age 60. Confirmation of the diagnosis depends on measuring elevated serum glucagon levels. CT scans demonstrate the tumor and sites of spread. Angiography is not essential but reveals a hypervascular lesion.

Glucagonomas arise from α_2 cells in the pancreatic islets. Most are large at the time of diagnosis. About 25% are benign and confined to the pancreas. The remainder have metastasized by the time of diagnosis, most often to the liver, lymph nodes, adrenal gland, or vertebrae. A few cases have been the result of islet cell hyperplasia.

Severe malnutrition should be corrected preoperatively with a period of total parenteral nutrition and treatment with somatostatin analogues. Surgical removal of the primary lesion and resectable secondaries is indicated if technically feasible. If the tumor is confined to the pancreas, cure is possible. Even if it is not possible to remove all the tumor deposits, considerable palliation may result from subtotal removal, so surgery is indicated in almost every case. Low-dose heparin therapy should be administered pre- and postoperatively because of a high risk of deep venous thrombosis and pulmonary embolism. Streptozocin and dacarbazine are the most effective chemotherapeutic agents for unresectable lesions. Somatostatin therapy normalizes serum glucagon and amino acid levels, clears the rash, and promotes weight gain. The clinical course generally parallels changes in serum levels of glucagon in response to therapy.

Bernstein M et al: Amino acid, glucose, and lipid kinetics after palliative resection in a patient with glucagonoma syndrome. Metabolism 2001;50:720.

Chastain MA: The glucagonoma syndrome: a review of its features and discussion of new perspectives. Am J Med Sci 2001;321:306.

El Rassi Z et al: Necrolytic migratory erythema, first symptom of a malignant glucagonoma: treatment by long-acting somatostatin and surgical resection. Report of three cases. Eur J Surg Oncol 1998;24:562.

Metz DC: Diagnosis of non-Zollinger-Ellison syndrome, non-carcinoid syndrome, enteropancreatic neuroendocrine tumours. Ital J Gastroenterol Hepatol 1999;31(Suppl 2):S153.

5. Somatostatinoma

Somatostatinomas are characterized by diabetes mellitus (usually mild), diarrhea and malabsorption, and dilation of the gallbladder (usually with cholelithiasis). Serum calcitonin and IgM concentrations may be elevated. The syndrome results from secretion of somatostatin by an islet cell tumor of the pancreas, half of which are malignant and accompanied by hepatic metastases. The lesion is usually large and readily demonstrated by CT scan. The diagnosis may be made by recognizing the clinical syndrome and measuring increased concentrations of somatostatin in the serum. Often, however, the somatostatin syndrome is unsuspected until histologic evidence of metastatic islet cell carcinoma has been obtained. When the disease is localized, resection is able to cure about 50% of cases. Enucleation is inappropriate for these tumors. Chemotherapy with streptozocin, dacarbazine, or doxorubicin is the best treatment for unresectable tumors. Small somatostatin-rich tumors of the duodenum or ampulla of Vater have also been reported, but none of these lesions have been associated with high serum levels of somatostatin or the clinical syndrome.

Metz DC: Diagnosis of non-Zollinger-Ellison syndrome, non-carcinoid syndrome, enteropancreatic neuroendocrine tumours. Ital J Gastroenterol Hepatol 1999;31(Suppl 2):S153.

Soga J, Yakuwa Y: Somatostatinoma/inhibitory syndrome: a statistical evaluation of 173 reported cases as compared to other pancreatic endocrinomas. J Exp Clin Cancer Res 1999;18:13.

Tanaka S et al: Duodenal somatostatinoma: a case report and review of 31 cases with special reference to the relationship between tumor size and metastasis. Pathol Int 2000;50:146.

Spleen

27

Douglas L. Fraker, MD

ANATOMY

The spleen is a dark purplish, highly vascular, coffee bean-shaped organ of mesodermal origin situated in the left upper quadrant of the abdomen at the level of the eighth to eleventh ribs between the fundus of the stomach, the diaphragm, the splenic flexure of the colon, and the left kidney (Figure 27–1). The adult spleen weighs 100–150 g, measures about 12 × 7 × 4 cm, and usually cannot be palpated. It is attached to adjacent viscera, the abdominal wall, and the diaphragm by peritoneal folds or "ligaments." The gastrosplenic ligament carries the short gastric vessels. The other ligaments are avascular except in patients with portal hypertension or myelofibrosis.

The splenic capsule consists of peritoneum overlying a 1- to 2-mm fibroelastic layer that contains a few smooth muscle cells. The fibroelastic layer sends into the pulp numerous fibrous bands (trabeculae) that form the framework of the spleen. Corrosion cast studies demonstrate that the spleen consists of specific segments based on arterial supply numbering between two and six separated by an avascular plane.

The splenic artery enters the hilum of the spleen, branches into the trabecular arteries, and then branches into the central arteries that course through the surrounding white pulp and send radial branches to the peripheral marginal zone and the more distant red pulp. The white pulp consists of lymphatic tissue, including T cells adjacent to the central artery (periarteriolar lymphoid sheets: PALS), with a surrounding area containing lymphoid follicles rich in B cells interspersed with dendritic and reticular cells important in antigen presentation. The vascular spaces of the marginal zone between the red and white pulp channel blood into the splenic Billroth cords and out to the associated sinuses. The red pulp vascular structures have a noncontiguous basement membrane that filters cells such as senescent erythrocytes into the macrophage-lined sinuses.

Accessory spleens (spleniculi) are seen in 10–15% of the normal population and are located primarily in the gastrosplenic, gastrocolic, and lienorenal ligaments, but they can also be found throughout the peritoneal cavity in the omentum, bowel mesentery, and pelvis. Accessory spleens probably result from a failure of infusion of splenic embryologic tissues. Ordinarily of no significance, they may play a role in recurrence of certain hematologic disorders for which splenectomy is performed. Removal of accessory spleens may lead to remission of disease in these patients. Accessory spleens are more difficult to identify with laparoscopic procedures, but the use of a hand port has allowed identification and resection of accessory spleens with a minimally invasive approach. Patients who fail to respond to initial splenectomy should undergo scanning with technetium 99m-labeled red cells or indium 111-labeled platelets to identify potential sites of missed accessory spleens.

Ectopic spleen (wandering spleen) is an unusual condition in which a long splenic pedicle allows the spleen to move within the peritoneum. It often resides in the lower abdomen or pelvis, where even a normal-sized spleen can be felt as a mass. The condition is 13 times more common in women than in men. Diagnostic radionuclide scan can diagnose the mass as a spleen. Acute torsion of the pedicle occurs occasionally, necessitating emergency splenectomy, and elective removal of pelvic spleens is recommended.

PHYSIOLOGY

The primary function of the spleen is filtration of the blood for clearance of cells, microorganisms, and other particulate matter as well as related immune and hematologic storage functions.

The spleen receives 5% of the total cardiac output, or approximately 150–300 mL/min, such that each red cell averages 1000 passes through the spleen each day. Normal blood cells pass rapidly through the spleen, while abnormal and senescent cells are retarded and entrapped. As they travel through the hypoxic, acidotic, glucose-deprived splenic cords and sinuses of the red pulp, senescent erythrocytes pass into the vascular spaces and are phagocytosed by macrophages in a process called "culling." Part of the membrane of erythrocytes can be removed through the gaps between endothelial cells lining the vascular spaces in a similar process called pitting. In the presence of splenomegaly and other disease states, the flow patterns of the spleen become more circuitous as the red pulp volume expands, so that even normal cells may be trapped.

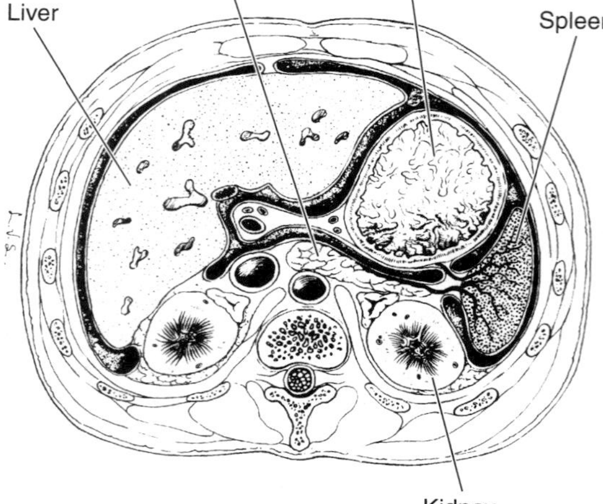

Figure 27–1. Normal anatomic relations of the spleen.

The adult spleen produces monocytes, lymphocytes, and plasma cells. Production of other blood elements occurs in patients with myeloid metaplasia and in the fetal spleen.

The spleen is considered to be a secondary organ of the immune system and represents the largest single collection of lymphoid tissue in the body. The white pulp of the spleen contains the various cellular components needed to generate an immune response, with structural and functional relationships similar to those of lymph nodes. Lymphocytes and circulating antigen-presenting cells enter the white pulp via the marginal zone capillaries and traverse the T cell–rich PALS before passing through bridging channels into the red pulp. Primary follicles or germinal centers with secondary follicles at the periphery of the white pulp are sites of B cell expansion and immunoglobulin production. Blood passing through the spleen is exposed to all the key cellular components necessary for both humoral and cellular immune responses. Moreover, the concentration of macrophages in the red pulp vascular spaces facilitates opsonization of particles coated with IgG and plays an important role in autoimmune hematologic diseases as well as explaining the increased risk of sepsis that follows splenectomy in children under 2 years of age. Even in adults, splenectomy leads to a slight but definite reduction in immune function.

Normally, about 30% of the total platelet pool is sequestered in the spleen. Splenomegaly typically involves expansion of the red pulp, which increases this sequestration to between 80% and 95% of the platelet cell mass. Storage of erythrocytes and granulocytes in the spleen is limited in humans, but newly formed reticulocytes released from the bone marrow concentrate in the spleen to undergo a maturational process.

Kraus MD: Pathology of the spleen. Introduction. Sem Diagn Pathol 2003;20:83.

Skandalakis PN et al: The surgical anatomy of the spleen. Surg Clin North Am 1993;73:747.

Were JM et al: The red cell revisited—matters of life and death. Cell Mol Biol 2004;50:139.

OPERATIVE INDICATIONS FOR SPLENECTOMY

To better describe and understand operative indications in surgery of the spleen, one could categorize the indications for splenectomy or procedures of the spleen into eight general areas:

(1) Hypersplenism is characterized by diffuse enlargement of the spleen by neoplastic disorders, hematopoietic disorders of the bone marrow, and metabolic or storage disorders. These various disease processes result in diffuse enlargement of the spleen and amplify the normal function of elimination of circulating blood cells resulting in general pancytopenia. Erythrocytes and platelets are most commonly affected. Hypersplenism also may cause symptoms of early satiety due to the splenic size.

(2) Autoimmune/erythrocyte disorders. Specific cytopenias are related either to antibodies targeting platelets, erythrocytes, or neutrophils. A second category of diseases relates to intrinsic structural changes within the erythrocyte that lead to a shortened red blood cell half-life with accelerated splenic clearance. There is nothing intrinsically wrong with the spleen, and splenic size is typically normal.

(3) Trauma or injury to the spleen.

(4) Vascular diseases. Splenic vein thrombosis and splenic artery aneurysm may require splenectomy for treatment.

(5) Cysts and primary splenic tumors and abscesses. This would include treatment of simple cysts, echinococcal cysts, splenic abscess, and various benign neoplasms including hamartomas, hemangiomas, lymphangiomas, and rare malignant lesions.

(6) Diagnostic procedures. This category of splenectomy occurs when the spleen is removed primarily to make a clinical diagnosis when none is available. A subcategory of this would be staging laparotomy for Hodgkin's disease, which has all but been eliminated based on alternative imaging techniques and current treatment regimens.

(7) Iatrogenic splenectomy. Splenectomy that is performed due to an incidental injury to the spleen during surgery within the general abdominal cavity or specifically, the left upper quadrant, can be categorized as iatrogenic splenectomy. This category is likely underreported and may be considered a subcategory of trauma.

(8) Incidental splenectomy. The spleen may be removed as part of a standard operation to remove the distal pancreas most commonly, and also for gastric cancers, left-sided renal cell carcinomas, adrenal cancers, and retroperitoneal sarcomas in the left upper quadrant. The spleen is removed in these instances due to direct tumor extension, vascular involvement, or the need for excision of splenic hilum lymph nodes.

When institutions analyze the most common reasons for splenectomy, trauma and incidental splenectomy account for the majority of the spleens removed. For elective splenectomy that is not incidental to removal of another organ or tumor, autoimmune disorders or other hereditary blood cell disease are the most common indication. Within this category, idiopathic thrombocytopenia purpura has the highest incidence for splenectomy. Each of these categories of disease will be discussed including the etiology and pathophysiology of the disorder, the specific indications for splenectomy, alternative treatments, and the results of splenectomy.

Kraus MD, Fleming MD, Vonderheide RH: The spleen as a diagnostic specimen: a review of 10 years' experience at two tertiary care institutions. Cancer 2001;91:2001.

Rose AT et al: The incidence of splenectomy is decreasing: lessons learned from trauma experience. Am Surg 2000;66:481.

HYPERSPLENISM

In the past, the term hypersplenism or increased splenic function has been used to denote the syndrome characterized by splenic enlargement, deficiency of one or more blood cell lines, normal or hyperplastic cellularity of deficient cell lines in the marrow, and increased turnover of affected cells. Increased understanding of the pathophysiology of specific disorders has shown that hypersplenism is not synonymous with splenomegaly. Some disorders in which there is spleen-dependent destruction of blood elements do not manifest all features of hypersplenism. For example, splenomegaly is rarely a feature of immune thrombocytopenic purpura, and splenectomy is not always curative. Conversely, other conditions that enlarge the spleen may not result in destruction or sequestration of blood elements with resultant cytopenias. In disorders with known pathogenesis, the recent trend has been to classify them as separate disease entities rather than as hypersplenic conditions.

The defects in hypersplenism are exaggerations of normal splenic functions primarily associated with the red pulp. The principal cause of cytopenias in hypersplenism is increased sequestration and destruction of blood cells in the spleen, which is hypertrophied or increased in volume in a variety of diseases. Etiologic factors include (1) neoplastic infiltration, (2) disease of the bone marrow in which the spleen becomes a site of extramedullary hematopoiesis, or (3) metabolic/genetic disorders such as Gaucher's disease. The hyperplastic spleen is not selective in its hyperfunction in most of these disorders. The splenomegaly can lead to an increased turnover in erythrocytes and platelets, with a lesser effect on leukocytes. For example, about 60% of patients with cirrhosis develop splenomegaly and 15% develop hypersplenism. The hypersplenism of cirrhosis is seldom of clinical significance; the anemia and thrombocytopenia are usually mild and rarely are indications for splenectomy.

Clinical Findings

A. Symptoms and Signs

The clinical findings depend largely on the underlying disorder or are secondary to the depletion of circulating blood elements caused by the hypersplenism (Table 27–1). Manifestations of hypersplenism usually develop gradually, and the diagnosis often follows a routine physical or laboratory examination. Some patients experience left upper quadrant fullness, discomfort (can be severe), or early satiety. Others have hematemesis due to gastroesophageal varices.

Purpura, bruising, and diffuse mucous membrane bleeding are unusual symptoms despite the presence of thrombocytopenia. Anemia may produce significant fatigue that may be the chief complaint in this patient population. Recurrent infections may be seen in patients with severe leukopenia.

Table 27–1. Disorders associated with secondary hypersplenism.

Congestive splenomegaly (cirrhosis, portal or splenic vein obstruction)
Neoplasm (leukemia, metastatic carcinoma)
Inflammatory disease (sarcoid, lupus erythematosus, Felty's syndrome)
Acute infections with splenomegaly
Chronic infection (tuberculosis, brucellosis, malaria)
Storage diseases (Gaucher's disease, Letterer-Siwe disease, amyloidosis)
Chronic hemolytic diseases (spherocytosis, thalassemia, glucose-6-phosphate dehydrogenase deficiency, elliptocytosis)
Myeloproliferative disorders (myelofibrosis with myeloid metaplasia)

B. Laboratory Findings

Patients with primary hypersplenism usually exhibit pancytopenia of moderate degree and generalized marrow hyperplasia. Anemia is most prominent, reflecting the destruction of erythrocytes in the hypertrophied red pulp of the spleen. Thrombocytopenia occurs due to sequestration of platelets but also possibly due to increased turnover. In most cases more immature cell types such as reticulocytes are present, reflecting the overactivity of the bone marrow to compensate for the pancytopenias. One exception is myeloid metaplasia, in which dysfunction of the bone marrow is the primary defect.

C. Evaluation of Splenic Size

Before it becomes palpable, an enlarged spleen may cause dullness to percussion above the left costal margin. Splenomegaly is manifested on supine x-rays of the abdomen by medial displacement of the stomach and downward displacement of the transverse colon and splenic flexure. CT scan is useful for differentiating the spleen from other abdominal masses and for demonstrating splenic enlargement or intrasplenic lesions. Some of the largest massive spleens (spleen weight > 1500 g) occur in these types of disease. Finding the edge of the spleen below the iliac crest and crossing the abdominal midline are frequently seen.

Differential Diagnosis

Leukemia and lymphoma are diagnosed by marrow aspiration, lymph node biopsy, and examination of the peripheral blood (white count and differential). In hereditary spherocytosis there are spherocytes, osmotic fragility is increased, and platelets and white cells are normal. The hemoglobinopathies with splenomegaly are differentiated on the basis of hemoglobin electrophoresis or the demonstration of an unstable hemoglobin level. Thalassemia major becomes apparent in early childhood, and the blood smear morphology is characteristic. In myelofibrosis, the bone marrow shows proliferation of fibroblasts and replacement of normal elements. In idiopathic thrombocytopenic purpura, the spleen is normal or only slightly enlarged. In aplastic anemia, the spleen is not enlarged and the marrow is fatty.

Treatment & Prognosis

The course, response to treatment, and prognosis of the hypersplenic syndromes differ widely depending on the underlying disease and its response to treatment and will be discussed for each particular disorder below. The indications for splenectomy are given in Table 27–2.

Splenectomy may decrease transfusion requirements, decrease the incidence and number of infections, prevent hemorrhage, and reduce pain. The course of congestive splenomegaly due to portal hypertension depends upon the degree of venous obstruction and liver damage. The hypersplenism is rarely a major problem and is almost always overshadowed by variceal bleeding or liver dysfunction.

Table 27–2. Indications for splenectomy.

Splenectomy always indicated
Primary splenic tumor (rare)
Hereditary spherocytosis (congenital hemolytic anemia)
Splenectomy usually indicated
Primary hypersplenism
Chronic immune thrombocytopenic purpura
Splenic vein thrombosis causing gastric varices
Splenic abscess (rare)
Splenectomy sometimes indicated
Splenic injury
Autoimmune hemolytic disease
Elliptocytosis with hemolysis
Nonspherocytic congenital hemolytic anemias
Hodgkin's disease (for staging)
Thrombotic thrombocytopenic purpura
Idiopathic myelofibrosis
Splenic artery aneurysm
Wiskott-Aldrich syndrome
Gaucher's disease
Mastocytosis-aggressive disease
Splenectomy rarely indicated
Chronic leukemia
Splenic lymphoma
Macroglobulinemia
Thalassemia major
Sickle cell anemia
Congestive splenomegaly and hypersplenism due to portal hypertension
Felty's syndrome
Hairy cell leukemia
Chédiak-Higashi syndrome
Sarcoidosis
Splenectomy not indicated
Asymptomatic hypersplenism
Splenomegaly with infection
Splenomegaly associated with elevated IgM
Hereditary hemolytic anemia of moderate degree
Acute leukemia
Agranulocytosis

NEOPLASTIC DISEASES

Neoplastic diseases in which splenectomy may play a role in management of hypersplenism include chronic lymphocytic leukemia (CLL), hairy cell leukemia, and non-Hodgkin's lymphoma. Lymphoma is discussed in detail in Chapter 46. Related neoplastic disorders of idiopathic myelofibrosis and mastocytosis are also discussed as precursors or variants of neoplastic diseases in which splenectomy are occasionally indicated.

1. Chronic Lymphocytic Leukemia

Chronic lymphocytic leukemia (CLL) is a low-grade neoplasm of B cell lineage characterized by accumulations of populations of lymphocytes that are mature morphologically but functionally incompetent. The clinical manifestations and natural history are variable, but initially the disease tends to be indolent. In more advanced stages, splenomegaly, which is frequently massive, is a common characteristic of CLL. Most symptoms related to the spleen are from thrombocytopenia and anemia due to secondary hypersplenism (80–90% of splenic symptoms). Ten to 20 percent of patients may have symptoms primarily related to pressure from the size of the enlarged spleen.

Other causes of cytopenia in CLL relate to decreased cellular production from the bone marrow. Bone marrow failure can be due to replacement with leukemic cells or to depletion of the bone marrow as a toxic effect of prior antitumor chemotherapy.

Splenectomy in patients with CLL corrects thrombocytopenia in 70–85% of cases and anemia in 60–75% of cases. The median duration of benefit for both platelets and red cell populations is well over 1 year. Patients with smaller spleens preoperatively, lower preoperative platelet counts, and extensive prior chemotherapy are less likely to respond to splenectomy. However, a positive bone marrow aspirate for leukemic cells is not a contraindication to splenectomy in CLL. Patients who do not have a good performance status should not undergo splenectomy, since patients in terminal stages have unacceptable operative morbidity.

Coad JE et al: Splenectomy in lymphoproliferative disorders: a report on 70 cases and review of the literature. Leuk Lymphoma 1993;10:245.

Delpero JR et al: Splenectomy for hypersplenism in chronic lymphocytic leukaemia and malignant non-Hodgkin's lymphoma. Br J Surg 1990;77:443.

Petroianu A: Subtotal splenectomy for the treatment of chronic lymphocytic leukemia. Ann Hematol 2003;82:708.

Ruchlemer R et al: Splenectomy in mantle cell lymphoma with leukemia: a comparison with chronic lymphocytic leukemia. Br J Haematol 2002;118:952.

2. Hairy Cell Leukemia

Hairy cell leukemia is a low-grade lymphoproliferative disorder with characteristic "hairy cells"—ie, B lymphocytes with irregular cytoplasmic protrusions—which infiltrate the bone marrow and spleen. Patients are typically male, and onset of the disease is in the fifth or sixth decade of life. Symptoms relate to pancytopenia, with anemia requiring transfusions; and to neutropenia, characterized by increased susceptibility to infections and increased bleeding tendencies. Some patients may have symptoms from splenomegaly, which is present in 80% of patients at the time of diagnosis of hairy cell leukemia. The cytopenias are due to a combination of bone marrow replacement and secondary hypersplenism.

The standard therapy for hairy cell leukemia between 1960 and 1995 was splenectomy, but recent advances in pharmacotherapy have superseded this surgical approach. Splenectomy is successful in improving cell counts in 80–90% of patients, but the duration of improvement is short-lived, with the majority of patients relapsing within 6–12 months. Chronic therapy with alpha interferon produced a higher proportion of responses of longer duration than splenectomy. First-line therapy is now treatment with purine nucleoside analogues (pentostatin or cladribine), with a complete response rate of 80–90%. It has never been shown that splenectomy offers survival benefit in this indolent disease, and the operation should be reserved for palliation of splenomegaly in patients who have failed treatment with purine analogues and alpha interferon.

Mey U et al: I. Advances in the treatment of hairy cell leukemia. Lancet Oncol 2003;4:86.

Pettit AR et al: Hairy-cell leukaemia: biology and management. Br J Haematol 1999;106:2.

Tallman MS: Current treatment strategies for patients with hairy cell leukemia. Rev Clin Exp Hematol 2002;6:389.

3. Idiopathic Myelofibrosis (Agnogenic Myeloid Metaplasia)

Myelofibrosis is a myeloproliferative disorder of unknown cause that is closely related to polycythemia vera and myelogenous leukemia. It appears to be a clonal disorder or a neoplasm originating from a stem cell that results in extensive bone marrow fibrosis, extramedullary hematopoiesis in the spleen and liver, and a leukoerythroblastic blood reaction.

The bone marrow is usually almost completely replaced by fibrous tissue, although in some cases it is hyperplastic and fibrosis is minimal. Extramedullary hematopoiesis develops mainly in the spleen, liver, and long bones. Symptoms are attributable to anemia (weakness, fatigue, dyspnea) and to splenomegaly (abdominal fullness and pain, which may be severe). Pain over the spleen from splenic infarcts is common. Spontaneous bleeding, secondary infection, bone pain, and a hypermetabolic state are frequent. Portal hypertension develops in some cases as a result of fibrosis of the liver, greatly increased splenic blood flow, or both.

Hepatomegaly is present in 75% of cases and splenomegaly with a firm and irregular spleen in all cases. Striking changes in the peripheral blood are referable to the combination of extramedullary hematopoiesis and hypersplenism. Patients are uniformly anemic, and red cells vary greatly in size and shape, many of them distorted and fragmented. The white count is usually high (20,000–50,000/μL). The platelet count may be elevated, but values less than 100,000/μL are seen in 30% of cases due to secondary hypersplenism. Bone marrow aspirates frequently result in a dry tap because marrow is replaced with fibrosis. It was once incorrectly thought that the spleen performed a crucial function of extramedullary hematopoiesis in this disease and that splenectomy could be lethal. In fact, many patients with myeloid metaplasia feel better if the massive spleen is removed, and their hypersplenism is often corrected.

About 30% of patients are asymptomatic at the time of initial diagnosis and require no therapy. When anemia and splenomegaly produce symptoms, transfusions, androgenic steroids, antimetabolites, and radiation therapy are indicated. Newer therapies include anti-angiogenesis treatments and immunosuppressive therapy. The bone marrow in this disease is the site of intense and inappropriate angiogenesis mediated by vascular endothelial growth factor (VEGF), and agents that block VEGF have shown benefit. A subset of patients with myeloid metaplasia has a component of autoimmune hemolytic anemia, and in this group of patients immunosuppressive therapy may be beneficial. Splenectomy is indicated in the following situations: (1) major hemolysis unresponsive to medical management, (2) severe symptoms of massive splenomegaly with mass effect of the spleen, (3) life-threatening thrombocytopenia, and (4) portal hypertension with variceal hemorrhage. This is one of the rare occasions when portal hypertension may be cured by splenectomy.

Splenectomy in myeloid metaplasia is associated with an 8–13% death rate and frequent complications often related to postsplenectomy hepatic morbidity. Splenectomy best relieves symptoms of splenomegaly and portal hypertension, but only about 50% of patients get relief from anemia and thrombocytopenia. Younger patients with normal platelet counts and symptoms are the best candidates for splenectomy in idiopathic myelofibrosis.

Cervantes F: Modern management of myelofibrosis. Br J Haematol 2005;128:583.

Raza A et al: Thalidomide produces transfusion independence in long-standing refractory anemias of patients with myelodysplastic syndrome. Blood 2001;98:958.

Saunthararajah Y et al: A simple method to predict response to immunosuppressive therapy in patients with myelodysplastic syndrome. Blood 2003;102:3025.

Teffer A: Myelofibrosis with myeloid metaplasia. N Engl J Med 2000;342:1255.

4. Systemic Mast Cell Disease

Systemic mast cell disease, or mastocytosis, is a rare condition characterized by mast cell infiltration of a number of tissues, including the spleen. There are two types: indolent and aggressive. In indolent systemic mass cell disease, there is no need for consideration of splenectomy. The aggressive type is associated with hematologic diseases with characteristics of lymphoma. Splenomegaly may occur, with the predominant symptoms resulting from thrombocytopenia due to hypersplenism. In this subgroup of patients with aggressive disease, splenectomy improves platelet counts and is associated with longer median survival time than for patients with aggressive disease who do not undergo splenectomy, although systemic therapy including alpha interferon has been shown to be effective.

Butterfield JH, Tefferi A, Kozuh GF: Successful treatment of systemic mastocytosis with high-dose interferon-alpha. Leuk Res 2005;29:131.

Hennessy B et al: Management of patients with systemic mastocytosis: review of the M.D. Anderson Cancer Center experience. Am J Hematol 2004;77:209.

METABOLIC DISORDERS

Metabolic disorders amenable to splenectomy are rare inherited diseases that include as a component splenic enlargement due to the pathologic deposition of material within the spleen. In Gaucher's disease, excess sphingolipid is deposited in the spleen. In sarcoidosis, the spleen becomes involved with noncaseating granulomas as can be seen in lymph nodes. Inherited disorders also include disease in which there is a specific immunologic target with associated destruction in the spleen.

1. Gaucher's Disease

Gaucher's disease is an autosomal recessive disorder characterized by a deficiency in beta-glucosidase, a lysosomal enzyme that degrades the sphingolipid glucocerebroside. There is an increased incidence of this disorder in Ashkenazi Jews. Three types of this disease exist, and the one amenable to splenectomy is type I, or the adult type. Pathologically, Gaucher's disease results in lipid accumulation within the white pulp of the spleen, the liver, or the bone marrow. Predominant symptoms relate to massive splenomegaly from either the direct effects of the size of the spleen or secondary to cytopenias from hypersplenism.

Treatment & Prognosis

Treatment by total splenectomy alleviates the symptoms but results in accelerated hepatic and bone disease as well as a significant increased risk of postsplenectomy infections. Treatment with partial or subtotal splenectomy has been studied over the past 10 years for both adults and children with Gaucher's disease. Removing most of the spleen corrects the symptoms of splenomegaly, but leaving a splenic remnant provides a site for further deposition of lipid that protects the liver and bone. The major problem with partial splenectomy is the eventual recurrence and enlargement of the splenic remnant accompanied by recurrent symptoms. As with hereditary spherocytosis, there is an increase incidence of pigmented gallstones occurring in up to two-thirds of female patients and one-third of male patients. The goal of subtotal splenectomy in Gaucher's disease is to leave a small fragment approximately the size of the fist of the patient. Replacement therapy with recombinant glucocerebrosidase enzyme has recently become available, but the cost of chronic treatment is prohibitive.

Ben Harosh-Katz M et al: Increased prevalence of cholelithiasis in Gaucher's Disease: association with splenectomy but not with Gilbert's Syndrome. J Clin Gastroenterol 2004;38:586.

Morgenstern L et al: Subtotal splenectomy for Gaucher's disease: a follow-up study. Am Surg 1993;59:860.

Zer M et al: Subtotal splenectomy in Gaucher's disease: towards a definition of critical splenic mass. Br J Surg 1992;79:742.

2. Wiskott-Aldrich Syndrome

Wiskott-Aldrich syndrome is an X-linked disease characterized by thrombocytopenia, combined B- and T-cell immunodeficiency, eczema, and a propensity to develop malignancies. Thrombocytopenia is the major feature of this rare disorder, with most patients presenting with bloody diarrhea, epistaxis, and petechiae at a young age. Platelet counts typically range between 20,000/μL and 40,000/μL, and the platelets that are present are between one-fourth and one-half of normal size. The spleen sequesters and destroys platelets in this disease, releasing "microplatelets" back into the circulation. The genetic defect in this disorder may be related to an abnormal adhesion molecule affecting immune as well as platelet cell-to-cell interaction.

Treatment & Prognosis

Splenectomy in Wiskott-Aldrich syndrome was at one time withheld, since the postoperative course was characterized by severe and fatal infections due to the underlying immune defect of this disorder combined with loss of the immune function of the spleen. However, splenectomy does normalize platelet shape, size, and numbers, and the use of prophylactic antibiotics after splenectomy has significantly increased survival rates. The optimal treatment of Wiskott-Aldrich syndrome is an HLA-matched sibling bone marrow transplantation. However, splenectomy with antibiotics results in better survival than an unmatched bone marrow transplantation. Patients who do not undergo bone marrow transplantation or splenectomy typically do not survive past the age of 5 years.

Verni W et al: The spleen in the Wiskott-Aldrich Syndrome: Histopathologic abnormalities of the white pulp correlate with the clinical phenotype of the disease. Am J Surg Pathol 1999;23:192.

3. Chédiak-Higashi Syndrome

Chédiak-Higashi syndrome is a rare autosomal recessive disease characterized by immunodeficiency that increases the susceptibility to bacterial and viral infections and is manifested by recurrent fever, nystagmus, and photophobia. Most patients experience widespread infiltration of tissues with histiocytes similar to a lymphoma. Secondary hepatosplenomegaly with lymphadenopathy, leukopenia, and bleeding complications occur in the accelerated phase of Chédiak-Higashi syndrome. Standard treatment includes chemotherapy, steroids, and ascorbic acid, but these patients have a poor prognosis. Splenectomy has been used in the accelerated phase with beneficial results.

Barton LM et al: Chediak-Higashi Syndrome. Br J Haematol 2004;125:2.

Harfi HA et al: Chédiak-Higashi syndrome: clinical, hematologic, and immunologic improvement after splenectomy. Ann Allergy 1992;69:147.

4. Sarcoidosis

Sarcoidosis is a granulomatous disease of unknown origin that can involve virtually any organ or area of the body. Pulmonary disease is most common, but autopsy studies have shown that the spleen is the second most common site, with enlargement by noncaseating granulomas in 50–60% of patients. However, most patients do not have massive splenomegaly. When this does occur, patients can have significant cytopenias related to hypersplenism as well as the constitutional symptoms and hypercalcemia of sarcoidosis. In this subgroup of patients, splenectomy is indicated as a potential curative procedure for each of these symptoms.

Kruithoff KL et al: Giant splenomegaly and refractory hypercalcemia due to extrapulmonary sarcoidosis. Arch Intern Med 1993;153:2793.

ERYTHROCYTE DISORDERS

In this category of diseases there is generally no intrinsic abnormality of the spleen, as opposed to hypersplenism, in which the spleen is primarily infiltrated by neoplasia or storage products and causes cytopenias due to increased volume of splenic tissue. In the autoimmune disorders, there is a humoral antibody response against proteins on circulating blood cells, resulting in depletion primarily within the spleen. Disorders involving platelets, erythrocytes, and neutrophils are listed in decreasing order of incidence. Erythrocyte disorders are genetic defects in structural components or hemoglobin that increase the clearance of red cells in the spleen, causing a significant decrease in erythrocyte half-life.

1. Hereditary Spherocytosis

ESSENTIALS OF DIAGNOSIS

- *Malaise, abdominal discomfort.*
- *Jaundice, anemia, splenomegaly.*
- *Spherocytosis, increased osmotic fragility of red cells, negative Coombs test.*

General Considerations

Hereditary spherocytosis (congenital hemolytic jaundice, familial hemolytic anemia), the most common congenital hemolytic anemia (affecting 1:5000 individuals), is transmitted as an autosomal dominant trait. It is caused by a variety of genetic defects related to abnormal cellular structural proteins, primarily spectrin and ankyrin, which alter binding of the cytoskeleton to the cellular membrane, causing a decreased cellular plasticity with membrane loss. The normal shape of the erythrocyte is changed from a biconcave disk into a sphere, and the decreased membrane-to-cell volume ratio causes a lack of deformability that delays passage through the channels of the splenic red pulp. Significant cell destruction occurs only in the presence of the spleen. Hemolysis is largely relieved by splenectomy.

The condition is seen in all races but is more frequent in whites than in blacks. When discovered early in infancy, it may resemble hemolytic disease of the newborn due to ABO incompatibility. In occasional instances the diagnosis is not made until later in adult life, but it is usually discovered in the first 3 decades.

Clinical Findings

A. Symptoms and Signs

The principal manifestations are splenomegaly, mild to moderate anemia, and jaundice. The patient may complain of easy fatigability. The spleen is almost always enlarged and may cause fullness and discomfort in the left upper quadrant. However, most patients are diagnosed during a family survey at a time when they are asymptomatic.

Periodic exacerbations of hemolysis can occur. The rare hypoplastic crises, which often follow acute viral illnesses, may be associated with profound anemia, headache, nausea, abdominal pain, pancytopenia, and hypoactive marrow.

B. Laboratory Findings

The red cell count and hemoglobin are moderately reduced. Some of the asymptomatic patients detected by family surveys have normal red cell counts when first seen. The red cells are usually normocytic, but microcytosis may occur. Macrocytosis may present during periods of marked reticulocytosis. Spherocytes in varying numbers, sizes, and shapes are seen on a Wright-stained smear. The reticulocyte count is increased to 5–20%.

The indirect serum bilirubin and stool urobilinogen are usually elevated, and serum haptoglobin is usually decreased to absent. The Coombs test is negative. Osmotic fragility is increased; hemolysis of 5–10% of cells may be observed at saline concentrations of 0.6%. A more accurate reflector of fragility is the cryohemolysis test, which has a sensitivity and specificity of almost 95% for spherocytosis. Occasionally, the osmotic fragility is normal but the incubated fragility test (defibrinated blood incubated at 37 °C for 24 hours) will show increased hemolysis. Autohemolysis of defibrinated blood incubated under sterile conditions for 48 hours is usually greatly increased (10–20%, compared to a normal value of < 5%). The addition of 10% glucose before incubation will decrease the abnormal osmotic fragility and autohemolysis. Infusion of the patient's own blood labeled with ^{51}Cr shows a greatly shortened red cell life span and sequestration in the spleen. Normal red cells labeled with ^{51}Cr have a normal life span when transfused into a spherocytotic patient, indicating that splenic function is normal.

Differential Diagnosis

At present there is no pathognomonic test for hereditary spherocytosis, although the cryohemolysis test is very promising. Spherocytes in large numbers may occur in autoimmune hemolytic anemias, in which osmotic fragility and autohemolysis may be increased but are usually not improved by incubation with glucose. The positive Coombs test, negative family history, and sharply reduced survival of normal donor red cells are diagnostic of autoimmune hemolysis. Spherocytes are also seen in hemoglobin C disease, in some alcoholics, and in some severe burns.

Complications

Pigment gallstones occur in about 85% of adults with spherocytosis but are uncommon under age 10. On the other hand, gallstones in a child should suggest congenital spherocytosis.

Chronic leg ulcers unrelated to varicosities are a rare complication but, when present, will heal only after the spleen is removed.

Treatment

Splenectomy is the sole treatment for hereditary spherocytosis and is indicated even when the anemia is fully compensated and the patient is asymptomatic. The longer the hemolytic process persists, the greater the potential risk of complications such as hypoplastic crises and cholelithiasis. At operation, the gallbladder should be inspected for stones and accessory spleens should be sought. When there is associated cholelithiasis, cholecystectomy should be performed along with the splenectomy. Unless the clinical manifestations are severe, splenectomy should be delayed in children until age 6 to avoid the risk of increased infection due to loss of reticuloendothelial function. For children under age 5 with severe disease and high transfusion requirements, a partial (80%) splenectomy may correct symptoms while maintaining the normal immune functions of the spleen.

Prognosis

Splenectomy cures the anemia and jaundice in all patients. The membrane abnormality, spherocytosis, and increased osmotic fragility persist, but red cell life span becomes almost normal. An overlooked accessory spleen is an occasional cause of failure of splenectomy. The presence of Howell-Jolly bodies in red cells makes the presence of accessory spleens unlikely.

Khoursheed M et al: Laparoscopic splenectomy for hematological disorders. Med Princ Pract 2004;13:122.

Stoehr GA, Stauffer UG, Eber SW: Near-total splenectomy: a new technique for the management of hereditary spherocytosis. Ann Surg 2005;241:40.

Tanoue K et al: Laparoscopic splenectomy for hematologic diseases. Surgery 2002;131:S318.

2. Hereditary Elliptocytosis

This autosomal dominant genetic disorder, also known as ovalocytosis, is usually of little clinical significance. Normally, up to 15% oval or elliptic red blood cells can be seen on a peripheral blood smear. In elliptocytosis, at least 25% and up to 90% of circulating erythrocytes are elliptic. As with hereditary spherocytosis, this disease is due to a variety of genetic defects in cytoskeletal proteins such as spectrin. The predominant abnormality is that this structural protein exists as a dimer instead of a tetramer, leading to change in the erythrocyte's shape, decreased plasticity, and a shortened life span of the cell.

Most affected individuals are asymptomatic; about 10% have clinical manifestations consisting of moderate anemia, slight jaundice, and a palpable spleen.

Symptomatic patients should have splenectomy, and cholecystectomy if gallstones are present. The red cell defect persists after splenectomy, but the hemolysis and anemia are cured.

Gallagher PG: Update on the clinical spectrum and genetics of red blood cell membrane disorders. Curr Hematol Rep 2004;3:85.

Silveira P et al: Red blood cell abnormalities in hereditary elliptocytosis and their relevance to variable clinical expression. Am J Clin Pathol 1997;108:391.

3. Hereditary Nonspherocytic Hemolytic Anemia

This is a heterogeneous group of rare hemolytic anemias caused by inherited intrinsic red cell defects that lead to oxidative hemolysis. Included in the group are pyruvate kinase deficiency and glucose 6-phosphate dehydrogenase (G6PD) deficiency. They are usually manifested in early childhood with anemia, jaundice, reticulocytosis, erythroid hyperplasia of the marrow, and normal osmotic fragility. As with other hemolytic anemias, there may be associated cholelithiasis.

Multiple blood transfusions are often required. Splenectomy, while not curative, may ameliorate some of these conditions, especially pyruvate kinase deficiency. In G6PD deficiency, splenectomy is not beneficial, and treatment consists of avoidance of dietary oxidants.

Baronciani L et al: Hematologically important mutations: red cell pyruvate kinase. Blood Cells Mol Dis 1998;24:273.

4. Thalassemia Major (Mediterranean Anemia; Cooley's Anemia)

In the most common form of this autosomal dominant disorder, a structural defect in the β-globin chain causes excess α chains to precipitate on the inner surface of the membrane of the erythrocyte and produces abnormal red cells (eg, target cells). Heterozygotes usually have mild anemia (thalassemia minor); however, starting early in infancy, homozygotes have severe chronic anemia accompanied by jaundice, hepatosplenomegaly (often massive), retarded body growth, and enlargement of the head. The peripheral blood smear reveals target cells, nucleated red cells, and a hypochromic microcytic anemia. Gallstones are present in about 25% of patients. A characteristic feature is the persistence of fetal hemoglobin (Hb F).

Since the anemia of thalassemia is due to both increased destruction of red cells and decreased hemoglobin production, splenectomy does not cure the anemia, as in spherocytosis, but it may reduce transfusion requirements by removing an enlarged, uncomfortable spleen. Treatment is by iron chelation and transfusion.

Al-Salem AH, Nasserulla Z: Splenectomy for children with thalassemia. Int Surg 2002;87:269.

Weatherall DJ: The thalassemias. BMJ 1997;314:1675.

AUTOIMMUNE DISORDERS

The production of IgG autoantibodies specific for cell membrane proteins on erythrocytes causes autoimmune hemolytic anemia; on platelets, it causes idiopathic thrombocytopenic purpura (ITP) and may cause neutropenia in Felty's syndrome. Macrophages express Fc receptors for IgG, and antibody-coated cells that pass through the splenic sinuses of the red pulp come into contact with these phagocytic cells. Furthermore, the microenvironment of the red pulp with slow flow of blood with a high cellular content through circuitous spaces facilitates opsonization of cells in the spleen. Production of autoantibodies in the white pulp germinal centers may also enhance cellular destruction, particularly in ITP. Understanding this pathophysiologic mechanism is important, since autoimmune hemolytic anemia caused by IgM autoantibodies (ie, cold agglutinin hemolytic anemia) does not respond to splenectomy because macrophages do not have Fc receptors for IgM. This mechanism also explains why treatment with high-dose intravenous immune globulin is beneficial in these diseases because it blocks the macrophage Fc receptor.

1. Acquired Hemolytic Anemia

ESSENTIALS OF DIAGNOSIS

- *Fatigue, pallor, jaundice.*
- *Splenomegaly.*
- *Persistent anemia and reticulocytosis.*

General Considerations

The **autoimmune hemolytic anemias** have also been classified according to the optimal temperature at which autoantibodies react with the red cell surface (warm or cold antibodies). This classification is particularly useful, since patients with cold antibodies will not benefit from splenectomy but those with warm antibodies may.

Although hemolysis without demonstrable antibody (Coombs test-negative) may occur in uremia, cirrhosis of the liver, cancer, and certain infections, in most cases the red cell membranes are coated with either immunoglobulin or complement (Coombs test-positive). The antibody in IgG autoimmune hemolytic anemia is specifically directed against the Rh locus on the erythrocyte. Initiation of this disease is either idiopathic (40–50%) or secondary to drug exposure, connective tissue disorders, or lymphoproliferative disorders. Cold agglutinin hemolytic anemia is due typically to an IgM directed against the I red cell antigen, and hemolysis occurs intravascularly by complement fixation and not within the spleen.

About 20% of cases of secondary immune hemolytic anemia are due to drug use, and hemolysis is usually mediated by warm antibodies. Penicillin, quinidine, hydralazine, and methyldopa have been most commonly implicated in this syndrome (Table 27–3).

Clinical Findings

A. Symptoms and Signs

Autoimmune hemolytic anemia may be encountered at any age but is most common after age 50; it occurs twice as often in women. The onset is usually acute, consisting of anemia, mild jaundice, and sometimes fever. The spleen is palpably enlarged in over 50% of patients, and pigment gallstones are present in about 25%. Rarely, a sudden severe onset produces hemoglobinuria, renal tubular necrosis, and a 40–50% death rate.

B. Laboratory Findings

Hemolytic anemia is diagnosed by demonstrating a normocytic normochromic anemia, reticulocytosis (over 10%), erythroid hyperplasia of the marrow, and elevation of serum indirect bilirubin. Stool urobilinogen may be greatly increased, but there is no bile in the urine. Serum haptoglobin is usually low or absent. The direct Coombs test is positive because the red cells are coated with immunoglobulins or complement (or both).

Treatment

Associated diseases must be carefully sought and appropriately treated. For drug-induced secondary hemolytic anemia, further exposure to the offending agent must be terminated. Corticosteroids produce a remission in about 75% of patients, but only 25% of remissions are

Table 27–3. Disorders associated with immune hemolysis.

Immune drug reaction (penicillin, quinidine, hydralazine, methyldopa, cimetidine)
Collagen vascular disease (lupus erythematosus, rheumatoid arthritis)
Tumors (lymphoma, myeloma, leukemia, dermoid cysts, ovarian teratoma)
Infection (*Mycoplasma*, malaria, syphilis, viremia)

permanent. Transfusion should be avoided if possible, since crossmatching may be extremely difficult, requiring washed red cells and saline-active antisera.

Splenectomy is indicated for patients with warm-antibody hemolysis who fail to respond to 4–6 weeks of high-dose corticosteroid therapy, for patients who relapse after an initial response when steroids are withdrawn, and for patients in whom steroid therapy is contraindicated (eg, those with active pulmonary tuberculosis). Patients who require chronic high-dose steroid therapy should also be considered for splenectomy, since the risks of long-term steroid administration are substantial.

Splenectomy is effective because it removes the principal site of red cell destruction. Occasionally, splenectomy discloses the presence of an underlying disorder such as lymphoma. About half of patients who fail to respond to splenectomy will respond to azathioprine or cyclophosphamide. Plasmapheresis has been employed as salvage therapy in patients with refractory hemolytic anemia.

Prognosis

Relapses may occur after splenectomy but are less frequent if the initial response was good. The ultimate prognosis in the secondary cases depends upon the underlying disorder.

Beutler E et al: Hemolytic anemia. Semin Hematol 1999;36:38.

Rice HE et al: Clinical and hematologic benefits of partial splenectomy for congenital hemolytic anemias in children. Ann Surg 2003;237:281.

2. Immune Thrombocytopenic Purpura (Idiopathic Thrombocytopenic Purpura, ITP)

ESSENTIALS OF DIAGNOSIS

- *Petechiae, ecchymoses, epistaxis, easy bruising.*
- *No splenomegaly.*
- *Decreased platelet count, prolonged bleeding time, poor clot retraction, normal coagulation time.*

General Considerations

Immune thrombocytopenic purpura is a hemorrhagic syndrome with diverse causes that can occur in an acute or chronic form and is characterized by marked reduction in the number of circulating platelets, abundant megakaryocytes in the bone marrow, and a shortened platelet life span. It may be idiopathic or secondary to a lymphoproliferative disorder, drugs or toxins, bacterial or viral infection (especially in children), systemic lupus erythematosus, or other conditions. An increased incidence of immune thrombocytopenic purpura has also been identified in homosexual males and appears to be associated with the acquired immunodeficiency syndrome (AIDS). Although responses to corticosteroids and to splenectomy in these patients are comparable to the responses observed in other patients with immune thrombocytopenic purpura, splenectomy should be reserved for those with signs of blood loss, since surgical complications are high and survival may be short. These patients may also have associated opportunistic infections, making corticosteroid treatment more hazardous.

The pathogenesis of both primary and secondary disorders involves a circulating antiplatelet IgG autoantibody usually directed against a membrane protein which is the fibrinogen receptor (glycoprotein IIb/IIIa). In this disorder, the spleen is primarily the site of platelet destruction and may also be a significant source of autoantibody production. Splenomegaly, present in only 2% of cases, is usually a manifestation of another underlying disease such as lymphoma or lupus erythematosus. Five to 15 percent of HIV-positive patients have thrombocytopenia independent of the immunologic state of their disease that is clinically indistinguishable from typical chronic ITP. The precise pathophysiologic mechanism in relation to HIV infection is not known.

Clinical Findings

A. Symptoms and Signs

The onset may be acute, with ecchymoses or showers of petechiae, and may be accompanied by bleeding gums, vaginal bleeding, gastrointestinal bleeding, and hematuria. Central nervous system bleeding occurs in 3% of patients. The acute form is most common in children, usually occurring before 8 years of age, and often begins 1–3 weeks after a viral upper respiratory illness.

The chronic form, which may start at any age, is more common in women. It characteristically has an insidious onset, often with a long history of easy bruisability and menorrhagia. Showers of petechiae may occur, especially over pressure areas. Cyclic remissions and exacerbations may continue for several years.

B. Laboratory Findings

The platelet count is moderately to severely decreased (always below 100,000/μL), and platelets may be absent from the peripheral blood smear. Although white and red cell counts are usually normal, iron deficiency anemia may be present as a result of bleeding.

The bone marrow shows increased numbers of large megakaryocytes without platelet budding.

The bleeding time is prolonged, capillary fragility (Rumpel-Leede test) greatly increased, and clot retraction poor. Partial thromboplastin time, prothrombin time, and coagulation time are normal. Specific determinations of antiplatelet antibody titers can now be routinely assessed to aid in diagnosis. Reduced red cell or platelet survival can be measured by labeling the patient's cells with ^{51}Cr or the platelets with indium-111 and measuring the rate of disappearance of radioactivity from the blood. The spleen's role in producing the anemia or thrombocytopenia can be determined by measuring the ratio of radioactivity that accumulates in the liver and spleen during destruction of the tagged cells; a spleen/liver ratio greater than 2 to 1 indicates significant splenic pooling and suggests that splenectomy would be beneficial.

Differential Diagnosis

Other causes of nonimmunologic thrombocytopenia must be ruled out, such as leukemia, aplastic anemia, and macroglobulinemia. Thrombocytopenia and purpura may be caused by ineffective thrombocytopoiesis (eg, pernicious anemia, preleukemic states) or by nonimmune platelet destruction (eg, septicemia, disseminated intravascular coagulation, or other causes of hypersplenism).

Treatment

Treatment of immune thrombocytopenic purpura depends on the age of the patient, the severity of the disease, the duration of the thrombocytopenia, and the clinical variant. Secondary immune thrombocytopenias are best managed by treating the underlying primary disorder (eg, if it is drug-induced, the drug should be stopped).

Patients with mild or no symptoms need no specific therapy but should avoid contact sports, elective surgery, and all nonessential medications. Corticosteroids are indicated in patients with moderate to severe purpura of short duration. Usually, 60 mg of prednisone (or equivalent) is required daily; this is continued until the platelet count returns to normal and then is gradually tapered after 4–6 weeks. Corticosteroids produce a response in 70–80%, but sustained remissions in only 20% of adults.

Splenectomy is the most effective form of therapy and is indicated for patients who do not respond to corticosteroids, for those who relapse after an initial remission on steroids, and for steroid-dependent patients. Corticosteroid therapy is not necessary in the immediate preoperative period unless bleeding is severe or the patient was receiving steroids before the operation. If indicated, platelet transfusions are given intraoperatively only after ligation of the splenic artery or removal of the spleen, since platelets from earlier transfusion would be rapidly sequestered in the spleen. For temporary treatment of the thrombocytopenia, intravenous immunoglobulin (IGIV) is effective.

Splenectomy produces a sustained remission in about 68% of patients. As with corticosteroids, success rates are better with acute than chronic immune thrombocytopenic purpura. Two factors associated with better outcomes are shorter duration of disease and younger age. The platelet count usually rises promptly following splenectomy (eg, it may double in 24 hours) and reaches a peak after 1–2 weeks. If the platelet count remains elevated after 2 months, the patient can be considered cured. When corticosteroids and splenectomy have failed, immunosuppressive drugs (azathioprine, vincristine) will achieve a remission in 25% of cases.

The benefit of splenectomy for HIV-associated ITP has been less clear. The risk of infection and the overall shortened survival in this population argue against splenectomy. However, in HIV patients without AIDS, clinically significant thrombocytopenia responds completely in 70% and there is partial improvement in 20% following splenectomy. Splenectomy does not appear to alter the overall natural history of HIV infection.

Prognosis

Acute immune thrombocytopenic purpura in children under age 16 has an excellent prognosis; approximately 80% of patients have a complete and permanent spontaneous remission. This occurs rarely in adults. Splenectomy is successful in about 80% of patients, but more often in idiopathic cases than in those secondary to another disorder.

Kojouri K et al: Splenectomy for adult patients with idiopathic thrombocytopenic purpura: a systematic review to assess long-term platelet count responses, prediction of response, and surgical complications. Blood 2003;104:2623.

McMillan R, Durette C: Long-term outcomes in adults with chronic ITP after splenectomy failure. Blood 2004;104:956.

Phom H et al: Comparative evaluation of Tc-99m-heat-denatured RBC and Tc-99m-anti-D IgG opsonized RBC spleen planar and SPECT scintigraphy in the detection of accessory spleen in postsplenectomy patients with chronic idiopathic thrombocytopenic purpura. Clin Nucl Med 2004;29:403.

Silver RM: Management of idiopathic thrombocytopenic purpura in pregnancy. Clin Obstet Gynecol 1998;41:436.

Stasi R, Provan D: Management of immune thrombocytopenic purpura in adults. Mayo Clin Proc 2004;79:504.

Tsereteli Z et al: Are the favorable outcomes of splenectomy predictable in patients with idiopathic thrombocytopenic purpura (ITP)? Surg Endosc 2001;15:1386.

Vesely SK et al: Treatment options for idiopathic thrombocytopenic purpura when splenectomy in ineffective. Ann Intern Med 2004;140:138.

3. Felty's Syndrome

Approximately 1% of patients with rheumatoid arthritis have splenomegaly and neutropenia—a triad known as Felty's syndrome. High levels of IgG have been identified on the surface of neutrophils with evidence of increased of granulopoiesis in the bone marrow. Pathologic analysis of the spleen in Felty's syndrome patients shows a larger proportionate increase in the white pulp as opposed to most conditions of splenomegaly. There is evidence of excess accumulation of neutrophils in both the T cell zone of the white pulp as well as the cord and sinuses of the red pulp.

Patients with severe neutropenia have clinical symptoms of recurring infections in Felty's syndrome. Symptomatic patients who have evidence of IgG on the surface of neutrophils should be considered for splenectomy. Neutropenia will improve in 60–70% of these patients, but relapse of neutropenia as well as recurrent infections in the presence of normal neutrophil counts may occur, and these untoward events have dampened enthusiasm for splenectomy in this disease.

Balint GP, Balint PV: Felty's syndrome. Best Pract Res Clin Rheumatol 2004;18:631.

Logue GL et al: Failure of splenectomy in Felty's syndrome. N Engl J Med 1981;304:580.

4. Thrombotic Thrombocytopenic Purpura

Thrombotic thrombocytopenic purpura (TTP) is a rare disease with a pentad of clinical features: (1) fever, (2) thrombocytopenic purpura, (3) hemolytic anemia, (4) neurologic manifestations, and (5) renal failure. The cause is unknown, but autoimmunity to endothelial cells or a primary platelet defect has been implicated, and its occurrence in patients with AIDS has been reported. It is most common between ages 10 and 40 years.

The thrombocytopenia is probably due to a shortened platelet life span. The microangiopathic hemolytic anemia is produced by passage of red cells over damaged small blood vessels containing fibrin strands. Rigid red cells are trapped and fragmented in the spleen, whereas those that escape the spleen may be more vulnerable to damage and destruction in the abnormal microvasculature. The anemia is often severe, and it may be aggravated by hemorrhage secondary to thrombocytopenia. Hepatomegaly and splenomegaly occur in 35% of cases.

Treatment & Prognosis

Until recently, there was no effective therapy for this disorder, and mortality rates as high as 95% were reported. Most patients died of renal failure or cerebral bleeding. Plasmapheresis with plasma exchange has recently emerged as an effective form of treatment that is superior to simple plasma infusion. The plasma supernatant after cryoprecipitation may be more effective than whole plasma. When combined with other therapies, including corticosteroids, dextran, splenectomy, and antiplatelet drugs, prolonged remission can be achieved in most patients.

Allford SL et al: Current understanding of the pathophysiology of thrombotic thrombocytopenic purpura. J Clin Path 2000;53:497.

Aqui NA et al: Role of splenectomy in patients with refractory or relapsed thrombotic thrombocytopenic purpura. J Clin Apheresis 2003;18:51.

Modic M, Cernelc P, Sver S: Splenectomy: the last option of immunosuppressive therapy in patients with chronic or relapsing idiopathic thrombotic thrombocytopenic purpura? Transplant Proc 2002;34:2953.

Rock GA: Management of thrombotic thrombocytopenic purpura. Br J Haematol 2000;109:496.

VASCULAR DISORDERS OF THE SPLEEN

Vascular disease of the spleen treated by splenectomy can occur both with the arterial inflow and the venous outflow. The most common disease is splenic vein thrombosis; this can be treated in a straightforward manner by splenectomy. Splenic artery aneurysms are one of the most common sites of visceral aneurysms and may require splenectomy (discussed in Chapter 34).

SPLENIC VEIN THROMBOSIS

Etiology

Thrombosis of the splenic vein can occur as an isolated event not due to any pathologic findings in the spleen but due to diseases that impact on the splenic vein as it travels along the superior border of the pancreas. The most common cause is acute or chronic pancreatitis or a pseudocyst of the body/tail of the pancreas, with the general inflammatory reaction in the pancreas resulting in thrombosis of the splenic vein. Inflammation from a posterior gastric ulcer is another cause. Direct extension of carcinoma of the pancreas or stomach into the lesser sac may cause splenic vein thrombosis, but the diagnosis is generally not subtle because of other manifestations of these malignancies. Idiopathic retroperitoneal fibrosis may be an alternative cause of splenic vein thrombosis.

Splenic vein thrombosis presents as upper gastrointestinal hemorrhage due to isolated gastric varices. With occlusion of the splenic vein, outflow of blood from the spleen is diverted into the short gastric veins as the remaining collateral vessels. These veins dilate and become varices primarily in the fundus of the stomach, resulting in bleeding.

Diagnosis

Splenic vein thrombosis is suspected when there are isolated varices of the stomach particularly in the proximal greater curvature without any esophageal varices. Since there is no portal hypertension, there are no associated signs or symptoms of cirrhosis. Definitive diagnosis is made by confirming that there is no blood flow in the main splenic vein. Invasive venography is no longer needed because this diagnosis can be confirmed by CT scan or MRI scans with contrast material or by high-resolution ultrasound. CT or MRI is preferred because the splenic vein may be hidden from ultrasound by bowel gas and CT or MRI allows characterization of the surrounding structures (pancreas, stomach) to assess for causative pathology.

Treatment & Prognosis

Splenectomy is curative in patients with splenic vein thrombosis. All of the symptoms relate to increased splenic blood flow through collateral vessels; eliminating that blood flow is curative. If a splenic vein thrombosis is diagnosed—even if the patients have not had an episode of upper gastrointestinal hemorrhage—an elective or prophylactic splenectomy is indicated if the patients are otherwise healthy. In patients with portal vein thrombosis, the magnitude of the disease and associated problems is greatly amplified, and splenectomy is almost never indicated because it is not curative.

Loftus JP et al: Sinistra portal hypertension. Splenectomy or expectant management. Ann Surg 1993;217:35.

CYSTS & TUMORS OF THE SPLEEN

Parasitic cysts are almost always echinococcal (see Chapter 8). They may be asymptomatic, but usually the patient notices splenomegaly. Calcification of the cyst wall may be seen on x-ray. Eosinophilia may be found, and serologic tests may confirm the diagnosis. The treatment of choice is splenectomy.

Other cysts are dermoid, epidermoid, endothelial, and pseudocysts. The latter are thought to be late results of infarction or trauma. Splenectomy may be indicated to exclude tumor; however, partial splenectomy or observation has been advocated.

The rare primary tumors of the spleen include lymphoma, sarcoma, hemangioma, and hamartoma. Hamartomas may be confused grossly with splenic lymphoma at laparotomy. These lesions are usually asymptomatic until splenomegaly causes abdominal discomfort or a palpable mass. The benign vascular tumors of the spleen (angiomas) can produce hypersplenism. Spontaneous rupture with massive hemorrhage can occur. Splenectomy is indicated if the tumor appears to be limited to the spleen. Inflammatory pseudotumors are benign lesions composed of a mixture of inflammatory cells and a granulomatous reaction that can occur in a variety of organs, including the spleen. Constitutional symptoms of lethargy, weight loss, and fatigue occur and can be alleviated by splenectomy.

The spleen is a common site for metastases in advanced cancers, especially of the lung and breast and melanoma. Splenic metastases are common autopsy findings but are rarely clinically significant.

Atmatzidis K et al: Splenectomy versus spleen-preserving surgery for splenic echinococcosis. Dig Surg 2003;20:527.

Du Plessis DG et al: Mucinous epithelial cysts of the spleen associated with pseudomyxoma peritonei. Histopathology 1999;35:551.

Kraus MD, Fleming MD, Vonderheide RH: The spleen as a diagnostic specimen: a review of 10 years' experience at two tertiary care institutions. Cancer 2001;91:2001.

Mackenzie RK, Youngson GG, Mahomed AA: Laparoscopic decapsulation of congenital splenic cysts: a step forward in splenic preservation. J Ped Surg 2004;39:88.

Scott GC et al: CT patterns of nodular hepatic and splenic sarcoidosis: a review of the literature. J Comput Assist Tomogr 1997;21:369.

Yu RS, Zhang SZ, Hua JM: Imaging findings of splenic hamartoma. World J Gastroent 2004;10:13.

INFECTIONS OF THE SPLEEN (Splenic Abscess)

Splenic abscesses are uncommon but are important because the death rate ranges between 40% and 100%. They may be caused by hematogenous seeding of the spleen with bacteria from remote sepsis such as endocarditis, by direct spread of infection from adjacent structures, or by splenic trauma resulting in a secondarily infected splenic hematoma. Splenic abscess is a complication of intravenous drug abuse. In 80% of cases, one or more abscesses exist in organs other than the spleen, and the splenic abscess develops as a terminal manifestation of uncontrolled sepsis in other organs. Enteric organisms are found in over two-thirds of splenic abscesses, with staphylococci and nonenteric streptococci comprising the majority of the remainder. In some patients, unexplained sepsis, progressive splenic enlargement, and abdominal pain are the presenting manifestations. The spleen may not be palpable, because of left upper quadrant tenderness and guarding. A left pleural effusion combined with unexplained leukocytosis in a septic patient suggests a splenic abscess. The finding of gas in the spleen on plain abdominal x-ray is pathognomonic of splenic abscess, but CT scan is the optimal way to define and diagnose a splenic abscess.

Most splenic abscesses remain localized, periodically seeding the bloodstream with bacteria, but spontaneous rupture and peritonitis may occur. Splenectomy is essential for cure if sepsis is localized to the spleen. Percutaneous drainage of large, solitary juxtacapsular abscesses may occasionally be feasible but is associated with an extremely high mortality rate and should be reserved for patients unable to withstand an operation.

Ooi LL et al: Splenic abscesses from 1987 to 1995. Am J Surg 1997; 174:87.

Phillips GS et al: Splenic abscess: another look at an old disease. Arch Surg 1997;132:1331.

DIAGNOSTIC SPLENECTOMY

One indication for splenectomy is for diagnosis in an otherwise asymptomatic patient. Splenectomy may be needed to make a diagnosis when an asymptomatic mass lesion is seen within the spleen on CT scan, ultrasound, or MRI scan for which a definitive diagnosis cannot be made radiographically. Another example is when a patient has either a palpable spleen on physical examination or an enlarged spleen by scan, and otherwise has no clear diagnostic disorder.

Splenic Mass Lesions

For the patients who have an isolated splenic mass, 60% turned out to be malignant lesions and 40% turned out to be benign lesions. Most malignant lesions are lymphoma; another large group is metastatic carcinomas, including some in which the primary diagnosis had not been made previously. In patients with benign lesions, more than half were cysts, and there were also splenic hamartomas and splenic hemangiomas.

In diagnosing an isolated splenic mass, most of these lesions could have been diagnosed by doing a fine-needle aspiration biopsy. Certain of these lesions—such as the cystic lesions or the hemangiomas—would have classic appearance on gadolinium-enhanced MRI scan, and these scans are another imaging modality that could be utilized to sort out mass lesions without tissue biopsy. Although there may be some hesitation to do fine-needle aspiration biopsies on splenic lesions due to the risk of bleeding, most mass lesions can be diagnosed with this minimally invasive technique. The risk of bleeding is significant in patients with hemangiomas. These benign tumors of endothelial cells can be definitively diagnosed with gadolinium-enhanced MRI, and this imaging test is optimal for characterizing an isolated splenic mass.

Splenomegaly without a Diagnosis

The second diagnostic indication for splenectomy is unexplained splenomegaly. Most of these enlarged spleens will be shown to have lymphoma. The minority will have benign diagnoses including benign lymphoid proliferation, benign vascular lesions, and granulomatous disease, as well as splenic infarction and hemorrhage. The role of the fine-needle aspiration and other percutaneous biopsies for undiagnosed splenomegaly is quite limited; there would be very low yield in terms of being able to make that diagnosis by that form of biopsy.

Staging Laparotomy for Hodgkin's Disease

Another type of diagnostic procedure would be a staging laparotomy for Hodgkin's disease. Discussion of this procedure is more of a historical note because it has limited use in today's current practice in treating this form of lymphoma.

A standard practice for pathologic staging between 1960 and 1990 was performance of a staging laparotomy in most patients with Hodgkin's disease. The reason for performing this invasive procedure was based on reports that laparotomy altered the clinical stage of disease in approximately 35% of patients. There are several reasons why the incidence of performing staging laparotomy has decreased over the past 10–15 years. The primary reason is that it does not alter treatment of Hodgkin's disease based on results of recent clinical series. Since systemic chemotherapy treats the whole patient, accurate pathologic staging makes no impact on the treatment outcome or treatment decisions.

Kraus MD, Fleming MD, Vonderheide RH: The spleen as a diagnostic specimen: a review of 10 years' experience at two tertiary care institutions. Cancer 2001;91:2001.

Linet MS et al: Risk of cancer following splenectomy. Int J Cancer 1996;66:611.

Rose AT et al: The incidence of splenectomy is decreasing: lessons learned from trauma experience. Am Surg 2000;66:481.

Swerdlow AJ et al: Risk of second primary cancer after Hodgkin's disease in patients in the British National Lymphoma Investigation: relationships to host factors, histology, and stage of Hodgkin's disease, and splenectomy. Br J Cancer 1993;68:1006.

Tura S et al: Splenectomy and the increasing risk of secondary acute leukemia in Hodgkin's disease. J Clin Oncol 1993;11:925.

IATROGENIC SPLENECTOMY

Procedures in which mobilization of the left upper quadrant is done (such as reflection of the spleen and pancreas medially to expose retroperitoneal tissue, left adrenalectomy, and left nephrectomy) put the spleen at risk for injury during the dissection. Simple mobilization of the splenic flexure of the colon can lead to bleeding from the inferior pole of the spleen that may be difficult to control. The ligaments that go directly from the omentum to the capsule of the spleen may be the most common cause of iatrogenic splenic trauma, as it is a common practice to aggressively retract the omentum as needed for exposure. If there are direct branches that sometimes may be sizable from the omentum to the splenic capsule, this could lead to capsular disruption and troublesome bleeding. A national database on antireflux procedures of 86,411 patients reported an incidence of iatrogenic splenectomy of 2.3%, which translates into 1987 iatrogenic splenectomies for that indication alone over a 6-year period.

Probably the best data for the incidence of iatrogenic splenectomy come from the recently reported series that listed 73 iatrogenic splenectomies over a 10-year period, or an average of 7 per year. This comprised 8.1% of all splenectomies performed during that time interval. There are probably several times that number of minor or moderate injuries to the spleen during unrelated operations in which the spleen was not removed but was repaired or salvaged. Just as in trauma to the spleen, the techniques of splenorrhaphy can be employed to preserve the spleen. A recent report indicates that use of a mesh wrap splenorrhaphy even in the setting of bowel surgery does not lead to an increased incidence of infection. For minor capsular disruption, the use of the argon beam coagulator for surface cautery is a helpful technique.

The primary teaching point regarding iatrogenic injuries is that the best way to preserve the spleen is to not damage it in the first place. This requires caution in mobilizing tissue in and around the spleen as well as visual inspection of the attachments of the spleen prior to blunt mobilization. Whenever possible, the spleen should be attempted to be preserved to decrease the risk of post-splenectomy sepsis.

Berry MF, Rosato EF, Williams NN: Dexon mesh splenorrhaphy for intraoperative splenic injuries. Am Surg 2003;69:176.

Brennan TV et al: Congenital cleft spleen with CT scan appearance of high-grade splenic laceration after blunt abdominal trauma. J Emerg Med 2003;25:139.

Cassar K, Munro A: Iatrogenic splenic injury. J Roy Coll Surg Edinburgh 2002;47:731.

Flum DR et al: The nationwide frequency of major adverse outcomes in antireflux surgery and the role of surgeon experience. J Am Coll Surg 2002;195:611.

INCIDENTAL SPLENECTOMY

In a recent large series evaluating reasons for splenectomy from tertiary institutions, the single most common indication for splenectomy was as an incidental procedure on operations on an adjacent organ. In these situations the spleen needs to be removed either for completeness of resection or because of division of the splenic vasculature. The actual primary treatments of those various disease entities in adjacent organs are subjects of multiple other chapters within this textbook, but a few comments need to be made regarding the reasons for splenectomy and whether splenic preservation procedures are possible.

One common indication for an incidental splenectomy is to remove tumors located in the distal pancreas. For decades, it was standard practice to remove the spleen when removing the body and tail of the pancreas because the splenic vein is intimately associated with the distal pancreas. Because of the interest in splenic preservation due to the incidence of post-splenectomy infection, operations have been developed to remove the distal pancreas without removing the spleen. The more technically challenging operation is a distal pancreatectomy with preservation of the splenic artery and vein. A second spleen-preserving distal pancreatectomy involves ligation of the splenic artery and vein but preservation of short gastric vessels and utilizing those vessels as collateral inflow and outflow to maintain splenic viability. Removal of the distal pancreas with splenic preservation has also been recently reported as a laparoscopic procedure. For patients with tumors that mandate removal of the lymph nodes of the splenic hilum or with direct association of the tumor with splenic parenchyma, certainly it is more appropriate to do an operation based on neoplastic principles and perform a distal pancreatectomy/splenectomy. In other indications, if the anatomy is appropriate and the completeness of tumor resection is not compromised, splenic preservation is certainly possible.

Additional procedures in which it is common to perform a splenectomy include proximal gastric cancers. The importance of complete nodal dissection in long-term results in gastric resections has been debated for several decades. Level X lymph nodes are located in the splenic hilum, and for 20–25% of proximal gastric cancers these nodes will have metastatic cancer mandating removal. Other tumors of the left upper quadrant and retroperitoneum may require splenectomy, including large renal cell carcinomas, left adrenal tumors, and retroperitoneal sarcomas that may infiltrate upward into the spleen. Although the asplenic state does make patients susceptible to infections (see Hyposplenism above), the spleen should be viewed as an expendable organ if necessary to accomplish complete resection of malignancies, and there should be no hesitation to remove the spleen in these situations to do an appropriate cancer operation.

Fernandez-Cruz L et al: Laparoscopic distal pancreatectomy combined with preservation of the spleen for cystic neoplasms of the pancreas. J Gastrointest Surg 2004;8:493.

Ikeguchi M, Kaibara N: Lymph node metastasis at the splenic hilum in proximal gastric cancer. Am Surg 2004;70:645.

Martin RC et al: Extended local resection for advanced gastric cancer: increased survival versus increased morbidity. Ann Surg 2002;236:159.

Martin RC et al: Achieving RO resection for locally advanced gastric cancer: is it worth the risk of multiorgan resection? J Am Coll Surg 2002;194:568.

SPLENOSIS (Splenic Autotransplantation)

In splenosis, multiple small implants of splenic tissue grow in scattered areas on the peritoneal surfaces throughout the abdomen. They arise from dissemination and autotransplantation of splenic fragments following traumatic rupture of the spleen. Splenic implants or intentional autotransplants are capable of cell culling, and some immunologic function appears to be exhibited in cases of intentional autotransplantation. Aggressive attempts at surgical excision are not warranted. Splenosis is usually an incidental finding discovered much later during laparotomy for an unrelated problem. However, the implants stimulate formation of adhesions and may be a cause of intestinal obstruction. They must be distinguished from peritoneal nodules of metastatic carcinoma and from accessory spleens. Histologically, they differ from accessory spleens by the absence of elastic or smooth muscle fibers in the delicate capsule.

Cothren CC et al: Radiographic characteristics of postinjury splenic autotransplantation: avoiding a diagnostic dilemma. J Trauma-Injury Infection & Crit Care 2004;57:537.

Pisters PWT et al: Autologous splenic transplantation for splenic trauma. Ann Surg 1994;219:225.

Resende V, Petroianu A: Functions of the splenic remnant after subtotal splenectomy for treatment of severe splenic injuries. Am J Surg 2003;185:311.

Timens W et al: Splenic autotransplantation and the immune system. Ann Surg 1993;215:256.

SPLENECTOMY

Preoperative preparation of patients undergoing elective splenectomy should correct coagulation abnormalities and deficits in red cell mass, treat infections, and control immune reactions. Because platelets are removed so rapidly from the circulation, they usually are not given for thrombocytopenia until after the splenic artery has been ligated. Antibodies in the patient's serum may complicate crossmatching of blood. Many patients with autoimmune disorders require corticosteroid coverage in the perioperative period. For emergency splenectomy, hypovolemia should be corrected by whole blood transfusions. For elective cases, prophylactic vaccination with a polyvalent pneumococcal vaccine that protects against a common encapsulated offending organism in postsplenectomy infection is recommended. Elective splenectomy is now most commonly performed as a laparoscopic procedure. This reduces the recovery period and is significantly better tolerated by most patients.

Details of surgical technique are not within the scope of this text, but it should be noted that there are two approaches to open splenectomy (Figure 27–2). In one, which is of value chiefly in traumatic rupture of the spleen, the organ is immediately mobilized and the splenic artery is secured from behind as it enters the hilum. In the other, which is of vital importance in the removal of massively enlarged spleens, the organ is left in situ. The gastrocolic ligament is opened, and the splenic artery is ligated as it courses along the upper edge of the pancreas. This permits blood to leave the spleen through the splenic vein while all other attachments (ie, the short gastric vessels and colic attachments) are divided before the spleen is delivered. This method permits the removal of massively enlarged vascular spleens with practically no loss of blood.

Splenorrhaphy is operative repair of the spleen following trauma. The principles of splenorrhaphy are to debride the devitalized tissue and to attempt to approximate the normal contour of the spleen with capsular sutures or external wraps of material. Partial splenic resections may be performed for trauma or for disease states in which splenic debulking is indicated. Partial splenectomy for Gaucher's disease, large cysts, or benign tumors has been reported using automatic stapling devices as well as microwave coagulators.

Massive splenomegaly is defined as a spleen weight of greater than 1500 g or eight to ten times the normal size. Disease processes leading to massive splenomegaly include lymphoma, leukemia, and metabolic storage diseases. The morbidity and mortality rates of splenectomy for massive splenomegaly are increased primarily as a result of the risk of severe and rapid intraoperative blood loss. The operative approach in these cases is initial ligation of the splenic artery through the lesser sac at the superior border of the pancreas. Next, ligation of the short gastric vessels along the greater curvature all the way to the gastroesophageal junction is performed, allowing the stomach and left lobe of the liver to be retracted away from the spleen. Only after decreasing the splenic arterial inflow by the above maneuvers should mobilization of the lateral and superior attachments be performed, leading to removal of the massive spleen.

Laparoscopic splenectomy is now the standard of care in most major centers with high volumes of splenic surgery. Virtually any indication for elective splenectomy

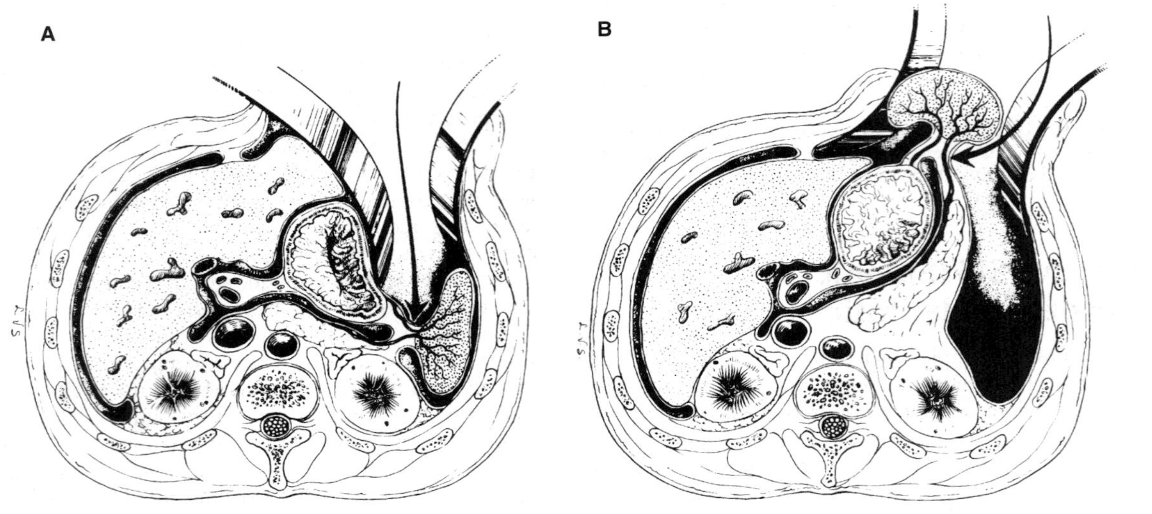

Figure 27–2. ***A:*** Anterior approach to splenic artery. ***B:*** Mobilization of spleen with posterior exposure of splenic artery.

qualifies for a laparoscopic approach, including patients with severe thrombocytopenia, patients with massive splenomegaly, patients needing partial splenectomy, and for the removal of accessory spleens and the wandering spleen.

Laparoscopic splenectomy is performed typically using four ports. Midline ports for the cannula as well as for retraction of the stomach away from the splenic hilum are placed. Left subcostal ports are used as operating sites for dissection of the splenic hilum. An angled laparoscope is required for visualization of the superior and lateral attachments of the spleen. Vessels are divided with clips, sutures, or stapling devices. Precise exposure of the hilum with gentle upward traction on the spleen to stretch and expose the vessels is preferred to blind stapling of the hilum. Clinical conditions such as idiopathic thrombocytopenic purpura and hereditary spherocytosis are the most common indications for laparoscopic splenectomy as the spleen is of normal size. Search via the laparoscope for accessory spleens is important in these procedures for a successful outcome, and this may be facilitated by the use of a hand port for palpation.

Borrazzo ED et al: Hand-assistant laparoscopic splenectomy for giant spleen. Surg Endosc 2003;17:918.

Kaban GK et al: Use of a laparoscopic hand-assist device for accessory splenectomy. Surg Endoscopy 2004;18:1001.

Katkouda N et al: Laparoscopic splenectomy: outcome and efficacy in 103 consecutive patients. Ann Surg 1998;228:568.

Machado MA et al: Exposure of splenic hilum increases safety of laparoscopic splenectomy. Surg Laparosc Endosc Percutan Tech 2004;14:23.

Rose AT et al: The incidence of splenectomy is decreasing: lessons learned from trauma experience. Am Surg 2000;66:481.

Smith L et al: Laparoscopic splenectomy for treatment of splenomegaly. Am J Surg 2004;187:618.

Terrosu G et al: The impact of splenic weight on laparoscopic splenectomy for splenomegaly. Surg Endosc 2002;16:103.

HEMATOLOGIC EFFECTS OF SPLENECTOMY

Absence of the spleen in a normal adult usually has few clinical consequences. Red cell count and indices do not change, but red cells with cytoplasmic inclusions may appear, eg, Heinz bodies, Howell-Jolly bodies, and siderocytes. Granulocytosis occurs immediately after splenectomy but is replaced in several weeks by lymphocytosis and monocytosis. Platelets are usually increased, occasionally markedly so, and may stay at levels of 400,000–500,000/μL for over a year. Even more striking thrombocytosis (eg, 2–3 million/μL) may develop after splenectomy for hemolytic anemia. A platelet count of over a million is not an indication for anticoagulants, but antiplatelet agents such as aspirin may help prevent thrombosis.

Horowitz J et al: Postsplenectomy leukocytosis: physiologic or an indicator of infection? Am Surg 1992;58:387.

Rutherford EJ et al: The white blood cell response to splenectomy and bacteraemia. Injury 1994;25:289.

POSTSPLENECTOMY SEPSIS & OTHER POSTSPLENECTOMY PROBLEMS

Complications related to splenectomy per se are relatively few, with atelectasis, pancreatitis, and postoperative hemorrhage being the most common. If splenectomy is done for thrombocytopenia, secondary bleeding may occur even though the platelet count usually rises promptly. Platelet transfusions should be given if primary hemostasis is abnormal (ie, oozing occurs) and the platelet count remains low. Thromboembolic complications may be more common following splenectomy, but this complication does not correlate with the degree of thrombocytosis. The risk of portal vein thrombosis is small but important, since this complication may be lethal if not recognized. Symptoms include fever, abdominal pain, diarrhea, and abnormal liver function tests. Treatment consists of anticoagulation plus antibiotics.

Individuals are more susceptible to fulminant bacteremia after splenectomy. This is a result of the following changes that occur after splenectomy: (1) decreased clearance of bacteria from the blood, (2) decreased levels of IgM, and (3) decreased opsonic activity. The risk is greatest in young children, especially in the first 2 years after surgery (80% of cases) and when the disorder for which splenectomy was required was a disease of the reticuloendothelial system. In general, the younger the patient undergoing splenectomy and the more severe the underlying condition, the greater the risk for developing overwhelming postsplenectomy infection. There is a low but significant risk of infection even in otherwise normal adults following splenectomy. Most of these infections occur after the first year, and nearly half occur more than 5 years after splenectomy. Lethal sepsis is very rare in adults. There is a distinct clinical syndrome: mild, nonspecific symptoms are followed by high fever and shock from sepsis, which may rapidly lead to death. *Streptococcus pneumoniae, Haemophilus influenzae,* and meningococci are the most common pathogens. Disseminated intravascular coagulation is a common complication. Awareness of this fatal complication has led to efforts to avoid splenectomy or to perform partial splenectomy or splenic repair for ruptured spleens (analogous to surgical management of liver trauma) to maintain adequate splenic function. Splenic autotransplantation may also achieve partial restoration of splenic function after splenectomy.

The risk of fatal sepsis is less after splenectomy for trauma than for hematologic disorders, probably due to splenic autotransplantation. Prophylactic vaccination against pneumococcal sepsis should be used in all surgically or functionally asplenic patients. Since splenic function may be important in the immune response to vaccine, early administration of polyvalent pneumococcal vaccine (Pneumovax) is advisable. The vaccine provides protection in adults and older children for 4–5 years, after which revaccination is advisable. Since the vaccine is only effective against about 80% of organisms, some authorities have recommended a 2-year course, treatment until age 16, or lifelong prophylaxis with penicillin following splenectomy. Others have advocated use of ampicillin to provide coverage for *H influenzae* as well as pneumococci. Antibiotic prophylaxis is essential in children under 2 years of age and should be continued until at least age 6. In general, splenectomy should be deferred until age 6 unless the hematologic problem is especially severe.

Brigden ML et al: Prevention and management of overwhelming postsplenectomy infection—an update. Crit Care Med 1999; 27:836.

Eber SW et al: Frequency of very late fatal sepsis after splenectomy for hereditary spherocytosis: impact of insufficient antibody response to pneumococcal infection. Ann Hematol 1999;78: 524.

Foss Abrahamsen A et al: Systemic pneumococcal disease after staging splenectomy for Hodgkin's disease 1969–1980 without pneumococcal vaccine protection: a follow-up study 1994. Eur J Haematol 1997;58:73.

Hansen K, Singer DB: Asplenic-hyposplenic overwhelming sepsis: postsplenectomy sepsis revisited. Pediatr Dev Pathol 2001; 4:105.

Lutwick LI: Life threatening infections in the asplenic or hyposplenic individual. Surr Clin Topics in Inf Dis 2002;22:78.

Park A et al: Laparoscopic vs open splenectomy. Arch Surg 1999; 134:1263.

Shatz DV: Vaccination practices among North American trauma surgeons in splenectomy for trauma. J Trauma-Injury Inf & Crit Care 2002;53:950.

Shatz DV et al: Antibody responses in postsplenectomy trauma patients receiving the 23-valent pneumococcal polysaccharide vaccine at 14 versus 28 days postoperatively. J Trauma-Injury Inf & Crit Care 2002;53:1037.

Appendix

28

Lawrence W. Way, MD

ANATOMY & PHYSIOLOGY

In infants, the appendix is a conical diverticulum at the apex of the cecum, but with differential growth and distention of the cecum, the appendix ultimately arises on the left and dorsally approximately 2.5 cm below the ileocecal valve. The taeniae of the colon converge at the base of the appendix, an arrangement that helps in locating this structure at operation. The appendix is fixed retrocecally in 16% of adults and is freely mobile in the remainder.

The appendix in youth is characterized by a large concentration of lymphoid follicles that appear 2 weeks after birth and number about 200 or more at age 15. Thereafter, progressive atrophy of lymphoid tissue proceeds concomitantly with fibrosis of the wall and partial or total obliteration of the lumen.

If the appendix has a physiologic function, it is probably related to the presence of lymphoid follicles. Reports of a statistical relationship between appendectomy and subsequent carcinoma of the colon and other neoplasms in humans are not supported by controlled studies.

Schumpelick V et al: Appendix and cecum. Embryology, anatomy, and surgical applications. Surg Clin North Am 2000;80:295.

ACUTE APPENDICITIS

ESSENTIALS OF DIAGNOSIS

- *Abdominal pain.*
- *Anorexia, nausea and vomiting.*
- *Localized right lower quadrant abdominal tenderness.*
- *Low-grade fever.*
- *Leukocytosis.*

General Considerations

Approximately 7% of people in Western countries have appendicitis at some time during their lives, and about 200,000 appendectomies for acute appendicitis are performed annually in the United States. The incidence has been steadily dropping over the past 25 years, however, while the incidence in developing countries—which in the past has been quite low—has been rising in proportion to economic gains and changes in lifestyle.

Obstruction of the proximal lumen by fibrous bands, lymphoid hyperplasia, fecaliths, calculi, or parasites has long been considered to be the major cause of acute appendicitis, though that theory is doubted by many experts. Evidence of temporal and geographic clustering of cases has suggested a primary infectious etiology. A fecalith or calculus is found in only 10% of acutely inflamed appendices.

As appendicitis progresses, the blood supply is impaired by bacterial infection in the wall and distention of the lumen by pus; gangrene and perforation occur at about 24 hours, though the timing is highly variable. Gangrene implies microscopic perforation and bacterial peritonitis (which may be localized by adhesions from nearby viscera).

Clinical Findings

Acute appendicitis has protean manifestations. It may simulate almost any other acute abdominal illness and in turn may be mimicked by a variety of conditions. Progression of symptoms and signs is the rule—in contrast to the fluctuating course of some other diseases.

A. Symptoms and Signs

Typically, the illness begins with vague midabdominal discomfort followed by nausea, anorexia, and indigestion. The pain is persistent and continuous but not severe, with occasional mild cramps. There may be an episode of vomiting, and within several hours the pain shifts to the right lower quadrant, becoming localized and causing discomfort on moving, walking, or coughing. The patient may feel constipated.

Examination at this point shows localized tenderness to one-finger palpation and perhaps slight muscular guarding. Rebound or percussion tenderness (the latter provides the same information more humanely) may be elicited in the same area. Peristalsis is normal or slightly reduced. Rectal and pelvic examinations are likely to be negative. The temperature is only slightly elevated (eg, 37.8 °C) in the absence of perforation.

Contrary to traditional teaching, tenderness on rectal examination is not a sign of acute appendicitis. If present, it more often points to another cause of the symptoms. Another common misconception is that inflammation in a retrocecal appendix produces an atypical syndrome. This too is incorrect; the clinical findings in this situation are the same as for ordinary (antececal) appendicitis.

Rarely, the cecum may lie on the left side of the abdomen, and appendicitis may be mistaken for sigmoid diverticulitis. An inflamed appendix in the right upper quadrant may mimic acute cholecystitis or perforated ulcer. Even when the cecum is normally situated, a long appendix may reach to other parts of the abdomen, and acute appendicitis in these circumstances may be very confusing indeed.

A couple of general points are worth remembering: (1) People with early (nonperforated) appendicitis often do not appear ill and may even apologize for taking your time. Finding localized tenderness over McBurney's point is the cornerstone of diagnosis. (2) A rule that will help considerably with atypical cases is never to place appendicitis lower than second in the differential diagnosis of acute abdominal pain in a previously healthy person.

B. Laboratory Findings

The average leukocyte count is 15,000/μL, and 90% of patients have counts over 10,000/μL. In three-fourths of patients, the differential white count shows more than 75% neutrophils. It must be emphasized, however, that one patient in ten with acute appendicitis has a leukocyte count indistinguishable from normal, and many have normal differential cell counts. Appendicitis in patients infected with HIV produces the same syndrome as in other people, but the white blood cell count is usually normal.

The urine is usually normal, but a few leukocytes and erythrocytes and occasionally even gross hematuria may be noted, particularly in retrocecal or pelvic appendicitis.

C. Imaging Studies

Localized air-fluid levels, localized ileus, or increased soft tissue density in the right lower quadrant is present in 50% of patients with early acute appendicitis. Less common findings are a calculus, an altered right psoas shadow, or an abnormal right flank stripe. The finding on plain films of a calculus in the right lower quadrant coupled with pain in this area strongly supports a diagnosis of appendicitis. Although perforated peptic ulcer is by far the most common cause of free intraperitoneal air, free air is also a rare manifestation of perforated appendicitis. In general, however, the findings on plain films are nonspecific and rarely of help in diagnosis. A suggestion that barium enema may contribute to the diagnosis has not been supported by experience.

A spiral CT examination of the appendix may be of help in diagnosis. An enlarged appendix with wall thickening or enhancement or periappendiceal fat stranding are the most useful CT findings of acute appendicitis. Other findings may be present including focal cecal thickening, appendicoliths, extraluminal air, intramural air, and pericecal phlegmon, but are less reliable. CT scans are of greatest value in patients with less than typical clinical and laboratory findings, where a positive study would be an indication for appendectomy. In the face of typical time course of disease, right lower quadrant pain and tenderness plus signs of inflammation (eg, fever, leukocytosis), a CT scan would be superfluous and, if negative, even misleading. Ultrasound imaging is much less reliable than CT. When appendicitis is accompanied by a right lower quadrant mass, an ultrasound or CT scan should be obtained to differentiate between a periappendiceal phlegmon and an abscess.

D. Appendicitis During Pregnancy

Appendicitis is the most common nonobstetric surgical disease of the abdomen during pregnancy. Pregnant women develop appendicitis with the same frequency as do nonpregnant women of the same age, and the cases are equally distributed through the three trimesters of pregnancy. By far the most common presentation is right lower quadrant pain and tenderness—the classic syndrome—but the enlarged uterus occasionally will have pushed the appendix into the right upper quadrant, which gives rise to pain in this location. Fever is less common than with appendicitis in the absence of pregnancy. Leukocytosis is typical, but it too may be absent. The main problem is to recognize the possibility of appendicitis and perform appendectomy promptly. Delay in operation runs a higher than usual risk of perforation and diffuse peritonitis, because omentum is less available to wall off the infection. The mother is in greater jeopardy of serious abdominal infection, and the fetus is more vulnerable to premature labor with complications. Laparoscopic appendectomy (specifically the pneumoperitoneum) is well tolerated by the mother and fetus, but the frequency of technical complications is higher than with the open approach. Appendectomy during pregnancy is often followed by preterm labor but rarely by preterm delivery. Early appendectomy has decreased the maternal death rate to under 0.5% and the fetal death rate to under 10%.

Diagnosis & Differential Diagnosis

The clinical diagnosis of appendicitis rests on a combination of localized pain and tenderness accompanied by signs of inflammation, such as fever, leukocytosis, and elevated C-reactive protein levels. Migration of pain from the periumbilical area to the right lower quadrant is also diagnostically significant. In the absence of signs of inflammation, the diagnosis is less certain (ie, falsely positive), and in this situation a CT scan might be of value. The best strategy in equivocal cases is to observe the patient for a period of 6 hours or more. During this time, patients with appendicitis experience increasing pain and signs of inflammation and those without appendicitis generally improve. False-positive diagnoses often involve cases where the surgeon has accorded more significance to the patient's pain than to the presence or absence of inflammatory signs. Anorexia, nausea, and rectal tenderness are not indicative of appendicitis. During the past 15 years, the overall false-positive rate for the diagnosis of appendicitis has dropped from 15% to 10% without an accompanying rise in the number of perforations. Thus, diagnostic accuracy appears to be improving.

The diagnosis of acute appendicitis is particularly difficult in the very young and in the elderly. These are the groups where diagnosis is most often delayed and perforation most common. Infants manifest only lethargy, irritability, and anorexia in the early stages, but vomiting, fever, and pain are apparent as the disease progresses. Classic symptoms may not be elicited in aged patients, and the diagnosis is often not considered by the examining physician. The course of appendicitis is more virulent in the elderly, and suppurative complications occur earlier.

The highest incidence of false-positive diagnosis (20%) is in women between ages 20 and 40 and is attributable to pelvic inflammatory disease and other gynecologic conditions. Compared with appendicitis, pelvic inflammatory disease is more often associated with bilateral lower quadrant tenderness, left adnexal tenderness, onset of illness within 5 days of the last menstrual period, and a history that does not include nausea and vomiting. Cervical motion tenderness is common in both diseases.

Complications

The complications of acute appendicitis include perforation, peritonitis, abscess, and pylephlebitis.

A. Perforation

Delay in seeking medical care appears to be the principal reason for perforations; the disease has just been allowed to progress according to its natural history. Perforation is accompanied by more severe pain and higher fever (average, 38.3 °C) than in appendicitis. It is unusual for the acutely inflamed appendix to perforate within the first 12 hours. The appendicitis has progressed to perforation by the time of appendectomy in about 50% of patients under age 10 or over age 50. Nearly all deaths occur in the latter group.

The acute consequences of perforation vary from generalized peritonitis to formation of a tiny abscess that may not appreciably alter the symptoms and signs of appendicitis. Perforation in young women increases the subsequent risk of tubal infertility about fourfold.

B. Peritonitis

Localized peritonitis results from microscopic perforation of a gangrenous appendix, while spreading or generalized peritonitis usually implies gross perforation into the free peritoneal cavity. Increasing tenderness and rigidity, abdominal distention, and adynamic ileus are obvious in patients with peritonitis. High fever and severe toxicity mark progression of this catastrophic illness in untreated patients.

C. Appendiceal Abscess (Appendiceal Mass)

Localized perforation occurs when the periappendiceal infection becomes walled off by omentum and adjacent viscera. The clinical presentation consists of the usual findings in appendicitis plus a right lower quadrant mass. An ultrasound or CT scan should be performed; if an abscess is found, it is best treated by percutaneous ultrasound-guided aspiration. Opinion differs about how small abscesses and phlegmons should be handled. Some surgeons prefer a regimen consisting of antibiotics and expectant management followed by elective appendectomy 6 weeks later. The purpose is to avoid spreading the localized infection, which usually resolves in response to the antibiotics. Other surgeons recommend immediate appendectomy, which some believe shortens the duration of the illness. However, the immediate surgery approach has significant complications in a higher percentage of patients. There is not currently a consensus.

When the surgeon encounters an unsuspected abscess during appendectomy, it is usually best to proceed and remove the appendix. If the abscess is large and further dissection would be hazardous, drainage alone is appropriate.

Appendicitis recurs in only 10% of patients whose initial treatment consisted of antibiotics or antibiotics plus drainage of an abscess. Therefore, when the presence of ancillary conditions increases the risks of surgery, interval appendectomy may be postponed unless symptoms recur.

D. Pylephlebitis

Pylephlebitis is suppurative thrombophlebitis of the portal venous system. Chills, high fever, low-grade jaundice, and, later, hepatic abscesses are the hallmarks of this grave condition. The appearance of shaking chills in a patient with acute appendicitis demands vigorous antibiotic therapy to prevent the development of pylephlebitis.

CT scanning is the best means of detecting thrombosis and gas in the portal vein. In addition to antibiotics, prompt surgery is indicated to treat appendicitis or other primary sources of infection (eg, diverticulitis).

Prevention

In the past it was common to perform an incidental appendectomy in people under age 50 during the course of an abdominal operation for another illness—as long as the exposure was adequate and there were no specific contraindications. The declining lifetime risk of appendicitis now calls this practice into question. A related question concerns the appropriate course when a laparoscopy is performed for presumptive appendicitis and the appendix looks normal. The trend in this case is to leave the appendix intact—not to remove it prophylactically or on the assumption that the visual assessment may be inaccurate.

Treatment

With few exceptions, the treatment of appendicitis is surgical (ie, appendectomy). The operation can be done open (see Figure 28–1) or laparoscopically. The results of clinical trials comparing the two methods show no clear-cut advantage of one method over the other, though patients treated laparoscopically return to work a few days earlier. A laparoscopic approach is desirable when the preoperative diagnosis is uncertain because the morbidity is less if the appendix is found to be uninflamed and an appendectomy is not done.

Prophylactic antibiotics are indicated preoperatively. A single-drug regimen, usually a cephalosporin, is as effective as more aggressive multiple-drug combinations. Routinely culturing abdominal fluid is of no practical value even when the appendix has perforated. The organisms obtained are the usual fecal flora.

Abdominal drains are called for only to treat established abscesses, not for diffuse inflammation or abdominal fluid.

If a patient with appendicitis cannot be taken to a modern surgical facility for care, treatment should consist of antibiotics alone. The complication-free success rate of this approach is high.

Prognosis

Although a death rate of zero is theoretically attainable in acute appendicitis, deaths still occur, some of which are avoidable. The death rate in simple acute appendicitis is approximately 0.1% and has not changed significantly since 1930. Progress in pre- and postoperative care—particularly the emphasis on fluid replacement before operation—has reduced the death rate from perforation to about 5%. Nonetheless, postoperative infections still occur in 30% of cases of gangrenous or perforated appendix. Although most of these patients survive,

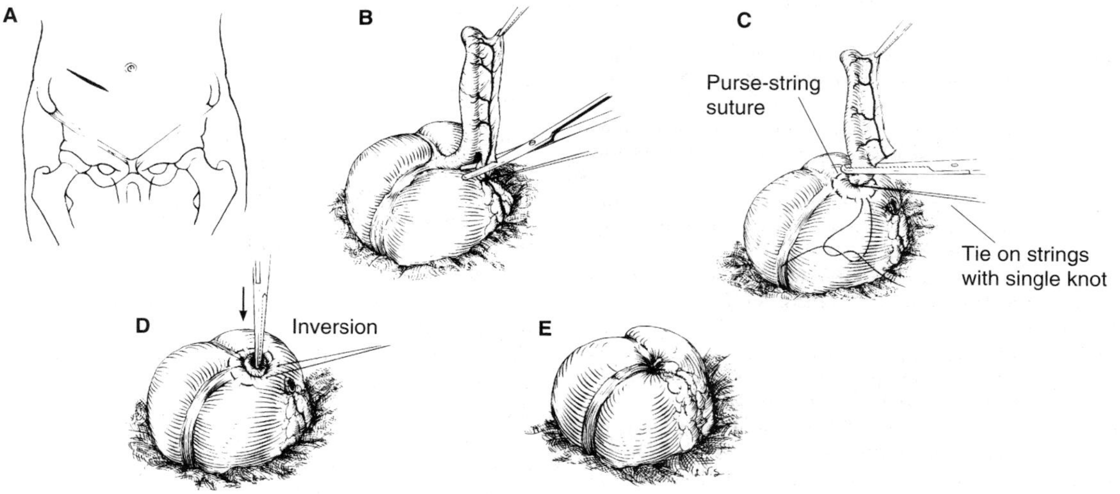

Figure 28–1. Technique of appendectomy. ***A:*** Incision. ***B:*** After delivery of the tip of the cecum, the mesoappendix is divided. ***C:*** The base is clamped and ligated with a simple throw of the knot. The next step—inversion of the stump—is optional. ***D:*** A clamp is placed to hold the knot during inversion with a purse-string suture of fine silk. ***E:*** The loosely tied inner knot on the stump assures that there is no closed space for the development of a stump abscess.

many near fatalities require prolonged hospitalization. The substantial increase in tubal infertility that follows perforation in young women is also avoidable by early appendectomy.

Andersson RE et al: Repeated clinical and laboratory examinations in patients with an equivocal diagnosis of appendicitis. World J Surg 2000;24:479.

Andersson RE et al: Why does the clinical diagnosis fail in suspected appendicitis? Eur J Surg 2000;166:796.

Andersson RE et al: Diagnostic value of disease history, clinical presentation, and inflammatory parameters of appendicitis. World J Surg 1999;23:133.

Asfar S et al: Would measurement of C-reactive protein reduce the rate of negative exploration for acute appendicitis? J R Coll Edinb 2000;45:21.

Bilik R et al: Is abdominal cavity culture of any value in appendicitis? Am J Surg 1998;175:267.

Blomqvist PG et al: Mortality after appendectomy in Sweden, 1987–1996. Ann Surg 2001;233:455.

Brown CV et al: Appendiceal abscess: immediate operation or percutaneous drainage? Am Surg 2003;69:829.

Carr NJ: The pathology of acute appendicitis. Ann Diagn Pathol 2000;4:46.

Choi D et al: The most useful findings for diagnosing acute appendicitis on contrast-enhanced helical CT. Acta Radiologica 2003;44:574.

Gronroos JM et al: Leucocyte count and C-reactive protein in the diagnosis of acute appendicitis. Br J Surg 1999;86:501.

Kokoska ER et al: Perforated appendicitis in children: risk factors for the development of complications. Surgery 1998;124:619.

Kraemer M et al: Perforating appendicitis: is it a separate disease? Acute Abdominal Pain Study Group. Eur J Surg 1999;165:473.

Laine S et al: Laparoscopic appendectomy: is it worthwhile? A prospective, randomized study in young women. Surg Endosc 1997;11:95.

Lee SL et al: Computed tomography and ultrasonography do not improve and may delay the diagnosis and treatment of acute appendicitis. Arch Surg 2001;136:556.

Long KH et al: A prospective randomized comparison of laparoscopic appendectomy with open appendectomy: clinical and economic analyses. Surgery 2001;129:390.

Mourad J et al: Appendicitis in pregnancy: new information that contradicts long-held clinical beliefs. Am J Obstet Gynecol 2000;182:1027.

Rucinski J et al: Gangrenous and perforated appendicitis: a meta-analytic study of 2532 patients indicates that the incision should be closed primarily. Surgery 2000;127:136.

Schuler JG et al: Is there a role for abdominal computed tomographic scans in appendicitis? Arch Surg 1998;133:373.

Stroman DL et al: The role of computed tomography in the diagnosis of acute appendicitis. Am J Surg 1999;178:485.

Watters JM et al: The influence of age on the severity of peritonitis. Can J Surg 1996;39:142.

Weyant MJ et al Interpretation of computed tomography does not correlate with laboratory or pathologic findings in surgically confirmed acute appendicitis. Surgery 2000;128:145.

CHRONIC APPENDICITIS

Chronic abdominal pain is a common problem, and when the complaints are confined to the right lower quadrant, the question of chronic appendicitis is usually raised. Patients with genuine chronic appendicitis experience pain that lasts for 3 weeks or more. The history usually includes an acute illness at some time in the past, compatible with acute appendicitis, which was managed nonoperatively. On examination, the appendix is chronically inflamed or fibrotic. The symptoms resolve with appendectomy.

Chronic intermittent pain in the right lower quadrant is most often caused by something other than appendicitis, such as Crohn's disease or renal disease. Barium x-rays are sometimes helpful, particularly in children. In many patients, the diagnosis is not obvious. Appendectomy relieves symptoms occasionally, but laparotomy for chronic abdominal pain is generally unproductive in the absence of objective findings (eg, localized tenderness, palpable mass, leukocytosis).

Mattei P et al: Chronic and recurrent appendicitis are uncommon entities often misdiagnosed. J Am Coll Surg 1994;178:385.

TUMORS OF THE APPENDIX

Benign tumors, including carcinoids, were found in 4.6% of 71,000 human appendix specimens examined microscopically. Benign neoplasms may arise from any cellular element and are usually incidental findings. Occasionally, a neoplasm obstructs the appendiceal lumen and produces acute appendicitis. No treatment other than appendectomy is indicated.

Malignant Tumors

Primary malignant tumors were found in 1.4% of appendices in the same large series. Carcinoid and argentaffin tumors comprise the majority of appendiceal cancers, and the appendix is the commonest location of carcinoid tumors of the gastrointestinal tract. Carcinoid tumors of the appendix are usually benign, but the uncommon tumor that is over 2 cm in diameter may exhibit malignant behavior. Most appendiceal carcinoids are found in the tip of the organ, while a few are at the base. About half of these tumors are discovered during an appendectomy for acute appendicitis, and the remainder are identified incidentally. Lesions less than 2 cm in diameter invade the appendiceal wall in 25% of cases, but only 3% metastasize to lymph nodes, and hepatic metastases and the carcinoid syndrome are truly rare. Appendectomy alone is adequate treatment unless the lymph nodes are visibly involved, the tumor is more than 2 cm in diameter, mucinous elements are present in the tumor (adenocarcinoid), or the mesoappendix or base of the cecum is invaded. Right hemicolectomy is recommended for these more aggressive lesions.

Adenocarcinoma of the colonic type can arise in the appendix and spread rapidly to regional lymph nodes or implant on ovaries or other peritoneal surfaces. Ten percent of patients have widespread metastases when first seen. Adenocarcinoma is virtually never diagnosed preoperatively; about half of cases present as acute appendicitis, and 15% have formed appendiceal abscesses. Right hemicolectomy should be performed if disease is localized to the appendix and regional lymph nodes. The 5-year survival rate is 60% after right hemicolectomy and only 20% after appendectomy alone, but the latter group includes patients with distant metastases at the time of diagnosis.

Mucocele

Mucocele of the appendix is a cystic, dilated appendix filled with mucin. Simple mucocele is not a neoplasm and results from chronic obstruction of the proximal lumen, usually by fibrous tissue. If the appendiceal contents distally are sterile, mucous cells continue to secrete until distention of the lumen thins the wall and interferes with nutrition of the lining cells; histologically, simple mucocele is lined by flattened cuboidal epithelium or no epithelium at all. Simple mucocele is cured by appendectomy.

Less commonly, mucocele is caused by a neoplasm—cystadenoma, or adenocarcinoma grade 1 in the older terminology. This lesion may arise de novo or (perhaps) in a preceding simple mucocele. In cystadenoma, the lumen is filled with mucin but the wall is lined by columnar epithelium with papillary projections. Tumor does not infiltrate the appendiceal wall and does not metastasize, although it may recur locally after appendectomy. Cystadenoma is believed to undergo malignant change in some instances. Appendectomy is adequate treatment.

Carr NJ et al: Epithelial noncarcinoid tumors and tumor-like lesions of the appendix. A clinicopathologic study of 184 patients with a multivariate analysis of prognostic factors. Cancer 1995;75:757.

Chiou YY et al: Rare benign and malignant appendiceal lesions: spectrum of computed tomography findings with pathologic correlation. J Comput Assist Tomogr 2003;27:297.

Connor SJ et al: Appendiceal tumors: retrospective clinicopathologic analysis of appendiceal tumors from 7,970 appendectomies. Dis Colon Rectum 1998;41:75.

Deans GT et al: Neoplastic lesions of the appendix. Br J Surg 1995;82:299.

Gouzi JL et al: Indications for right hemicolectomy in carcinoid tumors of the appendix. The French Associations for Surgical Research. Surg Gynecol Obstet 1993;176:543.

Kim SH et al: Mucocele of the appendix: ultrasonographic and CT findings. Abdom Imaging 1998;23:292.

Nitecki SS et al: The natural history of surgically treated primary adenocarcinoma of the appendix. Ann Surg 1994;219:51.

Roggo A et al: Carcinoid tumors of the appendix. Ann Surg 1993;217:385.

Soweid AM et al: Diagnosis and management of appendiceal mucoceles. Dig Dis 1998;16:183.

Sugarbaker PH et al: Results of treatment of 385 patients with peritoneal surface spread of appendiceal malignancy. Ann Surg Oncol 1999;6:727.

Small Intestine 29

Andrew A. Shelton, MD, George Chang, MD, & Mark Lane Welton, MD

The small intestine is the portion of the alimentary tract extending from the pylorus to the cecum. The structure, function, and diseases of the duodenum are discussed in Chapter 23; the jejunum and ileum are described in this chapter.

ANATOMY

Gross Anatomy

The small intestine in an adult is 5–6 m long from the ligament of Treitz to the ileocecal valve. The upper two-fifths of the small intestine distal to the duodenum are termed the **jejunum** and the lower three-fifths the **ileum**. There is no sharp demarcation between the jejunum and the ileum; however, as the intestine proceeds distally, the lumen narrows, the mesenteric vascular arcades become more complex, and the circular mucosal folds become shorter and fewer (Figure 29–1). In general, the jejunum resides in the left side of the peritoneal cavity and the ileum occupies the pelvis and right lower quadrant.

The small bowel is attached to the posterior abdominal wall by the mesentery, a reflection from the posterior parietal peritoneum. This peritoneal fold arises along a line originating just to the left of the midline and passing obliquely to the right lower quadrant. Although the mesentery joins the intestine along one side, the peritoneal layer of the mesentery envelops the bowel and is called the visceral peritoneum, or serosa.

The mesentery contains fat, blood vessels, lymphatics, lymph nodes, and nerves. The arterial blood supply to the jejunum and ileum derives from the superior mesenteric artery. Branches within the mesentery anastomose to form arcades (Figure 29–1), and small straight arteries travel from these arcades to enter the mesenteric border of the gut. The antimesenteric border of the intestinal wall is less richly supplied with arterial blood than the mesenteric side, so when blood flow is impaired, the antimesenteric border becomes ischemic first. Venous blood from the small intestine drains into the superior mesenteric vein and then enters the liver through the portal vein.

Submucosal lymphoid aggregates (Peyer's patches) are much more numerous in the ileum than in the jejunum. Lymphatic channels within the mesentery drain through regional lymph nodes and terminate in the cisterna chyli.

Parasympathetic nerves from the right vagus and sympathetic fibers from the greater and lesser splanchnic nerves reach the small intestine through the mesentery. Both types of autonomic nerves contain efferent and afferent fibers, but intestinal pain appears to be mediated by the sympathetic afferents only.

Microscopic Anatomy

The wall of the small intestine consists of four layers: mucosa, submucosa, muscularis, and serosa.

A. Mucosa

The absorptive surface of the mucosa is multiplied by circular mucosal folds termed plicae circulares (valvulae conniventes) that project into the lumen; they are taller and more numerous in the proximal jejunum than in the distal ileum (Figure 29–1). On the surface of the plicae circulares are delicate villi less than 1 mm in height, each containing a central lacteal, a small artery and vein, and fibers from the muscularis mucosae that lend contractility to the villus. Villi are in turn covered by columnar epithelial cells that have a brush border consisting of microvilli 1 μm in height (Figure 29–2). The presence of villi multiplies the absorptive surface about 8 times, and microvilli increase it another 14–24 times; the total absorptive area of the small intestine is 200–500 m^2.

The major cell types in the epithelium of the small intestine are absorptive enterocytes, mucous cells, Paneth cells, endocrine cells, and M cells. Absorptive enterocytes are responsible for absorption; they arise from continually proliferating undifferentiated cells in the crypts of Lieberkühn (Figure 29–3) and migrate to the tips of villi over a 3- to 7-day period. Peptide growth factors regulate this process. The life span of enterocytes in humans is 5–6 days.

Mucous cells originate in crypts and migrate to the tips of villi also; mature mucous cells are termed goblet cells. Paneth cells are found only in the crypts; their function is unknown but may be secretory. Endocrine cells have abundant cytoplasmic granules that contain 5-hydroxtryptamine and various peptides. Enterochromaf-

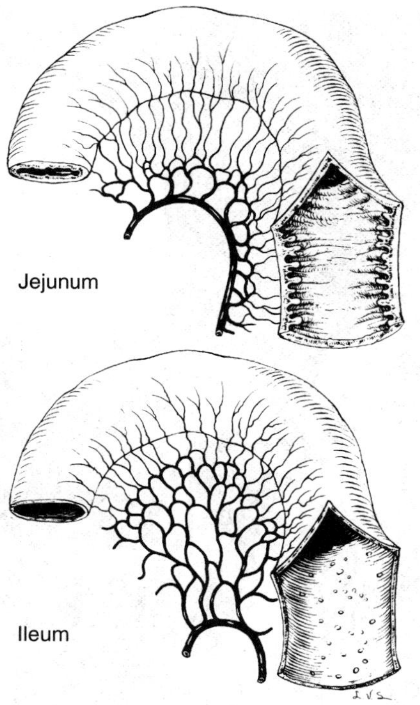

Figure 29–1. Blood supply and luminal surface of the small bowel. The arterial arcades of the small intestine increase in number from one or two in the proximal jejunum to four or five in the distal ileum, a finding that helps to distinguish proximal from distal bowel at operation. Plicae circulares are more prominent in the jejunum.

fin cells are the most numerous; N cells (containing neurotensin), L cells (glucagon), and other cells containing motilin and cholecystokinin are also present. M cells are thin membranous cells that cover Peyer's patches. They have the ability to sample luminal antigens such as proteins and microorganisms. Mucosal T lymphocytes of several phenotypes play an important role in mucosal cell-mediated immunity. Mast cells in the lamina propria are closely applied to nerve fibers, thus providing an anatomic basis for communication between these two structures in disease processes such as inflammation.

B. Other Layers

The submucosa is a fibroelastic layer containing blood vessels and nerves. Submucosa is the strongest component of bowel wall and must be included in intestinal sutures. The muscularis consists of an inner circular layer and an outer longitudinal coat of smooth muscle. The serosa is the outermost covering of the intestine.

Dignass AU et al: Fibroblast growth factors modulate intestinal epithelial cell growth and maturation. Gastroenterology 1994;106:1254.

Kagnoff MF: Immunology of the intestinal tract. Gastroenterology 1993;105:1275.

PHYSIOLOGY

The principal function of the small intestine is absorption.

Motility

Smooth muscles of the small intestine undergo spontaneous oscillations of membrane potential; these cyclic changes are termed pacesetter potentials or electrical control activity. Each segment of intestine has a characteristic frequency of pacesetter potentials; it is highest proximally, and it decreases progressively from duodenum to ileum. In intact intestine, higher-frequency pacesetter potentials can drive adjacent distal intestine so that both segments have the same frequency (said to be phase-locked). In humans, the duodenum determines the frequency of pacesetter potentials for the entire small intestine.

As pacesetter potentials spread distally, they bring the onset of action potentials and muscular contractions into phase. One type of muscular contraction (nonpropagating, or stationary) causes segmentation, which mixes chyme with digestive juices, repeatedly exposes the mixture to the absorptive surface, and moves chyme slowly in an aboral direction. Another type of muscular contraction (propagating) is peristaltic. Normal peristalsis is a short, weak propulsive movement that travels at about 1 cm/s for a distance of 10–15 cm before subsiding. Mean transit time for a solid meal is 4 hours from mouth to colon.

The enteric nervous system is a dominant regulator of all aspects of motility of the small intestine. The two major types of nerve plexuses in the enteric nervous system are the myenteric plexus, mainly responsible for control of peristaltic activity, and the submucosal plexus, which regulates secretion and absorption. The enteric nervous system contains four types of neurons: motor, secretory, sensory, and interneurons (which provide communication between neurons in the intestinal wall). Neurotransmitters found in the enteric nervous system include cholinergic, adrenergic, serotonergic, and peptidergic substances. Among the numerous peptides secreted by neurons in the enteric nervous system are cholecystokinin, vasoactive intestinal peptide (VIP), somatostatin, neurotensin, enkephalin, galanin, and substance P. In general, intestinal action potentials and muscular contractions are stimulated by substance P and galanin, and motility is inhibited by VIP, somatostatin, neurotensin, and enkephalin. Nitric oxide mediates neural inhibition in circular muscle of human small intestine.

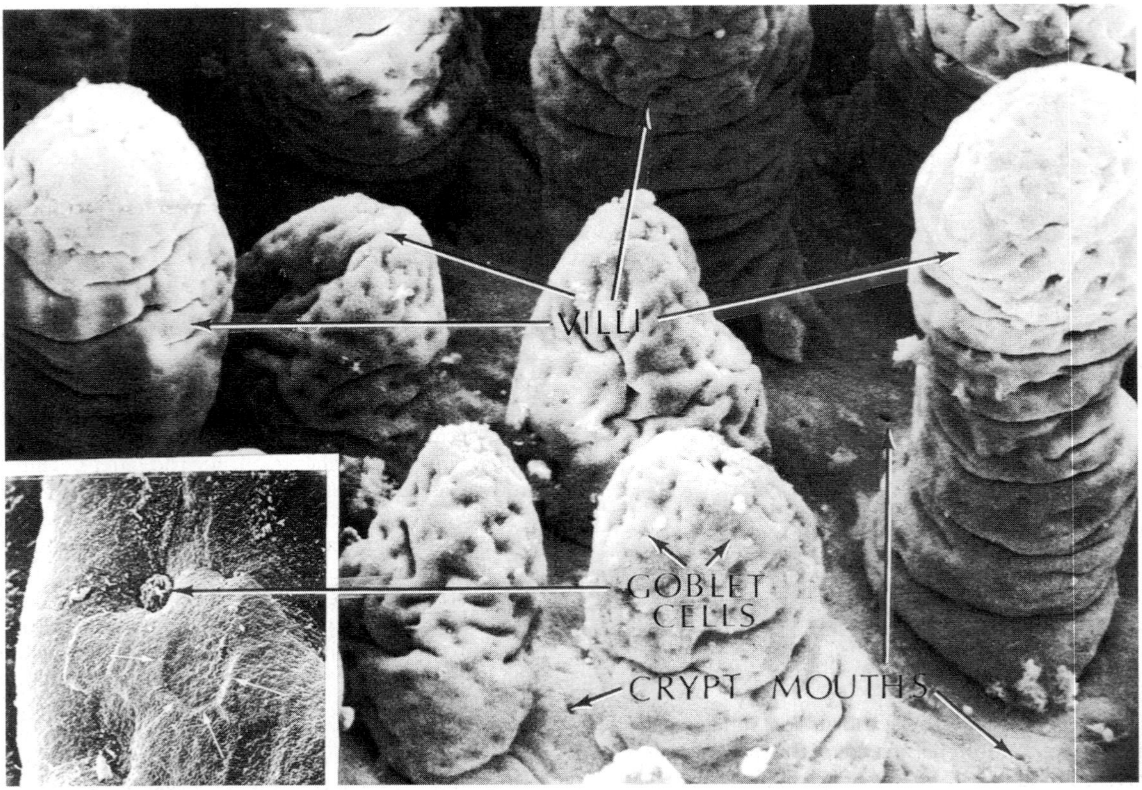

Figure 29–2. Scanning electron microscopic photo of small intestinal villi from the human terminal ileum. (Reduced from × 320.) ***Inset:*** Detail of a villous surface showing a mucous (goblet) cell surrounded by polygonal columnar cells. (Reduced from × 2100.) Epithelial cell borders are visible (white arrows). The pebbled columnar cell surface represents closely packed microvilli seen end-on. (Courtesy of Robert L. Owen, MD, and Albert L. Jones, MD.)

Peristalsis is initiated by stretch of the intestinal wall by a food bolus, and a dual reflex is set in motion. The circular smooth muscle orad to the bolus contracts; this reflex is mediated by enteric neurons with acetylcholine and substance P as neurotransmitters. Simultaneous relaxation of the intestinal circular muscle below is mediated by enteric neurons using VIP as the neurotransmitter.

The interdigestive migrating myoelectric complex (MMC) originates every $1^1/_2$–2 hours in the stomach and duodenum of fasting mammals. It is an aborally progressive front of action potentials and muscular contractions consisting of three successive phases: a quiescent phase 1 with slow waves only, phase 2 with increasing action potential activity, and phase 3 with action potentials on every slow wave. The MMC progresses aborally until it reaches the colon, and then another burst of potentials and contractions begins proximally. The MMC has been called the "intestinal housekeeper" because it cleans up remnants of the preceding meal and gets rid of microorganisms that escaped destruction by gastric acid. The MMC is controlled by the enteric nervous system; motilin and 5-hydroxytryptamine may play regulatory roles. The MMC is abolished by ingestion of food, and some features are altered by major abdominal operations or peritonitis.

Numerous peptides have been found to act in the brain to alter gastrointestinal motility. Hypothalamic hormones (eg, corticotropin-releasing factor and thyrotropin-releasing hormone), calcitonin, and nearly all of the enteric nervous system neurotransmitters have central nervous system actions that affect motility, at least in animals. Exogenous opioids, including codeine and loperamide, exert antidiarrheal action by inhibition or disruption of the pattern of circular muscle contraction; some of these effects are mediated by the μ-opioid receptor on the smooth muscle of the bowel wall. The vagus plays an important role in many of these phenomena.

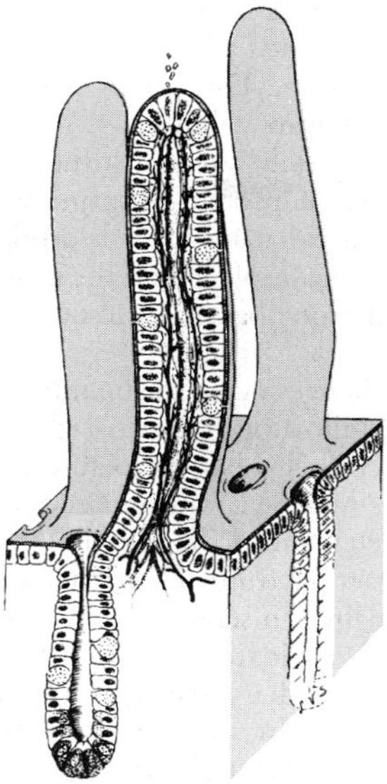

Figure 29–3. Schematic representation of villi and crypts of Lieberkühn.

Paralytic (adynamic) ileus is routine after abdominal operations, and it also accompanies inflammatory conditions in the abdomen, intestinal ischemia, ureteral colic, pelvic fractures, and back injuries. Abdominal surgery abolishes gastrointestinal motility for a period of time that varies with the type of operation; the MMC returns within 3 hours after cholecystectomy, the small intestine recovers in 12–24 hours, and the colon may not regain normal motility until the sixth postoperative day. The clinical manifestations of postoperative ileus do not correlate well with the myoelectric parameters, however, and the pathophysiology of ileus remains incompletely understood. Corticotropin-releasing factor may be an important mediator of postoperative ileus.

Orocecal transit time is an important indicator of small bowel function. Transit may be accelerated in patients with diarrhea and delayed in constipation; a variety of disease states are responsible. Orocecal transit time can be measured by the lactulose breath hydrogen test. An ingested solution of lactulose reaches the cecum in about 90 minutes; colonic fermentation of lactulose produces hydrogen, which is detected in the breath. Several techniques of gamma scintigraphy, including the use of isotopically labeled pellets, are alternative methods of estimating small bowel transit time.

Digestion, Secretion, & Absorption

With a few exceptions (eg, iron, calcium), the normal small intestine absorbs indiscriminately without regard to body composition. Absorption of fat, carbohydrate, and protein is just as complete in the obese patient as in the slender individual. The enteric nervous system regulates secretion and absorption in the small intestine; VIP is one mediator, and neuropeptide Y may be another.

A. Water and Electrolytes

Ingested fluid and salivary, gastric, biliary, pancreatic, and intestinal secretions present a total of 5–9 L of water to the absorptive surface of the small intestine each day, and 1–2 L are discharged from the ileum into the colon. Water is absorbed throughout the intestine, but the major site of absorption after a meal is in the upper tract.

The net flow of water and electrolytes across the intestinal mucosa is equal to the difference between absorption and secretion. The villi are mainly absorbing structures, and secretion of water and electrolytes is localized to the crypts. Much of the transfer of water and small solutes occurs via paracellular "shunt" pathways. The intercellular tight junctions between cells are actually rather loose, and it is through these "pores" that water moves passively in response to osmotic and hydrostatic pressures in the lumen and in the interstitial fluid. The pores are larger in the jejunum (0.7–0.9 nm) than in the ileum (0.3–0.4 nm). Hypertonic solutions in the duodenum and upper jejunum are rapidly brought into osmotic equilibrium with blood, and as the osmotic pressure of luminal contents is increased further by breakdown of large molecules into smaller ones, still more water enters the lumen. Net absorption of water accompanies active transport of ions and small molecules such as glucose and amino acids. If the lumen contains nonabsorbable solute, water is retained to maintain isotonicity.

Three mechanisms are responsible for sodium and chloride absorption in the small intestine: (1) active electrogenic transport of sodium, which establishes an electrical gradient for passive absorption of chloride, mostly through the paracellular pathway; (2) sodium absorption directly coupled to the absorption of water-soluble organic solutes such as hexoses, amino acids, and triglycerides, with passive absorption of chloride; and (3) neutral sodium chloride cotransport, in which a carrier at the mucosal membrane mediates the one-for-one entry of both ions into the cell. The ileum has low permeability to chloride, so that active absorption processes are needed for chloride in that part of the gut.

Potassium diffuses passively along electrical and concentration gradients. Calcium diffuses passively and also is actively transported, a process stimulated by vitamin D. Calcium absorption is most efficient in the duodenum, but because intestinal contents are in the jejunum and ileum longer, most calcium is absorbed in these areas. Magnesium is absorbed by all segments of the intestine, but relatively poorly. Iron is absorbed in the duodenum and jejunum, primarily as the ferrous ion.

Bicarbonate is absorbed by secretion of hydrogen ions in exchange for sodium ions; one bicarbonate ion is released into the interstitial fluid for every hydrogen ion secreted, and CO_2 is generated in the intestinal lumen. Phosphate is absorbed in all portions of the small bowel.

Epithelial transport of water and electrolytes is under partial control of the enteric nervous system. Ingestion of a meal increases the magnitude of jejunal water and electrolyte absorption by neuroendocrine mechanisms that have not been clarified. Intramural nervous reflexes elicited by luminal stimuli increase fluid secretion from the crypts. The afferent part of these reflexes is not well understood, but acetylcholine and perhaps substance P and VIP are secretory neurotransmitters on the efferent side. Absorption and secretion are influenced by other polypeptides such as somatostatin, corticosteroids, prostaglandins, neuropeptide YY, cAMP, various drugs, and bacterial toxins.

B. Carbohydrate

The polysaccharides starch and glycogen and the disaccharides sucrose and lactose comprise about half the calories ingested by humans. Digestion of starch is begun by salivary amylase and is completed by pancreatic amylase in the duodenum and upper jejunum. The products of hydrolysis are further hydrolyzed by contact with enzymes contained in the brush border of intestinal epithelial cells. The monosaccharides glucose, galactose, and fructose are actively transported against a concentration gradient by a carrier-mediated mechanism that is dependent on and coupled to the absorption of sodium. Monosaccharides are delivered directly into portal blood from the intestinal mucosa.

Although the entire small intestine has the capacity for carbohydrate digestion and absorption, under normal circumstances most absorption of monosaccharides occurs in the duodenum and proximal jejunum. About 10% of dietary starch passes unabsorbed into the colon.

Fiber is insoluble matrix substance of plant cells and is mostly indigestible by human enzymes. It is composed of the carbohydrates cellulose and hemicellulose and the noncarbohydrate lignin. Dietary fiber increases the osmotic load to the distal small intestine and colon and therefore increases stool mass.

C. Protein

Protein is denatured and partially digested in the stomach, but these steps are not essential. Pancreatic enzymes digest protein to form free amino acids and oligopeptides; oligopeptides are attacked by carboxypeptidases and aminopeptidases in the brush border, liberating amino acids, dipeptides, and tripeptides. Amino acids are absorbed by means of an active, carrier-mediated transport mechanism. Dipeptides and tripeptides are actively absorbed into columnar cells, where they are hydrolyzed completely to constituent amino acids. More than 80% of protein absorption occurs in the proximal 100 cm of jejunum. Absorption of ingested protein is virtually complete, and the protein excreted in feces is derived from bacteria, desquamated cells, and mucoproteins.

Important changes occur in the intestine during critical illness, eg, following trauma or abdominal surgery. The intestinal epithelial barrier to absorption of bacteria and endotoxins may be compromised, permitting translocation of bacteria into the circulation. Furthermore, glutamine extraction from the circulation by the small intestine is impaired in septic patients. Glutamine is the preferred fuel for oxidative metabolism by the enterocyte, and diminished uptake of this mucosal nutrient may be significant. In stressed states, glutamine deficiency is associated with mucosal atrophy.

D. Fat

Dietary fat is largely in the form of triglycerides, which are water-insoluble oil droplets until attacked by pancreatic lipase. Colipase, a protein in pancreatic juice, helps lipase adhere to the surface of these oil droplets as the triglycerides are partially hydrolyzed to fatty acids and 2-monoglycerides. These products of digestion are also water-insoluble, and their efficient absorption depends on the presence of bile acids. When the concentration of bile acids exceeds a certain level (the critical micellar concentration), they spontaneously aggregate to form micelles. Bile acids in micelles are arranged with the fat-soluble portion of the molecule toward the center of the aggregate and the water-soluble portion at the periphery; hydrophobic molecules such as fatty acids, monoglycerides, cholesterol, and fat-soluble vitamins are carried in the centers of the micelles.

Micelles release monoglycerides and fatty acids to enter the mucosal cells, where triglycerides are resynthesized, aggregated with phospholipid and cholesterol, and delivered to the lymph as chylomicrons. Medium-chain triglyceride is a synthetic substance that is hydrolyzed to water-soluble fatty acids that do not require bile acids for absorption. Also, these fatty acids are not reesterified to triglycerides in the mucosal cells; they pass directly into portal blood.

Normally, most of the ingested fat is digested and absorbed in the duodenum and proximal jejunum. Conjugated bile acids are actively absorbed in the distal ileum and returned via portal blood to the liver, where they again are secreted into the bile. Disease or resection of the terminal ileum disrupts this enterohepatic circulation, and increased amounts of bile acids enter the colon, where they induce net secretion of water and electrolytes and cause diarrhea (cholerrheic diarrhea). Malabsorbed fatty acids contribute to diarrhea by an effect similar to that of castor oil.

E. VITAMINS

Vitamin B_{12} (cyanocobalamin) is a water-soluble cobalt compound that requires a special mechanism for absorption, because of its large molecular weight. Dietary vitamin B_{12} complexes with intrinsic factor, a mucoprotein secreted by the gastric parietal cells. The complex dissociates at the surface of cells in the distal ileum, and vitamin B_{12} enters the cells, perhaps by receptor-mediated endocytosis. Folic acid, thiamin, and ascorbic acid are also absorbed by active transport. Other water-soluble vitamins diffuse passively across the mucosa.

Fat-soluble vitamins—notably vitamins A, D, E, and K—are dissolved in mixed micelles and absorbed like other lipids. Since they are totally nonpolar lipids, the absence of bile seriously impairs their absorption.

Agarwal R, Afzalpurkar R, Fordtran JS: Pathophysiology of potassium absorption and secretion by the human intestine. Gastroenterology 1994;107:548.

Ahluwalia NK et al: Human small intestinal contractions and aboral traction forces during fasting and after feeding. Gut 1994;35:625.

Ducerf C, Cuchamp C, Pouyet M: Postoperative electromyographic profile in human jejunum. Ann Surg 1992;215:237.

Fine KD et al: Mechanism by which glucose stimulates the passive absorption of small solutes by the human jejunum in vivo. Gastroenterology 1994;107:389.

Frantzides CT et al: Small bowel myoelectric activity in peritonitis. Am J Surg 1993;165:681.

Gleeson D: Acid-base transport systems in gastrointestinal epithelia. Gut 1992;33:1134.

Gorard DA, Libby GW, Farthing MJG: 5-Hydroxytryptamine and human small intestinal motility: effect of inhibiting 5-hydroxytryptamine reuptake. Gut 1994;35:496.

Inoue Y, Copeland EM, Souba WW: Growth hormone enhances amino acid uptake by the human small intestine. Ann Surg 1994;219:715.

Otterson MF, Sarr MG: Normal physiology of small intestinal motility. Surg Clin North Am 1993;73:1173.

Sanderson IR, Walker WA: Uptake and transport of macromolecules by the intestine: possible role in clinical disorders (an update). Gastroenterology 1993;104:622.

Stark ME et al: Nitric oxide mediates inhibitory nerve input in human and canine jejunum. Gastroenterology 1993;104:398.

von der Ohe MR, Camilleri M: Measurement of small bowel and colonic transit: indications and methods. Mayo Clin Proc 1992;67:1169.

BLIND LOOP SYNDROME

The normal concentration of bacteria in the small intestine is about 10^5/mL. Mechanisms that limit bacterial populations include the continual flow of luminal contents, resulting from peristalsis, the interdigestive migrating myoelectric complex, gastric acidity, local effects of immunoglobulins, and the prevention of reflux of colonic contents by the ileocecal valve. Disturbance of any of these mechanisms can lead to bacterial overgrowth and the blind loop (contaminated small bowel, intestinal bacterial overgrowth) syndrome. Strictures, diverticula, fistulas, or blind (poorly emptying) segments of intestine are anatomic lesions that cause stagnation and permit bacterial proliferation. In many patients, stasis of intestinal contents is the result of a functional abnormality of motility (eg, scleroderma). Bacterial overgrowth is observed in patients with immunodeficiency syndromes.

Steatorrhea, diarrhea, megaloblastic anemia, and malnutrition are the hallmarks of the blind loop syndrome. Steatorrhea is the consequence of bacterial deconjugation and dehydroxylation of bile salts in the proximal small bowel. Deconjugated bile salts have a higher critical micellar concentration, and micelle formation is inadequate to solubilize ingested fat in preparation for absorption. The presence of partially digested triglycerides in the distal ileum inhibits jejunal motility; nevertheless, the unabsorbed fatty acids enter the colon, where they increase net secretion of water and electrolytes, and diarrhea results. Hypocalcemia occurs because calcium is bound to unabsorbed fatty acids in the intestinal lumen. Macrocytic anemia is due to malabsorption of vitamin B_{12}, largely because of binding of the vitamin by anaerobic bacteria. Malabsorption of carbohydrate and protein is due partly to bacterial catabolism and partly to impaired absorption of these nutrients because of direct damage to the small intestinal mucosa. All of these mechanisms contribute to malnutrition in blind loop syndrome.

Quantitative culture of upper intestinal aspirates is valuable if properly performed; bacterial counts of more than 10^5 per milliliter are generally abnormal. Endoscopic biopsies of duodenum can be helpful in patients with suspected small intestinal malabsorption. Laboratory studies reveal impaired absorption of orally administered vitamin B_{12} (Schilling test), D-xylose, and ^{14}C triolein. Fecal fat measurement is an obsolete procedure. A large variety of breath tests have been studied, but most have proved to be unreliable. The ^{14}C-D-xylose breath test is the best of these methods available at present. Anaerobic bacteria in the small bowel metabolize xylose, releasing $^{14}CO_2$, which is detected in the breath.

Surgical treatment of the underlying neoplasm, fistula, blind loop, diverticula, or other lesion is carried out whenever possible. A majority of patients do not have a problem that is amenable to surgical correction, however, and treatment consists of broad-spectrum antibiotics and drugs to control diarrhea. It may be necessary to use different antibiotics in sequence, guided by culture results and response to therapy. Damage to enterocytes appears to be reversible with treatment. Octreotide (somatostatin analog) may reduce bacterial overgrowth and improved abdominal symptoms in patients with scleroderma according to a recent report.

Hughes JP et al: Scintigraphic demonstration of a blind loop following surgery for Crohn's disease: the value of Tc-99m HMPAO white cell scanning. Clin Nucl Med 1994;19:469.

Ladas SD et al: Effect of forceps size and mode of orientation on endoscopic small bowel biopsy evaluation. Gastrointest Endosc 1994;40:51.

Patel MC et al: Blind loop syndrome: diagnosis by In-111-labeled leukocyte scintigraphy. Clin Nucl Med 1999;24:623.

Rubesin SE, Rubin RA, Herlinger H: Small bowel malabsorption: clinical and radiologic perspectives. How we see it. Radiology 1992;184:297.

Strocchi A et al: Detection of malabsorption of low doses of carbohydrate: accuracy of various breath H_2 criteria. Gastroenterology 1993;105:1404.

Takahashi M et al: Use of the conjugate of disulphated ursodeoxycholic acid with *p*-aminobenzoic acid for the detection of intestinal bacteria. Gut 1993;34:823.

SHORT BOWEL SYNDROME

ESSENTIALS OF DIAGNOSIS

- *Extensive small bowel resection.*
- *Diarrhea.*
- *Steatorrhea.*
- *Malnutrition.*

General Considerations

The absorptive capacity of the small intestine is normally far in excess of need. The short bowel syndrome may develop after extensive resection of the small intestine for trauma, mesenteric thrombosis, regional enteritis, radiation enteropathy, strangulated small bowel obstruction, or neoplasm. Necrotizing enterocolitis and congenital atresia are the most common pediatric causes.

The ability of a patient to maintain nutrition after massive small bowel resection depends on the extent and site of resection, the presence or absence of the colon, the absorptive function of the intestinal remnant, adaptation of remaining bowel, and the nature of the underlying disease process and its complications. When 3 m or less of the small intestine remain, serious nutritional abnormalities can develop. With 2 m or less remaining, function is clinically impaired in most patients, and many patients with 1 m or less of normal bowel require parenteral nutrition at home indefinitely. Some patients with a very short small bowel are net absorbers, and others are net secretors—ie, they put out more intestinal fluid than they take orally.

If the jejunum is resected, the ileum is able to take over most of its absorptive function. Because transport of bile salts, vitamin B_{12}, and cholesterol is localized to the ileum, resection of this region is poorly tolerated (Figure 29–4). Bile salt malabsorption causes diarrhea, and steatorrhea occurs if 100 cm or more of distal ileum is resected. Abdominal gamma counting after oral administration of 23-selena-25-homocholyltaurine (^{75}SeHCAT) is a test of bile acid absorption in the distal ileum. Blind loop syndrome due to bacterial overgrowth in the shortened small bowel (see above) compounds the problems. Patients who undergo colectomy in addition to extensive small bowel resection are among the most difficult to manage.

Calcium oxalate urinary tract calculi form in 7–10% of patients who have extensive ileal resection (or disease) and an intact colon. This condition, called **enteric hyperoxaluria**, results from excessive absorption of oxalate from the colon. Two synergistic mechanisms are responsible: (1) Unabsorbed fatty acids combine with calcium, preventing the formation of insoluble calcium oxalate and allowing oxalate to remain available for absorption. (2) Unabsorbed fatty acids and bile acids increase the permeability of the colon to oxalate.

D-Lactic acidosis may result from colonic fermentation of unabsorbed carbohydrate; symptoms of confusion, loss of memory, slurred speech, unsteady gait, and inappropriate behavior resemble those associated with alcoholic intoxication. Treatment includes correction of the acidosis with bicarbonate infusion, thiamine replacement, and antibiotics to reduce colonic flora.

Some patients develop gastric hypersecretion after extensive small bowel resection. It is more marked after proximal resection, and it improves with time. The outpouring of gastric juice may damage the mucosa of the upper intestine, inactivate lipase and trypsin by lowering intraluminal pH, and present an excessive solute load to the intestinal remnant. The increased acid production results from loss of inhibitory hormones normally secreted by the small intestine. Elevated basal and postprandial serum gastrin levels have been detected in some cases.

Clinical Course

During the immediate postoperative period, more than 2 L of daily fluid and electrolyte losses from diarrhea are characteristic. The diarrhea is less severe after a few weeks, and eventually a reasonably normal existence is possible in most cases. The progression of a patient from strict depen-

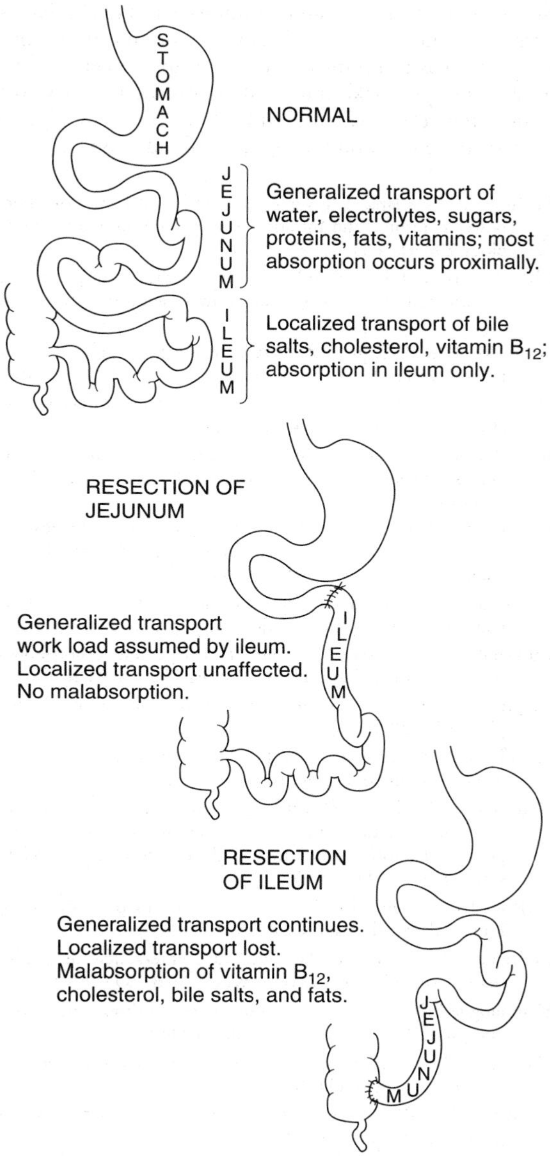
STOMACH
NORMAL
JEJUNUM
Generalized transport of water, electrolytes, sugars, proteins, fats, vitamins; most absorption occurs proximally.
ILEUM
Localized transport of bile salts, cholesterol, vitamin B12; absorption in ileum only.
RESECTION OF JEJUNUM
Generalized transport work load assumed by ileum. Localized transport unaffected. No malabsorption.
ILEUM
RESECTION OF ILEUM
Generalized transport continues. Localized transport lost. Malabsorption of vitamin B12, cholesterol, bile salts, and fats.
JEJUNUM

Figure 29–4. The consequences of complete resection of jejunum or ileum are predictable in part from the loss of regionally localized transport processes.

dence on intravenous feeding to nutritional maintenance by oral intake is possible because of intestinal **adaptation**, a compensatory increase of absorptive capacity in the intestinal remnant. The mucosa becomes hyperplastic, the villi lengthen and the crypts become deeper, the wall thickens, and the intestine elongates and dilates. The intensity of these responses is proportionate to the amount of intestine removed, the segment remaining (greater after proximal than after distal small bowel resection), and the presence of a luminal stream. Nutritional support is essential, and although nutrition must be provided intravenously at first, food in the lumen of the intestine is required for full adaptation. Short-chain fatty acids and long-chain triglycerides, sugars, and proteins are all important trophic nutrients. Glutamine is the principal fuel utilized by the small intestine, and gut glutamine extraction is increased in the first week after massive small bowel resection in animals, but it is not clear whether glutamine needs to be provided to patients to aid in adaptation. Circulating peptide factors no doubt are important. Enteroglucagon, epidermal growth factor (urogastrone), neurotensin, and insulin-like growth factors are implicated as trophic agents, and somatostatin and transforming growth factor-β (TGFβ) may play inhibitory roles.

Treatment

A. General Measures

Treatment of severe short bowel syndrome may be divided into three stages:

1. Stage 1 (intravenous feeding)—During this stage, which lasts 1–3 months, diarrhea is massive and patients should receive nothing by mouth. Careful intravenous fluid and electrolyte therapy and parenteral nutrition must be given. Catheter sepsis is a common complication in this setting. Other important measures include reduction of gastric secretion with intravenous H_2 blockers or proton pump inhibitors, control of diarrhea (eg, with loperamide, diphenoxylate, or deodorized tincture of opium), and protection of perianal skin from irritation. Somatostatin has limited value in reduction of fecal output.

2. Stage 2 (intravenous and oral feeding)—Oral feedings should not be initiated until diarrhea subsides to less than 2.5 L/d. Intravenous nutrition should continue while oral intake begins. Oral rehydration solutions that are used for diarrheal diseases in developing countries are applicable to short bowel syndrome as well. An oral solution of sodium and potassium salts and glucose takes advantage of the phenomenon of cotransport whereby sodium ions are absorbed with the hexose molecules across the intestinal epithelium. Other liquid diets are best tolerated if they are isotonic. Liquid polymeric diets are the next step, and then a more liberal selection of food is allowed. A diet with normal fat content is more palatable and just as effective as a low-fat diet.

Milk may aggravate diarrhea, because total intestinal lactase activity is severely reduced after extensive resection; cheese is tolerated because lactose has been digested in this product. There may be some advantage in making breakfast the largest meal of the day, because as a result of gallbladder filling during the overnight fast, morning may be the time when the greatest amount of bile salts are present in the proximal intestine.

3. Stage 3 (complete oral feeding)—After a few months, complete dependence on oral intake may be expected in patients with 1–2 m of remaining small bowel, but full adaptation may require up to 2 years. Maintenance of body weight at levels 20% or more below normal, acceptable bowel habits, and return to productive life are reasonable expectations in many patients. Chronic parenteral nutrition at home is required if oral intake is not tolerated.

Patients with extensive ileal resection require parenteral vitamin B_{12} (1000 μg intramuscularly every 2–3 months) for life. Hyperoxaluria often can be prevented by a diet low in fat and oxalate; supplementary oral calcium or citrate may be helpful. Oral cholestyramine to minimize diarrhea is usually rejected by patients due to texture and taste; loperamide (Imodium) and Lomotil are well tolerated. Pancreatic enzyme supplements may reduce diarrhea also. Deficiencies in magnesium, vitamins D, A, and K, and water-soluble vitamins should be prevented. Osteomalacia is common. Blind loop syndrome may require treatment. H_2 receptor antagonists or proton pump inhibitors reduce acid secretion and improve absorption in the early stages but probably are not needed long-term. The incidence of cholelithiasis is increased in patients with short bowel syndrome, and symptoms should be investigated. Interestingly, the stones may be composed of pigment rather than cholesterol.

B. Adjunctive Surgical Procedures

Surgical procedures to slow intestinal transit, reduce gastric acidity, or increase the absorptive surface are not recommended routinely and are rarely used. Reversed segments, recirculating loops, and construction of valve mechanisms have been tried in the hope of slowing transit and improving absorption. None of these methods have a clearly established role. By enhancing bacterial growth, damaging additional bowel, and obstructing the intestine, they are likely to make matters worse. Gastric hyperacidity is controlled by H_2 receptor antagonists, and operation is rarely necessary for this problem. A method of lengthening the small intestine by longitudinal division of the bowel and its mesentery has been described for certain pediatric situations.

C. Small Bowel Transplantation

Small bowel transplantation has become the treatment of choice for patients with life-threatening complications of intestinal failure. It is estimated that 15–20% of patients on chronic total parenteral nutrition for short bowel syndrome or intestinal failure will eventually require small bowel transplantation. Long-term parenteral nutrition frequently leads to liver failure, so a combined liver and small bowel transplantation is often necessary. Early attempts at intestinal transplantation were unsuccessful due to both technical and immunologic failure. However, the introduction of newer immunosuppressive drugs, such as tacrolimus, as well as improvement in surgical technique make intestinal transplantation a viable option for select patients with short bowel syndrome who are dependent on total parenteral nutrition.

Buchman AL, Scolapio J, Fryer J: AGA technical review on short bowel syndrome and intestinal transplantation. Gastroenterology 2003;124:1111.

Chris Anderson-Hill D, Heimburger DC: Medical management of the difficult patient with short-bowel syndrome. Nutrition 1993;9:536.

Georgeson K et al: Sequential intestinal lengthening procedures for refractory short bowel syndrome. J Pediatr Surg 1994;29:316.

Hines OJ et al: Up-regulation of Na^+, K^+ adenosine triphosphatase after massive intestinal resection. Surgery 1994;116:401.

Inoue Y et al: Effect of total parenteral nutrition on amino acid and glucose transport by the human small intestine. Ann Surg 1993;217:604.

Jeppesen PB: Glucagon-like peptide 2 improves nutrient absorption and nutritional status in short-bowel patients with no colon. Gastroenterology 2001;120:806.

Ko TC et al: Glutamine is essential for epidermal growth factor-stimulated intestinal cell proliferation. Surgery 1993;114:147.

Kurkchubasche AG, Rowe MI, Smith SD: Adaptation in short-bowel syndrome: reassessing old limits. J Pediatr Surg 1993;28:1069.

Langnas AN: Advances in small-intestine transplantation. Transplantation 2004;77:S75.

Nightingale JM, Lennard-Jones JE: The short bowel syndrome: what's new and old? Dig Dis 1993;11:12.

Nightingale JMD et al: Oral salt supplements to compensate for jejunostomy losses: comparison of sodium chloride capsules, glucose electrolyte solution, and glucose polymer electrolyte solution. Gut 1992;33:759.

Playford RJ et al: Effect of luminal growth factor preservation on intestinal growth. Lancet 1993;341:843.

Rodriguez DJ, Clevenger FW: Successful enteral refeeding after massive small bowel resection. West J Med 1993;159:192.

Shanbhogue LKR, Molenaar JC: Short bowel syndrome: metabolic and surgical management. Br J Surg 1994;81:486.

Thompson JS: Surgical considerations in the short bowel syndrome. Surg Gynecol Obstet 1993;176:89.

van der Hulst RRWJ et al: Glutamine and the preservation of gut integrity. Lancet 1993;341:1363.

OBSTRUCTION OF THE SMALL INTESTINE

ESSENTIALS OF DIAGNOSIS

Complete proximal obstruction:

- *Vomiting.*
- *Abdominal discomfort.*
- *Abnormal oral contrast x-rays or CT scan.*

Complete mid or distal obstruction:

- *Colicky abdominal pain.*
- *Vomiting.*
- *Abdominal distention.*
- *Constipation-obstipation.*
- *Peristaltic rushes.*
- *Dilated small bowel on x-ray.*
- *Transition point on CT scan.*

General Considerations

Obstruction is the most common surgical disorder of the small intestine.

Mechanical obstruction implies a physical barrier that impedes aboral progress of intestinal contents; it may be complete or partial. **Simple obstruction** occludes the lumen only; **strangulation obstruction** impairs the blood supply also and leads to necrosis of the intestinal wall. Most simple obstructions occur at only one point. Closed loop obstruction, in which the lumen is occluded in at least two places (eg, in a volvulus), is commonly associated with strangulation. Ileus is a term whose definition includes mechanical obstruction, but in the USA it usually refers to **paralytic ileus** (adynamic ileus), a disorder in which there is neurogenic failure of peristalsis to propel intestinal contents but no mechanical obstruction.

A. Etiology

1. Adhesions—Adhesions are by far the most common cause of mechanical small bowel obstruction (Table 29–1). Congenital bands are seen in children, but adhesions acquired from abdominal operations or inflammation are much more frequent in adults.

2. Neoplasms—Intrinsic small bowel neoplasms can progressively occlude the lumen or serve as a leading point in intussusception. Symptoms may be intermittent, onset of obstruction is slow, and signs of chronic anemia are present. Neoplasms extrinsic to small bowel may entrap loops, and strategically situated lesions of the colon—particularly those near the ileocecal valve—may present as small bowel obstruction.

3. Hernia—Incarceration of an external hernia is uncommon since prophylactic repair of hernias became routine. Inguinal, femoral, or umbilical hernias may have been present for years, or the patient may be unaware of the defect before the onset of obstructive symptoms. An incarcerated hernia may be overlooked by the examining surgeon, particularly if the patient is obese or if the hernia is of the femoral type, and a careful search for external hernias must be made during evaluation of every patient with acute abdominal illness. Internal hernias into the obturator foramen, foramen epiploicum (Winslow), or other anatomic defects are rare, but internal herniation is one of several mechanisms by which acquired adhesions produce obstruction. Surgical defects—lateral to an ileostomy, for example—also provide sites for internal herniation of small bowel loops.

4. Intussusception—Invagination of one loop of intestine into another is rarely encountered in adults and is usually caused by a polyp or other intraluminal lesion. Intussusception is more often seen in children; an organic lesion is not required, and the syndrome of colicky pain, passage of blood per rectum, and a palpable mass (the intussuscepted segment) is characteristic.

5. Volvulus—Volvulus results from rotation of bowel loops about a fixed point, often the consequence of congenital anomalies or acquired adhesions. Onset of obstruction is abrupt, and strangulation develops rapidly. Malrotation of the intestine is a cause of volvulus in infants and rarely in adults.

6. Foreign bodies—Bezoars and ingested foreign bodies may pass into the intestine and block the lumen.

7. Gallstone ileus—Passage of a large gallstone into the intestine through a cholecystenteric fistula may produce obstruction of the small bowel. Gallstone ileus is discussed in Chapter 25.

8. Inflammatory bowel disease—Inflammatory bowel disease (Crohn's disease) often causes obstruction when the lumen is narrowed by inflammation or fibrosis of the wall.

9. Stricture—Stricture due to ischemia or radiation injury or surgical trauma can result in mechanical obstruction.

10. Cystic fibrosis—Cystic fibrosis causes chronic partial obstruction of the distal ileum and right colon in adolescents and adults. It is equivalent to meconium ileus in newborns.

11. Hematoma—Hematoma may develop spontaneously in the intestinal wall in a patient taking anticoagulants.

Table 29–1. Causes of obstruction of the small intestine in adults.

Causes	Relative Incidence (%)
Adhesions	60
External hernia	10
Neoplasms	20
Intrinsic	3
Extrinsic	17
Miscellaneous	10

B. Pathophysiology

The small bowel proximal to a point of obstruction distends with gas and fluid. Swallowed air is the major source of gaseous distention, at least in the early stages, because nitrogen is not well absorbed by mucosa. When bacterial fermentation occurs later on, other gases are produced; the partial pressure of nitrogen within the lumen is lowered, and a gradient for diffusion of nitrogen from blood to lumen is established.

Enormous quantities of fluid from the extracellular space are lost into the gut and from the serosa into the peritoneal cavity. Fluid fills the lumen proximal to the obstruction, because the bidirectional flux of salt and water is disrupted and net secretion is enhanced. Mediator substances (eg, endotoxin, prostaglandins) released from proliferating bacteria in the static luminal contents are responsible. Somatostatin effectively inhibits secretion in animal models of intestinal obstruction, but it has no defined role in humans. Reflexly induced vomiting accentuates the fluid and electrolyte deficit. Hypovolemia leads to multi-organ system failure and is the cause of death in patients with nonstrangulating obstruction.

Audible peristaltic rushes are manifestations of attempts by the small bowel to propel its contents past the obstruction. The vomitus becomes feculent—particularly with distal obstruction—as the illness progresses. Bacterial translocation from lumen to mesenteric nodes and the bloodstream occurs even in simple obstruction. Abdominal distention elevates the diaphragm and impairs respiration, so that pulmonary complications are frequent.

Strangulation is a threat early in the course of closed loop obstruction but must be feared in any complete mechanical obstruction. Incarcerated inguinal hernia and volvulus are examples of obstructing mechanisms that occlude the vascular supply as well as the intestinal lumen. Strangulation rarely if ever results just from progressive distention. Venous drainage is more apt to be interrupted than arterial inflow when the mesentery is trapped. Gangrenous intestine bleeds into the lumen and into the peritoneal cavity, and eventually it perforates. The luminal contents of strangulated intestine are a toxic mixture of bacteria, bacterial products, necrotic tissue, and blood. Some of this fluid may enter the circulation by way of intestinal lymphatics or by absorption from the peritoneal cavity; septic shock is the result.

Clinical Findings

A. Simple Obstruction

1. Symptoms and signs—(Figure 29–5) Proximal (high) small bowel obstruction usually presents as profuse vomiting that seldom becomes feculent even in prolonged obstruction. Abdominal pain is variable and often is described as upper abdominal discomfort rather than cramping pain.

Obstruction of the mid or distal small intestine causes cramping periumbilical or poorly localized abdominal pain. Each episode of cramps has a crescendo-decrescendo pattern, lasts for a few seconds to a few minutes, and recurs every few minutes. Between cramps, the patient may be entirely free of pain. Vomiting follows the onset of pain after an interval that varies with the level of obstruction; it may not occur until several hours later. The more distal the obstruction, the more likely it is that vomitus will become feculent. Gas and feces present in the colon may be expelled after the onset of pain, but obstipation always occurs eventually in complete obstruction.

Vital signs may be normal in the early stages, but dehydration is noted with continued loss of fluid and electrolytes. Temperature is normal or mildly elevated. Abdominal distention is minimal to absent in proximal obstruction but is pronounced in more distal obstruction. Peristalsis in dilated loops of small bowel may be visible beneath the abdominal wall in thin patients. Mild tenderness may be elicited. Peristaltic rushes, gurgles, and high-pitched tinkles are audible in coordination with attacks of cramping pain in distal obstruction. Incarcerated hernias should be sought. Rectal examination is usually normal.

2. Laboratory findings—In the early stages, laboratory findings may be normal; with progression of disease, there are hemoconcentration, leukocytosis, and electrolyte abnormalities that depend on the level of obstruction and the severity of dehydration. Serum amylase is often elevated.

3. Imaging studies—Supine and upright plain abdominal films reveal a ladder-like pattern of dilated small bowel loops with air-fluid levels (Figure 29–6). These features may be minimal or absent in early obstruction, proximal obstruction, or closed loop obstruction or in some cases when fluid-filled loops contain little gas. The colon is often devoid of gas unless the patient has been given an enema, has undergone sigmoidoscopy, or has only a partial obstruction. Opaque gallstones and air in the biliary tree should be looked for. Administration of contrast media orally confirms the presence of mechanical obstruction and its completeness. CT scan is highly accurate in making the diagnosis of and determining the level of a small bowel obstruction.

B. Strangulation Obstruction

Although certain clinical features should make the surgeon suspicious of strangulation, no historical, physical, or laboratory findings entirely exclude the possibility of strangulation in complete small bowel obstruction. At least one-third of strangulation obstructions are unsuspected before operation, which underscores the need for early operation whenever obstruction is complete.

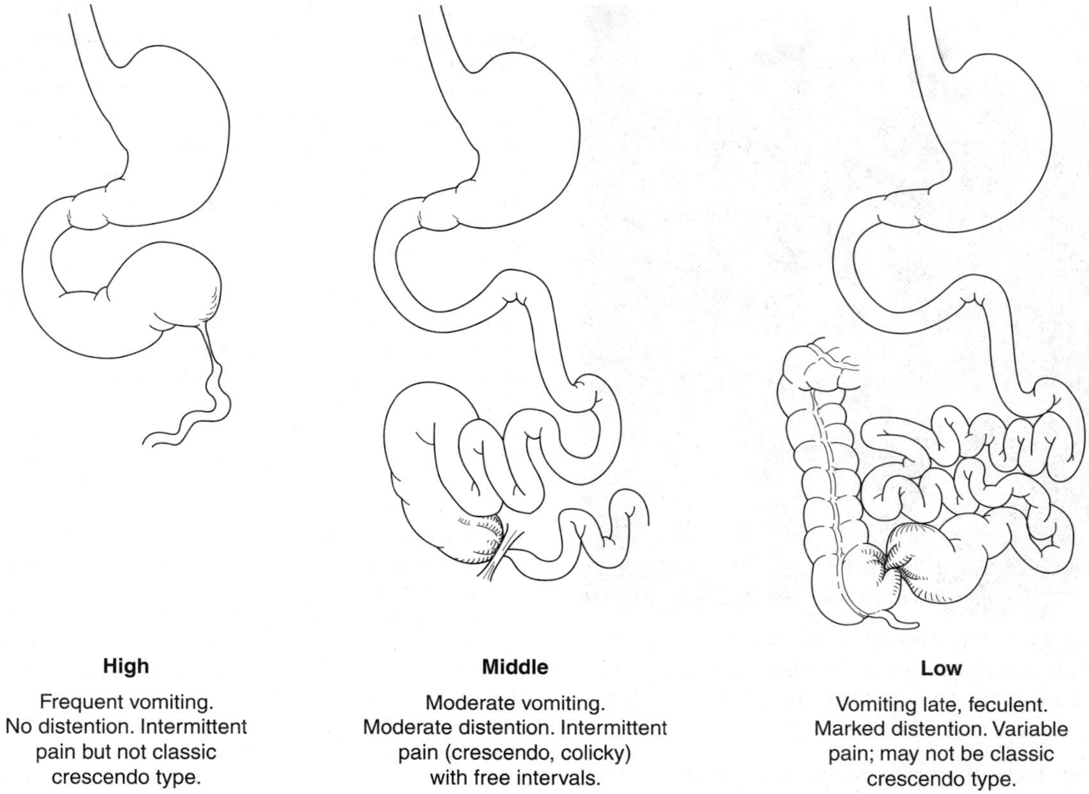

High
Frequent vomiting.
No distention. Intermittent
pain but not classic
crescendo type.
Middle
Moderate vomiting.
Moderate distention. Intermittent
pain (crescendo, colicky)
with free intervals.
Low
Vomiting late, feculent.
Marked distention. Variable
pain; may not be classic
crescendo type.

Figure 29–5. Small bowel obstruction. Variable manifestations of obstruction depend upon the level of blockage of the small bowel.

1. Symptoms and signs—Shock that appears early in the course of obstruction suggests a strangulated closed loop. When strangulation supervenes in simple obstruction, high fever may develop, previously cramping abdominal pain may become a severe continuous ache, vomitus may contain gross or occult blood, and abdominal tenderness and rigidity may appear.

2. Laboratory findings—Marked leukocytosis not accounted for by hemoconcentration alone should suggest strangulation, as does lactic acidosis that does not resolve with volume resuscitation.

3. Imaging studies—Intraperitoneal fluid is seen as widened spaces between adjacent loops of dilated bowel on plain films and is often found in simple obstruction as well as in strangulation. Thumbprinting, loss of mucosal pattern, and gas within the bowel wall or within intrahepatic branches of the portal vein may be seen in strangulation. Air-fluid levels outside the bowel indicate perforation. CT scanning is reported to have a sensitivity of 90% or higher in detecting complete or high-grade small bowel obstruction. It is also provides information as to the cause of the obstruction and the severity of bowel injury. The CT scan may reveal a whirling pattern in the mesentery of patients with a volvulus and closed loop obstruction as well as raise the suspicion of intestinal ischemia by documenting thickening and edema of the bowel wall or, in late cases, intramural air.

Differential Diagnosis

Pain from paralytic ileus is usually not severe but is constant and diffuse, and the abdomen is distended and mildly tender. If ileus has resulted from an acute intraperitoneal inflammatory process (eg, acute appendicitis), there should be symptoms and signs of the primary problem as well as the ileus. Plain films show gas mainly in the colon in uncomplicated postoperative ileus; gas in the small bowel suggests peritonitis. CT may be required in order to distinguish ileus from mechanical obstruction in postoperative patients.

Obstruction of the large intestine is characterized by obstipation and abdominal distention; pain is less often colicky, and vomiting is an inconstant symptom. X-rays

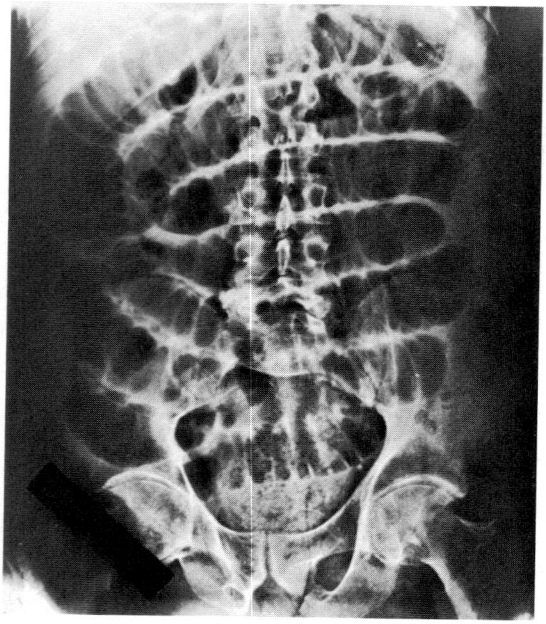

Figure 29–6. Small bowel obstruction. Note dilated loops of small bowel in a ladder-like pattern. Air-fluid levels are not obvious, because the patient is supine.

usually make the diagnosis by demonstrating colonic dilation proximal to the obstructing lesion. If the ileocecal valve is incompetent, the distal small bowel will be dilated, and a barium enema may be needed to determine the level of obstruction. This subject is covered in detail in Chapter 30.

Acute gastroenteritis, acute appendicitis, and acute pancreatitis can mimic simple intestinal obstruction. Strangulation obstruction may be confused with acute hemorrhagic pancreatitis or mesenteric vascular occlusion.

Intestinal pseudo-obstruction is a diverse group of disorders in which there are symptoms and signs of intestinal obstruction without evidence for an obstructing lesion. Acute pseudo-obstruction of the colon carries the risk of cecal perforation and is discussed in Chapter 30. Chronic or recurrent pseudo-obstruction affecting the small bowel with or without colonic involvement is often idiopathic. In other cases, pseudo-obstruction is associated with scleroderma, myxedema, lupus erythematosus, amyloidosis, drug abuse (eg, phenothiazine ingestion), radiation injury, or progressive systemic sclerosis. Several variations of familial visceral *myopathy* have been identified with seemingly distinct patterns of intestinal pseudo-obstruction. Patients with familial visceral *neuropathy* have degeneration of axons and neurons of the myenteric plexus of the gastrointestinal tract, and pseudo-obstruction results.

Patients with chronic pseudo-obstruction have recurrent attacks of vomiting, cramping abdominal pain, and abdominal distention. In some patients the esophagus, stomach, small bowel, colon, and urinary bladder all have abnormal motility, but in others one or more of these organs may be spared. Treatment is directed at the underlying disease if there is one. Management of idiopathic pseudo-obstruction is largely supportive.

Treatment

Partial small bowel obstruction can be treated expectantly as long as there is continued passage of stool and flatus. Plain abdominal x-rays show gas in the colon, and small bowel contrast x-rays prove the diagnosis. Decompression with a nasogastric tube is successful in 90% of such patients. Operation may be required if obstruction persists for several days even though it is incomplete. The decision of when—if ever—to operate for repeatedly recurring partial small bowel obstructions that resolve with nonoperative treatment can be a difficult one.

Complete obstruction of the small intestine is treated by operation after a period of careful preparation. The compelling reason for operation is that strangulation cannot be excluded with certainty, and strangulation is associated with high rates of complications and death. The surgeon must avoid being lulled into a false sense of security by the improvement in symptoms and signs that almost invariably occurs after resuscitation.

There are exceptions to the general rule that operation must be performed promptly: Incomplete obstruction, postoperative obstruction, a history of numerous previous operations for obstruction, radiation therapy, inflammatory bowel disease, and abdominal carcinomatosis are situations demanding mature judgment, and judicious nonoperative management may be in the patient's best interests. A long intestinal tube (eg, Miller-Abbott tube) may be passed in these cases to decompress the intestine.

A. Preparation

Proper timing of the operation is determined by the requirements of individual patients. The risk of strangulation must be weighed against the severity of fluid and electrolyte abnormalities and the need for evaluation and treatment of associated systemic diseases.

1. Nasogastric suction—A nasogastric tube should be inserted immediately upon admission to the emergency ward in order to relieve vomiting, avoid aspiration, and reduce the contribution of further swallowed air to the abdominal distention.

2. Fluid and electrolyte resuscitation—Depending upon the level and duration of obstruction, fluid and electrolyte deficits are mild to severe. Hemoconcentration induced by long-standing obstruction cannot be corrected by dextrose solutions alone. Fluid losses are isotonic, and resuscitation should begin with infusion of isotonic saline solution. Losses of gastrointestinal fluid also entail acid-base deficits, and since there is no neuroendocrine mechanism for correcting these deficits, the surgeon must do so. Serum electrolyte concentrations and arterial blood gas determinations are guides to electrolyte therapy; potassium is best withheld until urine output is satisfactory, but patients should not undergo operation until hypokalemia has been treated. The volume of fluid required and its exact electrolyte composition must be calculated for each patient, and careful monitoring of clinical signs and associated systemic diseases is imperative. Some patients—notably those with strangulation obstruction—require plasma or blood. Antibiotics should be given if strangulation is even remotely suspected.

B. Operation

Operation may commence when the patient has been rehydrated and vital organs are functioning satisfactorily. Occasionally, the toxic effects of strangulation may force operation at an earlier time.

A standard groin incision is used for patients with incarcerated inguinal or femoral hernias. Laparoscopic adhesiolysis may be performed in carefully selected patients by surgeons skilled in this procedure. Generally, however, an open procedure is performed through an incision that is partly dictated by the location of scars from previous operations.

Details of the operative procedure vary according to the cause of obstruction. Adhesive bands causing obstruction should be lysed; an obstructing tumor should be resected; and an obstructing foreign body should be removed through an enterotomy. Gangrenous intestine must be resected, but it may be difficult to determine whether obstructed bowel is viable or not. The loop should be wrapped in a warm saline-soaked pack and inspected for color, mesenteric pulsation, and peristalsis several minutes later. Intraoperative use of Doppler ultrasound is a method of determining viability of obstructed intestine. The qualitative fluorescein test may be helpful; 1000 mg of fluorescein is injected into a peripheral vein over a 30- to 60-second period, and the bowel is then inspected under ultraviolet (Wood's) light. If the loop appears nonviable, resection with end-to-end anastomosis is the safest course.

Extirpation of the obstructing lesion is not possible in some patients with carcinoma or radiation injury. Anastomosis of proximal small bowel to small or large intestine distal to the obstruction (bypass) may be the best procedure in these patients. Rarely, adhesions are so dense that the intestine cannot be freed and bypass cannot be accomplished. Prolonged decompression through a gastrostomy or jejunostomy tube and provision of nutrition via the parenteral route may allow spontaneous resolution over a period of a few weeks.

Decompression of massively dilated small bowel loops facilitates closure of the abdomen and may shorten the time for recovery of bowel function postoperatively. Decompression is accomplished by threading down a long tube passed orally or by needle aspiration through the bowel wall.

Attempts to prevent uncontrolled adhesion formation by suturing loops of bowel so that they are fixed in a suitable relation to one another (Nobel plication procedures) are unsuccessful. However, another procedure in which a long tube is inserted through a gastrostomy or jejunostomy for 10 days to provide intraluminal stenting has some proponents. Adhesion prevention with a hyaluronic acid methylcellulose bioabsorbable barrier has proved effective in decreasing adhesion formation and decreasing reoperative times. Studies proving efficacy in reducing the incidence of small bowel obstructions have shown a small benefit.

Prognosis

Nonstrangulating obstruction has a death rate of about 2%; most of these deaths occur in the elderly. Strangulation obstruction has a mortality rate of approximately 8% if operation is performed within 36 hours of the onset of symptoms and 25% if operation is delayed beyond 36 hours. Recurrent obstruction after lysis of adhesions is uncommon.

Assalia A et al: Therapeutic effect of oral Gastrografin in adhesive, partial small-bowel obstruction: a prospective randomized trial. Surgery 1994;115:433.

Balthazar EJ: George W. Holmes Lecture: CT of small-bowel obstruction. AJR Am J Roentgenol 1994;162:255.

Beck DE: The role of Seprafilm bioresorbable membrane in adhesion prevention. Eur J Surg (Acta Chirurgica) Suppl 1997;577:49.

Beck DE et al: A prospective, randomized, multicenter, controlled study of the safety of Seprafilm adhesion barrier in abdominopelvic surgery of the intestine. Dis Colon Rectum 2003;46:1310.

Beck DE et al: Incidence of small-bowel obstruction and adhesiolysis after open colorectal and general surgery. Dis Colon Rectum 1999;42:241.

Camilleri M, Balm RK, Zinsmeister AR: Determinants of response to a prokinetic agent in neuropathic chronic intestinal motility disorder. Gastroenterology 1994;106:916.

Cox MR et al: The operative aetiology and types of adhesions causing small bowel obstruction. Aust N Z J Surg 1993;63:848.

Fevang BT et al: Long-term prognosis after operation for adhesive small bowel obstruction. Ann Surg 2004;240:193.

Frager D et al: CT of small-bowel obstruction: value in establishing the diagnosis and determining the degree and cause. AJR Am J Roentgenol 1994;162:37.

Francois Y et al: Postoperative adhesive peritoneal disease: laparoscopic treatment. Surg Endosc 1994;8:781.

Jenkins JT: Secondary causes of intestinal obstruction: rigorous preoperative evaluation is required. Am Surg 2000;66:662.

Lazarus DE et al: Frequency and relevance of the "small-bowel feces" sign on CT in patients with small-bowel obstruction. AJR Am J Roentgenol 2004;183:1361.

Lo CY, Lorentz TG, Lau PWK: Obturator hernia presenting as small bowel obstruction. Am J Surg 1994;167:396.

Meagher AP, Moller C, Hoffmann DC: Non-operative treatment of small bowel obstruction following appendicectomy or operation on the ovary or tube. Br J Surg 1993;80:1310.

Merrett ND et al: Bacteremia associated with operative decompression of a small bowel obstruction. J Am Coll Surg 1994;179:33.

Miller G et al: Natural history of patients with adhesive small bowel obstruction. Br J Surg 2000;87:1240.

Ryan MD et al: Adhesional small bowel obstruction after colorectal surgery. ANZ J Surg 2004;74:1010.

Scaglione M et al: Helical CT diagnosis of small bowel obstruction in the acute clinical setting. Eur J Radiol 2004;50:15.

Seror D et al: How conservatively can postoperative small bowel obstruction be treated? Am J Surg 1993;165:121.

Zalcman M et al: Helical CT signs in the diagnosis of intestinal ischemia in small-bowel obstruction. AJR Am J Roentgenol 2000;175:1601.

ACQUIRED INTESTINAL DIVERTICULA*

Congenital diverticula of the jejunum are rare, but acquired diverticula are found in the jejunum (or ileum) in 1.3% of radiographic studies or autopsy series when specifically sought. Jejunal diverticula are wide-mouthed sacs measuring 1–25 cm in diameter. Most contain all layers of the intestinal wall (true diverticula), but some consist of mucosa and submucosa herniated through thickened muscularis (false diverticula). Diverticula in the small bowel are often multiple; they diminish in frequency from the ligament of Treitz to the ileocecal valve and are associated with diverticulosis of the duodenum or colon in 30% of cases. Most symptomatic patients are over age 60.

Jejunal diverticulosis is a heterogeneous disorder associated with abnormalities of smooth muscle or the myenteric plexus. Intestinal pseudo-obstruction is a common associated problem, also reflecting the presence of an underlying motility disorder such as familial visceral myopathy or progressive systemic sclerosis.

Symptoms may be due to pseudo-obstruction or to inflammation of the diverticula. Acute intestinal bleeding and diverticulitis leading to perforation may occur. Blind loop syndrome is caused by bacterial overgrowth in the stagnant bowel with pseudo-obstruction or in large diverticula.

Barium x-rays may outline the diverticula (Figure 29–7) and reveal the underlying motility disorder. The primary cause should be sought.

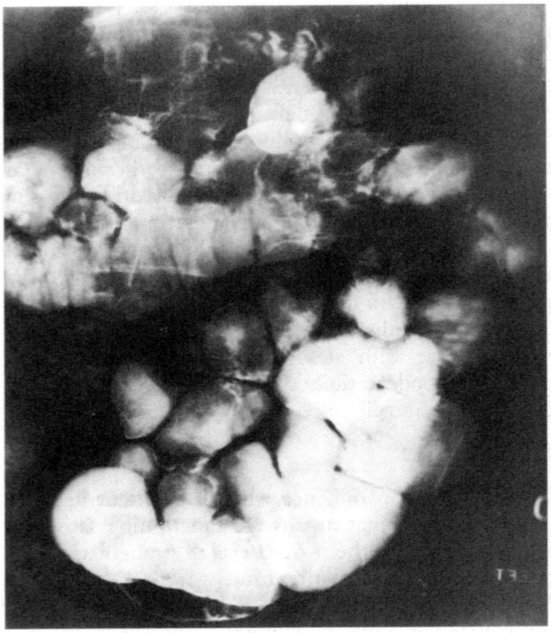

Figure 29–7. Jejunal diverticula.

Operation is required for perforation or bleeding. Symptoms of the underlying motility disorder are not improved by resection of the segment containing diverticula.

Akhrass R et al: Small-bowel diverticulosis: perceptions and reality. J Am Coll Surg 1997;184:383.

Benya EC, Ghahremani GG, Brosnan JJ: Diverticulitis of the jejunum: clinical and radiological features. Gastrointest Radiol 1991;16:24.

Longo WE, Vernava Ad: Clinical implications of jejunoileal diverticular disease. Dis Colon Rectum 1992;35:381.

Sibille A, Willcox R: Jejunal diverticulitis. Am J Gastroenterol 1992;87:655.

CROHN'S DISEASE* (Regional Enteritis)

ESSENTIALS OF DIAGNOSIS

- *Diarrhea.*
- *Abdominal pain and palpable mass.*

---

* Meckel's diverticulum and other congenital diverticula of the small intestine are discussed in Chapter 45.

* Crohn's disease of the colon is discussed in Chapter 30.

- *Low-grade fever, lassitude, weight loss.*
- *Anemia.*
- *Radiographic findings of thickened, stenotic bowel with ulceration and internal fistulas.*

General Considerations

Crohn's disease is a chronic progressive granulomatous inflammatory disorder of the gastrointestinal tract. From two to nine cases per 100,000 population are detected annually in Europe and the USA. The prevalence ranges broadly from 20 to 90 per 100,000 population. There is geographic variation (more common in urban dwellers and Northern residents of the USA), and there is a relatively high incidence among Ashkenazi Jews. The peak incidence occurs between the second and fourth decades. Cigarette smoking and a high intake of sugar are independent risk factors for Crohn's disease.

A. Etiology

Considerable progress has been made recently elucidating the underlying etiology of Crohn's disease. A complex interaction between genetic factors, environmental factors, host immune response, and inflammatory pathways is thought to result in inappropriate and ongoing activation of the mucosal immune system. A genetic influence is supported by several studies showing that first-degree relatives of patients with Crohn's disease have an incidence of Crohn's disease that is 4–20 times that of the general population. The cause of Crohn's disease is unknown; a number of candidate genes have been identified and are the subject of intense study. However, despite the role that genetics certainly plays in the development of Crohn's disease, environmental factors contribute as well, including the host immune response to luminal flora.

B. Pathology

Crohn's disease may affect any part of the gastrointestinal tract from the lips to the anus and may even spill over into the larynx or extend beyond the gut to the skin. "Metastatic" skin lesions have been described. The distal ileum is the most frequent site of involvement, eventually becoming diseased in about three-fourths of patients. The small bowel alone is involved in 15–30%, both the distal ileum and the colon in 40–60%, and the large bowel alone in 25–30%. Duodenal Crohn's disease is found in 0.5–7% of patients. Discontinuous areas of disease with segments of normal bowel between ("skip lesions") occur in 15% of patients. Subtle histologic changes can be seen in "normal," grossly uninvolved intestine of patients with Crohn's disease, suggesting that the mucosa of the entire bowel may be abnormal in this disorder.

The earliest Crohn's lesion is a focal accumulation of inflammatory cells adjacent to an epithelial crypt. Candidate mediators of inflammation include plasma activating factor, leukotrienes, complement, cytokines, enterotoxin, interleukins, tumor necrosis factor, phospholipase A_2, and neurotransmitters of the enteric nervous system. In a process similar to that seen in ischemia, reactive molecules such as oxygen radicals are generated; they propagate the inflammatory response and contribute to tissue damage. Erosions, crypt abscesses, and granulomas result.

Granulomas are seen in the bowel wall in 50–70% and in mesenteric lymph nodes in 25% of patients. The number of granulomas is related to the duration of disease and the site of involvement. It has been speculated that granuloma formation reflects efforts to localize or eliminate the causative agent of Crohn's disease. Mucosal lesions appear grossly as tiny (pinpoint) hemorrhagic spots or shallow ulcers with white bases and elevated margins (aphthous ulcers). Punched out ulcers are seen with progression of the disease. The next stage is development of fissures—knife-like clefts beginning in mucosa and extending deeply into the wall. These fissures and the serpiginous or linear ulcers surrounding islands of intact mucosa overlying edematous submucosa give a cobblestone appearance to the luminal surface. Crohn's disease ultimately becomes a transmural inflammatory process with thickening of the bowel wall, and it often progresses to stricture formation. The bowel and its mesentery are foreshortened in advanced cases, and on gross inspection mesenteric fat seems to have advanced over the surface of the bowel toward the antimesenteric border.

Clinical Findings

A. Symptoms and Signs

Crohn's disease has many modes of presentation:

1. Diarrhea—Continuous or episodic diarrhea is noted in about 90% of patients. Stools are liquid or semisolid and characteristically contain no blood if small bowel alone is diseased. One-third of patients with colonic involvement pass blood, and a few present with bloody diarrhea resembling that seen in ulcerative colitis.

2. Recurrent abdominal pain—Mild colic initiated by meals, centered in the lower abdomen, and relieved by defecation is common. These symptoms are due to chronic partial obstruction of the small bowel, colon, or both. Some patients progress to complete obstruction, and they have severe cramping, vomiting, and abdominal distention.

3. Abdominal symptoms and constitutional effects—Episodic attacks of abdominal pain and diarrhea accompanied by lassitude, malaise, weight loss, fever, and anemia are a common syndrome. A mass is often palpable in the right lower quadrant in these patients. Occasionally, fever of unknown origin is the only clinical finding.

4. Anorectal lesions—Chronic anal fissures, large ulcers, edematous skin tags, complex anal fistulas, or pararectal abscesses are seen in 15–25% of patients with Crohn's disease otherwise confined to small bowel and in 50–75% of those with colonic involvement. These problems may appear many years before the intestinal disease. Histologic features of Crohn's disease, including granulomas, are often found in biopsies of anorectal lesions even when the only other identifiable disease is located much higher in the gastrointestinal tract.

5. Anemia—Iron deficiency anemia or macrocytic anemia due to vitamin B_{12} or folate deficiency due to poor absorption from terminal ileal disease may occur in the absence of abdominal symptoms.

6. Malnutrition—Protein-losing enteropathy, steatorrhea, chronic obstruction, and diminished dietary intake from chronic illness contribute to malnutrition and weight loss. Mineral and vitamin deficiencies (especially vitamin D deficiency) are common. Deficiencies of water-soluble and fat-soluble vitamins are common in patients with Crohn's disease of the small intestine, but clinical symptoms of vitamin deficiency are rare. Zinc deficiency has been recognized. Children afflicted with extensive Crohn's disease fail to grow and may have severely retarded sexual maturation. Reversal of growth arrest by parenteral feeding emphasizes the importance of malnutrition as a cause of growth failure in Crohn's disease.

7. Acute onset—Acute abdominal pain and right lower quadrant tenderness mimicking acute appendicitis may be found at operation to be due to acute inflammation of the distal ileum. Only 15% of such cases evolve into chronic Crohn's disease, suggesting that most patients with acute ileitis have an infectious process unrelated to Crohn's disease. This condition is discussed further in the section on acute enteritis and mesenteric lymphadenitis.

8. Systemic complications—Any of the systemic complications described below may prompt the patient to seek medical advice.

B. Laboratory Findings

Test results are nonspecific and vary greatly according to the site of intestinal involvement, the severity of disease, and the presence of complications such as abscess or fistula. The sedimentation rate may not be elevated in patients with disease of the small intestine. Hypoalbuminemia, anemia, and steatorrhea are common. Abnormal D-xylose absorption suggests extensive disease or fistula formation, since carbohydrate is normally absorbed in the jejunum. Breath tests, as described in the section on blind loop syndrome, are abnormal if the ileum is diseased or if bacterial overgrowth has occurred, but are rarely used clinically.

C. Imaging Studies

Radiographic studies contribute substantially to the diagnosis of Crohn's disease. The appearance of small bowel during a barium small bowel follow-through is a composite of proliferative and destructive changes. The principal findings include thickened bowel wall with stricture ("string sign"), longitudinal ulceration that is shallow at first but becomes deep and undermining, deep transverse fissures resembling spicules, and cobblestone formation (Figure 29–8). Deformity of the cecum, fistulas, abscesses, and skip lesions are additional findings of importance. Enteroclysis provides excellent detail. CT scan, is useful for identifying thickened, abnormal loops of small bowel, strictured areas leading to obstruction, and abscesses due to contained perforation of the intestine.

D. Endoscopy

Upper gastrointestinal endoscopy diagnoses esophageal, gastric, and duodenal lesions. Colonoscopy reveals typical changes of Crohn's disease in the colon if it is involved or in the ileum if it can be examined. Ileoscopy after colectomy is accurate for the diagnosis of Crohn's disease in the ileum.

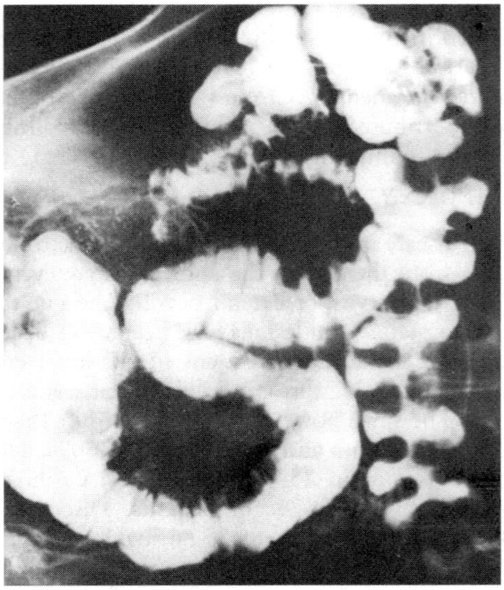

Figure 29–8. Barium x-ray showing spicules, edema, and ulcers in Crohn's disease.

E. Capsule Endoscopy

The capsule endoscope is a disposable plastic capsule that weighs 3.7 g and measures 11 mm in diameter and 26 mm in length. The contents include a silicon chip camera, a short focal-length lens, 4 white light emitting diode (LED) illumination sources, two silver oxide batteries, and a UHF band radio telemetry transmitter. Peristalsis propels the capsule through the intestine and pictures are received at a rate of 2 frames per second. Although the diagnostic yield of capsule endoscopy in Crohn's disease is high, its use has a positive impact on clinical outcome in only a small number of patients. Capsule endoscopy should not be used in the setting of a known stricture, as its use may lead to complete obstruction or perforation requiring surgery that may have otherwise not been needed.

Differential Diagnosis

A. Ulcerative Colitis

Crohn's disease of the colon may be difficult to distinguish from ulcerative colitis. This topic is covered in detail in Chapter 30.

B. Appendicitis

Acute ileitis may be the presenting manifestation, and differentiation from appendicitis may be impossible without operation.

C. Tuberculosis

Tuberculosis may affect any part of the gastrointestinal tract but is uncommon distal to the cecum. Small bowel tuberculosis is discussed elsewhere in this chapter.

D. Lymphoma

Radiographic findings help differentiate lymphoma from Crohn's disease, but histologic examination of the tissue is occasionally required before the diagnosis is certain. Rectal or colonic biopsies that show granulomas or colitis may support the diagnosis of Crohn's disease.

E. Other Diseases

Carcinoma, amebiasis, ischemia, eosinophilic gastroenteritis, nonsteroidal anti-inflammatory enteropathy, and other inflammatory conditions may simulate Crohn's disease.

Complications

A. Intestinal

Some intestinal complications, such as obstruction, abscess, fistula, and anorectal lesions, are so common that they are regarded as part of the characteristic clinical picture. Free perforation and massive hemorrhage are uncommon. The risk of cholelithiasis is increased. Oral manifestations of Crohn's disease may cause disabling pain. Carcinoma may occur in segments of small or large bowel that are involved with Crohn's disease, especially in segments excluded from the fecal stream by surgical bypass procedures.

B. Systemic

Systemic complications such as hepatobiliary disease, uveitis, arthritis, ankylosing spondylitis, aphthous ulcers, erythema nodosum, amyloidosis, thromboembolism, and vascular disorders are found both in Crohn's disease and in ulcerative colitis. These manifestations are described more fully in Chapter 30. "Metastatic" (distant cutaneous) Crohn's disease is a cutaneous ulcer with a granulomatous reaction at a site separated from gut by normal skin. Urinary complications include cystitis, calculi, and ureteral obstruction.

Treatment

A. Medical

The initial treatment of Crohn's disease is nonoperative. Physical rest, relief of emotional stress, and a confiding patient-doctor relationship have favorable effects. A low-residue, milk-free, high-protein diet may provide adequate nutrition. Malnourished patients benefit from elemental or polymeric diets if standard food is not tolerated, and total or supplementary parenteral nutrition is an important adjunct. As nutrition improves, infection is more successfully treated, and complications such as fistulas may be reversed. Chronic intermittent elemental diet improves growth failure in prepubertal children. Most clinicians prefer enteral feeding over the parenteral route when conditions permit, though comparative studies are inconclusive on this issue. Preoperative total parenteral nutrition prolongs the hospital stay and does not reduce the incidence or severity of postoperative complications. Chronic parenteral nutrition at home allows some patients with extensive disease to postpone operation, but it does not reduce the necessity of operation over the long term.

Enteral nutrition alone is insufficient therapy for active Crohn's disease compared with pharmacologic treatment. The standard drugs for Crohn's disease are aminosalicylates, immunosuppressive and immunoregulatory agents, antibiotics, steroids, and antitumor necrosis factor alpha (anti-TNF-α). Prednisone, prednisolone, and methylprednisolone are the most common corticosteroids for this purpose. Studies suggest that steroids are most effective for Crohn's disease of the small intestine, but they are applied to Crohn's colitis as well. Prednisone (0.25–0.75 mg/d) is superior to placebo in the control of acute disease over the short term but should not be used for long-term maintenance therapy. Relief of symptoms is seen in up to 70% of patients after 4 weeks of treatment. Steroids are then tapered once improvement is seen. The utility of prednisone is limited by side effects, including bone loss and osteopenia, cataract formation, weight gain, immunosuppression, and delayed wound healing. Sulfasalazine, an aminosalicylate, has been a cornerstone of therapy of Crohn's disease for many years. It is superior to placebo in control of acute disease, but its use is complicated by adverse reactions. The active principle of sulfasalazine is 5-aminosalicylic acid (5-ASA). Other aminosalicylates, including mesalamine, olsalazine, and balsalazide, are now used widely and are considered to be therapeutically equivalent to sulfasalazine. Not only are they beneficial for patients with active Crohn's colitis and ileocolitis, but oral aminosalicylates also may succeed in maintaining remission of Crohn's disease, a goal that has not been achieved by any other agents to date.

Azathioprine and mercaptopurine are the immunosuppressive drugs with the longest records. They are effective in Crohn's colitis and Crohn's disease of the small bowel; they spare steroids (allow reduction of steroid doses), help close fistulas, maintain remissions, and heal perianal disease. The disadvantage of azathioprine and mercaptopurine is their slow action. Bone marrow suppression may be seen in patients on these drugs, and monitoring of blood counts during therapy is necessary. Acute pancreatitis can also be a complication of therapy with 6-MP. 6-MP is also used to delay recurrence after surgical therapy of Crohn's disease. Various broad-spectrum antibiotics have been tried, most commonly metronidazole and ciprofloxacin for perianal disease. Infliximab (anti-TNFα monoclonal chimeric antibody) is now FDA approved for use in patients with active Crohn's disease. Infliximab is given as an intravenous infusion. Studies have shown prompt response to treatment with infliximab both for intestinal and perianal disease, although maintenance infusions are required. Despite medical advances in management, there is still no cure for Crohn's disease.

B. Surgical Therapy

Surgery is not curative for Crohn's disease, but its judicious use is often warranted to manage complications of the disease. The indication for operation in Crohn's disease of the small bowel is obstruction in about half of cases; perforation, internal fistula, external fistula, abscess, perianal disease, and growth failure in children are other reasons for operation. Over the long term, about 70% of patients with Crohn's disease undergo definitive surgery. Conservative resection of diseased bowel with a large side-to-side anastomosis is the preferred surgical procedure. The guiding principle in the surgical treatment of Crohn's disease is preservation of intestinal length. Increasingly, surgical resection of ileocolic Crohn's disease is being performed laparoscopically. Resection is usually limited to the area responsible for the complications that prompted operation. If multiple symptomatic strictures are encountered, they can be treated by "strictureplasty," a procedure in which the bowel is incised through the stricture and the wall is sutured or stapled in such a way that the lumen is widened. Strictureplasty is indicated for (1) diffuse involvement of the small bowel with multiple strictures; (2) stricture(s) in a patient who has previously undergone major resection of the small bowel; (3) rapid recurrence of Crohn's disease manifested as obstruction; and (4) a nonphlegmonous fibrotic stricture.

Prognosis

Crohn's disease is a chronic condition. It may progress to involve additional portions of bowel or may seem to spread no farther. Surgical procedures are palliative, not curative, but operations contribute greatly to rehabilitation of patients with refractory disease. The recurrence rate after resection of ileal or ileocolic disease increases with time. Symptomatic recurrence rates range from 25% to 50% at 5 years, from 35% to 80% at 10 years, and from 45% to 85% at 15 years. The marked variability is due to differences in patient populations, type of surgical procedures, and criteria for recurrence. Extensive confluent ulcers seen endoscopically in the ileum at the anastomosis within 1 year after ileocolectomy strongly predict symptomatic recurrence. Strictureplasty is effective for obstructive lesions, and there are few postoperative complications. Reoperation is needed in about 10% of patients within a year after strictureplasty and in one-third of patients by 10 years; surprisingly, however, the strictureplasty sites are usually not the source of symptoms.

Surgery should be used to manage complications in coordination with medical therapy. This team approach enables 80–85% of patients who require surgery to lead normal lives. Community-based studies have shown that long-term survival of people with Crohn's disease is similar to that of the general population irrespective of the age at diagnosis. There is little evidence that pregnancy affects the course of Crohn's disease or that inactive Crohn's disease alters the course of pregnancy.

Block GE et al: Crohn's disease. Curr Probl Surg 1993;30:173.

Cameron JL et al: Patterns of ileal recurrence in Crohn's disease: a prospective randomized study. Ann Surg 1992;215:546.

Dietz DW et al: Safety and long-term efficacy of strictureplasty in 314 consecutive patients with obstructing small bowel Crohn's Disease. J Am Coll Surg 2001;192:330.

Dixon PM, Roulston ME, Nolan DJ: The small bowel enema: a ten year review. Clin Radiol 1993;47:46.

Fazio VW et al: Evolution of surgery for Crohn's disease: a century of progress. Dis Colon Rectum 1999;42:979.

Geier DL, Miner PBJ: New therapeutic agents in the treatment of inflammatory bowel disease. Am J Med 1992;93:199.

Halligan S et al: The distribution of small bowel Crohn's disease in children compared to adults. Clin Radiol 1994;49:314.

Hay JW, Hay AR: Inflammatory bowel disease: costs-of-illness. J Clin Gastroenterol 1992;14:309.

Heimann TM et al: Prediction of early symptomatic recurrence after intestinal resection in Crohn's disease. Ann Surg 1993;218:294.

Kurata JH et al: Crohn's disease among ethnic groups in a large health maintenance organization. Gastroenterology 1992;102:1940.

Lavy A, Militianu D, Eidelman S: Diseases of the intestine mimicking Crohn's disease. J Clin Gastroenterol 1992;15:17.

Linn FV, Peppercorn MA: Drug therapy for inflammatory bowel disease: Part I. Am J Surg 1992;164:85.

Linn FV, Peppercorn MA: Drug therapy for inflammatory bowel disease: Part II. Am J Surg 1992;164:178.

Love JR, Irvine EJ, Fedorak RN: Quality of life in inflammatory bowel disease. J Clin Gastroenterol 1992;14:15.

Makowiec F et al: Intestinal stenosis and perforating complications in Crohn's disease. Int J Colorectal Dis 1993;8:197.

McLeod RS et al: Prophylactic mesalamine treatment decreases postoperative recurrence of Crohn's disease. Gastroenterology 1995;109:404.

Milsom JW et al: Prospective, randomized trial comparing laparoscopic vs. conventional surgery for refractory ileocolic Crohn's Disease. Dis Colon Rectum 2001;44:1.

Nwokolo CU et al: Surgical resections in parous patients with distal ileal and colonic Crohn's disease. Gut 1994;35:220.

Nyhlin H, Merrick MV, Eastwood MA: Bile acid malabsorption in Crohn's disease and indications for its assessment using SeHCAT. Gut 1994;35:90.

Olaison G, Smedh K, Sjodahl R: Natural course of Crohn's disease after ileocolic resection: endoscopically visualised ileal ulcers preceding symptoms. Gut 1992;33:331.

Podolsky DK: Inflammatory bowel disease. N Engl J Med 2002;347:417.

Prantera C et al: Oral 5-aminosalicylic acid (Asacol) in the maintenance treatment of Crohn's disease. Gastroenterology 1992;103:363.

Present DH et al: Infliximab for the treatment of fistulas in patients with Crohn's Disease. N Engl J Med 1999;340:1398.

Probert CSJ et al: Mortality from Crohn's disease in Leicestershire, 1972–1989: an epidemiological community based study. Gut 1992;33:1226.

Rastogi A, Schoen RE, Slivka A: Diagnostic yield and clinical outcomes of capsule endoscopy. Gastrointest Endosc 2004;60:959.

Ricart E et al: Infliximab for Crohn's disease in clinical practice at the Mayo Clinic: the first 100 patients. Am J Gastroenterol 2001;96:722.

Salomon P et al: How effective are current drugs for Crohn's disease? A meta-analysis. J Clin Gastroenterol 1992;14:211.

Stokes MA: Crohn's disease and nutrition. Br J Surg 1992;79:391.

Sutherland LR et al: Prevention of relapse of Crohn's disease. Inflamm Bowel Dis 2000;6:321.

Targan SR et al: A short-term study of chimeric monoclonal antibody cA2 to tumor necrosis factor (alpha) for Crohn's disease. N Engl J Med 1997;337:1029.

Tjandra JJ, Fazio VW, Lavery IC: Results of multiple strictureplasties in diffuse Crohn's disease of the small bowel. Aust N Z J Surg 1993;63:95.

OTHER INFLAMMATORY & ULCERATIVE DISEASES OF THE SMALL INTESTINE

Acute Enteritis & Mesenteric Lymphadenitis

Acute inflammation of the small intestine (enteritis) often also affects the stomach **(gastroenteritis)** or the colon **(enterocolitis)**. Involvement of regional lymph nodes is termed **mesenteric adenitis**. These usually self-limiting illnesses may be caused by viruses, bacteria, parasites, toxins, or unknown agents. These conditions are of importance to the surgeon when they mimic acute appendicitis or other problems that require operative treatment.

Achong DM, Oates E, Harris B: Mesenteric lymphadenitis depicted by indium 111-labeled white blood cell imaging. J Pediatr Surg 1993;28:1550.

Giannella RA: Enteric infections: 50 years of progress. Gastroenterology 1993;104:1589.

Kapikian AZ: Viral gastroenteritis. JAMA 1993;269:627.

HIV-Associated Enteropathy

Gastrointestinal infections are frequent in AIDS patients. Enteric pathogens recoverable from these patients include *Cryptosporidium,* cytomegalovirus, *Entamoeba histolytica, Giardia lamblia, Mycobacterium avium-intracellulare, Salmonella typhimurium, Shigella,* and *Campylobacter jejuni.*

Many symptomatic patients have no identifiable intestinal pathogen, and there is evidence to support the existence of an enteropathy caused by the human immunodeficiency virus itself. Intestinal perforation is a rare but devastating complication in these patients.

Batman PA et al: HIV enteropathy: comparative morphometry of the jejunal mucosa of HIV infected patients resident in the United Kingdom and Uganda. Gut 1998;43:350.

Giovanni B et al: HIV enteropathy: undescribed ultrastructural changes of duodenal mucosa and their regression after triple antiviral therapy. A case report. Dig Dis Sci 2005;50:617.

Kotler DP et al: Effects of enteric parasitoses and HIV infection upon small intestinal structure and function in patients with AIDS. J Clin Gastroenterol 1993;16:10.

Ullrich R et al: Gastrointestinal symptoms in patients infected with human immunodeficiency virus: relevance of infective agents isolated from gastrointestinal tract. Gut 1992;33:1080.

Yersinia Enteritis

Much attention has focused on *Yersinia enterocolitica;* this pathogen may cause acute gastroenteritis, terminal ileitis, enterocolitis, colitis, mesenteric lymphadenitis, hepatic and splenic abscesses, and autoimmune processes such as erythema nodosum and polyarthritis. *Y enterocolitica* has also been implicated in other disease (especially in women), including carditis, glomerulonephritis, Graves' disease, and Hashimoto's thyroiditis.

Acute gastroenteritis with fever, diarrhea, and sometimes vomiting is the most common clinical syndrome, especially in children. Acute mesenteric lymphadenitis and acute terminal ileitis are more frequent in adolescents and adults. These infections may cause enough abdominal pain and tenderness that appendicitis seems a likely diagnosis. If operation is performed, large inflamed lymph nodes are found in the mesentery of the distal ileum, and the bowel itself may be grossly inflamed. In these circumstances, appendectomy is usually performed. Organisms can be cultured from stool, and antibody titers may rise and then fall in some patients. *Y enterocolitica* may respond to trimethoprim-sulfamethoxazole or doxycycline, and complicated *Y enterocolitica* infections should be treated. Fatal septicemia has been reported. No patient with *Y enterocolitica* enteritis has progressed to classic Crohn's disease.

Saebø A, Lassen J: Acute and chronic gastrointestinal manifestations associated with *Yersinia enterocolitica* infection: a Norwegian 10-year follow-up study on 458 hospitalized patients. Ann Surg 1992;215:250.

Van Noyen R et al: Causative role of *Yersinia* and other enteric pathogens in the appendicular syndrome. Eur J Clin Microbiol Infect Dis 1991;10:735.

Campylobacter Enteritis

Campylobacter jejuni is a gram-negative rod that is now recognized as an important cause of human illness in all parts of the world. *C jejuni* infection is more common than infection by either salmonella or shigella. Raw milk, untreated drinking water, and undercooked poultry are recognized vehicles of transmission. Clinical features vary from mild abdominal pain, fever, emesis, and diarrhea indistinguishable from viral gastroenteritis to severe chronic or relapsing bloody diarrhea that resembles ulcerative or granulomatous colitis. *C jejuni* produces an enterotoxin that may play a role in causing diarrhea.

Darkfield or phase-contrast microscopy of stool samples may reveal the characteristic darting motility of *C jejuni* and allow for a presumptive diagnosis. Stool and occasionally blood cultures are positive. Colonoscopy may reveal colonic lesions, and x-rays show inflammation of the small bowel or colon.

Although *C jejuni* infection is self-limited in most patients and symptoms subside within a week, relapses occur in 20% of untreated patients. The appropriate antibiotic is erythromycin, ciprofloxacin, or doxycycline, depending on the results of in vitro sensitivity studies. Disease can be spread by symptomatic patients; once diarrhea subsides, transmission is unlikely.

Perkins DJ, Newstead GL: *Campylobacter jejuni* enterocolitis causing peritonitis, ileitis and intestinal obstruction. Aust N Z J Surg 1994;64:55.

Peterson MC: Clinical aspects of *Campylobacter jejuni* infections in adults. West J Med 1994;161:148.

Tuberculosis

Primary tuberculous infection of the intestine, caused by ingestion of the bovine strain of *Mycobacterium tuberculosis,* is rare in the USA. Secondary infection is due to swallowing the human tubercle bacillus. About 1% of patients with pulmonary tuberculosis have intestinal involvement. Recent immigration from endemic areas has increased the incidence. Tuberculosis is prevalent in individuals infected with HIV.

The distal ileum is the most common site of disease. The bacillus localizes in the mucosal glands and spreads to Peyer's patches, where inflammation, sloughing of tissue, and local attempts at walling off give rise to symptoms. The pathologic reaction is hypertrophic or ulcerative. Hypertrophic tuberculous enteritis results in stenosis, and the symptoms and signs are those of obstruction. The ulcerative form causes abdominal pain, alternating constipation and diarrhea, and, occasionally, progressive inanition. Free perforation, fistula formation, or hemorrhage may occur in severe untreated disease.

The diagnosis of intestinal tuberculosis can be difficult, but medical treatment should not be based on clinical suspicion alone, since carcinoma and Crohn's disease cause similar symptoms and signs. Less than half of patients in a recent study had an abnormality on chest x-ray, and none had a positive sputum result. Biopsy by colonoscopy, laparoscopy, or even laparotomy is needed to demonstrate the presence of the organism.

Antituberculosis chemotherapy is the mainstay of management. Surgery is required if the diagnosis is uncertain, if disease is resistant to chemotherapy, or if complications develop. Some surgeons recommend early operation because medical treatment results in healing by fibrosis with resultant obstruction. Resection is the preferred surgical procedure, and bypass is done only if abscesses or fistulas are present. The prognosis is good if the patient is operated on in the early stages of the illness.

Al-Quorain AA et al: Abdominal tuberculosis in Saudi Arabia: a clinicopathological study of 65 cases. Am J Gastroenterol 1993;88:75.

Engin G, Balk E: Imaging findings of intestinal tuberculosis. J Comput Assist Tomogr 2005;29:37.

Marshall JB: Tuberculosis of the gastrointestinal tract and peritoneum. Am J Gastroenterol 1993;88:989.

Misra SP et al: Endoscopic biopsies from normal-appearing terminal ileum and cecum in patients with suspected colonic tuberculosis. Endoscopy 2004;36:612.

Underwood MJ et al: Presentation of abdominal tuberculosis to general surgeons. Br J Surg 1992;79:1077.

Typhoid

Salmonella typhi may cause ulcers in the distal ileum or cecum. Bleeding or perforation presents a formidable surgical challenge. Early operation offers the best hope for survival.

Mandal BK: *Salmonella typhi* and other salmonellas. Gut 1994;35:726.

Mock CN, Amaral J, Visser LE: Improvement in survival from typhoid ileal perforation: results of 221 operative cases. Ann Surg 1992;215:244.

Enteropathy from Nonsteroidal Anti-Inflammatory Drugs

Nonsteroidal anti-inflammatory drugs increase intestinal permeability within hours after ingestion, exposing the mucosa to macromolecules and toxins in the lumen. Bacterial invasion may contribute to inflammation. Perhaps 70% of patients of any age and either sex who have taken these agents for 6 months or longer develop enteropathy, with subclinical intestinal inflammation and occult blood loss. Fewer than 1% of patients develop mucosal ulceration or transmural inflammation with submucosal fibrosis and circumferential diaphragmlike strictures. These patients may have obstruction, perforation, or anemia. The differential diagnosis includes Crohn's disease, ischemia, tuberculosis, and lymphoma.

The drug should be withdrawn. Strictures require resection.

Allison MC et al: Gastrointestinal damage associated with the use of nonsteroidal antiinflammatory drugs. N Engl J Med 1992;327:749.

Bjarnason I et al: Side effects of nonsteroidal anti-inflammatory drugs on the small and large intestine in humans. Gastroenterology 1993;104:1832.

Graham DY et al: Visible small-intestinal mucosal injury in chronic NSAID users. Clin Gastroenterol Hepatol 2005;3:55.

Henry D, Dobson A, Turner C: Variability in the risk of major gastrointestinal complications from nonaspirin nonsteroidal anti-inflammatory drugs. Gastroenterology 1993;105:1078.

Radiation Enteropathy

Aggressive radiation therapy for abdominal or pelvic cancer is almost always associated with some gastrointestinal injury, because proliferating intestinal epithelial cells are extremely radiosensitive. Degeneration of cells and edema of bowel wall may produce abdominal pain, nausea and vomiting, and sometimes bloody diarrhea during therapy or a few months later. Symptoms are usually minor and transient for most patients with modern irradiation techniques.

Injury to blood vessels in the bowel wall is far more serious than the early mucosal lesion. Endothelial proliferation and fibrosis in the media may gradually obliterate the vessel lumen over months or years, producing chronic intestinal ischemia. Carcinoma arising in irradiated small intestine is a rare late complication.

The incidence of significant bowel injury is dose-related and varies from 5% after 4500 cGy to 30% after 6000 cGy. Fixation of small bowel loops in the radiation field by adhesions from previous operations greatly increases the risk of intestinal complications. Absorbable polyglycolic acid mesh can be used to keep the small bowel out of the pelvis when radiation therapy is planned following pelvic surgery. Oral glutamine protects the small bowel mucosa from some of the morbidity of irradiation in preliminary animal studies.

Symptoms necessitating operation appear as early as 1 month or as late as 30 years after completion of therapy. Operation is required for obstruction due to stricture or entrapment in pelvic fibrosis, perforation with abscess or fistula formation, or hemorrhage from ulcerated mucosa. Symptoms should not be attributed to cancer until residual cancer is proved to be present.

The objective of operation is relief of symptoms. If resection of the involved segment is not possible, bypass is performed. It is imperative that normal bowel be used for anastomoses, because suture lines in irradiated bowel are likely to disrupt. The bowel is friable despite its thickness, and care must be taken in freeing adhesions. If the distal colon and rectum are involved, diverting colostomy is the safest course. Radiation proctitis is discussed in Chapter 31.

The operative death rate is 10–15%, and the prognosis thereafter depends on the extent of involvement and the presence of untreatable fistulas, short bowel syndrome, and cancer. Only 30–45% of patients with significant intestinal complications of radiation therapy are alive 5 years after operation.

Cross MJ, Frazee RC: Surgical treatment of radiation enteritis. Am Surg 1992;58:132.

Jain G et al: Chronic radiation enteritis: a ten-year follow-up. J Clin Gastroenterol 2002;35:214.

Johnson RJ, Carrington BM: Pelvic radiation disease. Clin Radiol 1992;45:4.

Nguyen NP et al: Current concepts in radiation enteritis and implications for future clinical trials. Cancer 2002;95:1151.

van Halteren HK et al: Surgical intervention for complications caused by late radiation damage of the small bowel: a retrospective analysis. Eur J Surg Oncol 1993;19:336.

Yeoh E et al: Effect of pelvic irradiation on gastrointestinal function: a prospective longitudinal study. Am J Med 1993;95:397.

SMALL INTESTINE FISTULAS

ESSENTIALS OF DIAGNOSIS

- *Fever and sepsis.*
- *Abdominal pain.*
- *Localized abdominal tenderness.*
- *External drainage of small bowel contents.*
- *Dehydration and malnutrition.*

General Considerations

External fistulas of the small bowel may form spontaneously as a result of disease, but about 95% are complications of surgical procedures (anastomotic dehiscence or injury to bowel during dissection). Fistulas are particularly prone to develop when the surgeon encounters extensive adhesions, inflamed intestine, or radiation enteropathy.

Fistulas can be classified according to anatomic site, characteristics of the tract (simple or complex), and volume of output (high or low). A high-output fistula produces more than 500 mL/24 h. Other descriptive terms are also used, eg, end fistula, which encompasses the entire diameter of the bowel, and lateral fistula, which arises from one side only.

Clinical Findings

A. Symptoms and Signs

Postoperative fistula formation is heralded by fever and abdominal pain until bowel contents discharge through the abdominal incision. Spontaneous fistulas from neoplasms or inflammatory disease usually develop in a more indolent manner. Most fistulas are associated with one or more abscesses, which often drain incompletely with fistulization, so that persistent sepsis is a common feature. Intestinal fluid escaping through the fistula may severely excoriate the skin and abdominal wall tissues. Fluid and electrolyte losses may be severe, especially if the fistula is large, if it is located in the upper tract, or if there is partial or complete intestinal obstruction distal to the fistula. Persistent sepsis and difficulty in nourishing the patient contribute to rapid weight loss.

B. Laboratory Findings

Routine laboratory tests reflect the severity of deficits in red cell mass, plasma volume, and electrolytes. Leukocytosis due to sepsis and hemoconcentration is common. Disease of other organs such as liver and kidneys may be detected.

C. Imaging Studies

Abscesses and intestinal obstruction may be evident on plain abdominal films. Contrast medium administered orally, per rectum, or through the fistula (fistulogram) delineates the abnormal anatomy, including intrinsic bowel disease, and demonstrates the location and number of fistulas, the length and course of fistula tracts, associated abscess cavities, and the presence of distal obstruction. Radiologists can manipulate catheters into tracts and provide detailed diagnostic information; this procedure may also be therapeutic (see below). Chest films, CT scans, ultrasound, endoscopy, and other special studies may be indicated in certain individuals.

Complications

Fluid and electrolyte losses, malnutrition, and sepsis contribute to multiple-organ failure and death unless effective therapy is instituted promptly.

Treatment

A systematic approach combining diagnostic, supportive, and operative procedures is essential in the management of patients with fistulas (Table 29–2). In few other conditions is the proper timing of operative intervention more critical.

A. Fluid and Electrolyte Resuscitation

Many fistula patients are profoundly depleted of intravascular and interstitial volume, and replacement of this fluid with isotonic saline solution takes first priority. Central venous pressure, urine output, and skin turgor

Table 29–2. Treatment of fistulas.

First:
Restore blood volume and begin correction of fluids and electrolyte imbalance.
Drain accessible abscesses.
Control fistula and measure losses.
Begin nutritional support.
Second:
Delineate anatomy of fistulas by radiographic studies.
Third:
Maintain caloric intake of 2000–3000 kcal or more per day, depending on status of nutrition and energy expenditure.
Drain abscesses as they appear.
Fourth:
Operate if fistula fails to close.

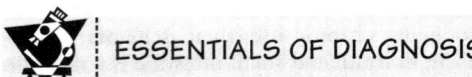

are guides to the progress of volume resuscitation. Blood is sent to the laboratory for measurement of serum electrolyte concentrations and arterial blood gases. Results of these studies assist in correcting electrolyte deficits and deranged acid-base balance. Body weight is recorded daily. Fluid and electrolyte resuscitation can usually be accomplished within the first day or two. Subsequent maintenance of homeostasis depends on accurately measuring losses and replacing them.

B. Control of Fistula

Fistula drainage fluid must be collected to avoid excoriation of skin and abdominal wall tissues and to record volume losses. An ostomy appliance may fit around the fistula or a catheter inserted by a radiologist under x-ray guidance may work best. Skilled and experienced nursing care is indispensable.

C. Control of Sepsis

Abscesses should be drained as soon as they are diagnosed. The source of sepsis is often obscure, and a continuous diligent search for abscesses must be made by repeated physical examination and imaging studies until the infection is located and treated. Blind therapy with broad-spectrum antibiotics is not a substitute for drainage of abscesses. In many cases, an incompletely drained abscess can be managed by an interventional radiologist, who passes a catheter through a fistula tract into the associated abscess cavity. Drainage is accomplished, and the fistula may close.

D. Delineation of Fistula

Radiographic contrast studies (see above) should be obtained as soon as feasible.

E. Nutrition

Adequate nutrition and control of sepsis make the difference between survival and death for these patients. A useful general rule is to avoid all oral intake at the outset. Nasogastric suction may be necessary temporarily. As soon as intravascular fluid and electrolytes are restored, parenteral nutrition should be instituted via a central intravenous catheter.

For many patients, total parenteral nutrition is the principal exogenous source of calories and nitrogen until the fistula heals or is closed surgically. For patients with low-output or distal fistulas, the enteral route for nutrition is preferred, and elemental or polymeric diets can be delivered into the distal gut in some patients with proximal fistulas.

F. Other Measures

H_2 receptor antagonists and proton pump inhibitors are useful adjuncts in patients with proximal fistulas. By reducing gastric acid secretion, fistula output is decreased and fluid and electrolyte management is simplified. Somatostatin analogues decrease fistula output and may accelerate fistula closure.

G. Operation

About 30% of fistulas close spontaneously; Crohn's disease, irradiated bowel, cancer, foreign body, distal obstruction, extensive disruption of intestinal continuity, and a short (< 2 cm) fistula tract are associated with failure of fistulas to heal. Fibrin glue has been effective in some small bowel fistulas, in particular it may be considered in complicated patients with a history of a hostile abdomen. Treatment may be successful if the fistula is long and the output is low. If they are going to heal spontaneously, fistulas usually close within a month after eradication of infection and institution of adequate nutritional support, and persistence much beyond a month indicates the need for surgical closure in most cases. Serum levels of short-turnover proteins, particularly transferrin, might be useful in predicting which patients are unlikely to close their fistulas. The operation should be postponed, however, until one can predict that intra-abdominal inflammation has resolved—typically 2–3 months or more after the last operation. The fistulous segment should be resected, associated obstruction relieved, and continuity reestablished by a functional end-to-end anastomosis.

Prognosis

The plan of management outlined above results in survival rates of 80–95% in patients with external fistulas. Uncontrolled sepsis is the chief cause of death.

Borison DI, Bloom AD, Pritchard TJ: Treatment of enterocutaneous and colocutaneous fistulas with early surgery or somatostatin analog. Dis Colon Rectum 1992;35:635.

Hollington P et al: An 11-year experience of enterocutaneous fistula. Br J Surg 2004;91:1646.

Kubshinoff BW et al: Serum transferrin as a prognostic indicator of spontaneous closure and mortality in gastrointestinal cutaneous fistulas. Ann Surg 1993;217:615.

Lynch AC et al: Clinical outcome and factors predictive of recurrence after enterocutaneous fistula surgery. Ann Surg 2004;240:825.

Spiliotis J et al: Treatment of fistulas of the gastrointestinal tract with total parenteral nutrition and octreotide in patients with carcinoma. Surg Gynecol Obstet 1993;176:575.

Torres AJ et al: Somatostatin in the management of gastrointestinal fistulas. A multicenter trial. Arch Surg 1992;127:97.

ACUTE VASCULAR LESIONS OF THE SMALL INTESTINE & MESENTERY

Lesions producing acute or chronic ischemia or hemorrhage may result from intrinsic vascular disease, systemic illness, pharmacologic agents, and surgical procedures. Chronic occlusion may be amenable to vascular reconstruction and is discussed in Chapter 34. Acute mesenteric ischemia is discussed here.

1. Acute Mesenteric Vascular Occlusion

ESSENTIALS OF DIAGNOSIS

- *Severe, diffuse abdominal pain.*
- *Gross or occult intestinal bleeding.*
- *Minimal physical findings.*
- *Radiographic findings (sometimes).*
- *Operative findings.*

General Considerations

Sudden occlusion of major small bowel arteries or veins is catastrophic. It is predominantly a disease of the elderly and is highly lethal. Mesenteric **arterial emboli** account for 50% of cases of acute mesenteric ischemia; they most commonly originate from mural thrombus in an infarcted left ventricle or clot in a fibrillating left atrium in patients with mitral stenosis. **Thrombosis of a mesenteric artery** (25% of cases) is the end result of atherosclerotic stenosis, and these patients often give a history of intestinal angina before the acute thrombosis occurs. Other causes of acute arterial occlusions, such as dissecting aortic aneurysm or fusiform aortic aneurysm, are rare. Occlusions of smaller mesenteric arteries often are associated with connective tissue or other systemic disorders. Cocaine ingestion is another cause. Nonocclusive disease (see below) is responsible for about 20% of patients with acute mesenteric ischemia.

Thrombosis of mesenteric veins (5% of cases) is associated with portal hypertension, abdominal sepsis, hypercoagulable states, or trauma, or there may be no apparent underlying disease. Mesenteric venous or arterial thrombosis can occur in women taking oral contraceptives. Some venous occlusions develop peripherally and progress insidiously, causing segmental infarction that resembles strangulation obstruction. Others have acute, severe, rapidly progressive ischemia.

The consequences of major vascular occlusion depend on the vessel involved, the level of occlusion, the status of other visceral vessels, the development of collaterals, the establishment of reperfusion, and other factors. Tissue injury is caused by events related to the ischemia itself (ischemic injury) and by return of blood flow, either spontaneous or as a result of treatment (reperfusion injury). Complete interruption of oxygen supply to the intestine produces necrosis first at the tips of villi. Mucosal slough begins within 3 hours after onset of ischemia, and ulceration and bleeding soon become extensive. Full-thickness infarction of bowel wall occurs as early as 6 hours after onset in total ischemia; in partial ischemia, it may take several days for this stage to be reached. Hemorrhage into the lumen, accumulation of bloody abdominal fluid, perforation, and death from sepsis are the end results of infarction. Sepsis and multiorgan system failure may develop even in the absence of full-thickness necrosis or perforation; bacteria proliferate in the necrotic segment; the mucosal barrier is disrupted; and bacteria and their toxic products translocate into the circulation. A variety of plasma substances including tumor necrosis factor and platelet-activating factor arise at the site of intestinal injury, enter the circulation, and damage target organs such as the lung and kidneys.

There is increasing recognition of the importance of reperfusion injury in the outcome of intestinal ischemia. Return of arterial blood flow from spontaneous events, lysis of clot by anticoagulants, or arterial reconstruction converts the enzyme xanthine dehydrogenase to xanthine oxidase, resulting in the release of superoxide and hydrogen peroxide. These oxygen radicals destabilize cell membranes, disrupt the mucosal barrier, and flood the systemic circulation with mediators of damage to other organs. Most of the data come from experimental animals, but there is little doubt that reperfusion injury is an important and potentially lethal phenomenon in patients.

Clinical Findings

A. Symptoms and Signs

The most constant symptom is severe, poorly localized abdominal pain that is often unresponsive to narcotics. Nausea and vomiting, diarrhea, and constipation are variable in occurrence.

In the early stages there is a striking paucity of abdominal findings; in fact, pain out of proportion to the objective findings is a hallmark of mesenteric vascular occlusion. Ischemia can also occur with much less severe pain, and serious illness may be recognized only when secondary toxicity develops. Later in the course, abdominal distention and tenderness occur. Shock and generalized peritonitis eventually develop, but by that time the opportunity for salvage has been lost. In some instances—particularly with a high venous occlusion—shock is an early finding. Stool or gastric contents contain blood in 75–95% of patients later in the course. Paracentesis does not help to establish the diagnosis in the reversible stages.

B. LABORATORY FINDINGS

There is no laboratory test to definitively rule in or out a diagnosis of mesenteric ischemia. Striking leukocytosis is present. Serum amylase is elevated in about half of patients, and creatine kinase (BB isoenzyme) correlates with intestinal infarction. Significant base deficits may be observed. Increased inorganic phosphate levels in serum and peritoneal fluid are a sign of irreversible ischemia. Hemoconcentration and the effects of hemorrhage into the lumen or mesentery are reflected in laboratory tests in the late stages. Antithrombin III deficiency and other abnormalities of coagulation should be sought.

C. IMAGING STUDIES

Plain abdominal films allow a presumptive diagnosis of vascular occlusion to be made in about 20% of patients. Absence of intestinal gas, diffuse distention with air-fluid levels, and distention of small bowel and colon up to the splenic flexure are nonspecific but suggestive. Blunt plicae, thickened bowel wall, and small bowel loops that remain unchanged over several hours are seen occasionally. Specific findings of intestinal necrosis, including intramural gas and gas in the portal venous system, which may be seen on either a CT scan or plain abdominal films, occur late. Barium studies may reveal "thumbprinting" and disordered motility (either slow or rapid). CT gives useful information in 50% of patients, though a specific diagnosis is possible in only 25% of cases. MRI may be useful. Mesenteric arteriography may be helpful but is logistically cumbersome in acutely ill patients and is not sensitive enough to rule out the diagnosis. It is important to recognize that short of mesenteric arteriography, imaging studies such as plain films, CT, and barium studies cannot be relied on to definitively rule out a diagnosis of acute mesenteric ischemia.

Differential Diagnosis

Acute pancreatitis and strangulation obstruction of the intestine may be difficult to distinguish from mesenteric vascular occlusion. A very high serum amylase early in the disease or an edematous pancreas on CT scan suggests pancreatitis. Differentiation from strangulation obstruction is less important, since both conditions require operation. Angiography may be definitive. Even surgeons with a special interest in this condition are unable to make an early diagnosis in more than half of cases.

Treatment

Survival depends upon diagnosis and operative treatment within 12 hours after onset of symptoms. Although acute occlusion of major arteries or veins requires operation, pre- and postoperative intra-arterial infusion of papaverine (30–60 mg/h) has been recommended if the angiogram demonstrates embolic occlusion of the superior mesenteric artery.

Acute venous thrombosis is diagnosed by the edematous mesentery and extrusion of clots when mesenteric veins are cut. Resection of all of the involved gut and its mesentery is the treatment of choice; direct mesenteric venous surgery (thrombectomy) is seldom successful. Administration of heparin postoperatively is recommended. Antithrombin III deficiency and other causes of hypercoagulability should be treated.

In arterial occlusion, there is segmental or diffuse ischemia or infarction of small bowel and colon in the distribution of the occluded vessel. Arterial pulsations are absent or reduced, and mesenteric edema is not so striking as in venous occlusion. Many methods of helping the surgeon judge viability have been suggested, but most have not proved their worth. The Doppler ultrasonic flowmeter is of some help, and the laser Doppler system is promising. The qualitative fluorescein test is not as sensitive as once believed. Quantitative fluorescence, as measured by a perfusion fluorometer, is under investigation.

Necrotic bowel should be resected unless the extent of damage is so great that satisfactory life could not be expected. With the availability of home parenteral nutrition, more patients are salvageable now than before. It is not clear how to integrate the new information about reperfusion injury into management of patients with reversibly ischemic bowel. Perhaps it is better to just resect the affected intestine, particularly in the elderly, even though vascular reconstruction may be technically possible by embolectomy, thromboendarterectomy, or arterial bypass. Vascular reconstruction was attempted in 10% or less of patients before reperfusion injury became recognized, and it is likely that even fewer patients will be treated by a direct approach to the vessels in the future.

Massive volume support and antibiotics are mandatory, and anticoagulants or drugs that inhibit platelet aggregation are given by some surgeons. A second-look operation is performed 24–48 hours later if marginally viable bowel was left in.

Percutaneous transluminal angioplasty and stent placement has been used to treat acute mesenteric ischemia, but its role is yet to be defined, and abdominal operation remains the standard treatment.

Prognosis

Acute mesenteric vascular occlusion is often lethal, because diagnosis and treatment are delayed, infarction is extensive, and arterial reconstruction is difficult. The overall mortality rate of arterial occlusion is about 45%, although a recent report of deaths occurring in only

24% is encouraging. If infarction is so extensive that over half of the small bowel must be resected, the death rate is 45–85%. Reconstruction of acutely thrombosed visceral arteries is often not feasible, and patency rates are poor. In a few patients, the acute ischemic episode goes unrecognized, and the process resolves spontaneously with stricture formation. The prognosis is excellent in this situation. Acute venous thrombosis has a death rate of 30%, and if long-term anticoagulants are not used, approximately 25% of patients have another episode of thrombosis. Administration of coumarin anticoagulants for at least 3 months is recommended to minimize the possibility of recurrence.

2. Nonocclusive Intestinal Ischemia

In about one-fourth of patients with intestinal ischemia, vascular occlusion does not involve a major artery or vein (although arterial stenosis is usually present). In the presence of some other acute disease such as a cardiac dysrhythmia or sepsis, splanchnic vasoconstriction occurs, and the intestine becomes ischemic because of low perfusion pressure and flow. Arterial blood is shunted away from the villi in these circumstances, and the ischemic villi are destroyed if the condition persists.

The diagnosis is suspected when a potentially susceptible patient develops acute abdominal pain. The clinical picture is similar to that of arterial thrombosis, but the onset is less often sudden. Arteriography documents the absence of major vascular occlusion but is not otherwise diagnostic in most cases.

Direct infusion of vasodilator agents into the superior mesenteric artery may reverse splanchnic vasoconstriction in selected cases. Papaverine is the drug of choice, but other drugs are under investigation. Operation is usually required to exclude other diseases that simulate intestinal ischemia and to resect infarcted bowel.

Patchy or diffuse ischemia varies in extent and severity. Ischemia is most pronounced on the antimesenteric border, and the mucosa may be extensively involved before abnormalities are visible on the serosal surface. There are often ischemic areas in other organs such as the liver and spleen. Vascular reconstruction is ineffective, and surgical procedures are limited to resection of infarcted bowel. Decisions about when to perform a primary anastomosis or second-look operation are individualized. The death rate was about 90% until recently, mainly because the underlying disease often could not be corrected. Intra-arterial vasodilator therapy has lowered this figure.

Angelelli G et al: Acute bowel ischemia: CT findings. Eur J Radiol 2004;50:37.

Cleveland TJ, Nawaz S, Gaines PA: Mesenteric arterial ischaemia: diagnosis and therapeutic options. Vasc Med 2002;7:311.

Boley SJ, Brandt LJ: Intestinal ischemia. Surg Clin North Am 1992;72:1.

Bulkley GB: Free radicals and other reactive oxygen metabolites: clinical relevance and the therapeutic efficacy of antioxidant therapy. Surgery 1993;113:479.

Kaleya RN, Boley SJ: Acute mesenteric ischemia: an aggressive diagnostic and therapeutic approach. 1991 Roussel Lecture. Can J Surg 1992;35:613.

Kam DM, Scheeres DE: Fluorescein-assisted laparoscopy in the identification of arterial mesenteric ischemia. Surg Endosc 1993;7:75.

Kempczinski RF et al: Intestinal ischemia secondary to thromboangiitis obliterans. Ann Vasc Surg 1993;7:354.

Kirschner RE, Fantini GA: Role of iron and oxygen-derived free radicals in ischemia-reperfusion injury. J Am Coll Surg 1994;179:103.

MacDonald PH et al: The use of oximetry in determining intestinal blood flow. Surg Gynecol Obstet 1993;176:451.

MacSweeney STR, Postlethwaite JC: "Second-look" laparoscopy in the management of acute mesenteric ischaemia. Br J Surg 1994;81:90.

Sarkar R: Evolution of the management of mesenteric occlusive disease. Cardiovasc Surg 2002;10:395.

Schoots IG et al: Systematic review of survival after acute mesenteric ischaemia according to disease aetiology. Br J Surg 2004;91:17.

Sheridan WG et al: Determination of a critical level of tissue oxygenation in acute intestinal ischaemia. Gut 1992;33:762.

Simpson R et al: Neutrophil and nonneutrophil-mediated injury in intestinal ischemia-reperfusion. Ann Surg 1993;218:444.

Stoney RJ, Cunningham CG: Acute mesenteric ischemia. Surgery 1993;114:489.

Wade TP, Jewell WR, Andrus CH: Mesenteric venous thrombosis: modern management and endoscopic diagnosis. Surg Endosc 1992;6:283.

3. Other Vascular Lesions

Vasculitis

Vascular lesions associated with systemic disorders such as polyarteritis nodosa and systemic lupus erythematosus may cause patchy infarction of the small intestine. Similar lesions have been seen in patients with a history of amphetamine abuse. The presenting manifestation is usually perforation with peritonitis or intraluminal bleeding, but strictures occur as well. The prognosis depends on the underlying pathologic process and the severity of peritoneal contamination. These patients are often on corticosteroid therapy and do not tolerate infection well. Survival is rare.

Kempczinski RF et al: Intestinal ischemia secondary to thromboangiitis obliterans. Ann Vasc Surg 1993;7:354.

Krant JD, Ross JM: Extracranial giant cell arteritis restricted to the small bowel. Arthritis Rheum 1992;35:603.

Kuehne SE, Gauvin GP, Shortsleeve MJ: Small bowel stricture caused by rheumatoid vasculitis. Radiology 1992;184:215.

Mesenteric Apoplexy

Mesenteric apoplexy is a rare disorder caused by spontaneous rupture of mesenteric arteries. The more general category of **abdominal apoplexy** includes spontaneous hemorrhage into the peritoneal cavity from tumors (particularly hepatomas), the spleen, or other organs. Arteriosclerotic lesions are the cause of arterial rupture in older individuals; the superior mesenteric, right colic, and branches of the celiac artery are the usual sites. Sudden hemorrhage from congenital aneurysms occurs in younger patients; the splenic artery is most commonly involved and is particularly prone to rupture during pregnancy (see Chapter 41). The typical picture is sudden onset of diffuse abdominal pain followed by hypotension. Operation is imperative.

Bellucci MJ, Burke MC, Querusio L: Atraumatic rupture of utero-ovarian vessels during pregnancy: a lethal presentation of maternal shock. Ann Emerg Med 1994;23:360.

Berera T et al: Spontaneous rupture of hepatocellular carcinoma. Ital J Gastroenterol 1992;24:461.

Jacobs PP et al: Haemoperitoneum caused by a dissecting aneurysm of the gastroepiploic artery. Eur J Vasc Surg 1994;8:236.

Bleeding Lesions

Arteriovenous malformations and other bleeding lesions in the small intestine are discussed under Acute Lower Gastrointestinal Hemorrhage in Chapter 30.

GAS CYSTS (Pneumatosis Cystoides Intestinalis)

Pneumatosis cystoides intestinalis is a rare condition characterized by gas-filled cysts in the wall of the gut and sometimes in the mesentery. When the process is limited to the large intestine, the term **pneumatosis coli** is used. Cysts vary in size from microscopic to several centimeters in diameter.

Pneumatosis may be primary or secondary. About 15% of cases are primary and idiopathic; the cysts are submucosal and usually are limited to the left colon. Secondary pneumatosis comprises 85% of cases. Cysts are subserosal and may be located anywhere in the gastrointestinal tract or its mesentery. Conditions that underlie secondary pneumatosis intestinalis or pneumatosis coli include inflammatory bowel disease, infectious gastroenteritis or colitis, steroid therapy, connective tissue disorders, intestinal obstruction, diverticulitis, chronic obstructive pulmonary disease, acute leukemia, lymphoma, AIDS, and organ transplantation.

The mechanism of cyst formation may not be the same in all patients. In some, anaerobic bacterial fermentation of carbohydrates leads to excess production of hydrogen gas, which enters the intestinal wall by diffusion. Some patients have greatly diminished activity of methanogenic and sulfate-reducing bacteria, which normally consume or metabolize hydrogen. Patients with impaired pulmonary function are less able to excrete excessive hydrogen gas through the lungs, and they are more prone to develop pneumatosis. Cysts are maintained because additional hydrogen is generated with each meal, thus replacing gas that may have diffused into the bloodstream since the previous meal. High breath hydrogen levels have been reported in pneumatosis patients even during fasting.

Symptoms are absent or nonspecific. In secondary pneumatosis, symptoms are due to the underlying disease. In the primary form, patients may complain of abdominal discomfort, distention, diarrhea with mucus, or passing of excessive amounts of gas. Rarely, perforation of a cyst, hemorrhage, obstruction, or malabsorption may bring benign pneumatosis to medical attention. **Fulminant pneumatosis** is associated with acute bacterial infection and necrosis of the bowel wall. Such patients are toxic and may have underlying impaired immunologic defenses. Gas may also be seen within the intestinal wall late in intestinal infarction. Pneumoperitoneum is sometimes present.

Treatment of secondary pneumatosis intestinalis is directed toward the underlying disease. Resolution of cysts can be accomplished in either primary or secondary pneumatosis by having patients breathe oxygen by mask for several days interrupted only at mealtime. Response to hyperbaric oxygen is more rapid. Recurrence of cysts after oxygen treatment reflects continued production of hydrogen, and in these patients it is necessary to reduce the amount of gas being generated. The amount of substrate can be controlled by dietary manipulation, and the fecal flora can be suppressed by antibacterial agents such as ampicillin or metronidazole. Surgical resection of bowel involved with benign primary pneumatosis is rarely required, but underlying disease may need operative treatment in the secondary form of this condition. Fulminant pneumatosis is treated surgically, but the mortality rate is high.

Christl SU et al: Impaired hydrogen metabolism in pneumatosis cystoides intestinalis. Gastroenterology 1993;104:392.

Collins CD et al: Case report: pneumatosis intestinalis occurring in association with cryptosporidiosis and HIV infection. Clin Radiol 1992;46:410.

Hoover EL et al: Avoiding laparotomy in nonsurgical pneumoperitoneum. Am J Surg 1992;164:99.

TUMORS OF THE SMALL INTESTINE

Neoplasms of the jejunum and ileum comprise 1–5% of all tumors of the gastrointestinal tract. The terminal ileum is the favored site, followed by proximal jejunum. Approximately 85% of patients are over age 40. There is a high correlation of small bowel tumors with primary neoplasms elsewhere.

Only 10% of small bowel tumors are symptomatic. Benign lesions are ten times as common as malignant ones. Lymphoma is now the most common primary malignant tumor of the small intestine. At least 75% of symptomatic neoplasms are malignant. Bleeding and obstruction, sometimes due to intussusception, are the most frequent symptoms.

1. Benign Tumors

Polyps

Adenomatous or villous polyps of the type seen in the colon are rare in the small bowel; they are usually solitary and cause symptoms by intussusception or bleeding.

Polypoid **hamartomas** may be solitary in patients who are free of associated anomalies. Hamartomas are multiple in 50% of cases, and 10% of these have **Peutz-Jeghers syndrome**, a familial disorder characterized by diffuse gastrointestinal polyposis and mucocutaneous pigmentation. The malignant potential of these polyps is very small. Operation is indicated only for symptoms (eg, obstruction, bleeding), at which time all polyps greater than about 1 cm should be removed. A combined surgical and endoscopic approach is the best strategy.

Familial adenomatous polyposis (familial polyposis coli, Gardner's syndrome; see Chapter 30) is characterized by multiple intestinal and colonic polyps, osteomas, and subcutaneous cysts or fibromas. The polyps are true neoplasms, and malignant degeneration of colonic polyps is common; there is a predilection for periampullary duodenal cancer as well.

Juvenile (retention) polyps may bleed or obstruct. They are more common in the colon than the small bowel and usually autoamputate before adolescence. Some pathologists regard these lesions as hamartomas.

Other Tumors

Leiomyomas, lipomas, neurofibromas, and fibromas may cause symptoms that require operation. Endometriosis can implant on the small bowel. Hemangiomas are discussed in the section on Acute Lower Gastrointestinal Hemorrhage in Chapter 30.

Ali J et al: Clinical presentations of gastrointestinal inflammatory fibroid polyps. Can J Surg 1992;35:194.

Bertoni G et al: Jejunal polyps in familial adenomatous polyposis assessed by push-type endoscopy. J Clin Gastroenterol 1993;17:343.

Buck JL et al: Peutz-Jeghers syndrome. Radiographics 1992;12:365.

Gall JA et al: Multiple benign stromal cell tumours of the small bowel. J Clin Pathol 1993;46:869.

Gourtsoyiannis NC et al: Radiological appearances of small intestinal leiomyomas. Clin Radiol 1992;45:94.

Hizawa K et al: Cancer in Peutz-Jeghers syndrome. Cancer 1993;72:2777.

Leggett BA et al: Exclusion of APC and MCC as the gene defect in one family with familial juvenile polyposis. Gastroenterology 1993;105:1313.

Serour F et al: Primary neoplasms of the small bowel. J Surg Oncol 1992;49:29.

2. Malignant Tumors

Primary

Adenocarcinoma is often asymptomatic or causes only minimal symptoms for prolonged periods. It usually arises in the proximal jejunum, except in Crohn's disease, in which bypassed distal ileum is at greatest risk. Metastases are present in 80% of cases at the time of operation. Segmental resection of bowel and adjacent mesentery is done when possible, but metastases near the superior mesenteric artery may make the procedure difficult. Five-year survival is 25% in patients undergoing intestinal resection.

Primary small intestinal lymphomas of the Western type arise focally. These lymphomas develop in the proximal jejunum in patients with celiac disease, and in another group of patients the lymphomas arise de novo in the distal ileum. Most primary lymphomas of the small intestine involve B-cell proliferation, but a few cases of primary T-cell lymphoma have been reported. In the Middle East, primary small bowel lymphoma is the most common form of extranodal lymphomatous disease. **Immunoproliferative small intestinal disease** is a geographic variant in that part of the world; it is characterized by diffuse infiltration of the small intestine by abnormal lymphoid cells. The infiltrate is probably benign in the initial phase of alpha-chain disease, but the other cases are malignant. AIDS-associated non-Hodgkin's lymphomas of B-cell origin can involve the small intestine; the prognosis in these patients is very poor.

Western-type lymphomas develop as a nodular, polypoid, or ulcerating mass. Lesions are multiple in 20% of patients. Obstruction, bleeding, and perforation bring the lesion to attention. Abdominal operation is often required to establish a histologic diagnosis by conservative resection of the intestinal lesion. Operation is followed by whole abdominal radiation, with or without chemotherapy, in some patients. The overall 5-year survival rate is about 40%.

Small bowel gastrointestinal stromal tumors (GIST) tend to ulcerate centrally and bleed. Other types of primary malignant neoplasm are rare.

Metastatic

Small bowel metastases are found in 50% of patients dying of malignant melanoma. Carcinomas of the cervix, kidney, breast, lung, etc, may also spread to bowel. Obstruction or hemorrhage may require operation if life expectancy is reasonably good. Significant palliation may be achieved, particularly in patients with solitary metastatic lesions.

Amer MH, El-Akkad S: Gastrointestinal lymphoma in adults: clinical features and management of 399 cases. Gastroenterology 1994;106:846.

Carbonnel F et al: Extensive small intestinal T-cell lymphoma of low-grade malignancy associated with a new chromosomal translocation. Cancer 1994;73:1286.

Chami TN et al: Angiosarcoma of the small intestine: a case report and literature review. Am J Gastroenterol 1994;89:797.

Delaunoit T et al: Pathogenesis and risk factors of small bowel adenocarcinoma: a colorectal cancer sibling? Am J Gastroenterology 2005;100:703.

DiSario JA et al: Small bowel cancer: epidemiological and clinical characteristics from a population-based registry. Am J Gastroenterol 1994;89:699.

Greenstein AJ et al: Lymphoma in inflammatory bowel disease. Cancer 1992;69:1119.

Kummar S, Ciesielski TE, Fogarasi MC: Management of small bowel adenocarcinoma. Oncology (Huntington) 2002;16:1364.

Nakamura S et al: Diagnostic value of push-type jejunal endoscopy in primary jejunal carcinoma. Surg Endosc 1993;7:188.

Ng E-H et al: Prognostic factors influencing survival in gastrointestinal leiomyosarcomas: implications for surgical management and staging. Ann Surg 1992;215:68.

Ruskone-Fourmestraux A et al: Primary digestive tract lymphoma: a prospective multicentric study of 91 patients. Gastroenterology 1993;105:1662.

Stemmermann GN, Goodman MT, Nomura AM: Adenocarcinoma of the proximal small intestine. A marker for familial and multicentric cancer? Cancer 1992;70:2766.

Stollman N et al: Intestinal lymphomatous polyposis in a patient with AIDS: an enteroscopic view and discussion. Am J Gastroenterol 1994;89:802.

3. Carcinoid Tumors & Carcinoid Syndrome

Carcinoid tumors are apudomas that arise from enterochromaffin cells throughout the gut. Carcinoids may be associated with multiple endocrine neoplasia (MEN) type 1 and type 2. Rare familial clustering not associated with MEN has been reported. Neoplasms of other organs—most commonly the colon, lung, stomach, or breast—are present in 15% of patients. Carcinoids occur in patients 25–45 years of age.

The origin of carcinoid tumors of the gastrointestinal tract is foregut, 5%; midgut, 88%; and hindgut, 6%. Most carcinoids associated with MEN are of foregut origin. Midgut carcinoids produce serotonin and substance P; neurotensin, gastrin, somatostatin, motilin, secretin, and pancreatic polypeptide are also common. Foregut and hindgut carcinoids do not produce serotonin, but they often contain gastrin, somatostatin, pancreatic polypeptide, and glucagon.

The appendix is the most common site of carcinoid tumors, and the small intestine is the second most common location; about ten times as many originate in the ileum as in the jejunum. Multiple tumors are present in 40% of cases. Grossly, carcinoids are firm, yellowish submucosal nodules. Special stains may demonstrate argentaffin or argyrophil reactions in microscopic sections.

Carcinoid of the small bowel should be regarded as "a malignant neoplasm in slow motion." At the time of surgical diagnosis, 40% of tumors have invaded the muscularis and 45% have metastasized to lymph nodes or liver. Of primary tumors less than 1 cm in diameter, fewer than 2% metastasize, but 80% of those larger than 2 cm have spread at the time of operation. Huge metastatic deposits emanating from a minute primary are sometimes encountered.

Clinical Findings

A. Symptoms and Signs

Small tumors are usually asymptomatic. Overall, 30% of small bowel carcinoids cause symptoms of obstruction, pain, bleeding, or the carcinoid syndrome. Obstruction due to sclerosis and kinking of the bowel may be related to elaboration of vasoactive materials by metastases in the mesentery. Intestinal ischemia has been reported.

About 10% of patients with small bowel carcinoids present with **carcinoid syndrome**, and others develop it later. The syndrome consists of cutaneous flushing, diarrhea, bronchoconstriction, and right-sided cardiac valvular disease due to collagen deposition. Biologically active substances secreted by carcinoids are usually inactivated in the liver, but hepatic metastases or primary ovarian or bronchial carcinoids release these compounds directly into the systemic circulation, where they produce symptoms. Serotonin production in large quantities occurs in almost all cases of carcinoid syndrome; it is responsible for much of the diarrhea. A host of other vasoactive substances may participate, including aminess (histamine, dopamine, 5-hydroxytryptophan, and 5-HIAA), tachykinins (kallikrein, substance P, and neuropeptide K), peptides (pancreatic polypeptide, chromogranins, neurotensin, and motilin), and prostaglandins.

B. Laboratory Findings

Some carcinoid tumors are detected by radiographic methods. Elevated urinary levels of 5-hydroxyindoleacetic acid (5-HIAA) or of serum chromogranin A are the diagnostic hallmark of carcinoid syndrome. An injection of pentagastrin can be used as a provocative test: Symptoms appear, and serum levels of serotonin and substance P increase.

Treatment

All accessible carcinoid tumor in small bowel, mesentery, and the peritoneal cavity should be removed. If intestinal obstruction is the principal serious manifestation of incurable abdominal disease, it should be treated aggressively because tumor growth is so slow. Extensive enterectomy followed by chronic total parenteral nutrition may even be justified in some cases. Patients are followed up postoperatively with CT and Octreotide scans.

Localized hepatic metastases should be resected. Unresectable hepatic metastases can sometimes be palliated by hepatic artery embolization or hepatic artery infusion chemotherapy. In some instances, long-standing, metastatic disease isolated to the liver has been successfully treated with liver transplantation. Octreotide can be used to suppress tumor growth and control the symptoms of carcinoid syndrome. Octreotide inhibits release of gastrointestinal hormones; in carcinoid syndrome, it relieves flushing, wheezing, and severe diarrhea refractory to other measures.

Prognosis

Carcinoid tumors grow slowly over months and years. The overall 5-year survival rate after resection of small bowel carcinoid is 70%; 40% of patients with inoperable metastases and 20% of those with hepatic metastases survive 5 years or longer. Median survival from the time of histologic diagnosis is 14 years, and from onset of the carcinoid syndrome it is 8 years.

Ahlman H et al: Clinical efficacy of octreotide scintigraphy in patients with midgut carcinoid tumours and evaluation of intraoperative scintillation detection. Br J Surg 1994;81:1144.

Basson MD et al: Biology and management of the midgut carcinoid. Am J Surg 1993;165:288.

Delcore R, Friesen SR: Gastrointestinal neuroendocrine tumors. J Am Coll Surg 1994;178:187.

Farahvash MJ et al: Jejunized colon: a rare complication of carcinoid tumor. Am J Gastroenterol 1994;89:429.

Horton KM, Fishman EK: Multidetector-row computed tomography and 3-dimensional computed tomography imaging of small bowel neoplasms: current concept in diagnosis. J Comput Assist Tomogr 2004;28:106.

Horton KM et al: Carcinoid tumors of the small bowel: a multitechnique imaging approach. AJR 2004;182:559.

Karatzas G et al: Gastrointestinal carcinoid tumors: 10-year experience of a general surgical department. Int Surg 2004;89:21.

Marshall JB, Bodnarchuk G: Carcinoid tumors of the gut: our experience over three decades and review of the literature. J Clin Gastroenterol 1993;16:123.

Moyana TN, Satkunam N: A comparative immunohistochemical study of jejunoileal and appendiceal carcinoids: implications for histogenesis and pathogenesis. Cancer 1992;70:1081.

Pyke CM et al: Carcinoid syndrome secondary to a primary tumour in a Meckel's diverticulum. Aust N Z J Surg 1993;63:732.

Søreide O et al: Surgical treatment as a principle in patients with advanced abdominal carcinoid tumors. Surgery 1992;111:48.

von der Ohe MR et al: Motor dysfunction of the small bowel and colon in patients with the carcinoid syndrome and diarrhea. N Engl J Med 1993;329:1073.

Yoshikane H et al: Carcinoid tumors of the gastrointestinal tract: evaluation with endoscopic ultrasonography. Gastrointest Endosc 1993;39:375.

Large Intestine

30

George J. Chang, MD, Andrew A. Shelton, MD, & Mark L. Welton, MD

ANATOMY

The colon extends from the end of the ileum to the rectum. The cecum, ascending colon, hepatic flexure, and proximal transverse colon comprise the **right colon**. The distal transverse colon, splenic flexure, descending colon, sigmoid colon, and rectosigmoid comprise the **left colon** (Figure 30–1). The ascending and descending portions are fixed in the retroperitoneal space, and the transverse colon and sigmoid colon are suspended in the peritoneal cavity by their mesocolons. The caliber of the lumen is greatest at the cecum and diminishes distally. The wall of the colon has four layers: mucosa, submucosa, muscularis, and serosa (Figure 30–2). The muscularis propria consists of an inner circular layer and an outer longitudinal layer. The longitudinal muscle completely encircles the colon in a very thin layer, and at three points around the circumference it is gathered into thick bands called taeniae coli. Sacculations (haustra) are the result of shortening of the colon by the taeniae and contractions of the circular muscle. The haustra are not fixed anatomic structures and may be observed to move longitudinally. There are fatty appendages (the appendices epiploicae) on the serosal surface. The wall of the colon is so thin that it becomes markedly distended when obstructed.

The **rectum** is 12–15 cm in length. The taeniae coli spread out at the rectosigmoid junction and are not apparent distal to that area. The upper rectum is invested by peritoneum anteriorly and laterally, but posteriorly it is retroperitoneal up to the junction with the sigmoid colon. The anterior peritoneal reflection dips low into the pelvis to approximately 6–8 cm above the anal verge—a fact to be noted when rectal lesions are biopsied or fulgurated; perforation into the peritoneal cavity can occur at a much lower level anteriorly than posteriorly. The anterior peritoneal reflection lies behind the bladder in males and behind the uterus (the rectouterine pouch of Douglas) in females. Tumor masses or abscesses in this location are readily palpated on digital rectal or pelvic examination. The rectum is normally capacious and distensible. When its capacity to distend is lost or impaired by surgery or disease, fecal urgency and frequency are noted.

The rectal valves of Houston are prominent spirally arranged mucosal folds within the rectum. Less than half of people have the so-called normal three valves, two on the left and one on the right. The valves are at variable distances from the anal verge in different individuals. Normally, the valves appear thin, with sharp edges, but they become thickened and blunted when inflamed. A rectal valve may hide a small lesion from endoscopic view, and during rigid sigmoidoscopy the valve must be "ironed out" so its superior surface can be examined.

In men, the prostate gland, the seminal vesicles, and the seminal ducts lie anterior to the rectum. The prostate usually is easily felt, but the seminal vesicles are not palpable unless distended, because the firm, unyielding rectovesical fascia of Denonvilliers intervenes. In women, the rectovaginal septum and uterus lie anterior and the uterine adnexa anterolateral to the rectum. The structures are easily palpated with one finger in the vagina and one in the rectum.

Blood Supply & Lymphatic Drainage

The arterial supply of the right colon, from the ileocecal junction to approximately the mid transverse colon, is from the superior mesenteric artery through its ileocolic, right colic, and middle colic branches.

The inferior mesenteric artery arises from the abdominal aorta and gives off the left colic and sigmoid branches before it becomes the superior hemorrhoidal artery. The vasa recta are the terminal arterial branches to the colon and run directly to the mesocolic wall or through the bowel wall to the antimesocolic border.

The colic arteries bifurcate and form arcades about 2.5 cm from the mesocolic border of the bowel, forming a pathway of communicating vessels called the **marginal artery of Drummond**. The marginal artery thus forms an anastomosis between the superior mesenteric and inferior mesenteric arteries. The configuration of the blood supply, however, varies greatly; the typical pattern is present in only 15% of individuals.

The middle hemorrhoidal artery arises on each side from the anterior division of the internal iliac artery or from the internal pudendal artery and runs inward at the level of the pelvic floor. The inferior hemorrhoidal arteries derive from the internal pudendal arteries and pass through Alcock's canal. The anastomoses between the superior hemorrhoidal vessels and branches of the

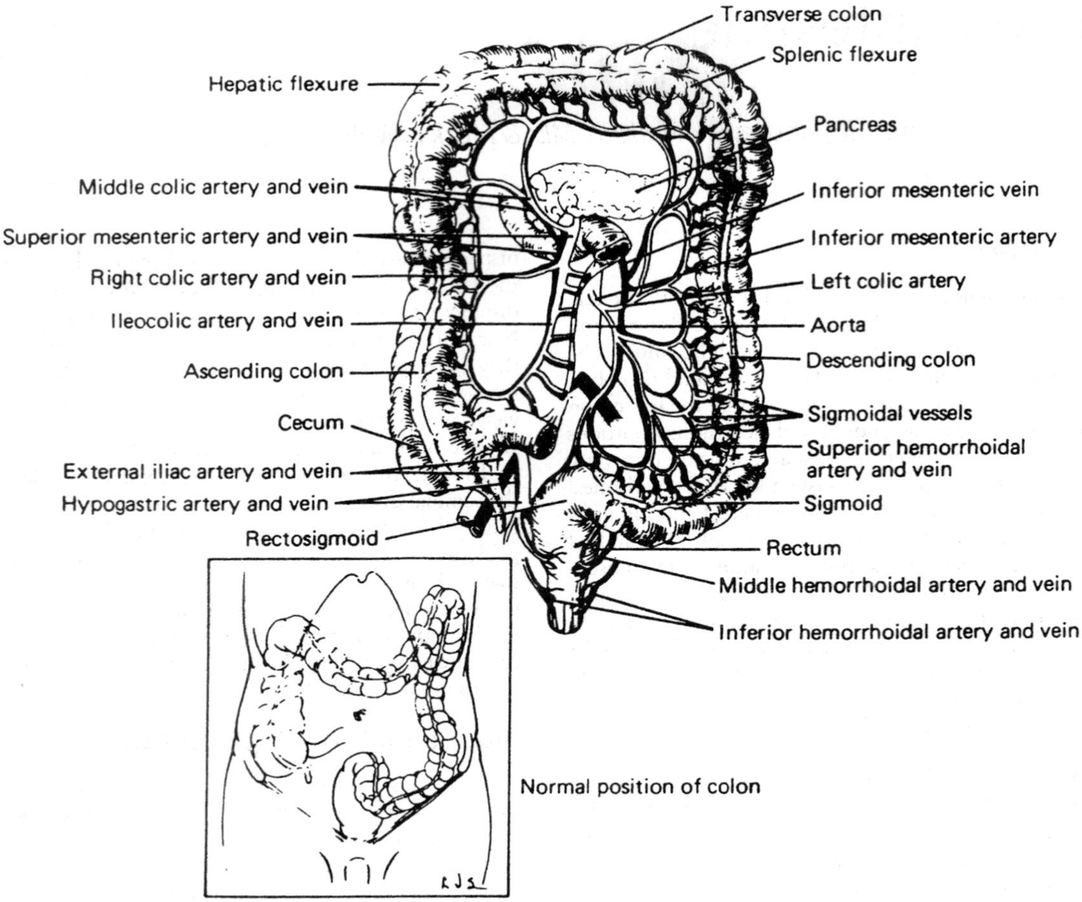

Figure 30–1. The large intestine: anatomic divisions and blood supply. The veins are shown in black. The insert shows the usual configuration of the colon.

internal iliac arteries provide collateral circulation; this is important after surgical interruption or atherosclerotic occlusion of the vascular supply of the left colon.

The veins accompany the corresponding arteries and drain into the liver through the portal vein or into the systemic circulation by way of the hypogastric veins. Continuous lymphatic plexuses in the submucous and subserous layers of the bowel wall drain into the lymphatic channels and lymph nodes that accompany the blood vessels.

Nerve Supply

The sympathetic nerves originating in T10–12 travel in the thoracic splanchnic nerves to the celiac plexus and then to the preaortic and superior mesenteric plexuses, from which postganglionic fibers are distributed along the superior mesenteric artery and its branches to the right colon. The left colon is supplied by sympathetic fibers that arise in L1–3, synapse in the paravertebral ganglia, and accompany the inferior mesenteric artery to the colon. The parasympathetic nerves to the right colon come from the right vagus and travel with the sympathetic nerves. The parasympathetic supply to the left colon derives from S2–4. These fibers emerge from the spinal cord as the nervi erigentes, which form the pelvic plexus and send branches to the transverse, descending, and pelvic portions of the large bowel.

Al-Fallouji MA, Tagart RE: The surgical anatomy of the colonic intramural blood supply and its influence on colorectal anastomosis. J R Coll Surg Edinb 1985;30:380.

Crowe R et al: Peptide-containing neurons in different regions of the submucous plexus of human sigmoid colon. Gastroenterology 1992;102:461.

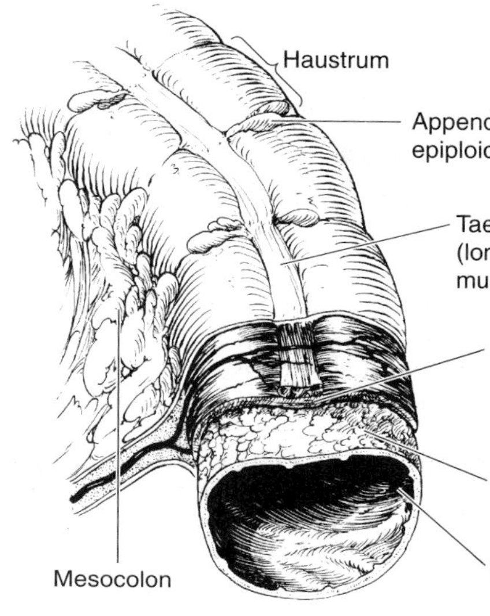

Figure 30–2. Cross section of colon. The longitudinal muscle encircles the colon but is thickened in the region of the taeniae coli.

Irving MH, Catchpole B: ABC of colorectal diseases: Anatomy and physiology of the colon, rectum, and anus. Br Med J 1992;304:1106.

Pace JL: The anatomy of the haustra of the human colon. Proc R Soc Med 1968;61:934.

Ward SM: Interstitial cells of Cajal in enteric neurotransmission. Gut 2000;47 (Suppl 4):40.

PHYSIOLOGY

The primary functions of the colon are absorption, secretion, motility, and intraluminal digestion. These interrelated phenomena process ileal effluent and convert it into semisolid feces that are stored until defecation is convenient. Regional variations in function are significant. The proximal colon absorbs electrolytes and water more efficiently than do the descending colon and rectum, and motility and intraluminal digestion differ by region also. Loss of colonic function through disease or surgery results in a continuous discharge of food wastes and increases daily intestinal losses of water and electrolytes, chiefly sodium and chloride.

The small intestine digests and absorbs most nutrients from ingested foods. The role of the colon in human nutrition is not well defined. Metabolism of carbohydrate to absorbable volatile fatty acids is probably important. Ureolysis—conversion of circulating urea to ammonia, which is reabsorbed and reused—may be significant. The colon also absorbs amino acids, bile acids, and vitamin K, but the contribution of the colon to homeostasis by these mechanisms has not been quantified.

Intestinal Gas

The volume and composition of intestinal gas vary greatly among normal individuals. The small intestine contains approximately 100 mL of gas and the colon somewhat more. Some gas is absorbed through the mucosa and excreted through the lungs, and the remaining 400–1200 mL/d are discharged as flatus.

Nitrogen (N_2) comprises 30–90% of intestinal gas. Swallowed air is the principal source of intestinal N_2, but N_2 also can diffuse across the mucosa from blood to lumen when other gases are produced in sufficient volume to lower the partial pressure of N_2 and establish a gradient for diffusion. Other intestinal gases include oxygen (O_2), carbon dioxide (CO_2), hydrogen (H_2), methane (CH_4), and odoriferous trace substances such as methyl sulfide, hydrogen sulfide, indole, and skatole. H_2 and CO_2 are generated by fermentation of ingested non-absorbed carbohydrate, especially carbohydrate present in polysaccharides (eg, fiber) and some starches. Lactose in milk provides the substrate in lactase-deficient persons. Mucus is the main endogenous source of carbohydrate in the colon; intestinal glycoproteins are 80% carbohydrate. Only about one-third of the population produces CH_4, which is a product of colonic bacteria that use hydrogen to reduce CO_2. Stools of CH_4 producers nearly always float, even in the absence of fecal fat. CH_4, like H_2, can be measured in the breath. H_2 and CH_4 are explosive gases, and caution must be exercised when using electrocautery in the bowel lumen.

Patients with "excessive gas" may complain of abdominal pain and distention, increased flatus, and watery stools. Some of these patients have irritable bowel syndrome. "Increased" flatus may reflect extreme sensitivity of the rectum to small volumes, resulting in frequent passage of gas. Alternatively, gas may be produced in excessive quantities in symptomatic patients. Almost invariably, hydrogen is the culprit. Measurement of breath hydrogen is a potentially useful test for malabsorption states. Treatment of overproduction of gas at present is directed toward elimination of lactose, legumes, and wheat from the diet.

Motility

Motor activity of the colon occurs in three patterns, and there is marked regional variation between the right and left colon. A pacemaker in the transverse colon has been postulated, perhaps pacing the proximal colon retrograde to facilitate storage and absorption while pacing the distal colon in the aborad direction to favor propulsion. **Retrograde peristalsis (antiperistalsis)**—annular contractions moving orad—dominates in the right colon. This kind of activity churns the contents and tends to confine them to the cecum and ascending colon. As ileal effluent continually enters the cecum, some of the column of liquid stool in the right colon is displaced and flows into the transverse colon. **Segmentation** is the most common type of motor activity in the transverse and descending colon. Annular contractions divide the lumen into uniform segments, propelling feces over short distances in both directions. Segmental contractions form, relax, and re-form in different locations, seemingly at random. **Mass movement** is a strong ring contraction moving aborad over long distances in the transverse and descending colon. It occurs infrequently—perhaps only a few times daily—most commonly after meals.

The enteric nervous system coordinates and programs motility (see Chapter 29). Eating produces a group of alterations in colonic myoelectrical and motor activity collectively termed the gastrocolic response. As a result, more fluid is emptied from the ileum into the colon; mass movements are increased; and the urge to defecate is perceived. The magnitude of the gastrocolic response depends on the caloric content of the meal. Dietary fat is the principal stimulus.

Physical activities such as changes in posture, walking, and lifting are physiologically important stimuli of movement of colonic contents. Colonic motility is also affected by emotional states. Transit through the colon is speeded by a diet containing large amounts of fiber from vegetables or bran. Fiber is defined as insoluble plant cell matrix and consists of cellulose, hemicellulose, and lignin. Dietary fiber slows transit through the jejunum.

Normal colonic movements are slow, complex, and extremely variable, making it difficult to define altered motility in disease states. The fecal stream itself does not move along in anything resembling orderly laminar flow. Some of the material entering the cecum flows past feces remaining from earlier periods. Portions of the stream enter the periphery of haustra, where they may fail to progress for 24 hours or more. In most persons with normal bowel function, residue from a meal reaches the cecum after 4 hours and the rectosigmoid by 24 hours. The transverse colon is the primary site for fecal storage. Mixing of bowel content in the colon results in passage of residue from a single meal in movements for up to 3–4 days afterward.

The urge to defecate is perceived when small amounts of feces enter the rectum and stimulate stretch receptors in the rectal wall or the levator muscles. Rectal distention elicits the rectoanal inhibitory reflex, the reflex relaxation of the internal anal sphincter, which allows the rectal contents to be "sampled" at the dentate line. Almost immediately after the internal sphincter relaxes, the external sphincter contracts, forcing the contents proximally into the rectum. This complex reflex mechanism is thought to allow the rectal contents to descend distally into the rectum, contacting the sensory fibers in the surgical anal canal. If it is a socially acceptable time and flatus is present, it may be expelled. If stool is present and defecation must be deferred, the rectum accommodates and the sense of rectal fullness abates. Defecation cannot be deferred indefinitely, and with continued rectal filling the urge to defecate is impossible to deny.

Defecation is facilitated by assuming the sitting position, performing a Valsalva maneuver, and relaxing the anal sphincters. The pelvic floor relaxes and the rectum loses its curves as the feces are discharged from the anus. Afterward, the sphincters resume their tone.

Absorption

The colon participates in maintaining the body economy by absorption of water and electrolytes, but the absorptive function of the colon is not essential to life. Although amino acids, fatty acids, and some vitamins can be absorbed slowly from the large bowel, only a small amount of these nutrients reaches the colon normally. Perhaps 10–20% of ingested starch, however, passes unabsorbed into the colon, where bacterial fermentation converts starch to short-chain volatile fatty acids (eg, acetate). Absorption of fatty acids contributes importantly to assimilation of calories. Dietary celluloses and hemicelluloses are degraded by colonic bacteria.

Approximately 1000–2000 mL of ileal effluent consisting of 90% water enters the cecum each day. This material is desiccated during transit through the colon, so that only 100–200 mL of water is excreted in the feces. Table 30–1 gives average values for the electrolyte and water composition of ileal effluent and feces; the differences provide a rough estimate of colonic absorption and secretion. Data are listed also for the estimated maximal absorptive capacity, which is greater in the right colon than in the left. This capacity depends on the rate at which fluid enters the cecum. Normally, formed feces are composed of 70% water and 30% solids. Almost half of these solids are bacteria; the remainder is food waste and desquamated epithelium.

Sodium is absorbed by an active transport mechanism that is enhanced by mineralocorticoids, glucocorticoids, and volatile fatty acids produced by bacteria. Volatile fatty acids may be essential mucosal nutrients for normal colonic absorption of electrolytes and water. There are segmental differences in the mode of absorption of sodium and water. Normally, sodium absorption is so efficient that a person can remain in balance on as little as 5 meq in the daily diet, but colectomy increases the minimum daily requirements to 80–100 meq to offset losses from the ileostomy. Potassium enters feces by passive diffusion and by secretion in mucus. Excessive mucus production may occur in colitis or with certain tumors such as villous adenomas and may lead to substantial potassium losses in the stool. Chloride is absorbed in exchange for bicarbonate.

Bowel Habits

The frequency of defecation is influenced by social and dietary customs. The average interval between bowel

Table 30–1. Mean values for electrolyte and water balance in the normal colon. A plus (+) sign indicates absorption from the colonic lumen; a minus (–) sign indicates secretion into the lumen.

	Ileal Effluent		**Fecal Fluid**		**Net Colonic Absorption (per 24 h)**	
	Concentration (meq/L)	***Quantity (per 24 h)***	***Concentration (meq/L)***	***Quantity (per 24 h)***	***Normal***	***Maximal Capacity***
Na^+	120	180 meq	30	2 meq	+178 meq	+400 meq
K^+	6	10 meq	67	5 meq	+5 meq	–45 meq
Cl^-	67	100 meq	20	1.5 meq	+98 meq	+500 meq
HCO_3^-	40	60 meq	50	4 meq	+56 meq	
H_2O		1500 mL		100 mL	+1400 mL	+5000 mL

movements among the population of Western countries is a little over 24 hours but may vary in normal subjects from 8–12 hours to 2–3 days. Dietary fiber content and physical activity influence stool frequency to a great extent. Many bedridden patients have infrequent, hard stools. Self-reported constipation in the general population of the USA has a prevalence of about 10% in men and 20% in women; gender differences in colonic function (slower transit and smaller fecal mass in women under controlled conditions) may be responsible for the difference in frequency of constipation. Diarrhea is reported by 5% of men and women. These complaints are more frequent with aging.

A change in bowel habits demands investigation for organic disease. Diarrhea may be debilitating and even fatal, because it is associated with loss of large amounts of water and electrolytes. Diarrhea is usually said to be present if stools contain more than 300 mL of fluid daily. Osmotic diarrhea results when excess water-soluble molecules remain in the bowel lumen, causing osmotic retention of water; this is one mechanism by which saline laxatives act. Colonic diseases that produce diarrhea usually cause excessive fluid secretion more so than impaired absorption. Bile salts, hydroxy fatty acids, and castor oil (ricinoleic acid) are a few of the many substances that stimulate secretion of fluid by the colon by increasing mucosal cAMP. Increased secretion by the small bowel may also cause diarrhea. Loss of absorptive surface (eg, after intestinal resection) and exudative diseases are other reasons for feces to contain excess fluid. Disordered intestinal motility is not primarily responsible for increased fecal excretion of water. The physician should be alert to surreptitious laxative abuse among patients who complain of diarrhea.

Constipation means infrequent stools (fewer than two per week), excessive straining, or incomplete evacuation. Recent onset of this complaint in an adult should prompt a search for obstructing lesions.

Severe idiopathic constipation refractory to usual remedies is more common in women; it often begins in adolescence and worsens during the 20s or 30s, or it may be precipitated by childbirth or hysterectomy. A heterogeneous group of disorders is responsible. Slow colonic transit (colonic inertia) is one mechanism of constipation. A decrease in the number of interstitial cells of Cajal has been implicated in this disorder. Failure of the pelvic floor to relax during defecation (obstructed defecation) is a separate category. A classification of disorders in which constipation and obstructed defecation are symptoms is given in Table 30–2. Conditions giving rise to obstructed

Table 30–2. Classification of constipation and obstructed defecation.[1]

Constipation
- Normal colon
  - Normal transit
  - Slow transit
- Megacolon/megarectum
  - Congenital
  - Acquired

Obstructed defecation
- Solitary rectal ulcer syndrome
- Descending perineum syndrome
- Rectal intussusception
- Complete rectal prolapse
- Anismus (inappropriate sphincter contraction)

[1]Modified from Bartolo DCG: Pelvic floor disorders: Incontinence, constipation, and obstructed defecation. Perspect Colon Rectal Surg 1988;1:1.

defecation are part of a larger group of abnormalities termed disorders of the pelvic floor.

A thorough history and physical examination may elucidate the origin of the symptoms, eg, depression, psychotropic or other drugs, or anatomic abnormalities. Further investigation of chronic idiopathic constipation requires assessment of colonic transit and study of pelvic floor function. Colonic transit is evaluated by obtaining serial plain abdominal x-rays after ingestion of tiny radiopaque markers or by scintigraphy after ingestion of radiolabeled solid pellets. Tests of pelvic floor function include defecography, anorectal manometry, electromyography, nerve conduction studies and dynamic magnetic resonance imaging.

Severe slow-transit constipation does not respond to dietary fiber; lactulose or an irritant laxative (eg, Senokot, Dulcolax) or retrograde enemas may be effective. Selected patients qualify for a surgical procedure (colectomy and ileorectal anastomosis). Although associated with a significant improvement in quality of life, postoperative persistence of abdominal pain and the development of incontinence or diarrhea are limitations. Obstructed defecation related to rectal prolapse responds to operative repair of the prolapse. Rectal intussusception is treated with fiber, water, and stimulating bowel movements with suppositories for mild to moderate situations. Patients are instructed to stimulate a bowel movement in the morning with a suppository and to ignore the urge to defecate during the day. The sense of rectal fullness that the patient experiences is a result of the proximal bowel prolapsing into the distal rectum. With this behavioral modification, the symptoms usually resolve. Biofeedback therapy may be a helpful adjunct. Surgical repair is reserved for severe cases of rectal intussusception.

Agarwal R, Afzalpurkar R, Fordtran JS: Pathophysiology of potassium absorption and secretion by the human intestine. Gastroenterology 1994;107:548.

Bassotti G et al: Colonic motility in man: features in normal subjects and in patients with chronic idiopathic constipation. Am J Gastroenterol 1999;94:1760.

Brown SR et al: Biofeedback avoids surgery in patients with slow-transit constipation: report of four cases. Dis Colon Rectum 2001;44:737.

FitzHarris GP et al: Quality of life after subtotal colectomy for slow-transit constipation: both quality and quantity count. Dis Colon Rectum 2003;46:433.

He CL et al: Decreased interstitial cell of Cajal volume in patients with slow-transit constipation. Gastroenterology 2000;118:14.

Knowles CH, Scott SM, Lunniss PJ: Slow transit constipation: a disorder of pelvic autonomic nerves? Dig Dis Sci 2001;46:389.

Locke GR 3rd, Pemberton JH, Phillips SF: AGA technical review on constipation. American Gastroenterological Association. Gastroenterology 2000;119:1766.

Mollen RM, Kuijpers HC, Claassen AT: Colectomy for slow-transit constipation: preoperative functional evaluation is important but not a guarantee for a successful outcome. Dis Colon Rectum 2001;44:577.

Monahan DW, Peluso FE, Goldner F: Combustible colonic gas levels during flexible sigmoidoscopy and colonoscopy. Gastrointest Endosc 1992;38:40.

Moran BJ, Jackson AA: Function of the human colon. Br J Surg 1992;79:1132.

Nordgaard I, Hansen BS, Mortensen PB: Colon as a digestive organ in patients with short bowel. Lancet 1994;343:373.

Pikarsky AJ et al: Long-term follow-up of patients undergoing colectomy for colonic inertia. Dis Colon Rectum 2001;44:179.

Robertson G et al: Effects of exercise on total and segmental colon transit. J Clin Gastroenterol 1993;16:300.

Scheppach W, Luehrs H, Menzel T: Beneficial health effects of low-digestible carbohydrate consumption. Br J Nutr 2001;85 (Suppl 1):S23.

Tack J, Vanden Berghe P: Neuropeptides and colonic motility: it's all in the little brain. Gastroenterology 2000;119:257.

Thakur A et al: Surgical treatment of severe colonic inertia with restorative proctocolectomy. Am Surg 2001;67:36.

MICROBIOLOGY

The colon of the fetus is sterile, and the bacterial flora is established soon after birth. The type of organisms present in the colon depends in part on dietary and environmental factors. It is estimated that stool contains up to 400 different species of autochthonous (native) bacteria.

Over 99% of the normal fecal flora is anaerobic. *Bacteroides fragilis* is most prevalent, and counts average 10^{10}/g of wet feces. *Lactobacillus bifidus,* clostridia, and cocci of various types are other common anaerobes. Aerobic fecal bacteria are mainly coliforms and enterococci. *Escherichia coli* is the predominant coliform and is present in counts of 10^7/g of feces; other aerobic coliforms include klebsiella, proteus, and enterobacter. *Streptococcus faecalis* is the principal enterococcus. *Methanobrevibacter smithii* is the predominant methane-producing organism in humans.

The fecal flora participates in numerous physiologic processes. Bacteria degrade bile pigments to give the stool its brown color, and the characteristic fecal odor is due to the amines indole and skatole produced by bacterial action. Fecal organisms deconjugate bile salts (only free bile salts are found in feces) and alter the steroid nucleus. Bacteria influence colonic motility and absorption, consume and generate intestinal gases, supply vitamin K to the host, and may be important in the defense against infection. Nutrition of colonic mucosal cells may be partially derived from fuels (eg, fatty acids) produced by bacteria. Intestinal bacteria participate in the pathophysiology of a variety of disease processes. Bacterial translocation from the small and large bowel in critically ill or traumatized patients is believed to contribute to multiple organ system failure. There is evidence that bacteria play a role in the pathogenesis of carcinoma of the large bowel.

Bourquin LD et al: Fermentation of dietary fibre by human colonic bacteria: disappearance of, short-chain fatty acid production from, and potential water-holding capacity of, various substrates. Scand J Gastroenterol 1993;28:249.

Chapman MA: The role of the colonic flora in maintaining a healthy large bowel mucosa. Ann R Coll Surg Engl 2001; 83:75.

Gibson GR, MacFarlane GT, Cummings JH: Sulphate reducing bacteria and hydrogen metabolism in the human large intestine. Gut 1993;34:437.

Pochart P et al: Pyxigraphic sampling to enumerate methanogens and anaerobes in the right colon of healthy humans. Gastroenterology 1993;105:1281.

Strocchi A et al: Methanogens outcompete sulphate reducing bacteria for H_2 in the human colon. Gut 1994;35:1098.

X-RAY EXAMINATION

Plain films of the abdomen depict the distribution of gas in the intestines, calcifications, tumor masses, and the size and position of the liver, spleen, and kidneys. In the presence of acute intra-abdominal disease, erect, lateral, and oblique projections and lateral decubitus views are helpful.

Although plain radiographs of the abdomen are generally nonspecific, they often give clues to the underlying problems. Free air in the abdominal cavity is best seen on upright views. An obstructing colon cancer may demonstrate dilation of the proximal colon with a paucity of gas distal to the mass. Air-fluid levels in the bowel in the absence of air within the rectum suggest a complete bowel obstruction. Volvulus of the sigmoid colon or cecum may demonstrate their characteristic radiographic findings.

The lumen of the colon can be seen radiographically by instilling a suspension of barium sulfate through the anus (barium enema) (Figure 30–3). Adequate preparation of the bowel is imperative before barium enema examination so that the colon will be as free as possible of fecal material and gas. Although many rectal lesions can be demonstrated by barium enema, x-rays are not as accurate here as with lesions above the rectosigmoid. Proctosigmoidoscopy is the best method for inspecting the rectum. Postevacuation films reveal the mucosal pattern and small lesions.

Barium enemas are performed as single-column or double-column studies. In the double-column (air contrast) barium enema, a higher-density, more viscous barium is used. After the mucosa is first coated with barium, carbon dioxide or air is insufflated to distend the colon and provide a second contrast medium. The double-column barium enema is more sensitive for detection of small lesions, but it is more strenuous and for that reason less well tolerated by frail or elderly patients.

Water-soluble contrast agents such as diatrizoate meglumine (Gastrografin) or diatrizoate sodium (Hypaque) may be used as alternatives to barium. Fine resolution with these

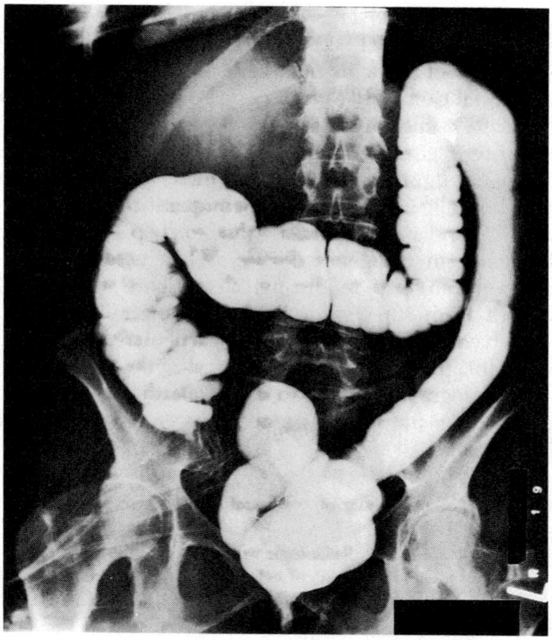

Figure 30–3. X-ray of normal colon. The colon has been rendered radiopaque by a barium enema (single-column technique).

agents is not as good as with barium; however, they can be used when barium is contraindicated, such as when there is a concern for perforation.

CT scan is useful in the diagnosis of masses (neoplasms and abscesses) and is also the most sensitive for detecting intra-abdominal free air and acute inflammatory processes such as appendicitis or diverticulitis. CT colography, or "virtual colonoscopy," is a new technique that utilizes 3D reconstruction of the air-distended colon. In a series of 1223 average-risk adults who subsequently underwent conventional (optical) colonoscopy, virtual colonoscopy was as good as or better at detecting relevant lesions. However, it may be less accurate in surveillance populations. Studies are ongoing to evaluate the efficacy of virtual colonoscopy in both screening and surveillance. Thus far, the major limitations include the need for full bowel preparation and follow-up colonoscopy for tissue diagnosis of radiographic abnormalities. Because virtual colonoscopy is considerably time- and labor-intensive from the standpoint of the radiologists, active investigations into methods of automating the evaluation process are ongoing.

MRI is proving reliable for staging of cancer. Sonography (external, endorectal, and endovaginal) is useful in the diagnosis of masses as well in the evaluation of anatomy, such as depth of penetration of rectal cancers or presence of pelvic nodal metastases. Positron emission tomography (PET) has emerged as an increasingly valuable tool in the management of patients with colon and rectal cancer. PET has been shown to be 95% sensitive, 98% specific, and 96% accurate in the detection of cancer recurrence. The technique utilizes the glucose analogue fluorodeoxyglucose, which accumulates in metabolically active tissues. Semiquantitative analysis uses a standardized uptake value to help discriminate benign from malignant disease. When used appropriately, it can help to distinguish patients who would benefit from surgery for recurrent cancer from those who have unresectable disease, particularly when the other imaging modalities fail to localize the disease.

Arteriography is used to detect bleeding sites and is discussed in the section on acute lower gastrointestinal hemorrhage.

Berlin JW et al: Staging of colorectal cancer. Semin Roentgenol 2000;35:370.

Dobos N, Rubesin SE: Radiologic imaging modalities in the diagnosis and management of colorectal cancer. Hematol Oncol Clin North Am 2002;16:875.

Fenlon HM et al: A comparison of virtual and conventional colonoscopy for the detection of colorectal polyps. N Engl J Med 1999;341:1496.

Freeman AH: CT and bowel disease. Br J Radiol 2001;74(877):4.

Hageman MJHH, Goei R: Cleansing enema prior to double-contrast barium enema examination: is it necessary? Radiology 1993;187:109.

Hunerbein M et al: Preoperative evaluation of colorectal neoplasms by colonoscopic miniprobe ultrasonography. Ann Surg 2000;232:46.

Jensen DM: What to choose for diagnosis of bleeding colonic angiomas: colonoscopy, angiography, or helical computed tomography angiography? Gastroenterology 2000;119:581.

Libutti SK et al: A prospective study of 2-[18F]fluoro-2-deoxy-D-glucose/positron emission tomography scan, 99m Tc-labeled arcitumomab (CEA-scan), and blind second-look laparotomy for detecting colon cancer recurrence in patients with increasing carcinoembryonic antigen levels. Ann Surg Oncol 2001;8:779.

Pickhart PJ et al: Computed tomographic virtual colonoscopy to screen for colorectal neoplasia in asymptomatic adults. N Engl J Med 2003;349:2191.

Suri S et al: Comparative evaluation of plain films, ultrasound and CT in the diagnosis of intestinal obstruction. Acta Radiol 1999;40:422.

Vernava AM 3rd et al: Lower gastrointestinal bleeding. Dis Colon Rectum 1997;40:846.

FIBEROPTIC COLONOSCOPY & SIGMOIDOSCOPY

The flexible colonoscope permits examination of the entire colon in most individuals, and biopsies or brushings (for cytologic examination) can be obtained under direct vision.

Table 30–3. Indications for colonoscopy.

Diagnostic indications
Age ≥ 50
Personal or family history of colorectal cancer, polyps, or specific familial cancer syndromes
Post abnormal or equivocal barium enema or episode of unexplained rectal bleeding
Post abnormal sigmoidoscopy (eg, polyps)
Inflammatory bowel disease
Therapeutic indications
Excision of polyps
Control of bleeding
Removal of a foreign body
Detorsion of volvulus
Decompression of pseudo-obstruction
Dilation of strictures
Destruction of neoplasms

Diagnostic colonoscopy is indicated in adults age 50 and over and repeated every 5–10 years if normal (Table 30–3). It is indicated also in those with a personal or family history of colorectal cancer, polyps, or specific familial cancer syndromes; after an abnormal or equivocal radiographic screening test or episode of unexplained rectal bleeding; after abnormal sigmoidoscopy (eg, polyps); and for any patient with a diagnosis of inflammatory bowel disease. Therapeutic uses of colonoscopy include excision of polyps, control of bleeding, removal of a foreign body, detorsion of volvulus, decompression of pseudo-obstruction, dilation of strictures, placement of endoluminal stents, and destruction of neoplasms. Relative contraindications to colonoscopy are fulminant colitis and suspected colonic perforation. The main complications of diagnostic colonoscopy procedures include perforation (0.1–0.2%) and bleeding (0.2%). Success may be limited by such technical difficulties as diverticular disease, strictures, sharp flexures, redundant colon, or previous pelvic surgery.

Flexible sigmoidoscopy uses an instrument 65 cm long. The diagnostic yield is two to six times greater than with the rigid sigmoidoscope because two to three times more colon can be seen. The complications of flexible sigmoidoscopy are similar to colonoscopy, although a higher rate of perforation (0.8%) has been reported. Flexible sigmoidoscopes have replaced the rigid variety for most but not all purposes.

Botoman VA, Pietro M, Thirlby RC: Localization of colonic lesions with endoscopic tattoo. Dis Colon Rectum 1994;37:775.

Hull T, Church JM: Colonoscopy: how difficult, how painful? Surg Endosc 1994;8:784.

Lieberman DA et al: Use of colonoscopy to screen asymptomatic adults for colorectal cancer. Veterans Affairs Cooperative Study Group 380. N Engl J Med 2000;343:162.

Sakanoue Y et al: Intraoperative colonoscopy. Surg Endosc 1993;7:84.

Sieg A, Hachmoeller-Eisenbach U, Eisenbach T: Prospective evaluation of complications in outpatient GI endoscopy: a survey among German gastroenterologists. Gastrointest Endosc 2001;53:620.

Winawer SJ et al: A comparison of colonoscopy and double-contrast barium enema for surveillance after polypectomy. National Polyp Study Work Group. N Engl J Med 2000; 342:1766.

DISEASES OF THE COLON & RECTUM

OBSTRUCTION OF THE LARGE INTESTINE

ESSENTIALS OF DIAGNOSIS

- *Constipation or obstipation.*
- *Abdominal distention and sometimes tenderness.*
- *Abdominal pain.*
- *Nausea and vomiting (late).*
- *Characteristic x-ray findings.*

General Considerations

Approximately 15% of intestinal obstructions in adults occur in the large bowel. The obstruction may be in any portion of the colon but most commonly is in the sigmoid. Complete colonic obstruction is most often due to carcinoma; volvulus, diverticular disease, inflammatory disorders, benign tumors, fecal impaction, and miscellaneous rare problems account for the remainder (Table 30–4). Adhesive bands seldom obstruct the colon, and intussusception is uncommon in adults.

Obstruction by a lesion at the ileocecal valve produces the symptoms and signs of small bowel obstruction. The pathophysiology of more distal colonic obstruction depends on the competence of the ileocecal valve (Figure 30–4). In 10–20% of individuals, the ileocecal valve is incompetent, and colonic pressure is relieved by reflux into the ileum. If the colon is not decompressed through the ileocecal valve, a "closed loop" is formed between the valve and the obstructing point. The colon distends progressively because the ileum continues to empty gas and fluid into the obstructed segment. If luminal pressure becomes very high, circulation is impaired and gangrene and perforation can result. The wall of the right colon is thinner than that of the left colon and its luminal caliber is larger, so the cecum is at greatest risk of perforation in these circumstances (law of Laplace). In general, if the cecum acutely reaches a diameter of 10–12 cm, the risk of perforation is great.

Table 30–4. Causes of colonic obstruction in adults.

Cause	Relative Incidence (%)*
Carcinoma of colon	65
Diverticulitis	20
Volvulus	5
Miscellaneous	10

*Obstruction due to diverticulitis is usually incomplete; volvulus is second to carcinoma as a cause of complete obstruction.

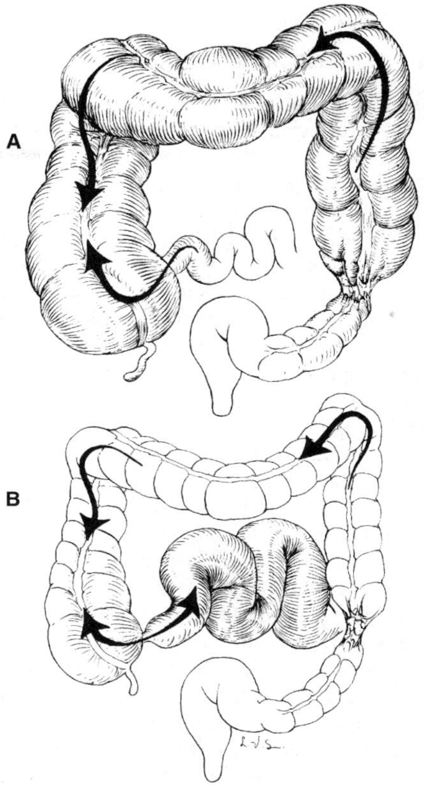

Figure 30–4. The role of the ileocecal valve in obstruction of the colon. The obstruction is in the upper sigmoid. ***A:*** The ileocecal valve is competent, creating a closed loop between the obstruction and the valve. Tension in the closed loop is increased further by emptying of gas and fluid from the ileum into the colon. ***B:*** The ileocecal valve is incompetent. Reflux into the ileum is permitted. The colon is relieved of some of its distention, and the small bowel has become distended.

Clinical Findings

A. Symptoms and Signs

Simple mechanical obstruction of the colon may develop insidiously. Deep, visceral, cramping pain from obstruction of the colon is usually referred to the hypogastrium. Lesions of the fixed portions of the colon (cecum, hepatic flexure, splenic flexure) may cause pain that is felt immediately anteriorly. Pain originating from the sigmoid is often located to the left in the lower abdomen. Severe, continuous abdominal pain suggests intestinal ischemia or peritonitis. Borborygmus may be loud and coincident with cramps. Constipation or obstipation is a universal feature of complete obstruction, though the colon distal to the obstruction may empty after the initial symptoms begin. Vomiting is a late finding and may not occur at all if the ileocecal valve prevents reflux. If reflux decompresses the cecal contents into the small intestine, the symptoms of small bowel as well as large bowel obstruction appear. Feculent vomiting is a late manifestation.

Physical examination discloses abdominal distention and tympany, and peristaltic waves may be seen if the abdominal wall is thin. High-pitched, metallic tinkles associated with rushes and gurgles may be heard on auscultation. Localized tenderness or a tender, palpable mass may indicate a strangulated closed loop. Signs of localized or generalized peritonitis suggest gangrene or rupture of the bowel wall. Fresh blood may be found in the rectum in intussusception and in carcinoma of the rectum or colon. Sigmoidoscopy may disclose a neoplasm. Colonoscopy may be diagnostic and perhaps therapeutic in some patients with strictures or neoplasms.

B. Imaging Studies

The distended colon frequently creates a "picture frame" outline of the abdominal cavity. The colon can be distinguished from the small intestine by its haustral markings, which do not cross the entire lumen of the distended colon. A contrast enema will confirm the diagnosis of colonic obstruction and identify its exact location. Water-soluble contrast medium should be used if strangulation or perforation is suspected. Once the obstruction is seen, the procedure should be discontinued. Barium must not be given orally in the presence of suspected colonic obstruction. A CT scan is the most useful single test as it can yield information regarding the location and etiology of the bowel obstruction.

Differential Diagnosis

A. Small Versus Large Bowel Obstruction

Large bowel obstruction is frequently slow in onset, causes less pain, and may not cause vomiting in spite of considerable distention. Elderly patients with no history of abdominal surgery or prior attacks of obstruction frequently have carcinoma of the large bowel. Plain abdominal x-rays and contrast studies are helpful in establishing the diagnosis.

B. Paralytic Ileus

Paralytic ileus may be a result of peritonitis or trauma to the back or pelvis. The abdomen is silent, and abdominal cramping is not present. There may be tenderness. Plain films show a dilated colon. Contrast enema may be required to exclude an obstruction.

C. Pseudo-obstruction

Acute pseudo-obstruction of the colon (**Ogilvie's syndrome**) is massive colonic distention in the absence of a mechanically obstructing lesion (Figure 30–5). It is a severe form of ileus and arises in bedridden patients who have serious extraintestinal illness (renal, cardiac, respiratory) or trauma (eg, vertebral fracture). Aerophagia and impairment of colonic motility by drugs are contributing factors. Abdominal distention without pain or tenderness is the earliest manifestation, but later symptoms mimic those of true obstruction. Plain x-rays of the abdomen show marked gaseous distention of the colon. Although the entire colon may contain gas, the distention is typically localized to the right colon, with a cutoff at the hepatic or splenic flexure. Contrast

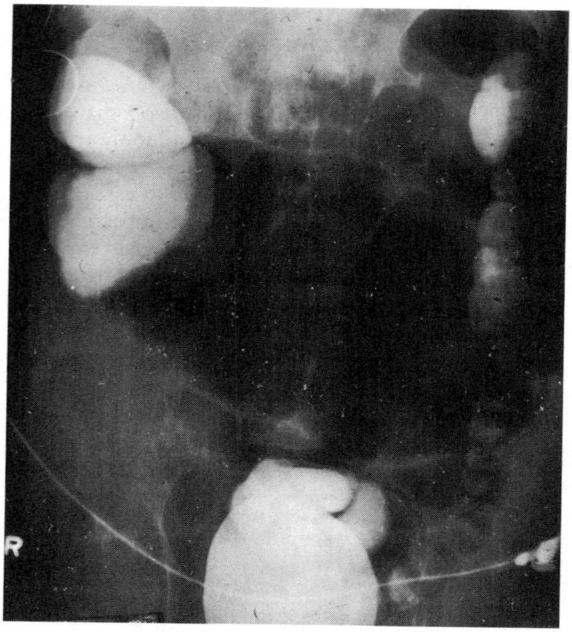

Figure 30–5. Plain radiograph demonstrating the dilated colon with pseudo-obstruction (Ogilvie's syndrome). (Courtesy of Dr. Santhat Nivatvongs.)

enema proves the absence of obstruction, but instillation of radiopaque material should cease as soon as the dilated colon is reached.

Conservative treatment with nasogastric suction and enemas may succeed in resolving colonic pseudo-obstruction. Neostigmine is highly effective in treating colonic pseudo-obstruction. It should be avoided in patients with a mechanical colonic obstruction, bradycardia, bronchospasm, or renal insufficiency. If the cecum is markedly dilated, the risk of perforation is high, and direct intervention must be prompt. Colonoscopic decompression is the method of choice if an expert is available. Initial success is claimed in 90% of patients, but recurrence is common (25% or more). Often it is possible to place a tube into the proximal colon during colonoscopy to maintain decompression. Placement of a decompressive tube per rectum under fluoroscopic guidance has been described recently. Another alternative is cecostomy, performed either in the standard open fashion or by an endoscopic percutaneous method, similar to the technique for gastrostomy, using laparoscopic assistance.

Complications

Cecal perforation, described above, is a potentially lethal complication. Partially obstructive lesions of the colon may be complicated by acute colitis in the bowel proximal to the obstruction; it is probably a form of ischemic colitis secondary to impaired mucosal blood flow in the distended segment.

Treatment

An operation is almost always required. The primary goals of treatment are resection of all necrotic bowel and decompression of the obstructed segment to prevent perforation. Removal of the obstructing lesion is a secondary goal, but a single operation to accomplish both objectives is preferred whenever possible.

Colonoscopic balloon dilation of obstructing benign strictures or neoplasms is applicable sometimes. However, stent placement has replaced balloon dilation for neoplasms, particularly of distal lesions in the sigmoid colon and rectum. Stent placement may allow for decompression of the obstruction as a bridge to elective resection. Stents should be considered also for palliation in patients whose life expectancy is less than 6 months, which is the expected patency of a colonic stent placed for malignancy. Laser photocoagulation of an obstructing cancer, especially in the rectum, may enlarge the lumen to permit an elective operation later under better circumstances, and occasionally a patient with advanced cancer may avoid operation entirely. Permanent diverting colostomy may be the only possible choice in a debilitated patient with unresectable obstructing rectal cancer.

Obstructing lesions of the right colon are resected in one stage, with ileotransverse colostomy if the patient's condition is good. If the patient's condition is precarious or if the colon has perforated, the bowel is resected but no anastomosis is done; an ileostomy is established, and anastomosis is performed at a second operation. Unresectable lesions may be bypassed.

Obstructing lesions of the left colon are best treated by resection in patients who seem likely to tolerate this procedure. There are three choices of operation after resection has been achieved. Anastomosis may be postponed and a temporary end colostomy created (two-stage procedure; Figure 30–6). Alternatively, intraoperative colonic lavage can be performed by inserting a tube into the cecum through the ileum or appendix; a large-bore tube is inserted into the colon proximal to the obstruction to allow effluent to drain out of the sterile field. This procedure may cleanse the colon well enough so that primary anastomosis can be performed safely. A primary anastomosis can be created with a proximal defunctioning (diverting) loop ileostomy. Two other options may be entertained. A colonic stent may be deployed preoperatively to decompress the obstructed bowel, allowing for an elective resection under better circumstances. Alternatively, in unfavorable circumstances, a diverting transverse colostomy may utilized. However, a serious disadvantage is the need for three operations if this approach is elected:

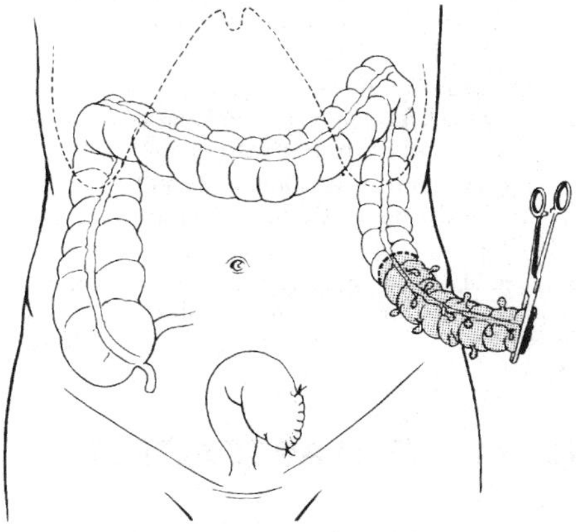

Figure 30–6. Primary resection for diverticulitis of the colon. The affected segment (shaded) has been divided at its distal end. If primary anastomosis is to be done, the proximal margin (dotted line) is transected, and the bowel is anastomosed end-to-end. If a two-stage procedure will be used, a colostomy is formed at the proximal margin, and the distal stump is oversewn (Hartmann procedure, as shown), or exteriorized as a mucous fistula. The second stage consists of colostomy takedown and anastomosis.

(1) colostomy, (2) resection of the obstructing lesion with anastomosis, and (3) closure of the colostomy.

Prognosis

The prognosis depends upon the age and general condition of the patient, the extent of vascular impairment of the bowel, the presence or absence of perforation, the cause of obstruction, and the promptness of surgical management. The overall mortality rate is about 20%. Cecal perforation carries a 40% mortality rate. Obstructing cancer of the colon has a worse prognosis than nonobstructing cancer because it is more likely to be locally extensive or metastatic to nodes or distant sites.

Baron TH: Expandable metal stents for the treatment of cancerous obstruction of the gastrointestinal tract. N Engl J Med 2001; 344:1681.

Bharucha AE et al: Acute, toxic, and chronic. Curr Treat Options Gastroenterol 1999;2:517.

Boorman P et al: Endoluminal stenting of obstructed colorectal tumours. Ann R Coll Surg Engl 1999;81:251.

Chapman AH, McNamara M, Porter G: The acute contrast enema in suspected large bowel obstruction: value and technique. Clin Radiol 1992;46:273.

Gooszen AW et al: Operative treatment of acute complications of diverticular disease: primary or secondary anastomosis after sigmoid resection. Eur J Surg 2001;167:35.

Gooszen AW et al: Prospective study of primary anastomosis following sigmoid resection for suspected acute complicated diverticular disease. Br J Surg 2001;88:693.

Ponec RJ, Saunders MD, Kimmey MB: Neostigmine for the treatment of acute colonic pseudo-obstruction. N Engl J Med 1999;341:137.

Stewart J, Diament RH, Brennan TG: Management of obstructing lesions of the left colon by resection, on-table lavage, and primary anastomosis. Surgery 1993;114:502.

Suri S et al: Comparative evaluation of plain films, ultrasound and CT in the diagnosis of intestinal obstruction. Acta Radiol 1999;40:422.

Tanaka T et al: Endoscopic transanal decompression with a drainage tube for acute colonic obstruction: clinical aspects of preoperative treatment. Dis Colon Rectum 2001; 44:418.

CANCER OF THE LARGE INTESTINE

ESSENTIALS OF DIAGNOSIS

Right colon:

- *Unexplained weakness or anemia.*
- *Occult blood in feces.*
- *Dyspeptic symptoms.*
- *Persistent right abdominal discomfort.*
- *Palpable abdominal mass.*
- *Characteristic x-ray findings.*
- *Characteristic colonoscopic findings.*

Left colon:

- *Change in bowel habits.*
- *Gross blood in stool.*
- *Obstructive symptoms.*
- *Characteristic x-ray findings.*
- *Characteristic colonoscopic or sigmoidoscopic findings.*

Rectum:

- *Rectal bleeding.*
- *Alteration in bowel habits.*
- *Sensation of incomplete evacuation.*
- *Intrarectal palpable tumor.*
- *Sigmoidoscopic findings.*

General Considerations

In Western countries, cancer of the colon and rectum ranks second after cancer of the lung in incidence and death rates. An estimated 150,000 new cases of colorectal cancer are diagnosed and 57,000 people die of this disease in the USA each year. The death rate from colorectal cancer in the USA has begun to decline for the first time, perhaps related to earlier detection. The incidence increases with age, from 0.39 per 1000 persons per year at age 50 to 4.5 per 1000 persons per year at age 80. Carcinoma of the colon, particularly the right colon, is more common in women, and carcinoma of the rectum is more common in men. The distribution of cancers of the colon and rectum is shown in Figure 30–7. An apparent "proximal shift" of cancer (increased incidence in the right colon and decreased incidence in the rectum) in recent decades is at least partially explainable by improved diagnostic accuracy for proximal lesions as a result of total colonoscopy. Multiple synchronous colonic cancers—ie, two or more carcinomas occurring simultaneously—are found in 5% of patients. Metachronous cancer is a new primary lesion in a patient who has had a previous resection for cancer. The cumulative risk of metachronous colorectal cancer was 6.3% at 18 years in one study and as high as 10% at a mean follow-up of 39 months in another series. Ninety-five percent of malignant tumors of the colon and rectum are adenocarcinomas.

Genetic predisposition to cancer of the large bowel is well recognized in persons with familial adenomatous polyposis (discussed in the Treatment section under Polyps of the Colon & Rectum). The most common form of hereditary colorectal cancer is **hereditary nonpolyposis**

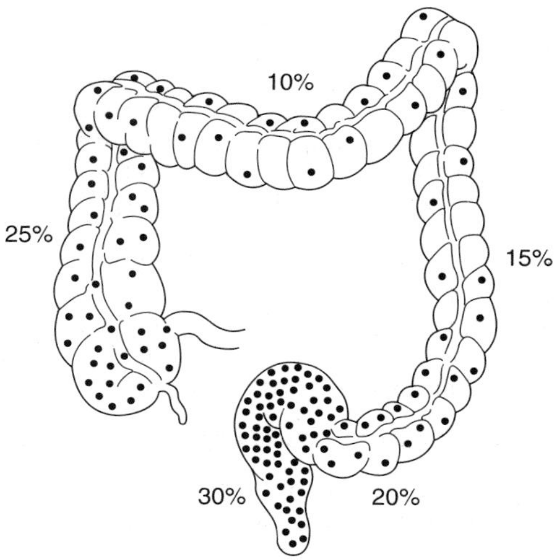

Figure 30–7. Distribution of cancer of the colon and rectum.

colorectal cancer (HNPCC), also referred to as the Lynch syndrome. There are 4 cardinal features of HNPCC: (1) earlier average age (45 years) at onset of cancer than in the general population, (2) the presence of associated cancers within the pedigree, (3) improved survival when compared stage for stage to sporadic cases, (4) the presence of a germ-line mutation in affected family members. The gene responsible for this syndrome has been localized to chromosome 2p and the genetic defect is in DNA mismatch repair genes (MLH1, MSH2, MSH6, PMS1, and PMS2. The defects occur in the setting of microsatellite instability. There may be other genes not as of yet identified. The Amsterdam I and II criteria (Table 30–5) were developed to identify patients with HNPCC. The presence of the Amsterdam criteria defines HNPCC by history alone. However, all patients with early-onset colorectal cancer, whether they meet Amsterdam criteria or not, should be offered a referral to a geneticist for screening for a familial cancer syndrome. First-degree relatives of patients with sporadic colorectal cancer have a twofold to threefold increased risk of large bowel cancer, and it is estimated that 15–20% of cancers of the large bowel are due primarily to an inherited genetic defect.

Ulcerative colitis, Crohn's colitis, schistosomal colitis, exposure to radiation, and the presence of an ureterocolostomy are conditions that predispose to cancer of the large bowel. Women with a history of breast cancer have a small increase in risk for colorectal adenomas and cancer. Also in women, gallstones (and the consequent cholecystectomy) are associated with colorectal cancer, especially in the right colon.

A high incidence of colorectal cancer occurs in populations that are economically prosperous. This observation has focused attention on environmental factors, particularly diet, in the etiology of this tumor. Increased intake of saturated fat, increased caloric intake, decreased dietary calcium, and decreased intake of fiber are among the possible dietary influences. Dietary fat enhances cholesterol and bile acid synthesis by the liver, and the amounts of these sterols in the colon increase. Anaerobic colonic bacteria convert these compounds to secondary bile acids, which are promoters of carcinogenesis. Other possible mechanisms by which saturated fat promotes colorectal cancer include changes in immunity, effects on lipid peroxidation, and modulation of prostaglandin synthesis through arachidonic acid metabolism. Experimental studies have suggested that dietary fish oil, rich in unsaturated fatty acids of the n-3 type, is protective against colorectal cancer, and the mechanism may be inhibition of prostaglandin synthesis from arachidonic acid.

The mechanism by which dietary fiber is protective remains elusive. Effects of fiber on fecal bulk, water content, transit time, and pH are less important than once thought. Plant lignans in fiber are fermented to a group of human lignans by colonic bacteria, and these substances may be important in some way. Metabolic activity of gut microflora is altered by dietary fiber, perhaps with important inhibitory effects on tumor promoters such as bile acids. Another possible mechanism is chelation of dietary iron by the phytate content of high-fiber foods. Iron catalyzes oxidation of lipid to

Table 30–5. AMSTERDAM I and II criteria.

Amsterdam I criteria: At least three relatives must have histologically verified colorectal cancer.	(1) One must be a first-degree relative of the other two. (2) At least two successive generations must be affected. (3) At least one of the relatives with CRC must have received the diagnosis before age 50.
Amsterdam II criteria: At least three relatives must have a cancer associated with hereditary nonpolyposis colorectal cancer (HNPCC): colorectal, endometrial, stomach, ovary, ureter or renal-pelvis, brain, small bowel, hepatobiliary tract, skin (sebaceous tumors)	(1) One must be a first-degree relative of the other two. (2) At least two successive generations must be affected. (3) At least one of the relatives with HNPCC-associated cancer must have received the diagnosis before age 50.

substances that are genotoxic, and iron has been associated with the initiating and promoting phases of carcinogenesis in experimental systems. Ingested calcium affects colonic epithelial cell proliferation topically and by absorption into the bloodstream. If these concepts are correct, reducing dietary saturated fat and calories and increasing the intake of calcium and fermentable fiber can minimize the risk of colorectal cancer. Populations with a high incidence of colon cancer tend to have low serum cholesterol levels, and average serum cholesterol levels are higher in groups with less cancer of the colon. In a study from Denmark, short stature and low body weight were strong predictors of rectal cancer development in men, and thin men had a higher risk of colon cancer than their obese counterparts. Cigarette smoking reportedly increases the risk of colorectal adenomas and cancer in both men and women.

Carcinogenesis in the large bowel and elsewhere is a long multistep process. Colorectal cancer involves multiple genetic alterations, ie, oncogene activation, including K-*ras* point mutation, c-*myc* amplification and overexpression, and c-*src* kinase activation. Tumor-suppressor gene inactivation is also important; these events may include point mutations in the *APC* gene (adenomatous polyposis coli, at chromosome 5q21), the *DCC* gene (deleted in colorectal carcinoma, on chromosome 18q), and *P53* (on chromosome 17). The *DCC* gene has been isolated. Genetic damage is initiated by carcinogenic agents. Promoters, such as bile acids, may stimulate growth of a benign neoplasm, and it may be that still other promoters cause malignant change to occur. There is evidence that female hormones are promoters, perhaps by influencing the availability of secondary bile acids in the colon. Estrogen and progesterone receptors are expressed in both normal and malignant colonic mucosa. Another series of changes, termed progression, makes cancer cells more aggressive in their behavior. This sequence is the basis for an enormous amount of current research in colorectal cancer. Aspirin and other NSAIDs, particularly the cyclooxygenase-2 inhibitors, may reduce the incidence of and mortality rate from colorectal cancer, by inhibition of the prostaglandins implicated in immune suppression and the promotion of metastasis. The use of such agents is the subject of several clinical trials for the chemoprevention of colon cancer.

Cancer of the colon and rectum spreads in the following ways:

A. Direct Extension

Carcinoma grows circumferentially and may completely encircle the bowel before it is diagnosed; this is especially true in the left colon, which has a smaller caliber than the right. It takes about 1 year for a tumor to encircle three-fourths of the circumference of the bowel. Longitudinal submucosal extension occurs with invasion of the intramural lymphatic network, but it rarely goes beyond 2 cm from the edge of the tumor unless there is concomitant spread to lymph nodes. As the lesion extends radially, it penetrates the outer layers of the bowel wall, and it may extend by contiguity into neighboring structures: the liver, the greater curvature of the stomach, the duodenum, the small bowel, the pancreas, the spleen, the bladder, the vagina, the kidneys and ureters, and the abdominal wall. Cancer of the rectum may invade the vaginal wall, bladder, prostate, or sacrum, and it may extend along the levators. Subacute perforation with inflammatory attachment of bowel to an adjacent viscus may be indistinguishable from actual invasion on gross examination.

B. Hematogenous Metastasis

Angiolymphatic invasion may allow tumor cells be carried via the portal venous system to establish hepatic metastases. Tumor embolization also occurs through lumbar and vertebral veins to the lungs and elsewhere. Rectal cancer spreads through tributaries of the hypogastric veins. Metastases to ovaries are mostly hematogenous; they are found in 1–10.3% of women with colorectal cancer. Venous invasion occurs in 15–50% of cases even though it does not always cause distant metastases. An attempt is made to avoid producing hematogenous metastases during operation by minimizing manipulation of the tumor prior to ligation of the blood supply.

C. Regional Lymph Node Metastasis

This is the most common form of tumor spread (Figure 30–8). Longitudinal spread via extramural lymphatics is an important mechanism. Rectal cancer metastasizes proximally to the mesorectal, iliac, and inferior mesenteric lymph nodes, and radially along lymphatics to the pelvic side walls, where obturator nodes can become involved. The lymphatic drainage of the tumor must be removed in curative operations, and some nodal involvement will be found in over half of the specimens. Recently, sentinel lymph node mapping for colorectal cancer has been under investigation in an effort to improve identification of candidates for adjuvant chemotherapy. However, a limitation is that positive nodes may be found at some distance from the primary site, with normal nodes intervening. Improved lymph node evaluation is associated with improved survival. The size of the lesion bears little relationship to the degree of nodal involvement. The more anaplastic the lesion, the more likely that lymph node metastasis will occur. Up to 10% of T1 rectal cancers may harbor occult lymph node metastases.

D. Transperitoneal Metastasis

"Seeding" may occur when the tumor has extended through the serosa and tumor cells enter the peritoneal

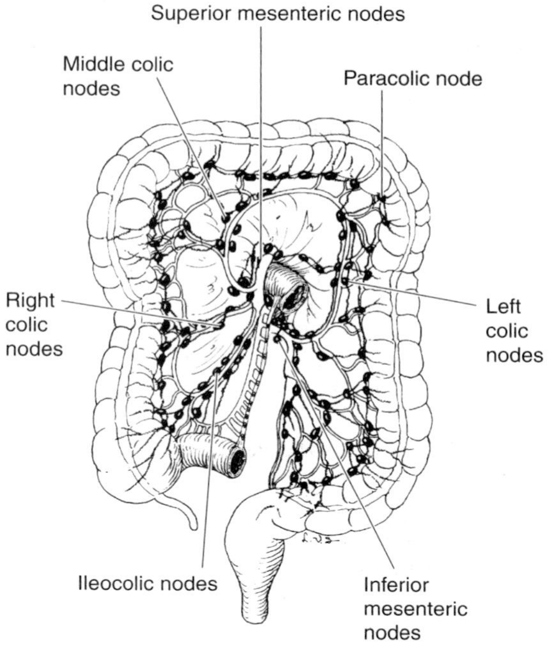

Figure 30–8. Lymphatic drainage of the colon. The lymph nodes (black) are distributed along the blood vessels to the bowel.

cavity, producing local implants or generalized abdominal carcinomatosis. Large metastatic deposits in the pelvic cul-de-sac are palpable as a hard shelf (Blumer's shelf).

E. Intraluminal Metastasis

Malignant cells shed from the surface of the tumor can be swept along in the fecal current. Implantation more distally on intact mucosa occurs rarely, if ever, but viable exfoliated cells presumably can be trapped in an anastomotic suture or staple line during operation.

Clinical Findings

A. Symptoms and Signs

Adenocarcinoma of the colon and rectum has a median doubling time (the time required for the tumor to double in volume) of 130 days, suggesting that at least 5 years—and often 10–15 years—of silent growth are required before a cancer reaches symptom-producing size. During this asymptomatic phase, diagnosis depends on routine examination.

The value of **routine screening** of asymptomatic populations who lack high-risk factors for development of large bowel cancer has been established. Screening should be initiated at age 50. The goals of screening are detection of early cancers and prevention of cancer by finding and removing adenomas. The screening recommendations of the American Society of Colon and Rectal Surgery are listed in (Table 30–6). There has been evidence for some time that screening for occult blood detects cancers at an earlier stage, but only recently has a survival benefit been shown in a USA prospective trial of occult blood testing followed by colonoscopy in those with positive tests. Improved survival in the screened group was related to a lower percentage of advanced cancers—the lesions that more commonly prove fatal. It is not clear whether the survival benefit in this study should be attributed mainly to the tests for occult blood or the colonoscopy, because the latter test alone might have achieved the same outcome. Four case-control studies have demonstrated that sigmoidoscopy is associated with a reduced mortality for colorectal cancer. However, its utility as a screening test for colorectal neoplasia is limited by the amount of colon visualized with a 70-cm sigmoidoscope. Cancer mortality is reduced for lesions within the reach of the sigmoidoscope but not in the area beyond the reach of the sigmoidoscope. Therefore, flexible sigmoidoscopy should be used in conjunction with radiographic evaluation of the more proximal colon or annual fecal occult blood testing. Dissatisfaction with the poor specificity of guaiac slide tests has led to development of alternative methods, including immunochemical FOBTs and fecal tests for DNA mutations. If fecal occult blood testing is positive, total colonoscopy should be performed. As a screening test, flexible sigmoidoscopy, when normal, should be repeated every 5 years. Alternatively, total colonoscopy can be performed as the initial examination, since all roads eventually lead to colonoscopy for diagnosis or therapy (as in the case of a lesion on barium enema).

The need for colonoscopic screening of patients in high-risk groups has been established, but the timing of initial evaluations must be individualized. Children with possible familial adenomatous polyposis should have annual or biannual sigmoidoscopy (then colonoscopy as indicated) starting at puberty. Biannual colonoscopy beginning at age 21 is the recommendation for members of families with HNPCC. Colonoscopy every year is probably the best advice for patients with ulcerative colitis for longer than 10 years. People with a history of colorectal cancer in one first-degree relative should undergo colonoscopy starting at age 50 or at age 10 years before age of onset in the index relative. People with a history of a colorectal cancer in a first-degree relative under the age of 55 should undergo colonoscopy at 40 or at age 10 years before the age of onset in the index relative.

Symptoms in patients with large bowel cancer depend upon the anatomic location of the lesion, its type and extent, and upon complications, including perforation,

Table 30–6. ASCRS guidelines for colorectal cancer screening.[1,2]

Risk	Procedure	Onset (Age, yr)	Frequency
I. Low Risk			
A. Asymptomatic—no risk factors	Fecal occult blood testing and flex-sig	50	FOBT yearly. Flex-sig every 5 years
B. Colorectal cancer in none of first-degree relatives	Total colon examination (colonoscopy or double-contrast barium enema and proctosigmoidoscopy)	50	Every 5–10 years
II. Moderate Risk (20–30% of people)			
A. Colorectal cancer in first-degree relative, age 55 or younger, or two or more first-degree relatives of any ages	Colonoscopy	40 or 10 years before the youngest case in the family, whichever is earlier	Every 5 years
B. Colorectal cancer in a first-degree relative over the age of 55	Colonoscopy	50, or 10 years before the age of the case, whichever is earlier	Every 5–10 years
C. Personal history of large (> 1 cm) or multiple colorectal polyps of any size	Colonoscopy	One year after polypectomy	If recurrent polyps—1 year If normal—5 years
D. Personal history of colorectal malignancy—surveillance after resection for curative intent	Colonoscopy	1 year after resection	If normal—3 years If still normal—5 years If abnormal—as above
III. High Risk (6–8 % of people)			
A. Family history of hereditary adenomatous polyposis	Flex-sig; consider genetic counseling; consider genetic testing	12–14 (Puberty)	Every 1–2 years
B. Family history of hereditary nonpolyposis colon cancer	Colonoscopy; consider genetic counseling; consider genetic testing	21–40 40	Every 2 years Every year
C. Inflammatory bowel disease			
1. Left-side colitis	Colonoscopy	15th	Every 1–2 years
2. Pancolitis	Colonoscopy	8th	Every 1–2 years

[1]FOBT = fecal occult blood testing; Flex-sig = flexible sigmoidoscopy.
[2]Used with permission from the ASCRS. http://www.fascrs.org/displaycommon.cfm?an=1&subarticlenbr=152.

obstruction, and hemorrhage. Marked systemic manifestations such as cachexia are indications of advanced disease. The average delay between the onset of symptoms and definitive therapy is 7–9 months; both patients and physicians are responsible.

The **right colon** has a large caliber and a thin and distensible wall, and the fecal content is fluid. Because of these anatomic features, carcinoma of the right colon may attain large size before it is diagnosed. Patients often see a physician for complaints of fatigue and weakness due to severe anemia. Unexplained microcytic hypochromic anemia should always raise the question of carcinoma of the colon. Gross blood may not be visible in the stool, but occult blood may be detected. Patients may complain of vague right abdominal discomfort, which is often postprandial and may be mistakenly attributed to gallbladder or gastroduodenal disease. Alterations in bowel habits are not characteristic of carcinoma of the right colon, and obstruction is uncommon. In about 10% of cases, the first evidence of the disease is discovery of a mass by the patient or the physician.

The **left colon** has a smaller lumen than the right, and the feces are semisolid. Tumors of the left colon can gradually occlude the lumen, causing changes in bowel habits with alternating constipation and increased frequency of defecation (not true watery diarrhea). Partial or complete obstruction may be the initial picture.

Bleeding is common but is rarely massive. The stool may be streaked or mixed with bright red or dark blood, and mucus is often passed together with small blood clots.

In **cancer of the rectum**, the most common symptom is the passage of bright red blood with bowel movements (hematochezia). Bleeding is usually persistent; it may be slight or (rarely) copious. Blood may or may not be mixed with stool or mucus. Predictions of an anal source of bleeding based on color and pattern are unreliable. *Whenever rectal bleeding occurs in a middle-aged or older individual, even in the presence of hemorrhoids, cancer must be ruled out.* There may be tenesmus (an ineffectual urge to evacuate the rectum).

Physical examination is important to determine the extent of local disease, to identify distant metastases, and to detect diseases of other organ systems that may influence treatment. The supraclavicular areas should be carefully palpated for metastatic nodes. Examination of the abdomen may disclose a mass, enlargement of the liver, ascites, or engorgement of the abdominal wall veins if there is portal obstruction. If a mass is palpated, its location and extent of fixation are important.

Distal rectal cancers can be felt as a flat, hard, oval or encircling tumor with rolled edges and a central depression. Its extent, the size of the lumen at the site of the tumor, and the degree of fixation should be noted. Blood may be found on the examining finger. Vaginal and rectovaginal examination will yield additional information on the extent of the tumor. Retrorectal nodes may be palpable.

B. Laboratory Findings

Urinalysis, leukocyte count, and hemoglobin determination should be done. Serum proteins, calcium, bilirubin, alkaline phosphatase, and creatinine should be measured if clinically indicated.

The most familiar chemical marker for cancer of the large bowel is **carcinoembryonic antigen (CEA)**, a glycoprotein found in the cell membranes of many tissues, including colorectal cancer. Some of the antigen enters the circulation and is detected by radioimmunoassay of serum; CEA is also detectable in various other body fluids, urine, and feces. Elevated serum CEA is not specifically associated with colorectal cancer; abnormally high levels are also found in sera of patients with other gastrointestinal cancers, nonalimentary cancers, and various benign diseases. CEA levels are high in 70% of patients with cancer of the large intestine, but less than half of patients with localized disease are CEA-positive. CEA does not, therefore, serve as a useful screening procedure, nor is it an accurate diagnostic test for colorectal cancer in a curable stage. CEA is helpful in detecting recurrence after curative surgical resection; if high CEA levels return to normal after operation and then rise progressively during the follow-up period, recurrence of cancer is likely.

C. Imaging Studies

Chest films should be obtained routinely. Barium enema examination is an important radiographic means of diagnosing cancer of the colon, but it is unnecessary in patients who have undergone complete colonoscopy. Carcinoma of the left colon appears as a fixed filling defect, usually 2–6 cm long, with an annular ("apple core") configuration (Figure 30–9). Lesions of the right colon may appear as a constriction or an intraluminal mass. The bowel wall is inflexible at the site of the lesion, and the mucosal pattern is destroyed. It is important to remember that this is the typical picture of locally advanced carcinoma. Earlier stages of the disease produce less characteristic filling defects that should be investigated with the colonoscope. Artifacts (stool, spasm) can resemble carcinoma. Barium should not be administered by mouth if there is evidence of carcinoma of the colon, especially on the left side, since it may precipitate acute large bowel obstruction. X-rays

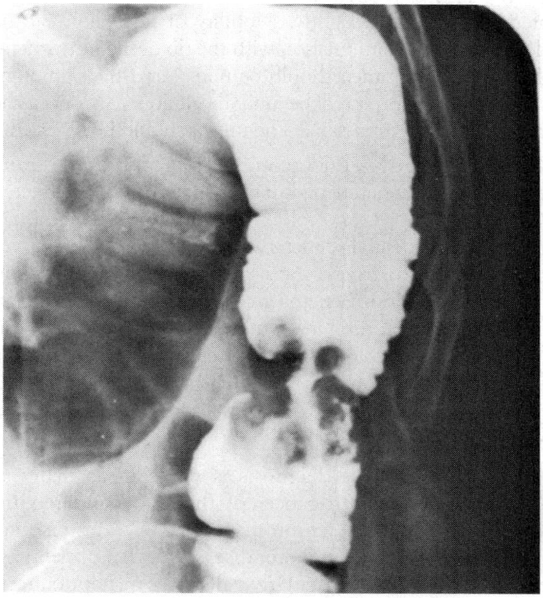

Figure 30–9. Barium enema roentgenogram of an encircling carcinoma of the descending colon presenting an "apple core" appearance. Note the loss of mucosal pattern, the "hooks" at the margins of the lesion owing to undermining by the growth, the relatively short (6-cm) length of the lesion, and its abrupt ends.

are unreliable in detecting cancer of the rectum. Such growths are more accurately diagnosed by palpation and endoscopy.

CT scans are not essential in patients with cancer of the colon, but they are helpful in assessing extramural extension in patients with rectal cancer and in detecting metastatic disease when a combined resection of the primary lesion with the metastatic lesion (eg, hepatic) can be performed. MRI may be useful for this purpose as well. PET scans are useful for detecting recurrences and metastatic disease but are probably not necessary as part of the routine initial evaluation. Detection of liver metastases by CT scan and other methods is discussed further in Chapter 24. Endorectal ultrasonography provides very accurate information about the depth of penetration of rectal cancer into or through the bowel wall. It also reveals the presence of enlarged pararectal lymph nodes but cannot at present distinguish between cancerous and reactive nodes. The T staging accuracy of endorectal ultrasound is 85% and 70% with CT scan. The nodal staging accuracy is 70% for both modalities.

D. Special Examinations

1. Proctosigmoidoscopy—Fifty to sixty-five percent of colorectal cancers are within the reach of a 60-cm flexible sigmoidoscope. Only 20% can be seen with a rigid sigmoidoscope. The typical cancer is raised, red, centrally ulcerated, and bleeding slightly. Mobility of the lesion can be determined by manipulation with the tip of the instrument. The size of the lumen should be noted, and the sigmoidoscope should be passed beyond the lesion to inspect the proximal bowel if possible. The tumor should be biopsied.

2. Colonoscopy—Endoscopic examination of the entire colon should be performed in every patient with suspected or known cancer of the colon or rectum if the intention is curative treatment. Preoperative colonoscopy is preferred, but when obstructing cancer or other circumstances do not allow it, barium enema may be used to visualize the proximal bowel to exclude synchronous lesions. However, increasingly CT colonography is replacing barium enema for incomplete colonoscopy.

Differential Diagnosis

An initial erroneous diagnosis is made in as many as 25% of patients with cancer of the colon and rectum after gastrointestinal symptoms appear. Symptoms may be attributed mistakenly to disease of the upper gastrointestinal tract, particularly gallstones or peptic ulcer. Chronic anemia may be attributed to a primary hematologic disorder if fecal occult blood testing is not done. Acute pain in the right side of the abdomen owing to carcinoma can simulate appendicitis.

Most errors are made when the clinical findings are ascribed to benign disease, and patients may even be operated upon for benign anorectal conditions in the presence of undetected cancer. Cancer must be sought out in every patient with recent onset of significant rectal bleeding even if there are obvious hemorrhoids.

Carcinoma may be difficult to distinguish from diverticular disease; colonoscopy is useful in these cases. Other colonic diseases—including ulcerative colitis, Crohn's colitis, ischemic colitis, and amebiasis—usually can be diagnosed by colonoscopy, sigmoidoscopy, or barium enema. Symptoms should be attributed to irritable bowel syndrome only after neoplasm has been ruled out.

Treatment

A. Cancer of the Colon

Treatment consists of wide surgical resection of the lesion and its regional lymphatic drainage after preparation of the bowel. Resection of the primary tumor may be indicated even if distant metastases have occurred, since prevention of obstruction or bleeding may offer palliation for long periods.

The abdomen is explored to determine resectability of the tumor and to search for distant metastases, and associated abdominal disease. Care is taken not to contribute to spread of the tumor by unnecessary palpation. The cancer-bearing portion of colon is mobilized and removed. Many surgeons irrigate the two open ends of bowel with saline solution or dilute povidone-iodine before anastomosis in the hope that tumor cells in the lumen will be washed away or destroyed. The extent of resection of the colon and mesocolon for cancers in various locations and the methods for restoration of continuity are shown in Figure 30–10.

B. Cancer of the Rectum

For cancer of the rectum, the choice of operation depends on the height of the lesion above the anal verge, the configuration (whether polypoid or infiltrative), the gross extent of the tumor, the degree of differentiation, and the patient's size, habitus, and general condition. Preoperative staging by digital rectal examination followed by CT, MRI, endorectal ultrasound, or some combination of these tests helps tailor the treatment to the patient. Preservation of the anal sphincter and avoidance of colostomy are desirable if possible.

The principal procedures for rectal tumors are as follows:

1. Low anterior resection of the rectum—This operation, performed through an abdominal incision, is the curative procedure of choice provided a margin of at least 2 cm of normal bowel—as estimated at operation—can be resected below the lesion. At least 10 cm of bowel proximal to the growth should also be removed along with the lymph node-bearing tissue. It is important to excise 5 cm of mesorectum distal to the

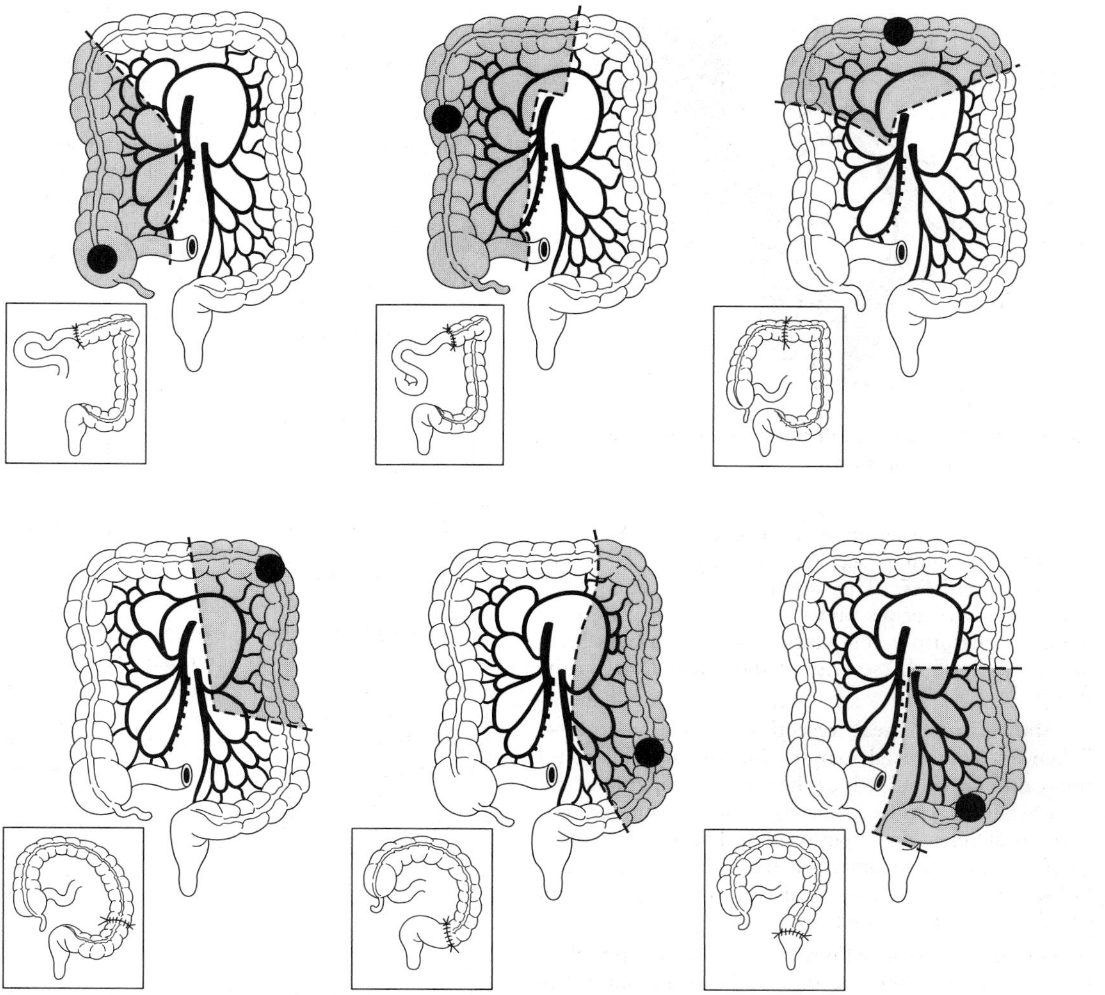

Figure 30–10. Extent of surgical resection for cancer of the colon at various sites. The cancer is represented by a black disk. Anastomosis of the bowel remaining after resection is shown in the small insets. The extent of resection is determined by the distribution of the regional lymph nodes along the blood supply. The lymph nodes may contain metastatic cancer.

tumor to minimize the chance of local recurrence from cancer in lymph nodes. The technique of **total mesorectal excision (TME)** reported by Heald in 1982 entails en bloc resection of the rectum as an intact unit with its lymphovascular drainage contained within the fascia propria (Figure 30–11). The mesorectum tapers and diminishes at the level of Waldeyer's fascia. However, this technique resulted in a high leak rate; therefore, surgeons now recommend a "tumor-specific" sharp mesorectal excision preserving the mesorectal fascia integrity for at least 4–5 cm distal to the tumor. Widespread acceptance of this technique has resulted in a decrease in recurrence rates of rectal cancer from 20–30% to 5–10%. Controversy surrounds the fact that prior to Heald's report, there were centers that reported very low recurrence rates for rectal cancer because they were already performing a "tumor-specific mesorectal excision" by following the natural plane of dissection when performing proctectomy. The descending or sigmoid colon is anastomosed to the rectum. This type of resection is likely to fail in patients with extensive carcinoma and local spread. The end-to-end stapling device facilitates very low anastomosis, sometimes even as low as the anal canal (coloanal anastomosis). Unfortunately,

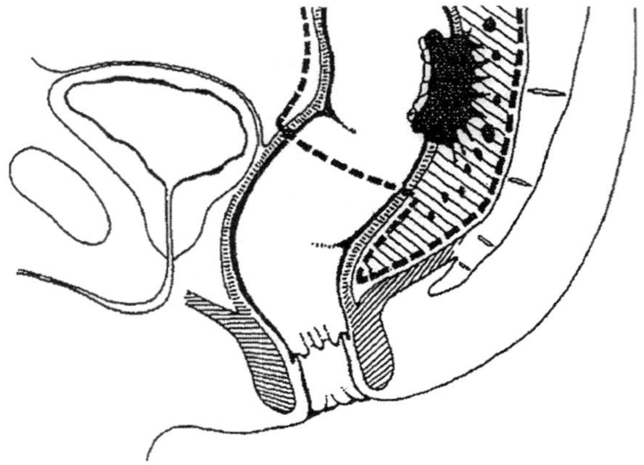

Figure 30–11. Total mesorectal excision as depicted in Heald's original publication.

such low reconstruction is associated with functional difficulties including seepage, urgency, and frequent bowel movements. This improves over time (1–2 years). Many surgeons prefer to construct a colonic J-pouch or perform a coloplasty, when technically feasible, to diminish the severity of these symptoms in the first year.

2. Abdominoperineal resection of the rectum—When adequate distal margins for low anterior resection cannot be obtained, or the patient's functional status obviates a sphincter-sparing approach, an abdominoperineal resection is performed. The distal sigmoid colon, rectum, and anus are removed through combined abdominal and perineal incisions. A permanent end colostomy is required.

3. Laparoscopic-assisted resection—Curative resections for cancer of the colon or rectum can be carried out by laparoscopic-assisted techniques. Initial enthusiasm for laparoscopic techniques was limited due to a high incidence of port site metastases in early reports. Contemporary reports demonstrate that with proper technique, port site metastases are no longer a concern. The final results of a prospective randomized, controlled, multi-institutional trial comparing conventional open resection with laparoscopic-assisted colectomy have just been published, and the data demonstrate patient benefits and oncologic efficacy of laparoscopic surgery for colon cancer when performed by qualified surgeons.

4. Local excision—In carefully selected patients with small, well-differentiated, superficial, mobile polypoid lesions, a disk of rectum containing the tumor can be excised as definitive therapy. This technique of resection should be limited to selected T1 lesions because patient survival with salvage radical surgery for recurrence after local excision of T2 and deeper lesions may be much poorer when compared to initial radical surgery. Lymph nodes are not sampled or treated by local excision, and success is based on adherence to strict criteria that predict a low likelihood of nodal spread. Even T1 tumors have been reported to be associated with a 7–14% chance of nodal metastasis. A strategy of chemoradiation and local excision has been reported in small case series for lesions more advanced than T1; however, the long-term results are not well documented and this approach should subject to clinical trials. **Transanal endoscopic microsurgery (TEM)** is a recently developed minimally invasive technique for the local resection of rectal tumors, best suited for more proximal rectal lesions. The same criteria are applied to patients for conventional local excision or TEM.

5. Palliative procedures—Unresectable rectal cancers can be palliated by fulguration (electrocoagulation) or laser photocoagulation. Fulguration requires general anesthesia, and the laser procedure does not. Unfortunately, symptom relief—of bleeding, tenesmus, and mucus discharge—in patients with these advanced lesions is often less than anticipated. A diverting colostomy can be performed for obstructing rectal cancer that cannot be resected. However, in such cases colonoscopically deployed endoluminal stents can provide relief of obstruction even when the lumen is too small to accommodate a pediatric colonoscope. Tumor ingrowth will cause stent occlusion within 6–9 months, but this can be prolonged with laser photocoagulation. The Hartmann procedure may be indicated in poor-risk patients—the bowel with its contained cancer is removed through the abdomen with permanent colostomy but without excision of the distal rectum, which is sutured closed.

6. Radiation therapy—Intracavitary, external, or implantation techniques are used alone or in combination with surgical excision for small rectal cancers. Preoperative external beam radiation therapy, often given with chemotherapy to enhance the radiation effect (**neoadjuvant therapy**), may shrink a rectal carcinoma, kill cells in regional lymphatics, and prevent pelvic recurrence. Complete clinical response has been reported to be as high as 30% after neoadjuvant treatment; however, many of these patients will still have pathologically detectable disease and therefore complete clinical response does not eliminate the need for surgical resection. Although the benefit of radiation on decreasing local recurrence rates has been well demonstrated, only one major randomized trial demonstrated a benefit in survival. External radiation therapy is widely employed in patients with bulky fixed lesions that do not seem to be resectable; after such treatment, some lesions can be removed. It should be noted, however, that the boundaries of resection for curative intent should be based on the pretreatment evaluation of tumor extent and not on the visible tumor after treatment. Intraoperative radiation therapy is a promising method of treatment of local pelvic recurrences.

C. Adjuvant Therapy

Chemotherapy and radiation therapy have been studied extensively as adjuvants to curative resection of cancer of the large intestine. It is apparent that strategies are different for cancer of the colon and cancer of the rectum. Patients with stage I lesions in either site do not benefit from adjuvant therapy. Some stage II and stage III rectal cancer patients have improved local control and survival with combined postoperative chemotherapy and radiation therapy. Poor functional results including frequent bowel movements, urgency, tenesmus, and incontinence with postoperative radiation can be avoided with preoperative therapy. Irradiation is not used for cancer of the colon. Stage III colon cancer patients may also enroll in clinical trials, but if that is not possible there are multiple regimens now available which include 5-FU, irinotecan, and oxaliplatin. It is anticipated that molecular markers and other innovative staging techniques discussed below will help select patients for adjuvant therapy in the future.

Treatment of Complications

A. Obstruction

Obstructing cancer of the left or right colon is treated by immediate resection in good-risk patients. (See Obstruction of the Large Intestine, above.)

B. Perforation

An aggressive approach to perforated cancer of the colon is advisable, but anastomosis is often delayed based on the degree of contamination and the health of the bowel. If contamination is severe or if bowel health is compromised, the proximal end is exteriorized as a colostomy (or ileostomy), and the distal end is exteriorized or closed. Secondary anastomosis is performed after inflammation subsides. Alternatively, the anastomosis may be performed and "covered" with a defunctioning loop ileostomy. Closure of a loop ileostomy is a simpler and less morbid procedure than reexploration and closure of an end stoma.

C. Direct Extension

When carcinoma of the colon has spread by contiguity to adjacent viscera such as the small intestine, spleen, kidney, uterus, prostate, or urinary bladder, the involved viscus—or a portion of it—should be resected en bloc with the colon.

Prognosis

The **clinicopathologic stage** of disease is the most important determinant of survival. In general the results of surgical treatment are better for cancer of the colon than for cancer of the rectum, and low rectal cancer has a worse prognosis than cancer higher in the rectum. The Dukes classification was introduced decades ago but has largely been replaced by the TNM system developed by the American Joint Committee for Cancer Staging and End Results Reporting. Table 30–7 lists the definitions of TNM and the stage grouping along with the corresponding Dukes classification. Clinical data are used for determination of M, and both clinical and pathologic information is included in assessment of T and N. Survival rates differ considerably in various series; actuarial rates are higher than crude survival rates. Before the wide application of adjuvant chemotherapy, average crude 5-year survival rates for colon and rectal cancer using the Dukes system were as follows: stage A, 80%; stage B, 60%; stage C, 30%; stage D, 5%. Adjuvant therapy, particularly with some of the newer agents in addition to improved surgical techniques, has led to 5-year survival rates approaching 80% for stage III (Dukes C) disease.

Up to 10% of lesions are not resectable at the time of operation, and an additional 20% of patients have liver or other distant metastases. Hence, operation for cure can be performed on only about 70% of patients. The operative mortality rate is 1–4%. The 5-year survival rate of patients undergoing resection is about 45–50% (all stages).

The prognosis is adversely affected by complications such as obstruction or perforation. The histologic features—including the degree of differentiation of the tumor, intravascular tumor cells, or malignant cells in the perineural space—also have a bearing on prognosis and may influence the decision to recommend adjuvant chemotherapy in node-negative patients.

In the view of many experts, clinicopathologic staging is not sufficiently discriminating for the purpose of selecting patients for adjuvant therapy because lesions of similar TNM stage may have widely different potentials for local recurrence and distant metastasis. Innovative staging techniques include immunohistochemistry for markers such as cytokeratins and reverse transcription polymerase chain reaction for CEA or p53 and genotypic subset analysis. Loss of heterozygosity at chromosome 18q (affecting expression of DCC, Smad4, and Smad2) is predictive of a poor outcome. Other markers of poor prognosis include loss of heterozygosity at chromosome 17p (affecting p53) and 8q, and a mutation in the BAX gene. Favorable prognostic factors include the presence of microsatellite instability in the genes of the mismatch repair family and increased expression of the cyclin-dependent kinase inhibitor $p21^{WAF1/CIP1}$ protein. Further study is required before clinicians can base therapeutic decisions on assays of these and other molecular markers.

Studies from several countries show that low-income people have more advanced disease when diagnosed and

Table 30–7. TNM classification of cancer of the colon and rectum.[1]

Primary Tumor (T)

TX	Primary tumor cannot be assessed
T0	No evidence of primary tumor
Tis	Carcinoma in situ
T1	Tumor invades submucosa
T2	Tumor invades muscularis propria
T3	Tumor invades through the muscularis propria into the subserosa, or into nonperitonealized pericolic or perirectal tissues
T4	Tumor perforates the visceral peritoneum, or directly invades other organs or structures

Regional Lymph Nodes (N)

NX	Regional lymph nodes cannot be assessed
N0	No regional lymph node metastasis
N1	Metastasis in one to three pericolic or perirectal lymph nodes
N2	Metastasis in four or more pericolic or perirectal lymph nodes
N3	Metastasis in any lymph node along the course of a named vascular trunk

Distant Metastasis (M)

MX	Presence of distant metastasis cannot be assessed
M0	No distant metastasis
M1	Distant metastasis

Stage Grouping

				Dukes	Modified Astler-Coller
Stage 0	Tis	N0	M0		
Stage I	T1	N0	M0	A	A
	T2	N0	M0	A	B1
Stage IIA	T3	N0	M0	B	B2
Stage IIB	T4	N0	M0	B	B3
Stage IIIA	T1-2	N1	M0	C	C1
Stage IIIB	T3-4	N1	M0	C2/C3	
Stage IIIC	Any T	N2	M0	C1/C2/C3	
Stage IV	Any T	Any N	M1		

[1]Used with the permission of the American Joint Committee on Cancer (AJCC), Chicago, IL. The original source for this material is *AJCC Cancer Staging Manual,* 6th ed. Lippincott-Raven, 2002.

that their stage-for-stage survival rates are worse; these observations have not been explained satisfactorily. An association of perioperative blood transfusions with poorer prognosis from colorectal cancer has been found by some but not all investigators; if it is genuine, the effect may reflect other effects—larger tumors requiring more extensive surgery and transfusions, for example—rather than some consequence of transfusion itself.

Follow-up after curative resection of cancer of the large bowel is controversial. There are good data to support the view that periodic colonoscopy to detect and remove adenomas after colonoscopic polypectomy prevents subsequent cancer, and colonoscopy at 3 years is just as beneficial as colonoscopy at 1 and 3 years after complete removal of the index adenoma. It is not known whether these observations can be extrapolated to follow-up after curative resection of cancer, but in the absence of data many clinicians perform surveillance colonoscopy periodically for the purpose of detecting adenomas and metachronous carcinomas. Other goals of follow-up are the diagnosis of recurrent cancer or metastatic cancer. The physician should tailor the follow-up strategy based on the patient's ability and interest in pursuing an aggressive approach should recurrent disease be discovered. Follow-up programs include a complete blood count, liver function tests, serum CEA levels, chest x-rays, and CT scans in addition to colonoscopy.

If recurrent cancer or metastatic cancer is discovered, the patient is evaluated for potential surgical resection of the lesions. This is particularly true for hepatic or pulmonary metastases where a survival benefit has been demonstrated. Local recurrences can be resected, sometimes in combination with intraoperative radiation therapy. The Mayo Clinic reported a 25% 5-year survival after multimodality therapy, including full-dose preoperative chemoradiation and surgical resection with intraoperative radiation, for recurrent rectal cancer. Unfortunately, the prognosis of patients with local recurrence is poor. If recurrent cancer is suggested on the basis of rising serum CEA levels and if the responsible lesion cannot be located by CT, MRI, or PET scan, a second-look laparotomy may be undertaken. Resectable cancer is found in 30% or more of patients.

Allison JE et al: A comparison of fecal occult-blood tests for colorectal-cancer screening. N Engl J Med 1996;334:155.

Arulampalam TH et al: Positron emission tomography and colorectal cancer. Br J Surg 2001;8:176.

Bruinvels DJ et al: Follow-up of patients with colorectal cancer. A meta-analysis. Ann Surg 1994;219:174.

Busch ORC et al: Blood transfusions and prognosis in colorectal cancer. N Engl J Med 1993;328:1372.

The Clinical Outcomes of Surgical Therapy Study Group (COST): A comparison of laparoscopically assisted and open colectomy for colon cancer. N Engl J Med 2004;350:2050.

Chu KC et al: Temporal patterns in colorectal cancer incidence, survival, and mortality from 1950 through 1990. J Natl Cancer Inst 1994;86:997.

Gann PH et al: Low-dose aspirin and incidence of colorectal tumors in a randomized trial. J Natl Cancer Inst 1993;85:1220.

Giardiello FM et al: The use and interpretation of commercial *APC* gene testing for familial adenomatous polyposis. N Engl J Med 1997;336:823.

Gryfe R et al: Tumor microsatellite instability and clinical outcome in young patients with colorectal cancer. N Engl J Med 2000;342:69.

Hecht JR: Dietary fat and colon cancer. Adv Exp Med Biol 1996;399:157.

Heys SD et al: Prognostic factors and survival of patients aged less than 45 years with colorectal cancer. Br J Surg 1994;81:685.

Howe GR et al: Dietary intake of fiber and decreased risk of cancers of the colon and rectum: evidence from the combined analysis of 13 case-control studies. J. Natl Cancer Inst 1992;84:1887.

Jessup JM et al: The National Cancer Data Base. Report on colon cancer. Cancer 1996;78:918.

Kapiteijn E et al: Preoperative radiotherapy combined with total mesorectal excision for resectable rectal cancer. Dutch ColoRectal Cancer Group. N Engl J Med 2001;345:638.

Lavery IC et al: Treatment of colon and rectal cancer. Surg Clin North Am 2000;80:535.

Lichtenstein P et al: Environmental and heritable factors in the causation of cancer—analyses of cohorts of twins from Sweden, Denmark, and Finland. N Engl J Med 2000;343:78.

Lieberman DA et al: Use of colonoscopy to screen asymptomatic adults for colorectal cancer. Veterans Affairs Cooperative Study Group 380. N Engl J Med 2000;343:162.

Lin KM et al: Colorectal and extracolonic cancer variations in MLH1/MSH2 hereditary nonpolyposis colorectal cancer kindreds and the general population. Dis Colon Rectum 1998;41:428.

Lynch HT, de la Chapelle A: Hereditary colorectal cancer. N Engl J Med 2003;348:919.

Macdonald JS, Astrow AB: Adjuvant therapy of colon cancer. Semin Oncol 2001;28:30.

Saha S et al: Sentinel lymph node mapping in colorectal cancer—a review. Surg Clinics North Am 2000; 80:1811.

Scholefield JH: ABC of colorectal cancer: screening. BMJ 2000;321:1004.

Simmang CL et al: American society of colon and rectal surgeons: Practice parameters for the detection of colorectal neoplasms.

Steinbach G et al: The effect of celecoxib, a cyclooxygenase-2 inhibitor, in familial adenomatous polyposis. N Engl J Med 2000;342:1946.

Swedish rectal cancer trial: Improved survival with preoperative radiotherapy in resectable rectal cancer. N Engl J Med 1997;336:980.

Watanabe T et al: Molecular predictors of survival after adjuvant chemotherapy for colon cancer. N Engl J Med 2001;344:1196.

Winawer SJ, Zauber AG: Colonoscopic polypectomy and the incidence of colorectal cancer. Gut 2001;48:753.

Weeks JC et al: Short-term quality-of-life outcomes following laparoscopic-assisted colectomy vs open colectomy for colon cancer. A randomized trial. JAMA 2002;287:321.

POLYPS OF THE COLON & RECTUM

ESSENTIALS OF DIAGNOSIS

- *Family history.*
- *Sigmoidoscopic, colonoscopic, or radiologic discovery of polyps.*

General Considerations

Colorectal polyps are masses of tissue that project into the lumen. They comprise a heterogeneous group of sessile or pedunculated, benign or malignant, mucosal, submucosal, or muscular lesions. "Polyp" is a morphologic term, and no histologic diagnosis is implied. The most common epithelial polyps of the colon and rectum are listed in Table 30–8. Most adenomas are tubular, tubulovillous, or villous. Hyperplastic polyps are diminutive lesions most often found in the left colon. Hamartomas are uncommon. Polyposis, discussed later in this section, is a term reserved for the presence of many polyps in the large bowel.

Estimates of the incidence of colonic and rectal polyps in the general population range from 9% to 60%—the higher figure includes small polyps found at autopsy. Polypoid adenomas are found in about 25% of asymptomatic adults who undergo screening colonoscopy. The prevalence of adenomas is 30% at age 50 years, 40% at age 60, 50% at age 70, and 55% at age 80. The mean age is 55 years, about 5–10 years younger

Table 30–8. Polyps of the large intestine.

Type	Histologic Diagnosis
Neoplastic	Adenoma Tubular adenoma (adenomatous polyp) Tubulovillous adenoma (villoglandular adenoma) Villous adenoma (villous papilloma) Carcinoma
Hamartomas	Juvenile polyp Peutz-Jeghers polyp
Inflammatory	Inflammatory polyp (pseudopolyp) Benign lymphoid polyp
Unclassified	Hyperplastic polyp
Miscellaneous	Lipoma, leiomyoma, carcinoid

than the mean age of patients with colorectal cancer. Approximately 50% of polyps occur in the sigmoid or rectum. About 50% of patients with adenoma have more than one lesion, and 15% have more than two lesions. An increased incidence of adenomas in breast cancer patients has been reported.

Inflammatory polyps have no malignant potential. Cancer developing in association with hamartomas is rare but has been reported. Hyperplastic polyps are not neoplastic and therefore do not become malignant. However, they may be difficult to distinguish from serrated adenomas, which do have malignant potential. It has been suggested that hyperplastic polyps in the left colon are markers for neoplastic polyps elsewhere in the colon, but the weight of evidence is against this concept.

Adenomas are a premalignant lesion. The vast majority of adenocarcinomas of the large bowel are believed to evolve through a series of genetic alterations from adenomas (adenoma-to-carcinoma sequence). In Western populations, both adenomas and cancer increase in incidence with age, and the distribution of adenomas and cancer in the bowel is similar. Approximately 25% of patients who have five or more adenomatous polyps have a synchronous colon cancer at the initial colonoscopy. About one-third of colonic and rectal specimens resected for cancer also harbor adenomas; if a surgical specimen contains two or more synchronous carcinomas, the incidence of associated adenomas is 75%. All gradations of malignancy—from total absence, to dysplasia, to a microscopic cytologic cancer, to invasive cancer, to a gross cancer with remnants of benign tumor at one margin—may be seen in colonic neoplasms; on the other hand, cancers that are smaller than 0.5 cm in diameter and contain no benign adenoma are extremely rare. Additional support for the malignant potential of adenomas is as follows: (1) Patients with familial adenomatous polyposis die of cancer at a young age unless the colon is removed. (2) Chemical carcinogens produce adenomas and cancers indiscriminately in the colons of experimental animals. (3) Routine removal of adenomas from the colon reduces the incidence of subsequent rectal cancer.

The malignant potential of an adenoma depends on size, growth pattern, and the degree of epithelial atypia. Cancer is found in 1% of adenomas under 1 cm in diameter, 10% of adenomas 1–2 cm in size, and up to 45% of adenomas larger than 2 cm. So-called flat adenomas, small flat or depressed tubular adenomas that tend to occur in the right colon, may be an exception to these guidelines; they may become malignant when still only a few millimeters in diameter. The three histologic patterns of adenoma are variations of one neoplastic process; about 5% of tubular adenomas, 22% of tubulovillous adenomas, and 40% of villous adenomas become malignant. The potential for cancerous transformation rises with increasing degrees of epithelial dysplasia. Sessile lesions are more apt to be malignant than pedunculated ones. It probably takes at least 5 years, and more often 10–15 years, for an adenoma to become malignant.

Clinical Findings

A. Symptoms and Signs

Most polyps are asymptomatic, but the larger the lesion, the more likely it is to cause symptoms. Rectal bleeding is by far the most frequent complaint. Blood is bright red or dark red depending on the location of the polyp, and bleeding is usually intermittent. Profuse hemorrhage from polyps is rare.

Alterations in bowel habits are more common in the presence of frank carcinoma, but large benign tumors may produce tenesmus, constipation, or increased frequency of bowel movements. Some polyps, notably large villous adenomas, may secrete copious amounts of mucus that are evacuated per rectum. Polypoid tumors may induce peristaltic cramps or varying degrees of intussusception, but most often obstructive symptoms are due to associated diverticular disease or irritable bowel syndrome and persist after polypectomy. Occasionally, a polyp on a very long pedicle will prolapse through the anus; this is most apt to occur with juvenile polyps.

General physical examination yields little information about the colonic polyps themselves, although other manifestations of diseases such as Peutz-Jeghers syndrome may be found. A polyp may be palpable by digital rectal examination, and proctosigmoidoscopy may disclose polyps in the rectum or sigmoid. Blood-tinged mucus strongly suggests the presence of a neoplasm situated farther proximally. Since polyps are often multiple and may occur synchronously with cancer, further investigation of the colon is mandatory even if a lesion is found by sigmoidoscopy.

B. Imaging Studies (Barium Enema)

A polyp appears as a rounded filling defect with smooth, sharply defined margins. Double-column technique is recommended. Thorough cleansing of the colon and careful examination are essential if small polyps are to be demonstrated.

C. Colonoscopy

This has been the most reliable way to diagnose colonic polyps. Polypectomy can be done at the same time. However, small polyps may still be missed at a rate of 5–10%. The entire colon should be examined by colonoscopy in every patient with known polyps or symptoms suggestive of their presence.

D. CT Colonography

CT colonography is emerging as a reliable and important technique for the diagnosis of colonic polyps in the screening population. The principal advantage is the potential for a more complete evaluation of the mucosal and extraluminal surfaces. The main disadvantage is the continued need for a bowel prep and the need for a subsequent colonoscopy should an abnormality be identified.

Differential Diagnosis

Artifacts seen on barium enema and CT colonography may be confused with polyps. Colonoscopy is essential in doubtful situations because polyps of various histologic types can be differentiated only by microscopic examination.

Treatment

Polyps of the colon and rectum are treated because they produce symptoms, because they may be malignant when first discovered, or because they may become malignant later. In a study of untreated colonic polyps, the cumulative risk of eventual cancer at the polyp site was 2.5% at 5 years, 8% at 10 years, and 24% at 20 years.

Small polyps can be removed with an electrocautery snare passed through a colonoscope. Large, sessile, soft, velvety lesions in the rectum are usually villous adenomas; these tumors have high malignant potential and must be excised completely. With the patient anesthetized, this can be accomplished through the anus in most instances. Only if histologic sections show invasive cancer at the margins of excision is further therapy necessary. Management of villous tumors by endoscopic Nd:YAG laser photocoagulation may be useful for extensive carpet-like tumors. Excision has the advantage of permitting histologic examination of the specimen.

Pedunculated polyps and small sessile lesions in the sigmoid and above should be removed with a hot biopsy forceps or an electrocautery snare passed through the colonoscope. Colonoscopic polypectomy is safer than laparotomy; the combined incidence of perforation and hemorrhage is less than 0.5%, and deaths are rare. Colonoscopy is less expensive and incurs much less disability than laparotomy.

Open or laparoscopic-assisted colonic resection should be considered if colonoscopy is unsuccessful, if the lesion is large and sessile, or if there are many polyps. Patients with HNPCC and others with multiple polyps may require total abdominal colectomy with ileorectal anastomosis.

From 2% to 4% of colonoscopically excised polyps contain invasive adenocarcinoma, and a decision must be made whether to resect the segment of colon or simply follow the patient. In 1985 Haggitt and coworkers proposed a morphologic classification for pedunculated malignant polyps (Table 30–9). The risk of lymph node metastasis in Haggitt level 1–3 lesions is < 1%.

Table 30–9. Haggitt classification.[1]

Level	Depth
0	Carcinoma in situ or intramucosal carcinoma
1	Carcinoma invading through muscularis mucosa into the submucosa but limited to the head of the polyp
2	Carcinoma invading the neck of the polyp
3	Carcinoma invading any part of the stalk
4	Carcinoma invading into the submucosa of the bowel wall below the stalk of the polyp but above the muscularis propria (T1)
Sessile	By definition, equivalent to level 4

[1]From Haggitt RC et al: Prognostic factors in colorectal carcinomas arising in adenomas: implications for lesions removed by endoscopic polypectomy. Gastroenterology 1985;89:328.

Haggitt level 4 and sessile lesions are associated with a 10% or greater risk for lymph node metastasis. In the case of malignant polyps, resection of the colon is not required if the following criteria are met: (1) Gross margin is clear at endoscopy; (2) microscopic margin is clear; (3) cancer is well-differentiated; (4) there is no lymphatic or venous invasion; and (5) cancer does not invade the stalk (Haggitt level 0–2). Other malignant polyps of the colon (eg, sessile) should be managed by resection of involved bowel. Molecular markers may help make this determination in the future. Since rectal cancers are sometimes treated definitively by local excision, it may not be necessary to do a radical resection if the malignant polyp arose in the distal rectum.

Familial adenomatous polyposis (adenomatous polyposis coli) is a rare but important disease because colorectal cancer develops before age 40 in nearly all untreated patients. The trait is autosomal dominant. Genetic advances have been explosive. The *APC* gene ("FAP" had already been used in the genetic lexicon) was localized to chromosome 5q21 in 1991, and since then more than 100 different mutations have been identified. Genetic testing of at-risk individuals is currently available. Patients present with hundreds to thousands of polyps of varying size and configuration in the colon and rectum. A subset of patients have attenuated FAP (previously known as hereditary flat adenoma syndrome) characterized by the presence of fewer polyps (usually < 100), usually less than 100, later onset of colon cancer, and characteristic different mutations of the APC gene. A long list of benign and malignant extracolonic manifestations are associated with familial adenomatous polyposis (Table 30–10). **Gardner's syndrome** (polyposis, desmoid tumors, osteomas of mandible or skull, and sebaceous cysts) and **Turcot's syndrome** (polyposis and childhood cerebellar medulloblastoma) are examples of familial adenomatous polyposis with variations in expression of the extracolonic manifestations; both syndromes are associated

Table 30–10. Extracolonic manifestations of familial adenomatous polyposis.[1]

Benign	Malignant
Endocrine adenoma	Duodenal carcinoma
Osteoma	Bile duct carcinoma
Epidermoid cyst	Pancreatic carcinoma
Hypertrophic retinal pigmentation	Desmoid tumor
	Carcinoma of the stomach
Gastric fundic gland polyp	Adrenal carcinoma
Duodenal adenoma	Medulloblastoma
Small bowel adenoma	Glioblastoma
	Thyroid carcinoma
	Small bowel carcinoma
	Carcinoid tumor of the ileum
	Osteogenic sarcoma
	Hepatoblastoma

[1]Reproduced, with permission, from Jagelman DG: The expanding spectrum of familial adenomatous polyposis. Perspect Colon Rectal Surg 1998;1:30.

with mutations in the APC gene, although Turcot's may also be associated with HNPCC and defects in mismatch repair genes (colon cancer with childhood or adult gliomas). Congenital hypertrophy of retinal pigment epithelium is present as early as at 3 months of age in affected members of two-thirds of families with familial adenomatous polyposis; this abnormality (always bilateral, more than four lesions on each side) predicts familial adenomatous polyposis with 97% sensitivity. Polyps begin to appear at puberty, at which time colonoscopy should be performed. Once the APC gene mutation or polyposis is diagnosed, colectomy should be done. Upper gastrointestinal endoscopy is performed to look for gastroduodenal lesions.

Although total proctocolectomy eliminates the risk of cancer, it leaves the patient with a permanent ileostomy. Abdominal colectomy ("subtotal colectomy") with ileorectal anastomosis may be favored when the number of rectal polyps is few, the patient is compliant with regular follow-up, and the patient is otherwise not a candidate for an ileoanal pouch procedure. It is hoped that cancer can be prevented by sigmoidoscopic destruction of the remaining rectal polyps every 6 months. The long-term success rate varies in different reports, and the incidence of cancer in the remaining rectum is low. Sulindac and celecoxib have both been reported to induce regression of polyps and may be used for chemoprevention in the remaining rectum. Total colectomy and the ileoanal pouch procedure (see Ulcerative Colitis, below) is preferred for patients if there are numerous adenomas in the rectum. If the rectal mucosa is excised completely, the risk of subsequent rectal neoplasia is essentially nil. Case reports of cancer arising in the anal canal after this operation may reflect incomplete excision of susceptible mucosa at the time of ileoanal anastomosis. Prophylactic colectomy does not alter the extracolonic manifestations. Desmoid tumor is a locally invasive nonmetastasizing fibrous tumor that occurs in the mesentery or abdominal wall of some patients after the colectomy. Results of attempts to excise desmoids are poor, with 80% recurrence. Sulindac, tamoxifen, prednisolone, and progesterone have been reported to halt the growth of desmoids. Combination chemotherapy with doxorubicin and dacarbazine may be helpful, but other chemotherapeutic regimens and radiation therapy have been ineffective. Desmoids grow slowly and capriciously, but they prove fatal in 10% of patients with familial adenomatous polyposis. Upper gastrointestinal tumors, specifically duodenal adenomas and duodenal and ampullary adenocarcinomas, occur in up to 10% of these patients, and medulloblastoma is also a significant risk.

Four syndromes of juvenile polyposis have been defined: (1) **juvenile polyposis syndrome** (1/100,000 population), (2) **Cronkhite-Canada syndrome** (juvenile polyposis and ectodermal lesions), (3) **Bannayan-Riley-Ruvalcaba syndrome** (juvenile polyposis and macrocephaly and genital hyperpigmentation), and (4) **Cowden's disease** (juvenile polyposis and facial trichilemmomas, thyroid goiter and cancer, and breast cancer). Although juvenile polyps are hamartomas with a low malignant potential, the risk of gastrointestinal cancer is increased in familial juvenile polyposis patients and their relatives. The lifetime risk of colorectal cancer with juvenile polyposis syndrome is 30–60%. Furthermore, hamartomas can coexist with adenomas, and one must not assume that a polyp is a hamartoma without proof. Colonoscopic excision is performed for large or symptomatic (bleeding, intussusception) lesions. Some juvenile polyps autoamputate. Colectomy is required in some patients with familial forms of juvenile polyposis.

Peutz-Jeghers syndrome is an uncommon autosomal dominant disease (1/200,000 population) in which multiple hamartomatous polyps appear in the stomach, small bowel, and colon. Affected individuals have melanotic pigmentation of the skin and mucous membranes, especially about the lips and gums. Until recently the Peutz-Jeghers hamartomas were thought to be without malignant potential, but adenomatous changes and the development of malignancy have been described. The lifetime risk of colorectal cancer has been reported to be 39%. Prophylactic colectomy has not been studied in the Peutz-Jeghers syndrome population and polyps are generally removed only if symptomatic, but patients should undergo continued surveillance. Carcinoma also develops at an increased rate in other tissues, eg, stomach, duodenum, pancreas, small intestine, and breast.

Prognosis

Villous adenomas recur at the excision site in about 15% of cases after local removal. Tubular adenomas seldom recur, but new ones may develop, and a patient who has had any type of adenoma is at greater risk of developing adenocarcinoma than the general population. The risk of metachronous neoplasms following excision of a colorectal adenoma is greatest if there were multiple index lesions or if an adenoma was sessile, villous, or over 2 cm in diameter. The risk is somewhat higher in men than in women. In one study, the cumulative risk of developing further adenomas was linear over time, reaching about 50% by 15 years after removal of one or more colorectal adenomas; the cumulative incidence of cancer in the same population rose to 7% at 15 years. Prospective studies show that if the colon is cleared by total colonoscopy at the time of excision of the index polyp, follow-up colonoscopy at 3 years is just as effective as colonoscopy at 1 and 3 years in preventing development of ominous neoplasms.

Boardman LA: Heritable colorectal cancer syndromes: recognition and preventive management. Gastroenterol Clin North Am 2002;31:1107.

Bond JH: Polyp guideline: diagnosis, treatment, and surveillance for patients with colorectal polyps. Practice Parameters Committee of the American College of Gastroenterology. Am J Gastroenterol 2000;95:3053.

Calland JF et al: Genetic syndromes and genetic tests in colorectal cancer. Semin Gastrointest Dis 2000;11:207.

Citarda F et al: Efficacy in standard clinical practice of colonoscopic polypectomy in reducing colorectal cancer incidence. Gut 2001;48:812.

Fahy B, Bold RJ: Epidemiology and molecular genetics of colorectal cancer. Surg Oncol 1998;7:115.

Frazier ML et al: Current applications of genetic technology in predisposition testing and microsatellite instability assays. J Clin Oncol 2000;18(21 Suppl):70S.

Gelfand DW: Decreased risk of subsequent colonic cancer in patients undergoing polypectomy after barium enema: analysis based on data from the preendoscopic era. AJR Am J Roentgenol 1997;169:1243.

Hawk E, Lubet R, Limburg P: Chemoprevention in hereditary colorectal cancer syndromes. Cancer 1999;86(11 Suppl):2551.

Helm JF, Sandler RS: Colorectal cancer screening. Med Clin North Am 1999;83:1403.

Lal G, Gallinger S: Familial adenomatous polyposis. Semin Surg Oncol 2000;18:314.

Lynch HT, de la Chapelle A: Genetic susceptibility to non-polyposis colorectal cancer. J Med Genet 1999;36:801.

Lynch HT, Smyrk T: An update on Lynch syndrome. Curr Opin Oncol 1998;10:349.

Macrae F: Wheat bran fiber and development of adenomatous polyps: evidence from randomized, controlled clinical trials. Am J Med 1999;106(Suppl 1A):38S.

Soravia C et al: Desmoid disease in patients with familial adenomatous polyposis. Dis Colon Rectum 2000;43:363.

Spagnesi MT et al: Rectal proliferation and polyp occurrence in patients with familial adenomatous polyposis after sulindac treatment. Gastroenterology 1994;106:362.

Villavicencio RT, Rex DK: Colonic adenomas: prevalence and incidence rates, growth rates, and miss rates at colonoscopy. Semin Gastrointest Dis 2000;11:185.

Winawer SJ, Zauber AG: Colonoscopic polypectomy and the incidence of colorectal cancer. Gut 2001;48:753.

OTHER TUMORS OF THE COLON & RECTUM

Carcinoids of the large bowel are uncommon, and most of them occur in the rectum. Lesions less than 2 cm in diameter usually are asymptomatic, behave benignly, and can be managed by local excision. Larger tumors arising in the colon (mainly the right side) or rectum cause local symptoms, often metastasize, and require standard cancer operations. Carcinoid syndrome appears in less than 5% of patients with metastatic carcinoid of the large bowel.

Lymphomas are the most common noncarcinomatous malignant tumors of the large bowel. Diffuse lymphomatous polyposis is a rare gastrointestinal manifestation. Non-Hodgkin's B cell lymphoma and Kaposi's sarcoma are two AIDS-related cancers that affect the colon and rectum. Lymphoma is often aggressive, but Kaposi's sarcoma may cause few colonic or systemic symptoms.

Lipomas may be difficult to distinguish with barium enema from mucosal neoplasms, but CT examination may demonstrate a mass with fat density and colonoscopy may demonstrate a soft "pillow" lesion often permitting accurate diagnosis. Lipomas are usually asymptomatic but can cause obstruction. Removal is recommended if they cause symptoms.

Leiomyomas are much less common in the colon than in the stomach or small intestine. Colonic tumors are less apt to cause significant hemorrhage than those of the upper bowel. Some leiomyomas become malignant. Fifteen percent of **gastrointestinal stromal tumors (GIST)**, previously known as leiomyosarcoma, may occur in the colon or rectum.

Endometriomas are masses of endometrial tissue that implant on the surface of the rectum, sigmoid colon, appendix, cecum, or distal ileum and may invade locally into the muscularis, submucosa, and even mucosa. Endoscopically they may even have the appearance of a primary colon cancer. The ectopic tissue responds to cyclic hormonal stimulation, causing inflammation and fibrosis. Intestinal symptoms of endometriosis include altered bowel habits, rectal pain, and rectal bleeding during menstruation. Tender nodularities are palpable in the pelvis in 90% of cases. Sigmoidoscopy, fiberoptic colonoscopy, and barium enema x-rays may make the diagnosis, but diagnostic laparoscopy may be necessary to be certain of the problem. Therapeutic laparoscopy is performed if symptoms are not controlled by endocrine therapy or if cancer cannot be excluded. Endometrial lesions on peritoneal surfaces in the pelvis may be excised or destroyed by laser or cautery; colonic or rectal lesions may be managed by partial or full-thickness resection of the bowel. Relief of intestinal symptoms is reported in 90–100% of patients who undergo surgical treatment.

Other benign colorectal tumors include neuro-fibromas associated with Recklinghausen's disease, teratomas, enterocystomas (duplication of rectum), lymphangiomas, and cavernous hemangiomas. Adenosquamous carcinoma, primary squamous cell carcinoma, and primary melanoma of the colon or rectum are extremely rare malignant tumors.

Henkel A, Christensen B, Schindler AE: Endometriosis: a clinically malignant disease. Eur J Obstet Gynecol Reprod Biol 1999;82:209.

Jerby BL et al: Laparoscopic management of colorectal endometriosis. Surg Endosc 1999;13:1125.

Kawamoto K et al: Colonic submucosal tumors: a new classification based on radiologic characteristics. AJR Am J Roentgenol 1993;160:315.

Londono-Schimmer EE, Ritchie JK, Hawley PR: Coloanal sleeve anastomosis in the treatment of diffuse cavernous haemangioma of the rectum: long-term results. Br J Surg 1994;81:1235.

Saclarides TJ, Szeluga D, Staren ED: Neuroendocrine cancers of the colon and rectum: results of a ten-year experience. Dis Colon Rectum 1994;37:635.

Soga J: Carcinoids of the colon and ileocecal region: a statistical evaluation of 363 cases collected from the literature. J Exp Clin Cancer Res 1998;17:139.

Spread C et al: Colon carcinoid tumors. A population-based study. Dis Colon Rectum 1994;37:482.

DIVERTICULAR DISEASE OF THE COLON

Diverticula are more common in the colon than in any other portion of the gastrointestinal tract. Colonic diverticula are acquired and are classified as false because they consist of mucosa and submucosa that have herniated through the muscular coats. True diverticula containing all layers of the bowel wall are rare in the colon. Colonic diverticula are pulsion (rather than traction) diverticula, because they are pushed out by intraluminal pressure. They vary from a few millimeters to several centimeters in diameter; the necks may be narrow or wide; and some contain inspissated fecal matter. Approximately 95% of patients with diverticula have involvement of the sigmoid colon. The descending, transverse, and ascending portions of the colon are involved in decreasing order of frequency. The presence of a solitary diverticulum of the cecum and the occurrence of multiple diverticula limited to the right colon are distinct entities often seen in Asian people but seldom encountered in other populations. Giant colonic diverticulum is a very rare lesion of huge dimensions, usually arising from the sigmoid colon.

In Western countries, perhaps 50% of individuals develop diverticula—10% by age 40 years and 65% by age 80 years. Diverticular disease is more common in Western nations than in Japan or in developing countries of the tropics. The prevalence of diverticulosis is 20%; in Singapore, 70% of the cases are right-sided. Cultural factors, especially diet, play an important etiologic role. Chief among the dietary influences is the fiber content of foods.

The pathogenesis of diverticula requires defects in the colonic wall and increased pressure in the lumen relative to the serosal surface. Small openings in the circular muscle layer for penetration of nutrient blood vessels are the sites of diverticula formation in many individuals (Figure 30–12). Diverticulosis of the colon comprises a spectrum with two extremes: (1) diverticulosis associated with hypermotility and (2) simple massed diverticulosis. In the first type, colonic musculature is shortened and thickened (myochosis coli); colonic pressures are high in response to meals or pharmacologic stimuli; patients may have pain and altered bowel habits; and diverticula are limited to the sigmoid, at least initially. It is hypothesized that myochosis reflects work hypertrophy from a lifetime of fiber-deficient diet and the consequent scybalous stools. High intraluminal pressures are possible because the colon forms closed compartments when opposite walls of the thickened bowel actually touch and occlude the lumen. The propensity for diverticula to develop in the sigmoid is explained by the law of Laplace, which states that pressure within a tube is inversely proportionate to the radius. It had been speculated that irritable bowel syndrome was a prediverticular state, but patterns of

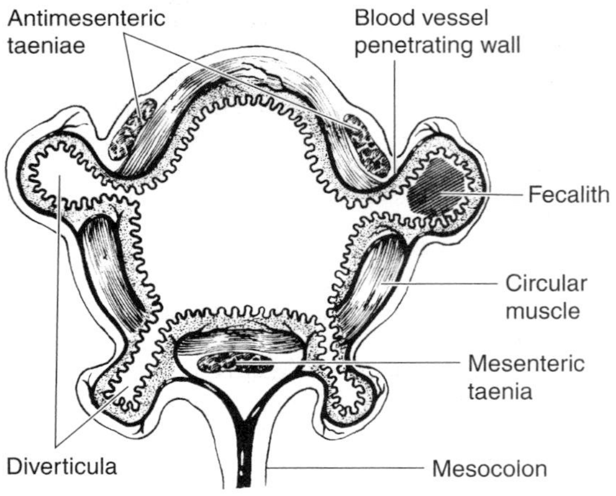

Figure 30–12. Cross section of the colon depicting the sites where diverticula form. Note that the antimesocolic portion is spared. The longitudinal layer of muscle completely encircles the bowel and is not limited to the taeniae as depicted here.

colonic motility are different in diverticular disease and irritable bowel syndrome. Moreover, it is clear that irritable bowel syndrome can affect the esophagus and small bowel in addition to the colon, so an etiologic link to colonic diverticula now seems unlikely. The two conditions can coexist, however, and irritable bowel syndrome may be the reason for symptoms.

Patients with simple massed diverticulosis have grossly normal colonic musculature, normal pressures, often no symptoms, and diverticula throughout the colon. Presumably, the primary abnormality is weakness of the colonic wall from aging or illness. It is of interest that Ehlers-Danlos syndrome and Marfan's syndrome, both of which involve abnormal connective tissue, are associated with colonic diverticulosis.

1. Diverticulosis

Diverticulosis is the presence of multiple false diverticula.

Clinical Findings

A. Symptoms and Signs

Diverticulosis probably remains asymptomatic in about 80% of people and is detected incidentally on barium enema x-rays or endoscopy if it is discovered at all. Symptoms attributable to the diverticula themselves are actually complications—bleeding and diverticulitis—each described in separate sections below. Symptoms (episodic pain, constipation, diarrhea) in patients with uncomplicated diverticulosis are due to the associated motility disorder, and the diverticula are coincidental. Physical examination may disclose mild tenderness in the left lower quadrant, and the left colon is sometimes palpable as a firm tubular structure. Fever and leukocytosis are absent in patients with pain but no inflammation.

B. Imaging Studies

In addition to diverticula, barium enema films may show segmental spasm and muscular thickening that narrow the lumen and give it a saw-toothed appearance.

C. Colonoscopy

There is little role for colonoscopy in the evaluation of diverticulosis. Its role in diverticulitis is discussed below.

Differential Diagnosis

Pain from the colonic muscular abnormality in the absence of inflammation can be difficult to differentiate from diverticulitis. The presence or absence of systemic signs of inflammation is the chief differential point, but the natural history of the acute episode may be the only way to make the distinction. Diverticulosis must be differentiated from other causes of rectal bleeding, especially carcinoma. Colonoscopy is essential in patients with bleeding.

Complications

Diverticulitis and massive hemorrhage are discussed below.

Treatment

A. Medical Treatment

Asymptomatic persons with diverticulosis may be given a high-fiber diet, though it is not certain that complications of diverticulosis can be avoided by dietary changes once the diverticula have formed. Symptomatic patients also can be treated with a high-fiber diet; constipation is improved, but abdominal pain is not. Wheat bran is the least expensive source of fiber; patients should take 10–25 g daily with cereal, soup, salad, or other food. Palatable bran products are now available. Other sources of wheat fiber include whole-grain bread and breakfast cereals. Commercial bulk agents (eg, psyllium seed or hemicellulose products) are also available at greater cost. One problem in prescribing bulk agents is that different types of fiber may have dissimilar effects on the colon. Anticholinergic agents, sedatives, tranquilizers, antidepressants, and antibiotics have no value. Analgesics should be avoided, but if pain relief is necessary, nonopioid medications are preferred. Education, reassurance, and a warm personal relationship between physician and patient are important to successful management.

B. Surgical Treatment

Operation is necessary for massive hemorrhage or to rule out carcinoma in some patients, but colonoscopy usually resolves the question of cancer. Colon resection for uncomplicated diverticular disease or irritable bowel syndrome is rarely necessary or advisable.

Prognosis

The natural history of diverticulosis has not been defined. Ten to 20 percent of patients with diverticulosis develop diverticulitis or hemorrhage when followed for many years. These patients are selected, however, and the incidence of complications in the population at large may be much lower. About 75% of complications of diverticular disease develop in patients with no prior colonic symptoms. Some evidence suggests that diverticulitis is more common with the hypermotility type of diverticulosis, and bleeding is the more frequent complication in simple massed diverticulosis. Irritable bowel syndrome is a chronic relapsing disorder distinct from diverticulosis that affects patients over long periods of their lives. There is hope that better understanding of the pathophysiologic mechanisms will soon lead to more rational therapy.*

2. Diverticulitis

ESSENTIALS OF DIAGNOSIS

- *Acute abdominal pain.*
- *Left lower quadrant tenderness and mass.*
- *Fever and leukocytosis.*
- *Characteristic radiologic signs.*

General Considerations

Acute colonic diverticulitis is the result of perforation of a diverticulum and may be due to intraluminal pressure. Only one diverticulum is involved at a time, usually in the sigmoid colon. Disease severity is a continuum from mild inflammation localized to a segment of the bowel wall to feculent peritonitis.

Contained perforation of a diverticulum leads to localized inflammation in the colonic wall or paracolic tissues and may progress to more serious complications including formation of a phlegmon, abscess, or fistula. Generally the original perforation seals quickly and the paracolic infection is isolated from the colonic lumen. An abscess may be confined by adjacent structures or may enlarge and spread; small abscesses may resorb with antibiotic treatment; others may drain spontaneously into the lumen of the bowel or into an adjacent viscus to form a fistula or require surgical drainage either percutaneously or by laparotomy. Free perforation results in purulent or feculent peritonitis. Chronic colonic obstruction can result from fibrosis in response to repeated episodes of microperforation (stricture). Also, small bowel may adhere acutely to an inflamed area and cause small bowel obstruction. Cecal diverticulitis resembles appendicitis clinically.

Clinical Findings

A. Symptoms and Signs

The acute attack consists of localized abdominal pain that is mild to severe, aching, and either steady or cramping; it resembles acute appendicitis except that it is situated in the left lower quadrant. Occasionally, pain is suprapubic, in the right lower quadrant, or throughout the lower abdomen. Constipation or increased frequency of defecation (or both in the same patient) is common, and passage of flatus may give some relief of pain. Inflammation adjacent to the bladder may produce dysuria. Nausea and vomiting depend on the location and severity of the inflammation. Physical findings characteristically include low-grade fever, mild abdominal distention, left lower quadrant tenderness, and a left lower quadrant or pelvic mass. Neither occult nor gross blood in the stools is common, and presence of blood may suggest malignancy. Leukocytosis is variably present.

The clinical picture described above is typical, but acute diverticulitis has other modes of presentation. Free perforation of a diverticulum produces generalized peritonitis rather than localized inflammation. An acute attack of diverticulitis may go unnoticed until a complication develops, and the complication may be the reason for the patient to seek help. The course of diverticulitis may be so insidious, particularly in old people, that vague abdominal pain associated with an abscess in the groin or a colovesical fistula is the initial presentation. In some cases, pain and inflammatory signs are not marked, but a palpable mass and signs of large bowel obstruction are present, so that carcinoma of the left colon seems the more likely diagnosis. In one series of women with proved diverticulitis, 38% were initially misdiagnosed as having a gynecologic pelvic mass because gastrointestinal symptoms and signs were mild or absent.

B. Imaging Studies

Plain abdominal films may show free abdominal air if a diverticulum has perforated into the general peritoneal cavity. If inflammation is localized, there is a picture of ileus, partial colonic obstruction, small bowel obstruction, or left lower quadrant mass.

CT scan is the preferred initial imaging study and should be obtained early in the patient's course, with intravenous and usually oral contrast to enhance the image. Stranding of pericolic fat is seen in diverticulitis, and complications such as abscess or fistula may be evident. In an effort to provide standardization for the discussion of perforated diverticulitis, Hinchey and coworkers described four stages of the disease: (1) pericolic abscess confined to the mesentery of the colon; (2) pelvic abscess resulting from an extension of a pericolic abscess; (3) purulent peritonitis; and (4) feculent peritonitis. Repeat CT or operative intervention is indicated when patients fail to improve or deteriorate over the initial 48 hours of medical therapy.

Barium enema is contraindicated during the initial stages of an acute attack of diverticulitis lest barium leak

*See references at end of next section.

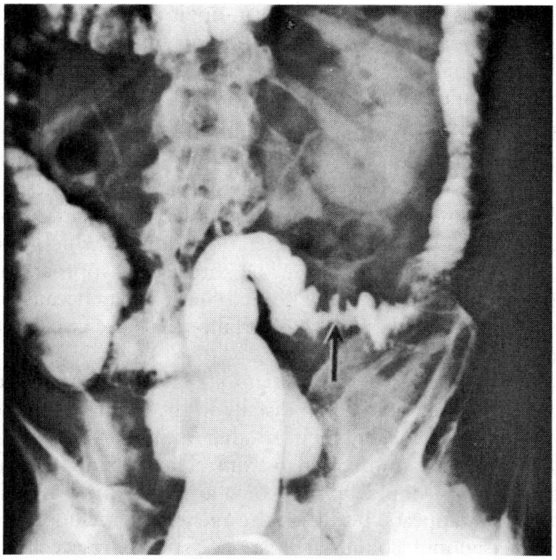

Figure 30–13. Barium enema x-ray showing upper sigmoid colon involved with diverticulitis. Note the long segment of narrowing, the spasm, and the deformity (arrow) produced by an intramural abscess.

into the peritoneal cavity, but water-soluble contrast media used under low pressure is safe. Barium enema can be performed a week or more after the attack began if the patient has recovered promptly. Radiographic signs include the following: (1) an abscess cavity or sinus tract outside the colonic wall communicating with the lumen; (2) an intramural abscess producing indentation of the barium column; (3) extrinsic compression by a paracolic mass; (4) intramural sinuses; and (5) fistulas. (See Figure 30–13.)

C. Special Examinations

The rigid sigmoidoscope usually cannot be passed beyond the rectosigmoid junction because of acute angulation and fixation at that level with a decrease in size of the lumen. Erythema, edema, and spasm may be noted. A purulent discharge can sometimes be seen coming from above. Flexible sigmoidoscopy or colonoscopy should be avoided during an acute attack but is helpful in ruling out cancer and evaluating strictures and other persistent abnormalities later. Small-bore upper tract instruments may be needed to examine narrow segments. Cystoscopy may reveal bullous edema of the bladder wall.

Differential Diagnosis

Free perforation of a diverticulum with generalized peritonitis often cannot be differentiated from the other causes of perforation, including foreign bodies and stercoraceous perforation. Acute diverticulitis with localized perforation may simulate appendicitis, perforated colonic carcinoma, obstruction with strangulation, mesenteric vascular insufficiency, Crohn's disease, and many other conditions. Differentiation from appendicitis is especially difficult when a redundant sigmoid colon lies in the right lower quadrant. A history of colonic symptoms on prior occasions, palpation of a mass, ultrasonography, CT, or water-soluble contrast enema may be helpful in differentiating these conditions. Colonoscopy may detect carcinoma, vascular insufficiency, or inflammatory disease of the colon. A difficult differential diagnosis lies between diverticulitis and carcinoma of the colon, particularly in the more silent forms of diverticulitis that present with a mass or fistula. Although barium enema and colonoscopy may clarify the issue, the diagnosis may not be known until the surgical specimen is examined by the pathologist.

Complications

The clinical spectrum of diverticulitis includes such complications as free perforation, abscess formation, fistulization, and partial obstruction. Colonic obstruction is usually slow in onset and incomplete. If acute, it generally resolves with nasogastric decompression and intravenous antibiotics, allowing for elective resection when necessary. Small bowel obstruction may result from the attachment of a loop of small intestine to the inflamed sigmoid.

Fistulas in males usually involve the bladder (see Colovesical Fistula, below). Fistulas may also occur to the ureter, urethra, vagina, uterus, cecum, small bowel, ovaries, fallopian tubes, perineum, and abdominal wall.

Treatment

A. Expectant Treatment

Patients with acute diverticulitis may need to be hospitalized. Details of management vary with the severity of the attack. Generally, nothing is given by mouth, nasogastric suction is instituted, intravenous fluids are given, and systemic broad-spectrum antibiotics are administered. Oral nonabsorbable antibacterial drugs are of little value. Opioid pain medications should be avoided. As acute manifestations subside, oral feeding is resumed gradually, and bulk-forming agents are prescribed if there is no stricture.

Colonoscopy is performed 4–6 weeks after the resolution of symptoms. Colonoscopy is mandatory in the presence of rectal bleeding or if x-rays show a possible neoplasm (stricture, mass, equivocal findings). The entire colon should always be evaluated for polyps or malignancy whenever elective resection for diverticular disease is planned. It is recommended—even if barium x-rays reveal only diverticula—in patients with abdominal pain or change in bowel habits attributed to diverticular disease. Colonoscopy will disclose a colonic neoplasm in about 30% of such patients.

B. Surgical Treatment

Indications for colectomy include perforation with generalized peritonitis or failure to improve with medical therapy. Elective resection is indicated for recurrent disease, a history of complicated disease (ie, phlegmon or abscess resolved with medical therapy or percutaneous drainage, stricture, or fistula), or the inability to rule out carcinoma. Age under 50 years is a relative indication for resection, but this is currently under debate. Obstruction and fistula seldom become indications for urgent operation during acute diverticulitis; both of these clinical problems are discussed separately in this chapter.

Percutaneous catheter drainage of well-localized paracolic abscesses can be performed by the interventional radiologist. This technique is especially useful because it converts a potential emergency operation to an elective one that can be performed when the acute inflammation has resolved. Colonic resection is indicated after an episode of complicated diverticulitis.

At laparotomy for severe acute diverticulitis, peritoneal fluid varies from turbid to purulent to grossly fecal. The sigmoid colon is involved in an inflammatory mass composed of large bowel, mesocolon, omentum, and sometimes small bowel. Except in cases of free perforation with generalized fecal peritonitis, the diseased diverticulum may not be visible. An abscess cavity may be hidden beneath colon or omentum and discovered when the bowel is mobilized; abscesses are commonly found lateral or medial to the colon, in the mesocolon, or in the pelvis. Microperforation of a diverticulum is not associated with a grossly apparent abscess. The extent of colonic inflammation, the amount of peritonitis, the patient's general condition, and the surgeon's experience and preferences determine the type of operation to be performed.

1. Primary resection with anastomosis—Resection of the diseased colon and primary colonic anastomosis has the advantage of solving the entire problem in one operation. It is not possible to anastomose the colon safely if there is gross infection in the surgical field after the diseased bowel has been removed, because the risk of anastomotic leakage is great. Intraoperative lavage of the colon may make it possible to perform primary anastomosis if other conditions permit.

2. Primary resection without anastomosis (two-stage procedure)—The diseased bowel is removed, the proximal end of the colon is brought out as a temporary colostomy, and the distal colonic stump is closed (Hartmann procedure; Figure 30–6) or exteriorized as a mucous fistula. Intestinal continuity is restored in a second operation after the inflammation subsides. Increasingly, percutaneous drainage of abscesses avoids the need for staged procedures.

3. Three-stage procedure—The three-stage procedure consists of a first operation during which a transverse colostomy is created and the paracolic abscess is drained; a second operation during which the left colon is resected; and a third operation during which the colostomy is taken down. The three-stage approach is uncommonly used in the United States today because it is associated with a higher mortality than the two-stage approach.

Definitive resection for sigmoid diverticulitis should include the sigmoid colon distally to the point where the taeniae become confluent so that anastomosis is performed to the uninvolved rectum. The proximal extent of resection should be the point at which the bowel is soft and appears healthy—this generally includes the entire sigmoid colon. It is unnecessary to resect additional bowel proximally; even if it is involved with diverticula, they are unlikely to become symptomatic in the absence of the sigmoid high-pressure zone. The laparoscopic approach may have advantages when compared to the open approach but may be difficult or technically not possible due to the persistence of inflammation.

Prognosis

Approximately 25% of patients hospitalized with acute diverticulitis require surgical treatment. The operative mortality rate is about 5% in recent reports, compared with 25% historically. Some of this improvement is attributable to the greater use of primary resection following percutaneous drainage of abscess.

Diverticulitis recurs in about one-third of medically treated cases. Most of these recurrences develop within the first 5 years. It is unknown whether recurrent attacks of diverticulitis can be prevented by increasing dietary fiber, although this measure is generally recommended. Recurrent diverticulitis after resection is unusual (about 3–7%) if the distal extent of the resection is at the rectum.

Aldoori WH et al: A prospective study of dietary fiber types and symptomatic diverticular disease in men. J Nutr 1998;128:714.

Ambrosetti P et al: Acute left colonic diverticulitis: a prospective analysis of 226 consecutive cases. Surgery 1994;115:546.

Baevsky R: Acute diverticulitis. N Engl J Med 1998;339:1082.

Brengman ML, Otchy DP: Timing of computed tomography in acute diverticulitis. Dis Colon Rectum 1998;41:1023.

Bruce CJ et al: Laparoscopic resection for diverticular disease. Dis Colon Rectum 1996;39(10 Suppl):S1.

Carbajo Caballero MA et al: The laparoscopic approach in the treatment of diverticular colon disease. J Soc Laparoendosc Surg 1998;2:159.

Desai DC et al: The utility of the Hartmann procedure. Am J Surg 1998;175:152.

Gooszen AW et al: Operative treatment of acute complications of diverticular disease: primary or secondary anastomosis after sigmoid resection. Eur J Surg 2001;167:35.

Janower ML: Acute diverticulitis. N Engl J Med 1998;339:1081.

Lee EC et al: Intraoperative colonic lavage in nonelective surgery for diverticular disease. Dis Colon Rectum 1997;40:669.

Miura S et al: Recent trends in diverticulosis of the right colon in Japan: retrospective review in a regional hospital. Dis Colon Rectum 2000;43:1383.

Nagorney DM, Adson MA, Pemberton JH: Sigmoid diverticulitis with perforation and generalized peritonitis. Dis Colon Rectum 1985;28:71.

Wong WD et al: Practice parameters for the treatment of sigmoid diverticulitis—supporting documentation. The Standards Task Force American Society of Colon and Rectal Surgeons. Dis Colon Rectum 2000;43:290.

Young-Fadok TM et al: Colonic diverticular disease. Curr Probl Surg 2000;37:457.

COLOVESICAL FISTULA

Colovesical fistula is the most common type of fistulous communication between the urinary bladder and the gastrointestinal tract. There is a 3:1 ratio of men to women with this condition, presumably because in women the uterus and adnexa are situated between the colon and the bladder.

Diverticulitis is the most common cause of colovesical fistula. This complication occurs in 2–4% of cases of diverticulitis, though an even higher incidence is reported from specialized referral centers. Carcinoma of the colon, cancer of other organs such as the bladder, Crohn's disease, radiation bowel injury, external trauma, foreign bodies, and iatrogenic injuries are other causes or underlying conditions.

A colovesical fistula may cause surprisingly little disturbance to the patient, and some patients remain completely asymptomatic. The appearance of a fistula from diverticulitis or colon cancer is seldom accompanied by dramatic or sudden abdominal symptoms; more typically, refractory urinary tract infection is the presenting complaint. Fecaluria and pneumaturia may have been obvious to the patient, or it may be recollected only in response to direct questioning. The episode of diverticulitis may have gone entirely unnoticed.

Physical examination may disclose a pelvic mass or no abnormalities. Leukocytosis is absent in most cases, and routine blood chemistries are normal. Urinalysis may reveal fecaluria or infected urine. Rigid sigmoidoscopy is usually unrevealing; flexible sigmoidoscopy or colonoscopy may disclose colon cancer or inflammation at the fistula site. Cystoscopy shows bullous edema, but the fistula is usually not visible. CT detects small amounts of air in the bladder in 90% of patients. Barium enema, sonography, and cystography may demonstrate the fistula, but small communications escape detection. In some cases, the fistula is not demonstrable because it has closed, at least temporarily.

Colovesical fistulas require surgical treatment if they persist, but there is no need for emergency or urgent operation. Patients may recover well from spontaneous drainage of a paracolic abscess through a fistula into the bladder, and operation can be delayed to be sure it is necessary and by then the conditions will be more favorable. Inability to rule out cancer may prompt earlier operation. If a fistula closes spontaneously, as it may do in up to 50% of patients with diverticulitis, requirements for resection depend on the nature of the underlying colonic disease. Some patients tolerate a colovesical fistula so well that operation is deferred indefinitely.

At operation, patients with diverticulitis or colonic carcinoma have mild to moderate inflammatory reaction around the sigmoid colon, which has dropped into the pelvis and adhered to the bladder; severe active diverticulitis with abscess or peritonitis is exceptional. If the fistula has been caused by cancer of the colon, the adherent bladder should not be separated from the colon lest tumor cells be spilled into the pelvis; a disk of bladder wall should be excised in continuity with the colon, the bladder closed primarily, and catheter drainage of the bladder provided for 7–10 days. Fortunately, most colovesical fistulas enter the bladder away from the trigone. Diverticulitis is managed by bluntly dissecting the colon from the bladder, resecting the colon, and performing a primary anastomosis. The bladder side of the fistula is sutured and the bladder is decompressed with a Foley catheter. It is rarely necessary to delay performance of the colonic anastomosis.

Lavery IC: Colonic fistulas. Surg Clin North Am 1996;76:1183.

Vasilevsky CA et al: Fistulas complicating diverticulitis. Int J Colorectal Dis 1998;13:57.

ACUTE LOWER GASTROINTESTINAL HEMORRHAGE

Acute hemorrhage per rectum can originate from lesions in the gastroduodenum, small bowel, colon, or anorectum. A source in the lower gastrointestinal tract is suggested by the passage of dark to bright red blood, but the color of evacuated blood is a function of the length of time it remained in the intestinal tract, and bright red blood may come from a duodenal ulcer or hemorrhoids as well as any point in between. If a patient passing bright red blood is not in shock, the bleeding site is probably in the distal small bowel or colon.

Exsanguinating hemorrhage from the colon in adults is caused by diverticular disease, angiodysplasia, solitary ulcer, ulcerative colitis, ischemic colitis, or a variety of uncommon lesions such as coagulation disorders, radiation injury, chemotherapeutic toxicity, and others. Bleeding occurs in the right colon about as often

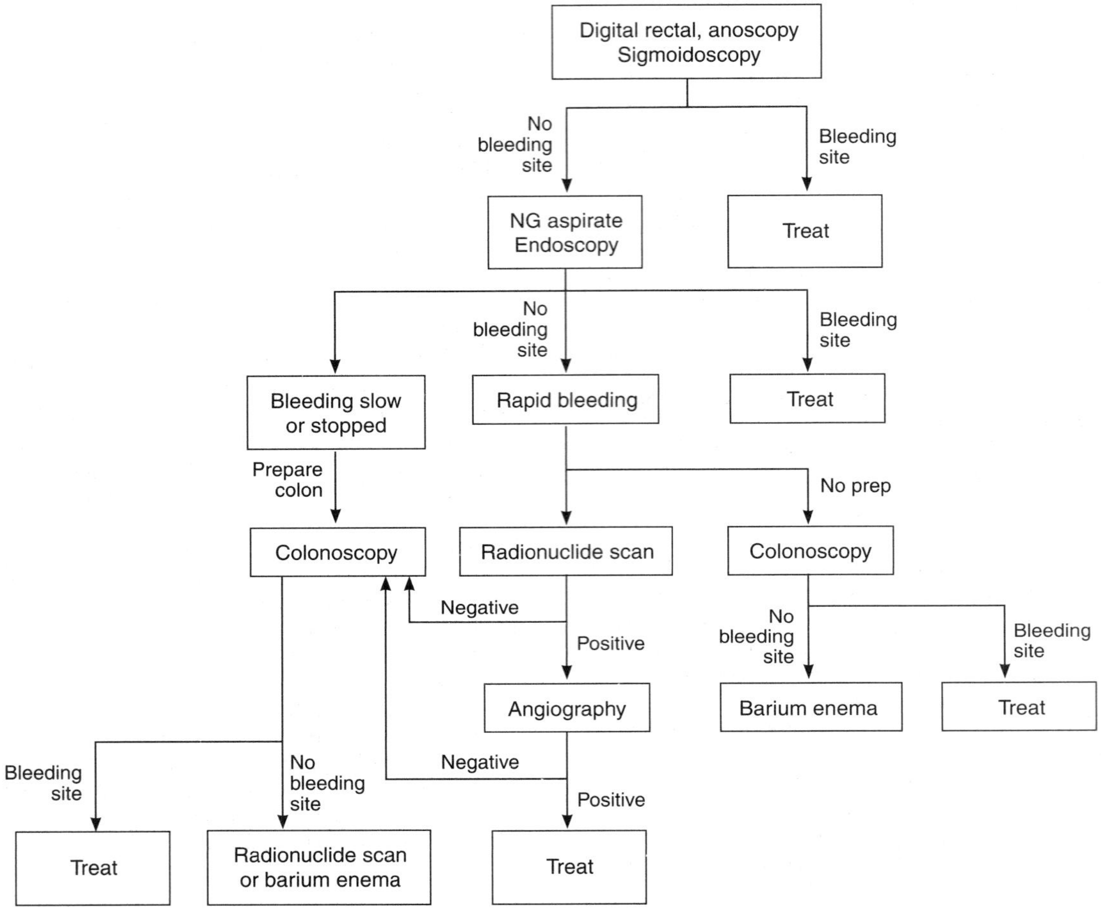

Figure 30–14. Plan for diagnosis and treatment of acute lower gastrointestinal hemorrhage. (NG = nasogastric.)

as in the left colon, probably because angiodysplasias are more prominent on the right side, but right-sided diverticula can also bleed. Bleeding lesions in the small intestine are rare and include hereditary hemorrhagic telangiectasia (Rendu-Osler-Weber syndrome).

Chronic rectal bleeding, typically seen in patients with cancer, polyps, hemorrhoids, fissures, and other conditions, does not require emergent evaluation. Anorectal examination, colonoscopy, and x-rays if indicated can be performed electively. Acute severe hemorrhage, however, is a potentially life-threatening problem, and prompt evaluation and treatment are critical. Some patients bleed rapidly, but the bleeding stops spontaneously after only a small amount of blood is lost, and these patients are never in danger. Usually, however, one cannot be sure that bleeding will not recur, so this type of bleeding must be taken seriously too, which means that aggressive evaluation is needed.

A plan of management of acute lower gastrointestinal hemorrhage is outlined in Figure 30–14. Many decisions depend on the rate of bleeding, which is difficult to include in an algorithm. Bleeding stops spontaneously in 90% of patients before transfusion requirements exceed two units.

The patient with severe rectal bleeding is resuscitated with intravenous fluids and transfusions while the diagnostic procedures are begun. Clotting parameters should be measured and deficits corrected, and associated medical conditions should be identified and treated as soon as possible. Digital rectal examination, anoscopy, and sigmoidoscopy should be performed with no attempt to prepare the bowel. If a bleeding lesion is found in the anorectum, it should be treated. Examples include hemorrhoids, polypoid neoplasm, and ulcerative proctitis.

A nasogastric tube should be inserted and the aspirate inspected for bile, gross blood, and occult blood.

Blood in the stomach is an indication of bleeding from a site proximal to the ligament of Treitz—ie, upper gastrointestinal bleeding—and esophagogastroduodenoscopy is performed. Occasionally, a patient bleeds from the duodenum but blood does not reflux back into the stomach; bile in the nasogastric aspirate would seem to eliminate this possibility, but in the absence of blood or bile, esophagogastroduodenoscopy should be done.

If esophagogastroduodenoscopy is negative and bleeding has presumably stopped or continues at a slow rate, the colon can be prepared and colonoscopy performed within a few hours. The bleeding site is identified in 25–94% of cases, depending in part on skill, experience, and, very importantly, the criteria for inclusion of a patient in this category of bleeding. Some bleeding lesions can be treated colonoscopically with a bipolar probe, heater probe, or laser. Colonoscopy with negative results probably means that bleeding has stopped. Barium enema discloses abnormalities such as diverticula but does not reveal which lesions have been bleeding.

The optimal method for evaluating patients who are bleeding rapidly is controversial, and the decision may hinge on available resources. A radionuclide "bleeding" scan after injection of 99m Tc-labeled red blood cells may show whether bleeding persists and can detect a 0.1 mL/min rate of bleeding. Localization of bleeding is not reliable, but valuable information may be obtained. Angiography is seldom successful in demonstrating an active bleeding site if the bleeding scan is negative, so colonoscopy should be undertaken. Active bleeding shown on radionuclide scan should be followed by angiography.

Selective mesenteric angiography identifies the bleeding site in 14–70% of patients (threshold 0.5 mL/min); here, too, enthusiasm of the angiographer is important. If the bleeding site is seen, intra-arterial infusion of vasopressin controls bleeding, at least transiently, in 35–90% of patients. Definitive treatment with highly selective arterial embolization may be performed with success in 75% of patients.

The other option for rapid bleeding is emergency colonoscopy without preliminary bowel cleansing. Blood is a cathartic, and the colon may be free of stool. Even so, colonoscopy in this situation is difficult. Experts are able to see the bleeding point in up to 50% of patients, and in 70% of cases bleeding can be localized to one region. Endoscopic therapeutic measures can be applied in up to 40% of patients, with success in half of them.

Operation is indicated for bleeding that persists or recurs despite angiographic and endoscopic therapeutic maneuvers. Operation is advisable also in good-risk patients who have stopped bleeding if the bleeding source is known and cannot be managed in some other way (eg, colonoscopic coagulation). Operation is limited to segmental colonic resection if the bleeding site has been localized conclusively. More extensive resection is usually warranted in patients who are bleeding from the right colon and have multiple diverticula in the left colon. If the surgeon has no preoperative localizing data and intraoperative examination is unrevealing, the stomach, small bowel, and colon can be endoscoped during the procedure to search for the source of blood. If all localizing efforts fail and the colon is the likely bleeding site, total abdominal colectomy (usually with primary anastomosis) may be the only recourse. Fortunately, extensive "blind" colectomy is seldom required today.

The mortality rate from lower gastrointestinal hemorrhage is about 10–15%.

Eisen GM et al: An annotated algorithmic approach to acute lower gastrointestinal bleeding. Gastrointest Endosc 2001;53:859.

Farrell JJ, Friedman LS: Gastrointestinal bleeding in the elderly. Gastroenterol Clin North Am 2001;30:377.

Gordon RL et al: Selective arterial embolization for the control of lower gastrointestinal bleeding. Am J Surg 1997;174:24.

Jensen DM: What to choose for diagnosis of bleeding colonic angiomas: colonoscopy, angiography, or helical computed tomography angiography? Gastroenterology 2000;119:581.

Luchtefeld MA et al: Evaluation of transarterial embolization for lower gastrointestinal bleeding. Dis Colon Rectum 2000;43:532.

The role of endoscopy in the patient with lower gastrointestinal bleeding. American Society for Gastrointestinal Endoscopy. Gastrointest Endosc 1998;48:685.

Suzman MS et al: Accurate localization and surgical management of active lower gastrointestinal hemorrhage with technetium-labeled erythrocyte scintigraphy. Ann Surg 1996;224:29.

ANGIODYSPLASIA

Angiodysplasia is an acquired condition most often affecting people over age 60. It is a focal submucosal vascular ectasia that has a propensity to bleed spontaneously. Most lesions are located in the cecum and proximal ascending colon, but in younger persons they are occasionally found in the small bowel, principally the jejunum. Multiple lesions occur in 25% of cases. Aortic stenosis is found in patients with angiodysplasias, but whether they are truly related is still being argued. Von Willebrand's disease is present in some patients, and it has been suggested that the two conditions may be reflections of a generalized tissue disorder. Bleeding is typically intermittent and is rarely massive; a typical episode requires transfusion of two to four units of blood and is not associated with hypotension. Angiodysplasia may also present clinically as melena or as iron deficiency anemia and guaiac-positive stools.

The diagnosis is made in some cases by colonoscopy, and colonoscopic therapy is often successful. Incidental angiomas should be ignored. The lesions are characterized angiographically by (1) an early-filling vein (ie, within 4–5 seconds after injection), (2) a vascular tuft, and (3) a delayed-emptying vein. It is generally thought that two of the three features should be seen for the diagnosis to be secure. Active bleeding (ie, extravasation) is rarely demonstrated by angiography. As many as 25% of persons over age 60 with no history of gastrointestinal bleeding have angiodysplasias of the cecum, so the finding of a lesion is not proof that it has caused bleeding.

The natural history of angiodysplasia is not well delineated, and in elderly, poor-risk patients who have bled only once, expectant management may be preferable to surgery if colonoscopic therapeutic methods are unsuccessful. Operation should consist of right hemicolectomy if the right colon was shown to be the bleeding site. It may be wise to resect the entire colon, with ileorectal anastomosis, in good-risk patients who also have extensive left-sided diverticulosis. In one series, 23% of patients who underwent operation for presumably bleeding colonic angiodysplasias were eventually found to have a small bowel lesion also.

Foutch PG: Colonic angiodysplasia. Gastroenterologist 1997;5:148.

Orsi P, Guatti-Zuliani C, Okolicsanyi L: Long-acting octreotide is effective in controlling rebleeding angiodysplasia of the gastrointestinal tract. Dig Liver Dis 2001;33:330.

Rockey DC: Occult gastrointestinal bleeding. N Engl J Med 1999;341:38.

Sharma R, Gorbien MJ: Angiodysplasia and lower gastrointestinal tract bleeding in elderly patients. Arch Intern Med 1995;155:807.

Veyradier A et al: Abnormal von Willebrand factor in bleeding angiodysplasias of the digestive tract. Gastroenterology 2001;120:346.

VOLVULUS

ESSENTIALS OF DIAGNOSIS

- *Colicky abdominal pain, usually with persistence of pain between spasms.*
- *Abdominal distention.*
- *Vomiting sometimes.*
- *Usually older age groups.*
- *Characteristic x-ray findings.*

General Considerations

Rotation of a segment of the intestine on an axis formed by its mesentery may result in partial or complete obstruction of the lumen and may be followed by circulatory impairment of the bowel (Figure 30–15). Volvulus of the colon involves the cecum (30%), sigmoid (65%), transverse colon (3%), or splenic flexure (2%). Volvulus of the colon accounts for 5–10% of cases of large bowel obstruction in the USA and is the second most common cause of complete colonic obstruction. In certain countries where the population consumes a high-residue diet, volvulus is the most frequent cause of large bowel obstruction. Volvulus—sigmoid more often than cecal—accounts for 25% of intestinal obstructions during pregnancy; it occurs most often in the last trimester, probably because the enlarging uterus displaces the colon.

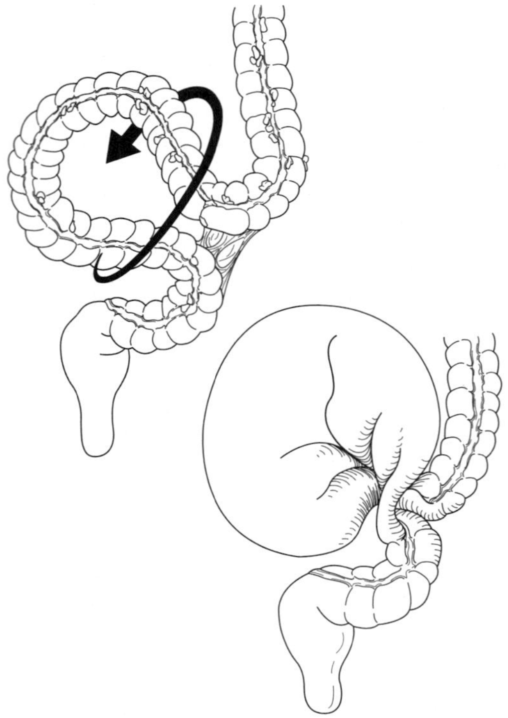

Figure 30–15. Volvulus of the sigmoid colon. The twist is counterclockwise in most cases of sigmoid volvulus.

Elongation of the sigmoid and rectosigmoid is a predisposing factor in sigmoid volvulus; 50% of patients are over age 70, and many patients are mentally ill or bedridden persons who do not evacuate stool with regularity. Chagas' disease of the colon is an important cause of sigmoid volvulus in South America. Formation of cecal volvulus requires a cecum that is hypermobile owing to incomplete embryologic fixation of the ascending colon. The bowel twists about the mesentery, forming a closed-loop obstruction as the entry and exit points of the twist engage; obstruction of the lumen usually occurs when the rotation is 180 degrees. When the twist is 360 degrees, the veins are occluded, and the circulatory impairment leads to gangrene and perforation if treatment is not instituted promptly. A related condition called **cecal bascule** involves folding of the ascending colon so that the cecum moves anteriorly and superiorly, causing obstruction at the site of the transverse fold. Patients may describe intermittent bloating, pain, and obstructive symptoms improved by lying down and massaging the abdomen. Since no axial twist of the mesentery is involved in this situation, early strangulation from occlusion of the main vessels is not a factor.

Clinical Findings

A. Cecal Volvulus

Not only the cecum but also the terminal ileum are involved in the rotation, so the symptoms generally include those of distal small bowel obstruction. Severe intermittent colicky pain begins in the right abdomen. Pain eventually becomes continuous, vomiting ensues, and passage of gas and feces per rectum decreases to the point of obstipation. Abdominal distention is variable; occasionally, a bulging tympanitic mass may be detected. There may be a history of similar but milder attacks, and valid examples of chronic intermittent cecal volvulus exist; they can be detected and operated on electively.

The diagnosis is seldom made without x-ray examination. Plain films show a hugely dilated ovoid cecum that may change position but favors the epigastrium or left upper quadrant. The distended loop may assume a "coffee bean" shape. In cecal volvulus, the concavity of the "coffee bean" points toward the right lower abdominal quadrant, and in sigmoid volvulus it points toward the left lower quadrant. In the early stages, there is a single fluid level that may be mistaken for gastric dilation, but large amounts of gas or fluid cannot be aspirated from the stomach, and the x-ray picture is not changed by this maneuver. Later, the radiologic findings of small bowel obstruction are superimposed on the cecal volvulus. The success rate of diagnosis based on plain abdominal films is extremely variable, ranging from 5% to 90%. Radiographic contrast enema may be diagnostic.

B. Sigmoid Volvulus

In volvulus of the sigmoid, there are intermittent cramplike pains, increasing in severity as obstipation becomes complete. Abdominal distention may be marked. There may be a history of transient attacks in which spontaneous reduction of the volvulus has occurred. On a plain film of the abdomen, a single greatly distended loop of bowel that has lost its haustral markings is usually seen

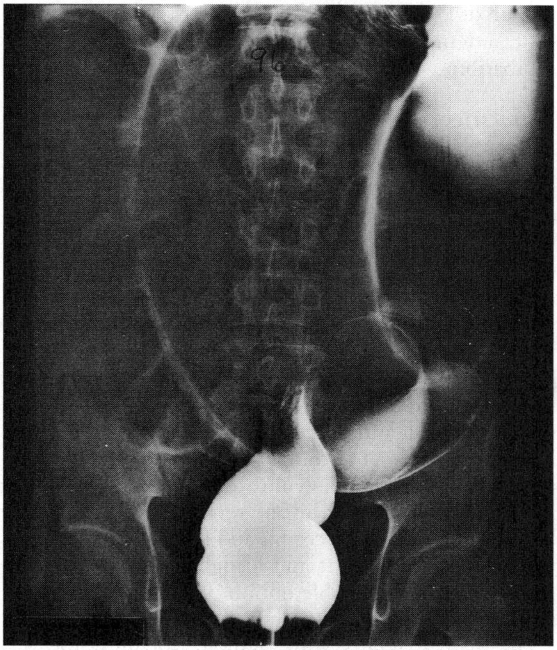

Figure 30–16. Volvulus of the sigmoid colon. Barium enema taken with the patient in the supine position. Note the massively dilated sigmoid colon. The distinct vertical crease, which represents juxtaposition of adjacent walls of the dilated loop, points toward the site of torsion. The barium column resembles a "bird's beak" or "ace of spades" because of the way in which the lumen tapers toward the volvulus.

rising up out of the pelvis, frequently as high as the diaphragm. On barium enema, a "bird's beak" or "ace of spades" deformity with spiral narrowing of the upper end of the lower segment is pathognomonic (Figure 30–16). Between attacks, barium enema may reveal sigmoid megacolon. The entire colon may be termed a megacolon in some cases.

Differential Diagnosis

Cecal volvulus must be differentiated from colonic pseudo-obstruction and from other causes of small bowel and colonic obstruction. Sigmoid volvulus mimics other types of large bowel obstruction. Alertness to the possibility and correct interpretation of x-rays are the essentials of diagnosis.

Complications

Early diagnosis and treatment are imperative because perforation may occur if circulation to the bowel is impaired. Delay may be due to incorrect diagnosis or to futile attempts at proximal decompression by gastric intubation.

Treatment

In cecal volvulus decompression is advisable as soon as the patient can be prepared by replacing fluid and electrolyte deficits. Colonoscopic detorsion and decompression may be attempted if an expert is available, especially in patients who have serious associated disease that would make operation hazardous. Resection and anastomosis is the preferred operation even if the bowel is viable, due to better long-term results than with lesser procedures. A laparoscopic or open approach may be utilized. Cecopexy (suture fixation of the bowel to the parietal peritoneum) has been reported and gives good immediate results, but the long-term success rate is controversial; recurrent volvulus developed in 29% of patients after cecopexy in one review. Tube cecostomy both decompresses the cecum and fixes it, but problems with tube management and a high risk for recurrence make this a less favorable option. Gangrenous colon or small bowel is found in about 20% of cases.

In many patients with sigmoid volvulus, the distended sigmoid can be decompressed by gentle insertion of a flexible colonoscope or sigmoidoscope. Decompression by passage of a tube through a rigid sigmoidoscope is also possible when flexible endoscopy is unavailable. Endoscopic decompression is contraindicated if there is evidence of strangulation or perforation. Percutaneous decompression of sigmoid volvulus has been reported, but it cannot be recommended for general use. If decompression is successful, good-risk young patients should be scheduled for elective resection of the affected bowel as soon as the colon can be prepared, because the recurrence rate after decompression alone is 50%. However, in patients with severe disease of other organ systems, one may need to tailor this approach. Emergency operation is performed if strangulation or perforation is suspected or if attempts to decompress the bowel per rectum are unsuccessful. Gangrenous bowel is found in about one-third of such patients and is treated by resection. If the sigmoid is viable, most surgeons proceed with resection, deferring anastomosis to a later time if the bowel is unprepared. If the entire colon is a megacolon, total abdominal colectomy should be considered. Recurrent volvulus in nonoperated patients is managed by transrectal decompression followed by a definitive surgical procedure in all patients but those with very severe associated disease.

Prognosis

The mortality rate after emergency operation in patients with cecal volvulus is 12%; if the bowel is gangrenous, 35% of patients die after resection. Recurrence after cecopexy or resection is very unusual.

Sigmoid volvulus is fatal in about 50% of patients with perforation; mortality rates are much lower with gangrene alone, and only 5% of patients die after operation if the bowel is viable. Elective resection after endoscopic decompression has a low mortality rate, and recurrent volvulus is rare. Nonresection therapies are ineffective at preventing recurrence.

Feldman D: The coffee bean sign. Radiology 2000;216:178.

Grossmann EM et al: Sigmoid volvulus in Department of Veterans Affairs Medical Centers. Dis Colon Rectum 2000;43:414.

Madiba TE, Thomson SR: The management of sigmoid volvulus. J R Coll Surg Edinb 2000;45:74.

COLITIS

Colitis is a nonspecific term. Patients have diarrhea, abdominal pain, systemic symptoms, and abnormal endoscopic, radiographic, and laboratory tests. The task of the clinician is to differentiate among the various causes of colitis discussed below.

1. Idiopathic Mucosal Ulcerative Colitis

ESSENTIALS OF DIAGNOSIS

- *Diarrhea, usually bloody.*
- *Abdominal cramps.*
- *Fever, weight loss, anemia.*
- *Absence of specific fecal pathogens.*
- *Endoscopic and radiographic abnormalities.*

General Considerations

The age at onset of ulcerative colitis has a bimodal distribution, with the first peak between ages 15 and 30 years and a second, lower peak in the sixth to eighth decades. Females are affected slightly more often than males. The annual incidence varies from 5 to 12 per 100,000 population, and the prevalence is 50–150 per 100,000 population. The disease is found worldwide but is more common in Western countries. It is uncommon in Asia. In the USA, Jews are more commonly affected than non-Jews, but in Israel the prevalence among new immigrants is low.

The cause of ulcerative colitis is not known. A combination of genetic, environmental, and host immune response factors appear to be important in the pathogenesis of inflammatory bowel disease. It is also possible that ulcerative colitis and Crohn's disease are different manifestations of a mechanistic continuum. Genetic factors contribute the susceptibility to inflammatory bowel disease but cannot be explained by simple Mendelian inheritance. In 15–40% of patients there is a family history of ulcerative colitis or Crohn's disease. Based on genome-wide screening and linkage analysis, the IBD1 locus on chromosome 16 appears to be important for Crohn's disease but not for ulcerative colitis. In addition, a locus within chromosome 5 appears to be associated with early-onset Crohn's disease. Chromosomes 3, 5, 7, and 12 have been linked to ulcerative colitis but not Crohn's disease.

Environmental factors are also important; only 45% of identical twins are concordant for Crohn's disease. Luminal flora is a requisite and perhaps central factor in the development of inflammatory bowel disease. This may explain the therapeutic benefits seen with broad-spectrum antibiotics and probiotics in specific subgroups of patients. Perhaps the best environmental association is seen with Crohn's disease and the use of nonsteroidal anti-inflammatory drugs, which can induce disease flares. Appendectomy is a protective factor against later development of ulcerative colitis. Cigarette smoking appears to be protective against ulcerative colitis, but it increases the risk of Crohn's disease.

The host immune response to mucosal antigens and environmental factors is also important. Differences may be on the basis of altered immune activation or a failure of counterregulation. The mucosa immune-cell population in Crohn's disease is dominated by CD4+ T lymphocytes with a type 1 helper T-cell (Th1), characterized by the production of interferon-γ and interleukin-2 (IL-2). In contrast, patients with ulcerative colitis exhibit a predominance of the type 2 helper T-cell (Th2) phenotype, characterized by the production of transforming growth factor β (TGF-β) and IL-5, but not IL-4. Ultimately, the activation of immune-cell populations results in the production of a variety of nonspecific inflammatory mediators that include cytokines, chemokines, and growth factors, as well as metabolites of arachidonic acid (eg, prostaglandins and leukotrienes). These mediators eventually play a critical role in the manifestation of inflammatory bowel disease.

Ulcerative colitis is a diffuse but contiguous inflammatory disease confined to the mucosa initially. Abscesses form in the crypts of Lieberkühn and penetrate the superficial submucosa, and by spreading horizontally cause the overlying mucosa to slough. Vascular congestion and hemorrhage are prominent. The margins of the ulcers are raised as mucosal tags that project into the lumen (pseudopolyps or inflammatory polyps). Except in the most severe forms, the muscular layers are spared; the serosal surface usually shows only dilated congested blood vessels. In fulminant disease, when the full thickness is involved, the colon may dilate or perforate. The colon is shortened, but the mesocolon remains thin—in contrast to Crohn's disease.

Ulcerative colitis can manifest as ulcerative proctitis (involvement limited to the rectum), ulcerative proctosigmoiditis (involvement limited to the rectum and sigmoid colon), left-sided ulcerative colitis (inflammation is distal to the splenic flexure), and pancolitis (inflammation extends proximal to the splenic flexure or involves the entire colon). A few centimeters of distal ileum are ulcerated in 10% of patients with pancolitis (backwash ileitis). The diseased areas are contiguous and extend proximally from the rectum. The presence of segmental involvement or skip lesions should prompt the evaluation for Crohn's disease.

Clinical Findings

A. Symptoms and Signs

The cardinal symptoms are rectal bleeding and diarrhea: frequent discharges of watery stool mixed with blood, pus, and mucus accompanied by tenesmus, rectal urgency, and even anal incontinence. Nearly two-thirds of patients have cramping abdominal pain and variable degrees of fever, vomiting, weight loss, and dehydration. The onset may be insidious or acute and fulminating, and the clinical findings differ accordingly. Mild disease may be manifested only by loose or frequent stools, and, paradoxically, a few patients complain of constipation. In isolated instances, the only symptoms may be from systemic complications such as arthropathy or pyoderma. Dairy products may aggravate diarrhea.

If the disease is mild, physical examination may be normal, but in severe disease the abdomen is tender, especially in the left lower quadrant, and the colon may be distended. As a rule, in contrast to Crohn's disease, the anus is spared in ulcerative colitis. However, severe rectal inflammation may result in considerable tenderness and spasticity during digital rectal examination. The examining finger may be covered with blood, mucus, or pus.

A simple classification of the severity of an attack was devised by Truelove and Witts. The assessment of disease severity is based on six simple clinical signs (Table 30–11).

Sigmoidoscopy is essential. The rectal mucosa is granular, dull, hyperemic, and friable, so that blood oozes where the mucosa is touched. The submucosal vascular pattern is lost because of edema. Gross ulcers are not visible in the rectum in ulcerative colitis because of the superficial nature of these lesions. In more advanced disease, the mucosa is purplish-red, velvety, and extremely friable. Blood mixed with mucopus is evident in the

Table 30-11. Ulcerative colitis disease severity (based on the Truelove and Witt classification).

Symptoms	Mild	Severe	Fulminant
Stools (per day)	< 4	> 6	> 10
Hematochezia	Intermittent	Frequent	Continuous
Temperature	Normal	> 37.5 °C	
Pulse (beats/min)	Normal	> 90	
Hemoglobin	Normal	< 75% of normal	Requires transfusion
ESR	< 30 mm/h	> 30 mm/h	

lumen. The disease is uniform in the affected bowel, and patches of normal mucosa are not seen. If the mucosa is not grossly diseased, biopsy may be helpful to confirm the diagnosis. In the recovery phase, mucosal hyperemia and edema subside and inflammatory polyps may be seen. The healing mucosa is typically dull and granular and has a neovascular pattern of telangiectatic vessels that differs from the normal pink mucosa.

B. Laboratory Findings

Anemia, leukocytosis, and an elevated sedimentation rate are usually present. Severe disease leads to hypoalbuminemia; depletion of water, electrolytes, and vitamins; and laboratory evidence of steatorrhea. Reduced plasma antithrombin III levels may contribute to thromboembolic complications. Smears of the stool should be examined for parasites, bacteria, and leukocytes, and stool should be sent for cultures.

C. Imaging Studies

Barium enema examination should not be preceded by catharsis in acute cases and should not be performed at all in severely ill patients, because it may precipitate acute colonic dilation. Plain films may reveal severe colonic dilation (megacolon) with fulminant disease.

Barium x-rays in acute ulcerative colitis show mucosal irregularity that varies from fine serrations to rough, ragged, undermined ulcers. As the disease progresses, haustrations are gradually effaced, and the colon narrows and shortens because of muscular rigidity (Figure 30–17). Pseudopolyposis signifies severe ulceration. Widening of the space between the sacrum and rectum is due either to periproctitis or to shortening of the bowel. The presence of a stricture should always arouse suspicion of cancer. An upper gastrointestinal contrast examination with small bowel follow through should be performed to rule out Crohn's disease.

CT may be helpful in assessing patients with severe disease. More recently evaluation of the small bowel by CT enterography has become useful.

D. Colonoscopic Findings

Colonoscopy should be performed in most situations. Usually the instrument need be inserted only into the sigmoid in order to make the initial diagnosis. Because of the danger of perforation, colonoscopy should be performed with great care if the disease is active, and it should not be done in the presence of colonic dilation. In chronic disease, colonoscopy with biopsies is valuable in surveillance for cancer. Strictures and other x-ray abnormalities can be investigated by colonoscopy also.

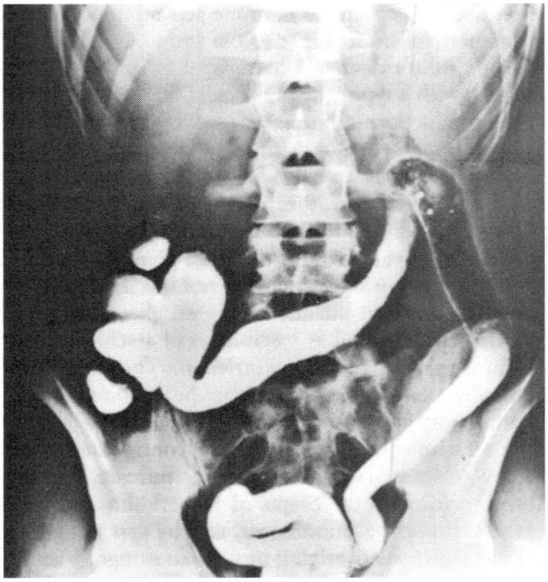

Figure 30–17. Ulcerative colitis. Barium enema x-ray of colon. Note shortening of colon, loss of haustral markings ("lead pipe" appearance), and fine serrations at the edges of the bowel wall that represent multiple small ulcers.

Differential Diagnosis

Malignant neoplasms of the colon (including lymphomas) and diverticular disease must be considered in the differential diagnosis. Salmonellosis and other bacillary dysenteries are diagnosed by repeated stool cultures. Shigellosis may be suspected on the basis of a positive methylene blue stain for fecal leukocytes. *Campylobacter jejuni* is a common cause of bloody diarrhea; the organisms can be cultured from the stool, and serum antibody titers rise during the illness. Hemorrhagic colitis—a syndrome of bloody diarrhea and abdominal cramps but no fever—is associated with infection by *Escherichia coli* O157:H7. Legionella infections can mimic ulcerative colitis. Gonococcal proctitis is detected by culture of rectal swabs. Herpes simplex virus is the most common cause of nongonococcal proctitis in homosexual men. *Chlamydia trachomatis* infections are also common in this group; the mucosa is markedly inflamed and resembles Crohn's disease; the organism can be cultured. It is most important in every case to rule out amebiasis (see Chapter 8) by microscopic examination of stool, rectal swabs, or rectal biopsies; serologic tests confirm that clinical infection has occurred. Corticosteroids must never be given to a patient with presumed idiopathic ulcerative colitis until amebiasis has been excluded.

Rare cases of histoplasmosis, tuberculosis, cytomegalovirus disease, schistosomiasis, amyloidosis, or Behçet's disease may be very difficult to diagnose. AIDS-related gastrointestinal infections are increasingly common. Colitis caused by antibiotics is discussed separately below; the history is important in this type of disease. NSAIDs can cause mucosal inflammation and even strictures in the large intestine. Collagenous colitis may or may not be related to NSAID usage. Watery diarrhea is the main symptom of this syndrome; endoscopy is grossly normal; and biopsies show a thickened band of collagen just beneath the surface. Treatment to date has been difficult, but most patients are not seriously troubled by this condition. Ischemic colitis has a segmental pattern of involvement quite unlike the contiguous distribution of ulcerative colitis. Functional diarrhea can mimic colitis, but organic disease must be excluded before it can be concluded that the diarrhea is functional. Malacoplakia is a rare chronic granulomatous disease that can cause colonic strictures and may resemble colitis.

Diversion colitis is inflammation of a previously normal segment of colon or rectum following construction of a temporary colostomy, eg, in a two-stage approach to diverticulitis. Deficiency of mucosal nutrients may be responsible, and inflammation may resolve with topical application of short-chain fatty acids. Restoration of intestinal continuity also solves the problem.

The most difficult differential diagnosis is between mucosal ulcerative colitis and Crohn's colitis (Table 30–12). None of the features are specific for one or the other disease, and often the differentiation can be made only after all the data have been assembled. About 10% of cases cannot be classified (indeterminate colitis).

Complications

The following **extracolonic manifestations** may occur in association with ulcerative colitis. There is an inexact relationship between the severity of the colitis and these complications: (1) lesions of the skin and mucous membranes, eg, erythema nodosum, erythema multiforme, pyoderma gangrenosum, pustular dermatitis, and aphthous stomatitis; (2) uveitis; (3) bone and joint lesions, eg, arthralgia, arthritis, and ankylosing spondylitis; (4) hepatobiliary and possibly pancreatic lesions, eg, fatty infiltration, pericholangitis, cirrhosis, sclerosing cholangitis, bile duct carcinoma, gallstones, and pancreatic insufficiency; (5) anemia, usually due to iron deficiency; (6) malnutrition and growth retardation; and (7) pericarditis. Sclerosing cholangitis may require liver transplantation.

Perianal diseases may affect patients with ulcerative colitis just as they do the general population. The presence of perianal findings in a patient with ulcerative colitis, however, should prompt a thorough reassessment of the patient's presentation to exclude Crohn's disease.

Perforation of the colon, which occurs in about 3% of hospitalized patients, is responsible for more deaths than any other complication of ulcerative colitis. The risk of perforation is highest in the initial attack of the disease and correlates well with its extent and severity. It occurs most commonly in the sigmoid or splenic flexure and may result in a localized abscess or generalized fecal peritonitis. Any severely diseased colon may perforate, but patients with toxic dilation (megacolon) are especially vulnerable. Systemic therapy (corticosteroids and antibiotics) may mask the development of this complication.

Acute colonic dilation (toxic megacolon) occurs in approximately 3–10% of patients and in about 9% of patients coming to emergency operation. The patients are severely ill (toxic) and usually have one or more of the following contributing factors: inflammation involving the muscular coats, hypokalemia, opioid use, anticholinergic use, or barium enema examination. Toxic megacolon is diagnosed by plain abdominal x-rays or barium enemas, which show a thickened bowel wall and dilated lumen (> 6 cm in the transverse colon); often, the luminal air outlines irregular nodular pseudopolyps (Figure 30–18). Placing the patient in the knee-elbow position and use of a rectal tube are recommended medical measures to help the colon decompress. Toxic dilation also occurs in Crohn's disease and in other types of colitis such as amebiasis and salmonellosis.

Massive hemorrhage is an uncommon but life-threatening complication.

Carcinoma of the colon or rectum begins to appear 8–10 years after onset of ulcerative colitis. The cumulative

Table 30–12. Comparison of various features of ulcerative colitis with those of granulomatous colitis.

	Ulcerative (Mucosal) Colitis	Crohn's (Granulomatous) Colitis
Signs and symptoms		
Diarrhea	Marked.	Present; less severe.
Gross bleeding	Characteristic.	Infrequent.
Perianal lesions	Infrequent, mild.	Frequent, complex; may precede diagnosis of intestinal disease.
Toxic dilatation	Yes (3–10%).	Yes (2–5%).
Perforation.	Free.	Localized.
Systemic manifestations (arthritis, uveitis, pyoderma, hepatitis	Common.	Common.
X-ray studies	Confluent, diffuse. Tiny serrations, coarse mucosa, mucosal tags. Concentric involvement. Internal fistulas very rare. Colon only except in backwash ileitis; may be limited to left side.	Skip areas. Longitudinal ulcers, transverse ridges, "cobblestone" appearance. Eccentric involvement. Internal fistula common. Any portion of intestinal tract may be involved; may be limited to ileum and right colon.
Morphology		
Gross	Confluent involvement. Rectum usually involved. Mesocolon not involved; nodes enlarged. Widespread ragged superficial ulceration. Inflammatory polyps (pseudopolyps) common. No thickening of bowel wall.	Segmental involvement with or without skip areas. Rectum often not involved. Thickened mesocolon; pronounced lymph node enlargement. Large longitudinal ulcers or transverse fissures. Inflammatory polyps not prominent. Thickened bowel wall.
Microscopic	Inflammatory reaction usually limited to mucosa and submucosa; only in severe disease are muscle coats involved; no fibrosis. Granulomas rare.	Chronic inflammation of all layers of bowel wall; damage to muscle layers usual; submucosal fibrosis. Granulomas frequent.
Natural history	Exacerbations, remissions; may be explosive, lethal.	Indolent, recurrent.
Treatment		
Response to medical treatment	Good response in 85% of cases.	Difficult to evaluate; less well controlled over long term.
Type of surgical treatment and response	Colectomy with ileoanal anastomosis; proctocolectomy with conventional or continent ileostomy. No recurrence.	Segmental colectomy; total colectomy with ileorectal anastomosis; proctocolectomy if rectum severely diseased. Recurrence common.

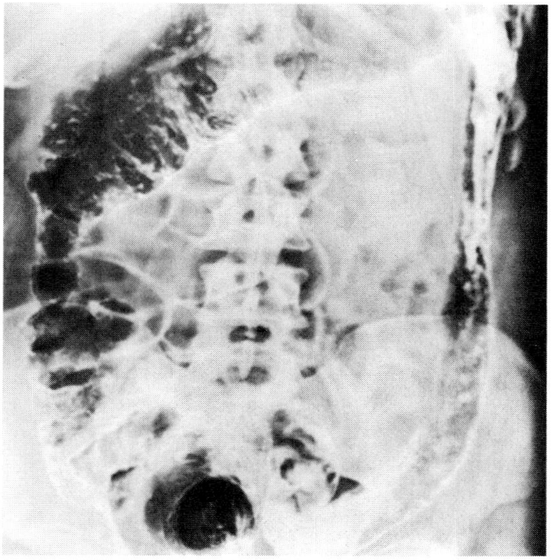

Figure 30–18. Barium enema showing acute colonic dilation in ulcerative colitis. Note dilation of the transverse colon, the multiple irregular densities in the lumen that represent pseudopolyps, and the loss of haustral markings.

incidence increases by about 1% per year after 10 years. Factors that are thought to identify patients at greatest risk for cancer are the extent of colitis, the severity of disease, the duration of active disease, and the presence of primary sclerosing cholangitis. Cancers in ulcerative colitis tend to be multicentric and may be difficult to recognize grossly by endoscopy or x-ray because they are small and flat. Periodic surveillance colonoscopy with multiple random biopsies is recommended to search for epithelial dysplasia. Dysplasia, low or high-grade, is an indication for colectomy, and the finding of a dysplasia associated lesion or mass (DALM) is particularly ominous. In the presence of high-grade dysplasia, the chances of finding cancer in the colon are 30–50%, and some of the cancers are advanced. There is an intensive search for a more sensitive marker, and one or more of the molecular markers may fill the need eventually. Meanwhile, the risks and benefits of colectomy should be weighed against those of repeated colonoscopy in patients with a long history of ulcerative colitis; with the availability of ileoanal anastomosis, colectomy is more appealing to physicians and their patients than in the past.

Treatment

A. Medical Therapy

The goals of conservative therapy are to terminate the acute attack as rapidly as possible and to prevent relapse. Management depends on the severity of the attack and the age group; children and the elderly present special problems.

1. Mild to moderate attack—Mild or insidious disease usually can be checked with outpatient management. Diet should be free of bovine milk products and any other food that exacerbates diarrhea in the individual patient. In controlled trials, sulfasalazine, 2–6 g/d orally, is effective for inducing and maintaining remission in mild to moderately active ulcerative colitis. Patients who are allergic to sulfonamide drugs can obtain similar benefit with oral mesalamine, 2–5 g/d. Other related drugs include olsalazine (1–3 g/d) and balsalazide (6.75 g/d). Drug-associated toxicity limits utility in up to 30% of patients treated with these regimens. Ulcerative proctitis and some cases of proctosigmoiditis can be treated with topical mesalamine or steroids. These agents can be delivered by suppository or foam if disease involves only 15–20 cm of distal bowel, and enemas can be used if colitis extends proximally for up to 60 cm; there are several choices of preparations.

Controlled trials have shown that high-dose oral corticosteroids, 100 mg/d cortisone or 40–60 mg/d prednisone, are effective for inducing remission in mild and severe ulcerative colitis. However, low-dose steroids are not effective at maintaining remission. Similar results have been obtained with rectally administered steroids for distal disease.

Azathioprine at doses of 1.5–2.5 mg/kg/day has been shown to be effective for steroid sparing in patients with steroid-dependent ulcerative colitis. It may also be useful for maintaining remission. There is no role for antibiotic therapy as primary treatment for ulcerative colitis.

2. Severe attack—Severe or fulminating ulcerative colitis requires hospitalization. Nasogastric suction is required in patients with colonic dilation or those at risk of developing this complication. Otherwise, "bowel rest" has no special benefit, and when the danger of dilation has passed, polymeric total enteral nutrition is just as safe and effective as total parenteral nutrition in patients with acute severe ulcerative colitis.

Corticosteroids are given intravenously initially as hydrocortisone (100–300 mg/d) or methylprednisolone (20–80 mg/d). Broad-spectrum antibiotics are often given to severely ill patients in an effort to prevent systemic sepsis from colonic bacterial translocation. Cyclosporine (4 mg/kg/d intravenously) is effective for severe colitis refractory to steroid therapy. Toxicity can be significant, however, and the long-term benefit of cyclosporine treatment is unknown. Hypokalemia is common and should be corrected. Caution should be exercised in administering anticholinergics and opioids because they may precipitate acute dilation of the colon.

3. Maintenance—Nightly mesalamine suppositories or oral mesalamine serves as maintenance therapy for patients with distal colitis. Oral mesalamine or 5-aminosalicylic acid reduces relapse rates of patients with more extensive colitis. Chronic steroid use should be avoided because of the systemic side effects even if the drug is administered topically. Furthermore, there are no studies that can demonstrate efficacy of low-dose steroids (prednisone 40 mg every other day, or hydrocortisone enema 100 mg twice a week) in maintaining remission in ulcerative colitis. Immunosuppressive therapy (azathioprine) is used by some physicians to treat ulcerative colitis in steroid-dependent patients. Transdermal nicotine reportedly has a therapeutic effect on ulcerative colitis, but clinicians are understandably reluctant to use this agent until more is learned about long-term safety and efficacy.

B. Surgical Treatment

1. Indications—

a. Acute disease—Emergency operation is indicated for proved or suspected perforation of the colon. Operation on an urgent basis is required for an acute problem (toxic megacolon, hemorrhage, or fulminating colitis) treated medically at first and then surgically if the response is inadequate. There are no firm guidelines for when to switch from medical to surgical therapy in these cases. If toxic megacolon does not respond to treatment, prompt operation is necessary to avoid perforation. Fulminating disease without megacolon should improve in 4–5 days or less; otherwise, operation may be advisable. Prolonged medical treatment may result in the need for a staged surgical approach, whereas earlier intervention may require only one operation.

b. Chronic disease—Intractable disease is difficult to define. Frequent exacerbations, chronic continuous symptoms, malnutrition, weakness, inability to work, incapacity to enjoy a full social and sexual life—all are elements of intractable disease. Exacerbation of disease when corticosteroids are tapered—and thus inability to discontinue these drugs over months or even years—is a compelling indication for colectomy. Children with chronic colitis may have impaired growth and development. Prevention or treatment of carcinoma is an important indication for operation. Severe extracolonic manifestations, such as arthritis or pyoderma gangrenosum, may respond to colectomy, but other problems (eg, ankylosing spondylitis or sclerosing cholangitis) do not improve after the diseased colon is removed.

2. Surgical procedures—Total colectomy with ileoanal anastomosis (restorative proctocolectomy, ileal pouch–anal anastomosis) is the elective operation of choice in most patients. Obesity and advanced age are limiting factors. In this procedure, the entire colon and rectum are excised, and the ileum (made into a reservoir or pouch) is brought into the pelvis and anastomosed to the anal canal just above the dentate line (Figure 30–19). Rectal

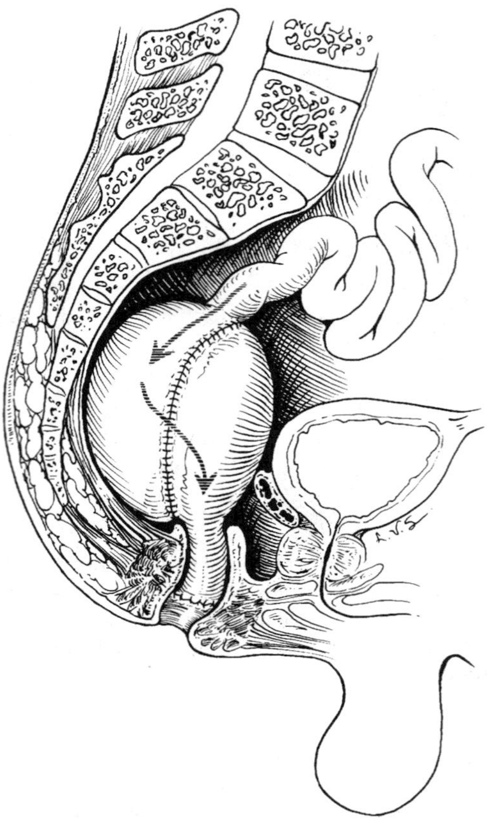

Figure 30–19. View of the pelvis after colectomy and ileoanal anastomosis in a male. The J pouch, shown here, is one of several types of reservoirs and is most commonly utilized. The pouch is anastomosed to the anal canal just above the dentate line.

mucosectomy was once routine, but many surgeons now do not strip the mucosa at all in patients with colitis; instead, the full thickness of rectum is excised to eliminate disease while preserving good rectal function. A temporary ileostomy to protect the ileoanal anastomosis for 2–3 months is not mandatory, but it is used if there is concern about the quality of the anastomosis or the patient's healing properties. Success is expected in 95% of patients. In a series of 1310 patients undergoing ileal pouch-anal anastomosis at the Mayo Clinic before 1994, overall operative mortality was 0.2% and the postoperative pelvic sepsis rate was 3% in the most recent 4 years. Pouch survival was 98% at 1 year and 91% at 10 years. Pouchitis (inflammation of the reservoir) occurs in up to 40% of patients and the risk increases with time; it usually responds to antibiotics such as metronidazole or ciprofloxacin.

Proctocolectomy with permanent conventional ileostomy is chosen in patients who may not be candidates for the ileoanal procedure. In an emergency operation, the rectum is preserved to minimize operative complications in an ill patient and to make it possible to do an ileoanal procedure later. This staged operation therefore consists of total abdominal colectomy (subtotal colectomy) and ileostomy with a distal mucous fistula or Hartmann procedure. Ileorectal anastomosis (ileoproctostomy, ileorectostomy) and continent ileostomies are seldom used for ulcerative colitis today.

Prognosis

The mortality rate of ulcerative colitis has dropped sharply in the past 2 decades. First attacks are seldom fatal when treated by specialists. In one large series, emergency colectomy was required in 25% of patients with severe first attacks; 60% responded rapidly to medical therapy; and 15% improved slowly on medications alone. Overall, the colitis-related mortality rate during the year after onset is about 1%. Emergency colectomy has a mortality rate of 6%; most of these deaths are due to perforation, a complication that has a fatal outcome in 40% of cases.

The long-term prognosis of ulcerative proctitis is good; about 10% of patients will develop colonic disease by 10 years, and the mortality rate is very low. If colitis involves the left colon, the prognosis is worse, and in patients with pancolitis, the likelihood of operation during the first year is about 25% and the mortality rate is 5% over 10 years. Colorectal cancer in ulcerative colitis is more often diagnosed at an advanced stage than is sporadic cancer, but the prognosis stage-for-stage is the same. Screening with colonoscopy and biopsies seems to have reduced the cancer mortality rate, but there are still too many patients who escape detection until the malignancy has progressed to incurability. The problem is lack of a sensitive marker that predicts cancer before it develops.

The operative mortality rate is less than 1% for elective colectomy. Quality of life after restorative proctocolectomy with an ileal pouch is excellent. Most patients who undergo the procedure are pleased with the outcome compared with their preoperative symptoms and treatment. In an estimated 90% of survivors, colectomy with ileostomy is consistent with normal life, but a few patients experience problems such as small bowel obstruction and ileostomy dysfunction. Altered sexual function after proctectomy occurs in about 12% of men overall, limited mostly to those over age 50. True impotence is found in 3% of men. Sexual dysfunction is common in the first few months in women.

Andersson RE et al: Appendectomy and protection against ulcerative colitis. N Engl J Med 2001;344:808.

Bernstein CN et al: Cancer risk in patients with inflammatory bowel disease: a population-based study. Cancer 2001;91:854.

Bernstein CN et al: The prevalence of extraintestinal diseases in inflammatory bowel disease: a population-based study. Am J Gastroenterol 2001;96:1116.

Blumberg D et al: Restorative proctocolectomy: Ochsner Clinic experience. South Med J 2001;94:467.

D'Haens G et al: Intravenous cyclosporine versus intravenous corticosteroids as single therapy for severe attacks of ulcerative colitis. Gastroenterology 2001;120:1323.

Eaden JA, Abrams KR, Mayberry JF: The risk of colorectal cancer in ulcerative colitis: a meta-analysis. Gut 2001;48:526.

Farmer M et al: Association of susceptibility locus for inflammatory bowel disease on chromosome 16 with both ulcerative colitis and Crohn's disease. Dig Dis Sci 2001;46:632.

Goudet P et al: Characteristics and evolution of extraintestinal manifestations associated with ulcerative colitis after proctocolectomy. Dig Surg 2001;18:51.

Hanauer SB: Inflammatory bowel disease. N Engl J Med 1996; 334:841.

Lawrance IC, Fiocchi C, Chakravarti S: Ulcerative colitis and Crohn's disease: distinctive gene expression profiles and novel susceptibility candidate genes. Hum Mol Genet 2001;10:445.

McIntyre PB et al: Comparing functional results one year and ten years after ileal pouch-anal anastomosis for chronic ulcerative colitis. Dis Colon Rectum 1994;37:303.

Melville DM et al: Surgery for ulcerative colitis in the era of the pouch: The St Mark's Hospital experience. Gut 1994;35:1076.

Robinson M: Medical therapy of inflammatory bowel disease for the 21st century. Eur J Surg Suppl 1998;582:90.

Shelton AA et al: Retrospective review of colorectal cancer in ulcerative colitis at a tertiary center. Arch Surg 1996;131:806.

Thomas GA et al: Transdermal nicotine as maintenance therapy for ulcerative colitis. N Engl J Med 1995;332:988.

2. Crohn's Colitis (Granulomatous Colitis)

The general features of Crohn's disease (regional enteritis, granulomatous colitis, transmural colitis) are described in Chapter 29. Approximately 40% of patients with Crohn's disease have both small and large bowel involvement; 30% have disease limited to the small bowel, 25% have colonic disease alone; and another 8% have anorectal involvement only. Diarrhea, cramping abdominal pain, constitutional effects, and extraintestinal manifestations are approximately the same in colonic and enteric disease. Internal fistulas and abscesses and intestinal obstruction are usually complications of small bowel disease. Anorectal complications (anal fistula, fissure, abscess, and rectal stricture) and hemorrhage are more common when the large bowel is affected, and toxic dilation is limited to patients with inflammation of the colon.

Typical anal lesions of Crohn's disease are large undermined indolent ulcers. The perianal skin has a violaceous hue, and if fistulas are present, they tend to be multiple and complex. Proctosigmoidoscopy discloses a normal rectum in 50% of patients with Crohn's colitis. Diseased mucosa is patchily involved, with irregular ulcerations separated by edematous or even normal-appearing mucosa. Biopsy may confirm the diagnosis. Radiographic features include sparing of the rectum, right colonic and ileal involvement, skip areas, transverse fissures, longitudinal ulcers, strictures, and fistulas. Features differentiating Crohn's disease from ulcerative colitis are summarized in Table 30–12. Ischemic colitis is another disease that may be confused with Crohn's colitis, and the differential diagnosis is discussed below. *Chlamydia trachomatis* infection is diagnosed by culture of the organism. Malacoplakia is a rare chronic granulomatous disease that can cause colonic strictures, and Behçet's disease is another rare condition that can mimic inflammatory bowel disease. Tuberculosis and amebiasis must be considered also.

Frank blood in the stools is observed in about one-third of patients with granulomatous colitis, but massive hemorrhage is unusual. Acute colonic dilation (toxic megacolon) occurs in 5%; it responds to nonoperative treatment more often than it does in ulcerative colitis.

Actuarial methods suggest that the risk of colonic cancer in granulomatous colitis patients is four to twenty times that of the general population, and it appears that segments of intestine excluded from the fecal stream (eg, an isolated rectal stump or bypassed ileum) are especially vulnerable. Carcinoma can also arise in anorectal or rectovaginal fistulas. The small bowel is at risk for development of cancer in patients with regional enteritis with or without colitis. Epithelial dysplasia is associated with cancer in Crohn's disease as well as in ulcerative colitis, but this indicator is not helpful for the areas at greatest risk (eg, bypassed segments of small bowel or colon) because they may not be able to be examined endoscopically. Surveillance colonoscopy may be worthwhile in colonic Crohn's disease, though it has not been routine in the past. Cancer should always be ruled out in colonic strictures.

Medical management of Crohn's disease of the small bowel is described in Chapter 29. Steroids are effective for acute attacks, but they are not advisable for maintenance therapy because of limited benefit and frequent complications. Oral 5-aminosalicylates (sulfasalazine, 4 g/d; or mesalamine, 2–5 g/d) are effective treatment for Crohn's colitis. Topical 5-aminosalicylates are beneficial for disease of the rectum and sigmoid. These agents are steroid-sparing, ie, they allow the dosage of steroids to be reduced. Metronidazole, 10–20 mg/kg/d orally in three to five doses, is used for treatment of anal complications of Crohn's disease. Abscesses and fistulas improve with less pain and drainage, but full permanent healing is unusual, and the disease worsens when the drug is discontinued. Immunosuppressants (azathioprine, mercaptopurine) are steroid-sparing drugs that seem to control Crohn's colitis well enough that surgery is delayed or avoided. There are mixed reports of effectiveness of cyclosporine in refractory Crohn's disease.

Surgical treatment is indicated for intractability, abscess or fistula, obstruction, fulminant disease, anorectal disease, hemorrhage, or cancer. Segmental colectomy with primary anastomosis is useful for limited colonic disease. Total colectomy with ileorectal anastomosis is done more frequently in Crohn's colitis than in ulcerative colitis. Proctocolectomy with ileostomy is needed if rectal disease is severe and the colon needs resection also. Diverting ileostomy or colostomy is only temporarily helpful. Perianal complications can be treated directly (eg, by fistulotomy) in carefully selected patients.

There is a high rate of recurrence at intestinal anastomoses (50–75% at 15 years). Recurrence is less common following proctocolectomy and ileostomy (about 15% at 15 years, but there is a wide disparity (3–46%) among different reports on this controversial topic). Cigarette smoking is an independent risk factor for recurrence of Crohn's disease after resection.

Surgical procedures—like medical therapy—should be regarded as palliative, not curative, in patients with Crohn's disease. Although recurrence rates are high and chronic disease is common, a productive life is usually possible with the aid of combined medical and surgical management. The mortality rate is about 15% over 30 years. Urolithiasis is a common sequela of resection for Crohn's disease.

Cellier C et al: Correlations between clinical activity, endoscopic severity, and biological parameters in colonic or ileocolonic Crohn's disease. A prospective multicentre study of 121 cases. Gut 1994;35:231.

Elton E, Hanauer SB: Review article: the medical management of Crohn's disease. Aliment Pharmacol Ther 1996;10:1.

Feagan BG et al: Methotrexate for the treatment of Crohn's disease. The North American Crohn's Study Group Investigators. N Engl J Med 1995;332:292.

Feagan BG et al: Low-dose cyclosporine for the treatment of Crohn's disease. N Engl J Med 1994;330:1846.

Guy TS, Williams NN, Rosato EF: Crohn's disease of the colon. Surg Clin North Am 2001;81:159.

McClane SJ, Rombeau JL: Anorectal Crohn's disease. Surg Clin North Am 2001;81:169.

Nwokolo CU et al: Surgical resections in parous patients with distal ileal and colonic Crohn's disease. Gut 1994;35:220.

Present DH et al: Infliximab for the treatment of fistulas in patients with Crohn's disease. N Engl J Med 1999;340:1398.

Rutgeerts P: Management of perianal Crohn's disease. Can J Gastroenterol 2000;14 Suppl C:7C.

Scott NA, Hughes LE: Timing of ileocolonic resection for symptomatic Crohn's disease: the patient's view. Gut 1994;35:656.

Slonim AE et al: A preliminary study of growth hormone therapy for Crohn's disease. N Engl J Med 2000;342:1633.

Thirlby RC, Sobrino MA, Randall JB: The long-term benefit of surgery on health-related quality of life in patients with inflammatory bowel disease. Arch Surg 2001;136:521.

3. Antibiotic-Associated Colitis

A spectrum of adverse colonic responses may develop in hospitalized patients during or after antibiotic therapy. There may be diarrhea without gross mucosal abnormality (antibiotic-associated diarrhea), gross inflammation of the mucosa, or whitish-green or yellow plaques on the inflamed mucosa (pseudomembranous colitis). It is not clear whether one or several pathologic processes are responsible. Patients may progress from mild to more severe disease. The differential diagnosis among these variations is based on endoscopic findings and the clinical picture.

Clostridium difficile is a resident of the gut in 3% of people in the general population and in about 10% of patients admitted to hospital. It is the major known cause of nosocomial antibiotic-associated diarrhea and colitis. Certain antibiotics allow the organism to proliferate, and it is then transmitted among patients and hospital personnel. Epidemics of *C difficile* infection have been noted on surgical wards. The organism can be transmitted by people caring for the patient, and gloving or hand-washing is essential. Infection with *C difficile* can be very severe in patients with AIDS.

C difficile may colonize the upper gastrointestinal tract as well as the colon, but the symptomatic infection appears at present to be colonic alone. The organism elaborates at least four toxins, including toxin A (an enterotoxin) and toxin B (a cytotoxin). Together these substances—and perhaps others—produce the symptoms and signs. Clindamycin causes watery diarrhea in 15–30% of patients and true pseudomembranous colitis in 1–10%, but all antibiotics that alter the gut flora including metronidazole may incite pathologic infections with *C difficile*. Colitis may develop as early as 2 days after beginning antibiotics or as late as many weeks after they are discontinued.

Symptoms and signs include diarrhea (usually watery, occasionally bloody), abdominal cramps, vomiting, fever, and leukocytosis. Sigmoidoscopy in pseudomembranous colitis shows elevated plaques or a confluent pseudomembrane, and the mucosa is erythematous and edematous. Biopsies reveal acute inflammation; the pseudomembrane is made up of leukocytes, necrotic epithelial cells, and fibrin. The rectum is spared in about one-fourth of cases, and colonoscopy may be necessary to detect the presence of pseudomembranous colitis. Demonstration of *C difficile* cytotoxin in stool is sensitive and specific. Stool culture is less efficient since some strains of *C difficile* are nontoxicogenic.

Management consists first of discontinuing the inciting antibiotic agent. In most patients, the colitis resolves in 1–2 weeks after the offending agent is withdrawn, but severe symptoms or persistent diarrhea calls for additional treatment. Vancomycin (125–500 mg orally four times daily for 7–10 days) is expensive but effective—though the relapse rate is 15–20% after vancomycin is discontinued. Vancomycin may also be effective as a retention enema. Metronidazole, 1.5–2 g/d orally for 7–14 days, is also effective and much less expensive. Paradoxically, however, metronidazole can also cause antibiotic-associated colitis. Bacitracin is an effective drug and, like vancomycin, is not absorbed from the gastrointestinal tract. Antidiarrheal drugs may prolong symptoms and should be avoided. Oral administration of *Saccharomyces boulardii,* a nonpathogenic yeast, has been successful in treatment of recurrent *C difficile* colitis in an experimental setting. In such refractory cases cholestyramine may be an effective adjunct by binding the toxin produced by *C difficile* bacteria.

The outcome of pseudomembranous colitis and the other forms of antibiotic-associated colonic disease is usually excellent if the disease is recognized and treated. Untreated pseudomembranous colitis, however, may lead to severe dehydration and electrolyte imbalance, toxic megacolon, or colonic perforation. Operation is required for perforation or toxic dilation. Chronic relapsing *C difficile* diarrhea has been treated by rectal instillation of mixed colonic bacteria (bacteriotherapy).

Cappell MS, Philogene C: *Clostridium difficile* infection is a treatable cause of diarrhea in patients with advanced human immunodeficiency virus infection: a study of seven consecutive patients admitted from 1986 to 1992 to a university teaching hospital. Am J Gastroenterol 1993;88:891.

Cozart JC et al: *Clostridium difficile* diarrhea in patients with AIDS versus non-AIDS controls: methods of treatment and clinical response to treatment. J Clin Gastroenterol 1993;16:192.

Fekety R, Shah AB: Diagnosis and treatment of *Clostridium difficile* colitis. JAMA 1993;269:71.

Herman BE et al: Antibiotic-associated fulminant pseudomembranous colitis without toxic megacolon. Am J Gastroenterol 1992;87:1816.

Kelly CP, Pothoulakis C, LaMont JT: *Clostridium difficile* colitis. N Engl J Med 1994;330:257.

Marts BC et al: Patterns and prognosis of *Clostridium difficile* colitis. Dis Colon Rectum 1994;37:837.

McFarland LV et al: A randomized placebo-controlled trial of *Saccharomyces boulardii* in combination with standard antibiotics for *Clostridium difficile* disease. JAMA 1994;271:1913.

Medich DS et al: Laparotomy for fulminant pseudomembranous colitis. Arch Surg 1992;127:847.

Qamar A et al: *Saccharomyces boulardii* stimulates intestinal immunoglobulin A immune response to *Clostridium difficile* toxin A in mice. Infect Immun 2001;69:2762.

4. Ischemic Colitis

Ischemic colitis is caused by mesenteric vascular occlusion or nonocclusive mechanisms. A common precipitating event is abdominal aortic reconstruction with interruption of a vital blood supply such as the inferior mesenteric artery. An entity that resembles ischemic colitis sometimes develops proximal to obstructing colonic carcinoma. Isolated ischemia of the right colon is seen in patients with chronic heart disease, especially aortic stenosis. Ischemic colitis most often afflicts the elderly (average age, 60 years), but it also occurs in younger adults in association with diabetes mellitus, systemic lupus erythematosus, or sickle cell crisis. Pancreatitis can occlude mesocolic vessels.

The most common location is the sigmoid colon (40%) followed by the transverse colon (17%), splenic flexure (11%), ascending colon (12%) and the rectum (6%). Ischemic colitis is categorized as reversible or irreversible. Reversible ischemia heals with nonoperative treatment, sometimes with stricture formation. Over half of the patients have a reversible injury. The severe form is fulminant from onset or may pursue an indolent course without resolution for weeks. Both of the severe forms require operation.

Patients with ischemic colitis have an abrupt onset of abdominal pain, diarrhea (commonly bloody), and systemic symptoms. The abdomen may be tender diffusely, in a localized area (eg, left lower quadrant), or not at all. Blood is seen coming from above at endoscopy; the mucosa of the involved segment is edematous, hemorrhagic, friable, and sometimes ulcerated. A grayish membrane may be present, resembling pseudomembranous colitis. Serum alkaline phosphatase is elevated in some cases. Plain abdominal x-rays are nonspecific. Barium enema x-rays show "thumbprints" or pseudotumors, typically limited to a 6- to 20-cm segment; 75% or more have involvement of the left colon. CT scan shows a thickened colonic wall and helps to exclude other conditions. Mesenteric arteriography may show major arterial occlusion or no abnormalities and is not usually recommended.

Differentiating ischemic colitis from carcinoma, ulcerative colitis, and diverticulitis should not be difficult, but Crohn's disease presents a greater diagnostic problem. Rectal bleeding—especially gross hemorrhage—is less common in Crohn's disease, and the rapid onset of ischemic colitis is also different from Crohn's disease. Radiographic findings and, in some cases, the colonoscopic appearance may be helpful, but the natural history of the acute attack is often the only way to make the distinction. Acute mesenteric ischemia may be difficult to exclude (see Chapter 29), but the more benign presentations of reversible ischemic colonic injury are not seen with ischemia of the small intestine. *C difficile* toxin is present in stool in pseudomembranous colitis.

Therapy for reversible ischemic colitis consists of intravenous fluids, antibiotics, and observation to be certain the problem is in fact reversible. Irreversible disease, whether fulminant from the beginning, becoming more severe over several days, or just failing to resolve after treatment, should be treated by operation. The diseased colon is resected; anastomosis is usually deferred if the colon is unprepared. Because patients with severe ischemia often have multiple other medical problems, the overall mortality rate is 50%.

Balthazar EJ, Yen BC, Gordon RB: Ischemic colitis: CT evaluation of 54 cases. Radiology 1999;211:381.

Houe T et al: Can colonoscopy diagnose transmural ischaemic colitis after abdominal aortic surgery? An evidence-based approach. Eur J Vasc Endovasc Surg 2000;19:304.

Hwang RF, Schwartz RW: Ischemic colitis: a brief review. Curr Surg 2001;58:192.

Hyun H, Pai E, Blend MJ: Ischemic colitis: Tc-99m HMPAO leukocyte scintigraphy and correlative imaging. Clin Nucl Med 1998;23:165.

Valentine RJ et al: Gastrointestinal complications after aortic surgery. J Vasc Surg 1998;28:404.

5. Neutropenic Colitis

Neutropenic colitis (neutropenic enterocolitis, neutropenic typhlitis, ileocecal syndrome, necrotizing enteropathy, agranulocytic colitis) occurs as colonic necrosis in neutropenic patients. Although the cecum and right colon are most often affected, all parts of the small or large bowel can be involved. Acute leukemia, aplastic anemia, and cyclic neutropenia are the underlying diseases in which this lesion occurs. Colonic perforation during treatment with interleukin-2 is probably related. The pathogenesis is not well understood, but responsible factors probably include mucosal ischemia, necrosis of intramural leukemic infiltrates, shock, hemorrhage into the bowel wall, chemotherapy, and corticosteroid therapy. *Clostridium septicum* has been implicated in some cases. The mucosa ulcerates, permitting bacterial invasion into the bowel wall, thrombosis of intramural vessels, necrosis, and perforation.

As many as 25% of patients with acute myeloblastic leukemia may develop typhlitis, and during induction chemotherapy the incidence may be much higher. Fever, watery or bloody diarrhea, abdominal discomfort and distention, and nausea are noted first. Pain and tenderness may then become localized to the right lower quadrant, and systemic toxicity increases. Careful examination and x-ray studies are required. Nasogastric suction, parenteral nutrition, and antibiotic therapy are instituted. Operation (resection of the involved segment of colon) is performed for persistent unresponsive sepsis, perforation, obstruction, severe bleeding, or abscess formation. Neutropenic colitis can recur after medical therapy.

Abbasoglu O, Cakmakci M: Neutropenic enterocolitis in patients without leukemia. Surgery 1993;113:113.

Gorbach SL: Neutropenic enterocolitis. Clin Infect Dis 1998;27:700.

Sayfan J et al: Acute abdomen caused by neutropenic enterocolitis: surgeon's dilemma. Eur J Surg 1999;165:502.

Song HK et al: Changing presentation and management of neutropenic enterocolitis. Arch Surg 1998;133:979.

INTESTINAL STOMAS (ILEOSTOMY & COLOSTOMY)

An intestinal stoma is an opening of the bowel onto the surface of the abdomen. It may be temporary or permanent. Esophagostomy, gastrostomy, jejunostomy, and cecostomy are usually temporary, but ileostomy, colostomy, and some urinary tract stomas are often permanent. Although "stoma" is the preferred medical term, "ostomy" is used by lay organizations devoted to the rehabilitation of these patients.

Few surgical alterations of anatomy are surrounded by as much misunderstanding as intestinal stomas, and few pronouncements by surgeons are as horrifying to patients as the indication that a stoma will be necessary. For these and other reasons, a paramedical profession, **enterostomy therapy**, has emerged. The enterostomal therapist (ET) is usually a registered nurse who has taken specialized training and is certified in the field. The enterostomal therapist provides the following services: (1) preoperative education and counseling of patient and family; (2) immediate postoperative care of the stoma; (3) training in the use of equipment and supervision of self-care; (4) fitting of a permanent appliance; (5) advice on day-to-day living with a stoma; (6) management of skin problems and odor control; (7) recognition of surgical stoma problems; (8) long-term emotional, moral, and physical support; and (9) information about the United Ostomy Association, an organization with chapters in many localities.

ILEOSTOMY

Permanent ileostomy is sometimes performed after proctocolectomy for ulcerative colitis; patients with Crohn's disease, familial polyposis, and other conditions may also require ileostomy. A temporary (loop) ileostomy often is used to divert the fecal stream for 3 months when ileoanal or coloanal anastomosis is performed. An ileostomy discharges small quantities of liquid material continuously; it does not require irrigation; and an appliance must be worn at all times.

The optimal position of the ileostomy is in the right lower quadrant (Figure 30–20). The ileum is brought through the rectus abdominis muscle and everted upon itself, and the mucosa is sutured to the skin (surgically matured). An appliance is placed immediately; it consists of a plastic bag attached to a square sheet of protective material containing a central opening for the stoma. A reusable appliance can be fitted after a few weeks, but modern disposable appliances are so satisfactory that most patients never do change to the other type. Appliances lie flat against the abdomen, adhere firmly to the skin, are inconspicuous and odor-proof, and in most cases need to be changed only every 3–5 days. They are drained at intervals during the day through an opening in the bottom of the pouch.

A **continent ileostomy** (reservoir ileostomy; Kock pouch) is designed to avoid the continual discharge of ileal effluent that necessitates construction of a protruding stoma and the wearing of an appliance at all times. A reservoir is constructed out of the distal ileum, and the outlet from the reservoir is arranged as a valve so that fluid cannot escape onto the abdominal wall. The reservoir is emptied several times a day by inserting a catheter into the stoma. Continent ileostomy is successful in 70–90% of patients. Problems with the valve, fistulas, and "pouchitis" (mucosal inflammation in the reservoir) are causes of failure. Crohn's disease is a contraindication, because of the risk of recurrence necessitating excision of the reservoir.

Physiologic changes after ileostomy are due to the loss of the water- and salt-absorbing capacity of the colon. If the small bowel is free of disease and extensive resection has not been done, an ileostomy puts out 1–2 L of fluid per day initially (Table 30–1). The volume of effluent diminishes to between 500 and 800 mL/d after a month or two. This loss of fluid is obligatory and is not reduced by manipulations of diet. Obligatory sodium losses are about 50 meq/d greater than in patients with an intact colon, and potassium losses are also increased. Healthy ileostomates (patients with ileostomies) have low total exchangeable sodium and potassium but normal serum electrolyte concentrations. The depletion, therefore, is primarily intracellular. The ileostomy patient is susceptible to acute or subacute salt and water depletion manifested by fatigue, anorexia, irritability, headache, drowsiness, muscle cramps, and thirst. Gastroenteritis or diarrhea from any cause and exposure to hot weather or vigorous exercise are situations that require caution; salt and water intake must be increased in these circumstances. Ileostomy patients must never be in a position where salt and water are unavailable, eg, on long hikes in the desert. Low-salt diets and diuretics may also induce salt depletion or dehydration. Patients should be counseled to salt food liberally, but salt tablets will not be required in usual circumstances. Patients with unusually high ileostomy outputs may need supplemental potassium in the form of bananas or orange juice. Water intake in response to thirst may not be adequate to maintain

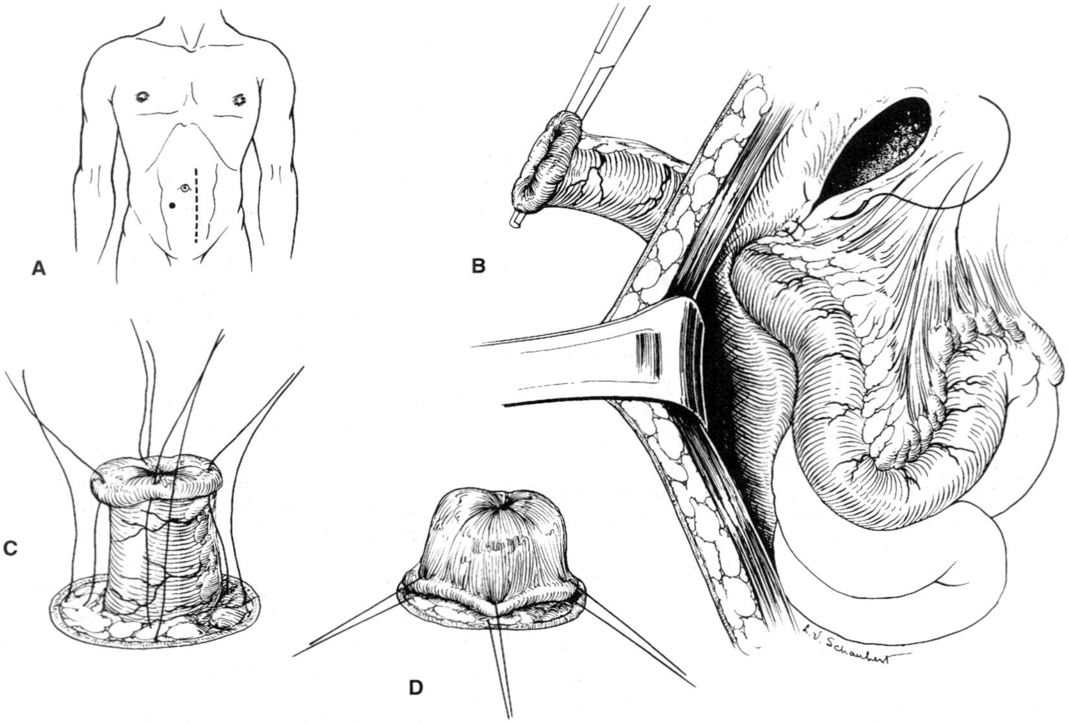

Figure 30–20. Ileostomy after colectomy. ***A:*** A midline incision for colectomy is indicated by the dotted line and the site of the ileostomy by the black dot. (A midline incision is favored by many surgeons.) ***B:*** The ileum has been brought through the abdominal wall. ***C and D:*** The ileostomy stoma has been everted and its margins sutured to the edges of the wound.

hydration, and patients should consume enough water to keep the urine pale or to maintain a urine output of at least 1 L/d.

Patients must be informed about these physiologic alterations and measures to compensate for them. Otherwise, instructions are simple, and ileostomy patients should live normally. A low-residue diet should be advised at least initially. Certain foods (eg, fish, eggs) may cause excessive odor or gas. Ordinary physical activity, employment, and social activities are encouraged. Bathing, swimming, sexual intercourse, and pregnancy and delivery are unrestricted.

Complications (Table 30–13) are reported in about 40% of patients with conventional ileostomy; about 15% require operative correction, usually minor.

In long-term follow-up of ileostomy patients, most return to their previous occupation and consider their health to be good to excellent. Continent ileostomy is preferable to conventional ileostomy in the view of some patients who have had both types of stoma.

Sexual consequences of proctocolectomy should be discussed before and after operation. Some degree of sexual impairment occurs in 10% of men after removal of the rectum for inflammatory bowel disease. Up to three-fourths of women report dyspareunia or reduced orgasmic sensation in the first few months after proctectomy and ileostomy but only 12% experience long-term sexual dysfunction. Infertility is more frequent among women after excision of the rectum, and cesarean delivery is necessary more often; both problems are related to pelvic fibrosis and not the ileostomy.

COLOSTOMY

Colostomies are made for the following purposes: (1) to decompress an obstructed colon; (2) to divert the fecal stream in preparation for resection of an inflammatory, obstructive, or perforated lesion or following traumatic injury; (3) to serve as the point of evacuation of stool when the distal colon or rectum is removed; and (4) to protect a distal anastomosis following resection. The colostomy may be temporary, in which event it is subsequently closed; or it may be permanent. Colostomies can be constructed by making an opening in a loop of colon

Table 30–13. Ileostomy complications.

Complication	Causes and Comment
Intestinal obstruction	May be due to adhesive bands, volvulus, or para-ileostomy herniation of bowel.
Stenosis	Circumferential scar formation at the skin or subcutaneous level is usually at fault. Stenosis may cause profuse watery discharge from the ileostomy. Treatment requires a minor local procedure to release the scar.
Retraction	The stoma should protrude 2–3 cm above the skin level to avoid leakage beneath the ileostomy pouch. A flush or retracted stoma functions poorly and should be revised.
Prolapse	Uncommon if the mesentery has been sutured to the parietal peritoneum.
Para-ileostomy abscess and fistula	Perforation of the ileum by sutures, pressure necrosis from an ill-fitted appliance, or recurrent disease may cause abscess and fistula.
Skin irritation	The single most common complication of ileostomy, due to leakage of ileal effluent onto the peristomal skin. Usually minor but can be severe if neglected. Treatment is directed toward the cause of leakage, usually an ill-fitted pouch. Protection of the skin by a barrier material (eg, karaya [*Sterculia*] gum) or a variety of synthetic products will resolve the problem. Enterostomy therapists manage these problems expertly.
Offensive odors	Odor-proof appliances, commercial deodorants placed in the appliance, and attention to diet usually control the problem.
Diarrhea	Excessive output should be reported to the physician promptly, and supplemental water, salt, and potassium should be given. Codeine, diphenoxylate with atropine, or loperamide may slow the output. Recurrent intestinal disease, bowel obstruction, or ileostomy stenosis should be looked for.
Urinary tract calculi	Uric acid and calcium stones occur in about 5–10% of patients after ileostomy and are probably the result of chronic dehydration due to inadequate fluid intake. Ileostomy is associated with lower urine pH and volume and higher urine concentration of calcium, oxalate, and uric acid than in patients with intact gastrointestinal tracts.
Gallstones	Cholesterol gallstones are three times more common in ileostomy patients than in the general population. Altered bile acid absorption preoperatively may be responsible.
Ileitis	Patients who develop inflammation of the ileum just proximal to the ileostomy usually have recurrence of their original inflammatory bowel disease. Stenosis of the stoma is another cause.
Varices	Varices develop around the stoma in patients with portal hypertension. Bleeding can be troublesome.

(**loop colostomy**) or by dividing the colon and bringing out one end (**end [terminal] colostomy**). A colostomy is double-barreled if a loop or both ends of a colon are exteriorized and single-barreled if only one end is brought out.

The most common permanent colostomy is a **sigmoid colostomy** made at the time of abdominoperineal resection for cancer of the rectum (Figure 30–21). Such a colostomy is compatible with a normal life except for the route of fecal evacuation. A sigmoid colostomy expels stool approximately once a day, but the frequency varies among individuals just as bowel habits vary in the general population. An appliance is not required, though many patients find that wearing a light pouch is reassuring. Some patients achieve a regular pattern of evacuation on their own; others require irrigation daily or every other day. Irrigation is performed by inserting a catheter into the stoma and instilling water, 500 mL at a time, by gravity flow from a reservoir held at shoulder height. A plastic olive-shaped tip on the catheter fits snugly into the stoma and greatly reduces the risk of perforation. Diet is individualized; generally, patients are able to eat the same foods they enjoyed preoperatively. Fresh fruits, fruit juices, and other foods may cause diarrhea. A properly functioning colostomy need not be dilated.

Transverse colostomy should not be constructed as a permanent stoma if it can be avoided. Unlike sigmoid colostomy, transverse colostomy is "wet"—ie, it discharges semiliquid waste frequently—and usually requires an appliance. These stomas are bulky, foul-smelling, and extremely difficult to manage. They are prone to leak under the appliance, and prolapse is common. The needs of most patients who require a permanent stoma are better served by an ileostomy than by a transverse colostomy.

The overall complication rate of colostomies is 20%, and 15% of complications require operative correction.

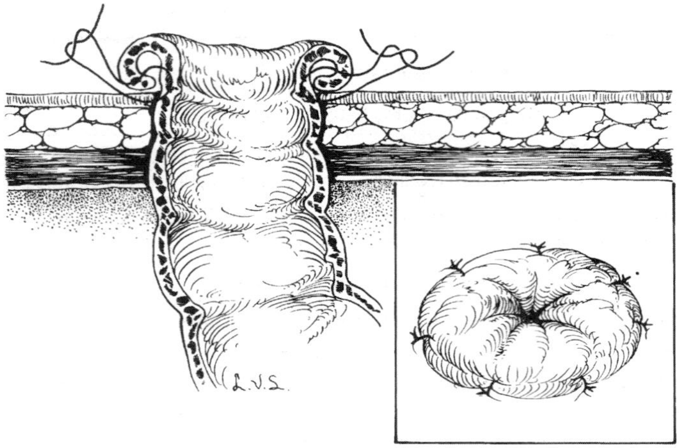

Figure 30–21. Single-barreled end colostomy. The margins of the stoma are fixed to the skin with sutures.

Chronic paracolostomy hernia is a frequent complication; it develops because the abdominal wall aperture enlarges with time, allowing colon, omentum, or small bowel to herniate adjacent to the colostomy. Hernia—and prolapse—are more apt to occur in obese patients. Stenosis may require revision. Necrosis and retraction are due to technical errors in constructing the stoma. Paracolostomy abscess occurs occasionally regardless of precautions. Perforation is avoided by the plastic catheter tip and by keeping the irrigation reservoir at no greater than shoulder height. Less serious complications include diarrhea, fecal impaction, and skin irritation.

Leong APK, Londono-Schimmer EE, Phillips RKS: Life-table analysis of stomal complications following ileostomy. Br J Surg 1994;81:727.

Lyons AS: Ileostomy and colostomy support groups. Mt Sinai J Med 2001;68:110.

Oliveira L et al: Laparoscopic creation of stomas. Surg Endosc 1997;11:19.

Rubin MS, Schoetz DJ Jr, Matthews JB: Parastomal hernia: is stoma relocation superior to fascial repair? Arch Surg 1994;129:413.

Rullier E et al: Loop ileostomy versus loop colostomy for defunctioning low anastomoses during rectal cancer Surgery. World J Surg 2001;25:274.

Sakai Y et al: Temporary transverse colostomy vs loop ileostomy in diversion: a case- matched study. Arch Surg 2001;136:338.

PREOPERATIVE PREPARATION OF THE COLON

Complications of colonic surgery such as wound infection and anastomotic dehiscence are partially related to the high bacterial content of the large bowel. It is widely accepted that elimination of the fecal mass and reduction of the numbers of bacteria prior to operation is desirable. Measures taken to achieve this purpose are known as the "bowel prep." Patients in good health can have preparation as an outpatient on the day before surgery and undergo operation on the day of admission.

Mechanical cleansing is employed except in patients with obstructing lesions or, perhaps, severe inflammatory bowel disease. There has been a strong trend toward whole-gut lavage, which involves ingestion (or instillation through a nasogastric tube) of large quantities of fluid; the absorptive capacity of the small bowel is overwhelmed, and the colon is cleared of fecal matter. A solution containing polyethylene glycol (PEG) minimizes the risk of fluid overload and excessive dehydration. Oral sodium phosphate compares favorably with PEG solutions. It requires only a small volume for ingestion but causes an osmotic diarrhea; therefore dehydration and electrolyte abnormalities are a concern.

Gut sterilization with oral antibiotics (neomycin and erythromycin base) remains controversial despite many years of study. An important reason for disparate opinions is the difficulty of performing prospective trials in which all the variables are strictly controlled. The wisdom of conventional bowel preparation as described above is currently being challenged. In meta-analyses of trials of mechanical bowel preparation prior to elective colon surgery, bowel preparation is associated with a significant increase in the incidence of wound infections. Furthermore, there is a trend toward a higher anastomotic leak rate. In fact, only the use of parenteral antibiotic prophylaxis given just prior to incision has been clearly associated with improved wound infection rates. Until a multicenter randomized trial of mechanical preparation can be performed, the debate is likely to continue.

Bleday R et al: Quantitative cultures of the mucosal-associated bacteria in the mechanically prepared colon and rectum. Dis Colon Rectum 1993;36:844.

Burke P et al: Requirement for bowel preparation in colorectal surgery. Br J Surg 1994;81:907.

Cohen SM et al: Prospective, randomized, endoscopic-blinded trial comparing precolonoscopy bowel cleansing methods. Dis Colon Rectum 1994;37:689.

Henderson JM et al: Single-day, divided-dose oral sodium phosphate laxative versus intestinal lavage as preparation for colonoscopy: efficacy and patient tolerance. Gastrointest Endosc 1995;42:238.

Matter SE, Rice PS, Campbell DR: Colonic lavage solutions: plain versus flavored. Am J Gastroenterol 1993;88:49.

Miettinen RP et al: Bowel preparation with oral polyethylene glycol electrolyte solution vs. no preparation in elective open colorectal surgery: prospective, randomized study. Dis Colon Rectum 2000;43:669.

Platell C, Hall J: What is the role of mechanical bowel preparation in patients undergoing colorectal surgery? Dis Colon Rectum 1998;41:875.

Santos JC Jr et al: Prospective randomized trial of mechanical bowel preparation in patients undergoing elective colorectal surgery. Br J Surg 1994;81:1673.

Zamora O, Pikarsky AJ, Wexner SD: Bowel preparation for colorectal surgery. Dis Colon Rectum 2001;44:1537.

Wolters U et al: Prospective randomized study of preoperative bowel cleansing for patients undergoing colorectal surgery. Br J Surg 1994;81:598.

Anorectum

31

Mark L. Welton, MD, George J. Chang, MD, & Andrew A. Shelton, MD

GENERAL ANATOMIC CONSIDERATIONS

The rectum, endodermal in origin, is the dorsal component of the cloaca, which is partitioned by the anorectal septum. The anal canal is an invagination of ectodermal tissue. The anorectum develops from fusion of the rectum and the anal canal, which occurs at 8 weeks, when the anal membrane ruptures. The dentate line marks the point of fusion and the transition from endodermal to ectodermal tissue.

The rectum is 12–15 cm long. It extends from the rectosigmoid junction, marked by the fusion of the tenia, to the anal canal, marked by the passage into the pelvic floor musculature (Figure 31–1). The rectum lies in the sacrum and forms three distinct curves, creating folds known as the **valves of Houston**. The proximal and distal curves are convex to the left and the middle curve is convex to the right. The middle curve roughly marks the anterior peritoneal reflection, which is 6–8 cm above the anus. The rectum gradually undergoes transition from intraperitoneal to extraperitoneal beginning 12–15 cm from the anus and becoming completely extraperitoneal 6–8 cm from the anus. The rectum is fixed posteriorly, laterally, and anteriorly by the presacral (Waldeyer's) fascia, the lateral ligaments, and Denonvilliers' fascia, respectively.

The anatomic anal canal starts at the **dentate line**, the junction of colorectal mucosa and anal mucosa, and ends at the **anal verge**, the junction of the anal mucosa with the perianal skin. However, for practical purposes, the surgical anal canal extends from the muscular diaphragm of the pelvic floor to the anal verge. The **anal canal** is a collapsed anteroposterior slit 3–4 cm long. The anal canal is supported by the surrounding **anal sphincter mechanism**, composed of the internal and external sphincters. The **internal sphincter** is a specialized continuation of the circular muscle of the rectum. It is an involuntary muscle that is normally contracted at rest. The structure and function of the **external sphincter** is the subject of some controversy, but it acts as a spout on a funnel of one continuous circumferential functional muscle mass that includes the external sphincter caudally and extends cranially to the conical puborectalis and levator ani muscles. The external sphincter is composed of voluntary striated muscle. The conjoined longitudinal muscle separates the internal and external sphincters. This intersphincteric plane is created by the continuation of the longitudinal muscle of the rectum joined by fibers from the levator ani and puborectalis, forming the conjoined muscle. Some fibers from this muscle become the corrugator cutis ani and insert on the perianal skin, creating rugal folds and a puckered appearance. Other fibers traverse the internal sphincter and support the internal hemorrhoids as the mucosal suspensory ligaments.

Familiarity with the histology of the rectum and anal canal is important in order to understand the disease processes of these areas. The rectum is composed of an innermost layer of mucosa that overlies the submucosa, two continuous sheaths of muscle—the circular and longitudinal muscles—and, in the proximal rectum, serosa. The mucosa is subdivided into three layers: (1) epithelial cells, (2) lamina propria, and (3) muscularis mucosae. The **muscularis mucosae** is a fine sheet of muscle containing a network of lymphatics. Lymphatics are essentially absent above this level, so the muscularis mucosae determines the metastatic potential of malignancies.

As the rectum enters the narrow musculature of the pelvic floor and becomes the anal canal, the tissue is thrown into folds known as the **columns of Morgagni**. At the lower end of the columns lie crypts, some of which communicate with anal glands lying in the intersphincteric plane. The epithelium of the anal canal is of three types: colorectal mucosa is present in the proximal 2–3 cm; transitional epithelium is at and just above the dentate line; and the anoderm is below the dentate line. The anoderm is squamous mucosa rich in nerve fibers. The anal verge marks the true mucocutaneous junction.

The pelvic floor is composed of the levator ani and puborectalis muscles. The levator ani, two broad, thin, symmetric muscular sheets that originate from the pelvic sidewall and sacrospinous ligament, form the principal support of the pelvic viscera. The puborectalis muscle originates on the posterior aspect of the pubis, forms a sling around the rectum, and returns to the posterior aspect of the pubis. The fibers of the puborectalis are situated immediately adjacent to and below the innermost component of the levator ani muscle, where they are intimately associated with the upper posterolateral

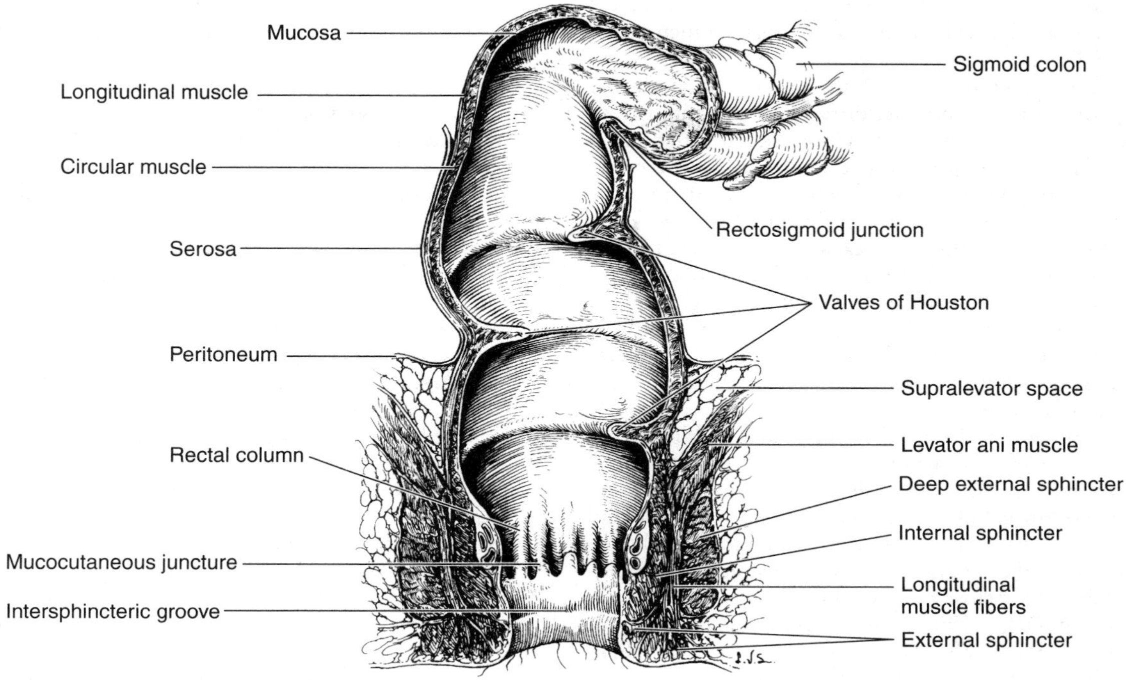

Figure 31–1. Anatomy of the anorectal canal.

fibers of the deep external anal sphincter. Thus, the puborectalis serves as a bridge between the broad sheet-like component of the funnel created by the levators and the narrow spout of the funnel created by the external anal sphincter. The puborectalis in the contracted state is responsible for the normal acute anorectal angle between the levators and the external sphincters. It is also responsible for the shelf that is normally palpable on digital examination as one passes from the distal narrow lumen of the anus to the more proximal capacious lumen of the rectum.

The innervation of the rectum is via the sympathetic and parasympathetic nervous systems. The sympathetic nerves originate from the lumbar segments L1–3, form the inferior mesenteric plexus, travel through the superior hypogastric plexus, and descend as the hypogastric nerves to the pelvic plexus.

The parasympathetic nerves arise from the second, third, and fourth sacral roots and join the hypogastric nerves anterior and lateral to the rectum to form the pelvic plexus, from which fibers pass to form the periprostatic plexus. Sympathetic and parasympathetic fibers pass from the pelvic and periprostatic plexuses to the rectum and internal anal sphincter as well as the prostate, bladder, and penis. Injury to these nerves can lead to impotence, bladder dysfunction, and loss of normal defecatory mechanisms.

The internal anal sphincter is innervated with sympathetic and parasympathetic fibers. Both are inhibitory and keep the sphincter in a constant state of contraction. The external sphincters are skeletal muscles innervated by the pudendal nerve with fibers that originate from S2–4. Above the dentate line, noxious stimuli are experienced as ill-defined dull sensations conducted through afferent fibers of the parasympathetic nerves. Below the dentate line, the epithelium is exquisitely sensitive. Cutaneous sensations of heat, cold, pain, and touch are conveyed through the inferior rectal and perineal branches of the pudendal nerve.

The arterial supply of the anorectum is via the superior, middle, and inferior rectal arteries. The superior rectal artery is the terminal branch of the inferior mesenteric artery and descends in the mesorectum. It supplies the upper and middle rectum. The middle rectal arteries arise from the internal iliac arteries and enter the rectum anterolaterally at the level of the pelvic floor musculature. They supply the lower two-thirds of the rectum. Collaterals exist between the middle and superior rectal arteries. The inferior rectal arteries—branches of the internal pudendal arteries—enter posterolaterally, do not anastomose with the blood supply to the middle rectum, and provide blood to the anal sphincters and epithelium.

The venous drainage of the anorectum is via the superior, middle, and inferior rectal veins draining into the portal and systemic systems. The superior rectal veins drain the upper and middle thirds of the rectum. They empty into the portal system via the inferior mesenteric vein. The middle rectal veins drain the lower rectum and the upper anal canal into the systemic system via the internal iliac veins. The inferior rectal veins drain the lower anal canal, communicating with the pudendal veins and draining into the internal iliac veins. Communication between the venous systems allows low rectal cancers to spread via the portal and systemic systems.

Lymphatic drainage of the upper and middle rectum is into the inferior mesenteric nodes. Lymph from the lower rectum may also drain into the inferior mesenteric system or into the systems along the middle and inferior rectal arteries, posteriorly along the middle sacral artery, and anteriorly through channels in the retrovesical or rectovaginal septum. These drain to the iliac nodes and ultimately to the periaortic nodes. Lymphatics from the anal canal above the dentate line drain via the superior rectal lymphatics to the inferior mesenteric lymph nodes and laterally to the internal iliac nodes. Below the dentate line, drainage occurs primarily to the inguinal nodes but can occur to the inferior or superior rectal lymph nodes.

NORMAL FUNCTION OF THE ANORECTUM

The normal function of the anorectum is storage and release of intestinal waste products. The rectum functions mainly as a capacitance storage vessel. The normal volume of the rectum is 650–1200 mL. Resting rectal pressure is approximately 10 mm Hg. Changes in intrarectal pressure are primarily a reflection of intra-abdominal pressure changes since the rectum itself has little peristaltic function.

The function of the pelvic floor is complex and poorly understood. The complexity of the interactions of the pelvic floor structures and the nature of material passed per rectum compromises the ability to study function with intraluminal monitors, as is done in the upper intestinal tract.

The levators ani form a funnel that suspends the rectum in a muscular sling which ends where the puborectalis angulates the rectum forward at the anorectal junction. The levators may contain sensory fibers that report pelvic fullness and thus may be important in the sensation of the urge to defecate. The acuity of the anorectal angle (created by the puborectalis) is critical for maintaining continence. The puborectalis contracts, increasing the angle during Valsalva maneuvers, where continence is maintained (coughing, straining), but relaxes, to open the angle during similar efforts performed as part of normal defecation.

The internal sphincter, composed of smooth muscle, accounts for 85% of the resting tone. It is innervated by sympathetic and parasympathetic fibers. Both are inhibitory and keep the sphincter in a constant state of contraction. The external sphincters are skeletal muscles innervated by the pudendal nerve with fibers from S2–4. The muscles provide 15% of the resting tone and 100% of the voluntary squeeze pressure. The external sphincter, pelvic floor, and cricopharyngeus muscles are unique skeletal muscles in being able to maintain a state of tonic contraction. The strength of contraction in the first two is increased by factors that increase intra-abdominal pressure such as erect posture, coughing, or Valsalva's maneuver. Voluntary contraction of the external sphincter doubles the resting pressure but it cannot be sustained longer than 3 minutes.

The normal hemorrhoidal pads are important participants in maintaining continence and minimizing trauma during defecation. They function as protective pillows that engorge with blood during the act of defecation, protecting the anoderm from direct trauma due to passage of stool. They also seal the anal canal and prevent leakage of gas and stool. The internal and external sphincters alone cannot close the anal canal, but when sphincter action is combined with interdigitating internal hemorrhoidal cushions, continence is achieved. Hemorrhoidal tissues become engorged when intra-abdominal pressure is increased (eg, obesity, pregnancy, lifting, and defecation).

Through complex mechanisms not clearly understood, the anal sphincters function as a unit in concert with the levator ani, the puborectalis, and the rectum, allowing defecation to be controlled. Continence is maintained when intrarectal pressures are lower than the pressures generated by the resting internal and external sphincters. In the resting state, the rectum is not completely empty but the contents are not sensed. Sensory fibers in the levators that initially signal the presence of pelvic fullness adapt and the rectum accommodates (decreases muscle tone), allowing the contents to remain. Periodically, the internal sphincter relaxes, allowing the rectal contents to drop down into the anal canal where the contents can be sensed by the anoderm. In response, the external sphincter contracts and the contents are pushed back into the rectum. This "sampling reflex," or **rectoanal inhibitory reflex**, also results from rectal distention, allowing determination of rectal contents as the rectum fills. The sampling reflex occurs up to seven times a day. Progressive distention of the rectum causes continuous inhibition of the internal sphincter and relaxation of the external sphincter, resulting in the urge to defecate. If solid waste is noted and one wishes to evacuate, a sitting or squatting position is assumed (straightening the anorectal angle), intra-abdominal pressure is increased by a Valsalva maneuver, the puborectalis relaxes, and reflex relaxation of the internal sphincter occurs as the contents enter the anal canal. As the puborectalis relaxes, the anorectal angle straightens, further shortening the anal canal and increasing the funnel shape of the musculature. The Valsalva maneuver is the principal force behind evacuation. Thus, normal defecation is a complex event involving multiple steps.

DYSFUNCTION OF THE ANORECTUM

INCONTINENCE

Continence is maintained through rectal compliance, anorectal sensation, anorectal reflexes, and anal sphincter function. The nature and quantity of stool and colonic transit are important as well. The incidence of fecal incontinence is difficult to determine because of underreporting and lack of a standard definition of the term. Obstetric trauma is the major cause of mechanical injury to the external sphincter and nerves. The incidence of incontinence is increased after third-degree perineal tears, multiple vaginal deliveries, and infection of an episiotomy repair. Prolonged labor may mechanically disrupt the sphincter and stretch of the pudendal nerve. Although incontinence is most common in parous women, the prevalence in men is also high.

Neurogenic causes of incontinence include pudendal nerve stretch from to prolonged labor or multiple births and a history of chronic straining to defecate. Vaginal deliveries are associated with reversible pudendal nerve injury in 80% of primigravida births. The injury may be unilateral or bilateral. If it is permanent or repeated multiple times, denervation and weakening of the external sphincter and pelvic floor result. The neuropathy and associated sphincter dysfunction progress with time. A weakened pelvic floor is less able to withstand increased intra-abdominal pressure, leading to further perineal descent and stretch injury.

Chronic straining at stool and a sense of incomplete evacuation are common features of the descending perineum syndrome. Straining leads to descent of the pelvic floor and straightening of the anorectal angle. This may result in folding in or prolapse of the anterior rectal wall and further obstruction of defecation. The resultant increased straining and perineal descent cause pudendal nerve injury as the nerve is stretched over the ischial spine, leading to idiopathic fecal incontinence sometimes associated with internal rectal prolapse (intussusception).

Incontinence may result from the treatment of cryptogenic abscess or fistula disease or of perianal Crohn's disease, where the external sphincter may be divided during fistulotomy. In women, the external sphincter is a thin band of muscle anteriorly and thus especially susceptible to complete transection in this location, resulting in incontinence.

Other causes of incontinence include systemic diseases affecting either the muscular or neurologic systems (eg, scleroderma, multiple sclerosis, dermatomyositis, diabetes) and causes unrelated to the function of the sphincter itself (severe diarrhea, fecal impaction with overflow incontinence, radiation proctitis with fibrosis, and tumors of the distal colon and rectum).

Clinical Findings

A. Symptoms and Signs

Complete incontinence is lack of control of gas, liquid, and solid stool. Inability to control liquid and gas or gas alone is **partial incontinence**. Urgency, seepage, and soiling may occur regularly or intermittently, depending on the nature of the stool presenting to the rectum. Elicitation of these symptoms is important in establishing the nature of the injury. Patients who complain of soiling with urgency may have a poorly distensible rectum and normal sphincters, whereas patients complaining of inability to sense stool until it has passed may have a neurologic injury. The physical signs of incontinence may include a patulous anus, focal loss of corrugation of the anal verge, flattening and maceration of the perineum, exaggerated descent of the perineum with straining, decreased sphincter tone, diminished voluntary squeeze pressures, and loss of anal sensation.

B. Laboratory and Imaging Studies

Anorectal manometry, transrectal ultrasound, pudendal nerve latency studies, electromyography, and defecography may all be part of the evaluation of the incontinent patient.

Anorectal manometry defines the limits of the injury by measuring the maximum resting pressure, the maximum squeeze pressure, the sphincter length and symmetry, the minimum sensory volume, the presence or absence of the rectoanal inhibitory reflex, and the ability to relax the puborectalis muscle. Maximal resting pressures normally range from 40 mm Hg to 80 mm Hg, while maximal squeeze pressures range from 80 mm Hg to 160 mm Hg. The internal sphincter gives rise to 85% of the resting maximal pressure, while the external sphincter provides 15% of the resting pressure and 100% of the maximal squeeze pressure. The sphincter is typically 3 cm long and asymmetric (longer in back), and the whole complex is shorter in women. The minimum sensory volume is about 10 mL. The rectoanal inhibitory reflex is manifested as a decrease in resting anal pressure when an air-filled balloon distends the rectum. Finally, pelvic floor function and the ability to relax the pelvic floor to achieve defecation are assessed with the balloon expulsion test. This requires the patient to expel a fully inflated 60-mL latex balloon.

Transrectal ultrasound provides useful anatomic images for evaluating internal and external anal sphincter defects. Electromyographic changes correlate closely with ultrasonographic evidence of sphincter injury, allowing transrectal ultrasound to largely replace the more painful electromyography.

Pudendal nerve latency studies further define the nature of the injury. If one or both nerves are injured, surgical or nonsurgical treatment of incontinence may be predictably unsuccessful. The study is performed by inserting a gloved finger with a stimulating electrode at the fingertip in the rectum and stimulating the pudendal nerve as it traverses the ischial spine. An electrode at the base of the examining finger records the delay between stimulation and contraction of the external sphincter. The normal delay is 2 ± 0.2 s. It may be prolonged with age, after childbirth, in individuals with a history of excessive straining to defecate and perineal descent, and in systemic diseases such as diabetes and multiple sclerosis.

Defecography is useful in patients with both constipation and incontinence, for in a few patients with incontinence, rectal intussusception occurs during the act of straining to defecate and the intussusception produces obstruction and an inability to evacuate, which is later followed by uncontrolled release of liquid stool after the straining is stopped.

Differential Diagnosis

Incontinence may result from obstructions to defecation caused by tumors or intussusception. Varying degrees of incontinence may also result from obstetric injury, either from excessive straining and pudendal nerve injury or disruption of the sphincter mechanism. Incontinence may occur immediately or after many years as the patient ages, sphincter tone decreases, and an occult injury is manifested. Chronic straining at defecation stretches the pudendal nerve over the ischial spine, leading to idiopathic fecal incontinence in the elderly. An extreme example of this is seen in rectal prolapse, where 30% of patients experience incontinence after repair because of stretch injury from chronic prolapse. Secondary effects of systemic diseases such as multiple sclerosis, dermatomyositis, and diabetes mellitus should be considered. Incontinence may also stem from disease that overwhelms a normally functioning sphincter. Examples are severe diarrhea, fecal impaction with overflow, inflammatory bowel disease of the rectum, radiation proctitis, and fibrosis.

Treatment

An algorithm for the diagnosis and treatment of incontinence is given in (Figure 31–2). In general biofeedback should be first-line therapy and in most series is reported to be highly effective in over two-thirds of patients. If a muscular defect is limited and there is no neurologic injury, surgical correction with an overlapping sphincter reconstruction restores continence by reestablishing a complete ring of muscle. Overlapping sphincteroplasty is associated with excellent results in about 75% of candidate patients. However, if there is extensive loss of sphincter muscle or severe neurologic injury, simple overlapping repair is not as successful, and consideration must be given to muscle flap procedures. The sacral nerve stimulator was initially designed for urinary incontinence and subsequently adapted for fecal incontinence. Ideal candidates have an anatomically intact sphincter and good results with a trial of "temporary" stimulation. The stimulating electrodes are applied to sacral nerve roots 2, 3, and 4 with a remotely implanted pulse generator. Excellent results with some improvement in virtually all patients can be achieved with appropriate patient selection. The main complications are lead dislodgement and the need for device explantation due to intractable pain.

The stimulated-gracilis, the gracilis, and the gluteal muscle flap procedures are reserved for patients with complete neurologic injury or extensive muscle loss who wish to avoid a colostomy. The stimulated-gracilis procedure (dynamic graciloplasty) is similar to the gracilis procedure with the exception that a pacemaker is used to retrain the gracilis. A recent international multicenter trial of dynamic graciloplasty reported an overall success rate of 58–74%. Most other series have reported similar degrees of success. The main limitation is a relatively high morbidity primarily due to infectious complications. An international multicenter trial and smaller single-institution trials of the artificial bowel sphincter have been completed. The multicenter trial reported a success rate of 53% based on an intent-to-treat analysis. However, a very high incidence of device-related adverse events and the need for revision surgery has limited its application.

Anal encirclement procedures with foreign material have been reserved for the critically ill or for patients with a short life expectancy. The anal canal is encircled with either a synthetic mesh or a silver wire. Patients are given daily enemas to evacuate the rectum, providing a form of continence involving artificial obstruction and stimulated evacuation. The obstructing foreign body is prone to infection and erosion into the rectum, often necessitating its removal.

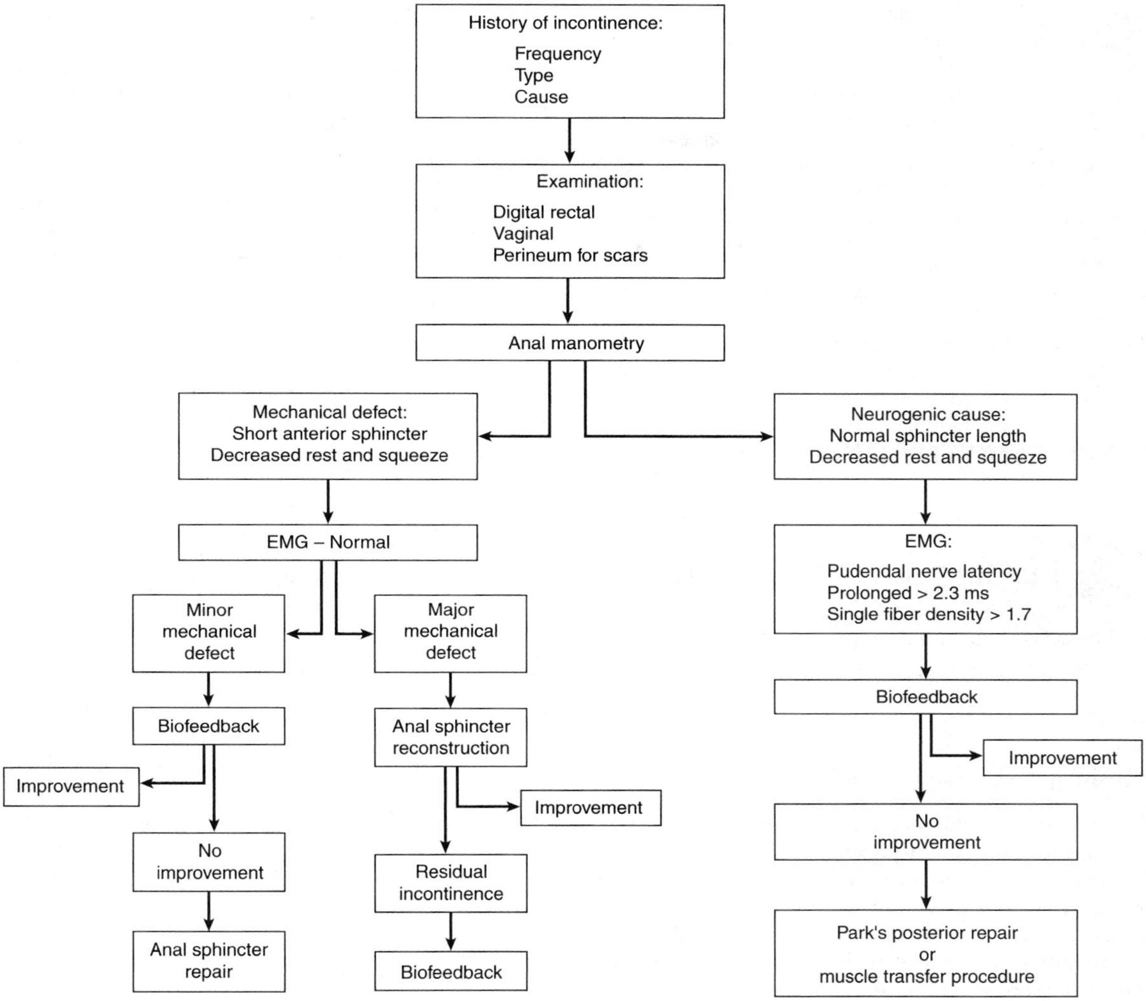

Figure 31–2. Algorithm for workup and treatment of fecal incontinence. (Reproduced, with permission, from Grendel JH, McQuaid KR, Friedman SL: *Current Diagnosis & Treatment in Gastroenterology.* Originally published by Appleton & Lange. Copyright © 1996 by The McGraw-Hill Companies, Inc.)

Prognosis

The incontinence associated with prolapse usually resolves after repair of the prolapse if there has not been severe nerve injury. Prior to repair, the prolapsing segment stimulates the rectoanal inhibitory reflex, decreasing internal sphincter pressure, fatiguing the external sphincter, and resulting in incontinence. The incontinence resolves after surgical repair in 70% of cases.

Baeten CG et al: Anal dynamic graciloplasty in the treatment of intractable fecal incontinence. N Engl J Med 1995;332:1600.

Cheong DM et al: Electrodiagnostic evaluation of fecal incontinence. Muscle Nerve 1995;18:612.

Falk PM et al: Transanal ultrasound and manometry in the evaluation of fecal incontinence. Dis Colon Rectum 1994;37:468.

Farouk R et al: Sustained internal sphincter hypertonia in patients with chronic anal fissure. Dis Colon Rectum 1994;37:424.

Hill JA et al: Pudendal neuropathy in patients with idiopathic fecal incontinence progresses with time. Br J Surg 1994;81:1492.

Johanson JF et al: Epidemiology of fecal incontinence: the silent affliction. Am J Gastroenterol 1996;91:33.

Ko CY et al: Biofeedback is effective therapy for fecal incontinence and constipation. Arch Surg 1997;132:829.

Lehur PA et al: Artificial anal sphincter: prospective clinical and manometric evaluation. Dis Colon Rectum 2000;43:1100.

Lestar B et al: The internal anal sphincter cannot close the anal canal completely. Int J Colorectal Dis 1992;7:159.

Madoff RD et al: Fecal incontinence. N Engl J Med 1992;326:1002.

Nelson R et al: Community-based prevalence of anal incontinence. JAMA 1995;274:559.

Osterberg A et al: Results of neurophysiologic evaluation in fecal incontinence. Dis Colon Rectum 2000;43:1256.

Ryhammer AM et al: Long-term effect of vaginal deliveries on anorectal function in normal perimenopausal women. Dis Colon Rectum 1996;39:852.

Sangwan YP et al: Fecal incontinence. Surg Clin North Am J 1994; 74:1377.

Sultan AH et al: Endosonography of the anal sphincters: normal anatomy and comparison with manometry. Clin Radiol 1994;49:368.

Wong WD et al: The safety and efficacy of the artificial bowel sphincter for fecal incontinence. Dis Colon Rectum 2002;45: 1139.

PELVIC FLOOR DYSFUNCTION

ESSENTIALS OF DIAGNOSIS

- *Inability to voluntarily evacuate rectal contents.*
- *Normal colonic transit time.*

General Considerations

Pelvic floor dysfunction, alternatively referred to as nonrelaxing puborectalis syndrome, anismus, or paradoxic pelvic floor contraction, is a functional disorder in that the muscle is normal but control is dysfunctional. In health, the puborectalis is contracted at rest, maintaining the anorectal angle. During defecation, the muscle relaxes and evacuation occurs. In nonrelaxing puborectalis syndrome, the muscle does not relax and maintains or increases (paradoxic contraction) the anorectal angle. The patient therefore performs a Valsalva maneuver against an obstructed outlet, and elimination does not occur or is significantly diminished.

Patients who chronically strain at stool, whether from colonic inertia or pelvic floor dysfunction, may develop lengthening of the attachments of the rectum to the sacrum or descending perineum syndrome. The increased mobility that results allows for internal prolapse (intussusception), solitary rectal ulcer, and rectal procidentia (see below).

Clinical Findings

A. Symptoms and Signs

Patients with pelvic floor dysfunction may complain of straining and anal or pelvic pain but also of constipation, incomplete evacuation, and a need to digitally evacuate rectal contents.

Digital examination of the patient with nonrelaxing puborectalis syndrome may reveal a tender pelvic muscular diaphragm. During the digital examination, if the patient is directed to squeeze to mimic holding in flatus, paradoxic relaxation and a Valsalva maneuver may occur. Similarly, if the patient is asked to bear down to simulate a bowel movement he may paradoxically contract the external sphincters and puborectalis muscles.

B. Laboratory and Imaging Studies

Patients with nonrelaxing puborectalis syndrome and internal intussusception should undergo defecography, colonic transit studies, anorectal manometry with the balloon expulsion test, and barium enema or colonoscopy.

The patient with isolated nonrelaxing puborectalis syndrome will have a normal colon on barium enema or colonoscopy and a normal colonic transit time to the rectosigmoid. Cinedefecography will demonstrate persistent anterior displacement of the rectum on the lateral view. The patient will be unable to expel the balloon during anorectal manometry evaluation.

Differential Diagnosis

Complaints suggestive of obstructed defecation occur in patients with both functional and anatomic abnormalities. A functional abnormality is exemplified by the nonrelaxing puborectalis syndrome. Anatomic abnormalities include rectocele, internal intussusception, fecal impaction, and rectal or anal cancer. The workup of these complex patients is outlined in Figure 31–3.

Treatment

A. Medical Treatment

Nonrelaxing puborectalis syndrome is best treated with biofeedback. The puborectalis is retrained to relax during the act of defecation, which allows the act to proceed without obstruction.

B. Surgical Treatment

Patients refractory to medical therapy may be offered a colostomy.

Prognosis

Patients with nonrelaxing puborectalis syndrome have excellent results with biofeedback training but may require periodic retraining.

Glia A et al: Constipation assessed on the basis of colorectal physiology. Scand J Gastroenterol 1998;33:1273.

Mertz H et al: Symptoms and physiology in severe chronic constipation. Am J Gastroenterol 1999;94:131.

```
                        ┌─────────────────────────┐
                        │ Symptoms:               │
                        │                         │
                        │ Constipation            │
                        │ Incomplete evacuation   │
                        │ Rectal pressure and pain│
                        │ Digital maneuvers       │
                        └─────────────────────────┘
                                   │
                                   ▼
                        ┌─────────────────────────┐
                        │ Defecography            │
                        │ Colonic transit times   │
                        │ Balloon expulsion       │
                        └─────────────────────────┘
```

Defecography	Nonrelaxing PR	Nonrelaxing PR	Internal intussusception	Internal intussusception
	+	+	+	+
Colonic transit	Normal	Outlet obstruction	Outlet obstruction	Outlet obstruction
	+	+	+	+
Balloon expulsion	Normal	Unable to expel	Normal	Unable to expel
	↓	↓	↓	↓
	Bulk forming agents with or without stool softeners	Psychological evaluation and biofeedback for nonrelaxing PR	Mild → Fiber Severe → Surgery	Psychological evaluation and biofeedback for nonrelaxing PR

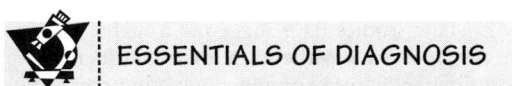

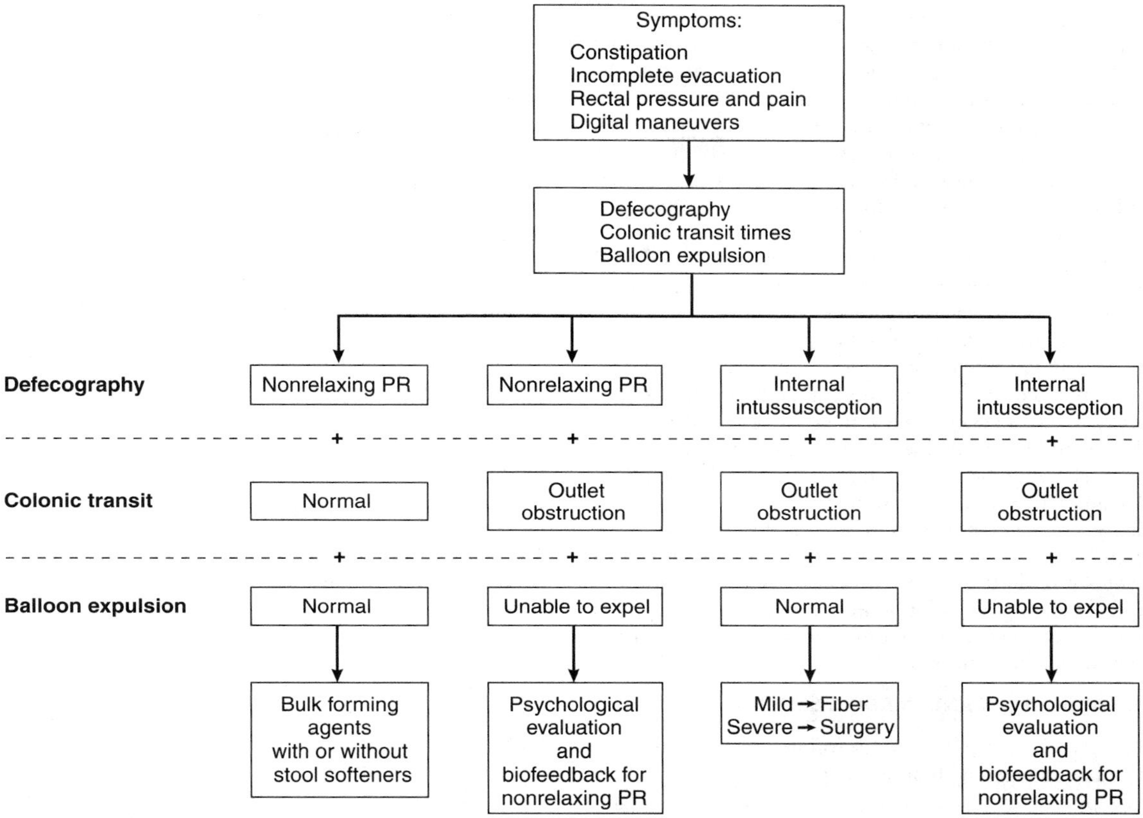

Figure 31–3. Algorithm for workup and treatment of obstructed defecation. (Reproduced, with permission, from Grendel JH, McQuaid KR, Friedman SL: *Current Diagnosis & Treatment in Gastroenterology.* Originally published by Appleton & Lange. Copyright © 1996 by The McGraw-Hill Companies, Inc.)

Nyam DC et al: Long-term results of surgery for chronic constipation. Dis Colon Rectum 1997;40:273. (Published erratum appears in Dis Colon Rectum 1997;40:529.)

ABNORMAL RECTAL FIXATION

ESSENTIALS OF DIAGNOSIS

- *Increased mobility of the rectum.*
- *Altered defecation (constipation, incontinence, or both).*

General Considerations

Abnormal rectal fixation is a group of diseases in which the attachment of the rectum to the sacrum has lengthened, allowing the rectum to block the act of defecation, to protrude into the vagina, or to prolapse through the anus. The reason for the increased mobility appears to be related to chronic straining. This may be secondary to colonic dysmotility or nonrelaxing puborectalis syndrome.

Clinical Findings

A. SYMPTOMS AND SIGNS

Internal intussusception leads to complaints of rectal fullness, an urge to defecate, incomplete evacuation, incontinence and, when associated with solitary rectal ulcers, rectal bleeding, mucus discharge, or tenesmus. Patients with rectal prolapse (rectal procidentia) complain of mucus discharge, progressive incontinence, pain, bleeding, and upon direct questioning they report that the rectum falls out.

Digital examination of the patient with internal intussusception may reveal a mass. This is the lead point of the intussusceptum and may be mistaken for a malignancy. The mass may be anterior and ulcerated (solitary rectal ulcer) or circumferential. The ulcer is 4–12 cm from the anal verge and is the ischemic traumatized lead point of the internal intussusceptum. Sigmoidoscopy may reveal the circumferential intussusceptum or an ulcerated mass that appears malignant. Pathologic examination reveals diffuse submucosal cysts with a characteristic fibrosis pattern and transverse smooth muscle cells within the lamina propria, distinguishing it from a malignancy. Physical examination of the patient with an acute rectal prolapse is not difficult. A large external mass of prolapsed tissue with concentric mucosal rings will be apparent. However, the diagnosis in a patient with a history of prolapse but without active prolapse may be more difficult. It may be necessary to give an enema, allow the patient to evacuate, and then examine the perineum. This often induces a prolapse, allowing for the diagnosis to be made in the office. An alternative is to demonstrate the prolapse on defecography. Digital examination may reveal decreased or absent sphincter tone. Anoscopy usually reveals a loss of normal hemorrhoidal tissue. The overlying distal rectal mucosa loses the dark plum color of the anal cushions and appears pink, resembling normal more proximal rectal mucosa right up to the dentate line.

B. Laboratory and Imaging Studies

Patients with internal intussusception and rectal prolapse may be evaluated with anorectal physiology testing, defecography or dynamic MRI, colonic transit studies, and barium enema or colonoscopy. Anorectal physiology testing may demonstrate obstructed defecation and exclude other causes of incontinence. Defecography or dynamic MRI will show the intussusceptum, making the diagnosis. Colonic transit time will be normal to the rectosigmoid, and barium enema or colonoscopy may document a normal colon. Rectal prolapse is usually diagnosed on physical examination without the need for further testing.

Differential Diagnosis

Internal intussusception must be differentiated from adenocarcinoma. The symptoms, physical appearance, and histologic characteristics of the ulcer may be confused with malignancy.

Rectal prolapse should be distinguished from hemorrhoidal disease. Rectal prolapse is seen as uninterrupted circumferential rings of mucosa, while hemorrhoidal prolapse will be seen as prolapsing tissue with deep grooves between areas of prolapsing edematous tissue.

Complications

The complications of intussusception and prolapse include progression of intussusception to prolapse, nerve injury from prolapse or chronic straining, descending perineum syndrome, bleeding, and incontinence. A severe rectal prolapse may become so edematous that it cannot be reduced, and it may progress to ischemia and gangrene.

Treatment

A. Medical Treatment

Mild to moderate intussusception is treated with bulk agents, modification of bowel habits, and reassurance. The patient is instructed to stimulate a bowel movement in the morning and avoid the urge to defecate the remainder of the day because the fullness they sense is the proximal rectum intussuscepting into the distal rectum. With time, the urge to defecate resolves and so does the intussusception.

B. Surgical Treatment

There are two classes of operations for rectal prolapse: abdominal and perineal. The abdominal procedures have a lower recurrence rate and preserve the reservoir capacity of the rectum but carry more risk and have a higher incidence of postoperative constipation. The perineal procedures avoid an intra-abdominal anastomosis but remove the rectum, thereby eliminating the rectal reservoir, but have higher recurrence rates. The abdominal procedures are generally preferred in low-risk active patients under age 50 and in those who require other abdominal procedures simultaneously.

The abdominal procedures for patients with severe intussusception or rectal prolapse with normal sphincter function are sigmoid resection with or without rectopexy and rectopexy alone. Both operations—rectopexy or resection—require complete mobilization of the entire rectum to the pelvic floor in order to avoid distal intussusception.

Rectopexy aims to secure the rectum to the sacral hollow. It may be performed with sutures or prosthetic materials such as polypropylene mesh (Marlex), Gore-Tex, or polyglycolic acid or polyglactin mesh (Dexon or Vicryl). Many studies have suggested a higher complication rate with the prosthetics, a lower continence rate, and no difference in recurrence, suggesting that suture rectopexy is preferable. Suture rectopexy is performed with heavy nonabsorbable sutures, attaching the rectum to the sacral hollow. The suture may be placed through the lateral ligaments or through the muscularis propria of the rectum.

The addition of a sigmoid resection at the time of rectopexy lowers the recurrence rate and the incidence of postoperative constipation without increasing the morbidity. Rectopexy corrects the mobility of the rectum but does not correct the underlying disorder for patients with pelvic floor dysfunction or chronic constipation. Sigmoid resection removes the intussusceptum and the mobile portion of colon. Thus, in the constipated patient or the patient with a redundant sigmoid colon, resection is preferable to fixation alone.

Laparoscopic methods for repair of rectal prolapse involve fixation, with or without resection. Patients may experience less pain and faster return of bowel function and have a shorter duration of hospitalization than with the open abdominal approach.

Perineal operations for rectal prolapse consist of anal encirclement, the transanal Delorme procedure, and the Altemeier procedure. Anal encirclement has limited application and should only be performed selectively in patients with a very high operative risk or a limited life expectancy. The original Thiersch procedure involved placing a silver wire around the external sphincter within the ischiorectal fat. Now synthetic mesh or silicone tubes are used instead of wire. The foreign body creates an outlet obstruction, and laxatives or enemas are required for rectal evacuation. Erosion of the foreign material into the rectum and infection are significant complications that limit the utility of this technique.

The Delorme procedure is essentially a mucosal proctectomy with plication of the prolapsing rectal wall. The dissection is started 1–2 cm above the dentate line and carried to the apex of the prolapsing segment, where the mucosa is amputated. The muscle is reefed in with four to eight heavy absorbable sutures, and the mucosa is reapproximated with sutures or a circular stapler.

The Altemeier procedure is a complete proctectomy and often a partial sigmoidectomy. The apex of the prolapsing segment is delivered and placed on traction, and a full-thickness incision is made approximately 1 cm above the dentate line. The rectum is everted. The dissection is carried into the deep cul-de-sac anteriorly. Laterally and posteriorly, the vascular supply to the rectum is taken with electrocautery or clamps when necessary. The dissection is carried up onto the midline mesorectum and sigmoid mesentery until the redundant segment of bowel has been completely mobilized. If a levatoroplasty is planned, it is most easily carried out at this time with heavy absorbable suture. A levatoroplasty plicates the pelvic floor musculature and adds to improved continence by increasing the anorectal angle. The bowel is transected proximally, excising the redundant portion, and a hand-sewn (heavy absorbable suture) or stapled anastomosis is performed.

Sphincter function returns and incontinence resolves in 65% of patients who were incontinent preoperatively, but there is no way to predict who will respond. Those who do not have return of sphincter function will not tolerate a sigmoid resection. Therefore, perineal proctectomy and posterior sphincter enhancement are recommended in these patients. The posterior reconstruction may alter the angle of the rectum or obstruct the outlet sufficiently to bring about continence. Individuals with severe intussusception and those who have rectal prolapse without sphincter dysfunction should do well with either the abdominal or the perineal approach.

Prognosis

The prognosis for patients with mild to moderate intussusception who are treated with bulking agents is excellent. Individuals with severe intussusception and those who have rectal prolapse without sphincter dysfunction should do well. Those with sphincter dysfunction have a 60–70% chance of regaining function. The abdominal approach is associated with approximately a 10% recurrence rate. The perineal approach is associated with a 20–30% recurrence rate. Reoperation for recurrence is possible after either approach but may be technically easier from the perineum if an abdominal resection has not been previously performed.

Athanasiadis S et al: The risk of infection of three synthetic materials used in rectopexy with or without colonic resection for rectal prolapse. Int J Colorectal Dis 1996;11:42.

Darzi A et al: Stapled laparoscopic rectopexy for rectal prolapse. Surg Endosc 1995;9:301.

Graf W et al: Laparoscopic suture rectopexy. Dis Colon Rectum 1995;38:211.

Huber FT et al: Functional results after treatment of rectal prolapse with rectopexy and sigmoid resection. World J Surg 1995;19:138; discussion 143.

Jacobs LK et al: The best operation for rectal prolapse. Surg Clin North Am 1997;77:49.

Mollen RM et al: Effects of rectal mobilization and lateral ligaments division on colonic and anorectal function. Dis Colon Rectum 2000;43:1283.

Novell JR et al: Prospective randomized trial of Ivalon sponge versus sutured rectopexy for full-thickness rectal prolapse. Br J Surg 1994;81:904.

Senagore AJ: Management of rectal prolapse: the role of laparoscopic approaches. Semin Laparosc Surg 2003;10:197.

Wexner SD et al: Laparoscopic colorectal surgery: analysis of 140 cases. Surg Endosc 1996;10:133.

HEMORRHOIDS

ESSENTIALS OF DIAGNOSIS

Internal hemorrhoids:

- *Painless bright red blood per rectum.*
- *Mucus discharge.*
- *Rectal fullness or discomfort.*

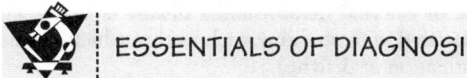

External hemorrhoids:

- *Sudden, severe perianal pain.*
- *Perianal mass.*

General Considerations

Hemorrhoidal tissues are part of the normal anatomy of the distal rectum and anal canal (Figure 31–1). **Internal hemorrhoids** are vascular and connective tissue cushions that originate above the dentate line and are lined with rectal or transitional mucosa. **External hemorrhoids** are vascular complexes underlying the richly innervated anoderm. Hemorrhoids function as protective pillows that become engorged with blood during the act of defecation, protecting the anal canal from direct trauma due to passage of stool. Hemorrhoidal tissues become engorged when intra-abdominal pressure is increased. This occurs with obesity, pregnancy, lifting, and straining for defecation.

Hemorrhoidal disease may involve the internal complex, the external complex, or both. Internal hemorrhoids become symptomatic when the internal complex becomes chronically engorged or the tissue prolapses into the anal canal due to laxity of the surrounding connective tissue and dilation of the veins. The external hemorrhoids become symptomatic with thrombosis, which leads to an acute onset of severe perianal pain. When the thrombosis resolves, the overlying skin becomes fibrotic, creating a skin tag.

Internal hemorrhoidal disease develops differently in older women and younger men. In older women the principal cause appears to be chronic straining, which leads to vascular engorgement and dilatation, resulting in stretching and disruption of the supporting connective tissue surrounding the vascular channels. The most common cause of prolonged straining is the act of defecation. Contrary to popular belief, the stool may be liquid or solid. Hemorrhoid pathology has no correlation with constipation (infrequent passage of stool) or portal hypertension. Pathologic hemorrhoids are not dilated vascular channels, varices, or vascular hyperplasias. The principal mechanism in younger men is increased resting pressure within the anal canal, leading to decreased venous return, venous engorgement, and disruption of the supporting tissues. The cause of external hemorrhoidal disease is unknown but is associated with straining such as that which occurs with constipation or diarrhea.

Internal hemorrhoidal disease is classified based on *history* as follows: first-degree hemorrhoids bleed; second-degree hemorrhoids bleed and prolapse, but reduce spontaneously; third-degree hemorrhoids bleed, prolapse, and require manual reduction; and fourth-degree hemorrhoids bleed, cannot be reduced, and may strangulate.

Clinical Findings

A. Symptoms and Signs

Pathologic internal hemorrhoids typically cause bright red bleeding per rectum, mucus discharge, and, when very large, a sense of rectal fullness or discomfort. Infrequently, internal hemorrhoids prolapse into the anal canal, where they may become incarcerated, thrombosed, and necrotic. In this instance, pain is common. Visual inspection may reveal a normal-appearing perineum, edema near the involved hemorrhoid, a prolapsed hemorrhoid, or an edematous, gangrenous, incarcerated hemorrhoid. The perineum may be macerated from chronic mucus discharge, the resulting moisture, and local irritation. Anoscopy may reveal tissue with evidence of chronic vascular dilatation, friability, mobility, and squamous metaplasia.

Acute intravascular thrombus may develop within external hemorrhoids associated with acute severe perianal pain. The pain usually peaks within 48–72 hours. An acutely thrombosed external hemorrhoid is a purple-black, edematous, tense subcutaneous perianal mass that is quite tender. The thrombus occasionally causes ischemia and necrosis of the overlying skin, resulting in bleeding.

B. Laboratory and Imaging Studies

Chronic bleeding from internal hemorrhoids may rarely cause anemia. However, until all other sources of blood loss have been ruled out, anemia must not be attributed to hemorrhoids regardless of the patient's age. Barium enema or colonoscopy is necessary to rule out malignancy and inflammatory bowel disease. Defecography is helpful in the patient in whom obstructed defecation and rectal prolapse is suspected.

Differential Diagnosis

Patients with perianal diseases often come to the surgeon with an inaccurate preliminary diagnosis of "hemorrhoids." A thorough history often suggests the correct diagnosis. Painless bleeding attributed to hemorrhoids must be distinguished from rectal bleeding from colorectal malignancy, inflammatory bowel disease, diverticular disease, and adenomatous polyps. Painful bleeding associated with a bowel movement is caused by a rectal ulcer or anal fissure. Straining at stool may be caused by obstructed defecation. Similarly, rectal prolapse must be distinguished from hemorrhoids because it is safe to band a hemorrhoid but not a prolapsed rectum. Moisture or maceration may be secondary to hemorrhoids or condylomata acuminata.

Complications

The complications of internal or external hemorrhoids are the indications for medical or surgical treatment:

bleeding, pain, necrosis, mucus discharge, moisture, and, rarely, perianal sepsis.

Treatment

A. Medical Treatment

Initial medical management is recommended for all but the most advanced cases. Dietary alterations, including elimination of constipating foods (eg, cheese, bananas) and the addition of bulking agents such as fiber, stool softeners, and increased intake of liquids, are advised. It is often beneficial to change daily routines by adding exercise and decreasing time spent on the commode.

B. Surgical Treatment

First- and second-degree hemorrhoids generally respond to medical management. Hemorrhoids that fail to respond to medical management may be treated with elastic band ligation, sclerosis, photocoagulation, cryosurgery, excisional hemorrhoidectomy, and many other local techniques that induce scarring and fixation of the hemorrhoids to the underlying tissues. The three classic techniques—elastic band ligation, sclerosis, and excisional hemorrhoidectomy—are discussed here along with the newer technique of stapled hemorrhoidopexy.

Elastic band ligation is safe and effective in the treatment of first-degree, second-degree, third-degree, and selected fourth-degree hemorrhoids. Hemorrhoidal tissue 1–2 cm above the dentate line is grasped, pulled into the barrel of an elastic band applicator, and two bands are placed at the base of the hemorrhoidal complex. After 7–10 days, the hemorrhoid sloughs away, removing a portion of the offending redundant tissue and leaving a scar that inhibits further prolapse and bleeding of the remaining tissue. If the band is placed in the transitional zone or below, the patient may experience severe pain, as this mucosa and skin are highly innervated. If that happens, the band should be removed immediately. Immunocompromised patients or those with unrecognized rectal prolapse have occasionally developed severe sepsis after banding, a complication heralded by inordinate pain, fever, and urinary retention. Treatment requires intravenous antibiotics, band removal, debridement of necrotic tissue, and observation. Patients are advised to avoid nonsteroidal anti-inflammatory agents and aspirin for 10 days after ligation, since significant bleeding may otherwise occur when the hemorrhoid sloughs.

Injection sclerotherapy is often tried for first-degree and second-degree hemorrhoids that continue to bleed despite medical measures. One to two milliliters of sclerosant is injected into the loose submucosal connective tissue above the hemorrhoidal complex, which causes inflammation and scarring. This inhibits prolapse and bleeding of the remaining hemorrhoidal tissue. The depth of injection is critical, since mucosal sloughing, infection, and full-thickness injury have been reported.

Excisional hemorrhoidectomy is reserved for the larger third- and fourth-degree hemorrhoids, mixed internal and external hemorrhoids not amenable to banding of the internal component, and incarcerated internal hemorrhoids requiring urgent intervention. The base of the hemorrhoid is inspected through an anoscope. The vascular pedicle may be suture-ligated with chromic catgut. The hemorrhoidal tissue is excised but care must be taken to avoid injuring the underlying internal sphincter while dissecting free the vascular cushion and overlying mucosa. The mucosal and skin defect may be left open, may be partially closed, or may be closed with the running the suture used to control the vascular pedicle.

Severe pain, urinary retention, bleeding, and fecal impaction are the most common complications of excisional hemorrhoidectomy. The incidence of these complications can be minimized with improved postoperative pain control, limited intraoperative intravenous fluid administration, attention to surgical technique, and stool bulking agents and stool softeners. Anal stenosis is a long-term complication that may be avoided by leaving enough anoderm between excised hemorrhoidal complexes.

Stapled hemorrhoidopexy is a technique that utilizes a circular stapling device to devascularize the hemorrhoidal tissue, reduce the mucosal prolapse, and perform an anopexy. The technique is safe, with improved postoperative pain control reported, but the cost of the device may limit its use. It is highly effective in the treatment of selected patients with circumferential advanced disease or mild rectal mucosal prolapse.

The acutely thrombosed external hemorrhoid may be treated with excision of the hemorrhoid or clot evacuation if the patient presents less than 48 hours after the onset of symptoms. Excision removes the clot and hemorrhoidal tissue, which decreases the chances of recurrence. However, many surgeons simply evacuate the thrombus, relieving the pressure and pain. If the patient presents over 48 to 72 hours after the symptoms begin, the thrombus will have started to organize and evacuation will be unsuccessful. Warm sitz baths, a high-fiber diet, stool softeners, and reassurance are appropriate at this point.

Prognosis

The prognosis for recurrence of hemorrhoidal disease is mostly related to success in changing the patient's bowel habits. Increasing dietary fiber, decreasing constipating foods, introducing exercise, and decreasing time spent on the toilet all decrease the amount of time spent straining in the squatting position. These behavioral modifications are the most important steps in preventing recurrence.

Arbman G et al: Closed vs. open hemorrhoidectomy—is there any difference? Dis Colon Rectum 2000;43:31.

Corman ML et al: Stapled haemorrhoidopexy: a consensus position paper by an international working party–indications, contra-indications and technique. Colorectal Dis 2003;5:304.

Galizia G et al: Lateral internal sphincterotomy together with haemorrhoidectomy for treatment of haemorrhoids: a randomised prospective study. Eur J Surg 2000;166:223.

Hayssen TK et al: Limited hemorrhoidectomy: results and long-term follow-up. Dis Colon Rectum 1999;42:909; discussion 914.

Ho YH et al: Randomized controlled trial of open and closed haemorrhoidectomy. Br J Surg 1997;84:1729.

Hoff SD et al: Ambulatory surgical hemorrhoidectomy—a solution to postoperative urinary retention? Dis Colon Rectum 1994;37:1242.

Komborozos VA et al: Rubber band ligation of symptomatic internal hemorrhoids: results of 500 cases. Dig Surg 2000;17:71.

Konsten J et al: Hemorrhoidectomy vs. Lord's method: 17-year follow-up of a prospective, randomized trial. Dis Colon Rectum 2000;43:503.

Lee HH et al: Multiple hemorrhoidal bandings in a single session. Dis Colon Rectum 1994;37:37.

Loder PB et al: Haemorrhoids: pathology, pathophysiology and aetiology. Br J Surg 1994;81:946.

MacRae HM et al: Comparison of hemorrhoidal treatment modalities. A meta-analysis. Dis Colon Rectum 1995;38:687.

O'Donovan S et al: Intraoperative use of Toradol facilitates outpatient hemorrhoidectomy. Dis Colon Rectum 1994;37:793.

Pescatori M: Urinary retention after anorectal operations. Dis Colon Rectum 1999;42:964.

Shalaby R, Desoky A: Randomized clinical trial of stapled versus Milligan-Morgan haemorrhoidectomy. Br J Surg 2001;88:1049.

ANAL STENOSIS

ESSENTIALS OF DIAGNOSIS

- *Obstructed defecation.*
- *Stenosis on rectal examination.*

General Considerations

Anal stenosis is typically an iatrogenic complication of scarring after anal surgery. In particular, hemorrhoidectomies, single quadrant or circumferential (Whitehead), when inexpertly performed, may lead to stenosis. Other causes include anal tumors, Crohn's disease, radiation injury, recurrent anal ulcers, infection, and trauma.

Clinical Findings

A. Symptoms and Signs

Anal stenosis causes increasing difficulty with—and straining at—defecation, thin and sometimes painful bowel movements, and bloating. Examination of the patient with anal stenosis may reveal postsurgical changes and a stenotic anal canal. Digital examination may be quite painful or impossible.

B. Laboratory and Imaging Studies

No additional studies of the patient with anal stenosis are required, although a contrast enema could help delineate the length of stenosis.

Differential Diagnosis

Patients with anal stenosis may complain of anal pain or obstructed defecation, and physical examination will assist with diagnosis. Other causes of anal pain include a fissure with or without concomitant stenosis, thrombosed external hemorrhoids, perirectal abscess, malignancy, foreign body, and proctalgia fugax. Proctalgia fugax (levator ani syndrome), a diagnosis of exclusion, is suggested when a patient complains of pain that awakens him or her from sleep. The pain is generally left-sided, short-lived, and relieved by heat, anal dilation, or muscle relaxants. The patient often has a history of migraine headaches and may report that the pain is triggered by stressful events.

Treatment

Mild anal stenosis may be treated successfully with gentle dilation and bulk-forming agents. Severe anal stenosis is treated surgically if there is no evidence of active disease (eg, Crohn's disease) and healthy tissue is available to perform the anoplasty. This can be achieved with a skin island or V-Y flap. Both procedures involve incision of the stenotic anus, mobilization of the surrounding skin, and advancement of the healthy tissue into the closure, relieving the stenosis. The prognosis for anal stenosis is excellent if there is no evidence of active disease of the anus.

ANAL FISSURE & ULCER

ESSENTIALS OF DIAGNOSIS

- *Tearing pain upon defecation.*
- *Blood on tissue or stool.*
- *Persistent perianal pain or spasm following defecation.*

- *Sphincter spasm.*
- *Disruption of anoderm.*

General Considerations

An anal fissure is a split in the anoderm. An anal ulcer is a chronic fissure. When mature, an ulcer is associated with a skin tag **(sentinel pile)** (Figure 31–4). Fissures typically occur in the midline just distal to the dentate line. Two studies have called into question Goligher's rule that 90% are posterior, 10% anterior, and less than 1% occur simultaneously in the anterior and posterior positions. Both studies found anterior fissures to be more common than expected, but the fissures were still in the midline.

Fissures result from forceful dilation of the anal canal, most commonly during defecation. The anoderm is disrupted, exposing the underlying internal sphincter muscle. The muscle goes into spasm in response to exposure and fails to relax with the next dilation (bowel movement). This leads to further tearing, deepening of the fissure, and increased muscle irritation and spasm. The persistent muscle spasm leads to relative ischemia of the overlying anoderm and inhibits healing. Ultraslow waves—low-frequency high-amplitude pressure changes—occur with increased frequency in patients with anal fissures and disappear with sphincterotomy and fissure healing, suggesting a relationship between spasm and persistent disease.

Classically, the initial insult is felt to be a firm bowel movement. The pain associated with the initial bowel movement is great and the patient therefore ignores the urge to defecate for fear of experiencing the pain again. This allows the formation of harder stool that tears the anoderm more as it passes due to its size and the poor relaxation of the sphincter. A self-perpetuating cycle of pain, poor relaxation, and reinjury is the result.

Factors that may predispose to fissure formation are previous anorectal surgery (hemorrhoidectomy, fistulotomy, destruction of condylomas) resulting in scarring of the anoderm with loss of elasticity, which increases the probability that the anoderm will tear.

Clinical Findings

A. Symptoms and Signs

Fissures cause pain and bleeding with defecation. The pain is often tearing or burning, worst during defecation, and subsides over a few hours. Blood is noted on the tissue and stool or dripping into the toilet water but it is not mixed in the stool. Constipation may develop because of fear of recurrent pain. Although less common, fissures may present as painless nonhealing wounds that bleed intermittently.

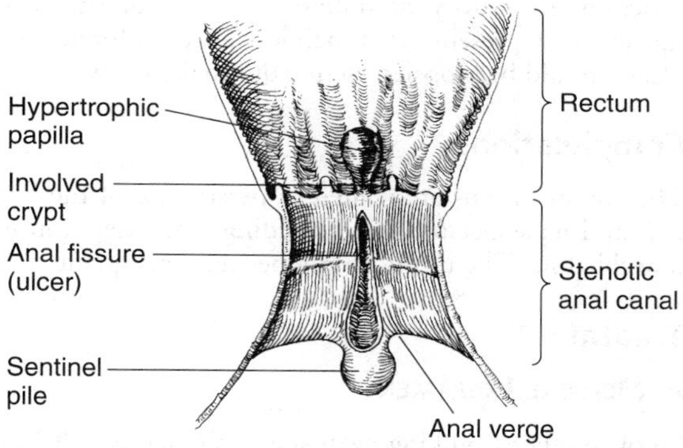

Figure 31–4. Diagram of the anorectum showing the fissure or ulcer triad.

Although anoscopy and sigmoidoscopy may not be tolerable in the initial evaluation of a patient with a fissure, they must be done later because associated anorectal malignancy or inflammatory bowel disease must be excluded. Any nonhealing midline fissure should be biopsied to exclude Crohn's disease or malignancy.

Physical examination by simple gentle traction on the buttocks will evert the anus enough to reveal a disruption of the anoderm in the midline at the mucocutaneous junction. This may be all there is in an acute fissure. In a chronic fissure, a sentinel pile may be seen at the inferior margin of the ulcer. Gentle, limited digital examination will confirm internal sphincter spasm. Anoscopy and proctosigmoidoscopy should be deferred until healing occurs, or alternatively the procedure can be performed under anesthesia. The classic triad of a proximal hypertrophied anal papilla above a fissure with the sentinel pile at the anal verge may be identified.

B. Laboratory and Imaging Studies

Anal manometry is unhelpful. Studies have shown increased anal pressures in patients with ulcers, but patients with high pressures have not been found to be at increased risk for fissure-ulcer disease.

Differential Diagnosis

Fissure-ulcer disease occurs in the anterior or posterior midline and involves the epithelium immediately distal to the dentate line. Ulcers occurring off the midline or away from the dentate line are suspect. Crohn's disease, anal tuberculosis, anal malignancy, abscess or fistula disease, cytomegalovirus, herpes, chlamydiosis, syphilis, AIDS, and some blood dyscrasias may all mimic fissure or ulcer disease. Initial manifestations of Crohn's disease are limited to the anal canal in 10% of patients. Anal tuberculosis will be associated with a previous or concomitant history of pulmonary tuberculosis. Anal cancer may present as a painless ulcer. Nonhealing ulcers should be biopsied to rule out malignancy.

Complications

The complications are related to persistence of the disease and its associated pain, bleeding, and alteration in bowel habits. The ulcers do not become malignant.

Treatment

A. Medical Treatment

Stool softeners, bulking agents, and sitz baths will heal 90% of anal fissures. A second episode has a 70% chance of healing with this regimen. Sitz baths after painful bowel movements soothe the muscle spasm. Patients are instructed to soak in a hot bath and contract the sphincters to identify the muscle in spasm and to then concentrate on relaxing that muscle. The effect is twofold: it decreases the pain associated with the spasm and improves blood flow to the fissure, which benefits healing. Stool softeners and bulking agents make the stool more malleable, decreasing the trauma of each successive bowel movement. Chronic (> 1 month history) or chronic-recurrent ulcers should be considered for surgery.

Botulinum toxin infiltration into the internal sphincters aids healing of anal fissures. This agent inhibits the release of acetylcholine from presynaptic nerve fibers, creating a reversible paralysis that lasts several months. This allows for improved perfusion of the disrupted anoderm and healing at rates higher than can be achieved with standard medical therapy or topical nitroglycerin ointment therapy.

0.2% nitroglycerin is also effective treatment. Nitroglycerin ointment is a nitric oxide source. Nitric oxide, an inhibitory neurotransmitter, relaxes the internal sphincter and improves blood flow to the anoderm. The major side effect, headache, persists at the lower therapeutic range (0.2% or 0.3%), causing some limitation of this therapy. An alternative approach is to use 0.3% nifedipine ointment. The calcium-channel blockade results in sphincter relaxation without the undesirable side effect of the headache associated with systemic absorption of nitroglycerin.

B. Surgical Treatment

Lateral internal anal sphincterotomy is the procedure of choice after conservative measures have failed. This may be performed open, where an incision is made in the skin and the hypertrophied distal one-third of the internal sphincter is divided under direct vision. It may also be done closed, where a scalpel is passed in the intersphincteric plane and swept medially, dividing the internal sphincter blindly. Both techniques give similar results. It is possible to disrupt the internal sphincter with a four-finger stretch, but this is an uncontrolled disruption that is associated with a higher recurrence rate and incontinence.

Prognosis

Lateral internal anal sphincterotomy is over 90% successful in the treatment of chronic anal fissure-ulcer disease. Fewer than 10% of patients so treated are incontinent of mucus and gas. The recurrence rate is less than 10%.

Altomare DF et al: Glyceryl trinitrate for chronic anal fissure–healing or headache? Results of a multicenter, randomized, placebo-controlled, double-blind trial. Dis Colon Rectum 2000;43:174.

Argov S et al: Open lateral sphincterotomy is still the best treatment for chronic anal fissure. Am J Surg 2000;179:201.

Brisinda G et al: A comparison of injections of botulinum toxin and topical nitroglycerin ointment for the treatment of chronic anal fissure. N Engl J Med 1999;341:65.

Cook TA et al: Oral nifedipine reduces resting anal pressure and heals chronic anal fissure. Br J Surg 1999;86:1269.

Fernández López F et al: Botulinum toxin for the treatment of anal fissure. Dig Surg 1999;16:515.

Garcia-Aguilar J et al: Open vs. closed sphincterotomy for chronic anal fissure: long-term results. Dis Colon Rectum 1996;39:440.

Jost WH: One hundred cases of anal fissure treated with botulin toxin: early and long-term results. Dis Colon Rectum 1997;40:1029.

Keck JO et al: Computer-generated profiles of the anal canal in patients with anal fissure. Dis Colon Rectum 1995;38:72.

Lund JN et al: A randomised, prospective, double-blind, placebo-controlled trial of glyceryl trinitrate ointment in treatment of anal fissure. Lancet 1997;349:11.

Maria G et al: Influence of botulinum toxin site of injections on healing rate in patients with chronic anal fissure. Am J Surg 2000;179:46.

Maria G et al: A comparison of botulinum toxin and saline for the treatment of chronic anal fissure. N Engl J Med 1998;338:217.

Nelson RL: Nonsurgical therapy for anal fissure. Cochrane Database Syst Rev 2003;4:CD003431.

Nelson RL: Meta-analysis of operative techniques for fissure-in-ano. Dis Colon Rectum 1999;42:1424; discussion 1428.

Nyam DC et al: Long-term results of lateral internal sphincterotomy for chronic anal fissure with particular reference to incidence of fecal incontinence. Dis Colon Rectum 1999;42:1306.

Oettle GJ: Glyceryl trinitrate vs. sphincterotomy for treatment of chronic fissure-in-ano: a randomized, controlled trial. Dis Colon Rectum 1997;40:1318.

Richard CS et al: Internal sphincterotomy is superior to topical nitroglycerin in the treatment of chronic anal fissure: results of a randomized, controlled trial by the Canadian Colorectal Surgical Trials Group. Dis Colon Rectum 2000;43:1048.

Schouten WR et al: Ischaemic nature of anal fissure. Br J Surg 1996;83:63.

INFECTIONS OF THE ANORECTUM

ANORECTAL ABSCESS & FISTULA

ESSENTIALS OF DIAGNOSIS

- *Severe anal pain.*
- *Palpable mass usually present on perineal or digital rectal examination.*
- *Systemic sepsis.*

General Considerations

Perirectal abscess and fistulous disease not associated with a specific systemic disease is most commonly cryptoglandular in origin. The anal canal has 6–14 glands that lie in or near the plane between the internal and external sphincters. Projections from the glands pass through the internal sphincters and drain into the crypts at the dentate line. Glands may become infected when a crypt is occluded, trapping stool and bacteria within the gland. Occlusion may follow impaction of vegetable matter or edema from trauma (firm stool or foreign body) or as a result of an adjacent inflammatory process. If the crypt does not decompress into the anal canal, an abscess may develop in the intersphincteric plane. The abscess may track within or across the intersphincteric plane. Abscesses are classified according to the space they invade (Figure 31–5). The most difficult to treat occurs when the abscess tracks proximally or circumferentially within the intersphincteric plane or within the ischiorectal fossa and deep postanal space. Regardless of location, the extent of an abscess may be difficult to determine without examination under anesthesia.

Antibiotics given while allowing the abscess to mature are not helpful. Early surgical operative drainage is the best way to avoid the potentially disastrous complications of undrained perineal sepsis. When the abscesses are drained, either surgically or spontaneously, 50% have persistent communication with the crypt, creating a fistula from the anus to the perianal skin (fistula-in-ano). A fistula-in-ano is not a surgical emergency.

Clinical Findings

A. Symptoms and Signs

An anorectal abscess typically causes severe and continuous throbbing pain that may worsen with ambulation and straining. Swelling and discharge are noted less frequently. Patients may present with fever, malaise, urinary retention, and life-threatening sepsis. People with diabetes mellitus or immune compromise are most vulnerable. A patient with fistula-in-ano may report a history of severe pain, bloody purulent drainage associated with resolution of the pain, and subsequent chronic mucopurulent discharge.

Physical examination reveals a tender perianal or rectal mass. The size is often difficult to assess until the patient is anesthetized. An apparently small abscess may extend high into the ischiorectal or supralevator space. A fistula is present when internal and external openings are identified. A firm connecting tract is often palpable.

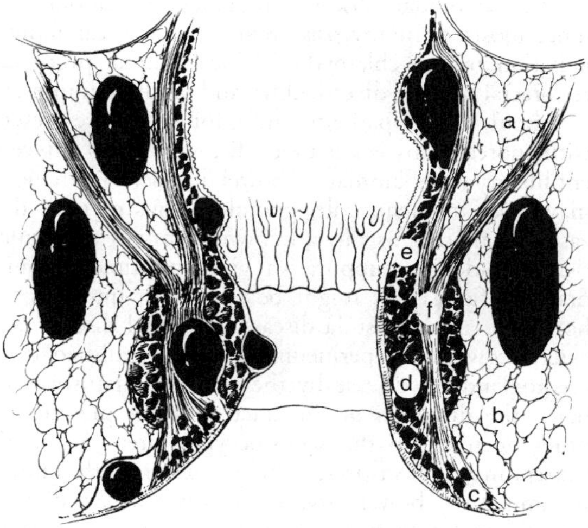

Figure 31–5. Composite diagram of acute anorectal abscesses and spaces. (a) Pelvirectal (supralevator) space. (b) Ischiorectal space. (c) Perianal (subcutaneous) space. (d) Marginal (mucocutaneous) space. (e) Submucous space. (f) Intermuscular space.

B. Laboratory and Imaging Studies

No imaging studies are necessary in uncomplicated abscess fistulous disease. Sinograms, transrectal ultrasound, CT, and MRI may be useful in the evaluation of complex or recurrent disease. Transrectal ultrasound can identify branching of fistulous tracts, persistent undrained sepsis, and extent of sphincter involvement. Hydrogen peroxide injection of the tract may improve sensitivity of the ultrasound. CT scan may be helpful in finding an undiagnosed supralevator abscess. MRI and MRI with endorectal coil may be of use in identifying and classifying fistulas.

Differential Diagnosis

Abscess and fistula disease of cryptoglandular origin must be differentiated from complications of Crohn's disease, pilonidal disease, hidradenitis suppurativa, tuberculosis, actinomycosis, trauma, fissures, carcinoma, radiation injury, chlamydiosis, local dermal processes, retrorectal tumors, diverticulitis, and urethral injuries.

About 10% of patients with Crohn's disease present with anorectal abscess fistulous disease with no antecedent history of inflammatory bowel disease. Tuberculosis may cause indolent, pale, granulomatous perianal disease, but there is usually a known history of tuberculosis. Hidradenitis suppurativa gives multiple chronic, draining fistulas, as might be seen with undiagnosed horseshoe abscess fistula disease. Pilonidal disease may extend toward the perineum; it is distinguished from cryptoglandular disease by the presence of inspissated hairs, the direction of the tract, and the presence of other openings in the sacrococcygeal area. A colonic source may be suspected in a patient with known inflammatory bowel disease or diverticular disease. Other less common causes include tumors, radiation, infections, and urologic injuries.

Complications

The complications of an undrained anorectal abscess may be severe. Unless drained, the infection may spread rapidly and result in extensive tissue loss, sphincter injury, and even death. In contrast, a fistula-in-ano, which develops when the abscess is drained, is not a surgical emergency. A chronic fistula may be associated with recurring perianal abscess formation and, rarely, with cancer of the fistulous tract.

Treatment

Abscesses should be drained surgically. It is best done in the operating room, where anesthesia allows adequate evaluation of the extent of disease. Abscesses thought to be superficial in the office may be found to extend above the levators. Intersphincteric abscesses are treated by an internal sphincterotomy that drains the abscess and destroys the crypt. Perirectal and ischiorectal abscesses should be drained by a catheter or with adequate excision of skin to prevent premature closure and reaccumulation of the abscess. If the internal opening of the fistula is identified and external sphincter involvement is minimal, a fistulotomy may be performed when the abscess is drained. However, the internal opening is often hard to find because of the inflammation, and drainage is all that can be achieved. In this instance, catheter drainage is preferred to skin excision since the catheter (1) establishes drainage with minimal disruption of normal perianal skin, (2) facilitates identification of the internal opening at subsequent evaluation, and (3) facilitates patient compliance by eliminating the need for packing or leaving the wound open.

Patients with chronic or recurring abscesses after apparent adequate surgical drainage often have an undrained deep postanal space abscess that communicates with the ischiorectal fossa via a horseshoe fistula. Treatment involves opening the deep postanal space and counter-draining the tract through the ischiorectal external opening. The horseshoe fistula almost always arises from a posterior midline cryptoglandular origin. Once the postanal space heals, the counter drain may be removed.

Immunocompromised patients are a particular challenge. With moderate compromise (eg, diabetes mellitus), urgent drainage in the operating room is required, as these patients are prone to necrotizing anorectal infections. With severe compromise (eg, patients receiving chemotherapy), infection may occur without an abscess due to neutropenia. In these patients it is important to attempt to localize the process, establish drainage, localize the internal opening, and obtain a biopsy for tissue examination and culture (to rule out leukemia and to select antibiotics).

The treatment of fistulas is dictated by the course of the fistula. The Salmon-Goodsall rule is of assistance in identifying the direction of the tract (Figure 31–6). If the tract passes superficially and does not involve sphincter muscle, a simple incision of the tract with ablation of the gland and saucerization of the skin at the external opening is all that is necessary. A fistula that involves a small amount of sphincter may be treated similarly. A tract that passes deep or that involves an undetermined amount of muscle is best treated with a mucosal advancement flap (described in the section on rectovaginal fistulas) because immediate or delayed (as with a seton) muscle division is associated with a risk for incontinence.

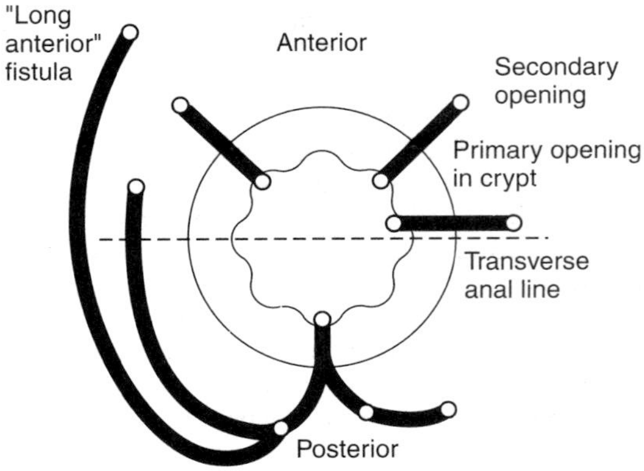

Figure 31–6. Salmon-Goodsall rule. The usual relation of the primary and secondary openings of fistulas. When there is an anterior and also a posterior opening of the same fistula, the rule of the posterior opening applies; the long anterior fistula is an exception to the rule.

Prognosis

The prognosis for cryptoglandular abscess and fistula disease is excellent once the source of infection is identified. Fistulas persist when the source has not been identified or adequately drained, when the diagnosis is incorrect, or when postoperative care is insufficient.

Brook I et al: The aerobic and anaerobic bacteriology of perirectal abscesses. J Clin Microbiol 1997;35:2974.

Chapple KS et al: Prognostic value of magnetic resonance imaging in the management of fistula-in-ano. Dis Colon Rectum 2000;43:511.

Cho DY: Endosonographic criteria for an internal opening of fistula-in-ano. Dis Colon Rectum 1999;42:515.

Cintron JR et al: Repair of fistulas-in-ano using fibrin adhesive: long-term follow-up. Dis Colon Rectum 2000;43:944.

Garcia-Aguilar J et al: Anal fistula surgery. Factors associated with recurrence and incontinence. Dis Colon Rectum 1996;39:723.

Ho YH et al: Marsupialization of fistulotomy wounds improves healing: a randomized controlled trial. Br J Surg 1998;85:105.

Jun SH et al: Anocutaneous advancement flap closure of high anal fistulas. Br J Surg 1999;86:490.

Knoefel WT et al: The initial approach to anorectal abscesses: fistulotomy is safe and reduces the chance of recurrences. Dig Surg 2000;17:274.

Miller GV et al: Flap advancement and core fistulectomy for complex rectal fistula. Br J Surg 1998;85:108.

Nelson RL et al: Dermal island-flap anoplasty for transsphincteric fistula-in-ano: assessment of treatment failures. Dis Colon Rectum 2000;43:681.

Park JJ et al: Repair of chronic anorectal fistulae using commercial fibrin sealant. Arch Surg 2000;135:166.

Practice parameters for treatment of fistula-in-ano—supporting documentation. The Standards Practice Task Force. The American Society of Colon and Rectal Surgeons. Dis Colon Rectum 1996;39:1363.

RECTOVAGINAL FISTULA

ESSENTIALS OF DIAGNOSIS

- *Passing stool and flatus through the vagina.*
- *Altered continence.*
- *Tract generally visible or palpable.*

General Considerations

Rectovaginal fistulas occur as a result of obstetric injury, Crohn's disease, diverticulitis, radiation, undrained cryptoglandular disease, foreign body trauma, surgical extirpation of anterior rectal tumors, and malignancies of the rectum, cervix, or vagina. The fistulas are classified as low, middle, or high. The location and cause of the fistula determine the operative approach.

Clinical Findings

A. Symptoms and Signs

Passing stool and flatus through the vagina is characteristic of rectovaginal fistulas. There may be varying degrees of incontinence. An opening in the vagina or rectum may be seen or felt on physical examination.

B. Laboratory and Imaging Studies

A vaginogram or barium enema may identify the fistula. If the fistula is not demonstrated on radiographic or physical examination, a dilute methylene blue enema may be administered with a tampon in the vagina. If a fistula is present, it should be confirmed by methylene blue staining of the tampon.

Differential Diagnosis

The signs and symptoms of a rectovaginal fistula are fairly unmistakable. The important differential is the cause of the fistula, as this affects management, as discussed below.

Complications

The major complication of a rectovaginal fistula is impaired hygiene and incontinence.

Treatment

The cause and location of the fistula determine the treatment. Involvement of surrounding tissue by the disease process that leads to the fistula may limit the surgical options. For example, in patients with active Crohn's disease or radiation injury of the surrounding tissue, the fistula cannot be repaired with local procedures; Crohn's disease must go into remission before a fistula can be repaired. Radiation injuries require that normal healthy tissue be brought from outside the irradiated field.

Low rectovaginal fistulas (rectal opening near the dentate line and vaginal opening just above the fourchette) commonly result from obstetric injuries, trauma from foreign bodies, cryptoglandular disease, or Crohn's disease. Obstetric injuries often heal within the first 3 months. Waiting 3 months allows inflammation to resolve, which facilitates repair and allows for closure of those fistulas that will spontaneously heal. Similarly, traumatic fistulas may be repaired most easily after inflammation resolves. Fistulas secondary to cryptoglandular disease may close spontaneously once the primary process is drained.

Fistulas secondary to Crohn's disease rarely heal spontaneously. Aggressive medical therapy and surgical control of perianal sepsis are necessary to conserve the sphincters. Once the disease is in remission, local advancement flap procedures may be performed. The principle is to bring fresh, uninvolved tissue down over the fistulous tract and excise the old rectal opening. This often delays proctectomy and preserves the anal sphincter and rectum. Patients with severe disease that does not respond to local measures may require a temporary diverting colostomy. After diversion, a single focus of disease is often found and an advancement procedure may be performed while the fecal stream is diverted. Extensive destruction of the rectum or sphincters may mandate immediate proctectomy without attempts at local preservation. Early surgical intervention and conservative drainage or diversion may postpone this situation.

Midrectal fistulas from cryptoglandular disease, Crohn's disease, or obstetric injury should be treated as outlined above. Those that occur secondary to radiation are not amenable to local procedures, as the surrounding tissue is similarly affected. Transabdominal resection and coloanal anastomosis is preferred. These are particularly challenging patients. Other surgical options are beyond the scope of this chapter.

High rectal fistulas result from Crohn's disease, diverticular disease, operative injury, malignancy, and radiation. High rectovaginal fistulas are best treated via a transabdominal approach. This allows for resection of the diseased bowel that created the fistula.

Prognosis

The prognosis is determined by the cause of the fistula.

Fry RD et al: Rectovaginal fistula. Surg Ann 1995;27:113.

Hull TL et al: Surgical approaches to low anovaginal fistula in Crohn's disease. Am J Surg 1997;173:95.

Hyman N: Endoanal advancement flap repair for complex anorectal fistula. Am J Surg 1999;178:337.

Khanduja KS et al: Reconstruction of rectovaginal fistula with sphincter disruption by combining rectal mucosal advancement flap and anal sphincteroplasty. Dis Colon Rectum 1999;42:1432.

Marchesa P et al: Advancement sleeve flaps for treatment of severe perianal Crohn's disease. Br J Surg 1998;85:1695.

Ozuner G et al: Long-term analysis of the use of transanal rectal advancement flaps for complicated anorectal/vaginal fistulas. Dis Colon Rectum 1996;39:10.

Simmang CL et al: Rectal sleeve advancement: repair of rectovaginal fistula associated with anorectal stricture in Crohn's disease. Dis Colon Rectum 1998;41:787.

Tsang CB et al: Anal sphincter integrity and function influences outcome in rectovaginal fistula repair. Dis Colon Rectum 1998;41:1141.

Tsang CB et al: Rectovaginal fistulas. Therapeutic options. Surg Clin North Am 1997;77:95.

Venkatesh KS et al: Fibrin glue application in the treatment of recurrent anorectal fistulas. Dis Colon Rectum 1999;42:1136.

Yee LF et al: Use of endoanal ultrasound in patients with rectovaginal fistulas. Dis Colon Rectum 1999;42:1057.

PILONIDAL DISEASE

ESSENTIALS OF DIAGNOSIS

- *Acute chronic recurring abscess or chronic draining sinus over the sacrococcygeal or perianal region.*
- *Pain, tenderness, purulent drainage, inspissated hair, induration.*

General Considerations

The incidence of pilonidal disease is highest in white males (3:1 male:female ratio) between ages 15 and 40, with a peak incidence between 16 and 20 years. It rarely occurs in patients more than 50 years old. It was once thought that pilonidal disease was a congenital condition that developed along an epithelialized tract of the natal cleft. It is now considered to be an acquired infection of natal cleft hair follicles, which become distended and obstructed and rupture into the subcutaneous tissues to form a pilonidal abscess. Hair from the surrounding skin is pulled into the abscess cavity by the friction generated by the gluteal muscles during walking.

Clinical Findings

Patients with pilonidal disease may present with small midline pits or abscesses on or off the midline near the coccyx or sacrum. The patients are generally heavy hirsute males who perspire profusely. The workup is limited to a physical examination unless one suspects Crohn's disease, in which case a more extensive evaluation may be necessary. Physical examination may reveal a spectrum of disease from acute suppuration and an undrained abscess or chronic draining sinuses with multiple mature tracts with hairs protruding from the pit-like openings.

Differential Diagnosis

The differential diagnosis includes cryptoglandular abscess-fistulous disease of the anus, hidradenitis suppurativa, furuncle, and actinomycosis.

Complications

Untreated pilonidal disease may result in multiple draining sinuses with chronic recurrent abscess, drainage, soiling of clothing, and, rarely, necrotizing wound infections or malignant degeneration.

Treatment

Pilonidal abscesses may be drained under local anesthesia. A probe may be inserted into the primary opening and the abscess unroofed. Granulation tissue and inspissated hair are pulled out, but definitive therapy is not required at the first procedure. Cure rates of 60–80% have been reported after primary unroofing and extraction of hair. For those that fail to heal after 3 months or develop a chronic draining sinus, definitive therapy may be considered.

Nonoperative therapy with meticulous skin care (shaving of the natal cleft, perineal hygiene) and drainage of abscesses will substantially reduce the need for surgery.

Conservative excision of midline pits with removal of hair from lateral tracts and postoperative weekly shaving has a 90% success rate. Excision with open packing, marsupialization, or primary closure with or without flaps have all been advocated. Either open packing or marsupialization leaves the patient with painful wounds slow to heal, and marsupialization has a reported recurrence rate of 10%. Simple primary closure often results in dehiscence because the midline skin has a poor blood supply, the wounds are closed under tension, and there is often dead space at the base of the defect that is susceptible to infection. Closure over suction drainage or the use of lateral incisions with excision of the tracts decreases the rate of wound dehiscence.

Prognosis

The prognosis after surgery is excellent. Recurrent or persistent disease has been reported to be 0–15% and is likely due to inadequate excision where external openings or occult tracts are missed. Inadequate postoperative hygiene with ingrowth of hair into the wound also leads to recurrence.

Abu Galala KH et al: Treatment of pilonidal sinus by primary closure with a transposed rhomboid flap compared with deep suturing: a prospective randomised clinical trial. Eur J Surg 1999;165:468.

Akinci OF et al: Simple and effective surgical treatment of pilonidal sinus: asymmetric excision and primary closure using suction drain and subcuticular skin closure. Dis Colon Rectum 2000;43:701.

Armstrong JH et al: Pilonidal sinus disease. The conservative approach. Arch Surg 1994;129:914.

Bozkurt MK et al: Management of pilonidal sinus with the Limberg flap. Dis Colon Rectum 1998;41:775.

Peterson S et al: Primary closure techniques in chronic pilonidal sinus: a survey of the results of different surgical approaches. Dis Colon Rectum 2002;45:1458.

Senapati A et al: Bascom's operation in the day-surgical management of symptomatic pilonidal sinus. Br J Surg 2000;87:1067.

Spivak H et al: Treatment of chronic pilonidal disease. Dis Colon Rectum 1996;39:1136.

PRURITUS ANI

ESSENTIALS OF DIAGNOSIS

- *Severe perianal itching, often at night.*
- *When chronic, skin becomes white, leathery, and thickened.*

General Considerations

Pruritus ani is usually idiopathic. Most patients have tried many over-the-counter preparations without relief. These agents may exacerbate the problem by keeping the perineum moist, causing further irritation, or by creating a contact dermatitis (especially local anesthetics). Poor cleansing of the perineum may lead to irritation of the exquisitely sensitive anoderm and subsequent pruritus. In contrast, frequent washing with soaps and detergents dries the skin, also leading to pruritus. Pinworms (*Enterobius vermicularis*) are the most common cause of perianal itching in children.

Clinical Findings

A. Symptoms and Signs

The patient experiences severe perianal itching, often worse at night. The skin is thickened, white, and leathery in the chronic state but may be normal to weeping in the acute stage. In children with pinworms, perianal itching is most severe at night, when the pinworm deposits its eggs on the perianal skin.

B. Laboratory and Imaging Studies

The diagnosis of pinworms is made by applying cellophane tape to the perianal skin, which collects the eggs and allows them to be viewed under a microscope. Scrapings of the perianal skin viewed microscopically may reveal fungi or parasites. Biopsy and histologic evaluation may be necessary in refractory cases to rule out underlying malignancy.

Differential Diagnosis

Pruritus may be associated with other perianal lesions that distort normal anal anatomy such as hemorrhoids, fistulas, fissures, tumors of the anorectum, previous surgery, and radiation therapy. As noted above, it may be secondary to excessive cleaning or application of ointments to the perianal region. Primary dermatologic diseases such as lichen planus, atopic eczema, psoriasis, and seborrheic dermatitis may all affect the perineum. Fungal (dermatophytosis, candidiasis), parasitic (*Enterobius vermicularis,* scabies, or pediculosis), and bacterial superinfection should be considered. Other causes include contact dermatitis from local anesthetic creams or soaps, recent antibiotic usage, systemic diseases (diabetes, liver disease), dietary factors, and perianal neoplasms (Bowen's disease and extramammary Paget's disease). Pruritus may result from tight clothing, obesity, and living in a hot climate. When a specific cause cannot be found, it is considered idiopathic.

Complications

Complications include severe excoriation, ulceration, and secondary infection of the perineum.

Treatment

Identifiable causes of pruritus ani such as hemorrhoids, yeast infection, or parasites should be treated. Patients should be educated about proper perineal care, and the use of soaps and topical ointments should be discouraged. The perineum should be kept dry. Use of a blow dryer on the perineum after bathing may be helpful. Alteration in dietary habits may be necessary. Coffee, tea, cola drinks, beer, chocolate, and tomatoes cause perianal itching and should be excluded from the diet for at least 2 weeks. Symptoms should resolve with alterations in dietary and cleaning habits. After symptoms resolve, each food group may be added sequentially to identify the causative agent. Pruritus refractory to the above measures may be treated by intradermal injection of 1% methylene blue solution.

Prognosis

Relapse is common, and reeducation is often effective. In refractory cases, dermatologic and psychiatric consultation may be necessary.

PROCTITIS & ANUSITIS

Proctitis and anusitis are nonspecific terms for varying degrees of inflammation due to infectious or inflammatory diseases. The causative agent or event determines the symptoms, signs, and appropriate management. In considering these diseases, particular attention should be paid to sexual practices and sexually transmitted diseases.

1. Herpes Proctitis

Lesions appear as vesicles, which rupture to form ulcers that may become secondarily infected. Patients may present early with anal pain and vesicles or later with ulcerations, discharge, rectal bleeding, tenesmus, and even fear of defecation because of severe pain. Fever and generalized malaise are often noted. No history of anoreceptive intercourse is required, as the disease may spread by extension from the vagina. Viral culture of the vesicle or biopsy of the ulcer is diagnostic. Herpes simplex type 2 is most common.

Oral acyclovir is the treatment of choice but is not curative. It decreases the duration of outbreaks and viral shedding and increases the interval between attacks. The first episode is associated with the most pain and longest duration of ulceration. Subsequent episodes are generally shorter and not as painful.

2. Anorectal Syphilis

The chancre is an indurated, nontender perianal ulcer at the site of inoculation. Proctitis, pseudotumors, and condylomata lata may also be present. Condylomata lata are contiguous hypertrophic papules associated with secondary syphilis. Darkfield microscopy of exudate for *Treponema pallidum* and serologic testing are the preferred methods of diagnosis. Serologic tests may initially be negative and should be repeated several months later.

Penicillin is the treatment of choice. The prognosis is good. Contacts must be sought and treated.

3. Gonococcal Proctitis

Symptoms range from none to painful defecation. Rectal bleeding and discharge, perianal excoriation, and fistulas may develop. The mucosa may appear friable and edematous. Cultures of the anus, vagina, urethra, and pharynx should be obtained and plated on Thayer-Martin medium. The gram-negative diplococcus *Neisseria gonorrhoeae* is the causative agent.

Intramuscular procaine penicillin G and oral probenecid is the treatment of choice. Resistant strains should be treated with spectinomycin. Follow-up examination and cultures should be performed to confirm adequate therapy. The prognosis is excellent.

4. Chlamydial Proctitis & Lymphogranuloma Venereum

As in gonococcal proctitis, the symptoms of chlamydial proctitis range from none to rectal pain, bleeding, and discharge. The small shallow ulcer of lymphogranuloma venereum (LGV) may go unnoticed, but the inguinal adenopathy may become quite marked. Late findings include hemorrhagic proctitis and rectal stricture. The causative agent is *Chlamydia trachomatis,* an intracellular parasite spread by anal intercourse or direct extension through the lymphatics of the rectovaginal septum.

The diagnosis is made with the LGV complement fixation test. Tissue cultures are also used.

Treatment with 21 days of tetracycline is recommended, but erythromycin is an acceptable alternative. Early strictures may be dilated. Although uncommon, strictures may cause bowel obstruction and require colostomy.

5. *Condylomata Acuminata*

Human papilloma virus (HPV) is the cause of condylomata acuminata. Multiple types have been identified. Types HPV-6 and HPV-11 are associated with the common benign genital wart, whereas HPV-16 and HPV-18 are associated with the development of high-grade anal dysplasia and anal cancer. In the United States, condyloma acuminatum is the most common sexually transmitted viral disease, with 1 million new cases reported per year. It is the most common anorectal infection of homosexual men and is particularly prevalent in HIV-positive patients. However, the disease is not limited to men or women who practice anoreceptive intercourse. In women, the virus may track down from the vagina, and in men it may pool and track from the base of the scrotum. Immunosuppression, either from drugs after transplantation or from HIV, increases susceptibility to condylomatous disease with prevalence rates of 5% and 85%, respectively.

Clinical Findings

A. Symptoms and Signs

The most frequent complaint is that of a perianal growth. Pruritus, discharge, bleeding, odor, and anal pain are present to a lesser degree. Physical examination reveals the classic cauliflower-like lesion, which may be isolated, clustered, or coalescent. The warts tend to run in radial rows out from the anus. The lesions may be surprisingly large at the time of presentation.

B. Laboratory and Imaging Studies

Anoscopy or proctosigmoidoscopy are essential because the disease extends internally in more than three-fourths of patients and because intra-anal disease is present in 95% of cases in homosexual men. Material for cultures and serologic tests for other venereal diseases may be taken from the penis, anus, mouth, and vagina.

Differential Diagnosis

These lesions must be distinguished from condylomata lata, the lesions of secondary syphilis, and anal squamous cell carcinoma. Condylomata lata are flatter, paler, and smoother than condylomata acuminata. Anal squamous cell carcinoma is generally painful and may be tender and ulcerated, whereas condylomas are not tender or ulcerated.

Complications

Squamous cell carcinoma of the anal canal is the major complication.

Treatment & Prognosis

The extent of the disease and the risk of malignancy determine the treatment. Minimal disease is treated in the office with topical agents such as bichloracetic acid or 25% podophyllum resin in tincture of benzoin. The former is preferred and there are fewer complications (scarring) because the latter must be washed off within 4–6 hours to limit pain. The warts respond promptly to therapy. Patients should be seen at regular intervals until resolution is complete. More extensive disease may require an initial treatment session under anesthesia so that random lesions can be excised for pathologic evaluation to rule out dysplasia and so that the remainder can be coagulated. Electrocautery coagulates the lesions. Care is taken to spare surrounding skin. Follow-up evaluation may reveal residual disease, but this is often easily treated with topical agents in the office.

Laser therapy is another method of condyloma destruction. Recurrence rates are low, but the equipment is expensive.

Recurrent disease may respond to repeat excision or destruction. Imiquimod is a topically applied immune modulator that induces interferon and cytokine release by the host tissues. It activates the host immune system to clear the HPV infection by both the innate and cell-mediated pathways. In select patients external wart clearance has been achieved in 72–84%. Imiquimod may also be a useful adjunctive therapy following excision.

The first description of autologous vaccines was reported in 1944, but it is only recently that vaccines have shown more promise. The current vaccines in trials target the late structural proteins of the viral capsid (E6, E7) to engender a cytotoxic T lymphocyte cell-mediated immune response.

Human papillomaviruses 16 and 18 are causally associated with squamous cell carcinomas of the anal canal. This association has led to new screening techniques to evaluate high-risk patients for occult disease. These techniques are discussed below in the section on anal cancer. Representative biopsies of clinically apparent condylomas should be sent for pathologic study because unsuspected low-grade or high-grade dysplasia or squamous cell carcinoma of the anal canal may be found.

Buschke-Löwenstein tumors are giant condylomata acuminata that are locally aggressive and exhibit malignant behavior but benign histology. Radical excision is often the only therapeutic option for either palliation or cure. Wide local excision and even surgery with adjuvant chemotherapy and radiotherapy have been used with success.

6. Chancroid

Haemophilus ducreyi causes a soft perianal ulcer that is painful, often multiple, and bleeds easily. Autoinoculation is common. Inguinal lymph nodes become fluctuant, rupture, and drain. Cultures are diagnostic.

Treatment options include azithromycin, 1 g orally in a single dose; or ceftriaxone, 250 mg intramuscularly in a single dose; or ciprofloxacin, 500 mg orally twice daily for 3 days; or erythromycin base, 500 mg orally four times daily for 7 days. All are effective.

7. Inflammatory Proctitis

Inflammatory proctitis is a mild form of ulcerative colitis that is limited to the rectum. Rectal bleeding, discharge, diarrhea, and tenesmus are common. The rectal mucosa is inflamed and friable, but the remainder of the colon appears normal on examination. The disease course is often self-limited. Only about 10% of patients ever develop colonic manifestations of ulcerative colitis. Biopsies are taken at endoscopy to rule out infectious processes and Crohn's disease.

An infectious process must be ruled out before initiating steroid therapy. Distinguishing between Crohn's disease and inflammatory proctitis may be difficult. Lack of response to appropriate therapy calls for reassessment of the patient.

Steroid retention enemas are given for 2 weeks. If there is no response, a short course of oral steroids may be given. In addition, mesalamine (5-aminosalicylic acid) may be given orally or rectally in an enema or suppository. Patients should avoid milk and milk products, fruit, and dietary fiber. The disease usually responds to these measures and resolves rapidly.

8. Radiation Proctitis

Radiation proctitis in a patient with a history of radiation to the rectum is manifested early by diarrhea, rectal bleeding, discharge, tenesmus, pain, and incontinence. Late disease may develop months to years after the injury. Symptoms of late disease are secondary to strictures, fistulas, and telangiectasias, which may present as recurrent urinary tract infections, vaginal discharge, fecal incontinence, rectal bleeding, changes in stool caliber, and constipation. The symptoms include bleeding, change in bowel habits, urinary tract infections, and vaginal discharge. Endoscopy may reveal friable edematous mucosa, telangiectasias, or strictures and may show internal openings of fistulas.

Initial therapy includes bulk-forming agents, antidiarrheals, and antispasmodics. Topical steroids, mesalamine preparations, misoprostol suppositories, and short-chain fatty acids have all been used in acute and chronic disease. Refractory hemorrhagic proctitis may be treated with the application of formalin to the rectal mucosa. Dilatation of strictures and laser coagulation of telangiectasias are useful in late disease. The key to surgical success in treating fistulas to the bladder or vagina is interposition or transposition of healthy nonirradiated tissue into the field. Only infrequently is the rectum so badly irradiated that it must be removed. The prognosis, therefore, is good.

Babb RR: Radiation proctitis: a review. Am J Gastroenterol 1996;91:1309.

Berry JM, Palefsky JM: A review of human papillomavirus vaccines: from basic science to clinical trials. Frontiers Biosci 2003;8:s333.

Bjork M et al: Giant condyloma acuminatum (Buschke-Löwenstein tumor) of the anorectum with malignant transformation. Eur J Surg 1995;161:691.

Breese PL et al: Anal human papillomavirus infection among homosexual and bisexual men: prevalence of type-specific infection and association with human immunodeficiency virus. Sex Transm Dis 1995;22:7.

Chang GJ, Welton ML: Human papillomavirus, condylomata acuminata, and anal neoplasia. Clin Colon Rectal Surg 2004;17:55.

Centers for Disease Control and Prevention: Sexually transmitted diseases treatment guidelines 2002. MMWR 2002;51.

Counter SF et al: Prospective evaluation of formalin therapy for radiation proctitis. Am J Surg 1999;177:396.

El-Attar SM et al: Anal warts, sexually transmitted diseases, and anorectal conditions associated with human immunodeficiency virus. Prim Care 1999;26:81.

Fantin AC et al: Argon beam coagulation for treatment of symptomatic radiation-induced proctitis. Gastrointest Endosc 1999;49(4 Part 1):515.

Farouk R, Lee PW: Intradermal methylene blue injection for the treatment of intractable idiopathic pruritus ani. Br J Surg 1997;84:670.

Hemminki K et al: Cancer in husbands of cervical cancer patients. Epidemiology 2000;11:347.

Khan AM et al: A prospective randomized placebo-controlled double-blinded pilot study of misoprostol rectal suppositories in the prevention of acute and chronic radiation proctitis symptoms in prostate cancer patients. Am J Gastroenterol 2000;95:1961.

Kobal B: Herpes simplex genitalis type 2: our experiences. Clin Exp Obstet Gynec 1999;26:123.

Palefsky JM: Anal squamous intraepithelial lesions in human immunodeficiency virus-positive men and women. Semin Oncol 2000;27:471.

Palefsky JM: Anal squamous intraepithelial lesions: relation to HIV and human papillomavirus infection. J Acquir Immune Defic Syndr 1999;21(Suppl 1):S42.

Pinto A et al: Short chain fatty acids are effective in short-term treatment of chronic radiation proctitis: randomized, double-blind, controlled trial. Dis Colon Rectum 1999;42:788.

Rompalo AM: Diagnosis and treatment of sexually acquired proctitis and proctocolitis: an update. Clin Infect Dis 1999; 28(Suppl 1):S84.

Saclarides TJ et al: Formalin instillation for refractory radiation-induced hemorrhagic proctitis. Report of 16 patients. Dis Colon Rectum 1996;39:196.

Tabet SR et al: Incidence of HIV and sexually transmitted diseases (STD) in a cohort of HIV-negative men who have sex with men (MSM). AIDS 1998;12:2041.

Talley NA et al: Short-chain fatty acids in the treatment of radiation proctitis: a randomized, double-blind, placebo-controlled, cross-over pilot trial. Dis Colon Rectum 1997;40: 1046.

Taylor JG et al: KTP laser therapy for bleeding from chronic radiation proctopathy. Gastrointest Endosc 2000;52:353.

FECAL IMPACTION

Fecal impaction may develop after excisional hemorrhoidectomy, in chronically debilitated patients, or from the use of constipating pain medications without stool softeners and fiber. In the hemorrhoidectomy population, preserving adequate anoderm between hemorrhoidal complexes minimizes the incidence of this complication. Postoperative pain control is essential because otherwise fear of defecation may develop. Limited use of constipating opioids, addition of nonsteroidal medications, stool bulking agents (fiber), and stool softeners will minimize the incidence of fecal impaction.

All hospitalized and postoperative patients are at risk for developing fecal impaction because of limitations on physical activity, disruption of dietary and bowel habits, and initiation of constipating medications (opioids, calcium-channel blockers, etc). Thus, patients at risk who do not suffer from diarrhea should be started on stool softeners and fiber bulking agents to avoid this complication. Enemas and laxatives may be given as needed.

Patients with fecal impaction commonly present with diarrhea, as only liquid stool is able to pass the obstructing inspissated fecal bolus. Some may complain of pelvic pain with episodic severe spasms from the pressure of the mass on the pelvic floor. Digital rectal examination may reveal hard, dry stool that obstructs the rectum. Abdominal examination may reveal a pelvic or abdominal mass much like a gravid uterus.

Once detected, a fecal impaction may be digitally dislodged at the bedside, but treatment in the operating room with local or regional anesthesia may be necessary to provide pelvic floor relaxation and pain control. At completion of disimpaction, sigmoidoscopy is necessary to rule out an obstructing inflammatory or malignant mass or rectal injury incurred during the procedure.

Prather CM et al: Evaluation and treatment of constipation and fecal impaction in adults. Mayo Clin Proc 1998;73:881.

Tiongco FP et al: Use of oral GoLytely solution in relief of refractory fecal impaction. Dig Dis Sci 1997;42:1454.

ANAL & PERIANAL NEOPLASMS

Tumors of the anal canal account for 1.5% of malignancies of the gastrointestinal tract, with about 3900 new cases annually in the United States. The incidence has been increasing over the last 30 years. Chronic anal irritation has historically been related to the development of anal cancer, but there is an etiologic relationship between chronic infection with the human papillomavirus and the development of anal cancer. Women are at increased risk for anal canal cancer, presumably because the virus may pool in the vagina and track down to the anus. Women also may practice anoreceptive intercourse in heterosexual relationships. Although in general women are at increased risk for anal cancer ($9{:}10^6$ versus $7{:}10^6$ women versus men, respectively), in HIV-negative and HIV-positive men who have sex with men the incidence is $360{:}10^6$ and $700{:}10^6$, respectively. Other factors associated with an increased risk for anal cancer are anogenital warts, a history of sexually transmitted disease, more than 10 sexual partners (but if one has HPV, only one is necessary), a history of cervical, vulvar, or vaginal cancer, immunosuppression (HIV-positive or transplantation), long-term corticosteroids, and cigarette smoking.

High-grade squamous intraepithelial lesions (HSIL) are the putative precursor lesion to invasive squamous cell cancer of the anus. It is an increasingly prevalent condition associated with HPV infection. Treatment consists of targeted excision of involved tissues with the aid of the operating microscope and the use of acetic acid and potassium iodide solutions to aid in the identification of high-grade dysplasia. Such an approach results in complete clearance of the dysplasia in immunocompetent patients. Immunocompromised patients are more likely to experience recurrence, but they can be safely retreated. In this way premalignant lesions can be controlled without radical surgery and with minimal morbidity.

Although women are at increased risk for anal canal cancer, this is not true of anal margin carcinoma, where men are at greater risk (4:1). This difference highlights the importance of classification based on anatomic landmarks such as the dentate line, the anal verge, and the anal sphincters. These landmarks distinguish tumors of the anal margin from tumors of the anal canal. Unfortunately, the literature is not clear with regard to these landmarks, and efforts have been made by the World Health Organization and the American Joint Committee on Cancer (AJCC) to establish anatomic landmarks to distinguish tumors of the anal canal from tumors of the anal margin. The definitions are as follows: The anal canal extends from the upper to the lower border of the internal anal sphincter (from the pelvic floor to the anal verge). Anal margin tumors occur outside the anal verge in the perianal skin but presumably within a 5- to 6-cm radius of the anus. Tumors of the anal canal tend to be aggressive, nonkeratinizing, and associated with HPV infection. Tumors of the anal margin are generally well-differentiated keratinizing tumors that behave similarly to other squamous cell carcinomas of the skin and are treated accordingly.

Staging of anal and perianal malignancies is clinical. Physical examination with digital rectal examination, paying attention to pararectal nodes, anoscopy, bilateral groin palpation, biopsy (examination under anesthesia, if necessary), endorectal ultrasound, CT, and MRI are used as needed to assess tumor size and establish nodal and distant disease. The AJCC staging classification for anal canal and anal margin tumors is presented in Table 31–1.

Table 31–1. Staging of anal cancer.

Anal Cancer	
Primary tumor (T stage)	
TX	Primary tumor cannot be assessed
T0	No evidence of primary tumor
Tis	Carcinoma in situ
T1	≤ 2 cm
T2	> 2 cm to 5 cm
T3	> 5 cm
T4	Invasion into adjacent organ(s)
Nodal involvement (N stage)	
NX	Regional nodes cannot be assessed
N0	No regional nodal involvement
N1	Perirectal nodal involvement
N2	Unilateral internal iliac/inguinal nodal involvement
N3	Perirectal and/or bilateral internal iliac/inguinal nodal involvement
Distant metastasis (M stage)	
MX	Distant metastasis cannot be assessed
M1	No distant metastasis
M2	Distant metastasis present

Stage Grouping			
Stage 0	Tis	N0	M0
Stage I	T1	N0	M0
Stage II	T2	N0	M0
	T3	N0	M0
Stage IIIA	T1	N1	M0
	T2	N1	M0
	T3	N1	M0
	T4	N0	M0
Stage IIIB	T4	N1	M0
	Any T	N2, N3	M0
Stage IV	Any T	Any M	M1

Adapted from *AJCC Cancer Staging Manual,* 6th ed. Springer, 2002.

TUMORS OF THE ANAL MARGIN

1. Squamous Cell Carcinoma

Patients complain of a mass, bleeding, pain, discharge, itching, and pain or tenesmus (complaints common to most lesions of this region). Typically the lesions are large and centrally ulcerated, with rolled, everted edges and have been present for over 2 years before detection. All chronic or nonhealing ulcers of the perineum should be biopsied to rule out squamous cell carcinoma. Squamous cell carcinoma is more common in men.

Small, well-differentiated lesions (≤ 4 cm) are treated by wide local excision. Deep lesions that involve the sphincters require abdominoperineal resection. Chemoradiation is used for less favorable lesions. Spread is to the inguinal lymph nodes, which are generally included in the radiation fields. Excision of inguinal nodal disease is reserved for palpable and symptomatic disease. Disease recurring in the skin may be treated with reexcision or abdominoperineal resection. The T stage determines survival, with reports of 100% 5-year and 10-year survivals for T1 lesions, compared with 60% and 40% survival rates for T2 lesions at 5 and 10 years, respectively.

2. Basal Cell Carcinoma

Bleeding, itching, and pain are the presenting symptoms of basal cell carcinoma. The superficial, mobile lesions have raised, irregular edges and central ulceration. They are more frequent in men.

As with squamous cell carcinoma of the margin, treatment is by wide local excision when possible. Deeply invasive lesions may require abdominoperineal resection. Metastasis is rare, but the local recurrence rate is 30%. Local recurrence is treated with reexcision.

3. Bowen's Disease

Bowen's disease (intraepithelial squamous cell carcinoma) is often associated with condylomas and can involve both the anal margin and the anal canal. Patients often complain of perianal burning, itching, or pain. Lesions are often found on routine histologic evaluation of specimens acquired during investigation of unrelated disorders. When grossly visible, the lesions appear scaly, discrete, erythematous, and sometimes pigmented. In immunocompromised patients (HIV-positive, transplantation), a Pap smear is a useful screening technique to detect dysplasia. If the Pap smear is positive, high-resolution anoscopy with acetic acid painting may reveal otherwise occult condyloma with dysplasia.

Wide local excision with four-quadrant biopsies to establish that no residual disease persists has been the treatment of choice. Skin grafts may be necessary for larger lesions. However, there is no histologic difference between Bowen's disease and HSIL, and radical skin excision ignores the intra-anal dysplastic lesions that may be even more aggressive than perianal disease. These intra-anal dysplastic lesions have been successfully managed with local excision or destruction, even in the immunocompromised host. Furthermore, fewer than 10% of patients with Bowen's disease will develop invasive squamous cell carcinoma of the anus. Therefore, the need to perform radical excision and flap procedures has been questioned.

4. Paget's Disease

Paget's disease (intraepithelial adenocarcinoma) occurs predominantly in women. Patients are usually in the seventh or eighth decade of life. Severe intractable anal pruritus is characteristic. On physical examination an erythematous, eczematoid rash is apparent. Biopsy of any nonhealing lesion should be taken to rule out this diagnosis. If Paget's disease is diagnosed, a thorough workup for an occult malignancy is indicated because up to 50% of patients have a coexistent gastrointestinal carcinoma.

Wide local excision is the treatment of choice. Abdominoperineal resection may be indicated for advanced disease. Lymph node dissection should be done only be for palpable adenopathy. The role of chemoradiation is less clear. The prognosis is good unless there is metastatic disease or an underlying neoplasm.

Beck DE: Paget's disease and Bowen's disease of the anus. Semin Colon Rectal Surg 1995;6:143.

Chang GJ et al: Surgical treatment of high-grade anal squamous intraepithelial lesions—a prospective study. Dis Colon Rectum 2002;45:453.

Frisch M et al: Sexually transmitted infection as a cause of anal cancer. N Engl J Med 1997;337:1350.

Fuchshuber PR et al: Anal canal and perianal epidermoid cancers. J Am Coll Surg 1997;185:494.

Marchesa P et al: Perianal Bowen's disease: a clinicopathologic study of 47 patients. Dis Colon Rectum 1997;40:1286.

Marchesa P et al: Long-term outcome of patients with perianal Paget's disease. Ann Surg Oncol 1997;4:475.

Peiffert D et al: Conservative treatment by irradiation of epidermoid carcinomas of the anal margin. Int J Radiat Oncol Biol Phys 1997; 39:57.

Sarmiento JM et al: Paget's disease of the perianal region—an aggressive disease? Dis Colon Rectum 1997;40:1187.

Touboul E et al: Epidermoid carcinoma of the anal margin: 17 cases treated with curative-intent radiation therapy. Radiother Oncol 1995;34:195.

TUMORS OF THE ANAL CANAL

1. Epidermoid (Squamous, Basaloid, Mucoepidermoid) Carcinoma

Clinical Findings

In most cases there is a long history of minor perianal complaints such as bleeding, itching, or discomfort. An indurated anal mass may be present. Disease may be extensive at presentation, with approximately half of the lesions extending beyond the bowel wall or perianal skin at presentation. Inguinal nodal metastases are found in 20% at diagnosis and another 15% over time. The workup is discussed in the section on perianal cancers.

Abdominal CT and chest radiographs may reveal liver or lung metastases. Endorectal ultrasound can determine the depth of invasion of the primary lesion and may identify pararectal nodes.

Treatment

Early lesions that are small, mobile, confined to the submucosa, and well differentiated may be treated with local excision. Overall reported recurrence rates with local excision alone are high, with an average survival rate of 70% at 5 years. Local excision of the most favorable lesions results in less than 10% recurrence and 5-year survival of 100%. Larger lesions of the anal canal call for radiation therapy or multimodality treatment with chemotherapy and radiation.

Chemoradiation has now replaced surgery as first-line therapy for all but the earliest lesions, and surgery is advised only as a salvage procedure for persistent or recurrent disease. The Nigro regimen consisted of 30 Gy to the primary tumor and to the pelvic and inguinal nodes. Mitomycin (15 mg/m^2 as an intravenous bolus) was delivered on day 1 of radiation therapy. Two 4-day infusions of fluorouracil (5-FU) (1000 mg/m^2 per day) were given starting on days 1 and 28 of chemoradiation therapy. Excellent tumor responses with 80% disease-free survivals have been reported. Because of the morbidity associated with this regimen, the amount and type of chemotherapy and radiation have been modified. Radiation only, without chemotherapy, has resulted in higher local recurrence rates in multicenter randomized trials. Much of the chemotherapy toxicity is related to the mitomycin, which has increasingly been replaced by cisplatin, which is effective and is associated with fewer side effects. External beam radiotherapy doses range from 35 Gy to 59 Gy; some centers use brachytherapy catheters as well.

Treatment failures occur most commonly in the pelvis at the primary site or in the locoregional lymph nodes, with disease occurring outside the pelvis in just 15% of patients. The most common site of extrapelvic failure is the liver. Salvage abdominal perineal resection for local failure with recurrent or persistent disease is associated with a 50% 5-year survival rate. Survival is related to the extent of disease at the time of failure and to nodal status before initiation of chemoradiation therapy.

Prophylactic groin dissection is not recommended, but some experts recommend that the groins be included in the radiation fields because the failure rate in the groins is 20% if they are not treated.

Prognosis

Tumor size is the single most important prognostic factor. Mobile lesions = 2 cm in diameter have cure rates of 80%, but tumors 5 cm or more in diameter are associated with a 50% mortality. There are reports of excellent 10-year survival for T1–3 node-negative disease (88%) and T1–3 node positive disease (50%). Metastatic disease is more likely to be present with increasing depth of invasion and size and worsening histologic grade. Distant disease is uncommon at the time of diagnosis but most commonly involves the liver when present. Subsequent metastasis out of the pelvis is not uncommon, and 40% of patients die with disease that has spread to distant sites. Lymph node involvement at the time of presentation is a bad prognostic sign.

2. Malignant Melanoma of the Anal Canal

Clinical Findings

Malignant melanoma of the anal canal accounts for less than 1% of all anal canal tumors, yet it is a common site of primary melanoma. As with other anal canal tumors there is often a delay in diagnosis that results in advanced stage disease at the time or presentation. Metastatic disease has been reported to be present in over one-third of patients at the time of diagnosis. The lesions can be located in the anal canal, rectum, or both. The overall prognosis has been poor, with 5-year survival rates of less than 25% in several series. Most patients will die of disseminated disease.

Treatment

Traditionally treatment of primary melanoma of the anal canal has been radical surgery to include an abdominoperineal resection (APR) with or without bilateral inguinal lymph node dissection, especially for localized small tumors. However, the uniformly poor prognosis of all patients has led many surgeons to question the appropriateness of this very morbid approach. The current approach favors wide local excision, reserving APR for those patients with bulky disease in whom a wide local excision is not possible. Very few patients present with isolated local recurrences; rather, most have disseminated disease at the time of recurrence.

Prognosis

Unfortunately, the prognosis for anorectal melanoma remains poor. It remains a biologically aggressive disease that is often systemic at the time of diagnosis. It is poorly responsive to chemotherapy or radiation; however, some encouragement has been noted in a recent series of adjuvant chemoradiation after sphincter-sparing local excision, borrowing on the lessons learned from other disease sites, with an actuarial 5-year survival of 31% and actuarial local control rate of 74%. The development of novel therapies to treat malignant melanoma will hopefully improve the outlook for these patients.

Allal AS et al: Effectiveness of surgical salvage therapy for patients with locally uncontrolled anal carcinoma after sphincter-conserving treatment. Cancer 1999;86:405.

Ballo MT et al: Sphincter-sparing local excision and adjuvant radiation for anal-rectal melanoma. JCO 2002;20:4555.

Brady MS et al: Anorectal melanoma. A 64-year experience at Memorial Sloan-Kettering Cancer Center. Dis Col Rectum 1995;38:146.

Doci R et al: Primary chemoradiation therapy with fluorouracil and cisplatin for cancer of the anus: results in 35 consecutive patients. J Clin Oncol 1996;14:3121.

Ellenhorn JD et al: Salvage abdominoperineal resection following combined chemotherapy and radiotherapy for epidermoid carcinoma of the anus. Ann Surg Oncol 1994;1:105.

Eng C et al: Chemotherapy and radiation of anal canal cancer: the first approach. Surg Onc Clinics N Am 2004;13:309.

Epidermoid anal cancer: results from the UKCCCR randomised trial of radiotherapy alone versus radiotherapy, 5-fluorouracil, and mitomycin. UKCCCR Anal Cancer Trial Working Party. UK Co-ordinating Committee on Cancer Research. Lancet 1996;348:1049.

Flam M et al: Role of mitomycin in combination with fluorouracil and radiotherapy, and of salvage chemoradiation in the definitive nonsurgical treatment of epidermoid carcinoma of the anal canal: results of a phase III randomized intergroup study. J Clin Oncol 1996;14:2527.

Klas JV et al: Malignant tumors of the anal canal: the spectrum of disease, treatment, and outcomes. Cancer 1999;85:1686.

Myerson RJ et al: Carcinoma of the anal canal. Am J Clin Oncol 1995;18:32.

Nilsson PJ et al: Salvage abdominoperineal resection in anal epidermoid cancer. Br J Surg 2002;89:1425.

Peiffert D et al: Preliminary results of a phase II study of high-dose radiation therapy and neoadjuvant plus concomitant 5-fluorouracil with CDDP chemotherapy for patients with anal canal cancer: a French cooperative study. Ann Oncol 1997; 8:575.

Pocard M et al: Results of salvage abdominoperineal resection for anal cancer after radiotherapy. Dis Colon Rectum 1998;41:1488.

Ryan DP et al: Carcinoma of the anal canal. N Engl J Med 2000;342:792.

Smith DE et al: Cancer of the anal canal: treatment with chemotherapy and low-dose radiation therapy. Radiology 1994;191:569.

Thibault C et al: Anorectal melanoma—An incurable disease? Dis Col Rectum 1997; 40:661.

Hernias & Other Lesions of the Abdominal Wall*

32

Karen E. Deveney, MD

I. HERNIAS

An external hernia is an abnormal protrusion of intra-abdominal tissue through a fascial defect in the abdominal wall. About 75% of hernias occur in the groin (indirect inguinal, direct inguinal, femoral). Incisional and ventral hernias comprise about 10%; umbilical 3%; and others about 3%. Generally, a hernial mass is composed of covering tissues (skin, subcutaneous tissues, etc), a peritoneal sac, and any contained viscera. Particularly if the neck of the sac is narrow where it emerges from the abdomen, bowel protruding into the hernia may become obstructed or strangulated. If the hernia is not repaired early, the defect may enlarge and operative repair may become more complicated. The definitive treatment of hernia is early operative repair.

A **reducible hernia** is one in which the contents of the sac return to the abdomen spontaneously or with manual pressure when the patient is recumbent.

An **irreducible (incarcerated) hernia** is one whose contents cannot be returned to the abdomen, usually because they are trapped by a narrow neck. The term "incarceration" does not imply obstruction, inflammation, or ischemia of the herniated organs, though incarceration is necessary for obstruction or strangulation to occur.

Though the lumen of a segment of bowel within the hernia sac may become **obstructed**, there may initially be no interference with blood supply. Compromise to the blood supply of the contents of the sac (eg, omentum or intestine) results in a **strangulated hernia**, in which gangrene of the contents of the sac has occurred. The incidence of strangulation is higher in femoral than in inguinal hernias, but strangulation may occur in other hernias as well.

An uncommon and dangerous type of hernia, a **Richter hernia**, occurs when only part of the circumference of the bowel becomes incarcerated or strangulated in the fascial defect. A strangulated Richter hernia may spontaneously reduce and the gangrenous piece of intestine be overlooked at operation. The bowel may subsequently perforate, with resultant peritonitis.

HERNIAS OF THE GROIN

Anatomy

All hernias of the abdominal wall consist of a peritoneal sac that protrudes through a weakness or defect in the muscular layers of the abdomen. The defect may be congenital or acquired.

Just outside the peritoneum is the **transversalis fascia**, an aponeurosis whose weakness or defect is the major source of groin hernias. Next are found the **transversus abdominis**, **internal oblique**, and **external oblique muscles**, which are fleshy laterally and aponeurotic medially. Their aponeuroses form investing layers of the strong **rectus abdominis muscles** above the semilunar line. Below this line, the aponeurosis lies entirely in front of the muscle. Between the two vertical rectus muscles, the aponeuroses meet again to form the **linea alba**, which is well defined only above the umbilicus. The subcutaneous fat contains Scarpa's fascia—a misnomer, since it is only a condensation of connective tissue with no substantial strength.

In the groin, an **indirect inguinal hernia** results when obliteration of the processus vaginalis, the peritoneal extension accompanying the testis in its descent into the scrotum, fails to occur. The resultant hernia sac passes through the **internal inguinal ring**, a defect in the transversalis fascia halfway between the anterior iliac spine and the pubic tubercle. The sac is located anteromedially within the spermatic cord and may extend partway along the **inguinal canal** or accompany the cord out through the subcutaneous (external) inguinal ring, a defect medially in the external oblique muscle just above the pubic tubercle. A hernia that passes fully into the scrotum is known as a **complete hernia**. The sac and the spermatic cord are invested by the **cremaster muscle**, an extension of fibers of the internal oblique muscle.

* See Chapter 45 for further discussion of hernias in the pediatric age group and Chapter 21 for a discussion of internal hernias.

Other anatomic structures of the groin that are important in understanding the formation of hernias and types of hernia repairs include the **conjoined tendon**, or falx inguinalis, a fusion of the medial aponeurotic transversus abdominis and internal oblique muscles that passes along the inferolateral edge of the rectus abdominis muscle and attaches to the pubic tubercle. Between the pubic tubercle and the anterior iliac spine passes the **inguinal (Poupart) ligament**, formed by the lowermost border of the external oblique aponeurosis as it rolls on itself and thickens into a cord.

Just deep and parallel to the inguinal ligament runs the iliopubic tract, a band of connective tissue that extends from the iliopsoas fascia, crosses below the deep inguinal ring, forms the superior border of the femoral sheath, and inserts into the superior pubic ramus to form the **lacunar (Gimbernat) ligament**. The lacunar ligament is about 1.25 cm long and triangular in shape. The sharp, crescentic lateral border of this ligament is the unyielding noose for the strangulation of a femoral hernia.

Cooper's ligament is a strong, fibrous band that extends laterally for about 2.5 cm along the iliopectineal line on the superior aspect of the superior pubic ramus, starting at the lateral base of the lacunar ligament.

Hesselbach's triangle is bounded by the inguinal ligament, the inferior epigastric vessels, and the lateral border of the rectus muscle. A weakness or defect in the transversalis fascia, which forms the floor of this triangle, results in a **direct inguinal hernia**. In most direct hernias, the transversalis fascia is diffusely attenuated, though a discrete defect in the fascia may occasionally occur. This **funicular** type of direct inguinal hernia is more likely to become incarcerated, since it has distinct borders.

A **femoral hernia** passes beneath the iliopubic tract and inguinal ligament into the upper thigh. The predisposing anatomic feature for femoral hernias is a small empty space between the lacunar ligament medially and the femoral vein laterally—the **femoral canal**. Because its borders are distinct and unyielding, a femoral hernia has the highest risk of incarceration and strangulation of groin hernias.

Surgeons must be familiar with the pathways of the nerves and blood vessels of the inguinal region to avoid injuring them when repairing groin hernias. The iliohypogastric nerve (T12, L1) emerges from the lateral edge of the psoas muscle and travels inside the external oblique muscle, emerging medial to the external inguinal ring to innervate the suprapubic skin. The ilioinguinal nerve (L1) parallels the iliohypogastric nerve and travels on the surface of the spermatic cord to innervate the base of the penis (or mons pubis), the scrotum (or labia majora), and the medial thigh. This nerve is the most frequently injured in anterior open inguinal hernia repairs. The genitofemoral (L1, L2) and lateral femoral cutaneous nerves (L2, L3) travel on and lateral to the psoas muscle and provide sensation to the scrotum and anteromedial thigh and to the lateral thigh, respectively. These nerves are subject to injury during laparoscopic hernia repairs. The femoral nerve (L2–L4) travels from the lateral edge of the psoas and extends lateral to the femoral vessels. It can be injured during laparoscopic or femoral hernia repairs.

The external iliac artery travels along the medial aspect of the psoas muscle and beneath the inguinal ligament, giving off the inferior epigastric artery, which borders the medial aspect of the internal inguinal ring. The corresponding veins accompany the arteries. These vessels can be injured during hernia repairs of all types.

Causes

Nearly all inguinal hernias in infants, children, and young adults are **indirect inguinal hernias**. Although these "congenital" hernias most often present during the first year of life, the first clinical evidence of hernia may not appear until middle or old age, when increased intra-abdominal pressure and dilation of the internal inguinal ring allow abdominal contents to enter the previously empty peritoneal diverticulum. An untreated indirect hernia will inevitably dilate the internal ring and displace or attenuate the inguinal floor. The peritoneum may protrude on either side of the inferior epigastric vessels to give a combined direct and indirect hernia, called a **pantaloon hernia**.

In contrast, **direct inguinal hernias** are acquired as the result of a developed weakness of the transversalis fascia in Hesselbach's area. There is some evidence that direct inguinal hernias may be related to hereditary or acquired defects in collagen synthesis or turnover. **Femoral hernias** involve an acquired protrusion of a peritoneal sac through the femoral ring. In women, the ring may become dilated by the physical and biochemical changes during pregnancy.

Any condition that chronically increases intra-abdominal pressure may contribute to the appearance and progression of a hernia. Marked obesity, abdominal strain from heavy exercise or lifting, cough, constipation with straining at stool, and prostatism with straining on micturition are often implicated. Cirrhosis with ascites, pregnancy, chronic ambulatory peritoneal dialysis, and chronically enlarged pelvic organs or pelvic tumors may also contribute. Loss of tissue turgor in Hesselbach's area, associated with a weakening of the transversalis fascia, occurs with advancing age and in chronic debilitating disease.

Classification of Groin Hernias

To facilitate comparison of results of their surgical repair, Nyhus has proposed a classification of groin hernias:

types 1 and 2, indirect inguinal hernias with a normal-sized (type 1) or enlarged (type 2) internal ring but with a normal inguinal floor; type 3, either direct (type 3A), indirect with a distorted inguinal floor (type 3B), or femoral hernias (type 3C); and type 4, recurrent hernias.

Lovett J, Kirgan D, McGregor B: Inguinal herniation justifies sigmoidoscopy. Am J Surg 1989;158:615.

Nyhus LM: Individualization of hernia repair: a new era. Surgery 1993;114:1.

Skandalakis JE et al: Embryologic and anatomic basis of inguinal herniorrhaphy. Surg Clin North Am 1993;73:799.

INDIRECT & DIRECT INGUINAL HERNIAS

Clinical Findings

A. Symptoms

Most hernias produce no symptoms until the patient notices a lump or swelling in the groin, though some patients may describe a sudden pain and bulge that occurred while lifting or straining. Frequently, hernias are detected in the course of routine physical examinations such as preemployment examinations. Some patients complain of a dragging sensation and, particularly with indirect inguinal hernias, radiation of pain into the scrotum. As a hernia enlarges, it is likely to produce a sense of discomfort or aching pain, and the patient must lie down to reduce the hernia.

In general, direct hernias produce fewer symptoms than indirect inguinal hernias and are less likely to become incarcerated or strangulated.

B. Signs

Examination of the groin reveals a mass that may or may not be reducible. The patient should be examined both supine and standing and also with coughing and straining, since small hernias may be difficult to demonstrate. The external ring can be identified by invaginating the scrotum and palpating with the index finger just above and lateral to the pubic tubercle (Figure 32–1). If the external ring is very small, the examiner's finger may not enter the inguinal canal, and it may be difficult to be sure that a pulsation felt on coughing is truly a hernia. At the other extreme, a widely patent external ring does not by itself constitute hernia. Tissue must be felt protruding into the inguinal canal during coughing in order for a hernia to be diagnosed.

Differentiating between direct and indirect inguinal hernia on examination is difficult and is of little importance since most groin hernias should be repaired regardless of type. Nevertheless, each type of inguinal hernia has specific features more common to it. A hernia that descends into the scrotum is almost certainly indirect. On inspection with the patient erect and straining, a direct hernia more commonly appears as a symmetric, circular swelling at the external ring; the swelling disappears when the patient lies down. An indirect hernia appears as an elliptic swelling that may not reduce easily.

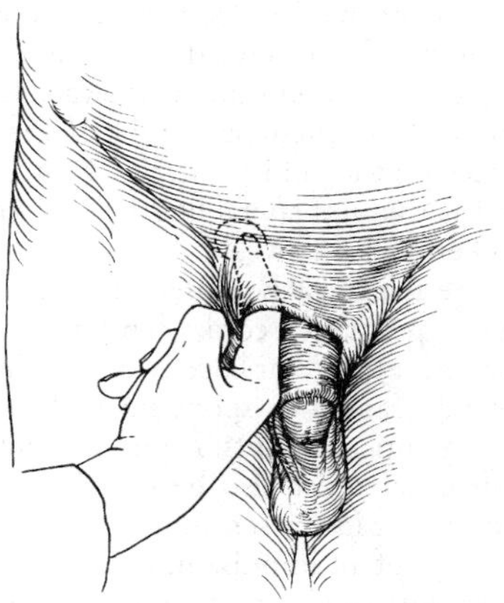

Figure 32–1. Insertion of finger through upper scrotum into the external inguinal ring.

On palpation, the posterior wall of the inguinal canal is firm and resistant in an indirect hernia but relaxed or absent in a direct hernia. If the patient is asked to cough or strain while the examining finger is directed laterally and upward into the inguinal canal, a direct hernia protrudes against the side of the finger, whereas an indirect hernia is felt at the tip of the finger.

Compression over the internal ring when the patient strains may also help to differentiate between indirect and direct hernias. A direct hernia bulges forward through Hesselbach's triangle, but the opposite hand can maintain reduction of an indirect hernia at the internal ring.

These distinctions are obscured as a hernia enlarges and distorts the anatomic relationships of the inguinal rings and canal. In most patients the type of inguinal hernia cannot be established accurately before surgery.

Differential Diagnosis

Groin pain of musculoskeletal or obscure origin may be difficult to distinguish from hernia. Herniography, in which x-rays are obtained after intraperitoneal injection of contrast medium, may aid in the diagnosis in cases of groin pain when no hernia can be felt even after multiple maneuvers to increase intra-abdominal pressure.

Herniation of preperitoneal fat through the inguinal ring into the spermatic cord ("lipoma of the cord") is commonly misinterpreted as a hernia sac. Its true nature may only be confirmed at operation. Occasionally, a femoral hernia that has extended above the inguinal ligament after passing through the fossa ovalis femoris may be confused with an inguinal hernia. If the examining finger is placed on the pubic tubercle, the neck of the sac of a femoral hernia lies lateral and below, while that of an inguinal hernia lies above.

Inguinal hernia must be differentiated from hydrocele of the spermatic cord, lymphadenopathy or abscesses of the groin, varicocele, and residual hematoma following trauma or spontaneous hemorrhage in patients taking anticoagulants. An undescended testis in the inguinal canal must also be considered when the testis cannot be felt in the scrotum.

The presence of an impulse in the mass with coughing, bowel sounds in the mass, and failure to transilluminate are features which indicate that an irreducible mass in the groin is a hernia.

Treatment

Inguinal hernias should always be repaired unless there are specific contraindications. The same advice applies to patients of all ages; the complications of incarceration, obstruction, and strangulation are greater threats than are the risks of operation.

Elderly patients tolerate elective repair of a groin hernia very well, especially when other medical problems are optimally controlled and local anesthetic is used. Emergency operation carries a much greater risk for the elderly than carefully planned elective operation.

If the patient has significant prostatic hyperplasia, it is prudent to solve this problem first, since the risks of urinary retention and urinary tract infection are high following hernia repair in patients with significant prostatic obstruction.

Although most direct hernias do not carry as high a risk of incarceration as indirect hernias, the difficulty in reliably differentiating them from indirect hernias makes the repair of all inguinal hernias advisable. Direct hernias of the funicular type, which are particularly likely to incarcerate, should always be repaired.

Because of the possibility of strangulation, an incarcerated, painful, or tender hernia usually requires an emergency operation. Nonoperative reduction of an incarcerated hernia may first be attempted. The patient is placed with hips elevated and given analgesics and sedation sufficient to promote muscle relaxation. Repair of the hernia may be deferred if the hernia mass reduces with gentle manipulation and if there is no clinical evidence of strangulated bowel. Though strangulation is usually clinically evident, gangrenous tissue can occasionally be reduced into the abdomen by manual or spontaneous reduction en masse. It is therefore safest to repair the reduced hernia at the earliest opportunity.

At surgery, one must decide whether to explore the abdomen to make certain that the intestine is viable. If the patient has leukocytosis or clinical signs of peritonitis or if the hernia sac contains dark or bloody fluid, the abdomen should be explored.

A. Principles of Operative Treatment of Inguinal Hernia

1. Successful repair requires that any correctable aggravating factors be identified and treated (chronic cough, prostatic obstruction, colonic tumor, ascites, etc) and that the defect be reconstructed with the best available tissues that can be approximated without tension.

2. An indirect hernia sac should be anatomically isolated, dissected to its origin from the peritoneum, and ligated (Figure 32–2). In infants and young adults in whom the inguinal anatomy is normal, repair can usually be limited to high ligation, removal of the sac, and reduction of the internal ring to an appropriate size. For most adult hernias, the inguinal floor should also be reconstructed. The internal ring should be reduced to a size just adequate to allow egress of the cord structures. In women, the internal ring can be totally closed to prevent recurrence through that site.

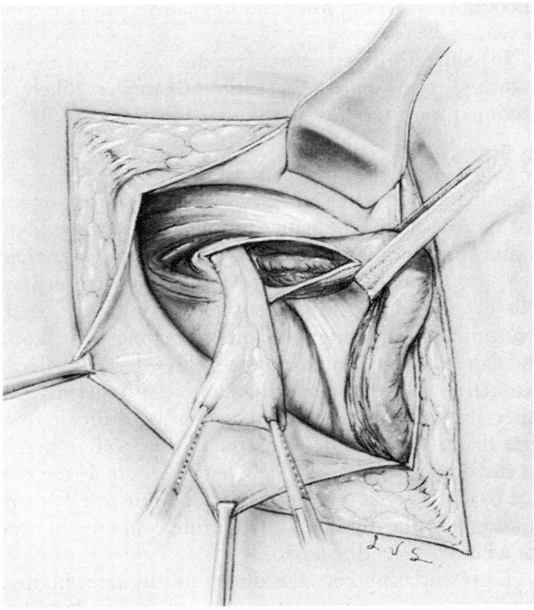

Figure 32–2. Indirect inguinal hernia. Inguinal canal opened, showing spermatic cord retracted medially and indirect hernia peritoneal sac dissected free to above the level of the internal inguinal ring.

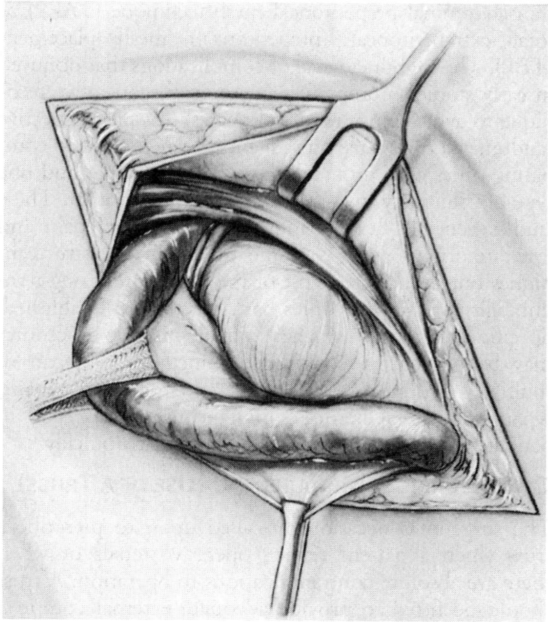

Figure 32–3. Direct inguinal hernia. Inguinal canal opened and spermatic cord retracted inferiorly and laterally to reveal the hernia bulging through the floor of Hesselbach's triangle.

3. In direct inguinal hernia (Figure 32–3), the inguinal canal may be so wide and its floor so weak that the repair appears to be under tension. In such cases, a vertical relaxing incision in the anterior rectus abdominis sheath has traditionally been used, though recent experience favors the use of mesh so that a tension-free repair can be accomplished.

4. Even though a direct hernia is found, the cord should always be carefully searched for a possible indirect hernia as well.

5. In patients with large hernias, bilateral repair has traditionally been discouraged under the assumption that greater tension on the repair would result and therefore would increase the recurrence rate and surgical complications. If open mesh repair or laparoscopic methods are used, however, bilateral repairs can be done with low risk of recurrence. In children and adults with small hernias, bilateral hernia repair is usually recommended because it spares the patient a second anesthetic.

6. Recurrent hernia within a few months or a year of operation usually indicates an inadequate repair, such as overlooking an indirect sac, missing a femoral hernia, or failing to repair the fascial defect securely. Any repair completed under tension is subject to early recurrence. Recurrences two or more years after repair are more likely to be caused by progressive weakening of the patient's fascia. Repeated recurrence after careful repair by an experienced surgeon suggests a defect in collagen synthesis. Because the fascial defect is often small, firm, and unyielding, recurrent hernias are much more likely to develop incarceration or strangulation than unoperated inguinal hernias, and they should nearly always be repaired again.

If recurrence is due to an overlooked indirect sac, the posterior wall is often solid and removal of the sac may be all that is required. Occasionally, a recurrence is discovered to consist of a small, sharply circumscribed defect in the previous hernioplasty, in which case closure of the defect suffices. More diffuse weakness of the posterior inguinal wall or repeated recurrences occasionally require more elaborate repair using fascia lata from the thigh or a nonabsorbable patch such as polypropylene or polytetrafluoroethylene (PTFE).

B. Types of Operations for Inguinal Hernia

The goal of all hernia repairs is to eliminate the peritoneal sac (in the case of an indirect hernia) and to close the fascial defect in the inguinal floor. Traditional repairs approximated native tissues using permanent sutures. More recently, a permanent mesh has been used with greater frequency to decrease tension on the repairs. As surgeons have gained more experience with the techniques, laparoscopic approaches have increased in frequency as well as in their success.

Simple high ligation of the sac through an inguinal incision is the key to the repair of indirect hernias in infants and children. Combined with a tightening of the internal ring, it is called the **Marcy repair**.

Inguinal hernias in adults can be repaired successfully through an inguinal, preperitoneal, or abdominal approach, though inguinal repairs are most widely used today. While a given repair may be championed by a particular surgeon or group, comparative studies do not conclusively demonstrate the superiority of any one type; in fact, it seems likely that all the methods in common use give equivalent results when properly performed. Details of technique and the experience and skill of the surgeon are more likely to account for the success of the procedure than is the type of repair.

Though most methods of repairing indirect inguinal hernias in adults emphasize high ligation of the sac, as in children, elimination of the sac by reducing it may suffice. The factor common to all successful methods of inguinal hernia repairs in adults is repair of the inguinal floor. Over the past 15–20 years, mesh repairs have gradually gained in popularity and have become the most commonly employed method. Comparative studies show a clear superiority of open mesh repairs over the more traditional repairs using native tissues alone.

Over the past decade, increased experience has been gained with laparoscopic and other minimally invasive techniques. Although laparoscopic approaches offer less pain and more rapid return to work or normal activities, no long-term studies are yet available to assure that hernia recurrence rates are as low as those seen with open mesh hernia repairs. Operative time and procedure costs are generally higher for laparoscopic repair. As with open hernia repairs, surgeons with the most experience performing laparoscopic herniorrhaphies have lower hernia recurrence rates.

Among the traditional autologous tissue repairs, the **Bassini repair** was the most widely used method. In this repair, the conjoined tendon is approximated to Poupart's ligament and the spermatic cord remains in its normal anatomic position under the external oblique aponeurosis. The **Halsted repair** places the external oblique beneath the cord but otherwise resembles the Bassini repair. **Cooper's ligament (Lotheissen-McVay) repair** brings the conjoined tendon farther posteriorly and inferiorly to Cooper's ligament. Unlike the Bassini and Halsted methods, McVay's repair is effective for femoral hernia but always requires a relaxing incision to relieve tension. Recurrence rates after these open nonmesh repairs vary widely according to skill and experience of the surgeon, but range around 10%. Though the **Shouldice repair** has a low reported recurrence rate, it is not widely used, perhaps because of the more extensive dissection required and a belief that the skill of the surgeons may be as important as the method itself. In the Shouldice repair, the transversalis fascia is first divided and then imbricated to Poupart's ligament. Finally, the conjoined tendon and internal oblique muscle are also approximated in layers to the inguinal ligament.

The **preperitoneal approach** exposes the groin from between the transversalis fascia and peritoneum via a lower abdominal incision to effect closure of the fascial defect. Because it requires more initial dissection and is associated with higher morbidity and recurrence rates in less experienced hands, it has not been widely favored. For recurrent or large bilateral hernias, a preperitoneal approach using a large piece of mesh to span all areas of potential herniation has been described by Stoppa. Laparoscopic preperitoneal approaches have demonstrated excellent success, with low recurrence and complications in experienced hands.

A desire to decrease the recurrence rate of hernias has prompted an increased use of prosthetic materials in repair of both recurrent and first-time hernias. Methods include "plugs" of mesh inserted into the internal ring and sheets of mesh to create a tension-free repair. The most widely used technique is that of Lichtenstein, an open mesh repair that allows an early return to normal activities and a low complication and recurrence rate.

Virtually all laparoscopic approaches utilize mesh in the repair. Several methods have been explored, from a transabdominal intraperitoneal onlay of mesh (IPOM) to a transabdominal preperitoneal mesh technique (TAPP) to total extraperitoneal (preperitoneal) mesh placement (TEP). The high incidence of complications that occurred in early studies prompted revisions in the operative technique to avoid injury to lateral nerves. Several prospective randomized trials have subsequently been conducted comparing open with minimally invasive techniques and one type of minimally invasive technique with another. These studies generally have demonstrated decreased pain and faster return to work with the minimally invasive techniques but at increased cost of the procedure. Long-term durability of the procedures has not yet been established. Specific situations in which minimally invasive procedures may be particularly advantageous include the repair of multiply recurrent hernias after anterior open repairs, repair of bilateral hernias simultaneously, and repair in patients who must return to work particularly quickly.

C. Nonsurgical Management (Use of a Truss)

The surgeon is occasionally called upon to prescribe a truss when a patient refuses operative repair or when there are absolute contraindications to operation. A truss should be fitted to provide adequate external compression over the defect in the abdominal wall. It should be taken off at night and put on in the morning before the patient arises. The use of a truss does not preclude later repair of a hernia, although it may cause fibrosis of the anatomic structures, so that subsequent repair may be more difficult.

Pre- & Postoperative Course

The preoperative evaluation should be completed before hospitalization. The patient usually enters the hospital on the morning of operation. The anesthetic may be general, spinal, or local. Local anesthetic is effective for most patients, and the incidence of urinary retention and pulmonary complications is lowest with local anesthesia. Recurrent hernias are more easily repaired with the patient under spinal or general anesthesia, since local anesthetic does not readily diffuse through scar tissue. In the past, the patient was routinely kept in the hospital for a few days after operation, but "come-and-go" hernia repair has been shown to be safe and effective and is now routine. A sedentary worker may return to work within a few days; heavy manual labor has traditionally not been performed for up to 4–6 weeks after hernia repair, though recent studies document no increase in recurrence when full activity is resumed as early as 2 weeks after surgery, particularly when open or laparoscopic mesh repairs have been used.

Prognosis

In addition to chronic cough, prostatism, and constipation, poor tissue quality and poor operative technique may contribute to recurrence of inguinal hernia. Because tissue is often more attenuated in direct hernias, recurrence rates are higher than for indirect hernias. Placing the repair under tension and using absorbable suture are technical errors that lead to recurrence. Failure to find an indirect hernia, to dissect the sac high enough, or to adequately close the internal ring may lead to recurrence of indirect hernia. Postoperative wound infection is associated with increased recurrence. The recurrence rate is considerably increased in patients receiving chronic peritoneal dialysis—in one report, the rate was as high as 27%.

Recurrence rates after indirect hernia repair in adults are reported at best to be 0.6–3%, though the incidence is more probably 5–10%. Inadequate sac reduction or internal ring closure and failure to identify a femoral or direct hernia contribute to recurrence, as does inadequate repair of the inguinal canal. A wide range of figures is quoted for recurrence after repair of direct hernias, from less than 1% to as high as 28%. The point of recurrence is most often just lateral to the pubic tubercle, implicating excessive tension on the repair and adding evidence to favor mesh repairs or the use of a relaxing incision in the rectus sheath if a traditional autologous tissue method is used in the repair of a direct hernia. The use of mesh in hernia repairs decreases the recurrence risk by 50–75%.

Amid PK et al: Open "tension-free" repair of inguinal hernias: the Lichtenstein technique. Eur J Surg 1996;162:447.

Cheek CM et al: Trusses in the management of hernia today. Br J Surg 1995;82:1611.

The EU Hernia Trialists Collaboration: Repair of groin hernia with synthetic mesh: Meta-analysis of randomized controlled trials. Ann Surg 2002;235:322.

Kark AE et al: 3175 primary inguinal hernia repairs: advantages of ambulatory open mesh repair using local anesthesia. J Am Coll Surg 1998;186:447.

Liem MSL et al: Comparison of conventional anterior surgery and laparoscopic surgery for inguinal hernia repair. N Engl J Med 1997;336:1541.

McCormack K et al: Laparoscopic techniques versus open techniques for inguinal hernia repair. The Cochrane Database of Systematic Reviews 2004;Vol. 4.

Neumayer L et al: Open mesh versus laparoscopic mesh repair of inguinal hernia. N Engl J Med 2004;350:1819.

Scott NW et al: Open mesh versus non-mesh for groin hernia repair. The Cochrane Database of Systematic Reviews 2004;Vol. 4.

Zieren J et al: Prospective randomized study comparing laparoscopic and open tension-free inguinal hernia repair with Shouldice's operation. Am J Surg 1998;178:330.

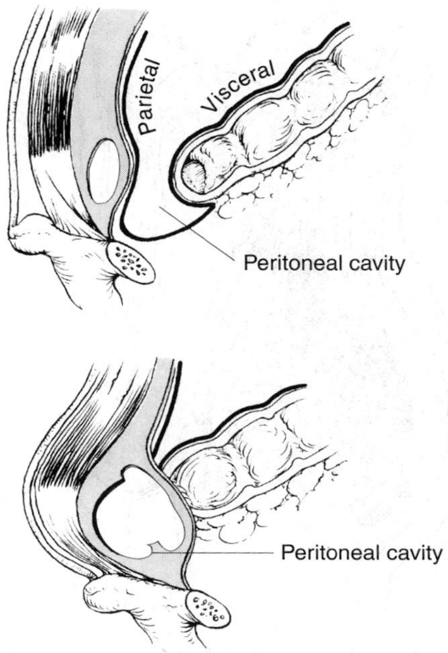

Figure 32–4. Right-sided sliding hernia, sagittal view. *Top:* Note cecum and ascending colon sliding on fascia of posterior abdominal wall. *Bottom:* Hernia has entered internal inguinal ring. Note that one-fourth of the hernia is not related to the peritoneal sac.

SLIDING INGUINAL HERNIA

A sliding inguinal hernia (Figures 32–4 and 32–5) is a type of indirect inguinal hernia in which the wall of a viscus forms a portion of the wall of the hernia sac. On the right side the cecum is most commonly involved, and on the left side the sigmoid colon. The development of a sliding hernia is related to the variable degree of posterior fixation of the large bowel or other sliding components (eg, bladder, ovary) and their proximity to the internal inguinal ring.

Clinical Findings

Though sliding hernias have no special signs that distinguish them from other inguinal hernias, they should be suspected in any large hernia that cannot be completely reduced or whenever a large scrotal hernia is seen in an elderly man. Finding a segment of colon in the scrotum on barium enema strongly suggests a sliding hernia. Recognition of this variation is of great importance at operation, since failure to recognize it may result in inadvertent entry into the lumen of the bowel or bladder.

Treatment

It is essential to recognize the entity at an early stage of operation. As is true of all indirect inguinal hernias, the

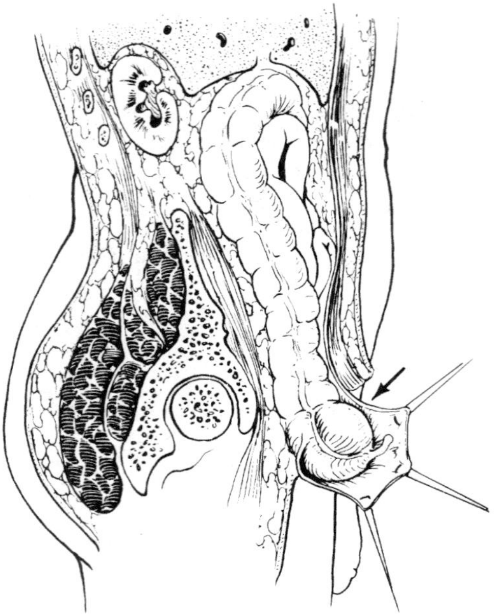

Figure 32–5. Right-sided sliding hernia seen in sagittal section. (After Linden in Thorek.) At arrow, the wall of the cecum forms a portion of the hernia sac.

sac will lie anteriorly, but the posterior wall of the sac will be formed to a greater or lesser degree by colon or bladder.

After the cord has been dissected free from the hernia sac, most sliding hernias can be reduced by a series of inverting sutures (Bevan technique) and one of the standard types of inguinal repair performed. Very large sliding hernias may have to be reduced by entering the peritoneal cavity through a separate incision (La Roque), pulling the bowel back into the abdomen, and fixing it to the posterior abdominal wall. The hernia is then repaired in the usual fashion.

Prognosis

Sliding hernias have a higher recurrence rate than uncomplicated indirect hernias.

The surgical complication most often encountered following sliding hernia repair is bowel injury. Rarely, other retroperitoneal structures such as the bladder or ureter may accompany the viscus into the hernia and are at risk of injury. Injury can best be avoided by simply reducing the hernia and sac into the preperitoneal space and repairing the hernia defect.

Bendavid R: Sliding hernias. Hernia 2002;6:137.

FEMORAL HERNIA

A femoral hernia descends through the femoral canal beneath the inguinal ligament. Because of its narrow neck, it is prone to incarceration and strangulation. Femoral hernia is much more common in women than in men, but in both sexes femoral hernia is less common than inguinal hernia. Femoral hernias comprise about one-third of groin hernias in women and about 2% of groin hernias in men.

Clinical Findings

A. Symptoms

Femoral hernias are notoriously asymptomatic until incarceration or strangulation occurs. Even with obstruction or strangulation, the patient may feel discomfort more in the abdomen than in the femoral area. Thus, colicky abdominal pain and signs of intestinal obstruction frequently are the presenting manifestations of a strangulated femoral hernia, without discomfort, pain, or tenderness in the femoral region.

B. Signs

A femoral hernia may present in a variety of ways. If it is small and uncomplicated, it usually appears as a small bulge in the upper medial thigh just below the level of the inguinal ligament. Because it may be deflected anteriorly through the fossa ovalis femoris to present as a visible or palpable mass at or above the inguinal ligament, it can be confused with an inguinal hernia.

Differential Diagnosis

Femoral hernia must be distinguished from inguinal hernia, a saphenous varix, and femoral adenopathy. A saphenous varix transmits a distinct thrill when a patient coughs, and it appears and disappears instantly when the patient stands or lies down—in contrast to femoral hernias, which are either irreducible or reduce gradually on pressure.

Treatment

A. Principles

The principles of femoral hernia repair are as follows: (1) complete excision of the hernia sac, (2) the use of nonabsorbable sutures, (3) repair of the defect in the transversalis fascia that is responsible for the hernia, and (4) use of Cooper's ligament for the repair, since it gives a firm support for sutures and forms the natural line for closure of the defect.

B. Types of Repair for Femoral Hernia

A femoral hernia can be repaired through an inguinal, thigh, preperitoneal, or abdominal approach, though the inguinal approach is most commonly used. No matter what the approach, the hernia is often difficult to reduce. Reduction may be facilitated by carefully incising the iliopubic tract, Gimbernat's ligament, or even the inguinal ligament. Occasionally, a counterincision in the thigh is required to free attachments below the inguinal ligament.

Irrespective of the approach used, successful femoral hernia repair must close the femoral canal. The Lotheissen-McVay repair, also used for inguinal hernia, is most commonly employed.

If the hernia sac and mass reduce when the patient is given opiates or anesthesia and if bloody fluid appears in the hernia sac when it is exposed and opened, one must strongly suspect the possibility of nonviable bowel in the peritoneal cavity. In such cases, it is mandatory to open and explore the abdomen, usually through a separate midline incision. The laparoscopic approach is well-suited for repair of femoral hernias.

Prognosis

Recurrence rates usually approximate the middle range for direct inguinal hernia, ie, about 5–10%.

Berliner SD et al: The Henry operation for incarcerated and strangulated femoral hernias. Arch Surg 1992;127:314.

Glassow F: Femoral hernia: review of 2,105 repairs in a 17 year period. Am J Surg 1985;150:353.

Hernandez-Richter T: The femoral hernia: an ideal approach for the transabdominal preperitoneal technique (TAPP). Surg Endos 2000;14:736.

OTHER TYPES OF HERNIAS

UMBILICAL HERNIAS IN ADULTS

Umbilical hernia in adults occurs long after closure of the umbilical ring and is due to a gradual yielding of the cicatricial tissue closing the ring. It is more common in women than in men.

Predisposing factors include (1) multiple pregnancies with prolonged labor, (2) ascites, (3) obesity, and (4) large intra-abdominal tumors.

Clinical Findings

In adults, umbilical hernia does not usually obliterate spontaneously, as in children, but instead increases steadily in size. The hernia sac may have multiple loculations. Umbilical hernias usually contain omentum, but small and large bowel may be present. Emergency repair is often necessary, because the neck of the hernia is usually quite narrow compared to the size of the herniated mass and incarceration and strangulation are common.

Umbilical hernias with tight rings are often associated with sharp pain on coughing or straining. Very large umbilical hernias more commonly produce a dragging or aching sensation.

Treatment

Umbilical hernia in an adult should be repaired expeditiously to avoid incarceration and strangulation. Repairs utilizing mesh result in the lowest recurrence rate. The laparoscopic approach is associated with less postoperative pain and faster recovery than open techniques. Mesh should be used for all but the smallest umbilical hernias.

The presence of cirrhosis and ascites should not discourage repair of an umbilical hernia, since incarceration, strangulation, and rupture are particularly dangerous in patients with these disorders. If significant ascites exists, however, it should first be controlled medically or by peritoneovenous shunt if necessary, since mortality, morbidity, and recurrence are higher after hernia repair in patients with ascites. Preoperative correction of fluid and electrolyte imbalance and improvement of nutrition will improve the outcome in these patients.

Prognosis

Factors that may lead to high rates of complication and death after surgical repair include large size of the hernia, old age or debility of the patient, and the presence of related intra-abdominal disease. In healthy individuals, surgical repair of the umbilical defects gives good results with a low rate of recurrence.

Arroyo A et al: Randomized clinical trial comparing suture and mesh repair of umbilical hernia in adults. Br J Surg 2001;88:1321.

Hansen J et al: Danish nationwide cohort study of postoperative death in patients with liver cirrhosis undergoing hernia repair. Br J Surg 2002;89:805.

Lau H et al: Umbilical hernia in adults. Surg Endos 2003;17:2016.

EPIGASTRIC HERNIA

An epigastric hernia (Figure 32–6) protrudes through the linea alba above the level of the umbilicus. The hernia may develop through one of the foramina of egress of the small paramidline nerves and vessels or through an area of congenital weakness in the linea alba.

About 3–5% of the population have epigastric hernias. They are more common in men than in women and most common between the ages of 20 and 50. About 20% of epigastric hernias are multiple, and about 80% occur just off the midline.

Clinical Findings

A. Symptoms

Most epigastric hernias are painless and are found on routine abdominal examination. If symptomatic, their presen-

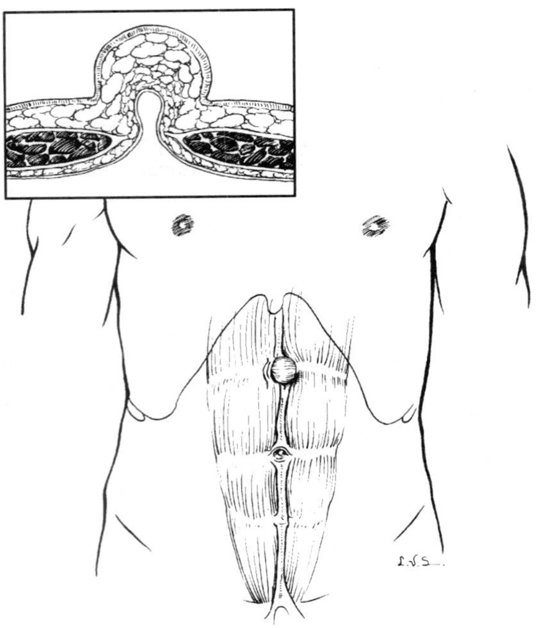

Figure 32–6. Epigastric hernia. Note closeness to midline and presence in upper abdomen. The herniation is through the linea alba.

tation ranges from mild epigastric pain and tenderness to deep, burning epigastric pain with radiation to the back or the lower abdominal quadrants. The pain may be accompanied by abdominal bloating, nausea, or vomiting. The symptoms often occur after a large meal and on occasion may be relieved by reclining, probably because the supine position causes the herniated mass to drop away from the anterior abdominal wall. The smaller masses most frequently contain only preperitoneal fat and are especially prone to incarceration and strangulation. These smaller hernias are often tender. Larger hernias seldom strangulate and may contain, in addition to preperitoneal fat, a portion of the nearby omentum and, occasionally, a loop of small or large bowel.

B. Signs

If a mass is palpable, the diagnosis can often be confirmed by any maneuver that will increase intra-abdominal pressure and thereby cause the mass to bulge anteriorly. The diagnosis is difficult to make when the patient is obese, since a mass is hard to palpate; ultrasound, CT, or tangential radiographs may be needed in the very obese patient.

Differential Diagnosis

Differential diagnosis includes peptic ulcer, gallbladder disease, hiatal hernia, pancreatitis, and upper small bowel obstruction. On occasion, it may be impossible to distinguish the hernial mass from a subcutaneous lipoma, fibroma, or neurofibroma.

Another condition that must be distinguished from an epigastric hernia is **diastasis recti**, a diffuse widening and attenuation of the linea alba without a fascial defect. On examination, this condition appears as a fusiform, linear bulge between the two rectus abdominis muscles without a discrete fascial defect. Although this condition may be unsightly, repair should be avoided since there is no risk of incarceration, the fascial layer is weak, and the recurrence rate is high.

Treatment

Most epigastric hernias should be repaired, since small ones are likely to become incarcerated and large ones are often symptomatic and unsightly. The defect can usually be closed primarily. Herniated fat contents are usually dissected free and removed. Intraperitoneal herniating structures are reduced, but no attempt is made to close the peritoneal sac.

Prognosis

The recurrence rate is 10–20%, a higher incidence than with the routine inguinal or femoral hernia repair. This high recurrence rate may be partly due to failure to recognize and repair multiple small defects.

Hodgson TJ et al: Anterior abdominal wall hernias: diagnosis by ultrasound and tangential radiographs. Clin Radiol 1991;44:185.

INCISIONAL HERNIA (VENTRAL HERNIA)

About 10% of abdominal operations result in incisional hernias. The incidence of this iatrogenic type of hernia is not diminishing in spite of an awareness of the many causative factors.

Etiology

The factors most often responsible for incisional hernia are listed below. When more than one factor coexists in the same patient, the likelihood of postoperative wound failure is greatly increased.

(1) Poor surgical technique. Inadequate fascial bites, tension on the fascial edges, or too tight a closure are most often responsible for incisional failure.

(2) Postoperative wound infection.

(3) Age. Wound healing is usually slower and less solid in older patients.

(4) General debility. Cirrhosis, carcinoma, and chronic wasting diseases are factors that affect wound healing ad-

versely. Any condition that compromises nutrition increases the likelihood of incision breakdown.

(5) Obesity. Fat patients frequently have increased intra-abdominal pressure. The presence of fat in the abdominal wound masks tissue layers and increases the incidence of seromas and hematomas in wounds.

(6) Postoperative pulmonary complications that stress the repair as a result of vigorous coughing. Smokers and patients with chronic pulmonary disease are therefore at increased risk of fascial disruption.

(7) Placement of drains or stomas in the primary operative wound.

(8) Intraoperative blood loss greater than 1000 mL.

(9) Failure to close the fascia of laparoscopic trocar sites over 10 mm in size.

Treatment

Small incisional hernias should be treated by early repair since they may cause bowel obstruction. If the patient is unwilling to undergo surgery or is a poor surgical risk, symptoms may be controlled by an elastic corset.

Defects too large to close easily may be left without surgical repair if they are asymptomatic, since they are unlikely to incarcerate.

A. Small Hernias

Small incisional hernias usually require only a direct fascia-to-fascia repair for satisfactory closure. Interrupted or continuous closure may be used, but the sutures should be nonabsorbable. Sutures tied too tightly or tension on the repair will predispose to recurrence.

B. Large Hernias

Although no specific diameter distinguishes a small from a large hernia, a hernia can be considered large when the fascial edges cannot be approximated without tension.

In performing the repair, excess and scarred skin and subcutaneous tissues over the hernia are removed. The hernia sac is then carefully dissected free from the underlying muscles and fascial tissues. If there are no adherent intraperitoneal structures, the sac may be inverted and the repair done over the inverted sac. If there is incarceration or adhesion of intraperitoneal contents, the abdominal contents should be dissected free from the sac and dropped back into the abdomen. The edges of the fascial defect should be cleaned so that the closure will be to solid fascial tissue rather that to scar.

Primary closure of a large defect is not advisable, since tension on the closure increases the risk of hernia recurrence. Increasingly, repair of large or recurrent defects is performed using nonabsorbable mesh. Although a variety of techniques exist for placement of the mesh, a retrorectus inlay or sandwich technique achieves a lower recurrence rate than an edge-to-edge or onlay placement. If a large dead space persists, a closed drainage system is usually employed in the space above the fascia. A primary fascial closure should be used only if the fascia can be brought together without tension.

Laparoscopic techniques are also currently being used to repair incisional hernias and perform adhesiolysis electively. A sheet of synthetic material is secured to the abdominal wall as an inlay graft; the intraperitoneal placement of the graft enhances the durability of the repair, though it also increases the risk of bowel adhesions or fistula formation.

Alternative methods to close the fascial defect using the patient's native tissues, such as a sliding myofascial flap or lateral counterincisions in the anterior rectus sheath to allow primary closure in the midline, are increasingly used to avoid the need for mesh.

Prognosis

The recurrence rate for first-time incisional hernia repairs varies directly with the size of the fascial defect. Small hernias have a recurrence rate of 2–5%; medium-sized hernias recur in 5–15% of cases; and large hernias, too often closed under tension, have a recurrence rate approaching 50%. Repair of recurrent incisional hernias is even less likely to succeed, with a recurrence rate exceeding 50%. Results with mesh placed laparoscopically are lower than those seen with open repairs.

Burger JWA et al: Long-term follow-up of a randomized controlled trial of suture versus mesh repair of incisional hernia. Ann Surg 2004;240:578.

DiBello J Jr et al: Sliding myofascial flap of the rectus abdominus muscles for the closure of recurrent ventral hernias. Plast Reconstr Surg 1996;98:464.

Israelsson LA et al: Suture technique and wound healing in midline laparotomy incisions. Eur J Surg 1996;162:605.

Leber GE et al: Long-term complications associated with prosthetic repair of incisional hernias. Arch Surg 1998;133:378.

McLanahan D et al: Retrorectus prosthetic mesh repair of midline abdominal hernia. Am J Surg 1997;173:445.

Sugerman HJ et al: Greater risk of incisional hernia with morbidly obese than steroid-dependent patients and low recurrence with prefascial polypropylene mesh. Am J Surg 1996;171:80.

VARIOUS RARE HERNIATIONS THROUGH THE ABDOMINAL WALL

Littre's Hernia

A Littre hernia is a hernia that contains a Meckel diverticulum in the hernia sac. Although Littre first described the condition in relation to a femoral hernia, the relative distribution of Littre's hernias is as follows: inguinal, 50%; femoral, 20%; umbilical, 20%; and miscellaneous, 10%. Littre's hernias of the groin are more common in men and on the right side. The clinical findings are similar to those of Richter's hernia; when strangulation is present, pain, fever, and manifestations of small bowel obstruction occur late.

Treatment consists of repair of the hernia plus, if possible, excision of the diverticulum. If acute Meckel's diverticulitis is present, the acute inflammatory mass may have to be treated through a separate abdominal incision.

Trupo FJ et al: Meckel's diverticulum in femoral hernia: a Littre's hernia. South Med J 1987;80:655.

Spigelian Hernia

Spigelian hernia is an acquired ventral hernia through the linea semilunaris, the line where the sheaths of the lateral abdominal muscles fuse to form the lateral rectus sheath. Spigelian hernias are nearly always found above the level of the inferior epigastric vessels. They most commonly occur where the semicircular line (fold of Douglas) crosses the linea semilunaris.

The presenting symptom is pain that is usually localized to the hernia site and may be aggravated by any maneuver that increases intra-abdominal pressure. With time, the pain may become more dull, constant, and diffuse, making diagnosis more difficult.

If a mass can be demonstrated, the diagnosis presents little difficulty. The diagnosis is most easily made with the patient standing and straining; a bulge then presents in the lower abdominal area and disappears with a gurgling sound on pressure. Following reduction of the mass, the hernia orifice can usually be palpated.

Diagnosis is often made more difficult because the hernial defect may lie beneath an intact external oblique layer and therefore not be palpable. The hernia often dissects within the layers of the abdominal wall and may not present a distinct mass, or the mass may be located at a distance from the linea semilunaris. Patients with spigelian hernias should have a tender point over the hernia orifice, though tenderness alone is not sufficient to make the diagnosis. Both ultrasound and CT scan may help to confirm the diagnosis.

Spigelian hernias have a high incidence of incarceration and should be repaired. These hernias are quite easily cured by primary aponeurotic closure. Laparoscopic repair may decrease morbidity and hospital stay.

Broughton G 2nd et al: Repair of a spigelian hernia. J Am Coll Surg 1997;185:490.

Moreno-Egea A et al: Open vs laparoscopic repair of spigelian hernia: a prospective randomized trial. Arch Surg 2002;137:1266.

Lumbar or Dorsal Hernia

Lumbar or dorsal hernias (Figure 32–7) are hernias through the posterior abdominal wall at some level in the lumbar region. The most common sites (95%) are the superior (Grynfeltt's) and inferior (Petit's) lumbar triangles. A "lump in the flank" is the common complaint, associated with a dull, heavy, pulling feeling. With the patient erect, the presence of a reducible, often tympanitic mass in the flank usually makes the diagnosis. Incarceration and strangulation occur in about 10% of cases. Hernias in the inferior lumbar triangle are most often small and occur in young, athletic women. They present as tender masses producing backache and usually contain fat. Lumbar hernia must be differentiated from abscesses, hematomas, soft tissue tumors, renal tumors, and muscle strain.

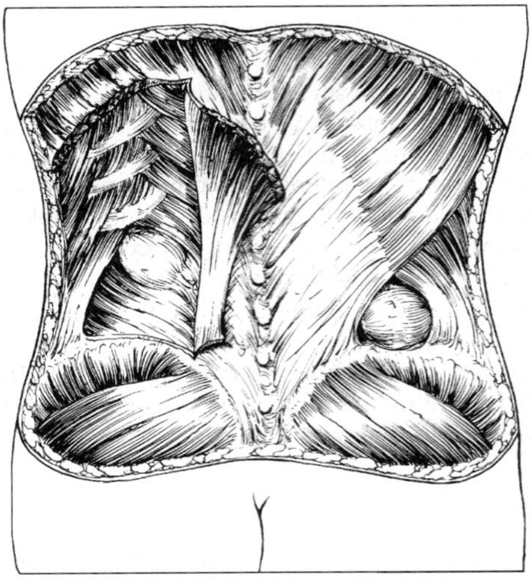

Figure 32–7. Anatomic relationships of lumbar or dorsal hernia. (Adapted from Netter.) On the left, lumbar or dorsal hernia into space of Grynfeltt. On the right, hernia into Petit's triangle (inferior lumbar space).

Acquired hernias may be traumatic or nontraumatic. Severe direct trauma, penetrating wounds, abscesses, and poor healing of flank incisions are the usual causes. Congenital hernias occur in infants and are usually isolated unilateral congenital defects.

Lumbar hernias increase in size and should be repaired when found. Repair is by mobilization of the nearby fascia and obliteration of the hernia defect by precise fascia-to-fascia closure. The recurrence rate is very low.

Heniford BT et al: Laparoscopic inferior and superior lumbar hernia repair. Arch Surg 1997;132:1141.

Killeen KL et al: Using CT to diagnose traumatic lumbar hernia. AJR Am J Roentgenol 2000;174:1413.

Thor K: Lumbar hernia. Acta Chir Scand 1985;151:389.

Obturator Hernia

Herniation through the obturator canal is more frequent in elderly women and is difficult to diagnose preoperatively. The mortality rate (13–40%) of these hernias makes them the most lethal of all abdominal hernias. These hernias most commonly present as small bowel obstruction with cramping abdominal pain and vomiting. The hernia is rarely palpable in the groin, though a mass may be felt on pelvic or rectal examination. The most specific finding is a positive Howship-Romberg sign, in which pain extends down the medial aspect of the thigh with abduction, extension, or internal rotation of the knee. Since this sign is present in fewer than half of cases, diagnosis should be suspected in any elderly debilitated woman without previous abdominal operations who presents with a small bowel obstruction. Though diagnosis can be confirmed by CT scan, operation should not be unduly delayed if complete bowel obstruction is present.

The abdominal approach gives the best exposure; these hernias should not be repaired from the thigh approach. The Cheatle-Henry approach (retropubic) may also be used. Simple repair is most often possible, though bladder wall, pectineal muscle, peritoneum, or mesh has been used when the defect cannot be approximated primarily.

Naude G et al: Obturator hernia is an unsuspected diagnosis. Am J Surg 1997;174:72.

Perineal Hernia

A perineal hernia protrudes through the muscles and fascia of the perineal floor. It may be primary but is usually acquired following perineal prostatectomy, abdominoperineal resection of the rectum, or pelvic exenteration.

These hernias present as easily reducible perineal bulges and usually are asymptomatic, but may present with pain, dysuria, bowel obstruction, or perineal skin breakdown.

Repair is usually done by an abdominal approach, with an adequate fascial and muscular perineal repair. Occasionally polypropylene (Marlex) mesh or flaps using the gracilis or gluteus may be necessary, when the available tissues are too attenuated for adequate primary repair.

So JB et al: Post operative perineal hernia. Dis Colon Rectum 1997;40:954.

Interparietal Hernia

Interparietal hernias, in which the sac insinuates itself between the layers of the abdominal wall, are usually of an indirect inguinal type but, rarely, may be direct or ventral hernias. Although interparietal hernias are rare, it is essential to recognize them, because strangulation is common and the mass is easily mistaken for a tumor or abscess. The lesion usually can be suspected on the basis of the physical examination provided it is kept in mind. In most cases, extensive studies for intra-abdominal tumors have preceded diagnosis. A lateral film of the abdomen will usually show bowel within the layers of the abdominal wall in cases with intestinal incarceration or strangulation, and an ultrasound or CT scan may be diagnostic.

As soon as the diagnosis is established, operation should be performed, usually through the standard inguinal approach.

Sciatic Hernia

Sciatic hernia is the rarest of abdominal hernias and consists of an outpouching of intra-abdominal contents through the greater sciatic foramen. The diagnosis is made after incarceration or strangulation of the bowel occurs. The repair is usually made through the abdominal approach. The hernia sac and contents are reduced, and the weak area is closed by making a fascial flap from the superficial fascia of the piriformis muscle.

TRAUMATIC HERNIA

Abdominal wall hernias occur rarely as a direct consequence of direct blunt abdominal injury. The patient presents with abdominal pain. On examination, ecchymosis of the abdominal wall and a bulge are usually present. The existence of a hernia may not be obvious, however, and the patient may require CT scan to confirm it. Because of the high incidence of associated intra-abdominal injuries, laparotomy is usually required. The defect should be repaired primarily if possible.

Gill IS et al: Traumatic ventral abdominal hernia associated with small bowel gangrene: case report. J Trauma 1993;35:145.

Otero C et al: Injury to the abdominal wall musculature: the full spectrum of traumatic hernia. South Med J 1988;81:517.

Wood RJ et al: Traumatic abdominal hernia: a case report and review of the literature. Am Surg 1988;54:648.

II. OTHER LESIONS OF THE ABDOMINAL WALL

CONGENITAL DEFECTS

Congenital defects of the abdominal wall other than hernias or lesions of the urachus and umbilicus are rare.

The important ones involving the urachus and umbilicus are discussed in Chapter 46.

TRAUMA TO THE ABDOMINAL WALL

Hematoma of the Rectus Sheath

This is a rare but important entity that may follow mild trauma to the abdominal wall or may occur secondary to disorders of coagulation, blood dyscrasia, or degenerative vascular diseases.

Abdominal pain, usually in the right lower abdomen, is a presenting sign. It may be sudden and severe in onset or slowly progressive. The key to diagnosis is the physical examination. Careful palpation will reveal an exquisitely tender mass within the abdominal wall. If the patient tenses the rectus muscles by raising the head or body, the swelling becomes more tender and distinct on palpation, in contrast to an intra-abdominal mass or tenderness that disappears when the rectus muscles are contracted (Fothergill's sign). In addition, there may be detectable discoloration or ecchymosis. If the physical signs are not diagnostic, ultrasound or CT scan can demonstrate the hematoma in the abdominal wall.

Usually, the condition can be treated without operation. The acute pain and discomfort should disappear within 2 or 3 days, although a residual mass may persist for several weeks. If pain is severe, an acceptable alternative is evacuation of the clot and control of the bleeding.

Edlow JA et al: Rectus sheath hematoma. Ann Emerg Med 1999;34:671.

PAIN IN THE ABDOMINAL WALL

A number of conditions are characterized by pain in the abdominal wall without a demonstrable organic lesion. Pain from a diaphragmatic, supradiaphragmatic, or spinal cord lesion may be referred to the abdomen. Herpes zoster (shingles) may present as abdominal pain, in which case it will follow a dermatomal distribution.

Scars may be sensitive or painful, particularly in the first 6 months after surgery.

Entrapment of a nerve by a nonabsorbable suture may cause persistent incisional pain, sometimes quite severe. Hyperesthesia of the skin over the involved dermatome may provide a clue to the cause.

In all cases of epigastric pain in the abdominal wall, careful search should be made for a small epigastric hernia, as noted earlier.

ABDOMINAL WALL TUMORS

Tumors of the abdominal wall are quite common, but most are benign, eg, lipomas, hemangiomas, and fibromas. Musculoaponeurotic fibromatoses (desmoid tumors), which often occur in abdominal wall scars or after parturition in women, are discussed in more detail in Chapter 47. Most malignant tumors of the abdominal wall are metastatic. Metastases may appear by direct invasion from intra-abdominal lesions or by vascular dissemination. The sudden appearance of a sensitive nodule anywhere in the abdominal wall that is clearly not a hernia should arouse suspicion of an occult cancer, the lung and pancreas being the more likely primary sites.

Adrenals

33

Quan-Yang Duh, MD, Chienying Liu, MD, & J. Blake Tyrrell, MD

Operations on the adrenal glands are performed for primary hyperaldosteronism, pheochromocytoma, hyperadrenocorticism (Cushing's disease or Cushing's syndrome), and adrenocortical carcinoma. Less commonly, surgery may also be performed for nonfunctioning tumors or metastases. These conditions are usually characterized by hypersecretion of one or more of the adrenal hormones.

Anatomy & Surgical Principles

The normal combined weight of the adrenals is 7–12 g. The right gland lies posterior and lateral to the vena cava and superior to the kidney (Figure 33–1). The left gland lies medial to the superior pole of the kidney, just lateral to the aorta and immediately posterior to the superior border of the pancreas. An important surgical feature is the remarkable constancy of the adrenal veins. The right adrenal vein, 2–5 mm long and several millimeters wide, connects the anterior aspect of the adrenal gland with the posterolateral aspect of the vena cava. The left adrenal vein is several centimeters long and travels inferiorly from the lower pole of the gland, joining the left renal vein after receiving the inferior phrenic vein. The adrenal arteries are small, multiple, and inconstant. They usually come from the inferior phrenic artery, the aorta, and the renal artery.

With the exception of rare nonsecreting cancers, indications for adrenal surgery result from hypersecretory states. Diagnosis and treatment begin with confirmation of a hypersecretory state (ie, measurement of excess cortisol, aldosterone, or catecholamines in blood or urine). In order to determine whether the problem originates in the adrenal, levels of the trophic hormone in question (ie, ACTH or renin) must be measured. If levels of the trophic hormone are suppressed but hormone secretion is excessive, autonomous secretion is proved. The next step, except in pheochromocytoma, is to determine the degree of autonomy, a process that usually distinguishes hyperplasias (which respond to most but not all controlling mechanisms) from adenomas and adenomas from cancers. In general, cancers are under little if any feedback control. If the primary problem is not in the adrenal, as in Cushing's disease, treatment must be directed elsewhere when possible.

Adrenal masses are usually detected and localized by CT scan or MRI. Functioning tumors of the adrenal can be localized by adrenal scintigraphy, ^{131}I-6β-iodomethylnorcholesterol (NP-59) for cortical tumors and ^{131}I-metaiodobenzylguanidine (MIBG) for medullary tumors. Functioning adrenal or pituitary tumors can also be localized by demonstrating a gradient of hormone levels between their venous drainage and a peripheral vein.

The major principles of adrenal surgery are as follows:

(1) Whenever possible, the surgeon must be certain of the diagnosis and the location of the lesion before undertaking the operation.

(2) The patient must be thoroughly prepared so he or she can withstand any metabolic problems caused by the disease or by the operation.

(3) The surgeon and consultants must be able to detect and treat any metabolic crisis that occurs during or after operation.

Surgical Approaches

Currently, almost all adrenal tumors are identified preoperatively by localization studies such as CT and MRI, so very few operations require general exploration of the abdomen. This permits the use of minimally invasive surgery. Almost all adrenal tumors can be removed laparoscopically. Traditional open adrenalectomy is only necessary when the tumor is especially large (eg, > 12 cm, depending on the surgeon's experience) or for locally invasive adrenocortical cancer where resection of lymph nodes or adjacent organs may be required.

Laparoscopic adrenalectomy can be performed using a transabdominal or retroperitoneal approach, but the former is preferable in most cases. This involves medial rotation of the spleen and pancreas (on the left) or the liver (on the right), using gravity to drop the viscera away from the adrenal.

The traditional open surgical approach should be used only when laparoscopic expertise is not available or when required by the size and nature of the tumor. The advantages of the laparoscopic operation are so great that it is strongly preferred.

The open anterior (transperitoneal) approach through a long vertical midline incision or a bilateral subcostal incision allows wide exposure of the abdominal organs and the retroperitoneum. Unfortunately, this incision also causes more pain, ileus, and atelectasis and a much

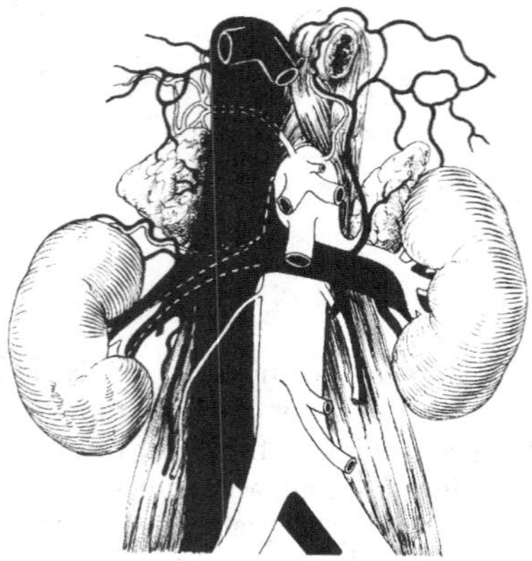

Figure 33–1. Anatomy of the adrenals, showing venous return.

longer period of recovery. The risks of poor wound healing, (Table 33–1) are greater—especially for patients with Cushing's syndrome.

Table 33–1. Frequency of manifestations of hyperadrenocorticism.

	Percentage
Obesity	95%
Hypertension	70%
Glucose tolerance	80%
Centripetal distribution of fat	80%
Weakness	20%
Muscle atrophy in upper and lower extremities	70%
Hirsutism	80%
Menstrual disturbance or impotence	75%
Purple striae	50%
Plethoric facies	85%
Easy bruisability	35%
Acne	40%
Psychological symptoms	40%
Edema	20%
Headache	15%
Back pain	60%

The open posterior approach, performed through incisions on each side of the spine and the bed of the 11th or 12th rib with the patient lying prone, is better tolerated postoperatively but provides a more limited exposure. It is adequate only for lesions smaller than 4–5 cm and has been superseded by the laparoscopic approach. An open lateral approach through the bed of the 11th rib to expose the adrenals retroperitoneally or a thoracoabdominal incision may be considered for large or invasive tumors.

DISEASES OF THE ADRENALS

PRIMARY HYPERALDOSTERONISM

ESSENTIALS OF DIAGNOSIS

- *Hypertension with or without hypokalemia.*
- *Elevated aldosterone secretion and suppressed plasma renin activity.*
- *Metabolic alkalosis, relative hypernatremia.*
- *Weakness, polyuria, paresthesias, tetany, cramps due to hypokalemia.*

General Considerations

Aldosterone, the most potent mineralocorticoid secreted by the adrenal cortex, regulates the body's electrolyte composition, fluid volume, and blood pressure. Excess aldosterone increases total body sodium, decreases potassium levels, increases extracellular fluid volume (without edema), and increases blood pressure. Under normal conditions, aldosterone secretion is regulated by the renin-angiotensin system in a feedback fashion and is also stimulated transiently by ACTH.

In primary hyperaldosteronism, aldosterone levels are elevated and renin levels are suppressed. In secondary hyperaldosteronism, increased aldosterone is due to increased renin secretion. Examples of secondary hyperaldosteronism include renal vascular disease, renin-secreting tumors, and cirrhosis with low intravascular volume. Among the subtypes of primary hyperaldosteronism, aldosterone-producing adenoma (aldosteronoma) and idiopathic hyperaldosteronism with adrenal hyperplasia are the most common types. Unilateral primary adrenal hyperplasia, aldosterone-producing adrenocortical carcinoma, and familial hyperaldosteronism (eg, glucocorticoid-remediable hyperaldosteronism) are rare. Surgery is beneficial only in patients with aldosterone-producing adenomas and in patients with unilateral primary adrenal hyperplasia.

Primary hyperaldosteronism in its classic form is characterized by hypertension, hypokalemia, increased aldosterone secretion, and suppressed plasma renin activity. However, hypokalemia is not required to make the diagnosis; recent studies have shown that many patients have a normal potassium level. Primary hyperaldosteronism was once thought to be present in about 1% of patients with hypertension, but its prevalence has increased to 5–13% based on various studies when plasma aldosterone concentration-to-plasma renin activity was used to screen for hyperaldosteronism in patients with hypertension who were not hypokalemic. Although rare, normotensive primary hyperaldosteronism has been described.

Aldosteronomas are usually solitary and small (0.5–2 cm). They have a characteristic chrome color when sectioned. Tumor cells typically have heterogeneous cytomorphology, resembling those of all three zones of the adrenal cortex, including hybrid cells having cytologic features of the zona glomerulosa and zona fasciculata. Hyperplasia is also often seen in glands harboring adenomas.

Clinical Findings

Aldosterone facilitates the exchange of sodium for potassium and hydrogen ions in the distal nephron. Therefore, when aldosterone secretion is chronically increased, serum potassium and hydrogen ion concentrations fall (hypokalemia and alkalosis), total body sodium rises, and hypertension results.

A. Symptoms and Signs

Symptoms if present are usually those of hypokalemia and depend on the severity of potassium depletion. Patients complain of a sense of malaise, muscle weakness, polyuria, polydipsia, cramps, and paresthesias. Tetany and hypokalemic paralysis occur rarely. Headaches are common. Hypertension is usually moderate to severe and may be refractory to medical therapy, but advanced retinopathy is rare. Although extracellular fluid volume is increased, edema is not seen unless renal failure occurs.

B. Laboratory Findings

1. Screening test—Primary hyperaldosteronism should be suspected in patients with hypertension and hypokalemia—either spontaneous or following the administration of diuretics—and in patients with refractory hypertension. The diagnostic evaluation should start with screening tests. A simple ambulatory test determines the ratio of plasma aldosterone concentration (in ng/dL) to plasma renin activity (in ng/mL/h). A ratio of > 20 with a plasma aldosterone concentration > 15 ng/dL suggests primary hyperaldosteronism and warrants confirmatory biochemical studies. Hypertensive individuals without primary hyperaldosteronism usually have ratios of < 20. If the patient is taking spironolactone, the data are uninterpretable, and estrogens increase plasma aldosterone concentrations by increasing angiotensinogen. Both should be discontinued for 6 weeks before the workup. Many other medications, such as diuretics, angiotensin-converting enzyme inhibitors, prostaglandin synthetase inhibitors, cyproheptadine, and vasodilators, can also affect the renin-angiotensin-aldosterone axis and confuse the results. These medications should be discontinued for 2 weeks before the workup. Peripheral alpha-adrenergic blockers are the preferred antihypertensive agents during evaluation. In many patients, it is unwise to withdraw antihypertensive medications, and one must be content with imperfect data. Beta-blockers and calcium-channel blockers cause few problems.

2. Confirmatory test—If the screening test is positive, failure to suppress aldosterone secretion with sodium loading will confirm the diagnosis of primary hyperaldosteronism in most patients. Aldosterone can be suppressed by oral salt loading or intravenous sodium chloride infusion. The patient should consume a high-sodium diet for 3 days, supplemented with NaCl tablets (2–3 g with each meal) if necessary. A 24-hour urine sample is collected for aldosterone, sodium, and potassium determinations on the third day. Urinary aldosterone excretion > 12 μg/24 h distinguishes most patients with primary hyperaldosteronism from those with essential hypertension. If sodium intake has been as high as desired, urinary sodium excretion should exceed 200 meq/24 h. Supplemental potassium chloride should be given to avoid hypokalemia because the high-salt diet increases kaliuresis. Hypokalemia may interfere with the test results by decreasing aldosterone secretion, and it may also cause cardiac arrhythmias. Alternatively, a plasma aldosterone concentration > 10 ng/mL after an infusion of 2 L of normal saline over 4 hours is also consistent with primary hyperaldosteronism. However, the variability of aldosterone secretion throughout the day in patients with aldosteronomas makes this method less desirable than oral salt loading.

Differential Diagnosis

Once the diagnosis is established, the surgically correctable forms—aldosterone producing adenoma (aldosteronoma) and the rare unilateral primary adrenal hyperplasia—should be distinguished from idiopathic hyperaldosteronism due to bilateral adrenal hyperplasia, for which medical therapy is the best management. Aldosteronoma and idiopathic hyperaldosteronism are the most common subtypes. Compared with those with idiopathic hyperaldosteronism, patients with aldosteronoma have more severe hypertension, more severe hypokalemia, higher aldosterone secretion (> 20 ng/dL), higher 18-hydroxycorticosterone concentrations (> 100 ng/dL), and are younger.

The postural stimulation test may be helpful. The test is based on the observation that aldosteronomas are usually unaffected by the renin-angiotensin system but retain sensitivity to ACTH stimulation. Therefore, the plasma aldosterone concentration follows the diurnal variation of ACTH and cortisol. In contrast, idiopathic hyperaldosteronism is characterized by enhanced sensitivity to small changes in the renin-angiotensin axis but is unaffected by ACTH. Thus, if the patient remains upright for 4 hours, plasma aldosterone levels fall and renin remains suppressed in patients with aldosteronoma. In patients with idiopathic hyperaldosteronism, plasma aldosterone increases in response to a small increase in plasma renin.

Unfortunately, these features do not absolutely distinguish the two types. Combined biochemical studies and imaging studies are frequently necessary.

High-resolution, thin-section CT identifies most adenomas and should be performed once the diagnosis of primary hyperaldosteronism is established. Adrenal vein sampling is indicated if the CT scan is equivocal or negative. Adrenal vein sampling is the most certain way to differentiate aldosteronoma from idiopathic hyperaldosteronism and to diagnose and localize an aldosteronoma. Routine use of selective adrenal venous sampling is advocated by some centers. Nevertheless, it is technically difficult, and failure to cannulate the adrenal veins, especially the right adrenal vein, is common.

Aldosterone-secreting adrenocortical carcinoma should be suspected if the tumor is larger than 4 cm. Glucocorticoid-remediable hyperaldosteronism (familial hyperaldosteronism type 1) is inherited in an autosomal dominant fashion. The genetic defect results in a chimeric gene. The mutated gene juxtaposes the promoter for expression of the 11α-hydroxylase gene, which is ACTH-responsive, with the coding sequence of the aldosterone synthase gene. This leads to aldosterone production under ACTH stimulation in the zona fasciculata. Glucocorticoid therapy reverses this type of hyperaldosteronism. These patients have a family history of onset of hypertension at an early age. The diagnosis can be established by measuring elevated 24-hour urine 18-hydroxycortisol and 18-oxocortisol levels or by genetic testing.

Tumor Localization

An aldosterone-producing adenoma can usually be demonstrated by high-resolution CT or MRI scanning. Some small aldosteronomas can be missed, and in such cases a patient with a small aldosteronoma not seen on CT may be misdiagnosed as having adrenal hyperplasia. Aldosteronomas that coexist with nonfunctional adenomas can be mislabeled as adrenal hyperplasia because of multinodularity or bilateral masses on CT. Small abnormalities on CT scans may represent hyperplasia rather than true aldosteronomas. Therefore, unless an unequivocal unilateral tumor, preferably > 1 cm, is present on the CT scan and the contralateral gland is normal, the diagnosis and localization of aldosteronoma cannot be considered certain. The clinical features and results of the postural stimulation test may offer clues but are not always predictive. When in doubt, adrenal vein sampling should be done; it is 95% accurate in identifying an aldosteronoma. Blood is sampled from the adrenal veins and the inferior vena cava for aldosterone and cortisol levels at baseline and after ACTH infusion. Proper catheter placement is confirmed by finding high cortisol levels in adrenal venous blood compared with the inferior vena cava. Corrected aldosterone levels are calculated from the ratio of aldosterone to cortisol in each venous sample. A lateralization ratio of the corrected aldosterone level > 4 indicates unilateral aldosterone secretion, thereby confirming a diagnosis of aldosteronoma in most patients. Adrenal vein sampling is invasive and requires considerable skill and experience. The success rate for cannulating both adrenal veins is about 90%. Unilateral catheterization of the left adrenal vein alone does not give useful information.

Complications

Uncontrolled hypertension can lead to renal failure, stroke, and myocardial infarction. Severe hypokalemia can cause weakness, paralysis, and arrhythmia especially in patients taking digitalis.

Treatment

The goal of therapy is to prevent the complications of hypertension and hypokalemia. Unilateral adrenalectomy is recommended for patients with aldosteronoma and medical therapy for those with idiopathic hyperaldosteronism or those with aldosteronoma who are poor candidates for surgery.

A. Surgical Treatment

1. Preoperative preparation—Blood pressure and hypokalemia should be controlled before surgery. Spironolactone, a competitive aldosterone antagonist, has been the drug of choice. It blocks the mineralocorticoid receptor, promotes potassium retention, restores normal potassium concentrations, and reduces the extracellular fluid volume, thereby controlling blood pressure. Furthermore, it reactivates the suppressed renin-angiotensin-aldosterone system in the contralateral adrenal gland, reducing the risk of postoperative hypoaldosteronism. Initial dosages of 200–400 mg/d may be required to control hypokalemia and hypertension. Once blood pressure has normalized and hypokalemia is corrected, the dose can be tapered and maintained at about 100–150 mg/d. Spironolactone may have antiandrogenic side effects, such as impotence, gynecomastia, menstrual irregularity, and gastrointestinal disturbances.

Amiloride, 20–40 ng/d, a potassium-sparing diuretic, may be used alternatively or as a supplement to spironolactone. Other medications such as calcium-channel blockers and diuretics may be required to control hypertension. These agents can be continued to the day of operation. Hypokalemia and hypertension should be controlled preoperatively, and most patients require a minimum of 1–2 weeks of treatment with spironolactone. Glucocorticoids are unnecessary for patients undergoing unilateral adrenalectomy for aldosteronoma. Unlike spironolactone, which also blocks androgen and progesterone receptors, eplerenone is a selective mineralocorticoid receptor antagonist and has fewer endocrine side effects. It has been approved for treatment of hypertension and for heart failure after myocardial infarction. Eplerenone may become the treatment of choice for primary hyperaldosteronism if it is proven as efficacious as spironolactone.

2. Surgery—Because aldosteronomas are almost always small and benign, laparoscopic adrenalectomy is the procedure of choice. It can be performed safely and with equally good results by several approaches. The lateral transabdominal approach uses gravity to help medially rotate the viscera (liver on the right and spleen and pancreas on the left) and exposes the adrenal gland. It is the most versatile approach and is preferred by most surgeons. The retroperitoneal approach, either laterally or posteriorly, is used occasionally. It may be best in patients with prior upper abdominal operations, but the working space is cramped. Although some surgeons perform a subtotal resection for aldosteronoma, most excise the adrenal gland with the tumor. The surrounding adrenal tissue frequently appears hyperplastic. A few small aldosteronomas may not be visible intraoperatively, so accurate preoperative localization is important. Bilateral adrenalectomy is not indicated, since patients with idiopathic hyperaldosteronism should be treated medically, and bilateral aldosteronomas are extremely rare.

3. Postoperative care—Occasional patients may develop transient aldosterone deficiency because of suppression of the contralateral adrenal gland by the hyperfunctioning adenoma. This is rare in patients treated with spironolactone preoperatively. Symptoms include postural hypotension and hyperkalemia. Adequate sodium intake is usually sufficient for treatment; rarely, short-term fludrocortisone replacement (0.1 mg/d orally) is required.

B. Medical Treatment

The goal is to control hypertension and hypokalemia. Spironolactone is the preferred agent, though amiloride may be better tolerated. Angiotensin-converting enzyme inhibitors and calcium-channel blockers have been used with some success. A combination of antihypertensive agents may be necessary.

Prognosis

Hyperaldosteronism usually follows a prolonged and subtly changing course. Untreated hypertension may cause stroke, myocardial infarction, or renal failure.

Removal of an aldosteronoma normalizes potassium levels, but the hypertension is not always cured. About one-third of patients have persistent mild hypertension that is usually easier to control than before the operation. Essential hypertension and atherosclerosis due to chronic hypertension are contributing factors. Although patients with idiopathic hyperaldosteronism should be treated medically, adrenalectomy is indicated for those with aldosteronoma because the tumor may grow and because side effects of the medications and compliance make long-term medical treatment undesirable. The low morbidity, short hospitalization, and high success rate of laparoscopic adrenalectomy have made surgery preferable to long-term medical therapy.

Al Fehaily M, Duh QY: Clinical manifestation of aldosteronoma. Surg Clin North Am 2004;84:887.

Ghose RP, Hall PM, Bravo EL: Medical management of aldosterone-producing adenomas. Ann Intern Med 1999;131:105.

Magill SB et al: Comparison of adrenal vein sampling and computed tomography in the differentiation of primary aldosteronism. J Clin Endocrinol Metab 2001;86;1066.

Mulatero P et al: Increased diagnosis of primary aldosteronism, including surgically correctable forms, in centers from five continents. J Clin Endocrin Metab 2004;89:1045.

Shen WT et al: Laparoscopic vs open adrenalectomy for the treatment of primary hyperaldosteronism. Arch Surg 1999;134:628.

Weinberger MH, Fineberg NS: The diagnosis of primary aldosteronism and separation of two major subtypes. Arch Intern Med 1993;153:2125.

Young WF: Minireview: primary aldosteronism-changing concepts in diagnosis and treatment. Endocrinology 2003;114:2208.

Young WF Jr et al: Role for adrenal venous sampling in primary aldosteronism. Surgery 2004;136:1227.

PHEOCHROMOCYTOMA

ESSENTIALS OF DIAGNOSIS

- *Episodic headache, excessive sweating, palpitation, and visual blurring.*
- *Hypertension, frequently sustained, with or without paroxysms.*

- *Postural tachycardia and hypotension.*
- *Elevated urinary catecholamines or their metabolites, hypermetabolism, hyperglycemia.*

General Considerations

Pheochromocytomas are tumors of the adrenal medulla and related chromaffin tissues elsewhere in the body that secrete epinephrine or norepinephrine, resulting in sustained or episodic hypertension and other symptoms of catecholamine excess.

Pheochromocytoma is found in less than 0.1% of patients with hypertension and accounts for about 5% of adrenal tumors incidentally discovered by CT scanning. Most pheochromocytomas occur sporadically without other diseases, but they may be associated with various familial syndromes such as MEN 2A (medullary thyroid carcinoma, pheochromocytoma, and hyperparathyroidism), MEN 2B (medullary thyroid carcinoma, pheochromocytoma, mucosal neuromas, marfanoid habitus, and ganglioneuromatosis), Von Recklinghausen's disease (café au lait spots, neurofibromatosis, pheochromocytoma), and von Hippel-Lindau disease (retinal hemangioma, hemangioblastoma of the central nervous system, renal cysts and carcinoma, pheochromocytoma, pancreatic cysts, and epididymal cystadenoma). These syndromes should be considered especially in young patients and in patients with multifocal tumors. Family members of patients who have been diagnosed with these syndromes also need screening to determine whether they are gene carriers and are at risk for developing the various tumors, including pheochromocytoma.

On pathologic examination, pheochromocytoma appears reddish-gray and frequently has areas of necrosis, hemorrhage, and sometimes cysts. The usual size is about 100 g or 5 cm in diameter, but they can be as small as 2–3 cm or as large as 12–16 cm. Cells are pleomorphic, showing prominent nucleoli and frequent mitoses. Cytologic findings cannot be used to determine whether a pheochromocytoma is malignant or benign. The veins and capsules may also be invaded even in clinically benign tumors. Malignancy can only be diagnosed in the presence of metastases or invasion into surrounding tissues.

Clinical Findings

A. Symptoms and Signs

The clinical findings of pheochromocytoma are variable, and mild cases may only come to attention because of an incidental finding of an adrenal tumor (incidentaloma) on CT or MR scans performed to evaluate other diseases. Classically, the patient has episodic hypertension associated with the triad of palpitation, headache, and sweating. The patient may also complain of anxiety, tremors, weight loss, dizziness, nausea and vomiting, abdominal discomfort, constipation, and visual blurring. Some patients have diarrhea, which may be secondary to secretion of vasoactive intestinal peptide. The physical examination may be unremarkable except during an attack, when pallor and excess sweating may be observed. Tachycardia, postural hypotension, and hypertensive retinopathy are other signs. Flushing can occur but is not typical.

Hypertension, the most common feature of pheochromocytoma, occurs in 90% of patients. More than half have sustained hypertension, which may be mild to moderate, with or without other signs and symptoms of catecholamine excess, and the diagnosis may be missed. In some cases, basal blood pressure may not be elevated, and severe hypertension occurs only while the patient is under stress, such as general anesthesia or trauma. Patients with diastolic hypertension and postural hypotension, who are not receiving antihypertensive medications, may have pheochromocytoma. Epinephrine raises blood glucose and norepinephrine decreases insulin secretion, and hyperglycemia may occur.

Traditionally, catecholamine-secreting tumors have been said to be 10% malignant, 10% familial, 10% bilateral, 10% multiple, and 10% extra-adrenal. In children, hypertension is less prominent, and about 50% have multiple or extra-adrenal tumors. Malignancy may be more common in extra-adrenal pheochromocytomas. Pheochromocytomas occur in 40–50% of patients with MEN 2; they tend to be bilateral and multiple but are rarely extra-adrenal or malignant. Screening of MEN 2 patients and family members who are *ret* proto-oncogene mutation carriers by measuring urinary catecholamines and metanephrines or plasma free metanephrines may diagnose pheochromocytomas before they produce clinical manifestations. Plasma free metanephrines (metanephrine and normetanephrine) is the most sensitive test for pheochromocytoma in familial syndromes.

B. Laboratory Findings

The diagnosis of pheochromocytoma is best confirmed either by fractionated 24-hour urinary catecholamines and metanephrines measured in the same collection or by fractionated plasma free metanephrines. Both tests have high diagnostic sensitivity and specificity. However, plasma free metanephrines are not widely available, and although the test is more sensitive than the urine test, it has a higher false-positive rate especially in elderly patients. Controversies exist as to which biochemical test is best (Figure 33–2). Urinary output of metanephrines or free catecholamines is elevated in 99% of patients with pheochromocytoma. In 80% of patients, the level exceeds twice normal. Measurement of urinary vanillylmandelic acid (VMA) is less sensitive. Assays using high-performance liquid chromatography (HPLC) reduce interference by drugs and diets, but not all HPLC

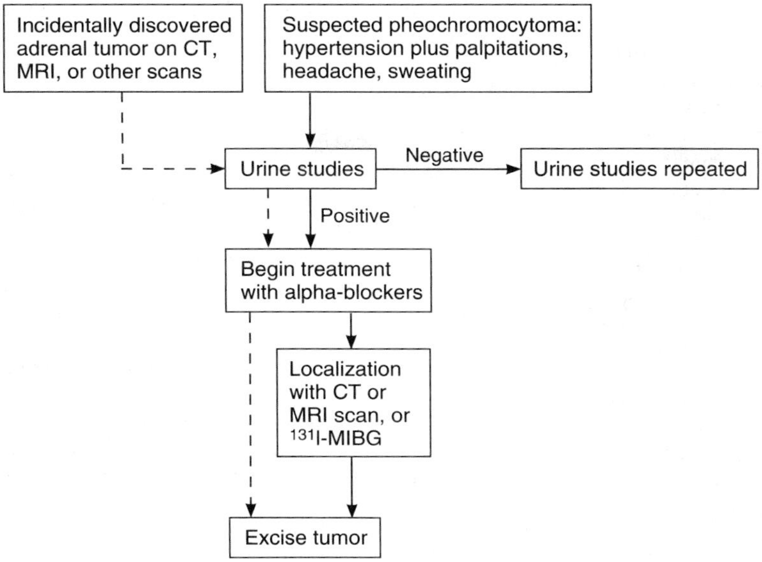

Figure 33–2. Scheme for evaluation of a patient with suspected pheochromocytoma.

assays are the same and many drugs and diets can potentially interfere with certain HPLC assays or affect the secretion and metabolism of catecholamines. Examples include acetaminophen, beta-blockers (especially labetalol), vasodilators (such as nitroglycerin), alpha-blockers, calcium-channel blockers (nifedipine, verapamil), theophylline, stimulants (amphetamine, caffeine, nicotine, methylphenidate), antipsychotics (clozapine, chlorpromazine), antidepressants (fluvoxamine, venlafaxine), prochlorperazine, and methyldopa. The assays may also be affected by ethanol, bananas, radiographic dyes, drugs that contain catecholamines, and withdrawal from clonidine. These agents should be discontinued for 2 weeks before measuring urinary catecholamines and metanephrines. The interfering substances vary depending on the specific assays used, so a list and protocol for preparing the patient should be obtained from the specific laboratory. Liquid chromatography-tandem mass spectrometry is a new assay that has been shown to minimize drug interferences in the measurement of urinary metanephrines and may prove to improve diagnostic accuracy of urinary metanephrines in the future.

Overnight urinary collection and short collection periods following a paroxysm, indexed to creatinine, have also been used. Measuring plasma free metanephrines is 97–100% sensitive and 85–95% specific. The assays are not yet widely available. Depending on the particular assay, acetaminophen and phenoxybenzamine may interfere with the assay. Plasma epinephrine and norepinephrine should only be measured under standard, controlled conditions, since their levels may be falsely elevated if the patient is under stress. The levels may be low if the tumor secretes episodically. Provocative tests—using glucagon, histamine, or tyramine—are not accurate, are potentially dangerous, and are no longer used. Clonidine suppression tests are rarely used. Clonidine does not decrease plasma catecholamine levels in patients with pheochromocytoma, as it may in normal anxious individuals or in patients with essential hypertension.

C. Tumor Localization

Localization studies should be performed only after biochemical studies have confirmed the diagnosis of a catecholamine-secreting tumor. Ninety percent of pheochromocytomas are found in the adrenal glands and most are > 3 cm in diameter. Of the extra-adrenal pheochromocytomas (also called paragangliomas), 75% are in the abdomen, 10% in the bladder, 10% in the chest, 2% in the pelvis, and 3% in the head and neck. Both CT and MRI can localize most pheochromocytomas. CT scan is less expensive and gives better anatomic details for the surgeons, but MRI avoids radiation exposure. Pheochromocytoma usually has a characteristic bright appearance on T2-weighted MRI. MIBG may be helpful for localizing extra-adrenal pheochromocytomas, and it should be considered when searching for extra-adrenal, multiple, malignant or metastatic pheochromocytomas. MIBG is more specific but less sensitive compared with CT or MRI for localization. Arteriography and fine-needle aspiration biopsy can precipitate a hypertensive crisis. They do not contribute to the diagnosis, and are not indicated. Venous sampling for catecholamines is no longer indicated.

Differential Diagnosis

The differential diagnosis includes all causes of hypertension. Hyperthyroidism and pheochromocytoma have many features in common (weight loss, tremor, and tachycardia). The diagnosis of pheochromocytoma is easier if episodic hypertension is present. Acute anxiety attacks mimic the symptoms and may precipitate hypertensive episodes, but anxiety alone rarely produces severe hypertension. Carcinoid syndrome causing episodes of flushing may also be mistaken for pheochromocytoma. Urinary 5-HIAA level is usually markedly elevated, and CT scan may show liver metastases in patients with carcinoid syndrome. Labile essential hypertension is not associated with elevated catecholamine levels.

Pheochromocytoma in pregnancy, if not recognized, will kill half of the fetuses and nearly half of the mothers. Hypertension in pregnancy is usually ascribed to preeclampsia-eclampsia. The diagnosis of pheochromocytoma requires the same biochemical studies; radiation (CT) and radioisotopes (MIBG) are usually not used; MRI is indicated to localize the tumor when a biochemical diagnosis has been established. Alpha- and beta-adrenergic blockers appear to be well tolerated. Timing of the operation is individualized. If recognized early, the tumor is best removed early in the second trimester. Otherwise, alpha-adrenergic blockade is continued and then followed by a planned cesarean section at term. The pheochromocytoma can be resected either at the time of cesarean section—if easily accessible through the same incision—or electively a few weeks postpartum laparoscopically.

Pheochromocytoma crisis may develop in patients with pheochromocytoma, usually precipitated by trauma, surgery, or other procedures. Crisis usually occurs when alpha-adrenergic blockade has not been instituted. These patients may develop multisystem failure, mimicking severe sepsis. If the disease is not recognized, death is the usual result. Once pheochromocytoma is diagnosed, the patient should be stabilized and alpha-adrenergic blockade started. Emergent operation may be necessary. Otherwise, resection during the same hospitalization after the patient is stabilized is preferred.

Complications

Pheochromocytoma causes complications because of hypertension, cardiac arrhythmia, and hypovolemia. The sequelae of hypertension are stroke, renal failure, myocardial infarction, and congestive heart failure. Sudden death can result from ventricular tachycardia or fibrillation. Alpha-adrenergic stimulation by the catecholamines causes vasoconstriction and a low total blood volume. The patient is therefore unable to compensate for a sudden loss of blood volume (bleeding) or catecholamines (tumor removal) and at risk of cardiovascular collapse. Preoperative alpha-adrenergic blockade and restoration of blood volume can prevent these complications.

Treatment

A. Medical Treatment

Treatment with alpha-adrenergic blocking agents should be started as soon as the biochemical diagnosis is established. The aims of preoperative therapy are (1) to restore the blood volume, which has been depleted by excessive catecholamines; (2) to prevent a severe crisis, with its potential complications; and (3) to allow the patient to recover from cardiomyopathy. Close control of hypertension is necessary in order to keep blood volume normal.

Phenoxybenzamine, a nonselective alpha-adrenergic antagonist, has a long duration of action and is the preferred drug. It should be started at a dosage of 10 mg per 12 hours, and the dose should be increased—as postural hypotension allows—until signs of excess catecholamine stimulation have disappeared and blood volume is clinically normal. Usual doses are 100–160 mg/d; however, dosages as high as 300 mg/d may be necessary. Most patients require 10–14 days of treatment, as judged by stabilization of blood pressure and reduction of symptoms. Nasal stuffiness is usually present when alpha blockade is well established.

Metyrosine inhibits tyrosine hydroxylase and reduces catecholamine synthesis and can be added to phenoxybenzamine as preoperative therapy. Calcium-channel blockers and competitive selective alpha-adrenergic blocking agents such as prazosin are effective.

Beta-adrenergic blocking agents are often useful to treat arrhythmias and tachycardia but should only be given after alpha blockade has been achieved. Otherwise, a hypertensive crisis may be precipitated because of the unopposed alpha-adrenergic effect of the catecholamines. Opioids should be avoided because they may stimulate histamine release and precipitate a crisis.

B. Surgical Treatment

The definitive treatment of pheochromocytoma is excision. It was once recommended that both adrenal glands and other areas likely to harbor extra-adrenal tumors should be examined at the time of surgery, but that practice is now outmoded even for patients clinically at risk for bilateral or multiple tumors, because CT, MRI, and MIBG scans are so sensitive in finding all lesions.

Smaller (< 5–6 cm) adrenal pheochromocytomas can be safely resected by laparoscopic adrenalectomy. Very large (> 8–10 cm) and extra-adrenal tumors are technically more difficult and may require laparotomy.

During surgery, an arterial line is necessary for continuous blood pressure monitoring. Monitoring of pulmonary artery pressure is rarely necessary in patients who are well blocked.

Nitroprusside should be immediately available to treat sudden hypertension and beta-blockers to treat the cardiac dysrhythmias that may occur when the tumor is manipulated. Manipulation of the gland is less with laparoscopic than with open adrenalectomy, which minimizes fluctuations in plasma catecholamine levels.

Very large malignant tumors may require a thoracoabdominal incision. Malignant pheochromocytomas may invade the adrenal vein or vena cava. Extra-adrenal pheochromocytomas are usually found along the abdominal aorta and in the organ of Zuckerkandl near the aortic bifurcation. However, tumors have been found in widely scattered sites such as the bladder, the vagina, the mediastinum, the neck, and even the skull and pericardium. In general, extra-adrenal tumors should be localized with MIBG, CT, or MRI preoperatively to avoid a blind exploration.

In patients with MEN 2 and bilateral pheochromocytomas, cortical-sparing subtotal adrenalectomy on the side of the smaller tumor may avoid postoperative adrenal insufficiency, though it increases the risk for recurrence. In patients with MEN 2 and a unilateral pheochromocytoma, prophylactic resection of the contralateral normal-appearing adrenal gland is contraindicated, since bilateral adrenalectomy leads to lifelong hypoadrenalism requiring cortisol replacement. These patients should be followed with biochemical evaluations, and the contralateral adrenal gland should be resected only if pheochromocytoma develops.

Many patients undergoing resection of pheochromocytoma who are not adequately prepared preoperatively will have hypertensive crises, cardiac arrhythmia, myocardial infarction, or acute pulmonary edema. In addition, these patients may experience intractable hypotension and die in shock after tumor removal. If the patient has been properly prepared with alpha-blockers, the changes in blood pressure will not be severe. Otherwise, intravenous infusion of large amounts of saline and vasopressors may be necessary to maintain blood pressure after the tumor is removed. Although not common, hypoglycemia may develop after tumor removal.

Prognosis

The outlook for patients with untreated pheochromocytoma is grim, whereas the operative mortality rate was decreased to 0–3% from 30% following the introduction of alpha-adrenergic blockade. Mild to moderate essential hypertension may persist after surgery. Second tumors in the remaining adrenal or metastatic tumors can occur years after excision of the primary pheochromocytoma; long-term follow-up is mandatory. Metastatic or recurrent malignant pheochromocytoma should be resected if possible to reduce the catecholamine load. Treatment with high-dose ^{131}I-MIBG may be helpful in these patients.

Bravo EL, Tagle R: Pheochromocytoma: state-of-the-art and future prospects. Endocr Rev 2003;24:539.

Duh Q-Y: Editorial: Evolving surgical management for patients with pheochromocytoma. J Clin Endocrinol Metab 2001;86:1477.

Eisenhofer G et al: Plasma normetanephrine and metanephrine for detecting pheochromocytoma in von Hippel-Lindau disease and multiple endocrine neoplasia type 2. N Engl J Med 1999; 340:1872.

Kebebew E et al: Benign and malignant pheochromocytoma: diagnosis, treatment, and follow up. Surg Oncol Clin N Am 1998;7:765.

Kudva et al: The laboratory diagnosis of adrenal pheochromocytoma: the Mayo clinic experience. J Clin Endocrinol Metab 2003;88:4533.

Lenders JW et al: Biochemical diagnosis of pheochromocytoma. Which test is best? JAMA 2002;287:1427.

Mannelli M, Bemporad D: Diagnosis and management of pheochromocytoma during pregnancy. J Endocrinol Invest 2002; 25:567.

Peaston RT et al: Overnight excretion of urinary catecholamines and metabolites in the detection of pheochromocytoma. J Clin Endocrinol Metab 1996;81:1378.

Prys-Roberts C: Phaeochromocytoma—recent progress in its management. Br J Anaesth 2000;85:44.

Rose B et al: High dose ^{131}I-metaiodobenzylguanidine therapy for 12 patients with malignant pheochromocytoma. Cancer 2003;98:239.

Young WF: Pheochromocytoma and primary aldosteronism: diagnostic approaches. Endocrinol Metab Clin North Am 1997;26:801.

HYPERADRENOCORTICISM

(Cushing's Disease & Cushing's Syndrome)

ESSENTIALS OF DIAGNOSIS

- *Facial plethora, dorsocervical fat pad, supraclavicular fat pad, truncal obesity, easy bruisability, purple striae, acne, hirsutism, impotence or amenorrhea, muscle weakness, and psychosis.*
- *Hypertension and hyperglycemia.*

General Considerations

Cushing's syndrome is due to chronic glucocorticoid excess. It may be caused by excess ACTH stimulation or by adrenocortical tumors that secrete glucocorticoids independently of ACTH stimulation. Excess ACTH may be produced by pituitary adenomas (Cushing's disease), or extrapituitary ACTH-producing tumors (ectopic ACTH syndrome). Cushing's syndrome not dependent on ACTH is usually caused by primary adrenal diseases such as adrenocortical adenoma and micro- or macronodular hyperplasia or carcinoma.

The natural history of Cushing's syndrome depends on the underlying disease and varies from a mild, indolent disease to rapid progression and death.

Clinical Findings

A. Symptoms and Signs

(See Table 33–1.) The classic description of Cushing's syndrome includes truncal obesity, hirsutism, moon facies, acne, buffalo hump, purple striae, hypertension, and diabetes, but other signs and symptoms are common. Weakness and depression are striking features. Weakness and other features are also seen after prolonged and excessive administration of adrenocortical steroids.

In children, Cushing's syndrome is most commonly caused by adrenal cancers, but adenomas and nodular hyperplasia have been described. Cushing's syndrome in children also causes growth retardation or arrest.

B. Pathologic Examination

The pathologic features of the adrenal gland depend on the underlying disease. Normal adrenal glands weigh 7–12 g combined. The hyperplastic adrenal glands in patients with Cushing's disease weigh below 25 g combined. In ectopic ACTH syndrome, the combined adrenal weight is greater—from 25 g to 100 g.

Adrenal adenomas in Cushing's syndrome range in weight from a few grams to over 100 g, usually over 3 cm in diameter, and are larger than aldosterone-producing adenomas. The typical cells usually resemble those of the zona fasciculata. Variable degrees of anaplasia are seen, and differentiation of benign from malignant tumors is often difficult on the basis of cytology alone. These adrenal adenomas occur in women and are very rare in men. Adrenal cancers are frequently very large—almost always over 5 cm in diameter. They are undifferentiated, invade the surrounding tissues, and metastasize via the blood stream.

Rare forms of ACTH-independent Cushing's syndrome include macronodular hyperplasia, which in some cases is due to aberrant expression of receptors in the adrenals that respond to stimuli other than ACTH. In these cases, the adrenal glands can be massively enlarged. Pigmented micronodular hyperplasia is associated with the syndrome of Carney's complex that also includes cardiac myxoma and lentigines.

Rarely, ectopic adrenal tissue can be the source of excessive cortisol secretion. It has been found in various locations, most commonly near the abdominal aorta.

Cushing's disease is most commonly caused by pituitary adenomas.

Ectopic ACTH syndrome is usually caused by small-cell lung cancers and carcinoid tumors, but tumors of the pancreas, thymus, thyroid, prostate, esophagus, colon, and ovaries—as well as pheochromocytoma and malignant melanoma—may also secrete ACTH.

C. Laboratory Findings

Since no one test is specific, a combination of tests must be used.

Normal subjects have a circadian rhythm of ACTH secretion that is paralleled by cortisol secretion. Levels are highest in the early morning and decline during the day to their lowest levels in the late evening. In Cushing's disease, the circadian rhythm is abolished, and total secretion of cortisol is increased. In mild cases, the plasma cortisol and ACTH levels may be within the normal range during much of the day but abnormally high in the evening.

When Cushing's syndrome is suspected, the first objective is to establish the diagnosis; the second is to establish the cause. An algorithm for the diagnosis is presented in Figure 33–3. When hyperadrenocorticism is suspected, an **overnight dexamethasone suppression test**—or measurement of 24-hour urinary free cortisol—is the first diagnostic step. Dexamethasone, 1 mg orally (equivalent to about 30 mg of cortisol), will suppress ACTH secretion and stop cortisol production. This low-dose dexamethasone, however, will not suppress excessive cortisol production from autonomous adrenocortical tumors or adrenals that are being stimulated by excess ACTH. Since dexamethasone does not cross-react in the assay for plasma cortisol, suppression of endogenous circulating cortisol is easily demonstrated. The test is done as follows: At 11 PM, the patient is given 1 mg of dexamethasone by mouth. A fasting plasma cortisol is measured the following morning between 8 and 9 AM. Suppression of plasma cortisol to 1.8 μg/dL (50 nmol/L) or less excludes Cushing's syndrome. Higher cutoff levels have been recommended, but some patients with mild ACTH-dependent Cushing's syndrome may be suppressed easily; thus, the response is falsely negative and the diagnosis of Cushing's syndrome is missed. On the other hand, this low cutoff level increases the likelihood of a false-positive result. False-positive results are more common in patients with depression, alcoholism, physiologic stress, marked obesity, or renal failure and in those taking estrogens or drugs that accelerate dexamethasone metabolism, such as phenytoin, rifampin, and phenobarbital. Estrogens increase cortisol-binding globulin and elevate total plasma cortisol concentrations. In these situations, measurement of 24-hour urinary free cortisol is preferred.

The results of the dexamethasone test should be confirmed with a measurement of 24-hour urinary excretion of free cortisol. It directly measures the physiologically active form of circulating cortisol, integrates the daily variations of cortisol production, and is very

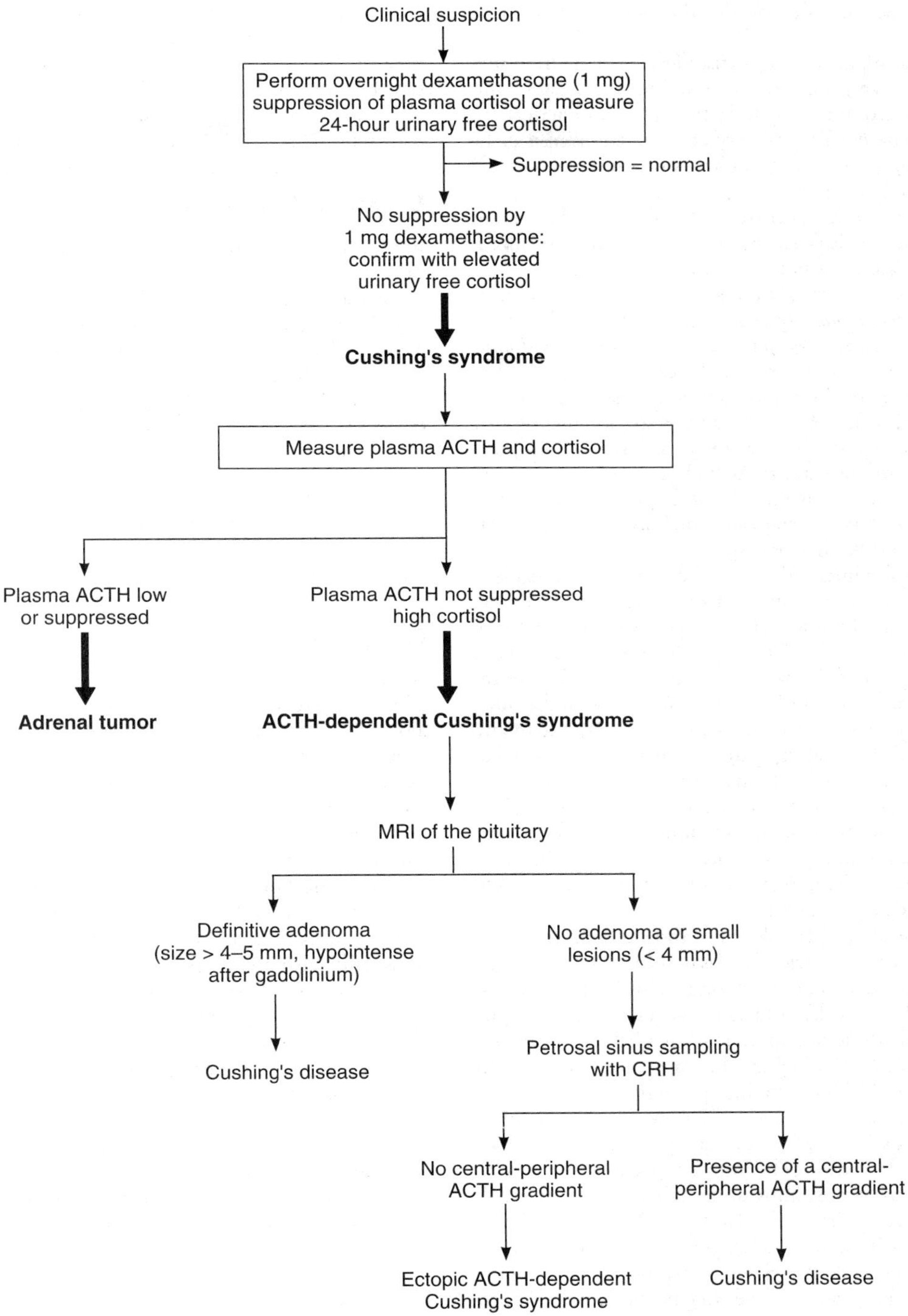

Figure 33–3. Cushing's syndrome: diagnosis and differential diagnosis.

sensitive and specific for the diagnosis of Cushing's syndrome.

The midnight plasma cortisol level also distinguishes Cushing's syndrome from non-Cushing states, but because it requires hospitalization it is impractical. In contrast, late-evening salivary cortisol sampling can be easily accomplished at home without stress. The procedure involves chewing a cotton tube for 2–3 minutes. Salivary cortisol levels correlate highly with plasma and serum free cortisol levels. The test is underutilized, mainly because it is not generally available.

If the plasma cortisol level is not suppressed by the overnight dexamethasone suppression test and the urinary free cortisol is elevated, the patient has Cushing's syndrome. The next step is to determine the cause. Plasma ACTH measurement by immunoradiometric assay (IRMA) is the most direct method. A normal to elevated ACTH level is diagnostic of hyperadrenocorticism due to pituitary adenoma or ectopic ACTH secretion. Suppressed ACTH levels are diagnostic of hyperadrenocorticism due to a primary adrenal cause such as adenoma, carcinoma, or nodular hyperplasia.

The differential diagnosis of ACTH-dependent Cushing's syndrome can be challenging. No test is perfect, and a combination of tests may be necessary. Since 90% of patients have Cushing's disease, pituitary MRI is the first test to identify the source of ACTH secretion. However, 10% of normal adults have focal pituitary lesions 3–6 mm in diameter on MRI, and many patients with Cushing's disease have no detectable lesions. Lesions smaller than 3–4 mm are more likely to represent normal variation, artifacts, volume averaging, incidental nonfunctional adenomas, or cysts. An unequivocal pituitary lesion (ie, > 4–5 mm in diameter with decreased signal intensity on gadolinium) strongly suggests Cushing's disease.

If the pituitary MRI does not show a definite lesion, the next step is inferior petrosal sinus sampling with corticotropin-releasing hormone (CRH) stimulation. Compared with other biochemical tests, such as high-dose dexamethasone suppression or CRH stimulation, petrosal sinus sampling is the most accurate way to identify an ACTH-secreting pituitary adenoma; the diagnostic accuracy is close to 100%. The test requires simultaneous bilateral venous sampling from the inferior petrosal sinuses. The inferior petrosal sinus connects the cavernous sinus and drains the pituitary. A central to peripheral ACTH ratio of 2 or greater without CRH stimulation is diagnostic of pituitary adenoma. CRH, 100 μg given intravenously as a bolus injection, can increase the diagnostic sensitivity to 100%; a peak central to peripheral ACTH ratio of 3 or greater is diagnostic of pituitary adenoma. The lack of a central to peripheral ACTH gradient is diagnostic of an ectopic ACTH-secreting tumor.

In Cushing's syndrome caused by primary adrenal diseases, the plasma ACTH level is completely suppressed. Adenomas are usually 3–5 cm in diameter and secrete only cortisol. Adrenal carcinomas are typically > 5 cm in diameter, are usually rapidly progressive, and cosecrete other hormones, such as adrenal androgens, deoxycorticosterone, aldosterone, and estrogens.

D. Imaging Studies

For Cushing's syndrome caused by primary adrenal diseases, thin-section CT or MRI is able to detect virtually all of the adrenal tumors and hyperplasia. MRI of the sella is the imaging study of choice for pituitary adenomas. If a definitive adenoma is not seen, inferior petrosal sinus sampling with CRH stimulation can differentiate Cushing's disease from ectopic Cushing's syndrome. For ectopic Cushing's syndrome, CT or MRI of the chest and abdomen may detect ACTH-secreting tumors. Bronchial carcinoids may be very small and difficult to find; high-resolution, thin-cut CT of the chest is indicated. Occasionally, the source of an ectopic ACTH-secreting tumor cannot be determined (occult ectopic ACTH syndrome).

Complications

Severe or lethal complications may result from sustained hypercortisolism, including hypertension, cardiovascular disease, stroke, thromboembolism, infection, severe debilitating muscle wasting, and weakness. Psychosis is common. Death may also be caused by the underlying tumors, such as adrenal carcinoma, small cell lung cancer, and others causing ectopic ACTH Cushing's syndrome.

The truncal obesity and muscle weakness in patients with Cushing's syndrome predispose them to postoperative pulmonary complications. Atrophic skin and easy bruisability also predict poor wound healing.

Nelson's syndrome, the progression of an ACTH-secreting pituitary adenoma following bilateral adrenalectomy for Cushing's disease, occurred in as many as 30% of patients in the era when bilateral adrenalectomy was used as primary therapy. However, since transsphenoidal resection has become the initial procedure of choice for Cushing's disease and since MRI now allows accurate diagnosis of pituitary adenomas larger than 5 mm, Nelson's syndrome occurs in < 5% of patients.

These tumors in patients with Nelson's syndrome are among the most aggressive of pituitary tumors, causing sellar enlargement and extrasellar extension. Plasma ACTH levels are markedly elevated. Patients are frequently hyperpigmented and hypopituitary and have symptoms of mass effects including headaches, visual field deficits, and even blindness from optic nerve compression. Removal of feedback control from hypercortisolism at the pituitary level probably explains the aggressiveness of these tumors.

Treatment

Resection is the best treatment for cortisol-producing adrenal tumors or ACTH-producing tumors. Medical treatment may be necessary to temporarily control hypercortisolism—or for patients not cured by resection or when complete resection is impossible.

A. Medical Treatment

Drugs are mainly used as adjuvant therapy. Hypercortisolism may be controlled with ketoconazole, metyrapone, or aminoglutethimide, all of which inhibit steroid biosynthesis. Ketoconazole is usually the first choice. A combination of drugs may be necessary to control hypercortisolism and to decrease dose-related side effects. Mifepristone (RU 486), a progesterone and glucocorticoid receptor antagonist, is also effective, but it raises cortisol and ACTH levels, making it difficult to monitor the patient.

Mitotane is a DDT derivative that is toxic to the adrenal cortex. It has been used with modest success in the treatment of adrenal hypersecretory states, especially adrenocortical carcinoma. Unfortunately, serious side effects are common at effective doses.

B. Excision of Pituitary Adenoma

Patients with Cushing's disease are usually treated by transsphenoidal microsurgical excision of the pituitary adenomas. Relief of symptoms is rapid, and the prognosis for adequate residual pituitary-adrenal function is good. Total or subtotal hypophysectomy may be performed in older patients if a discrete tumor is not found. Pituitary procedures fail in about 15–25% of patients because of failure to find the adenoma, pituitary hyperplasia, or recurrence of adenoma. When pituitary surgery fails, the disease may respond to pituitary irradiation. In some patients, medical therapy or total adrenalectomy will be necessary. Because of the effectiveness of pituitary microsurgery, radiotherapy is usually not recommended as primary treatment for Cushing's disease.

C. Adrenalectomy

Compared with patients with other adrenal tumors, those with severe Cushing's syndrome are at higher risk for postoperative complications such as wound infection, hemorrhage, peptic ulceration, and pulmonary embolism. Adrenalectomy, however, is usually successful in reversing the devastating effects of hypercortisolism.

Laparoscopic adrenalectomy causes less morbidity than open adrenalectomy and is preferred for benign hyperplasia or adenomas. Laparoscopic adrenalectomy for adrenocortical carcinoma is technically challenging. Local recurrence may be more common after laparoscopic resection for large and invasive cancer, especially if the capsule is breached during dissection.

Unilateral adrenalectomy is indicated for adrenal adenomas or carcinomas that secrete cortisol. The contralateral adrenal gland and the hypothalamic-pituitary-adrenal axis will usually recover from the suppression 1–2 years after the operation.

Total bilateral adrenalectomy is indicated for selected patients with Cushing's disease or ectopic ACTH syndrome in whom the ACTH-secreting tumor cannot be found or resected. It is also indicated for patients with bilateral primary adrenal disease, such as pigmented micronodular hyperplasia or massive macronodular hyperplasia.

Bilateral adrenalectomy can almost always be accomplished by the laparoscopic approach.

Subtotal resection is not recommended in patients with Cushing's syndrome, because it usually leaves inadequate adrenocortical reserve initially, and the disease frequently recurs with continuing ACTH stimulation. Total bilateral adrenalectomy with adrenal gland autotransplantation is rarely successful and offers little advantage over pharmacologic replacement.

D. Postoperative Maintenance Therapy

After total adrenalectomy, lifelong corticosteroid maintenance therapy becomes necessary. The following schedule is commonly used: No cortisol is given until the adrenals are removed during surgery. On the first day, give 100 mg of hydrocortisone intravenously every 8 hours. On the second day, give 50 mg every 8 hours. Thereafter, the dose should be tapered as tolerated. The same tapering process is used after excision of a unilateral cortisol-secreting adenoma, because the remaining adrenal may not function normally for months.

As the hydrocortisone dose is reduced below 50 mg/d, it is often necessary to add fludrocortisone (a mineralocorticoid), 0.1 mg daily orally. The usual maintenance doses are about 20–30 mg of hydrocortisone and 0.1 mg of fludrocortisone daily. More than half the hydrocortisone dose is given in the morning.

Patients who have had a total bilateral adrenalectomy and are on maintenance therapy can develop addisonian crisis when under stress, such as general anesthesia or infection. Adrenal insufficiency causes fever, hyperkalemia, abdominal pain, and hypotension and should be promptly recognized and treated with saline infusion and cortisol.

Prognosis

The prognosis is good after resection of benign adrenal adenomas, pituitary adenomas, or benign ACTH-secreting tumors. Symptoms and signs of hypercortisolism resolve, usually over months. Short-term adrenal insufficiency after surgery requires cortisol replacement. Cushing's disease can recur after excision of a pituitary adenoma. An occult ACTH-secreting tumor may become apparent later and require removal.

Residual adrenal tissue or embryonic rests are present in up to 10% of patients after total adrenalectomy. Cushing's syndrome can then recur if stimulation with ACTH continues.

The prognosis is extremely poor in patients with adrenocortical carcinoma and in those with malignant tumors causing ectopic ACTH syndrome.

Doherty GM et al: Time to recovery of the hypothalamic-pituitary-adrenal axis after curative resection of adrenal tumors in patients with Cushing's syndrome. Surgery 1990;108:1085.

Findling JW, Raff H: Newer diagnostic techniques and problems in Cushing's disease. Endocrinol Metab Clin North Am 1999;28:191.

Hall WA et al: Pituitary magnetic resonance imaging in normal human volunteers: occult adenomas in the general population. Ann Intern Med 1994;120:817.

Hawn MT et al: Quality of life after bilateral adrenalectomy for Cushing's disease. Surgery 2002;132:1064.

Kemink L et al: Residual adrenocortical function after bilateral adrenalectomy for pituitary-dependent Cushing's syndrome. J Clin Endocrinol Metab 1992;75:1211.

Liu C et al: Cavernous and inferior petrosal sinus sampling in the evaluation of ACTH-dependent Cushing's syndrome. Clin Endocrinol (Oxf) 2004;61:478.

Papanicolaou DA et al: A single midnight serum cortisol measurement distinguishes Cushing's syndrome from pseudo-Cushing's states. J Clin Endocrinol Metab 1998;83:1163.

Raff H et al: Late-night salivary cortisol as a screening test for Cushing's syndrome. J Clin Endocrinol Metab 1998;83:2681.

Tyrrell JB et al: Cushing's disease. Therapy of pituitary adenomas. Endocrinol Metab Clin North Am 1994;23:925.

Walz MK: Extent of adrenalectomy for adrenal neoplasm: cortical sparing (subtotal) versus total adrenalectomy. Surg Clin North Am 2004;84:743.

VIRILIZING ADRENAL TUMORS

In adults, hormonally active benign adrenal adenomas usually secrete aldosterone or cortisol. Virilizing tumors in women are more likely to be caused by ovarian tumors. Virilizing adrenal tumors are rare, and virilization is usually due to hypersecretion of adrenal androgens, mainly dehydroepiandrosterone (DHEA), its sulfate derivative (DHEAS), and androstenedione, all of which are converted peripherally to testosterone and 5α-dihydrotestosterone. Very rarely, virilizing adrenal tumors secrete only testosterone.

The differentiation of benign from malignant adrenocortical tumors may be difficult when based on histologic features; some patients with histologically benign tumors may develop metastases, and others with histologically malignant tumors may never have recurrent disease. Malignancy is only definitely diagnosed from local or distant spread. Seventy percent of virilizing adrenal tumors exhibit malignant behavior. Adrenocortical carcinomas are usually large tumors with local spread or distant metastases. They often secrete multiple steroids, most commonly cortisol and androgens, leading to Cushing's syndrome and virilization.

In children, adrenocortical tumors are rare, but virilization with or without hypercortisolism is the most frequent feature. Virilizing adrenal tumors are less likely to be malignant in children than in adults. Histologic features of malignancy do not always predict malignant behavior. Large tumors (> 100 g) have a worse prognosis.

Signs and symptoms of virilization include hirsutism, male-pattern baldness, acne, deep voice, male musculature, irregular menses or amenorrhea, clitoromegaly, and increased libido. Rapid linear growth with advanced bone age is common in children.

CT and MRI are used to image virilizing adrenal tumors. Resection is the only successful treatment.

Virilization can also be caused by congenital adrenal hyperplasia, an autosomal recessive disorder. The mutated genes encode enzymes essential for cortisol and mineralocorticoid synthesis. 21-Hydroxylase deficiency accounts for 90% of cases. The inhibition of cortisol synthesis leads to stimulated ACTH secretion, accumulation of precursors, and overproduction of androgens. Administration of glucocorticoids is the mainstay of treatment in patients with classic congenital adrenal hyperplasia. Mineralocorticoid replacement is required in the salt-wasting forms of congenital adrenal hyperplasia. Antiandrogens, aromatase inhibitors, and lower-dose glucocorticoid replacement may be useful. Adrenalectomy with lifelong steroid replacement is another approach.

Cordera F et al: Androgen-secreting adrenal tumors. Surgery 2003;134:874.

Latronico AC et al: Extensive personal experience—adrenocortical tumors. J Clin Endocrinol Metab 1997;82:1317.

Liou LS et al: Adrenocortical carcinoma in children. Review and recent innovations. Urol Clin North Am 2000;27:403.

Merke DP et al: New approaches to the treatment of congenital adrenal hyperplasia. JAMA 1997;277:1073.

Michalkiewicz EL et al: Clinical characteristics of small functioning adrenocortical tumors in children. Med Pediatr Oncol 1997;28:175.

Moreno S et al: Profile and outcome of pure androgen-secreting adrenal tumors in women: experience of 21 cases. Surgery 2004;136:1192.

Pang S: Congenital adrenal hyperplasia. Endocrinol Metab Clin North Am 1997;26:853.

FEMINIZING ADRENAL TUMORS

Estrogens are not normally synthesized by the adrenal cortex. Feminizing adrenal tumors are extremely rare and are almost always carcinomas. They are usually seen in men with feminization or in girls with precocious puberty. Vaginal bleeding may be the presenting symptom in adult women. Feminizing adrenal carcinomas frequently hypersecrete other hormones. The diagnosis is based on a finding of increased plasma estrogens. Ovarian tumors and administration of exogenous estrogen should be ruled out.

Definitive treatment is by excision of the tumor. The prognosis is guarded.

Goto T et al: Oestrogen producing adrenocortical adenoma: clinical, biochemical and immunohistochemical studies. Clin Endocrinol 1996;45:643.

ADRENOCORTICAL CARCINOMA

Adrenal cortical carcinomas are rare. Fifty percent of patients have symptoms related to hypersecretion of hormones, most commonly Cushing's syndrome and virilization. Feminizing and purely aldosterone-secreting carcinomas are rare. In some cases, hormone hypersecretion is subclinical and only found by biochemical studies. A palpable abdominal mass is common. The mean diameter of adrenal carcinoma is 12 cm (range, 3–30 cm). Adrenocortical carcinoma invades the surrounding tissues, and about half of the patients have metastases (lung, liver, and elsewhere) at the time of diagnosis. In those without local spread or distant metastases, a diagnosis of carcinoma based on cytologic features may be wrong.

The median survival is 25 months, and 5-year actuarial survival is 25%. Tumor stage at the initial operation predicts the prognosis. Surgery is the only treatment that can cure or prolong survival; however, beneficial outcomes are confined to patients with localized disease. When grossly complete resection is possible, the 5-year survival is 50%. Thus, recurrence is common despite apparent complete resection. Laparoscopic adrenalectomy is technically more difficult for adrenocortical carcinomas than for other adrenal tumors because the tumor is fragile and adjacent organs may have to be removed. Where the adrenal tumor is small, malignancy is uncertain, and the surgeon is technically capable, starting the operation laparoscopically is acceptable, but the abdomen should be opened if there is any question about whether a better operation could be accomplished that way. For local recurrent disease, reoperation is the only effective therapy and may prolong life. Patients with distant metastases at initial presentation usually die within 1 year. Resecting the adrenal tumor in these patients may decrease survival.

Mitotane, an adrenolytic agent, has been used as an adjuvant to surgery in patients with adrenocortical carcinoma. It controls endocrine symptoms in 50% of patients, and the tumor regresses in some. Nevertheless, survival is not generally affected, though a few cases of prolonged remission have been reported. Dose-related side effects (eg, gastrointestinal symptoms, weakness, dizziness, and somnolence) limit its use. A variety of other chemotherapeutic agents have been tried with limited success. The role of radiation is limited and usually is for palliation, especially for bony metastases.

Ahlman H et al: Cytotoxic treatment of adrenocortical carcinoma. World J Surg 2001;25:927.

Allolio B et al: Management of adrenocortical carcinoma. Clin Endocrinol (Oxf) 2004;60:273.

Barnett CC et al: Limitations of size as a criterion in the evaluation of adrenal tumors. Surgery 2000;128:973.

Bellantone R et al: Role of reoperation in recurrence of adrenal cortical carcinoma: results from 188 cases collected in the Italian National Registry for Adrenal Cortical Carcinoma. Surgery 1997;122:1212.

Dackiw AP et al: Adrenal cortical carcinoma. World J Surg 2001;25:914.

Icard P et al: Adrenocortical carcinomas: surgical trends and results of a 253-patient series from the French Association of Endocrine Surgeons study group. World J Surg 2001;25:891.

Stratakis CA et al: Adrenal cancer. Endocrinol Metab Clin North Am 2000;29:15.

Vassilopoulou-Sellin R, Schultz PN: Adrenocortical carcinoma. Clinical outcome at the end of the 20th century. Cancer 2001;92:1113.

Wajchenberg BL et al: Adrenocortical carcinoma—clinical and laboratory observations. Cancer 2000;88:711.

INCIDENTALOMAS

Adrenal tumors have traditionally been diagnosed after presentation with clinical symptoms of excess hormone secretion. However, the increased use of ultrasonography, CT, and MRI for various diseases in the abdomen has led to the discovery of what are referred to as adrenal incidentalomas. Most are small nonfunctioning adrenal cortical adenomas; some are functioning adenomas or pheochromocytomas with subclinical secretion of hormones; and some are adrenocortical carcinomas or metastases.

Incidentalomas are found in 1–4% of CT scans and 6% of random autopsies. The incidence increases with age. Preclinical Cushing's syndrome, pheochromocytoma, and adrenocortical carcinoma each account for about 5% of cases, metastatic carcinoma for 2%, and aldosteronoma for 1% (Table 33–2). Thus, over 80% of patients have presumed nonfunctioning cortical adenomas. Simple adrenal cysts, myelolipomas, and adrenal hemorrhages can be identified by the CT characteristics alone. Adrenal cysts can be large but are rarely malignant. Adrenal hemorrhage may occur in preexisting adrenal tumors.

The major issues in managing a patient with an incidentaloma is to determine whether the tumor is hormonally active and whether it is a cancer; either would be an indication for resection. Since most incidentalomas are

Table 33–2. Adrenal incidentalomas.

Tumor Types	Percentage
Preclinical Cushing's	5%
Pheochromocytoma	5%
Adrenocortical carcinoma	5%
Metastatic carcinoma	2%
Aldosterone-producing adenoma	1%
Presumed nonfunctional adenoma	82%
Total	100%

[1]Based on data reported in Endocrinol Metab Clin North Am 2000; 29:159.

nonfunctioning adenomas, the workup should be selective to avoid unnecessary expense and procedures.

The workup should include a complete history and physical examination with specific reference to a history of previous malignancy and signs and symptoms of Cushing's syndrome or pheochromocytoma. Hyperaldosteronism, pheochromocytoma, and virilizing or feminizing adrenocortical carcinoma should be investigated. Further laboratory studies may be indicated depending on the clinical presentation.

The management of an incidentaloma depends on its functional status and the size and imaging characteristics of the tumor. All functioning tumors should be excised. Large nonfunctioning tumors also should be excised because of the increased risk of cancer. Small nonfunctioning tumors are almost always benign adenomas; they can be followed with serial CT scans checking for changes in size.

All patients—even those who do not have hypertension—should have a 24-hour urine collection for fractionated catecholamines and metanephrines or fractionated plasma metanephrines to search for pheochromocytoma; the risk of unrecognized pheochromocytoma is high, and the hypertension may be absent or episodic. Most pheochromocytomas are over 2 cm in diameter and characteristically bright on T2-weighted MRI. *Thirty percent of pheochromocytomas are found incidentally because of CT or MRI scans obtained for other indications.*

All patients should also have a 24-hour urine collection for cortisol and an overnight dexamethasone suppression test. Patients with subclinical Cushing's syndrome may subsequently become cushingoid and may experience an addisonian crisis if the tumor is resected and glucocorticoid replacement is not adequate.

Patients who are hypertensive should also have plasma aldosterone and plasma renin activity measured to screen for primary hyperaldosteronism.

If the above studies show that the tumor is nonfunctional, the size and imaging characteristics of the tumor and the patient's overall medical condition should determine the appropriate treatment. Nonfunctioning adrenal tumors larger than 5 cm in diameter should usually be removed because of higher risk of cancer. Nonfunctioning adrenal tumors smaller than 3 cm that are homogeneous and have low density on CT or MRI are unlikely to be cancers and can be safely followed. The patient's age and overall medical condition and the CT scan findings (will usually determine whether a tumor 3–5 cm in size should be resected. (High density, irregular borders, and heterogeneity make pheochromocytoma, adrenocortical carcinoma, and metastases more likely.)

In patients with a previously treated malignancy such as lung or breast cancer, an adrenal mass larger than 3 cm is very likely a metastasis. Once the possibility of pheochromocytoma is excluded, a CT-guided fine-needle aspiration biopsy can be used to distinguish an adrenocortical tumor from metastatic cancer. This is the only situation when the result of fine-needle aspiration biopsy influences management of an adrenal tumor. Resection of a solitary adrenal metastasis from a primary lung cancer may improve long-term survival if there are no other clinically obvious metastases. Patients with a metachronous solitary adrenal metastasis are more likely to benefit from adrenalectomy than are those with a synchronous metastasis. Patients with adrenal metastases from melanoma or renal cell carcinoma also benefit from resection. Adrenal metastasis can be resected laparoscopically with minimal risk of local recurrence.

REFERENCES

Bailey RH et al: The diagnostic dilemma of incidentalomas. Working through uncertainty. Emerg Med Clin North Am 2000;29:91.

Barzon L et al: Risk factors and long-term follow-up of adrenal incidentalomas. J Clin Endocrinol Metab 1999;84:520.

Emral R et al: Prevalence of subclinical Cushing's syndrome in 70 patients with adrenal incidentaloma: clinical, biochemical and surgical outcomes. Endocr J 2003;50:399.

Sippel RS, Chen H: Subclinical Cushing's syndrome in adrenal incidentalomas. Surg Clin North Am 2004;84:875.

Young WF: Management approaches to adrenal incidentalomas: a review from Rochester, Minnesota. Endocrinol Metab Clin North Am 2000;29:159.

RELEVANT WEB SITES

[National Institutes of Health State-of-the-Science Conference Statement: Management of the clinically inapparent adrenal mass (incidentaloma), Final Statement July 16, 2002] http://consensus.nih.gov/ta/021/021_statement.htm

Arteries

34

*Joseph H. Rapp, MD, Charles M. Eichler, MD, William C. Krupski, MD,**
& Louis M. Messina, MD

ATHEROSCLEROSIS

Atherosclerosis is the major disease of human arteries. Early lesions are confined to the intima. In advanced lesions both intima and media are involved but the adventitia is spared. Preservation of the adventitia is essential for the vessel's structural integrity and is the basis for all cardiovascular interventions. Significant luminal narrowing with reduced flow occurs late in the disease process and may lead to thrombotic occlusion or distal embolization. Depending upon the vascular bed involved, symptoms include stroke, myocardial infarction, and ischemic gangrene with limb loss.

Atherosclerotic plaques most commonly develop in areas of low shear stress such as arterial bifurcations and the posterior wall of the aortoiliac arterial segment. The common exception is the superficial femoral artery, which is often affected where the vessel passes through the adductor hiatus, a restricting fascial sling. The restriction may limit arterial enlargement, a key compensatory mechanism in early lesion development.

Although atherosclerosis can be seen in any artery, there are patterns of distribution that have clinical implications. Smokers who present with premature atherosclerosis (age < 55 years) have an accelerated disease process most commonly involving the aortoiliac segments. In contrast, diabetics are far more likely to have disease involving the tibioperoneal artery. Lesions are often symmetrically distributed, although the rate of progression may vary.

Multiple risk factors for atherosclerosis have been identified. Controlling these risk factors may slow the progress of atherosclerosis and have significant clinical impact.

Major risk factors:
Cigarette smoking
Age
Diabetes
Hyperlipidemia (hypercholesterolemia and hypertriglyceridemia)
Hypertension
Positive family history
Homocysteinemia
Hyperfibrinogenemia
Lipoprotein(a)
Minor risk factors:
Obesity
Sedentary lifestyle
Male gender
Hypercoagulable states
Race (nonwhite)
Excessive alcohol use
C-reactive protein

Clinical Manifestations

Clinical manifestations of atherosclerosis include arterial insufficiency, aneurysm formation, and embolism. Usually, manifestations of only one of these conditions are present, but they may coexist.

Arterial insufficiency results from atherosclerotic plaques that have become large enough to narrow the arterial lumen. In medium-sized and large arteries, a 50% reduction in arterial diameter on an arteriogram roughly correlates with a 75% stenosis of cross-sectional area and enough resistance to decrease downstream flow and pressure.

The hemodynamic circuit consists of the diseased major artery, a parallel system of collateral vessels, and the peripheral runoff bed. Collateral vessels are much smaller, more circuitous, and always have a higher resistance than the original unobstructed artery. The stimuli for collateral development include the presence of an abnormal pressure gradient across the collateral system and an increased velocity of flow through intramuscular channels that connect to reentry vessels. Patients with good collateral circulation can expect excellent results with conservative therapy alone.

The final event in atherosclerosis is thrombosis. The clot propagates in the stagnant column of blood both proximally and distally to the first major tributaries. Persistent flow at these sites halts the propagation of clot (Figure 34–1). The presence of additional arterial stenoses further reduces blood flow. Severe ischemia is

* Deceased.

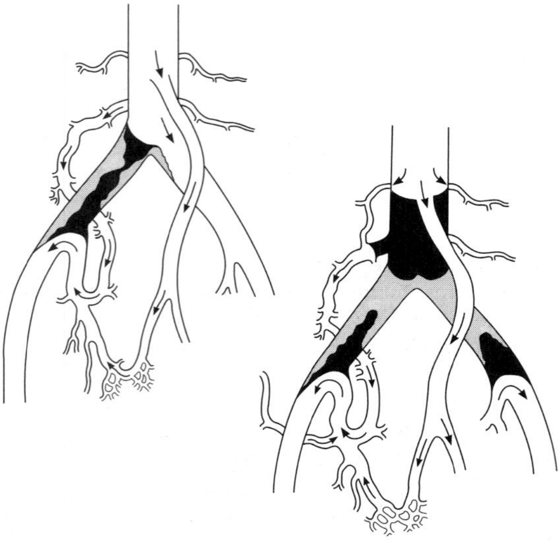

Figure 34–1. Development of collateral channels in response to occlusion of the right common iliac artery and the aortic bifurcation.

nearly always due to multiple sites of occlusion of the major vessels proximal to the affected tissues.

Although atherosclerosis generally causes narrowing of the artery, it may be associated with **degenerative aneurysms**. The link between these diseases is not clear. Although alterations in the architecture or metabolism of the arterial wall may be the primary cause of the dilation, patients with arterial aneurysms have many of the same risk factors as patients with atherosclerosis, and the aneurysmal wall is often lined with atherosclerosis.

Emboli, fragments of plaque or thrombus, can create distal arterial occlusion. Symptoms produced by emboli depend on their size and the affected organ and its arterial anatomy. Emboli are the primary mechanism of stroke from carotid atherosclerosis.

Boger RH et al: Biochemical evidence for impaired nitric oxide synthesis in patients with peripheral arterial occlusive disease. Circulation 1997;95:2068.

Chengpei X, Zarins CK, Glagov S: Aneurysmal and occlusive atherosclerosis of the human abdominal aorta. J Vasc Surg 2001;33:91.

Dormandy J, Heeck L, Vig S: Peripheral arterial occlusive disease. Clinical data for decision making. Semin Vasc Surg 1999;12:93.

Kadar A, Glasz T: Development of atherosclerosis and plaque biology. Cardiovasc Surg 2001;9:109.

McMillan WD, Pearce WH: Increased plasma levels of metalloproteinase-9 are associated with abdominal aortic aneurysms. J Vasc Surg 1999;29:122.

Muluk SC et al: Outcome events in patients with claudication: a 15-year study in 2777 patients. J Vasc Surg 2001;33:251.

Rosenfeld ME et al: Chlamydia, inflammation, and atherogenesis. J Infect Dis 2000;181(Suppl 3):5492.

Taylor LM Jr et al: Prospective blinded study of the relationship between plasma homocysteine and progression of symptomatic peripheral arterial disease. J Vasc Surg 1999;29:8.

Tegos TJ et al: The genesis of atherosclerosis and risk factors: a review. Angiology 2001;52:89.

PERIPHERAL ARTERIAL INSUFFICIENCY

ESSENTIALS OF DIAGNOSIS

- *Intermittent claudication.*
- *Ischemic rest pain.*
- *Decreased pulses.*
- *Nonhealing wounds.*
- *Pallor of foot on elevation, rubor on dependency.*
- *Necrosis and atrophy.*
- *Low ankle-brachial index.*

General Considerations

Peripheral arterial insufficiency is predominantly a disease of the lower extremities. Upper extremity arterial lesions are uncommon and confined mostly to the subclavian arteries. Stenoses of the radial and ulnar arteries occur primarily in patients with long-standing diabetes mellitus. Even when present, upper extremity atherosclerosis rarely produces symptoms due to abundant collateral pathways. In the lower extremities, however, obstructive lesions are distributed widely (Figure 34–2), although involvement of the femoropopliteal vessels is most common. Symptoms are related to the location and number of obstructions.

Peripheral arterial disease affects at least 20% of individuals older than 70 years. Although most patients with this disorder do not develop gangrene or require amputations, adverse outcomes of systemic atherosclerosis, including death, are common. Even after adjustment for known risk factors, individuals with peripheral arterial disease exhibit a higher mortality rate than a healthy population. A low ankle-brachial index is one of the strongest risk factors for all-cause mortality (Figure 34–3). Peripheral arterial disease is more a marker for early death than an indicator of imminent limb loss; thus, recognition and treatment of associated atherosclerotic risk factors is essential.

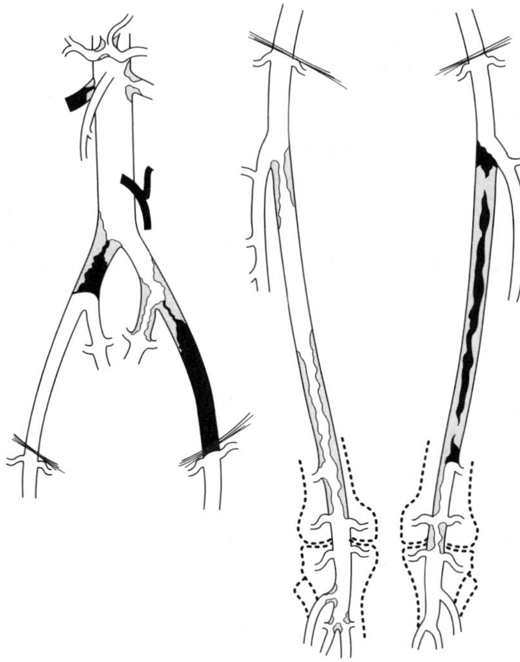

Figure 34–2. Common sites of stenosis and occlusion of the visceral and peripheral arterial systems.

Clinical Findings

A. Symptoms

1. Intermittent claudication—Intermittent claudication refers to pain or fatigue in muscles of the lower extremity caused by walking and relieved by rest. Claudication is derived from the Latin word for "limping, lame"; strictly speaking, the term should be used only for symptoms in the lower extremities. The pain is a deep-seated ache usually in the calf muscle, which gradually progresses until the patient is compelled to stop walking. Patients occasionally describe "cramping" or "tiredness" in the muscle. Typically, symptoms are completely relieved after 2–5 minutes of inactivity. Claudication is distinguished from other types of pain in the extremities in that some exertion is always required before it appears; it is reproducible; it does not occur at rest; and it is relieved by cessation of walking. Relief of symptoms is not dependent upon sitting or other positional change. The distance a patient can walk varies with the rate of walking, the level of incline, and the degree of arterial obstruction. The average patient with involvement of a single arterial segment can walk 90–180 meters on a level terrain at a moderate pace before pain appears. The presence of additional lesions may reduce the walking tolerance to a few meters. The degree of claudication is traditionally expressed in terms of city blocks, a poorly defined and variable unit that should be defined to clarify walking distance.

Regardless of which arterial segment is involved, claudication most commonly involves the calf muscles due to their high workload with normal walking. Occlusions proximal to the origin of the profunda femoris can extend the pain to involve the thigh. Gluteal pain is added by lesions in or proximal to the hypogastric arteries; impotence often accompanies these symptoms. Leriche's syndrome occurs in men as a result of aortoiliac disease and includes claudication of calf, thigh, and buttock muscles, impotence, and diminished or absent femoral pulses. Occasionally, patients describe transient numbness of the extremity accompanying the pain and fatigue of claudication as nerves become ischemic as well as muscles.

The two conditions that most often mimic claudication are osteoarthritis of the hip or knee, and neurospinal compression due to congenital or osteophytic narrowing of the lumbar neurospinal canal (spinal stenosis). Osteoarthritis can be differentiated from claudication because pain occurs predominantly in joints; the amount of exercise required to elicit symptoms varies; symptoms are characteristically worse in the morning; rest does not relieve symptoms promptly; and the severity of symptoms

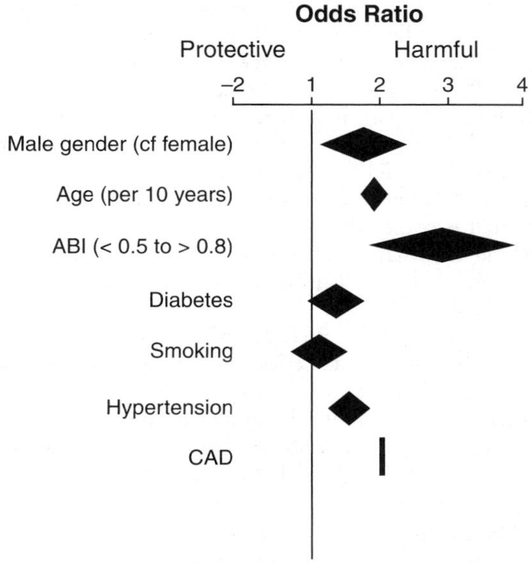

Figure 34–3. Odds ratios for risk factors for all-cause mortality. ABI, ankle-brachial index; CAD, coronary artery disease. (Reproduced, with permission, from TASC Working Group: Management of peripheral arterial disease: epidemiology, natural history, risk factors. J Vasc Surg 2000;31[1 Suppl]:S22. © 2000 Society for Vascular Surgery. Reprinted with permission from Elsevier.)

changes from day to day and anti-inflammatory agents may relieve the pain. Neurospinal compression symptoms are produced by impinging on the spinal canal or nerve root; therefore, standing as well as walking causes symptoms, and symptoms may occur while sitting. Neurospinal pain may follow a dermatomal distribution, which can be identified.

There are uncommon conditions that can mimic symptoms of arterial insufficiency such as coarctation of the aorta, chronic compartment syndrome, popliteal artery entrapment, and vasculitis, although age at presentation and associated findings may aid in diagnosing these unusual conditions.

The correct diagnosis should be easily established by determining the location of pain (calf), the quality of the pain, the length of time required for relief of symptoms, the reproducibility of symptoms, the distance walked before symptoms begin (initial claudication distance), and the type of rest or position required for symptom relief.

2. Ischemic rest pain—Ischemic rest pain—a grave symptom caused by ischemic neuritis—indicates advanced arterial insufficiency that usually terminates in gangrene and amputation of the extremity if arterial reconstruction cannot be performed. This is a severe burning pain usually confined to the forefoot distal to the metatarsals. It may be localized to the vicinity of an ischemic ulcer or pregangrenous toe. It is aggravated by elevation of the extremity or by bringing the leg to the horizontal position. Thus, it appears at bed rest (hence the name) and may prevent sleep. Because gravity aids the delivery of arterial blood, classically, the patient with rest pain can obtain relief by simply hanging the leg over the side of the bed. This simple maneuver will not relieve pain caused by peripheral neuropathy, the most common cause of foot pain at rest. If the foot is constantly kept dependent to relieve pain, the leg and foot may be swollen, causing some confusion in diagnosis. Ischemic neuritis pain is severe and resistant to opioids for relief.

Rest pain may be preceded by claudication but may occur de novo in diabetics with distal tibial disease, embolic occlusion of the distal tibial arteries, and patients whose walking is limited by other conditions (eg, angina pectoris). Differentiating ischemic rest pain from neuropathy in diabetics may be difficult and require vascular testing.

3. Nonhealing wounds or ulcers—Patients with severe lower extremity arterial insufficiency often develop ulcers or wounds on the feet even from seemingly trivial trauma. These lesions are most commonly located on the distal foot and toes, but on occasion they can be in the upper foot and ankle. Typically, the wounds are excruciatingly painful, deep, and devoid of any evidence of healing such as contraction or formation of granulation tissue. Frank gangrene eventually affects these ulcerations.

4. Erectile dysfunction—Inability to attain or maintain an erection may be produced by lesions that obstruct blood flow through both hypogastric arteries, and is commonly found in association with narrowing of the terminal aorta or common iliac arteries. Vasculogenic erectile dysfunction is less common than that due to most other causes (see Chapter 40).

5. Sensation—Although the patient may report numbness in the extremity, sensory abnormalities are generally absent on examination. If decreased sensation is found in the foot, peripheral neuropathy should be suspected.

B. Signs

Physical examination is of paramount importance in assessing the presence and severity of vascular disease. The physical findings of peripheral atherosclerosis are related to changes in the peripheral arteries and to tissue ischemia.

1. Arterial palpation—Decreased amplitude of the pulse denotes proximal stenosis. It is unusual for collateral flow to be sufficient to produce a pulse distal to an occluded artery. The authors generally use the right common carotid as "normal" for that patient and the 4+ denominator in the traditional 4+/4+ grading system (Table 34–1).

2. Bruits—A bruit is the sound produced by dissipation of energy as blood flows through a stenotic arterial segment. It is heard loudest during systole and, with greater stenosis, may extend into diastole. The bruit is transmitted distally along the course of the artery. Thus, when a bruit is heard through a stethoscope placed over a peripheral artery, stenosis is present *at* or *proximal* to that level. The pitch of the bruit rises as the stenosis becomes more marked, until a critical stenosis is reached or the vessel becomes occluded, when the bruit may disappear. Thus, absence of a bruit does not indicate insignificant disease.

3. Pallor—Pallor of the foot on elevation of the extremity indicates advanced ischemia. Pallor on elevation does not occur unless advanced ischemia is present.

Table 34–1. Grading of pulses.

Traditional		Basic	
4+	Normal	2+	Normal
3+	Slightly reduced	1+	Diminished
2+	Markedly reduced	0	Absent
1+	Barely palpable		
0	Absent		

4. Reactive hyperemia—The ischemia produced by elevation results in maximum cutaneous vasodilation. When the extremity is returned to a dependent position, blood returning to the dilated vascular bed produces an intense red color in the foot, called reactive hyperemia, and denotes advanced disease. Reactive hyperemia occurs only if ischemia is provoked. The rate of return of skin color when the extremities return to a dependent position is proportionate to the efficiency of the collateral circulation; the more delayed the reactive hyperemia, the more severe the impairment in circulation.

5. Rubor—In advanced atherosclerotic disease, the skin of the foot displays a characteristic dark red cyanosis on dependency. Because of reduced inflow, the blood in the capillary network of the foot is relatively stagnant, oxygen extraction is high, and the capillary blood becomes the color of the venous blood. The concurrent vasodilation due to ischemia causes blood to suffuse the cutaneous plexus, imparting a purple color to the skin. The purple discoloration due to chronic congestion from venous insufficiency does not become pallid on elevation.

6. Response to exercise—Exercise in a normal individual increases the pulse rate without producing arterial bruits or changes in pulse amplitude. In an individual who complains of claudication but who has minimal findings at rest, exercise will sometimes produce an audible bruit and a decrease in pulse strength and distal arterial pressure, unmasking a significant stenosis. This is best used in vascular testing (see below).

7. Skin temperature—With chronic ischemia, the temperature of the skin of the foot decreases. Coolness can best be detected by palpation with the back of the examiner's hand against the dorsum of the patient's foot.

8. Ulceration—Ischemic ulcers are usually very painful and accompanied by rest pain in the foot. They occur in toes or at a site where trauma from a shoe or bedding causes additional ischemia or infection. The margin of the ulcer is sharply demarcated or punched-out, and the base is devoid of healthy granulation tissue. The surrounding skin is pale and mottled, and signs of chronic ischemia are invariably present.

9. Necrosis—Tissue necrosis first becomes apparent in the most distal portions of the extremity, often at an ulcer site. Necrosis halts proximally at a line where the blood supply is sufficient to maintain viability and results in dry gangrene. If the necrotic portion is infected (wet gangrene), necrosis may extend into tissues that would normally remain viable.

10. Atrophy—Moderate to severe degrees of chronic ischemia produce gradual soft tissue and muscle atrophy and loss of strength in the ischemic zone. Joint mobility may be reduced in the forefeet as atrophy of the muscles of the feet produces increasing prominence of the interosseous spaces. Subsequent changes in foot structure and gait increase the possibility of developing foot ulceration.

11. Integumentary changes—Chronic ischemia commonly produces loss of hair over the dorsum of the toes and foot and may be associated with thickening of the toenails (onychomycosis) due to slowed keratin turnover. With more advanced ischemia, there is atrophy of the skin and subcutaneous tissue so that the foot becomes shiny, scaly, and skeletonized. Hence, a quick glance at a foot can identify the presence or absence of serious arterial insufficiency.

C. Noninvasive Vascular Tests

Noninvasive assessment is helpful to determine the severity of hypoperfusion and the sites of hemodynamically significant stenoses or occlusions.

The **ankle-brachial index (ABI)** is a quick screening test and the cornerstone of diagnosis. It consists of measurement of resting systolic blood pressure in the brachial artery and the posterior tibial or dorsalis pedis artery. The ABI is determined by dividing the systolic pressure obtained by Doppler insonation at the ankle by the brachial arterial pressure. Normally, the ABI is 1.0 or greater; a value below 1.0 indicates occlusive disease proximal to the point of measurement. ABIs correlate roughly with the degree of ischemia; eg, rest pain usually appears when the ratio is 0.3 or lower.

In elderly patients or diabetics, the tibial artery wall may be calcified. Since such a vessel cannot be compressed, an elevated pressure is recorded even though the intraluminal pressure may be low, leading to a false-negative examination. Wall calcification should be suspected whenever the ABI is above 1.2 or when the value is out of proportion to the patient's clinical status. This pitfall can be avoided by listening to the quality of the Doppler signal, ie, a monophasic signal indicates significant disease, or by obtaining toe pressures by plethysmography.

Additional noninvasive studies are useful in localizing disease or determining its severity. Segmental limb pressure measurement using both Doppler and plethysmography accurately detects and segmentally localizes hemodynamically significant large vessel occlusive lesions by determining pressures and pulse volume changes at the high thigh, low thigh, upper calf, and lower calf levels in addition to ankle pressures. A sphygmomanometer cuff is placed at a given level with a Doppler probe over one of the pedal arteries. The location of the occlusive lesions and their relative severity can be ascertained from these measurements.

Blood pressures can also be measured at rest and after exercise in the ankle and the effect of exercise can be monitored. This type of functional testing confirms and quantitates the diagnosis of claudication. To perform exercise testing the patient walks on a treadmill at a standard speed and grade until claudication pain is experienced or a time limit is reached. A graded treadmill with a slowly rising walking platform is often used. With significant arterial occlusive disease there will be a decrease in the ABI between the resting and postexercise time, usually measured 1 minute after cessation of walking. If the pain is not due to arterial stenosis, no fall in pressure will occur. This test is particularly useful in differentiating neurogenic pain with walking from vascular insufficiency.

D. Imaging Studies

Color duplex imaging is a mainstay of vascular imaging. It is a painless, relatively inexpensive, and (in experienced hands) accurate method for developing anatomic and functional information (eg, velocity gradients across stenoses) about arterial insufficiency and arterial aneurysms. Although the accuracy of this study is operator-dependent, it can supply sufficient information to permit intervention in selected cases.

Arteriography provides detailed anatomic information about peripheral arterial disease. It is reserved for patients warranting invasive intervention such as percutaneous transluminal angioplasty (PTA) or vascular surgery. Complications of angiography are related to technique and contrast media. Technical complications such as puncture site hematomas, arteriovenous fistulas, and false aneurysms are rare (about 1% risk). Contrast agents may precipitate allergic reactions (about 0.1% risk). Use of nonionic agents, carbon dioxide instead of contrast, and digital subtraction angiography lessens symptoms and the risk of adverse outcomes. Both standard and nonionic agents cause a transient decrease in renal blood flow and increased vascular resistance. In a small proportion of patients, angiography induces acute renal insufficiency. Patients with renal failure, proteinuria, diabetes, and dehydration are at increased risk for contrast-induced renal failure. Adequate hydration of patients before and after angiography, acetylcysteine, and periprocedural infusions of sodium bicarbonate infusions have dramatically reduced the incidence of this complication.

Magnetic resonance angiography (MRA) can delineate arteries without using contrast agents. The basic principle of MRA is that the vector of the proton spin becomes aligned with the brief application of a magnetic field. The MRA signal is generated as the protons return to a nonexcited or random alignment. The use of gadolinium as a contrast agent has dramatically improved MRA resolution and reduced imaging time. Recent studies using a gadolinium contrast agent that is attached to albumin shows that MRA compares favorably to arteriography in the identification of aortoiliac stenoses. This coupled with the fact that MRA has reduced toxicity compared to angiography has led to MRA replacing angiography as the first-line imaging technique (Figure 34–4).

The introduction of multiplanar CT scanners has allowed high-resolution images of the arterial tree. Although CT-angiography (CTA) still requires the administration of contrast material, it avoids an arterial puncture, and 3D reconstructions are an excellent alternative to arteriography. Current management and surgery of aortic aneurysms is done with CT alone, with arteriography rarely needed.

Calcification in the walls of atherosclerotic arteries is often visible on standard x-ray films and may occur without narrowing of the arterial lumen; for this reason, it is not an index of the functional status of the artery.

Treatment & Prognosis

The objectives of treatment for occlusive disease are relief of symptoms, prevention of limb loss, and maintenance of bipedal gait. This treatment is often in response to symptoms. For cerebrovascular atherosclerosis, prevention of stroke is the objective, while in aneurysmal disease it is prevention of rupture and death. Treatment is ideally done prophylactically, and outcomes depend on diagnosis of an asymptomatic lesion prior to a catastrophic event.

The operative risk must be assessed for each patient. Recognition of coexistent cardiac and respiratory systems is particularly relevant, because many patients with peripheral vascular disease also have ischemic heart disease, chronic pulmonary disease associated with tobacco use, or both.

In general, patients with peripheral vascular disease have shortened life expectancies. Nondiabetic patients with ischemic disease of the lower extremity have a 5-year survival rate of 70%. The survival rate is 60% in patients with associated ischemic heart disease or cerebrovascular insufficiency. Patients with peripheral vascular disease and renal failure have a 2-year survival rate of less than 50%. Most deaths are due to myocardial infarctions and strokes. Only 20% of deaths are due to nonatherosclerotic causes.

A. Conservative Treatment

Conservative treatment consists of (1) reducing risk factors, (2) exercise rehabilitation, (3) foot care, and (4) pharmacotherapy.

1. Reduction of risk factors—Cigarette smoking is the single most important risk factor for atherosclerosis, and all patients should stop smoking. Hypertension should be controlled, although the effects of its treatment on the natural history of peripheral arterial disease have not been evaluated. In peripheral arterial disease, elevated triglyceride levels and low HDL cholesterol levels are more prevalent than elevated levels of LDL

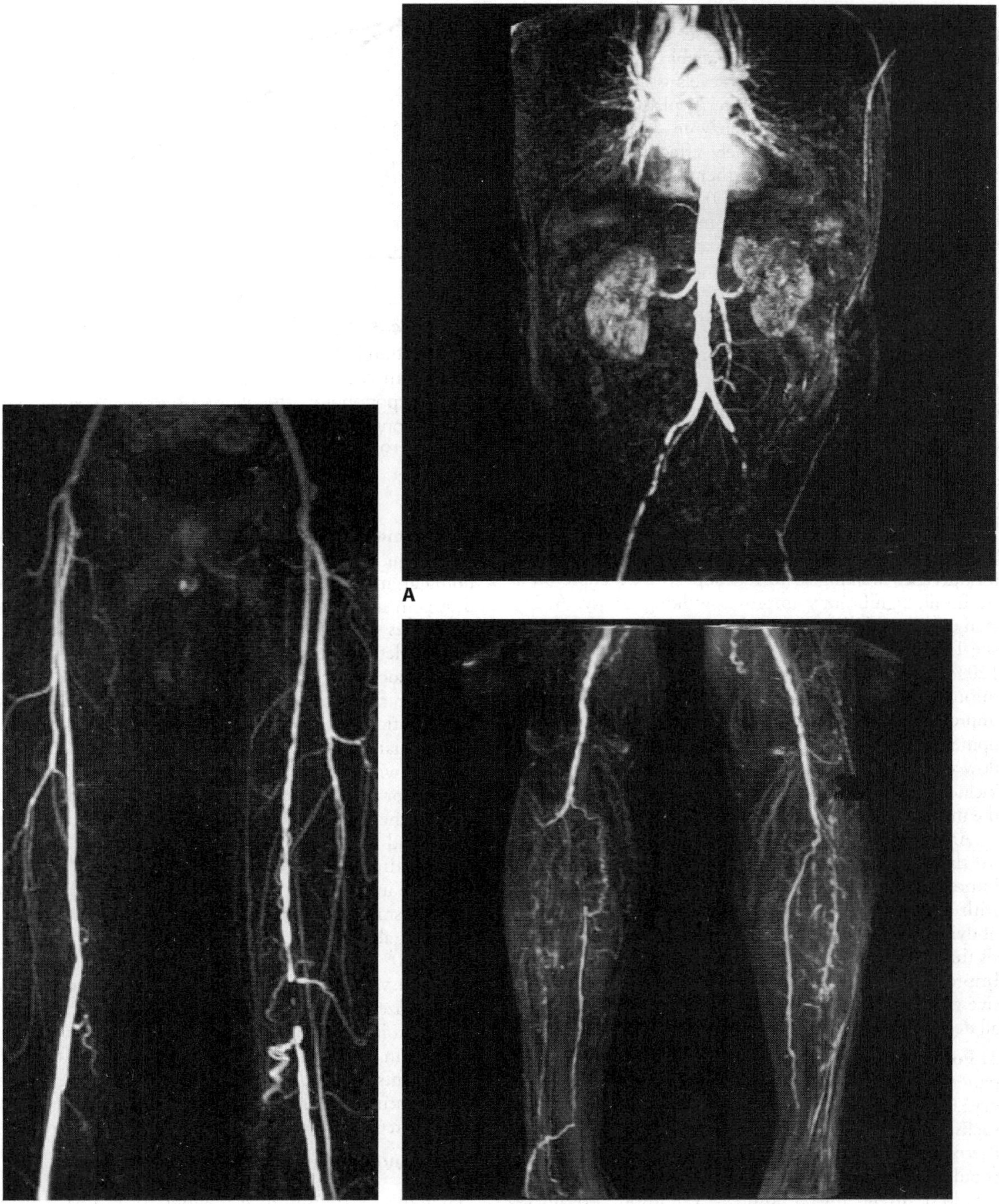

A
B
C

Figure 34–4. MRA studies showing the three most common levels of lower extremity atherosclerotic disease. ***A:*** Aortoiliac disease with segmental stenoses of the right common and external iliac arteries and occlusions on the left. ***B:*** SFA disease with occlusion at the adductor canal on the left. ***C:*** Tibial disease with bilateral tibial artery occlusions.

cholesterol. Lipoprotein(a) may be an independent risk factor for peripheral arterial disease, but accurate level determinations are not widely available.

Reduction of elevated lipid levels is associated with stabilization or regression of arterial plaques. Inhibitors of hydroxymethylglutaryl coenzyme A (HMG-CoA) reductase (statins) are extremely effective in reducing LDL cholesterol, and goals of therapy for patients with peripheral vascular disease (PVD) are to maintain cholesterol levels at less than 100 mg/dL (2.6 mmol/L). Other antihyperlipidemic medications, including niacin and fibrates (gemfibrozil), may be used to lower hypertriglyceridemia, which increases HDL cholesterol.

Both type 1 and type 2 diabetes increase the prevalence and severity of cardiovascular disease. Intensive glycemic control reduces the incidence of nephropathy, neuropathy, and retinopathy in diabetes, but it does not correlate with the severity or progression of peripheral arterial disease. In order to reduce all-cause mortality, however, it is recommended that fasting blood sugars should range from 80 to 120 mg/dL and that postprandial blood sugar levels be < 180 mg/dL; hemoglobin A_{1c} levels should be less than 7%.

2. Exercise rehabilitation—Exercise, ranging from unsupervised walking to formal supervised exercise on a treadmill, significantly improves walking ability. A 21-study meta-analysis of exercise programs showed an average 180% increase in initial claudication distance and a 120% increase in maximal walking distance achieved through exercise. The precise mechanism behind this improvement is not firmly established. Collateral development seems unlikely because ankle pressures and limb flow do not increase substantially. Possible explanations include improved metabolic capacity and conditioning of the muscles.

An additional benefit of improving exercise tolerance in these patients is that their overall prognosis is improved by restoring their ability to walk. Patients with claudication are at a two to four times greater risk of dying from complications of generalized atherosclerosis than people without claudication. (See Figure 34–5.) Improvement in walking distance as part of an aggressive risk factor modification regimen results in an overall decrease in cardiovascular risk.

3. Foot care—The feet of neuropathic or ischemic patients should be inspected and washed daily and kept dry. Clean cotton socks should be worn beneath dress socks, and shoes must fit properly. Mechanical and thermal trauma to the feet should be avoided. Toenails should be trimmed carefully, and corns and calluses should be attended to promptly. Even minor foot infections or injuries should be treated aggressively. Educating the patient to understand neuropathy, peripheral vascular insufficiency, and the importance of foot care is a central aspect of treatment.

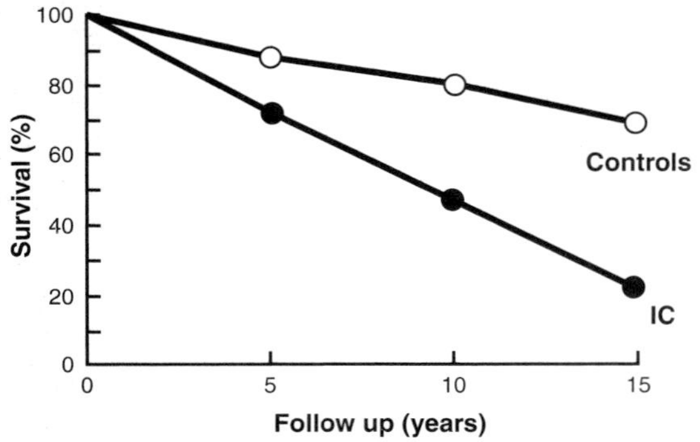

Figure 34–5. Survival of patients with intermittent claudication (IC) and matched controls. (Reproduced, with permission, from TASC Working Group: Management of peripheral arterial disease: epidemiology, natural history, risk factors. J Vasc Surg 2000;31[1 Suppl]:S19.)

4. Pharmacotherapy—The Antiplatelet Trialists Collaboration found an overall 25% decrease in fatal and nonfatal myocardial infarctions, strokes, and vascular deaths in those treated with antiplatelet agents. Aspirin at dosages ranging from 75 to 350 mg/d is the first-line antiplatelet agent recommended, though clopidogrel, which blocks the activation of platelets by ADP, is useful in aspirin-intolerant patients or those with large atherosclerotic burdens (ie, coronary artery disease, cerebrovascular disease, and peripheral arterial disease). All patients with peripheral arterial disease, whether symptomatic or asymptomatic, should be considered for antiplatelet therapy to reduce the risk of cardiovascular morbidity and mortality.

Two drugs have been approved by the FDA for treatment of intermittent claudication. **Pentoxifylline** produces a small improvement in both initial claudication distance (about 20%) and absolute claudication distance (about 10%). **Cilostazol** is a phosphodiesterase III inhibitor with vasodilator, antiplatelet, and antilipid activity. Randomized, placebo-controlled, blinded trials have shown an increase of about 50% in absolute claudication distance in patients treated with cilostazol. Quality-of-life assessments also improved significantly. Gene therapy for cardiovascular disease is also being investigated, but conclusions regarding safety and efficacy are premature.

B. Endovascular Therapy

Percutaneous transluminal angioplasty (PTA) consists of dilation of a stenotic arterial segment using an inflatable balloon catheter. As the balloon expands, it stretches the media and adventitia, fracturing plaque and expanding the artery to widen the lumen. Because energy losses associated with a stenosis are inversely proportionate to the fourth power of the radius at that point, small increases in radius can result in substantial increases in blood flow. Angioplasty has increasing become a first-line treatment for arterial stenoses.

Angioplasty may be used as primary therapy or, more commonly, as an adjunct to stenting. As noted above, the success rate for angioplasty with stenting is highest in the treatment of short stenoses of large proximal arteries. The 1-year success rate is 85% in common iliac disease, 70% in external iliac disease, and only 50% in femoral and popliteal artery disease. The use of angioplasty for tibial vessels is currently limited but growing with the introduction of small catheters and wires. In all vascular beds, the success of angioplasty is inversely related to the number and length of stenoses treated.

Since disease may recur more frequently after angioplasty than after bypass surgery, the patient should be closely followed up using noninvasive tests. Repeat angioplasty may be indicated for recurrent disease. The apparent cost savings afforded by angioplasty instead of operative treatment of arterial disease may be offset by the need for multiple repeat procedures, but patient satisfaction remains high.

Stent technology is rapidly evolving. In addition to balloon-expandable (Palmaz type) and self-expanding (Wallstent type) types, there are alterations in internodal design and flexibility that have improved the delivery and use of these devices. Only below the femoral artery is angioplasty alone still considered desirable.

Atherectomy is an endovascular procedure in which plaque is removed by shaving with a cutting or rotating catheter. In theory, removing the plaque should be more effective than angioplasty in treating stenosis, and it does not produce thermal injury as does laser angioplasty. The short-term results of atherectomy have been satisfactory, but restenosis has been a major problem for long surgical atherectomies in the past. If durability is reasonable, this may be an excellent tool for high-risk patients with distal arterial lesions.

C. Surgical Treatment

Intervention, open or endovascular, is performed both for limb salvage and for incapacitating claudication. The choice of operative procedure depends upon the location and distribution of arterial lesions and the presence of associated cardiac, pulmonary, or other disease. Direct revascularization procedures are applicable for patients with obstructive lesions located anywhere from the abdominal aorta to the arteries of the calf, providing there is demonstrable patency of the arteries distal to the segment to be revascularized. All patients undergoing vascular surgery should have preoperative risk assessments (see Chapter 2). Recent trials have shown that perioperative beta-blocker administration is mandatory for most patients to reduce cardiac morbidity.

1. Aorta, iliac, and femoral interventions—Endovascular techniques have replaced operative intervention for many lesions involving the aorta and common iliac artery. When stenoses or even occlusions are relatively short and localized, PTA with placement of intraluminal stents (Figure 34–6) is the treatment of choice, for patency rates of such "less invasive" procedures approach the results of operative treatment; moreover, if disease recurs, repeat interventions are possible. Newer devices have improved outcomes after PTA and stenting of the external iliac artery, but lesions of the common femoral artery, where greater degrees of flexion may occur, are treated with open procedures.

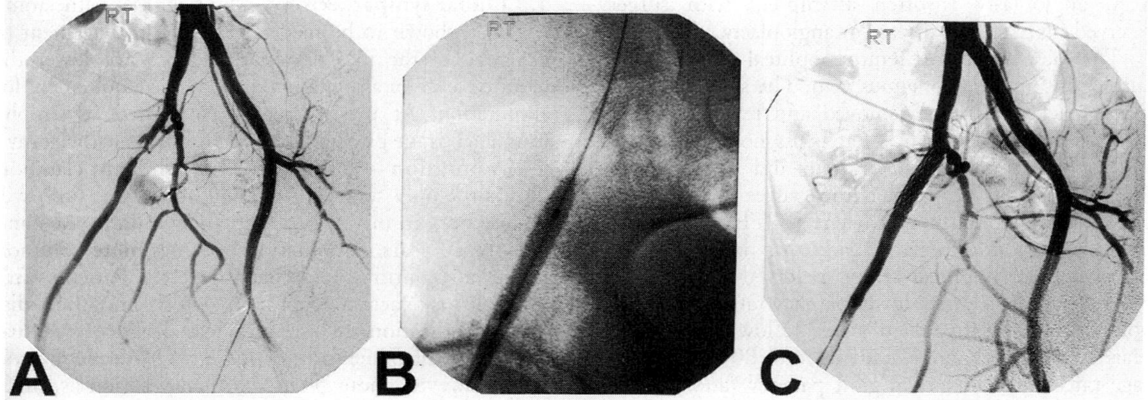

Figure 34–6. Percutaneous treatment of iliac artery stenosis: ***A:*** Preoperative arteriogram showing focal iliac artery stenosis. ***B:*** Percutaneous transluminal dilation of lesion. ***C:*** Widely patent arterial segment with stent in place.

Open operations are required for aortoiliofemoral occlusive disease when there are multiple lesions. An inverted Y-shaped prosthesis is interposed between the infrarenal abdominal aorta and the femoral arteries. The goal of operation is restoration of blood flow to the common femoral artery or, when occlusive disease of the superficial femoral artery is present, to the profunda femoris artery. The clinical results of aortofemoral reconstruction are excellent, although the mortality and morbidity clearly are higher than for endovascular therapy. The operative death rate is 5%; early patency rate, 95%; and late patency rate (5–10 years postoperatively), about 80%. Late complications may be as high as 10% and include graft-intestinal fistula formation, anastomotic aneurysm formation, renal failure, and erectile dysfunction.

Although the risks of aortoiliac reconstruction are acceptably low in the average patient, simpler procedures may be preferable in high-risk patients. If the clinically important lesions are confined to one side, a femorofemoral or iliofemoral bypass graft can be used. A graft from the axillary to the femoral artery (ie, axillofemoral graft) can be used for patients with aortoiliac disease when an abdominal operation is to be avoided, as in patients with excessive adhesions, infected abdominal aortic Dacron grafts, or aortoenteric fistulas. These "extra-anatomic" methods of arterial reconstruction are more prone to late occlusion and infection than are direct reconstructions.

2. Femoropopliteal reconstruction—When disease affects both the aortoiliac and femoropopliteal segments of the arterial tree, aortofemoral bypass (with profundoplasty if indicated) is generally adequate. When disease is confined to the femoropopliteal segment, femoropopliteal bypass is used. The principal indication for these operations is limb salvage. In patients with claudication alone, the indications for femoropopliteal bypass are more difficult to define but must include substantial disability from claudication. For limited lesions of the SFA, angioplasty is often attempted, with surgery reserved for extensive disease or angioplasty failure.

The best graft for femoropopliteal bypass is an autologous greater saphenous vein. The saphenous vein may be left in situ or removed and reversed. In the former instance the vein is left in its normal position, the venous tributaries are ligated, and special instruments are used to render the valves incompetent. Expanded polytetrafluoroethylene (PTFE) may also be used as a conduit, particularly for bypass to the supragenicular popliteal artery. Below the knee PTFE conduits produce much lower patency rates than saphenous veins. Operative death rates are low (2%), and 5-year patency rates range from 60% to 80%. Limb salvage rates are higher than graft patency rates. Patients undergoing femoropopliteal bypass for limb salvage have a 5-year survival rate of approximately 50%.

When profundaplasty alone is performed for limb salvage, the goal is improvement of flow through collaterals to the popliteal and tibial arteries. Limb salvage in patients undergoing profundaplasty is 80% when the suprageniculate popliteal artery is patent and 40–50% when the popliteal artery is occluded. Isolated profundaplasty is rarely helpful for treating claudication.

As noted above, percutaneous transluminal angioplasty with or without stent placement also can be performed for patients with infrainguinal occlusive arterial disease, especially if they are at high risk for surgical complications. Most patients with limb-threatening ischemia have extensive disease, and long-term patency rates are lower for these procedures. However, the use of flexible stents, cryo-balloons, and atherectomy devices has shown promise in this area.

3. Distal arterial reconstruction—Reconstruction of distal arteries (ie, bypass to the tibial, peroneal, or pedal vessels) is performed only for limb salvage. Endovascular techniques are not widely used in the tibial vessels, and bypass remains the primary mode of therapy for these patients. Autogenous saphenous vein is the best graft material, and either in situ or reversed technique may be used. If the greater saphenous vein is unavailable, a composite graft of lesser saphenous or arm veins is the next best choice. Prosthetic conduits have high failure rates. The operative death rate for these procedures is about 5%. Five years after operation, only approximately one-half of the grafts at risk are still functioning, but the limb salvage rate is substantially higher.

Successful revascularization results in lower costs than primary amputation and an infinite improvement in quality of life. Occasionally, primary amputation may be preferable to revascularization if the likelihood of successful bypass is low, extensive foot infection is present, or the architecture of the foot is compromised so that ambulation is unlikely.

4. Lumbar sympathectomy—Lumbar sympathectomy has been shown to be ineffective in the management of gangrene of the toes or foot and does not lower the required level for amputation or delay the requirement for amputation. At present, reflex sympathetic dystrophy (causalgia) is the principal indication for sympathectomy.

5. Amputation—Fortunately, if intermittent claudication is the only symptom, amputation of the limb will be necessary in only 5% of patients within 5 years and 10% in 10 years. Amputation becomes more common if patients continue to smoke cigarettes. Patients with multiple risk factors for atherosclerosis and short-distance claudication are also at increased risk for eventual limb loss. Of patients who present with ischemic rest pain, however, about 5% require amputation as initial therapy, and most will require amputation within 5 years, if not revascularized.

Ballard JL et al: Aortoiliac stent deployment versus surgical reconstruction: analysis of outcome and cost. J Vasc Surg 1998;28:1.

Beebe HG et al: A new pharmacological treatment for intermittent claudication: results of a randomized, multicenter trial. Arch Intern Med 1999;159:2041.

Byrne J et al: Infrainguinal arterial reconstruction for claudication: is it worth the risk? An analysis of 409 procedures. J Vasc Surg 1999;29:259.

Chew DK et al: Autogenous composite vein bypass graft for infrainguinal arterial reconstruction. J Vasc Surg 2001;33:259.

Conti CR: Current status of medical therapy of peripheral arterial disease. Clin Cardiol 1999;22:331.

Cronenwett JL, Birkmeyer JD (editors): *The Dartmouth Atlas of Vascular Health Care.* AHA Press, 2000.

de Virgilio C et al: Dipyridamole-thalhum/sestamibi before vascular surgery: a prospective blinded study in moderate-risk patients. J Vasc Surg 2000;32:77.

Donnelly R et al: ABC of arterial and venous disease: vascular complications of diabetes. BMJ 2000;320:1062.

Dormandy J et al: The fate of patients with critical leg ischemia. Semin Vasc Surg 1999;12:142.

Feinglass J et al: Measures of success and health-related quality of life in lower-extremity vascular surgery. Annu Rev Med 2000;41:101.

Golledge J et al: Outcome of femoropopliteal angioplasty. Ann Surg 1999;229:146.

Gordon IL et al: Three-year outcome of endovascular treatment of superficial femoral artery occlusion. Arch Surg 2001;136:221.

Hill SL, Holtzman G: Vascular surgeons—do they make a difference in peripheral vascular disease? Surgery 2001;129:136.

Jarvis B et al: Clopidogrel: a review of its use in the prevention of atherothrombosis. Drugs 2000;60:347.

Johnson WC et al: A comparative evaluation of polytetrafluoroethylene, umbilical vein, and saphenous vein bypass grafts for femoral-popliteal above-knee revascularization: a prospective randomized Department of Veterans Affairs cooperative study. J Vasc Surg 2000;32:268.

Krupski WC et al: Negative impact of cardiac evaluation before vascular surgery. Vasc Med 2000;5:3.

McDermott MM: Ankle brachial index as a predictor of outcomes in peripheral arterial disease. J Lab Clin Med 1999;133:33.

Merten GJ et al: Prevention of contrast-induced nephropathy with sodium bicarbonate. JAMA 2004;291:2334.

Mills JL et al: The natural history of intermediate and critical vein graft stenosis: recommendations for continued surveillance or repair. J Vasc Surg 2001;33:273.

Nelemans PJ et al: Peripheral arterial disease: meta-analysis of the diagnostic performance of MR angiography. Radiology 2000;217:105.

Oppat WF et al: Natural history of composite sequential bypass: ten years' experience. Arch Surg 1999;134:754.

Poldermans D et al: The effect of bisoprolol on perioperative mortality and myocardial infarction in high-risk patients undergoing vascular surgery. N Engl J Med 1999;341:1789.

Powell RJ et al: The durability of endovascular treatment of multisegment iliac occlusive disease. J Vasc Surg 2001;31:1178.

Quinn SF et al: Aortic and lower-extremity arterial disease: evaluation with MR angiography versus conventional angiography. Radiology 1998;206:693.

Rutherford RB et al: Recommended standards for reports dealing with lower extremity ischemia: revised version. J Vasc Surg 1997;26:517.

Savander SJ et al: The Legs for Life screening for peripheral vascular disease. J Vasc Interv Radiol 2001;12:33.

Strandness DE Jr et al: Peripheral vascular disease. Circulation 2000;102(Suppl 4):46.

Tan KH et al: Exercise training and peripheral vascular disease. Br J Surg 2000;87:553.

TASC Working Group: Management of peripheral arterial disease (PAD). J Vasc Surg 2000;31:S1.

Taylor LM et al: The incidence of perioperative myocardial infarction in general vascular surgery. J Vasc Surg 1992;15:52.

Tetterroo E et al: Randomised comparison of primary stent placement versus primary angioplasty followed by selective stent placement in patients with iliac artery occlusive disease. Dutch Iliac Stent Trial Study Group. Lancet 1998;351:1153.

Veith FJ et al: Six-year prospective multicenter randomized comparison of autologous saphenous vein and expanded polytetrafluoroethylene grafts in infrainguinal arterial reconstructions. J Vasc Surg 1986;3:104.

Wain RA et al: Can duplex scan arterial mapping replace contrast arteriography as the test of choice before infrainguinal revascularization? J Vasc Surg 1999;29:100.

ACUTE ARTERIAL OCCLUSION

Sudden occlusion of a previously patent artery is a dramatic event characterized by the abrupt onset of severe pain, coldness, numbness, motor weakness, and absent pulses in the involved extremity. Tissue viability depends on the extent to which flow is maintained by collateral circuits or surgical intervention. When ischemia persists, motor and sensory paralysis, muscle infarction, and cutaneous gangrene become irreversible in a matter of hours. If left untreated, a line of demarcation will develop between viable and nonviable tissue. Flow in the distal arteries is reduced progressively by propagating intraluminal thrombus, and surgical restoration of blood flow to the ischemic portion of the extremity eventually becomes impossible.

Acute major arterial occlusion may be caused by an embolus, thrombosis, trauma, or dissection. The heart is the source of embolus in 80–90% of episodes, with the remainder from proximal arterial lesions. Aortic aneurysms often contain thrombi but they rarely embolize. In contrast, femoral and particularly popliteal aneurysms embolize frequently. Ulceration in atherosclerotic plaques also can lead to formation of thrombus, which may fragment. Miscellaneous infrequent sources of emboli include cardiac tumors (including cardiac myxoma) and paradoxic emboli (venous thrombi migrating through a patent foramen ovale). Up to 5–10% of spontaneous emboli originate from a source that remains unidentified despite thorough diagnostic interrogation.

It may be difficult to differentiate between sudden thrombosis of an atherosclerotic peripheral artery and embolic occlusion. The former patients have preexisting atherosclerotic stenosis and low blood flow, which predisposes to stagnation and thrombosis. One should also keep in mind the clinical setting and a history of preexisting symptoms such as atrial fibrillation (embolus) or claudication (primary thrombosis).

Clinical Findings

Acute arterial occlusion is characterized by the five *P*s: pain, pallor, pulselessness, paresthesias, and paralysis. Severe sudden pain is present in 80% of patients, and its onset usually indicates the time of vessel occlusion. Pain is absent in some patients because of prompt onset of anesthesia and paralysis and portends a poor prognosis.

On examination, pallor may be replaced by mottled cyanosis as deoxygenated blood gradually suffuses the extremity. It is important to determine if sensitivity to light touch is maintained. These fibers are highly susceptible to ischemia and their dysfunction heralds the beginning of irreversible ischemic changes. The onset of motor paralysis implies impending gangrene. Early intervention is critical. Swelling with acute tenderness of a muscle belly—usually in the calf following acute femoral artery occlusion—generally denotes irreversible muscle infarction. Skin and subcutaneous tissues have greater resistance to hypoxia than nerves and muscles, which may demonstrate irreversible histologic changes after as little as 3–4 hours of ischemia.

Treatment & Prognosis

A. Embolism and Thrombosis

Immediate anticoagulation by intravenous heparin slows the propagation of thrombus and allows time for assessment of adequacy of collateral flow and preparation for operation. If light touch is intact, arteriography may be performed to define the anatomy and assist in planning the operation. Diagnosis of acute embolic occlusion is based upon an abrupt block of the artery with little accompanying arterial disease; conversely, acute in situ thrombosis is associated with extensive atherosclerosis and a well-established collateral network. The operative treatment of an embolus differs from that of preexisting atherosclerosis, which may require bypass.

Nonoperative management is reserved for emboli to major arteries in the upper extremities, where collateral circulation is outstanding, and for the rare event in the lower extremities when skin color improves or neural function returns quickly after an initial ischemic episode. If the initial ischemia recedes, the decision for removal of the embolus is based upon an estimate of the disability that will be produced by chronic occlusion of the involved artery. Chronic occlusion of the axillary or brachial arteries is usually well tolerated, whereas chronic occlusion of lower extremity vessels causes claudication, if not rest pain, and should be removed.

Therapeutic options include catheter-directed thrombolysis, percutaneous mechanical thrombectomy, and surgical embolectomy. For patients with severe acute ischemia, operative therapy is preferable because it is usually associated with the least delay in reestablishing perfusion. Surgical embolectomy may be performed through an arteriotomy at the site of the embolus or, most commonly, by extraction with a balloon (Fogarty) catheter inserted through a proximal arteriotomy. Successful embolectomy requires removal of the embolus and the "tail" of thrombus that extends distally or proximally from it. If operation is not performed within the first few hours, the clot may become adherent and subsequent revascularization is less successful. Intraoperative infusion of thrombolytic agents is often a useful adjunct to embolectomy.

Fasciotomy is normally required after prolonged acute ischemia to treat the compartment syndrome that may accompany the reperfusion injury. Renal insufficiency from myoglobin release should be anticipated after reperfusion of ischemic muscle. Treatment consists of vigorous hydration and alkalinization of the urine. Administration of free radical scavengers may be helpful in this disorder.

Patients with clearly irreversible limb ischemia should undergo amputation without an attempt at revascularization, as revascularization may expose the patient to the serious hazards of the reperfusion syndrome caused by release of acidotic and hyperkalemic venous blood from the dying extremity.

In patients who will tolerate a delay in revascularization, ie, those who do not have neural changes on examination, intra-arterial thrombolysis should be considered. The usual regimen involves selective intra-arterial infusion of low doses of thrombolytic agent (eg, tPA) directly into the clot. This activates thrombus plasminogen efficiently, allows high concentrations in the clot while limiting systemic effect, and has acceptable complication rates. In cases of thrombosis on preexisting atherosclerotic lesions, thrombolysis will reveal the underlying lesions. These should be treated to prevent recurrent thrombosis.

B. Traumatic Arterial Occlusion

Traumatic arterial occlusion must be corrected within a few hours to avoid development of gangrene. Repair of arterial injury is usually performed in conjunction with repair of other injuries. The general principles are described in Chapter 13.

Campbell WB, Ridler BM, Szymanska TH: Current management of acute leg ischaemia: results of an audit by the Vascular Surgical Society of Great Britain and Ireland. Br J Surg 1998;85: 1498.

Greenberg R et al: The role of thrombolytic therapy in the management of acute and chronic lower extremity ischemia. J Endovasc Ther 2000;7:72.

Ouriel K et al: Acute lower limb ischemia: determinants of outcome. Surgery 1998;124:336.

Suggs WD et al: When is urokinase treatment an effective sole or adjunctive treatment for acute limb ischemia secondary to native artery occlusion? Am J Surg 1999;178:103.

Swischuk JL et al: Transcatheter intraarterial infusion of rt-PA for acute lower limb ischemia: Results and complications. J Vasc Interv Radiol 2001;12:423.

PERIPHERAL MICROEMBOLI

The most common source of microembolization is cardiac valvular disease. However, if no cardiac valvular lesions are found, a careful examination of the proximal arterial tree must be done to identify an arterial source.

Recurrent microemboli in the extremities can arise from occlusive lesions already described, particularly if the lesion develops an excoriated or ulcerated surface. Other lesions noted for shedding emboli are the peripheral aneurysms, most commonly the popliteal and subclavian aneurysms. The mural thrombus in the wall of popliteal aneurysms is particularly susceptible to fragmentation with flexion of the knee joint.

Microemboli are most damaging when they occlude a digital artery. This causes sudden pain, cyanosis, and coldness or numbness in the affected digit. These changes characteristically improve over several days. If there are multiple emboli, these symptoms may reappear perhaps in a different area of the hand or foot. In the lower extremity this clinical entity has been called **blue toe syndrome**, or **trash foot**. The sudden onset of pain and purple discoloration of a toe in the presence of palpable pulses is recognized as a potentially limb-threatening arterial problem. With each succeeding episode, recovery is slower and less complete.

Sudden onset differentiates peripheral atheroembolism from other causes of blue toes, such as vasculitis, thromboangiitis obliterans, trauma, or chronic ischemia. It is important to remember that a patent proximal artery is required to serve as a conduit for the embolus, so pulses are intact. Furthermore, a normal blood supply is present in adjacent tissue segments. The appearance of a normally perfused foot with a cyanotic toe should not be misdiagnosed. However, the waxing and waning symptoms of repeated emboli can make the diagnosis difficult. Unless the syndrome is recognized and the lesion of origin corrected, survival of the foot or hand may be in peril.

Once discovered, the source of microemboli must be removed by appropriate valvular or arterial reconstruction. Catheter-directed thrombolytic therapy may be used to dissolve distal emboli in selected cases. Acute anticoagulation is nearly always indicated and chronic anticoagulation may be necessary, particularly with valvular disease.

Farooq MM et al: Penetrating ulceration of the infrarenal aorta: case reports of an embolic and an asymptomatic lesion. Ann Vasc Surg 2001;15:255.

Matchett WJ et al: Blue toe syndrome: treatment with intraarterial stents and review of therapies. J Vasc Interv Radiol 2000;11: 585.

Sharma PV et al: Changing patterns of atheroembolism. Cardiovasc Surg 1996;4:573.

SMALL ARTERY OCCLUSIVE DISEASE

Obstructing lesions may occur in arteries less than 3 mm in diameter (eg, the radial, ulnar, tibial, or peroneal arteries), most commonly in patients with diabetes mellitus. Less common causes are recurrent microembolization (see above), vasculitis, and thromboangiitis obliterans (Buerger's disease). Hand, foot, or digital ischemia can result from these conditions, and amputation is sometimes required.

DIABETIC VASCULAR DISEASE

Atherosclerotic arterial disease in patients with diabetes mellitus is more diffuse and more severe than in nondiabetics. In diabetic patients the tibioperoneal vessels frequently contain atherosclerotic changes and the vessels may be heavily calcified. The degree of ischemia is often severe and extensive, and noninvasive tests (ABIs) may be falsely normal. Fortunately, in many diabetics the small arteries in the foot are relatively spared, making distal bypass to these arteries possible and allowing foot salvage in cases of threatened limb loss.

Diabetic patients also have a high incidence of neuropathy and are more apt to ignore minor foot injuries, which can develop into ulcerations. Daily foot inspections are essential to avoid progression of minor injuries. Neuropathy is also responsible for loss of tone of intrinsic foot muscles that leads to subluxation of the metatarsal phalangeal joints, resulting in a "rocker-bottom" foot and ultimately producing complete joint destruction termed a "Charcot foot." These architectural changes also make skin breakdown more likely to occur.

Akbari CM et al: Diabetes and peripheral vascular disease. J Vasc Surg 1999;30;373.

Bouton AJ et al: The diabetic foot: the scope of the problem. J Fam Pract 2000;49:S3.

LoGerfo FW, Coffman JD Current concepts. Vascular and microvascular disease of the foot in diabetes. Implications for foot care. N Engl J Med 1984;311:1615.

Nehler MR et al: Intermediate-term outcome of primary digit amputations in patients with diabetes mellitus who have forefoot sepsis requiring hospitalization and presumed adequate circulatory status. J Vasc Surg 1999;30;509.

NONATHEROSCLEROTIC DISORDERS CAUSING LOWER LIMB ISCHEMIA

Thromboangiitis Obliterans

Thromboangiitis obliterans **(Buerger's disease)** is characterized by multiple segmental occlusions of tibial and pedal arteries. Migratory phlebitis may be present. In contrast to atherosclerosis, which involves the intima and media, thromboangiitis obliterans is manifested by infiltration of round cells in all three layers of the arterial wall. The disease occurs almost exclusively in young male smokers. It is essential that the patient stop smoking to avoid progression of the disease. Patients with Buerger's disease may have specific cellular immunity against arterial antigens, specific humoral antiarterial antibodies, and elevated circulatory immune complexes, but a precise diagnosis can only be made by tissue histology. Arteriographic findings are distinctive but not pathognomonic. Sympathectomy decreases arterial spasm and is useful in some patients. Amputation is indicated for persistent pain or gangrene and can be performed adjacent to the line of demarcation with satisfactory primary healing.

The disease may become dormant if the patient can stop smoking. Unfortunately, this seems particularly difficult in these patients and many ultimately require multiple amputations.

Popliteal Artery Entrapment Syndrome

This rare cause of popliteal artery stenosis or occlusion occurs as a result of an anomalous course of the popliteal artery. The popliteal artery normally passes between the two heads of the gastrocnemius muscle as it enters the lower leg. In the entrapment syndrome, the artery passes medial to both heads of the gastrocnemius, causing compression of the popliteal artery when the knee is extended. There are five anatomic variants of popliteal artery entrapment, but all produce similar clinical effects. Fibrous thickening of the intima occurs at the site of compression and gradually progresses to total occlusion. Symptoms vary from calf claudication to those of more severe ischemia depending on lesion severity and embolization. Popliteal artery entrapment should be considered when a young, otherwise healthy patient presents with calf claudication. Until the artery becomes occluded, the only finding is a decrease in strength of the pedal pulses, most evident when using provocative maneuvers like foot dorsiflexion and plantar flexion. MRI studies are most useful in confirmation of the diagnosis. Atherosclerotic changes are notably absent. Treatment consists of returning the popliteal artery to its normal anatomic course.

Cystic Degeneration of the Popliteal Artery

Arterial stenosis is produced by a mucoid cyst in the adventitia, usually located in the middle third of the artery. Calf claudication is the most common symptom, and the only finding is a decrease in the strength of the peripheral pulses. Rarely, a mass can be palpated. Arteriography shows a sharply localized zone of popliteal stenosis with a smooth concentric tapering having an hourglass appearance. Ultrasound or CT scans can be used to demonstrate the cyst within the vessel wall. The stenosis may be missed on conventional anteroposterior films and may appear only on lateral exposures. The cyst and the affected artery should be excised because of the possibility of recurrence with evacuation of the cyst only.

Abdominal Aortic Coarctation

Coarctation of the thoracic or abdominal aorta may be congenital and developmental or may result from an inflammatory large vessel arteritis such as Kawasaki's disease or Takayasu's disease. These rare disorders may produce symptoms of lower extremity, mesenteric, or renal ischemia depending on the location of the constriction. The congenital variant of this condition is best managed surgically when it is recognized; autogenous repair may be preferable to the use of prosthetic grafts. Surgical repair in the presence of ongoing inflammation is not recommended, as those patients do poorly. However, if the disease is quiescent with a normal sedimentation rate, standard surgical operations appear to produce satisfactory results.

Blank M et al: Monoclonal anti-endothelial cell antibodies from a patient with Takayasu arteritis activate endothelial cells from large vessels. Arthritis Rheum 1999;42:1421.

Eichorn J et al: Antiendothelial cell antibodies in thromboangiitis obliterans. Am J Med 1998;315:17.

Levien LJ et al: Popliteal artery entrapment syndrome: more common than previously recognized. J Vasc Surg 1999;30:587.

Levien LJ et al: Adventitial cystic disease: a unifying hypothesis. J Vasc Surg 1998;28:193.

Mickley V et al: Coarctations of descending and abdominal aorta: long-term results of surgical therapy. J Vasc Surg 1998:28:206.

O'Hara N et al: Surgical treatment for popliteal artery entrapment syndrome. Cardiovasc Surg 2001;9:141.

Ring DH Jr et al: Popliteal artery entrapment syndrome: arteriographic findings and thrombolytic therapy. J Vasc Interv Radiol 1999:10:713.

Teoh MK: Takayasu's arteritis with renovascular hypertension: results of surgical treatment. Cardiovasc Surg 1999;7:626.

Tsolakis IA et al: Cystic adventitial disease of the popliteal artery: diagnosis and treatment. Eur J Vasc Endovasc Surg 1998;15:188.

ARTERIAL ANEURYSMS

ESSENTIALS OF DIAGNOSIS

- *Pulsatile mass.*
- *Rupture, hypotension, and possible death.*
- *Emboli/thrombosis with peripheral aneurysms.*

General Considerations

An aneurysm is a permanent, localized dilation of an artery to at least one and one-half times its normal diameter. Arterial aneurysms may be classified according to etiology (eg, degenerative (atherosclerotic), inflammatory, congenital, dissecting); shape (eg, saccular, fusiform); location (eg, aortic, peripheral, splanchnic, cerebral); or structure (eg, true, false). A **true aneurysm** involves primary dilation of the artery including all vessel wall layers (intima, media, and adventitia). The expanding vessel usually elongates as well as dilates. A **false aneurysm** or **pseudoaneurysm** is characterized by a disruption of the artery wall, and actually is a pulsatile hematoma not contained by the artery wall but by a fibrous capsule. A **mycotic aneurysm** is a false aneurysm caused by infection.

False aneurysms of the femoral artery secondary to catheterization are the most numerous of all aneurysms. Aortic aneurysms are the most common of the true aneurysms. In descending order, other arteries affected are the iliac arteries, the popliteal artery (Figure 34–7), the common femoral artery, the arch and descending portions of the thoracic aorta, the carotid arteries, and other peripheral arteries. There are other rare causes of true aneurysms, which include Marfan's syndrome, Ehlers-Danlos syndrome, Behçet's disease, cystic medial necrosis, and the gradual dilation after aortic dissection.

ABDOMINAL AORTIC ANEURYSMS

At present abdominal aortic aneurysms (AAAs) are found in 2% of the elderly male population, and the incidence is increasing. In selected groups the incidence is higher—5% of patients with coronary artery disease and as many as 50% of patients with femoral or popliteal aneurysms have aortic aneurysms. Males are four times as likely to be affected as females. Ruptured aortic aneurysms are the thirteenth leading cause of death in the United States, resulting in 15,000 deaths per year. In Great Britain, 1:70 men between the age of 60 and 84 years die of a ruptured AAA.

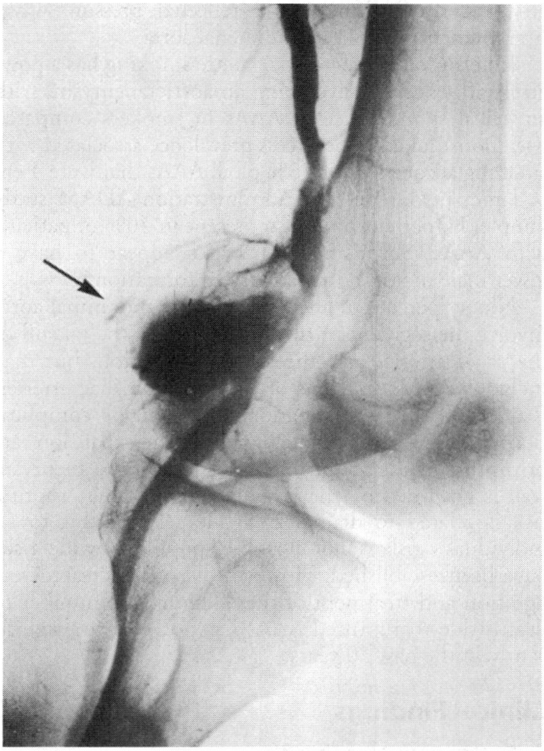

Figure 34–7. Arteriogram showing aneurysm of the popliteal artery (arrow).

Numerous mechanisms have been proposed for the cause of AAAs. Structural issues may contribute; reductions in the number of elastic lamellae and virtual absence of vasa vasorum in the media of the distal abdominal aorta compared with the thoracic aorta may favor aneurysmal degeneration. Whereas collagen makes up about 25% of the wall of an atherosclerotic aorta, it comprises only 18% of an aneurysmal aortic wall. Excessive protease activity or local reductions in the concentration of protease inhibitors also have been implicated in aneurysm formation. Studies have shown that lysyl oxidase, a sex-linked enzyme that helps regulate collagen cross-linking, is mutated in families in which every male has been diagnosed with an aneurysm. A hereditary deficiency of pyridinoline cross-linkage in collagen also has been found in some patients with aneurysms. This speaks to a genetic predisposition for this disorder. Indeed, a positive family history of aortic aneurysms infers a 20% chance that a first-degree family member will have an aneurysm. There may be hemodynamic factors as well, owing to large pulsatile stresses because of tapering geometry, increased stiffness, and reflected pressure waves from branch vessels in the infrarenal aorta.

In terms of risk factors, cigarette smoking has a powerful influence on developing an aortic aneurysm, with an 8:1 preponderance of AAAs in smokers compared with nonsmokers. The excess prevalence associated with smoking accounted for 78% of all AAAs that were 4 cm or larger in the Veteran Administration ADAM study sample. Hypertension is also present in 40% of patients with AAAs. Surprisingly, diabetics appear to have a lower incidence of aortic aneurysm formation.

Ninety percent of aneurysms of the abdominal aorta involve the segment of the aorta between the takeoff of the renal arteries and the aortic bifurcation, but may include variable portions of the common iliac arteries. Rupture with exsanguination is the major complication of AAAs. Unfortunately, neither the expansion rate or rupture risk is predictable. Tension on the aneurysm wall is governed by the law of Laplace. Thus, rupture risk is related to diameter. While relating this to an individual's risk is not possible, populationwide risks have been established. However, despite increased recognition and treatment of these lesions, the number of deaths due to ruptured AAAs has not changed significantly in the past 20 years.

Clinical Findings

A. Symptoms and Signs

The vast majority of unruptured aneurysms are asymptomatic. Rarely, intact AAAs produce back pain due to pressure on nerves or erosion into vertebral bodies. Severe pain in the absence of rupture characterizes the rare inflammatory aneurysm that is surrounded by 2–4 cm of perianeurysmal retroperitoneal inflammatory reaction.

Usually, the sole physical finding of abdominal aneurysms is a palpable fusiform or globular pulsatile abdominal mass. Lederle and colleagues found that 80% of 5-cm AAAs are palpable (Figure 34–8). Usually the AAA is centered in the mid-abdomen just above and to the left side of the umbilicus, which corresponds to the infrarenal portion of the abdominal aorta. Physical examination for an AAA is less reliable in obese patients or older individuals whose aortas may have become tortuous. The aneurysm may be slightly tender to palpation. Severe tenderness suggests a "symptomatic aneurysm" and is found in inflammatory aneurysms, after rupture has occurred, or if the aneurysm has recently expanded. A truly noninflammatory, symptomatic aneurysm demands urgent imaging and usually urgent surgery.

B. Imaging Studies

Plain films of the abdomen reveal calcification in the outer layers of about 20% of degenerative abdominal aneurysms, and are not good screening studies. CT scans provide valuable information about aneurysm architecture and have been used to predict aneurysm expansion rates. In addition, CT scans show important adjacent structures that affect AAA repair, such as colonic or pancreatic masses, horseshoe kidneys or other renal abnormalities, and venous anomalies, including retroaortic renal veins, circumaortic renal

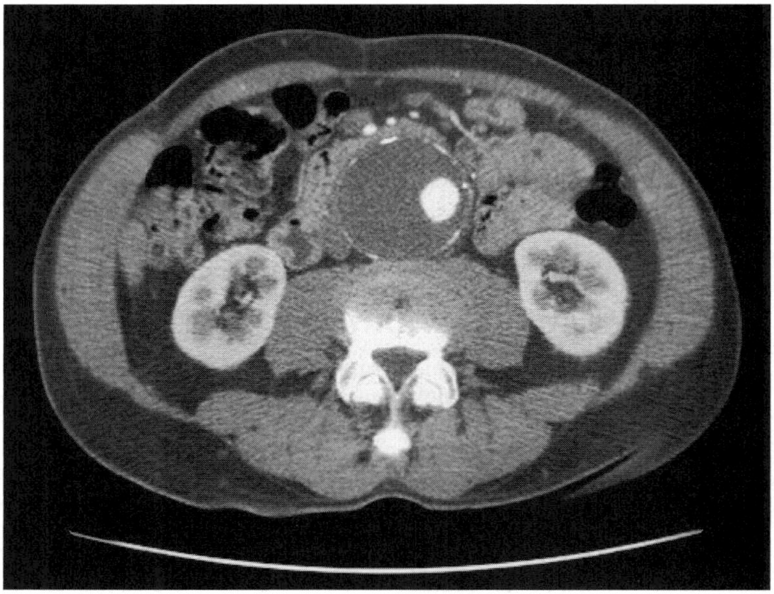

Figure 34–8. CT showing the typical position of a 5.5-cm AAA and its proximity to the abdominal wall.

veins, and left-sided or duplicated vena cavas. If the patient has a multiplanar CT scan, aortograms, once routine studies in planning operative management of AAAs, are rarely needed.

Ultrasound is the least expensive method for measuring the size of infrarenal aortic aneurysms. Repeated ultrasound examinations are cost-effective for observing small AAAs and are generally used for this purpose. However, ultrasound examinations do not reliably detect perigraft collections of blood or fluid and should not be used to diagnose ruptured AAAs. CT scan or MRI with 3D reconstructions are both accurate methods for assessing aneurysm diameter, although the ADAM trail showed that there can be substantial inter-reader variability in size determinations.

Natural History

The expansion rate of an AAA is variable and unpredictable. Most aneurysms continue to enlarge and will eventually rupture if left untreated. The average expansion rate for an AAA is 0.4 cm per year. The rate of expansion correlates with diastolic blood pressure, initial aneurysm diameter, and the degree of obstructive pulmonary disease.

Aneurysm size is currently the best determinant of rupture risk. About 40% of aneurysms 5.5–6 cm or larger in diameter will rupture within 5 years if untreated, and the average survival of an untreated patient is 17 months (Table 34–2). In contrast, the ADAM study found a 0.5% per year rupture rate in AAAs 4–5.4 cm, an overall rate remarkably similar to a comparable trial in the United Kingdom. Thus, surgery is recommended for nearly all aneurysms 5.5 cm or more in size, but small aortic aneurysms can be safely observed using serial ultrasound examinations to assess expansion. Regardless of size, repair is mandatory for an aneurysm that is symptomatic or enlarging rapidly (> 0.5–1 cm/yr).

Table 34–2. Probable AAA rupture rate by presenting diameter.

	Follow-Up (Years)	
Diameter of Aneurysm (cm)	***1***	***2***
5.5–5.9	9.4%	22.1%
≥ 7.0	32.5%	43.4%

Data extracted from Lederle FA et al: Veterans Affairs Cooperative Study #417 Investigators. Rupture rate of large abdominal aortic aneurysms in patients refusing or unfit for elective repair. JAMA 2002;287:2968.

Treatment

As with occlusive disease, endovascular repair of AAA has lower perioperative mortality and morbidity. Conventional operative repair, introduced in 1951, is a well-established and successful intervention but entails a major surgical procedure with substantial morbidity and mortality. Endovascular repair, introduced in 1991, is gaining in popularity. The repair is achieved with a synthetic graft to which metal stents have been attached. This stent-graft device is then introduced through a small femoral arteriotomy. AAA repair using a stent-graft reduces ICU and hospital stays and procedure-related morbidity and mortality. However, it may be associated with higher failure rates and definitely has higher device-related expense.

Conventional operative AAA repair consists of replacing the aneurysmal segment with a synthetic fabric graft. Tubular or bifurcation grafts of Dacron or PTFE are preferred. The proximal anastomosis is made to the aorta above the aneurysm. The site of the distal anastomosis is determined by the extent of aneurysmal involvement of the iliac arteries (Figures 34–9 and 34–10). Traditionally, a transperitoneal approach via midline laparotomy has been used for AAA repair, but retroperitoneal operations via flank incision may decrease perioperative pulmonary and gastrointestinal complications.

Elective infrarenal abdominal aneurysmectomy has a 2–4% operative death rate and a 5–10% rate of complications, such as bleeding, renal failure, myocardial infarction, graft infection, limb loss, bowel ischemia, and erectile dysfunction. Paraplegia is a very rare complication due to involvement of an abnormally low artery of Adamkiewicz, a major collateral of the anterior spinal artery. Malignant tumors are encountered unexpectedly in about 4% of cases, although that rate is now dwindling with the routine use of multiplanar CT scans. If bowel cancer is discovered while one is doing an aneurysm resection, the aneurysm resection should be done first unless the malignancy is preocclusive.

Long-term results of aneurysmectomy are excellent: the graft failure rate is low, and false aneurysm formation at the anastomoses is rare. The long-term survival of these patients is determined principally by their extent of coronary artery disease.

Endovascular Repair

Endovascular repair requires that the aorta proximal to the aneurysm have a cylindrical configuration for at least 1.5 cm and iliac arteries of sufficient size and have limited tortuosity. Devices for endovascular repair of AAAs are introduced through femoral arteriotomies using a system of guidewires and delivery systems with large-bore sheaths. Several devices are available with

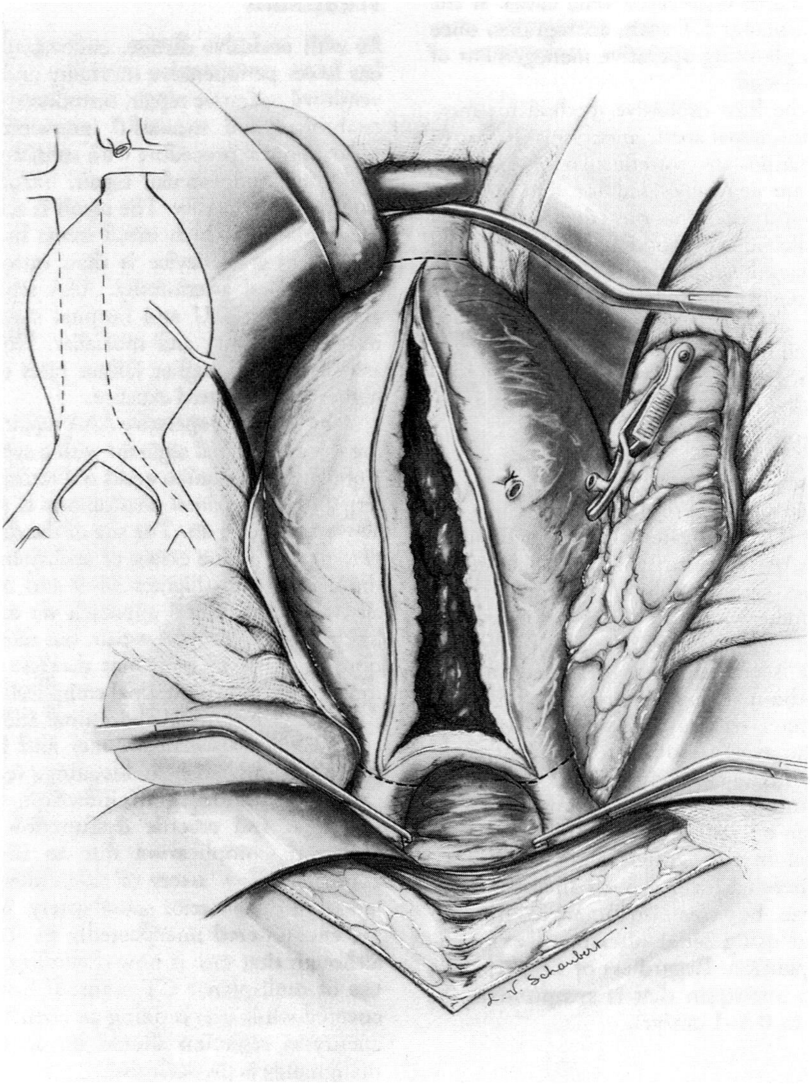

Figure 34–9. Exposure of an infrarenal abdominal aortic aneurysm. Arterial clamps are placed at the neck of the aneurysm below the left renal vein and on the common iliac arteries.

unique design features. The authors have the most experience with the Zenith Endograft (Cook), which guards against migration by aggressive fixation of the graft with bare metal stents extending above the renal arteries (Figure 34–11). In series of comparable patients, patients with endovascular repair have less operative blood loss, shorter hospital stays, and reduced operative morbidity compared to those undergoing conventional repair.

The most important intermediate or long-term adverse outcome is persistent perfusion of the aneurysm ("endoleak"). These are divided into types denoting clinical importance. A Type 1 endoleak denotes ineffective proximal or distal sealing with pressurization of the aneurysm sac and should be fixed immediately. A Type 2 endoleak results in persistent flow through the aneurysm between small aortic branches, usually from the inferior mesenteric

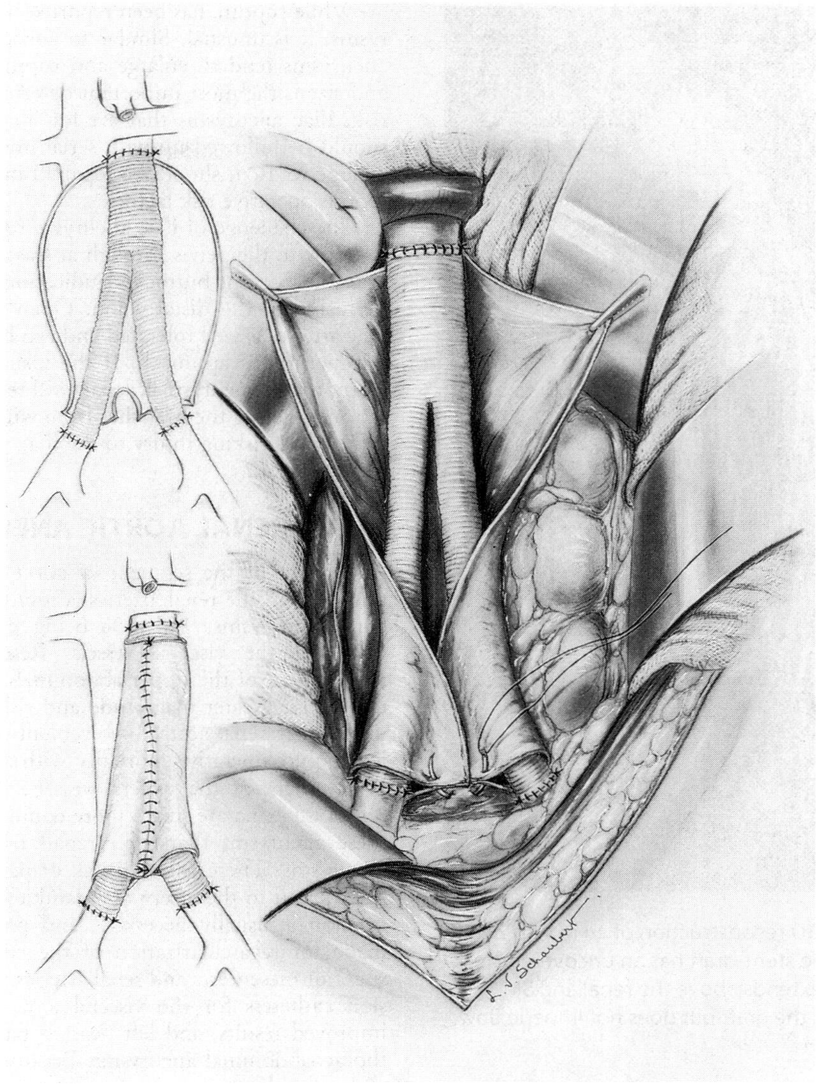

Figure 34–10. Replacement of an aortic aneurysm with a synthetic bifurcation graft. The laminated clot within the aneurysm has been removed and the outer wall is closed over the graft.

artery to a patent lumbar artery. These have relatively low pressures and, unless the aneurysm is enlarging, are not obliterated. Pressurization of the aneurysm through the graft itself is a Type 3 endoleak. The graft should be replaced if the aneurysm continues to enlarge over time.

Rupture has occurred after endovascular aortic aneurysm repair. The rate of late ruptures is low but underscores that patients need extended follow-up to ensure the durability of endovascular aneurysm repair. The devices are expensive (~$10-15,000). Add to this the cost of extended follow-up with CT scans to identify graft movement or endoleak, and endograft repair may be more expensive than open repair in spite of the lower periprocedural morbidity and shorter hospital stays.

ILIAC ANEURYSMS

Iliac artery aneurysms generally occur in conjunction with AAAs. Isolated iliac aneurysms are unusual (Figure

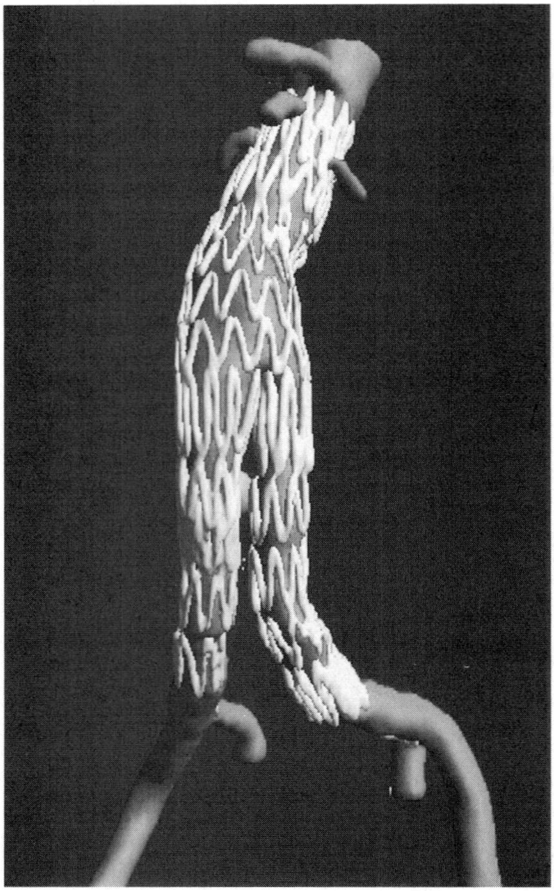

Figure 34–11. A 3D reconstruction of an in vivo Zenith graft. Note that the stent-graft has an uncovered stent component that extends above the renal and SMA arteries and secures the graft but does not impede flow.

34–12), but in some cases the iliac segment of the aneurysmal artery may enlarge at a greater rate than the aortic segment and is the primary reason for repair. As with aortic aneurysms, most iliac aneurysms are asymptomatic. However, they may present with symptoms related to compression or erosion of surrounding structures, such as obstructive uropathy with ureteral obstruction, neuropathy from compression of local nerves, and unilateral leg swelling from compression of the adjacent iliac vein.

Physical examination can suggest the diagnosis of large (> 4 cm) iliac artery aneurysms if the physician is alert to that possibility. Most symptomatic iliac aneurysms can be palpated as pulsatile masses on abdominal or rectal examinations. However, iliac aneurysms are usually found incidentally on ultrasound or CT.

While rupture has been reported in small iliac aneurysms, it is unusual. Similar to aortic aneurysms, iliac aneurysms tend to enlarge and rupture unpredictably, and size is the most important determinant for rupture risk. Iliac aneurysms that are less than 3.5 cm in size should be followed up with serial imaging. Those that enlarge to 4 cm should be repaired in patients without serious operative risk factors.

The challenge of iliac aneurysm repair is in preserving flow to the pelvis through at least one internal iliac artery to prevent buttock claudication, impotence, and perfusion of the distal colon. Open repair of isolated iliac arteries is well tolerated and can be done through a retroperitoneal approach. If the ipsilateral hypogastric artery is also aneurysmal, repair will require opening the sac and ligating the branches from within the aneurysm rather than risking injury to the iliac veins surrounding the aneurysm.

SUPRARENAL AORTIC ANEURYSMS

Aneurysms of the segment of aorta between the diaphragm and the renal arteries account for only 10% of aortic aneurysms, with 6% being pararenal and 4% involving the visceral vessels. Resection and graft replacement of the upper abdominal aorta is an operation of far greater magnitude and risk than operations on the infrarenal aorta. Involvement of the renal arteries doubles operative mortality with additional risk for involvement of the visceral vessels. Renal failure and bowel ischemia are much more common after repair of these aneurysms than after repair of infrarenal aortic aneurysms. There is also a risk of paraplegia if flow is interrupted to the artery of Adamkiewicz. An extended incision is usually necessary, and provisions must be made for revascularization of the celiac axis and the superior mesenteric and renal arteries. The use of perfusion catheters for the visceral and renal arteries has improved results, and left heart bypass is used in true thoracoabdominal aneurysms. Because of the mortality and morbidity of repair of suprarenal aneurysms, there has been considerable interest in endovascular repair of these aneurysms using branched systems. Initial reports have been encouraging from these technically demanding procedures.

RUPTURED AORTIC ANEURYSMS

With increasing aneurysm size, lateral pressure within the aneurysm will eventually lead to spontaneous rupture of the aneurysm wall. Although immediate exsanguination may ensue, there is often an interval of several hours between the first episode of bleeding and death from exsanguination. This initial bleed is contained in the periaortic, and later retroperitoneal tissues, and constitutes a "contained rupture." When the peri-

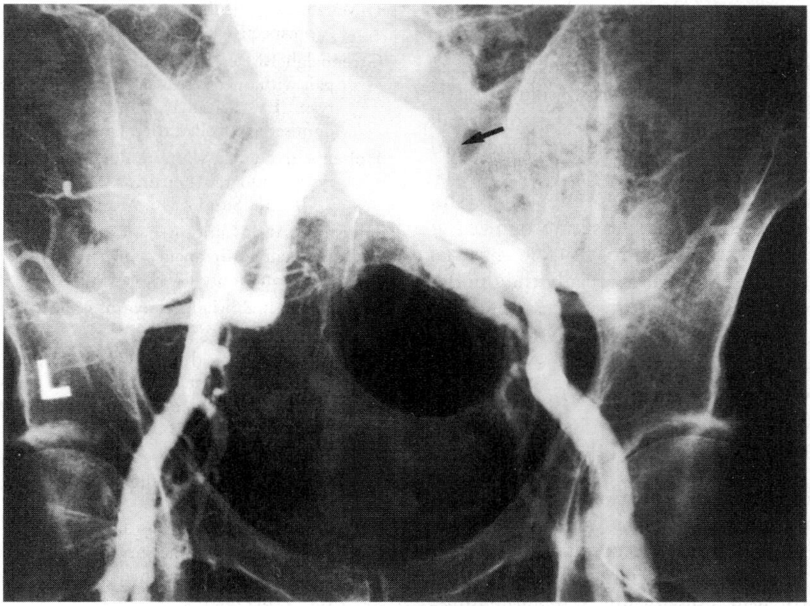

Figure 34–12. Arteriogram of isolated iliac artery aneurysm.

aortic tissue can no longer contain the expanding hematoma, "free rupture" occurs with exsanguination into the free peritoneal cavity.

Clinical Findings

The patient presents with sudden severe abdominal pain that usually radiates into the back and occasionally into the inguinal region. Lightheadedness or syncope results from blood loss. Pain may lessen and lightheadedness may disappear after the first hemorrhage, only to reappear and progress to shock if bleeding continues. When bleeding remains contained in the periaortic tissue, a discrete, pulsatile abdominal mass may be felt. In contrast with an intact aneurysm, the ruptured aneurysm at this stage is painful to palpation. Signs of an acute abdomen may be present. As bleeding continues—usually into the retroperitoneum, the discrete mass is replaced by a poorly defined mid-abdominal fullness, often extending toward the left flank.

Shock can be profound, manifested by peripheral vasoconstriction, hypotension, and anuria. Unfortunately, the classic triad of pain, a pulsatile abdominal mass, and hypotension is not always present, and precious time may be lost while confirming the diagnosis. An abdominal ultrasound performed in the emergency room will confirm the presence of an aortic aneurysm but may not disclose hemorrhage. CT scans reliably confirm hemorrhage from an aneurysm, but the delay in obtaining them usually precludes their use in unstable patients. It is best to follow the adage that a patient with an AAA, signs of an acute abdomen, and hypotension belongs in the operating room with the diagnosis to be confirmed by laparotomy.

Treatment & Prognosis

Laparotomy should be performed as soon as intravenous fluids have been started, the airway has been secured, and blood has been sent for crossmatching. Attempts to control the proximal aorta through the chest have been associated with poor outcomes. Control of the aorta proximal and distal to the aneurysm must be obtained immediately. A successful outcome of the operation is related to the patient's condition on arrival, the promptness of diagnosis, and the speed of operative control of bleeding and blood replacement. The operative death rate is between 30–80%, with an average of approximately 50%. Because many patients with ruptured aneurysms die before reaching the hospital, the overall death rate approaches 80%. Without operation, the outcome is uniformly fatal.

INFLAMMATORY ANEURYSMS

Inflammatory aneurysms are degenerative aneurysms that elicit a unique inflammatory response adjacent to the external calcified layer of the aneurysmal wall. Although similar to retroperitoneal fibrosis, the inflammation is usually confined to the anterior aorta and iliac arteries. The aneurysm is tender to palpation. One-fourth of patients have some degree of ureteral obstruction. CT scanning reliably demonstrates the characteristic thick wall and confirms the diagnosis. Characteristic pathologic changes include infiltration of the aortic wall by lymphocytes, plasma cells, occasional multinucleated giant cells, and lymphoid follicles with germinal centers. Inflammation resolves in most cases after successful repair. Inflammatory aneurysms are easily recognized at operation by the dense, shiny, white, fibrotic material that envelops the adjacent viscera, especially the duodenum, left renal vein, and inferior vena cava. Those structures therefore are especially vulnerable to operative injury. Endovascular repair is ideal and is the procedure of choice for inflammatory aneurysms.

INFECTED (MYCOTIC) ANEURYSMS

The confusing term "mycotic aneurysm" is commonly used to denote infected aneurysms in general, not just fungal infections. The aneurysm is secondary to a microbial aortitis, in which virulent bacteria infect the aorta and destroy the aortic wall. Historically, *Salmonella* infection was the most common cause. In the current era, staphylococcus is the more common infection due to intravenous drug use. These organisms may involve every major artery, but aortic involvement predominates.

The typical patient presents with a rapidly enlarging, tender pulsatile mass that may feel warm, if palpable. Fever is present, and half the patients have positive blood cultures. Alternatively, the aneurysm may be discovered late, after successful treatment of the infection. Angiography of these patients may show a *saccular* false aneurysm. Treatment consists of excision and remote bypass grafting if possible. Direct repair has been successful when done after a course of antibiotics. A prolonged course of antibiotics should be given to guard against recurrence.

Abraham CZ et al: A modular multi-branched system for endovascular repair of bilateral common iliac artery aneurysms. J Endovasc Ther 2003; 10:203.

Beebe HG et al: Results of an aortic endograft trial: impact of device failure beyond 12 months. J Vasc Surg 2001;33 (2 Suppl): S55.

Chuter TA et al: Multi-branched stent-graft for type III thoracoabdominal aortic aneurysm. J Vasc Interv Radiol 2001;12:391.

Curci JA et al: Preoperative treatment with doxycycline reduces aortic wall expression and activation of matrix metalloproteinases in patients with abdominal aortic aneurysms. J Vasc Surg 2000;31:342.

Dardik A et al: Results of elective abdominal aortic aneurysm repair in the 1990s: a population-based analysis of 2335 cases. J Vasc Surg 1999;30:985.

Dardik A et al: Surgical repair of ruptured abdominal aortic aneurysms in the state of Maryland: factors influencing outcome among 527 recent cases. J Vasc Surg 1998;28:413.

DiMarzo L et al: Inflammatory aneurysm of the abdominal aorta. A prospective clinical study. J Cardiovasc Surg 1999;40:407.

Greenhalgh RM et al: Comparison of endovascular aneurysm repair with open repair in patients with abdominal aortic aneurysm (EVAR trial 1), 30 day operative mortality results: randomised controlled trial. Lancet 2004;364:818.

Holzenbein T et al: Midterm durability of abdominal aortic aneurysm endograft repair: a word of caution. J Vasc Surg 2001;33(2 Suppl):S46.

Johnston KW: Multicenter prospective study of nonruptured abdominal aortic aneurysm: part II. Variables predicting morbidity and mortality. J Vasc Surg 1989;9:437.

Kanazawa S et al: Management of isolated iliac artery aneurysms. J Cardiovasc Surg 2000;41:513.

Lederle FA et al: Yield of repeated screening for abdominal aortic aneurysm after a 4-year interval. Aneurysm Detection and Management Veterans Cooperative Study Investigators. Arch Intern Med 2000;160:1117.

Lederle FA et al: Prevalence and associations of abdominal aortic aneurysm detected through screening. Ann Intern Med 1997;126:441.

Mortality results for randomized controlled trial of early elective surgery or ultrasonic surveillance for small abdominal aortic aneurysms. The UK Small Aneurysm Trial Participants. Lancet 1998;352:1649.

Rasmussen TE et al: Inflammatory aortic aneurysms. A clinical review with new perspectives in pathogenesis. Ann Surg 1997;225:155.

Safi HJ et al: Progress in the management of type I thoracoabdominal and descending thoracic aortic aneurysms. Ann Vasc Surg 1999;13:457.

Santilli SM et al: Expansion rates and outcomes for iliac artery aneurysms. J Vasc Surg 2000;31:114.

Scheinert D et al: Treatment of iliac artery aneurysms by percutaneous implantation of stent grafts. Circulation 2000;102(19 Suppl 3):III,253.

Smoking, lung function, and the prognosis of abdominal aortic aneurysm. The UK Small Aneurysm Trial Participants. Eur J Vasc Endovasc Surg 2000;19:636.

Sternbergh WC 3rd et al: Hospital cost of endovascular versus open repair of abdominal aortic aneurysms. J Vasc Surg 2000;31:237.

Zarins CK et al: The AneuRx stent graft: four-year results and worldwide experience 2000. J Vasc Surg 2001;33:5129.

PERIPHERAL ARTERIAL ANEURYSMS

Popliteal artery aneurysms account for 70% of peripheral arterial aneurysms. Like aortic aneurysms, they are silent until critically symptomatic. However, unlike aortic aneurysms, they rarely rupture. The presenting manifestations are due to peripheral embolization and thrombosis. Popliteal aneurysms may embolize repetitively over time and occlude distal arteries. Due to the redundant parallel arterial supply to the foot, ischemia does not occur until a final embolus occludes flow. Acute ischemia caused by popliteal aneurysms has a poor prognosis due to the chronicity of the process. Approximately one-third of patients will require an amputation. The results of both chemical and mechanical thrombolysis may be disappointing because of clot age and adherence to the artery wall. To prevent limb loss, popliteal artery aneurysms should be repaired if greater than 2 cm in diameter or if lined with thrombus at any size.

Primary aneurysms of the femoral artery are much less common than aneurysms of the popliteal artery. However, pseudoaneurysms of the femoral artery following arterial punctures for arteriography and cardiac catheterization occur with an incidence ranging from 0.05% to 6%. Thrombosis and embolization are the main risks of femoral true or false aneurysms and, like popliteal aneurysms, should be repaired when greater than 2 cm in diameter.

These same complications can occur in a rare anomaly, **persistence of the sciatic artery**. In this anomaly, the large embryonic sciatic artery originates from the internal iliac artery and communicates directly with the popliteal artery. Persistent sciatic arteries have a propensity for aneurysmal degeneration, presenting as painful, pulsatile buttock masses. There is no femoral artery. The diagnosis of a persistent sciatic artery is suggested by the absence of a femoral pulse with intact popliteal and pedal pulses. The prevalence is 0.25:1000 patients studied by angiography.

Clinical Findings

A. Symptoms and Signs

Until progressive stenosis or thrombosis occurs, peripheral artery aneurysms are usually asymptomatic. The patient may be aware of a pulsatile mass when the aneurysm is in the groin, but popliteal aneurysms are often undetected by the patient and physician. Peripheral aneurysms may produce symptoms by compressing the local vein or nerve, but this is unusual. In most patients, the first symptom is due to ischemia of acute arterial occlusion. The pathologic findings range from rapidly developing gangrene to moderate ischemia that slowly lessens as collateral circulation develops. Symptoms from recurrent embolization to the leg are often transient if they occur at all. Sudden ischemia may appear in a toe or part of the foot, followed by slow resolution, and the true diagnosis may be elusive. The onset of recurrent episodes of pain in the foot or hand, particularly if accompanied by cyanosis, suggests embolization and requires investigation of the heart and proximal arterial tree.

Because popliteal pulses are somewhat difficult to palpate even in normal individuals, a particularly prominent or easily felt pulse is suggestive of aneurysmal dilation and should be confirmed by ultrasound. Since popliteal aneurysms are bilateral in 60% of cases, the diagnosis of thrombosis of a popliteal aneurysm is often aided by the palpation of a pulsatile aneurysm in the contralateral popliteal space. Approximately 50% of patients with popliteal aneurysms have an aneurysmal abdominal aorta.

B. Imaging Studies

Arteriography may not demonstrate aneurysms accurately, because mural thrombus reduces the apparent diameter of the lumen. Nevertheless, arteriography is advised—especially when operation is considered—to define the status of the arteries distal to the aneurysm.

Duplex color ultrasound is the most efficient investigation to confirm the diagnosis of peripheral aneurysm, to measure its size and configuration, and to demonstrate mural thrombus.

Treatment

Early operation is indicated for any peripheral embolization, size greater than 2 cm or an aneurysm with mural thrombus. Immediate or urgent operation is indicated when acute embolization or thrombosis has caused acute ischemia. Intra-arterial thrombolysis may be done in the setting of acute ischemia, if examination (light touch) suggests that immediate surgery is not imperative. Bypass with saphenous vein may include either excision or exclusion, by proximal and distal ligation, depending upon location. If exclusion rather than resection is performed, the geniculate "feeder" arteries within the aneurysm must be ligated or progressive enlargement can still occur.

Acute pseudoaneurysms of the femoral artery due to arterial punctures can be successfully treated using ultrasound-guided compression. Open surgery with prosthetic interposition grafting is preferred for primary aneurysms of the femoral and popliteal arteries. Endovascular repair with small stent-grafts has been done but is reserved for high-risk patients.

Persistent sciatic artery aneurysms are treated by exclusion of the aneurysm by surgical or endovascular techniques and a femoral-popliteal bypass.

Prognosis

The long-term patency of bypass grafts for femoral and popliteal aneurysms is generally excellent but depends on the adequacy of the outflow tract. Late graft occlusion is less common than in similar operations for occlusive disease.

Diwan A et al: Incidence of femoral and popliteal aneurysms in patients with abdominal aortic aneurysms. J Vasc Surg 2000;31:863.

Duffy ST et al: Popliteal aneurysms: a 10-year experience. Eur J Vasc Endovasc Surg 1998;16:218.

Henry M et al: Percutaneous endovascular treatment of peripheral aneurysms. J Cardiovasc Surg 2000;41:871.

Levi N et al: Arteriosclerotic femoral artery aneurysms: a short review. J Cardiovasc 1997;38:335.

Steinmetz E et al: Preoperative intraarterial thrombolysis before surgical revascularization for popliteal artery aneurysm with acute ischemia. Ann Vasc Surg 2000;14:360.

UPPER EXTREMITY ANEURYSMS

Subclavian Artery Aneurysms

Subclavian artery aneurysms are less common than aneurysms of the lower extremity; most supraclavicular pulsatile masses represent tortuous vessels. Pseudoaneurysms due to injections by drug addicts are becoming increasingly frequent. An interesting anomaly, an aberrant right subclavian artery (incidence 0.5%), arises from the aorta distal to the left subclavian and courses behind the esophagus. As found in other aberrant arteries, enlargement is common and may compress the esophagus against the trachea and causing difficulty swallowing (termed dysphagia lusoria). This anomaly also is the most common cause of a nonrecurrent laryngeal nerve.

A true subclavian artery aneurysm is usually due to poststenotic dilation in a patient with thoracic outlet syndrome or a large callous from a fractured clavicle. As with popliteal aneurysms, the most common manifestations result from embolization. Treatment consists of resection of the restricting structures at the time of arterial replacement.

Radial Artery False Aneurysms

The incidence of radial artery false aneurysms has increased as a result of increasing use of radial artery catheters. Occasionally, the aneurysm is infected. If the Allen test is normal and adequate collateralization is confirmed with imaging, treatment consists of excision and ligation. If the ulnar collaterals are insufficient to preserve viability of the hand, excision and replacement with vein should be performed.

Cina CS et al: Kommerell's diverticulum and aneurysmal right-sided aortic arch: a case report and review of the literature. J Vasc Surg 2000;32;1208.

Gray RJ et al: Management of true aneurysms distal to the axillary artery. J Vasc Surg 1998;28:606.

Witz M et al: Subclavian artery aneurysms. A report of 2 cases and a review of the literature. J Cardiovasc Surg 1998;39:429.

EXTRACRANIAL CAROTID ARTERY ANEURYSMS

Aneurysms of the extracranial carotid arteries are rare. True aneurysms of the carotid are usually degenerative but occasionally may be caused by cystic medial necrosis, Marfan's syndrome, or fibromuscular dysplasia. False aneurysms may occur rarely after carotid endarterectomy, or as a result of trauma or infection. Pharyngeal abscess may cause false aneurysms of the carotid artery if not appropriately treated, and pharyngeal abscess drainage must be done realizing that the internal carotid artery is in close proximity.

Clinical Findings

A. Symptoms and Signs

In patients with a pulsatile neck mass, a coiled or redundant carotid or subclavian artery is the most common diagnosis and must be differentiated from aneurysm. On rare occasion, a carotid aneurysm protrudes into the oropharynx, where it produces symptoms of dysphagia. Pain from the aneurysm may radiate to the angle of the jaw. About 30% of patients will have had a transient neurologic event before presentation. Rupture is common with false aneurysms but rare with true aneurysms.

B. Imaging Studies

Duplex ultrasound can differentiate redundant and coiled arteries from aneurysms and should be used as the initial test. Doppler also is useful in demonstrating coexistent occlusive disease. Further imaging should be done if an aneurysm is found and is necessary to plan the operation. True aneurysms may be fusiform or saccular. False aneurysms assume bizarre shapes, depending on location and containment by neck tissues. Size, extent, and the presence of laminar thrombus can be best determined using CTA.

Treatment

Most accessible true aneurysms that are 2.5 to 3 times the proximal artery diameter should be resected and replaced with a PTFE or autogenous graft. All false aneurysms should be repaired. A large aneurysm extending to the skull base is best treated with a covered endovascular stent graft. Carotid ligation can be done safely if, after proximal clamping, the pressure in the internal carotid (*back pressure* from the circle of Willis) is greater than 65 mm Hg. Temporary carotid artery balloon occlusion can also be used to assess potential neurologic consequences during conscious arteriography. If the back pressure is low or the patient experiences neurologic symptoms during provocative temporary occlusion, a superficial temporal-to-middle cerebral bypass may be required at the time of internal carotid ligation.

El-Sabrout R et al: Extracranial carotid artery aneurysms: Texas Heart Institute experience. J Vasc Surg 2000;31:702.

May J et al: Endoluminal repair of internal carotid artery aneurysm: a feasible but hazardous procedure. J Vasc Surg 1997;26:1055.

Rosset E et al: Surgical treatment of extracranial internal carotid artery aneurysms. J Vasc Surg 2000;31:713.

Carotid Body Tumors

These unusual tumors cause pulsatile masses in the neck that on examination appear to be carotid aneurysms. The normal carotid body is a 3- to 6-mm nest of chemoreceptor cells of neuroectodermal origin located on the posterior medial side of the carotid bifurcation and responds to decreased oxygen tension and blood pH. Histologically, the tumors resemble the normal carotid body. While the tumor is capable of metastatic behavior, this only occurs in about 10% of cases. Extension into local structures is the most common complication.

A solitary midlateral pulsatile neck mass that is firm and rubbery should always suggest carotid body tumor. Because it is attached to the underlying artery, the mass is more mobile in the horizontal than the vertical plane. Bruits are present over the mass in about half of cases. Rarely, cranial nerve dysfunction occurs from tumor extension.

Angiography shows a characteristic tumor blush at the carotid bifurcation, with characteristic separation of the internal and external carotid arteries (Figure 34–13). Noninvasive color duplex scanning is also often diagnostic. Percutaneous needle biopsy or incisional biopsy is inaccurate and dangerous because of the risk of serious hemorrhage.

Complete excision—the preferred treatment—occasionally requires arterial reconstruction when the lesion is large and complex. Radiation therapy and chemotherapy have no value. Preoperative angiographic embolization of large tumors decreases vascularity but carries a risk of stroke; it is rarely employed. The incidence of cranial nerve injury from operative removal of carotid body tumors is high and increases with larger masses and prior attempts at resection.

Kohn JS et al: Familial carotid body tumors: a closer look. J Vasc Surg 1999;29:649.

Westerband A et al: Current trends in the detection and management of carotid body tumors. J Vasc Surg 1998;28:84.

VISCERAL ARTERY ANEURYSMS

The etiology of this interesting group of aneurysms is generally unknown. Most often they occur as single lesions in a younger age group than those at risk for aortic aneurysms. Rupture is the primary danger and is one cause of "abdominal apoplexy."

Splenic Artery Aneurysms

Aneurysms of the splenic artery account for more than 60% of splanchnic artery aneurysms. Women are affected four times more commonly than men and often during childbearing years. Arterial fibrodysplasia and portal hypertension predispose to formation of splenic artery aneurysms. Rupture, the major complication, has been reported in less than 2% of splenic aneurysms; it rarely occurs with lesions smaller than 2–3 cm in diameter. Rupture during pregnancy tends to occur in the third trimester and is associated with a 75% maternal death rate and 90% fetal death rate. Diagnosis is most often made from plain x-ray films of the abdomen, showing concentric calcification in the upper left quadrant.

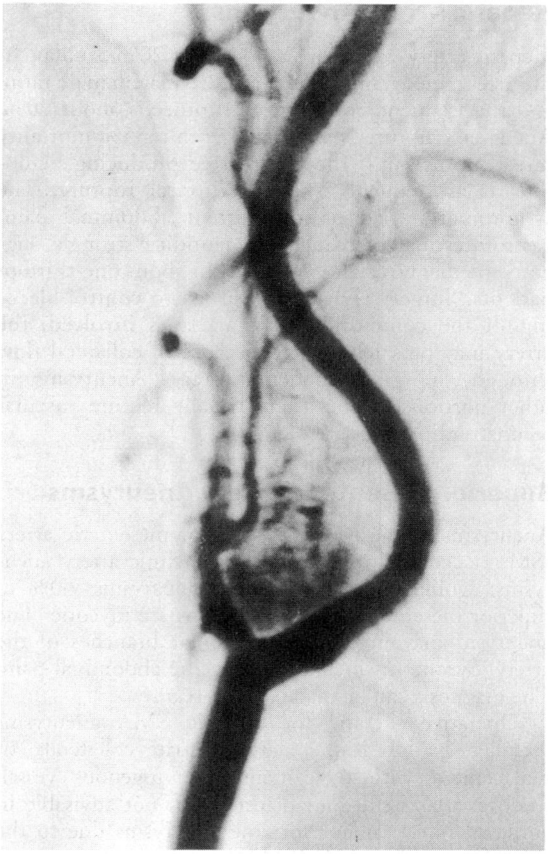

Figure 34–13. Carotid body tumor.

Operation is indicated for patients with symptomatic aneurysms, aneurysms in pregnant women, and patients who have a low operative risk profile and whose aneurysm is greater than 3 cm in diameter. Endovascular repair with covered stent grafts is ideal, but is limited by delivery of the device through the often tortuous splenic artery. Laparoscopic ligation of the artery is also feasible.

Hepatic Artery Aneurysms

Hepatic artery aneurysms account for 20% of splanchnic artery aneurysms. There is a 2:1 male:female ratio, and the frequency of reported rupture is about 20%. Aneurysm rupture is associated with a 35% mortality rate. Rupture into the biliary tree producing hemobilia is as frequent as intraperitoneal rupture. The symptomatic triad of intermittent abdominal pain, gastrointestinal bleeding, and jaundice strongly suggests the diagnosis and is present in about one-third of patients. Surgery is usually required to control bleeding. If the common hepatic artery is involved, the artery may be safely ligated because of collateral flow through the gastroduodenal artery. Aneurysms in other portions of the artery usually require vascular reconstruction.

Superior Mesenteric Artery Aneurysms

Aneurysms of the proximal superior mesenteric artery (SMA) account for 5% of all splanchnic artery aneurysms. Unlike splenic or hepatic aneurysms, 60% of superior mesenteric artery aneurysms are mycotic. The aneurysm may involve the origin or branches of the artery. Symptoms include nonspecific abdominal pain. The diagnosis can be made on CT scan.

Operative therapy for mycotic SMA aneurysms includes ligation if there are adequate collaterals, or replacement with a segment of autogenous vessel. Endovascular stent graft placement is not advisable in an acute infection nor for true aneurysms due to the risk of covering critical SMA branches proximal and distal to the aneurysm. For distal branch aneurysms, bowel resection may be necessary.

RENAL ARTERY ANEURYSMS

This uncommon aneurysm occurs in less than 0.1% of the population and is often associated with hypertension. The aneurysm is usually saccular and located at a primary or secondary bifurcation of the renal arteries. Women are affected slightly more frequently than men. There are three principal categories: (1) idiopathic, (2) aneurysms associated with medial fibrodysplastic disease, and (3) arteritis-related microaneurysms.

Most aneurysms are asymptomatic and are discovered on plain abdominal films or during an investigation of hypertension.

Renovascular hypertension may occur in 30% of patients due to distortion of the involved or nearby vessels by the aneurysm. Spontaneous rupture of renal artery aneurysms is rare except during pregnancy. Bleeding may tamponade in Gerota's fascia, but nephrectomy is recommended. Emboli from the aneurysm to the distal renal vessels occur rarely. Renal artery aneurysms that are small relative to the vessel involved can be managed nonoperatively if blood pressure is controlled. CT scans or digital subtraction angiography should be performed to monitor enlargement. Operation is indicated in women of childbearing age or in patients with associated renal artery disease, uncontrolled hypertension, or large aneurysms. Most renal artery aneurysms can be repaired in situ, but ex vivo repair is occasionally required.

Area MJ et al: Splenic artery aneurysms: methods of laparoscopic repair. J Vasc Surg 1999;30:184.

Carr SC et al: Visceral artery aneurysm rupture. J Vasc Surg 2001; 33:806.

Dave SP et al: Splenic artery aneurysm in the 1990s. Ann Vasc Surg 2000;14:223.

Messina LM et al: Visceral artery aneurysms. Surg Clin North Am 1997;77:425.

VASOCONSTRICTIVE DISORDERS

Vasoconstrictive disorders are characterized by abnormal activity of the sympathetic nervous system that reduces peripheral blood flow, causing tissue ischemia.

Raynaud's disease/syndrome consists of sequential pallor, cyanosis, and rubor of fingers or toes after exposure to cold. Excessive vasoconstriction, sluggish flow, and reflex vasodilation produce the characteristic white-blue-red color changes. Raynaud's disease, this response without underlying arterial lesions, is quite common and benign.

Sudden onset or progression of symptoms suggests underlying arterial lesions that exaggerate the reduction in blood flow caused by vasoconstriction. This is termed Raynaud's phenomenon, a more virulent entity, associated primarily with immunologic and connective tissue disorders (eg, scleroderma, systemic lupus erythematosus, polymyositis, or drug-induced vasculitis). However, other disorders, occupational trauma (vibration injury, cold injury), and other disorders (cold agglutinins, chronic renal failure, and neoplasia) also have been reported. Repeated microembolization to the hand may present with Raynaud's phenomenon.

Hyperreactivity to cold stimuli may be the initial presentation of arterial pathology. In new-onset or severe cases of Raynaud's-type symptoms, a search for underlying pathology is required. All patients with Raynaud's syndrome should avoid cold exposure, tobacco, oral contraceptives, beta-adrenergic blocking agents, and ergotamine preparations. Calcium-channel blockers are generally prescribed but may cause hypotension. Transdermal prostaglandins, ketanserin, and cilostazol also have been used, with relief of symptoms in some patients. In rare cases symptoms progress to tissue loss. Finger amputation is necessary once gangrene has developed.

Acrocyanosis is a common chronic, benign vasoconstrictive disorder related to Raynaud's syndrome that is largely restricted to young females. It is characterized by persistent cyanosis of the hands and feet. The changes disappear with exposure to a warm environment. Examination in a cool room shows diffuse symmetric cyanosis, coldness, and occasionally hyperhidrosis of the hands and feet. Cyanosis of the skin of the calf, thigh, or forearm usually displays a reticulated pattern and has been called **livedo reticularis** and **cutis marmorata**. The peripheral pulses may diminish in the cold but return to normal with rewarming.

Gasbanini A et al: *Helicobacter pylori* eradication ameliorates primary Raynaud's phenomenon. Dig Dis Sci 1998;43:1641.

Knapid-Kordecka M et al: Clinical spectrum of Raynaud's phenomenon in patients referred to a vascular clinic. Cardiovasc Surg 2000;8:457.

Maricq HR et al: An objective method to estimate the severity of Raynaud phenomenon: digital blood pressure response to cooling. Vasc Med 1998;3:109.

McLafferty RB et al: Raynaud's syndrome in workers who use vibrating pneumatic air knives. J Vasc Surg 1999;30:1.

Melone CP Jr et al: Surgical management of the hand in scleroderma. Curr Opin Rheumatol 1999;11:514.

REFLEX SYMPATHETIC DYSTROPHY

The pathophysiology of posttraumatic pain syndromes remains poorly understood. A number of terms are used to refer to the same condition, including causalgia, posttraumatic sympathetic dystrophy, Sudeck's atrophy, shoulder-hand syndrome, traumatic neuralgia, and Mitchell's causalgia. Reflex sympathetic dystrophy occurs with equal frequency in the upper and lower extremities and in men and women. The type or severity of the initial injury does not predict the development of this syndrome.

The most distinctive and dramatic feature of the syndrome is severe pain. It is a burning pain involving the entire hand or foot. The slightest stimuli can produce a sudden increase in the severity of pain. Pain with increased sympathetic nervous system activity characterizes the syndrome. Marked vasoconstriction causes the extremity to become cold, cyanotic, and moist. If left untreated, the limb shows dystrophy, and atrophy.

Initial management consists of a diagnostic sympathetic block with local anesthetic agents. This is successful in relieving pain in the majority of cases. If the patient has long-lasting relief after the block, it should be repeated, as this alone will result in a permanent cure in about one-third of patients. Surgical sympathectomy is indicated for patients who have only short-lived pain relief after sympathetic blockade. Spinal cord stimulation and intrathecal baclofen may also provide temporary (sometimes permanent) pain relief.

Ciccone DS et al: Psychological dysfunction in patients with reflex sympathetic dystrophy. Pain 1997;71:323.

Kemler MA et al: Spinal cord stimulation in patients with chronic reflex sympathetic dystrophy. N Engl J Med 2000;343:618.

Schwartzman RJ: New treatments for reflex sympathetic dystrophy. N Engl J Med 2000;343:654.

van Hilten BJ et al: Intrathecal baclofen for the treatment of dystonia in patients with reflex sympathetic dystrophy. N Engl J Med 2000;343;6256.

THORACIC OUTLET SYNDROME

The term thoracic outlet syndrome refers to the variety of disorders caused by abnormal compression of arterial, venous, or neural structures in the base of the neck. Numerous mechanisms for compression have been described, including cervical rib, anomalous ligaments, hypertrophy of the scalenus anticus muscle, and positional changes that alter the normal relation of the first rib to the structures that pass over it. Patients may describe a history of cervical trauma.

Symptoms rarely develop until adulthood. For this reason, it has been assumed that an alteration of normal structural relationships that occurs with advancing years is the primary factor. Even anomalous cervical ribs seem well tolerated during childhood and adolescence.

Inclusion of these syndromes in discussions of vascular disease originates from a former view that many of the symptoms were the result of intermittent compression of the subclavian or axillary arteries. This assumption was reinforced by the frequent finding that certain postural manipulations could produce depression of the radial pulse. The present view holds that whereas transient circulatory changes may indeed occur, the primary cause of symptoms in most patients is intermittent compression of one or more trunks of the brachial plexus. Thus, neurologic symptoms predominate over those of ischemia or venous compression. However, compression of the subclavian artery and vein in the thoracic outlet also can produce severe sequelae. Compression of the subclavian artery can produce stenosis and reflex poststenotic dilation of the artery, leading to arterial occlusion or emboli, as discussed above. Compression of the vein can produce thrombosis, which can result in severe upper extremity pain and swelling. Compression may be exaggerated with exercise precipitating an occlusion. This syndrome is termed effort thrombosis or Paget-Schroetter syndrome.

Clinical Findings

A. Symptoms and Signs

Neural symptoms consist of pain, paresthesias, or numbness in the distribution of one or more trunks of the brachial plexus (usually in the ulnar distribution). Most patients associate their symptoms with certain positions of the shoulder girdle. These may occur from prolonged hyperabduction, as in house painters, hairdressers, and truck drivers. Others may relate their symptoms to the downward traction of the shoulder girdle produced by carrying heavy objects. Numbness of the hands often wakes the patient from sleep. On physical examination, motor deficits are rare and usually indicate severe compression of long duration. Muscular atrophy may be present in the hand. The radial pulse can be weakened by abduction of the arm with the head rotated to the opposite side **(Adson's test)**, though pulse reduction by this maneuver often occurs in completely asymptomatic persons. Light percussion over the brachial plexus in the supraclavicular fossa produces peripheral sensations **(Tinel's test)** and reproduces the symptoms in patients with chronic neurologic impingement.

Arterial symptoms are less common and often the result of emboli. A bruit may be heard over the subclavian artery with abduction of the arm, but this is not a specific finding. Venous occlusion results in unilateral arm swelling. There are good collaterals around the shoulder girdle, but symptoms may be debilitating in young active patients.

B. Diagnosis

Neurogenic thoracic outlet compression must be differentiated from other disorders that mimic this condition (eg, carpal tunnel syndrome and cervical disk disease). Cervical x-rays and peripheral nerve conduction studies are not diagnostic but are valuable to eliminate other possibilities. Unfortunately, there is no recognized objective study to unequivocally confirm the diagnosis of neurogenic thoracic outlet syndrome. Arteriograms may demonstrate subclavian or axillary artery stenosis when the arm is in abduction. This finding is not diagnostic, but poststenotic dilation of the artery is distinctly abnormal and indicates a definite lesion.

Treatment

Most patients benefit from postural correction and a physical therapy program directed toward restoring the normal relation and strength of the structures in the shoulder girdle. Surgical techniques for decompression of the thoracic outlet are reserved for patients who have not responded after 3–6 months of conservative treatment. Some surgeons prefer transaxillary first rib resection, while others prefer a supraclavicular approach. With either operation, the anterior scalene muscle and any associated fibrous bands should be excised.

Symptomatic arterial stenoses require decompression of the thoracic outlet in combination with arterial reconstruction. Effort thrombosis of the subclavian vein is usually best treated by catheter-directed thrombolysis of the venous occlusion followed by thoracic outlet decompression with or without operative venous reconstruction or intraluminal stent placement. Insertion of intraluminal venous stents without rib resection is ineffective because the stents themselves are compressed and narrowed by the underlying anatomy.

Angle N et al: Safety and efficacy of early surgical decompression of the thoracic outlet for Paget-Schroetter syndrome. Ann Vasc Surg 2001;15:37.

Kreienberg PB et al: Long-term results in patients treated with thrombolysis, thoracic inlet decompression, and subclavian vein stenting for Paget-Schroetter syndrome. J Vasc Surg 2001;33:5100.

Sharp WJ et al: Long-term follow-up and patient satisfaction after surgery for thoracic outlet syndrome. Ann Vasc Surg 2001;15:32.

Wilbourn AJ: Thoracic outlet syndromes. Neurol Clin 1999;17:477.

ARTERIOVENOUS FISTULAS

Arteriovenous fistulas, often called "malformations," may be congenital or acquired. Abnormal communications between arteries and veins occur in many diseases and affect vessels of all sizes and in many locations. In congenital fistulas, the systemic effect is often not great, because although the communications may be multiple, they are small. The effects of AV fistulas depend upon their size and location—for example, when a limb is involved, extensive A-V communications may exist with increased flow and increased muscle mass and bone length.

Acquired fistulas are usually the result of trauma, violent or iatrogenic. Spontaneous fistulas are uncommon. These communications can have considerable flow and high-output heart failure can occur. Surgically created fistulas for hemodialysis access are a unique class of AF fistulas.

Arteriovenous malformations in the gastrointestinal tract may cause hemorrhage. Osler-Weber-Rendu disease or syndrome (also termed hereditary hemorrhagic telangiectasia) is an autosomal dominant disorder characterized by gastrointestinal bleeding and epistaxis due to large arteriovenous anomalies in the gastrointestinal tract and lungs. Pulmonary lesions cause recirculation with lower PO_2, polycythemia, clubbing, and cyanosis.

Penetrating injuries either from trauma or iatrogenic ones from arterial punctures are the most common causes of acquired fistulas. Blunt trauma, erosion of an atherosclerotic or mycotic arterial aneurysm into adjacent veins, communication with an arterial prosthetic graft, or neoplastic invasion can all cause AV fistulas as well. When large vessels are involved, the presentation is dramatic. For example, an aortic aneurysm can rupture into the inferior vena cava. These large fistulas enlarge rapidly and result in cardiac dilation and failure when shunting is excessive.

AV Fistula for Hemodialysis

A successful AV fistula for hemodialysis access requires a large vein (≥ 5 mm) that lies close to the skin for at least 20 cm. The cephalic vein is ideal for this purpose, and radial artery to cephalic vein AV fistula **(Cimino fistula)** is the classic hemodialysis access fistula. If no suitable vein is available for an autogenous fistula, prosthetic grafts are used, most commonly of PTFE. These are most commonly placed subcutaneously in a loop configuration. The poor patency rates of these grafts, 40% at 2 years, and potential for infection, have driven national guidelines to encourage a higher rate of autogenous fistula formation. To maximize autogenous vein utilization, current practice includes transposing deep veins such as the basilic vein in the upper arm to the subcutaneous tissue. All veins used for access require "arterialization" of the wall, which takes at least 6 weeks prior to cannulization for dialysis. Transposed veins may take even longer to mature.

Flow rates of 300 cc/min or greater are necessary for efficient dialysis. Patients with a newly created AV access should be watched carefully for arterial steal and distal ischemia. Diabetics are the most vulnerable to this complication due to calcified proximal arteries or intrinsic arterial lesions of the hand. High-output cardiac failure does not occur.

Clinical Findings

A. Symptoms and Signs

A typical continuous machinery murmur can be heard over most acquired arteriovenous fistulas and is often associated with a palpable thrill and locally increased skin temperature. Proximally, the arteries and veins dilate and the pulse distal to the lesion diminishes. There may be signs of venous insufficiency, coolness, and hypertrophy distal to the communication on the involved extremity. Tachycardia occurs in some patients as a feature of increased cardiac output. When the fistula is occluded by compression, the pulse rate slows **(Branham's sign)**.

In contrast, venous malformations rarely produce hemodynamic effects. In this disorder, the presence of a mass, which may or may not be tender, is the principal finding. Because flow rates are low, bruits and thrills are absent.

B. Imaging Studies

MRI has become the imaging study of choice for the evaluation and follow-up of peripheral arteriovenous malformations, but CTA also gives excellent anatomic information. Precise delineation of arteriovenous fistulas can be done with selective arteriograms.

Treatment

Not all arteriovenous connections require treatment. Most venous malformations should be treated conservatively. In addition, small peripheral fistulas may be observed and will often remain asymptomatic. Some are surgically inaccessible.

The indications for intervention include hemorrhage, local expansion, severe venous or arterial insufficiency, cosmetic deformity, and heart failure.

Most fistulas are now managed by embolization under radiographic control. The embolic material used includes blood clot, glass beads, Gelfoam, and muscle. Arteriovenous malformations of the head and neck and of the pelvis appear particularly well suited for this form of therapy. Direct injection of sclerosant compounds into venous malformations under fluoroscopic control also has been successful.

Surgical options are generally reserved for large acquired fistulas. Covered stent grafts are now being used for a variety of traumatic fistulas. Surgery should be avoided in most cases of congenital arteriovenous malformations, as cure requires en bloc resection of all tissue involved. When the fistulous connections involve substantial portions of an extremity, local ligation is invariably followed by recurrence, and only temporary palliation can be expected.

Prognosis

The results of therapy vary according to the extent, location, and type of fistula. In general, traumatic fistulas have the most favorable prognosis. Congenital fistulas are more difficult to eradicate, due to the numerous arteriovenous connections usually present.

Hisamatsu K et al: Peripheral arterial coil embolization for hepatic arteriovenous malformation in Osler-Weber-Rendu disease. Intern Med 1999;38:962.

Iqbal M et al: Pulmonary arteriovenous malformations: a clinical review. Postgrad Med J 2000;76:390.

Jacobowitz GR et al: Transcatheter embolization of complex pelvic vascular malformations: results and long-term follow-up. J Vasc Surg 2001;33:51.

Mattle HP et al: Dilemmas in the management of patients with arteriovenous malformations. J Neurol 2000;247:917.

Mulliken JB et al: Vascular anomalies. Curr Probl Surg 2000;37:517.

White RI Jr et al: Long-term outcome of embolotherapy and surgery for high-flow extremity arteriovenous malformations. J Vasc Interv Radiol 2000;11:1285.

CEREBROVASCULAR DISEASE

ESSENTIALS OF DIAGNOSIS

- *Episodic motor and sensory dysfunction; unilateral vision loss, stroke; aphasia, and ataxia.*
- *Cervical arterial bruits, pulse deficits, or blood pressure differences in the arms.*
- *Duplex ultrasound confirmation of carotid stenosis.*
- *Selective MRA, CTA or arteriography.*

General Considerations

Symptoms of extracranial cerebrovascular disease are most often the result of emboli and less often the result of hypoperfusion. Arterial emboli account for approximately one-quarter of strokes in Europe and North America, and 80% of these originate from atherosclerotic lesions in a surgically accessible artery in the neck or mediastinum (Figures 34–14, 34–15, and 34–16). The most common lesion is at the bifurcation of the carotid artery. Transcranial Doppler (TCD) studies have shown that the cerebral cortex with its extensive collateral network can tolerate multiple microemboli before developing local ischemia. Emboli are seen on TCD in approximately 20% of patients with moderate (> 50% stenosis) lesions at the carotid bifurcation. The incidence and frequency of emboli is dramatically increased in recently symptomatic patients. Thus, **transient ischemic attacks** (TIAs) and strokes from emboli may not be single events but multiple small emboli that obliterate the collateral reserve of the cerebral cortex.

Characteristically, lesions of atherosclerosis in the internal carotid artery occur along the wall of the carotid bulb opposite to the external carotid artery. The enlargement of the bulb just distal to this major branch point creates an area of low wall shear stress, flow separation, and loss of unidirectional flow. Presumably this allows greater interaction of atherogenic particles and the vessel walls at this site.

Since most microemboli originate from a lesion in the internal carotid artery, neurologic dysfunction is confined to the carotid territory and may appear as

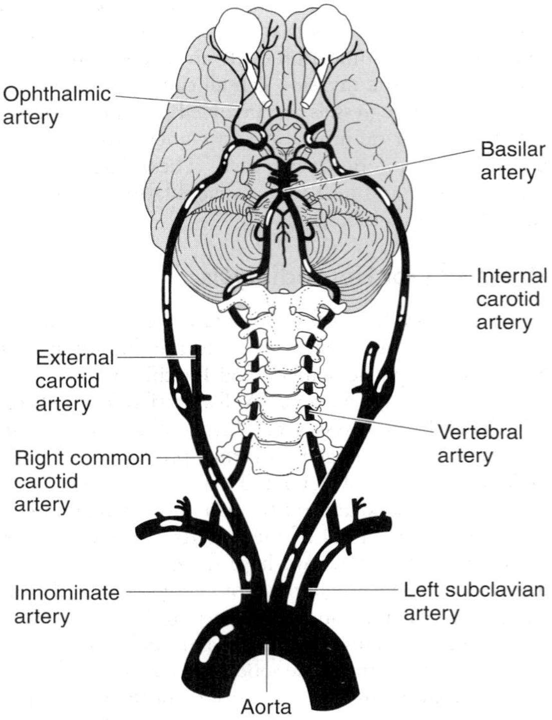

Figure 34–14. Diagram of arterial blood supply to the eyes and brain.

"short-lived" paresis or numbness of the contralateral arm or leg. This is a transient ischemic attack. The onset is swift, and most TIAs are brief (minutes). By convention, 24 hours is the arbitrary limit of a TIA. A microembolus to the ophthalmic artery, the first branch of the internal carotid artery, produces a temporary monocular loss of vision called **amaurosis fugax**. Emboli may be visible as small bright flecks **(Hollenhorst plaques)** lodged in arterial bifurcations in the retina.

Without treatment, over 30% of patients with TIAs will eventually develop permanent neurologic impairment either from dislodgement of a macroembolus or thrombotic occlusion of the internal carotid artery. The risk of stroke is lower (20%) for patients presenting with amaurosis fugax.

Clinical Findings

A. Symptoms

Patients with cerebrovascular disease can be grouped into five categories based on symptoms at presentation.

1. Asymptomatic disease—An audible bruit heard in the neck may be the only manifestation of cerebrovascu-

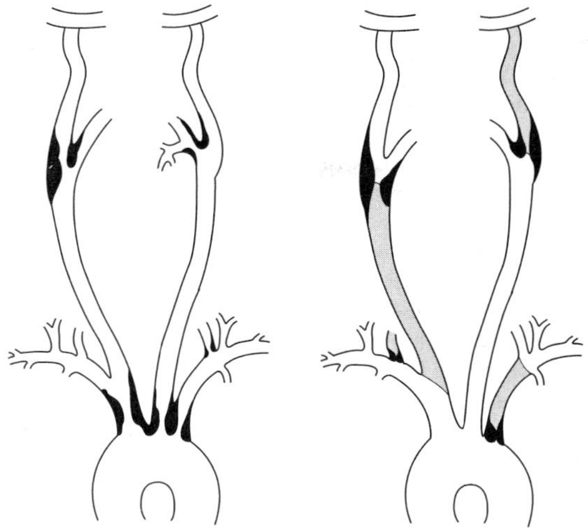

Figure 34–15. Diagram showing common sites of stenosis and occlusion of the extracranial cerebral vasculature.

lar disease. Severe carotid stenosis may also occur in the absence of a bruit with markedly reduced blood flow. Ultrasound screening also can identify these patients.

2. Transient neurologic or visual episodes—Symptoms depend upon the ischemic area of the brain; size of the embolus, and the condition of collaterals to the affected area. Hypoperfusion less commonly causes transient neurologic and visual attacks. In symptomatic patients, stroke risk after TIA correlates with severity of internal carotid artery stenosis.

3. Acute unstable neurologic deficits—Patients in this category have multiple (crescendo) TIAs, stroke in evolution, or waxing and waning neurologic deficits. These patients must be treated urgently, as even with anticoagulation over half of these patients will progress to completed stroke.

4. Stroke—Intervention is indicated for patients after stroke who have mild to moderate deficits, as over one-half will suffer another stroke with further loss of neural function. The timing of intervention is controversial. If the infarct is large, a healing period prior to revascularization may be advisable to prevent hemorrhage into the necrotic area. In these patients the risk of stroke with intervention is higher than in patients post TIA.

5. Vertebrobasilar disease—In the posterior circulation, emboli are less common and hypoperfusion is the dominant pathology. Reduction of flow in the vertebral and basilar arteries causes drop attacks, clumsiness, and a variety of sensory phenomena. Frequently, the symptoms are bilateral. Vertigo, diplopia, dysphagia, or dysequilibrium occurring *individually* is rarely due to vertebrobasilar disease, but when these symptoms occur in combination the diagnosis becomes more likely. It is unusual for dizziness alone to be due to cerebrovascular disease.

B. Signs

Auscultation of the carotid and subclavian arteries may delineate the sites of hemodynamically significant dis-

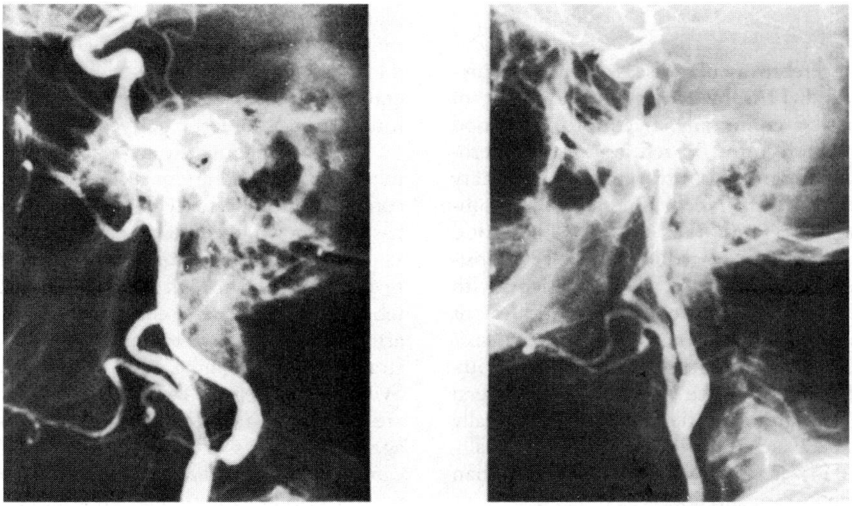

Figure 34–16. *Left:* Preoperative carotid arteriogram showing stenosis of the proximal internal carotid artery. *Right:* Postoperative carotid arteriogram showing restoration of normal luminal size following endarterectomy.

ease. However, bruits are nonspecific findings correlating more with overall risk for cardiovascular disease than with stroke. Pulse deficits are unusual in the neck but common in the arms. Although there is little chance that palpation will release an embolus, it should be confined to the lower neck in symptomatic patients.

C. Noninvasive Tests

The most useful test for the diagnosis of extracranial carotid artery disease is the duplex ultrasound. Imaging demonstrates plaque morphology, whereas Doppler spectral velocity analysis determines the degree of stenosis rapidly and accurately. New color-flow duplex devices have further improved the utility of this technology.

Determination of the degree of luminal narrowing is based on velocity criteria. As the stenosis encroaches on the lumen of the vessel, the velocity of blood increases in the area of the stenosis to maintain distal flow. Ultrasound is better than arteriography and at least as accurate as MRA at determining severe to critical stenosis, and many clinicians now recommend intervention based solely on color-duplex scanning.

D. Imaging Studies

Cerebral arteriography is performed in many patients with symptomatic and asymptomatic cerebrovascular disease who are candidates for surgery. Arteriography is invasive and has a low but significant risk of stroke (0.5–1.0%). Preoperative studies are now commonly done with MRA, which is minimally invasive and gives excellent delineation of the anatomy from aortic arch to intracranial arteries. Multiplanar CTA also is used for this purpose.

Treatment

The treatment of cerebrovascular disease focuses on preventing strokes and TIAs by removing the source of atheroemboli or, less commonly, by improving blood flow. Carotid endarterectomy, ie, removal of the atherosclerotic lesion at the carotid bifurcation, is the primary operation performed. In the North American Symptomatic Carotid Endarterectomy Trial (NASCET), carotid endarterectomy was shown to reduce incidence of ipsilateral stroke from 26% to 9% at 2 years in patients with presenting with either TIA or stroke and carotid lesions of 70% stenosis or greater. The results also favored surgery in patients with moderate carotid stenosis (50–69%), but less dramatically. The 5-year risk of ipsilateral stroke was 15.7% among patients treated surgically (n = 1108) and 22.2% among those treated medically (n = 1118; $P = .045$). Patients with stenoses of less than 50% did not benefit from surgery.

Large clinical trials have also shown a benefit of surgery for asymptomatic carotid stenosis. Both the Asymptomatic Carotid Atherosclerosis Study (ACAS) in North America and the Asymptomatic Carotid Surgery Trial in Europe showed that stroke incidence is halved (12% to 6%) by carotid endarterectomy versus best medical therapy, which included antiplatelet agents, in patients with substantial carotid narrowing at 5 years of follow-up. While ACAS did not show a benefit for endarterectomy in women, the larger European study did.

Stenting of the carotid artery has shown promise with the introduction of protection devices, devices placed in the internal carotid artery during stenting to filter the debris released by plaque manipulation. Stenting has already become the primary treatment option for occlusive lesions of the origins of the arch vessels and for lesions that recur after treatment. Stenting appears to offer similar protection from stroke and reduced periprocedural morbidity for high-risk patients. It is currently the subject of a large randomized trial (CREST) to determine its place for patients judged to be candidates for endarterectomy. The early results from CREST have shown that stenting has a higher morbidity in patients over 80 years of age.

For lesions not amenable to stenting due to tortuosity or calcification, endarterectomy also is the preferred technique for the removal of lesions of the proximal vertebral artery (Figure 34–17). Proximal stenoses of the carotid and subclavian arteries can be managed by transplanting the obstructed artery (after thromboendarterectomy) to the side of the adjacent patent artery. A prosthetic graft can also be placed between the subclavian and common carotid arteries beyond the stenosis or occlusion (subclavian-carotid bypass).

As noted above, caution must be exercised when planning intervention after a completed stroke. If the infarct on MRI is relatively small, urgent treatment has a low risk of worsening the deficit or creating an intracranial hemorrhage. However, with a large infarct, intervention should be delayed approximately 6 weeks.

Thromboendarterectomy cannot be performed when the internal carotid artery is completely occluded, because complete thrombectomy is not possible and residual clot has been shown to embolize.

The **subclavian steal syndrome** is characterized by reversal of flow through the vertebral artery, ie, the vertebral artery serves as a collateral to supply blood to the arm. While this *anatomic* arrangement is often demonstrated on angiograms, clinical sequelae are very rare. Symptoms of effort fatigue in the involved extremity are more common than neurologic complaints. Management consists of bypass grafting from the common carotid to the subclavian artery distal to the lesion, or transposition of the subclavian artery beyond the lesion to the side of the nearby common carotid artery.

When patients have coexistent severe **coronary and carotid atherosclerosis** requiring treatment, there has

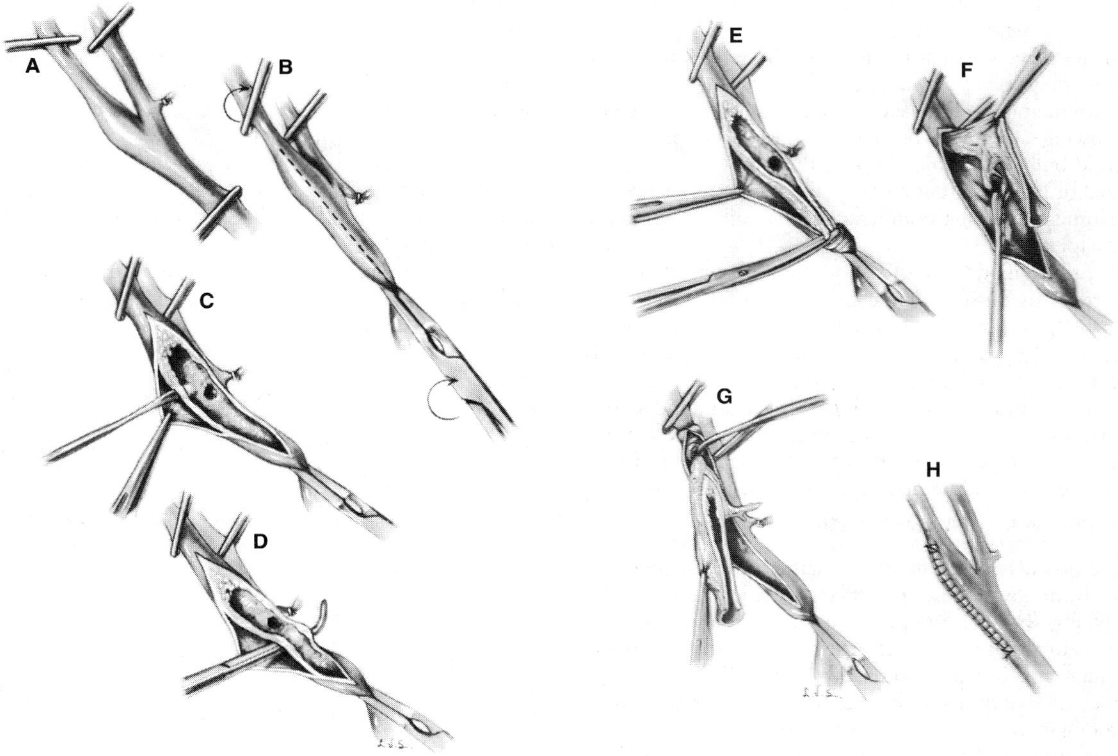

Figure 34–17. Technique of carotid endarterectomy. The common, internal, and external carotid arteries are occluded ***(A)***, and a longitudinal arteriotomy is created ***(B)***. Plaque is removed ***(C–F)*** with careful attention to achieve a smooth end point ***(G)***. The arteriotomy is closed, using continuous suture technique ***(H)***.

been controversy as to which lesion should be addressed first. Since most strokes during cardiac procedures are from atheromatous emboli from the aortic arch, not from low flow through a carotid stenosis, our policy has been to perform combined procedures only in patients with symptomatic carotid stenosis or when critical bilateral asymptomatic stenoses occur. Stenting of the coronary and carotid stenoses would obviously be preferable if the lesions were appropriate for this procedure. Carotid stenting in these high-risk patients should be done with an anesthesia team in attendance.

Other Causes of Cerebrovascular Symptoms

Other than atherosclerosis, primary disease of the extracranial arteries is rare.

A. Takayasu's (Giant Cell) Arteritis

Takayasu's arteritis is an obliterative arteriopathy principally involving the aortic arch vessels that often affects young women. The pararenal abdominal aorta and pulmonary arteries also may be affected. High-dose corticosteroids and cyclophosphamide have been shown to arrest and in some cases reverse the progress of the disease. Operative treatment of nonspecific arteritis should be avoided when the arteritis is active, but it may be successful in quiescent disease.

B. Dissecting Aortic Aneurysms

Dissecting aortic aneurysms may extend into the arch branches, producing obstruction and cerebral symptoms. These are discussed in Chapter 19, Part I.

C. Internal Carotid Dissection

Dissection originating in the internal carotid artery and localized to its extracranial segment occurs as an acute event that may narrow or obliterate the internal carotid lumen. The primary lesion is an intimal tear at the distal end of the carotid bulb. It may follow various types of neck trauma or, more commonly, severe hypertension. Dissection may also develop spontaneously, most frequently in young adults.

Cerebral symptoms are the result of ischemia in the ipsilateral hemisphere. Acute neck pain in association with localized cervical tenderness adjacent to the angle of the mandible is a frequent finding.

Arteriography shows a characteristic pattern of tapered narrowing at or just beyond the distal portion of the carotid bulb. The lumen beyond this point may be obliterated or may persist as a barely visible narrow shadow. If the lumen persists, it resumes a normal caliber beyond the bony foramen.

Anticoagulation is the treatment of choice for this disorder. In most patients, the intramural clot will be resorbed, restoring a normal lumen. Intervention is indicated for patients with recurrent TIAs. Stenting is the procedure of choice and will restore the normal carotid contour. If stenting is not successful and symptoms persist, ligation can be performed if the carotid back pressure exceeds 65 mm Hg. Extracranial to intracranial bypass will be needed if the pressure is low.

D. Fibromuscular Dysplasia

Fibromuscular dysplasia is a nonatherosclerotic angiopathy of unknown cause that affects specific arteries chiefly in young women. Symptoms of cerebrovascular disease can occur when the carotid artery is affected. It is usually bilateral and involves primarily the middle third of the extracranial portions of the internal carotid artery. Several pathologic variants of the disease have been described, but in most of them the primary lesion is overgrowth of the media in a segmental distribution, producing irregular zones of arterial narrowing. The most common result is a series of concentric rings, producing the radiologic appearance of a *string of beads* in a long internal carotid artery. Approximately one-third of patients are hypertensive due to renal artery involvement.

The prevalence of fibromuscular dysplasia and the portion of patients who develop symptoms are not known. Once symptoms develop, transient neurologic events are the most common manifestation. However, more than 20% of patients have had a stroke by the time of presentation. Because of the high incidence of neurologic disability, the lesion should be corrected by angioplasty with distal protection when patients develop symptoms. Surgery with dilation of the carotid with graduated dilators or balloon dilation has given excellent results.

Surgical Results

Late restenosis or occlusion is uncommon after carotid endarterectomy and appears equally uncommon after carotid stenting. For endarterectomy, restenosis can be reduced by using a prosthetic patch for closure of the arteriotomy.

The main complication of cerebrovascular interventions is stroke, which occurs in 2–6% of patients depending on the operative indications and cerebrovascular anatomy. Higher stroke rates occur in the setting of symptomatic stenosis or contralateral carotid occlusion. Lower stroke rates occur with asymptomatic stenosis. The operative death rate for all extracranial cerebrovascular interventions is less than 1%.

Transient cranial nerve injury occurs in about 10% of cases after endarterectomy and may cause tongue weakness, hoarseness, mouth asymmetry, earlobe numbness, and dysphagia. Less than 5% of peripheral nerve deficits are permanent, although this number goes up with surgery for recurrent disease, making stenting all the more attractive for this indication.

Abou-Zamzam AM Jr et al: Is a single preoperative duplex scan sufficient for planning bilateral carotid endarterectomy? J Vasc Surg 2000;31:282.

Baker WH et al: Effect of contralateral occlusion on long-term efficacy of endarterectomy in the asymptomatic carotid atherosclerosis study (ACAS). ACAS Investigators. Stroke 2000;31;2330.

Barnett HJJM et al: Benefit of carotid endarterectomy in patients with symptomatic moderate or severe stenosis. N Engl J Med 1998;339:1415.

Beneficial effect of carotid endarterectomy in symptomatic patients with high-grade stenosis. North American Symptomatic Carotid Endarterectomy Trial Collaborators. N Engl J Med 1991;325:445.

Darling RC 3rd et al: Analysis of the effect of asymptomatic carotid atherosclerosis study on the outcome and volume of carotid endarterectomy. Cardiovasc Surg 2000;8:436.

Endarterectomy for asymptomatic carotid artery stenosis. Executive Committee for the Asymptomatic Carotid Atherosclerosis Study (ACAS). JAMA 1995;273;1421.

Ferguson GG et al: The North American Symptomatic Carotid Endarterectomy Trial: surgical results in 1415 patients. Stroke 1999;30:1751.

Halliday A et al: Prevention of disabling and fatal strokes by successful carotid endarterectomy in patients without recent neurological symptoms: randomized controlled trial. Lancet 2004;363:1491.

Hobson RW: Carotid angioplasty-stent: clinical experience and role for clinical trials. J Vasc Surg 2001;33:5117.

Kresowik TF et al: Improving the outcomes of carotid endarterectomy: results of a statewide quality improvement project. J Vasc Surg 2000;31:918.

Moore WS et al: Indications, surgical technique, and results for repair of extracranial occlusive lesions. In: *Vascular Surgery,* 5th ed. Rutherford RB (editor). Saunders, 2000.

A randomised, blinded, trial of clopidogrel versus aspirin in patients at risk of ischaemic events (CAPRIE). CAPRIE Steering Committee: Lancet 1996;348:1329.

Rothwell PM et al: Interrelation between plaque surface morphology and degree of stenosis on carotid angiograms and the risk of ischemic stroke in patients with symptomatic carotid stenosis. On behalf of the European Carotid Surgery Trialists' Collaborative Group. Stroke 2000;342:1693.

Roubin GS et al: Immediate and late clinical outcomes of carotid artery stenting in patients with symptomatic and asymptomatic carotid artery stenosis: a 5-year prospective analysis. Circulation 2001;103:532.

Schievink WI: Spontaneous dissection of the carotid and vertebral arteries. N Engl J Med 2001;344:898.

Yadav JS et al: Stenting and angioplasty with protection in patients at high risk for endarterectomy Investigators. Protected carotid-artery stenting versus endarterectomy in high risk patients. N Engl J Med 2004;351:1493.

RENOVASCULAR HYPERTENSION

ESSENTIALS OF DIAGNOSIS

- *Severe hypertension.*
- *Declining renal function*
- *Renal insufficiency with ACE inhibitor use.*
- *Flank bruits.*

General Considerations

More than 23 million people in the USA have hypertension, and renovascular disease is a causative factor in 2–7% of cases. Atherosclerosis of the aorta and renal artery (two-thirds of cases) and fibromuscular dysplasia account for nearly all cases of renovascular hypertension. Less common causes of hypertension include renal artery emboli, renal artery aneurysms, renal artery dissection, hypoplasia of the renal arteries, and stenosis of the suprarenal aorta.

Atherosclerosis characteristically produces stenosis at the orifice of the main renal artery. The lesion usually consists of an atheroma that originates in the aorta and extends into the renal artery. Less commonly, the atheroma arises in the renal artery itself. Renal artery stenosis is more common in males over age 45 years and is bilateral in about 95% of cases.

Fibromuscular dysplasia (FMD) usually involves the middle and distal thirds of the main renal artery and may extend into the branches (Figure 34–18). Medial fibroplasia is the most common variety of FMD, accounting for 85% of these lesions. It is bilateral in 50% of cases. The arterial stenoses are caused by concentric rings of hyperplasia that project into the arterial lumen. Renal artery aneurysms frequently coexist. FMD occurs mainly in women, with onset of hypertension usually occurring before age 45 years. It is the causative disorder in 10% of children with hypertension. Developmental renal artery hypoplasia, coarctation of the aorta, and Takayasu's aortitis are other vascular causes of hypertension in childhood.

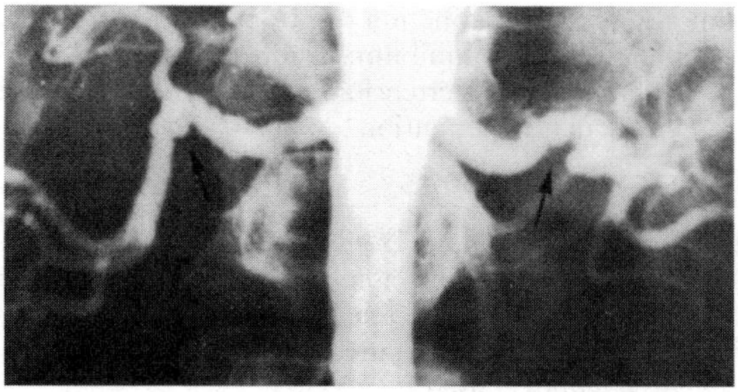

Figure 34–18. Renal arteriogram showing bilateral fibromuscular hyperplasia of the renal arteries (arrows).

Hypertension due to renal artery stenosis results from the kidney's response to reduced blood flow. Cells of the juxtaglomerular complex secrete renin, which acts on circulating angiotensinogen to form angiotensin I, which is rapidly converted to angiotensin II by angiotensin-converting enzyme (ACE). This octapeptide constricts arterioles, increases aldosterone secretion, and promotes sodium retention. Due to the excess aldosterone, hypertension becomes volume-dependent. Over time pathologic changes occur in the uninvolved kidney and the hypertension is no longer sensitive to ACE inhibition. However, with sodium restriction and volume reduction (diuretics), the hypertension becomes once again sensitive to ACE inhibition. If both kidneys have renal artery stenoses, or if the disease exists in a solitary kidney, renal insufficiency may occur with ACE inhibitor administration due to a reduction of angiotensin II constriction of the efferent arteriole.

Clinical Findings

A. Symptoms and Signs

Most patients are asymptomatic, but irritability, headache, and emotional depression are seen in a few. Persistent elevation of the diastolic pressure is usually the only abnormal physical finding. A bruit is frequently audible to one or both sides of the midline in the upper abdomen. Other signs of atherosclerosis may be present when this is the cause of the renal artery disease.

Other clues to the presence of renovascular hypertension include absence of a family history of hypertension; early onset of hypertension (particularly during childhood or during early adulthood); marked acceleration of the degree of hypertension; resistance to control with antihypertensive drugs; and rapid deterioration of renal function. One should suspect renovascular hypertension if initial diastolic pressure is greater than 115 mm Hg, or if renal function deteriorates while a patient is being given ACE inhibitors. Sudden onset of pulmonary edema with hypertension also is highly suggestive of renovascular hypertension.

B. Diagnostic Studies

In the past, there have been several diagnostic tests devised to diagnose renovascular hypertension. Divided urinary excretion studies, selective renin determinations from renal vein samples, and captopril renal scintigraphy are now rarely used.

Noninvasive or minimally invasive imaging of the renal arteries is justified when the patient has a precipitous drop in blood pressure, decreased renal function with an ACE inhibitor, difficult-to-control hypertension, unexplained deteriorating renal function, or all of these.

C. Imaging Studies

In experienced hands, duplex ultrasound scanning has an overall agreement with angiography of over 90%. Renal artery stenosis is characterized by peak systolic velocities in the range of 180–200 cm/s, and the ratio of these velocities to those in the aorta approaches 3.5. Magnetic resonance angiography, especially with gadolinium enhancement, may provide high-resolution images of diseased renal arteries. Its lack of nephrotoxicity and noninvasiveness have made it the preferred diagnostic test in most centers.

Renal arteriography is the most precise method for delineating the obstructive lesion (Figure 34–19). Since atherosclerotic disease most often involves the origins of the renal arteries, a midstream aortogram should be obtained in addition to selective renal artery catheterization. The presence of collateral vessels circumventing a renal artery stenosis suggests a hemodynamically significant renal artery lesion.

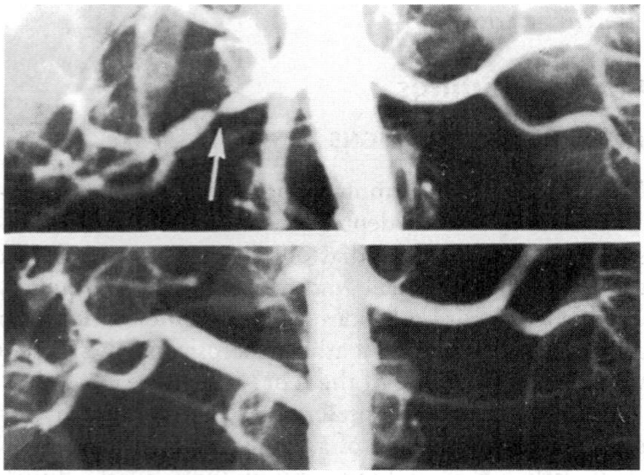

Figure 34–19. *Top:* Preoperative renal arteriogram of a patient with stenosis of the mid portion of the right renal artery (arrow). *Bottom:* Postoperative renal arteriogram after renal artery bypass with an autograft of the hypogastric artery.

Nonionic contrast agents should be used and the patient should be prepared with overnight hydration. Administration of *N*-acetylcysteine and periprocedural sodium bicarbonate infusion dramatically reduces the incidence of acute tubular necrosis with angiography and should used routinely.

Treatment

A. Surgical Treatment

Surgical repair is reserved for failed angioplasty and stenting, renal revascularization during a procedure on the aorta, and lesions that are in branch vessels. As with any operation, the indications for arterial reconstruction are influenced by the extent of disease, the patient's life expectancy, and the anticipated morbidity associated with operation. Nephrectomy may be considered when arterial repair is impossible or especially hazardous and the disease is unilateral.

Options include endarterectomy, which is most easily accomplished through an incision into the adjacent aorta, or bypass using prosthetic or autogenous conduits. An alternative is "nonanatomic" bypass such as a hepatorenal or splenorenal procedure. The celiac and splenic arteries often have coexistent occlusive atherosclerotic disease that mandates preoperative arteriographic assessment of these vessels.

Extracorporeal techniques have been developed for distal branch aneurysms or extensive FMD. These require removal of the kidney from the abdomen (ex vivo arterial reconstruction), continuous cold perfusion of its vascular tree, and microvascular techniques for arterial replacement. The kidney is then either returned to a site near its original position or transplanted to the ipsilateral iliac fossa.

B. Percutaneous Transluminal Angioplasty

The adjunctive use of stents after renal percutaneous transluminal angioplasty has improved success and durability of this procedure. This is the preferred procedure for most patients. In the very young surgery is still the primary mode of treatment due to concern regarding the long-term durability of angioplasty and stenting.

Prognosis

Procedures for revascularization of the renal artery are successful in lowering blood pressure in over 90% of patients with fibromuscular hyperplasia. Operation for atherosclerotic stenosis results in improvement or cure of hypertension in about 60%. The results for angioplasty and stenting are not as good. There is atheroembolization to the kidney during angioplasty, and current trials with protection devices to catch emboli, as done during carotid stenting, are evaluating whether this will improve the results of angioplasty.

The results of intervention for salvage of renal function are even better. Results are better in patients whose only clinical manifestation of atherosclerosis is secondary hypertension than in those with clinically overt systemic atherosclerosis. The operative mortality rate of renovascular surgery in children is almost nil, whereas it increases to 2–8% in adults with diffuse atherosclerosis.

Ballard JJ: Renal artery endarterectomy for treatment of renovascular hypertension combined with infrarenal aortic reconstruction: analysis of surgical results. Ann Vasc Surg 2001;15:260.

Cambria RP et al: Surgical renal artery reconstruction without contrast arteriography: the role of clinical profiling and magnetic resonance angiography. J Vasc Surg 1999;29;1012.

Darling RC 3rd et al: Outcome of renal artery reconstruction: analysis of 687 procedures. Ann Surg 1999;230:524.

Giroux MF et al: Percutaneous revascularization of the renal arteries: predictors of outcome. J Vasc Interv Radiol 2000;11:713.

Hansen KJ et al: Management of ischemic nephropathy: dialysis-free survival after surgical repair. J Vasc Surg 2000;32:472.

Helin KH et al: Predicting the outcome of invasive treatment of renal artery disease. J Intern Med 2000;247:105.

Hua HT et al: The use of colorflow duplex scanning to detect significant renal artery stenosis. Ann Vasc Surg 2000;14:118.

Iglesias JI et al: The natural history of incidental renal artery stenosis in patients with aortoiliac vascular disease. Am J Med 2000;109:642.

Safian RD et al: Renal-artery stenosis. N Engl J Med 2001;344:431.

Teoh MK: Takayasu's arteritis with renovascular hypertension: results of surgical treatment. Cardiovasc Surg 1999;7:626.

Textor SC et al: Renal artery stenosis: a common, treatable cause of renal failure? Annu Rev Med 2001;52:421.

Travis JA et al: Aneurysmal degeneration and late rupture of an aortorenal vein graft: case report, review of the literature, and implications for conduit selection. J Vasc Surg 2000;32:612.

van Jaarsveld BC et al: The effect of balloon angioplasty on hypertension in atherosclerotic renal-artery stenosis. Dutch Renal Artery Stenosis Intervention Cooperative Study Group. N Engl J Med 2000;1342:1007.

van Rooden CJ et al: Long-term outcome of surgical revascularization in ischemic nephropathy: normalization of average decline in renal function. J Vasc Surg 1999;29:1037.

Woolfson RG: Renal failure in atherosclerotic renovascular disease: pathogenesis, diagnosis, and intervention. Postgrad Med J 2001;77:68.

Wong JM et al: Surgery after failed percutaneous renal artery angioplasty. J Vasc Surg 1999;30:468.

GASTROINTESTINAL ISCHEMIA SYNDROMES

ESSENTIALS OF DIAGNOSIS

- *Postprandial pain.*
- *Fear of eating.*
- *Weight loss.*
- *Epigastric bruit.*
- *Pain out of proportion to physical findings.*

General Considerations

The celiac axis and the superior and inferior mesenteric arteries are the principal sources of blood supply to the stomach and intestines, with the two internal iliac arteries adding collateral flow to the distal colon. The anatomic collateral interconnections between these arteries are numerous. Single or even multiple visceral artery lesions are generally well tolerated, because collateral flow is readily available (Figure 34–20).

Atherosclerosis is the cause of obstructive lesions in the visceral arteries in the vast majority of cases. Vasculitis (eg, lupus erythematosus, Takayasu's disease) is the second most common cause. When atherosclerosis is the cause, the usual lesion is a collar of plaque that creates a proximal stenosis or occlusion. Associated atherosclerosis in the aorta and its other branches is common.

Acute mesenteric ischemia is a complex, highly morbid disorder. Patients classically present with excruciating diffuse abdominal pain with a surprising absence of physical findings such as abdominal tenderness or distention—unless actual bowel perforation produces a surgical abdomen. The cause is either embolic or thrombotic. The diagnosis can be difficult and its recognition is often delayed, resulting in irreversible bowel ischemia. The mortality rate from acute mesenteric ischemia remains high. Patients who require massive bowel resection rarely survive or, if they survive, can develop incapacitating short-gut syndrome. The prognosis improves dramatically if revascularization can be achieved prior to intestinal infarction. This obviously requires early diagnosis, which will only occur if the practitioner has a high index of suspicion.

Visceral ischemia due to external compression of the celiac artery, or **median arcuate ligament syndrome**, is an unusual cause of visceral ischemia. It generally

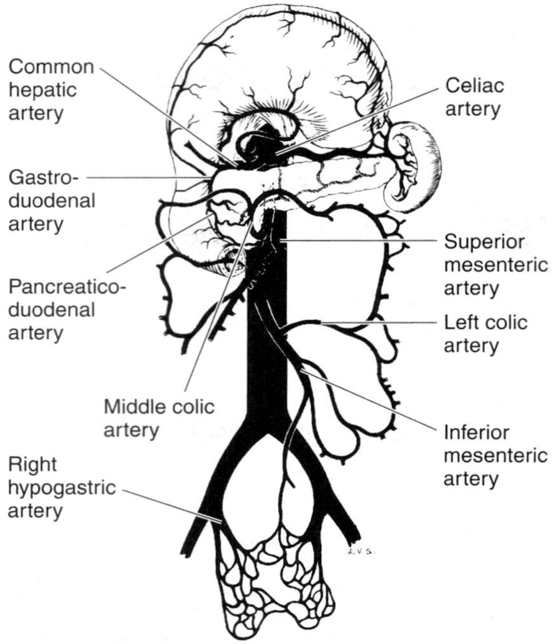

Figure 34–20. Visceral arterial circulation and interconnections.

affects young adults, with women more commonly affected than men. The artery is scarred and must be repaired in conjunction with release of the compressing ligament. The diagnosis is difficult to make with certainty as some compression of the celiac artery by the arcuate ligament is common. Surgery should be advised only after a search for other causes of postprandial pain.

Clinical Findings

The principal complaint is postprandial abdominal pain, which has been labeled abdominal or **visceral angina**. Pain characteristically appears 15–30 minutes after the beginning of a meal and lasts for an hour or longer. Pain is occasionally so severe and prolonged that opiates are required for relief. Pain occurs as a deep-seated steady ache in the epigastrium, occasionally radiating to the right or left upper quadrant. Weight loss results from reluctance to eat, although mild degrees of malabsorption can occur. Thus, gastrointestinal absorption studies are not helpful. Diarrhea and vomiting have been described. An upper abdominal bruit may be heard in over 80% of patients.

Arteriography in the anteroposterior and especially the lateral projections demonstrates both the arterial lesion and the patterns of collateral blood flow (Figure 34–21). Patients should be well hydrated before angiography because this procedure can precipitate hypercoagulability and osmotic diuresis with dehydration, vascular occlusion, and bowel infarction. Duplex scanning and MRA are used with increasing frequency because they are less invasive methods of screening.

Treatment

When the obstruction is atherosclerotic, surgical revascularization of the superior mesenteric and celiac axes may be performed by either endarterectomy or graft replacement. During endarterectomy, a sleeve of aortic intima and the orifice lesions in the celiac or superior mesenteric arteries are removed. The operation is performed by a retroperitoneal approach to the aorta through a left thoracoabdominal incision. Alternatively, a Dacron graft may be brought from the lower thoracic aorta to the celiac axis or superior mesenteric artery—an operation that is performed from within the abdomen. External compression of the celiac artery by the median arcuate ligament may be relieved by simple division of the ligament in 50% of cases, but simultaneous arterial reconstruction produces the best results. Operation should be avoided in patients with acute vasculitis as the underlying cause of mesenteric ischemia; high-dose steroids and immunosuppressive agents are indicated instead.

In addition, PTA and stenting has gained acceptance as an alternative form of therapy for both chronic and acute mesenteric ischemia. Results are best for focal, nonorificial stenoses.

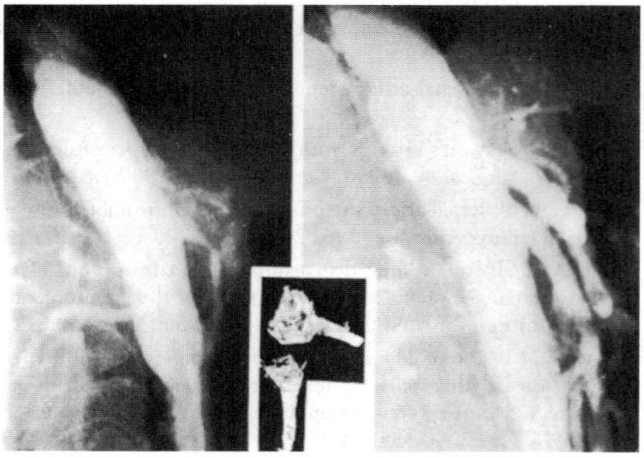

Figure 34–21. *Left:* Preoperative visceral arteriogram showing severe stenosis of the celiac and superior mesenteric arteries. *Right:* The postoperative visceral arteriogram shows wide patency of the celiac and superior mesenteric arteries after transaortic endarterectomy. The inset shows the atherosclerotic stenotic lesions removed by endarterectomy.

Prognosis

Surgery for atherosclerotic visceral artery insufficiency almost always results in relief of symptoms if a technically adequate operation is accomplished. If operation is not performed, death will occur from inanition or massive bowel infarction.

Patients with median arcuate ligament compression respond favorably to operation in the majority of instances; however, some of these patients are not improved even though a technically adequate operation is performed.

Farber MA et al: Distal thoracic aorta as inflow for the treatment of chronic mesenteric ischemia. J Vasc Surg 2001;33:281.

Foley MI et al: Revascularization of the superior mesenteric artery alone for treatment of intestinal ischemia. J Vasc Surg 2000;32:37.

Geelkerken RH et al: Duplex ultrasound examination of splanchnic vessels in the assessment of splanchnic ischaemic symptoms. Eur J Vasc Endovasc Surg 1999;18:371.

Kazmers A: Operative management of chronic mesenteric ischemia. Ann Vasc Surg 1998;12:299.

Leduc FJ et al: Acute mesenteric ischaemia: minimal invasive management by combined laparoscopy and percutaneous transluminal angioplasty. Eur J Surg 2000;166:345.

Mateo RB et al: Elective surgical treatment of symptomatic chronic mesenteric occlusive disease: early results and late outcomes. J Vasc Surg 1999;29:821.

Meaney JF: Non-invasive evaluation of the visceral arteries with magnetic resonance angiography. Eur Radiol 1999;9:1267.

Schulte KM et al: Coral reef aorta: a long-term study of 21 patients. Ann Vasc Surg 2000;14:626.

Vicente DC et al: Acute mesenteric ischemia. Cuff Opin Cardiol 1999;14:453.

INTRA-ARTERIAL INJECTIONS & IATROGENIC ARTERIAL TRAUMA

Intra-arterial injections are seen frequently among intravenous drug abusers. Brachial and femoral injections are most frequent. The patient experiences severe burning pain in the affected arterial distribution, followed by intense vasoconstriction and in many cases thrombosis with gangrene of digits or of the entire extremity. In lesser insults, after the period of vasospasm, the extremity becomes swollen and discolored. When intra-arterial injection is recognized, the artery should be irrigated immediately with copious amounts of heparinized saline. However, the patient usually presents late with chemical endarteritis well established. At present, heparinization is the recommended immediate management. Intra-arterial vasodilators (eg, nitroglycerin, papaverine, tolazoline) may be useful to alleviate vasospasm. Various therapeutic regimens have been advocated—anticoagulants, sympathectomy, dextran, corticosteroids—with mixed results. Late complications such as infected pseudoaneurysm formation are often best treated by excision and ligation—in many cases without extra-anatomic revascularization—but with reliance on collateral blood flow to maintain tissue viability.

The marked increase in performance of percutaneous catheter-based vascular interventions combined with anticoagulation regimens has resulted in a greater frequency of peripheral arterial pseudoaneurysms and arteriovenous fistulas (see above). Most of these iatrogenic injuries are self-limited and will resolve spontaneously over time, especially after systemic anticoagulation is discontinued. Emergent operation is rarely indicated unless the iatrogenic arterial trauma results in distal ischemia, major hemorrhage, or local integumentary or neurologic compromise.

Hye RJ: Compression therapy for acute iatrogenic femoral pseudoaneurysms. Semin Vasc Surg 2000;13:58.

Nehler MR et al: Iatrogenic vascular injuries from percutaneous vascular suturing devices. J Vasc Surg 2001;33:943.

Nehler MR et al: Iatrogenic vascular trauma. Semin Vasc Surg 1998;11:283.

O'Sullivan GJ et al: A review of alternative approaches in the management of iatrogenic femoral pseudoaneurysms. Ann R Coll Surg Engl 1999;81:226.

Reddy DJ et al: Infected femoral artery false aneurysms in drug addicts: evolution of selective vascular reconstruction. J Vasc Surg 1986;3:718.

Ting AC et al: Femoral pseudoaneurysms in drug addicts. World J Surg 1997;21:783.

Vermeulen EG et al: Percutaneous duplex-guided thrombin injection for treatment of iatrogenic femoral artery pseudoaneurysms. Eur J Vasc Endovasc Surg 2000;20:302.

Amputation

35

*William C. Krupski, MD**

Amputations are sometimes necessary as part of surgical care for disorders involving the upper and lower extremities. Amputation may have several goals depending on the indications for operation and the condition or functional status of the patient. These goals have variable success rates and priorities—again contingent on the indication for surgery and the patient population. Amputations have four aims: (1) The removal of all diseased tissue—but this is not always achieved with the initial amputation, particularly when performed for ischemic or infectious disease. (2) The relief of pain is critical—but this may not be achieved because of healing failures and chronic pain syndromes (eg, phantom limb pain and reflex sympathetic dystrophy). (3) Primary healing of the amputation wound is desirable but may not be accomplished because of infection or efforts to maintain limb length. (4) Construction of a stump that will permit the most useful function with or without prosthetic fitting is most consequential in functional patients. Many minimally functional elderly patients develop breakdown and pressure necrosis of their distal lower extremities primarily from inactivity in combination with ischemia. Amputations in these patients are often performed more proximally to ensure healing.

Toe amputations and major leg amputations (transtibial and transfemoral) are common surgical procedures. In contrast, more proximal leg amputations (hip disarticulations, hemipelvectomy) and upper extremity amputations are uncommon. Toe amputations are performed by surgeons of varied specialties, including podiatrists, orthopedic surgeons, and vascular surgeons. Transtibial and transfemoral amputations are usually performed by vascular or orthopedic surgeons. Orthopedic or plastic reconstructive surgeons customarily perform more proximal lower extremity amputations and major upper extremity amputations.

As the average age of the population has risen, the incidence of peripheral arterial disease and diabetes mellitus has increased. More than 90% of the 110,000 amputations performed in the USA each year are for ischemic or infective gangrene. More than half of lower extremity amputations are performed for vascular and infectious complications of diabetes mellitus, and 15–50% of diabetic amputees will lose a second leg within 5 years. This risk is about two times higher for men than for women. Other indications for amputations are nondiabetic infection with ischemia (15–25%), ischemia without infection (5–10%), osteomyelitis (3–5%), trauma (2–5%), and frostbite, tumors, neuromas, and other miscellaneous causes (5–10%).

Many patients facing amputation are near the end of life because of systemic cardiovascular disease. Approximately 20–30% of patients undergoing major amputation (below-knee or above-knee) will be dead within 2 years. The prevalence of many comorbidities in this population is also reflected in the perioperative mortality rates for major amputation, ranging from 5% to 10% for below-knee amputations to 10% or higher for above-knee amputations. In addition, failure of primary below-knee amputation healing ranges from 30% to 90%. Although major amputations do not receive the notoriety of higher-profile operations, they are difficult procedures with higher morbidity and mortality rates than many of the other commonplace major operations.

Level of Amputation

The level of amputation is determined by assessing the likelihood of healing of the limb in association with the functional potential of the patient. Extensive myocutaneous free flap grafting to maintain a below-knee amputation and preserve the use of the knee joint may be appropriate in a young patient with limb loss related to extensive trauma. Conversely, a demented elderly nursing home patient with mild ischemia and heel pressure necrosis may be better treated with a primary above knee amputation to avoid a knee flexion contracture despite adequate blood supply for healing of a below knee-amputation. In general, the knee joint should be preserved if possible in patients who can be rehabilitated. The clinical conundrum in patients with limb ischemia is twofold: (1) determining which limbs have adequate blood supply to heal at the below-knee level and (2) determining which patients with vascular disease have reasonable rehabilitation potential. There is no way of answering either question with confidence.

Technical decisions regarding amputation level are based on adequacy of blood flow, extent of tissue necro-

*Deceased.

sis, and location of tumor. In the upper extremities, circulatory impairment is rare. In the lower extremities, in which impairment is more likely to occur, the circulatory status at different levels may be determined by measurement of the peripheral pulses and the capillary refill time and by noting the presence of rubor, the condition of the skin, and the presence of ischemic atrophy. At present, no single measurement of blood flow can reliably predict the best level of healing. Extremely low or absent blood flow predicts nonhealing, and normal flow predicts healing. However, in most cases the prediction falls in between. The best predictions are based on clinical assessment by an experienced surgeon, assisted by one of the several techniques for determining amputation level. In patients with distinct lines of demarcation (eg, with gangrene) and in those with tumors, the amount of tissue that must be removed is usually more obvious.

For most patients with ambulatory potential, as long a limb as possible should be preserved in order to maintain nearly normal walking with the least expenditure of energy. Compared with normal walking, energy expenditure is increased 10–40% with a transtibial prosthesis, 50–70% with a transfemoral prosthesis, and 60% with crutches. One obvious way to reduce energy cost is to reduce the velocity. The average speed of ambulation for a normal adult is 4.8 km/h, compared with 3.2–4 km/h for a transtibial amputee and 2.4 km/h for a transfemoral amputee.

Determination of Amputation Level

A. Clinical Examination

The presence of palpable pedal pulses in a warm, pink limb is a reliable indicator that arterial flow is adequate to support healing of a below-knee amputation. Conversely, an absent ipsilateral femoral pulse is associated with an 80% chance of failure of a primary below-transtibial amputation. In general, the presence of a palpable pulse in the major artery immediately above the amputation site (eg, femoral pulse for above-knee, popliteal pulse for below-knee) indicates a high probability of amputation primary healing, and absence of a palpable pulse in these locations significantly reduces the likelihood of amputation healing.

B. Measurement of Blood Pressure

In addition to clinical assessment, measurement of blood pressure in the thigh and ankle with a Doppler ultrasound device and pneumatic cuffs is a useful technique for determining the level of amputation. Readings are not accurate enough, however, to be the sole basis for decision making. Segmental blood pressures are fallible, and blood pressure in the ankle is an unreliable guide to healing in the foot if the tibial vessels are calcified and cannot be compressed by the cuff, a condition reported in at least 20–25% of diabetics. In addition, significant lower extremity edema hinders accurate measurements. The notion that above-knee amputation is mandatory if the blood pressure in the ankle is below 60 mm Hg is unwarranted. This technique does not adequately demonstrate collateral circulation, and healing is common even when ankle pressures are extremely low or undetectable. Absence of an arterial flow signal in the popliteal space, however, reliably predicts that transtibial amputation will fail to heal.

C. Oxygen Tension Measurements

Transcutaneous measurement of oxygen tension (using a modified Clark-type oxygen electrode) is another guide to healing. A transcutaneous PaO_2 of zero indicates a high probability that healing will be unsatisfactory at that site, whereas a PaO_2 above 40 mm Hg indicates that good healing is likely. Intermediate values do not correlate closely with the degree of healing. Transcutaneous PaO_2 measurement is noninvasive and very reproducible. Disadvantages of the technique are the expense of the equipment and the time required for examination (about 30 minutes per site). It is important to heat the skin to 44 °C, which causes a temperature-dependent microstructural change in the lipid phase of the stratum corneum from solid to liquid.

D. Other Measures of Skin Perfusion

Multiple techniques are available to assess the skin perfusion for determination of the optimal amputation level. Most of these methods have not gained widespread use in clinical practice. Problems with these techniques include impracticality, expense, and technical difficulty—and inconsistent confirmatory studies.

1. Laser Doppler studies—Laser Doppler is a noninvasive technique to determine the velocity of blood flow in the skin microcirculation. This method is popular in Europe but has not been extensively used in North America. Absence of flow reliably predicts nonhealing, but specific flow velocities have not been differentiated.

2. Skin fluorescence—Intravenous injection of fluorescein dye followed by measurements of skin fluorescence with a fluorometer have been reported to predict healing with 80% accuracy. Fluorometers are commercially available, but this technique has not gained widespread application.

3. Skin perfusion pressure—Photoelectric measurement of skin perfusion pressure involves positioning a blood pressure cuff over a photoelectric detector that is connected to a plethysmograph. The external pressure required to prevent skin hyperemia after blanching is recorded. A skin perfusion pressure of 20 mm Hg or higher predicts healing with 80% accuracy.

4. Skin temperature—Infrared thermography has been correlated with skin blood flow. A single report demonstrated a 94% positive predictive value but only an 11% negative predictive value.

E. Arteriography

Arteriography provides anatomic, not physiologic, information. It assesses feasibility of vascular reconstructions but is of little value in selecting the amputation site because findings do not correlate with circulation to the skin. Arteriography provides anatomic information, not physiologic data.

Preparation for Amputation

No pharmacologic treatment can forestall amputation; however, patients must be adequately prepared for operation. Diabetes mellitus, heart failure, and infection should be controlled. Material from sites of potential infection should be cultured and appropriate antibiotics administered preoperatively. In the presence of infection or a necrotic tumor, the first step should be a debriding (guillotine-type) amputation and continued antibiotics. A definitive amputation with primary closure of the wound can be performed 5–7 days later.

Malnutrition adversely affects the healing of amputation sites, and serum albumin levels and total lymphocyte counts correlate with success rates. Assuming that the amputation level is appropriate, healing occurs in 80% of patients when serum albumin is at least 3.5 g/mL and total lymphocyte count is at least 1500 cells/μL, but in less than 30% of patients when values are lower.

When patients are so critically ill that they cannot tolerate a general or regional anesthetic, a "medical amputation" can be used as a temporary measure. This involves placing a tourniquet at the level of amputation and packing the distal extremity in ice, thereby diminishing the systemic metabolic effects of profound ischemia.

Urgent or Emergency Amputation

A. Acute Arterial Occlusion

Arterial flow can be restored surgically in most patients with acute arterial occlusion, but when flow cannot be restored or when the patient's presentation or the diagnosis is delayed beyond viability, urgent or emergency amputation is required. The most reliable sign of nonviability on physical examination is rigor of the involved muscle bed. The degree of urgency is determined by the extent of ischemia, the mass of ischemic muscle, the amount of pain, and the presence of systemic toxicity and infection. If there is little ischemic or necrotic tissue, amputation may be deferred until demarcation between viable and nonviable tissue becomes evident; this usually takes a day or two. This allows for maximum development of collateral circulation and increases the chances that a limited amputation will heal. When circulatory improvement stops or if toxicity develops, amputation should be performed promptly. With more extensive tissue destruction, there is greater risk of serious toxicity when amputation is delayed. Myoglobinuria and renal dysfunction are early signs of toxicity. Mental confusion, sepsis, and deterioration of vital signs are late findings. All should mandate emergency amputation, usually above or through the knee.

B. Injury

In patients with massively injured or crushed extremities, early amputation may greatly shorten the time required for successful rehabilitation. There are several scoring systems for determining the advisability of immediate amputation after major extremity trauma. The most popular is designated MESS (Mangled Extremity Severity Score). In brief, severe major nerve injury in conjunction with bone, soft tissue, and vascular injury warrants consideration of primary amputation, because a neurologically useless extremity is not worth salvaging. In addition, the incidence of postamputation chronic phantom pain syndrome increases the longer a chronically painful posttraumatic limb goes without proper treatment. Whereas plantar sensation is the minimum degree of neural function required for the lower extremity to function, a compromised upper extremity can frequently function better than currently available prostheses. Although severity scores are helpful, the decision to amputate in marginal cases can be postponed until the extremity is clearly nonviable or insensate.

SPECIFIC TYPES OF AMPUTATIONS

LOWER EXTREMITY AMPUTATIONS

All patients and physicians wish to avoid limb loss. However, with modern prosthetic equipment, improvements in the functional usefulness of wheelchairs, and legislation (Americans With Disabilities Act) mandating wheelchair access to most public facilities, an amputee can be more mobile after than before the procedure. The goals of amputation vary depending on the functional status of the patient.

Lower extremity amputations are done most commonly at one of the following levels: toe (called digit amputations, which may be extended to include resection of the metatarsal and called ray amputations), transmetatarsal, below-knee, and above-knee. Amputations at other levels (Syme's amputation, Chopart's amputation, knee disarticulation, and hip disarticulation) are infrequently performed, usually to treat conditions other than vascular disease.

1. Toe & Ray Amputations

Toes are the most frequently amputated parts of the body. Over two-thirds of amputations in diabetics involve the toes and forefoot. The indications include gangrene, infection, neuropathic ulceration, frostbite, and osteomyelitis limited to the middle or distal phalanx. Good blood flow is required.

Contraindications to digit amputation include indistinct demarcation, infection at the metatarsal level, dependent rubor, and ischemia of the forefoot. Important principles pertaining to digit and ray amputations include the following:

(1) The first metatarsal head is important for patient balance and should be preserved if possible.

(2) Amputation that leaves only one or two remaining digits (unless the first) does not facilitate normal foot function but complicates functional footwear. Patients often develop pressure lesions of the remaining digits due to neuropathy.

(3) Resection of metatarsal heads in diabetic patients with malperforans ulcers often transfers the pressure point responsible for the initial lesion to the adjacent metatarsal head. Therefore, without adequate protection with orthotic shoes or inserts (along with patient compliance), recurrence of these lesions is the rule rather than the exception. This is particularly likely in obese diabetic patients. Several clinical series of toe amputations in diabetic patients have demonstrated the necessity of another toe amputation in up to two-thirds of cases, and below-knee amputation was eventually required in 15–20% of patients.

(4) Digit and ray amputations should be carried out through the shafts of bones because joint cartilage will secrete fluid into the wound and retard healing.

(5) Tendons are avascular structures and should be divided as proximally as possible.

For dry, uninfected gangrene of one or more toes, **autoamputation** may be allowed to occur. During this process, epithelialization occurs beneath the eschar, and the toe spontaneously detaches, leaving a clean residual limb at the most distal site. Although preferable in many patients (and especially frostbit patients), autoamputation sometimes requires months to complete.

Ray or wedge amputation includes removal of the toe and metatarsal head; occasionally, two adjacent toes may be amputated by this method. As with toe amputation, there is modest cosmetic deformity and a prosthesis is not required. Ray amputation of the great toe leads to unstable weight bearing and some difficulty with ambulation resulting from loss of the first metatarsal head.

The extents of toe and ray amputations are shown in Figure 35–1. For distal resections, a circular incision is made at the midpoint of the proximal phalanx, and the phalanx is resected at about its midpoint. If it is necessary to remove the entire phalanx or to excise the distal portion of the metatarsal, the incision is extended proximally over the metatarsal, and the bone is divided behind the metatarsal head. Not uncommonly, the incision must be left open to heal by second intention owing to the presence of local infection.

Complications that may require amputation at higher levels include infection, osteomyelitis of remaining bone, and nonhealing of the incision. These complications have been reported in up to one-third of diabetic patients.

2. Transmetatarsal Amputation

Transmetatarsal forefoot amputations preserve normal weight bearing. The principal indication is gangrene of several toes or the great toe, with or without soft tissue infection or osteomyelitis. The gangrene should have spread beyond a level that could be treated by a two-ray

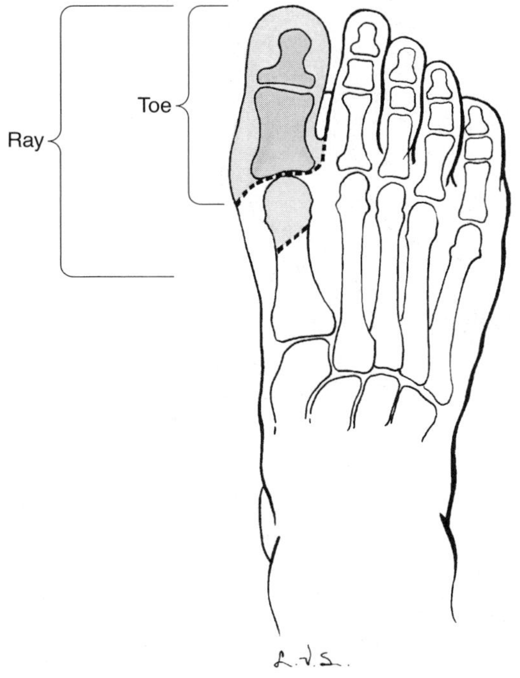

Figure 35–1. Toe and ray amputation.

amputation; there must be no evidence of spreading infection within the foot; and the plantar skin must be healthy. Patients who do not meet these criteria require a higher amputation.

The incision creates a generous plantar flap (Figure 35–2). There is no dorsal flap. On the plantar surface, the incision is continued medially to laterally just proximal to the metatarsophalangeal crease. The metatarsal bones are divided with the medial and lateral shafts cut shorter than those in the middle to preserve the normal architecture of the foot and assist with orthotic fitting postoperatively, and the tendons are pulled down and transected as high as possible.

Transmetatarsal amputation produces an excellent functional result. Walking requires no increase in energy expenditure, and the gait is usually smooth. A prosthesis is not mandatory, but to achieve optimal gait, the shoes must be modified. Lamb's wool or custom-molded foam can be used to fill the toe portion of the shoe. A spring steel shank in the sole of the shoe approximates the action of the longitudinal foot arch during the toe-off phase of walking.

Open transmetatarsal amputations are occasionally necessary in the presence of infection. After the wound has contracted, a split-thickness skin graft may be used for skin coverage. The prosthetic fitting and rehabilitation of these patients are delayed and more difficult, because preservation of the skin graft becomes a primary concern. An ankle-foot orthosis may be necessary.

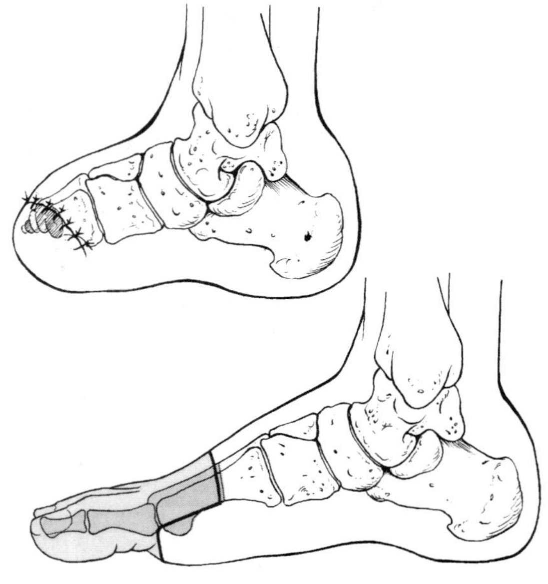

Figure 35–2. Transmetatarsal amputation.

Chopart's amputation (transtarsal amputation of the forefoot through the talonavicular-calcaneo-cuboid joint), **Lisfranc's amputation** (through the tarsometatarsal joint), and **Piroff's amputation** (removal of the talus and rotation of the calcaneus) are unpopular procedures because they produce an imbalance in the remaining muscles of the foot. This results in equinovarus deformity of the foot, with a tender scar and unsatisfactory weight bearing. The Achilles tendon can be transected in an attempt to improve the situation. Ambulation in these patients is somewhat limited. However, limb salvage may be greater when unconventional foot amputations are used.

3. Syme's Amputation

Syme's amputation is a modification of disarticulation through the ankle joint. Trauma of the forefoot with good vascularity of the heel and ankle are the chief indications for this procedure. It is rarely performed except in young trauma patients. Spreading infection in the spaces of the foot, gangrene involving the heel pad, advanced ischemia of the foot, and a neurotropic foot with absence of heel sensation are contraindications to Syme's amputation.

Syme's amputation is the most technically demanding lower extremity amputation, and strict attention to surgical detail is crucial for success. The incision is shown in Figure 35–3. During the operation, particular attention must be paid to preserving the posterior tibial vessels, which supply the heel pad and inferior margins of the wound. The calcaneus must be dissected from the heel pad with great care in order to avoid injury to the soft tissues of the heel flap. The malleoli are resected flush with the joint surface, and the bones are trimmed so there are no pressure points. These last steps may be delayed for 6–8 weeks and performed as a second-stage procedure.

Syme's amputation produces an end-bearing residual limb and leaves a lower extremity only several inches shorter than normal, thus allowing the patient to walk short distances on safe surfaces without a prosthesis. A prosthesis is not essential, and the patient can wear a cup slipper around the house. A cosmetic prosthesis employs a lightweight foot with a plastic shell into which the amputated limb fits. It is more difficult to fit than a conventional transtibial prosthesis and therefore requires an experienced prosthetist for ultimate success. Walking speed is decreased, but energy consumption is increased very little.

4. Major Leg Amputation

Despite efforts to preserve limb length for rehabilitation purposes, the ratio of above-knee to below-knee amputations is roughly 1.0 and has not changed in several

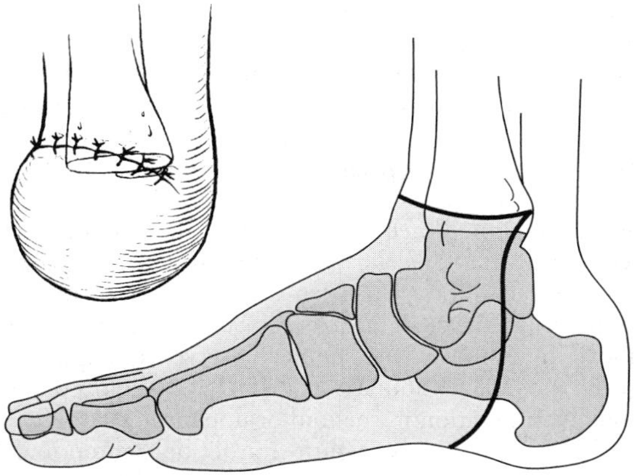

Figure 35–3. Syme's amputation.

decades. Preservation of the knee joint reduces the oxygen consumption required to ambulate from 60% above baseline levels to 40%. Although young trauma patients undergoing an above-knee amputation may eventually be able to walk, an elderly patient after transfemoral amputation rarely does so. An attempt at performing a below-knee amputation is warranted in almost any patient who appears to be a potential candidate for rehabilitation.

The morbidity and mortality for major limb amputation is substantial, primarily due to the systemic disease burden of the patient population. Mortality rates range from 5% to 30% and are generally highest in patients undergoing above-knee amputations since these patients are the least functional and most ill. Perioperative myocardial infarction is the most common cause of death. Deep venous thrombosis occurs in 10–15% of patients and may be present prior to amputation because of the sedentary state of these patients both preoperatively and postoperatively.

Difficulty in accurately predicting healing has led to a discrepancy in reported healing rates—ranging from 30% to 90%—for below-knee amputations. One-third of patients having below-knee amputations require reamputation. Approximately half of the below-knee amputations that do not heal will require conversion to the above-knee level. Patients undergoing amputation for acute severe infections have wound infections or breakdown of the amputation stump in up to two-thirds of cases. These patients should have primary guillotine amputation as a preliminary step to clear the infectious process before a definitive below-knee stump is created.

Absolute indications for primary above-knee amputation include contracture at the knee joint (observed in debilitated patients with long-standing extremity pain who have been in a prolonged withdrawal posture with the knee flexed) and nonviable calf muscle or skin for creation of the below-knee flap. Primary above-knee amputation is relatively contraindicated in patients who are not candidates for rehabilitation. The frequent failure of healing of below-knee amputation, the higher perioperative morbidity and mortality in this population (making secondary operations more dangerous), and the modest functional benefit of preserving the knee joint in a nonambulatory patient are the major arguments in favor of primary above-knee procedures in such cases.

Amputations can be performed using proximal tourniquets. This offers the advantage of minimizing blood loss, particularly in an infected hyperemic limb. Regional anesthesia is frequently used, but there is scant evidence that this decreases perioperative mortality compared with general anesthesia. Blood transfusions are rarely required since the potential for significant hemorrhage is modest.

Guillotine amputations are simple circular incisions usually just above the ankle (which can be more proximal if necessary) that are carried through sharply to divide all structures at that level (hence the name). Absolute indications for guillotine amputation include severe foot infections that preclude limb salvage. Necrotizing diabetic foot infections with or without gross purulence are the most frequent indication. Removing the grossly infected foot allows the lymphatics to be cleared of infection and reduces the risk of below-knee stump infection. Most surgeons do not perform guillotine amputations prior to an above-knee amputation because the distance from the infection source is felt to be relatively protective. The calf muscles should be compressed to reveal purulence that may have tracked proximally, most commonly in the anterior compartment. The major tibial vessels are oversewn at the end of the stump, and the wound is dressed. Controlling the tibial vasculature can be difficult, particularly in young diabetic patients with normal circulation. The wound is then examined in 48 hours to determine if the infectious process has been controlled. If that is so, a formal below-knee amputation is then performed.

The most common procedure for below-knee amputation is the Burgess technique, which utilizes a long posterior flap.

The blood supply to a posterior flap is generally better than the supply to an anterior flap or to sagittal flaps, because the sural arteries (which supply the gastrocnemius and soleus muscles) arise high on the popliteal artery, an area not often diseased, whereas the more distal popliteal artery or tibial arteries are often diseased, especially in diabetics.

The use of rigid dressings and immediate postoperative prostheses has proved advantageous. Application of a rigid cast bandage has several potential advantages:

(1) It controls postoperative edema, which may reduce pain; (2) it protects the stump from trauma, particularly when a patient falls during attempts at mobilization; and (3) it allows the patient to be ambulatory with a temporary prosthesis much sooner. The disadvantages include cost and personnel time to apply the rigid bandages and lack of patient compliance. A single randomized trial in vascular patients did not demonstrate a difference in wound complications with rigid dressings compared with standard bandages.

Use of immediate postoperative prostheses provides two advantages: (1) a rigid dressing and (2) early ambulation. The rigid dressing controls edema, improves healing, prevents joint contractures, and protects from trauma. Early ambulation decreases hospital stay, increases rates of rehabilitation, decreases complications of prolonged bed rest (eg, decubitus ulcers, pneumonia, pulmonary emboli), and improves the patient's psychologic outlook.

The skin flaps are shown in Figure 35–4. The anterior incision is made approximately 7–10 cm below the tibial tuberosity and carried to the midpoint of the leg both medially and laterally. After the muscles of the anterior compartment have been transected, the fibula and tibia are divided, and the tibia is beveled to avoid a sharp projection beneath the skin. The posterior flap is wedge-shaped and contains soleus muscle, gastrocnemius muscle, and skin; it is fashioned to avoid tension when the wound is closed and to provide a generous pad over the distal residual limb. Drains are generally not required for amputations performed for vascular disease, because bleeding is minimal, but they are often necessary for amputations performed for trauma or tumor.

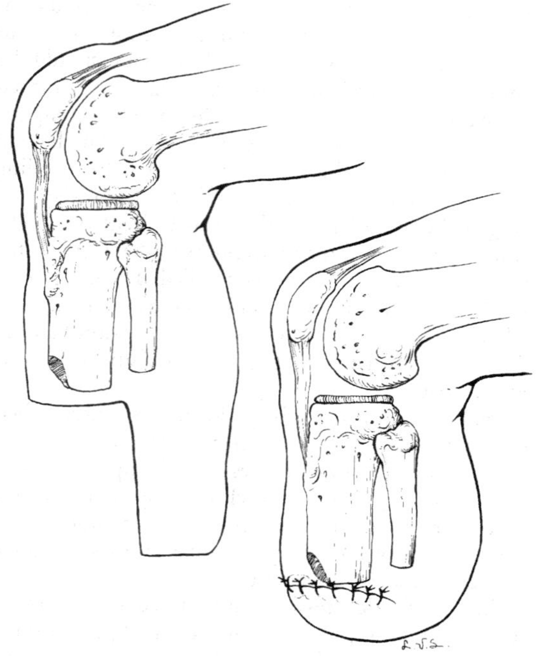

Figure 35–4. Below-knee amputation.

Above-knee amputation may be performed at several levels, including knee disarticulation; the patient is left without a functional knee. Knee disarticulation amputation is technically more demanding than transfemoral amputation at a higher level. When fashioning an above-knee stump, one should preserve as long a lever arm as possible; amputation in the lower thigh is preferable to amputation in the mid or upper thigh.

The technique is straightforward. Short anterior and posterior flaps, sagittal flaps, or a circular incision may be used. The bone is divided slightly higher than the skin and soft tissue to avoid tension when the wound is closed. A simple dressing is then applied.

5. Hip Disarticulation

Most dysvascular patients requiring high amputations can be successfully treated with transfemoral amputation. Hip disarticulation is reserved for the few dysvascular patients in whom transfemoral amputation fails or who have tumors of the thigh or lower femur. Life-threatening infection that cannot be controlled by hip disarticulation is almost uniformly fatal.

An anterior racket-shaped incision or a long posterior flap can be developed to cover the large defect created by a hip disarticulation. In the presence of vascular insufficiency, the flaps may have to be modified to achieve a closure that heals primarily. The muscles, nerves, and capsule of the hip joint are incised, and the disarticulation is completed by division of the ligamentum teres.

Most of these patients cannot be rehabilitated, but vigorous efforts should be made to rehabilitate selected well-motivated individuals, especially young patients who have undergone operation for tumor.

6. Hemipelvectomy

Hemipelvectomy (hindquarter amputation) is reserved for patients with malignant tumors of the lower extremity or pelvis that cannot be removed by lesser procedures. The classic operation involves removal of the entire lower extremity and varying amounts of the innominate bone (Figure 35–5). If the iliac bone is removed completely, the procedure is termed radical; in conservative hemipelvectomy, part of the iliac bone attached to the sacrum is left in place. Internal hemipelvectomy is the procedure in which the innominate bone and surrounding musculature are removed and the lower extremity is preserved.

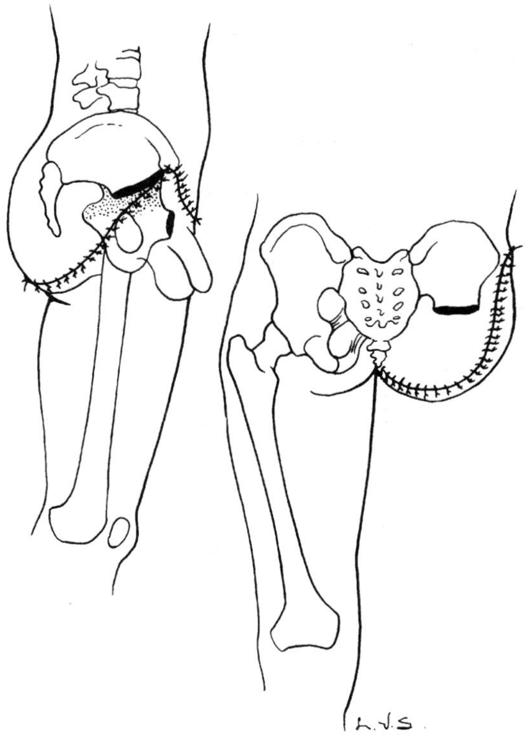

Figure 35–5. Hemipelvectomy.

The incision for hemipelvectomy is determined by the site of the tumor. For posteriorly placed tumors, an anterior flap of skin, subcutaneous tissue, and fascia lata based on the femoral vessels is appropriate. Alternatively, quadriceps muscle can be used for a myocutaneous flap. Rectus abdominis island flaps and thigh flaps based on the femoral vessels have also been used to close the defect after a hindquarter amputation. In some cases, a combination of Marlex mesh and skin graft may be applied over such defects.

The operative mortality rate for hindquarter amputation is about 3%, but complications occur in about 50% of cases. Five-year survival rates depend on the kind of tumor and stage of disease at the time of operation. The 5-year survival rate is 75% after hemipelvectomy for fibrosarcomas and chondrosarcomas; few patients with malignant melanoma are alive after 5 years.

UPPER EXTREMITY AMPUTATIONS

The indications for amputation of upper extremities are much different from those of lower extremities because advanced atherosclerosis is unusual in the upper extremity. Upper extremity amputations are most often performed for severe trauma or malignant tumors. Conditions causing arterial ischemia in upper extremities that may require amputation include thromboangiitis obliterans, connective tissue disorders, accidental intra-arterial injection of drugs, and diabetic patients with long-standing end-stage renal disease.

Microsurgical techniques now allow previously hopeless cases of traumatic amputation to be treated by **replantation**. Function following replantation of the thumb and other digits is good; after replantation of the palm, wrist, or forearm, function is less satisfactory, but an attempt at limb salvage is warranted in selected cases, especially in children. The advantages and disadvantages of amputation and replantation must be weighed: with amputation, there is a cosmetic defect but a relatively short period of rehabilitation; with replantation, there is normal appearance but a long, costly rehabilitation period.

It is advisable to preserve as much length as possible when performing amputations in the upper extremity. Good skin coverage must be obtained, but length should not be sacrificed for the sake of skin closure; split-thickness skin grafts, musculocutaneous flaps, and skin traction can all help in complex situations. In the hand, maintenance of length should be based on functional considerations (Figure 35–6).

Usefulness of the upper extremity prosthesis is limited by diminished sensory and proprioceptive feedback; thus, auditory and visual control of the prosthesis is required. Limited "gadget tolerance" and high costs due to low demand reduce the availability of electric-

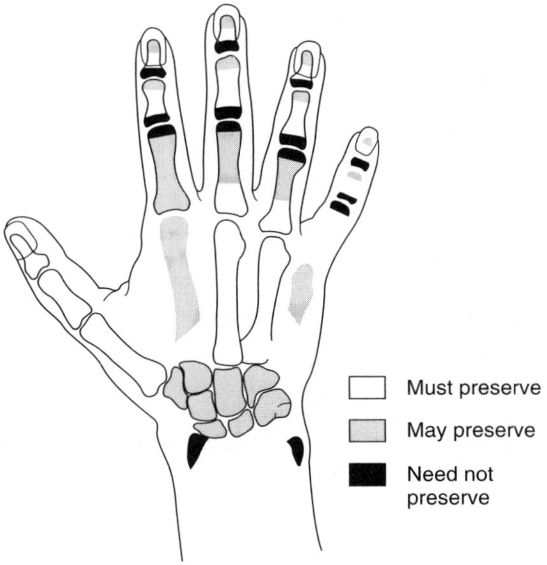

Figure 35–6. Amputation in the hand.

powered prostheses. Prostheses with elbow joints and terminal devices activated by body power are generally more acceptable to amputees.

Traumatic amputations do not have to be treated definitively at the initial debridement. Expectant management will permit questionably viable tissues to demarcate and thereby allow maximal preservation of length. When deciding whether to amputate an injured extremity, the physician should assess the status of five structures: skin, tendons, nerves, bones, and joints. If three or more are compromised, amputation is usually favored over attempts at preserving the part.

1. Wrist Disarticulation

After amputation below the elbow, only about 50% of the ability to perform pronation and supination can be transmitted to a prosthesis, because of the bulk of the proximal forearm and the length of the remaining radius and ulna. The more proximal the amputation, the less pronation and supination is possible. Amputations through the wrist permit the most pronation and supination and provide for better prosthetic control than higher amputations do.

2. Forearm Amputation

Even if only a short residual limb can be achieved, forearm amputation is preferable to above-elbow amputation. As much muscle function as possible should be preserved to maximize control of a prosthesis. Several innovative reconstructive procedures are available that allow upper arm muscles to assist in controlling a prosthesis when a very short residual limb precludes pronation and supination by forearm muscles.

3. Transhumeral Amputation

Every effort should be made to preserve length. Even if a very high amputation is necessary, the head of the humerus should be spared, since it serves as a support for a prosthesis and maintains shoulder width.

4. Forequarter Amputation

Malignant tumor is the usual indication for forequarter amputation. The operation is easiest if done from a posterior approach, but the location and size of the mass may require an anterior approach (Figure 35–7). A thoracotomy or partial neck dissection may be necessary to resect the tumor completely. After the wound has healed, a Silastic foam shoulder cap held in place with straps provides a cosmetically acceptable shoulder.

SPECIAL PROBLEMS OF AMPUTEES

Thromboembolism

The amputee is at great risk for deep venous thrombosis (15%) and pulmonary embolism (2%) postoperatively because (1) amputation often follows prolonged immobilization during treatment of the primary disease and (2) the operation involves ligation of large veins, causing stagnation of blood, a situation that predisposes to thrombosis. If immediate-fit prosthetic techniques are not employed, an additional period of inactivity follows the operation, further increasing the risk of thromboembolism.

Pain & Flexion Contracture

Flexion contractures of the knee or hip occur rapidly in the painful limb because of the natural tendency to assume a flexed posture. Measures to prevent contracture are indicated preoperatively, and application of a rigid dressing postoperatively decreases the incidence of this complication.

Persistent pain in a residual limb and phantom limb pain are common. If the cause of pain is residual limb ischemia, higher amputation is the treatment. A neuroma in a residual limb can be treated by injection of a local anesthetic or excision of the neuroma. Causalgia may respond to sympathectomy. Continuous nerve sheath block using catheters placed adjacent to the transected nerve trunks at the time of surgery may reduce early postoperative pain and late phantom pain. However, introduction of infection by the catheters is a concern.

Phantom limb pain is the sensation that a painful limb is present after amputation. Most amputees experience this phenomenon to some degree. Hypotheses concerning etiology include the gate theory (loss of sensory input decreases self-sustaining neural activity of the gate, causing pain), the peripheral theory (nerve endings in the residual limb represent parts originally innervated by the severed nerve), and the psychologic theory (hostility, guilt, and denial are interpreted as pain). Treatment is difficult; improvement has been reported using tricyclic antidepressants, transcutaneous electrical nerve stimulation (TENS), and calcitonin. The incidence and severity of phantom limb pain are increased if there has been prolonged ischemia before amputation and decreased if postoperative rehabilitation has been rapid.

Increased Mortality Rate

Five-year survival for all lower extremity amputees is less than 50%, compared with 85% for an age-matched

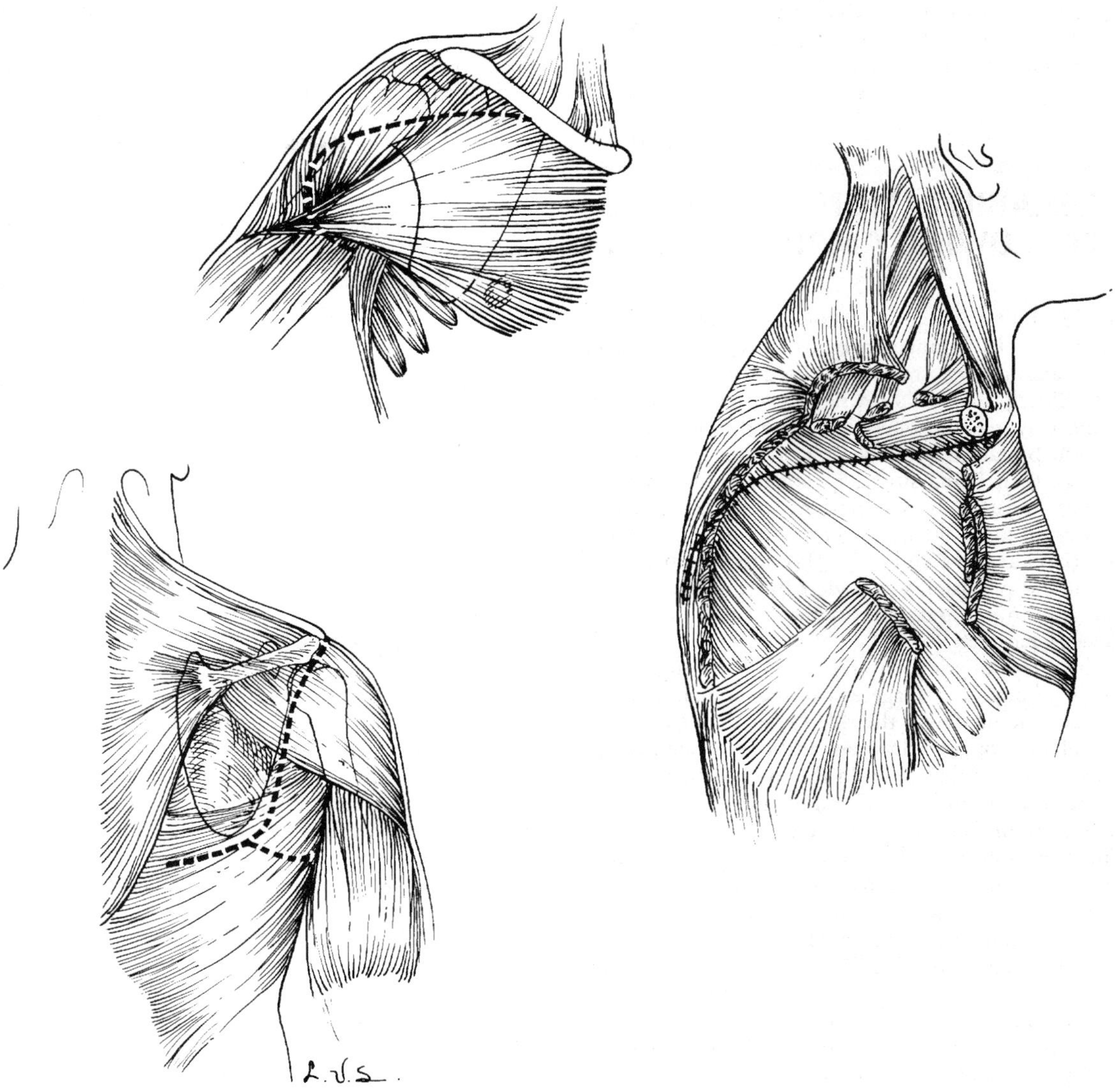

Figure 35–7. Forequarter amputation.

population. Diabetic amputees have only a 40% 5-year survival. Two-thirds of all deaths are due to cardiovascular disease.

Trauma to the Residual Limb

Because their gait is relatively unstable, amputees are at increased risk for falls that may lead to fractures or other injury to the residual limb. Disruption of the wound or skin should usually be allowed to heal by secondary intent. About 3–5% of amputees experience fractures at some time, principally of the distal femur and hip. The diagnosis of fracture is overlooked or delayed in 25% of cases. Although most fractures can be successfully treated, one-half of amputees who were ambulatory before injury become wheelchair-bound afterward.

Ischemia in Residual Limbs

Progressive vascular disease results in ischemia of about 8% of transfemoral amputations and 1% of transtibial amputations. Operations are often required to improve arterial flow when gangrene develops in a residual limb. The mortality rate of this condition is high.

REHABILITATION FOLLOWING AMPUTATION

The rehabilitation goals following amputation are highly variable. Younger patients universally want to regain ambulatory status and frequently return to work. Elderly patients with significant comorbid conditions may remain wheelchair-bound, and much of their rehabilitation is focused on providing wheelchair access in their living situations and working on independent transfers. It is important to understand that amputation in an elderly patient is frequently an event that occurs near the end of life. For these people, relief of pain and provision for modest function may be the most appropriate outcome in the limited amount of time they have left.

The rehabilitation strategy for a young lower extremity amputee is aggressive and straightforward. Eventual ambulation is the rule rather than the exception. The use of rigid dressings and immediate postoperative prostheses has reduced the interval from operation to the beginning of ambulation to 1 month. Patients are instructed in the use of a compressive garment (stump shrinker) to control edema and are taught massage techniques to soften the scar and decrease its sensitivity. A temporary prosthesis allows gait training.

The rehabilitation strategy for older amputees is much different. Only half of elderly patients undergoing amputation are considered rehabilitation candidates. Because of delays in wound healing, the mean time from amputation to prosthetic fitting averages 9 months. Although up to 80% of patients considered candidates for rehabilitation are fitted with a prosthesis, only one-third are ambulatory outside the home. At 2 years, only two-thirds of the ambulatory patients who initially walk remain ambulatory (primarily as a result of contralateral limb disease or cardiopulmonary restrictions). Therefore, independent ambulation after major limb amputation in an elderly vascular patient is the exception rather than the rule.

The rehabilitation of a major upper extremity amputee is more complicated. Most of these patients are young, since trauma is the most common reason for upper extremity amputation. Loss of an upper extremity has greater functional impact on the patient. In addition, the psychologic effects are frequently more severe. For example, the highest suicide rate for amputees in the Vietnam War was reported in those with major upper extremity loss. The variety of functions performed in daily activities using the upper extremity is far greater than for the lower extremity. Effective prostheses for upper extremity amputees utilizing neuromuscular feedback are currently available. However, owing to cost and cosmesis, up to one-third of upper extremity amputees do not wear the prosthesis at all and a larger number wear their prostheses only intermittently. Finally, because of the traumatic etiology for most major upper extremity amputations, the incidence of postamputation pain syndromes is greater than in patients with major lower limb loss.

The length of the residual limb correlates well with regaining the ability to walk. Cardiopulmonary disease and physical weakness make walking an overwhelming effort for some patients; this emphasizes the importance of preserving as long a residual limb as possible, so that walking will require the least possible amount of energy.

PROSTHESES

The patellar tendon-bearing prosthesis is used for 90% of lower extremity amputees. It provides total contact with the residual limb, avoiding excessive pressure in any one area. A cuff suspension strap above the knee maintains close contact between the limb and prosthesis. The solid ankle cushion heel (SACH) prosthesis, the most frequently prescribed foot used for transfemoral and transtibial prostheses, is rugged and adequately simulates ankle motion at heel-strike and toe-off. It is a good initial foot even for the younger, more athletic individual who may go on to a newer, dynamic energy-storing foot after becoming accustomed to the SACH foot.

The most commonly prescribed transfemoral prosthesis is the total-contact suction socket. For older, dysvascular amputees, a single-axis constant friction knee or single-axis "stabilizing" (friction lock) knee is best because it is lightweight. Younger, more athletic transfemoral amputees can tolerate heavier prostheses with hydraulic or pneumatic knees, which permit changes in cadence.

More efficient prostheses requiring less energy are constantly being developed. Components fashioned from new types of plastics, fiberglass casting tapes, and carbon fiber polymers allow construction of ultra-lightweight strong and durable prostheses. They are useful both in elderly amputees (who have less energy reserve) and in young amputees who want to participate in sports.

Gait Analysis

The gait of both transfemoral and transtibial amputees is markedly different from normal gait. The forward velocity of walking is significantly lower in amputees and is lower in transfemoral than transtibial amputees. The time-distance parameters of velocity, cadence, strike length, and gait cycle are 1 SD below normal in transtibial amputees and 2 SD below normal in transfemoral amputees. The normal symmetry of walking is not present, as has been documented by measurements of single-limb support time and motion analyses of the lower extremities, head, arms, and trunk. This asymmetry of motion increases the excursion of the center of mass during each gait cycle and thereby increases the amount of energy used in ambulation.

LONG-TERM CARE FOLLOWING AMPUTATION

Patients who have undergone amputation require periodic checks of the prosthesis and residual limb, physical therapy, and in many cases psychologic support for life. Shrinkage of the residual limb requires replacement of the initial prosthesis after about 6 months and again 1 year after amputation. Thereafter, well-made transtibial prostheses should have a useful life of approximately 2 years. Patients must be educated to care for the residual limb, with utmost attention to cleanliness, and shown how to protect areas of pressure, trauma, or insensitivity.

After amputation for vascular disease or complications of diabetes mellitus, symptoms in the opposite leg should be anticipated and reported promptly, and ulcers or other changes in the residual limb should be brought to the attention of the physician as early as possible.

Adunsky A et al: Non-traumatic lower limb older amputees: a database survey from a geriatric center. Disabil Rehabil 2001;20:80.

Cutson TM, Borgiorni DR: Rehabilitation of the older lower limb amputee: a brief review. J Am Geriatr Soc 1996;44:1388.

Dirschl DR, Dahners LE: The mangled extremity: when should it be amputated? J Am Acad Orthop Surg 1996;4:182.

Fletcher DD et al: Rehabilitation of the geriatric vascular amputee patient: a population-based study. Arch Phys Med Rehabil 2001;82:776.

Huang ME, Levy CE, Webster JB: Acquired limb deficiencies. 3. Prosthetic components, prescriptions, and indications. Arch Phys Med Rehabil 2001;82:S17.

Kent R, Fyfe N: Effectiveness of rehabilitation following amputation. Clin Rehabil 1999;13(Suppl I):43.

Levy CE et al: Acquired limb deficiencies. 4. Troubleshooting. Arch Phys Med Rehabil 2001;82:S25.

Manord JD et al: Management of severe proximal vascular and neural injury of the upper extremity. J Vasc Surg 1998;27:43.

Mayfield JA et al: Trends in lower limb amputations in the Veterans Health Administration, 1989–1998. J Rehabil Res Dev 2000;37:22.

Nehler MR et al: Intermediate term outcome of primary digit amputations in diabetic patients with forefoot sepsis and adequate circulatory status. J Vasc Surg 1999;30:509.

Pohjolainen T, Alarnta H: Ten-year survival of Finnish lower limb amputees. Prosthet Orthot Int 1998;22:10.

Sewell P et al: Developments in the trans-tibial prosthetic socket fitting process: a review of past and present research. Prosthet Orthot Int 2000;24:97.

Trautner C et al: Incidence of lower limb amputations and diabetes. Diabetes Care 1996;19:1006.

White SA et al: Lower limb amputation and grade of surgeon. Br J Surg 1997;84:509.

Veins & Lymphatics

36

Thomas W. Wakefield, MD, & Louis M. Messina, MD

I. THE VEINS

VENOUS ANATOMY

Veins of the lower extremity (Figure 36–1) consist of superficial and deep systems joined by venous perforators. The greater and lesser saphenous veins are superficial—veins, the name "saphenous" aptly derived from the Greek word for "manifest, clear," ie, "visible." They contain many valves and show considerable variation in their location and branching points. In up to 10% of patients, the greater saphenous vein may be duplicated. Typically, it originates from the superficial arch of the foot and is found anterior to the medial malleolus at the ankle. As it ascends in the calf just beneath the superficial fascia, it is joined by two major tributaries: an anterior vein, which crosses the tibia; and a posterior arch vein, which arises posterior to the medial malleolus beside the posterior tibial artery. The greater saphenous vein then enters the fossa ovalis to empty into the deep femoral vein.

The saphenofemoral junction is marked by four or five prominent branches of the greater saphenous vein: the superficial circumflex iliac vein, the external pudendal vein, the superficial epigastric vein, and the medial and lateral accessory saphenous veins. Another important anatomic landmark is the relationship of the greater saphenous vein to the saphenous branch of the femoral nerve; as it emerges from the popliteal space, the nerve follows a course parallel to the vein. Injury during saphenous vein stripping or saphenous vein harvest for bypass produces neuropathic pain or numbness along the medial calf and foot. The lesser saphenous vein arises from the superficial dorsal venous arch behind the lateral malleolus at the ankle and curves toward the midline of the posterior calf, ascending to join the popliteal vein behind the knee.

Deep veins of the leg parallel the courses of the arteries. Two or three venae comitantes accompany each tibial artery. At the knee, these paired high-capacitance veins merge to form the popliteal vein, which continues proximally as the superficial femoral vein. At the inguinal ligament, the superficial and deep (profunda) femoral veins join medial to the femoral artery to form the common femoral vein. In the pelvis, external and internal iliac veins join to form common iliac veins that empty into the inferior vena cava. The right common iliac vein ascends almost vertically to the inferior vena cava, while the left common iliac vein takes a more transverse course. For this reason, the left common iliac vein may be compressed between the right common iliac artery and lumbosacral spine, a condition known as May-Thurner (Cockett) syndrome.

Muscular sinusoids represent another component of the deep veins of the leg. These thin-walled, nonvalved venous lakes run longitudinally within soleus muscle bellies and then coalesce to join the posterior tibial and peroneal veins. Blood empties from these sinusoids during muscle contraction; inactivity leads to stasis and may contribute to the development of deep venous thrombosis.

Blood flow is directed from superficial to deep veins of the leg via valved perforating (communicating) veins. Perforators are located below the medial malleolus (inframalleolar perforator), in the medial calf (Cockett perforators), at the level of the adductor canal (Hunterian perforator), and just above (Dodd's perforator) and below (Boyd's perforator) the knee.

Delicate bicuspid venous valves prevent reflux and direct the flow of blood from the foot and leg toward the heart. Valves are more numerous in the distal part of the extremity, decrease in number proximally, and are virtually absent in the inferior vena cava itself.

The inferior vena cava ascends in the abdomen and ends at the right atrium. It lies to the right of the midline, lateral to the aorta, and receives a number of lumbar veins that connect with the vertebral and paravertebral venous plexuses. The inferior vena cava and its tributaries are derived in the sixth to tenth week of life from the fusion and obliteration of several paired embryonic veins: the anterior and posterior cardinal veins, the subcardinal veins, the supracardinal veins, and the sacrocardinal veins. Because of this complex embryonic development, anomalies in the venous system are not uncommon. The most common abnormality is a circumaortic left renal vein (1.5–8.7% incidence), followed by a retroaortic left renal vein (1.2–2.4% incidence), duplication of the inferior vena cava (0.2–3% incidence), and left-sided inferior vena cava (0.2–0.5% incidence). An unsuspected retroaortic or

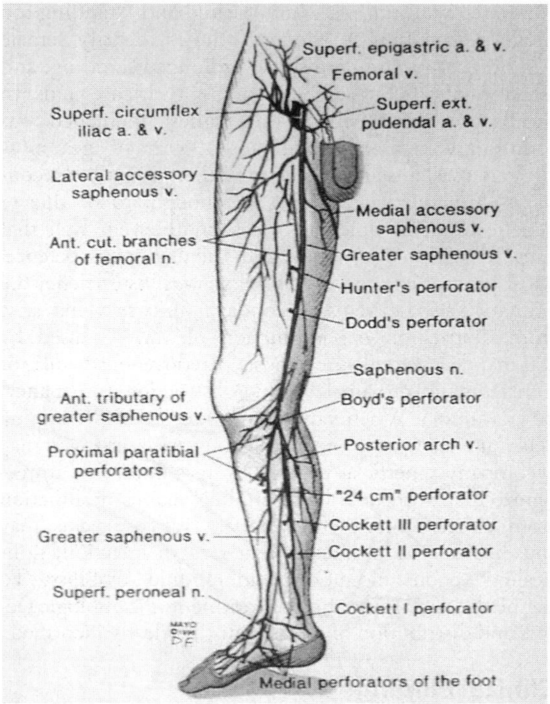

Figure 36–1. Anatomy of the superficial and perforating veins of the lower extremity. (From Rutherford RB, Cronenwett JL, Gloviczki P: *Vascular Surgery.* Philadelphia: Saunders, 2000. Reproduced by permission from Elsevier.)

circumaortic renal vein can be inadvertently injured during aortic cross-clamping.

Veins of the upper extremity are also divided into superficial and deep groups, though direction of flow from superficial to deep is not as distinct as in the lower extremity. Dorsal veins of the hand empty into the cephalic vein ("intern vein") on the radial aspect and into the basilic vein on the ulnar aspect of the forearm. The cephalic vein ascends lateral to the biceps muscle into the deltopectoral groove, where it passes through the clavipectoral fascia to join the axillary vein. The cephalic vein is useful for arteriovenous fistulas because it is superficial and lateral in the arm, allowing easy access for hemodialysis needles. The basilic vein, which runs medially in the arm to become the axillary vein, is deeper and thicker-walled than the cephalic vein. Its many branches make it tedious to harvest, but it can be used for a bypass conduit or for a laterally tunneled upper arm dialysis fistula (basilic vein transposition). The median cubital vein links the cephalic and basilic veins in the antecubital space.

Paired brachial veins comprise the deep system of veins. They accompany the brachial artery and join the basilic vein as it becomes the axillary vein. The axillary vein continues medially as the subclavian vein, which passes through a tight space anterior to the first rib and anterior scalene muscle and posterior to the clavicle. The subclavian vein and the internal jugular vein join behind the clavicular head to form the brachiocephalic vein, which empties into the superior vena cava.

Caggiati A et al: Nomenclature of the veins of the lower limbs: an international interdisciplinary consensus statement. J Vasc Surg 2002;36:416.

Giordano JM et al: Anomalies of the vena cava. J Vasc Surg 1986;3:924.

Scultetus AH et al: Facts and fiction surrounding the discovery of venous valves. J Vasc Surg 2001;33:435.

VENOUS PHYSIOLOGY

Knowledge of lower extremity venous anatomy is essential to understanding the physiology of venous flow. The volume of blood in the lower extremities may increase by one-half liter when an individual moves from a reclining to an erect position (Figure 36–2). Increased blood volume is accommodated by increased venous

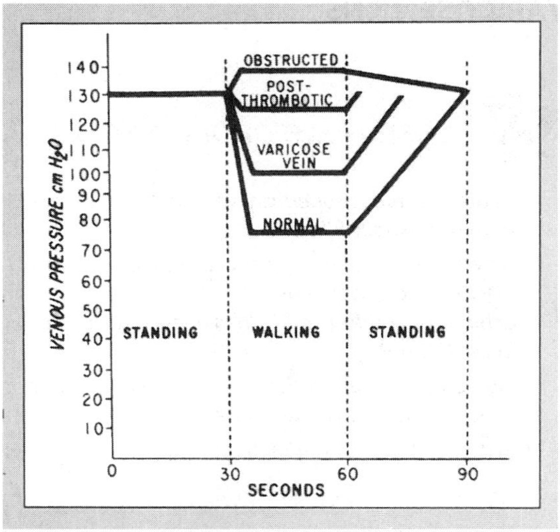

Figure 36–2. Pedal venous pressure measurements with exercise. The normal drop in pressure associated with ambulation is impaired by deep vein incompetence and proximal venous obstruction. (Reproduced, with permission, from DeWeese JA: Venous and lymphatic disease. In: *Principles of Surgery,* 4th ed. Schwarz S [editor]. McGraw-Hill, 1983.)

capacitance, which is regulated by smooth muscle contractility in the vein walls. Erect posture creates a vertical column of blood, exerting a hydrostatic pressure equal to the distance from the toes to the right atrium (about 100–120 mm Hg). The hydrostatic pressure must be overcome to avoid pooling of blood in the legs and to provide venous return to the heart. Several aspects of the venous system make it possible to move blood against the force of gravity. Because the circulation is a closed system, venous return is affected by arterial inflow and by the negative intrathoracic pressure created during inspiration. Valves assure unidirectional movement of blood from superficial to deep systems and from the foot back to the heart. Hydrostatic pressure is dissipated by lack of simultaneous opening of the valves. Soleal venous sinusoids are another central component to the system. When the muscle contracts during exercise, blood empties from the sinusoid into the deep veins of the calf and leg. This high-velocity flow siphons blood from deep veins of the foot upward into the calf, analogous to smoke being drawn up a smokestack by wind blowing past the chimney (Venturi effect).

DISEASES OF THE VENOUS SYSTEM

VARICOSE VEINS

ESSENTIALS OF DIAGNOSIS

- *Dilated, tortuous superficial veins in the lower extremities, usually bilateral.*
- *May be asymptomatic or may be associated with bleeding, localized pain, nocturnal cramps, or aching discomfort and "heaviness" with prolonged standing.*
- *Pigmentation, ulceration, and edema suggest concomitant venous stasis disease.*
- *Increased frequency after pregnancy.*

General Considerations

Varicose veins are very common, afflicting 10–20% of the world's population. Abnormally dilated veins occur in several locations in the body: the spermatic cord (varicocele), esophagus (esophageal varices), and the anorectum (hemorrhoids). Varicosities of the legs were described as early as 1550 BC, and in the 1600s AD were correlated with trauma, childbearing, and "standing too much before kings." Modern studies identify female sex, pregnancy, family history, prolonged standing, and a history of phlebitis as risk factors for varicose veins. In the Framingham Study, the highest incidence was found in women between 40 and 49 years of age.

Varicose veins are classified as either primary or secondary. Primary varicose veins are thought to be due to genetic or developmental defects in the vein wall that cause diminished elasticity and valvular incompetence. Most cases of isolated superficial venous insufficiency are primary varicose veins. Secondary varicose veins arise from destruction or dysfunction of valves caused by trauma, deep venous thrombosis, arteriovenous fistula, or nontraumatic proximal venous obstruction (pregnancy, pelvic tumor). When valves of the deep and perforating veins are disrupted, chronic venous stasis changes may accompany superficial varicosities. It is important to recognize that untreated, long-standing venous dysfunction from either primary or secondary varicose veins may cause chronic skin changes that lead to infection, nonhealing venous ulceration, and chronic disability. To define the optimal method of treatment, the etiologic factors and distribution of disease must be clearly identified.

Clinical Findings

The clinical presentation of patients with varicose veins can be quite variable. Most varicose veins are asymptomatic and come to medical attention because of aesthetic concerns. If symptomatic, varicose veins may be associated with localized pain, a burning sensation over the vein, a diffuse ache or "heaviness" in the calf (particularly with prolonged standing), or phlebitis. Mild ankle edema may occur. Symptoms generally improve with leg elevation.

The varicosities appear as dilated, tortuous, elongated veins predominantly on the medial aspect of the lower extremity along the course of the greater saphenous vein. Overlying skin changes may be absent even in the presence of extensive large varicosities. Smaller flat, blue-green reticular veins, telangiectasias, and spider veins may accompany varicose veins and are further evidence of venous dysfunction. A cluster of telangiectasias below the inframalleolar perforator is termed a corona phlebectatica paraplantaris. Secondary varicose veins can cause symptoms characteristic of chronic venous insufficiency, including edema, hyperpigmentation, stasis dermatitis, and even venous ulcerations.

Physical examination begins with inspection of all extremities to determine the distribution and severity of the varicosities. Bimanual circumferential palpation of the thighs and calves is helpful. Palpation of a thrill or auscultation of a bruit indicates the presence of an arteriovenous fistula as a possible etiologic factor. The **Brodie-Trendelenburg test** is a maneuver for identifying sites of valvular incompetence. Today, tourniquet tests have been virtually replaced by venous duplex ultrasound imaging, identifying points of venous reflux.

Differential Diagnosis

Ulceration, brawny induration, and hyperpigmentation often indicate accompanying chronic deep venous insufficiency. This is important to recognize because the changes generally do not resolve with saphenous vein stripping, and wound healing following surgery may be jeopardized by failure to treat the venous stasis disease.

If extensive varicose veins are encountered in a young patient, especially if unilateral and in an atypical distribution (lateral leg), Klippel-Trenaunay syndrome must be considered. The classic triad is varicose veins, limb hypertrophy, and a cutaneous birthmark (port wine stain or venous malformation). Because the deep veins are often anomalous or absent, saphenous vein stripping can be hazardous. Standard treatment for patients with Klippel-Trenaunay syndrome is graduated support stockings, limited stab avulsion of symptomatic varices after thorough duplex ultrasound vein mapping, and occasional surgery for correction of limb length discrepancy.

Treatment

A. Nonsurgical Treatment

Treatment for both primary and secondary varicose veins initially involves a program directed at management of venous insufficiency, including elastic stocking support, periodic leg elevation, and regular exercise. Prolonged sitting and standing are discouraged. For most patients, knee-high or thigh-high gradient compression stockings of 20–30 mm Hg are sufficient, although some patients require 30–40 mm Hg pressure. The compression stockings are worn all day to diminish venous distention during standing and are removed at night.

B. Surgical Treatment

Indications for surgical treatment (Figure 36–3) include persistent or disabling pain, recurrent superficial thrombophlebitis, erosion of the overlying skin with bleeding, and manifestations of chronic venous insufficiency (particularly ulceration).

The operative plan is dependent on determination of the competency of the deep and perforating veins and the location of sites of venous reflux. Surgery can then be tailored to the pattern of disease. High ligation and stripping of the saphenous system is performed for patients with an incompetent valve at the saphenofemoral junction and varicosities throughout the length of the greater saphenous vein. This is performed by ligating the saphenofemoral junction and the major proximal saphenous vein branches through a small incision in the groin. Then the saphenous vein is removed to the point of clusters of varicosities. These clusters of varicose veins are then removed by the stab-avulsion technique. Stab incisions 1.5–2 mm long are made along premarked varicosities, and specially designed vein hooks are then used to loop the vein segments, which are then delivered through the incisions. With careful patient selection and properly selected operative techniques, the recurrence rate should be approximately 10%. Complications include hematoma formation, infection, and saphenous nerve irritation.

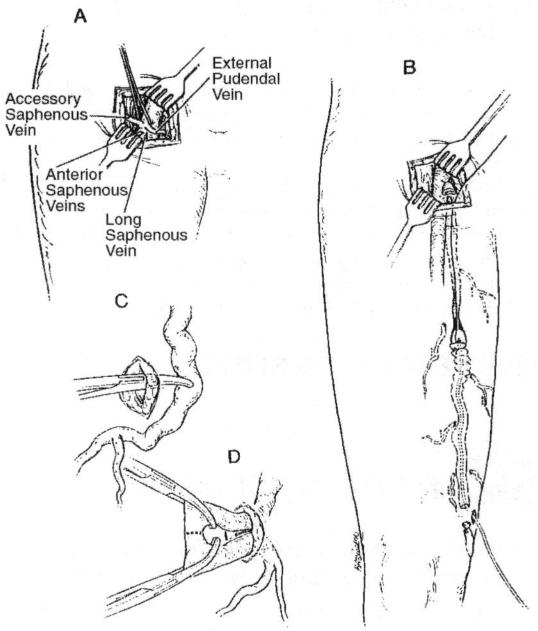

Figure 36–3. Technique of varicose vein stripping. (From Bergan JJ, Kistner RL: *Atlas of Venous Surgery.* Saunders, 1992. Reproduced by permission from Elsevier.)

C. Compression Sclerotherapy

Compression sclerotherapy is usually applied to telangiectasias, spider veins, and small varicosities that persist after vein stripping. With the patient supine, a small volume of sclerosing solution (0.2–3% sodium tetradecyl sulfate or hypertonic saline) is injected into a varix isolated by proximal and distal digital venous occlusion. Direct pressure with compression stockings is maintained for 1 week afterward. The goal is to obliterate the abnormal vein by inducing localized endothelial destruction and fibrosis. More than one treatment is often required. Complications, including allergic reactions, thrombophlebitis, neoangiogenesis, and skin necrosis or hyperpigmentation, are rare.

Belcaro G et al: Endovascular sclerotherapy, surgery, and surgery plus sclerotherapy in superficial venous incompetence: a randomized, 10 year follow-up trial—final results. Angiology 2000;51:529.

Bradbury A et al: The relationship between lower limb symptoms and superficial and deep venous reflux on duplex ultrasonography: the Edinburgh Vein Study. J Vasc Surg 2000;32:921.

Dwerryhouse S: Stripping the long saphenous vein reduces the rate of reoperation for recurrent varicose veins: five year results of a randomized trial. J Vasc Surg 1999;29:589.

DEEP VEIN THROMBOSIS

ESSENTIALS OF DIAGNOSIS

- *Pain in the thigh or calf sometimes accompanied by edema. Half of patients are asymptomatic.*
- *History of recent surgery, trauma, cancer, prolonged immobilization, or oral contraceptive use.*
- *Clinical impression is accurate in 50% of cases.*
- *Venous duplex ultrasound is the diagnostic modality of choice.*

General Considerations

Deep venous thrombosis (DVT) affects more than 250,000 people per year in the USA and its incidence increases with age. Treatment is estimated to cost billions of dollars per year, not even including expenditures associated with long-term sequelae of this disease.

Virchow's triad (stasis, vascular injury, and hypercoagulability) should be the cornerstone for assessment of risk factors for DVT. In the majority of cases, the cause is multifactorial.

Acquired risk factors include older age, cancer, surgery, trauma, immobilization, hormone replacement therapy, oral contraceptive use, pregnancy, neurologic disease, cardiac disease, and antiphospholipid antibodies. Approximately 20–30% of patients with a new DVT (both upper and lower extremity) have an occult or known malignancy. One-fourth of these are lung cancers, although hypercoagulability may also be seen in patients with cancer of the pancreas, prostate, colon, breast, and ovary. Most of these malignancies are associated with increased fibrinogen or thrombocytosis.

Endothelial injury can result from direct trauma (severed vein, venous cannulation, or transvenous pacing) or local irritation secondary to infusion of chemotherapy, previous DVT, or phlebitis. Damaged endothelium leads to platelet aggregation, degranulation, and formation of thrombus as well as vasoconstriction and activation of the coagulation cascade. Thrombin activation from release of tissue factor and diminished fibrinolysis mediated by plasminogen activator inhibitor are intraoperative events that may be related to endothelial disruption.

Hypercoagulable states may also be inherited. Genetic causes include deficiencies of natural coagulation inhibitors (antithrombin III, protein C, protein S), factor V Leiden, prothrombin 20210A gene variant, blood group non-O, elevated homocysteine levels, plasminogen abnormalities, elevated levels of coagulation factors (such as factor VIII), and reduced heparin cofactor II activity. Hematologic disorders associated with DVT include disseminated intravascular coagulation, heparin-induced thrombocytopenia, antiphospholipid antibody syndrome, thrombotic thrombocytopenic purpura, hemolytic uremic syndrome, polycythemia vera, and essential thrombocythemia. Inflammatory bowel disease, systemic lupus erythematosus, and obesity are additionally associated with DVT.

Deep venous thrombosis occurs most frequently in the calf veins, though it may arise in the femoral or iliac veins. Thrombi originate in soleal sinusoids or in valve sinuses, where there are flow eddies. Treatment of isolated calf vein thrombosis is controversial, as it is associated with a low risk of pulmonary embolism. However, if untreated, up to 25% may progress to proximal deep veins of the leg, where the incidence of chronic venous insufficiency is 25% and that of pulmonary embolism is 10%. These observations and the improved safety profile of low-molecular-weight heparin are compelling practitioners to treat isolated calf DVTs aggressively.

Clinical Findings

A. Symptoms and Signs

The diagnosis of DVT cannot be made solely on the basis of presenting symptoms and signs, as up to half of patients with acute thromboses have no abnormality detectable in the involved extremity. Homans' sign (pain on passive dorsiflexion of the ankle) is positive in only half of cases and is so nonspecific that it is not useful. Some patients present with acute pulmonary embolism unaccompanied by leg edema or pain.

Symptomatic patients most often complain of a dull ache or pain in the calf or leg associated with mild edema. With extensive proximal DVT, there can be massive edema, cyanosis, and dilated superficial collateral veins. Low-grade fever and tachycardia occasionally occur. Iliofemoral venous thrombosis can result in phlegmasia. In phlegmasia alba dolens, the leg is pulseless, pale, and cool, which may progress to phlegmasia cerulea dolens, characterized by cyanosis of the limb and a precursor to gangrene.

B. Imaging Studies

Because DVT is difficult to diagnose on the basis of physical signs or symptoms, some objective diagnostic study is required before treatment is started. Historically, the standard for diagnosis was ascending phlebography, accomplished by fluoroscopic imaging during contrast injection into an intravenous line on the dorsum of the foot. The patient stands but is non-weight-bearing on the extremity studied. An abrupt cutoff of the contrast column indicates DVT. The complications of this procedure include risk of contrast allergy, contrast-induced nephropathy, and phlebitis.

Duplex ultrasound has now become the test of choice. It is a noninvasive examination, does not expose the patient to radiation, is easily reproducible, and has specificity and sensitivity of greater than 95%. It is also useful to detect other potential pathologic processes such as Baker's cyst. The examination includes both a B-mode image and Doppler flow analysis. Each venous segment is assessed for the presence of thrombosis, indicated by venous dilation and incompressibility during light probe pressure. Doppler findings suggestive of acute DVT are absence of spontaneous flow, loss of flow variation with respiration, and failure to increase flow velocity after distal augmentation. The criteria for the presence of chronic venous thrombosis are less well established. The chronically occluded vein is often narrowed, and there are prominent nearby collaterals. Chronic thrombi are highly echogenic, while acute thrombi are anechoic (and, therefore, not visible) on the B-mode image. Duplex ultrasound is less accurate in detection of calf thromboses and is highly operator-dependent.

Magnetic resonance venography shows promise as a diagnostic study for this disorder. The sensitivity and specificity of magnetic resonance venography are 100% and 96%, respectively. The injection of gadolinium is useful for determining the age of the thrombus.

Measurement of D-dimer levels is too nonspecific for use alone and scanning with radiolabeled fibrinogen too sensitive in the pelvis for use in the acute clinical setting. Additionally, fibrinogen scanning carries with it a risk of transmission of infectious disease. Older tests, such as impedance plethysmography and venous pressure measurements, do not achieve the same accuracy as duplex ultrasound and have been largely abandoned.

Differential Diagnosis

Localized muscle strain or contusion or Achilles tendon rupture can often mimic the symptoms of DVT. Cellulitis may cause edema, localized pain, and erythema. Unilateral leg swelling can also result from lymphedema, obstruction of the popliteal vein by Baker's cyst, or obstruction of the iliac vein by retroperitoneal mass or idiopathic fibrosis. Bilateral leg edema suggests heart, liver, or kidney failure or inferior vena cava obstruction by tumor or pregnancy.

Treatment

Treatment is aimed at reducing the incidence of complications associated with DVT, which include varicose veins, chronic venous insufficiency, recurrent DVT, or pulmonary thromboembolism. The primary treatment of DVT is systemic anticoagulation. This reduces the risk of pulmonary embolism and extension of venous thrombosis and also decreases the rate of recurrent DVT by 80%. Systemic anticoagulation does not directly lyse thrombi but stops propagation and allows natural fibrinolysis to occur. Heparin is initiated immediately and dosed to a goal PTT of 1.5–2.5 times normal. Achieving therapeutic heparinization within the first 24 hours after diagnosis is shown to reduce the rate of recurrent DVT.

Warfarin is started after therapeutic heparinization. The two therapies should overlap to diminish the possibility of a hypercoagulable state, which can occur during the first few days of warfarin administration, because warfarin also inhibits the synthesis of natural anticoagulant proteins C and S. The recommended treatment for a first episode of uncomplicated DVT is 3–6 months of warfarin, maintained at a goal international normalized ratio (INR) of 2.0–3.0. After a second episode of DVT, the usual recommendation is lifelong warfarin. The risk for recurrent venous thrombosis is increased markedly in the presence of homozygous factor V Leiden mutations, antiphospholipid antibody, and antithrombin III and protein C or protein S deficiencies, so lifelong anticoagulation is usually recommended for these conditions as well.

Low-molecular-weight heparin (LMWH) has been shown to be as safe and effective as standard unfractionated heparin in the treatment of DVT. It is administered once or twice daily by subcutaneous injection. LMWH does not require monitoring of its anticoagulant effect because of its predictable dose-response relationship, and this feature of the drug has made feasible the outpatient treatment of DVT. Standard unfractionated heparin inhibits thrombin because it is large enough to make a three-way complex between thrombin, antithrombin, and itself. LMWHs are much smaller than standard heparin molecules and do not inhibit thrombin; their main therapeutic effect comes from inhibition of factor Xa activity. The advantages of LMWHs over standard heparin preparations include a lower risk of bleeding complications and thrombocytopenia, less interference with proteins C and S, less complement activation, and a lower risk of osteoporosis.

Moreover, recent randomized trials have shown regression of thrombus with LMWH. In many situations, standard heparin is being replaced by LMWH.

Two new areas of treatment that have demonstrated significant promise include direct thrombin inhibitors and specific factor Xa inhibitors. Regarding direct thrombin inhibitors, ximelagatran/melagatran has shown considerable promise for both the prophylaxis and treatment of DVT. This drug can be taken orally and may be an alternative to warfarin without the need for monitoring and with no increase in bleeding. In a large prospective study comparing orally administered ximelagatran (which is metabolized to the active melagatran) to placebo for 18 additional months after 6 months of standard anticoagulation for DVT in 1223 patients, the recurrent DVT/pulmonary embolism (PE) rate was reduced from approximately 13% to 3%. Likewise, this agent has been found to be effective in the prophylaxis of DVT in orthopedic surgery patients. The specific factor Xa inhibitor pentasaccharide has also shown significant promise for the prophylaxis and treatment of DVT. This drug potentiates by approximately 300-fold the neutralization of factor Xa by antithrombin III, without inactivating thrombin. In orthopedic surgical indications, this agent has shown superiority to the best currently available DVT prophylaxis using LMWH. Regarding DVT treatment, large prospective randomized studies for both DVT and PE have been conducted. For DVT, in 154 centers, 23 countries, and with 2205 patients (> 30% outpatients), the recurrent DVT rate/major hemorrhage rate was 3.9%/1.1% for pentasaccharide versus 4.1%/1.2% for LMWH. For PE, in 214 centers, 20 countries, and with 2213 patients (with 15% outpatients), the recurrent PE/major hemorrhage rate was 3.8%/1/3% for pentasaccharide and 5%/1.1% for standard unfractionated heparin. Mortality rates were equal. These two agents, alone with others in development, likely will revolutionize the prophylaxis and treatment (acute and chronic) of DVT.

Many studies have evaluated the efficacy of fibrinolytic agents in the treatment of DVT. Recombinant tissue plasminogen activator (rt-PA; alteplase) has generally superseded urokinase and streptokinase in clinical use, although urokinase (which had been withdrawn from the market) is again available for use. Although faster clot lysis and increased venous patency are observed with alteplase versus heparin, this has not translated to a decreased incidence of long-term sequelae such as chronic venous insufficiency. The risk of bleeding complications is higher with alteplase and does not appear to be reduced by selective catheterization for local administration. To be effective, alteplase should be instituted within 1 week after clot formation, before extensive fibrin cross-linking can occur. There has been no demonstrable benefit to selective administration of alteplase, but theoretically this technique may allow medication dose reduction. One possible application for LMWH is acute iliofemoral venous thrombosis complicated by massive extremity edema, cyanosis, or calf compartment syndrome. Iliofemoral thrombectomy achieves a clinical success rate of 40–90% for this disorder, with most treatment failures being due to residual distal thrombosis, stenosis or obliteration of the proximal vein, or recurrent thrombosis.

Prevention

Surgery increases the risk of DVT 21-fold. This disorder is a reported complication for approximately 20–25% of patients admitted for a general surgical procedure, 20–30% of those undergoing an elective neurosurgical procedure, and 50–60% of those undergoing hip or knee arthroplasty. These statistics emphasize the need for routine DVT prophylaxis in the surgical patient. The most commonly used measures are elastic stockings, pneumatic sequential compression devices (PCD), low-dose unfractionated heparin (5000 units given by subcutaneous injection), or LMWH given at a prophylactic dose subcutaneously (either once or twice daily).

For general surgical patients, the incidence of DVT is high without prophylaxis, and the risk of PE is 1.6%, 0.9% fatal. Patients have been categorized into levels of risk. In low-risk patients, no specific thromboembolism prophylaxis is indicated other than early ambulation. In moderate-risk patients, prophylaxis includes low-dose standard unfractionated heparin (LDH), LMWH, PCD, or elastic stockings. For higher-risk patients, LDH, LMWH, or PCD should be used, whereas for very high-risk patients, LDH or LMWH plus PCD is recommended. Full-dose warfarin may also be used, but few general surgeons use full-dose warfarin during surgery because of the risk of significant bleeding. Aspirin alone is not recommended for general surgery patients.

For orthopedic patients without prophylaxis, the incidence of DVT is as high as 45–57% for total hip replacement, 40–84% for total knee replacement, and 36–60% for hip fracture surgery patients. For these groups, total PE incidence is 0.7–30%, 1.8–7%, and 4.3–24%, respectively, and fatal PE incidence is 0.1%–0.4%, 0.2–0.7%, and 3.6–12.9%, respectively. For total hip replacement, LMWH, adjusted-dose warfarin, or adjusted-dose standard unfractionated heparin has been recommended. Adjuvant physical modalities may provide additional benefit. For total knee replacement, LMWH, adjusted-dose warfarin, or PCD should be used. For both total hip and knee surgery, mechanical measures are indicated when anticoagulation cannot be used due to the risk of bleeding. For hip fracture surgery, preoperative or postoperative LMWH or adjusted-dose warfarin is suggested. Prolonged post-hospital prophylaxis may improve both total DVT and PE rates, as studies suggest that up to one-third of these episodes occur after discharge.

For trauma patients evidence is lacking, and randomized studies are needed. Without DVT prophylaxis, DVT may occur > 50% of cases. PE is the third most common cause of death in trauma patients surviving past the first day. Trauma risk factors include lower extremity or pelvic fractures, surgical procedures, advanced age, femoral vein lines or major venous repairs, prolonged immobility, spinal cord injury, and prolonged duration of hospital stay. Acceptable prophylaxis includes LMWH and PCD (when bleeding risk is high). Duplex ultrasound screening is appropriate when standard methods cannot be used. Inferior vena cava filters are recommended in patients when anticoagulation is contraindicated. The benefits of combined therapy are unknown. Contraindications to the initiation of LMWH include intracranial bleeding, incomplete spinal cord injury with perispinal hematoma, severe uncorrected coagulopathy, and uncontrolled bleeding.

In neurosurgery, DVT and PE occur equivalent to rates in general surgery patients, and risk factors include intracranial surgery, prolonged surgery, malignant tumors, the presence of leg weakness, and increased age. PCD with or without elastic stockings is recommended when anticoagulation cannot be used, although combining LDH or postoperative LMWH with PCD with or without stockings may be more effective than either technique alone. Overall rates of DVT and proximal DVT are reduced approximately 50% by combined treatment. For those with spinal cord injury, PE is a frequent cause of death. LMWH with or without mechanical measures is recommended for 3 months or at least until the completion of rehabilitation. LDH, PCD, and elastic stockings are inadequate alone, whereas adjusted-dose warfarin or LMWH have been suggested in the rehabilitation phase. Although IVC filters have been recommended in high-risk trauma and orthopedic patients to prevent PE with good results in small series, no large randomized prospective studies comparing prophylactic filters with more standard methods is available.

Bauer KA, Rusendaal FR, Heit JA: Hypercoagulability: too many tests, too much conflicting data. Hematology 2002;1:353.

Breddin HK et al: Effects of a low-molecular-weight heparin on thrombus regression and recurrent thromboembolism in patients with deep-vein thrombosis. N Engl J Med 2001;344:626.

Douglas MG, Sumnar DS: Duplex scanning for deep vein thrombosis: has it replaced both phlebography and non-invasive testing? Sem Vasc Surg 1996;9:3.

Ferrari E et al: Travel as a risk factor for venous thromboembolic disease: a case-control study. Chest 1999;115:440.

Forster A et al: Tissue plasminogen activator for the treatment of deep venous thrombosis of the lower extremity: a systematic review. Chest 2001;119:572.

Geerts WH et al: Prevention of venous thromboembolism. Chest 2001;119:132S.

Heit JA et al: The epidemiology of venous thromboembolism in the community. Thromb Haemost 2001;86:452.

Hirsh J et al: Clinical trials that have influenced the treatment of venous thromboembolism: a historical perspective. Ann Intern Med 2001;134:409.

Hyers TM et al: Antithrombotic therapy for venous thromboembolic disease. Chest 2001;119(Suppl):176S.

The Matisse Investigators: Subcutaneous Fondaparinux versus intravenous unfractionated heparin in the initial treatment of pulmonary embolism. N Engl J Med 2003;349:1695.

Prandoni P et al: The long term clinical course of acute deep venous thrombosis. Ann Intern Med 1996;125:1.

Schulman S et al: Secondary prevention of venous thromboembolism with the oral direct thrombin inhibitor Ximelagatran. N Engl J Med 2003;349:1713.

AXILLARY-SUBCLAVIAN VENOUS THROMBOSIS

ESSENTIALS OF DIAGNOSIS

- *History of strenuous, repetitive upper extremity activity or recent venous cannulation.*
- *Aching pain, cyanosis, and edema of the anterior chest wall, axilla, shoulder, arm, and hand.*
- *Prominent distended venous collaterals.*
- *Subclavian vein obstruction at the thoracic outlet.*

General Considerations

Thrombosis of the axillary or subclavian vein is a relatively uncommon event, accounting for less than 5% of all cases of DVT. Only 12% result in pulmonary thromboembolism, but local symptoms of upper extremity thrombosis can cause significant disability.

There are two major etiologies. Primary axillary-subclavian thrombosis, also known as Paget-Schroetter syndrome or "effort thrombosis," occurs as a result of intermittent transient obstruction of the vein in the costoclavicular space during repetitive or strenuous activities involving the upper extremity (Figure 36–4). This condition was first described in independent reports by Paget and von Schroetter in the late 19th century. During strenuous repetitive

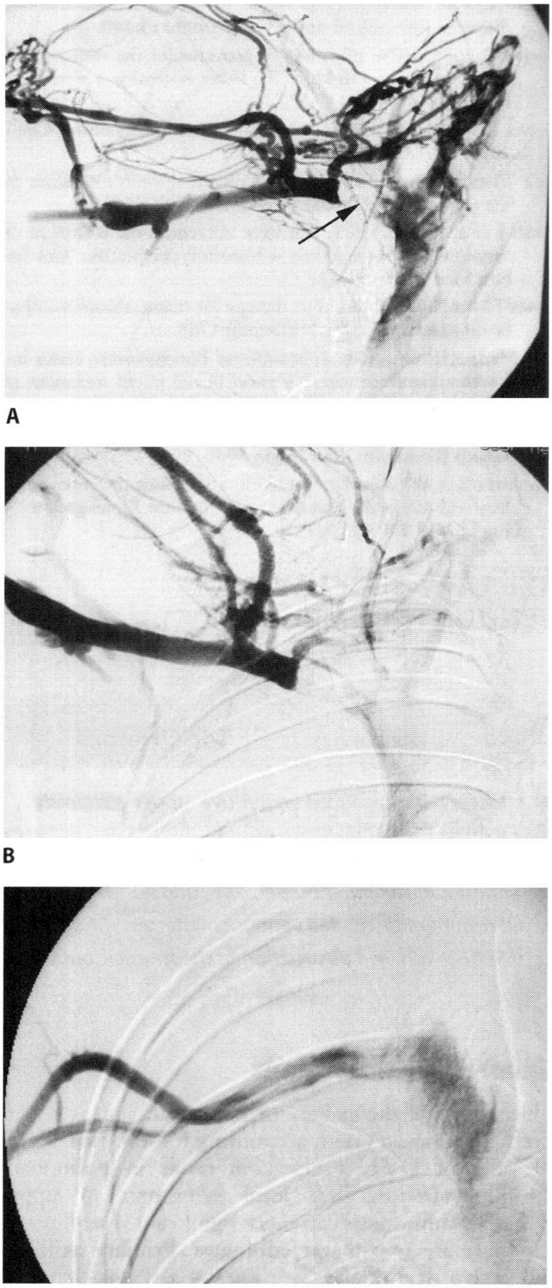

Figure 36–4. A: Effort thrombosis in a 13-year-old wrestler. Arrow marks subclavian vein thrombosis refractory to rt-PA thrombolysis. ***B:*** Arm in abduction. Note disappearance of prominent venous collaterals. ***C:*** Immediate postoperative venogram following scalenectomy, first rib resection, and thrombectomy.

movements of the upper extremity, the subclavian vein is compressed between the first rib and the anterior scalene muscle posteriorly and the clavicle—with underlying subclavius muscle and fibrous costocoracoid ligament—anteriorly. Primary subclavian vein thrombosis can also occur in patients with hypercoagulable states such as antiphospholipid antibody syndrome or factor V Leiden mutation. Secondary subclavian vein thrombosis results from venous injury by indwelling central venous catheters, external trauma, or pacemaker wires.

Clinical Findings

A. Symptoms and Signs

Primary axillary-subclavian vein thrombosis usually occurs in healthy young athletes and people who perform heavy manual labor. Men outnumber women 4:1. Most often patients give a history of repetitive arm activity, but sometimes a single strenuous exercise, such as wrestling or weight lifting, can precipitate thrombosis. Most patients present with an aching pain most severe in the axilla, accompanied by edema and cyanosis of the upper extremity. Significant superficial venous distention is usually apparent in the arm, forearm, shoulder, and anterior chest wall. Symptoms may abate somewhat with the arm elevated.

Paget-Schroetter syndrome may also be accompanied by symptoms of neurogenic thoracic outlet syndrome: tingling, numbness, and pain in the hand and anterior chest wall caused by compression of the brachial plexus between hypertrophied or anomalous anterior and middle scalene muscles. Some patients may have a positive Adson test, signifying impingement of the subclavian artery in the thoracic outlet. This test is positive if diminishment of the radial pulse is noted on abducting and externally rotating the arm while turning the head away from the arm examined. Thoracic outlet syndrome involving the arterial circulation is manifested by effort fatigue of the arm and hand, coolness, and digital embolization.

B. Imaging Studies

Upper extremity venous duplex ultrasound is a good screening modality for patients with suspected axillary-subclavian vein thrombosis. If this study is positive, upper extremity venography and thrombolysis should be considered. It is important that the patient undergo positional venography, abducting the arm 120 degrees to confirm extrinsic compression of the subclavian vein at the thoracic outlet. Venous compromise is further evidenced by prominent collateral veins.

Chest x-ray should be obtained on all patients to exclude the presence of cervical rib, which can also cause compression of the subclavian vein.

Treatment

Any indwelling central venous lines or pacemaker wires in the thrombosed vein should be removed if possible. Arm elevation, pain control, and intravenous fluid resuscitation should be instituted.

Distinguishing these types of thoracic outlet syndrome is important in selecting the appropriate mode of therapy. A new standard of care for patients with acute axillary-subclavian vein thrombosis is emerging. Selective catheterization with thrombolytic infusion is performed at diagnosis. Lytic agent is infused over 12–24 hours through a multi-sideholed catheter centered in the thrombosed vein. Positional venography is repeated after lysis of the clot is achieved. If short-segment stenoses resulting from venous catheterization are identified, these can be corrected by angioplasty. Compression of the vein with the appearance of large venous collaterals when the arm is abducted suggests venous thoracic outlet syndrome, involving the venous circulation, which is best treated with early surgery. A 35–65% risk of rethrombosis and chronic venous stasis is expected without surgery. Delaying surgery to allow endothelial remodeling while the patient receives anticoagulation has not been proved to enhance outcome.

Because the etiology of venous thoracic outlet syndrome is compression of the vein between the first rib-anterior scalene muscle origin and the clavicle, surgery consists of anterior scalenectomy, first rib resection, and venolysis (release of the vein from constricting scar). This operative plan may be modified if there is residual thrombus in the vein (thrombectomy with primary closure or patch angioplasty, interposition graft, internal jugular turndown, or jugular-subclavian bypass), or concomitant neurogenic thoracic outlet syndrome (anterior and middle scalenectomy with neurolysis) or arterial thoracic outlet syndrome (anterior and middle scalenectomy with resection of subclavian aneurysm). Positional venography is performed postoperatively, with angioplasty and stenting reserved for tight residual venous stenoses. Warfarin is continued for 1–3 months, and aspirin is then continued indefinitely afterward.

It is the general practice at our institution to evaluate patients for hypercoagulable states. As many as 50–60% of patients presenting with acute axillary-subclavian vein thrombosis are found to have a hypercoagulable state, the most common of which are mutations in coagulation factor V and antithrombin III. Because of a 40–60% rate of recurrent thrombosis, these patients are maintained indefinitely on warfarin.

Prognosis

The prognosis after axillary-subclavian vein thrombosis is dependent upon the cause of the condition. Most patients experience fairly rapid resolution of their initial presenting symptoms. For patients with secondary forms of this disease, the outcome is dependent upon resolution of the underlying condition. For patients with Paget-Schroetter syndrome who undergo thoracic outlet decompression, excellent outcomes in terms of continued venous patency and avoidance of symptoms of chronic venous insufficiency can be expected. In contrast, chronic axillary-subclavian vein thrombosis with symptoms persisting for over 3 months does not often respond to thrombolysis, mechanical thrombolysis, or prolonged anticoagulation and may cause significant long-term disability.

Angle N et al: Safety and efficacy of early surgical decompression of the thoracic outlet for Paget-Schroetter syndrome. Ann Vasc Surg 2001;15:37.

Hingorani A et al: Upper extremity deep venous thrombosis: an under-recognized manifestation of a hypercoagulable state. Ann Vasc Surg 2000;14:421.

Schneider DB et al: Management of vascular thoracic outlet syndrome. Chest Surg Clin N Am 1999;9:781.

Urschel HC et al: Paget-Schroetter syndrome: what is the best management? Ann Thorac Surg 2000;69:1663.

PULMONARY THROMBOEMBOLISM

ESSENTIALS OF DIAGNOSIS

- *Acute onset of dyspnea, chest pain, and hemoptysis.*
- *Tachypnea and a widened arterial-alveolar oxygen difference.*
- *Abnormal findings on a ventilation-perfusion lung scan, spiral CT scan, or magnetic resonance angiogram.*

General Considerations

Pulmonary thromboembolism is responsible for up to 50,000 deaths each year in the United States. It is the third leading cause of death among hospitalized patients, yet only 30–40% of those with pulmonary thromboembolism have suspected deep venous thrombosis. Efforts directed at reduction in the mortality rate of pulmonary thromboembolism demand an aggressive approach to diagnosis of this problem in patients identified to be at high risk.

Pulmonary thromboembolisms arise from a number of sources. Air embolism can occur during the placement or removal of central venous catheters. Amniotic fluid emboli may occur during active labor. Fat emboli from long bone fractures cause a syndrome characterized by respiratory insufficiency, coagulopathy, encephalopathy, and an upper body petechial rash. Other less common causes of pulmonary emboli include septic emboli, tumor emboli from atrial myxoma or inferior vena cava extension of renal cell carcinoma, and parasitic emboli. However, DVT remains the most common source of pulmonary thromboemboli. Up to 60% of patients with untreated proximal lower extremity DVT may develop pulmonary thromboembolism.

Fewer than 10% of pulmonary thromboemboli will produce pulmonary infarction. The pathophysiology of pulmonary embolism depends on the size and frequency of the emboli as well as the condition of the underlying lung. Obstruction of large pulmonary arteries results in increases in pulmonary artery pressure and acute right ventricular failure, but many of the clinical manifestations of pulmonary thromboembolism result from release of vasoactive amines that cause severe pulmonary vasoconstriction. Vasoconstriction leads to increased physiologic dead space and systemic hypoxia from a right-to-left shunt. Reflex bronchial vasoconstriction is also common.

Clinical Findings

A. Symptoms and Signs

Dyspnea and chest pain are present in up to 75% of patients with pulmonary thromboembolism. However, these symptoms are nonspecific, especially in patients who may have underlying cardiopulmonary disease. Tachycardia, tachypnea, and altered mental status are highly suggestive findings in an at-risk population. The classic triad of dyspnea, chest pain, and hemoptysis is present in only 15% of patients with pulmonary thromboembolism. Pleural friction rub and the S1Q3T3 morphology on electrocardiography are even less common findings.

B. Imaging and Other Diagnostic Studies

Chest x-ray is most often normal but may show a pleural cap. Electrocardiography may reveal new-onset atrial fibrillation or ischemic changes, but in most cases only acute sinus tachycardia and nonspecific ST and T wave changes are identified. Arterial blood gas determination reveals hypoxia and often a respiratory alkalosis or increased arterial-alveolar oxygen gradient. Plasma D-dimer levels are elevated in the presence of both pulmonary thromboembolism and acute DVT, but this test lacks sufficient specificity to be of primary diagnostic value.

Until recently, the most common studies used to diagnose pulmonary embolism were ventilation-perfusion (VQ) scan and pulmonary angiogram (Figure 36–5). Ventilation-perfusion scans have sensitivity and specificity that approach 90% if results of the scan correlate with clinical risk factor assessment. For example, treatment can be started in a patient with a high-probability scan and a highly suggestive examination. Unfortunately, two-thirds of studies are inconclusive. Pulmonary angiography remains the most reliable test for diagnosis, but it is invasive, time-consuming, and expensive.

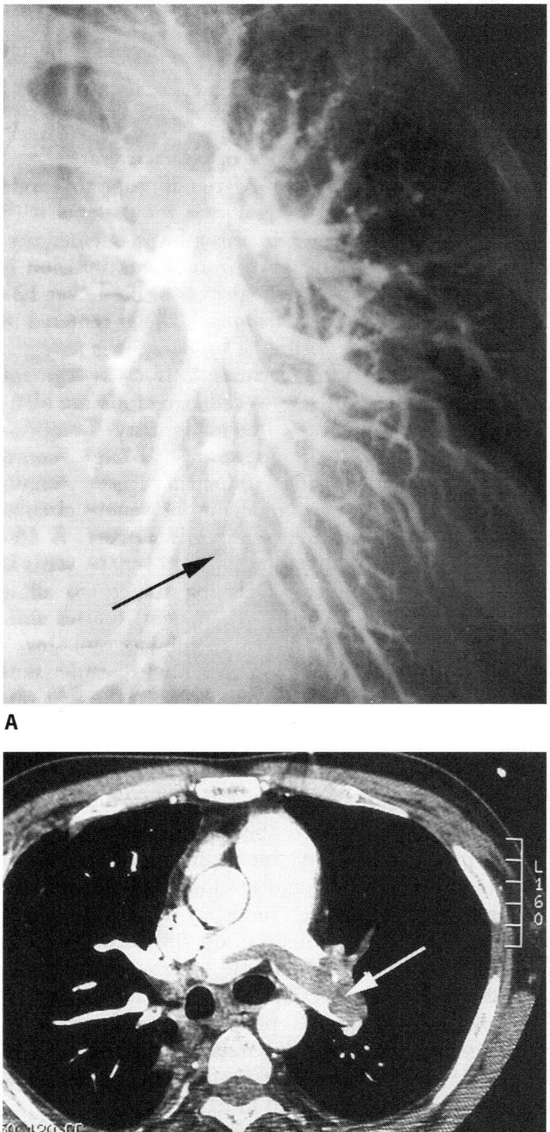

Figure 36–5. Pulmonary embolism. ***A:*** Pulmonary angiogram. Arrow marks location of left lower lobe emboli. ***B:*** Spiral CT. Arrow marks location of large embolus in left main pulmonary artery.

Two newer modalities have improved the accuracy and safety of the diagnosis of pulmonary thromboembolism. Spiral CT scan has virtually replaced VQ scan in the diagnosis of pulmonary thromboembolism. Accuracy supersedes that of VQ scan and does not require clinical correlation. Magnetic resonance angiography has also demonstrated excellent sensitivity and specificity and is now being used in many institutions.

Treatment

A. Anticoagulation

Heparin or LMWH anticoagulation is started as soon as the diagnosis is made after initial stabilization with ventilatory support and vasopressor medications. Thrombolysis is considered for large clot burden, severe respiratory compromise, or hemodynamic instability. When compared with heparin alone, thrombolytic therapy speeds the resolution of pulmonary emboli in the first 24 hours. The disadvantages of lytic therapy include its greater cost and higher risk of significant bleeding complications.

B. Inferior Vena Cava Interruption

Inferior vena cava interruption is considered in patients who have extension of venous thrombus on adequate heparin therapy, patients in whom heparin anticoagulation is contraindicated, or in those who have had a complication of anticoagulation. More recently, temporary or permanent inferior vena cava filters have been placed prophylactically in high-risk patients such as those with unresectable cancer or major trauma.

Historically, inferior vena cava interruption was performed as an open surgical procedure, involving ligation or plication of the infrarenal vena cava or placement of a serrated clip to "strain" blood returning to the right atrium. The Greenfield filter developed in 1973 was initially deployed by venous cutdown. Multiple devices are now available for fluoroscopically guided percutaneous placement through a 12F sheath introduced into the common femoral vein or, in cases of femoral thrombus, into the internal jugular vein. The presence of a duplicated inferior vena cava must be excluded by venography at the time of filter placement because lower extremity DVT might still serve as a source of emboli. Newer devices being developed today include those used for only a temporary period of time (retrievable filter). Additionally, devices are being deployed under ultrasound guidance.

C. Surgical Treatment

Hemodynamically unstable patients in whom thrombolytic therapy has failed or cannot be instituted require percutaneous or open surgical extraction of the thrombus. Open surgical pulmonary embolectomy is reserved for patients who develop intractable hypotension, those who fail transcatheter pulmonary embolectomy, and those who have tumor or foreign body emboli. Catheter techniques involve mechanical thrombolysis or removal of intact pulmonary emboli using a suction cup embolectomy device.

Prognosis

Pulmonary embolism is one of the most frequent causes of preventable hospital death. Prevention by use of DVT prophylaxis and early diagnosis by selective testing of high-risk patients are essential steps to reducing the morbidity of this disease.

Anderson FA et al: A population-based perspective of the hospital incidence and case-fatality rates of deep vein thrombosis and pulmonary embolism: the Worcester DVT Study. Arch Intern Med 1991;151:933.

Cross JJ et al: A randomized trial of spiral CT and ventilation perfusion scintigraphy for the diagnosis of pulmonary embolism. Clin Radiol 1998;53:177.

Dalen JD et al: Thrombolytic therapy for pulmonary embolism. Is it effective? Is it safe? When is it indicated? Arch Intern Med 1997;157:2550.

Greenfield LJ, Proctor MC: Vena caval filters for the prevention of pulmonary embolism. N Engl J Med 1998;339:47.

Hull RD: Low-molecular-weight heparin vs. heparin in the treatment of patients with pulmonary embolism: American-Canadian Thrombosis Study Group. Arch Intern Med 2000;160: 229.

Meaney JF: Diagnosis of pulmonary embolism with magnetic resonance angiography. N Engl J Med 1997;336:1422.

Mohan CR et al: Comparative efficacy and complications of vena caval filters. J Vasc Surg 1995;21:235.

Value of the ventilation/perfusion scan in acute pulmonary embolism: results of the prospective investigation of pulmonary embolism diagnosis (PIOPED). The PIOPED Investigators. JAMA 1990;263:2753.

SUPERFICIAL THROMBOPHLEBITIS

ESSENTIALS OF DIAGNOSIS

- *Erythema, induration, and tenderness along the superficial vein.*
- *Usually spontaneous but can follow venous cannulation.*

General Considerations

Superficial thrombophlebitis may appear spontaneously in patients with varicose veins, in pregnant or postpartum women, or in patients with thromboangiitis obliterans or Behçet's disease. It may also occur after intravenous therapy or in an area of localized trauma. The presence of superficial phlebitis, particularly if it occurs in a migratory manner, suggests the presence of an abdominal cancer such as carcinoma of the pancreas (Trousseau's thrombophlebitis). The most common vein affected is the greater saphenous vein and its branches. In up to 20% of cases, a simultaneous DVT exists. Pulmonary emboli are rare unless extension into the deep venous system occurs.

Clinical Findings

The patient usually presents complaining of localized extremity pain and redness. Areas of induration, erythema, and tenderness correspond to dilated and often thrombosed superficial veins. Over time, a firm cord may develop. Generalized edema is absent unless the deep veins are involved. The presence of fever and shaking chills suggests septic or suppurative phlebitis, which occurs most commonly as a complication of intravenous cannulation.

Differential Diagnosis

Superficial thrombophlebitis must be distinguished from ascending lymphangitis, cellulitis, erythema nodosum, erythema induratum, and panniculitis. Unlike these other disorders, superficial phlebitis tends to be well localized over a superficial vein.

Treatment

The primary treatment of superficial venous thrombophlebitis is the administration of nonsteroidal anti-inflammatory drugs, local heat, elevation, and support stockings or ACE wraps. Ambulation is encouraged. In most cases, symptoms will resolve within 7–10 days. Excision of the involved vein is recommended for symptoms that persist over 2 weeks despite treatment or for recurrent phlebitis in the same vein segment. If there is progressive proximal extension with involvement of the saphenofemoral junction or cephalic-subclavian junction, ligation and resection of the vein at the junction should be performed. Alternatively, full-dose anticoagulation can be utilized. Ligation and resection is most effective treating pain, while anticoagulation is most effective treating thrombus extension/embolization.

Septic thrombophlebitis requires treatment with broad-spectrum intravenous antibiotics. If rapid resolution of the cellulitis occurs, no treatment beyond a short course of antibiotics is required. However, if the patient becomes septic, excision of the entire infected vein is required. With positive blood cultures, an extended course of antibiotics specific for the identified organism is indicated.

Prognosis

Most episodes of uncomplicated superficial thrombophlebitis respond to conservative management. Cases in which extension into the deep venous system occurs can be associated with thromboembolism.

Belcaro G et al: Superficial thrombophlebitis of the legs: a randomized, controlled, follow-up study. Angiology 1999;50:523.

Lucia MA et al: Images in clinical medicine: superficial thrombophlebitis. N Engl J Med 2001;344:1214.

Sullivan V et al: Ligation versus anticoagulation: treatment of above-knee superficial thrombophlebitis not involving the deep venous system. J Am Coll Surg 2001;193:556.

CHRONIC VENOUS INSUFFICIENCY

The basic physiologic abnormality in patients with chronic venous insufficiency is chronic elevation of venous pressure. The normal venous capacitance can accommodate large-volume changes that occur during exercise with only minimal changes in venous pressure. However, with calf muscle pump dysfunction and valvular reflux, blood pools in the lower extremities and venous hypertension occurs, leading to venous hypertension. Outflow obstruction from proximal obstruction can also produce venous hypertension, resulting in "venous claudication" as the deep venous system fills with blood during exercise. The leg becomes painful, swollen, and heavy (especially with exercise), mimicking arterial insufficiency.

Valvular incompetence of the deep veins can be congenital or result from damage following phlebitis, varicose veins, or deep venous thrombosis. The best estimate for the incidence of chronic venous insufficiency is approximately 30% after 8-year follow-up. Chronic venous stasis changes are centered in the "gaiter areas" around the ankles. This is the location of the commonly affected perforator veins and is a region with sparse soft tissue support to withstand elevated venous pressures. Brawny edema is produced by extravasation of plasma fluid, red blood cells, and plasma proteins. Lysis of red blood cells results in deposition of hemosiderin, which creates a brownish discoloration. Leukocytes become sequestered in the microcirculation, leading to capillary occlusion and release of superoxide radicals, proteolytic enzymes, and growth factors. Macrophages and T lymphocytes are primary mediators of this inflammatory response, which results in fibroblast activation and scarring and fibrosis of the subcutaneous tissues. Ultimately, this fibrosis results in compromised skin perfusion and ulceration.

Clinical Findings

A. Symptoms and Signs

Both isolated saphenous vein incompetence and deep venous insufficiency can lead to chronic venous stasis changes. The first symptom to develop is usually ankle and calf edema. Involvement of the foot and toes suggests lymphedema. Typically, the edema is worse at the end of the day and improves with leg elevation. Long-standing disease is characterized by stasis dermatitis, hyperpigmentation, brawny induration, and ulceration. Venous stasis ulcers are large, painful, and irregular in outline. They have a shallow, moist granulation bed, occur in the gaiter area on the medial or lateral aspects of the ankle, and are often accompanied by stasis dermatitis and stasis pigmentation changes.

B. Imaging and Other Diagnostic Studies

Duplex ultrasound can identify the presence and location of incompetent perforating veins and has been used to evaluate the function of individual venous valves. However, it does not easily assess calf muscle pump function or the presence of proximal obstruction. These concerns are addressed with use of other tests, such as air plethysmography, which gives a quantitative assessment of venous reflux (by the venous filling index), calf muscle pump function (by the ejection fraction), and overall venous function (by residual volume function). These measurements help to stratify patients into treatment groups.

Determination of functional outflow obstruction requires venography with or without pressure measurement, although intravascular ultrasound is also very useful to determine the presence or absence of venous obstruction. Descending phlebography involves injection of contrast media into the common femoral vein to test the valves during normal breathing and with a forced Valsalva maneuver. Using this technique, pathologic reflux can be identified in patients with postthrombotic damage.

Differential Diagnosis

Congestive heart failure and chronic liver and kidney disease must be considered in the differential diagnosis of bilateral lower extremity edema. Lymphedema is characterized by nonpitting edema of the dorsum of the foot and toes as well as the calf and generally is not associated with ulceration. Severe arterial insufficiency produces ulcers that are painful, well circumscribed, and located over pressure points on the distal end of the extremity and foot. Ulcers due to autoimmune diseases, erythema nodosum, and fungal infections are distinguished by appearance and distribution.

Treatment

Venous insufficiency is an incurable but manageable problem. Most patients respond well to a conservative treatment program composed of intermittent leg elevation, regular exercise to improve calf muscle pump function, and the use of surgical elastic graduated compression stockings. Although the mechanism by which elastic compression improves the symptoms of chronic venous insufficiency has not been clearly established, recent work suggests that external compression may restore competency of dilated valve cusps and affect venoarterial reflex. Most venous ulceration will improve with leg elevation, external compression, and local wound care. Compression can be achieved with either an inelastic bandage such as a Unna's boot or with an occlusive wound dressing covered by ACE bandage wrapping or surgical support stockings.

Surgery is indicated for a small percentage of patients with nonhealing ulcers or disabling symptoms refractory to conservative management. The two main categories of procedures are antireflux procedures and bypass operations for obstruction. The pathology must be accurately characterized so that an appropriate operative strategy can be developed. The most common abnormality in patients with chronic venous insufficiency is incompetence of the popliteal or tibial veins; 50–60% of patients have incompetent perforators.

Perforating vein ligation is used in patients with recurrent or recalcitrant venous ulcers with demonstrated incompetence of perforating veins under the area of ulceration. It is performed to reverse the local wound complication of venous ulceration and does nothing to change the underlying deep venous hemodynamics of the leg. Therefore, patients must understand that for maximal effectiveness after perforator ligation, standard treatment for chronic venous insufficiency must be continued. Patients who have proximal venous obstruction should have this problem corrected prior to perforator interruption. The incidence of ulcer recurrence after perforator ligation is 15–20%, but the wound complication rate secondary to impaired incisional healing with severe stasis disease ranges from 12% to 55%. Wound complications have been reduced to 5% with the introduction of subfascial endoscopic perforator surgery, which achieves an ulcer recurrence rate of 12–28% at 2 years, equal to the rate following open surgery.

Direct venous reconstructive surgery is indicated for (1) venous reflux not amenable to a conservative treatment regimen, (2) failure to relieve symptoms after vein stripping or perforator ligation, or (3) intractable disabling venous claudication associated with venous outflow obstruction. Procedures for reflux include valvuloplasty, valvular transplantation, and venous segment transposition. The best results with valvuloplasty are achieved when it is combined with perforator ligation. The reported success rate is approximately 80% in one recent study of 155 extremities with a 1- to 13-year follow-up. Valvuloplasty can be performed by placement of external cuffs or bands, vein wall plication, angioscopic repair, or open valve repair. Venous valve transplantation involves replacing a refluxing segment of vein with a healthy segment of autologous axillary vein with functional valves. Transplantation of individual valves at the level of the popliteal vein is a technique with reported good clinical results in 60–70% of cases and an improvement in venous hemodynamics by air plethysmography. Alternatively, a competent segment of profunda vein can be used to replace an incompetent segment of superficial femoral or greater saphenous vein in a vein transposition. Although initial results of these procedures are good, the effect is apparently not long-lasting.

Bypasses and angiographic procedures can be performed for venous obstruction. The Palma procedure is a cross-femoral bypass first described in 1958 for iliac vein obstruction. In this procedure, the proximal saphenous vein from the contralateral leg is tunneled suprapubically to the femoral vein on the side of the iliac obstruction. This allows for venous flow to bypass across the pelvis and empty through the patent contralateral iliac vein. Prosthetic material has also been used. Overall 5-year graft patency averages 75–80%. Historically, distal femoral arteriovenous fistulas were constructed to improve iliofemoral vein graft patency, but more current experience does not support their continued use in many cases. Patients with short-segment iliac vein obstruction from May-Thurner syndrome (left iliac vein compression) have also been successfully treated by angioplasty and stenting.

Saphenopopliteal bypass (May-Husni procedure) can be considered for patients with occlusion of the superficial femoral vein. In this procedure, calf blood flow is shunted around the obstructed superficial femoral vein through the patent saphenous vein. Approximately 75% of patients are reported to show clinical improvement postoperatively.

Criado E et al: The role of air plethysmography in the diagnosis of chronic venous insufficiency. J Vasc Surg 1998;27:660.

DePalma RG et al: Target selection for surgical intervention in severe chronic venous insufficiency: comparison of duplex scanning and phlebography. J Vasc Surg 2000;32:913.

Gloviczki P et al: Mid-term results of endoscopic perforator vein interruption for chronic venous insufficiency: lessons learned from the North American Subfacial Endoscopic Perforator Surgery registry. J Vasc Surg 1999;29:489.

Gruss JD, Heimer W: Bypass procedures for venous obstruction. In: *Surgical Management of Venous Disease.* Raju S, Villavicencio JL (editors). Williams & Wilkins, 1997.

Heit JA et al: Trends in the incidence of venous stasis syndrome and venous ulcer: a 25-year population based study. J Vasc Surg 2001;33:1022.

Iafrati MD et al: Is the nihilistic approach to surgical reduction of superficial and perforator vein incompetence for venous ulcer justified? J Vasc Surg 2002;36:1167.

Mohr DN et al: The venous stasis syndrome after deep venous thrombosis or pulmonary embolism: a population-based study. Mayo Clin Proc 2000;75:1249.

Raju S: Technical options in venous valve reconstruction. Am J Surg 1997;173:301.

II. THE LYMPHATICS

LYMPHEDEMA

ESSENTIALS OF DIAGNOSIS

- *Can be developmental or acquired.*
- *Painless edema of one or both lower extremities, usually involving the ankle, the dorsum of the foot, and the toes.*
- *Edema is usually pitting at first and then becomes firm, rubbery, and nonpitting due to fibrosis.*
- *Frequent episodes of lymphangitis and cellulitis may occur.*

General Considerations

Much less is known about the fluid dynamics of the lymphatic system than of the venous or arterial system. Most energy for lymph propulsion arises from the intrinsic lymphatic smooth muscle contractions that occur rhythmically. Lymphatic luminal pressures are usually 30–50 mm Hg and can exceed arterial pressure under special circumstances. The lymphatic system carries interstitial fluid and macromolecular proteins lost from the capillaries, as well as infectious agents and foreign material, back into the central circulation. Two to 4 liters a day of lymph drain into the subclavian vein.

The fundamental mechanism responsible for lymphedema formation is impairment of lymph flow out of the extremity. Primary lymphedema is caused by abnormal lymphatic development, most often hypoplasia resulting in severe reduction in the number of lymphatics and the lymphatic diameters. It is classified by age at onset of the disease. Congenital lymphedema develops before 1 year of age, is usually bilateral, and affects males more than females; if familial, it is known as Milroy's disease. More often, lymphedema develops during adolescence (lymphedema praecox) and is unilateral; there is a 10:1 female predominance. Lymphedema occurring after age 35 is referred to as lymphedema tarda.

Secondary lymphedema results from a wide variety of disease processes that cause obstruction to the lymphatic system. The most common of these is surgical excision and radiation to the axillary or inguinal lymph nodes as part of the treatment of breast cancer, cervical cancer, prostate cancer, melanoma, and soft tissue tumors. Less common causes of secondary lymphedema are bacterial and fungal infections, trauma, and lymphoproliferative diseases. In many developing countries, lymphatic obstruction due to filariasis is caused by three different parasites: *Wuchereria bancrofti, Brugia malayi,* and *Brugia timori.*

Clinical Manifestations

A. Symptoms and Signs

The history of the disease process will usually define the cause of the lymphedema. Development of painless edema in an adolescent girl with a family history of lymphedema would indicate primary lymphedema as a diagnosis. A history of lymph node dissection, irradiation, or the presence of a parasitic infection suggests secondary lymphedema.

Lymphedema development is usually slowly progressive and painless. In the early stages the edema is pitting, but as the disease progresses, chronic fibrosis occurs and the edema becomes nonpitting. The distribution of edema is also characteristic. It is usually centered around the ankle (Figure 36–6) and is most pronounced on the dorsum of the foot, producing a buffalo hump appearance. Unlike edema of venous stasis disease, lymphedema also often involves the toes. In the early stages the skin is normal, but skin thickening and hyperkeratosis occurs with long-standing disease. A chronic eczematous dermatitis may ensue.

Rarely, lymphangiosarcoma or angiosarcoma may develop as a complication of chronic lymphedema. This neoplastic transformation of blood vessels and lymphatics is called Stewart-Treves syndrome.

B. Imaging Studies

Venous duplex scans are performed to rule out venous insufficiency. Lymphangiography is rarely used now, as it can further damage the lymphatics and is unnecessary to establish the diagnosis. Lymphoscintigraphy is a specialized test used for the detection of lymph node metastasis that may confirm the diagnosis. CT and MRI are useful tests in patients with suspected secondary lymphedema from unknown malignancy.

Differential Diagnosis

A variety of diseases can result in bilateral lower extremity edema. These include congestive heart failure, chronic renal or hepatic insufficiency, and hypoproteinemia. In patients with unilateral leg edema, differential diagnosis includes congenital vascular malformations, chronic venous insufficiency, and reflex sympathetic dystrophy.

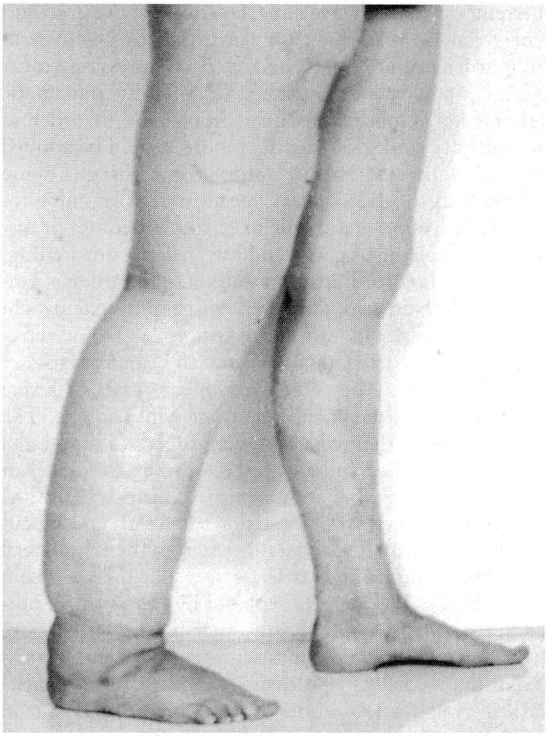

Figure 36–6. Acquired lymphedema. Edema is centered at the ankle and involves the foot and toes.

Treatment

Lymphedema is a chronic disease for which there is no complete cure. However, a variety of conservative measures can substantially reduce the risk of further complications and disability.

No drug therapy is effective. Use of benzopyrones (coumarins) and steroid injections to increase lymphatic transport has not shown consistent benefit. Diuretics can be useful for acute exacerbation of edema secondary to infection or for coexisting venous stasis disease, but these agents are not recommended for long-term use in lymphedema.

The mainstay of treatment is external compression and meticulous skin care. Mechanical reduction of lymphedema can best be achieved with a program of frequent leg elevation, manual lymphatic drainage massage, low-stretch wrapping techniques, and intermittent pneumatic compression. Sequential pneumatic compression devices are traditionally the first line of treatment. Many different devices are available for use on the leg, and sleeves can be custom fit for patients with postmastectomy arm lymphedema. Graduated compression stockings maintain the limb after reduction by pneumatic compression. Good skin care is imperative in order to prevent infection. Moisturizing lotions should be applied regularly, especially after showering or bathing. Drying and cracking of the skin can create portals of entry for bacteria. Infection is difficult to eradicate because of disordered lymphatic drainage and can be limb-threatening.

The psychologic impact of chronic lymphedema cannot be underestimated. However, with appropriate patient education that results in the prevention of chronic infection or massive edema, this problem can be manageable.

Operation may be considered in rare cases of severe functional impairment and recurrent lymphangitis. The primary goals of these operations are to reduce limb bulk, either by ablative techniques (excision of excess tissue) or physiologic techniques (lymphatic reconstruction). The Charles procedure involves excision of all skin and subcutaneous tissue from the tibial tuberosity to the lateral head of the fibula and wound coverage by a split-thickness skin graft. This has been largely replaced by the Sistrunk procedure, which is a staged subcutaneous tissue excision. Wide skin flaps are raised for excision of subcutaneous tissues in the medial leg and then 3 months later in the lateral leg. Ablative techniques have been less successful in the upper extremity than in the lower extremity.

The Thompson procedure is an indirect lymphatic reconstruction. A flap of dermis is buried in the muscle compartment to promote formation of communications between subdermal and deep lymphatics. Omental free flaps are similarly designed to encourage new lympholymphatic channels. Direct lymphatic reconstruction by creation of lymphovenous anastomoses or lymphatic interposition grafting is achievable by microsurgical techniques and has had limited success in some centers. Long-term efficacy is not yet known. Again, the use of any of these operative procedures for lymphedema is limited to rather rare situations.

Ko DS et al: Effective treatment of lymphedema of the extremities. Arch Surg 1998;133:452.

Pain SJ et al: Lymphoedema following surgery for breast cancer. Br J Surg 2000;87:1128.

Singh I, Burnand KG: Lymphoedema. Surgery 2002;20:42.

LYMPHANGITIS

ESSENTIALS OF DIAGNOSIS

- *Red streaks traveling longitudinally up an extremity toward regional lymph nodes.*
- *Shaking chills, fever, and malaise.*

General Considerations

Lymphangitis is usually caused by a hemolytic streptococcal or staphylococcal infection that arises in an area of cellulitis near an open wound. Multiple long red streaks can be seen coursing toward the regional lymph nodes. Severe systemic manifestations include tachycardia, fever, chills, and malaise, which untreated can lead to sepsis and death.

Clinical Findings

A. Symptoms and Signs

Pain at the site of the initial wound is present. High fevers develop rapidly. The streaks may be faint in appearance initially, especially in dark-skinned patients. Regional lymph nodes are often enlarged and tender.

B. Laboratory Findings

An elevated white blood cell count associated with a left shift is almost universally present. Blood and wound cultures should be obtained routinely.

Differential Diagnosis

Lymphangitis should be distinguished from superficial thrombophlebitis, which is usually localized to a single venous segment often with a palpable cord. Patients with thrombophlebitis usually do not appear toxic, as do patients with lymphangitis. Cat-scratch fever should always be considered when lymphadenitis is present. It is also important to differentiate cellulitis and severe soft tissue infections from lymphangitis. In general, lymphangitis is characterized by its superficial location and the linear pattern of erythema.

Treatment

The extremity should be elevated and warm compresses applied. Analgesics and intravenous antibiotics should be instituted immediately. Examination of the wound should be made to determine the need for debridement or incision and drainage of an abscess.

Prognosis

Delayed or inadequate therapy can lead to overwhelming sepsis and death. Aggressive institution of appropriate antibiotic therapy and wound care will usually control the infection within 48–72 hours.

Neurosurgery & Surgery of the Pituitary

37

Mitchel S. Berger, MD

DIAGNOSIS & MANAGEMENT OF DEPRESSED STATES OF CONSCIOUSNESS

Cornelia S. von Koch, MD, PhD, & Julian T. Hoff, MD

Definitions

The clinical definition of consciousness ranges from alert wakefulness to deep coma. An **alert**, awake patient responds immediately and appropriately to all stimuli. A **stuporous** patient responds only when aroused by vigorous stimulation. **Coma** implies failure to respond to stimulation. Most cases of depressed states of consciousness lie between these extremes and are best categorized by accurate descriptions of their responses to specific stimuli—eg, auditory, visual, and tactile (touch or pain).

The Neurologic Examination

The most reliable index for assessing the level of consciousness at any moment is the patient's response to external stimuli. (How quick and how accurate are the patient's responses to questions, to touch, to pain, etc?) Brain stem reflexes also allow an accurate estimate of the level of consciousness—pupillary responses to light, corneal reflexes, oculocephalic and caloric responses, cough and gag reflexes, pattern of breathing, etc. Motor activity of the extremities, either spontaneous or induced by the examiner's stimulus, provides assessment of the entire neuraxis. Does the patient move the extremities purposefully, equally, and briskly, or is there failure to move at all? Which extremities do not move? Nonpurposeful or reflex movement of the arms and legs may also establish the level of neuraxis function, though less reliably (eg, decorticate or decerebrate posturing).

Depressed consciousness may occur abruptly (eg, cerebral concussion) or gradually (eg, barbiturate overdose), often with fluctuations in the level of consciousness (eg, waxing-waning consciousness associated with subdural hematoma). Accurate and repeated examinations will establish not only the level of consciousness but also its changing course. The urgency of diagnosis depends largely upon the rate of change in the patient's course as determined by repeated examinations.

Diagnostic Possibilities

Depressed states of consciousness may be due to many causes. Trauma is usually obvious, both from the history and upon examination of the patient. **Metabolic disorders** (eg, diabetes mellitus, uremia, poisoning, electrolyte imbalance, hypoxia) may similarly alter the state of consciousness. In addition to an accurate history and physical examination, laboratory investigations are required to establish a diagnosis of metabolic coma.

Patients with **intracranial neoplasms** may be alert, comatose, or at any level of consciousness in between. A progressive, unrelenting history is a valuable criterion of this initial diagnosis. **Central nervous system infections** (eg, encephalitis, meningitis) are usually accompanied by systemic signs of infection and a progressively worsening course. Cerebral abscess, on the other hand, behaves more like an expanding neoplasm than a fulminating infection.

Vascular occlusions (emboli, thrombosis) usually cause abrupt neurologic deficits without grossly impaired consciousness, whereas cerebral hemorrhage typically causes abrupt coma with profound neurologic deficits. Conversely, subarachnoid hemorrhage may occur without any alteration of wakefulness. **Degenerative diseases** are usually slowly progressive, dementing illnesses that dull consciousness but characteristically do not produce coma.

Diagnostic Tools

Laboratory and radiographic tests help to establish the clinical diagnosis. Routine examinations should include a complete blood count, urinalysis, plasma glucose, blood urea nitrogen, and serum electrolytes.

Urine and blood for toxicologic study are essential if poisoning is a possibility. Head CT and spinal x-rays or

CT scans as well as chest x-ray are obvious aids after trauma. Cerebrospinal fluid analysis is an essential step toward diagnosis of meningitis or subarachnoid hemorrhage. Lumbar puncture is rarely helpful in the assessment of head trauma and probably is contraindicated during the initial workup after injury.

Although most patients are unconscious for a single reason, some may have combined or additive reasons. A severe head injury may have been caused by abrupt coma induced by cerebral hemorrhage in a hypertensive patient, or a diabetic patient with glioblastoma multiforme may be in coma from an insulin overdose and not from the expanding neoplasm. The physician must be aware of these possible—though uncommon—complexities.

The administration of intravenous hypertonic glucose (50%, 50 mL) is occasionally diagnostic but should be done only after blood has been taken for glucose measurement and before an intravenous glucose drip has been started.

Most patients with depressed consciousness should undergo CT scanning or MRI to establish the presence or absence of an intracranial mass lesion. Appropriate therapy depends on the early recognition of the specific intracranial problem.

Management

Protection of the airway and control of shock are fundamental principles of management of patients with depressed consciousness. Most complications of coma can be attributed to failure to follow these basic rules. Responsive patients with good cough reflexes can often protect their own airways. Other patients, usually stuporous or comatose, require endotracheal intubation in order to (1) reduce the likelihood of aspiration of gastric contents and (2) ensure unrestricted gas exchange (PO_2, PCO_2).

Adequate tracheal suctioning, frequent changes in position, pulmonary physiotherapy, and intermittent positive pressure breathing help maintain good pulmonary function once the airway is secure.

Shock must be controlled. If it is due to hypovolemia, blood and fluids must be given intravenously. In the absence of trauma, other causes of hypotension must be sought and treated specifically (eg, gram-negative sepsis).

A nasogastric tube (to sample ingested drugs, to remove gastric contents that might be aspirated into the lungs, etc), intravenous cannulas to administer drugs and fluids, and an indwelling bladder catheter to assess fluid balance are necessary steps in the early management of comatose patients.

ELEVATED INTRACRANIAL PRESSURE

The skull contains brain, cerebrospinal fluid, and blood (Figure 37–1). At normal intracranial pressures of 10–15 mm Hg (120–180 mm H_2O), these three components maintain volumetric equilibrium. Increased volume of one component will elevate intracranial pressure unless the volume of the other two components decreases proportionately (Monro-Kellie doctrine). Because compensatory volumetric changes have physical and physiologic limits, the ability of the skull's contents to maintain normal pressure can be exceeded by a change of volume that is either too fast or too great.

The compensatory properties of the intracranial contents follow a pressure-volume exponential curve (Figure 37–2). Increased volume of any of the three components can be accommodated to a certain point without change in intracranial pressure. Once that critical volume is reached, however, additional volume increase produces an increase in intracranial pressure.

Increased intracranial pressure exerts its deleterious effect (1) by distorting and shifting the brain as pressure gradients develop, and (2) by reducing the effective perfusion pressure of the brain (cerebral perfusion pressure [CPP] = mean arterial pressure [MAP] minus intracranial pressure [ICP]). Common examples of a significant volumetric change in one or more of the three normal intracranial components are cerebral edema (brain), hydrocephalus (cerebrospinal fluid), and cerebral venous occlusion (blood).

An intracranial mass (eg, tumor, hematoma) represents a fourth component, and its presence initiates compensatory adjustments of the other three: (1) Intracranial vessels are compressed, reducing the amount of intracranial blood; (2) cerebrospinal fluid volume is reduced by increased absorption or reduced production (at high intracranial pressure); and (3) intracranial bulk is reduced by brain creeping out of adjacent foramina (eg, transtentorial herniation, tonsillar herniation). Children with expandable skulls due to unfused sutures have an additional compensatory mechanism to accommodate expanding intracranial volume and are thereby partially protected from extreme rises of intracranial pressure.

Clinical Findings

Most brain insults, whether from trauma, ischemia, poisoning, or other sources, are accompanied by raised intracranial pressure. Following head trauma, intracranial pressure may rise quickly to very high levels as a result of vascular congestion, extravasation, and cerebral edema. Intracranial pressure may also rise substantially when a neoplasm occupies the intracranial cavity. Intracranial hypertension may occur after cerebrovascular occlusions (stroke), during central nervous system infections, and following cerebral hypoxia. Intracranial pressure by itself is rarely a clinical problem when coma is the result of a metabolic disorder (eg, uremia, hepatic coma).

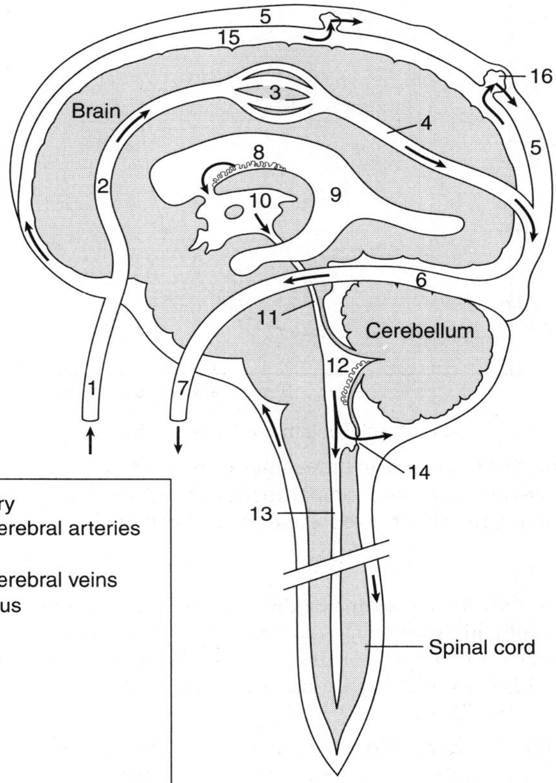

1. Internal carotid artery
2. Cortical and deep cerebral arteries
3. Capillary network
4. Cortical and deep cerebral veins
5. Superior sagittal sinus
6. Transverse sinus
7. Internal jugular vein
8. Choroid plexus
9. Lateral ventricles
10. Third ventricle
11. Cerebral aqueduct
12. Fourth ventricle
13. Central canal of spinal cord
14. Foramina of Magendie and Luschka
15. Subarachnoid space
16. Arachnoid granulations

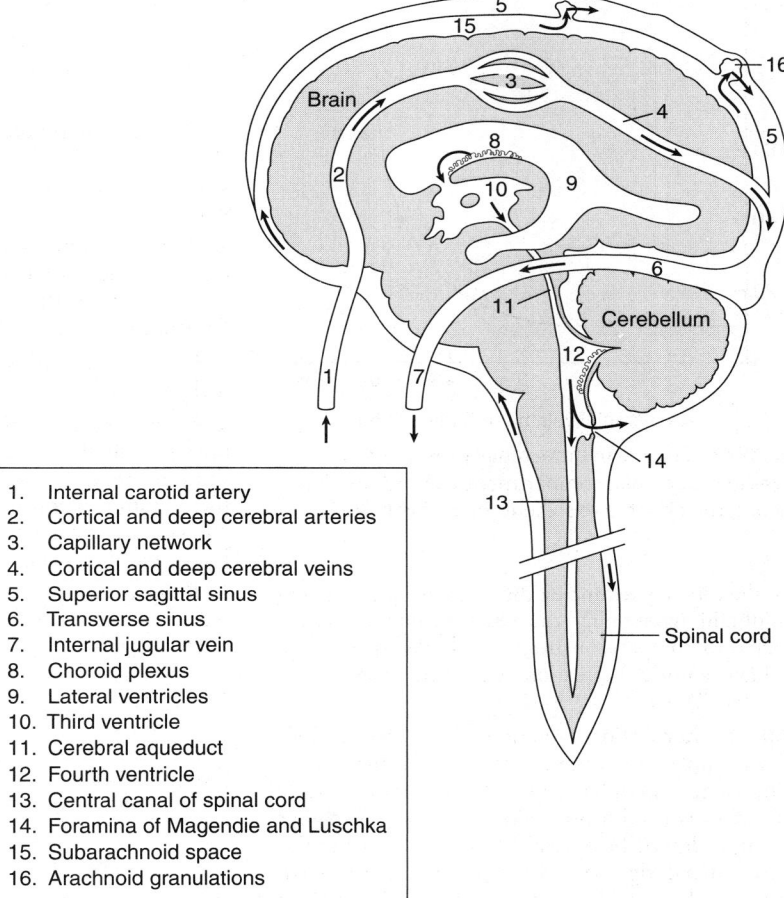

Figure 37–1. Intracranial compartments and circulation of cerebrospinal fluid.

A. Specific Signs of Raised Intracranial Pressure

While any of the following clinical signs may result from causes other than raised intracranial pressure, most will appear during raised intracranial pressure if the elevation is severe or prolonged.

1. Cardiovascular—Blood pressure elevation accompanied by bradycardia and respiratory slowing classically results from raised intracranial pressure. This "Cushing response," however, usually appears only when intracranial hypertension is severe.

2. Gastrointestinal—Hemorrhage from gastric ulcerations (Cushing's ulcer) may accompany raised intracranial pressure.

3. Pulmonary—Hemorrhagic pulmonary edema may result from severe elevation of intracranial pressure as well as from other brain insults. The lung lesion is the end product of a pathophysiologic sequence mediated by the sympathetic nervous system. Few patients survive this hemodynamic storm of neurogenic origin unless intracranial pressure is reduced.

4. Neurologic—Papilledema, abducens nerve paresis (unilateral occasionally; bilateral often), and depressed consciousness are the most common signs associated with generalized intracranial pressure elevations. Loss of visual acuity may occur as a late consequence of optic nerve atrophy. In children, decreased upward gaze is common.

B. Specific Syndromes

Specific syndromes may appear when intracranial pressure is raised by the presence of an intracranial mass.

1. Transtentorial herniation—A laterally placed supratentorial mass may push the uncus and hippocampus medially into the tentorial incisure. The oculomotor

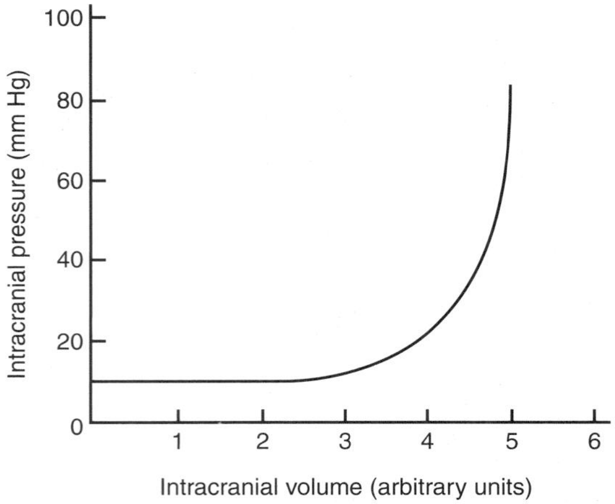

Figure 37–2. Change in intracranial pressure with changes in intracranial compartment volume. The figures along the abscissa represent units of volume.

nerves, the cerebral peduncles, the cerebral aqueduct, and the midbrain (containing the reticular formation) are vulnerable to compression from the displaced temporal lobe. Transtentorial herniation may then appear clinically (Table 37–1).

2. Tonsillar herniation—Herniation of the cerebellar tonsils into the foramen magnum causes compression of the medulla. The hallmark of medullary compression is respiratory failure: slow and irregular breathing followed by apnea. Earlier signs of herniation are nuchal rigidity, intermittent opisthotonos, and depressed gag and cough reflexes. Consciousness may be retained until the patient becomes severely hypoxic.

Although raised intracranial pressure usually becomes obvious clinically, it may go undetected for months. Patients with benign intracranial hypertension (pseudotumor cerebri) often have no symptoms despite severe papilledema and intracranial hypertension. Similarly, patients with obstruction of cerebrospinal fluid pathways may tolerate intracranial pressure elevation for weeks or months without developing overt clinical signs. Failing mentation may provide the only clue to progressive hydrocephalus in the latter circumstance.

Treatment

A. Specific Treatment

Management of specific causes of raised intracranial pressure is effective treatment. Removal of intracranial masses, shunting of obstructed cerebrospinal fluid, and removal of toxins (eg, lead, in lead encephalopathy) are examples of specific forms of treatment.

B. Nonspecific Treatment

When raised intracranial pressure as such must also be managed, the following nonspecific measures are useful:

1. Control of respiration—Accumulation of CO_2 ($PaCO_2 > 40$ mm Hg) will increase cerebral blood flow and raise intracranial pressure. A therapeutic goal is maintenance of $PaCO_2$ in the range of 30–40 mm Hg.

2. Control of body temperature—Hypothermia reduces cerebral metabolism and lowers intracranial pressure. Hyperthermia increases intracranial pressure. Thus, fever must be controlled.

3. Osmotic diuretics—Mannitol can reduce intracranial pressure by cerebral dehydration.

4. Cerebrospinal fluid drainage—Reduction of cerebrospinal fluid volume by repeated spinal taps or by shunting may control raised intracranial pressure from pseudotumor. Ventricular drainage of cerebrospinal fluid reduces intracranial pressure transiently in severe head injury and in patients with obstructive hydrocephalus.

5. Bony decompression—This nonspecific method of reducing intracranial pressure may be employed when other measures fail.

Duff D: Altered states of consciousness, theories of recovery, and assessment following a severe traumatic brain injury. Axone 2001;23:18. Review.

Giacino JT et al: The minimally conscious state: definition and diagnostic criteria. Neurology 2002;58:349.

Table 37–1. Clinical manifestations of transtentorial herniation.

Compressed Structure	Clinical Manifestations
Cranial nerve III	Ipsilateral mydriasis
Midbrain physiologic functional transection	Decerebrate rigidity
Reticular formation	Coma
Ipsilateral cerebral peduncle	Contralateral hemiparesis
Contralateral cerebral peduncle	Ipsilateral hemiparesis (false localizing sign)
Cerebral aqueduct (of Sylvius)	Headache and vomiting due to acute hydrocephalus
Posterior cerebral artery	Contralateral hemianopsia (false localizing (sign)[1]

[1]This sign is a consequence of herniation and does not indicate the localization of the primary process; in this sense, the sign falsely localizes the primary lesion.

King BS et al: The early assessment and intensive care unit management of patients with severe traumatic brain and spinal cord injuries. Surg Clin North Am 2000;80:855.

Marshall LF: Head injury: recent past, present, and future. Neurosurgery 2000;47:546.

Wilkins RH, Rengachary SS (editors): *Neurosurgery,* 2nd ed. McGraw-Hill, 1996.

Youmans J: *Neurological Surgery,* 4th ed. Saunders, 1996.

NEURODIAGNOSTIC PROCEDURES

William P. Dillon, MD

Magnetic resonance (MR) imaging is the study of choice for the evaluation of most lesions affecting the brain and spine. It has gradually replaced computed tomography (CT) for many indications and has also reduced the need for invasive neuroimaging techniques such as myelography and angiography. CT is more sensitive than MR imaging in visualizing fine osseous detail such as temporal bone anatomy fractures. Recent developments such as helical CT, CT angiography (CTA), MR angiography (MRA), and interventional neuroradiologic procedures have continued to advance the diagnosis and guide the therapy of neurologic disorders.

PLAIN FILM RADIOGRAPHY

CT and MR have largely replaced plain films, especially in cases with neurologic deficits. Plain films of the skull and spine are useful in the initial assessment of spinal trauma and in suspected infection but are rarely indicated otherwise. Plain films are also no longer indicated in the setting of head trauma, as CT or MR reveals more critical information regarding the intracranial contents.

ULTRASOUND

High-resolution ultrasound (US) may image intracranial and spinal anatomy when an acoustic window (bony defect) is present. It is noninvasive, does not involve x-rays, and can be performed with portable equipment. Ultrasound has found wide application in the evaluation of intracranial anatomy in infants with open fontanelles. In the neonatal intensive care unit, ultrasound is the standard technique for evaluating the premature infant for intraventricular hemorrhage and hydrocephalus. Ultrasound examination of the infant spine can delineate normal and abnormal anatomy, although MR imaging is now the standard imaging technique for evaluation of children with suspected spinal cord anomalies and aids in the diagnosis of central nervous system anomalies such as anencephaly, hydrocephalus, and myelomeningocele. Intrauterine MR imaging may confirm fetal anomalies shown by US. Intraoperative ultrasound can also be used to help position the ventricular catheter during shunting and is used to evaluate intracranial anatomy.

COMPUTED TOMOGRAPHY (CT)

The CT image is a computer-generated cross-sectional representation of anatomy created by analysis of the attenuation of x-ray beams that have been passed through various points around a section of the body or brain. The x-ray source is collimated to the desired slice thickness. Sensitive x-ray detectors are aligned 180 degrees from the x-ray source and detect x-rays that are not attenuated by the patient's anatomy. A computer calculates a "back projection" image from the attenuation profile. Greater x-ray attenuation, as caused by bone, results in areas of high "density," while soft tissue structures, which attenuate x-rays less, appear lower in density. The resolution of an image depends on the radiation dose, the collimation (slice thickness), the field of view, and the matrix size of the display. Recent developments in slip ring helical scanners have increased the speed of CT acquisition to as short as 0.5–1 second per scan, or 1–2 minutes for a typical head CT. In the helical scan mode, the table moves continuously through the rotating x-ray beam, generating a "helix" of information that can be reformatted into various slice thicknesses. Advantages of helical CT include shorter scan times, reduced patient and organ motion, and the ability to acquire dynamic CT images during the infusion of intravenous contrast. Dynamic contrast images can be used to construct CT angiograms (CTAs) of vascular structures as well as physiologic maps of vascular perfusion. CTA has proved useful in assessment of the intracranial and extracranial carotid arteries, especially in acute stroke victims (Figure 37–3). "Multidetector" CT scanners acquire multiple sections with each revolution of the gantry, further decreasing the time per examination and improving the spatial and temporal assessment of vascular anatomy and physiology.

CT is safe and reliable. Radiation exposure is between 3 cGy and 5 cGy per examination. The most frequent complications are associated with use of intravenous contrast agents. Two broad categories of contrast media—ionic and nonionic—are in use. Nonionic agents are preferred; ionic agents are less expensive but are associated with a higher incidence of toxicity and allergic reactions than nonionic agents.

The indications for CT have narrowed since the development of MR imaging. CT is useful in imaging osseous structures of the spine, skull base, and temporal bones. CT is also more sensitive and specific than MR for acute subarachnoid hemorrhage. In the spine, CT is

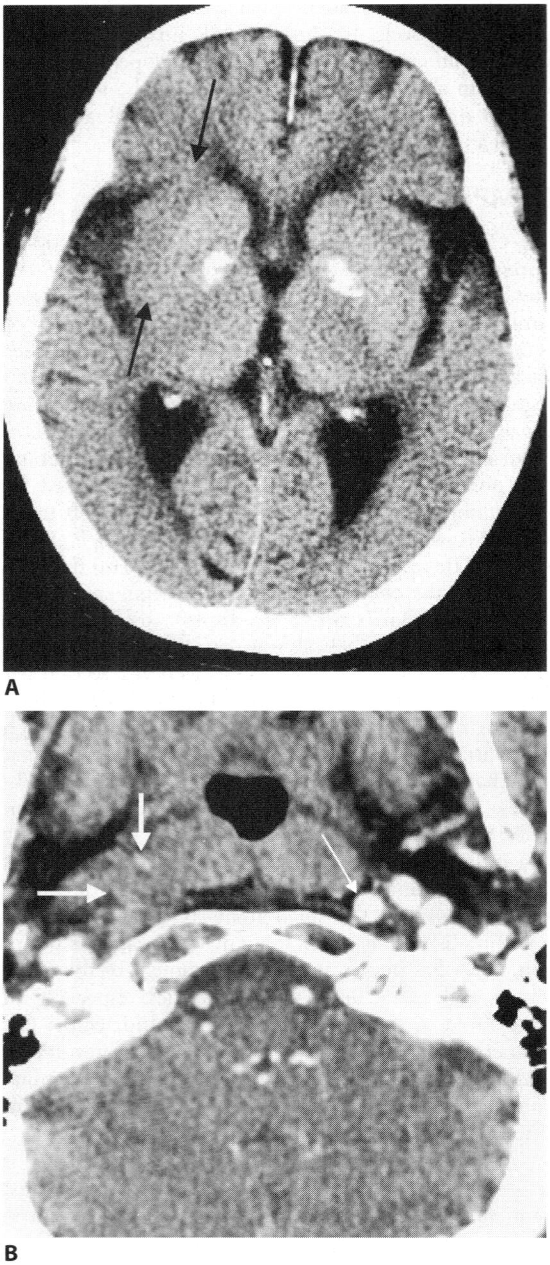

Figure 37–3. ***A:*** A 50-year-old patient presents with acute left hemiparesis. Noncontrast CT scan demonstrates the "insular string sign"—low density involving the insular cortex—a finding consistent with acute middle cerebral arterial infarction (arrows). ***B:*** Partition from a contrast-enhanced CT angiogram. Note the normally enhancing left internal carotid artery (thin arrow) and nonfilling of the thrombosed right internal carotid artery (thick arrows).

often useful in the evaluation of patients with traumatic spinal injury, osseous spinal stenosis, and spondylosis, but MR is preferred for patients with neurologic deficits. CT obtained following instillation of intrathecal contrast (CT myelography) is useful to evaluate the intracranial cisterns for cerebrospinal fluid fistula, as well as the spinal subarachnoid space in patients with ambiguous MR results. Conditions that are identified with a high degree of accuracy by CT include intracerebral, subdural, and epidural hematomas, cerebral atrophy, and hydrocephalus. Patients with suspected cerebral infarction are also candidates for CT scan, though MR is more sensitive to early infarction. Lesions situated near the calvarium or skull base are more difficult to delineate with CT because of beam-hardening artifacts from adjacent bone. Use of thin sections orthogonal to the area can minimize these artifacts. MR is, however, ideal for detecting and delineating lesions adjacent to the calvarium, as bone artifacts are minimized. Intravenous administration of iodinated contrast media may improve the sensitivity of CT by enhancing the density of lesions with an increased blood pool (eg, meningioma, arteriovenous malformations) or a deficient blood-brain barrier (eg, metastatic tumor and inflammatory lesions).

MAGNETIC RESONANCE IMAGING

The phenomenon of magnetic resonance (MR) is a complex interaction between protons in biologic tissues, static and alternating magnetic field (the magnet), and energy in the form of radiofrequency (Rf) waves of a specific frequency, introduced by coils placed next to the body part of interest. The images that are created reflect the density of hydrogen protons as well as their relaxation rates. The relaxation rate of protons is different for different normal and pathologic tissues. T1- and T2-weighted images can be obtained in order to highlight certain aspects of disease processes. The surrounding molecular environment and atomic neighbors influence the relaxation rates of a hydrogen proton in a tissue. MR images can be generated in sagittal, coronal, axial, and oblique planes without changing the patient's position. Each plane obtained requires a separate sequence lasting 2–10 minutes. Unlike CT, movement of the patient during a sequence will distort all of the images; therefore, patient cooperation is important. Approximately 5% of the population experience claustrophobia in the MR environment, but this can be reduced by mild sedation. MR may be obtained in 2D or 3D modes. Three-dimensional volumetric imaging results in a volume of data that can be reformatted in any plane and manipulated in a real-time fashion to highlight certain disease processes. Fluid-attenuated inversion recovery (FLAIR) is a pulse sequence that produces T2-weighted images in which the cerebrospinal fluid signal is suppressed. FLAIR images are more sensitive than standard spin echo images for cortical lesions and meningeal processes (Figure 37–4). Echo-planar imaging (EPI) techniques permit rapid MR imaging on the order of milliseconds. EPI is the basis for diffusion imaging, which is the most sensitive technique for identifying acute infarction and perfusion imaging (Figure 37–5).

The heavy-metal element gadolinium forms the basis of all current intravenous MR contrast agents. Gadolinium is a paramagnetic substance, which reduces the T1 and T2 relaxation times of nearby water protons, resulting in a high signal on T1-weighted images. Gadolinium contrast does not cross a normal blood-brain barrier and thus causes enhancement of brain tissue only at sites of abnormalities in the barrier or lesions with slow vascular flow. Allergic reactions and renal dysfunction are extremely rare side effects of gadolinium agents. These agents can be administered safely to children as well as adults and are often use to increase the sensitivity of MR to various disease states that disrupt the blood-brain barrier.

MR is particularly useful—compared with CT—for identifying lesions in the posterior fossa and the spinal cord. MR imaging has replaced myelography and CT as the initial diagnostic procedure for most conditions of the spine and spinal cord.

Magnetic resonance angiography (MRA) delineates the major extracranial and intracranial vessels without the need for contrast agents, though recent fast scan techniques during a bolus of contrast material have improved the detection of vascular disorders (Figure 37–6). It is important to understand that MRA is a **vascular flow map** and not an anatomic map as revealed by conventional angiography. Two MRA techniques—time-of-flight (TOF) and phase-contrast—are currently in use. TOF, currently the technique used most frequently, relies on the suppression of nonmoving tissue to provide a background for the high signal intensity of flowing blood. A typical TOF angiography sequence results in a series of contiguous thin MR sections (0.9 mm thick) that can be viewed as a maximum intensity projection (MIP), which can be reformatted or viewed in various planes and angles to reveal vascular relationships. Either arterial or venous structures can be obtained (Figures 37–7 and 37–8). The ability to delineate intracranial vascular lesions noninvasively is useful in screening for aneurysms and vascular occlusive disease. MRA has supplanted routine diagnostic angiography for many purposes, with the exception of patients suspected of vasculitis or other small vessel diseases.

MYELOGRAPHY

Myelography is a radiographic study that outlines the spinal canal and its contents. Water-soluble nonionic contrast material is injected into the subarachnoid space

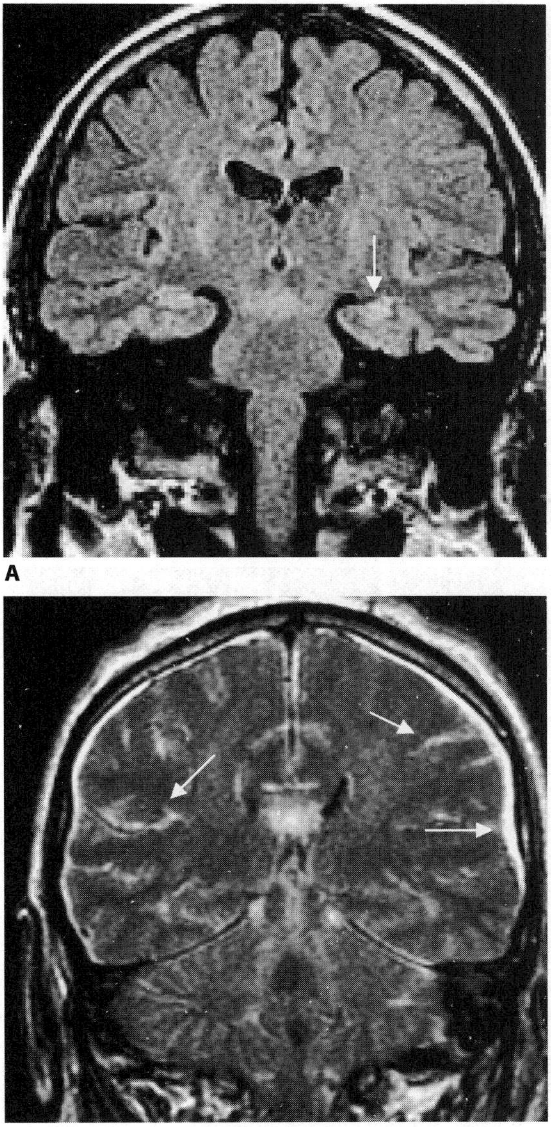

A

B

Figure 37–4. FLAIR MR imaging. Two examples of the utility of FLAIR imaging. ***A:*** Coronal T2-weighted FLAIR image in a patient with intractable epilepsy demonstrates high signal intensity of the hippocampus consistent with mesial temporal sclerosis (arrow). Note the normal low signal intensity of cerebrospinal fluid in the cisterns and ventricles. ***B:*** Coronal FLAIR in a patient with subarachnoid hemorrhage. High signal blood replaces the normal low signal blood in the cisterns and in the left hemispheric subdural hematoma.

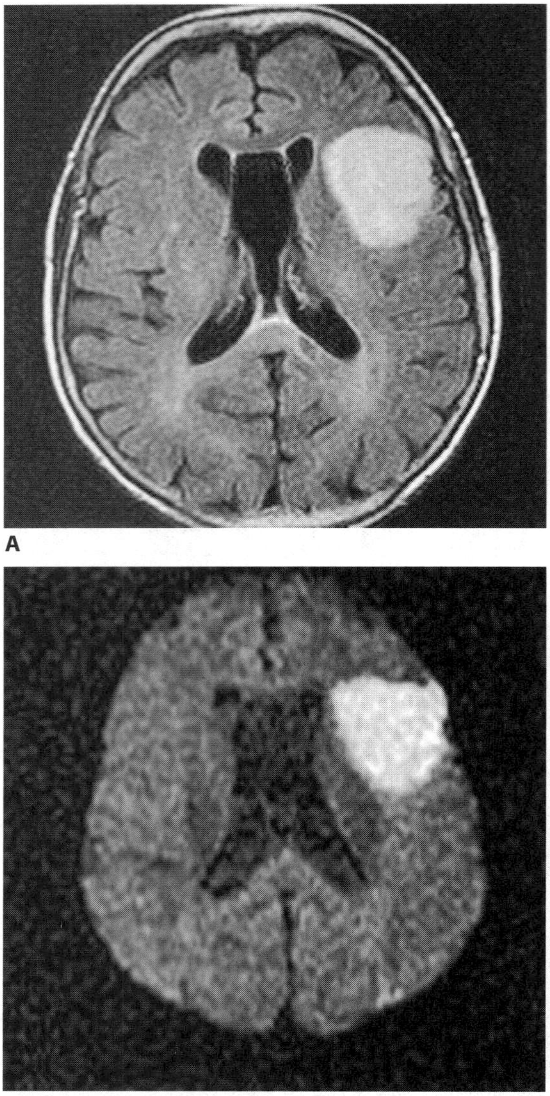

Figure 37–5. Diffusion imaging in acute stroke. ***A:*** FLAIR image demonstrates a nonspecific mass of high signal intensity. The differential diagnosis is stroke and tumor. ***B:*** Diffusion-weighted image shows the lesion with high intensity, or restricted, diffusion signal consistent with acute cerebral infarction.

via a lumbar or cervical puncture. The hyperbaric contrast material mixes with cerebrospinal fluid and is manipulated within the spinal canal by tilting the patient into various positions. The flow of contrast material is monitored by fluoroscopy, and radiographs are taken in desired projections to record and preserve with more detail the areas of interest. The agent is excreted by the renal system. CT scanning following subarachnoid instillation of contrast material—"CT myelography"—increases the amount of information obtained compared with routine plain film myelography. Low-dose CT myelography has replaced conventional myelography in most instances; however, CT myelography is still necessary in patients with metallic spinal prostheses or other conditions where MR imaging is contraindicated. Myelography is also useful in detecting cerebrospinal fluid fistula.

DIGITAL SUBTRACTION ANGIOGRAPHY

Radiographic visualization of the arterial and venous systems of the neck, brain, and spinal cord is accomplished by intra-arterial injection of a water-soluble iodinated contrast agent. Injections are made via a long catheter placed into the femoral artery and positioned into the artery of interest. Extremely small catheters

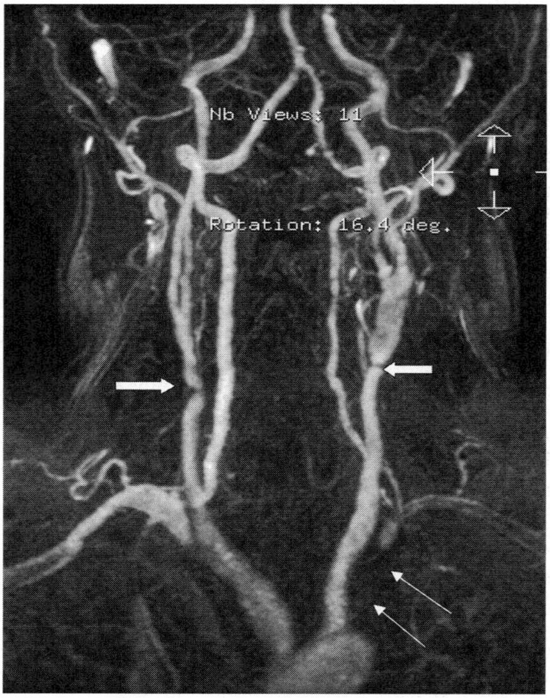

Figure 37–6. Contrast-enhanced MR angiography. Coronal view of contrast-enhanced MRA of the cervical vasculature acquired in 30 seconds during infusion of intravenous gadolinium contrast material. The patient suffered from subclavian artery occlusion and steal syndrome (arrows).

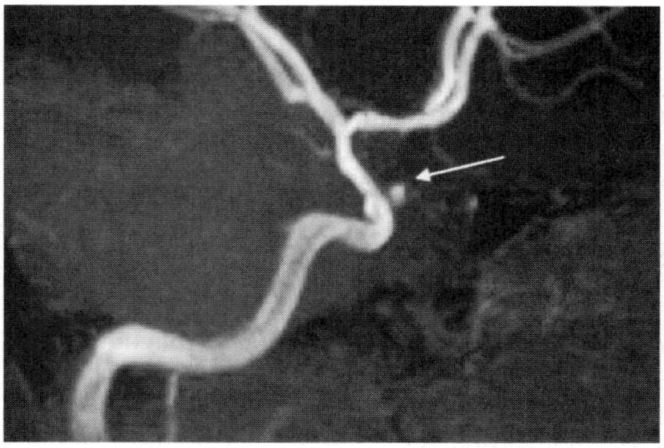

Figure 37–7. MRA of aneurysm. 3D time of flight MRA of the circle of Willis demonstrates a small carotido-ophthalmic artery aneurysm (arrow).

have allowed supraselective catheterization of cerebral arteries, permitting endovascular therapies with various devices. Endovascular placement of electrolytically detachable coils has become a standard therapy for certain cerebral aneurysms and assists in the preoperative management of arteriovenous malformations. Digital subtraction angiography is the best procedure for characterizing aneurysms and arteriovenous malformations; however, MRA and CTA have improved in recent years, making possible noninvasive assessment of many of these vascular disorders. Conventional angiography is reserved for cases in which small-vessel detail is essential for diagnosis. Digital subtraction angiography (DSA) permits the use of smaller amounts of contrast material and decreases radiation exposure to the patient. Newer contrast materials and careful attention to technique have reduced the rate of side effects to less than 1%.

RADIONUCLIDE IMAGING

Short half-life gamma-emitting isotopes such as technetium Tc 99m pertechnetate or indium In 113m diethylenetriamine pentaacetic acid (DTPA) are excluded by the intact blood-brain barrier. The isotopes will cross defects in the blood-brain barrier such as those caused by neoplasms or vascular accidents, which appear as an area of increased activity. Intravenous injection of the isotope as a bolus followed by rapid-sequence imaging can give qualitative information about extracranial carotid artery and supratentorial cerebral blood flow.

Isotope cisternography can give qualitative information about cerebrospinal fluid flow and absorption characteristics. An isotope such as indium In 113m DTPA is injected into the subarachnoid space, followed by scanning at intervals of up to 48 hours. This technique is useful for the evaluation of hydrocephalus, cerebrospinal fluid shunt function, and cerebrospinal fluid fistulas (leaks).

Xenon CT is a technique that quantifies regional cerebral blood flow. Inhalation of xenon gas (25–28%)

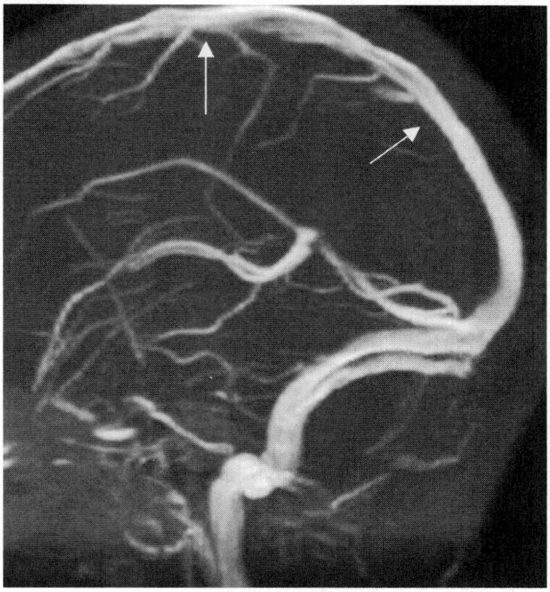

A

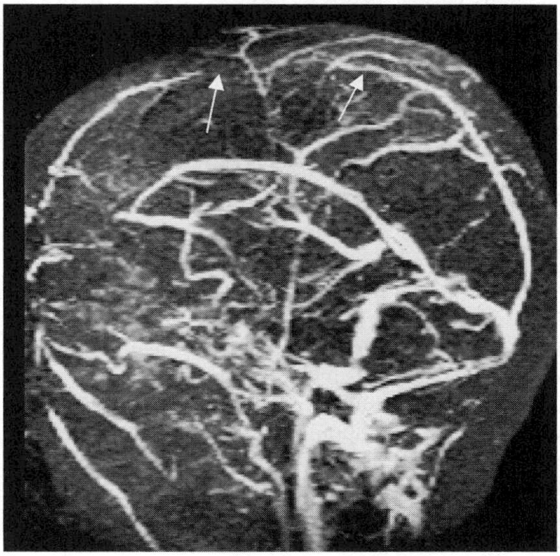

B

Figure 37–8. MR venography. ***A:*** Normal lateral view of MRV demonstrates the normal sagittal sinus (arrows). ***B:*** A patient with acute headaches demonstrates thrombosis of the sagittal sinus (arrows).

during CT scanning increases the density proportionate to blood flow. This technique may be combined with the administration of acetazolamide, which normally increases cerebral blood flow, to assess circulatory reserve.

Positron emission tomography (PET) relies on the detection of positrons emitted during the decay of a radionuclide that has been injected into a patient. The most frequently used moiety is 2-[^{18}F]fluoro-2-deoxy-D-glucose (FDG), which is an analogue of glucose and is taken up by cells competitively with 2-deoxyglucose. Multiple images of glucose uptake activity are formed after 45–60 minutes. Images reveal differences in regional glucose activity among normal and pathologic brain structures. FDG PET scanning has been used to assist in differentiating radiation necrosis from active neoplasm following therapy, in localizing temporal lobe epileptic foci, and in detecting metastatic disease and determining cardiac viability. A lower activity of FDG in the parietal lobes has been associated with Alzheimer's disease.

MAGNETOENCEPHALOGRAPHY (MEG)

Magnetoencephalography (MEG) is a technique that detects the magnetic dipoles intrinsic to the brain during task activation such as sensory stimulation, language tasks, or auditory stimuli. The foci of activity may be mapped onto MRI scans to reveal anatomic localization of somatosensory function.

INTRAOPERATIVE NEUROPHYSIOLOGIC MONITORING

Charles D. Yingling, PhD

The last decade has seen a rapid growth in the development of techniques for intraoperative neurophysiologic monitoring. Examples include monitoring cranial nerves during skull base surgery, assessing cerebral perfusion during aneurysm clipping or carotid endarterectomy, monitoring both ascending and descending pathways during spinal surgery, and mapping sensory, motor, and language regions of the cerebral cortex. Most major medical centers now have personnel and equipment dedicated to intraoperative monitoring, and there are many private groups offering monitoring services on a contract basis to smaller hospitals nationwide. Neural monitoring specialists now have national certification offered by the American Board of Neurophysiological Monitoring (supervisory level) and the American Board of Registered Electrodiagnostic Technologists (technologist level). Neurophysiologic monitoring has become an integral part of many neurosurgical procedures as well as of a wide range of orthopedic, otolaryngologic, vascular, pediatric, and neurointerventional radiology procedures.

SKULL BASE SURGERY

One of the first applications of intraoperative neurophysiology was monitoring facial nerve function during acoustic neuroma resection, a technique actually pioneered in the late 19th century that came into widespread use during the 1980s. Small needle electrodes are placed within facial muscles to record electromyographic potentials, and electrical stimulation is used to map the nerve in relation to the tumor by eliciting electromyographic responses when the nerve is contacted. The threshold and amplitude of the responses can be used to quantify facial nerve function and predict postoperative outcome. Electromyographic responses may also be elicited by surgical events such as traction on the nerve and can alert the surgeon to the location of the nerve in the surgical field, which can then be confirmed with stimulation. Conversely, the absence of a response to suprathreshold stimulation indicates an area in which resection can proceed safely. This technique has been shown to dramatically lower the incidence of facial nerve palsy following acoustic neuroma resection, and its routine use has been recommended in an NIH Consensus Conference report.

Similar techniques can be used to monitor other cranial motor nerves by appropriate placement of recording electrodes. For anterior skull base surgery, such as removal of prepontine or cavernous sinus region tumors, the nerves to the extraocular muscles can be monitored by placing fine hookwire electrodes into the inferior rectus, superior oblique, and lateral rectus muscles. The motor component of the trigeminal nerve can be monitored with electrodes in the temporalis or masseter muscles. Lower cranial nerves can be identified with electrodes in the trapezius and genioglossus for tumors of the jugular foramen or foramen magnum region. By intubating with a special electromyographic endotracheal tube (Xomed-Treace), electromyography can be recorded from the vocalis muscles, innervated by the recurrent laryngeal component of the tenth cranial nerve. In all of these cases, electromyographic reactions to surgical manipulations may alert the surgeon to the location of a specific nerve, and electrical stimulation can be used for confirmation.

Development of techniques for monitoring sensory nerves has been more difficult. Visual evoked potentials (VEP), which have long been used in the diagnostic clinic and which are an obvious means of monitoring optic nerve function, are notoriously unstable under anesthesia. Despite repeated efforts with different anesthetic agents, this problem has remained intractable, and optic nerve function is for that reason rarely monitored. Excessive stimulus artifact due to short response latencies has limited the applicability of somatosensory evoked potentials (SEPs) for monitoring trigeminal sensory function. The only sensory cranial nerve that is routinely monitored is the cochlear nerve, which can readily be assessed with only slight modifications of the auditory brain stem response (ABR) technique routinely used in the audiology clinic. However, the small amplitude of this response limits its utility, since signal averaging over 1 or 2 minutes is often necessary to obtain a repeatable response—too slow to be of much use in the surgical context. Direct recordings from the cochlear nerve are much faster but require an invasive electrode, which can be difficult to place so that it is stable and not in the way. Digital signal processing techniques show promise for speeding ABR collection times but have yet to come into widespread use. Despite these limitations, ABR monitoring has a place in management of smaller acoustic tumors with good residual hearing. It is also useful in detecting excessive stretching of the cochlear nerve during cerebellar retraction for microvascular decompression or other posterior fossa procedures.

Anesthetic requirements for cranial nerve monitoring are straightforward: No muscle relaxants should be used except for intubation, since electromyographic responses must be unaffected. Otherwise, any desired technique can be used, since the ABR is almost unaffected by normal concentrations of commonly used agents such as N_2O, halogenated vapors, opioids, barbiturates, or propofol.

SPINAL CORD SURGERY

One of the earliest applications of intraoperative neurophysiologic monitoring was the use of somatosensory evoked potentials (SEPs) during scoliosis correction. SEPs are recorded with methods similar to those used in the diagnostic clinic: Appropriate peripheral nerves (usually the median, ulnar, common peroneal, or posterior tibial) are electrically stimulated and averaged responses are obtained from scalp electrodes near somatosensory cortical regions as well as from more peripheral sites. However, since SEPs are mediated primarily by the dorsal columns, it is possible for isolated anterior spine injury or ischemia to remain undetected. There has thus been great interest in development of techniques for monitoring spinal motor pathways as well. An early technique involved stimulation of the cord itself via percutaneous needles placed adjacent to the spinal lamina rostrad to the incision and recording from electrodes placed over peripheral motor nerves. This so-called "neurogenic motor evoked potential" (nMEP) had the advantage that the patient could be maintained on neuromuscular blocking agents to prevent movement in response to stimulation.

Unfortunately, subsequent studies demonstrated that the nMEP response is primarily mediated by antidromic conduction in the dorsal columns, so it is not a true motor evoked potential. The technique now preferred is transcranial electrical stimulation with electrodes placed over the primary motor cortex. A series of brief high-voltage pulses (typically 300–500 volts, four to seven pulses at intervals of 2–3 ms) is delivered through scalp electrodes, and responses are recorded from upper and lower extremity muscles such as abductor pollicis brevis, tibialis anterior, and gastrocnemius. Since antidromic activity cannot cross the somatosensory synapses in the thalamus and dorsal column nuclei, the response is thought to be mediated by corticospinal tracts. Multiple pulses are necessary to elicit the response under general anesthesia, which affects the synapse to the motor nerve in the anterior horn of the spinal cord. The responses are large in amplitude and can thus be seen in single trials without the need for signal averaging. Owing to the predominance of upper extremity representation in the cortical motor areas, lower extremity transcranial MEPs typically have higher thresholds and lower amplitudes than responses in upper extremity muscles. This transcranial motor evoked potential (tcMEP) is quite sensitive to changes in spinal cord perfusion and has been successfully employed not only in scoliosis surgery but also in many other procedures where the spinal cord or its vascular supply is at risk. Spinal tumors, decompressive procedures (both anterior and posterior), and thoracoabdominal aortic aneurysms have all benefited from tcMEP monitoring, which is usually done in conjunction with SEP recording so as to monitor both ascending and descending pathways.

The anesthetic requirements for spinal cord monitoring are much more constraining than for cranial nerve monitoring. The tcMEP technique requires that no muscle relaxants be used, since EMG activity is being recorded. The stimulus causes contractions in scalp muscles, which are activated directly, so a bite block must be used to prevent tongue injuries. Some patient movement may be seen in the surgical field, but this is usually minimal; since the responses can be seen in single trials, the surgeon only need pause for a few seconds to allow the pathways to be checked. Both tcMEPs and SEPs are greatly diminished or abolished by high concentrations of commonly used agents such as nitrous oxide or halogenated vapors. The most marked responses are usually obtained with a total intravenous technique based on propofol and narcotics, which can usually be supplemented by low doses of desflurane or similar agents.

Surgery in the lumbar and sacral levels (eg, for tethered cord, myelomeningocele, or lumbosacral tumors) requires a different approach than for cervical or thoracic level surgery. Since the spinal cord terminates at approximately T12 in adults, issues of cord compression, distraction, or perfusion are less relevant than the status of sensory and motor roots in the cauda equina. While it is desirable to preserve innervation of the legs, the most devastating complications of surgery in this region are loss of bowel and bladder control by interruption of lower sacral roots. Motor roots in the cauda equina can be easily monitored using procedures very similar to those developed for cranial motor nerves; the electrodes are simply placed in different muscles. Depending on the level of interest, quadriceps, tibialis anterior, hamstring, gastrocnemius, or intrinsic foot muscles can be easily recorded, as can the external anal sphincter. The urethral sphincter can also be monitored by means of a special ring electrode placed over a standard Foley catheter. The course of roots in relation to lumbosacral tumors can be easily mapped in the same way the facial nerve is mapped in acoustic neuroma. For tethered cord, the filum terminale is identified and stimulated before being transected to ensure that no roots are adherent to its ventral surface, which is a common finding. After all roots are dissected free, stimulation of the filum will produce no responses at intensities from 10 times to 100 times those necessary to activate motor roots. For lumbosacral root monitoring, anesthetic management is simplified since the only constraint is that no muscle relaxants can be employed.

ANEURYSM SURGERY

Treatment of cerebral aneurysms carries risks of ischemia to structures downstream from the aneurysm. Aneurysm clips may occlude parent vessels or perforators arising from them, and temporary occlusion of a major vessel is often necessary. The risk is particularly high for aneurysm of the posterior communicating or basilar arteries because of the large number of perforators supplying critical brain stem and thalamic structures. Thus, a means of monitoring perfusion in these territories is desirable.

In principle, electroencephalographic recordings could be used to detect cortical ischemia since hypoperfusion causes electroencephalographic slowing, which can be detected readily with digital electroencephalographic techniques. However, because of the risk of ischemia, many vascular neurosurgeons prefer to administer barbiturates prior to clipping or occlusion for cerebral protection. By lowering the cerebral metabolic rate of oxygen consumption ($CMRO_2$), the risk of damage due to cerebral hypoperfusion is reduced; however, since barbiturates produce significant effects on the EEG, such recordings can no longer be used to detect hypoperfusion or ischemia. Fortunately, SEP recordings are also sensitive to decreased cerebral blood flow and can still be recorded even when the EEG is rendered isoelectric by barbiturate administration.

In practice, EEGs and SEPs can be recorded from the same scalp electrodes by directing the signals to separate amplifiers with appropriate filter settings. Electrodes are placed over midline and bilateral parietal and frontal sites. The exact electrode position may have to be altered from standard clinical placements in order to avoid the craniotomy site; since intraoperative changes are assessed rather than comparisons to normative data, this generally does not pose a problem. Baseline recordings under standard anesthesia are obtained first in order to confirm system function and avoid any problems due to positioning; baseline problems are often detected if there is concurrent cervical stenosis and should be corrected by adjusting patient position before proceeding with the craniotomy.

Barbiturates should be administered a few minutes before clipping or occlusion since a new SEP baseline will be necessary. Thiopental sodium is typically administered in a dose comparable to that which would be used for anesthetic induction. The EEG is used to titrate the level of barbiturate to obtain a burst-suppression pattern, in which periods of isoelectricity alternate with higher-amplitude bursts. A burst/suppression ratio of about 20% burst activity is adequate; more than this provides no further cerebral protective effect and will make it more difficult to extubate the patient after the procedure. A new SEP baseline is then obtained; it will typically exhibit prolonged latency and decreased amplitude but will still have a high enough signal/noise ratio to effectively assess intraoperative changes.

For middle cerebral artery aneurysms, either ulnar or median nerve SEPs can be employed. For anterior cerebral or anterior communicating artery aneurysms, posterior tibial nerve SEPs should be used since the lower extremity somatosensory area is in the distal anterior cerebral artery territory. For posterior communicating or basilar artery aneurysms, both upper and lower extremity SEPs should be recorded since occlusion of perforating arteries into the brain stem or thalamus can affect either or both of these pathways. Unilateral changes in SEP amplitude can usually be detected within 2–4 minutes after inadvertent occlusion and are a signal for repositioning clips as necessary to restore baseline values. Such changes are relatively rare in treatment of uncomplicated middle or anterior cerebral artery aneurysms but are encountered more frequently in treatment of posterior circulation aneurysms. This is presumably due to the higher number of small perforating arteries, which are more difficult to visualize with the longer reach from a standard pterional or orbitozygomatic craniotomy.

MAPPING MOTOR PATHWAYS

Surgery for tumors near the central sulcus or internal capsule poses risks of compromised motor function. However, patient survival is enhanced if the most complete resection possible is obtained. In order to locate both cortical and subcortical motor regions, electrical stimulation mapping is employed. For dominant hemisphere tumors resected under local anesthesia, verbal reports from the patient can be used to determine any sensory or motor responses accompanying stimulation. Areas critical for language or memory function can similarly be mapped using appropriate behavioral testing during stimulation. However, when surgery is performed under general anesthesia, this is not possible. If light surgical anesthesia is maintained without the use of muscle relaxants, gross movement of the contralateral body can often be observed in response to direct stimulation of the exposed cortex. However, the sensitivity of this method can be greatly enhanced by simultaneous recording of electromyographic activity from multiple muscles. Consistent electromyographic responses are often observed without any overt motion being detected. This technique is particularly valuable when resecting tumors near subcortical motor pathways, since there is no obvious topography to indicate where a response is likely to be observed. It is much easier to scan multiple electromyographic channels at a slow sweep speed than to simultaneously observe the entire contralateral body. Since mapping takes little time, it can be repeatedly employed as tumor resection proceeds until responses are obtained. Use of such mapping techniques allows maximal tumor resection to be obtained without compromising motor function.

CRANIOCEREBRAL TRAUMA

Martin C. Holland, MD

ESSENTIALS OF DIAGNOSIS

- *Pathogenesis*
- *Clinical findings*
- *Radiographic findings*
- *Initial assessment*
- *Medical management*
- *Surgical treatment*

General Considerations

Trauma is the leading cause of death among persons younger than 45 years of age, with craniocerebral trauma constituting a major portion of deaths within this group. Craniocerebral trauma is also second only to stroke as a cause of death from injury to the central nervous system. Though precise numbers are difficult to obtain, it is estimated that the incidence of traumatic brain injury (TBI) falls between 132 and 367 cases per 100,000 population. The 1985–1987 National Health Interview Survey estimated that 1.975 million Americans annually sought medical attention for head injuries. Of these, 373,000 were admitted to hospitals for their injury, and 75,000 subsequently died.

Not surprisingly, TBI is primarily a disease of young men, with the male:female ratio falling between 2 and 2.8:1. Motor vehicle accidents are the most common cause of serious injury, with approximately 30–55% of admissions belonging to this group. Falls constitute 15–35%, assaults and gunshot wounds 2–25%, and sports-related injuries 5–20% of injuries. As patients get older, the risk of developing a TBI increases—-specifically, the incidence of falls and pedestrians-hit-by-automobiles rises after the seventh decade of life.

Craniocerebral trauma can involve injury to the scalp, skull meninges, or brain. Most are not life threatening, though lifelong sequelae are not uncommon. Fifty to 90 percent of TBI-related hospital admissions are for mild injuries, while 10–30% are for moderate injuries and 5–25% for severe ones. These numbers must be taken with caution, however, as the definition of "mild" varies considerably. Nevertheless, it is important to note that a minority of hospital admissions following TBI are for severe injuries.

Pathogenesis

One of the easiest classification schemes for TBI is based on the mechanism of injury. Injuries can be classified as acceleration/deceleration, impact, or penetrating.

A. Acceleration/Deceleration Injury

Typically seen following high-speed motor vehicle accidents, these injuries involve sudden acceleration or deceleration of the brain. Usually, the skull and brain accelerate differentially, causing the brain to slosh back and forth within the skull. As it does, the brain impacts against intracranial bony irregularities such as the floor of the frontal fossa, the sphenoid wing or the petrous ridge, leading to the development of superficial cortical contusions. A further consequence of this differential movement between skull and brain is the stretching of cortical draining veins as they cross the subdural space before penetrating the dural sinuses. If stretched enough, these veins tear and bleed into the subdural space, thus forming subdural hematomas

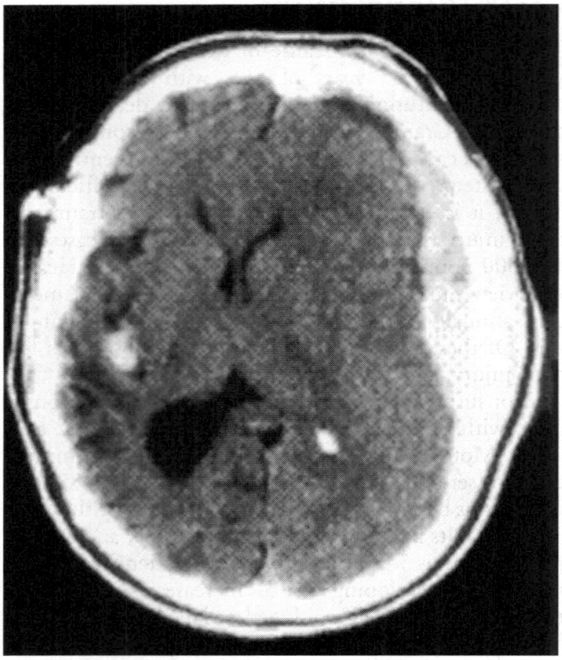

Figure 37–9. Subdural hematoma resulting from tearing of bridging cortical veins. The hematoma roughly follows the contour of the brain and causes significant left-to-right brain shift. Subdural hematoma is often associated with acceleration/deceleration-type injuries and the underlying brain injury is often quite severe.

(Figure 37–9). The final consequence of acceleration/deceleration is the transmission of kinetic forces to the brain that cause shear injury to neurons (axons particularly) and blood vessels. This leads to diffuse axonal injury (DAI) and the development of subcortical, pericentral, and posterolataral mesencephalic hematomas.

B. Impact Injuries

Impact injury is often seen following assaults with blunt objects such as bats or pipes. As such, the skull absorbs much of the object's kinetic force, though the brain often absorbs enough to cause a concussion. Skull fractures are common in this type of injury and dural injury often follows. This also results in the development of epidural hematomas as the meningeal vessels under the fracture tear (Figure 37–10). Since the skull absorbs much of the impact, the severity of brain injury per se is less severe than that following acceleration/deceleration injuries. Thus, the classic clinical picture is that of initial loss of consciousness at the time of impact followed by a lucid period as the patient recovers from the concussion. In some cases, a second period of decreased mentation develops after the lucid period, as the epidural hematoma expands to compress the brain stem or other vital brain areas. The thin temporal squamosa is the skull bone most likely to fracture. Thus, the underlying middle meningeal artery is the most vulnerable to injury and a temporal epidural hematoma the most likely to form.

C. Penetrating Injuries

Penetrating brain injuries can be divided into high-velocity and low-velocity injuries. The cutoff is somewhat arbitrary but is generally defined as missile velocity of 300 feet per second at impact. Since the energy (E) transmitted to the brain equals $^1/_2$ the missile mass (M) times its velocity (V) squared ($E = {}^1/_2 \times M \times V^2$), the higher the velocity or the greater the missile mass,

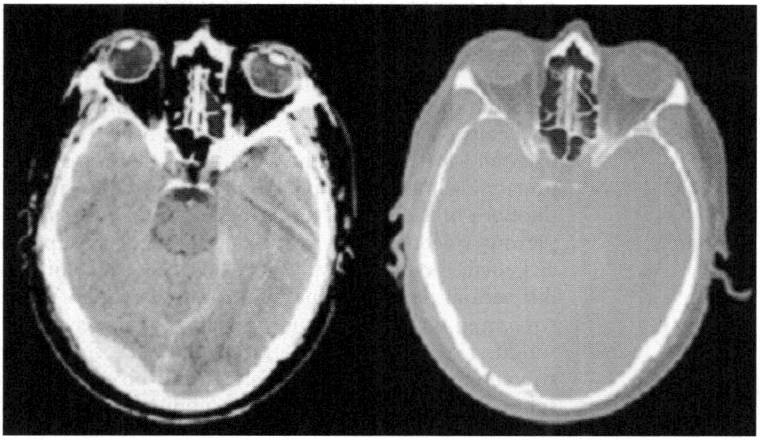

Figure 37–10. Epidural hematoma. CT of the head windowed for brain (left) and bone (right) shows an epidural hematoma resulting from an underlying occipital skull fracture. This injury was caused by a blow to the back of the head. Notice the classic lens-shaped hematoma. The brain window also shows a thin left tentorial subdural hematoma appearing as a white line running from the midline posteriorly and curving towards the left of the pons.

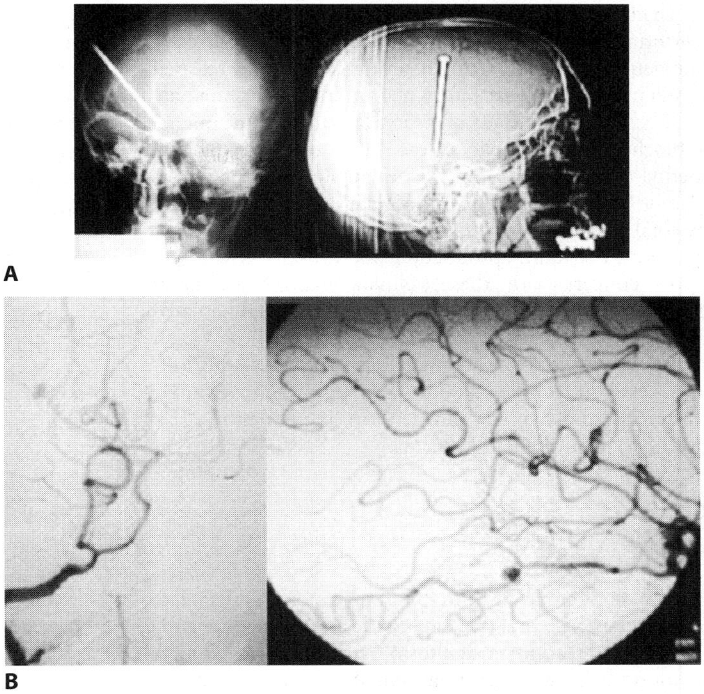

Figure 37–11. ***A:*** AP and lateral skull x-ray showing a nail injury to the brain. The patient had a GCS of 15 and minimal diplopia on initial examination. An axial noncontrast CT showed the tip of the nail within the right perimesencephalic cistern. The patient's diplopia was secondary to injury of the right fourth cranial nerve. ***B:*** AP right vertebral artery injection (left) and lateral right internal carotid artery injection (right) demonstrating a traumatic pseudoaneurysm of the right PCA after removal of the nail.

the greater the energy transmitted to the brain. Since energy varies with the square of the velocity, V has greater impact than M in determining the energy absorbed by the brain.

Since low-velocity missiles often cannot penetrate the thick cranial vault, most low-velocity injuries occur though the relatively thin skull base—particularly the orbitocranial window—causing damage to structures along the path of entry, with the cerebral vasculature being particularly vulnerable (Figure 37–11). A multitude of low-velocity missiles have been described including pens, pencils, chopsticks, branches, arrows, darts, and needlefish.

High-velocity injuries are of a different nature. Though structures along the path of entry are certainly injured, much of the damage occurs away from the missile tract. This is because the missile's kinetic energy is absorbed by the skull and brain as it slows. The resulting transfer of energy to the brain precipitates a diffuse injury similar to that imparted to the brain following acceleration/deceleration injuries. As such, the morbidity and mortality of high-velocity injuries is significantly higher than that of low-velocity injuries. The increased use of military-style assault weapons in United States urban centers has increased the lethality of gunshot wounds (Figure 37–12), as these weapons are designed to fire with much higher muzzle velocities than conventional firearms.

Pathobiology

Regardless of mechanism, all injuries to the brain share some common physiologic characteristics. The initial impact leads to a number of biochemical alterations, many

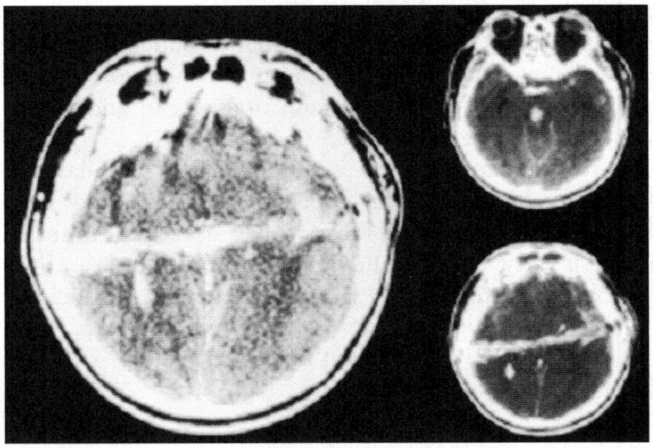

Figure 37–12. Through-and-through gunshot wound to the head. The entrance is on the right and the exit on the left. The small right upper-hand image shows a distant Duret hemorrhage within the brain stem, 2 cm caudal to the bullet tract. The patient was admitted with a GCS of 3 and was subsequently declared brain-dead. (Reprinted with permission from Elsevier.)

of which are thought to involve the unregulated release of neurotransmitters from traumatic depolarization of cerebral neurons. Though many neurotransmitters are released simultaneously, the excitatory neurotransmitter glutamate is released in the greatest quantity. It is thought to initiate a biochemical cytotoxic cascade mediated through *N*-methyl-D-aspartate (NMDA) glutamate receptors. This cascade leads to alterations in cellular energy metabolism, cerebral blood flow, transmembrane ion concentration gradients, free radical production, and cytokine release.

In concert with these cellular changes are gross changes such as the development of intracranial hematomas, cerebral edema, and hydrocephalus—all of which can contribute to intracranial hypertension. Additionally, systemic problems such as hypotension, seizures, infections, and hypoxia can develop, increasing the risk of further neurologic injury.

Clinical Findings

A. Symptoms & Signs

The range of clinical findings and neurologic deficits following craniocerebral trauma is wide and varied, depending on the location, mechanism, and severity of injury. Confounding factors such as spinal cord injury, shock, and the presence of drugs or alcohol can also mask neurologic deficits, making accurate assessment difficult. Finally, the neurologic examination can change drastically—especially in the acute setting—a situation that warrants frequent and careful neurologic assessments.

The initial general trauma assessment should focus on the ABCs (airway, breathing, and circulation), and steps should be taken to stabilize the patient hemodynamically. At the same time, an initial trauma neurologic examination is done, focusing on the patient's mental status, cranial nerve reflexes, and motor function—thus, a quick assessment of the brain, brain stem, and spinal cord can be done.

Mental status is best assessed using the Glasgow Coma Scale (GCS), developed by Teasdale and Jennette in 1976. It is the most widely used neurotrauma scale, is easy to use, and has excellent interexaminer concordance. Based on a scale from 3 to 15, three clinical parameters (eye opening, verbal response, and motor response) are assessed to determine the patient's level of consciousness.

1. Eye-opening—Graded from 1 to 4, this component assesses the level of stimulus required for a patient to open his or her eyes. Eye-opening to ambient stimulus is graded as a 4; eye-opening to directed verbal stimulus, a 3; eye-opening to pain, a 2; and no eye-opening at all is graded a 1.

2. Verbal response—This parameter grades the level or complexity of spontaneous verbal output on a scale of 1–5. Normal speech with normal content is graded a 5; normal speech with inappropriate content receives a 4; words without sentence structure is graded a 3; sound without word structure is a 2, and absence of verbal output is graded as a 1.

3. Motor response—The most sensitive indicator of neurologic dysfunction and best predictor of outcome, motor response is graded on a scale from 1 to 6. The highest grade (6) is given to patients who follow verbal commands. All other grades are scored in response to painful stimulus. Patients who localize pain receive a 5; those who withdraw from it are graded as a 4; flexor posturing (also called decorticate posturing) grades as a 3; and extensor posturing (decerebrate posturing) as a 2. No response to painful stimulus receives a 1.

All three components are added up to give a composite score. Coma is technically considered at a grade of 8 or less—this is also considered a severe injury. Moderate injuries are generally considered at a GCS score of 9–12 and mild from 13–15.

The detail and extent of cranial nerve examination depends on the patient's level of consciousness. Awake, cooperative patients presumably can follow commands, allowing full examination of cranial nerve function. Comatose patients, however, can only elicit cranial nerve reflexes. The most simple and directed cranial nerve examination focuses on three reflexes—the pupillary reflex, the corneal reflex, and the gag reflex. The first assesses pupillary response to light, carrying afferent information via cranial nerve (CN) II (optic nerve) and efferent information via CN III (occulomotor). The corneal reflex carries afferent information via CN V (ophthalmic portion of the trigeminal nerve) and efferent information via CN VII (facial). Finally, the gag reflex afferent and efferent signals are carried via the glossopharyngeal (CN IX) and vagus nerves (CN X), respectively. With these three reflexes, the entire brain stem can be quickly assessed as the pupillary reflex is localized in the midbrain, the corneal reflex in the pons, and the gag reflex in the medulla. The presence of a unilaterally dilated or fixed pupil in the comatose patient is of considerable concern as it often indicates transtentorial herniation of the ipsilateral temporal uncus due to supratentorial intracranial hypertension. The loss of the corneal or gag reflex is of much more concern as it indicates severe brain stem injury.

Other cranial reflexes include the occulovestibular reflex (caloric reflex) and occulocephalic reflex (doll's eye), though these are not usually assessed in the trauma bay, as they are impractical in the case of the former and unsafe in the latter (due to the potential presence of a cervical injury).

The initial motor examination should be limited to a qualitative assessment of movement of all four extremities. It is often impossible to formally examine motor strength due to resuscitation efforts and pelvic or long-bone fractures. As such, it is enough to establish the presence of a paresis or plegia and which limbs are affected. More detailed examination can wait until the initial resuscitation has stabilized the patient. The awake, cooperative, hemodynamically stable patient can be examined more formally and at leisure. A rectal examination assessing tone is mandatory in the acute period.

Assessment of sensation, deep tendon reflexes, and coordination is completely useless in the comatose patient and can generally be performed along with the more formal motor examination in the awake, cooperative patient.

In addition to assessing the patient's neurologic function, it is imperative to closely monitor the vital signs. Hypotension in the presence of tachycardia most frequently indicates hypovolemia, though this picture can also be due to a high to mid thoracic spinal cord injury. Hypotension with a normal or low pulse can indicate a cervical injury or primary cardiac pathology such as sick sinus syndrome or junctional rhythm. Hypertension and bradycardia (Cushing's reflex) in the comatose patient usually indicates the presence of intracranial hypertension. This can manifest in subtle ways. Even trends toward hypertension and bradycardia can be harbingers of intracranial hypertension. As such, the neurosurgeon must be alert to gradually increasing blood pressure with downwards drift in heart rate even if the patient remains nominally normotensive and tachycardiac.

B. Imaging Studies

This section will focus exclusively on the radiographic evaluation of craniocerebral trauma, as evaluation of spinal trauma is beyond the scope of this chapter. Since the advent of computed tomography (CT) in the mid 1970s, the radiographic evaluation of craniocerebral trauma has changed dramatically. No longer are plain skull films, pneumoencephalography, or cerebral angiography mainstays of trauma evaluation. Head CT has for all practical purposes supplanted them. It is fast, easy, readily available in any trauma center, and exceedingly sensitive to intracranial blood or air and bony (skull) injury. Most modern CT scanners can obtain a complete head CT with 5-mm-thick sections in less than 2 minutes, and the images are of excellent quality and resolution.

Cerebral angiography is still used occasionally if vascular injury is suspected. An example is the patients who present with massive epistaxis and have a head CT indicating a basilar skull fracture involving the carotid canal. This situation calls for emergent angiographic assessment of the petrous carotid with possible endovascular occlusion of the injured vessel.

If the patient is stable, magnetic resonance imaging (MRI) can be used to establish the severity of any intracranial pathologic process not clearly visualized on CT. This is often the case in the posterior fossa, where bone can cause significant artifact on CT images, potentially obscuring cerebellar or brain stem pathology. MRA (magnetic resonance angiography) is a viable alternative to conventional angiography in the hemodynamically and neurologically stable patient. The biggest disadvantages of MRI and MRA is that studies take considerably longer than CT scans and they cannot be performed in patient with implanted metallic objects such as cardiac pacers, some intracranial pressure monitors, and some older aneurysm clips.

Treatment

The heterogeneous and dynamic nature of craniocerebral trauma makes it impossible to address treatment options as a strict algorithm. However, we can address the two major issues that, if left untreated, can lead to severe disability or death—hemodynamic and neurologic instability.

A. Hemodynamic Instability

Signs of hemodynamic instability should be treated with rapid and aggressive volume resuscitation. Crystalloid solutions such as 0.9% ssodium chloride (NaCl) solution or lactated Ringer's solution are the fluid of choice. The author prefers the former to keep the patient mildly hypernatremic (serum sodium 146–148 mmoles/L). This both raises the seizure threshold and helps control intracranial hypertension. Packed red blood cells (O-negative or type-specific) and whole blood infusions should be given if the patient has suffered significant blood loss. At least four units of blood products should be ready and available for immediate use during the initial resuscitation period. Trauma patients also commonly develop coagulopathies such as diffuse intravascular coagulopathy, which must be treated aggressively with fresh frozen plasma. Pressor agents such as Neo-Synephrine, dopamine, or norepinephrine must be used judiciously and never before the patient's intravascular volume has been repleted.

In addition to hemodynamic support, the patient's airway ventilation and oxygenation must be rapidly assessed and secured. In some cases, this involves endotracheal intubation or, if necessary, placement of a transcutaneous tracheal airway (via cricothyrotomy or tracheotomy). In any case, the patient's cervical spine should not be widely manipulated in order to minimize risk of injury (or further injury) to the spinal cord. The term "in-line traction" is often used to describe the maneuver used to maintain cervical stability during intubation. This is somewhat of a misnomer, since the spine is rarely placed in traction per se. Essentially, all that is needed is to maintain normal cervical alignment during intubation.

B. Neurologic Instability

Neurologic instability is almost always the result of intracranial hypertension, and in the acute setting is most likely due to an intracranial mass lesion. Seizures, drugs, and systemic hypotension can also present as neurologic instability and must be considered in the differential diagnosis.

1. Seizures—Patients with craniocerebral trauma are at risk for developing seizures. Some patients present actively seizing and should be treated with anticonvulsant medications—phenytoin (or fosphenytoin) 15–20 mg/kg intravenous (IV) load, followed by a maintenance dose of 300–400 mg/d in adults for 7 days. The advantage of fosphenytoin is that it can be infused more quickly than phenytoin without the risk of inducing hypotension—it is, however, considerably more expensive. Status epilepticus should be treated with benzodiazepines such as Ativan or Valium, though, occasionally, barbiturates or even general anesthesia are needed to control the seizures. Patients with intracranial pathology such as intraparenchymal contusions, subdural hematomas, or large epidural hematomas should also be given anticonvulsants, as they are at risk for developing posttraumatic seizures. In the absence of seizures, anticonvulsants can be discontinued at 7 days. This approach decreases the incidence of early posttraumatic seizures yet minimizes the patient's exposure to anticonvulsants. If the patient develops seizures after anticonvulsants are stopped, these should be reinstituted for at least 6 months. Patients who are chronic alcoholics are also at risk for developing alcohol-withdrawal seizures and should be treated primarily with benzodiazepines such as chlordiazepoxide (if taking oral medications) or diazepam (if nothing by mouth) until they have completed their withdrawal—usually in 5–7 days.

2. Intracranial hypertension—Normal intracranial contents include brain parenchyma, cerebrospinal fluid (CSF), and intracranial blood. Since intracranial volume is fixed, volume changes in of any of the three components affect intracranial pressure (ICP). The pressure-volume curve described by Langfitt and coworkers demonstrates a curvilinear relationship between intracranial volume and changes in ICP. As intracranial volume increases, so does intracranial pressure. Initially, the rise in ICP is barely noticeable and the slope of the curve approximates zero. As intracranial volume accumulates, the curve becomes increasingly steeper, eventually approaching the vertical. Thus, ICP varies exponentially with intracranial CSF, brain, or blood volume. The treatment of intracranial hypertension essentially relies on this relationship and aims at lowering intracranial CSF, brain, and blood volume. It follows that ICP management mandates the use of intracranial pressure monitors.

Two basic types of ICP monitors are currently available: **drainage** and **nondrainage types**. The former can be placed in the ventricle, subarachnoid, or subdural space. The latter is usually placed within the brain parenchyma, though it can be placed in virtually any intracranial compartment. Because of its potential therapeutic role, the external ventricular drain is the ICP monitor of choice at our institution. Not only does it provide information on ICP, it also allows the physician to drain ventricular CSF, thus lowering ICP. If the ventricular catheter cannot be placed, then a nondraining ICP monitor is used. We use fiberoptic ICP monitors at our institution due to their ease of placement.

The major risks associated with these monitors are infection and hemorrhage. The infection rates for external ventricular drain versus fiberoptic catheters are 0–27% (average, 8%) and 0–1.7%, respectively. The risk of hemorrhage with either type is similar (0–1%). The incidence of malfunction, on the other hand, is considerably higher with fiberoptic technology. Malfunction or obstruction rates for intraventricular, subdural, and subarachnoid drains are 2.5%, 2.7%, and 16%, respectively. The risk of malfunction with the fiberoptic catheter, on the other hand, is 10–30%. In addition, the cost difference between fiberoptic and drainage catheters is enormous, with nondraining monitors costing an order of magnitude more than external ventricular drains. All things considered, the accuracy, reliability, therapeutic value, and cost make the external ventricular drain the most useful ICP monitor available.

Though the risk of placing either hydrostatic or fiberoptic monitors is small, it is clear that not all traumatic brain injury patients require invasive monitoring. Generally speaking, patients who have a GCS from 9 to 15 are at low risk for developing intracranial hypertension, while those with a GCS of 8 or less are at higher risk. Naryan has shown that patients with a GCS of 8 or less with abnormalities on head CT have a 53–63% chance of developing intracranial hypertension compared with a 13% risk in patients with a normal CT. Interestingly, patients with a normal CT but with at least two of the following clinical features—systolic blood pressure < 90 mm Hg, extensor or flexor posturing, or age over 40 years—run a risk of developing intracranial hypertension equal to that of patients with abnormal head CTs.

Treatment

Intracranial hypertension is treated by decreasing intracranial CSF, brain, or blood volume. Both surgical and nonsurgical approaches are available, though not all are useful in the acute setting.

A. Cerebrospinal Fluid Volume

Cerebrospinal fluid volume is generally lowered via use of a ventriculostomy. This can be done in one of two ways—either by keeping the drain constantly open or by keeping it to monitor, draining only if the ICP reaches a set threshold. For most trauma situations, the author finds it most useful to keep the drain to monitor with intermittent drainage, as this allows for close monitoring of ICP spikes that otherwise might not be captured by leaving the drain constantly open. When no amount of drainage controls ICP, other ICP-lowering modalities should be started. Medical management of CSF volume is impractical in the trauma setting, as medications such as steroids or acetazolamide are slow in acting and have significant side effects that make their use undesirable.

B. Brain Volume

The surgical approach to decreasing brain volume is crude and generally unsatisfactory, as it requires the performance of a lobectomy. This is sometimes necessary in order to buy some extra space into which the remaining brain can swell, but generally, lobectomies are bloody affairs to be avoided if possible. Medical management of brain volume is more satisfying as it essentially boils down to giving IV mannitol and keeping serum sodium (Na^+) at or slightly above the high end of normal. Mannitol does not cross the blood-brain barrier and as such establishes an osmotic gradient across the blood-brain barrier, drawing interstitial water out of the brain and into the vasculature. There are two practical limits to mannitol: hypotension and serum osmolality. Mannitol not only draws water across the blood-brain barrier, but it also is a powerful osmotic diuretic that can drop a patient's blood pressure. Hypotension, therefore, is a contraindication to mannitol infusion. The second limit is serum osmolality—as it increases, so does viscosity. At levels above 320 mosm/kg, its deleterious effects on blood viscosity supersede the benefits of giving mannitol to lower ICP.

Hypernatremia helps control cerebral edema by normalizing the Na^+ gradient across cellular membranes. As noted earlier, glutamate initiates a series of biochemical changes thought to be mediated through NMDA receptors. One of these changes involves intracellular Na^+ accumulation, which leads to cellular swelling. Increasing serum Na^+ presumably decreases cerebral (cytotoxic) edema by ameliorating intracellular water accumulation. The main issues of concern associated with hypernatremia are two—hyperchloremia and diabetes insipidus. The former results from infusion of large volumes or 0.9% NaCl solution. High serum chloride facilitates renal excretion of serum bicarbonate, which then leads to a metabolic acidosis. This can be reversed somewhat by changing from sodium chloride to a sodium bicarbonate solution.

C. Blood Volume

Of the three components, intracranial blood volume is the most interesting and challenging to manage. The surgical approach is fairly straightforward—its aim is to evacuate intracranial blood clots. The exact approach depends on the type and location of the hematoma and will be described in detail below. Nonsurgical management focuses on the intravascular compartment. This is comprised of arterial, capillary, and venous volumes, which we will deal with individually.

1. Capillary volume—This compartment is passive and cannot be manipulated to any significant degree.

2. Venous volume—Though also passive, intracranial venous volume can be altered in a number of ways. The main goal is to lower ICP by decreasing venous volume. This can be accomplished simply by elevating the head of the bed. This facilitates intracranial venous drainage by increasing the pressure differential between intracranial venous pressure and central venous pressure. Another approach is simply to prevent increased intrathoracic pressure, as this would inhibit intracranial venous outflow and increase ICP. Causes of increased intrathoracic pressure include Valsalva maneuvers (ie, seizures, coughing, agitation, vomiting, straining) and primary pulmonary issues (ie, ARDS, pneumonia). By treating the underlying cause of each, we can sometimes control ICP. Sedatives, paralytics, anticonvulsants, and stool softeners all decrease Valsalva maneuvers; and optimizing ventilator parameters and treating pneumonias can also help control ICP.

3. Arterial volume—This compartment is essentially manipulated by taking advantage of cerebral autoregulatory mechanisms. These couple cerebral blood flow to cerebral metabolic demands. First, *metabolic autoregulation* alters local cerebral blood flow to match changes in local cerebral metabolism. Second, *pressure autoregulation* is designed to keep a constant cerebral blood flow over a wide range of blood pressures. Third, *osmotic autoregulation* keeps blood flow constant with changes in blood viscosity—all other things being equal. They all essentially work through tissue pH as a means of detecting ischemia. As tissue pH drops, autoregulatory mechanisms see this as the tissue becoming ischemic and respond by vasodilating upstream arterioles in order to increase local blood flow. Though vasodilatation increases local tissue perfusion, it also increases arterial blood volume—which increases ICP. Conversely, increasing tissue pH leads to vasoconstriction and, consequently, lowers ICP.

The most common way of inducing cerebral vasoconstriction is to decrease serum PCO_2 though mechanical hyperventilation. Serum PCO_2 and pH are closely interrelated—decreasing PCO_2 increases serum pH—and by hyperventilating, we essentially fool the cerebral vasculature into believing that the local cerebral blood flow is too high, thus causing vasoconstriction and decreased ICP. It is easy to see that this approach has the theoretical disadvantage that it can actually cause cerebral ischemia—a notion supported by data suggesting that hyperventilation below a P_{CO_2} of 30 leads to worse neurologic outcome.

As long as autoregulation remains intact, we can also decrease ICP through induced systemic hypertension. This maneuver transiently increases cerebral blood flow and causes the brain to respond by inducing cerebral vasoconstriction. This then leads to a lowering of ICP. Finally, we can decrease cerebral metabolism through medications such as barbiturates and propofol. As the cerebral metabolic rate falls, so does metabolic demand. In response, the cerebral vasculature naturally constricts, thus lowering ICP. The biggest problem with the last approach is that both barbiturates and, to a lesser degree, propofol can lower blood pressure and decrease cardiac function. Therefore, these medications need to be used with caution.

Surgical Treatment

The surgical treatment of trauma is fairly straightforward—the most difficult aspect, really, is not technical, but knowing when to operate and when not to. The actual surgical approach depends on the location and effects of the pathology. As such we will discuss the treatment of epidural hematomas, subdural hematomas, intraparenchymal contusions, open skull fractures, and scalp lacerations separately. All trauma patients get a complete head shave at our institution prior to incision and if time permits (and skull integrity permits) are put in three-point fixation.

A. Epidural Hematoma

Epidural hematomas almost always underlie a skull fracture. The most common location is the temporal fossa, since the temporal squamosa is the thinnest part of the cranial vault and the most likely to fracture and can easily lacerate the underlying middle meningeal artery. Other less common locations include the frontal and parietal convexity as well as the occipital and infratentorial compartments. Occasionally, a skull fracture will cross a venous sinus—the superior sagittal sinus and transverse sinuses being the most susceptible—causing the formation of a venous epidural hematoma.

The general approach is to make a curvilinear scalp incision to expose the entire skull overlying the hematoma (or as much as possible). Usually, one encounters a skull fracture on turning the skin flap. If the temporalis muscle is overlying the site, this should also be reflected inferiorly, leaving a thin rim of temporalis fascia attached to the superior temporal line (if possible) to which the muscle can be attached at the end of surgery. Once the bone is exposed, a single burr hole is made with a cutting burr somewhere near the edge of the underlying hematoma. The cranial flap can then be turned using the drill's footplate attachment. The hematoma is then evacuated, any dural bleeding stopped, and the dura secured to the craniotomy edge using 4-0 braided nylon sutures. The authors usually make a small dural incision to inspect the subdural space to rule out the presence of a coincident subdural hematoma. Once hemostasis is ensured, the bone flap is reattached using three "dog-bone" titanium plates at the edge of the craniectomy. The musculocutaneous flap is then closed using 2-0 Vicryl sutures for the galeal layer and staples for the skin. An ICP monitor is frequently placed at this time, prior to transport to the ICU.

A special note about venous epidural hematoma should be offered: These injuries can cause massive exsanguination in a very short period of time. What makes them so difficult is the state of the underlying venous dural sinus. Exposing the sinus is very difficult as this is usually criss-crossed by multiple comminuted scull fractures that make localization of the dural sinus tear difficult. Massive blood loss occurring at the time of opening makes visibility even more difficult. The key is to run the craniotomy parallel to and just lateral to the sinus (and, if possible, both sides) and place multiple dural tack-up stitches along its edge. Trying to expose the entire sinus is usually futile and fatal.

B. Subdural Hematoma

The approach to subdural hematoma is really no different than that for epidural hematoma except that the craniotomy is usually much larger and the dura is opened. The scalp incision is usually a very large curvilinear incision beginning at the hairline in the midline and continuing along the midline to approximately lambda. From here, the incision continues parallel to the lambdoid suture to the level of the asterion and then continues anteriorly just above the ear and curves anterior to the ear to end 1 cm inferior to the root of the zygoma. The temporalis muscle is removed as above, but no time is wasted in preserving the fascial attachment to the superior temporal line. This distinction is in contrast to the approach to epidural hematoma since the author often does not replace the bone flap following the evacuation of the hematoma because the brain is much more likely to swell significantly, causing ICP management problems. In any case, the skull is removed as described above but hugging the periphery of the skin incision and extending the craniotomy down to the frontal floor and pole and the temporal floor and pterion. Though this seems like a lot of surgery, it rarely takes more than 5 minutes to complete the craniotomy from the time of first skin incision. Once the skull is off, the dura is rapidly and widely opened using tenotomy scissors. At this point, the hematoma is evacuated.

Subdural hematomas result from tearing of cortical draining veins. These typically drain into six areas—the superior sagittal sinus at (1) the frontal pole, (2) along the frontoparietal junction and (3) the occipital pole, (4) the sphenoparietal sinus at the temporal pole, (5) the transverse sigmoid junction, and (6) along the superior petrosal sinus. These areas should be inspected to ensure that any active bleeding has stopped. Once hemostasis is ensured, a ventriculostomy is passed through the exposed frontal lobe into the lateral ventricle. A subdural drain is placed and both catheters are tunneled through the skin outside the musculocutaneous flap. The brain is then covered with Gelfoam and the skin flap closed with 2-0 Vicryl and staples. If the bone is replaced, it is done so as described above.

C. Intraparenchymal Contusion

The approach to intraparenchymal contusion depends on the presence of an overlying subdural hematoma and the degree of cerebral swelling. In the absence of subdural hematoma and significant global cerebral swelling, an approach akin to that of epidural hematoma is used. If not, the subdural hematoma approach is used. Once the brain is exposed, a small cortical incision is made where the contusion is closest to the surface of the brain—avoiding eloquent areas such as the primary motor cortex. Once the contusion is encountered, it usually delivers itself with minimal effort. Hemostasis is ensured and the wound closed as above.

D. Open Skull Fractures and Scalp Lacerations

These can be discussed together as their surgical approach is similar. The main surgical objective is to clean the area to minimize the risk of infection and optimize wound closure. In the case of skull fractures, attention must be paid to the possibility of underlying dural lacerations or hematomas. If either is present, a more extensive exploration may be necessary. Much emphasis has been placed on the need for meticulous dural repair. In the author's opinion, this is not necessary as long as the area has been cleaned and debrided well. Experience from treatment of penetrating injuries has shown that even these do not require aggressive surgical debridement and dural repair. Scalp wounds require mainly that devitalized tissue be removed, wound edges cleaned, and the galea be closed as completely as possible.

Outcome

The subject of outcome is a difficult one to discuss given the constraints of this chapter. However, a brief description of outcome measures and predictors is warranted.

There are many outcome scales used for the long-term assessment of traumatic brain injury. Some measure cognitive function, others physical disability, still others emotional, neuropsychological, psychosocial, or behavioral function. There are no outcome scales that fully cover the spectrum of neurologic dysfunction that follows traumatic brain injury.

Some of the more common are the Galveston Orientation and Amnesia Test (GOAT), which assesses orientation and degree of amnesia; the Paced Auditory Serial Addition Test (PASAT), which assesses attention; and the Trail Making Test B for assessing mental processing. Three others are the Disability Rating Scale, the Rancho Los Amigos Cognitive Functioning Scale, and the Glasgow Outcome Scale (GOS)—all of which assess the patient's disability and handicap. To some degree, the choice of test depends on the patient's disability. Moderately and severely injured patients are most often assessed with the Glasgow Outcome Score—usually administered at 3, 6, and 12 months after injury. This scale places patients into one of five categories: Death, Persistent Vegetative State, Severe Disability (conscious but disabled), Moderate Disability (disabled but independent), and Good Recovery.

As is true of any functional scoring system, those that are most comprehensive are the most difficult to use and those that are the easiest to administer are the least comprehensive. For example, the Halstead-Reitan Neuropsychological Battery (a common standardized neuropsychological battery) consists of 12 individual tests and can take up to 9 hours to administer. Similarly, the Luria-Nebraska Neuropsychological Battery consists of 248 individual items that can take up to 6 hours to administer. The Glasgow Outcome Score, on the other hand, is reliable, is easily used, and takes minutes to score, but is relatively insensitive to neurocognitive and behavioral deficits.

The outcome following traumatic brain injury primarily depends on the initial severity of injury and correlates fairly well with the postresuscitation Glasgow Coma Score. Other factors that influence outcome are patient age and presence of physiologic alterations that can cause secondary brain injury.

A. Outcome Following Mild Traumatic Brain Injury

Patients who present with a Glasgow Coma Score between 13 and 15 generally do well in the long run. The most significant sequelae are designated postconcussive symptoms and include headache, fatigue, dizziness, nausea, blurred vision, diplopia, memory difficulties, tinnitus, irritability, and difficulty concentrating (among others). Approximately 50% of patients complain of at least one of these 6 weeks after injury, while 14% still complain of symptoms at 1 year. Generally speaking, persistent symptoms are less severe and less frequent with time. The presence of more symptoms at 1 year compared to 6 weeks is associated with a higher incidence of pending litigation.

B. Outcome Following Moderate Traumatic Brain Injury

Of patients with a Glasgow Coma Score of 9–12, only 60% make a good recovery, while 26% remain moderately disabled, 7% severely disabled, and 7% are either vegetative or dead. Factors that influence outcome within this group are Glasgow Coma Score, patient age greater than 40, abnormality on admission CT scan, and progressive changes on CT scan.

C. Outcome Following Severe Traumatic Brain Injury

Outcome following severe injury is particularly difficult to predict—particularly early within the patient's hospital course. Patients in this group are often hemodynamically and neurologically unstable and can suffer significant secondary injury. Factors contributing to bad outcome are many, but as is true of moderate injury, postresuscitation Glasgow Coma Score (particularly motor score) and age are the most significant. Other significant predictive factors presenting in the acute postinjury period include pupillary response, pupillary size, midline shift, and intracranial pressure. Some data have shown that early, aggressive intensive care management with focus on hemodynamic and intracranial pressure monitoring, control of ventilation and oxygenation, and prevention of causes of secondary injury has some effect on the Glasgow Outcome Score following severe traumatic brain injury.

Summary

Traumatic brain injuries are a heterogeneous group of injuries that require early, aggressive treatment, intensive and constant hemodynamic and intracranial monitoring, and frequent and critical reassessment of all physiologic and clinical parameters. As we learn more about the physiology of the disease itself, monitoring parameters and treatment modalities are bound to change. What is dogma today will be anathema tomorrow. As long as we keep this in mind and are willing to change our preconceptions, we are in a great position to advance the treatment of traumatic brain injury.

Alberico AM et al: Outcome after severe head injury. Relationship to mass lesions, diffuse injury, and ICP course in pediatric and adult patients. J Neurosurg 1987;67:648.

Annegers JF et al: Seizures after head trauma: a population study. Neurology 1980;30(7 Pt 1):683.

Artru F et al: Monitoring of intracranial pressure with intraparenchymal fiberoptic transducer. Technical aspects and clinical reliability. Ann Fr Anesth Reanim 1992;11:424.

Aucoin PJ et al: Intracranial pressure monitors. Epidemiologic study of risk factors and infections. Am J Med 1986;80:369.

Becker DP et al: The outcome from severe head injury with early diagnosis and intensive management. J Neurosurg 1977;47:491.

Bobo H et al: Delayed intracerebral hematoma at the site of a subarachnoid bolt pressure monitor. Case report. J Neurosurg 1986;64:673.

Bowers SA, Marshall LF: Outcome in 200 consecutive cases of severe head injury treated in San Diego County: a prospective analysis. Neurosurgery 1980;6:237.

Brandvold B et al: Penetrating craniocerebral injuries in the Israeli involvement in the Lebanese conflict, 1982–1985. Analysis of a less aggressive surgical approach. J Neurosurg 1990;72:15.

Bruce DA et al: Outcome following severe head injuries in children. J Neurosurg 1978;48:679.

Choi SC et al: Prediction tree for severely head-injured patients. J Neurosurg 1991;75:251.

Clark WC et al: Complications of intracranial pressure monitoring in trauma patients. Neurosurgery 1989;25:20.

Collins JG: Types of injuries by selected characteristics. Vital Health Stat 10 1990;(175):1.

Dikmen S, McLean A, Temkin N: Neuropsychological and psychosocial consequences of minor head injury. J Neurol Neurosurg Psychiatry 1986;49:1227.

Fife D: Head injury with and without hospital admission: comparisons of incidence and short-term disability. Am J Public Health 1987;77:810.

Fife D et al: Incidence and outcome of hospital-treated head injury in Rhode Island. Am J Public Health 1986;76:773.

Foy PM et al: Do prophylactic anticonvulsant drugs alter the pattern of seizures after craniotomy? J Neurol Neurosurg Psychiatry 1992;55:753.

Friedman WA, Vries JK: Percutaneous tunnel ventriculostomy. Summary of 100 procedures. J Neurosurg 1980;53:662.

Gambardella G, d'Avella D, Tomasello F: Monitoring of brain tissue pressure with a fiberoptic device. Neurosurgery 1992;31:918; discussion 921.

Gronwall DM: Paced auditory serial-addition task: a measure of recovery from concussion. Percept Mot Skills 1977;44:367.

Ivan LP, Choo SH, Ventureyra EC: Intracranial pressure monitoring with the fiberoptic transducer in children. Childs Brain 1980;7:303.

Jagger J et al: Epidemiologic features of head injury in a predominantly rural population. J Trauma 1984;24:40.

Jennett B, Bond M: Assessment of outcome after severe brain damage. Lancet 1975;1:480.

Jennett B et al: Prognosis of patients with severe head injury. Neurosurgery 1979;4:283.

Kanter RK et al: Infectious complications and duration of intracranial pressure monitoring. Crit Care Med 1985;13:837.

Klauber MR et al: Prospective study of patients hospitalized with head injury in San Diego County, 1978. Neurosurgery 1981;9:236.

Kraus JF et al: The incidence of acute brain injury and serious impairment in a defined population. Am J Epidemiol 1984;119:186.

Langfitt TW, Weinstein JD, Kassell NF: Cerebral vasomotor paralysis as a cause of brain swelling. Trans Am Neurol Assoc 1964;89:214.

Levin AB: The use of a fiberoptic intracranial pressure transducer in the treatment of head injuries. J Trauma 1977;17:767.

Levin HS, O'Donnell VM, Grossman R.G: The Galveston Orientation and Amnesia Test. A practical scale to assess cognition after head injury. J Nerv Ment Dis 1979;167:675.

Levin HS et al: Neurobehavioral outcome following minor head injury: a three-center study. J Neurosurg 1987;66:234.

MacKenzie EJ, Edelstein SL, Flynn JP: Hospitalized head-injured patients in Maryland: incidence and severity of injuries. Md Med J 1989;38:725.

Miller JD et al: Further experience in the management of severe head injury. J Neurosurg 1981;54:289.

Muizelaar JP et al: Cerebral blood flow and metabolism in severely head-injured children. Part 1: Relationship with GCS score, outcome, ICP, and PVI. J Neurosurg 1989;71:63.

Narayan RK et al: Intracranial pressure: to monitor or not to monitor? A review of our experience with severe head injury. J Neurosurg 1982;56:650.

North B, Reilly P: Comparison among three methods of intracranial pressure recording. Neurosurgery 1986;18:730.

North JB et al: Phenytoin and postoperative epilepsy. A double-blind study. J Neurosurg 1983;58:672.

Ostrup RC et al: Continuous monitoring of intracranial pressure with a miniaturized fiberoptic device. J Neurosurg 1987;67:206.

Pazzaglia P et al: Clinical course and prognosis of acute post-traumatic coma. J Neurol Neurosurg Psychiatry 1975;38:149.

Rappaport M et al: Disability rating scale for severe head trauma: coma to community. Arch Phys Med Rehabil 1982;63:118.

Rutherford WH: Sequelae of concussion caused by minor head injuries. Lancet 1977;1:1.

Rutherford WH, Merrett JD, McDonald JR: Symptoms at one year following concussion from minor head injuries. Injury 1979;10:225.

Smith RW, Alksne JF: Infections complicating the use of external ventriculostomy. J Neurosurg 1976;44:567.

Sundbarg G, Nordstrom CH, Soderstrom S: Complications due to prolonged ventricular fluid pressure recording. Br J Neurosurg 1988;2:485.

Teasdale G, Jennett B: Assessment and prognosis of coma after head injury. Acta Neurochir 1976;34:45.

Whitman S, Coonley-Hoganson R, Desai BT: Comparative head trauma experiences in two socioeconomically different Chicago-area communities: a population study. Am J Epidemiol 1984;119:570.

Winfield JA et al: Duration of intracranial pressure monitoring does not predict daily risk of infectious complications. Neurosurgery 1993;33:424; discussion 430.

Winn HR, Dacey RG, Jane JA: Intracranial subarachnoid pressure recording: experience with 650 patients. Surg Neurol 1977;8:41.

Wyler AR, Kelly WA: Use of antibiotics with external ventriculostomies. J Neurosurg 1972;37:185.

Yablon JS et al: Clinical experience with a fiberoptic intracranial pressure monitor. J Clin Monit 1993;9:171.

SPINAL CORD INJURY

Geoffrey T. Manley, MD, PhD, Guy Rosenthal, MD, Alexander M. Papanastasio, MD, & Larry H. Pitts, MD

ESSENTIALS OF DIAGNOSIS

- *Neck or back pain following injury.*
- *Numbness or tingling in the trunk or extremities.*
- *Weakness or paralysis.*
- *Loss of bowel or bladder function.*
- *Imaging studies.*

General Considerations

Spinal cord injury remains one of the most devastating of all survivable traumatic injuries. Each year, more than 11,000 new spinal cord injuries occur in the USA as a result of motor vehicle accidents, falls, sports injuries, assaults, and various other mechanisms. Today, more than 200,000 Americans are living with spinal cord injury. Most of the injured are between 16 and 30 years of age at the time of injury, and males are much more likely than females to be injured. While most victims are employed at the time of injury, only 30–40% will be able to return to work. From the time of injury to death, the average cost of care of one patient exceeds $500,000, and the annual cost for acute and chronic care of spinal cord-injured patients is estimated to be $4 billion.

In the past, management of acute spinal cord injury focused on conservative care. The finding that pharmacologic treatment with intravenous methylprednisolone resulted in modest improvements in the National Acute Spinal Cord Injury Studies (NASCIS-1, 2, and 3) has provided new hope that future pharmacologic therapies may further diminish neurologic deficits. Recently, significant advances have also been made in the safety and efficacy of surgical decompression, stabilization, and fixation of the spine, paving the way for potentially repairing the damage resulting from the spinal injury. It is likely that future treatments will combine pharmacologic and surgical approaches to improve the outcome of this devastating injury.

Pathogenesis

In general, injury to the spinal cord follows compression or severe angulation of the vertebral spine. In rare instances, severe hypotension will lead to cord infarction, or axial distraction of elements of the vertebral column will result in a stretch injury of the cord. Most cord injuries follow subluxation with or without rotation of adjacent vertebral bodies that compress the cord between dislocated bone. Less often, axial compression of the spine will crush or wedge a vertebral body, and either bone or intervertebral disk fragments can be extruded into the spinal canal and compress the spinal cord or the anterior spinal artery. Another injury, seen usually in older patients with degenerative arthritis and stenosis of the cervical spine, involves neck hyperextension with infolding of the ligamentum flavum located in the spinal canal posterior to the cord. The spinal cord is trapped between arthritic bony spurs anteriorly and the ligamentum flavum posteriorly, producing a characteristic injury known as the central cord syndrome.

Early after spinal cord injury, there is a temporary loss of function with little or no demonstrable pathologic change. However, the initial trauma initiates a cascade of injury mechanisms that includes accumulation of excitatory amino acids, neurotransmitters, vasoactive eicosanoids, oxygen free radicals, and by-products of lipid peroxidation. Activation of programmed cell death pathways occurs. Loss of the "blood-cord barrier" causes edema and increased tissue pressure that, along with cord hemorrhage, limit the blood supply, with the result that cell ischemia may further damage the cord. The distribution of cord edema, hemorrhage, and infarction dictates the neurologic symptoms and signs elicited at the time of evaluation.

Clinical Findings

A. Symptoms, Signs, and Syndromes

In complete spinal cord injuries, there is no voluntary nervous function below the injury site. There is an initial phase of spinal shock, a loss of *all reflexes* below the injured segment, including bulbocavernosus, cremasteric, anal contraction to perianal stimulation, and deep tendon reflexes. This phenomenon may be temporary because of ionic and blood flow changes at the injury site. In incomplete spinal cord injuries, some function is present below the injury site, accounting for a much more favorable overall prognosis. Cord function may improve rapidly as spinal shock clears, or function may improve slowly in the months or years after injury.

The sites of damage within the cord and nerve root will determine what function is lost and what remains:

1. Anterior cord syndrome—This disorder results from damage to spinothalamic tracts and corticospinal tracts with relatively intact dorsal columns and preservation of touch and position sense, often related to injury to the spinal artery.

2. Brown-Séquard's syndrome—A lesion involving the spinal cord extensively on one side of the midline results in ipsilateral motor weakness and loss of proprioception and contralateral loss of pain perception below the level of injury.

3. Central cord syndrome—Injury to the central portions of the cervical spinal cord often follows a brief concussive injury. Because distal leg and sacral motor and sensory fibers are located most peripherally in the cervical cord, the perianal sensation and some lower extremity movement and sensation may be preserved.

4. Nerve root injury—This can occur at the level of vertebral body dislocation. Direct root compression may be relieved by reduction of the dislocation or by removal of fractured bone or disrupted disk.

5. Conus medullaris syndrome—Injuries at the thoracolumbar region may cause injury to nerve cells of the tip of the spinal cord, descending corticospinal fibers, and lumbosacral nerve roots with a mixed upper motor neuron and lower motor neuron dysfunction.

6. Cauda equina syndrome—This syndrome may arise from bony dislocation or disk extrusions in the lumbar or sacral regions, with compression of lumbosacral nerve roots below the conus medullaris. Bowel and bladder dysfunction as well as leg numbness and weakness occur commonly in this syndrome.

B. Physical Examination

Evaluation and initial treatment must be started at the scene of the injury. Early recognition of a spine or spinal cord injury will dictate preventive measures to preserve remaining neurologic function. Patients suspected to have spinal cord injuries must be immobilized with rigid cervical collars and backboards. At the receiving medical facility, care must be taken to treat hypoventilation, hypoxia, and hypercapnia (found with high cervical cord injuries). Hypotension accompanied by bradycardia may be present. This results from the loss of sympathetic innervation to the heart in injuries to the cervical cord and is known as **neurogenic shock**. The loss of sympathetic innervation may also lead to paralytic ileus with abdominal sequestration of fluid, bladder distention, and hypothermia.

Until x-rays show otherwise, the examiner should assume that any comatose patient has an unstable spine fracture. Concern about combined injury *must not delay resuscitation* of hypotension and hypoventilation. If the patient is awake, a history should be taken as soon as possible, including information about the specific nature of the injury and what pain or neurologic symptoms followed. Complaints of numbness and weakness should be noted carefully. Severe headache, particularly occipital pain, is common with odontoid fracture or hangman's fracture (bilateral fracture of the C2 pedicles). Palpation of the spine by sliding the hands under the patient with minimal spine movement can reveal focal bone tenderness or deformity. To assess weakness, the patient is asked to move hands and feet spontaneously and against resistance. Deep tendon reflexes must be evaluated in arms and legs; depression or absence of these reflexes will help localize the level of injury (Figure 37–13). Absence of abdominal reflex contraction to skin stimulation of the lower abdomen will localize a lesion in the T9–11 region. Absence of the cremasteric reflex (contraction of scrotal musculature in response to pinching of the medial thigh) indicates a lesion in the T12–L1 region of the cord. An intact bulbocavernosus reflex (anal sphincter contraction to penile or clitoral compression or downward pressure on the bladder trigone by a Foley catheter balloon when the catheter is gently pulled) indicates that sacral motor and sensory pathways are present; absence of the bulbocavernosus reflex is consistent with spinal shock or with sacral nerve root injury. Sensory testing of the extremities, anterior trunk, neck, and face should be done to define a sensory level below which sensation is absent or decreased. Sensation in the sacral region should always be noted as sparing at this level may provide evidence of an incomplete injury.

When the patient must be transferred to an x-ray table or bed, the transfer should be done with a fireman's carry, with at least three people *on each side* of the patient, with a fourth person, who directs the move, keeping the head in a *neutral position* by gentle axial traction (4–7 kg) applied with one hand on the chin and the other on the occiput.

C. Imaging Studies

Along with the physical examination, x-rays are essential for the evaluation of spine injuries. The lateral film is the most informative and should be examined for alignment of the anterior and posterior aspects of adjacent vertebral bodies and for angulation of the spinal canal at any level. Paravertebral or prevertebral soft tissue swelling usually indicates hemorrhage into these areas from fractures or ligamentous disruption. Anterioposterior spine films of the thoracic region and other levels permit assessment of lateral displacement of the vertebral bodies or widening or disruption of the pedicles. An odontoid view should be included in the evaluation of a patient suspected of having a cervical injury. Oblique views in the cervical and lumbar regions will demonstrate facet fractures or dislocations. Frontal and lateral tomography can further identify bony abnormalities, but this procedure requires movement of the patient onto special tables for study.

MRI gives excellent views of the spine, disks, and spinal cord and is the diagnostic procedure of choice in patients with spinal cord injuries. Increased T2 signal in the spinal cord indicates injury to the cord (Figure 37–14). CT scanning provides superior visualization of the bony spine and paraspinal soft tissues that often provides additional insights regarding the management of spinal injury. Instillation of intrathecal metrizamide can outline the spinal cord and demonstrate cord compression.

Differential Diagnosis

A detailed neurologic examination of motor and sensory function allows for the classification of a spinal cord injury and differentiation from other pathologic entities. Often, the principal diagnostic obstacle in the setting of trauma is the inability to assess a patient due to altered mental status from associated brain injury or intoxication. Other complicating factors in the differential diagnosis include peripheral nerve injuries secondary to fractures of the extremities. Here again, a detailed neurologic examination and an understanding of the anatomy of the peripheral nervous system is essential for making the correct diagnosis. The possibility of factitious symptoms should also be considered, especially when there is a question of psychiatric illness or secondary gain. This diagnosis can be addressed by detailed serial neurologic examinations. The potential for other related traumatic injuries must be considered, as nearly 60% of patients with spinal cord injury have other organ system injuries and 10% have additional spinal fractures.

Treatment

Injuries of bony and neural elements of the spine often coexist, and the treatment of both should be coordinated to ensure the best possible outcome. Anatomical transection of the spinal cord almost never occurs in spinal cord injury in humans. Thus, strict adherence to the following principles is imperative to protect surviving spinal tissue: First, the injury must be recognized. Second, care must be exercised to prevent further damage ("secondary" injury) and to detect deteriorating neurologic function so that corrective measures can be taken. Third, the patient must be maintained in optimal condition to allow the greatest possible nervous system repair and recovery. Fourth, evaluation and rehabilitation of the patient must be actively pursued to maximize the function of surviving but dysfunctional nervous tissue. These principles must be followed in order to diminish the economic, social, and emotional cost of spinal cord injury.

Emergency resuscitation of the spinal cord-injured patient parallels that of any major trauma, with the modification that alignment of the spine must be

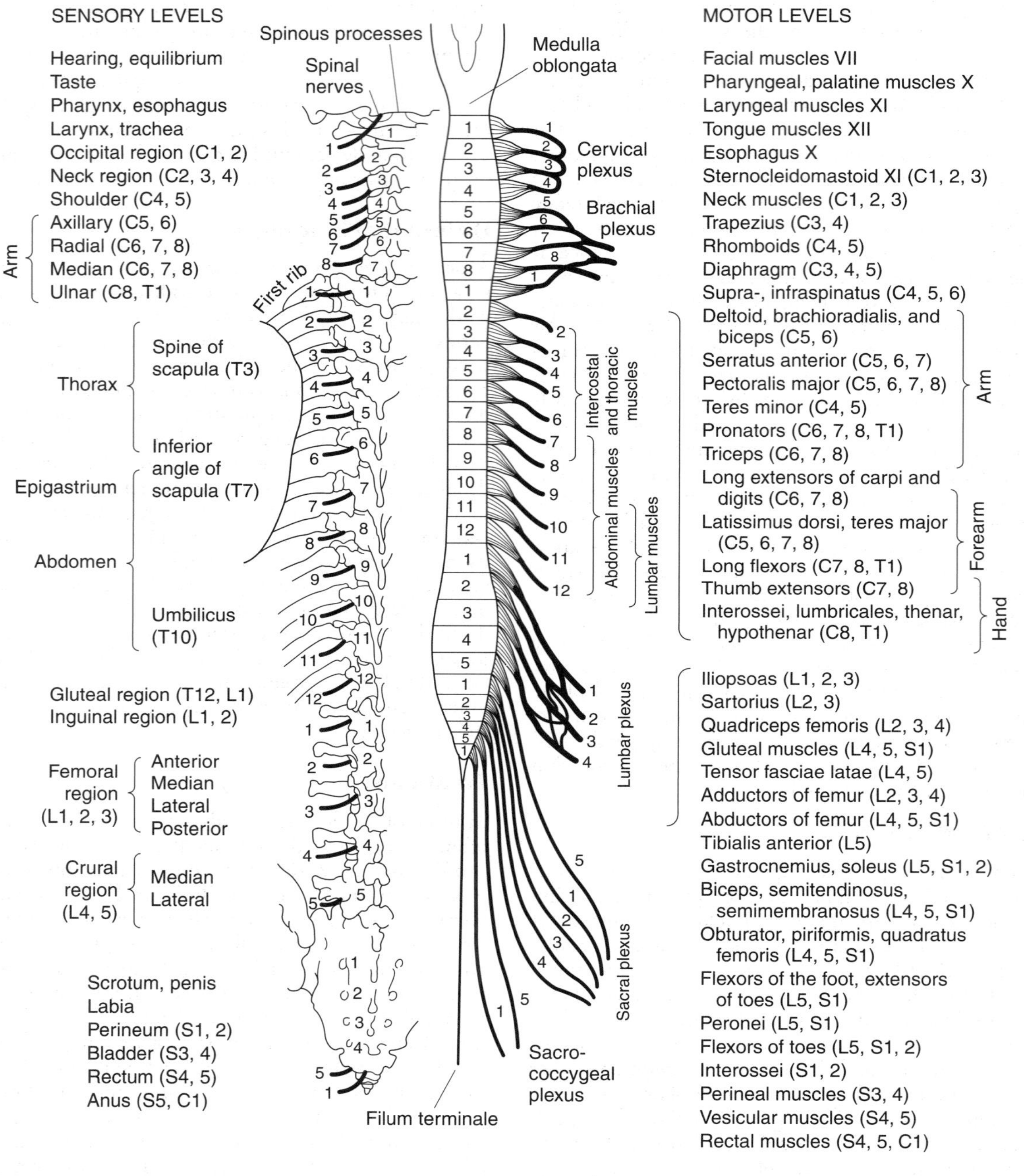

Figure 37–13. Motor and sensory levels of the spinal cord. (Reproduced, with permission, from Waxman SG: Correlative Neuroanatomy, 24th ed. originally published by Appleton & Lange. Copyright © 2000 by McGraw-Hill Companies, Inc.) (Reprinted with permission from Elsevier.)

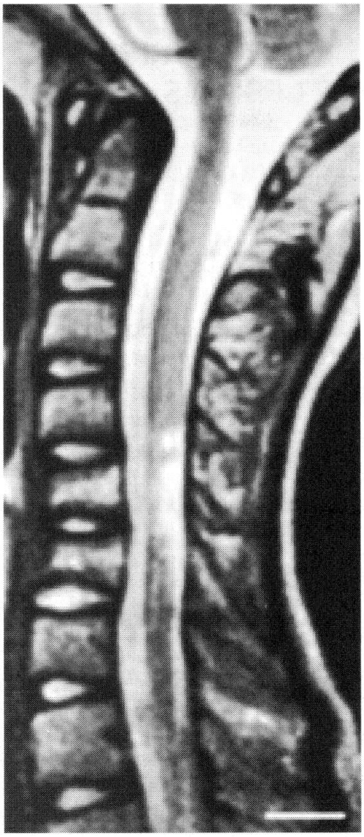

Figure 37–14. MRI demonstrates increased T2 signal in the cervical spinal cord at the C4 to C6 level, indicating injury at this location.

scrupulously maintained. Based on evidence from the NASCIS-2 and NASCIS-3 studies, adult patients with acute, nonpenetrating spinal cord injury can be treated with methylprednisolone immediately after recognition of spinal cord injury. Patients should be given 30 mg/kg of methylprednisolone intravenously within 8 hours, and preferably within 3 hours after injury, followed by a continuous infusion of 5.4 mg/kg/h. Those patients that received the initial bolus of methylprednisolone between 3 and 8 hours after injury should receive a 48-hour infusion instead of the standard 24-hour regimen used for patients treated within 3 hours.

Maintenance of adequate ventilation is critical. Patients with upper cervical cord injuries rely primarily on diaphragmatic activity for breathing. If paralytic ileus with abdominal distention occurs—or if the patient becomes fatigued—initially adequate ventilation may deteriorate. The patient will become hypoxic, requiring intubation and mechanical ventilation. Because of the loss of spinal cord sympathetic pathways, blood pressure may be low and may contribute to secondary injury. A mean arterial blood pressure between 85 and 90 mm Hg should be maintained for the first 7 days after spinal cord injury to improve perfusion of the injured cord. If urinary output is inadequate after catheterization, patients with mild hypotension will respond to low doses of pressors such as ephedrine, but these should be used only after unsuspected sources of hemorrhage in the chest or abdomen have been excluded.

Unstable cervical fractures should be managed initially with external immobilization. Skeletal fixation with Gardner-Wells tongs or halo traction can be achieved in most emergency rooms, or halter traction can be used temporarily. Thoracic and lumbar fractures are managed by keeping the patient in a neutral position, "logrolling" as necessary for skin care or pulmonary management. Oscillating beds also improve skin and pulmonary care.

Operative management of spinal cord injury must take into account two major considerations: **decompression** and **stability**. Realignment of the spinal canal can be achieved by proper application of traction, postural adjustment, and spine manipulation done by experienced physicians. Surgical exploration for bony realignment may be necessary in some patients. Surgery may also be indicated if bone or a foreign body is in the spinal canal or if the injury is followed by a progressive neurologic deficit that may be the result of a spinal epidural or subdural hematoma. Management of spine instability may include spinal fusion with metal plates, rods, and screws in combination with bone fusion.

Complications

The primary causes of death after spinal cord injury are potentially avoidable. Renal failure following repeated urinary tract infections is best prevented by carefully performed intermittent bladder catheterization, which often can be done by the patient. Decubitus ulcers form easily over bony prominences in anesthetic areas and can be prevented with intermittent turning of patients and rotary beds. The patient with a motor deficit following a spinal cord injury is at high risk for deep vein thrombosis. These patients require prophylaxis with low-molecular-weight heparin, pneumatic compression stockings, or both.

Prognosis

The neurologic examination and age of the patient are the most critical prognostic factors for short-term and long-term recovery. In the acute trauma setting, spinal cord injury mortality is 20%. Long-term, patients with complete motor and sensory loss at 72 hours are unlikely to recover function beyond one root level below the level of the injury, but up to 90% of patients with incomplete lesions can ambulate 1 year after injury. Recovery is more likely with limited lesions and in younger patients. Of the incomplete cord syndromes, the central cord syndrome and the Brown-Séquard's syndrome have relatively good prognoses, while patients with anterior cord syndrome improve less. Excluding the first 18 months, patients' 25-year survival rate is 70–80%. The most frequent causes of death include respiratory and cardiac disease, as well as a tenfold increased risk of suicide.

The team approach provided by centers that specialize in the spinal cord injury has been very successful and has shown that hospital stays can be shortened, complications can be reduced, and costs lowered. Rehabilitation also requires emotional support and patient education for the activities of daily living and job retraining. Exciting new insights into molecular mechanisms involved in spinal cord injury hold great promise for improved pharmacologic treatments. Emerging surgical procedures that incorporate advances in bioengineering and functional neurosurgery suggest that restorative neurosurgery will also have an increasing role in improving the functional abilities of patients with spinal cord injuries. It is likely that the evolving multidisciplinary approach will lead to improved treatment, recovery, and outcome for patients with spinal cord injuries.

Belanger E et al: The acute and chronic management of spinal cord injury. J Am Coll Surg 2000;190:603.

Bracken MB et al: Administration of methylprednisolone for 24 or 48 hours or tirilazad mesylate for 48 hours in the treatment of acute spinal cord injury. Results of the Third National Acute Spinal Cord Injury Randomized Controlled Trial. National Acute Spinal Cord Injury Study. JAMA 1997;277:1597.

Chen TY et al: The role of decompression for acute incomplete cervical spinal cord injury in cervical spondylosis. Spine 1998;23:2398.

DeVivo MJ: Causes and cost of spinal cord injury in the United States. Spinal Cord 1997;35:809.

Hadley MN et al: Guidelines for the management of acute cervical spine and spinal cord injuries. Clin Neurosurg 2002;49:407.

Kirshblum SC, O'Connor KC: Predicting neurologic recovery in traumatic cervical spinal cord injury. Arch Phys Med Rehabil 1998;79:1456.

Nesathurai S: Steroids and spinal cord injury: revisiting the NASCIS 2 and NASCIS 3 trials. J Trauma 1998;45:1088.

Vale FL et al: Combined medical and surgical treatment after acute spinal cord injury: results of a prospective pilot study to assess the merits of aggressive medical resuscitation and blood pressure management. J Neurosurgery 1997;87:239.

TRAUMATIC PERIPHERAL NERVE LESIONS

Nicholas M. Barbaro, MD

ESSENTIALS OF DIAGNOSIS

- *History of trauma (blunt, laceration, or surgical) followed by neurologic deficit.*
- *Neurologic findings may consist of partial or complete loss of function in one or more nerves.*
- *Electrodiagnostic studies are helpful only after 2–3 weeks.*

General Considerations

Peripheral nerves contain sensory or motor axons (or both), most of which are myelinated. Each axon is surrounded by fine collagen fibers, the endoneurium. Groups of axons called fasciculi are bound together by the perineurium, which consists of Schwann cells and fine collagen fibrils. The epineurium, made of thicker collagen fibrils, surrounds the fasciculi. This layer is thought to elaborate the fibroblastic reaction that is the primary cause of fibrosis subsequent to nerve injury.

The four major causes of nerve injury are laceration, contusion, stretch, and compression. Less commonly, nerves may be injured inadvertently when an injection is given. Irrespective of cause, localized injuries fall into one of three categories: neurotmesis, axonotmesis, and neurapraxia. In **neurotmesis** (eg, nerve laceration), axons and endoneurial tubes are disrupted. The proximal nerve end first swells and then, to a variable degree, undergoes retrograde degeneration. Subsequently, a neuroma develops, composed of connective tissue and a tangle of regenerating axons. The axons in the distal end die (wallerian degeneration), the endoneurial tubes shrink, collagen is deposited, and an end-bulb glioma forms. In **axonotmesis**, there is wallerian degeneration, but because the endoneurial tubes are retained, effective axonal regeneration can occur unless it is impeded by a connective tissue fibroblastic reaction (neuroma in continuity). In **neurapraxia**, there is temporary failure of conduction without loss of axonal continuity.

Clinical Findings

Following nerve injury, the history suggests the type of pathology while the neurologic examination localizes the lesion. A standard neuroanatomy textbook should be available for review of specific motor and sensory innervation and possible anatomic variations. A complete neurologic examination must be done, with emphasis on the nerves involved. Motor, sensory, and reflex deficits must be correlated to determine severity and distribution of involvement. The sensory findings are the least reliable because of overlap from adjacent uninjured nerves. Electromyography and nerve conduction studies establish a baseline for monitoring subsequent recovery but are not helpful until 2–3 weeks after an acute injury.

Differential Diagnosis

An accurate history and a meticulous examination are the key elements. The history will help differentiate traumatic neuropathies from those of infectious origin (diphtheria, mumps, influenza, malaria, syphilis, typhoid, typhus, dysentery, tuberculosis, gonorrhea) or toxic or metabolic origin (diabetes, rheumatic fever, gout, leukemia, vitamin deficiency, polyarteritis nodosa, drug reaction, heavy metals, carbon monoxide).

Complications

Pain resulting from nerve injury (neuropathic pain) can be caused by neuroma formation, by involvement of the sympathetic nervous system (complex regional pain syndrome; CRPS), or by alterations in peripheral and central processing of sensory information. Painful neuromas produce pain when pressure is applied locally. Pain associated with CRPS (formerly known as causalgia or sympathetically maintained pain) is burning and dysesthetic and is associated with hyperpathia and trophic skin and joint changes. Early aggressive treatment of CRPS is essential to avoid permanent disability. Local anesthetic blocks of the peripheral and sympathetic nerves may be helpful in diagnosing and treating these problems. Medical management includes tricyclic antidepressants, anticonvulsants (carbamazepine or gabapentin), mexiletine, or sympathetic blocking agents. Surgical treatment includes neurolysis, resection of the neuroma away from sites of mechanical trigger, sympathectomy, or electrical stimulation of the proximal nerve or the spinal cord.

Treatment & Prognosis

The choice of treatment depends on the nature of the nerve injury. Early exploration and repair should be used for clean lacerations. When associated injuries are present (major arterial laceration, shock) or when there is gross contamination, it is better to tag the nerve endings with nonabsorbable suture to prevent excessive retraction and to facilitate subsequent repair. Such injuries should be approached within 10 days if the patient's condition warrants. Patients with nerves injured by stretch or contusion should be followed for clinical signs of recovery. If no recovery is seen within 3 months, exploration is indicated. Intraoperative electrical studies help distinguish between axonotmetic injuries in the process of recovery (compound nerve action potential present) and those with no evidence of recovery. Recovering nerves should be left intact, but in those with no evidence of function, the damaged segment should be resected. Although this approach sometimes results in exploration when the nerves would have recovered spontaneously, initiation of early repair is important in nerve that will not recover. Because nerve regeneration is relatively slow (1 inch per month) and because intraneural fibrosis eventually prevents axonal growth (approximately 18 months), waiting too long may eliminate the chance for recovery.

The techniques of nerve anastomosis depend on whether the primary nerve endings are in close proximity; if so, epineurial repair should be performed with microscopic magnification and fine (8-0 or finer) suture. Nerve repair must be done without tension. If the gap between endings is too long for primary repair, nerve grafts (usually sural) should be used in an interfascicular repair.

Some lesions resulting from contusion or compression are improved by neurolysis. The same is true of some injection neuropathies (depending upon the substance injected).

Prompt institution of physical therapy for improvement of muscle function and maintenance of joint range of motion is indicated. The denervated portion of the limb is subject to muscle atrophy and fibrosis, joint stiffness, motor end-plate atrophy, and trophic skin changes. The longer the denervation persists, the less likely it is that a good functional result will ultimately be achieved.

Only careful grading of sensorimotor function following injury will allow accurate evaluation of recovery, especially after surgical repair. Intraoperative factors such as axial orientation of fasciculi, proper coaptation, suture material, hemostasis, and especially suture line tension determine the outcome. In axonotmetic and neurotmetic injuries, regeneration occurs at a rate of 1 inch per month. Thus, improvement may not be noted for many months, and the patient must be psychologically prepared. Recovery of function should proceed smoothly from proximal to distal; maximum recovery may take 1–2 years. Factors that adversely affect the return of function are the type of nerve injured (mixed), the age of the patient, proximal nerve injury, large nerve defect, and associated tissue injury.

Patients must understand that their role in treatment is an active one, and their motivation must be maintained. Early rehabilitation is important to maintain full joint range of motion while awaiting functional return. Later, physical therapy will help maximize the return of useful function. Neurologic recovery is often incomplete, and the use of tendon transfers may be helpful as a means of improving the functional outcome.

Carter GT et al: Electrodiagnostic evaluation of traumatic nerve injuries. Hand Clin 2000;16:1.

Noble J et al: Analysis of upper and lower extremity peripheral nerve injuries in a population of patients with multiple injuries. J Trauma 1998;45:116.

Penkert G et al: Diagnosis and surgery of brachial plexus injuries. J Reconstr Microsurg 1999;15:3.

Spinner RJ, Kline DG: Surgery for peripheral nerve and brachial plexus injuries or other nerve lesions. Muscle Nerve 2000;23:680.

BRAIN TUMORS

Michael W. McDermott, MD, Sandeep Kunwar, MD, & Mitchel S. Berger, MD

ESSENTIALS OF DIAGNOSIS

- *Headache.*
- *Seizures.*
- *Progressive neurologic deficit.*
- *Change in personality or behavior.*

General Considerations

Tumors of the central nervous system are considered either primary or metastatic (secondary). Among primary brain tumors a useful surgical classification is into intra-axial and extra-axial lesions. Intra-axial tumors are those that are within the brain parenchyma, and extra-axial ones are those arising outside the parenchyma, usually attached to leptomeninges or involving the skull or skull base. Primary malignant brain tumors are among the most difficult malignancies to eradicate with treatment. Even low-grade astrocytomas of the cerebral hemispheres or brain stem are generally considered to behave in a "malignant" manner because of their infiltrating and progressive nature and because they lead to death if not treated. There are a few well localized primary brain tumors, such as cerebellar astrocytomas, juvenile pilocytic astrocytomas, and gangliogliomas, and dysembryoplastic neuroepithelial (primitive neuroectodermal) tumors (PNETs), that can be removed surgically with long-term control rates without adjunctive therapy (Figures 37–15 and 37–16).

The intracranial compartment is a fixed space, and for that reason growing brain tumors produce nonspecific

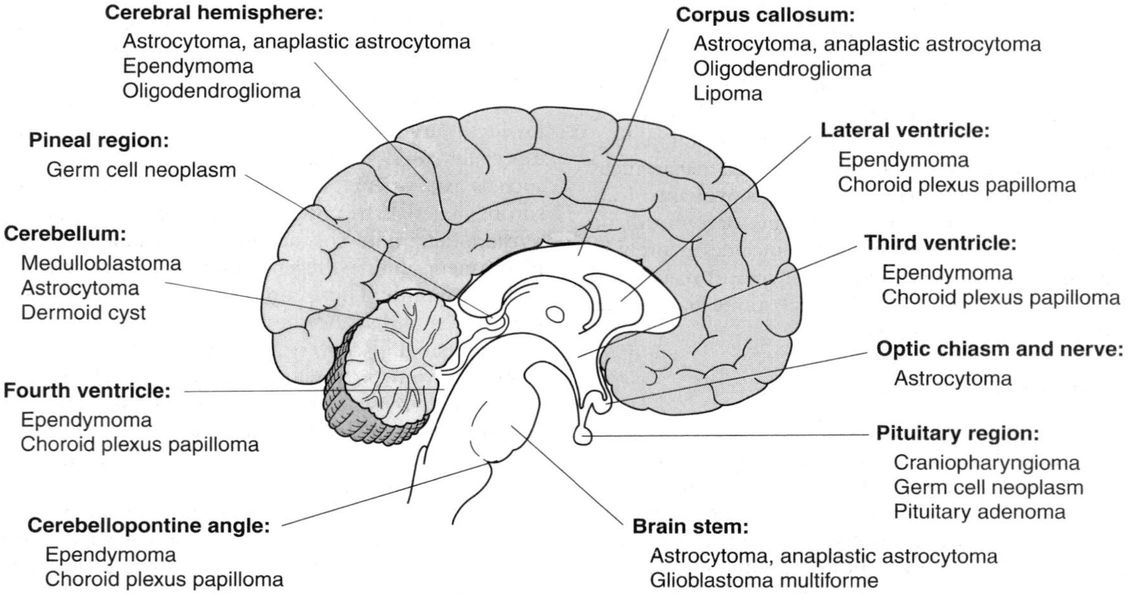

Figure 37–15. Distribution of intracranial tumors in children. (Reproduced, with permission, from Burger PC, Scheithauer BW, Vogel FS: Surgical Pathology of the Nervous System and Its Coverings, 3rd ed. Churchill Livingstone, 1990.)

symptoms as they increase the intracranial pressure. The most common symptom is generalized headache, usually worse in the morning and sometimes relieved by vomiting. Papilledema is a clinical sign that confirms the presence of long-standing increased intracranial pressure. Specific localizing signs are created by invasion or compression of functioning neural tissue such as the speech and language cortices, the motor or primary sensory cortices, or the visual cortex. Given that most primary brain tumors of the astrocytic series arise within the frontal lobe, it is not surprising that one of the most common presenting symptoms is change in personality or behavior. Irritation of cortical tissue or its deafferentation may produce focal or secondarily generalized seizures.

The most recent data from the Central Brain Tumor Registry of the United States indicates that the overall incidence of primary and central nervous system tumors is 12.7 per 100,000 person years. (See Tables 37–2, 37–3, and 37–4.) For the period of data collection between 1992 and 1997, among 38,848 tumors reported, 35.9% occurred in the supratentorial compartment, 6.5% primarily within the infratentorial compartment, and in 17.6% there was an overlap between the two. By histology, neuroepithelial tumors were the most common, accounting for 36% of all primary brain tumors, followed by meningiomas (26%), nerve sheath tumors (7%), and pituitary adenomas (6%). The mean age at diagnosis for all tumors in this study was 54 years. The incidence rates for most primary tumors were higher in males or similar to the rates in females with the exception of meningiomas, which was twice as common in women. Overall, the incidence for brain tumors was highest among persons aged 75–84 years. In children, brain tumors are the second most common cause of cancer-related deaths; in adolescents and young adults between the ages of 15 and 34, brain tumors are the third leading cause of cancer-related deaths. In the pediatric age group from birth to 19 years, astrocytomas, medulloblastomas, and ependymomas are the most common diagnoses.

In adults, it is generally considered that 70% of primary brain tumors arise in the supratentorial compartment, with the remainder in the infratentorial compartment. In children the distribution is reversed, with 70% of tumors within the posterior fossa. The Central Brain Tumor Registry data show that 61% of primary

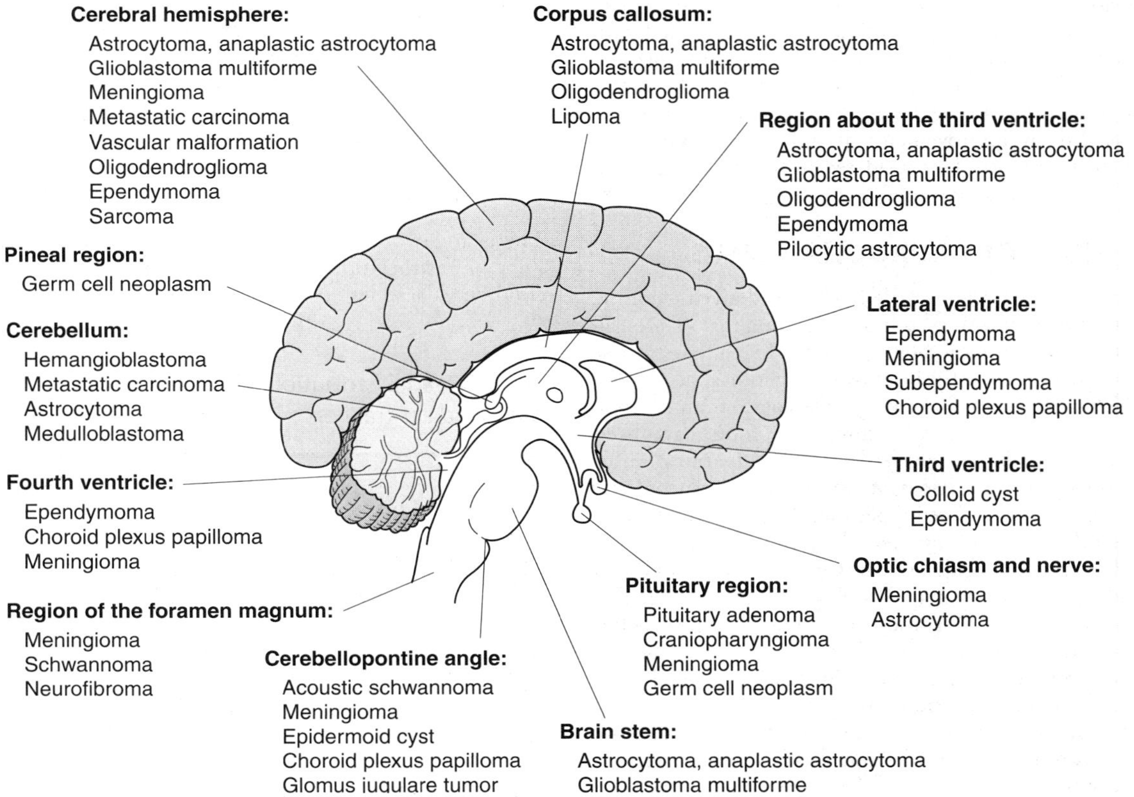

Figure 37–16. Distribution of intracranial tumors in adults. (Reproduced, with permission, from Burger PC, Scheithauer BW, Vogel FS: Surgical Pathology of the Nervous System and Its Coverings, 3rd ed. Churchill Livingstone, 1990.)

Table 37–2. Distribution of all primary brain and central nervous system tumors by site.[1]

Site	Percentage of Total[2]
Supratentorial	35.9%
Infratentorial	6.5%
Intraventricular	1.3%
Pituitary	7.2%
Pineal region	0.5%
Overlapping and not otherwise specified	17.6%
Other central nervous system tumors	31.0%

[1]Central Brain Tumor Registry of the United States, 1992–1997.
[2]Total number of cases = 38,848.

Table 37–3. Distribution of all primary brain and central nervous system tumors by histology.[1]

Histology	Percentage of Total[2]
Glioblastoma	23%
Astrocytomas	13%
Meningioma	26%
Schwannoma	7%
Pituitary adenoma	6%
All others[3]	25%

[1]Central Brain Tumor Registry of the United States, 1992–1997.
[2]Total number of cases = 38,848.
[3]Includes lymphoma, germ cell tumors, hemangioblastoma, craniopharyngioma, epidermoid and dermoid cysts, hemangioma, and chordoma.

tumors are located within the brain (intra-axial) and 31% within the leptomeninges (extra-axial).

In recent years, advances in molecular biology have identified specific oncogenes or, more commonly, loss of tumor suppressor genes that may be associated with development of a primary brain tumor. Advances in surgical instrumentation and technique and the use of surgical navigation systems for intracranial operations have led to improvements in safety and outcomes. These aspects will be considered further under the specific diagnostic groups.

TUMORS OF NEUROGLIAL CELLS

Neuroglial cell tumors arise from cells derived from the primitive neuroepithelium and account for 50% of all intracranial primary brain tumors. In the past these tumors were collectively known as gliomas, a category which now includes several histologic tumor types. Many classifications for neuroglial tumors have been proposed, and most are based on the identification of reasonably precise etiologic features linking neoplastic elements to normal cell types found both in the mature and in the developing central nervous system. In the widely used World Health Organization (WHO-2) grading system, the main histologic subtypes are graded from one to four. Astrocytomas and oligodendrogliomas—the most common gliomas—are widely distributed throughout the brain, brain stem, and spinal cord. Ependymomas arise from ependymal cells that line the ventricle walls and central canal, which is where they are most commonly located. Medulloblastomas (primitive neuroectodermal tumors of the cerebellum) presumably originate from fetal cells residing in the cerebellum and occur primarily in children. Gliomas represent a very complex set of tumors in classification as well as in treatment. The cardinal property of gliomas is their propensity to undergo anaplastic change to a more malignant lesion, ie, to increase in histologic grade over time. Most of the gliomas are known for their ability to infiltrate into normal tissue, and for that reason patients commonly present with seizures, focal neurologic deficits, or increased intercranial pressure.

1. Astrocytomas & Oligodendrogliomas

There are two categories of low-grade astrocytomas. Pilocytic astrocytomas are most commonly found in children. These lesions are most commonly found in

Table 37–4. Distribution of pediatric primary brain and central nervous system tumors.[1]

Histology	Percentage of Total[2]
Embryonal[3]	15.9%
Pilocytic astrocytoma	15.5%
Astrocytomas	21.7%
Ependymoma	6.3%
Malignant glioma not otherwise specified	8.5%
All others	32%

[1]Central Brain Tumor Registry of the United States, 1992–1997.
[2]Total number of cases = 38,848.
[3]Includes medulloblastoma.

the cerebellum and less commonly in the hypothalamus, then the optic nerve and chiasm, and at times in the brain stem and spinal cord. Pilocytic astrocytomas are well-circumscribed and often cystic neoplasms composed of varying compact and loose-textured astrocytes associated with Rosenthal fibers.

The second type of low-grade astrocytoma is the low-grade fibrillary astrocytoma, or WHO-2 astrocytoma. Fibrillary astrocytomas favor the cerebral hemispheres of young to middle-aged adults and the brain stems of children.

Among patients with low-grade astrocytomas, seizures are more common than functional deficits owing to the absence of cortical destruction, which is more commonly seen with higher-grade lesions. These slow-growing neoplasms occur predominantly in the third and fourth decades. Grade II astrocytomas over time can progress to grade III or grade IV tumors.

Anaplastic Astrocytomas

This group of fibrillary astrocytic tumors is intermediate in differentiation between the better-differentiated astrocytoma and the poorly differentiated glioblastoma. Anaplastic astrocytomas are considered WHO-2 grade III tumors and occur primarily within the cerebral hemispheres. They most frequently occur a decade later than the grade II astrocytomas, peaking in the fifth and sixth decades. These tumors can also appear in the pons, typically in children (diffuse pontine hypertrophy). Unlike differentiated astrocytomas, anaplastic astrocytomas tend to be more infiltrative and diffuse lesions. A particular variant results in gliomatosis cerebri, a condition in which the tumor infiltrates most of one or both hemispheres.

Glioblastoma Multiforme

The most common glioma, accounting for 23% of primary brain tumors, is biologically and histologically the most malignant of the fibrillary astrocytomas. Histologically, these tumors show pseudopalisading necrosis, endothelial proliferation, and multiple mitotic figures. Some tumors are so poorly differentiated that they provide no histologic evidence of an astrocytic precursor lesion, and most have histologic heterogeneity within different regions of the tumor. More recently, glioblastomas have been classified as primary or secondary glioblastomas. In general, glioblastomas that contain distinct large areas of differentiated astrocytic tumor or have been documented previously as low-grade lesions are classified as secondary glioblastomas and are due to malignant transformation of lower-grade lesions. Primary glioblastomas are believed to arise de novo as malignant tumors. Studies using biologic markers support the notion that primary and secondary glioblastomas are cytogenetically different. By the WHO-2 grading system this is a grade 4 tumor and is extremely infiltrative. Biopsies of adjacent normal tissue up to 2 cm beyond the radiographic boundaries of the tumor show evidence on neoplastic cells intermixed with normal parenchyma. Because of the rapid growth and the degree of adjacent cerebral edema, patients commonly present with symptoms of increased intracranial pressure or focal neurologic deficits.

Oligodendrogliomas

Oligodendrogliomas are infiltrative gliomas composed of oligodendrocytes, which occur primarily in the cerebral hemispheres, especially the frontal lobes. These tumors usually present in adulthood and are often associated with a long history of seizures—sometimes a decade or more. Many of these lesions have mineralization, which is visible on a CT scan. On histologic examination these tumors have perinuclear halos, giving them a "fried egg" appearance. Oligodendrogliomas vary in aggressiveness from low-grade (WHO-2 grade II) to anaplastic oligodendrogliomas (WHO-2 grade III). Tumors can also have a mixed component of oligodendroglial as well as astrocytic components, which are graded separately.

2. Ependymomas

Most ependymomas are slow-growing, well-circumscribed neoplasms arising throughout the neuraxis in intimate relationship with the ependyma or its remnants. Intracranial lesions most often occur in children and adolescents, though adults are also affected. The primary site of ependymomas is heavily age-dependent. The fourth ventricle is the most common site and accounts for up to 60% of these tumors. Among adults, the location in intracranial ependymomas appears to be evenly divided between infratentorial and supratentorial locations. In contrast, the vast majority of spinal ependymomas occur in adults and comprise the main glioma of the spinal cord and phylum terminale (over 60%). Although most ependymomas are slow-growing lesions, because of their location they can produce clinical and radiographic signs of increased intracranial pressure or obstruction of the cerebrospinal fluid pathways. The prognosis of these tumors is markedly improved if total resection can be accomplished. Tumors arising from the floor of the fourth ventricle (dorsal surface of the brain stem) constitute a poor operative risk for gross total resection, resulting in incomplete resections and an increased likelihood of recurrence. Because of the location of these tumors, they may descend along the cerebrospinal fluid pathways.

3. Medulloblastomas

Medulloblastoma is a small-cell neuroectodermal tumor of the cerebellum and is the most common brain tumor of childhood. Over 50% occur in the second half of the first decade, and one-third occur in adolescence and early adulthood. Symptoms may be a reflection of cerebellar dysfunction, increased intracranial pressure, or craniospinal dissemination. The genesis of medulloblastoma is controversial, but it is believed that these cells are bipotential (neuronal and glial) and may arise from immature cells residing in the external granular layer or cells in the posterior medullary velum. Histologically, these tumors are highly malignant, with populations of dense small cells lacking apparent stroma or distinctive architectural features. Medulloblastomas have a propensity to seed throughout the cerebrospinal fluid pathways. These tumors are highly radiosensitive and, depending on tumor stage, 10-year survival rates of 40–50% have been achieved by aggressive resection and radiotherapy.

Choroid Plexus Papilloma & Carcinoma

These tumors are papillary neoplasms derived from choroid plexus epithelium. Choroid plexus neoplasms in children usually arise within the lateral ventricles and most frequently the third ventricles. Plexus tumors in adults are nearly all papillomas, many of which arise within the fourth ventricle or its lateral recess. These tumors can cause hydrocephalus secondary either to obstruction of cerebrospinal fluid flow or to overproduction of cerebrospinal fluid. Malignant variants (choroid plexus carcinomas) occur and carry a very poor prognosis. Most carcinomas are frankly infiltrative and are likely to recur or result in craniospinal dissemination.

NON-GLIAL CELL TUMORS

These tumors arise from a variety of tissues, including the skull base, leptomeninges, pituitary gland, and pineal region. Nerve sheath tumors—most commonly schwannomas—are also included in this group. For the most part, these tumors are benign and produce symptoms by compression of brain rather than invasion as well as by elevation of intracranial pressure.

1. Meningiomas

Meningiomas account for 26% of all primary brain tumors and arise from arachnoid cap cells. At operation they are usually attached to the dura although they do not arise from it. Many are globular in shape, and 85% are histologically benign. They most commonly occur along the faux (falx, parasagittal), sphenoid wing, and convexity dura. In 10% of patients the tumors are multiple, and this may be associated with neurofibromatosis type 2. In children there is a tendency for meningiomas to be histologically and clinically more aggressive. Hyperostosis of bone may occur either in the skull base or in the convexity and usually relates to stimulation of bony activity by invading meningioma. A characteristic clinical picture is of a middle-aged woman with unilateral painless proptosis that usually is seen with a hyperostotic sphenoid wing meningioma.

Meningiomas are known to be induced by radiation therapy with latent intervals of 10–40 years between radiation exposure and tumor appearance. Radiation-induced meningiomas are commonly more atypical or aggressive on histology and have a more aggressive clinical behavior. A possible role of sex steroid hormones has been investigated in an attempt to explain the female preponderance of meningiomas, but no causal relationship has been established. Multiple meningiomas are the hallmark of neurofibromatosis type 2, which develops in response to loss of the tumor suppresser gene on chromosome 22. The most common karyotypic abnormality in meningiomas is monosomy of 22 or loss of the long arm of 22. Other allelic losses on chromosome arms 1-p, 6-q, 9-q, 10-q, 14-q, 17-p, and 18-q may well be important in development and progression of these tumors.

The World Health Organization has classified meningiomas on the basis of the likelihood of recurrence and grade. Brain invasion alone is no longer sufficient for the diagnosis of malignant meningioma (Table 37–5).

2. Nerve Sheath Neoplasms

These benign tumors originate from Schwann cells and have a predilection for the eighth, fifth, and tenth nerves. Clinically, the most common intracranial schwannoma is the vestibular schwannoma, or acoustic neuroma, which arises from the superior or inferior portion of the vestib-

Table 37–5. Classification of meningiomas.[1]

Grade I: Low risk of recurrence
Meningothelial
Fibrous
Transitional
Psammomatous
Angiomatous
Microcystic
Secretory
Lymphoplasmacyte-rich
Metaplastic
Grade II: Intermediate risk of recurrence
Atypical
Clear cell
Choroid
Grade III: High risk of recurrence
Rhabdoid
Papillary
Anaplastic

[1]World Health Organization, 2000.

ular nerve in the internal auditory canal. As the tumor enlarges, it expands the bony canal and extends into the cerebellopontine angle. Patients who present with unilateral hearing loss confirmed by audiogram more commonly are imaged with magnetic resonance studies, and the diagnosis of these tumors is being made earlier. The presence of bilateral vestibular schwannomas is diagnostic of neurofibromatosis type 2. All age groups are affected, but there is a peak incidence in the fourth to sixth decades. Pathologically, the tumors are composed of spindle-shaped neoplastic Schwann cells with alternating areas of compact stroma with loose, less cellular areas. Most schwannomas are sporadic tumors, and almost all have a mutation of a tumor suppresser *NF2* gene, which encodes for the protein merlin. By Western blotting or immunohistochemistry, almost all tumors appear to have loss of merlin expression. This may be an essential step in schwannoma tumorigenesis.

3. Cranial Meningiomas

These benign tumors of epithelial origin are found in the region of the sella or suprasellar cistern. They account for 1.2–4% of adult intracranial tumors and 6–10% of pediatric brain tumors. The sex incidence is equal. Cranial meningiomas are thought to originate from epithelial rests found within the infundibular stalk or pituitary. During the fourth week of gestation, Rathke's pouch forms as a diverticulum and migrates to meet the infundibulum, which is a downgrowth from the floor of the diencephalon. Two pathologic types are identified: the adamantinomatous craniopharyngioma and papillary craniopharyngioma. The tumors are confined to the sella in only 5% of cases, while the majority involve both the sella and the suprasellar regions. Clinically, patients most often present with visual pathway disturbances, followed in frequency by endocrinopathy or hydrocephalus. The tumors can be solid or cystic (or both). On CT imaging, the adamantinomatous form may show intratumoral calcification. In adult patients, this calcification can be the most prominent imaging characteristic of the tumor. Cystic portions of the tumor may displace the third ventricle and cause obstructive hydrocephalus. While the goal of treatment is complete surgical resection, tumor location around the vital structures makes this goal difficult to achieve.

4. Congenital Tumors

Epidermoid Tumors

Epidermoid tumors were formerly called "pearly tumors" because of the findings at surgery of a smooth, glistening mother-of-pearl appearance related to the accumulation of desquamated epithelium. Epidermoid cysts occur along the basal cisterns, most commonly in the suprasellar or parasellar regions as well as in the cerebellopontine angle. The capsule of these tumors is frequently adherent to adjacent cranial nerves and vascular structures. The aim of surgery is evacuation of the central portion of the cyst in order to eliminate surrounding mass effect. Epidermoid cysts in the sellar region usually present with visual or endocrine disturbances or hydrocephalus. Patients with these cysts have repeated attacks of aseptic meningitis, presumably related to leakage of cyst contents into the cerebrospinal fluid pathways. MRI studies are extremely useful, particularly in the noncontrast T1, proton density, and FLAIR sequences. As compared with arachnoid cysts, epidermoid tumors typically have increased signal intensity in the FLAIR images.

Dermoid Tumors

Dermoid tumors are less common than epidermoid cysts, but they generally grow more quickly and thus present at a younger age than epidermoids. While epidermoid cysts are generally found laterally in basal cistern compartments, dermoid cysts tend to be located in the midline. One-third occur in the region of the fourth ventricle. Obstruction of cerebrospinal fluid pathways and a presentation with hydrocephalus is more common. Dermoid tumors contain adnexal elements as hair, hair follicles, or sebaceous glands. They may be associated with a dermal sinus tract, which may present anywhere on the occipital scalp along the midline. Repeated bouts of bacterial meningitis associated with dermoid tumors should arouse suspicion of such a tract. On imaging studies there is a much higher incidence of calcification in dermoids than in epidermoid tumors. Treatment consists of excision.

Central Nervous System Germ Cell Tumors

This histologically heterogeneous group of tumors is derived from all three germ layers. They tend to occur in the midline, most commonly in the region of the third ventricle or the pineal gland. They constitute less than 1% of all primary intracranial neoplasms and only 3% of those encountered in childhood or adolescence. Their incidence is much higher in East Asian countries for some reason. Approximately 90% of patients with germ cell tumors are under age 20. Because of their location in the pineal or third ventricular regions, they obstruct cerebrospinal fluid pathways and cause hydrocephalus with intracranial hypertension. Positioned within the pineal region along the posterior of the midbrain, they can compress the tectal plate and cause characteristic paralysis of upward gaze and impaired conversions with absence of pupillary light reflex (Parinaud's syndrome). Involvement of the hypothalamic region and pituitary stalk produces diabetes insipidus. Many of these tumors have a propensity for spread within the cerebrospinal fluid, which must be examined in the workup prior to treatment. Oncoproteins are also secreted by some of these tumors, and the most useful markers are alpha-fetoprotein, human chorionic gonadotropin, and placental alkaline phosphatase. Elevation of any of these markers constitutes presumptive evidence that the tumor is a germ cell tumor.

5. Pituitary Tumors

The incidence of pituitary adenomas in autopsy studies is greater than 20%. Most are benign adenomas. They are classified as endocrine-active or endocrine-inactive (nonfunctioning) depending on whether the adenoma secretes a hormone resulting in a hypersecretory syndrome. Of the endocrine-active tumors, those that secrete growth hormone (somatotropic adenomas) result in acromegaly (or gigantism in children), excess secretion of adrenocorticotropic hormone (corticotropic adenomas) results in Cushing's disease, excess secretion of thyroid-secreting hormone (thyrotropic adenomas) results in hyperthyroidism, and hyperprolactinemia results in galactorrhea-amenorrhea in women. Hyperprolactinemia is related to prolactin secretion from the adenoma or to loss of the dopaminergic suppression by the hypothalamus of prolactin from the normal gland, the latter occurring when the pituitary stalk is distorted. Gonadotropic adenomas (secreting FSH or LH) present in a fashion similar to that of endocrine-inactive adenomas.

Pituitary tumors are also divided by size into microadenomas (< 1 cm) or macroadenomas (> 1 cm). Secretory tumors commonly present as microadenomas, whereas endocrine-inactive tumors and prolactinomas in men present as macroadenomas. Macroadenomas result in pituitary dysfunction, with the initial loss of growth hormone and gonadotropin release resulting in diminished libido. Although these tumors are benign, they result in progressive pituitary dysfunction and can compress the optic chiasm, resulting in a bitemporal visual field cut (tunnel vision).

Treatment of pituitary adenomas is excision with the exception of prolactinomas, which can be treated with dopamine agonists to prevent tumor growth and cause shrinkage. Surgery entails either a transsphenoidal approach by a sublabial or transseptal incision or a purely endonasal approach. Postoperative hospitalization is usually 1–2 days, with relatively rapid recovery. Complete resection is curative, but the likelihood of complete resection depends on the size of the tumor and whether there has been invasion of adjacent cavernous sinus or bone. The treatment of prolactinomas by surgery or medical therapy depends on the size and extent of the tumor, the serum prolactin level, and the patient's desires. Radiotherapy for pituitary adenomas is reserved for tumor recurrence or for tumors incurable by surgery alone.

6. Tumors Within the Skull Base

Primary skull neoplasms include both benign and malignant variants. These tumors generally produce symptoms by direct compression of brain tissue or cranial nerves. Benign tumors are often found incidentally in the course of investigation for other processes. These include osteoma, hemangioma, and aneurysmal bone cyst. Malignant primary skull tumors commonly include chordoma and chondrosarcoma. Chordomas are thought to arise from notochordal remnants and usually occur along the clivus. They are slowly growing and histologically benign, though clinically they have a very high rate of recurrence in spite of complete surgical removal. Their location within the skull base surrounding basal blood vessels and cranial nerves makes complete removal difficult. Chondrosarcomas have a more benign course and usually present in men in the fourth decade. They frequently arise in the upper third of the clivus or parasellar region and present with local compressive cranial neuropathy. Treatment both of these tumors is excision plus radiotherapy to reduce the rate of recurrence.

7. Metastatic Tumors

Autopsy studies have revealed the presence of intracranial metastases in one-fourth of cancer patients. Tumors of the lungs, breast, and skin account for over 90% of brain metastases. Choriocarcinoma, renal cell carcinoma, and metastatic melanoma are the most common hemorrhagic metastases. Eighty percent of brain metastases are located within the vascular distribution of the middle cerebral artery. They typically occur near the junction of the gray and white matter and can also occur within the pituitary, the pineal gland, or the choroid plexus. Involvement of the leptomeninges is common and is universally fatal. Approximately 30% of brain metastases are solid at the time of presentation, and a characteristic of these lesions is the abundant vasogenic edema they produce in surrounding brain. Metastases affecting the spinal cord occur in the epidural space, in the leptomeninges, or within the spinal cord. Epidural metastases are the most common clinical pattern of presentation.

Clinical Findings

Symptoms produced by brain tumors are largely related to their site, size, and rate of growth. The clinical manifestations may be divided into two broad categories: those related to elevated intracranial pressure and those related to tumor location.

A. Generalized Symptoms and Signs

Symptoms and signs may be due to elevation of intracranial pressure related to tumor growth, associated cerebral edema, obstruction of cerebrospinal fluid pathways with development of hydrocephalus, obstruction of cerebrospinal fluid absorption mechanisms, or intratumoral hemorrhage. The most common symptom of increased intracranial pressure is headache, which is typically generalized and relatively constant but worse in the morning. Morning headache may be relieved by vomiting. Exacerbation of headache in the early hours of the day may be related to increased venous pressure in the supine position. Any change in the pattern of a preexisting headache syndrome or new onset of severe headache or persistent syndrome should arouse suspicion of brain tumor.

Personality change, easy fatigability, listlessness, mental slowing, and problems with attention and concentration are commonly noted by patients or family when there is a rapidly growing tumor. Without intervention or diagnosis, continued elevation of intracranial pressure leads to deterioration to unconsciousness and ultimately to coma and death.

Signs of increased intracranial pressure may be subtle or marked. In its most obvious form, disturbed level of attentiveness, alertness, or frank coma may be observed. Elevated intracranial pressure that has been present for days, weeks, or months may lead to the development of papilledema. In severe cases this is associated with frank hemorrhages in the nerve fiber layer. Long-standing untreated papilledema eventually leads to loss of nerve fibers with the development of optic atrophy and blindness. A nonlocalizing sign of elevated intracranial pressure is the development of a sixth nerve palsy, resulting in paralysis of the lateral rectus muscle of the eye and inturning of the involved eye. Patients complain of double vision, most marked on looking toward the side of the affected nerve. This is thought to be related in part to the long intradural course of the sixth nerve after it exits the pons to enter a dural fold in the upper third of the clivus. Following treatment of the underlying associated problem, this nerve palsy resolves over weeks to months and in the interim can be corrected with prism glasses.

Seizures, while not a direct manifestation of increased intracranial pressure, are a nonspecific presenting symptom in adults with brain tumors. Tumors of the frontal, temporal, and parietal lobes are more likely to present with seizures than those involving the basal ganglia, brain stem, or cerebellum. Tumors within the occipital lobe may present with irritative phenomena such as nonformed visual hallucinations or a visual field defect.

It should be noted that in children, before closure of the cranial sutures, progressive enlargement of the head and bulging of the anterior fontanelle is a sign of elevated intracranial pressure. This may be due to a number of intracranial conditions including, but not limited to, brain tumor.

B. Focal Symptoms and Signs

Intra-axial tumors involving the cerebral hemispheres, basal ganglia, brain stem, or cerebellum may present with specific clinical constellations of symptoms and signs. Extra-axial non-glial neoplasm may also present with focal neurologic symptoms. Focal symptoms and signs are usually due to interference with function of a specific local area of brain. Clinical localization may be assisted by knowledge of the function localized to any of these areas. Some general comments can be made.

1. Cerebral hemispheres—Tumors of the frontal lobe commonly present with alterations in personality, behavior, motivation, mood, and memory. Within the dominant hemisphere, laterally located (usually left) frontal tumors may produce expressive language difficulties. Posterior frontal tumors bordering the primary motor cortex may produce irritative phenomena such as focal simple seizures with motor phenomena or secondary generalization. Direct invasion by glial neoplasms or compression by extra-axial tumors may produce frank loss of function. Initially this will begin in the contralateral extremity and progress in both severity and degree. Face, hand, and arm motor cortices are represented over the lateral frontal cortex, while trunk and legs are represented mesially.

2. Parietal lobe—Within the dominant hemisphere, anterior inferior parietal tumors produce receptive language difficulties. Patients have difficulty with left-right orientation and comprehension of the spoken or written word. Difficulties may also be present with naming, calculating, and reading. It is uncommon for patients with parietal tumors to complain of focal sensory deficits, but they will say that an entire side of the body is numb. Specific to the nondominant parietal lobe are functions related to three-dimensional constructional abilities as well as common daily activities such as dressing. Disturbances in these areas may be indicative of tumor location. There may also be contralateral inattention to both the visual and tactile stimulation.

3. Temporal lobe—In the dominant hemisphere, posterior temporal lobe tumors may produce difficulties with naming, calculation, and reading. Anterior and mid temporal lobe tumors may produce a contralateral quadrant visual sphere defect. Seizures not uncommonly are the presenting manifestation of temporal lobe tumors.

4. Occipital lobe—Occipital lobe tumors usually present with a visual field defect manifested by bumping into objects on the contralateral side of extrapersonal space. They may have irritative visual phenomena with nonformed visual hallucinations as simple as scintillating scotomas. Generalized seizure is not a common presentation of occipital lobe tumors.

5. Sellar and parasellar regions—Tumors in and about the optic nerve chiasm, tract, hypothalamus, and cavernous sinus may produce either visual or endocrine disturbances. Lesions of the optic nerve produce unilateral visual loss while those of the chiasm produce a bitemporal field defect. Disturbance of hypothalamic function results in autonomic disturbances and endocrinopathy. Extension of any process into the third ventricle may produce noncommunicating hydrocephalus. Involvement in structures coursing through the cavernous sinus—ie, cranial nerves III, IV, V, and VI—may produce double vision and facial numbness. Trigeminal neuralgia may be a feature of cerebellopontine angle or skull base extra-axial tumors.

6. Pineal region—Tumors of the pineal region produce symptoms related to elevated intracranial pressure from hydrocephalus and disturbance of coordinated eye movements. Hydrocephalus is usually noncommunicating, related to obstruction or compression of the cerebral aqueduct with enlargement of the third and lateral ventricles. Compression of the midbrain tectum produces problems with upward gaze and convergence. Typically, there is an absence of the pupillary light reflex.

7. Posterior fossa—Tumors of the brain stem typically cause multiple cranial nerve palsies—usually cranial nerves V, VI, and VII—followed by ataxia and long tract sensory and motor signs. Tumors of the midline cerebellum may produce a midline truncal ataxia or ipsilateral limb ataxia or incoordination when involved in the cerebral hemispheres. In many cases there is associated noncommunicating hydrocephalus.

8. Cerebellopontine angle—Vestibular and trigeminal schwannomas as well as petroclival meningiomas are the most common tumors in this location. These tumors produce a combination of specific cranial nerve dysfunction plus cerebellar disturbances and, later, hydrocephalus related to kinking of the cerebral aqueduct.

SPECIAL INVESTIGATIONS FOR SUSPECTED BRAIN TUMORS

Most patients with primary brain tumors do not have specific laboratory findings on routine blood work. However, for germ cell tumors, serum levels of alpha-fetoprotein, human chorionic gonadotropin, carcinoembryonic antigen, and placental alkaline phosphatase may be elevated. Patients with malignant primitive neuroectodermal tumors require examination of cerebrospinal fluid for central nervous system axis staging that may direct further treatment. For patients with metastatic tumors, evaluation of the primary organ system with appropriate imaging studies is necessary in order to adequately stage the primary tumor locally.

Most patients with intracranial brain neoplasms are imaged using MRI as the standard. The addition of intravenous paramagnetic contrast agents preoperatively helps predetermine the possible grade and the site for the most definitive biopsy. Anatomic detail derived from MRI is superior to that of CT scanning. Functional localization of eloquent areas of brain and their relationship to the associated tumor is also possible with functional MRI techniques using blood oxygen level-dependent (BOLD) contrast imaging. In addition, magnetic resonance spectroscopy can also help define the metabolism of volumes of tumor that are independent from static imaging features. MR imaging of the spinal axis is another important feature for staging those malignant tumors with a propensity for leptomeningeal spread, such as medulloblastoma and germinoma.

Following tumor tissue biopsy or removal, standard histologic and immunohistochemical techniques are used for distinguishing different tumor cell types. The proliferative potential for tumors can be derived by MIB-1 (evaluating Ki-67 expression) or proliferating cell nuclear antigen (PCNE) labeling studies. Molecular markers such as *P53* status and loss of heterozygosity of genes on portions of chromosomes (-1p, -19q for oligodendrogliomas) may have important therapeutic implications.

DIFFERENTIAL DIAGNOSIS OF BRAIN TUMORS

Because brain tumors can cause focal neurologic signs and increased intracranial pressure, many conditions may be simulated by brain tumor. In infants and adolescents, unexplained seizures usually herald the onset of idiopathic epilepsy. In adults, the onset of seizures is usually the first manifestation of a brain tumor. Vascular malformations, degenerative diseases, subdural hematoma, brain abscess, encephalitis, meningitis, and toxic states may mimic a tumor. Parasitic infections with a combination of solid and cystic components may mimic a benign brain tumor. Opportunistic infections in immunocompromised patients may present as mass lesions. Multiple small ring-enhancing lesions, seen with some forms of pyogenic brain abscess, may mimic intracranial metastases from a systemic primary. Even with the advent of modern imaging techniques that now are able to evaluate the metabolic "fingerprint" of a tumor, the final diagnosis still rests with tissue examination of the imaged lesion.

MEDICAL TREATMENT OF BRAIN TUMORS

The medical treatment of patients with brain tumors involves correction of metabolic abnormalities such as hyponatremia, administration of steroids to reduce vasogenic edema, and possibly administration of antiepileptic drugs in patients who present with seizures, to reduce the likelihood of further events.

In patients with elevated intracranial pressure, the syndrome of inappropriate antidiuretic hormone (SIADH) secretion may lead to the development of hyponatremia. Patients should be cautioned against drinking excessive amounts of water in order to flush out metabolic tumor toxins. We generally limit patients who have intra-axial neoplasms with surrounding edema to 1800 mL of fluid per day. No specific dietary restrictions are recommended, though patients scheduled for biopsy or open craniotomy are asked to stop aspirin-containing compounds 10 days prior to the procedure. Other anti-inflammatory agents are stopped 3 days before the procedure.

No agent is more effective than dexamethasone at reversing vasogenic edema related to intracranial tumor. Standard doses for symptomatic patients with elevations of intracranial pressure are 4 mg orally four times daily. This is tapered over time as the clinical condition allows. Patients are cautioned to observe for side effects, which include tremors, sleeplessness, excessive appetite, weight gain, and exacerbation of underlying glucose intolerance. Steroid medications can generally be reduced 1–2 weeks after operation for an intracranial tumor. In this way, long-term complications of excessive steroid use are avoided.

A variety of new antiepileptic drugs are currently available for the treatment of patients who present with epilepsy. As yet there is no good information that prophylaxis prior to surgery is warranted for patients with intra-axial brain neoplasms who did not present with a seizure. Standard agents to be used are carbamazepine, phenytoin, and valproic acid. Serum levels of any antiepileptic drug should be monitored after intravenous or oral loading and after waiting five half-lives of the drug before a steady state is reached. Modification of drug dosages is necessary in order to achieve a therapeutic serum concentration so that further seizures can be avoided.

SURGICAL TREATMENT OF BRAIN TUMORS

Prior to any operative treatment, the options of simple observation, stereotactic biopsy, or attempt at gross total tumor removal with open craniotomy should be presented to the patient. Realistic steps should be discussed with appropriate risks. The major objectives of surgical treatment are (1) to confirm the pathologic diagnosis in order to recommend appropriate further therapy; (2) to remove as much tumor as possible without increasing neurologic deficits or compromising quality of life; (3) to remove tumor for relief of symptoms of increased intracranial pressure; and (4) to remove tumor for relief of focal neurologic symptoms related to compression about the cortex by adjacent tumor.

For intra-axial glial neoplasms of the cerebral hemispheres, apart from pilocytic astrocytomas, total tumor removal is not always possible. Significant debulking of the tumor can now be accomplished safely through increased use of surgical navigation systems and intraoperative neurophysiologic monitoring and testing. Some data exist supporting the role of cytoreductive surgery for both low-grade and high-grade glial neoplasms. However, some patients live better—though perhaps not longer—after debulking surgery that reduces intracranial pressure and reduces focal mass effect, allowing for improved neurologic function.

For some posterior fossa tumors, complete tumor excision is the goal. For primitive neuroectodermal tumors, the residual volume of the tumor influences the patient's prognosis. Complete removal of lower-grade neoplasms such as ependymoma and choroid plexus papilloma obviates the need for further therapies and allows for simple imaging follow-up.

For extra-axial non-glial tumors such as meningiomas, complete surgical removal of the tumor is the goal. For convexity meningiomas, the excision of a tough normal dura surrounding the globular mass may reduce the chance for a later marginal occurrence. However, marginal excisions of dura cannot be accomplished safely in the region of the falx, major renal sinuses, the skull base, or the parasellar and posterior fossa regions. In these cases, subtotal removal of tumor may be followed by radiotherapy techniques. Fractionated external beam radiotherapy and radiosurgery offer the patient a good chance of extended tumor control not requiring further treatment.

Benign nerve sheath neoplasms of the fifth and eighth cranial nerves are best treated by surgical excision. Depending on their size, fifth nerve schwannomas can either be removed via a lateral subtemporal, anterolateral, or orbitozygomatic craniotomy or a posterolateral combined supratentorial or infratentorial approach. Vestibular schwannoma, when small and when functional hearing is still present, can be removed by a middle fossa approach. Larger tumors with preserved hearing and without a significant internal auditory canal component can be removed via a suboccipital approach. Large tumors in patients with no useful hearing are usually best managed via a translabyrinthine approach. Radiosurgery remains an option for vestibular schwannomas smaller than 2.5 cm in diameter. We have generally reserved this for the older patient population, but younger patients are now also being treated in this way. This treatment involves the application of a stereotactic head frame for imaging and treatment in a single session. Fractionated stereotactic radiotherapy techniques are also being employed with the hope of reducing facial neuropathy and increasing the chance of preserving useful hearing.

Craniopharyngiomas present a special surgical challenge because of their proximity to the optic apparatus, infundibulum, and hypothalamus. When tumors are almost completely intrasellar, a transsphenoidal approach can be used. However, when there is a significant suprasellar component, a supratentorial approach is usually required through a pterional, unilateral, frontal, or midline subfrontal approach. Residual tumors are best controlled through fractionated external beam radiotherapy.

Benign tumors of the basal cisterns such as epidermoid cysts are approached with standard neurosurgical techniques. In the case of epidermoid tumors, while it is possible to remove the desquamated epithelium from the center of the tumor, removal of the cyst capsule is usually not possible. For dermoid tumors, excision of any associated sinus tract is mandatory, accompanied by repair of the involved dura. These cyst walls may also be adherent to the cranial nerves, arteries, or adjacent brain surface. For pineal region tumors, open surgical approaches are preferred to stereotactic biopsy techniques because of the confluence of deep veins in this region. Supracerebellar infratentorial, occipital transtentorial, and interhemispheric transventricular approaches are used depending on the size, shape, and distribution of tumor.

Bone tumors of the skull base such as chordoma and chondrosarcoma are approached with multiple surgical disciplines, usually involving neurosurgery, neuro-otology, ophthalmology, and plastic surgery. These complicated and prolonged procedures require that the surgeons be skilled in a variety of aspects of neurosurgical care, including vascular neurosurgery.

Postoperative Complications

Surgical risks include those related to general anesthesia and those specific to the procedure. Anesthetic risks include bronchial pneumonia, urinary tract infection, venous thrombosis, skin pressure sores, air embolization, compression neuropraxia of peripheral nerves, and other benign reversible conditions. The risks of intraoperative cardiac death are exceedingly low, usually less than 1%. Risks specific to intracranial operation include the risks of infection of cerebrospinal fluid, brain, or the bone flap. Postoperative intracerebral, subdural, or epidural hematomas are uncommon, occurring in only 2–4% of patients postoperatively. Risks of increased neurologic deficit are related to a number of factors, most importantly tumor location and proximity to major arteries, veins, and venous sinuses. The risks of neurologic deficit when operating close to the functional cortex may be reduced by intraoperative neurophysiologic monitoring and testing. Wound complications are more common in patients who have been given long-term steroids, those who have had prior operations or radiotherapy, or those who have a persistent cerebrospinal fluid leak after surgery.

RADIATION THERAPY FOR BRAIN TUMORS

Fractionated external beam radiotherapy is usually administered to patients with malignant primary brain tumors even after the total excision. For low-grade tumors, it remains an option after biopsy or subtotal excision. Techniques from malignant tumors usually include once-a-day treatment, 5 days per week, 180–200 Gy per day to a total of 6000 Gy. Craniospinal axis treatment for primitive neuroectodermal tumors usually requires a dose of 2500–3500 Gy to the entire head and spinal access with a boost to the primary tumor site. Malignant primary brain tumors that receive fractionated radiation therapy as part of a standard treatment protocol include glioblastoma, anaplastic astrocytoma, anaplastic oligodendroglioma, malignant ependymoma, choroid plexus carcinoma, medulloblastoma, malignant meningioma, malignant germ cell tumors, and metastatic tumors. With respect to metastatic brain tumors, persuasive data exist supporting the use of external beam radiation therapy of the entire brain after excision of the lesion. The survival of patients is improved with this combination when compared with whole-brain radiation therapy alone.

Radiosurgery is a technique defined by the use of stereotactic methods for target localization and delivery of treatment and involves a single treatment session. Radiosurgery can be delivered with a variety of systems, including linear accelerator, gamma knife, and proton beam units. A great deal of clinical work with radiosurgery has centered on treatment of benign conditions such as vascular malformations and intracranial schwannomas and meningiomas. Control rates of the benign tumors appear to be excellent—above 90% at 5–8 years posttreatment. Further follow-up is required to determine the long-term results of this treatment.

CHEMOTHERAPY FOR BRAIN TUMORS

The therapeutic efficacy of antineoplastic agents against primary or metastatic brain tumors has been disappointing. This is due to several factors, including the presence of a blood-brain barrier that inhibits the transport of chemotherapeutic drugs to the interstitium of the brain. In addition, the endothelial cells within the brain have a high concentration of P-glycoprotein, which actively transports many chemotherapeutic agents out of the brain. Despite these difficulties, there are a few chemotherapeutic agents that have made it to general clinical practice for the treatment of glial neoplasms. These drugs are able to achieve reasonable concentrations within the brain because of their lipophilic nature. The most widely used antineoplastic agent for the treatment of grade III and grade IV astrocytomas are nitrosourea-based compounds. More recently, temozolomide has been shown to have some activity against grade III astrocytomas. Most chemotherapeutic trials have shown the greatest effects in younger patients. In order to overcome the difficulties of drug delivery, several systems have been developed, including the use of biodegradable polymers locally implanted into the tumor cavity, hyperosmotic blood-brain barrier disruption, and direct interstitial microinfusion for convection-enhanced delivery. Since conventional chemotherapy agents yield only marginal improvement in survival for glioma patients when compared with radiation therapy alone, new therapeutic strategies are being developed, including monoclonal antibodies, recombinant toxins, and gene transfer therapy.

PROGNOSIS

1. Glial Neoplasms

The prognosis for glia-based neoplasms is strongly dependent on the histology. Among astrocytomas, histologic grade, age, Karnofsky status, and in certain cases the extent of resection influence overall survival. For grade II astrocytomas, median survival varies from 7 years to 10 years. For grade III anaplastic astrocytomas, the median survival ranges from 3 years to 5 years, and for glioblastoma multiforme the median survival is approximately 12–18 months. Longer survival is most often noted in younger patients, and the outlook is especially poor in elderly patients with glioblastoma. Tumors with oligodendroglial components tend to have better survival rates. In general, these tumors are more radiation-sensitive as well as chemotherapy-sensitive. Among anaplastic oligodendrogliomas, there is a clear association between chemosensitivity and loss of chromosome-1p. Long-term survival has been seen in patients with low-grade oligodendroglioma. Medulloblastomas treated by gross total resection and radiation therapy can be associated with 10-year survivals of 40–50%. Significant residual disease postresection or dissemination carries a worse prognosis. Ependymomas, when completely resected, have long-term survival rates, with some patients being cured. Choroid plexus papillomas are cured following complete resection.

2. Non-Glial Tumors

Meningiomas

The prognosis of patients treated for intracranial meningioma depends upon the pathologic type and whether the tumor is benign or malignant. The degree of surgical resection also has a significant influence on the probability of recurrence. The recurrence rate ranges from 9% for excision of all tumor and adjacent dura to 39% for partial tumor removal without excision of the dural attachment or involved bone. Recurrence of tumor usually requires consideration of reoperation or external beam radiation therapy. For benign meningiomas recurrent after subtotal resection, the control rates with fractionated external beam radiation therapy are excellent—nearly 90% at 5 years and 80% 10 years after treatment. For malignant meningiomas, the prognosis is poor even with combined treatment, with median survivals of approximately 30% at 3 years posttreatment.

Trigeminal & Vestibular Schwannomas

The prognosis for these patients depends primarily on whether or not their complications are associated with surgical treatment. These tumors are slowly growing, and recurrences can be treated with reoperation or radiosurgery. Unlike meningiomas, subtotal resections are often followed by a prolonged period of no tumor growth and the enhancing mass seen on the scans remains dormant for many years. Recurrence rates after microsurgical resection vary in the literature but are less than 5%. Recurrence rates after radiosurgery are 10–12% at 5–10 years.

Craniopharyngioma

Most of the tumors that can be totally removed are reported to have 80–90% 10-year survivals. Significant endocrine or hypothalamic complications after surgery reduce these numbers. After subtotal removal and radiation therapy, survival figures are similar to those of completely removed tumors, though controversy exists as to which approach gives the best outcome.

Chordoma & Chondrosarcoma

It is rare to accomplish complete surgical excision of these tumors of the skull base. After particle beam radiation therapy, tumor control rates at 5 years are 63% and 78% for chordoma and chondrosarcoma, respectively.

Germ Cell Tumors

Radiotherapy responses for germinoma are excellent, with 5-year survivals of over 90%. With malignant neoplasms such as embryonal cell carcinoma, yolk sac tumor, and choriocarcinoma, 5-year survivals are much worse—on the order of 20–40%.

3. Metastatic Tumors

Survival of patients with metastatic brain tumors depends also to a great extent on the status of their systemic disease and whether or not it is progressive or controlled. Studies of patients with progressive systemic disease within 3 months of diagnosis of their brain metastases have found no benefit for combined surgical and radiotherapy treatment over whole-brain radiation therapy alone. Most patients survive somewhere between 8 and 12 months after the original diagnosis, but survival can be very long with some tumors such as renal cell carcinoma that have an indolent course and are responsive to radiosurgical techniques.

Brandes AA, Pasetto LM, Monfardini S: The treatment of cranial germ cell tumours. Cancer Treat Rev 2000;26:233.

Cho BK et al: Pineal tumors: experience with 48 cases over 10 years. Childs Nerv Syst 1998;14:53.

Chung WY et al: Gamma knife radiosurgery for craniopharyngiomas. J Neurosurg 2000;93(Suppl 3):47.

Habrand JL et al: The role of radiation therapy in the management of craniopharyngioma: a 25-year experience and review of the literature. Int J Radiat Oncol Biol Phys 1999;44:255.

Hader WJ et al: Intratumoral therapy with bleomycin for cystic craniopharyngiomas in children. Pediatr Neurosurg 2000;33: 211.

Mainprize TG, Taylor MD, Rutka JR: Pediatric brain tumors: a contemporary prospectus. Clin Neurosurg 2000;47:259.

Maira G et al: Craniopharyngiomas of the third ventricle: trans-lamina terminalis approach. Neurosurgery 2000;47:857.

McDermott MW: Current treatment of meningiomas. Curr Opin Neurol 1996;9:409.

McElveen JR et al: A review of facial nerve outcome in 100 consecutive cases of acoustic tumor surgery. Laryngoscope 2000;110:1667.

Prasad D, Steiner M, Steiner L: Gamma surgery for vestibular schwannoma. J Neurosurg 2000;92:745.

Rosenberg SI: Natural history of acoustic neuromas. Laryngoscope 2000;110:497.

TUMORS OF THE SPINAL CORD

Philip R. Weinstein, MD

The clinical diagnosis of spinal cord tumor should be considered when signs and symptoms suggest or localize an intraspinal lesion. These may consist of pain or numbness in a nerve root distribution, bilateral arm or leg weakness and numbness, Brown-Séquard's hemicord syndrome (weakness on one side and numbness on the other), a sensory level on the torso, or weakness and muscle atrophy with loss of the appropriate deep tendon reflexes at the level of the lesion. In cases in which long tract findings such as spasticity, hyperreflexia, and loss of proprioception predominate, a search for signs of segmental anterior or posterior horn cell loss may indicate the upper level of involvement. Horner's syndrome, when present in conjunction with other signs or symptoms of cervical cord involvement, is helpful in localization of an intramedullary lesion. If, in addition, the history is one of progression not associated with severe pain, and if bladder function has been impaired, the suspicion of a mass lesion takes precedence over other possibilities such as disk herniation or spinal stenosis. However, valuable time is lost if one expects and waits for the full picture to develop, since decompensation of function begun by compression may accelerate rapidly because of the added effect of spinal cord ischemia. Intramedullary tumors may grow to a large size while producing only mild sensory loss with sacral sparing, or localized weakness with mild long tract signs such as hyperreflexia and extensor plantar response.

Certain spinal cord tumors occur in clinical settings that should increase the suspicion of their presence. For example, signs and symptoms of thoracic cord involvement in a middle-aged woman should raise the probability of meningioma. If there is a history of Recklinghausen's disease, one must consider neurofibroma, schwannoma, meningioma, or ependymoma, as well as multiple tumors as likely possibilities. A mass in the posterior mediastinum seen on chest x-ray may have an intraspinal dumbbell extension of a neurofibroma. A patient with lymphoma or Hodgkin's disease who develops impairment of bladder function may have an otherwise asymptomatic extradural tumor implant at the level of the thoracic cord or conus. Cervico-occipital pain with weakness progressing downward on one side of the body and then upward on the other, with nystagmus and atrophy of the intrinsic muscles of the hands, suggests meningioma of the foramen magnum. Subarachnoid hemorrhage for which no intracranial cause can be found may be due to spinal cord tumor or arteriovenous malformation. The rare patient with papilledema or communicating hydrocephalus and elevated cerebrospinal fluid protein levels without evidence of a brain tumor on MRI scans may have a thoracolumbar neoplasm. Kyphoscoliosis, pain, and weakness occurring in infancy and childhood should suggest the possibility of a spinal cord glioma or neuroblastoma. If the child is known to have an intracranial medulloblastoma or an ependymoma, meningeal seeding may have taken place. A cutaneous hairy mole or fat pad overlying the vertebral column may be associated with a dermoid or lipomeningocele.

Metastatic disease of the spine must always be kept in mind. Intercostal neuralgia may be the first sign of myeloma that has invaded the bone marrow and destroyed the pedicle adjacent to the affected root. Since spinal metastases are most commonly due to lung carcinoma, a chest x-ray should be obtained in every patient suspected of a diagnosis of spinal tumor with cord compression.

Imaging Studies

On plain x-rays of the spine, one may see the following changes consistent with intraspinal tumor: destruction of bone or erosion and widening of the pedicles with scalloping of the posterior surfaces of the vertebral bodies, or enlargement of the intervertebral foramina. Calcification is sometimes seen with meningiomas. In general, destructive bony changes and pathologic compression fracture of the vertebral body are due to metastatic tumor, whereas more localized erosions are seen with neurofibroma, epidermoid tumor, and ependymoma. Neurofibroma has a predilection for the C1–2 interlaminar space and is characterized by marked thinning of the posterior arches. If a thoracic neurofibroma is suspected, one should check for deviation of the mediastinal pleural reflection at the involved level, which is indicative of a dumbbell tumor. CT scans or MRI of the spine may differentiate between extramedullary tumors, syrinx, hemangioblastoma, and lipoma, but not between astrocytoma or ependymoma. Myelography was once the definitive test, but MRI with gadolinium enhancement has superseded it as the examination of choice. Occasionally, angiography may provide information of diagnostic value (eg, in hemangioblastoma or arteriovenous malformation and fistula).

Tumors are distributed along the spinal axis as follows (in order of decreasing frequency): thoracic, lumbar, cervical, and sacral. About two-thirds of primary tumors are extramedullary-intradural and are benign (meningioma, neurofibroma, epidermoid), a fact that makes early diagnosis imperative in order to prevent irreversible loss of function due to spinal cord compression. The common intramedullary tumors, for which treatment is less satisfactory, are astrocytoma, ependymoma, hemangioblastoma, and lipoma. Some can be totally or partially resected using microsurgical technique and intraoperative neurophysiologic monitoring.

Treatment

An attempt should be made to completely excise all neurofibromas, schwannomas, and meningiomas with their respective attachments to spinal roots or dura. However, because some extend extradurally into the foramen and beyond the spinal canal, this attempt may require facetectomy and extraspinal exposure by thoracotomy or a retroperitoneal abdominal approach. A dumbbell tumor protruding discretely through a thoracic intervertebral foramen into the posterior mediastinum should be removed through a curved paraspinal incision that will allow both laminectomy and costotransversectomy to be done.

Arthrodesis with internal spinal fixation may be necessary to accomplish or maintain vertebral column stability. Intramedullary ependymomas and hemangioblastomas that can be demarcated from the surrounding spinal cord after myelotomy may be removed with microsurgical and microbipolar techniques. Infiltrating gliomas may be radically but subtotally resected and then treated with radiation therapy. Recurrence is to be expected, and progression of paralysis is inevitable when the tumor is malignant.

Ultrasonic aspiration is used to aid in excision of intramedullary tumors such as ependymomas, with excellent results. Intraoperative ultrasonography is very useful for localization of tumors and cysts. Syringopleural shunts are used when necessary to drain persistent syringomyelia caused by intramedullary tumors.

Metastatic vertebral tumors not associated with pathologic fracture causing cord compression by bone fragments may be treated with x-ray therapy, which is to be administered on an emergency basis in the presence of epidural intraspinal tumor mass if there is beginning loss of function and a pathologic diagnosis has previously been made. The indications for operation to treat metastatic spine tumors are as follows: (1) rapid progressive loss of function; (2) presence of a known radioresistant tumor; (3) undiagnosed mass, especially with the possibility of another diagnosis, such as abscess or hematoma; (4) recurrence or progression of symptomatic tumor growth after radiation therapy; and (5) presence of progression of symptomatic spinal deformity due to vertebral instability. Radiation therapy may be used in conjunction with operative decompression and stabilization to retard or prevent recurrence. Radiation therapy alone should be used to relieve pain when spinal cord function is intact and there is no evidence of bony compression. Lesion-directed surgical approaches have improved the outcome of operation for metastatic disease. Thus, when a metastatic tumor lies anterior to the spinal cord and involves the vertebral body, it is to be approached by anterior vertebrectomy or wide posterolateral laminectomy to allow transpedicular removal of any anterior tumor. Not only compression, but also vertebral column stabilization, in some cases with both anterior and posterior instrumentation extending over multiple levels, must also be done. Chemotherapy may be a useful adjunct to radiotherapy in the treatment of myeloma or lymphoma, including Hodgkin's disease.

Byrne TN: Metastatic epidural cord compression. Curr Neurol Neurosci Rep 2004;3:191. Review.

Cohen-Gadol AA et al: Spinal meningiomas in patients younger than 50 years of age: a 21-year experience. J Neurosurg 2003; 98(Suppl):258.

Conti P et al: Spinal neurinomas: retrospective analysis and long-term outcome of 179 consecutively operated cases and review of the literature. Surg Neurol 2004;61:34; discussion 44. Review.

Houten JK et al: Intramedullary ependymomas: clinical presentation, surgical treatment strategies and prognosis. J Neuro-Oncol 2004;7:211.

Janjan NA: Radiotherapeutic management of spinal metastases. J Pain Symptom Manage 1996;11:47.

Koeller KK et al: Neoplasms of the spinal cord and filum terminale: radiologic-pathologic correlation. Radiographics 2000;20:1721.

TUMORS OF PERIPHERAL NERVES

Nicholas M. Barbaro, MD, & Charles B. Wilson, MD, DSc, MSHA

ESSENTIALS OF DIAGNOSIS

- *A mass along the course of a peripheral nerve.*
- *Evidence of motor or sensory dysfunction confined to a single peripheral nerve.*
- *Pain distributed along a single peripheral nerve.*
- *Magnetic resonance imaging (MRI) showing gadolinium-enhancing mass within a peripheral nerve.*

General Considerations

Peripheral nerve tumors may be removable or diffusely invasive. The most common of the former type is the nerve sheath tumor, variously called perineurial fibroblastoma, neurilemmoma, or schwannoma. These tumors may displace a major portion of the nerve to one side and often can be totally or almost totally excised. They are found in patients with neurofibromatosis more often than in the general population. Rarely, these tumors may become malignant, metastasizing to other portions of the body and invading surrounding tissues.

Schwannomas are typically benign tumors that arise from the supporting cells within a nerve. They usually arise from a single fascicle within a nerve, displacing the other fascicles. Symptoms occur when the tumor gets big enough to be felt through the skin or when pressure within the nerve causes pain, numbness, or weakness in the distribution of the parent nerve.

Neurofibromas are characterized by general neoplastic activity within the nerve sheath. A wide spectrum of connective tissue and endoneurial cells intermixed with axons is seen histologically. These diffuse growths usually cannot be excised without resecting a segment of the involved nerve; at times they may spread in a plexiform fashion along all of a nerve's branches. Neurofibromas are most often found in patients with neurofibromatosis.

Nerve sheath tumors tend to be less than 1 mm in diameter but may become quite large—eg, to involve the entire sciatic nerve in the thigh. They may be excruciatingly painful even early in development or may become gigantic before being noted—especially, for example, when deep within an extremity or the abdomen. Growth activity is often associated with puberty.

Clinical Findings

The symptoms and signs are those of peripheral nerve dysfunction, irritative or paralytic. The nature and distribution of this dysfunction show that it is related to a specific nerve rather than tracts in the spinal cord or brain. Sensory disturbances or muscular atrophy may be noted. Nerve conduction tests and precise electromyography may be of assistance. MRI with gadolinium will image the lesions.

Differential Diagnosis

Peripheral neuropathies, including those that are the result of pressure (entrapment), may mimic peripheral nerve tumors, but a tumor that produces symptoms is usually large enough to be felt. Nerve tumors may occur anywhere along the course of the nerve, whereas entrapment occurs at characteristic locations. Generalized sensitivity along a nerve is more characteristic of neuritis than dysfunction caused by a primary nerve tumor.

Treatment & Prognosis

The operative approach to peripheral nerve tumors depends on the type of lesion. Schwannomas can almost always be removed with little permanent increase in the preoperative neurologic deficit. Typically, an operating microscope is used, and the lesion is separated from surrounding normal nerve fascicles. Complete resection is curative in these benign lesions. Amputation of the extremity may be necessary for an invasive malignant schwannoma unless it is so advanced that long-term survival is unlikely. Neurofibromas cannot usually be resected without loss of function in the parent nerve. For this reason, true neurofibromas should only be biopsied to ensure that they are not malignant and should be left in place unless the parent nerve can be sacrificed without producing significant neurologic deficit.

In patients with neurofibromatosis, the growths are often multiple, so only the tumors that cause clinical signs and symptoms (eg, pain or sensorimotor loss) should be removed. In this disease, tumors not causing dysfunction should be left alone unless cosmetic deformity is substantial or they are subject to repeated trauma or irritation.

Because most peripheral nerve tumors can be completely removed or are slowly growing lesions confined to a single nerve, the overall prognosis is good. However, moderate disability can be produced by unresectable lesions of major nerves. In addition, patients with neurofibromatosis may have multiple lesions, including those in the craniospinal axis, which can produce progressive and severe neurologic deficits. Malignant peripheral nerve tumors can be fatal if not treated aggressively in their early stages.

Artico M: Benign neural sheath tumours of major nerves: characteristics in 119 surgical cases. Acta Neurochir (Wien) 1997; 139:1108.

Hems TE, Burge PD, Wilson DJ: The role of magnetic resonance imaging in the management of peripheral nerve tumours. J Hand Surg (Br) 1997;22:57.

Vauthey JN, Woodruff JM, Brennan MF: Extremity malignant peripheral nerve sheath tumors (neurogenic sarcomas): a 10-year experience. Ann Surg Oncol 1995;2:126.

Wong WW et al: Malignant peripheral nerve sheath tumor: analysis of treatment outcome. Int J Radiat Oncol Biol Phys 1998;42:351.

PITUITARY TUMORS

Sandeep Kunwar, MD

ESSENTIALS OF DIAGNOSIS

- *Hypopituitarism: hyposecretion of one or more pituitary tropic hormones.*
- *Syndrome of pituitary hypersecretion: acromegaly and gigantism, Cushing's disease, amenorrhea-galactorrhea.*
- *Visual impairment: typically bitemporal hemianopia.*

General Considerations

The pituitary gland is often considered the "master gland" regulating most of the body's hormonal balance. It is composed of the adenohypophysis (anterior lobe) and the neurohypophysis (posterior lobe) sitting within the sella turcica ("Turkish saddle"). The anterior lobe is responsible for the secretion of prolactin, growth hormone, FSH and LH, thyroid stimulating hormone (TSH), and ACTH. The posterior lobe is a storage depot for antidiuretic hormone (ADH) and oxytocin. The majority of pituitary tumors arise from the anterior lobe and represent benign pituitary adenomas. Pituitary tumors are classified by their secretory state as endocrine-active or endocrine-inactive, and by size. Microadenomas are tumors with a diameter of less than 1 cm, whereas larger tumors are macroadenomas. Endocrine-active tumors are further classified based on the hormone they secrete and the clinical syndrome they cause.

Clinical Findings

Endocrine-active adenomas result in characteristic syndromes caused by hypersecretion or dysregulated secretion of a hormone by the tumor (Table 37–6). Endocrine-inactive adenomas and large endocrine-active adenomas can present with symptoms associated with anterior pituitary gland compression, resulting in hypopituitarism, or with elevation of the optic chiasm, resulting in bitemporal hemianopia (chiasmatic syndrome). Progressive compression of the anterior lobe causes progressive loss of glandular function with GH, FSH, and LH being affected early, and TSH and ACTH affected later. The earliest symptom in adult males is loss of libido or infertility and in premenopausal women, oligomenorrhea or amenorrhea. Central hypogonadism can be caused by primary compression of the pituitary gland, causing diminished LH/FSH

Table 37–6. Classification of pituitary adenomas.[1]

	Secretory Product	Clinical Syndrome
Endocrine-active		
Somatotropic	Growth hormone (GH)	Acromegaly (adult), gigantism
Corticotropic	Adrenocorticotropic hormone (ACTH)	Cushing's disease, Nelson's syndrome[2]
Prolactinoma	Prolactin (PRL)	Amenorrhea/galactorrhea, diminished libido
Thyrotropic	Thyroid-stimulating hormone	Hyperthyroidism
Gonadotropic	Follicle-stimulating (FSH), luteinizing hormone (LH)	Behave as endocrine-inactive
Endocrine-inactive	Alpha subunit	Hypopituitarism, chiasmatic compression

[1]Some tumors secrete more than one hormone, most often GH-PRL and ACTH-PRL.
[2]Can occur after adrenalectomy.

secretion, or by loss of tonic inhibition of prolactin secretion, resulting in hyperprolactinemia (stalk effect) and subsequent physiologic suppression of gonadotropins. Diabetes insipidus, a result of direct hypothalamic or pituitary stalk involvement, is rarely caused by pituitary adenomas. As pituitary adenomas enlarge, they grow outside the sella turcica and result in suprasellar extension. This elevates the optic chiasm and will lead to distortion of the decussating nasal fibers, causing bitemporal hemianopia. With progressive compression of the optic chiasm and nerves, decreased visual acuity can occur, eventually leading to blindness. Endocrine-inactive adenomas grow slowly and thus present when they are relatively large, particularly in males and postmenopausal women. In rare cases, intratumoral hemorrhage or infarction may occur, resulting in a sudden increase in tumor size and intrasellar pressure (pituitary apoplexy). With apoplexy, patients present with severe headaches, sudden vision loss (including acute blindness), and panhypopituitarism.

The sudden loss of pituitary function can result in addisonian crisis, with patients developing headaches, nausea, electrolyte abnormalities, and hypotension. In cases of pituitary apoplexy, immediate correction of the hypocortisolemia and surgical decompression of the optic nerves to preserve visual function is necessary.

Elevated growth hormone levels result in acromegaly after puberty (when the epiphyseal plates have fused) or gigantism prior to puberty. The clinical findings of an enlarged protruding jaw (macrognathia)—with associated overbite, separation of the teeth, enlarged tongue (macroglossia), enlarging hands or feet, coarse facial features, arthralgias, skin tags, hyperhidrosis, hirsutism, deepening of the voice, and nerve entrapment syndromes—are common in acromegaly. Cardiovascular disease with left ventricular hypertrophy, hypertension, and diabetes mellitus result in an increased risk of cardiovascular morbidity in patients with acromegaly. There is also a significant increased risk of colonic polyps that mandates colonoscopy in patients with this diagnosis.

Hyperprolactinemia is among the most common of pituitary disorders and may be seen in a variety of medical conditions through different mechanisms. Prolactinomas (pituitary adenomas that secrete excess prolactin) are the most common type of pituitary adenomas and are primarily diagnosed in young women. Since the hyperprolactinemia can result in primary or secondary amenorrhea early on, these tumors are typically diagnosed as microadenomas. The elevated prolactin causes physiologic suppression of FSH/LH with subsequent hypogonadism and also causes galactorrhea and gynecomastia, hence the syndrome of galactorrhea/amenorrhea in women. In postmenopausal women and men, the hypogonadism is often undiagnosed; thus, these tumors typically present as macroadenomas. Hyperprolactinemia up to 150 ng/dL can also be caused by loss of the tonic inhibition of prolactin secretion from the normal anterior lobe as a result of pituitary stalk distortion or compression of the gland ("stalk effect").

Hypercortisolemia can be due to Cushing's *syndrome* (as in adrenal adenomas) or Cushing's *disease* (ACTH-secreting pituitary adenoma). The clinical syndrome is the same, with centripetal fat deposition resulting in moon facies and a buffalo-hump, facial plethora, diabetes mellitus, abdominal striae, hirsutism, osteoporosis, myopathy, and often psychic disturbances including depression. Cushing's disease can also be associated with hyperpigmentation. The diagnosis can be confirmed by laboratory testing, MRI imaging, and occasionally inferior petrosal sampling of ACTH levels.

Elevated TSH causes hyperthyroidism and can be associated with thyrotoxicosis and osteoporosis. TSH-secreting adenomas are extremely rare, comprising 1% of pituitary adenomas. An elevated TSH in the presence of an elevated free T4 is suggestive of a TSH-secreting adenoma.

Differential Diagnosis

For endocrine-inactive adenomas presenting with hypopituitarism, headaches, or chiasmatic syndrome, an MRI focused on the sella will confirm the diagnosis and extent of tumor involvement. Current MRI with coronal and sagittal views will identify all but the smallest (< 2 mm) intrasellar tumors. Occasionally, an incidental adenoma may be seen on MRI and complete hormonal evaluation will confirm whether the tumor is asymptomatic, as are most endocrine-inactive microadenomas. Other sellar and perisellar masses include a Rathke's cleft cyst (a congenital cyst typically between the anterior and posterior lobe), craniopharyngioma, tuberculum sella meningioma, cavernous sinus meningioma, chordoma, or rarely metastatic lesion. The presence of diabetes insipidus would raise the suspicion of a lesion affecting the pituitary stalk such as germ cell tumor, Langerhans histiocytosis X, lymphocytic hypophysitis, or sarcoidosis.

For endocrine-active adenomas, the diagnosis is established by laboratory tests of pituitary hormones and clinical features. Dynamic studies such as the physiologic regulation of hormone secretion can be helpful (eg, loss of GH suppression with an oral glucose challenge seen in acromegaly or loss of cortisol suppression with low-dose dexamethasone seen with Cushing's syndrome). In some patients with Cushing's disease, a tumor too small to detect from standard imaging may be present and require further investigation with inferior petrosal sinus sampling. Hyperprolactinemia can result from many causes, including pregnancy, emotional or physical stress, medications (such as phenothiazines, antipsychotics, and certain antidepressants), or hypothyroidism, which must be excluded before making the diagnosis of a prolactinoma.

Treatment

The treatment of symptomatic endocrine-inactive adenomas is surgical resection. This is usually accomplished through a transsphenoidal approach. Despite several variations including sublabial, transnasal/transseptal, endonasal, and endoscopic transsphenoidal approaches, all are associated with low morbidity and short hospital stays when performed in experienced centers. The surgical goal is an attempt for complete resection of the tumor with preservation of the remaining normal pituitary gland. In many large adenomas, invasion into the cavernous sinus will preclude a gross total resection. In such cases, radiotherapy may be necessary. With the advent of stereotactic radiosurgery, it is possible to treat residual surgically inaccessible tumors with radiation therapy without sacrificing pituitary function. Although standard fractionated external beam radiotherapy is highly effective in the treatment of pituitary adenomas, the risk of hypopituitarism remains high. Therefore, in patients with adequate pituitary function, either stereotactic radiosurgery should be utilized when possible or radiotherapy should be deferred until recurrent tumor growth can be documented. Rarely, a transcranial approach may be necessary if the anatomy of the tumor is atypical or the radiographic diagnosis suggests a nonpituitary pathology.

Prolactinomas are the only pituitary adenoma where an effective medical therapy is available. An MRI is imperative before medical therapy is started to assess whether the cause is an endocrine-inactive macroadenoma with stalk effect or a prolactinoma. The use of dopamine analogues such as bromocriptine or, more recently, cabergoline can normalize the prolactin level, cause shrinkage of the tumor, and prevent future tumor growth while patients receive therapy. With bromocriptine, lifelong therapy is required; however, cabergoline, which is a selective D2 agonist, may have more longer-acting effects.

Currently, patients may undergo withdrawal of cabergoline therapy with close monitoring. In women with large prolactinomas, tumor control during pregnancy may be complicated when medical therapy needs to be halted. Patients with small prolactinomas that do not have involvement of the cavernous sinus are typically treated with medical therapy; however, surgical resection can be offered as an alternative because of the low morbidity and elimination of lifelong medical therapy. In patients with invasive prolactinomas or macroadenomas, medical therapy is the primary treatment and surgery is reserved for tumors that fail to respond or patients who are intolerant of medical therapy. The primary treatment for acromegaly and Cushing's disease is surgical resection of the tumor. For patients with acromegaly who are not cured by surgery, medical therapy with somatostatin analogues can inhibit GH release. Persistent Cushing's disease may necessitate radiotherapy to control the primary tumor or bilateral adrenalectomy to control the hypercortisolemia.

Abosch A et al: Transsphenoidal microsurgery for growth hormone-secreting pituitary adenomas: initial outcome and long-term results. J Clin Endocrinol Metab 1998;83:3411.

Freda PU et al: Long-term treatment of prolactin-secreting macroadenomas with pergolide. J Clin Endocrinol Metab 2000; 85:8.

Kovacs K, Horvath E: *Atlas of Tumor Pathology,* Second Series, Fascicle 21. Armed Forces Institute of Pathology, 1986.

Littley MD et al: Hypopituitarism following external radiotherapy for pituitary tumours in adults. Q J Med 1989;70:145.

Mampalam TJ, Tyrrell JB, Wilson CB: Transsphenoidal microsurgery for Cushing's disease: a report of 216 cases. Ann Intern Med 1988;109:487.

Munari C et al: Long term results of stereotactic endocavitary beta irradiation of craniopharyngioma cysts. J Neurosurg Sci 1989; 33:99.

Peck WW et al: High-resolution MR imaging of pituitary microadenomas at 1.5 T: experience with Cushing's disease. AJR Am J Roentgenol 1989;152:145.

Peillon F et al: Receptors and neurohormones in human pituitary adenomas. Horm Res 1989;31:13.

Pinzone JJ et al: Primary medical therapy of micro- and macroprolactinomas in men. J Clin Endocrinol Metab 2000;85:3053.

Rush SC, Newall J: Pituitary adenoma: the efficacy of radiotherapy as the sole treatment. Int J Radiat Oncol Biol Phys 1989;17:165.

Samaan NA et al: Multiple endocrine syndrome type I. Clinical, laboratory findings, and management in five families. Cancer 1989;64:741.

Semple PL et al: Transsphenoidal surgery for Cushing's disease: outcome in patients with a normal magnetic resonance imaging scan. Neurosurgery 2000;46:553.

Tyrrell JB, et al: Transsphenoidal microsurgical therapy of prolactinomas: initial outcomes and long-term results. Neurosurgery 1999;44:254.

Wass JA et al: The treatment of acromegaly. Clin Endocrinol Metab 1986;15:683.

Wilson CB: Endocrine-inactive pituitary adenomas. Clin Neurosurg 1992;38:10.

Wilson CB: Role of surgery in the management of pituitary tumors. Neurosurg Clin North Am 1990;1:139.

PEDIATRIC NEUROSURGERY

Nalin Gupta, MD, PhD, & Warwick J. Peacock, MD

Most neurosurgical problems in infancy and childhood are due to one of four causes: congenital malformations, neoplasms, infections, or trauma. They represent a distinct group of disorders that require management tailored to the needs of the developing nervous system. Trauma and infections are discussed elsewhere in this chapter and will be discussed only briefly in reference to specific pediatric problems.

CONGENITAL MALFORMATIONS

Congenital malformations occur frequently in the nervous system and are exceeded only by prematurity as a cause of death in infants. In most cases, no specific cause can be demonstrated, although a number of teratogenic factors are recognized: (1) maternal infections, eg, rubella, toxoplasmosis, cytomegalic inclusion disease, and syphilis; (2) drugs ingested by the mother during gestation, eg, thalidomide, LSD, methotrexate; (3) ionizing radiation; (4) maternal anesthesia; and (5) systemic disease, electrolyte imbalance, and dietary deficiencies. Although specific genes responsible for some congenital defects have been identified, it is reasonable to assume that the final phenotype results from a complex interplay of genetic predisposition and various intrauterine factors.

1. Malformations of the Skull or Vertebral Column

A spectrum of anomalies can result from either improper ossification of bony elements or failed segmentation during early development. Children may be asymptomatic or profoundly disabled.

Craniosynostosis is defined as the premature closure or absence of one or more of the sutures that normally separate the individual bones of the skull (Table 37–7). The majority of these cases involve a single suture and are isolated. The incidence is 4:10,000 births. Sutural closure prevents radial and symmetric growth of the head and is manifest as a secondary deformation of head shape with compensatory growth occurring parallel to the plane of the fused suture. Single suture synostosis is rarely associated with abnormal neurologic function. When the process involves two or more sutures, growth and development of the brain can be affected, particularly during the first year of life when the brain triples its volume. Primary craniosynostosis must be differentiated from the secondary approximation and fusion of sutures in microcephaly and that which sometimes follows operative procedures on the skull or shunting for hydrocephalus. Premature closure of a specific suture results in a characteristic visual appearance.

Treatment consists of excision of the fused suture and sometimes reconstruction of the skull. Most procedures are performed between 3 months and 6 months of age, when the growing brain is still able to mold the relatively thin cranial vault into a "normal" shape.

Craniofacial syndromes such as Crouzon's and Apert's involve closure of several sutures resulting in cranial vault and midface abnormalities such as hyper- or hypotelorism, maxillary hypoplasia, and proptosis. Treatment may require multiple osteoplastic techniques at the skull base to achieve an acceptable result.

Chiari malformations are related by the presence of abnormalities of the posterior fossa and cerebellum. Chiari type 1 is characterized by a small posterior fossa and caudal displacement of the cerebellar tonsils through the foramen magnum and may be associated with hydrocephalus or syringomyelia (a central cavity in the spinal cord). Chiari type 2 is usually seen in patients with myelomeningocele. In addition to cerebellar herniation, there are other abnormalities such as kinking of the cervicomedullary junction, cortical malformations, and agenesis of the corpus callosum. Types 3 and 4 are rare.

Split cord malformations (also known as diastematomyelia) are characterized by a bony spur or fibrous band projecting through the middle of the spinal canal dividing and spinal cord into two compartments. They are usually accompanied by other skeletal anomalies and varying degrees of spinal cord dysfunction. Surgical removal of the midline abnormality is needed to untether the spinal cord and prevent progression of neurologic deficits.

Table 37–7. Types of craniosynostosis.

Suture	Cranial abnormality	Features	Frequency
Sagittal	Scaphocephaly	AP elongation, reduced biparietal distance	40–60%
Unilateral coronal	Anterior plagiocephaly	Recession of the forehead, elevation of the ipsilateral eye	20–30%
Bilateral coronal	Brachycephaly	"Tower-like" pointed head, reduced overall size, flattened forehead	10%
Metopic	Trigonocephaly	Pointed frontal bone, hypotelorism	5–10%
Lambdoid	Posterior plagiocephaly	Flattening of the occipital area, prominence of the contralateral frontal area	1–3%

Basilar impression is the upward displacement of the cervical spine into the base of the skull. It results in reduced capacity of the posterior fossa and stenosis of the foramen magnum, leading to compression of the brain stem and spinal cord.

2. Incomplete Formation of the Neural Tube

Failure of the neuroectoderm to fuse in the midline during the third and fourth week of fetal life leads to secondary failure of formation of overlying mesoderm and ectoderm. These defects may be small and concealed or they may be exposed and involve large areas of the spinal cord, meninges, vertebral column, overlying muscles, and skin. The most frequently involved anatomic level is the lumbosacral area; the least frequently involved is the thoracic area. (Cervical myelomeningoceles are very rare.)

Spina bifida occulta is a defect in fusion of the spinous processes and lamina that is present in up to 10% of the population, is asymptomatic, and does not require treatment. Cases that involve multiple levels and those associated with skin abnormalities (eg, hemangioma, patches of hair, dermal sinus, or subcutaneous lipoma) may produce neurologic dysfunction by tethering of the spinal cord. The clinical picture includes progressive weakness, scoliosis, gait instability, urinary or bowel difficulties, and sometimes pain. MRI is the diagnostic procedure of choice. In newborn infants, spinal ultrasound can assist in determining the position of the conus medullaris and associated spinal cord anomalies. Surgical correction of the tethered cord usually halts progression of symptoms in most patients and may improve neurologic and urologic function in up to 25% of patients.

Myelomeningocele (spina bifida aperta) (see Figure 37–17) is protrusion of nerve roots or cord elements along with the meninges. It occurs at least ten times more often than simple meningocele and always causes some degree of neurologic deficit. Findings range from mild weakness and slight sphincteric disturbance to complete sensory and motor paralysis below the lesion and incontinence. Hydrocephalus is associated with at least 80% of lumbosacral myelomeningoceles; Chiari malformation type 2 is always present and may cause brain stem dysfunction. The term lipomyelomeningocele is used when the neural tube defect is associated with a lipoma that is continuous with the spinal cord.

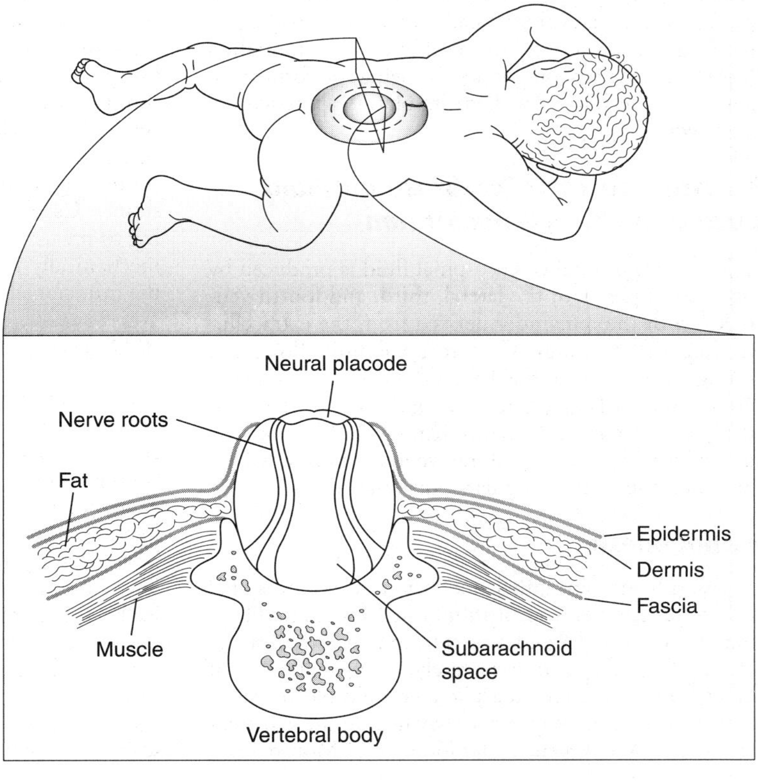

Figure 37–17. Diagrammatic representation of a myelomeningocele. The neural placode is superficial and not covered by any ectodermal or mesodermal elements. Laterally, the dermis fuses with the dura, which is then continuous with the thin lateral edge of the placode. The actual neural placode is usually easily visualized as the most central portion of the defect.

Meningocele consists of herniation of the meninges through a spina bifida without abnormality of the spinal cord or nerve roots. Neurologic function is usually preserved in these patients.

Encephalocele is a much less common midline protrusion of the meninges through the skull. It is usually occipital or at the base of the nose. The extent of brain tissue within the encephalocele often determines the functional outcome.

Treatment

For all open spina bifida lesions, the fundamental surgical principle is reconstitution of the neural tube by layered closure of the dura, skin, and sometimes fascia usually within a few days of birth. The goals of early repair are prevention of meningitis, preservation of neurologic function, and facilitation of nursing care. For lesions that are covered by normal skin, repair can be delayed for several months, unless symptoms develop. Early recognition and treatment of hydrocephalus is essential.

A team approach is required to manage a broad range of orthopedic (spasticity, club feet, scoliosis), urologic (urinary reflux, neurogenic bladder, hydronephrosis), and rehabilitation (orthoses, therapy, special schooling) concerns. Entry into a normal school, completion of education, and physical independence are the ultimate goals. Urosepsis and shunt malfunction remain the primary causes of long-term morbidity and mortality. Repair of myelomeningoceles is being performed in utero, but the long-term benefits of this approach are unknown.

3. Disturbances of Cerebrospinal Fluid Circulation (CSF) & Absorption

At least 50% of total cerebrospinal fluid is produced by the choroid plexus of the lateral, third, and fourth ventricles, with the remainder derived from the extracellular fluid of the brain. Cerebrospinal fluid flows out through foramina at the base of the fourth ventricle into the subarachnoid spaces, along the spinal cord, and finally over the cerebral hemispheres to be absorbed via the arachnoid villi into dural venous sinuses, which drain into the internal jugular veins (Figure 37–1).

Pathogenesis

Hydrocephalus, an imbalance between cerebrospinal fluid production and absorption, usually leads to dilatation of the ventricles and results from either an obstruction to CSF flow; or very rarely, overproduction of cerebrospinal fluid secondary to a choroid plexus papilloma. Obstruction may occur anywhere in the ventricular system (eg, interventricular foramen of Monro, cerebral aqueduct of Sylvius, or outlet foramina of the fourth ventricle). Hydrocephalus arising from these causes is termed obstructive. Hydrocephalus arising from interference of CSF absorption at the arachnoid villi is termed communicating.

Obstruction of the cerebral aqueduct is the most frequent cause of congenital hydrocephalus. Gliomas in critical locations, especially those found adjacent to the cerebral aqueduct, may present with cerebrospinal fluid obstruction as their only manifestation. Intraventricular hemorrhage secondary to prematurity or infections often cause gliosis (scarring) of the aqueduct or the outlet of foramina of the fourth ventricle, with similar results. Scarring (arachnoiditis) in the basal cisterns or over the cerebral convexities may result from meningitis, intracranial hemorrhage, meningeal carcinomatosis, or, rarely, tumors blocking the foramen magnum or basal cisterns.

Treatment

CT scans and other tests (eg, MRI flow studies, cerebrospinal fluid drainage, nuclear isotope studies, intracranial pressure monitoring) are used to determine the cause of hydrocephalus by identifying the site of cerebrospinal fluid flow obstruction. Although endoscopic fenestration of the floor of the third ventricle (third ventriculocisternostomy) is successful in treating a subset of patients, thereby avoiding shunt insertion, most cases of hydrocephalus are treated by diverting cerebrospinal fluid to an alternate site. Cerebrospinal fluid shunts consist of a silicon tube leading from one of the cerebral ventricles to a distal site. In the vast majority of cases, shunts are placed into the peritoneal cavity (VP shunt), right atrium (VA shunt), or pleural space (VPl shunt). Usually, a valve is placed in series with the tubing to prevent overdrainage of CSF. Most valves have a mechanically fixed pressure point and only open when the intracranial pressure rises above that pressure.

4. Vascular Malformations

The most common type found in children are **arteriovenous (AV) malformations** (see section later in the chapter). These lesions contain a direct arterial-to-venous shunt that creates symptoms by gradual enlargement of the mass, cerebral ischemia caused by hypoperfusion of the surrounding brain, seizures, or hemorrhage. The hemorrhage can be either small, with few symptoms, or massive and at times, fatal. Pathologically, the involved vessels have thin walls with defective muscular and elastic layers and thus have a propensity to bleed. A loud bruit can be heard over the cranium in some infants with large lesions. The diagnosis is suggested by the history and confirmed by CT scan, MRI, MRA, and conventional angiography.

Rupture of intracranial arterial **saccular aneurysms** leading to subarachnoid hemorrhage are rare in children. Vein of Galen aneurysms (a misnomer since the primary abnormality is an arterial-to-venous fistula) are more common in young children and can present with severe congestive heart failure as the result of high-output cardiac failure. **Cavernous malformations** do not contain high flow AV shunts but are composed of thin-walled sinusoidal vessels that can rebleed over time. If surgically accessible, most are removed.

Treatment

Treatment of AV malformations varies depending on the symptoms, the age and condition of the patient, and size and location of the malformation. Interventional neuroradiologic procedures can be used to reduce the size of AV malformations and thus allow safer excision. Total excision is preferred but should not be attempted if a severe neurologic deficit is likely. Deep or residual lesions can be treated using tightly collimated radiation (gamma knife or LINAC), which usually results in obliteration of the lesion over months to years.

NEOPLASMS

Neoplasms of the central nervous system are the most common solid tumors of childhood (3.3:100,000), exceeded in frequency only by lymphoma and leukemia. They differ from those found in adults by their sites of origin and histologic type. Twenty percent of pediatric nervous system tumors are located in the spinal cord and 80% in the brain. Of the latter, 50% arise in the posterior fossa and 50% in the supratentorial compartment (Table 37–8). Meningiomas, pituitary tumors, and metastatic tumors—among the more common adult tumors—are rare in children.

1. Brain Tumors

Brain tumors produce symptoms by increasing intracranial pressure (through occupying space or obstructing cerebrospinal fluid pathways) or by directly invading or compressing neural tissues. In infants and children, the symptoms and signs of increased intracranial pressure are vomiting, headache, papilledema, mental dysfunction, personality changes, and cranial nerve palsy. Symptoms and signs of direct brain involvement are ataxia, incoordination, nystagmus, weakness of extremities, seizures, and head tilt to the side of the lesion (seen with cerebellar hemisphere lesions).

For most common brain tumors (medulloblastoma, ependymoma, and astrocytoma), the extent of surgical resection is a positive predictive factor for survival. In addition, for other less frequently encountered tumors (hemangioblastoma, dermoid cyst, craniopharyngioma, or unilateral optic nerve glioma), gross total removal is curative. Therefore, for most patients a definitive surgical procedure is the initial step. For unresectable tumors, cerebrospinal fluid pathways are reopened or bypassed, and radiation therapy or chemotherapy is given. Radiation is avoided in children younger than 3 years of age due to sequelae such as cognitive decline, visual loss, endocrine dysfunction, and second malignancies. A current trend is the use of intensive chemotherapy to delay radiation treatment as long as possible.

Specific Types

Astrocytomas (Figure 37–18) are the most common primary brain tumor in children and fortunately are either benign or low-grade by histology. Astrocytomas arising in the cerebellar hemispheres (about 15% of all brain tumors) are almost always benign and can be cured by gross total resection. Approximately 10% of all tumors are astrocytomas arising from the hypothalamus or optic

Table 37–8. Types of central nervous system tumors in children and their location.

Cell Type	Incidence	Supratentorial	Infratentorial
Astrocytoma	40%	Common, especially suprasellar	Cerebellar hemisphere
Primitive neuroectodermal tumor	20%	Rare	Midline cerebellum (medulloblastoma)
Ependymoma	10%	Rare	Fourth ventricle
Craniopharyngioma	5%	Suprasellar	Rare
Brain stem glioma	5%	N/A	Pons
Neuronal tumors	3%	Cause seizures	Rare
Dermoid tumors	3%	Rare	Rare
Other	10%		

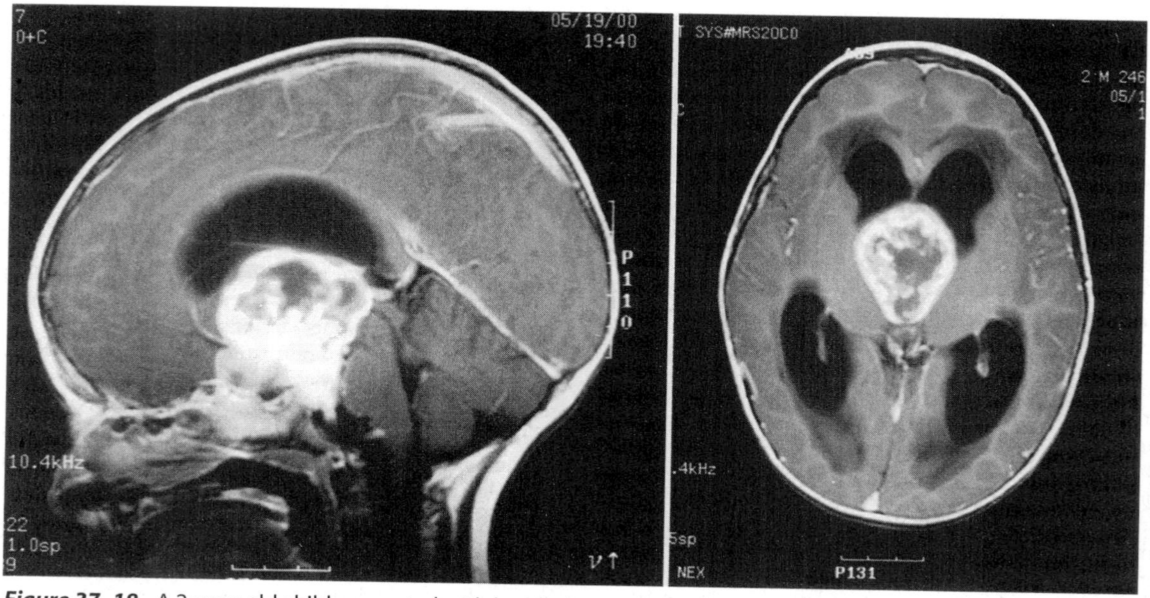

Figure 37–18. A 2-year-old child presented with headaches and vomiting. Post-gadolinium MR images demonstrate a large hypothalamic astrocytoma filling the third ventricle (sagittal plane on left) and leading to obstruction of cerebrospinal fluid flow and marked enlargement of the lateral ventricles (axial plane on right).

apparatus. This location prevents radical resection. Patients with neurofibromatosis type 1 are predisposed to the development of optic pathway gliomas. Some astrocytomas are malignant and these tumors—particularly those that arise in the brain stem—are infiltrative by nature and have a very poor prognosis regardless of treatment.

Medulloblastoma

This tumor is composed of small, poorly differentiated cells that are identical to those found with pineoblastoma, Ewing's sarcoma, and other primitive tumors. Some pathologists group these tumors under the umbrella of **primitive neuroectodermal tumors (PNETs)**. Medulloblastomas are tumors of children and young adults, with the majority arising in the posterior fossa. Gross total excision followed by radiation carries the best long-term prognosis. High-risk patients include those whose have residual tumor after surgery, central nervous system spread at diagnosis, and age younger than 3 years. For patients without these features, the 5-year survival is 60–70%.

Craniopharyngiomas

These histologically benign tumors arise in the suprasellar area and are composed of epithelial tissue with a central cystic area containing desquamated material. Their proximity to vital structures in the suprasellar area makes their management a formidable challenge. Visual, endocrine, and neurologic complications are commonly encountered following either surgery or adjunctive treatment.

2. Spinal Cord Tumors

Spinal cord tumors are uncommon. The clinical presentation is insidious, with gradual progression of symptoms such as back pain, leg weakness, gait instability, torticollis, or bowel and bladder dysfunction. Tumors are classified by the site of origin. Intramedullary tumors include gliomas such as astrocytomas and ependymomas and undifferentiated tumors such as medulloblastomas. The congenital group (eg, dermoids, teratomas, and neurofibromas) are usually intradural but not within the spinal cord. Extradural tumors are generally metastatic (ie, neuroblastomas and lymphosarcoma) and cause spinal cord compression.

Diagnostic evaluation in the current era requires a detailed contrast MRI study of the spine. Other studies are of limited value. Depending upon the nature of the lesion, the surgical goal is total removal, although in certain cases only a biopsy is possible. For these tumors, radiation therapy or chemotherapy (or both) is the treatment of choice.

TRAUMA

1. Head Injuries

Head injury is the most common cause of death and disability in children. In general, management follows the same principles used in adult trauma patients. A few injuries are seen in children. Nonaccidental trauma has a number of synonyms (eg, shaken baby syndrome) and represents a spectrum of injuries including intracranial hemorrhage or contusion, retinal hemorrhage, and extremity fractures. Often, there is no relevant history or at best a vague history. Most jurisdictions have legal requirements for reporting these injuries, if suspected, to the appropriate authorities. **Greenstick skull** fractures occur in infants when the skull is pushed inward without fragmenting. These fractures can usually be elevated by leverage through a small burr hole.

2. Spine Injuries

A child's spine develops the biomechanical features of the adult spine by the early teen years. Prior to this, the relatively large size of the head with respect to the body, the immaturity of ligamentous structures, and the orientation of the facet joints predisposes children to cervical spine injures, and to C1–C2 injuries in particular. **Spinal cord injury without radiologic abnormality (SCIWORA)** is the syndrome of a neurologically apparent spinal cord injury in the absence of a detectable vertebral column injury. These injuries are often delayed in onset and are presumed to be caused by hypermobility of the spine or a delayed ischemic event.

FUNCTIONAL DISORDERS

1. Spastic Cerebral Palsy

Extreme prematurity is often the prelude to the later development of spastic cerebral palsy. Spasticity is due to the loss of descending inhibition on the spinal reflex arc. Selective posterior rhizotomy has proved to be a safe and effective method of reducing the muscular hypertonicity that interferes with the acquisition of motor skills in the developing child. By dividing selected posterior spinal rootlets, excitatory influence on the anterior horn cells is reduced, leading to improved muscle tone and motor function and normalization of gait patterns. More recently, implantation of a constant infusion pump delivering intrathecal baclofen has been found to be helpful in some children with spastic cerebral palsy.

2. Surgery for Intractable Seizures in Childhood

Whereas epilepsy surgery in adults is mainly limited to temporal lobectomy, a variety of procedures are extremely helpful in controlling intractable seizures in children. The pathologic basis of seizures and the seizure types found in children differ from those in adults. Resective procedures such as hemispherectomy, lobectomy, and focal resection are often helpful but when resection is not feasible disconnective surgery is an option. Division of the corpus callosum may eliminate drop attacks, and multiple subpial resections can be used in a seizure focus that is also the site of an important cortical function such as speech or movement. In children with intractable seizures where neither resection nor disconnection is possible, the implantation of a vagus nerve stimulator is useful in significantly reducing seizure frequency.

American Association for the Surgery of Trauma et al: Guidelines for the acute medical management of severe traumatic brain injury in infants, children, and adolescents. J Trauma 2003; 54(6 Suppl):S235.

Botto LD et al: Neural-tube defects. N Engl J Med 1999;341:1509.

Bruner JP et al: Fetal surgery for myelomeningocele and the incidence of shunt-dependent hydrocephalus. JAMA 1999;17: 282:1819.

Davis FG et al: Survival rates in patients with primary malignant brain tumors stratified by patient age and tumor histological type: an analysis based on Surveillance, Epidemiology, and End Results (SEER) data, 1973–1991. J Neurosurg 1998; 88:10.

Pollack IF: Pediatric brain tumors. Sem Surg Oncol 1999;16:73.

Rankin J et al: The changing prevalence of neural tube defects: a population-based study in the north of England, 1984–96. Paediatr Perinat Epidemiol 2000;14:104.

INTRACRANIAL ANEURYSMS

Philip V. Theodosopolous, MD, &
Michael T. Lawton, MD

ESSENTIALS OF DIAGNOSIS

- *Clinical symptoms or signs of aneurysm rupture: sudden, severe headache with associated stiff neck, nausea and vomiting, impaired consciousness, seizures, or coma.*
- *Clinical symptoms or signs of an expanding intracranial mass: progressive oculomotor nerve palsy, visual field cut, lower cranial nerve dysfunction, brain stem deficits, or hydrocephalus.*
- *Radiographic evidence of subarachnoid hemorrhage on CT scan (ruptured aneurysms) or the aneurysm itself on CT scan or MRI (unruptured aneurysms). In either case, four-vessel cerebral angiography is needed to confirm the diagnosis and elucidate aneurysm anatomy.*

General Considerations

An aneurysm is a saccular dilation of an artery that typically occurs at a branch point or curve in the artery's course and generally points in the direction of blood flow. Usual aneurysm morphology consists of a neck (where the aneurysm originates from the parent artery), the body or fundus, and the dome. Small perforating branches that supply adjacent brain arise from the neck at some aneurysm sites (anterior communicating artery, internal carotid artery [ICA] bifurcation, and basilar apex). Aneurysms enlarge and rupture at the dome, where walls are thinnest and there is frequently a daughter sac or lobe. Saccular aneurysms are thought to be acquired degenerative defects that develop in response to relentless hemodynamic stress. However, defects in the media or internal elastic lamina may be genetically or congenitally influenced.

Aneurysms are named by their associated branch artery or, when not associated with a discrete branch, by their anatomic location. Aneurysms in the anterior circulation—in order from proximal to distal—include petrous ICA, cavernous ICA, clinoidal ICA, ophthalmic artery (OphA), superior hypophysial artery (SHA), Posterior communicating artery (PCoA), anterior choroidal artery (AChA), ICA bifurcation, anterior communicating artery (ACoA), pericallosal artery, and middle cerebral artery (MCA) aneurysms. Aneurysms in the posterior circulation, in anatomic order from proximal to distal, include vertebral artery (VA), posterior inferior cerebellar artery (PICA), vertebrobasilar junction (VBJ), anterior inferior cerebellar artery (AICA), superior cerebellar artery (SCA), basilar tip, and posterior cerebral artery (PCA) aneurysms. The most common aneurysms are ACoA, PCoA, MCA, and basilar tip aneurysms.

The prevalence rate of intracranial saccular aneurysms is between 0.1% and 9%, with rates around 0.5–1% in angiographic series and around 1–6% in autopsy studies. Approximately 25% of patients have multiple aneurysms. Intracranial arteries lie in the subarachnoid space between the pia and arachnoid layers, a space filled with cerebrospinal fluid and compartmentalized into interconnecting cisterns. Consequently, aneurysms also lie in the subarachnoid space (except for petrous, cavernous, and clinoidal ICA aneurysms), and ruptured aneurysms produce subarachnoid hemorrhage (SAH). In the USA, the annual incidence of SAH is 11 per 100,000, with an estimated 30,000 new cases each year. It accounts for 5–10% of all strokes and afflicts women more than men and blacks more than whites. SAH occurs most commonly in patients between the ages of 40 and 60 years. Aneurysm rupture is a potentially devastating event. The 30-day mortality rate for SAH is around 45%. Half of these patients die before arriving at a hospital from the effects of the initial hemorrhage, and many of the remainder die later of rebleeding or the effects of vasospasm. Survivors experience neurologic deficits in about 30% of cases.

While saccular aneurysms are the most common type, other nonsaccular aneurysms include fusiform (atherosclerotic), dissecting, traumatic, infectious, and neoplastic aneurysms. Fusiform aneurysms are tortuous, elongated, dilated arteries with separate inflow and outflow, most commonly seen in elderly patients with generalized atherosclerosis. Traumatic aneurysms are the result of direct arterial injury, with rupture of all three arterial layers (intima, media, and adventitia) and fibrous organization of the surrounding hematoma. In contrast, dissecting aneurysms result from tears through—but no deeper than—intima and internal elastic lamina. Infectious and neoplastic aneurysms develop from circulation of infectious material or tumor cells, often from a focus within the heart (eg, bacterial endocarditis, or atrial myxoma). Infectious emboli lodge in small distal cerebral arteries and occlude flow, after which intense inflammation in the adventitia and media destroys the integrity of the wall and weakens it. Neoplastic aneurysms have a similar pathogenesis except that arterial invasion is directly from tumor cells. The resulting aneurysms are typically fusiform, eccentric, and at distal sites.

Clinical Findings

A. Symptoms and Signs

Most aneurysms present with rupture. The classic presentation is a sudden, unusually severe headache that may be associated with nausea, vomiting, painful nuchal rigidity, and photophobia. The critical features that distinguish this headache from other headaches are its instantaneous onset and its severity. When asked to evaluate severity on a scale from 1 to 10, patients typically respond with a number off the scale. They describe their headaches as "the worst headache of my life" and can remember vivid details of events surrounding its onset. These symptoms are characteristic of a "sentinel hemorrhage," a small contained leak from the aneurysm without frank rupture. Misdiagnosis of a sentinel hemorrhage can be catastrophic because patients have the highest risk of rehemorrhage in the following 24 hours. An estimated 60% of SAH patients who seek medical attention are misdiagnosed and for that reason have worse outcomes than those who are properly diagnosed.

More severe hemorrhages produce seizures, neurologic deficits, impaired consciousness, and death. These more devastating presentations are often due to intraparenchymal or intraventricular extension of the hemorrhage or sustained elevation of intracranial pressure (ICP). Several grading scales are used to evaluate the severity of hemorrhage, providing a "shorthand" description of a patient's clinical condition and also some guidance in treatment decisions and prognosis. The Hunt-Hess Scale is the most common one (Table 37–9), but others include the Glasgow Coma Scale (GCS) and the World Federation of Neurological Surgeons (WFNS) Scale.

Table 37–9. Classification scales for subarachnoid hemorrhage.

A. Hunt-Hess Scale[1]

Grade	Criteria
I	Asymptomatic, or minimal headache, nuchal rigidity
II	Moderate to severe headache, no neurologic deficit except for cranial nerve palsy
III	Drowsiness, confusion, mild focal deficit
IV	Stupor, moderate to severe hemiparesis, early decerebrate posturing
V	Deep coma, decerebrate posturing, moribund

B. Glasgow Coma Scale

Points	Eye Opening	Verbal	Motor
6			Obeys commands
5		Oriented	Localizes pain
4	Spontaneous	Confused	Withdraws to pain
3	To voice	Inappropriate	Flexes (decorticate)
2	To pain	Incomprehensible	Extends (decerebrate)
1	None	None	None

C. World Federation of Neurological Surgeons Scale

Grade	Glasgow Coma Scale	Motor Deficit
I	15	None
II	13–14	None
III	13–14	Present
IV	7–12	Any
V	3–6	Any

D. Fisher Scale

Grade	Subarachnoid Blood
I	No blood detected
II	Diffuse, < 1 mm thick
III	Localized clot or thick layer, > 1 mm thick
IV	Diffuse or none, with intracerebral or intraventricular blood

[1]Reproduced, with permission, from Hunt WE, Hess RM: Surgical repair as related to time of intervention in the repair of intracranial aneurysms. J Neurosurg 1968;28:14.

Unruptured aneurysms are typically diagnosed incidentally during the evaluation of unrelated problems such as headaches or other neurologic symptoms. Still, unruptured aneurysms can present with symptoms related to mass effect or cerebral ischemia. The cranial nerve most frequently involved is the oculomotor nerve, which runs parallel to the posterior communicating artery and can be compressed by PCoA and basilar apex aneurysms. A patient presenting with a new oculomotor palsy (unilateral dilated pupil with deviation of the eye downward and laterally) should be considered to have an aneurysm until proved otherwise. With PCoA aneurysms, the dilated pupil usually precedes the diplopia because of the greater sensitivity and peripheral location of the parasympathetic fibers within the nerve. Cavernous ICA aneurysms may also present with oculomotor palsy but in addition may involve the trochlear, abducens, and trigeminal nerves. These patients have an immobile eye, retro-orbital pain, and facial numbness or dysesthesias. AChA aneurysms rarely cause oculomotor deficits but can impinge on the mesial temporal lobe to produce epilepsy or can compress the optic tract. ICA bifurcation aneurysms can also compress the optic tract and, when giant, the internal capsule to produce a contralateral hemiparesis.

Ophthalmic artery aneurysms lie under the optic nerve, and their growth to giant sizes (≥ 25 mm) causes progressive visual field loss, initially a unilateral inferior nasal field defect that may enlarge to involve the entire ipsilateral nasal field and the superior temporal loss in the contralateral eye (junctional scotoma). SHA aneurysms project medially toward the sella and produce bitemporal hemianopsias similar to those associated with pituitary tumors.

Large or giant basilar aneurysms can cause pressure on the midbrain, causing a contralateral hemiparesis from compression of the cerebral peduncle or hydrocephalus from occlusion of the cerebral aqueduct. The oculomotor deficits from basilar aneurysms tend to spare the pupil and cause ipsilateral ptosis and weakness of upgaze. Large basilar trunk, vertebrobasilar, and vertebral artery aneurysms can compress lower cranial nerves or nuclei with corresponding dysphasia, dysarthria, hoarseness, gait instability, and incoordination.

Giant aneurysms with intraluminal thrombus can present with ischemic symptoms if clot from the aneurysm embolizes downstream. This is particularly true with ICA and MCA aneurysms, manifesting with symptoms of aphasia and contralateral motor and sensory deficits. Ischemic symptoms account for 5–25% of symptoms from unruptured aneurysms.

B. Imaging Studies

The diagnosis of SAH requires the confirmation of blood in the subarachnoid space, which can be accomplished best with CT scan. Blood is easily seen on noncontrast CT scan, with a sensitivity of greater than 95%. In addition, the location of blood provides clues to the aneurysm location and identifies associated intracerebral and intraventricular hemorrhage. Hydrocephalus is a common finding in these patients because subarachnoid blood interferes with the normal circulation and reabsorption of cerebrospinal fluid. Often this associated hydrocephalus is more responsible for a patient's depressed level of consciousness than the hemorrhage itself and is reversible with ventriculostomy.

Ultimately, the diagnosis of an intracranial aneurysm depends on its identification with catheter angiography. A complete angiogram includes injections of all four major intracranial arteries (both ICAs and both VAs), filmed in two orthogonal views (anteroposterior and lateral). Additional views of the aneurysm are often needed to fully visualize its anatomy. Pre- and postinjection images are digitally subtracted to visualize just the vascular structures, removing shadows cast by the skull, skull base, and overlying opacities. These digital subtraction angiograms provide detailed information about the aneurysm location, anatomy, hemodynamics, other aneurysms, and collateral circulation. It should be remembered that angiographic images show the internal anatomy of an aneurysm, which may be much smaller than the external diameter of the aneurysm if it is filled with thrombus or coil material or thickened with calcium or atherosclerotic changes.

Catheter angiography has its disadvantages, namely, it is invasive, time-consuming, costly, and associated with increased risks (dissection, embolization, aneurysm rupture, and groin hematomas). Still, it is the most definitive test for the diagnosis of aneurysms. Angiograms generated with MR or CT data (MRA and CTA, respectively) are newer imaging modalities that currently do not provide all the information that catheter angiography does. Both CTA and MRA are noninvasive and easier to obtain. CTA results are available quickly and may play a role in unstable patients with ruptured aneurysms who need to get to the operating room right away. MRA is slower and lacks the resolution of CTA or conventional angiography, missing small aneurysms less than 3 mm in diameter. However, MRI or MRA is becoming a common method of detecting unruptured aneurysms in patients with other neurologic issues that have to be dealt with.

C. Laboratory Findings

Lumbar puncture is the only laboratory study that needs to be considered in the evaluation of an aneurysm patient. It is used in those cases where the patient's history is strongly suggestive of subarachnoid hemorrhage but the CT scan is normal. There are two explanations for this inconsistency. The first explanation is a sentinel hemorrhage that has leaked so little blood that it is not radiographically apparent. In this case, cerebrospinal fluid may be blood-tinged and will not clear in successive tubes. The second explanation is a delayed CT scan performed days after the subarachnoid hemorrhage. A delay in seeking medical attention or in ordering the CT scan allows subarachnoid blood to disperse, making it difficult to detect on the imaging study. In this case, cerebrospinal fluid will be xanthochromic, indicating that blood has been present for days and is being metabolized. If the fluid from a lumbar puncture is positive for new or old blood, further evaluation with an angiogram is indicated. It should be noted that so-called "traumatic taps" yield fluid that initially is bloody but clears in successive tubes. This finding should not be mistaken for true SAH.

Treatment

A. Rationale

Once an aneurysm has been diagnosed, a decision needs to be made about treatment. The primary cause of death and disability from aneurysms is the brain injury produced by the initial hemorrhage, and there is no treatment that can reverse it. Existing treatments are aimed instead at preventing the initial rupture or rerupture and reversing the effects of SAH, eg, vasospasm. There is little controversy about the need to treat ruptured aneurysms because of their high risk of rerupture (4% in the first 24 hours and 20% by the first 2 weeks after the initial hemorrhage). Furthermore, the mortality rate associated with rebleeding is 40%. Therefore, treatment is undertaken quickly after diagnosis, usually within 72 hours of the initial bleed. The only treatment controversy arises in poor-grade patients (Hunt-Hess grades IV and V), since these patients have a poor prognosis to begin with and aggressive management will yield good outcomes in only 25–40%. Patients with minimal neurologic function, uncontrollable ICP, or who are moribund are managed expectantly. Still, it is difficult to predict outcome, and an aggressive treatment policy is generally more prudent. In addition to protecting against rerupture, early treatment of ruptured aneurysms enables aggressive postoperative management of delayed vasospasm with induced hypertension.

The treatment of unruptured aneurysms is more controversial because of the difficulty of accurately determining the risks of rupture and the risks of treatment. The annual risk of aneurysm rupture is between 0.05% and 2%. Factors that contribute to rupture risk are the size and location, the presence of another aneurysm that has ruptured, and possibly hypertension and smoking. While there is no critical size or cutoff value, there are prospective data showing increased rupture risk in aneurysms 10 mm or more in diameter. The cumulative natural history risk of an aneurysm is determined by estimating the patient's life expectancy in years and extrapolating the annual rupture risk over this interval. Therefore, a patient's age and general health impact the treatment decision. In making a choice between treating an aneurysm or observing it, one must compare this natural history risk with the treatment risk. Morbidity and mortality rates associated with surgery for unruptured aneurysms vary from 4 to 15% and 0–4%, respectively. Many factors influence surgical outcome, including aneurysm size, location, and morphology; patient age, symptoms, and medical condition; and the experience of the surgical team and hospital staff. Weighing these factors together, treatment is generally recommended for patients with large or symptomatic aneurysms or another previously ruptured aneurysm. Treatment is favored in young patients with long life expectancies, a family history of aneurysm rupture, multiple aneurysms, or documented growth. Conservative management is favored in older patients, those with small aneurysms and short life expectancies, or severe comorbid medical conditions. Ultimately, patient preferences will determine the final decision with unruptured aneurysms.

B. Initial Management of SAH

After a ruptured aneurysm is diagnosed, the aneurysm is secured as quickly as possible. In the meantime, efforts are made to stabilize the patient and minimize the risk of rerupture. Most important is blood pressure control. Rebleeding is caused by absolute elevations in blood pressure and also rapid variations. Blood pressure should be carefully monitored with invasive arterial lines in an ICU setting where intravenous agents or drips can be administered. Hydrocephalus is present in approximately one-fourth of SAH patients and resolves with the insertion of a ventriculostomy. External ventricular drainage can improve the clinical status of patients dramatically and is recommended in all obtunded or comatose patients. In addition, ventriculostomy allows ICP to be transduced and can guide preoperative management of increased pressures. In poor-grade patients, intubation and mechanical ventilation is usually needed to protect the airway and sometimes to hyperventilate the patient for ICP management. Other comfort measures such as bed rest, sedation, and analgesics help minimize agitation that might precipitate rerupture. Seizures can precipitate rerupture, and anticonvulsants are given in the immediate post-SAH period.

C. Surgical Management

Clipping of the aneurysm neck effectively closes the aneurysm and keeps blood from flowing into it. The clip application is done under direct visualization under an operating microscope, allowing preservation of flow in the parent and perforating arteries around its base. Once clipped, an aneurysm can be deflated or opened to removed blood and thrombus that might be compressing neural structures. Blood in the subarachnoid spaces can also be removed directly or diluted with irrigation, which may have some beneficial effects on subsequent vasospasm. Microsurgical clipping provides an immediate, durable cure for aneurysms. The recurrence rate after clipping is less than 1%, and after an immediate postoperative angiogram no follow-up imaging is required.

Surgical clipping requires exposure of the aneurysm. There are many surgical approaches for aneurysms, but the most common is the pterional or frontotemporal craniotomy. It provides direct exposure of the internal carotid artery from its entry into the subarachnoid space to its terminus, working in the space between the frontal and temporal lobes. Extensive removal of bone from the skull base (pterion, sphenoid ridge, and orbital roof), as well as opening the lateral cerebral sulcus to further separate the frontal and temporal lobes, creates ample room to access all ICA, ACoA, MCA, and basilar apex aneurysms. Additional exposure can be gained by removing the orbital rim with the orbitozygomatic approach, commonly used for giant anterior circulation aneurysms and basilar apex aneurysms. Posterior circulation aneurysms are accessed through the far-lateral approach (PICA aneurysms), one of the transpetrosal approaches (VBJ, AICA, and midbasilar artery aneurysms), or a combined transpetrosal-subtemporal approach that communicates the regions above and below the tentorium in front of the sigmoid sinus.

The vast majority of aneurysms (> 95%) can be treated with direct surgical clipping. However, aneurysms that are giant-sized, fusiform in shape, or lacking a defined neck may require alternative techniques such as trapping or proximal occlusion. These techniques can be performed safely if trial arterial occlusion with a balloon-tipped catheter is tolerated by the patient without ischemic deficits. Hypotensive challenge or cerebral blood flow studies increase the accuracy of balloon test occlusion. Bypass procedures are indicated in those patients who do not tolerate their balloon test occlusion, and a variety of bypasses are available to meet the flow demands of the involved vascular territory. The superficial temporal artery (STA) is a commonly used donor artery that can revascularize the middle cerebral artery territory. Saphenous vein grafts can also be used to bypass aneurysms along the ICA as it travels through the skull base and cavernous sinus, providing flows equal to the native ICA. Intracranial arteries such as the distal MCA, ACA, or PICA can be used as donor arteries to revascularize adjacent arteries with proximal aneurysms. Wrapping an aneurysm with cotton is another surgical alternative used as a last resort, externally reinforcing the walls with a material that elicits an inflammatory reaction to promote scarring and thickening of the aneurysm.

D. Endovascular Management

Endosaccular occlusion of intracranial aneurysms has become an acceptable alternative to microsurgical clipping during the past decade. This technique is performed using electrolytically detachable Guglielmi coils (GDC) deployed through transfemoral intra-aneurysmal catheters and angiographic visualization. In general, aneurysm coiling appears to have lower morbidity and mortality rates than surgery but higher rates of incomplete obliteration and higher rates of recurrence, making its long-term efficacy still unproved. Complications from endovascular coiling are different from those associated with surgery and include arterial dissection, intraoperative aneurysm rupture, parent artery occlusion, distal embolization, and groin hematomas. Although overall complication rates are around 8%, permanent neurologic morbidity is observed in around 4%. Mortality rates are up to 2%. The rates of complete aneurysm occlusion vary according to aneurysm size and morphology and range between 35% and 80%. Consequently, incompletely coiled aneurysms may not be protected from rehemorrhage risk, and new hemorrhages in patients treated with coils have been reported to be around 3–4%. Furthermore, endosaccular coils remain exposed to hemodynamic forces that can shift or compact the coils or promote growth of the aneurysm around the coils. Aneurysm recurrence after coiling has been reported in 5–45% of cases. Therefore, surveillance angiography is required and recurrences can pose complicated treatment issues.

Currently in North America, endovascular coils are used as a primary treatment for elderly patients, those considered to have high surgical risk, and those who are medically unsuitable for surgery. The minimally invasive appeal of this treatment is increasing patient interest and demand. In addition, new deployment techniques that use balloons to protect the parent artery from coil herniation and new devices such as three-dimensional coils and stents make aneurysms with unfavorable anatomy treatable with endovascular methods. For example, stent-supported coil embolization lays a stent across a wide aneurysm neck and deploys coils through the interstices of the stent. Endovascular techniques have become an integral part of multimodality therapy for aneurysms and will be increasingly utilized in the future.

E. Vasospasm

Vasospasm is the narrowing of cerebral arteries from smooth muscle cell contraction in the vessel walls, leading to diminished cerebral perfusion, ischemia, and infarction. Vasospasm typically occurs during a time period 4–14 days after SAH and resolves spontaneously thereafter. The pathogenesis is unclear but is related to the amount and distribution of blood in the subarachnoid space. The Fisher Grading Scale is a useful predictor of a patient's likelihood of developing vasospasm. Approximately 70% of patients experience some degree of vasospasm, with 20–30% developing ischemic symptoms. The mortality from vasospasm alone has been estimated between to be 5% and 15%, and the neurologic morbidity has been estimated at around 6%.

Patients at risk of developing vasospasm are monitored closely in an ICU. All patients are given nimodipine, a calcium-channel blocker that inhibits vascular smooth muscle cell contraction and platelet aggregation. It is started within 4 days of SAH and continued for 21 days, regardless of admission grade, at a dose of 60 mg every 4 hours. Vasospasm is detected with angiography, transcranial Doppler ultrasonography (TCD), or changes in the neurologic examination. Angiography is the optimal diagnostic study but is limited by its invasiveness. TCD measures velocity of blood flow in cerebral arteries, which increases as arteries narrow with vasospasm. Therefore, measuring TCD velocities indirectly monitors vasospasm. TCD is noninvasive and can be done repeatedly to detect trends. Rising TCD velocities guide the timing of more aggressive measures, like hypertensive therapy and angioplasty.

The mainstay of medical management is hypervolemia, hypertension, and hemodilution (HHH therapy). Volume expansion is achieved with packed red blood cells, albumin solution, or hypertonic saline solution. Invasive monitoring with either a central venous pressure line or a pulmonary artery catheter is required to guide fluid management. Volume expansion to central venous pressures greater than 8 mm Hg or diastolic pulmonary artery pressures of greater than 14 mm Hg is usually enough to dilute the hematocrit to under 35%. In addition, volume expansion may increase systolic blood pressure to desired end points. As the patient's clinical condition demands, the blood pressure is elevated further with pressor agents to systolic values between 180 mm Hg and 220 mm Hg.

Endovascular therapies for vasospasm are becoming increasingly utilized when aggressive medical management fails, when TCD velocities rise, or when there are multiple risk factors for severe vasospasm. Transluminal balloon angioplasty (TBA) mechanically dilates segments of large cerebral arteries that are in spasm, usually restoring the normal caliber of the lumen. This intervention immediately improves blood flow to ischemic brain and typically results in clinical improvement. Furthermore, the effects of angioplasty appear to last up to a week, which corresponds to the duration of vasospasm. The success of this intervention has largely to do with timing. Early angioplasty before or immediately after neurologic deterioration enhances its efficacy.

TBA is limited to large cerebral arteries such as ICA, MCA, and ACA. Transluminal balloon angioplasty is limited to large vessels such as the internal, middle, and anterior cerebral arteries. Smaller distal arteries are not amenable to angioplasty and instead can be treated with intra-arterial papaverine infusion. Superselective infusion of papaverine, a potent vasodilator, can improve the caliber of vasospastic arteries, but the effects are short-lived (< 12 hours). Repeated treatments may be needed for severe distal vasospasm, which limits its utility.

Prognosis

Outcome depends on the extent of damage done by the initial aneurysm hemorrhage or subsequent rehemorrhage, complications resulting from treatment, and complications resulting from vasospasm. Of these factors, the initial injury is most important. The patient's preoperative status as assessed by the Hunt-Hess Scale is perhaps the best predictor of outcome. Good recovery, as defined by Glasgow Outcome Scores, can be expected in 97% of grade I patients, 88% of grade II patients, and 81% of grade III patients. In these low-grade patients, 55% resumed in their normal living conditions, 67% returned to full-time work, and 23% reported physical disabilities. In contrast, poor-grade patients (Hunt-Hess grade IV and grade V) have less favorable outcomes. Left untreated, more than 90% of grade V patients will die or be severely disabled. When treated aggressively, between one-fourth and one-third of poor-grade patients will have a favorable outcome.

Brilstra EH et al: Treatment of intracranial aneurysms by embolization with coils: a systematic review. Stroke 1999;30:470.

Chyatte D, Porterfield R: Nuances of middle cerebral artery aneurysm microsurgery. Neurosurgery 2001;48:339.

Dovey Z et al: Guglielmi detachable coiling for intracranial aneurysms: the story so far. Arch Neurol 2001;58:559.

Hacein-Bey L et al: Complex intracranial aneurysms: combined operative and endovascular approaches. Neurosurgery 1998;43:1304.

Thornton J et al: What percentage of surgically clipped intracranial aneurysms have residual necks? Neurosurgery 2000;46:1294.

Tregiarie-Venzi MM, Suter PM, Romand JA: Review of medical prevention of vasospasm after aneurysmal subarachnoid hemorrhage: a problem of neurointensive care. Neurosurgery 2001;48:249.

ARTERIOVENOUS MALFORMATIONS

G. Edward Vates, MD, PhD, & Michael T. Lawton, MD

ESSENTIALS OF DIAGNOSIS

- *Arteriovenous malformations (AVMs) present with seizures, spontaneous subarachnoid or intracerebral hemorrhage, or progressive neurologic deficit.*
- *AVMs can present at any age but more commonly become symptomatic during the second or third decades of life.*
- *CT and MRI often suggest the diagnosis and can provide important information about the location of the lesion in relation to critical brain structures; cerebral angiography is diagnostic and essential for planning therapy.*

General Considerations

Arteriovenous malformations (AVMs) occur within the central nervous system as congenital anomalies that allow blood to be shunted directly from arteries to veins without an interposed capillary network. Afferent and efferent vessels are dilated, and they lead to and from a tangle of malformed channels (the nidus) containing arterial blood. Because these abnormal vessels receive blood at arterial pressure, bleeding can result. AVMs can also grow over time through a combination of vessel enlargement and recruitment of new vessels, perhaps involving mechanisms of angiogenesis. Congestion of draining veins with arterial blood flow can also lead to neurologic symptoms by causing venous hypertension and reduced perfusion in adjacent brain areas. Excision of the malformation will restore normal perfusion to the uninvolved brain.

AVMs can be small, with only a single feeding artery, or they can encompass several lobes of the brain and have arterial feeders from multiple sources. They can occur in virtually any portion of the nervous system but are most common in the cerebral hemispheres (90% of AVMs). Cerebral AVMs are usually conical, with the apex near the ventricles and a broad base at the cortical surface; large cortical AVMs commonly present with seizures caused by irritation of adjacent cortical tissue. Small AVMs are more likely to present with spontaneous hemorrhage, causing headache, neurologic deficits, coma, or even death. AVMs can be associated with flow-related aneurysms on feeding arteries or can have aneurysms on vessels within the nidus of the AVM itself. If aneurysms are present, they are usually the source of hemorrhage. AVMs can occur in the cerebellum or brain stem but are much less common. Rarely, AVMs occur within the spinal cord, or they may involve only the dura (intracranial or intraspinal).

Patients with AVMs usually develop symptoms before age 40 (but usually not during childhood). The most common presentation is hemorrhage (50–65%), followed by seizures (15–35%). Mortality and morbidity with each hemorrhage are 10–30% and 15–50%, respectively. For the first year after a hemorrhage, the risk of another hemorrhage is 6%, but for all subsequent years the annual risk drops to 2%, which is the risk of hemorrhage in an unruptured AVM that presents with other signs or symptoms.

Clinical Findings

A. Symptoms and Signs

Hemorrhage may cause symptoms ranging from headaches to focal neurologic deficits to coma, or the defect can be clinically silent. The site of the hemorrhage will determine the neurologic deficit but the size of a hemorrhage is often irrelevant, as small hematomas in eloquent areas cause more impairment than large ones in silent areas of the brain. Hemorrhage into the ventricles of the brain can cause hydrocephalus that must be managed with ventricular drainage. Hemorrhage into the subarachnoid space can cause headache and nuchal rigidity, much like subarachnoid hemorrhage from an aneurysmal hemorrhage. However, the subsequent risk of vasospasm is usually much less after AVM-related subarachnoid hemorrhage than after aneurysmal subarachnoid hemorrhage; this is probably due to differences in the amount and distribution of subarachnoid blood found after AVM versus aneurysmal rupture. (AVMs leak less blood that is distributed over the convexities, while aneurysms leak more blood into the basilar cisterns, adjacent to the origins of the major brain arteries as they emerge from the skull base.)

Seizures can be focal or general and may cause temporary postictal neurologic deficits. The clinical importance of AVM presentation with seizures is that it may allow for treatment of an AVM prior to symptomatic hemorrhage. There are insufficient data in the literature to predict either the seizure frequency or the prognosis of seizure control based on the size or location of an AVM, though frontal or temporal lobe AVMs are more commonly associated with seizures.

Headaches are common in patients with AVMs, but headache is one of the most common neurologic complaints. It is difficult to show a precise relationship between headache and AVMs, and the literature is inconclusive on the subject of which (if any) headache syndromes reliably predict an underlying AVM.

Focal neurologic deficits can occur in the absence of hemorrhage or seizure in patients with AVMs. These symptoms were once thought to be due to "steal" of arterial blood from adjacent areas of functional brain by the high-flow arteriovenous shunt of an AVM. However, recent studies using measurements of intra-arterial and intravenous pressure and blood flow in AVMs and adjacent cortical territories in patients suggest that focal neurologic symptoms may be produced by venous congestion leading to venous hypertension and ischemia in adjacent cortical territories.

It is worth noting one uncommon but well-known complication of large AVMs in infants and children: arteriovenous shunting leading to left ventricular dysfunction and high-output cardiac failure. Frequently, these children will have an audible cranial bruit and can present with noncommunicating hydrocephalus due to obstruction of the cerebral aqueduct by enlarged basal veins surrounding the midbrain.

B. Laboratory Findings

If a patient presents with sudden-onset headache or neurologic deficits, a CT scan is usually all that is required for diagnosis of an intracranial or subarachnoid hemorrhage (see below). However, if this is not diagnostic, lumbar puncture may be required to establish the presence of subarachnoid blood that would prompt rigorous search for a cause.

C. Imaging Studies

Any young adult presenting with new-onset severe headache, neurologic deficits, coma, or seizures should first be studied by noncontrast CT scan, which will routinely demonstrate intracerebral or subarachnoid blood if a hemorrhage has occurred and, in the absence of bleeding, may suggest a mass lesion without contrast. CT scans also help to guide immediate management decisions such as the need for emergency hematoma evacuation or ventriculostomy for hydrocephalus and intraventricular hemorrhage. MR imaging with intravenous gadolinium contrast defines the relationships of the AVM to surrounding brain structures and can be critical in assessing the surgical risks and choosing the appropriate surgical approach.

Four-vessel cerebral arteriography (both carotid arteries and both vertebral arteries) is the standard test used to define the vascular anatomy of AVMs. This procedure identifies all feeding arteries, all compartments of the nidus, and all draining veins. In addition, angiography can identify associated aneurysms within the nidus or those on feeding arteries far removed from the nidus. Selective external carotid artery injections should be performed on the side of large lesions because many will have feeding artery contributions from the dura or from external-to-internal carotid anastomoses that can be embolized easily. If surgical resection is planned, angiography with endovascular embolization of large feeding arteries can significantly reduce arterial supply to an AVM prior to surgery and thereby make resection much less difficult.

It should be noted that any or all of the studies described above can fail to detect an AVM nidus immediately after acute hemorrhage because the intraparenchymal clot can compress the nidus and close it off, making it radiographically "silent." Therefore, in any patient suspected of having an AVM-related hemorrhage but in whom MRI and angiography are not diagnostic, these studies should be repeated 1–3 months after the hemorrhage. By this time, the hematoma will have been absorbed and any underlying vascular pathology should be evident. On occasion, bleeding may be due to a cavernous malformation, another kind of vascular malformation whose characteristic appearance on MRI is described below.

Differential Diagnosis

Hemorrhage—intracerebral or subarachnoid—can be caused by hypertension, amyloid angiopathy, diabetes mellitus, or hemorrhagic conversion of an ischemic stroke, but these diseases are unlikely in the age group usually affected by AVM-related hemorrhage. Therefore, in the absence of blood dyscrasia, spontaneous intracranial hemorrhage in a child or young adult is the hallmark of an AVM. Other diagnostic considerations include an intracranial aneurysm or a primary brain neoplasm or secondary metastatic lesion within the brain that has bled spontaneously. Each of these has a characteristic appearance on MRI or angiography and can be easily differentiated from an AVM. Cavernous malformations ("cryptic" vascular malformations) are the second most frequently seen cerebrovascular malformation but are nonetheless much less common than AVMs. They are composed of small-caliber venous sinusoidal vascular channels that are commonly thrombosed, and because of their slow flow they are usually angiographically "silent." Their low flow also makes them less likely to bleed (annual risk of 0.7%) and less likely to cause neurologic deficits when they do. These defects have a characteristic "mulberry" appearance on MRI and are usually surrounded by a ring of T2-weighted susceptibility that makes them easy to distinguish from AVMs. They typically present with seizures unless they are located in the brain stem, where even a small venous hemorrhage can cause a profound and sudden neurologic deterioration. These are treated with surgical removal.

A wide range of structural and biochemical disorders can cause seizures although, as noted before, they usually give rise to a radiographic evaluation that can suggest or prove the presence of an AVM.

Treatment

A. Medical Treatment

Medical treatment is only effective for relieving symptoms or for reducing posthemorrhagic sequelae. Anticonvulsants can control AVM-incited seizures, and blood pressure control is important after a hemorrhage, especially if the hemorrhage is due to an AVM-related aneurysm.

B. Surgical Treatment

The ideal treatment of an AVM is excision and removal of any associated hematoma. However, treatment must be guided by two basic principles: (1) The AVM should be removed completely, because any residual nidus can still bleed; and (2) neurologic function should be preserved. Some malformations cannot be removed with reasonable risk, and some of these can be treated by endovascular embolization or focused irradiation (stereotactic radiosurgery; see below).

In an attempt to determine which patients should or should not be offered surgery, a number of grading systems have been developed. AVM grading systems are important for estimating the risk of operation compared with the risks associated with the natural history of the lesion, and for these reasons they should be simple but comprehensive enough to grade all AVMs, address all factors that influence treatment risk, and predict these treatment risks. Most grading systems are based on radiographic features of the lesion. The most widely accepted grading system is the Spetzler-Martin system, which attempts to predict the risk of surgical resection based on three variables: AVM size, pattern of venous drainage, and location in relation to eloquent brain (Table 37–10). Size is scored by measuring the greatest diameter of the AVM on angiography, MRI, or CT and relates to the number of feeding arteries and the degree of flow. Venous drainage is scored by determining whether the AVM empties into the superficial cortical venous system or into the deep venous system (internal cerebral veins, basal veins of Rosenthal, or vein of Galen); this relates to the depth of the AVM and surgical accessibility. Eloquence is scored by the proximity of the AVM nidus to areas of brain that have easily identifiable neurologic function and, when injured, produce dis-

Table 37–10. Spetzler-Martin grading system for AVMs.

Factor	Point Weight
Factor 1: AVM size	
Small (< 3 cm)	1
Medium (3–6 cm)	2
Large (> 6 cm)	3
Factor 2: Functional eloquence of location	
Noneloquent	0
Eloquent	1
Factor 3: Pattern of venous drainage	
Surface cortical only	0
Deep drainage component	1

Total grade = sum of all three factors (grades 1–5).

abling neurologic deficits (motor and sensory cortex, deep gray matter, corticospinal tracts, or brain stem). A numerical AVM grade is then assigned by adding the scores for size, venous drainage, and eloquence. AVMs can then be stratified into five grades, with grade 1 lesions being small, superficial, and in noneloquent brain and grade 5 lesions being large and deep in eloquent brain.

Prospective analysis of AVM grade and surgical results in 120 patients showed minimal risk associated with surgical resection of AVMs in patients with grade 1 or grade 2 lesions, with no new neurologic deficits after surgery. We therefore recommend aggressive surgical excision of these lesions. In contrast, surgical resection of grade 4 and grade 5 AVMs resulted in 15–20% incidence of new deficits. Patients with grade 4 and grade 5 AVMs are recommended for surgical treatment only when they suffer repeated hemorrhages or are experiencing a rapid and progressive neurologic decline. Grade 3 lesions remain ambiguous in that some studies suggest these lesions can be resected with low surgical morbidity while others report an unacceptable surgical risk. This may be due to the variability in the nature of these lesions as prescribed by the Spetzler-Martin grading system, and patients with grade 3 malformation should therefore be evaluated on an individual basis. Patients whose neurologic condition is deteriorating are typically ready to accept surgical risks, whereas patients who are neurologically intact may prefer to postpone treatment until absolute indications are present and the surgical risks become more acceptable relative to the natural history of the AVM. Because the risk of hemorrhage accrues annually, young patients are exposed to substantial cumulative risk during their lifetimes and may be more amenable to a strategy of surgical excision.

Endovascular embolization as sole treatment of AVMs is usually unacceptable because complete occlusion rates are low and the long-term occlusion rates are unknown. Therefore, embolization should be used as part of a multimodality approach to either devascularize a large lesion before surgery or reduce its size before radiosurgery. In this context, embolization can significantly simplify surgical resection or can convert a large AVM into a much smaller one that can be more effectively treated with radiosurgery.

Stereotactic radiosurgery is rapidly gaining attention as an alternative treatment for AVMs and has been shown to work well for small defects. However, radiosurgical obliteration is inversely related to AVM size, with larger lesions showing a lower rate of occlusion after delivery of radiation. In addition, there is a lag-time in the onset of effectiveness; generally, radiosurgery takes up to 2 years to achieve full effect, and during that time studies suggest that the risk of hemorrhage from an irradiated AVM may actually increase compared with an untreated AVM. Therefore, we do not currently recommend stereotactic radiosurgery for small AVMs, as these lesions can be surgically resected with no morbidity and with immediate elimination of the risk of hemorrhage. Instead, stereotactic radiation can be used as part of a multimodal treatment plan for deep AVMs located in critical brain structures where there is no easy surgical access. Such an AVM can be reduced in size, either by endovascular embolization or partial surgical resection, and then obliterated with stereotactic radiation therapy applied to the much smaller residual nidus.

Postoperative Complications

The complication rates associated with resection of AVMs of different grades are reviewed above. The most important postoperative complication relates to a phenomenon called "normal perfusion pressure breakthrough." Once an AVM has been resected, the shunting of blood through the nidus is gone, thus restoring normal perfusion and normal arterial pressure within vessels of adjacent brain. Because shunting through the AVM has altered the autoregulation of these vessels, these arteries are ill-suited for accommodation of the new influx of arterial blood and can hemorrhage. The actual risk of normal perfusion pressure hemorrhage is unknown, but because of the theoretical risk, blood pressure control is critical during the first 24–48 hours after surgery while arteries adjacent to the AVM nidus reestablish their normal autoregulation.

Postoperative hemorrhage should also sound the alarm for a possible residual AVM nidus. Nothing short of complete AVM resection will protect the patient from further hemorrhage, and all patients should therefore undergo postoperative angiography to verify complete obliteration of the AVM nidus. Intraoperative angiography should be considered in selected cases of either large or deep AVMs where it can be difficult to determine if resection is complete. In addition, any patient treated with stereotactic radiation should undergo follow-up angiography 2–3 years after treatment; if there is residual nidus, this may need to be treated with further stereotactic radiotherapy (staged radiosurgery) or with conventional microsurgical removal.

Prognosis

The annual risk of hemorrhage from an unruptured AVM is approximately 2%. This risk doubles during the first year after a hemorrhage but then drops back to the prehemorrhage annual rate for all subsequent years. The morbidity associated with each hemorrhage is 15–50%, and the mortality is 10–30%. Because the lesion is present at birth, there is a lifelong risk of serious complications from bleeding and neurologic deficits. In contrast, the overall morbidity from AVM treatment is less than 10%, and the overall mortality is less than 5%, though this varies widely depending on the grade of AVM, as described above. The patient's preoperative neurologic condition is also important. Patients who present with devastating hemorrhage may not deteriorate with treatment but will be left with disabling deficits that require prolonged rehabilitation. Age is also an important factor because young patients are much more resilient after treatment than elderly ones. However, with adequate time, full recovery is usually possible; studies have demonstrated that most early neurologic deficits after surgery will resolve.

Drake CG: Cerebral arteriovenous malformations: considerations for and experience with surgical treatment in 166 cases. Clin Neurosurg 1979;26:145.

Hamilton MG, Spetzler RF: The prospective application of a grading system for arteriovenous malformations. Neurosurgery 1994;34:2.

Heros RC, Morcos J, Korosue K: Arteriovenous malformations of the brain. Surgical management. Clin Neurosurg 1993;40:139.

Lawton MT, Hamilton MG, Spetzler RF: Multimodality treatment of deep arteriovenous malformations: thalamus, basal ganglia, and brain stem. Neurosurgery 1995;37:29.

Lunsford LD et al: Stereotactic radiosurgery for arteriovenous malformations of the brain [see comments]. J Neurosurg 1991;75:512.

Steiner L et al: Microsurgery and radiosurgery in brain arteriovenous malformations [editorial] [see comments]. J Neurosurg 1993;79:647.

MOVEMENT DISORDERS RESPONSIVE TO SURGERY

Philip Starr, MD

Recently, there has been a resurgence of interest in subcortical brain surgery for movement disorders. Movement disorders amenable to surgical treatment include Parkinson's disease (PD), essential tremor, and generalized dystonia.

PARKINSON'S DISEASE

ESSENTIALS OF DIAGNOSIS

- *Idiopathic Parkinson's disease is diagnosed clinically, as there is no laboratory test short of brain examination at autopsy by which it can be diagnosed with certainty. The criteria for diagnosis are as follows:*
- *At least 2 of the following 4 cardinal clinical signs: rigidity, bradykinesia, tremor, and postural instability.*
- *Symptomatic improvement in response to oral administration of levodopa.*
- *Exclusion, by MRI and clinical history, of atypical parkinsonism.*

General Considerations

Surgery for Parkinson's disease has a long history. Beginning in the 1950s, thalamotomy (lesioning of the motor thalamus) and pallidotomy (lesioning of the globus pallidus) were performed before a solid scientific basis for these procedures was established. When treatment of Parkinson's disease with oral levodopa became widespread in the 1960s, surgical treatment declined. In the 1990s, several factors combined to produce a resurgence of interest in surgery for Parkinson's disease:

- Improved surgical techniques, including MRI and CT-guided stereotaxy
- Recognition of the limitations of long-term medical therapy as the disease advances
- Understanding of the theoretical basis for basal ganglia surgery in Parkinson's disease
- The development of chronic deep brain stimulation as a reversible, adjustable alternative to lesioning surgery.

Pathogenesis

Parkinson's disease is an idiopathic, progressive neurodegenerative disorder involving loss of dopaminergic cells in the substantia nigra pars compacta (SNc). Loss of dopaminergic neurons of the SNc results in excessive and abnormally patterned activity in the subthalamic nucleus (STN) and in its major target nuclei, the internal segment of the globus pallidus (GPI) and the substantia nigra, pars reticulata (SNr). Since GPi and SNr have inhibitory projections to motor regions of the thalamus, thalamocortical activity is suppressed. This is thought to be the basis for many of the motor abnormalities in Parkinson's disease. As predicted by this model, inactivation of brain tissue in STN or GPi—effectively decreasing the inhibitory influence on the motor thalamus and, thus, "normalizing" thalamocortical activity—was found to be effective in treating parkinsonism in animal models. This provided the theoretical basis for pallidal and subthalamic surgery for Parkinson's disease in humans.

Differential Diagnosis

Idiopathic Parkinson's disease must be distinguished from a variety of atypical parkinsonian symptoms, which include multisystem atrophy and progressive supranuclear palsy. While the symptoms may be similar, atypical parkinsonism should be suspected if the symptoms have never responded robustly to oral dopamine replacement. The distinction is important to neurosurgeons since atypical parkinsonism is unresponsive to basal ganglia surgery.

Medical Treatment

A variety of pharmacologic treatments are initially effective in reducing the symptoms of Parkinson's disease. Treatment with levodopa in combination with carbidopa (Sinemet) is the mainstay of pharmacotherapy. Sinemet is usually supplemented with dopamine agonists such as pergolide or pramipexole. The activity of levodopa may be prolonged by inhibitors of catechol-*O*-methyl transferase (COMT) such as entacapone. After 5–15 years of treatment, Sinemet continues to produce a beneficial response, but its utility is compromised by peak-dose dyskinesias and a shorter, more unpredictable duration of action. When patients develop these complications of medical therapy, they are considered for surgery.

Surgical Treatment

Three types of surgery for Parkinson's disease are in current practice or under clinical investigation:

- Lesioning surgery
- Deep brain stimulation (DBS)
- "Restorative" therapies such as intrastriatal transplantation of dopamine-secreting cells or intrastriatal delivery of growth factors

Lesioning and deep brain stimulation procedures attempt to compensate for, rather than correct, the brain defect in Parkinson's disease, by interruption of abnormal basal ganglia output. Deep brain stimulation has similar effects on motor function as lesioning, but has several advantages: It is reversible in the event of an unwanted stimulation induced-effect, it can be adjusted as symptoms change, and it is safer for bilateral use.

In contrast, cell transplantation and growth factor infusion strategies attempt to correct the biochemical defect of Parkinson's disease by replacing lost dopaminergic brain cells. Human fetal substantia nigra allografts can survive in the human brain without long-term immunosuppression. However, in two randomized, placebo-controlled clinical trials of intrastriatal fetal dopaminergic allograft transplantation, alleviation of parkinsonian signs was modest and uncontrollable involuntary movements occurred in a subset of patients. A more promising strategy at present is intrastriatal infusion of glial-derived neurotrophic factor (GDNF), which is entering phase III clinical trials.

Outcomes of surgery are measured by changes in the Unified Parkinson's Disease Rating Scale (UPDRS), a quantitative rating scale of overall function in Parkinson's disease. At this time, bilateral deep brain stimulation of the globus pallidus or subthalamic nucleus appears to offer the greatest symptomatic relief for Parkinson's disease, producing 40–60% improvements in the motor subscore of the UPDRS in the off-medication state, with efficacy persisting at 5 years after surgery. The best results of intrastriatal human allograft transplantation were only a 20–30% improvement. In a pilot study, intrastriatal infusion of GDNF produced a 39% improvement in the UPDRS motor subscore.

Surgical Techniques

Because the basal ganglia are deep structures, they are approached through small skull openings without direct visualization of the target structures, rather than by open craniotomy. Target localization is performed by the method of stereotaxis. In stereotactic neurosurgery, a stereotactic frame is fixed to the patient's head to provide both an external coordinate system and a mechanical platform on which to mount instruments and direct them to known coordinates in the patient's brain. A brain image, such as CT or MR, is then obtained to visualize both the frame and the target within the patient's brain. The coordinates of the brain target, in the coordinate system defined by the frame, are calculated. In the operating room, instruments are mounted on the frame and directed toward the image-defined stereotactic target. Correct identification of the target is confirmed by intraoperative physiological studies, such as neuronal recording with microelectrodes. The neurologic status of the patient (such as strength, vision, and improvement of motor function) must be monitored frequently during the procedure.

Postoperative Complications

Hemorrhagic stroke occurs in 1–5% of patients undergoing stereotactic neurosurgery for movement disorders. Transient postoperative confusion is common in elderly patients or following bilateral surgery. For deep brain stimulation implants, perioperative infection of the device occurs in 3–5% of cases.

Prognosis

Idiopathic Parkinson's disease is progressive, with slow worsening of all motor symptoms, and in late-stage Parkinson's disease, cognitive decline. It is currently unknown whether any of the surgical treatments alters the course of Parkinson's disease. One of the investigational therapies, intrastriatal infusion of GDNF, has shown a neuroprotective effect in animal models of Parkinson's disease, but it is not yet known if this will be proved in clinical trials.

ESSENTIAL TREMOR

Essential tremor is characterized by tremor of the arms, head, or voice, without other neurologic signs. The arm tremor is more prominent with outstretched postures and action than at rest. In about 50% of cases there is a clear family history. It is not a degenerative disease, as the brain MRI and pathologic examination of the brain are normal.

Three classes of drugs can be used to treat essential tremor: beta-blockers such as propranolol, barbiturate derivatives such as primidone, and benzodiazepines such as clonazepam. Surgery should be considered if the tremor interferes with activities of daily living and fails to respond to these medications. Lesioning or deep brain stimulation of the ventralis intermedius nucleus (Vim) of the motor thalamus are both effective for essential tremor, though in a randomized study thalamic stimulation was associated with slightly lower complication rate.

DYSTONIA

Dystonia is a movement disorder defined as a syndrome of sustained muscle contractions, frequently causing twisting and repetitive movements, and abnormal postures. Electromyographic studies show abnormal cocontraction of agonist and antagonist muscles, prolongation of the electromyographic bursts, and overflow of electromyographic activity into muscle groups outside the area of intended movement. Reciprocal inhibition in spinal and brain stem reflexes is diminished. Dystonia may be classified according to body part (focal, segmental, or generalized), age of onset, or according to presumed etiology. Four etiologic subcategories of dystonia are now recognized: primary dystonia, dystonia-plus syndromes, secondary dystonia, and heredodegenerative dystonias.

Medical therapy with anticholinergic drugs such as trihexyphenidyl, or injection of botulinum toxin into the affected muscles, should be the initial treatment. Lesioning or deep brain stimulation of the GPi have been shown to be effective for primary generalized dystonia, particularly in cases associated with a mutation in the *DYT1* gene. The efficacy of pallidal surgery for secondary dystonias, such as those due to stroke or cerebral palsy, is less than in primary dystonias but may still be clinically useful. Surgical techniques and complications are similar to those described above for Parkinson's disease.

Bergman H, Wichmann T, DeLong MR: Reversal of experimental parkinsonism by lesions of the subthalamic nucleus. Science 1990;249:1436.

Coubes P et al: Treatment of *DYT1*-generalized dystonia by stimulation of the internal globus pallidus. Lancet 2000;355:2220.

Deep brain stimulation for Parkinson's disease study group. Deep-brain stimulation of the subthalamic nucleus or the pars interna of the globus pallidus in Parkinson's disease. N Engl J Med 2001;345:956.

Eltahawy HA et al: Primary dystonia is more responsive than secondary dystonia to pallidal interventions: outcome after pallidotomy or pallidal deep brain stimulation. Neurosurgery 2004;54:613.

Fahn S, Bresman SB, Marsden CD: Classification of dystonia. Adv Neurol 1998;78:1.

Freed CR et al: Transplantation of embryonic dopamine neurons for severe Parkinson's disease. N Engl J Med 2001;344:710.

Gash DM et al: Functional recovery in parkinsonian monkeys treated with GDNF. Nature 1996;380:252.

Gill SS et al: Direct brain infusion of glial cell line-derived neurotrophic factor in Parkinson disease. Nat Med 2003;9:589.

Guridi J, Lozano AM: A brief history of pallidotomy. Neurosurgery 1997;41:1169.

Koller WC et al: Long-term safety and efficacy of unilateral deep brain stimulation of the thalamus in essential tremor. Mov Disord 2001;16:464.

Kordower JH et al: Neuropathological evidence of graft survival and striatal reinnervation after the transplantation of fetal mesencephalic tissue in a patient with Parkinson's disease. N Engl J Med 1995;332:1118.

Krack P et al: Five year follow-up of bilateral stimulation of the subthalamic nucleus in advanced Parkinson's disease. N Engl J Med 2003;349:1925.

Krauss JK et al: Bilateral stimulation of the globus pallidus internus for treatment of cervical dystonia. Lancet 1999;354:837.

Limousin P, Speelman JD, Gielen F: Multicentre European study of thalamic stimulation in parkinsonian and essential tremor. J Neurol Neurosurg Psychiatry 1999;66:289.

Olanow CW et al: A double-blind controlled trial of bilateral fetal nigral transplantation in Parkinson's disease. Ann Neurol 2003;54:403.

Ondo WG et al: Pallidotomy for generalized dystonia. Mov Disord 1998;13:693.

Shuurman PR et al: Comparison of continuous thalamic stimulation and thalamotomy for suppression of severe tremor. N Engl J Med 2000;342:461.

Starr PA: Placement of deep brain stimulators into the subthalamic nucleus or globus pallidus internus: technical approach. Stereotact Funct Neurosurg 2003;79:118.

Starr PA, Vitek JL, Bakay RA: Ablative surgery and deep brain stimulation for Parkinson's disease. Neurosurgery 1998;43:989; discussion 1013.

PAIN

Nicholas M. Barbaro, MD

Pain has been defined as "an unpleasant sensory and emotional experience associated with actual or potential tissue damage, or described in terms of such damage." This definition takes into account that pain is a well-recognized signal of damage and, as such, an important symptom of numerous diseases. Pain resulting from injury to the nervous system (neuropathic pain) may not indicate tissue damage and thus may not be a useful sensory phenomenon; rather, it may constitute a pathologic process in itself. The above definition of pain also takes into account the emotional aspects of pain, which can be all-consuming for a patient, and suggests the importance of psychologic factors in evaluation and treatment.

Patients with pain can be divided into two groups: those with diseases that limit life expectancy, such as malignant tumors (malignant or cancer pain); and those with normal life expectancy (chronic benign pain). For practical purposes, patients expected to live 2 years or less are put into the malignant pain group. The medical and surgical management of these two groups is very different.

In general, the approach to treating pain begins with an attempt to diagnose the cause. The natural history of the underlying problem must also be considered. For example, pain in a region recently operated on is expected to resolve with wound healing. When possible, the source of the pain should be treated directly (eg, removal of a herniated disk, treatment of a primary tumor). If the pain cannot be treated directly or if the source of the pain is unknown, efforts are made to treat the pain as such.

MALIGNANT PAIN

The main goal in treating patients with malignant pain is to reduce suffering during a terminal illness. Therapies that might be inappropriate in patients with normal life expectancies can be considered. Opioids, for example, can be used in high doses unless excessive sedation, respiratory depression, severe constipation, or other significant adverse effects occur. Any dose that relieves pain and maximizes useful function can be used. Other medications, such as tricyclic antidepressants, anticonvulsants, and nonsteroidal anti-inflammatory agents, may provide additional relief. When medical management fails to reduce the pain sufficiently, surgical treatment is indicated. Surgical management of malignant pain involves two approaches: (1) epidural or intrathecally administered morphine and (2) ablation to interrupt pain transmission.

The spinal cord contains opioid receptors which, when activated by locally administered morphine, produce rather profound pain relief. Temporary percutaneous catheters can be used to test this therapy; if significant pain relief is demonstrated, prolonged spinal administration of morphine is indicated. This can be accomplished by implanting a subcutaneous reservoir attached to an epidural or intrathecal catheter; morphine can be injected into the reservoir by the patient or caregiver. Although this technique provides useful pain relief, it is impractical because repeated skin punctures are required and there is a risk of infection. If the patient's life expectancy is more than a few months, implantation of an infusion pump is recommended. Spinal morphine is most effective for midline and multifocal pain problems, such as sacral pain associated with prostate tumors, pelvic pain from carcinoma of the cervix, and multifocal bone pain from widely metastatic disease. Other drugs such as bupivacaine and clonidine may relieve pain related to nerve invasion.

Cancer pain that is unilateral and focal may be treated with cordotomy, creating a lesion in the spinothalamic tract designed to interrupt pain transmission. An open cordotomy, which requires laminectomy, produces excellent analgesia and can be done in the thoracic region for leg pain. Percutaneous cordotomy using a radiofrequency needle is done at the C1–2 level. This is less traumatic for the patient and may produce analgesia in both the arm and the leg. Bilateral high cervical cordotomy is not recommended because of the risk of respiratory depression.

Other ablative techniques for treating cancer pain are used relatively rarely. These include midline myelotomies, rhizotomies (open or percutaneous), and neurectomies.

POSTOPERATIVE PAIN

Some pain is experienced by nearly every patient after invasive surgical procedures. The amount and duration of pain varies with the type of procedure, with the individual patient, and with many other factors, including the rapidity of healing and associated complications such as infection. The fact that pain is expected after surgical procedures does not mean it should not be treated aggressively. Reducing postoperative pain not only lessens the most unpleasant aspect of the procedure for the patient, it also reduces the incidence of other types of morbidity, such as pneumonia and deep vein thrombosis. For these reasons, appropriate doses of opioids and other pain-reducing drugs such as anti-inflammatory agents are an essential part of postoperative care.

The treatment of postoperative pain has improved substantially in recent years. These improvements include the use of epidural or intrathecal opioids and the use of long-acting nerve blocks at the end of a procedure. In addition, new delivery techniques such as patient-controlled analgesia, in which the patient self-administers small incremental doses of opioid analgesic, reduce overall postoperative pain and actually decrease the amount of analgesic required during the postoperative period.

CHRONIC BENIGN PAIN

Patients with a life expectancy longer than 2 years who have pain that cannot be eliminated by treating the underlying cause are considered to have chronic benign pain. Such patients should be evaluated by a team of individuals experienced in pain treatment (pain clinic), including specialists in anesthesiology, psychology, psychiatry and neurology or neurosurgery, physical therapy, and pharmacology. This multidisciplinary approach takes into account the multifactorial cause of long-standing pain.

The medical management of such patients is beyond the scope of this chapter. In general, drugs with little or no potential for addiction or significant dependence should be used. When opioids are used, long-acting drugs on a time-contingent rather than pain-contingent schedule are preferred, and short-acting opioids should be avoided. Anticonvulsant and tricyclic antidepressant drugs may be effective and are best administered by physicians with experience in their use.

When medical management fails to reduce pain adequately, surgical treatment can be considered. Ablative techniques such as rhizotomy (cutting of nerve roots), neurectomy, and cordotomy are inappropriate in these cases except as noted below. Techniques of neuromodulation that do not cause neural injury should be used instead.

Neuromodulation techniques take advantage of the capacity of the nervous system to reduce the access of painful stimuli to higher central nervous system centers. Transcutaneous electrical nerve stimulation, the least invasive of these techniques, uses skin electrodes to activate the large fibers in peripheral nerves. This selective activation reduces the ability of nociceptive fibers (A δ and C) to activate spinal neurons, which transmit pain signals to higher centers. This technique is limited by the inability to stimulate large painful areas and by the inconvenience of wearing electrodes for long periods.

A more invasive approach to neuromodulation involves direct or percutaneous implantation of electrodes into the spinal canal to electrically stimulate the dorsal columns. Spinal cord stimulation is most effective for pain in the extremities, such as pain after nerve injury, peripheral neuropathies, and complex regional pain syndromes. In patients with ischemic pain, spinal cord stimulation not only reduces the pain but may also improve blood flow in the involved extremities as well.

SPECIFIC PAIN SYNDROMES

1. Trigeminal Neuralgia

Trigeminal neuralgia is an episodic lancinating facial pain that conforms to one—or perhaps two—divisions of the trigeminal nerve. It is more common in elderly patients except when seen as a manifestation of multiple sclerosis, and is slightly more common in women. The mainstay of treatment is the anticonvulsant drug carbamazepine and, more recently, gabapentin. Patients who do not respond to medical management may be treated with a percutaneous, open, or radiosurgical procedure. Percutaneous approaches involve placing a needle through the foramen ovale at the skull base. The trigeminal nerve is then partially damaged with glycerol, a mildly toxic alcohol, a radiofrequency-induced heat lesion, or by balloon compression of the trigeminal ganglion. The percutaneous approaches are minimally invasive and require very short hospitalization, but the recurrence rate is higher than with an open approach, and patients are left with some loss of facial sensation, perhaps including protective corneal sensation.

Many cases of trigeminal neuralgia are caused by irritation of the trigeminal nerve at the brain stem by blood vessels, such as the superior cerebellar and anterior inferior cerebellar arteries. This syndrome can often be cured by moving the offending vessel away from the nerve. When the trigeminal nerve is exposed and such a neurovascular relationship cannot be demonstrated, partial rhizotomy (nerve sectioning) can provide excellent pain relief. A recent addition to the surgical treatment of trigeminal neuralgia is radiosurgery, a stereotaxic technique used to deliver high levels of radiation to precise brain regions. Typically, a single dose of radiation (70–80 Gy) is delivered to the trigeminal nerve between its entrance in the pons and the gasserian ganglion behind the cavernous sinus. Such treatment is very effective in reducing or eliminating the pain of trigeminal neuralgia, but longer follow-up is required to determine whether it will become the treatment of choice for this condition.

2. Pain After Amputation

A variety of pain syndromes may follow limb amputation. Most patients experience sensory phenomena in the amputated limb. In a minority of cases, these so-called phantom sensations are painful. Phantom limb pain is described as a continuous pain, as if fingernails were digging into the palm or the limb were being twisted into painful postures. Some patients have painful neuromas at the cut ends of peripheral nerves; the pain is usually electrical and occurs each time the stump is pressed. Injury to the cutaneous nerves may cause painful skin sensitivity in the stump. Medications such as tricyclic antidepressants and anticonvulsants may be effective in these cases, but opioids usually are not. Surgical options include revision and burying of painful neuromas and, in refractory cases, spinal cord or brain stimulation.

3. Spinal Nerve Root Avulsion Pain

Injuries that radically displace the head and shoulder can avulse the spinal nerves from the spinal cord. This commonly occurs after motorcycle accidents in which the head and shoulder are rapidly and severely distracted. This type of brachial plexus injury is not surgically reparable and usually is not painful. In some cases, however, the pain is severe; typically, it is a burning pain and may include a phantom-like pain sensation. When such pain is refractory to medical management, it can be alleviated in 80% of cases by a dorsal root entry zone lesion. In this procedure, the spinal cord is exposed, and the region where dorsal roots formerly entered the spinal cord is identified. Lesions are made either with small needles (radiofrequency) or with a laser. Care must be taken to avoid damaging nearby spinal tracts.

4. Spinal Cord Injury Pain

Most patients with severe spinal cord injury experience some pain. In some cases, it is severe and requires specific medical treatment. Pain after spinal cord injury may occur at the border zone between normal and abnormal sensation or may affect large areas of the body with little or no sensory function. The former may be treated with the dorsal root entry zone procedure described above; lesions are created at the region immediately above and below the spinal cord injury. More diffuse spinal cord injury pain is very difficult to treat and does not respond well to any surgical procedures. Such patients should be referred to multidisciplinary pain clinics.

Barker FG 2nd et al: The long-term outcome of microvascular decompression for trigeminal neuralgia. N Engl J Med 1996; 334:1077.

Dickenson AH: Central acute pain mechanisms. Ann Med 1995;27:223.

Kondziolka D et al: Gamma knife radiosurgery for trigeminal neuralgia: results and expectations. Arch Neurol 1998;55:1524.

North RB, Roark GL: Spinal cord stimulation for chronic pain. Neurosurg Clin North Am 1995;6:145.

Stanton-Hicks M, Salamon J: Stimulation of the central and peripheral nervous system for the control of pain. J Clin Neurophysiol 1997;14:46.

Taha JM, Tew JM Jr: Comparison of surgical treatments for trigeminal neuralgia: reevaluation of radiofrequency rhizotomy. Neurosurgery 1996;38:865.

Wasner G, Backonja MM, Baron R: Traumatic neuralgias: complex regional pain syndromes (reflex sympathetic dystrophy and causalgia): clinical characteristics, pathophysiological mechanisms and therapy. Neurol Clin 1998;16:851.

INTERVERTEBRAL DISK DISEASE

Philip R. Weinstein, MD

Anatomic Considerations

A. The Intervertebral Disk

The intervertebral disk has three parts: the circumferential annulus, which consists of dense fibrous tissue and is very strong; the central nucleus, which consists of gelatinous fibrocartilage and has little tensile strength but great elasticity; and the vertebral body end-plates, which are composed of dense and firm cartilage and form the interface between bone and disk above and below each joint. Fibrocartilage may be fragmented acutely or may degenerate gradually with time. It heals poorly because of limited blood supply. Nutrient arteries atrophy with age beginning in the second decade. The nucleus contains approximately 80% water at birth; it gradually dehydrates and loses its elasticity with advancing age. The annulus, however, has more capacity to heal and is buttressed by thick anterior and posterior longitudinal ligaments that add strength and contribute vascular supply.

Intervertebral disk disease may occur at any level from C2 to L5. The midcervical and lower lumbar areas are affected most often. Thoracic disk disease is uncommon, but it may cause severe neurologic deficit if herniation results in spinal cord compression.

B. The Spinal Cord and Nerve Roots

Knowledge of the anatomic and physiologic relationships of the spinal cord, nerve roots, vertebrae, and neural foramina is useful for understanding the principles for diagnosis of intervertebral disk disease.

The cervical spinal cord occupies between one-half and two-thirds of the cross-sectional area of the normal spinal canal, is centrally placed, and moves rostrally and caudally a few millimeters during flexion and extension of the neck. Anteroposterior and lateral motion is restricted by the tethering effect of the intradural dentate ligaments and paired nerve roots.

The spinal cord terminates as the conus medullaris at approximately the L1–2 level. Posterior and anterior nerve roots emerge from the conus separately, passing within the lumbar sac to their respective intervertebral foramina, where they exit from the spinal canal. The roots join to form a peripheral nerve within the neural foramen, which also contains the dorsal root ganglion. In the cervical and lumbar areas, the roots merge to form the brachial or lumbosacral plexus. Sacral nerve roots are medial and central within the lumbar sac adjacent to the filum terminale, the meningeal structure that attaches the conus to the caudal end of the spinal canal. In the neck, the C1 root emerges from the spinal canal above the C1 vertebra; the C2 root emerges below C1. Thus, the nerve root that emerges from the spine between the C5 and C6 vertebrae is the C6 root. C8 emerges between C7 and T1, and the T1 root emerges below the pedicle of the T1 vertebra crossing through the T1–T2 foramen.

Sensation around the deltoid area is basically related to the C5 root; sensation in the thumb and possibly in the index finger is a C6 root function. Sensation in the third and fourth fingers is a C7 root function, whereas the fifth finger is supplied by C8. Biceps muscle strength and the biceps tendon reflex require an intact C6 root; triceps reflex and strength are dependent upon the C7 root. Intrinsic muscles of the hand allowing abduction and adduction of the fingers are innervated by C8 and T1.

Lumbosacral nerve roots carry on the same relationships to the vertebrae determined by emergence of the T1 nerve root below the T1 vertebra. That is, the L4 nerve root emerges below the L4 pedicle, and the S1 root emerges below the S1 pedicle in the S1-S2 foramen. Each root (eg, L4) passes laterally toward the neural foramen as it descends within the spinal canal. It crosses the adjacent intervertebral disk (eg, L4–5) and the extreme lateral edge of the disk after exiting the spinal canal below the pedicle of the L4 vertebra inferolaterally. The nerve root (eg, L5) that descends to the next lowest foramen passes across the same intervertebral disk (eg, L4–5) more medially within the lateral recess of the neural canal, in a location that is more vulnerable to diseases involving intraspinal displacement of the disk.

The sensory distribution of L5 is on the medial aspect of the foot and the great toe. S1 sensation is experienced over the lateral aspect of the foot, the fifth toe, and the lateral sole of the foot. Pain or sensory deficit in those dermatomal areas implies involvement of either L5 or S1 fibers. Plantar flexion is primarily an S1 motor function; dorsiflexion of the foot is an L5 function. Knee extension by the quadriceps muscle group is subserved primarily by the L3 and L4 motor roots. The ankle jerk is primarily dependent upon the S1 root, whereas the knee jerk depends upon L3 and L4. The L5 fibers may contribute to both reflexes or to neither one. The L5 nerve root selectively supplies the great toe extensor muscle (extensor hallucis longus).

The sensory distribution of the remaining sacral roots, S2–5, is in the "saddle" area over the buttocks and on the soles of the feet. Voluntary motor control of the urinary bladder and anal sphincters is subserved by the S2–4 nerve roots. Thus, the cauda equina syndrome, a rare complication of massive extrusion of a lumbar disk, is associated with sensory loss over the perineal area and buttocks and with urinary and fecal incontinence.

CERVICAL DISK SYNDROME

ESSENTIALS OF DIAGNOSIS

SUBJECTIVE:

- *Pain in the suboccipital, cervical, interscapular, thoracic, and shoulder areas radiating into the upper extremities.*
- *Discomfort aggravated by neck movement.*
- *Pain, paresthesias, and dysesthesias radiating into the cervical dermatomes.*

OBJECTIVE:

- *Straightening of cervical lordosis, limitation of cervical movements, and paraspinous muscle spasm.*
- *Weakness, fasciculations, muscle atrophy, depression of deep tendon reflexes, and dermatome sensory change in the upper extremities.*
- *Spasticity, weakness, and extensor plantar sign in the lower extremities.*
- *Spastic bladder dysfunction.*
- *Radiologic evidence of narrowed disk spaces, formation of osteophytes, and spinal stenosis.*
- *MRI, CT, or myelographic evidence of extradural cervical cord or root displacement or compression, often at multiple levels.*

General Considerations

If the cervical intervertebral disk ruptures and extrudes through the annulus and posterior longitudinal ligament, adjacent neural structures may be compressed. Compression of the spinal cord may result in paraplegia or quadriplegia, depending on the segment involved. Compression of a spinal root may cause weakness and sensory loss in structures of the upper extremity innervated by that root. The severity of the clinical syndrome depends upon the site and severity of compression by the displaced disk fragment. Often, intrinsic disruption of the disk occurs, but the adjacent ligaments hold, preventing complete extrusion of the fragmented cartilage. The annulus may separate from its attachment to the vertebral body margin or tear sufficiently to allow the disk to bulge into the spinal canal or foramina. Thus, neural structures also may be compressed by protrusion of an injured or degenerated disk.

After trauma or spontaneously, the annulus may rupture and the nucleus may herniate into the spinal canal or neural foramen acutely. Often, however, the nucleus does not extrude but simply becomes desiccated and progressively degenerates, losing its biomechanical function and elasticity. The disk space gradually narrows, the joint becomes looser, and the cartilaginous end-plates of the adjacent vertebra touch, stimulating reactive osteogenesis. Bony spurs develop at the vertebral body margins adjacent to the disk joint in reaction to the increased mobility and stress. If a bony spur (osteophyte) forms in the neural foramen, the nerve root passing through may be chronically irritated and compressed. If the osteophyte forms within the spinal canal, spinal cord compression may result in the development of myelopathy, with signs and symptoms of impaired cord function. Formation of osteophytes around the joints of vertebrae is termed **spondylosis**.

Degenerative thickening with ossification of the posterior interlaminar ligament (ligamentum flavum) or the posterolateral facet joint capsule may further contribute to compression of the cord and roots in cases of spondylostenosis.

Cervical spondylosis is common and may even be "normal" in aging persons. Radiographic evidence of cervical spondylosis exists in 85% of people over 65 years of age. It may not be associated with symptoms of cord or root compression, however, unless the neural canal or foramina are narrowed. Developmental reduction of canal dimensions, resulting in spinal stenosis, may contribute to the appearance of symptoms that are the result of entrapment of neural elements.

Clinical Findings

A. Symptoms and Signs

The onset of symptoms and signs of an extruded disk fragment may be acute or insidious. Acute symptoms may follow trauma or be unrelated to injury. Neck and radicular pain radiating down the arm occur simultaneously, but spinal cord symptoms are rare. There is usually limitation of neck motion, tenderness over the brachial nerves, and straightening of the normal cervical lordosis. Decrease in a deep tendon reflex (biceps or triceps jerk) is common with or without weakness in the muscles supplied by the compressed root. With foraminal osteophytes, episodes of cervical discomfort may recur over many months or years before radicular symptoms occur. Interscapular aching and suboccipital headaches are common associated complaints that may be explained as episodes of sequential radiation of referred skeletal pain. The signs and symptoms of cervical spondylosis are those of progressive cervical radiculopathy and, in advanced cases, spastic paraparesis with mild to moderate sensory deficit on the torso and in the lower extremities as well as in a cervical dermatome pattern. Neck and arm pain may or may not be present along with some limitation of cervical spine movement.

B. Imaging Studies

Plain x-rays may be normal except for straightening of the cervical lordosis. The lateral view may demonstrate narrowing of one or more disk spaces. X-rays may show osteophyte formation at the appropriate neural foramen in association with disk narrowing. This is usually best seen on oblique views. In symptomatic cervical spondylosis, there is usually x-ray evidence of osteophytes and disk narrowing at several levels, and in most cases with neurologic symptoms and signs. The sagittal diameter of the cervical spinal canal may also be congenitally narrowed. When the diameter of the canal is 10 mm or less, clinically significant spinal cord compression can be expected to occur.

MRI is now being used with increasing success as the initial diagnostic study for patients with cervical radiculomyelopathy. Subarachnoid cerebrospinal fluid spaces, spinal cord, nerve roots, and vertebral structures can be visualized without injection of contrast material, but resolution of osseous anatomic details may not always be as clear as is obtained with CT scanning, especially for visualization of vertebral fractures. CT scans of the spine are useful for evaluating the diameter of the canal and the foramina in patients with cervical spine stenosis. Osteophytes and posttraumatic deformities of the vertebral bodies and facet joints can be identified on CT scans, especially if they are calcified or ossified. Soft tissue lesions such as displaced disk or hypertrophied ligaments and joint capsules that may cause compression of neural elements in patients with spondylosis are less well visualized in the cervical and thoracic areas by CT.

Following acute disk herniation, MRI may show a small ventral extradural defect, displacing or compressing the nerve root. In cervical spondylosis, the sagittal image shows bar-like ventral defects at the disk space, usually at several levels and sometimes associated with apparent widening of the cord shadow on the axial projection if the spinal diameter is narrowed. CT scanning in conjunction with myelography also provides images of the relationship between vertebral and neural elements in the axial plane or in the sagittal and oblique planes using reformatted views. With contrast material demonstrating the size and configuration of the subarachnoid space, compression or atrophy of the cervical cord and nerve roots can be clearly visualized and the lesions identified.

Differential Diagnosis

Cervical disk disease must be differentiated from traumatic and inflammatory disease affecting the soft tissues and joints of the neck and pectoral girdle, such as deltoid or acromial bursitis and cervical intervertebral or shoulder joint sprains. Nerve entrapment syndromes in the upper extremities such as cervical rib and scalenus anticus syndrome, carpal tunnel syndrome, and tardy ulnar palsy may also cause neck and arm pain, weakness, and numbness. Other conditions that must be considered include coronary insufficiency and angina pectoris; neoplasms of the pulmonary apex (eg, Pancoast tumors); primary peripheral or central nervous system tumors of the brachial plexus, cervical cord, or cervicomedullary junction; fractures, dislocations or subluxations of the cervical spine; and inflammatory disease of the cervical theca such as arachnoiditis, sarcoidosis, and Pott's disease. The condition that is most difficult to distinguish from cervical radiculopathy is brachial neuritis, an idiopathic inflammatory disease that affects the brachial plexus.

The disorder that most frequently mimics cervical disk disease is invasion of the cervical spine by metastatic tumor. Biopsy and surgical decompression or radiation therapy are indicated as emergency procedures, especially when a pathologic fracture or epidural mass lesion threatens spinal cord function.

Complications

Permanent damage to the nerve roots and spinal cord may occur, with loss of motor and sensory function. This is particularly true in cervical stenosis and spondylosis, in which both direct pressure on the spinal cord and compression of its vascular supply may produce a severe, progressive irreversible myelopathy with spastic paraplegia or quadriplegia that does not respond to surgical decompression. Such patients are also vulnerable to acute onset of paraparesis or quadriparesis initiated by relatively mild cervical hyperextension injuries sustained during a fall or motor vehicle accident.

Treatment

A. Medical Measures

Initially, cervical disk disease should be treated medically unless there is evidence of spinal cord compression or radicular motor loss in an extremity from severe neural compression. Medical therapy for patients suffering from radiculitis includes immobilization of the neck with a cervical collar. Physical therapy to pain sites, including mild traction with the cervical spine in a neutral position, may be helpful. Analgesics, anti-inflammatory agents, muscle relaxants, and local heat are frequently used in combination with physical therapy.

B. Surgical Treatment

There are two methods of treating cervical disk disease surgically: (1) posterior decompression of the nerve roots, spinal cord, or both, with or without fusion; and (2) anterior decompression of nerve roots, spinal cord, or both, with or without fusion. The choice is based on consideration of a particular patient's anatomic lesions as demonstrated with MRI, CT, and dynamic flexion-extension radiographs. It may be necessary to use both an anterior and a posterior approach in separate stages if satisfactory recovery is not observed within 3–6 months after the initial operation.

Prognosis

Seventy-five percent of patients with cervical radiculopathy will recover following an adequate trial (10–14 days) of medical therapy, even though some continue to have cervical or interscapular discomfort or mild paresthesias. In some patients, radicular or myelopathic symptoms recur upon return to full activity. Although many patients with cervical disk disease can be managed symptomatically for years with intervals of physical therapy and a cervical collar, others eventually require surgical therapy. For the 25% who do not respond to conservative therapy, operation is required. Even after surgery, symptoms may reappear, perhaps because of residual or recurrent disease at the same or adjacent disk levels. In some instances, reevaluation for additional surgery is indicated. Improvement follows operative treatment of a cervical disk in approximately 80% of patients. Surgical treatment of cervical spondylosis with myelopathy results in improvement in 70% of cases and arrest of progression in many of the remainder.

THORACIC DISK DISEASE

Although the disorder is rare, knowledge of thoracic disk disease is essential, because it is associated with significant deficit when it does occur. Occasionally, the nucleus of a thoracic disk extrudes into the spinal canal as a result of forceful trauma. Because the thoracic canal is small in relation to the spinal cord within it, severe cord compression often results from disk rupture. The onset of paraplegia is often abrupt, and paralysis may be permanent. More often, however, osteophyte formation due to a degenerated thoracic disk accounts for spinal canal narrowing. The occurrence of cord compression is then more gradual and progressive.

Treatment for ruptured thoracic disk associated with intractable pain or disabling neurologic deficit is primarily surgical and consists of removal of the offending disk or discogenic osteophyte by the anterior thoracotomy, lateral extracavitary costo-transversectomy, or posterolateral transpedicular approach. Posterior decompression by laminectomy is the least effective approach in the thoracic area and has the highest risk of complications.

LUMBAR DISK SYNDROME

ESSENTIALS OF DIAGNOSIS

- *History of back injury or stress or a discrete episode of spontaneous onset.*
- *Low back pain.*
- *Pain aggravated by activity and relieved by bed rest.*
- *Signs of root compression, associated with the onset of radicular radiation to the legs, eg, sciatica.*
- *Abnormal straight leg-raising test.*
- *Neurologic findings variable; usually mild.*

General Considerations

If the nucleus of a lumbar intervertebral disk extrudes through the annulus and elevates or tears the posterior longitudinal ligament, lumbosacral nerve roots may be displaced or compressed. Sensory loss, dermatomal pain, motor loss in the myotomes innervated by those roots, and loss of the knee or ankle tendon jerks may result. The severity of the syndrome produced depends upon the site and severity of nerve root compression. Occasionally, the entire cauda equina may be compressed, resulting in paraplegia and loss of motor and sensory function below the lesion, including anal and urethral sphincter control. Disk rupture may occur in the midline, compressing centrally placed sacral nerve roots preferentially, without involvement of laterally placed lumbar roots at the level of herniation.

Disruption of a lumbar disk may occur without extrusion of the nucleus. In that event, elasticity of the joint is reduced and mobility is increased. Degeneration of the facet joint and its capsule follows. The annulus may bulge without tearing. As time passes, osteophytes form around the degenerated disk or facet joint and may encroach upon the spinal canal and foramina anteriorly, posteriorly, or both. Lumbar spondylosis, a condition common in the elderly, is the end result. Stenosis of the lumbar canal and foramen may also present as a developmental defect, aggravating the compressive effects of degenerative disk disease and spondylosis.

Clinical Findings

Over 90% of problems arise at the L4–5 and L5–S1 intervertebral disk levels, with most of the remainder occurring at L3–4. Lumbar disk disease rarely involves higher levels.

A. Symptoms and Signs

Although pain is usually acute when associated with frank herniation, it may also be chronic. There may be back pain, leg pain, or both. The radiation of low back pain into the buttock, posterior thigh, and calf is usually the same with disease at the L4–5 or L5–S1 interspaces. This radiating pain may be aggravated by coughing, sneezing, or the Valsalva maneuver. Bending or sitting accentuates the discomfort, whereas lying down characteristically relieves it. Most commonly, the back pain is described as deep, aching, and constant (lumbago) with a sharp shooting element traveling from the buttock down the leg posteriorly to the foot or toes (sciatica). Sometimes pain and paresthesias radiate in localizing patterns to the groin (L3), medial thigh and calf (L4), big toe (L5), or little toe (S1).

Palpation of the paravertebral area (less frequently, over the vertebral spinous processes or facets) reveals tenderness at the affected disk level. Palpation under the buttock may elicit radiating pain from the sciatic notch. Palpation of the sciatic nerve in the popliteal fossa may also elicit tenderness or referred pain. The paravertebral musculature may be in spasm, and reactive scoliosis may be present. Straight-leg raising produces back or leg pain that may be accentuated with further stretching of the sciatic nerve (by ankle dorsiflexion). Pain produced when the leg opposite the affected side is raised is highly suggestive of disk extrusion.

Weakness of the anterior calf musculature (with the extensor hallucis longus being the first affected) is a common finding, especially with L4–5 disk herniation and L5 radiculopathy. Foot drop can occur in advanced cases. Weakness of the gastrocnemius-soleus muscle group suggests L5–S1 disk herniation. Weakness of the quadriceps may occur with L3–4 herniation. Atrophy may be present in cases of long-standing radiculopathy. Comparison of knee and ankle reflexes is important.

Depression of the ankle jerk is common with L5–S1 disease but is also present in a significant number of cases of L4–5 disease. The knee jerk may be depressed in L3–4 disease, or, rarely, because of L2-3 herniation.

Sensory patterns are variable. Numbness or paresthesias in the legs are present in fewer than one-third of patients. When sphincter dysfunction is reported in association with unilateral radicular pain, a large central disk herniation should be suspected as a cause of bilateral sacral root compression. Hypesthesia on the dorsum of the foot is common; sensory deficit on the little toe and the lateral surface of the foot is more frequent with L5–S1 disease, and deficit on the big toe and medial aspect of the foot is more frequent with L4–5 disease.

B. Imaging Studies

Plain films of the lumbosacral spine should be taken to identify congenital or acquired vertebral abnormalities. Narrowing of the disk spaces occurs with equal frequency in symptomatic and asymptomatic patients and therefore has no diagnostic value.

MRI scans are useful to image the thecal sac, disks, and vertebral elements. Thoracolumbar tumors can be excluded and, in some instances, peridural scar tissue can be distinguished from recurrent disk herniation in postoperative patients by administration of a paramagnetic contrast agent that enhances signal intensity in scar or granulation tissue but not in disk. When certain imaging parameters are selected, the cerebrospinal fluid can be demonstrated, and the need to inject contrast material into the lumbar subarachnoid space is eliminated. Lumbar puncture is not necessary. MRI of the lumbar spine is rapidly replacing both myelography and CT as the initial diagnostic procedure of choice.

CT scanning of the lumbar spine may provide adequate diagnostic information if disk protrusion or rupture has occurred when MRI is not available or feasible. Because the neural canal is larger in the lumbar area, slowly expanding lesions may remain asymptomatic until a critical degree of nerve root compression has occurred. Tumors or cysts as well as spinal canal stenosis may be identified, but MRI will be required for definitive diagnosis. Sagittal and coronal section reformatting of axial CT scans provides images showing the longitudinal configuration of the lumbar thecal sac. In patients with an appropriate history of disk rupture and a neurologic deficit that correlates anatomically with the level of abnormality shown in the CT scan, MRI may not be necessary. However, if more than one level is involved or if previous disk disease has been treated surgically, CT scanning without MRI will not provide sufficient diagnostic information.

MRI is diagnostic in 80–90% of cases and is important in localizing the disease and ruling out intraspinal tumors. The scan must include the lower thoracic cord and conus in order to eliminate the possibility of more rostral compression of the lumbosacral nerve roots by tumor or disk. Since false-positive and false-negative results may occur, myography followed by CT scanning may be necessary in complex cases.

C. Special Examinations

Electromyography may demonstrate denervation of the muscles in the appropriate nerve root distribution and can be used as an adjunct to neurologic examination when diagnosis is difficult. Electromyography alone is not diagnostic of disk rupture.

Although rarely indicated for initial diagnosis, discography may demonstrate an abnormal and inflamed or painful disk. Radiopaque contrast material is injected under fluoroscopic control into the disk space, and volume accepted and pressure reached are measured, pain response is recorded by severity and similarity to the patient's complaint, and a CT scan is obtained. Degenerated and extruded disks may be identified. Internal disruption or degeneration of the annulus without dislocation of the nucleus into the neural canal can be demonstrated by discography. Such information can often be obtained with MRI without injection of contrast material. Report by the patient of concordant pain typical of the predominant symptoms at one level that is also anatomically abnormal and not during injection of adjacent levels may localize the site of incapacitating discogenic back pain.

Differential Diagnosis

Back pain with radiation to the leg has many causes: (1) bony abnormalities such as spondylolisthesis, spondylosis, spinal stenosis, or Paget's disease; (2) primary and metastatic tumors of the cauda equina or the pelvic region; (3) inflammatory disorders, including abscess in the epidural space or retroperitoneal lumbosacral plexus, postinfectious or posttraumatic arachnoiditis, and rheumatoid spondylitis; (4) degenerative lesions of the spinal cord and peripheral neuropathies; and (5) peripheral vascular occlusive disease.

Treatment

A. Medical Measures

A trial of medical treatment is indicated in all patients who do not demonstrate progressive weakness or sphincter dysfunction. This consists initially of bed rest with application of hot packs to the pain site, anti-inflammatory medications, analgesics, and skeletal muscle relaxants. External immobilization by bracing, bed rest, or pelvic traction may help relieve muscle spasm and nerve root irritation. Physical therapy and graded exercise are indicated in chronic cases or after an acute episode subsides. A lumbar corset or back brace that provides external support may allow patients to return to activity earlier. An external plastic body jacket may be required in cases where subacute or chronic pain is relieved by external immobilization.

B. Surgical Treatment

Surgical treatment is indicated in patients with progressive neurologic deficits and chronic or recurrent disabling pain due to radiculopathy or, less frequently, to severe intervertebral joint degeneration. Acute onset of symptoms associated with muscle weakness or sphincteric disturbance must be treated with urgent decompression.

A simple laminotomy and foraminotomy is opened posteriorly at the appropriate interspace, taking care to protect the nerve root and dura. Microsurgical technique allows adequate exposure through a smaller incision that reduces muscle dissection. Endoscopic instrumentation is also available and in use. If disk extrusion has occurred, the surgeon attempts to remove this piece and diligently searches for other detachable portions of the disk. When herniation without extrusion has occurred, the surgeon makes a window in the posterior longitudinal ligament and annulus and removes all accessible degenerated material from the intervertebral space.

Some surgeons recommend that a fusion be done primarily or as a secondary procedure in chronic back pain cases where preoperative immobilization has relieved symptoms of joint instability. Total diskectomy through bilateral posterior laminotomies or an anterior lumbar transperitoneal approach by laparotomy can be followed by interbody fusion that replaces the disk with iliac crest bone grafts and titanium, carbon fiber, or bone dowel cages for relief of intractable discogenic pain syndromes and stabilization of the intervertebral joint. Posterior pedicle screw fixation may also be added for circumferential arthrodesis of the motion segment.

Transcutaneous injection of enzymes (eg, chymopapain, collagenase) into lumbar disks has been used in the past to dissolve fibrocartilage or collagen material to relieve pain and radiculopathy without surgery. Needle or probe placement is guided by fluoroscopy. Although satisfactory results were reported in 60% of patients, complications related to nerve root injury, transverse myelitis, and systemic anaphylaxis occurred. Patients with fragments of disk material that detach and extrude into the spinal canal are unlikely to benefit from such treatments. Percutaneous coagulation or aspiration of degenerative disk material has been attempted through a radiofrequency electrode, an ultrasonic nucleotome cannula, or a laser probe inserted into the intervertebral space as a safer method for relieving painful in situ disk protrusions. Fragmentation and excision of pieces of degenerated fibrocartilage can also be accomplished through a fiberoptic arthroscopic cannula using microsurgical instruments under fluoroscopic or fiberoptic videoscope control. Further studies are in progress to evaluate long-term results with these techniques.

Prognosis

With medical treatment, most patients improve sufficiently to return to full activity. Lumbar disk syndrome may ultimately be treated surgically, often successfully.

About 10–20% of cases of lumbar discogenic radiculopathy require surgical management. The best results are obtained in patients with extrusion of disk material and acute radiculopathy. Those with chronic poorly localized discogenic pain and no neurologic deficit are less likely to benefit from diskectomy. If joint instability is demonstrated at one or two levels, spinal fusion with or without discectomy may be indicated.

Thus, if the syndrome has resulted from an extruded disk fragment and is accompanied by an unequivocally positive radiographic study that correlates with clinical findings, 85% of patients will recover completely after surgical treatment. If the syndrome is not associated with a ruptured disk and a positive scan or myelogram, intensive physiotherapy for postural correction and strengthening of spinal and abdominal support musculature is indicated. Emotional and economic factors, including litigation and compensation for injury, play an important role in outcome, regardless of whether treatment is medical or surgical.

Biyani A, Andersson GB: Low back pain: pathophysiology and management. J Am Acad Orthop Surg 2004;12:106. Review.

Joanes V: Cervical disc herniation presenting with acute myelopathy. Surg Neurol 2000;54:198.

Khanna AJ et al: Magnetic resonance imaging of the cervical spine. Current techniques and spectrum of disease. J Bone Joint Surg (Am) 2002;84-A(Suppl 2):70.

Leufven C, Nordwakk A: Management of chronic disabling low back pain with 360 degrees fusion. Results from pain provocation test and concurrent posterior lumber interbody fusion, posterolateral fusion, and pedicle screw instrumentation in patients with chronic disabling low back pain. Spine 1999;24:2042.

Levi N, Gjerris F, Dons K: Thoracic disc herniation. Unilateral transpedicular approach in 35 consecutive patients. J Neurosurg Sci 1999;43:37.

Modic MT: Degenerative disc disease and back pain. Magn Reson Imaging Clin N Am 1999;7:481.

Sitzmann A, Hejazi N, Krasznai L: Posterior cervical foraminotomy. A follow-up study of 67 surgically treated patients with compressive radiculopathy. Neurosurg Rev 2000;23:213.

Wang JC et al: The outcome of lumbar discectomy in elite athletes. Spine 1999;24:570.

SURGICAL INFECTIONS OF THE CENTRAL NERVOUS SYSTEM

Cornelia S. von Koch, MD, PhD, &
Mark L. Rosenblum, MD

BRAIN ABSCESS

ESSENTIALS OF DIAGNOSIS

- *History of predisposing factors such as sinusitis, dental abscess, otitis, systemic infection (especially pulmonary infection or endocarditis), congenital cyanotic heart disease, or brain damage from trauma or surgery.*
- *Headache, localized neurologic signs, seizures, fever.*
- *Positive CT or MRI brain scan.*
- *Acute or subacute course (days to weeks).*
- *Immune status.*

General Considerations

Brain abscess is a relatively rare disease; large medical centers see only four to six cases each year. In patients with normal immune systems, brain abscesses usually occur secondary to intracranial extension of infections of the paranasal sinuses, middle ear, lungs, heart, and teeth. Congenital cyanotic heart disease resulting in right-to-left shunting and open cranial wounds from trauma or surgical procedures are predisposing factors for abscess formation; however, in 10–60% of patients, no cause can be identified. The organisms most commonly responsible for infections are streptococcus, staphylococcus, and enteric gram-negative rods. However, brain abscess in neonates and infants is caused exclusively by proteus and citrobacter species. Anaerobic organisms are found in 50%, with bacteroides and fusobacterium being the most common, and multiple microbes in up to 69% of cultures from abscesses; 3–50% are sterile.

Abscesses arising from frontal and ethmoid sinusitis usually occur in the frontal lobes, whereas those arising from middle ear disease occur in the posterior temporal lobe. Hematogenous abscesses commonly involve the middle cerebral artery distribution.

Immunosuppressed patients and patients with AIDS are predisposed to brain abscesses caused by fungi and protozoal infections. AIDS patients are especially vulnerable to toxoplasma, cryptococcus, nocardia, and mycobacteria.

Clinical Findings

A. Symptoms and Signs

The usual presenting symptoms depend on the location of the abscess and the immune status of the patient and include low-grade fever (40–70%), headache (60–90%), focal neurologic deficits (50–75%), seizures (10–50%), and an altered level of consciousness due to increased intracranial pressure (10–70%).

B. Laboratory Findings

Blood studies may show mild polymorphonuclear leukocytosis and an elevated sedimentation rate. *Lumbar puncture should not be performed with suspected abscess unless CT scan or MRI shows only a small mass or no mass.* Cerebrospinal fluid analysis is rarely helpful and often normal, with negative cultures or nonspecific results.

C. Imaging Studies

The diagnosis of brain abscess is made on CT or MRI scans, which show a discrete mass with a smooth, symmetric contrast-enhancing ring, low-density center, and variable surrounding edema. Magnetic resonance spectroscopy has recently been used to better distinguish brain abscesses from ring-enhancing brain tumors.

Differential Diagnosis

Brain abscess must be differentiated from brain tumor, cerebral infarction, resolving intracranial hemorrhage, subdural empyema, extradural abscess, and encephalitis.

Complications

The major complications of brain abscess are rupture into the ventricles or subarachnoid space, obstruction of cerebrospinal fluid pathways, and transtentorial herniation, because of the mass effect of the abscess and the reactive brain swelling.

Treatment

A. Medical Treatment

Before starting antibiotic therapy, obtain cultures of blood, nasopharyngeal secretions, sputum, urine, or draining material from paranasal sinuses or wounds, as may be indicated by the suspected source of infection. Culture of the cerebrospinal fluid should only be performed when no mass effect is seen on imaging and symptoms of meningitis are present. Whenever possible, antibiotics should not be started prior to abscess aspiration, since doing so preoperatively results in cultures that frequently do not grow out organisms.

Vancomycin, a third-generation cephalosporin, and metronidazole are started when the diagnosis is made. As soon as the organism is identified, specific antibiotics that are cytotoxic and can cross the blood-brain barrier are instituted. The duration of administration of parenteral antibiotics is largely empiric and can range from 4 weeks to 8 weeks. Infectious disease consultation is strongly advised. Toxoplasma abscesses will usually respond to treatment with pyrimethamine and sulfadiazine. Treatment of fungal abscesses relies on the use of agents such as amphotericin B, but the results have been discouraging.

Since new antibiotics with improved activity and ability to cross the blood-brain barrier are being developed every year, the reader is referred to the infectious disease literature for the most recent updates.

If there is an extracerebral focus of infection (sinus, mastoid, wound, etc), it should be drained surgically.

B. Surgical Treatment

Surgical treatment consists of excision of the abscess or aspiration through a burr hole. CT-guided stereotaxic aspiration, performed under local anesthesia, is the procedure of choice for most abscesses, especially small, deep abscesses or diseases found in patients who are poor candidates for surgery. Solitary abscesses larger than 1.5 cm in diameter and multiple abscesses larger than 3 cm in diameter should be aspirated without delay. Medical treatment is justified only if the patient has a known predisposing factor, a CT scan that suggests the presence of an abscess, is alert and either clinically stable or improving with antibiotic therapy, if the abscess is small (less than 1.5 cm in diameter), and if there is little associated mass effect or if the patient has a bleeding diathesis. Aspiration of the abscess may be necessary if the organism is not otherwise identifiable and is essential if the patient deteriorates or if CT or MRI shows an increase in abscess size. After the organism is identified, antibiotics are adjusted appropriately. Corticosteroids are given only when there is significant mass effect from the abscess and surrounding edema, both of which may put the patient at significant risk. Anticonvulsants should be used. An abscess will occasionally resolve with antibiotic treatment alone, as shown by serial CT or MRI scans. In patients with multiple abscesses, small lesions can be followed with antibiotics after the organism has been identified by aspiration of the largest lesion. The decision to treat with antibiotics alone requires frequent follow-up visits, with CT or MRI scans and treatment planning by a neurosurgeon who is ready to operate whenever the patient's condition deteriorates or serial imaging demonstrates an increase in abscess size or no change after 4 weeks of antibiotic therapy.

Postoperative CT or MRI scans are done for early detection and management of complications such as hemorrhage and recurrent abscess. Monitoring for 1 year is indicated to make certain that no recurrence develops.

LESS COMMON PYOGENIC INFECTIONS

Epidural Abscess

Epidural abscess in the cranial or spinal epidural space produces focal neurologic deficit by pressure on the underlying neural tissues. In the cranium, it is usually secondary to adjacent osteomyelitis or head trauma or to cranial operations. In the spine, epidural abscesses are usually metastatic from a remote infection in the pelvis or lower extremities, or from bacteremia usually caused by urinary tract infection or illicit intravenous drug use.

Treatment consists of immediate drainage of the pus and appropriate treatment of the primary infection with antibiotics. Operations should also be performed on the primary focal sites of infection.

Subdural Abscess

Subdural abscess or empyema, a serious complication of sinus and ear infections and of meningitis in infants, progresses rapidly and has a high death rate. Immediate MRI scan followed by surgical drainage and antibiotic therapy are indicated.

Cerebral Thrombophlebitis

Cerebral thrombophlebitis is a rare complication of meningitis, epidural and subdural abscesses, and thrombophlebitis of facial veins. The lateral, cavernous, and superior sagittal sinuses are most commonly involved, producing neurologic deficit by venous infarction. Treatment is with specific antibiotics and surgical drainage of the original site of infection. If marked cerebral edema is associated, treatment with glucocorticoids, diuretics, and mannitol should be considered.

CLOSED DISK SPACE INFECTIONS FOLLOWING REMOVAL OF LUMBAR INTERVERTEBRAL DISK

Closed disk space infection is seen in approximately 1–3% of patients following lumbar diskectomy and is thought to be due to pyogenic infection confined to the disk space. The most common organism is *Staphylococcus aureus.* Symptoms usually occur 1–3 weeks or longer after operation. Preoperative sciatica has usually resolved when the patient complains of severe pain localized in the back and thighs, aggravated by any motion. The patient may run a low-grade fever or be afebrile; the white count may be normal or slightly elevated. The erythrocyte sedimentation rate and C-reactive protein are elevated. Starting at about 4 weeks, plain films reveal destruction of the vertebral end-plates and narrowing and eventual bony fusion of the disk space. MRI shows characteristic changes in disk spaces and vertebral bodies as early as 3–5 days after onset of symptoms.

Treatment consists of immobilization with a brace and analgesics. A needle biopsy of the interspace should be performed before antibiotic therapy is planned; antibiotics should be given for 6–8 weeks. Surgery consisting of disk space debridement and fusion is indicated if conservative treatment fails.

TUBERCULOSIS OF THE SPINE (POTT'S DISEASE)

Tuberculous infections of the spine have recently become more prevalent in the United States due to the emergence of multidrug-resistant strains. The thoracic cord is most commonly involved, followed by the cervical cord and the lumbar cord segments. Radiographically, there is usually destruction of one or more intervertebral disks, apposition of the adjacent vertebral bodies, and destruction of one or more vertebral bodies. Soft tissue swelling is usually evident around the affected area, and a soft tissue mass of varying size is commonly present.

Treatment consists of isoniazid, rifampin, and pyrazinamide with or without ethambutol, depending on the susceptibility of the organism. Continuation of antibiotic treatment for up to 12 months may be indicated. For advanced disease and unstable spines, surgical drainage and anterior or posterior fusion is necessary. The affected area must be immobilized.

Bockova J et al: Intracranial empyema. Pediatr Infect Dis J 2000;19:735.

Khan IA et al: Management of vertebral diskitis and osteomyelitis. Orthopedics 1999;22:758.

Luk KD: Tuberculosis of the spine in the new millennium. Eur Spine J 1999;8:338.

Saez-Llorens X: Brain abscess in children. Semin Pediatr Infect Dis 2003;14:108. Review.

Sampath P et al: Spinal epidural abscess: a review of epidemiology, diagnosis, and treatment. J Spinal Disord 1999;12:89.

Tay BK, Deckey J, Hu SS: Spinal infections. J Am Acad Orthop Surg. 2002;10:188.

Otolaryngology—Head & Neck Surgery

38

Lee D. Rowe, MD

Otolaryngology is a regional surgical specialty devoted to diseases of the head and neck. An understanding of head and neck anatomy, physiology, and pathology is necessary to manage diverse disorders of head and neck structures, ranging from hearing and communication impairments to disorders calling for facial plastic and reconstructive surgery.

EAR

Sound waves travel as alternating compressions and rarefactions of the elastic medium through which they are transmitted (sound travels at about 1100 ft/s [346 m/s]). Sound waves exhibit several physical characteristics, including amplitude and frequency, which are related to the subjective psychoacoustic attributes of loudness and pitch. The intensity range of human hearing is great—the most intense tone that can be perceived as sound is several million times louder than the faintest detectable one.

The auricle serves to localize sound in space and to amplify sound waves impinging on the tympanic membrane through the resonance capabilities of the external auditory canal. Sound waves strike the tympanic membrane and produce in-and-out vibrations that transmit sound energy to the ossicular chain. The tympanic membrane protects the round window from simultaneous sound exposure by interposing an air-filled middle ear space. With large perforation of the tympanic membrane, sound simultaneously strikes the round window and the tympanic membrane, decreasing the energy transmitted to the oval window.

Acoustic energy at the tympanic membrane is transformed by the malleus, incus, and stapes into energy within the oval window perilymph. Sound is amplified by the lever mechanism of the ossicular chain and also as a function of the large ratio of the tympanic membrane area to the area of the small stapes footplate. Therefore, the middle ear and ossicular system act as an efficient device for transferring acoustic energy from one elastic medium (air) to another medium of different impedance (fluid).

Movement of the stapes footplate produces a traveling wave in the scala vestibuli perilymph that is propagated along the basilar membrane of the cochlea from the base to the apex and down the scala tympani to the round window. Vibration of the basement membrane produces a shearing movement between the tectorial membrane and the hairs of the hair cells, generating electrical activity within the cochlea and auditory nerves. The point of maximal displacement of the basilar membrane is dependent upon the frequency (or pitch) of the wave. High-frequency tones cause maximal displacement near the base of the cochlea, and low-frequency tones cause maximal stimulation near the apex.

Cochlear frequency encoding involves depolarization of afferent neurons that synapse in the cochlear nuclei in the brain stem. The attendant perception of loudness and pitch depends upon the total number of neurons activated and their frequency specificities. The central auditory pathway is a complex system with many crossovers and relay stations to the auditory cortex.

CLINICAL AUDIOLOGY

Audiology is the study of hearing and disorders in sound recognition. Sound carried by air to the ear and perceived in the normal way represents hearing by **air conduction**. Tests of hearing by air conduction provide information about the patency of the external auditory canal, the efficiency of sound transmission by the tympanic membrane and the ossicular chain, and the integrity of the cochlea, acoustic nerve, and central auditory pathway. A defect in the auditory system from the external auditory canal to but not including the cochlea causes conductive hearing loss and raises the intensity threshold for perception of sound. The conductive hearing loss applies only to air conduction. Otitis media with effusion is the most common cause of conductive hearing loss in children. Other causes include ceruminous impactions in the external auditory canal, large tympanic membrane perforations, ossicular chain discontinuities from trauma or infection, otosclerosis, and temporal bone neoplasms involving the external auditory canal or middle ear.

If the sound source is placed on the skull or teeth, the vibration will directly stimulate the cochlear perilymph and bypass the external and middle ear. **Bone conduction** hearing tests thus examine the integrity of the cochlea, the eighth nerve, and the central auditory pathway. Bone conduction hearing losses are secondary to lesions of the sensory (cochlea) and neural (acoustic nerve) components of the auditory system and are designated **sensorineural** hearing losses. The most common cause of sensorineural hearing loss is aging (presbycusis), which is associated with progressive loss of outer hair cells within the organ of Corti and neural degeneration. However, noise exposure (especially industrial noise), ototoxic drugs including neomycin and other aminoglycosides, temporal bone fractures, labyrinthine infections, and arterial insufficiency may also produce sensorineural hearing disorders. Composite or mixed losses have both conductive and sensorineural elements.

Hearing is clinically evaluated by a careful history and physical examination that includes tuning fork testing, whispered voice assessment, and audiometric analysis. Because of the importance of hearing in speech acquisition and intellectual maturation, it is critical to diagnose disorders early. By noting the verbal responses to spondaic words or phrases (eg, "football," "hot dog," "childhood," "heartbreak"—taking care to sustain the accent on both syllables), the examiner can grossly establish the level of hearing loss in each ear. The degree of loss may be estimated from Table 38–1 by determining the voice level at which the words are no longer perceived.

Table 38–1. Estimation of hearing loss by voice level.[1]

Examiner's Voice Level	Decibel Equivalent	Degree of Loss
Soft whispered voice (inaudible to examiner)	25 dB	None
Moderate whispered voice (just audible to examiner)	25–40 dB	Mild
Loud whispered voice	40–55 dB	Moderate
Moderately loud spoken voice	70–90 dB	Moderately severe
Loud spoken voice	90–120 dB	Profound

[1]The degree of hearing loss may be estimated by determining the voice level at which the patient understands the examiner's voice. If the patient hears the examiner's whispered voice distinctly, hearing is probably normal.

It is important to provide masking (noise) by rubbing the tragus or hair in front of the ear not being tested when the loud whispered level is reached. Otherwise, sound or speech may cross over to the nontested ear, yielding a false result.

Further characterization of the type of hearing loss requires the use of tuning forks to differentiate a conductive from a sensorineural defect. In the **Weber test**, placement of a 512-Hz tuning fork on the skull in the midline or on the teeth stimulates both cochleae simultaneously. If the patient has a conductive hearing loss in one ear, the sound will be perceived loudest in the affected ear (ie, it will lateralize). When a unilateral sensorineural hearing loss is present, the tone is heard in the unaffected ear. The **Rinne test** compares air conduction (AC) with bone conduction (ie, AC > BC) in one ear, and commonly utilizes the 256-Hz and 512-Hz tuning forks. Sound stimulation by air in front of the pinna is normally perceived twice as long as sound placed on the mastoid tip (ie, AC > BC). With conductive hearing loss, the duration of air conduction is less than bone conduction (ie, BC > AC; negative Rinne test). In the case of sensorineural hearing loss, the duration of both air conduction and bone conduction are reduced; however, the 2:1 ratio remains the same (ie, AC > BC; positive Rinne test). The results of these two tuning fork tests are assessed to determine the type of hearing loss.

Further quantification of the type and degree of hearing loss and the ability to hear and understand speech requires pure tone audiometry, speech reception threshold testing, and speech discrimination analysis. An audiometer is an electronic device capable of delivering pure sound frequencies by both air and bone conduction from 125 Hz to 8000 Hz at intensities ranging from 0 to 110 decibels (dB) in 5-dB steps. The decibel is a logarithmic ratio of two sound pressure levels or intensities that are related to a reference intensity, measured in dynes per square centimeter. The threshold intensity of sound perception in a normal individual is 0–25 dB within the speech frequencies (300–4000 Hz). The ear has the greatest sensitivities between these frequencies, because the tympanic membrane and ossicular chain transmit sound most efficiently in this range. Pure tone audiometry will demonstrate normal thresholds at all frequencies for both air and bone conduction (Figure 38–1). A conductive hearing loss raises the threshold for sound perception in air. With air conduction hearing loss of 60 dB, for example, the threshold is 10,000-fold greater than normal (Figure 38–2). Sensorineural hearing losses result in equal increases in the threshold for air conduction and bone conduction and produce a characteristic audiogram (Figure 38–3).

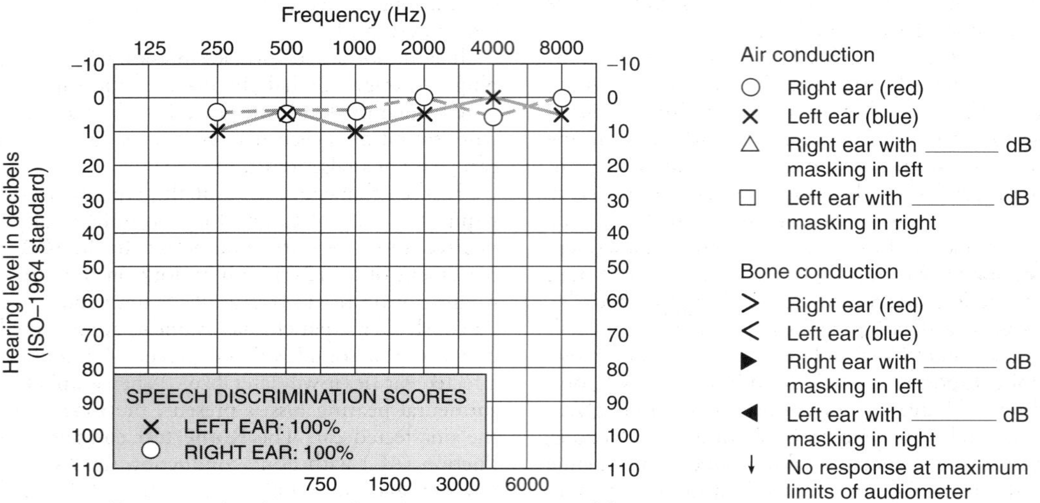

To convert the above readings based on the 1964 ISO reference thresholds to readings based on the 1951 ASA reference thresholds, subtract the following (rounded) difference in dB:

125	250	500	1000	2000	4000	8000
10	15	15	10	10	5	10

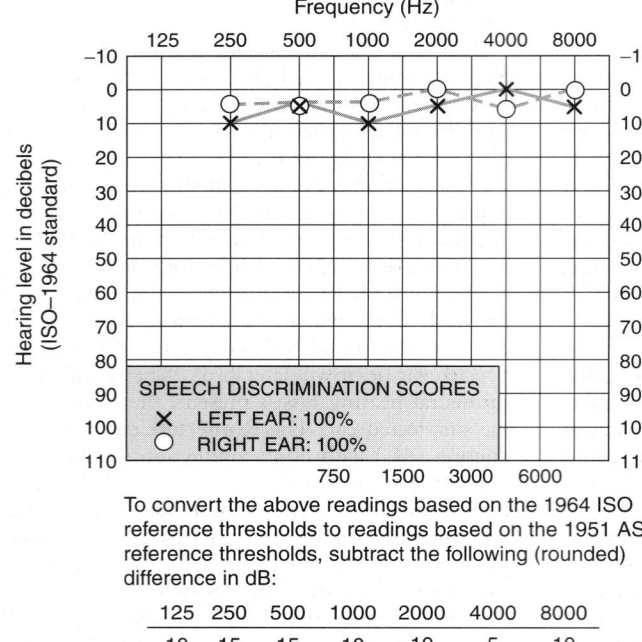

Figure 38–1. Normal hearing.

Speech perception can be evaluated by presenting the patient with a list of spondaic words at an intensity corresponding to 50% comprehension. The resulting speech reception threshold should approximate the average hearing levels for the speech frequencies of 500 Hz, 1000 Hz, and 2000 Hz. These frequencies are extremely important for understanding conversation in English and fall within the 300-Hz to 3000-Hz transmission range of the telephone. The ability to discriminate speech is ascertained by presenting a list of 50 phonetically balanced monosyllabic words 30–40 dB above the speech reception threshold. The percentage of words the patient repeats correctly is called the **discrimination score** and should normally be between 90%

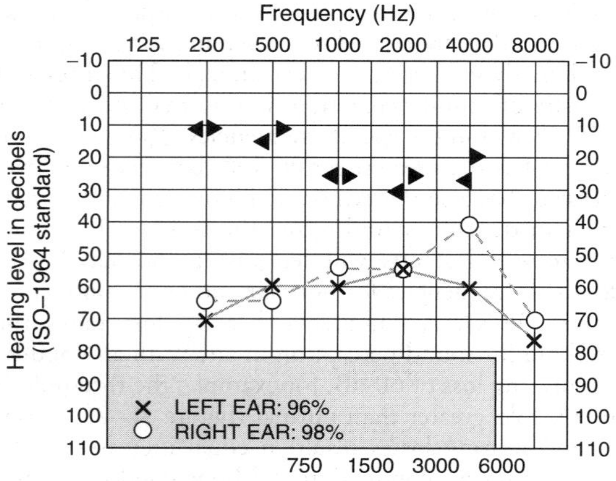

Figure 38–2. Bilateral severe conductive hearing loss due to otosclerosis.

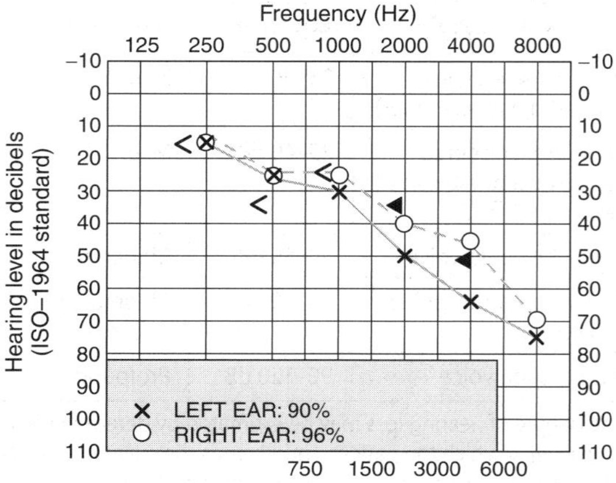

Figure 38–3. Bilateral high-frequency sensorineural hearing loss.

Table 38–2. High-risk criteria for hearing loss.[1]

1. Family history of childhood hearing impairment
2. Congenital perinatal infection, eg, cytomegalovirus, rubella, herpes, toxoplasmosis, syphilis, TORCH
3. Anatomic malformation of the head or neck
4. Birth weight < 1500 g
5. Hyperbilirubinemia at level exceeding indications for exchange transfusion
6. Bacterial meningitis, especially *Haemophilus influenzae*
7. Severe asphyxia, including infants with Apgar scores of 0–3 who fail to start spontaneous respiration by 10 minutes and those with hypotonia persisting to 2 hours of age

[1]Joint Committee on Infant Hearing, 1982.

and 100%. In conductive hearing loss, the discrimination score is normal; in sensorineural hearing losses, the discrimination score decreases with progressive cochlear and neuronal impairment.

Because the tests described above require a voluntary response, they are of little use if age or illness prevents the patient from performing the required tasks. For example, infants with a high risk of hearing loss (eg, congenital rubella) are unable to give voluntary responses; therefore, an objective method of determining auditory thresholds is necessary to fully evaluate a suspected hearing loss. **Evoked response** or **brain stem audiometry** measures electrical responses to sound stimuli (clicks) from the acoustic nerve, cochlear nuclei, and inferior colliculi from the surface of the scalp and the mastoid prominence or ear lobe of the test ear. These techniques are particularly useful in evaluating patients with suspected sensorineural hearing losses secondary to acoustic neuroma, cerebellopontine angle tumor, or a brain stem lesion. **Brain stem evoked response audiometry (BSERA)** is especially important in newborn nurseries for identifying infants at risk of hearing impairment. These include low-birth-weight infants (< 1500 g), infants with low Apgar scores, infants with hyperbilirubinemia (> 20 mg/dL) or neonatal meningitis, or infants with the TORCH (toxoplasmosis, rubella, chlamydia) complex (Table 38–2). Accordingly, a protocol for audiologic screening of at-risk newborn infants (Table 38–3) is indicated using BSERA. If hearing loss is identified, habilitation should begin by age 6 months. BSERA is also used for evaluating potential candidates for pediatric cochlear implantation.

Gelfand SA et al: Apparent auditory deprivation in children: implications of monaural versus binaural amplification. J Am Acad Audiol 1993;4:313.

CONDUCTIVE HEARING LOSS

1. Otitis Media With Effusion

Otitis media with effusion is the leading cause of hearing loss in childhood. More than 30% of all children have had three or more episodes of otitis media by their second birthday. Although otitis media with effusion occurs in all age groups, it is most common from the newborn period to age 7. The term **nonsuppurative otitis media** denotes a broad range of middle ear effusions characterized by an inflammatory exudate and various amounts of mucus. Several distinct types are recognized: (1) serous otitis media—a sterile, pale, low-viscosity transudate; (2) secretory otitis media—a chronic **glue ear** with infiltration of lymphocytes, histiocytes, plasma cells, leukocytes, and markedly increased glandular production of mucus; and (3) aerotitis media secondary to barotrauma or direct temporal bone injury. Chronic otitis media with effusion is unsterile in 50% of cases; *Haemophilus influenzae, Streptococcus pneumoniae, Moraxella catarrhalis,* and *Streptococcus pyogenes* are the organisms most often found. Although many factors may be implicated, including rhinoviruses, upper respiratory bacteria, passive smoking, and inflammatory mediators of arachidonic acid metabolism, the common denominator appears to be auditory tube (eustachian tube) dysfunction. The physiologic role of the auditory tube is to protect the middle ear from nasopharyngeal secretions, clear middle ear secretions into the nasopharynx, and, more importantly, ventilate the middle ear space. Auditory tube dysfunction develops from barotrauma when the nasopharyngeal pressure exceeds middle ear pressure during rapid descent in an airplane or from adenoidal hypertrophy that produces lymphatic or mechanical obstruction of the auditory tube. In addition, over half of children with cleft palate deformities manifest auditory tube dysfunction secondary to malfunction of the tensor veli palatini muscle, resulting in inefficient opening of the auditory tube.

If auditory tube function is compromised—as it frequently is in young children—early diagnosis and treatment are critical to prevent impairment of speech development. On physical examination, the tympanic membrane

Table 38–3. Protocol for screening infants at risk for hearing loss.

1. Newborn infants with no risk factors are not screened unless the parent is concerned about auditory behavior or speech and language development. Parents of infants not at risk are to be given information and education.
2. Infants at risk are screened by BSERA prior to discharge. Parents of at-risk infants are to be given information and education.
   a. Infants who passed the screening procedure are provided with follow-up as needed for medical and developmental consideration.
   b. Infants who pass the screening procedure but are at risk for progressive hearing impairment are monitored audiologically and managed as needed.
   c. Infants who fail the screening procedure are evaluated, given follow-up, and provided with a management system.

is retracted, the short process of the malleus is extremely prominent, and the light reflex is frequently lost. Pneumatic otoscopy discloses marked reduction of tympanic membrane mobility, and a characteristic yellow or amber color is often seen in the middle ear space. Middle ear effusions can be confirmed by the presence of an air-fluid level in the middle ear.

Otoscopy is not a reliable method of assessing middle ear effusions. Impedance audiometry (tympanometry) is a more accurate means of diagnosing otitis media with effusion. The overall compliance of the tympanic membrane and middle ear system, which varies inversely with its impedance, is measured by delivering to the tympanic membrane a continuous 220-Hz tone signal via a sealed probe tip and recording the amount of energy reflected from the surface. The pressure in the external auditory canal is varied from +400 mm H_2O to –400 mm H_2O, and the reflected energy is recorded. The resulting tympanogram correlates well with the presence or absence of effusion. A normal type A tympanogram is characterized by peak compliance at 0 mm H_2O pressure; the absence of a peak of maximal compliance is commonly encountered in middle ear effusion (type B tympanogram). By contrast, type C tympanograms exhibits a peak of maximal compliance of less than –100 mm of H_2O and are chiefly associated with a retracted tympanic membrane with or without effusion.

Initial management of otitis media with effusion consists of identifying the cause. In adults, a malignant neoplasm of the nasopharynx such as carcinoma or lymphoma should be carefully excluded. Unilateral hearing loss secondary to otitis media with effusion is a common manifestation of obstruction of the auditory tube by tumor. Allergy and enlargement of the adenoids may play a causative role in children. Group day care settings are associated with a high risk of otitis media with effusion. Conservative treatment with sympathomimetic amines and antihistamines is often attempted first, though there is no evidence that they alter the clinical course. Nonoperative therapy also includes antibiotics, autoinflation (Valsalva's maneuver), and control of etiologic factors (nasal infections, sinusitis, allergy, etc). Many consultants would start with a course of amoxicillin in doses twice the current recommendations of 40 mg/kg/d in three divided doses. Some patients may respond to a 3- to 4-week course of antibiotics. Failure of medical treatment necessitates myringotomy and insertion of ventilating tubes (Figure 38–4). Usually this is defined as 3 months of chemoprophylaxis with amoxicillin-clavulanate potassium, amoxicillin, or sulfisoxazole. Current indications for sustained middle ear ventilation with tubes include (1) significant conductive hearing loss; (2) persistent tympanic membrane atelectasis and negative middle ear pressure of less than 150 mm H_2O; (3) cleft palate; and (4) impending cholesteatoma. Approximately 80% of intubated patients respond after one insertion and require no further treatment. Surgical treatment immediately corrects the conductive hearing loss, reduces the incidence of recurrent infections, and improves the child's learning capacity. Adenoidectomy, which is recommended for children requiring more than one set of myringotomy tubes, reduces recurrent middle ear infections, since chronically infected adenoids obstruct the auditory tube and serve as a persistent source of infection in the middle ear. Otitis media-prone children carry nontypable *H influenzae* at an unusually high prevalence.

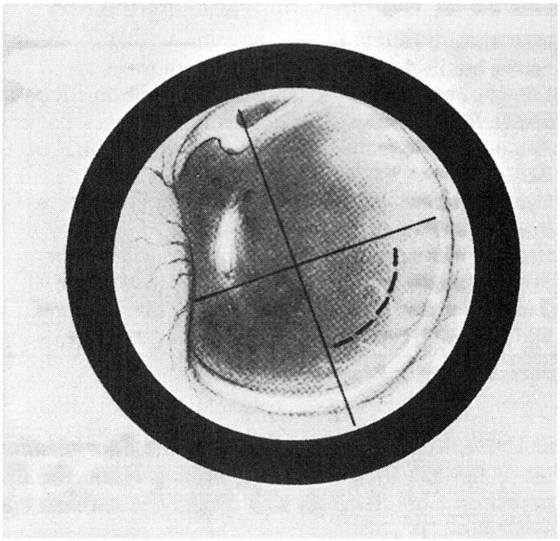

Figure 38–4. Site of myringotomy.

Bluestone CD et al: "Appropriateness" of tympanostomy tubes: setting the record straight. Arch Otolaryngol Head Neck Surg 1994;120:1051.

Grundfast KM: Management of otitis media and the New Agency for Health Care Policy and Research Guideline. Arch Otolaryngol Head Neck Surg 1994;120:797.

Managing otitis media with effusion in young children. Arch Otolaryngol Head Neck Surg 1994;120:793.

Rosenfeld RM: Comprehensive management of otitis media with effusion. Otolaryngol Clin North Am 1994;27:443.

2. Chronic Otitis Media

The long-term sequela of chronic auditory tube dysfunction is chronic otitis media, which involves chronic perforation of the tympanic membrane that may or may not be associated with recurrent acute suppuration, destruction of the ossicular chain, or both. The perforation of the tympanic membrane may take two forms: (1) a central (or safe) perforation, in which a remnant of the tympanic membrane is interposed between the rim of the perforation and the annulus of the tympanic membrane (Figure

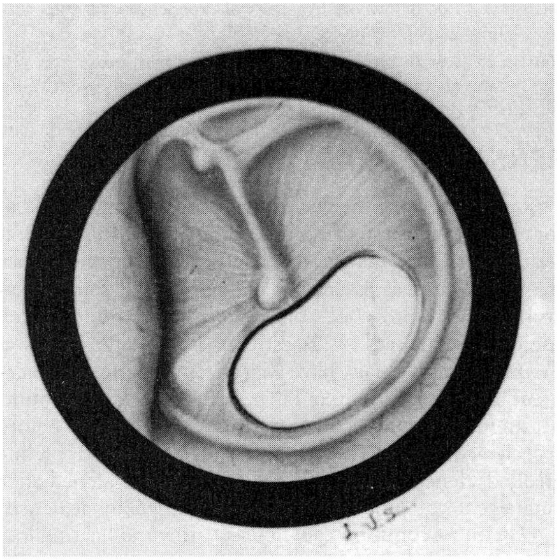

Figure 38–5. Perforation of eardrum.

38–5); and (2) marginal (or dangerous) perforation, in which the annulus of the tympanic membrane has been destroyed, primarily in the posterosuperior quadrant. In the former case, the middle ear is usually dry; in the latter, suppuration commonly occurs. The pars flaccida is frequently involved in marginal perforations, and central perforations are restricted to the pars tensa. However, suppuration may develop in either situation as a result of the introduction of staphylococci or gram-negative rods (commonly *Pseudomonas aeruginosa,* klebsiellae, and Enterobacteriaceae) via the auditory tube or external auditory canal. Foul-smelling otorrhea characteristic of anaerobic streptococcal infection should be treated by vacuum drainage of the external auditory canal and instillation of neomycin plus polymyxin otic drops with or without an oral fluoroquinolone such as ciprofloxacin, norfloxacin, grepafloxacin, or ofloxacin. These are avoided, however, in children aged 16 and younger and in infants. Alternative therapy may be instituted with gentamicin drops plus clindamycin orally, or tobramycin with hydrocortisone topically. Some clinicians add metronidazole to this regimen. In recalcitrant cases, parenteral azlocillin, ticarcillin, or ceftazidime may prove beneficial if no cholesteatoma is present. Intravenous ciprofloxacin or grepafloxacin may also be considered in adults.

Complications of chronic otitis media such as seventh nerve paralysis, labyrinthitis, lateral semicircular canal fistula, petrositis (Gradenigo's syndrome), or intracranial suppuration are less frequently associated with central perforations than with marginal ones. If squamous epithelium migrates into the middle ear or mastoid, a keratinizing aural cholesteatoma develops. The desquamating epithelium produces bone-destroying collagenase and tends to remain infected. The associated middle ear inflammation interferes with the tenuous blood supply to the stapes and the long process of the incus, resulting in ossicular destruction with a conductive hearing loss of 50–60 dB. White amorphous debris is often observed in the pars flaccida. If untreated, a cholesteatoma may progressively destroy the ossicular chain and erode into the inner ear, producing profound hearing loss. Computed tomography is essential in the management of chronic otitis media in determining the extent of the disease, the presence of any associated complications, and the degree of pneumatization of the mastoid. For example, the finding of a large radiolucent defect secondary to bone destruction may imply an aggressive cholesteatoma.

Bacterial invasion of the cranium from an infected cholesteatoma may occur as a result of osteitis, thrombophlebitis, bony erosion, or along a preformed pathway such as the oval or round windows, perilymphatic duct, or endolymphatic duct. In the preantibiotic era, the onset of severe temporoparietal headache and nuchal rigidity in a patient with chronic otitis media was an ominous sign. The most common intracranial complication of chronic otitis media is meningitis secondary to pneumococcal or other streptococcal infection. Additional potential problems include epidural abscesses, temporal lobe abscess, cerebellar abscess, lateral sinus thrombosis, subdural empyema, and otitic hydrocephalus. Fortunately, these complications are now rare and can be prevented by early surgical treatment of chronic otitis media and cholesteatoma. Intracranial complications of chronic otitis media are best evaluated by MRI with or without CT. Management includes drainage, mastoidectomy, and penicillin or clindamycin (for anaerobic bacteria) and ceftazidime (for pseudomonas, staphylococcus, and most gram-negative species) as initial agents. An alternative antibiotic choice is tobramycin and ticarcillin/clavulanate.

Simple central tympanic membrane perforations are repaired by grafting the tympanic membrane with temporalis fascia or canal wall skin. In the absence of cholesteatoma, associated ossicular discontinuity is repaired with an autogenous homograft or alloplastic materials to reestablish the sound-transforming capability of the middle ear. With advanced middle ear and mastoid disease and associated cholesteatoma, more radical surgery is required. In a radical mastoidectomy, the remnants of the tympanic membrane, ossicles, and cholesteatoma are removed and the mastoid air cells, antrum, and middle ear are converted into an open cavity that is periodically inspected and cleaned. If the cholesteatoma lies above and superficial to the tympanic membrane and middle ear ossicles, either a canal wall-up mastoidectomy or canal wall-down mastoidectomy is performed depending on the location of the cholesteatoma. The primary goal of each is to eradicate infection and provide a temporal bone free of cholesteatoma.

Merfield DO et al: Therapeutic management of chronic suppurative otitis media with otic drops. Otolaryngol Head Neck Surg 1993;109:77.

Naguib MB et al: Surgical management of epitympanic cholesteatoma with intact ossicular chain: the modified Bondy Technique. Otolaryngol Head Neck Surg 1994;111:545.

3. Otosclerosis

In otosclerosis, a unique localized disease of the otic capsule, new spongy bone replaces normal bone, producing ankylosis or fixation of the stapes footplate. The resulting primarily conductive hearing loss starts insidiously in the third and fourth decades of life and progressively involves both ears in 80% of individuals. Otosclerosis is an inherited disease, more common in whites, with an incidence of approximately 12% in temporal bone series. Bilateral otosclerosis is present more commonly in women by a ratio of 2:1. In adults with normal-appearing tympanic membranes, it is the most common cause of progressive conductive hearing loss. Evaluation of the hearing loss requires tuning fork and audiometric testing, including air conduction, bone conduction, and speech audiometry. The patient with a significant hearing loss secondary to otosclerosis has several options. If the hearing loss is unilateral, no treatment may be necessary. Hearing aids or surgery can be offered to improve hearing. The complete-in-the-canal hearing aid, which fits close to the tympanic membrane of the ear canal, is extremely effective for patients with otosclerosis. The hearing loss may be treated in selected cases by microsurgical removal of the stapes and reconstruction with a metallic prosthesis (3.7–4.5 mm in length) crimped over the long process of the incus. The medial end of the prosthesis is placed over vein or fascia inserted in the oval window. Alternatively, a small hole is created in the footplate of the stapes with a pick or microdrill (stapedotomy) and a Teflon wire or platinum ribbon prosthesis (4.25–0.5 mm) inserted. Argon, KTP (potassium titanyl phosphate), and CO_2 lasers can be used for small-fenestra stapedotomy. Stapedectomy or stapedotomy corrects the conductive hearing loss in most patients and may cause partial or total sensorineural hearing loss in fewer than 1% of patients. Revision stapedectomy may be necessary because of recurrent conductive hearing loss or because of a suspected oval window fistula associated with vertigo, fluctuating hearing loss, or tinnitus.

Emmett JR: Physical examination and clinical evaluation of the patient with otosclerosis. Otolaryngol Clin North Am 1993; 26:353.

Glasscock M et al: Twenty-five years of experience with stapedectomy. Laryngoscope 1995;105:899.

Vartiainen E et al: Hearing levels of patients with otosclerosis 10 years after stapedectomy. Otolaryngol Head Neck Surg 1993;108:251.

SENSORINEURAL HEARING LOSS

Disorders affecting the cochlea and auditory neurons distort the perception of sound, producing sensorineural hearing loss. The deficit is generally greater in the higher frequencies and is associated with decreased speech discrimination scores (ie, ability to understand complex speech is impaired). It is estimated that one out of a thousand individuals have significant hearing impairment at birth. Children born with bilateral profound hearing loss or who acquire profound hearing loss before speech acquisition (2 years of age) are termed prelingually deafened. Those children and adults deafened after language development are termed postlingually deafened.

The most common cause of sensorineural hearing loss is presbycusis, a gradual deterioration that starts after 20 years of age in the highest frequencies and often involves all speech frequencies by the sixth and seventh decades. The impaired hearing stems from degenerative changes in the hair cells, auditory neurons, and cochlear nuclei. Tinnitus (ringing in the ear) is a common complaint. Hearing rehabilitation includes physician counseling and formal aural rehabilitation, encompassing the range from assisted listening devices, in-the-canal aids, in-the-ear aids, behind-the-ear aids, body aids, and bone conduction aids up to cochlear implants. Profound bilateral sensorineural hearing loss in adults who are postlingually deaf and unresponsive to conventional amplification may benefit from cochlear implants. A cochlear implant provides sound awareness, permits identification of environmental sounds, and improves ability to communicate through auditory clues such as prosody, rhythm, and intensity. A cochlear implant has two components: an external component, consisting of a small microphone to pick up auditory information, a speech processor that changes the mechanical acoustical sound energy into an electrical transmitter coil to send the information via radiofrequency through the skin; and an internal component, consisting of one or more electrodes implanted directly into the cochlea as well as a signal receiver and stimulator that interprets the electrical signal sent by the processor.

Injury to the inner ear or acoustic trauma from a sudden very loud noise (ie, painful, > 140 dB) may produce a permanent sensorineural hearing loss. More importantly, prolonged exposure (8 hours daily or more) to intense nonpainful sound such as industrial noise above 90 dB may result in destruction of the outer hair cells of the organ of Corti and a sensorineural hearing loss that characteristically initially affects perception at 4000 Hz. These patients may also experience tinnitus. Up to 10 million Americans are routinely exposed to potentially hazardous noise levels. Further noise exposure should be prevented with ear protectors (earmuffs or earplugs) and a hearing conservation program initiated at work.

Additional causes of sudden sensorineural hearing loss include diabetes mellitus, hypothyroidism, cochlear artery insufficiency, aminoglycosides, ototoxic diuretics (eg, ethacrynic acid), antimetabolites such as cisplatin and mechlorethamine, tumors of the vestibular nerve (vestibular schwannoma) or cerebellopontine angle, perilymph fistulas, trauma, autoimmune inner ear disorders such as Cogan's syndrome, Wegener's granulomatosis and systemic lupus erythematosus, congenital inner ear malformations, multiple sclerosis, and AIDS. Rubella in the first trimester of pregnancy, Rh incompatibility, birth trauma, hyperbilirubinemia, prematurity, congenital syphilis, meningitis, treatment of postnatal infection with ototoxic drugs such as kanamycin, gentamicin, tobramycin, and streptomycin, and congenital anomalies are often associated with profound bilateral prelingual deafness, and infants at risk should be tested immediately with brain stem evoked response audiometry (BSERA). Over 90% of infants with congenital sensorineural hearing loss have no known risk factors. Genetic causes for sensorineural hearing loss in children resulting in pre- and postlingual deafness represent approximately 50% of the cases. The remainder is divided equally among environmental and idiopathic causes. Profoundly impaired children with puretone averages at 500, 1000, and 2000 Hz greater than 90 dB who are unable to detect speech at 60 dB or greater with an appropriately fitted hearing aid should be considered for cochlear implantation. Children must be at least 2 years of age at most centers to be considered for implantation.

In cases of sudden sensorineural hearing loss when no cause can be identified, viruses such as mumps, measles, influenza, and adenoviruses are the most likely cause. Laboratory testing, which is essential to determine the cause, may include a complete blood count, erythrocyte sedimentation rate, determination of rheumatoid arthritis factor and antinuclear antibody levels, quantitative serum immunoglobulin levels, FTA-ABS, fasting blood glucose, serum cholesterol and triglycerides, and thyroid functions tests. In addition, MRI with gadolinium testing should be done. Prednisone (60 mg daily for 9 days and then tapering over 5 days) may be beneficial in preventing permanent hearing loss.

Callanan V et al: Cochlear implantation for children and adults. Lancet 1996;347:412.

Dodds A et al: Cochlear implantation after bacterial meningitis: the dangers of delay. Arch Dis Child 1997;76:139.

Langman AW et al: Cochlear implants in children. Pediatr Clin North Am 1996;43:1217.

OTALGIA

Ear pain may be caused by a primary disorder of the ear or may be referred from structures with a common sensory innervation. Inflammation of tissues innervated by the fifth cranial nerve—including the nose, paranasal sinuses, nasopharynx, mandible, and salivary glands—may produce otalgia. Inflammatory lesions of the oropharynx, the larynx, and the base of the tongue are commonly associated with otalgia. Neoplastic lesions usually do not produce otalgia until they are significantly advanced.

Inflammation of the external auditory canal (otitis externa) is commonly caused by bacteria (*Proteus mirabilis, Pseudomonas aeruginosa,* staphylococci) and occasionally by otomycoses *(Aspergillus niger, Candida albicans).* Predisposing causes are water immersion, high humidity, instrumentation in the external auditory canal, and ceruminous impaction. Patients complain of otalgia, pruritus, otorrhea, and decreased hearing and intermittent blockage of the canal. Pain on traction of the pinna or tragus differentiates otitis externa from acute otitis media. Hyperemia, edema, and otorrhea are seen on inspection of the external auditory canal. Treatment consists of early precise debridement, topical broad-spectrum antibiotics (eg, polymyxin B, bacitracin, neomycin), and hydrocortisone to reduce canal wall inflammation. In neomycin-sensitive individuals, topical 2% aqueous acetic acid is effective. Contact with water should be avoided, and dry heat hastens resolution. Diabetics are particularly at risk of developing invasive pseudomonas otitis externa. If untreated, invasive otitis externa can progressively involve the underlying skin, cartilage, or bone, leading eventually to osteomyelitis of the skull, multiple cranial nerve palsies, and death. Patients with invasive otitis externa are treated with immediate debridement and intravenous semisynthetic penicillin such as ticarcillin with clavulanate, mezlocillin, piperacillin, or azlocillin, and an aminoglycoside (tobramycin or amikacin) for 4–6 weeks. Some clinicians choose imipenem, meropenem, or ceftazidime as primary therapy. Two fluoroquinolones, ciprofloxacin (available for intravenous use) and ofloxacin, administered orally may be effective for invasive pseudomonas otitis externa. Most clinicians would switch to oral antibiotics only when pain, drainage, and granulation tissue are substantially decreased. After 4 weeks of therapy a gallium scan can aid in the evaluation for ongoing inflammation. If the patient is symptom-free and the scan is negative, antibiotics are discontinued and the patient is followed clinically. If symptoms persist and the scan remains positive, treatment for an additional 2–3 weeks is continued. A repeat scan is obtained. Late to advanced malignant external otitis requires more than 6 weeks of intravenous antibiotics, reserving surgery for abscess drainage or dead bone that serves as a nidus of continuing infection.

Inflammation that progresses to involve the auricular appendage may result in **perichondritis** and then **chondritis** with cartilaginous necrosis. Perichondritis or chondritis of the pinna may also follow auricular trauma and hematoma, frostbite, or surgical drainage of a furuncle of the external auditory canal. It is manifested by edema, erythema, and tenderness of the pinna. Treatment consists of systemic antistaphylococcal penicillin or, as an alternative, cephalothin or clindamycin and incision and drainage of any hematoma or abscess. Cotton soaked in an antiseptic solution (eg, povidone iodine) is placed within the recesses of the auricle, and a mastoid dressing is applied. Failure to adequately drain an auricular hematoma or abscess will result in a **cauliflower ear** deformity secondary to cartilaginous destruction and fibrosis.

Paradise JL: Managing otitis media: a time for change. Pediatrics 1995;96:712.

Poole MD: Otitis media complications and treatment failures: implications of pneumococcal resistance. Pediatr Infect Dis J 1995;14(4 Suppl):S23.

ACUTE OTITIS MEDIA

Acute suppurative otitis media is a very common problem in pediatric and family practice, with otalgia the most common ear complaint in childhood. Twenty percent of children under 8 years of age experience at least one episode. The peak prevalence is between 6 and 11 months of age. Recurrence is common, especially if the initial episode occurs during the first 12 months of life. Viruses may cause otitis media, but suppuration is predominantly caused by bacteria, especially *S pneumoniae. H influenzae, M catarrhalis, S pyogenes* (group A) or *S aureus,* and anaerobes are also seen. *H influenzae* (non-type B) infection occurs more commonly in the age group under 5 years. In the newborn, gram-negative infections with *Escherichia coli, Klebsiella pneumoniae,* Enterobacter species, *P aeruginosa,* and *P mirabilis* predominate.

The presenting clinical signs and symptoms are variable: In adults, otalgia and a conductive hearing loss are most common; infants may exhibit only fever, lethargy, or irritability. The tympanic membrane is commonly red, bulging, and extremely painful. Spontaneous perforation of the tympanic membrane with purulent otorrhea and hemorrhage is often present in infants when first seen by a physician. Prompt antibiotic therapy hastens resolution of the disease and prevents the development of temporal bone and intracranial complications. Topical vasoconstrictors such as phenylephrine should be instilled into the nasal cavities, and systemic vasoconstrictors, including ephedrine, pseudoephedrine, or phenylpropanolamine, may be prescribed to improve auditory tube function. In nonallergic low-risk patients over 6 weeks of age, amoxicillin may be recommended, and erythromycin and sulfisoxazole may be used in penicillin-allergic individuals. Patients who fail to respond may have an infection caused by β-lactamase-producing *H influenzae* type B and should be given cefpodoxime, cefprozil, loracarbef, cefuroxime, or cefixime. In infants under 1 month of age, therapy must also be directed against gram-negative enteric organisms.

Emerging *S pneumoniae* resistance to penicillin secondary to alterations of penicillin-binding proteins may require limiting choices to amoxicillin or amoxicillin and clavulanate at doses of 80–100 mg/d in divided doses, based upon the amoxicillin component. When penicillin-resistant pneumococci cause bacteremia or other more serious infections, vancomycin with or without ceftriaxone is the treatment of choice. In infants with impending otologic or intracranial complications such as meningitis, labyrinthitis, or lateral sinus thrombosis, ceftriaxone is recommended. In children over 4–6 weeks of age, *H influenzae* type B is the most common cause of meningitis. Because of this organism's high resistance to ampicillin and rare resistance to chloramphenicol, ceftazidime or ceftriaxone is recommended. Early administration of dexamethasone in children with meningitis in a dosage of 0.15 mg/kg four times a day for 4 days may lower the incidence of severe hearing loss. Myringotomy is indicated to relieve severe pain unresponsive to opioids or to identify antibiotic-resistant organisms. The development of sudden facial paralysis is an indication for emergency myringotomy. The incision should be made in the posteroinferior quadrant, midway between the umbo and the annulus. When repeated episodes of acute otitis media occur, it is important to rule out associated infection such as chronic adenoiditis or chronic sinusitis. Occasionally it is necessary to do serum IgG subclass testing to identify immune system immaturity. Children who continue to have episodes of otitis media in spite of adequate chemoprophylaxis and who do not clear their middle ear effusions between episodes should undergo tympanostomy tube placement.

Alho OP et al: Which children are being operated on for recurrent acute otitis media? Arch Otolaryngol Head Neck Surg 1994;120:807.

Haddad J: Treatment of acute otitis media and its complications. Otolaryngol Clin North Am 1994;27:431.

ACUTE MASTOIDITIS

Acute mastoiditis is a complication of acute otitis media and develops as a result of pus retention in the mastoid. It is most likely caused by *S pneumoniae; H influenzae* and *S aureus* are also commonly identified. The destruction of bony septa results in a coalescence of mastoid air cells and subsequent erosion of the cortices of the mastoid process of the temporal bone. Otalgia, aural discharge, and fever are characteristically observed 2–3 weeks after an episode of acute suppurative otitis media. Examination reveals severe mastoid tenderness, lateral displacement of the pinna, or postauricular mastoid swelling secondary to subperiosteal abscess. Ceftriaxone with or without metronidazole is given, and if a subperiosteal abscess develops, the mastoid and its air cells must be surgically drained. Alternative antibiotic choices include imipenem or chloramphenicol plus vancomycin or nafcillin. A complete mastoidectomy through a postauricular incision includes exenteration of the infected bone and pus and inspection of the dura of the posterior and middle cranial fossae to exclude epidural abscess.

FOREIGN BODIES IN THE EAR

Foreign bodies of the external auditory canal frequently traumatize the epithelium and may also perforate the tympanic membrane or disrupt the ossicular chain, producing a conductive hearing loss. Oval or round window injury may cause a concomitant sensorineural hearing loss. All kinds of objects are inserted into the external canal, especially by children. In addition, insects such as cockroaches may enter the canal, attaching their pincers to the tympanic membrane. Most foreign bodies can be removed with a right-angled hook or forceps if they are not lodged significantly medial to the isthmus of the external auditory canal. Gentle expulsion of nonvegetable matter with a soft rubber syringe (similar to the removal of cerumen) is effective. In young children or adults with firmly embedded objects, a general anesthetic is necessary to avoid injuring the tympanic membrane or ossicular chain. Insects may be suffocated by instilling mineral oil or lidocaine into the external auditory canal.

Bressler K et al: Ear foreign body removal: a review of 98 consecutive cases. Laryngoscope 1993;103:367.

TINNITUS

Tinnitus is the subjective sensation of noise in the ear or head not of psychogenic origin. Tinnitus is extremely common, affecting an estimated 10 million Americans. It is reported by patients as a constant or intermittent buzzing, ringing, or humming sound. Tinnitus originates from the inner ear when localized loss of outer hair cells occurs while the inner hair cells are still functional. An accompanying decrease of neuronal signals coming from the outer hair cell system leads to compensatory mechanisms within the auditory pathways that enhance tinnitus-related neuronal activity. The presence of depression and anxiety increases the perception of tinnitus. It has been estimated that up to 50% of tinnitus sufferers are depressed. Tinnitus is experienced by patients with presbycusis, noise-induced hearing loss, ceruminous impaction, otosclerosis, temporomandibular joint disorders, and otitis media (acute and chronic). Exposure to ototoxic drugs, closed head trauma, endolymphatic hydrops (Meniere's disease), and vestibular schwannoma (acoustic neuroma) are other causes. Highly vascular lesions of the temporal bone less commonly may elicit pulsatile tinnitus; examples are glomus jugulare or tympanicum tumors (non-chromaffin-producing neoplasms of paraganglionic cell origin). Aneurysms or arteriovenous malformations are rare causes of true tinnitus. In fact, pulsatile tinnitus can emanate from any arterial or venous structure within the cranial cavity, head and neck region, and thoracic cavity. The venous type can originate from jugular bulb anomalies but also occurs in young morbidly obese women suffering from benign intracranial hypertension.

Comprehensive management includes assessment of hypertension, blood lipids, thyroid function, and allergies and informing patients of factors that aggravate tinnitus, including stress, caffeine, nicotine, and aspirin. Treatment is determined by the primary disease, but since most cases are caused by presbycusis, effective therapy is often unavailable. Attempts at symptomatic relief have included diuretics, antihistamines (eg, dexchlorpheniramine maleate), anticonvulsants (eg, clonazepam), anxiolytics such as alprazolam and diazepam, and antidepressants (eg, nortriptyline, amitriptyline). Masking of tinnitus with frequency-specific hearing aids or extraneous noise such as a radio or stereo—especially before sleep—may be helpful in motivated patients. Biofeedback therapy has been used successfully in anxious patients. Cochlear nerve section may be offered when hearing acuity is severely diminished, and in rare circumstances microvascular decompression of the intracranial portion of the auditory nerve may provide relief from incapacitating tinnitus. Recent success has been reported with an electrical radiofrequency transmitter transmitting audio frequencies across the skin. Other modalities, including acupuncture, psychotherapy, and hypnotherapy, have given inconsistent results and are not recommended. Currently, habituation training aimed at habituating the reactions induced by tinnitus and blocking out the perception of tinnitus is being studied.

Brooke GB: Vascular decompression surgery for severe tinnitus. Am J Otol 1996;17:569.

Jastreboff PJ et al: Neurophysiological approach to tinnitus patients. Am J Otol 1996;17:236.

Nodar RH: Tinnitus reclassified: new oil in an old lamp. Otolaryngol Head Neck Surg 1996;114:582.

TEMPORAL BONE FRACTURES

Fractures of the skull base from blunt trauma commonly involve the temporal bone. Hemorrhagic otorrhea, ecchymosis of the postauricular area (Battle's sign), and disturbances in cochlear or vestibular function may be encountered. Eighty percent of fractures of the temporal bone are longitudinal to the petrous ridge; the remainder are transverse or perpendicular. Longitudinal fractures are chiefly secondary to parietal blows with the fracture line extending across the floor of the middle cranial fossa and through the roof of the external auditory canal, rupturing the tympanic membrane. The incudostapedial joint is frequently disrupted and requires ossiculoplastic reconstruction. The labyrinth is often spared, and only 35% of patients develop a sensorineural hearing loss. Twenty percent of patients develop delayed seventh nerve paralysis caused by ischemia and compression rather than neural disruption.

Transverse fractures, on the other hand, are caused by a blow to the occiput and are associated with a higher death rate. The fracture may involve the foramen magnum, pass through or near the jugular foramen, and cross the internal auditory canal to reach the foramen lacerum or foramen spinosum. Often the fracture line will splinter to reach the medial wall of the inner ear. The tympanic membrane remains intact, with a blue-black hemotympanum, and cerebrospinal fluid rhinorrhea is not uncommon. In one-third to one-half of cases, the seventh nerve is lacerated or transected, typically in the labyrinthine or mastoid segment, resulting in immediate facial paralysis. In addition, disruption of the membranous labyrinth leads to complete loss of cochlear-vestibular function and subsequent sensorineural hearing loss and vertigo.

If there is a cerebrospinal fluid leak, it is treated with head elevation, fluid restriction, and diuretics. In 85% of cases, the leak stops by 7 days and no repair is necessary. If the leak continues beyond several weeks, surgical repair is indicated. The development of progressive facial paralysis and loss of greater than 90% electrical stimulability of the facial nerve within 2 weeks requires immediate neuronal decompression of the facial canal. If the nerve has been anatomically disrupted, debridement and end-to-end anastomosis or nerve grafting will be necessary.

NEOPLASMS OF THE SKULL BASE

Squamous cell and **basal cell carcinomas** are the most common malignant tumors of the pinna, occurring in sun-exposed individuals. Small lesions may be removed by V-wedge excision while those complex morpheaform neoplasms require MOHS (microscopically oriented histologic surgical) technique for primary control. Adjunctive radiation therapy is considered for recurrent or deeply invasive tumors. Tumors invading the cartilage require wide surgical excision. Melanoma of the pinna is a dangerous neoplasm that can spread to the cervical lymph node chain as well as distantly. Most melanomas can be removed with wedge resection while some require partial or total auriculectomy. A functional elective neck dissection is considered for lesions over 1.5 mm thick. Squamous cell or basal cell carcinomas arising in the external auditory canal require wide excision for the best chance of cure. MRI is important to define surgical limits, as it better visualizes infiltration of the infratemporal fossa, parotid, dura, and temporomandibular joint than CT scanning. En bloc resection of the external auditory canal is possible for lesions not involving the middle ear or mastoid, whereas more invasive tumors require parotidectomy, partial or total temporal bone resection, and, for tumors extending beyond the temporal bone, skull base surgery. Squamous cell carcinomas arising in the middle ear should be treated by resection of the temporal bone combined with full-course radiation therapy (6000–7000 cGy).

Glomus jugulare and **glomus tympanicum** tumors are vascular neoplasms that usually arise from the jugular bulb and tympanic plexus, respectively. Both tumors spread cephalically and posteriorly into the middle ear and mastoid. Both are non-chromaffin-producing paragangliomas and are histologically the same as carotid body tumors, the most common chemodectomas of the neck. In addition, a **glomus vagale** neoplasm arising in the skull base and neck may extend superiorly into the cranial vault. The natural history of these tumors is one of slow, progressive growth and gradual invasion of the jugular foramen and its nerves (cranial nerves IX, X, XI) as well as cranial nerves VII, XII, and VIII. The overall incidence of central nervous system invasion is less than 20%.

The principal manifestation of a tumor of the middle ear is conductive hearing loss and a violaceous retrotympanic mass; pulsatile tinnitus is often present if the tumor is highly vascular. **Brown's sign** may be present (pulsation of the tympanic membrane that is inhibited by positive pressure applied to the tympanic membrane by a pneumatic otoscope). Thin-section, high-resolution CT scanning in combination with gadolinium-enhanced MRI is used to delineate the extent of tumor. Angiography is used for preoperative assessment of tumors requiring embolization. The treatment of choice is lateral cranial base surgical removal if the lesion does not involve the carotid siphon and has not spread by distant metastases. Small glomus tympanicum tumors may be cured by total surgical removal. When intracranial extension is present, a neurosurgical approach is required in addition to the neuro-otologist's lateral skull-based surgery. Radiotherapy causes tumor shrinkage but not eradication and is best combined with surgical excision of the tumor.

Benign facial nerve schwannoma is another skull base and temporal bone neoplasm. This fusiform lesion typically is elongated to involve more than one segment of the nerve. MRI with gadolinium is the current standard screening procedure for suspected tumors because of the high false-negative rate associated with BSERA testing. Microsurgical excision is the procedure of choice via either a translabyrinthine, middle fossa, or retrosigmoid approach depending on the tumor size and level of hearing. Observation is the best choice for management of patients with smaller tumors who have limited life expectancy.

Jackson CG et al: Hearing conservation in surgery for glomus jugulare tumors. Am J Otol 1996;17:425.

Prasad S et al: Efficacy of surgical treatments for squamous cell carcinoma of the temporal bone: a literature review. Otolaryngol Head Neck Surg 1994;110:270.

Thomas SS et al: Squamous cell carcinoma of the pinna: a six year study. Br J Plast Surg 1994;47:81.

CONGENITAL DEFORMITIES OF THE EAR

Lop-ear, the most common congenital deformity of the auricle, is the result of failure of development of the antihelical fold or excessive protrusion of the conchal cartilage. Treatment consists of otoplasty, the surgical creation of an antihelical fold or reduction of conchal cartilage projection (or both). Treatment before 5 or 6 years of age, when the auricle is three-fourths adult size, avoids ridicule of the child by its peers.

Preauricular cysts and sinus tracts are common unilateral or bilateral congenital defects found anterior to the upper helix or tragus. They develop following incomplete fusion of the auricular hillocks. Many subsequently become infected, requiring complete excision, which may be hazardous because of ramification of the sinus tracts near facial nerve branches. Congenital aural atresia varies widely in severity from mild narrowing of the external auditory canal—with or without dysplasia of the tympanic membrane and middle ear space—to entire absence of the middle ear cleft and auricle and bony atresia of the external auditory canal. Complete congenital aural atresia is rare, occurring in one in 10,000 births, with males affected more commonly than females. In the presence of complete bony atresia, anomalies of the middle ear cavity and structures are more common. Congenital aural atresia can occur in isolation or in association with microtia and other craniofacial dysplasias such as Treacher Collins', Crouzon's, Goldenhar's, Möbius', and Pierre Robin syndromes. Additional congenital anomalies include colobomas, heart defects, atresia of the choana, retarded growth or development, and genital hypoplasia, which have been observed in a unique group of patients afflicted with the so-called CHARGE association. Facial nerve palsies and laryngotracheal abnormalities are also common in this group. Initial treatment requires first establishing the presence of adequate hearing in the opposite ear. If hearing in the opposite ear is normal, surgical repair is not recommended, because the potential risk to the seventh nerve, which takes an anomalous course through the temporal bone, is too great. However, the use of a nerve monitoring unit during external ear canal and middle ear reconstruction will help reduce the risk of injury to the seventh nerve. If there is a profound conductive hearing loss on both sides, however, surgical reconstruction of the middle ear is indicated if feasible; if not, bilateral bone conduction hearing aids should be used. Auricular reconstruction for severe microtia or complete atresia is a challenging cosmetic surgical problem, often requiring soft tissue flaps and autogenous cartilaginous grafts, and should be done prior to middle ear reconstruction typically at 6 years of age when rib length is large enough to allow an adequate cartilage block for auricular sculpting. Four stages are required, beginning with the autogenous cartilage framework and construction of a cutaneous pocket, leading to transposition of lobular remnants, elevation of the auricular framework, and tragal reconstruction with conchal bowl definition.

Briggs RJS et al: Correction of conductive hearing loss in children. Otolaryngol Clin North Am 1994;27:607.

Cressman WR et al: Surgical aspects of congenital aural atresia. Otolaryngol Clin North Am 1994;27:621.

Hayes D: Hearing loss in infants with craniofacial anomalies. Otolaryngol Head Neck Surg 1994;110:39.

Nagata S: Secondary reconstruction for unfavorable microtia results utilizing temporoparietal and innominate fascia flaps. Plast Reconstr Surg 1994;254.

SYSTEMIC DISORDERS AFFECTING THE EAR

A variety of systemic illnesses are associated with hearing loss, including diabetes mellitus, hypothyroidism, renal disease, Paget's disease of the bone, and others. It is now well recognized that the human immunodeficiency virus (HIV) can cause hearing loss and vestibular complaints. Indeed, 50% of HIV-positive patients have abnormal auditory and vestibular testing. Patients with AIDS are subject to reactivation of otosyphilis and sudden sensorineural hearing loss secondary to cryptococcal meningitis and *Pneumocystic carinii* infection

Immune-mediated inner ear disease can cause progressive hearing loss with or without vestibular symptoms secondary to the production of autoantibodies directed toward inner ear structures. Although many patients do not exhibit signs of autoimmune disease, some may have other evidence of autoimmune illnesses such as systemic lupus erythematosus, Sjögren's syndrome, rheumatoid arthritis, Wegener's syndrome, and Cogan's syndrome. Treatment is with steroids and occasionally antimetabolites.

Osteogenesis imperfecta, an autosomal dominant inherited disorder, may appear with ossicular abnormalities, including otosclerosis with stapes fixation. Four different types (I–IV) are recognized and are associated with varying degrees of systemic skeletal involvement, multiple fractures, and growth retardation. Conductive hearing loss and sensorineural hearing loss can occur in osteogenesis imperfecta, and the stapes abnormality does not respond as well to stapedectomy as in otosclerosis.

Chen AY et al: Otolaryngologic disease progression in children with human immunodeficiency virus infection. Arch Otolaryngol Head Neck Surg 1996;122:1360.

VESTIBULAR SYSTEM

The vestibular system serves to maintain balance, posture, and spatial orientation in concert with vision and peripheral proprioception. Loss of two of these three sensory modalities is severely incapacitating. The vestibular end organs are dynamic structures that respond to linear acceleration (saccule and utricle) and to angular acceleration (semicircular canals). Angular acceleration of the head displaces endolymph and deflects hair cell cupulae in the cristae. Hair cell deflection results in either an increase or a decrease in neuronal impulses to the vestibular nuclei. Because the six semicircular canals are arranged in three pairs with one member of a pair (right) lying in a plane parallel to the plane of the other member (left), differences in acceleration between the right and left sides of the body are monitored in the vestibular nuclei. Normally, when a person is resting or moving at a constant rate, sensory input from the paired horizontal semicircular canals and two pairs of posterior and superior semicircular canals is balanced. Angular acceleration with subsequent hair cell deflection results in unilateral increased vestibular output and increased muscle tone in the extraocular and skeletal muscles, maintaining balance, posture, and spatial orientation. Failure of the vestibular apparatus to sustain the organism's balance produces vertigo, nystagmus, falling, and past-pointing. Sudden unilateral diminution of function in the vestibular system, in Meniere's disease, perilymph fistula, acute labyrinthitis, or temporal bone fracture, causes an imbalance of neuronal information arriving in the temporal lobe cortex. The cortical interpretation is constant motion or vertigo aggravated by head movement. Similarly, neuronal imbalance arriving at the extraocular motor nuclei and reticular formation produces rapid nystagmus, nausea and vomiting, and parasympathetic discharge. In response to overwhelming vestibular dysequilibrium, the cerebellum inhibits vestibular nuclei, but only incompletely. Ultimately, restoration of balance will require (1) functional repair of the diseased end organ, requiring hours or days; (2) central nervous system suppression of the normally functioning side, requiring months; or (3) generation of new neuronal output in the hypofunctioning labyrinth.

Clinical Assessment of the Dizzy Patient

Nowhere in medicine and surgery is a carefully taken history more important than in evaluating patients with dizziness. Nonvertiginous or extravestibular dizziness is far more common than otogenic or true vertiginous imbalance. The sensation of lightheadedness or syncope points to nonvestibular causes of dizziness such as cardiac arrhythmias, vasovagal episodes, orthostatic hypotension, or hyperventilation, which are not associated with the perception of the room spinning around. The clinical evaluation of the vestibular system includes examination of cerebellar function (gait, Romberg, two-step Fukuda, finger-to-nose, dysdiadochokinesis, and dysmetria testing) and the cranial nerves and observation of spontaneous positional nystagmus. The vestibular ocular reflex can be evaluated qualitatively at the bedside with doll's-eye, dynamic visual acuity, and ice water caloric tests. Because visual fixation with the eyes open may suppress nystagmus, it is important to record eye movements with electronystagmography. This is a technique for recording changes in the corneoretinal potential with skin electrodes and an electronic apparatus. Spontaneous, positional, and positioning nystagmus may be recorded to determine whether the vertigo is peripheral or central in origin.

Additional information is obtained with the Hallpike caloric stimulation test. Caloric stimulation of the labyrinth via the tympanic membrane induces convection currents within the horizontal semicircular canal, producing cupular deflection in one direction with 30 °C water and in the opposite direction with 44 °C water. With the patient supine and the head elevated 30 degrees, irrigation of the external auditory canal with cold water (30 °C) produces the rapid component of nystagmus to the opposite side; warm water (44 °C) produces nystagmus to the same side. The mnemonic device is COWS ("cold to the opposite" and "warm to the same"). Decreased vestibular response to caloric stimulation (canal paresis) indicates a vestibular end organ, vestibular nerve, or brain stem lesion.

Baloh RW: Approach to the evaluation of the dizzy patient. Otolaryngol Head Neck Surg 1995;112:3.

Honrubia V: Contemporary vestibular function testing: accomplishments in future prospective. Otolaryngol Head Neck Surg 1995;112:64.

Lindstrom CJ: Office management of the dizzy patient. Otolaryngol Clin North Am 1992;25:745.

MENIERE'S DISEASE (ENDOLYMPHATIC HYDROPS)

Meniere's disease is characterized by a tetrad of symptoms of unknown cause: episodic vertigo, fluctuating sensorineural hearing loss, a sensation of aural fullness, and tinnitus. The tinnitus is usually low-pitched and roaring. The hearing loss is more severe in the lower frequencies, in many cases progresses over several years, and remains confined to one ear in most patients. The attacks are associated with nausea, vomiting, and prostration. Pathologically, there is generalized dilation of the membranous labyrinth that includes the scala media and endolymphatic sac and is associated with occasional membrane breaks and intermingling of endolymph and perilymph. Circulating immune complexes may be involved in the pathogenesis of Meniere's disease.

Patients with severe hydrops should be treated with diuretics, salt restriction, a low-caffeine diet, avoidance of nicotine, and labyrinthine sedatives such as diazepam, 5 mg three times daily, to prevent recurrent attacks. Antihistamines such as meclizine, dimenhydrinate, and cyclizine are used to reduce the severity of vertigo. Associated vertigo, nausea, and vomiting are controlled without antiemetics by combining the synergistic effects of a cholinergic antagonist (scopolamine) and an adrenergic agonist (dextroamphetamine).

Surgical treatment is currently reserved for patients with severe incapacitating vertigo or tinnitus or to prevent further deterioration of hearing. In patients with useful hearing, decompression of the endolymphatic sac and insertion of a shunt between the membranous labyrinth and subarachnoid space improves symptoms in over half of cases. Vestibular neurectomy through either a middle cranial fossa or retrolabyrinthine approach may conserve hearing. With severe loss of hearing and speech discrimination, a total transmastoid labyrinthectomy is used, which relieves vertigo in over 90% of patients. Unilateral chemical ablation of vestibular function has been accomplished with the intratympanic installation of gentamicin once or twice weekly for 2 or 3 weeks. The main complication has been sensorineural hearing loss, which occurs in 5–25% of patients depending upon the protocol used.

Cohen H et al: Disability in Meniere's disease. Arch Otolaryngol Head Neck Surg 1995;121:29

Goycooleh MV et al: Overall view and rationale for surgical alternatives for incapacitating peripheral vertigo. Otolaryngol Clin North Am 1994;27:283.

Hirsh BE et al: Intratympanic gentamicin therapy for Meniere's disease. Am J Otol 1997;18:44.

Santos PM: Diuretic and diet effect on Meniere's disease evaluated by the 1993 committee on hearing and equilibrium guidelines. Otolaryngol Head Neck Surg 1993;109:680.

Telischi FF et al: Long-term efficacy of endolymphatic sac surgery for vertigo in Meniere's disease. Otolaryngol Head Neck Surg 1993;109:83.

Wackym PA: Histopathologic findings in Meniere's disease. Otolaryngol Head Neck Surg 1995;112:90.

VESTIBULAR SCHWANNOMA

Vestibular schwannomas account for about 8% of intracranial tumors and arise twice as often from the vestibular division of the eighth nerve as from the auditory division. They develop in one per 100,000 individuals yearly. Growth varies according to the patient's age. Although vestibular schwannomas account for about 80% of all cerebellopontine angle neoplasms, other lesions in the cerebellopontine angle may produce a nearly identical clinical picture. These include meningiomas, primary cholesteatomas, metastatic tumors, and aneurysms. Vestibular schwannomas, which are derived from Schwann cells, initially produce a high-frequency sensorineural hearing loss. Tinnitus is less common, and true vertigo is unusual. However, unsteadiness or balance disorders may develop as the tumor enlarges. Hallpike caloric testing commonly reveals canal paresis on the affected side. MRI with gadolinium is the current standard for screening for suspected vestibular schwannomas because of the high false-negative rate associated with BSERA.

Management of acoustic neuromas depends on the tumor's size and growth rate, the patient's age, and the state and prognosis of bilateral hearing. For patients under 65, small intracanalicular tumors (within the internal auditory canal) may be surgically removed through the transmastoid labyrinthine route if no useful hearing remains; a middle cranial fossa or retrosigmoid approach is utilized to preserve serviceable hearing for tumors 1.5 cm or less if the puretone average is less than 30 dB and the discrimination score is greater than 70%. Both routes maintain the integrity of the facial nerve. Larger tumors (> 3 cm) are associated with an increased incidence of hearing loss, dysequilibrium, headache, facial numbness, and diplopia and are removed via a suboccipital craniotomy; huge ones can only be removed via a combined suboccipital and translabyrinthine approach if the facial nerve is to be preserved. For patients over age 65 with slowly growing tumors, observation is the preferred treatment.

Dornhoffer JL et al: Presentation and diagnosis of small acoustic tumors. Otolaryngol Head Neck Surg 1994;111:232.

Grey PL et al: Audio vestibular results after surgery for cerebellopontine angle meningiomas. Am J Otol 1996;17:634.

Kartush JM et al: Acoustic neuroma update. Otolaryngol Clin North Am 1996;29:377.

Sekhar LN et al: The best treatment for vestibular schwannoma (acoustic neuroma): microsurgery or radiosurgery? Am J Otol 1996;17:676.

LABYRINTHITIS

In the preantibiotic era, acute suppurative labyrinthitis developing as a complication of acute otitis media or meningitis was not rare. More common today, however, is viral inflammation of the labyrinth or inner ear, causing vestibular neuritis or labyrinthitis. The clinical picture is a sudden onset of vertigo lasting days to a week, with gradual resolution of unsteadiness over weeks or months. Unilateral hearing loss can occur, and an electronystagmogram will often show reduced caloric response in one ear. Initial treatment with vestibular suppressants such as meclizine or diazepam are helpful. These should be removed as soon as possible and a vestibular rehabilitation program started to facilitate central cerebellar compensation.

BENIGN PAROXYSMAL POSITIONAL VERTIGO

Benign paroxysmal positional vertigo is associated with brief (< 30 seconds) episodes of sudden onset of intense vertigo precipitated by head or body movement. Hallpike positional testing often reveals horizontal rotatory nystagmus toward the involved undermost ear in the lateral decubitus position. The disorder is believed to result from degenerative otoconia from the utricular macula in the posterior semicircular canal. These particles may float free and, because they have a higher specific gravity than endolymph, produce abnormal cupular deflection in the semicircular canal with certain head movements.

Vestibular rehabilitation exercise programs have been prescribed for this problem. The particle repositioning maneuver developed by Epley appears to be the most effective form of therapy and is designed to disperse the otoconia back into the utricle, where they cannot cause cupular deflection.

GERIATRIC DYSEQUILIBRIUM

There are many vestibular disorders in the elderly, including vascular disease with ischemia (vertebral basilar insufficiency) or infarction (lacunar, brain stem, or cerebellar), endolymphatic hydrops, and benign paroxysmal positional vertigo (see above). Vertebral basilar insufficiency usually results from atherosclerosis involving the subclavian, vestibular, or basilar arteries and is associated with visual changes, weakness, paresthesias, and drop attacks. In addition, degenerative changes and loss of otoconia, vestibular epithelium, vestibular nerves, Scarpa's ganglion, and cerebellum occur with aging. The resulting dizziness and falls that are common among persons over age 65 are usually caused by central discoordination, but positional vertigo not uncommonly plays a central role. Because these peripheral vestibular aging changes are compensated by visual input, more dysequilibrium occurs at night. Gait abnormalities and a positive Romberg test, especially with the eyes closed, predominate. The vestibular rehabilitation exercises are most helpful. The morbidity and mortality associated with falls in the elderly are substantial and increase with age.

Blakley BW: Randomized controlled assessment of the canalith repositioning maneuver. Otolaryngol Head Neck Surg 1994;110:391.

Herdman SJ et al: Single treatment approaches for BPPV. Arch Otolaryngol Head Neck Surg 1993;119:450.

FACIAL NERVE PARALYSIS

Paralysis of the seventh nerve immobilizes the muscles of facial expression: The eye fails to close, the forehead does not wrinkle (as opposed to central or supranuclear facial paralysis with forehead sparing), and the angle of the mouth droops, so the patient drools. Peripheral seventh nerve paralysis suggests serious disease, such as tumor of the cerebellopontine angle, acoustic neuroma, facial nerve neuroma, neoplasm of the middle ear, or parotid gland neoplasm. Acute otitis media, temporal bone fracture, and chronic otitis media with or without cholesteatoma may produce facial paralysis. Other causes include surgical trauma, Guillain-Barré syndrome, Lyme disease, AIDS, and herpes zoster oticus (Ramsay Hunt's syndrome). When the cause is unknown, the condition is known as Bell's palsy. Although Bell's palsy is the commonest cause of peripheral seventh nerve paralysis, the pathogenesis is mysterious. Current theories implicate vascular ischemia and compressive edema within the facial canal as the cause of neurapraxia and cessation of axoplasmic flow. There is evidence that Bell's palsy is part of a viral cranial polyneuropathy that usually resolves in 6–12 weeks. Recent herpes simplex viral DNA has been clearly demonstrated in the geniculate ganglion of a patient with Bell's palsy.

All patients with facial paralysis should have a thorough history and physical examination. In addition, a high-resolution CT scan of the temporal bones and gadolinium-enhanced MRI should be obtained. The latter frequently demonstrates better soft tissue visualization and gadolinium enhancement in Bell's palsy, herpes zoster oticus, facial neuromas and vestibular schwannomas. MRI is indicated in patients experiencing weakness lasting more than 2 months or with progressive or recurrent palsies. The following special diagnostic tests should be performed: pure-tone audiometry, speech reception thresholds and speech discrimination; glucose tolerance tests to rule out diabetes mellitus; and Lyme titers; supramaximal electroneurography nerve excitability testing over the peripheral branches and main trunk of the seventh nerve is often used to predict the need for surgical decompression. With electroneurography, a supramaximal stimulus is delivered to the seventh nerve trunk and a compound action potential is recorded using surface electrodes. In patients with a greater than 90% loss of compound action potential prior to day 14 after the onset of paralysis, middle cranial fossa decompression is indicated.

The initial medical management of Bell's palsy is controversial. However, routine eye care with petroleum-based ocular lubricants (eg, Lacrilube) at night and artificial tears every 2–3 hours during the day is not. Approximately 70% of patients recover completely, but the prognosis for complete recovery falls to 10% in the presence of dry eye. Early treatment with corticosteroids (eg, 60–80 mg of prednisone daily with gradual tapering over 7–10 days) is felt by some experts to hasten resolution of edema and improve the outcome (ie, prevent permanent paralysis or synkinesis). Acyclovir, 800 mg orally five times a day, or valacyclovir, 500 mg orally twice daily, is recommended. In patients with herpes zoster oticus, intravenous acyclovir with prednisone is helpful. Nonpregnant adults with facial paralysis secondary to Lyme disease are best treated with doxycycline; amoxicillin, erythromycin, ceftriaxone, and cefuroxime may be used as substitutes.

Rehabilitation of the paralyzed face exhibiting no recovery is a challenging problem. Unilateral facial paralysis is unlikely to recover if a year has passed since the injury and no voluntary motion is noted. If paralysis persists, placement of a gold weight eyelid implant will be necessary to provide adequate ocular closure and thus prevent exposure keratitis. Nerve crossover procedures using a hypoglossal to seventh nerve anastomosis are recommended for restoring resting facial tone in cases of complete paralysis where a proximal facial nerve stump is not available for grafting or repair. For traumatic lesions, immediate neural repair or interposition grafting of the damaged segment with a greater auricular or sural nerve graft may be efficacious. Occasionally, decompression of the facial nerve combined with rerouting through the temporal bone is sufficient. Finally, neuromuscular transfer techniques utilizing either temporalis or masseter muscle pedicles or microvascular free muscle transfer are effective for facial reanimation in patients who are not candidates for cable nerve grafts or hypoglossal nerve transposition.

Adour KK: Bell's palsy treatment with acyclovir and prednisone compared with prednisone alone. Ann Otol Rhinol Laryngol 1996;105:371.

Burgess RC et al: Polymerase chain reaction of herpes simplex viral DNA from the geniculate ganglion of a patient with Bell's palsy. Ann Otol Rhinol Laryngol 1994;103:775.

Seiff SR et al: Management of ophthalmic complications of facial nerve palsy. Otolaryngol Clin North Am 1992;25:669.

NOSE & PARANASAL SINUSES

NASAL FOREIGN BODIES

Nasal foreign bodies are common in children, who frequently place pebbles, beads, seeds, buttons, or paper into the nares. A severe inflammatory reaction ensues, especially with organic matter, and this is associated with a foul-smelling unilateral nasal discharge. Chronic foreign bodies may encrust with calcium and magnesium to form rhinoliths. Removal of foreign body requires topical vasoconstrictors such as phenylephrine and topical anesthesia with lidocaine or cocaine. General anesthesia may be needed in uncooperative children.

NASAL VESTIBULITIS

Inflammation of the nasal vestibule may assume two forms: a localized acute furunculitis or a chronic diffuse dermatitis. Acute staphylococcal furunculitis of the pilosebaceous follicles in the vestibule may develop into a spreading cellulitis of the tip of the nose. Treatment includes hot soaks and oral cephalexin. Incision and drainage of a localized abscess is rarely necessary, since the majority of cases drain spontaneously. Diffuse nasal vestibulitis is treated with antibiotic ointments containing polymyxin B, bacitracin, and neomycin. Early treatment of all acute infections of the nose, paranasal sinuses, and face is important to prevent the occurrence of retrograde thrombophlebitis and cavernous sinus thrombosis, as well as facial cellulitis. If these complications occur, intravenously therapy with a broad-spectrum agent such as ampicillin-sulbactam or ceftriaxone plus clindamycin is essential.

ACUTE RHINITIS (CORYZA, COMMON COLD)

Acute rhinitis is often secondary to infection with respiratory viruses, including rhinoviruses, coronaviruses, and papillomaviruses. It is associated with sneezing, watery rhinorrhea, tearing, malaise, and headache. The incidence of colds increases during the fall, remains elevated during the winter, and generally declines during the spring. Examination of the nasal mucous membrane reveals hyperemia, edema, and watery mucosal discharge. Later, the secretions may become thick and yellow-green in color. Tenderness to palpation over the paranasal sinuses may be found. Nonnarcotic analgesics such as aspirin, decongestants, and antihistamines as well as fluids and rest will alleviate symptoms. Topical vasoconstrictors such as oxymetazoline and phenylephrine provide symptomatic relief. Antibiotic therapy is not necessary unless secondary bacterial invasion occurs. The condition usually resolves within 5–10 days.

ALLERGIC RHINITIS

Antigens inhaled and deposited on the mucous membranes of the nasal cavities of hypersensitive individuals elicit an IgE-mediated rhinitis. This perennial or seasonal disorder is often associated with other respiratory allergies

Table 38–4. Oral antihistamines for allergic rhinitis.

Drug	Usual Adult Dose
Alkylamines	
Brompheniramine maleate	4 mg every 4–6 hours
Chlorpheniramine maleate	4 mg every 4–6 hours
Ethanolamines	
Clemastine fumarate	1.34–2.68 mg every 12 hours
Diphenhydramine hydrochloride	20–50 mg every 4–6 hours
Others	
Fexofenadine	60 mg every 12 hours, or 180 mg daily
Azatadine maleate	1–2 mg every 12 hours
Cyproheptadine hydrochloride	4 mg every 6–8 hours
Pheniramine tartrate	25 mg every 4–6 hours
Terfenadine	60 mg every 12 hours
Astemizole	10 mg daily
Loratadine	10 mg daily
Cetirizine	5–10 mg daily

such as asthma, chronic laryngitis, or tracheobronchitis. Allergens such as animal danders, molds, dust, and pollens are commonly implicated, and sensitivity to them may be confirmed by skin end point titration, skin prick testing, or in vitro radioallergosorbent testing (RAST). Allergic rhinitis is characterized by sneezing, watery rhinorrhea, tearing, dysosmia, and nasal obstruction. The mucous membrane appears edematous and pale, with a thin discharge. Individuals with chronic allergic rhinitis commonly develop nasal polyps and acute or chronic sinusitis. Polyps may arise from the middle meatal region at the sinus ostia and appear as pale gray, glistening edematous masses within the nasal cavity. Occasionally, a large antrochoanal polyp arises from the maxillary sinus ostia in conjunction with chronic maxillary sinusitis and presents as a long pedunculated mass in the nasopharynx. Treatment requires removal of the polyp and drainage of the maxillary sinus.

Treatment for mild allergic rhinitis is started with an antihistamine (Table 38–4) and avoidance of the allergen if possible. Topical nasal steroids in the form of beclomethasone dipropionate, triamcinolone acetonide, budesonide, fluticasone, mometasone, or flunisolide or the use of topical cromolyn sodium delivered intranasally is effective in reducing or eliminating moderate symptoms in some patients. These nasal sprays are given in concert with saline nasal rinses. For severe conditions, oral glucocorticoids or intramuscular steroids are employed in addition to antihistamines, nasal steroids, and oral decongestants. Desensitization immunotherapy should be considered if pharmacotherapy insufficiently controls symptoms or produces undesirable side effects; if there are positive skin tests or serum specific IgE that correlates with rhinitis symptoms; if there is a history of allergic rhinitis for at least two seasons or 6 months (perennial); or if appropriate measures to avoid indoor allergens fail to control symptoms. Finally, surgical removal of nasal polyps associated with allergic rhinitis combined with endoscopic surgical drainage of obstructed maxillary and ethmoid sinuses is performed for severe nasal obstruction and chronic sinusitis unresponsive to medical therapy.

Baraniuk JN: Pathogenesis of allergic rhinitis. J Allergy Clin Immunol 1997;99:S763.

Durham SR et al: Changes in allergic inflammation associated with successful immunotherapy. Int Arch Allergy Immunol 1995;107:282.

Ferguson BJ: Allergic rhinitis. Options for pharmacotherapy and immunotherapy. Postgrad Med 1997;101:117.

Fornadley JA et al: Allergic rhinitis: clinical practice guidelines. Otolaryngol Head Neck Surgery 1996;115:115.

Nightingale CH: Treating allergic rhinitis with second-generation antihistamines. Pharmacotherapy 1996;16:905.

RHINITIS MEDICAMENTOSA

Misuse or abuse of intranasal vasoconstrictors (eg, phenylephrine, cocaine) may lead to mucosal edema, hyperemia, and watery rhinorrhea. The resulting nasal obstruction is severe, prompting the individual to increase the use of topical decongestants and thus perpetuate the cycle. Successful treatment requires complete cessation of intranasal medications for 2–3 weeks, and an oral decongestant such as pseudoephedrine must be used. A short course of systemic corticosteroid therapy or the gradual substitution of topical steroids for topical decongestant therapy seems to assist the withdrawal process. The complex of nasal septal perforation, palatal retraction, pharyngeal wall ulceration, and nasal collapse secondary to cocaine abuse that mimics midline granuloma does not respond to this management. Invariably, these lesions are colonized with *S aureus* and require intravenous antistaphylococcal penicillin and, in rare cases, external beam radiation therapy.

VASOMOTOR RHINITIS

Vasomotor rhinitis results from hyperreactivity of parasympathetic control of the nasal vasculature and glands. The vasomotor reaction is characterized by vascular engorgement mediated by the release of acetylcholine (a powerful vasodilator) at parasympathetic nerve endings. This commonly occurs in response to changes in external temperature and humidity and is not caused by allergens. Exposure to inhalant irritants such as tobacco smoke, perfume, and industrial pollutants may provoke parasympathetic activity. There is often a history of trauma. The patient complains of nasal obstruction, sneezing, and watery rhinorrhea. Systemic decongestants such as pseudoephedrine and phenylpropanolamine give some relief. Antihistamines help combat the problem through their anticholinergic action. Corticosteroid nasal spray is occasionally effective, while the use of intranasal cromolyn sodium may benefit the patient by preventing the release of mediators from mast cells. A recent option for control of vasomotor rhinitis is the application of nasal ipratropium bromide at either 0.03% or 0.06% concentration (two puffs three times a day) for control of congestion and rhinorrhea. Septoplasty to correct traumatic nasal septal obstruction with or without bilateral partial inferior turbinectomy is successful in relieving nasal airway obstruction.

PARANASAL SINUSITIS

Inflammation of the paranasal sinuses is commonly precipitated by an acute upper respiratory tract infection of viral origin. Edema of the nasal mucosa produces obstruction of the sinus ostia, resulting in secondary bacterial invasion and localized pain and tenderness. Headache that is exacerbated by changes in position and barometric pressure is very common. Other common symptoms are auditory tube dysfunction with otalgia, rhinorrhea, nasal congestion, postnasal discharge, and sometimes anosmia in adults. Acute sinusitis is defined by persistence of upper respiratory tract symptoms beyond the usual 7-day course of the predisposing viral illness. Microorganisms responsible for acute sinusitis are most often *S pneumoniae, M catarrhalis,* and *H influenzae.* Because β-lactamase production is common among strains of *H influenzae* and particularly *M catarrhalis,* therapy with amoxicillin-clavulanic acid, cefuroxime, or erythromycin and trimethoprim-sulfamethoxazole for 2–3 weeks is preferred initial management of acute sinusitis. In persons allergic to penicillin, erythromycin plus a sulfonamide is recommended. Therapy also includes oral decongestants, antihistamines for patients who have a substantial component of allergic rhinitis, immunotherapy with IgE desensitization, and corticosteroids in the form of topical nasal sprays, systemic agents, or both. Chronic sinusitis in adults is defined as 12 weeks of persistent signs and symptoms or four episodes per year of recurrent acute sinusitis. If there is no improvement with previous antibiotic treatment, anaerobic and *S aureus* coverage should be included with either amoxicillin-clavulanate and metronidazole or cefuroxime plus metronidazole. In HIV-infected patients who develop pseudomonas infections, ciprofloxacin plus clindamycin or an aminoglycoside has proved effective. For chronic sinusitis, first-line antibiotics include amoxicillin-clavulanate, second-generation cephalosporins, and the newer macrolides and fluoroquinolones. Cefixime is an excellent choice when resistant *H influenzae* and *Moraxella* are implicated but fails in managing *S pneumoniae* infection. Treatment is continued for 3 weeks.

Endoscopic sinus surgery is indicated for patients with persistent facial pain, headache, or nasal congestion and those who fail to respond to aggressive medical management. CT scans should be obtained in the axial and coronal planes to evaluate the persistence of chronic sinusitis and the presence of sinus abnormalities such as nasal septal deformity, pneumatization of the middle turbinates (concha bullosa), inferior turbinate hypertrophy, or substantial obstruction of the osteomeatal complex. Because the flow of mucus in the sinuses is toward the natural ostium, relief of obstruction of the osteomeatal complex (hiatus semilunaris and ethmoid infundibulum) is indicated to restore drainage from the sinuses and prevent persistent symptoms. Reestablishment of ethmoid and maxillary sinus ventilation and elimination of foci of ethmoid disease are necessary for success. The introduction of the nasal endoscopy combined with articulating video cameras and video imaging allows removal of just enough mucosa to restore drainage. The commonest site of infection in chronic sinusitis is the anterior ethmoid air cells. Endoscopic sinus surgery is most effective in controlling localized disease, recurrent acute sinusitis, and sinusitis secondary to anatomic obstruction, particularly in patients with no previous sinus surgery or in those who have a maxillary sinus mycetoma. The prognosis is unfavorable in patients with immunodeficiencies, immotile cilia syndrome, severe allergy, triad asthma with nasal polyposis and aspirin sensitivity, sarcoidosis, multiple prior operations, diffuse severe polypoid disease, or polyposis with diffuse extramucosal fungal infection.

Patients undergoing successful endoscopic sinus surgery show the greatest improvement with respect to resolution of facial pain. Frequently, simultaneous septoplasty and partial inferior turbinectomies is necessary for adequate exposure and endoscopic drainage of the sinuses. Patients with opacification of the sphenoid sinus have a poorer outcome, whereas those who have no purulent drainage or reformation of polypoid mucosa postoperatively have a dramatic resolution of facial pain, nasal obstruction, postnasal discharge, rhinorrhea, and improvement in their history of recurrent asthma. If maxillary sinus disease remains after this approach, a Caldwell-Luc procedure through an incision in the gingival labial sulcus may be necessary. For patients who have persistent ethmoid disease, external ethmoidectomy is indicated via a Lynch incision midway between the dorsum of the nose and the medial canthal ligament of the eye.

Complications of acute sinusitis are rare in infancy and childhood. Acute maxillary sinusitis and, more commonly, ethmoiditis may be complicated by orbital cellulitis and abscess formation. The progressive development of chemosis, scleral erythema, proptosis, and ophthalmoplegia points to orbital infection and potential intracranial invasion. A CT scan with contrast enhancement will detect an orbital abscess and evaluate other causes of unilateral proptosis. Treatment consists of intravenous ceftriaxone and clindamycin or ampicillin-sulbactam. In patients developing an orbital abscess, drainage through a Lynch incision must be performed early to avoid serious intracranial complications such as meningitis, epidural abscess, subdural abscess, cerebral abscess, and cavernous sinus thrombosis. Several factors in pediatric sinusitis are critical: (1) Chronic purulent rhinosinusitis in children has an immunologic (IgG subclass deficiencies) or anatomic origin. (2) Children under age 7 with nasal polyposis and chronic sinusitis must be considered to have cystic fibrosis or ciliary abnormalities causing poor mucus transport until proved otherwise. (3) Sinusitis exacerbates asthma. (4) Atopic children are more likely to develop sinusitis. (5) Allergy must be suspected in the age group from 3 years to 5 years, particularly when the symptoms include eczema, colic, and a family history of allergy.

Acute frontal sinusitis is more common in adults and frequently occurs following nasal trauma involving the nasal frontal duct. In the adolescent, it is the major source of orbital infection. In cases refractory to medical management, treatment consists of trephination of the anterior floor of the frontal sinus in the medial portion of the eyebrow. Chronic frontal sinusitis unresponsive to medical treatment and development of a mucocele are additional indications for operation. Endoscopic removal of frontal sinus mucoceles is now possible. A mucocele results from mucosal membrane duplication and obstruction of the sinus ostium secondary to chronic infection or trauma. It gradually enlarges to destroy the frontal bone and encroach upon the orbit or anterior cranial fossa. In large mucoceles of the frontal sinus that cannot be approached endoscopically, a bicoronal incision with an osteoplastic flap is used to excise and obliterate the sinus with fat or muscle. Finally, if patients have persistent postendoscopic drainage with facial pain, headache, or recurrent asthma, a repeat CT scan is indicated.

Gungor A et al: Pediatric sinusitis: a literature review with emphasis on the role of allergy. Otolaryngol Head Neck Surg 1997;116:4.

Kennedy DW et al: Functional endoscopic sinus surgery: theory and diagnosis. Arch Otolaryngol 1995;11:576.

Kuhn FA et al: Postoperative care following functional endoscopic sinus surgery. Otolaryngol Clin North Am 1997;30:479.

EPISTAXIS

The nasal cavity is a common site of spontaneous hemorrhage. The blood supply to the nose is derived both from the external and the internal carotid artery systems. In 90% of cases, the epistaxis originates in the anterior nasal septum in the rich vascular plexus (Kiesselbach's plexus) in Little's area. The terminal septal branches of the anterior and posterior ethmoidal arteries arising from the internal carotid artery (via the ophthalmic artery) anastomose in this area along with branches from the superior labial artery (via the external facial) and the sphenopalatine artery (via the internal maxillary artery). Both originate from the external carotid artery system. Because of their location, vessels on the anterior septal mucosa are readily susceptible to trauma from nasal picking, drying, crusting, and infection. Severe caudal septal deformities may lead to mucosal drying over the point of deflection, causing spontaneous hemorrhage. In addition, the concomitant use of alcohol, aspirin, or other NSAIDs interferes with platelet function, increasing the risk of epistaxis.

Mild epistaxis from the anterior septum is readily controlled with digital pressure for 5–10 minutes. Persistent hemorrhage requires topical cocainization and cauterization with a silver nitrate applicator or electrocautery. If hemorrhage is still not controlled, 14-inch gauze packing impregnated with petrolatum should be placed atraumatically in the nasal cavity. Bleeding associated with leukemia, uremia, hepatic failure, coagulopathies, or hereditary hemorrhagic telangiectasia (Rendu-Osler-Weber syndrome) should be treated with absorbable gelatin sponge (Gelfoam) soaked in topical thrombin, oxidized regenerated cellulose (Surgicel), microfibrillar collagen hemostat (Avitene Hemostat), or a compressed Merocel sponge inserted into the nasal cavity for 4–5 days. All packing should be coated or saturated with an antibiotic to prevent toxic shock, which is caused when the pack is colonized by *S aureus* strains that express TSS toxin-1, enterotoxin B, or enterotoxin C. Treatment of underlying coagulopathy, leukemia, uremia, or liver disorder is obviously important. Moderate long-term success in hemorrhagic hereditary telangiectasia has been achieved with estrogen derivatives and septal dermoplasty. Septal dermoplasty involves removing the diseased mucosa together with subepithelial telangiectasias and replacing it through a lateral rhinotomy with a skin graft. The YAG laser is currently used in recalcitrant cases for photocoagulation of nasal hemorrhagic telangiectasias.

Posterior epistaxis from the terminal branches of the sphenopalatine and internal maxillary arteries is more serious and is frequently associated with hypertension, diabetes, or major systemic vascular disorders. It arises from a plexus of vessels located in the posterior 1 cm of the nasal floor, inferior meatus, inferior turbinate, and middle turbinate. Successful treatment requires the use of

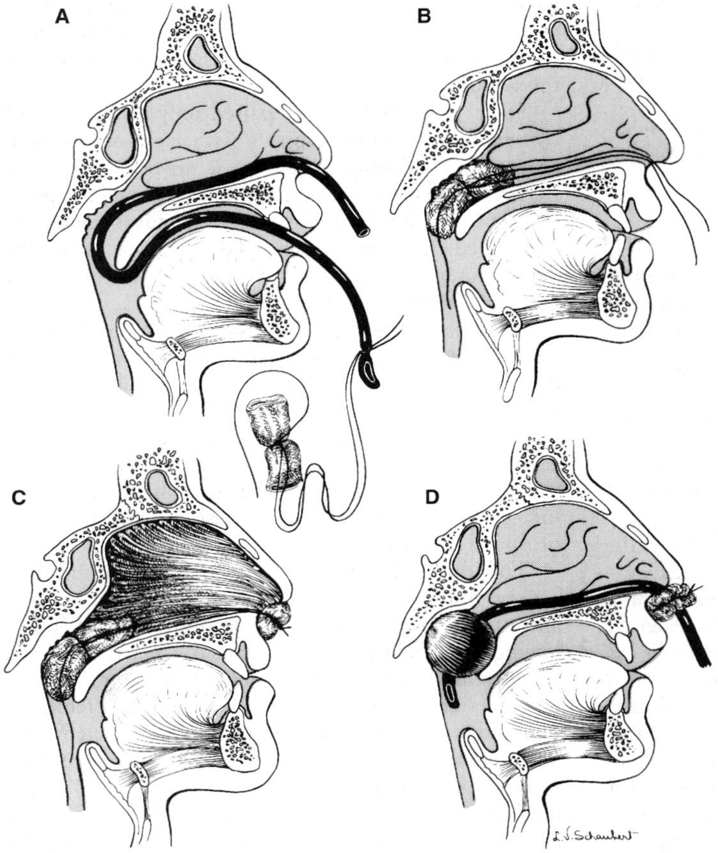

Figure 38–6. Packing to control bleeding from the posterior nose. ***A:*** Catheter inserted and pack attached. ***B:*** Pack drawn into position as catheter is removed. ***C:*** Strip tied over a bolster to hold pack in place with anterior pack installed "accordion pleating" style. ***D:*** Alternative method using balloon catheter instead of a gauze pack.

both anterior and posterior packing, inserted with topical 4% cocaine anesthesia. The posterior pack is made by tying folded 4 × 4 gauze squares to the end of a catheter that has been passed transnasally and brought out through the mouth. Two strings are tied to the pharyngeal end of the catheter and brought out through the nares. They are then tied over an anterior nasal pack and bolster (Figure 38–6). The remaining third string is brought out through the mouth and taped to the cheek, where it can be grasped and removed in 4–5 days. These techniques are extremely uncomfortable, lower arterial oxygen saturation, and may induce dysrhythmias or an acute myocardial infarction in patients with severe cardiovascular disease. Because toxic shock syndrome has been reported with the use of nasal packs, patients are started on intravenous cephalothin. Packing is left in place for 3–5 days. If bleeding fails to respond to posterior packing or posterior endoscopic cauterization under general anesthesia, transantral ligation of the internal maxillary artery through a Caldwell-Luc approach with or without anterior ethmoid artery ligation or angiographic embolization will be required. Currently, both ligation and embolization are specifically indicated for epistaxis secondary to vascular anomalies, bleeding disorders, trauma, or tumor. This practice has the advantage that it can be conducted under local anesthesia with conscious sedation. Its most frequently reported complication is facial paralysis. Transantral internal maxillary ligation, on the other hand, is associated with risk of dental injury, oral antral fistula, facial pain and paresthesias, postoperative sinusitis, and intraoperative bleeding. Unlike embolization, internal maxillary ligation requires a general anesthetic, which may place a patient at significant cardiovascular risk.

Elahi MN et al: Therapeutic embolization in the treatment of intractable epistaxis. Arch Otolaryngol Head Neck Surg 1995;121:65.

Elden L et al: Angiographic embolization for the treatment of epistaxis: review of 108 cases. Otolaryngol Head Neck Surg 1994;111:44.

Hartley C et al: The Foley catheter in epistaxis management—a scientific appraisal. J Laryngol Otol 1994;108:399.

McGarry GW et al: Idiopathic epistaxis, hemostasis and alcohol. Clin Otolaryngol 1995;20:174.

Strong EB et al: Intractable epistaxis: transantral ligation versus embolization: efficacy review and cost analysis. Otolaryngol Head Neck Surg 1995;113:674.

Winstead W: Sphenopalatine artery ligation: An alternative to internal maxillary artery ligation for intractable posterior epistaxis. Laryngoscope 1996;106:667.

NASAL TRAUMA

Nasal bone fractures are the most common fractures of the maxillofacial skeleton and frequently are associated with septal fractures and epistaxis. Clinical findings commonly include periorbital edema and ecchymosis, displacement of the bony dorsum to the right with depression of the left nasal bone (secondary to a "right hook" fisticuffs injury), crepitus, and, occasionally, laceration of the dorsum. In severe facial trauma, because the other facial bones are often broken, the entire facial skeleton should be assessed by x-ray.

Early reduction under local anesthesia before significant swelling appears produces an excellent result. Elevation with a periosteal elevator— combined with laterally applied digital pressure—is usually effective. An external plaster of Paris splint or commercially available splint is applied and removed in 1 week. It may be necessary to reduce severely impacted nasal bones with a Walsham forceps, one blade placed intranasally and the other extranasally. If the nasal fracture is encountered after severe edema has developed, it is better to postpone reduction for several days to allow resolution of edema. In children, the facial skeleton heals so fast that fracture must be reduced within 4–5 days to avoid malunion. Malunion in adults is treated by rhinoplasty and often concomitant septoplasty to repair the deviated nasal septum.

Complications of nasal trauma include septal hematoma and abscess formation, septal perforation, septal deviation, and cerebrospinal fluid rhinorrhea secondary to fracture of the cribriform plate, the roof of the ethmoid sinus, the posterior table of the frontal sinus, or the sphenoid sinus.

A septal hematoma is a collection of blood underneath the mucoperichondrium or mucoperiosteum of the septum. Physical examination discloses a bulging red septum, and nasal obstruction is usually complete and bilateral. Unless the hematoma is immediately incised and drained, a staphylococcal abscess may develop that results in cartilaginous necrosis and saddle nose deformity. Intravenous nafcillin, oxacillin, cefazolin, or clindamycin should be given to prevent cavernous sinus thrombosis and meningitis.

A septal deviation, especially along the nasal floor, produces varying degrees of nasal obstruction depending upon the severity of deflection into the nasal cavity. The caudal end of the septum may be deflected into the nasal vestibule, causing obstruction or external deformity. Nasal septoplasty through a caudal submucoperichondrial incision is used to reconstruct and straighten the septum.

Septal perforations are repaired only if complicated by persistent epistaxis, crusting with nasal obstruction, or, rarely, whistling. The repair involves an open transcolumellar rhinoplastic approach, using a temporalis fascial or perichondrial graft and advancement of two bipedicled mucoperichondrial flaps to cover the defect. Alternatively, an alloplastic septal button can be created to close the perforation.

Fractures of the nasal bones, nasoethmoidal region, and frontal region may occur in association with a dural defect and cerebrospinal fluid rhinorrhea. This provides a potential route for ascending infection and meningitis. The dural defect may communicate with the nasal cavity via the ethmoidal, frontal, or sphenoidal sinuses or the cribriform plate. A basilar skull fracture with an intact tympanic membrane may also present with cerebrospinal fluid rhinorrhea.

The diagnosis should be suspected upon finding watery rhinorrhea with an increased glucose content and may be confirmed by thin-section coronal CT following subarachnoid instillation of metrizamide by intrathecal injection. Fluid should be sent for β_2-transferrin determination, which is found only in cerebrospinal fluid and aqueous humor. The source of cerebrospinal fluid leak may be demonstrated in many cases by placing fluorescein dye (0.5 mL of 5% solution) in the lumbar subarachnoid space. Thirty minutes later, the nose can be endoscopically examined to determine the fistula site—front sinus, sphenoid sinus, roof of the ethmoid (fovea ethmoidalis), cribriform plate, or middle ear (via the auditory tube). Cerebrospinal fluid appears as a yellowish-green fluid using a xenon light source, and Wood's lamp is not necessary.

Acute posttraumatic cerebrospinal fluid rhinorrhea is treated conservatively with bed rest in the semisitting position, fluid restriction, lumbar drainage, and diuretics for 5–7 days. The patient should avoid straining, blowing the nose, sneezing, or vigorous coughing. Indications for surgery are persistent cerebrospinal fluid leakage of more than 6 weeks' duration, recurrent meningitis, pneumoencephalos, or intermittent leakage. In sinusitis or osteitis, intravenous ceftriaxone is indicated.

Small defects of the cribriform plate, fovea ethmoidalis, and sphenoid sinus have been successfully repaired through an external ethmoidectomy incision using a variety of septal or middle turbinate mucoperiosteal flaps. However, an endoscopic approach using free grafts of fascia, nasal mucoperichondrium, muscle, fascia lata, or fibrin glue is preferred. Fibrin glue, composed of 10% calcium chloride and topical thrombin, added to cryoprecipitate in separate syringes, becomes gelatinous when combined and effectively seals the leak. The fibrin glue will last about 7–10 days and then dissolve. In all cases, the graft and glue are held in position by an absorbable packing such as Gelfoam, Surgicel, or Oxycel. Alternatively, Avitene paste may be used. Small defects of the posterior table of the frontal sinus are best managed by a bicoronal incision, osteoplastic flap approach, and obliteration of the frontal sinus with abdominal fat. Large defects will necessitate anterior fossa craniotomy and repair. Bone fragments are stabilized with low-contour titanium plates and screws.

Other soft tissue facial injuries and fractures of the zygoma, maxilla, orbit, and mandibles are discussed in Chapter 43.

Dodson EE et al: Transnasal endoscopic repair of cerebral spinal fluid rhinorrhea and skull base defects: a review of 29 cases. Otolaryngol Head Neck Surg 1994;111:600.

El Jamel MS: Fractures of the middle third of the face and cerebral spinal fluid rhinorrhea. Br J Neurosurg 1994;8:289.

Teichgradber JF et al: The management of septal perforations. Plast Reconstr Surg 1993;91:229.

El Jamel MS et al: Localization of inactive cerebral spinal fluid fistulas. J Neurosurg 1995;83:795.

CONGENITAL NASAL MALFORMATIONS

Congenital malformations of the nose and central face are unusual. Facial clefts, such as cleft lip and palate or a bifid nose, commonly result from genetic or teratogenic factors operating in the second month of fetal life. Although atresia and stenosis of the anterior nares are rare, they should be suspected in any infant who has difficulty breathing. Bilateral bony posterior choanal atresia is more commonly the cause of congenital neonatal respiratory impairment. Because they are obligatory nasal breathers during the first several weeks of life, newborns develop apnea and cyanosis when crying stops and the mouth is closed. The definitive diagnosis is confirmed by inability to pass a catheter transnasally.

Initial treatment includes either an oral endotracheal tube or McGovern nipple (which allows mouth breathing), followed by early transnasal or transpalatal correction of the atresia. The atretic plate can be successfully removed endoscopically with diamond burrs, powered oscillating blades, or the CO_2 laser. The surgically created posterior choana is kept patent with a 16F or 18F polyvinyl chloride (Portex) endotracheal tube that is removed in 6–8 weeks. Unilateral choanal atresia, on the other hand, is usually not diagnosed until later in childhood or early adulthood and is associated with unilateral nasal obstruction or rhinorrhea. Repair is best performed when the nasal cavities and hard palate have reached adult size.

Other congenital lesions that may produce nasal obstruction include nasal gliomas, encephaloceles, meningoceles, and teratomas (dermoids, teratoids, true teratomas, and epignathi). Nasal gliomas are composed of neural and glial elements. Similarly, meningoceles and encephaloceles that have intracranial connections through the cribriform plate, fovea ethmoidalis, or sphenoid bone may present as a nasal mass that may be mistaken for a nasal polyp. Not infrequently, these heterotopic brain elements are seen as a mass on the nasal dorsum that is frequently confused with a midline dermoid cyst. CT scans or MRI of the anterior cranial fossa and cribriform plate must be obtained to rule out intracranial connections. Treatment of heterotopic brain elements with an intracranial connection requires a combined craniotomy and transfacial approach. If the diagnosis remains in doubt, frontal craniotomy is performed before transfacial excision to avoid development of cerebrospinal fluid rhinorrhea and meningitis. Other surgical approaches for complete excision of congenital nasal masses include open rhinoplasty and transnasal, endoscopic, or combined transcranial-endoscopic techniques.

Koltai PJ: The external rhinoplasty for the correction of unilateral choanal atresia in young children. Ear Nose Throat J 1991; 70:450.

ORAL CAVITY

WHITE LESIONS OF THE ORAL CAVITY

The mucous membrane of the oropharynx resembles the skin in that individual cells arise from the germinal layer and mature, but they do not keratinize. Mechanical, thermal, and chemical trauma (eg, alcohol; nicotine, including smokeless tobacco products) may lead to thickening of the germinal layer and later development of a nonnucleated keratinized layer that appears as gray-white nonulcerated plaques on the oral cavity mucosa (leukoplakia). Because the histologic appearance varies considerably and up to one-half of these lesions may exhibit malignant transformation, biopsy is indicated to rule out early carcinoma. The treatment is surgical excision of small lesions with a knife or with a CO_2 or KTP laser and avoidance of further exposure to irritants. Laser excision has a lower recurrence rate plus the advantages of better precision, bloodless field, excellent tissue healing, and less pain and discomfort.

Lichen planus, though primarily a dermatologic disorder affecting up to 2% of the population, may involve any mucous membrane exposed to trauma or chronic irritation such as tobacco—eg, the buccal mucosa frequently develops white papules or striae from repetitive biting. Hyperkeratosis, acanthosis, and subepithelial edema complete the histologic picture. Because of the clinical similarities between lichen planus and discoid lupus erythematosus and lichenoid stomatitis—and because of its relationship to liver disease and oral cancer—biopsy of representative lesions is indicated to confirm the diagnosis and rule out other disorders. Topical triamcinolone is often useful for associated submucosal inflammation. In some cases, this may undergo malignant degeneration into squamous cell carcinoma.

Finally, ill-fitting dentures may elicit raised folds of white tissue in the gingivolabial sulcus that histologically consist of fibrous tissues proliferation and overlying epithelial hyperplasia. An inflammatory papillary hyperplasia on the hard palate may occur as a result of improperly fitting dentures. These polypoid lesions are hyperemic, soft, and mobile. Surgical removal is often necessary, followed by denture readjustment.

Bagan JV et al: Oral lichens planus and chronic liver disease: a clinical and morphometric study of the oral lesions in relationship to transaminase elevation. Oral Surg Oral Med Oral Pathol 1994;78:337.

Banard NA et al: Oral cancer development in patients with oral lichen planus. J Oral Pathol Med 1993;22:421.

INFLAMMATORY DISEASES OF THE GINGIVA

Inflammation of the gums (gingivitis) frequently develops as a result of poor oral hygiene, heavy smoking, and lowered resistance. **Acute necrotizing ulcerative gingivitis** (Vincent's gingivitis) is due to an overgrowth of the normal oral bacterial symbionts. Clinically, it is characterized by painful hemorrhagic gums, ulceration, fever, lymphadenopathy, and a yellow-gray gingival pseudomembrane. Treatment consists of topical hydrogen peroxide, proper oral hygiene with removal of plaque and tartar at the tooth margins, and oral penicillin. Clindamycin is an acceptable antibiotic alternative, especially for penicillin-resistant anaerobic infections.

Although not limited to the gingivae, recurrent **aphthous stomatitis** (canker sores) frequently presents on the gingivae as round or ovoid, discrete, erythematous macules 2–30 mm in diameter that rapidly indurate and ulcerate but do not vesiculate (as do herpetic lesions). They are the most commonly reported oral ulcers, occurring in approximately one-fourth of the population. They may elicit enough pain to interfere with mastication and speaking. Tetracycline solution, 250 mg held in the mouth for 20 minutes four to six times a day and the analgesic dyclonine 0.5%, plus diphenhydramine elixir are effective treatment. Alternative therapy includes an emollient paste such as 0.1% triamcinolone acetonide in sodium carboxymethylcellulose or an aqueous 0.1% or 0.2% suspension alone or combined with initial bursts of prednisone (40–60 mg). The application of silver nitrate to the ulceration base is also useful. The cause is uncertain, but evidence suggests that aphthous stomatitis is a noninfectious inflammatory mucosal disease that may have multiple causes, including stress and gastroesophageal reflux. Severe recurrent aphthous stomatitis may also respond to oral colchicine and dapsone.

Trauma to the tooth may provoke inflammation of the periodontal membrane **(acute periodontitis)**, rendering it tender to touch. If the traumatic stimulus is removed, the inflammation resolves. Recurrent gingivitis coupled with poor dental hygiene may cause chronic periodontitis, pyorrhea, and regression of the periodontal ligament from the neck of the tooth. The gingival sulcus deepens, pockets form between the roots of the teeth and the surrounding gingivae, and debris and tartar accumulate. Mild periodontitis is characterized by gingival erythema, edema, tenderness, and hemorrhage. Severe periodontitis is associated with gingival necrosis, halitosis, and loss of unstable teeth. Unless the cycle is broken, periapical abscess formation and tooth devitalization will continue. Frequent flossing and regular professional dental care are recommended.

HERPETIC STOMATITIS

Herpetic lesions of the oral cavity are divided into primary gingivostomatitis, herpes labialis, and intraoral herpes—all caused by human herpes virus type 1 (HHV-1) and presenting as small vesicles that rupture, yielding a yellow-white superficial ulcer surrounded by a red halo. They are usually located on the labial and buccal mucosa, gingivae, and tongue. In contrast to recurrent aphthous ulcers, recurrent HHV-1 lesions are limited to the attached gingiva and hard palate. In severe cases, the gingivae are edematous and bleed readily. The primary form is accompanied by fever, pain, malaise and cervical lymphadenopathy. Although the primary disease is self-limiting, virus may be reactivated by physical trauma and endogenous stress. Treatment is supportive, including topical anesthetics in solution or troche form. If herpetic stomatitis occurs as part of a disseminated infection or in an immunocompromised patient, systemic acyclovir (200 mg five times daily) is prescribed. Newer antiviral agents—valacyclovir and famciclovir—have been used successfully. Topical acyclovir has limited usefulness in treating herpes labialis but can be effective if prescribed early in the prodromal stage. Penciclovir cream has also been reported to be effective in reducing the clinical signs and symptoms of recurrent herpes labialis.

Spruance SL et al: Penciclovir cream for the treatment of herpes simplex labialis. A randomized, multicenter, double-blind, placebo-controlled trial. JAMA 1997;277:1374.

ORAL CANDIDIASIS

Oral candidiasis (thrush) is caused by the yeast-like fungus *C albicans* and characterized by a white pseudomembranous lesion closely adherent to the mucous membrane, which bleeds and ulcerates when it sloughs. It also occurs in a hyperplastic form, characterized by superficial fungal invasion of the epithelium and leukoplakia; in an erythematous or atrophic form; and as angular cheilitis. Candida is normally a part of the oral biota but may become pathogenic after prolonged administration of antibiotics; radiation therapy to the cavity or pharynx; immunotherapy for carcinoma, leukemia, or lymphoma; or immune deficiency associated with corticosteroid therapy, diabetes, hepatic disease, etc. In addition, candidiasis along with oral hairy leukoplakia (nontender, caused by Epstein-Barr virus) is identified in patients with AIDS. Other local causative factors include xerostomia, smoking, smokeless tobacco, and mechanical changes in the oral environment such as dentures or poor oral hygiene. Oral nystatin, clotrimazole, or miconazole is effective treatment. For immunocompromised hosts who develop systemic candidal infections, amphotericin B is recommended. Ketoconazole administered orally is the drug of choice for chronic mucocutaneous candidiasis. The treatment of chronic mucocutaneous candidiasis may also include immunologic therapy with thymic transplants and infusion of lymphocytes from immunocompetent donors. Severely immunocompromised patients may benefit from the protracted use of prophylactic fluconazole. Chlorhexidine rinses have proved useful in treating oral candidiasis in children with leukemia.

Como JA et al: Oral azole drugs as systemic antifungal therapy. N Engl J Med 1994;330:263.

Lynch DP: Oral candidiasis: history, classification and clinical presentation. Oral Surg Oral Med Oral Pathol 1994;78:189.

Scully C et al: Candida and oral candidosis: a review. Crit Rev Oral Biol Med 1994;5:125.

CONGENITAL ORAL CAVITY MALFORMATIONS

Torus Palatinus & Torus Mandibularis

Torus palatinus, a common developmental abnormality of the oral cavity, consists of a bony exostosis of varying size and shape in the midline of the palate. Clinically, it may interfere with proper fitting of dentures and require surgical removal. It must be distinguished from tumors of the minor salivary glands and fissural cysts of the palate.

Torus mandibularis, like its palatal counterpart, is a bony exostosis usually situated on the lingual surface of the mandible adjacent to the cuspid and first bicuspid teeth. It is asymptomatic until an attempt is made at fitting a denture.

Macroglossia

Isolated macroglossia is rare and may be seen in cretinism, Down's syndrome, and acromegaly. It may also be caused by lymphangiomatous invasion of the tongue. Relative macroglossia is encountered in Pierre Robin syndrome (micrognathia and cleft palate). The relatively large tongue may obstruct the upper airway, necessitating insertion of an oral airway or tongue-lip adhesion. The tongue base is sutured over an anterior neck button to assist in anterior displacement of the tongue. These measures are only necessary until the oral cavity enlarges enough to accommodate the tongue. Tracheostomy is rarely necessary.

Ankyloglossia

Tongue-tie or partial ankyloglossia is manifested by an abnormally short and thick lingual frenulum. Various degrees of ankyloglossia occur, ranging from mild restriction with only a mucous membrane band to those in which both the frenulum and the underlying fibers of the genioglossus muscle are markedly fibrosed. Rarely, complete ankyloglossia with fusion of the tongue to the floor of the mouth may be encountered. Limitation of movement of the tongue tip results in malocclusion with an anterior "open bite" deformity, early prognathism, and swallowing and speech difficulties. Children with severe ankyloglossia meeting any of these criteria require frenulectomy, genioglossus myotomy, and mucous membrane closure with multiple Z-plasties.

Ranula

A ranula is a transparent retention cyst in the floor of the mouth arising from the sublingual salivary glands. The cyst enlarges gradually, penetrating the deep structures of the floor of the mouth above the mylohyoid muscle. It should be excised if it is small; marsupialization is necessary for large cysts, owing to the multiple ramifications.

SALIVARY GLANDS

There are three pairs of major salivary glands (parotid, submandibular, and sublingual) responsible for the secretion of saliva and stimulated by swallowing. Hundreds of minor salivary glands maintain resting levels of saliva necessary for moisturizing, lubrication, cleansing, digestion, and immunologic protection of the mouth.

ACUTE BACTERIAL SIALADENITIS

Acute bacterial sialadenitis may develop secondary to obstruction, stasis of saliva, or decreased secretion. There is diffuse painful enlargement of the gland, often with erythema and tenderness. Typically this occurs in the older patient who is taking diuretics or is dehydrated. The most common organism responsible, especially in acute parotitis, is *S aureus.* Other organisms include streptococci, *E coli,* and anaerobes. Antibiotic therapy is with a first-generation cephalosporin (cephalothin or cephalexin) or dicloxacillin. Alternatives are clindamycin, amoxicillin-clavulanate, or ampicillin-sulbactam.

VIRAL SIALADENITIS

Mumps is the most common viral cause of acute salivary inflammation. Young children 4–10 years of age are most commonly affected, developing bilateral swelling of the parotid glands 2–3 weeks after exposure. Symptoms last 7–10 days. Cytomegalovirus (CMV) is the second most common cause of acute viral sialadenitis and may mimic infectious mononucleosis clinically and hematologically.

CHRONIC SIALADENITIS

Chronic or recurrent bacterial sialadenitis or submandibular sialadenitis may develop as a result of antecedent acute suppuration or viral inflammation. More commonly, however, there is a history of ductal obstruction. Recurrent bacterial invasion of the parotid gland or submandibular gland leads to destruction and fibrosis of acini with ductal ectasia. The subsequent decrease in salivary flow creates a cycle of ascending sialadenitis, ductal ectasia, acinar atrophy, and obstructive fibrosis. Clinically, the patient complains of recurrent parotid pain and swelling, typically while eating. Initial treatment should be conservative, utilizing sialagogues (lemon balls or chewing gum), adequate oral hydration to stimulate salivary flow, and amoxicillin-clavulanate or cephalexin. In patients with recalcitrant disease, an extended course of clindamycin, cefoxitin, nafcillin, or vancomycin plus metronidazole may be necessary if methicillin-resistant *S aureus* and penicillin-resistant streptococci are considered. Superficial parotidectomy is recommended if prolonged conservative management fails.

White AK: Salivary gland diseases in infancy and childhood: non-malignant lesions. J Otolaryngol 1992;21:422.

SIALOLITHIASIS

Salivary gland stones are both a cause and a consequence of chronic sialadenitis. In addition, they may produce acute suppurative sialadenitis. The stones are composed of inorganic calcium and sodium phosphate salts that are deposited in the duct on an organic nidus of mucus or cellular debris. Eighty to ninety percent of salivary calculi occur in the submandibular gland and may lead to complete acute obstruction of the gland, with most stones occurring in the ducts rather than the gland itself. The patient complains of painful swelling, especially with meals, and may report extrusion of gravel from the duct.

The diagnosis is confirmed by palpation of a stone or by demonstration of decreased salivary flow from the duct. Soft tissue films may reveal a radiodense stone, and CT may show sialoliths, though 20–40% of calculi are radiolucent on plain films. Treatment consists of intraoral removal of stones that are close to the duct orifice by ductal dilation and massage. Stones in the hilum of the submandibular gland necessitate excision of the gland if associated with chronic pain and swelling. Parotid sialoliths are managed in a similar fashion.

SALIVARY GLAND TRAUMA

Injuries to the salivary glands may be intraoral or extraoral, blunt or lacerating. The parotid gland is most commonly injured along with associated structures, including the facial nerve, Stensen's duct, soft tissues, mandible, or zygoma. Laceration of the parotid duct may occur with a facial laceration posterior to the anterior edge of the masseter muscle and results in simultaneous injury to the buccal branch of the facial nerve. The severed duct is repaired over a small polyethylene catheter using fine interrupted sutures. The associated seventh nerve injury is repaired by anastomosing the cut ends with 10-0 monofilament suture. All lacerations in the parotid gland region must be examined for seventh nerve injury. Injury may occur either to the main trunk proximal to the pes anserinus or to one of the branches within the parotid gland. Facial injuries anterior to a vertical line from the lateral canthus of the eye generally do not require exploration, and the nerve will regenerate spontaneously. However, some surgeons advocate microscopic repair to offer a better chance of complete recovery without development of synkinesis (mass movement of the face). If injury to the nerve is suspected, each of the five major branches is assessed by observing voluntary movements and responses to nerve excitability testing. If transection of the facial nerve is likely, exploration and precise repair through a parotidectomy incision with the operating microscope is crucial. The greater auricular or sural nerve may be used as a cable graft for avulsed segments of the facial nerve. An exception to this approach would be an extensively contaminated wound such as a shotgun injury. In this situation, it is better to explore and debride the wound, tag the proximal and distal branches of the injured nerve with metal clips, and delay nerve repair until wound healing is more complete. This should be performed within 30 days after injury to achieve the best results.

May M et al: Managing segmental facial nerve injuries by surgical repair. Laryngoscope 1990;100:1062.

PHARYNX

PHARYNGITIS

Acute pharyngitis is usually caused by viruses (especially the adenoviruses and rhinoviruses) or group A beta-hemolytic streptococci. Clinically, erythema, edema, and occasional membrane formation are present, and the patient complains of pain on swallowing. In bacterial pharyngitis, the white count and fever are higher and cervical adenopathy is more marked. Pneumococci, *H influenzae, M catarrhalis, Neisseria gonorrhoeae,* and coagulase-positive staphylococci are the primary pathogens. Pharyngeal cultures are obtained. Antibiotic treatment is primarily directed toward group A beta-hemolytic streptococcus with penicillin or erythromycin, even in the face of a negative rapid strep test because of the potential sequelae of rheumatic fever and glomerulonephritis. The goal of antibiotic therapy is to eliminate infections, avoid suppurative complications, hasten recovery, and prevent rheumatic fever. Other bacterial agents, including *Mycoplasma pneumoniae* and chlamydia species, may account for a third of bacterial pharyngitis in adults. Treatment is with a macrolide (erythromycin, clarithromycin, or azithromycin). Gonococcal pharyngitis occurs in 1–2% of the sexually active population and is treated with a single dose of intramuscular ceftriaxone or oral cefixime. Concurrent treatment for chlamydia is required.

One must differentiate acute bacterial pharyngitis from diphtheritic pharyngitis and infectious mononucleosis. *Corynebacterium diphtheriae* is a potentially lethal bacterium in a nonimmunized host. Characteristic features are odynophagia, fever, and the development of a gray pseudomembrane on the oropharynx associated with a fetid odor. The membrane bleeds easily when removed and may gradually involve the larynx, producing acute upper airway obstruction. Infectious mononucleosis may mimic diphtheria, exhibiting faucial arch edema, a pharyngeal pseudomembrane, and laryngeal edema. A positive heterophil agglutination or Monospot test, absolute lymphocytosis, generalized lymphadenopathy, and hepatosplenomegaly differentiate this disease from diphtheria. Tonsilloadenoidal hyperplasia may be so marked as to obstruct the upper airway, necessitating intubation and tonsilloadenoidectomy.

Acute tonsillitis secondary to group A beta-hemolytic streptococcal infection commonly occurs in children under 10-years of age and may occasionally present in epidemic form. Clinically, pyrexia, odynophagia, referred otalgia, and malaise predominate. The usual signs of viral upper respiratory tract infection—cough, coryza, and conjunctivitis—are absent. The tonsils appear hyperemic and edematous with or without a purulent exudate filling the tonsillar crypts that coalesces to form a yellow-white pseudomembrane. A 7- to 10-day course of penicillin or cephalexin is adequate therapy, but amoxicillin is frequently substituted because of its dosing schedule. An alternative choice is erythromycin in patients allergic to penicillin. Clindamycin, amoxicillin-clavulanate, or dicloxacillin is indicated for those who do not respond to these drugs. With emerging worldwide *S pneumoniae* resistance to penicillin, clinicians must consider culturing in order to guide treatment when treatment failures occur. The mechanism of streptococcal resistance primarily involves alterations in penicillin-binding proteins responsible for binding β-lactam antibiotics in general rather than the production of β-lactamase enzymes. Amoxicillin, 80–100 mg/kg/d in divided doses, plus amoxicillin-clavulanate may be necessary.

Chronic tonsillitis may follow acute or subacute episodes of tonsillitis, especially in older children, and is associated with recurrent odynophagia, cough, and findings of tonsillar enlargement, debris in tonsillar crypts, and cervical lymphadenitis. There is increasing evidence that *H influenzae* plays a major role in this disorder as well as in the pathogenesis of tonsillar hypertrophy. In addition, *S aureus* has become a more prominent offender, along with actinomycetes. In view of the high incidence of β-lactamase-producing organisms, amoxicillin-clavulanate, clindamycin, or an antistaphylococcal penicillin is recommended. Tonsillectomy is indicated if there are four to six documented episodes of acute tonsillitis per year, three to four episodes in each of the preceding 2 years or three episodes in each of the preceding 3 years.

Acute tonsillitis may in some instances extend beyond the tonsillar tissue into the space between the anterior and posterior tonsillar pillars into the soft palate, producing a **peritonsillar abscess**, or quinsy, which is frequently associated with *S pyogenes* infection. Physical examination reveals an edematous, bulging, anterior tonsillar pillar with medial displacement of the soft palate and uvula. Immediate therapy includes incision and drainage of the abscess through the anterior tonsillar pillar or needle aspiration, intravenous penicillin or clindamycin, hydration, and antipyretics followed by either immediate tonsillectomy or an interval tonsillectomy in 6 weeks. The advantages of immediate tonsillectomy in carefully selected patients include complete abscess drainage without recurrence, rapid relief of symptoms, greater technical simplicity with less hemorrhage, less severe illness, and shorter hospitalization.

Pulmonary hypertension, cor pulmonale, and congestive heart failure (Noonan's syndrome) secondary to chronic hypoxia have been reported in young children with hyperplasia of Waldeyer's ring. More recently, chronic hypersomnolence and periodic apnea have been recognized in children with upper airway obstruction secondary to tonsilloadenoidal hyperplasia. During sleep, these patients experience episodes of hypopnea and periods of cessation of nasal-oral air flow of longer than 10 seconds, persistent chest wall movement, and subsequent hypoxia and hypercapnia. The obstructive sleep apnea syndrome is characterized by frequent arousals during sleep and more subtle clinical findings such as weight loss, behavioral disturbances, learning disabilities, daytime somnolence, and enuresis. Tonsillectomy and adenoidectomy are indicated to relieve upper respiratory tract obstruction.

Isolated adenoidal hypertrophy secondary to physiologic enlargement of the adenoids or chronic viral nasopharyngitis may produce nasal airway obstruction. These children exhibit chronic rhinorrhea, mouth breathing, dental abnormalities, an elongated face, and snoring during sleep. Adenoidectomy is curative.

The obstructive sleep apnea syndrome in adults (Pickwickian syndrome) is commonly seen in obese middle-aged men and spans a wide range of severity. It is defined as daytime sleepiness with altered cardiopulmonary function associated with frequent obstructive apneas or hypopneas during sleep. It is characterized by loud, stertorous snoring. Snoring is caused by high-frequency oscillation of the soft palate, resulting in intermittent narrowing of the pharyngeal airway. An estimated 25% of the adult male population snores every night. The degree of severity of airway obstruction is ascertained by obtaining a polysomnogram that measures the number, frequency, and duration of apneic episodes, the degree of arterial oxygenation saturation, the presence of cardiac arrhythmias associated with apnea, and the degree of daytime impairment. There are many forms of treatment, including behavioral, surgical, medical, and mechanical, some of which can be used in combination. In mild sleep apnea, behavioral treatment—particularly weight reduction—is sufficient. Alcohol consumption should be reduced in the evening hours, and sedative medications that can worsen sleep apnea should be avoided. Mechanical treatment is the best choice for many patients. Nasal continuous positive airway pressure (CPAP) is given by a silicone mask over the nose that is attached by tubing to an air pump. It acts as a pneumatic splint to maintain the patency of the airway. Alternative systems include the use of bi-level pressure (BiPAP). If this is not tolerated, the upper airway obstruction can be corrected with nasal septoplasty and turbinectomy to reduce nasal resistance plus a uvulopalatal pharyngoplasty (UPPP) and tonsillectomy for patients with collapse at either the retropalatal or the velopharyngeal level.

April MM et al: The effect of intravenous dexamethasone in pediatric adenotonsillectomy. Arch Otolaryngol Head Neck Surg 1996;122:117.

Deutsch ES: Tonsillectomy and adenoidectomy. Changing indications. Pediatr Clin North Am 1996;43:1319.

Doern GV et al: Antimicrobial resistance of Streptococcus pneumonia recovered from out patients in the United States during the winter months of 1994 to 1995: results of a 30-center national surveillance study. Antimicrob Agents Chemother 1996;40:1208.

Kiselica D: Group A beta-hemolytic streptococcal pharyngitis: current clinical concepts. Am Fam Physician 1994;49:1147.

Riley RW et al: Obstructive sleep apnea in the hyoid: a reviewed surgical procedure. Otolaryngol Head Neck Surg 1994; 111:717.

Sherae et al: The efficacy of surgical modifications of the upper airway in adults with obstructive sleep apnea syndrome. Sleep 1996;19:156.

Strollo PJ et al: Obstructive sleep apnea. N Engl J Med 1996;334:99.

Wood AJ: Antimicrobial drug resistance. N Engl J Med 1996; 335:1415.

BENIGN NEOPLASMS OF THE PHARYNX

The most common benign tumor of the nasopharynx is the juvenile angiofibroma, a highly vascular, nonencapsulated, invasive neoplasm with a propensity to occur in adolescent males. The hormone-dependent tumor is stimulated by testosterone and in vitro its growth rate is reduced by antiandrogens such as cyproterone and flutamide.

Onset of clinical signs and symptoms may be at any time from 7 years to 21 years of age. Epistaxis occurs in 75% of cases in addition to nasal obstruction and rhinorrhea. Anosmia is common. Preoperative digital subtraction angiography and CT scanning should be performed to evaluate the blood supply and the anatomic extent of the tumor. The major blood supply is from the internal maxillary artery. Preoperative embolization of the tumor and estrogen therapy markedly decrease blood loss at surgical resection. For lesions confined to the nasopharynx, a transpalatal approach is satisfactory. Larger tumors with involvement of the nasal cavity, the maxillary sinus, the ethmoid sinus, or the sphenoid sinus require a lateral rhinotomy and transpalatal or Caldwell-Luc approach (or both) for complete excision. Although these neoplasms are only moderately responsive to radiation therapy, such therapy is often the treatment of choice for orbital or intracranial invasion.

Hagen R et al: Juvenile nasopharyngeal fibroma: androgen receptors and their significance for tumor growth. Laryngoscope 1994;104:1125.

PHARYNGEAL FOREIGN BODIES

Irregular foreign bodies entering the pharynx are likely to lodge in the lingual or palatine tonsils, valleculae, or piriform sinuses. Smooth round or ovoid objects commonly lodge at the opening to the esophagus or the cricopharyngeus muscle, especially in children. Dysphagia, odynophagia, or aphagia may result. In a young child or infant, drooling is a characteristic sign. Dyspnea, wheezing, or persistent cough may develop secondary to compression of the larynx or trachea. If the esophagus is penetrated by a sharp object such as a pin or fish bone, subcutaneous emphysema can be palpated in the neck. Foreign bodies lodging more distally in the esophagus such as at the level of the aortic arch, left main bronchus, or gastroesophageal junction generally do not produce early symptoms.

Chest x-ray, anteroposterior and lateral neck films, and occasionally a barium swallow are necessary to delineate the site of a foreign body. Foreign bodies of the palatine and lingual tonsils are removed directly with a curved hemostat: objects located in the hypopharynx or esophagus require direct laryngoscopy or esophagoscopy under general anesthesia.

LARYNX

The larynx has four functions: (1) protection of the lower airway, (2) phonation, (3) respiration, and (4) fixation of the chest. Laryngeal dysfunction can therefore lead to abnormalities such as aspiration, weak cry, hoarseness, stridor, and poor cough. These problems point to laryngeal dysfunction and should prompt an inspection of the larynx with a laryngeal mirror (indirect laryngoscopy) or fiberoptic nasopharyngolaryngoscopy during phonation, swallowing, and deep inspiration. Cinefluoroscopy with barium sulfate allows assessment of the competency of the larynx during swallowing. Neoplasms and traumatic lesions of the larynx are effectively evaluated by CT scan or MRI. In any individual with hoarseness of more than 2–3 weeks' duration, the larynx should be inspected as described above. If the larynx cannot be inspected in this way, transnasal fiberoptic laryngoscopy or direct laryngoscopy under general anesthesia is required. A specimen of larynx is obtained at direct laryngoscopy for biopsy examination for suspected neoplasms.

FOREIGN BODIES OF THE LARYNX & TRACHEOBRONCHIAL TREE

For children, a variety of objects, including seeds, beans, pins, and tiny toys, may be aspirated into the tracheobronchial tree. In adults, meat is the most common cause of obstruction and is associated with a number of factors: (1) large, poorly chewed pieces of food, (2) elevated blood alcohol, and (3) upper and lower dentures. The development of a **café coronary** is frequently confused with a myocardial infarction.

Foreign bodies entering the tracheobronchial tree must pass (1) the epiglottis, (2) the upper laryngeal inlet, (3) the false cords (ventricular bands), (4) the true vocal cords, and (5) the cough reflex. If a foreign body lodges in the larynx, there is immediate pain and laryngospasm, dyspnea, and inspiratory stridor proportionate to the degree of upper airway obstruction. The voice may be hoarse or aphonic.

If partial airway obstruction is present and the victim can exchange air and cough, no attempt should be made to move the foreign body at that time. If the victim is aphonic, unable to cough or exchange air, and is clutching his or her neck, complete airway obstruction is present. If equipment is not at hand for emergency tracheotomy or cricothyrotomy, the Heimlich maneuver is recommended for relieving foreign body airway obstruction: a series of four manual thrusts are administered to the upper abdomen, exerting downward pressure on the diaphragm and compressing the lung. Finally, if the foreign body remains in the larynx or pharynx after these maneuvers, manual removal with the finger probe may be successful.

In the conscious adult patient with adequate air exchange, indirect laryngoscopy supplemented with anteroposterior and lateral x-rays of the neck and chest will confirm the position of the foreign body. Removal of a laryngeal foreign body necessitates general anesthesia and a laryngoscope and alligator forceps. Foreign bodies in the tracheobronchial tree also require general anesthesia and open bronchoscopy with forceps removal.

The reaction of the tracheobronchial tree to a foreign body depends upon the degree of obstruction and the physical nature of the foreign body. For example, a bean acts as a ball valve, rising with expiration and occluding the distal airway on inspiration. Vegetable matter produces a violent bronchitis that may be associated with chronic suppurative pneumonitis; and nonobstructive metallic objects may remain within the tracheobronchial tree for an extended period causing little tissue damage.

Tracheal foreign bodies produce inspiratory and expiratory wheezing. With distally located objects, three different patterns may occur: (1) partial (bypass valve) bronchial obstruction, in which the foreign body permits the passage of air during both inspiration and expiration; (2) expiratory check valve obstruction, where ingress of air is minimally impaired but egress is checked, resulting in obstructive emphysema; and (3) stop valve obstruction, in which no air enters the subjacent lung, resulting in atelectasis. Radiographic evaluation is invaluable. The recommended protocol includes anteroposterior and lateral neck and chest films, inspiratory and expiratory films, and, in selected cases, fluoroscopy and decubitus films. Currently, open (rigid) bronchoscopy is the standard way to remove foreign bodies of the tracheobronchial tree and will result in fewer complications and missed foreign bodies. Flexible fiber optic bronchoscopy is reserved for removing peripheral foreign bodies in patients being maintained on mechanical ventilators or in patients with cervical or maxillofacial trauma.

Hayashi AH et al: Management of foreign body bronchial obstruction using endoscopic laser therapy. J Pediatr Surg 1990;25:1174.

Inglis AF et al: Lower complication rates associated with bronchial foreign bodies over the last 20 years. Ann Otol Rhinol Laryngol 1992;101:61.

Limper AH et al: Tracheobronchial foreign bodies in adults. Ann Intern Med 1990;112:604.

Mu L et al: The causes and complications of late diagnosis of foreign body aspiration in children. Report of 210 cases. Arch Otolaryngol Head Neck Surg 1991;117:876.

Sataloff RT: Office evaluation of dysphonia. Otolaryngol Clin North Am 1992;25:843.

LARYNGEAL TRAUMA

Trauma to the larynx and trachea may occur from iatrogenic causes (prolonged endotracheal intubation or inappropriate tracheotomy, laryngotomy, or cricothyrotomy) or extrinsic injuries (automobile accidents, neck blows, strangulation, etc). The passenger in the front seat of an automobile is particularly vulnerable to hyperextension injury of the neck. This results in compression of the larynx, hyoid bone, and upper trachea between the dashboard and the cervical spine. Injuries of the larynx are less common in children because of the higher position of the larynx in the neck and the resulting protection provided by the mandible. Severe laryngotracheal injury may occur, however, in children riding bicycles, motor bikes, snowmobiles, etc, who strike a horizontal cable or fall against the handlebars.

The most common injury to the larynx is vertical fracture of the thyroid cartilage with or without fracture of the cricoid cartilage. Because the cricoid cartilage is the only complete cartilaginous ring in the respiratory tract, its functional integrity is critical in maintaining a patent airway. An unreduced fracture of the cricoid may result in subglottic stenosis. Associated injuries of the pharynx, trachea, esophagus, soft tissues, and neurovascular structures of the neck are common. Escape of air into the mediastinum may produce tension pneumothorax.

Clinical findings in laryngotracheal trauma include (1) subcutaneous emphysema or crepitus, (2) dysphonia, (3) loss of the laryngeal prominence (Adam's apple), (4) dysphagia, (5) odynophagia, (6) stridor, (7) hemoptysis, and (8) cough.

Conservative treatment with cool mist, intravenous fluids, cefazolin, and parenteral corticosteroids will suffice for laryngeal soft tissue edema without significant airway obstruction or impaired vocal cord mobility. CT scanning is done to evaluate the laryngeal skeleton for fracture and determine the subsequent course of treatment. It is not performed in patients with an obvious penetrating wound who will require immediate tracheotomy and exploration. More severe laryngotracheal injury requires endotracheal intubation or tracheotomy. In an emergency, an endotracheal tube may be introduced through an open laryngotracheal wound. Ideally, tracheotomy should be performed after the airway is controlled by intubation or open bronchoscopy. However, this may not be possible in cases of complete laryngotracheal separation. If a high tracheotomy or a cricothyrotomy has been performed, it should be revised as soon as possible to the third or fourth tracheal ring to prevent vocal cord paralysis and subglottic stenosis. Open reduction and stabilization of all cartilaginous, mucosal, and soft tissue defects with internal fixation and a soft stent is done immediately if the patient's general condition permits. This is recommended within 24 hours. Late laryngeal stenosis may be successfully treated in some patients with the CO_2 laser. Ultimately, the following factors affect wound healing within the larynx and trachea and determine the success or failure of therapy: (1) mechanical loss of lumen-supporting structures, (2) loss of blood supply to cartilaginous structures, (3) presence of chondritis, and (4) degree of progressive fibrosis and stenosis.

Bent JP et al: Acute laryngeal trauma: a review of 77 patients. Otolaryngol Head Neck Surg 1993;109:441.

Schaefer SD: The acute management of external laryngeal trauma. A 27-year experience. Arch Otolaryngol Head Neck Surg 1992;118:598.

Weymuller EA et al: Problems associated with prolonged intubation in the geriatric patient. Otolaryngol Clin North Am 1990;23:1057.

PEDIATRIC AIRWAY OBSTRUCTION

Airway obstruction at birth or in the first several months of life is commonly secondary to congenital and neoplastic disorders. At birth, immediate differentiation must be made between respiratory depression, with cyanosis and shallow, slow respirations; and respiratory tract obstruction, producing tachypnea, stridor, and suprasternal and subcostal retractions.

Stridor (noisy breathing) is the most prominent symptom and is an expression of partial respiratory tract obstruction secondary to external compression or partial occlusion within the airway. The character and intensity of stridor depend upon the site and degree of obstruction and the airflow velocity and pressure gradient across the point of obstruction. Obstruction at the level of the true vocal cords produces high-pitched inspiratory stridor. By contrast, stridor that occurs chiefly during expiration and is lower in pitch is commonly associated with tracheal obstruction. The quality of the cry remains normal in most infants with airway obstruction who do not have a laryngeal lesion. A weak or absent cry at birth suggests neurogenic vocal cord impairment. In addition to evaluating the cry and breathing patterns, the physician should also assess swallowing function in all infants with stridor. Mediastinal tumors and vascular rings producing extrinsic esophageal and tracheal compression cause feeding difficulties and failure to thrive. The presence of recurrent pneumonitis and aspiration suggests a laryngeal lesion or tracheoesophageal fistula. All infants with stridor should have an anteroposterior and lateral chest film and barium swallow followed by endoscopy.

Newborns & Small Infants

The most common cause of infantile stridor is **laryngomalacia**, or **congenital flaccid larynx**. During inspiration, there is extreme infolding of the omega-shaped epiglottis and aryepiglottic folds owing to inadequate cartilaginous support. The presence of staccato stridor with expiration helps identify laryngomalacia. The supine position or head flexion aggravates the stridor, whereas patency of the airway is improved by the prone position and head extension. The stridor gradually resolves in most infants within 2–3 months. Endoscopic inspection is necessary in infants with persistent or progressive stridor.

Congenital subglottic stenosis is the second most frequently encountered laryngeal lesion and may become evident several weeks or more after birth, following an upper respiratory tract infection. Because the subglottic region is the narrowest point in the upper respiratory tract (4.5–5.5 mm at full term, 3.5 mm when premature), a small amount of edema will critically narrow this conduit. Subglottic stenosis is present when the subglottic airway measures less than 4 mm in a full-term infant or 3 mm in a preterm infant. Isolated congenital subglottic stenosis may involve soft tissue stenosis or cartilaginous stenosis of the cricoid cartilage (or both). **Pediatric laryngotracheal stenosis** may be more commonly caused by neonatal intubation as well as external trauma, high tracheotomy, infections, inflammation or burns. It may be isolated to the subglottic space or may occur in combination with supraglottic, glottic, or subglottic stenosis. It often extends into the upper trachea. The subglottis is almost universally involved. A grading system from grade 1, which represents no obstruction, to grade 4, when no detectable lumen can be found, can be used to plan therapy. For grade 1 and 2 stenosis, which ranges from less than 50% obstruction to 70% obstruction, endoscopic CO_2 laser techniques may be the primary therapy for isolated supraglottic, glottic, or subglottic pathology, while anterior laryngotracheal split with either costal or auricular cartilage may be necessary for grade 2 lesions. In grades 3 and 4, where the obstruction ranges from 71% to 100%, anterior and posterior laryngotracheal splits or cricotracheal resection with thyrotracheal anastomosis are required. In most cases, concomitant tracheotomy or stenting of the airway will be necessary until an adequate airway with vocal cord movement is confirmed by microlaryngoscopy and bronchoscopy.

Progressive laryngeal stridor and a croup-like illness in the first several months of life suggest a lesion simulating subglottic stenosis, ie, the **subglottic hemangioma**. The neoplasm is a soft, compressible, bluish tumor below the level of the true vocal cords that is frequently poorly delineated from surrounding tissue. There is a 2:1 female to male preponderance, and 50% of the lesions are associated with cutaneous hemangiomas. The lateral neck film confirms the presence of a localized subglottic soft tissue mass.

Mechanical airway obstruction is treated with tracheotomy; however, early therapy with systemic corticosteroids may decrease the need for tracheotomy. Hemangiomas producing severe airway obstruction that do not respond to corticosteroids or regress spontaneously should be surgically removed. Because they are so vascular, these lesions are best excised with the neodymium:YAG or CO_2 laser in a staged manner.

Larger Infants & Children

Supraglottitis is an acute inflammatory disorder of the larynx secondary to infection with *H influenzae* type B that affects the epiglottis, aryepiglottic folds, arytenoids, and ventricular bands (Table 38–5). There is usually no prodromal phase, and dysphagia, odynophagia, and shortness of breath rapidly progress to drooling, inspiratory stridor, and a muffled but clear voice. The disease affects principally children 2–6 years of age. Most children are extremely toxic, with fever, tachycardia, and tachypnea. The child sits erect, anxious and increasingly exhausted, drooling, and hungry for air. Lateral neck films confirm the diagnosis and reveal massive edema of the epiglottis (Figure 38–7). However, an x-ray is not essential for the diagnosis. It should not delay immediate treatment.

Immediate control of the airway is mandatory and lifesaving. Children are given 100% humidified oxygen and taken immediately to the operating room, where rapid halothane and oxygen anesthetic induction is followed by atraumatic peroral endotracheal intubation. Pharyngeal and epiglottic blood cultures are obtained, and an intravenous line is started. A course of parenteral antibiotics consisting of ceftriaxone, cefotaxime, or cefuroxime is initiated pending culture and sensitivity reports. Many consultants today prefer ceftriaxone. If a history of penicillin allergies is obtained, aztreonam or chloramphenicol alone is begun. Direct laryngoscopy is performed to rule out other potential causes of acute laryngeal obstruction. Direct inspection of the larynx reveals a cherry-red swollen epiglottis. At this time, the endotracheal tube is changed to a nasotracheal tube (one or two sizes smaller than normal). A tracheotomy set should be available in case the nasal tracheal tube cannot

Table 38–5. Laryngotracheobronchitis and supraglottitis.

Laryngotracheobronchitis	Supraglottitis
Onset and history	
Relatively slow in onset as the terminal event of a 4- or 5-day respiratory tract infection	Rapid in onset and progressive, advancing to severe airway obstruction within 6–8 hours. Usually no antecedent respiratory infection.
Etiology	
Usually viral but may be bacterial	Usually bacterial (*Haemophilus influenzae*) but may be viral
Symptoms	
Stridor, barking cough, sometimes hoarseness	Stridor preceded by severe sore throat and dysphagia (drooling)
X-ray findings	
Narrowing of the subglottic airway ("steeple sign")	Enlarged epiglottis on soft tissue lateral to the pharynx and larynx (thumbprint sign)
Treatment	
Early: Moist oxygen, corticosteroids, antibiotics, and nebulized epinephrine Late: Endoscopic intubation with or without tracheostomy	Immediate moist oxygen and early establishment of an airway by endoscopic intubation. This is followed by administration of intravenous antibiotics.

be properly positioned. Within 72 hours, the infant is generally afebrile and coughing around the tube during suctioning and may be successfully extubated. Of interest is a shifting trend in supraglottitis toward the older pediatric patient and adult. Since the introduction of the Hib vaccine in 1985, a marked decrease in pediatric supraglottitis has occurred. As a result, a relative increase in adult supraglottitis has developed, with two to nine cases per 100,000 in adults and only one per 100,000 in children. Unlike children, adults with supraglottitis have a more gradual onset of symptoms of 36–48 hours, with odynophagia, dysphagia, fever, and leukocytosis—and fewer requiring intubation. Nevertheless, patients should be admitted to an ICU for airway monitoring, intravenous hydration, and intravenous antibiotics aimed at *H influenzae* with equipment available for rapid intubation if necessary.

By contrast, **acute laryngotracheobronchitis** is a viral illness which is far more common than acute supraglottitis (Table 38–5). This illness occurs chiefly in late autumn and winter, with parainfluenza virus the most common cause and adenovirus, rhinovirus, and respiratory syncytial virus also responsible. The principal lesion is subglottic edema, with a variable component of tracheobronchial inflammation. Infants 3 months to 2 years of age are principally affected, exhibiting a 2:1 male:female ratio. The symptoms of a seal-like barking cough, hoarseness, inspiratory and expiratory stridor, and substernal retractions are frequently preceded by an insidious upper respiratory tract illness lasting 1–7 days. In contrast to children with supraglottitis, the infant appears sick but not toxic. Anteroposterior neck films confirm the clinical impression of marked subglottic narrowing (steeple sign) and assist in excluding aerodigestive tract foreign bodies, mediastinal tumors, laryngotracheal neoplasms, and vascular compression of the trachea (Figure 38–8). Initial treatment in the emergency room includes high humidification, oxygenation, hydration, and parenteral corticosteroids (dexamethasone, 0.5–1 mg/kg). Racemic epinephrine is administered by nebulizer with or without intermittent positive pressure, decreasing airway obstruction within 10–30 minutes after administration with the

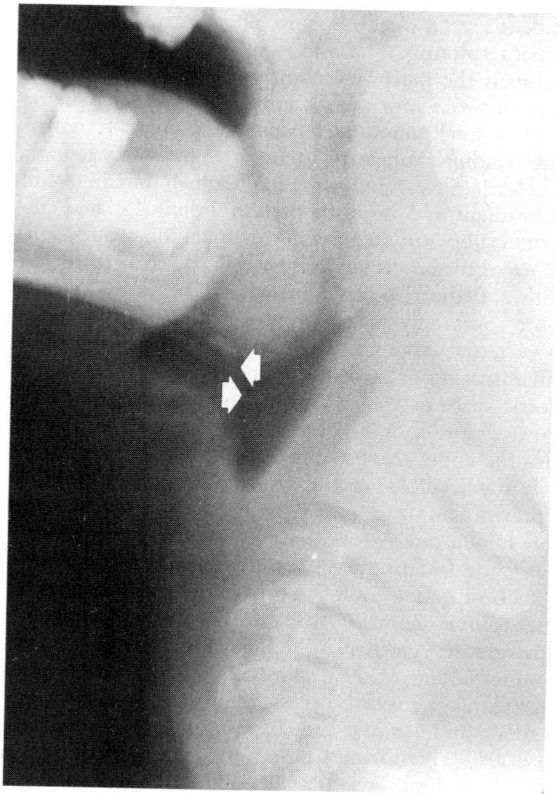

Figure 38–7. Lateral neck film in child with acute supraglottitis. Note the enlarged epiglottis (arrows).

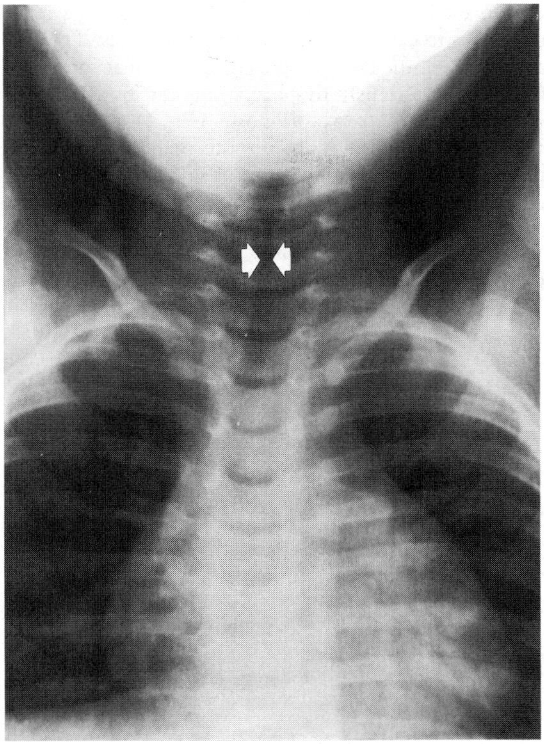

Figure 38–8. Anteroposterior chest film in infant with laryngotracheobronchitis. Marked narrowing of the subglottic space is seen (arrows).

effect waning after 2 hours. The L-isomer is more effective, and the recommended dosage is 0.25 mL of 1:1000 epinephrine if the patient is less than 6 months of age and 0.5 mL of 1:1000 epinephrine if the patient is older. Patients with progressive hypoxia, cyanosis, hypercapnia, and increasing tachypnea and tachycardia who do not respond to medical management should be intubated. The choice of tracheotomy versus oral or nasal intubation is controversial. The rationale against intubation is that in 5% of patients who are intubated subglottic stenosis occurs. This may, however, be reduced by the use of an endotracheal tube that is at least 0.5 mm smaller than the predicted size.

Barrow HN et al: Adult supraglottitis. Otolaryngol Head Neck Surg 1993;109:474.

Carey MJ: Epiglottitis in adults. Am J Emerg Med 1996;14:421.

Frantz TD et al: Acute epiglottitis: changing epidemiologic patterns. Otolaryngol Head Neck Surg 1993;109:457.

Senior BA et al: Changing patterns in pediatric supraglottitis: a multi-institutional review, 1980–1992. Laryngoscope 1994; 104:1314.

RECURRENT RESPIRATORY PAPILLOMATOSIS

The most common benign laryngeal neoplasm is the papilloma. The term juvenile laryngeal papillomatosis was at one time used to describe this condition, but currently the term recurrent respiratory papillomatosis is preferred because it reflects the involvement of the entire upper respiratory tract and its tendency to recur. Caused by human papillomavirus types 6 and 11, one-half of the cases are of juvenile onset, occurring from early infancy through 12 years of age. Adult-onset disease has a peak incidence during the third and fourth decades of life. A history of maternal condylomas is found in up to one-half of patients with juvenile-onset disease. Adult-onset recurrent respiratory papillomatosis is presumed to occur on the basis of sexual contact—primarily oral and genital exposure.

Clinically, because the vocal fold is the first and predominant site of a papilloma lesion, hoarseness is the primary symptom in both juvenile-onset and adult-onset cases. Upper airway obstruction of varying degrees of severity may worsen or initially occur during an intercurrent upper respiratory tract infection. In preschool children and infants, the first presentation of the disorder may occur as a sudden airway crisis.

The clinical course is unpredictable. However, in general, juvenile-onset recurrent respiratory papillomatosis is more severe than adult-onset disease, based upon the clinical extent or on the number of operations required to control dysphonia and airway obstruction. Microendoscopic CO_2 laser excision of papillomas at fixed intervals (2, 4, 6 months) tailored to individual needs fulfills the two main objectives of elimination of disease and maximal preservation of normal epithelium. Secondly, interferon alfacon-1 adjunctive therapy is considered in patients with moderately severe disease or those with uncontrolled or progressive disease in spite of repeated microendoscopic excision. Of the wide variety of additional nonsurgical adjuvants available, including vitamin A derivatives, hematoporphyrin derivatives with concomitant photodynamic therapy, and aerosolized fluorouracil, the most effective appears to be podophyllin, which is applied at the time of conventional excision. Tracheotomy is to be avoided if possible because of the increased risk of spread of papillomas in the lower respiratory tract.

Avidano MA et al: Adjuvant drug strategies in the treatment of recurrent respiratory papillomatosis. Otolaryngol Head Neck Surg 1995;112:197.

Derkay CS: Task force on recurrent respiratory papillomas: a preliminary report. Arch Otolaryngol Head Neck Surg 1995;121:1386.

Doyle DJ et al: Recurrent respiratory papillomatosis: juvenile versus adult forms. Laryngoscope 1994;104:523.

Eicher SA: Isotretinoin therapy for recurrent respiratory papillomatosis. Arch Otolaryngol Head Neck Surg 1994;120:405.

Hartley C et al: Recurrent respiratory papillomatosis—the Manchester experience, 1974–1992. J Laryngol Otol 1994;108: 226.

Kashima H et al: Sites of predilection in recurrent respiratory papillomatosis. Ann Otol Rhinol Laryngol 1993;102(8 Part 1): 580.

Kashima HK et al: Recurrent respiratory papillomatosis. Obstet Gynecol Clin North Am 1996;23:699.

LARYNGITIS

Acute laryngitis often occurs in association with a general viral upper respiratory tract infection caused mainly by rhinoviruses, respiratory syncytial virus, and adenoviruses. However, if hoarseness persists for more than several days, the possibility of secondary bacterial invasion by *M catarrhalis, H influenzae,* or *S pneumoniae* must be considered. Hoarseness, cough, and odynophagia are often marked, with minimal edema or erythema of the true vocal folds. Treatment includes voice rest, hydration, humidification, and oral cefuroxime, amoxicillin-clavulanate, or a macrolide (clarithromycin, azithromycin).

Chronic laryngitis culminating in polypoid chorditis, on the other hand, is related to many factors, including voice misuse, inhalation of irritants, gastroesophageal reflux, and chronic allergies. Pathologically, fluid accumulates in the subepithelial space of the vocal cords (Reinke's space) on the superior surface of the musculomembranous fold. In some individuals, large sessile polyps may develop and occupy the entire vocal cord or a portion thereof. The voice is severely affected, having a hoarse and breathy character with an abnormally low pitch. Females present with these complaints more frequently than males. In adults, polyps and chronic laryngitis are managed by voice rest, cessation of smoking, avoidance of chronic irritants, and speech therapy. Microdirect laryngoscopy and surgical excision with microforceps or the CO_2 laser are necessary for polyps not responding to conservative management. In patients with gastroesophageal reflux disease, nocturnal heartburn, chronic throat pain, dysphonia, wheezing, and cough are common complaints. The origin is multifactorial: smoking, large meals; drugs such as theophylline, diazepam, and calcium-channel blockers; and dietary factors, including caffeine, alcohol, chocolate, fats, and mints contribute to the problem. The resulting chronic posterior laryngitis is related to reflux of acid into the pharynx and may occur without the classic symptoms of gastroesophageal reflux disease. The diagnostic evaluation of GERD-induced posterior laryngitis includes flexible endoscopic examination of the larynx and barium esophagography. Medical therapy includes dietary and lifestyle changes with total acid suppression. Two classes of drugs that are effective are histamine H_2 receptor antagonists (cimetidine, ranitidine, famotidine, nizatidine) and the proton pump inhibitors (omeprazole, lansoprazole). Many clinicians would concomitantly consider esophagogastroduodenoscopy to establish a diagnosis of GERD and stage reflux esophagitis to exclude other esophageal diseases. This permits biopsy of the distal esophagus if columnar metaplasia (Barrett's esophagus), dysphagia, or carcinoma is suspected. As an alternative diagnostic test, 24 hour double-probe pH monitoring and pressure manometry may be appropriate if the patient fails to improve with symptomatic treatment. Omeprazole or lansoprazole for over 6 months may be effective in recalcitrant cases.

Hanson DJ et al: Outcomes of antireflux therapy for the treatment of chronic laryngitis. Ann Otol Rhinol Laryngol 1995;104:550.

Kahrilas PJ: Gastroesophageal reflux disease. JAMA 1996;276:983.

Shaker R et al: Esophagopharyngeal distribution of reflux gastric acid in patients with reflux laryngitis. Gastroenterology 1995; 109:1575.

Thompson AR: Pharmacological agents with effects on voice. Am J Otolaryngol 1995;16:1218.

VOCAL NODULES

Misuse of the voice, particularly shouting or roaring in a very high or very low tone of voice, will result in condensation of hyaline connective tissue at the junction of the anterior and middle thirds of the true vocal cords. Vocal nodules occur in both children and adults and produce a hoarse and breathy voice. In children, most nodules regress with voice therapy, and surgical removal is unnecessary. In both children and adults, however, voice therapy must be instituted for persistent nodules before they are endoscopically removed with the laser or microforceps.

VOCAL CORD PARALYSIS

The recurrent laryngeal nerves of the vagus nerves are the primary innervators of the abductors and adductors of the vocal folds. Isolated injury of the recurrent laryngeal nerve results in paralysis of the vocal cord in the paramedian position on one side 2–3 mm lateral to the laryngeal midline. Combined injury of the recurrent and superior laryngeal nerves paralyzes the vocal cord in the intermediate position several millimeters lateral to the paramedial position.

Vocal cord paralysis may be unilateral or bilateral, central or peripheral. Unilateral left vocal cord paralysis is most common. Fewer than 20% of cases are bilateral. Thyroidectomy is by far the most common cause of bilateral vocal cord paralysis. Central causes include brain stem and supranuclear lesions and account for only 5% of all cases. Supranuclear or cortical causes of vocal cord paralysis are exceedingly rare, owing to the bilateral crossed neural innervation to the brain stem medullary centers in the nucleus ambiguus. The most frequent central cause is vascular insufficiency or a stroke affecting the brain stem. Cortical lesions usually do not produce spastic or flaccid paralysis. The patients present with aphonia or speech apraxia. Brain stem lesions, on the other hand, cause flaccid paralysis of the vocal muscles, producing severe dysfunction with weakness of the larynx, pharynx, or tongue and accompanying sensory deficits. Congenital central lesions are usually secondary to Arnold-Chiari malformation or brain stem dysgenesis and are often associated with additional cranial neuropathies.

Most cases of peripheral vocal cord paralysis are secondary to thyroidectomy or nonlaryngeal neoplasms, including bronchogenic, esophageal, and thyroid carcinoma. Other less common lesions causing paralysis of a vocal cord include tumors of the deep lobe of the parotid gland, carotid body tumors, glomus jugulare vagale tumors, and neurogenic neoplasms of the tenth nerve and jugular foramen. External penetrating wounds to the neck or prolonged endotracheal intubation may also traumatize the recurrent laryngeal nerve, producing vocal cord paralysis. Finally, toxic neuropathy and idiopathic causes account for the remaining cases. Idiopathic vocal cord paralysis is a diagnosis of exclusion and is considered to be a viral mononeuropathy. In the majority of these cases, spontaneous recovery occurs within 4–6 months.

In adults, unilateral recurrent laryngeal nerve paralysis generally produces hoarseness and a weak, breathy voice with varying amounts of aspiration of liquids, vocal fatigue, and dysphagia. The normal vocal cord may cross the midline to approximate the paralyzed vocal cord in the paramedian position. In children, varying degrees of inspiratory stridor may also be present. Bilateral vocal cord paralysis is commonly associated with inspiratory stridor, shortness of breath, and dyspnea on exertion.

Diagnostic assessment of vocal cord paralysis includes flexible fiberoptic examination of the larynx and vocal cord movement, examination of the head and neck for neoplasms, chest x-ray, CT scan of the base of the skull to the carina, and perhaps endoscopic evaluation of the aerodigestive tract. Stroboscopic examination of the vocal fold vibratory pattern as well as laryngeal electromyography may be helpful to assess recurrent laryngeal nerve function, determine prognosis for recovery, and evaluate treatment outcomes. In cases of laryngeal trauma, thin-cut (2 mm) CT scanning of the larynx should be obtained to look for arytenoid dislocation or laryngeal fracture.

Management of unilateral vocal cord paralysis due to lesions of the recurrent laryngeal nerve includes observation, speech therapy, and surgery. Compensation by the opposite cord over the first 3–6 months may be sufficient in many patients to preclude the necessity for operation. The options for surgical management are medialization and reinnervation of the paralyzed cord. Medialization options include injection into the paralyzed vocal cord of Teflon paste or Gelfoam under local anesthesia, mobilizing it medially. Medialization is valuable in the therapy of aspiration and results in dramatic improvement in voice quality. Other injection options for glottic insufficiency include bovine collagen, and autologous medialization of the paralyzed cord may also be accomplished externally via a thyroidotomy and placement of a Silastic wedge implant inside the thyroid cartilage in a small pocket deep to the paralyzed vocal cord. An additional external medialization approach—arytenoid adduction through the posterior border of the thyroid lamina—is ideal for correction of a glottic gap involving the posterior and mid portion of the vocal cord. In the past, bilateral paramedian vocal cord paralysis was commonly managed by permanent tracheotomy. Medial arytenoidectomy through an endolaryngeal approach using the CO_2 laser is performed leaving the phonatory glottis intact. This procedure may be complicated by loss of adequate voice production and exacerbation of aspiration. Attempts to treat bilateral abductor vocal cord paralysis with nerve-muscle transposition of the ansa hypoglossi nerve and the omohyoid muscle to the posterior cricoarytenoid muscle have met with qualified success. This reinnervation technique attempts to provide inspiratory neuronal input to the sole abductor of the vocal cord, the posterior cricoarytenoid muscle. Direct anastomosis of the ansa cervicalis to the recurrent laryngeal nerve may reinnervate the larynx and allow the tracheostomy tube to be removed.

Berninger MS: Evaluation and treatment of the unilateral paralyzed vocal cord. Otolaryngol Head Neck Surg 1994;111:497.

Crumley RL: Endoscopic laser medial arytenoidectomy for airway management in bilateral laryngeal paralysis. Ann Otol Rhinol Laryngol 1993;102:81.

McCaffrey TV: Transcutaneous Teflon injection for vocal cord paralysis. Otol Laryngol Head Neck Surg 1993;109:54.

Netterville JL et al: Silastic medialization and arytenoid adduction: the Vanderbilt experience. A review of 116 phonosurgical procedures. Ann Otol Rhinol Laryngol 1993;102:413.

Shindo ML et al: Autologous fat injection for unilateral vocal cord paralysis. Ann Otol Rhinol Laryngol 1996;105:602.

INFLAMMATORY NECK MASSES

Acute suppurative lymphadenitis usually occurs in infants and children with viral upper respiratory tract infections. In adults with AIDS or who are immunocompromised for any reason, it may initially present with painful lymphadenopathy in the neck. Bacterial lymphadenitis commonly develops secondary to infection with group A streptococci, *S aureus, S pneumoniae,* or mouth anaerobes and may evolve into a deep neck abscess forming a lateral neck mass. These abscesses are most commonly mixed infections, with anaerobic organisms predominating. Mixed infections are synergistic, and β-lactamase production is common. High fever, neck stiffness, odynophagia, trismus, and leukocytosis characterize this complication. Material obtained from a deep neck infection should be routinely submitted to the laboratory for Gram stain, culture, and sensitivity testing. Deep neck abscesses may develop in the prevertebral, sublingual, submandibular, submental, or retropharyngeal spaces as well as in the lateral neck region. Abscesses of the neck are compartmentalized by two of the three envelopes of the deep cervical fascia—the superficial, middle, and deep layers. Infections may spread from one space to another or extend downward into the mediastinum. In addition, cellulitis or abscess formation in the retropharyngeal space or sublingual space (Ludwig's angina) can obstruct the airway. Infection around the carotid sheath may also produce serious hemorrhage by necrosis of the great vessels and their branches. Necrotizing cervical fasciitis is a particularly virulent form of deep neck infection and is invariably polymicrobial and of dental origin with a significant role played by anaerobes.

Patients with deep neck infections should be hospitalized immediately. Broad-spectrum antibiotic therapy directed against β-lactamase-resistant organisms and anaerobic bacteria is started. Treatment includes ampicillin-sulbactam or clindamycin or cefuroxime plus metronidazole. Methicillin-resistant *S aureus* is often found in patients with deep neck infections secondary to drug abuse. Vancomycin should be considered in these cases. Preoperative localization of the abscess is performed with CT scanning. MRI may be superior to CT in some cases. The presence of free gas in the neck should warn of a possible necrotizing fasciitis. The airway should be controlled with an endotracheal tube or tracheostomy before the abscess is incised and drained. The surgical approach to a deep neck abscess depends on the space involved. Proximal control of the carotid artery should be obtained. The lateral pharyngeal space is approached through an incision parallel to the anterior border of the sternocleidomastoid muscle. Most well-localized retropharyngeal abscesses are drained intraorally. A more conservative approach is transcervical. Submandibular abscesses are approached through an incision 2 cm below the inferior border of the mandible.

Chronic granulomatous infections, which may involve the cervical lymph nodes, include tuberculosis, cat-scratch disease, infections with atypical mycobacteria, and occasionally actinomycosis. Tuberculous adenitis commonly develops following pulmonary tuberculosis and usually responds to triple-drug chemotherapy. Persistently enlarged or suppurative nodes should be excised. Atypical mycobacterial adenitis, on the other hand, is seldom associated with pulmonary disease, and routine tuberculin skin tests are either negative or weakly positive. In contrast to tuberculous adenitis, these atypical infections do not respond well to chemotherapy alone and frequently must be excised or curettaged. Neck masses may result from intravenous cervical drug abuse. *S aureus* is the most common pathogen, and treatment with incision and drainage and intravenous nafcillin or cephalothin is recommended.

Finally, actinomycosis may present as an abscess with multiple draining sinuses near the angle of the mandible, discharging pus with characteristic sulfur granules. Often there is underlying dental disease or osteomyelitis of the adjacent bone. Long-term (3–4 weeks) intravenous penicillin in high doses is necessary; surgical excision should be reserved for persistent disease.

Armstrong M Jr et al: Radiographic imaging of sinusitis and HIV infection. Otolaryngol Head Neck Surg 1993;108:36.

Beitler JJ et al: Low-dose radiotherapy for multicystic benign lymphoepithelial lesions of the parotid gland in HIV-positive patients: long-term results. Head Neck 1995;17:31.

Bielamowicz SA et al: Spaces and triangles of the head and neck. Head Neck 1994;16:383.

Brook I et al: Clinical and microbiological features of necrotizing fasciitis. J Clin Microbiol 1995;33:2382.

Carbone A et al: Head and neck lymphomas associated with human immunodeficiency virus infection. Arch Otolaryngol Head Neck Surg 1995;121:210.

Friedman M et al: Treatment of aphthous ulcer in AIDS patients. Laryngoscope 1994;104:566.

Kennedy TL: Curettage of nontuberculous mycobacterial cervical lymphadenitis. Arch Otolaryngol Head Neck Surg 1992; 118:759.

Lazor JB et al: Comparison of computed tomography and surgical findings in deep neck infections. Otolaryngol Head Neck Surg 1994;111:746.

Lee KC et al: Contemporary management of cervical tuberculosis. Laryngoscope 1992;102:60.

Singh B et al: Kaposi's sarcoma of the head and neck in patients with acquired immunodeficiency syndrome. Otolaryngol Head Neck Surg 1994;111.

Stuart MG et al: Nontuberculous mycobacterial infection of the head and neck. Arch Otolaryngol Head Neck Surg 1994; 120:873.

AIDS IN OTOLARYNGOLOGY

Because of AIDS, the otolaryngologist is encountering previously rare diseases more often. Examples include cranial and cervical herpes zoster, oral hairy leukoplakia, and oral candidiasis. There are many similarities between AIDS and primary immunodeficiency disorders, including ataxia-telangiectasia, common variable immunodeficiency disease, Wiscott-Aldrich syndrome, and severe combined immunodeficiency disease. As immunosuppressed patients survive longer, they are beginning to manifest cancers such as lymphomas and squamous cell carcinomas in addition to Kaposi's sarcoma.

The most common manifestations of AIDS in the head and neck region are sinusitis and postnasal discharge. Maxillary sinusitis is more common and more severe in AIDS patients than in the general population. In the mouth, Kaposi's sarcoma may occur, primarily on the hard palate, but is also now seen in the larynx. Overall, 15% of AIDS patients present with Kaposi's sarcoma of the head and neck. Lymphoma and oral candidiasis are also common. Oral candidiasis is treated with nystatin or clotrimazole. Oral ketoconazole and fluconazole are alternative agents. Hairy leukoplakia, a nontender lesion caused by the Epstein-Barr virus, is frequently seen with major aphthous ulcers. These ulcers are treated with intralesional injection of triamcinolone acetonide (20–40 mg/mL) depending upon the size of the ulcers. Ulcers are reinjected biweekly as needed. An oral mixture of diphenhydramine, dexamethasone, nystatin, and tetracycline may also prove beneficial. In the cervical region, Kaposi's sarcoma, lymphoma, and *Mycobacterium avium-intracellulare* infections are also encountered.

The otologic manifestations of AIDS are primarily hearing loss, otalgia, otorrhea, vertigo, and tinnitus. Sensorineural hearing loss is the most common finding, with the loss greater in high frequencies. Most commonly, Kaposi's sarcoma presents as a flat lesion involving the auricle. Kaposi's sarcoma of the ear canal is easily managed with the argon laser. *Pneumocystis carinii* granuloma of the ear canal is treated by resection and trimethoprim-sulfamethoxazole. There is no evidence of increased external ear canal fungal infection in AIDS. However, serous otitis media due to auditory tube dysfunction secondary to benign lymphoid hyperplasia is frequent.

Herpes zoster oticus syndrome (Ramsay Hunt's syndrome) is associated with facial paralysis, vertigo, and hearing loss and is best treated with either acyclovir or famciclovir for acyclovir-resistant varicella-zoster virus. Ototoxic drugs used in the treatment of AIDS include acyclovir (which produces vertigo), trimethoprim-sulfamethoxazole (which produces vertigo and tinnitus), and zidovudine (which causes vertigo and hearing loss). HIV infection may alter the natural course of latent syphilis, and patients may present with otosyphilis that is difficult to treat because of the poor vascularity of the otic capsule and its isolation from cerebrospinal fluid. Early treatment with zidovudine (AZT) may help control progression of the disease. Alternatively, didanosine (ddI) or zalcitabine (ddC) may be used for patients unresponsive to AZT or for concurrent use with AZT in advanced cases. Treatment for Kaposi's sarcoma and non-Hodgkin's lymphoma is combination chemotherapy or chemotherapy plus erythropoietic support drugs. Multicystic benign lymphoepithelial lesions of the parotid gland are increasingly seen in patients with HIV and can produce considerable physical discomfort as well as cosmetic deformity. Low-dose radiation therapy provides reliable and temporary palliation for these large lesions.

Armstrong M Jr et al: Radiographic imaging of sinusitis in HIV infection. Otolaryngol Head Neck Surg 1993;108:36.

Beitler JJ et al: Low-dose radiotherapy for multicystic benign lymphoepithelial lesions of the parotid gland in HIV-positive patients: long-term results. Head Neck 1995;17:31.

Carbone A et al: Head and neck lymphomas associated with human immunodeficiency virus infection. Arch Otolaryngol Head Neck Surg 1995;121:210.

Weber PC, Adkins WY Jr: The differential diagnosis of Meniere's disease. Otolaryngol Clin North Am 1997;30:977.

The Eye & Ocular Adnexa 39

Linda M. Tsai, MD, & Stephen A. Kamenetzky, MD

EXAMINATION OF THE EYE

Evaluation of the eye and its adnexa requires a good history, physical examination of the eyes, and assessment of visual function. The history should include general information about the patient's age, occupation, and health status as well as ocular complaints. Occasionally, special examinations may be required to identify specific ocular disorders or to establish the presence of associated systemic disease.

The basic office equipment required for a routine eye examination by a nonophthalmologist includes the following: (1) a hand-held flashlight, (2) a binocular magnifying loupe, (3) an ophthalmoscope, (4) a visual acuity chart, and (5) a tonometer.

The basic medications required for an eye examination are (1) a local anesthetic such as proparacaine 0.5% or tetracaine 0.5%; (2) fluorescein strips; and (3) dilating drops, such as phenylephrine 2.5% or tropicamide 0.5–1%.

Visual Acuity Testing

Central visual acuity should be part of the routine examination of the eye in all patients. The Snellen chart is most commonly used. The patient faces the test chart at a distance of 6 meters (20 feet). The patient is tested by occluding one eye at a time and reading the chart with the unoccluded eye. Visual acuity corresponds to the smallest line the patient can read and is recorded as 20/20, 20/30, 20/40, 20/50, etc. The patient who is unable to read the large letters at the top of the chart should be moved progressively closer until the characters can be read, whereupon the distance between the patient and the chart should be recorded as the numerator. If the patient wears eyeglasses for distance, the visual acuity should be repeated with the glasses on and the results recorded as uncorrected vision and corrected vision. Preschool children or illiterates should be properly instructed and then tested with the illiterate E chart.

Visual Field Testing

Confrontation visual fields can be used to grossly detect visual field defects such as quadrantanopia, hemianopia, or severe visual field constriction. With one eye occluded, the patient is asked to fixate on the examiner's face and detect finger count or hand motion in each quadrant. Formal visual field testing (perimetry) is used to more carefully examine the central and peripheral visual fields. The technique is performed separately for each eye. It is used to measure the function of the retina, the optic nerve, and intracranial visual pathway. Because perimetry relies on subjective patient responses, the results will depend on the patient's alertness and cooperation. Several methods are used to assess visual field functions, including the tangent screen, Goldmann perimetry, and computerized automated perimetry.

Tonometry

Tonometry measures intraocular pressure. The most common instruments used are the Tono-Pen and the Goldmann applanation tonometer. Tonometers measure the amount of corneal indentation produced by a preset amount of weight or force. The softer the eye, the less force required to indent the cornea. The normal intraocular pressure varies between 10 mm Hg and 20 mm Hg.

Inspection of Anterior Segment & Adnexa

Inspection of the external ocular structures—lids, conjunctiva, cornea, sclera, and lacrimal apparatus—should include everting the upper eyelids for inspection of the conjunctival surface with the patient looking down. The exposed surfaces are inspected for anatomic defects, foreign bodies, lacerations, inflammation, discharge, tearing, dryness, or other abnormalities. In patients who are unconscious or in coma, the degree of lid closure and the presence of Bell's phenomenon—upward position of the cornea during sleep—are significant findings. Corneal sensation and reflexes in each eye should be noted before any anesthetic drops are used. With the aid of a hand-held flashlight and magnifying loupe or with a biomicroscope (slit lamp), the eye and adnexa can be inspected.

A direct ophthalmoscope focused on the ocular surface may provide some magnification. In addition, considerable detail of the ocular surface can be observed using a +20 diopter lens and a hand-held flashlight. The depth of the anterior chamber should be noted by shining a light across the eye.

Assessment of Pupillary Functions

Examination of the pupils should be performed before any dilating drops are instilled. Both direct and consensual light reflexes of the pupils should be assessed. The reaction of the pupils with accommodation should be noted. The size of the pupil should be noted, and any differences between the size of the right and left pupil should be recorded and described. In hospitalized patients and those with neurologic disorders, pupils should be dilated with discretion and only with short-acting mydriatics.

Eye Movements

Ocular motility should be assessed in different directions of gaze. In examining eye movements, one should note random movements, the position of the eyes in primary gaze, latent nystagmus, the convergence of the eyes, and ductions in the cardinal positions of gaze. The oculocephalic reflex (doll's head) may be tested, and the response to forced eyelid closure (Bell's phenomenon) should be noted. The light reflection ("reflex") on the cornea from a penlight is at the same point in each eye when the eyes are straight.

Ophthalmoscopy

Ophthalmoscopy is important for the diagnosis of both ocular and systemic conditions. It can be critical in neurologic and neurosurgical contexts. In most instances, the optic nerve head can be clearly seen without dilating the pupils. In hospitalized patients with neurologic and neurosurgical disorders, dilation of the pupils should be avoided unless absolutely necessary. In exceptional cases, short-acting mydriatics such as tropicamide 0.5% should be used to dilate the pupils.

SYMPTOMS & SIGNS OF OCULAR DISORDERS

Visual disturbances or decrease in visual acuity may be due to a number of ocular and systemic diseases.

Decrease in Visual Acuity

Decrease in visual acuity may be unilateral or bilateral, painful or painless, and persistent or transient. The duration of the decrease in visual acuity is important. Was the change noted recently? Was it gradual or sudden? Was it binocular or monocular? Was it discovered accidentally? Unilateral acute painful loss of vision may be due to angle-closure glaucoma, endophthalmitis, or uveitis. Painless unilateral loss of vision may be due to ischemic optic neuropathy, optic neuritis, central retinal artery or vein occlusion, retinal detachment, vitreous hemorrhage, or retinal hemorrhages. Transient painless acute loss of vision in one eye may be due to migraine or amaurosis fugax. Bilateral acute loss of vision may be due to pituitary abnormality, ophthalmic migraine, conversion reaction, or intracranial occipital vascular occlusion.

Disturbances in Vision

Disturbances in vision may consist of image distortion, photophobia, color change, spots before the eyes, visual field defects, night blindness, momentary loss of vision, or halos around lights. Distortion of normal shape is most often due to astigmatism or macular lesions. Photophobia is commonly due to corneal inflammation, iritis, ocular albinism, or aniridia. Changes in color (chromatopsia) such as yellow vision are due to retinal lesions or the use of systemic medications such as digoxin. Spots before the eyes are reported by patients with vitreous opacities or in association with intraocular inflammation. Visual field defects may be due to lid edema, retinal and optic nerve lesions, visual pathway lesions, or cortical abnormalities. Night blindness may be genetic, as in patients with retinitis pigmentosa, or acquired—for example, as a result of vitamin A deficiency, glaucoma, optic atrophy, cataract, or retinal degeneration. Transient loss of vision may imply impending cerebrovascular accident or partial occlusion of the internal carotid artery. Colored halos around lights or bright objects are associated with acute angle-closure glaucoma. Fortification images or scintillating scotomas are common in ocular migraine. Incipient cataract may also cause halos (colorless) around point light sources.

Double Vision

Double vision (diplopia) can be constant or intermittent and may occur suddenly in certain positions of gaze or only at certain distances. It is important to differentiate between horizontal diplopia and vertical diplopia, because the nerve pathways are different. Monocular diplopia occurs with refractive error, lenticular changes, macular lesions, malingering, or conversion reactions. Binocular double vision is most often due to misalignment of the eyes from extraocular muscle dysfunction or neurologic abnormalities.

Ocular & Orbital Pain

Ocular pain may result from corneal lesions, inflammation, sudden increase in intraocular pressure, anterior uveitis, cyclitis, scleritis, or optic neuritis. Other causes of pain include inflammation of the orbital contents or tumors in the orbit. Dacryocystitis may also cause severe pain. Eyelid pain may arise from infections of the meibomian glands and the glands of Zeis and Moll.

Redness of the Eye

Acute redness (injection) of the eye not associated with trauma may be due to conjunctivitis, acute anterior uveitis, acute angle-closure glaucoma, corneal infection, or corneal abrasion (Table 39–1). Subconjunctival hemorrhage may also present as a red eye, but this is usually painless and otherwise asymptomatic. Conjunctivitis is the most frequent cause of red eye and can be due to bacterial, chlamydial, viral, or allergic causes. Nonspecific irritation by exogenous agents or a foreign body may also cause redness of the eye. Physical (thermal and irradiation), chemical, and mechanical injury to the eye may lead to redness of the eye and swelling of the periocular and adnexal structures. "Dry eye" or ocular surface anomalies will cause redness, a foreign body sensation, and variable degrees of decreased vision.

Discharge

Ocular discharge may be noted as watery, mucopurulent, purulent, or chronic crusting of the lid margins. When the discharge is watery and not associated with redness or pain, it may be due to excessive tear formation or obstruction of the lacrimal passages. Watery discharge with photophobia, pain, or irritation may be due to keratitis or keratoconjunctivitis. Purulent discharge is a sign of bacterial infection, severe inflammation of the conjunctival surface, or bacterial infection of the lacrimal sac or canaliculus. Mucopurulent discharge may be due to infections with bacterial organisms (eg, pseudomonas or haemophilus species). When the discharge forms mucoid strings, it is characteristic of allergic disorders involving the conjunctiva or dry eye syndrome.

Swelling of the Eyelids

Swelling of the eyelids may be unilateral or bilateral. In unilateral swelling, the patient may suffer from infection of the glands of Meibom, Zeis, or Moll; bilateral swelling may indicate blepharitis or allergic dermatitis. Systemic diseases associated with water retention, hyperthyroidism, or hypothyroidism may also be associated with swelling or puffiness of the eyelids.

Displacement of the Eyes

Forward displacement of the eyes (exophthalmos, proptosis) may be due to abnormalities of the thyroid gland or to tumors of the orbit.

Strabismus

Strabismus results from misalignment of the eyes due to muscle imbalance and may be in the form of tropia (manifest deviation) or phoria (latent deviation). Ocular deviations may be lateral (exotropia) or medial (esotropia) and upward (hypertropia) or downward (hypotropia).

Table 39–1. Differential diagnosis of common causes of inflamed eye.

	Acute Conjunctivitis	Acute Iritis[1]	Acute Glaucoma[2]	Corneal Trauma or Infection
Incidence	Extremely common	Common	Uncommon	Common
Discharge	Moderate to copious	None	None	Watery or purulent
Vision	No effect on vision	Slightly blurred	Markedly blurred	Usually blurred
Pain	None	Moderate	Severe	Moderate to severe
Conjunctival injection	Diffuse; more toward fornices	Mainly circumcorneal	Diffuse	Diffuse
Cornea	Clear	Usually clear	Steamy	Change in clarity related to cause
Pupil size	Normal	Small	Moderately dilated and fixed	Normal
Pupillary light response	Normal	Poor	None	Normal
Intraocular pressure	Normal	Normal	Elevated	Normal
Smear	Causative organisms	No organisms	No organisms	Organisms found only in corneal ulcers due to infection

[1]Acute anterior uveitis.
[2]Angle-closure glaucoma.

Leukocoria

A white pupil in a child indicates a serious eye disorder. The most frequent cause of leukocoria is congenital cataract, which requires urgent management to prevent amblyopia. Other causes include retinoblastoma, retrolental fibroplasia (retinopathy of prematurity), toxocariasis, persistent hyperplastic primary vitreous, vitreous hemorrhage, retinal detachment, retinal dysplasia, incontinentia pigmenti, Coats' disease, and Norrie's disease.

Other Symptoms

Patients may present with other symptoms such as burning, itching, gritty and foreign body sensations, or a "sandy" feeling. These symptoms in elderly patients are suggestive of dry eye syndrome. Itching is frequently associated with allergic disorders.

DISEASES OF THE EYE & ADNEXA

ACUTE HORDEOLUM

Acute hordeolum (sty) is a common infection of the glands of the eyelids involving the glands of Zeis or Moll (external hordeolum). The meibomian glands may be infected, leading to internal hordeolum. The usual causative agent is *Staphylococcus aureus.* Acute hordeolum is characterized by pain, swelling, and redness of the eyelid. A large hordeolum is infrequently associated with a preauricular lymph node but may lead to an abscess in the eyelid.

If pus is localized and pointing out to the skin or conjunctiva, treatment consists of making a local horizontal (skin) or vertical (conjunctiva) incision. If there is no evidence of abscess formation, the patient can be treated with warm compresses three times daily and topical antibiotic drops such as tobramycin or sulfacetamide 10% three or four times daily for 5–7 days. Ophthalmic ointments such as erythromycin or bacitracin may alternatively be used twice daily for 5–7 days. Oral antibiotics, especially tetracycline derivatives, may be required as an adjunct in patients with acne rosacea.

CONJUNCTIVITIS

Acute conjunctivitis is the most frequent cause of red eye. Infectious causes include bacterial, viral, chlamydial, fungal, and parasitic agents. Less common causes of conjunctivitis include chemical irritation, allergy, hypersensitivity to topical medications, vitamin A deficiency, dry eye syndrome, and injury.

Clinical Findings

A. Symptoms and Signs

Patients with conjunctivitis complain of redness, irritation, a foreign body sensation, and conjunctival discharge. One or both eyes may be affected. In patients with bacterial conjunctivitis, the eyelids may be stuck together in the morning. Examination reveals conjunctival hyperemia with purulent or mucopurulent discharge and variable degrees of lid swelling.

B. Laboratory Findings

If bacterial conjunctivitis is suspected, conjunctival swabs and scrapings should be taken for culture on blood agar and chocolate agar and for staining with Gram and Giemsa stains.

Treatment

In patients with suspected bacterial conjunctivitis and until laboratory reports are received, topical broad-spectrum antibacterial agents can be prescribed, eg, sulfacetamide 10% eye drops or ciprofloxacin 0.3% eye drops four times daily during the day plus erythromycin or bacitracin ophthalmic ointment at bedtime.

Viral conjunctivitis does not need to be treated and is self-limited. However, if the diagnosis is unclear, topical antibiotics are often used. Contact precautions are useful in all situations of bacterial and viral conjunctivitis since spread of disease is through contact with tears, either directly or through fomites.

Treatment of patients with allergic conjunctivitis consists of topical decongestants (naphazoline 0.1%), and H_1 receptor blocker (levocabastine), or a mast cell stabilizer (cromolyn). Combination mast cell and antihistamine drops such as olopatadine are also available. In severe cases of allergic conjunctivitis, topical corticosteroids may be used with the assistance of an ophthalmologist.

CORNEAL ULCERS

Corneal infections leading to ulceration may be due to bacteria (including chlamydia), viruses, fungi, or protozoa. The most serious infection of the cornea is caused by pseudomonas species.

Clinical Findings

A. Symptoms and Signs

Patients with corneal ulcers complain of pain, photophobia, and blurring of vision. Patients develop conjunctival hyperemia and chemosis, with ulceration of the cornea and whitish or yellowish infiltrate. Hypopyon (pus in the anterior chamber) may be present in cases due to bacterial or fungal infections.

B. Laboratory Findings

Laboratory studies include culture and cytologic inspection of corneal scrapings.

Treatment

Corneal ulceration is a serious condition that should be managed carefully and followed closely. The most severe and devastating infection of the cornea is caused by *Pseudomonas aeruginosa.* Topical and subconjunctival antibiotics should be given on an empirical basis until the results of culture and sensitivity tests are obtained. Organism-specific antimicrobial treatment should then be given. Central corneal ulcers may leave corneal scars, causing loss of vision. Patients severely affected may require penetrating keratoplasty (corneal transplant).

Patients wearing contact lenses should be advised to stop wearing them. Patients using topical corticosteroids should stop using them.

HERPES SIMPLEX

Herpes simplex is a DNA virus that can affect the eye in a primary ocular reaction as well as in a reactivated state when latent virus travels down the axon of the sensory nerve to its target tissue. Herpes simplex virus (HSV) is extremely common and about 90% of the population is seropositive for HSV antibodies. HSV-1 predominantly causes infection above the waist (face, lips, and eyes), and HSV-2 typically causes infection below the waist. Very occasionally HSV-2 is transmitted to the eye through infected genital secretions during birth, but most ocular infections are HSV-1.

Clinical Findings

A. Symptoms and Signs

Primary infections usually occur in children between ages 6 months and 5 years and may be associated with generalized symptoms of a viral illness. HSV is usually self-limited, and the most common symptoms are blepharoconjunctivitis and keratitis, which is classically in a dendritic pattern.

B. Laboratory Findings

A clinical diagnosis can be made with the classic dendritic presentation. However, definitive diagnosis is made using viral culture or Giemsa-stained smears of corneal scrapings that reveal mononuclear cells, polymorphonuclear neutrophil leukocytes, multinucleated giant epithelial cells, and eosinophilic Lipschütz inclusion bodies in the cell nuclei. ELISA can be used to detect whether live viral particles are present.

Treatment

The mainstays of treatment are topical and oral antiviral medications. Antibiotic ointment may be used at night to help prevent bacterial superinfection. Topical Viroptic 1% (trifluorothymidine) or vira-A ointment (acycloguanosine) is used to treat keratitis. Oral acyclovir, 400 mg five times a day, is also used for ocular herpetic disease. Topical steroids may be used to treat corneal scarring or uveitis, but must be used carefully with concurrent topical or systemic antiviral therapy or both.

HERPES ZOSTER

Herpes zoster is a caused by a reactivation of latent varicella (chickenpox) virus dormant in the dorsal root ganglion. Approximately 15% of herpes zoster cases arise from the ophthalmic division of the trigeminal nerve, which is then referred to as "herpes zoster ophthalmicus" (HZO). Hutchinson's sign (involvement of the nasociliary nerve, which supplies the tip of the nose) occurs in about one-third of patients with HZO; if present, it suggests intraocular involvement. Reactivation is associated with decreased cell-mediated immunity, and patients with HIV, blood dyscrasias, neoplasms, or other forms of immunosuppression are more at risk.

Clinical Findings

HZO can involve virtually all ocular and adnexal tissues. Reactivation often starts with headache, malaise, fever, and ocular pain, followed within 24–48 hours by the classic vesicular lesions in a dermatomal, unilateral pattern. Corneal involvement may occur with either the acute event or following it by months or years. A corneal pseudodendritic pattern is common. Conjunctivitis, keratitis, episcleritis/scleritis, and uveitis can also occur.

Treatment

Treatments of skin lesions include warm compresses and topical antibiotic ointment. Oral antiviral medication is the standard of care. Oral acyclovir, 800 mg five times daily for 7–10 days, initiated within 72 hours of symptoms, has been demonstrated to accelerate the resolution of skin rash and the healing of skin lesions, reduce lesion formation and viral shedding, and reduce the incidence of episcleritis, keratitis, and iritis. Oral acyclovir also appears to reduce acute zoster-associated pain and may decrease postherpetic neuralgia. Topical antiviral medication and steroids may be indicated in certain situations to treat corneal lesions or uveitis. See Table 39–2.

DRY EYE

Dry eye is a disorder of the tear film due to either deficiency of production or excess tear evaporation. The

Table 39–2. Herpes simplex virus (HSV) versus herpes zoster virus (HZV).

	HSV	HZV
Rash	Clear vesicles on erythematous base; crusting	Vesicular rash along dermatomal distribution, not crossing midline; Hutchinson's sign (nasociliary branch of V1) may be present
Epithelial lesion	Dendritic epithelial lesions with heaped edges	Pseudodendrites (mucous plagues without true terminal bulbs)
Staining	Edges stain with rose bengal; central ulceration stains with fluorescein	Minimal fluorescein staining
Patient population	Young	Older or immunocompromised

tear film is composed of mucin and aqueous and lipid components, and abnormalities of any layer lead to a wide variety of symptoms.

Primary lacrimal deficiency from disease such as Riley-Day syndrome and hypoplastic lacrimal glands is rare, and most patients with dry eye have a secondary lacrimal deficiency. This has been seen post radiation and in lymphoma, sarcoidosis, graft-versus-host disease, HIV, hemochromatosis, and amyloidosis. Systemic medications such as anticholinergics (including antihistamines and antidepressants), antiadrenergics, and diuretics can also cause decreased tear production. Dry eye has also been associated with menopause, presumably due to decreased androgens, and women have a much higher incidence of symptomatic dry eye.

Evaporative dry eye problems are most often associated with meibomian gland dysfunction (MGD). The protective lipid and mucin layers that normally keep the aqueous layer of tears stable are reduced, leading to a poor-quality tear film that breaks up easily.

Clinical Findings

Symptoms of tear deficiency often include foreign body sensation, redness, decreased vision, and even reflex tearing. These symptoms tend to vary with time and eye usage; symptoms are usually worse at the end of the day.

Symptoms of evaporative tear loss include a chronic "film" over the vision, redness, burning, and itching of the eyelid margin; these symptoms are often worse in the morning. The quick breakup time of the tear film leads to difficulty reading and prolonged eye usage.

Post-LASIK (laser in-situ keratomileusis) patients have decreased corneal sensation, lower tear production, and diminished blink rate, which may cause dry eye symptoms for 6–18 months or more postoperatively.

Treatment

Treatment for aqueous deficiency includes lubricant tear supplementation and punctal occlusion to retard normal drainage. In meibomian gland disease, eyelid hygiene is extremely important. Hot compresses with eyelid scrubs can improve tear quality and prevent evaporative tear loss. Mild topical corticosteroids or systemic tetracycline may also be used, especially if the patient has associated signs of acne rosacea. Recently topical cyclosporine A, because of its anti-inflammatory action, has been found to dramatically improve dry eye symptoms, although it may take up to 6 weeks for symptomatic improvement.

DACRYOCYSTITIS

Dacryocystitis is a common infection of the lacrimal sac. It may be acute or chronic and occurs most often in infants and in persons over age 40 years. It is usually unilateral and always secondary to obstruction of the nasolacrimal duct. In rare instances, the nasolacrimal duct may be obstructed by a tumor.

Normally, the nasolacrimal duct opens spontaneously during the first month of life. Failure of canalization leads to obstruction of the sac and secondary dacryocystitis.

The cause of acquired nasolacrimal duct obstruction is usually unknown, but trauma to the nose or infection may be responsible. In infants, dacryocystitis leading to obstruction may be due to *Haemophilus influenzae,* staphylococci, or streptococci. In patients with trachoma, nasolacrimal and canalicular obstruction is common. The cause of acute dacryocystitis in adults is usually *Staphylococcus aureus* or beta-hemolytic streptococci. In chronic dacryocystitis, *Streptococcus pneumoniae* is a common pathogen.

Clinical Findings

A. Symptoms and Signs

Acute dacryocystitis is characterized by pain, swelling, tenderness, and redness in the tear sac area; pus may be expressed. In chronic dacryocystitis, tearing and discharge are the principal signs. Mucus or pus may be expressed from the tear sac.

B. Laboratory Findings

Pus can be expressed from the upper or lower puncta and should be examined by Gram stain and culture and sensitivity testing.

Treatment

A. Adults

Acute dacryocystitis responds well to systemic antibiotic therapy, but recurrences are common if the obstruction is not surgically relieved.

B. Infants

When ductal obstruction is due to failure of canaliculization in the first month of life, daily forceful massage of the tear sac is indicated, and topical antibiotics should be instilled in the conjunctival sac four or five times daily. If this is not successful, probing of the nasolacrimal duct is indicated. Most ophthalmologists postpone probing until the age of 6 months since in most cases the ducts that will open spontaneously have opened by that time. The probe should be passed through both the upper and the lower canaliculi.

ORBITAL CELLULITIS

Orbital cellulitis is manifested by an abrupt onset of swelling and redness of the lids, accompanied by proptosis, decreased vision, diplopia, and fever. It is usually caused by staphylococci or streptococci. Immediate treatment with intravenous antibiotics is indicated to prevent abscess formation and rapid increase in the orbital pressure, which may interfere with the blood supply to the eye. The response to antibiotics is excellent, but surgical drainage may be required if an abscess forms. CT is indicated to rule out abscess formation. Preseptal cellulitis is limited to the area anterior to the orbital septum and may be treated with oral antibiotics while monitoring closely for progression to orbital infection.

PTERYGIUM

Pterygium is a fleshy, triangular encroachment of the conjunctiva onto the nasal side of the cornea and is usually associated with excessive exposure to wind, sun, sand, and dust. Pterygium may be either unilateral or bilateral. There may be a genetic predisposition, but no hereditary pattern has been described. Excision is indicated if the growth threatens vision by approaching the visual axis, though recurrence is common.

Treatment is by superficial excision. After excising large or recurrent pterygia, autologous conjunctival tissue transplantation is indicated. A thin layer of conjunctiva is obtained from the upper bulbar conjunctiva and sutured to the area where the pterygium was removed. This leads to rapid restoration of anatomic integrity of the epithelial surface and may prevent further recurrences. Patients should be advised to wear sunglasses out of doors. Topical mitomycin eye drops have been used to prevent recurrences of the disease, but serious complications such as scleral thinning and keratitis have been reported.

CATARACT

Cataract is opacity in the lens that may lead to a decrease in vision when it occupies the visual axis. Cataract is the leading cause of curable blindness in the world.

There are three types: (1) congenital cataract, (2) cataract associated with other disorders, and (3) age-related (senile) cataract. Some cataracts are rapidly progressive, while others may show slow progression.

1. Congenital Cataract

Congenital cataract may be genetically determined or may be caused by intrauterine factors that interfere with normal development of the lens. Intrauterine viral infections (the most common is rubella), for example, can lead to congenital cataract.

Congenital cataract may be unilateral or bilateral and complete or incomplete. Dense cataract present at birth is an indication for urgent operative management to prevent amblyopia. Phacoemulsification or simple aspiration with central posterior capsulotomy and limited anterior vitrectomy is recommended for congenital cataract. Preservation of the peripheral posterior capsule and zonules is important for future implantation of intraocular lenses. If the cataract is aspirated, leaving the posterior capsule intact, the posterior capsule becomes opaque, requiring capsulotomy at a later stage. Correction with soft contact lenses can be started immediately after surgery. Posterior chamber intraocular lenses may be implanted when the child is older, although children as young as 2 years are being given primary intraocular lens implants. Restoration of true binocular vision in very young children is seldom achieved after removal of unilateral congenital cataracts.

2. Cataracts Associated with Other Disorders

Many systemic conditions may be associated with cataracts, including diabetes mellitus, galactosemia, hypocalcemia, myotonic dystrophy, Down's syndrome, and cutaneous disorders such as atopic dermatitis. Certain systemic medications and eye drops containing corticosteroids can also cause cataracts. Other disorders of the eye such as retinal detachment or chronic uveitis may also be associated with cataracts. Physical, mechanical, and thermal injury or ionizing radiation may also lead to cataract.

The treatment of such cataracts is similar to that of senile cataract.

3. Age-Related (Senile) Cataract

This is the most common type of cataract. The rate of progression is variable. Diagnosis is by slitlamp examination. Nuclear changes of the lens produce a brunescent color. In advanced cortical cataracts, a white opacity may be seen in the pupillary area upon gross inspection.

Treatment

Once the cataract leads to visual impairment, treatment is by surgical removal of the lens. Clinical trials of agents that may delay or prevent the formation of cataracts are under way, but no pharmacologic means of prevention is available at present.

Cataract surgery can be done in three different ways. All three methods give restoration of visual acuity, although in most modern countries, phacoemulsification is the procedure of choice. Primarily, lens implant is preferred, although in rare cases where intraocular lenses are contraindicated, such as certain forms of uveitis, optical correction can be achieved with eyeglasses or contact lenses.

A. Intracapsular Lens Extraction

Intracapsular extraction, rarely used today, removes the lens entirely with its capsule either by forceps or a cryoprobe. This procedure cannot be performed on children or young adults because of the adhesion between the lens and the vitreous.

B. Extracapsular Extraction

With standard extracapsular cataract extraction, the anterior capsule of the lens is removed, the nucleus of the cataract is expressed, and the residual cortical material is aspirated from the eye through a 9–11 mm incision. The posterior capsule is left intact and an intraocular lens is placed in the capsular bag. The incision is then sutured with 10-0 nylon. In 25–35% of patients undergoing extracapsular cataract extraction, the posterior capsule may become opacified. This is treated by Nd:YAG laser capsulotomy. If such a laser is not available, surgical incision of the opaque posterior capsule is required.

C. Phacoemulsification

See Figure 39–1.

Phacoemulsification, now the most common form of extracapsular cataract extraction, involves fragmenting the nucleus of the lens with a high-frequency ultrasonic probe and simultaneously aspirating the nuclear fragments from the eye. The advantage of phacoemulsification is that the incision size can be reduced and the patient more quickly rehabilitated. The cortical material is removed by irrigation and aspiration. The use of foldable or injectable intraocular

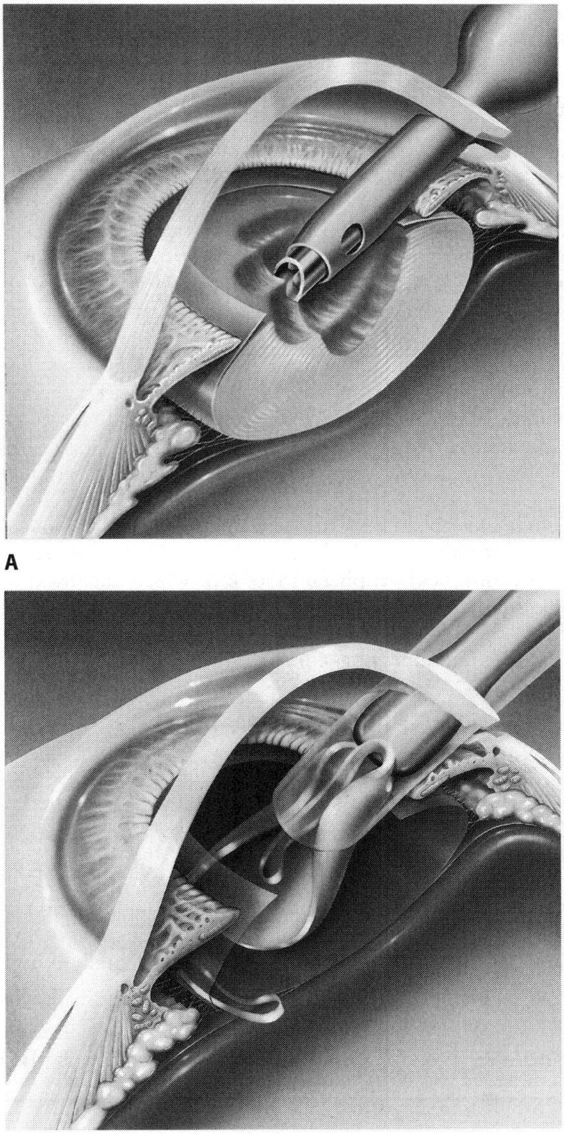

A

B

Figure 39–1. Phacoemulsification. ***A:*** Phacoemulsification probe removing lens nucleus through a clear corneal incision. ***B:*** Implantation of an injectable intraocular lens implant into the capsular bag through a small incision. (Photos, Courtesy of Alcon Laboratories, Inc.)

lenses allows placement of the lens implant through the small incision, and in many cases no suture is required.

ANGLE-CLOSURE GLAUCOMA

About 1% of people over age 35 have anatomically narrow anterior chamber angles. In such patients, if the pupil dilates spontaneously or is dilated with a mydriatic or cycloplegic agent, the angle may close and an attack of acute glaucoma may be precipitated. For this reason, it is a wise precaution to estimate the depth of the anterior chamber angle before instilling these drugs.

Acute angle-closure glaucoma is manifested by an acute onset of pain, headache, and blurring of vision. Some patients develop nausea and vomiting. The eye is red, the cornea is hazy, and the pupil is mid-dilated and does not react to light. Intraocular pressure is elevated.

The attack is aborted by use of topical pilocarpine, beta-blockers, apraclonidine and latanoprost drops, systemic acetazolamide, and, if necessary, an intravenous hyperosmotic agent such as mannitol. Definitive treatment consists of peripheral iridotomy, which establishes a communication between the posterior and anterior chambers. This is usually done with an argon or Nd:YAG laser. Rarely, surgical peripheral iridectomy is required.

OPEN-ANGLE GLAUCOMA

In open-angle glaucoma, the intraocular pressure is usually consistently elevated. Over a period of months or years, this results in optic atrophy, with loss of vision varying from slight constriction of the upper nasal peripheral visual fields to complete blindness. The cause of the decreased rate of aqueous outflow in open-angle glaucoma has not been clearly demonstrated. The disease is bilateral but can be asymmetric and is probably genetically influenced. African Americans are particularly at risk.

Clinical Findings

Patients with open-angle glaucoma are initially asymptomatic. On examination, there may be slight cupping of the optic disk. The visual fields gradually constrict, but central vision remains good until late in the disease. Tonometry, evaluation of the optic nerve, and visual field testing are the three principal tests used for the diagnosis and continued clinical evaluation of glaucoma.

The normal intraocular pressure is about 10–20 mm Hg. The diagnosis is never made on the basis of a single tonometric measurement. Transient elevations of intraocular pressure do not constitute glaucoma for the same reason that periodic or intermittent elevations of blood pressure do not constitute hypertensive disease. All persons over age 20 should have tonometric and ophthalmoscopic examinations every 3–5 years. If there is a family history of glaucoma or other risk factors, annual examination is indicated. Low tension glaucoma is an uncommon condition characterized by visual field changes and optic nerve cupping in the presence of normal ocular pressure.

Treatment

See Table 39–3.

Most patients can be controlled with topical beta-blockers (eg, timolol maleate 0.25–0.5%, 1 drop twice daily), topical alpha-adrenergic agonists (eg, brimonidine 0.2%, 1 drop twice daily), topical carbonic anhydrase inhibitors (eg, dorzolamide 2%, 1 drop twice daily), or topical prostaglandins (eg, latanoprost 0.005%, 1 drop once daily). Oral carbonic anhydrase inhibitors (eg, acetazolamide) are used in patients with persistently uncontrolled high intraocular pressures. Mitotic (eg, pilocarpine 1–4%, 1 drop four times daily) and epinephrine eye drops (0.5–2.0%, 1 drop twice daily) are less commonly used. (*Caution:* Epinephrine is contraindicated if the anterior chamber angle is narrow.)

Table 39–3. Types of glaucoma medications and side effects.

Class	Mechanism	Side Effects	Pregnancy Class
Beta-blockers (eg, timolol)	Decrease aqueous production	Hypotension, bradycardia, asthma exacerbation	C
α_2-adrenergic agonist (eg, brimonidine, Propine)	Decrease aqueous production	Allergy, tachyphylaxis, CNS depression	B
Cholinergics (eg, pilocarpine)	Increase outflow	Brow ache, cataract formation, retinal detachment	C
Carbonic anhydrase inhibitors (eg, acetazolamide, dorzolamide)	Decrease aqueous production	Sulfa allergy, systemic metabolic acidosis, tingling, aplastic anemia, metallic taste	C
Prostaglandin analogues (eg, latanoprost)	Increase outflow	Bitter taste, iris color change, red eye	C

Argon laser trabeculoplasty can be helpful in decreasing the intraocular pressure in some patients. In those with persistent pressure elevation, surgery is indicated. The most common filtering procedure is trabeculectomy. The success of this procedure has been improved by the use of intraoperative application of mitomycin or 5-fluorouracil to inhibit the fibrosis and closure of the filtering channels. In certain types of glaucoma such as neovascular glaucoma or aphakic glaucoma with failed filtering procedures, valves can be used.

OCULAR MIGRAINE

Migraine is a disorder with multiple clinical presentations. Recurrent headaches are classic and ocular symptoms are often associated. The pathophysiology of migraine is unknown. There may be a genetic component. The differential diagnosis of migraine headache include stress-tension headache, cluster headache, sinus congestion/pathology, elevated intracranial pressures, orbital inflammation, orbital neoplasia, and rarely, temporal arteritis. A thorough headache history and neurologic examination helps to diagnosis migraine.

In ocular migraine, ocular symptoms predominate. Headache and nausea, if present, follow the episode. Ocular symptoms can mimic retinal disease and a dilated ocular examination is needed to rule out retinal pathology. Prophylaxis of ocular symptoms with beta-adrenergic blockers, calcium-channel blockers, and tricyclic antidepressants may be used.

Classical Migraines

Classical migraines are headaches preceded by visual auras lasting about 20 minutes. The aura may consist of bright or dark spots, zigzag lines (fortification scotoma), heat haze distortions, scintillating scotomata, and tunnel vision. Homonymous or altitudinal hemianopias may rarely occur. The headaches that follow may be trivial or very severe. Ocular symptoms without subsequent headache also occur **(acephalgic migraine)**.

Retinal Migraine

Retinal migraine is characterized by acute but transient unilateral loss of vision that can be identical to that seen in amaurosis fugax. Vascular etiologies must be ruled out with thorough ocular and medical examination.

Ophthalmoplegic Migraine

Ophthalmoplegic migraine is very rare and typically starts before the age of 10 years. It is characterized by a recurrent transient 3rd nerve palsy that begins after the headache.

Complicated Migraine

Complicated migraine is associated with neurologic deficits such as tingling in the extremities, hemisensory disturbance, or partial visual loss, and rarely, the deficit persists after the headache has resolved. Antiplatelet therapy with aspirin is often recommended.

DIABETIC RETINOPATHY

Diabetes is the number one cause of new blindness in most industrialized countries. Diabetic retinopathy develops in almost half of all diabetics and is a major cause of blindness. There are two clinical classifications: **(1) nonproliferative or background diabetic retinopathy** and **(2) proliferative diabetic retinopathy**. The prevalence of retinopathy increases with the duration of diabetes. Patients who have had type 1 for 5 years or less are at low risk of retinopathy. However, 27% of those with diabetes for 5–10 years and 71–90% of those with diabetes for longer than 10 years have diabetic retinopathy. After 20–30 years, the prevalence rises to 95%, with 30–50% of those patients having proliferative changes.

Diabetes may have other effects on the eye. Poor corneal healing and decreased corneal sensation have been noted. Neovascular glaucoma may occur in patients with proliferative disease. Patients with diabetes also have a higher incidence of concurrent primary open-angle glaucoma. Optic neuropathy and cranial neuropathies may occur.

Clinical Findings

Microaneurysms, intraretinal hemorrhages, cotton wool spots, and lipid deposits due to vascular leakage are retinal changes seen in early diabetic retinopathy. Later stages include retinal ischemia and neovascularization with subsequent vitreous hemorrhage. Rhegmatogenous and tractional retinal detachments are late complications from proliferative disease. Diabetic retinopathy may be asymptomatic until vision decreases, usually from macular edema or vitreous hemorrhage. Renal disease (microalbuminuria, elevated blood urea and creatinine levels) is an excellent predictor of the presence of retinopathy.

Treatment

Careful control of blood sugar and blood pressure appears to reduce the incidence of diabetic retinopathy. Recent epidemiologic studies show that many diabetics fail to have the recommended yearly eye examinations. However, if patients are followed up closely and retinopathy is treated according to the guidelines of the Early Treatment Diabetic Retinopathy Study (ETDRS), the risk of severe visual loss is less than 5%. Treatment consists of photocoagulation, either of the macula to reduce edema or the retinal periphery to reduce ischemic neovascular changes (see "Laser Treatments for Ocular Disease").

AGE-RELATED MACULAR DEGENERATION (AMD)

Age-related macular degeneration (AMD) is the leading cause of central visual loss among individuals aged 65 and above. The cause of AMD is unknown, although it appears to have a genetic component. Regardless of the mechanism, the disease appears to affect the retinal pigment epithelium (RPE) at the level of Bruch's membrane. Drusen are caused by the thickening, hyalinization, and calcification of the RPE and are characteristic of AMD.

1. Atrophic ("Dry") Macular Degeneration

Atrophic ("dry") macular degeneration is the most common form, occurring in approximately 80% of those with AMD. Drusen, pigment changes, and atrophy are present, but there is no leakage of fluid. Usually only minimal to moderate visual loss is present.

2. Exudative ("Wet") Macular Degeneration

Exudative ("wet") macular degeneration is when choroidal neovascular membranes develop and serous detachments of the (RPE) occur. Vision loss can be devastating.

Clinical Findings

Visual loss is caused by geographical atrophy, serous detachment of the RPE, or choroidal neovascularization. Although central vision is heavily affected, peripheral vision usually remains intact. Metamorphopsia, or distortion of the central vision, is classic.

Treatment

The Age-Related Eye Disease Study (AREDS) is the first large, prospective clinical trial to show the benefit of antioxidant and zinc supplementation on the progression of AMD and associated visual loss. In evaluating the rate of progression to advanced visual loss, nutritional supplements statistically significantly benefited patients who had moderate to severe disease. Supplements were not found to prevent the development of AMD or to prevent progression in patients with mild disease.

Treatment of exudative AMD is more difficult. Standard laser photocoagulation can be useful in treating certain neovascular complexes. Photodynamic therapy (PDT) is a method of more selective laser therapy using verteporferin to enhance treatment success.

Smoking cessation is extremely important. Exercise and control of other systemic diseases such as hypertension and hypercholesterolemia may also help.

RETINAL DETACHMENT

Detachment of the retina is usually spontaneous but may be secondary to trauma. Spontaneous detachment occurs most frequently in persons over 50 years of age, and often after vitreous detachments.

Clinical Findings

Retinal tears or holes are the most important predisposing factors. Increased risk of retinal detachment is also associated with cataract surgery and high myopia. In the presence of a retinal tear or hole, fluid from the vitreous cavity enters the defect and transudation from choroidal vessels and detaches the retina from the pigment epithelium. The superior temporal area is the most common site of detachment. The area of detachment rapidly increases, causing progressive visual loss. Central vision remains intact until the macula becomes detached. On ophthalmoscopic examination, the retina is seen as an elevated gray membrane. One or more retinal tears may be seen.

Treatment

All cases of retinal detachment should be referred immediately to an ophthalmologist. If the patient must be transported a long distance, the head should be positioned so that the detached portion of the retina will recede with the aid of gravity.

Retinal detachment is a true emergency if the macula is threatened. If the macula is detached, permanent loss of central vision may occur even though the retina is eventually successfully reattached by surgery. Treatment consists of closure of retinal tears by cryosurgery, laser, or scleral buckling. This produces an inflammatory reaction that causes the retina to adhere to the choroid. The laser can create an inflammatory adhesion between the choroid and the retina. Its main use is in the prevention of detachment by sealing small retinal tears before detachment occurs.

In uncomplicated retinal detachment with a superior retinal tear and healthy vitreous, pneumoretinopexy may be performed. The procedure consists of injection of air or certain gases into the vitreous cavity through the pars plana, and positioning the patient to augment sealing of the retinal hole and permit spontaneous reabsorption of the subretinal fluid.

About 85% of uncomplicated cases can be cured with one operation; an additional 10% will need repeated operations; and the remainder never reattach. The prognosis is worse if the macula is detached, if there are many vitreous strands, or if the detachment is of long duration.

Without treatment, retinal detachment almost always becomes total in 1–6 months. Spontaneous detachments are ultimately bilateral in 20–25% of cases.

STRABISMUS

Any child under age 7 (especially infants and young children) with strabismus should be seen without delay to prevent amblyopia and to treat it at an early stage. In adults, the sudden onset of strabismus usually follows head trauma, microvascular infarct, intracranial hemorrhage, or brain tumor. About 3% of children are born with or develop strabismus. In descending order of frequency, the eyes may deviate inward (esotropia), outward (exotropia), upward (hypertropia), or downward (hypotropia).

Clinical Findings

Children with frank strabismus first develop diplopia. They soon learn to suppress the image from the deviating eye, and the vision in that eye therefore fails to develop. This is the first stage of amblyopia. Most cases of strabismus are obvious, but if the angle of deviation is small or if the strabismus is intermittent, the diagnosis may be missed.

Amblyopia due to strabismus can be detected by routine visual acuity examination of all preschool children. Visual acuity testing with an illiterate E card can be used by those who cannot be tested with a standard eye chart.

Treatment

The objectives in treatment of strabismus (Figure 39–2) are to achieve good visual acuity in each eye; straight eyes, for cosmetic purposes; and coordinate function of both eyes (fusion). The best time to initiate treatment is at about age 6 months. If treatment is delayed beyond this time, the child will favor the straight eye and suppress the image in the other eye. This results in failure of visual development (amblyopia) in the deviating eye.

If the child is under age 6 years and has an amblyopic eye, vision may be improved by occluding the good eye. At age 1 year, patching may be successful within 1 week; at 6 years, it may take a year to achieve the same result, ie, to equalize the visual acuity in both eyes. Surgery to align the eye is usually performed after the visual acuity has been equalized. The prevention of blindness by these simple diagnostic and treatment procedures is one of the most rewarding experiences in medical practice.

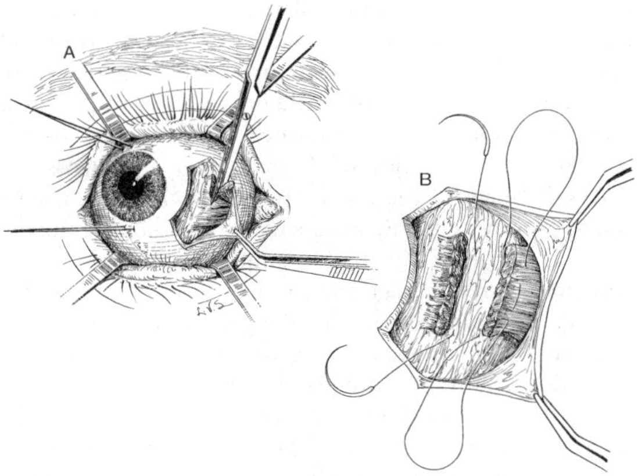

Figure 39–2. ***A:*** Exposure of an extraocular muscle in surgery for strabismus. ***B:*** Recession of the muscle behind its original insertion followed by suturing to the sclera with absorbable suture.

Surgery for correction of strabismus consists of weakening or strengthening the extraocular muscles. For correction of exotropia, the lateral rectus muscles in each eye are weakened by recession. The muscle is detached at its insertion and then resutured posteriorly to the sclera at a distance not to exceed 8 mm from the original insertion. Alternatively, a lateral rectus muscle may be recessed and the medial rectus muscle in the same eye cut at its insertion and a part of the muscle not to exceed 6 mm resected. The muscle is then resutured to its original insertion. The amount of recession and resection and the number of extraocular muscles resected or recessed is determined by the degree of ocular deviation. In patients with esotropia, both medial recti are recessed or a single medial rectus is recessed in combination with resection of the lateral rectus in the same eye. For vertical deviation, the vertical muscles are recessed, resected, tucked, or weakened by myectomy (usually the inferior oblique).

OCULAR BURNS

CHEMICAL BURNS

Apart from the history, the diagnosis of chemical eye burns is usually based on the presence of swelling of the eyelids and marked conjunctival hyperemia and chemosis. The limbus may show blanched patchy areas and conjunctival sloughing, especially in the interpalpebral area. There is usually corneal stromal haze and diffuse edema, with wide areas of epithelial cell loss and corneal ulcerations. Defects in the cornea can be better visualized with the instillation of fluorescein.

Alkali burns of the eye are serious because the agents tend to rapidly penetrate intraocularly and damage the tissue. Retained particles in the conjunctival fornices may cause progressive damage and must be promptly removed. Patients are managed by instilling a topical anesthetic agent and then promptly irrigating copiously with isotonic saline solution. Double eversion of the upper eyelid should be performed to look for and remove material lodged in the superior fornix. This can be easily done by using a forceps or moist cotton applicator. A lid speculum is placed after the instillation of tetracaine 0.5% eye drops, and the eye is irrigated with saline. Topical dilating drops such as atropine 1% or homatropine 5% are instilled and a topical antibiotic ointment such as ophthalmic erythromycin and bacitracin should be applied.

Acid burns cause rapid damage but are in general less serious than alkali burns. Management consists of immediate irrigation with sterile isotonic saline solution, water, or whatever safe liquid is available. A topical anesthetic agent is instilled to minimize pain during irrigation. The patient is then given an analgesic and the eye is patched. Topical antibiotic ointment may also be used.

THERMAL BURNS

The treatment of thermal burns of the eyes is similar to the treatment of burns elsewhere on the body. Systemic analgesia should be provided. A topical anesthetic agent such as proparacaine 0.5% or tetracaine 0.5% is used to minimize pain during manipulation. In cases of burns involving the cornea, topical dilating drops such as atropine 1% or homatropine 5% are instilled. Antibiotic drops are often prescribed for 3–5 days.

BURNS DUE TO ULTRAVIOLET RADIATION

Injuries to the corneal epithelium by ultraviolet rays may be mild or severe. This is referred to as actinic keratitis, snow blindness, welder's arc burn, or flash burn, depending on the source of ultraviolet radiation. Patients present with severe pain and photophobia. The examination reveals diffuse punctate staining of the cornea, best seen with fluorescein staining, proper magnification, and a cobalt blue light.

A topical antibiotic such as ophthalmic erythromycin or bacitracin ointment is instilled. Topical nonsteroidal drops such as diclofenac or ketorolac tromethamine may be used for pain.

OCULAR TRAUMA

Ocular trauma may be classified as penetrating or nonpenetrating. Trauma can lead to permanent reduction or loss of vision. Eye injuries are common in spite of the protection afforded by the bony orbit. The use of safety goggles at work helps prevent most serious occupational injuries to the eye.

Clinical Evaluation

A careful history of the injury should be obtained from the patient or someone who knows what happened. Visual acuity should be measured with and without glasses. The eyelids, conjunctiva, cornea, anterior chamber, iris, lens, vitreous, and fundus should be inspected for lacerations, breaks, or hemorrhage. Detection of corneal damage (such as abrasions) can be performed by instilling fluorescein dye and examining the eye using a cobalt blue light under magnification. X-ray examination is helpful in looking for fractures of the orbital bones and trying to rule out radiopaque foreign bodies. CT scan is performed when available. Patients with severe injuries should have immediate ophthalmic consultation. Further damage can be caused by manipulation, which for that reason should be avoided.

PENETRATING OR PERFORATING INJURIES

Penetrating or perforating ocular injuries require immediate careful attention and prompt surgical repair to prevent functional loss.

Many facial injuries—especially those occurring in automobile accidents—are associated with penetrating ocular trauma. Some injuries may be undetected because of eyelid swelling or because the patient's other injuries have demanded the attention of the emergency room staff. Such injuries, if not promptly attended to or adequately managed by an ophthalmologist, may lead to loss of vision. Accurate records and a description of how the injury occurred should be obtained. The eye and ocular adnexa should be examined, including vision testing and testing of ocular motility. *Do not apply pressure on the globe.* X-ray examination and CT scan are performed to rule out fractures of orbital bones or the presence of intraocular foreign bodies.

Careful repair and approximation of corneal and scleral lacerations should be performed in the operating room. Metallic intraocular foreign bodies can often be removed with a magnet at the time of suturing of the corneal or scleral lacerations. The major objectives in management of ocular penetrating or perforating injuries are to relieve pain, preserve or restore vision, and achieve good cosmetic results. Pain relief may be achieved by the administration of morphine, 2–4 mg intravenously or subcutaneously, or meperidine, 50–75 mg intramuscularly as needed. Sedatives such as diazepam, 5 mg, may be given orally as required.

The injured eye should be covered gently with sterile gauze or an eye pad and a protective Fox shield, but no pressure should be applied. Parenteral broad-spectrum antibiotics such as cefazolin or gentamicin should be given. Antiemetics—ondansetron, 4 mg intravenously—should be given to patients who are vomiting to prevent further injury.

LACERATIONS OF THE OCULAR ADNEXA

Lacerations of the eyelids and the periorbital skin should be carefully evaluated and inspected. Superficial laceration of the skin can be sutured by approximation. In cases of deep eyelid lacerations, intraocular or orbital damage should be ruled out. The skin of the eyelids has good elasticity, is loosely attached to underlying tissue, and in adults is frequently present in surplus quantities. This facilitates the development of flaps and grafts. Small linear skin lacerations may be easily sutured and the wound secured with interrupted 6-0 nylon suture. Because of the good blood supply, the sutures may be removed in 3–5 days. In deep lacerations of the eyelids, if the wound divides the orbicularis muscle parallel to its fibers, only skin sutures are generally required. When the muscle fibers are transversely divided they should be approximated with absorbable sutures using 6-0 Vicryl or Dexon sutures. The skin can be approximated with fine silk or nylon sutures. In patients with lacerations resulting in round or oval losses of skin, the skin is undermined and the laceration approximated. In larger defects, reconstruction with flaps may be required. Flaps used in reconstruction of the eyelids are advancement flaps, rotational flaps, transposition flaps, island flaps, and Z-plasty flaps.

In large defects, when flaps cannot be used, free skin grafts may be obtained from behind the ear or from the skin of the inner upper arm.

The main problem that complicates suturing of the lower eyelid is retraction or eversion from vertical tension, which for that reason should be avoided.

BLUNT TRAUMA TO THE OCULAR ADNEXA & ORBIT

See Table 39–4.

Contusions of the eyeball and ocular adnexa may result from blunt trauma. The outcome of such an injury cannot always be determined, and the extent of damage may not be obvious upon superficial examination. Careful eye examination is needed, along with x-ray or CT scan.

BLOWOUT FRACTURE OF THE FLOOR OF THE ORBIT

Blowout fracture of the floor of the orbit can be associated with enophthalmos, double vision in primary position or in upper gaze, limitation of ocular movement in upper gaze, hypotropia, and decreased or absent sensation over the maxillary area. CT scan of the orbit shows orbital floor displacement.

The management of patients with blowout fractures of the orbital floor should be carefully assessed by both an ophthalmologist and an otolaryngologist because of potential associated fractures of the maxilla or zygoma. The patients is usually treated with a systemic antibiotic (cephalothin or amoxicillin/potassium clavulanate), told not to blow his nose, and reassessed within 1 week by an ophthalmologist. Operative management is recommended if there is significant enophthalmos, continued diplopia in primary gaze, or significant instability of the orbital floor.

CORNEAL & CONJUNCTIVAL FOREIGN BODIES

Patients may give a history of working with high-speed tempered steel tools, or drilling, or hammering against a hard object. There may be no history of trauma to the eye, and the patient may not be aware of a foreign body. In most cases, however, the patient complains of foreign body sensation in the eye or under the eyelid, pain, tearing, and photophobia.

Table 39–4. Types of ocular injury associated with blunt trauma.

Eyelids	Ecchymosis, swelling, laceration, abrasions, conjunctival or subconjunctival hemorrhages.
Cornea	Edema, lacerations.
Anterior chamber	Hyphema, recession of angle, secondary glaucoma.
Iris	Iridodialysis, iridoplegia, rupture of iris sphincter.
Ciliary body	Hyposecretion of aqueous humor.
Lens	Cataract, dislocation.
Vitreous	Vitreous hemorrhage.
Ciliary muscle	Paralysis.
Retina	Commotio retinae, retinal edema, choroidal breaks in Bruch's membrane, choroidal hemorrhage.

A corneal foreign body can be seen with the aid of a loupe and diffuse light. Conjunctival foreign bodies often become embedded in the conjunctiva under the upper eyelid; the lid must be everted to facilitate inspection and removal. Sterile fluorescein should be instilled to visualize small foreign bodies not readily visible with the naked eye or loupe. A topical anesthetic such as proparacaine 0.5% or tetracaine 0.5% is applied. Some loose foreign bodies can be removed with a moist cotton applicator, while superficial foreign bodies can be removed with the tip of a hypodermic needle. Topical prophylactic antibiotic ointment should be instilled, eg, erythromycin or bacitracin. The eyes should be covered overnight. ***Note:*** If there is any suspicion of penetrating trauma, appropriate ultrasound and radiologic tests should be performed.

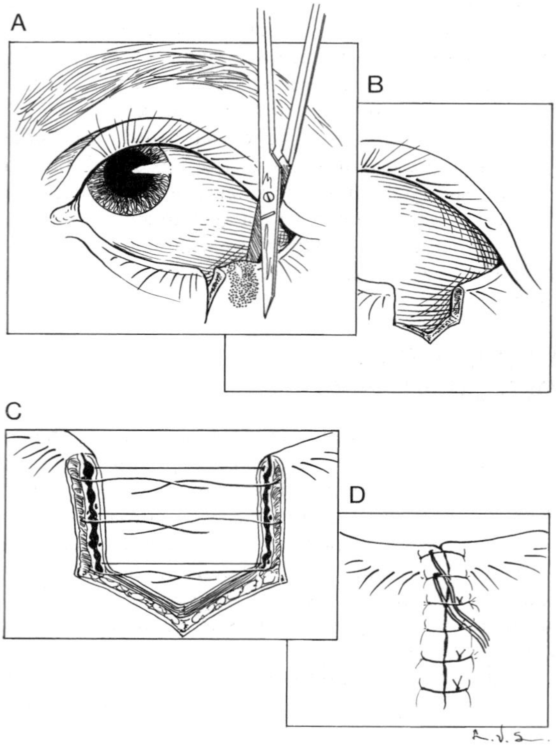

Figure 39–3. Tumor of the left lower eyelid involving the lid margin. ***A:*** Two vertical incisions are made. ***B:*** The defect after removal of the tumor. ***C:*** Suturing of the tarsus and orbicularis with absorbable sutures. ***D:*** Approximation of the eyelid margin. Skin is approximated with 6-0 silk sutures.

OCULAR TUMORS

Tumors of the eye and its related adnexal structures can be recognized and diagnosed early because they are visible and cause local disfigurement, changes in color, interference with vision, or displacement of the globe. In children, ocular tumors such as retinoblastoma affecting visual function may lead to strabismus or leukocoria. Tumors of the eye may be primary, affecting only the ocular or adnexal tissues; or secondary to metastasis of tumors from other organs. In the eye, the most frequent site of metastasis is the choroid, and the tumors that most frequently metastasize to the eye are carcinoma of the breast and carcinoma of the lung.

The history of growth of the lesion is extremely important, as well as recent changes in its size or appearance. Excisional biopsy of lesions of the skin or conjunctiva is indicated if cancer is suspected.

LID TUMORS

Benign Tumors of the Eyelids

The most frequent benign tumors of the eyelids are **melanocytic nevi**. Excision is indicated for cosmetic reasons (Figure 39–3). Xanthelasmas represent lipid deposits in histiocytes in the dermis of the skin of the eyelid. In such patients, serum lipid and serum cholesterol levels should be determined. Treatment is indicated for cosmetic reasons and consists of simple excision. Recurrences are common.

Hemangiomas of the eyelids are of two types: capillary and cavernous. **Capillary hemangiomas** consist of dilated capillaries and proliferation of endothelial cells. The lesions appear as bright red spots. They may show rapid growth in early childhood but later undergo involution and subside spontaneously. **Cavernous hemangiomas**, on the other hand, are venous channels in the subcutaneous tissue. They appear bluish in color and are distended. Treatment of hemangiomas in infancy and early childhood is not indicated unless the lesion causes interference with vision, which may lead to amblyopia. Low-dose oral steroids or local injection of steroids may cause rapid involution of capillary hemangiomas. Surgical excision may be required. Radiation is not recommended because it leads to excessive scarring of the eyelid.

Other benign tumors of the eyelids include verrucae and molluscum contagiosum. These lesions are caused by viruses.

Malignant Tumors of the Eyelids

Squamous cell carcinoma has a tendency to grow slowly and painlessly. It begins as a small lesion covered by a layer of keratin. The lesion may erode, causing an ulcer with hyperemic edges. It may enlarge to form a fungating mass and may invade the orbital cavity. Early excision may result in cure. If early treatment is not provided, squamous cell carcinoma may spread via the lymphatic system to the preauricular and submandibular lymph nodes.

Basal cell carcinoma begins as a slowly growing, locally invasive tumor forming the so-called rodent ulcer with raised nodular borders. Inner canthal basal cell carcinoma may invade locally and extend into the orbit. Treatment should include complete excision to prevent recurrence.

Malignant melanomas of the eyelids are similar to malignant melanomas of the skin elsewhere on the body.

CONJUNCTIVAL TUMORS

Benign tumors of the conjunctiva include melanocytic nevi (pigmented or nonpigmented), papillomas, granulomas, dermoid tumors, and lymphoid hyperplasia. Malignant tumors of the conjunctiva include carcinoma, malignant melanoma, and, rarely, lymphoma. Carcinoma of the conjunctiva arises frequently at the limbus or the inner canthus in the exposed area of the bulbar conjunctiva. Early in the course of the disease, the lesion may resemble a pterygium. The tumor is slightly elevated, with a gelatinous surface, and may spread over the corneal surface. The growth of this lesion is slow. Treatment is by excisional biopsy.

INTRAOCULAR TUMORS

Benign Intraocular Tumors

Melanocytic nevi of the iris, ciliary body, or choroid are common. No treatment is required for these lesions. Retinal angioma may be seen in patients with phacomatoses (eg, Bourneville's disease). Choroidal hemangioma is another less frequently encountered benign intraocular tumor.

Malignant Intraocular Tumors

Malignant intraocular tumors include malignant melanoma of the uvea, retinoblastoma, and a rare tumor of the ciliary body known as diktyoma or medulloepithelioma.

Malignant melanoma of the uvea is most common primary intraocular tumor in adults. It typically occurs in the fifth or sixth decade and is almost always unilateral. The most frequent site is the choroid, but malignant melanoma may occur also in the ciliary body or iris. Malignant melanomas of the choroid may cause a decrease in vision and may undergo necrosis, leading to intraocular inflammation. Histopathologic examination shows spindle-shaped cells with or without prominent nuclei and large epithelioid tumor cells. Intraocular malignant melanomas may spread directly through the sclera by local invasion or directly into the central nervous system via optic nerve extension.

Malignant melanomas can be detected by ophthalmoscopy after pupillary dilation.

Treatment of malignant melanoma consists of enucleation or radiotherapy, using radioactive plaques or charged particles. Extension outside the eye may require exenteration of the orbit. Patients with small melanomas—less than 10 mm in diameter—can be observed by serial photography of the fundus. Similarly, small melanomas of the iris that have not invaded the iris root can be safely followed and observed until growth is documented. If there is growth of the iris tumor, treatment is by local iridectomy. If the iris malignant melanoma invades the root and ciliary body, it can be removed surgically by iridocyclectomy.

Retinoblastoma is a rare but life-threatening condition in childhood. It is the most frequent intraocular malignant tumor in children arising from embryonic cone cells of the photoreceptor layer. Most patients with retinoblastoma present in the first or second year of life. Patients may present with leukocoria or strabismus. Retinoblastoma may be multifocal, and both sporadic and inherited forms occur. It may grow slowly to fill the intraocular space and undergo necrosis, leading to calcific deposits. Tumor cells may seed on the iris and in the anterior chamber, causing fluffy whitish exudates.

Spontaneous remission of retinoblastoma has been reported. Treatment options include radiotherapy, cryotherapy, chemotherapy, and enucleation.

ORBITAL TUMORS

Orbital tumors may be of two types: those arising from orbital tissues (primary orbital tumors) and those invading the orbit from adjacent structures (secondary orbital tumors). Primary orbital tumors include benign tumors such as dermoid cysts, hemangiomas, lipomas, fibromas, osteomas, chondromas, neurofibromas, and lacrimal gland tumors. Malignant tumors of the orbit include rhabdomyosarcoma, adenocarcinoma of the lacrimal gland, and lymphomas. Invading tumors include malignant melanoma and retinoblastoma from the intraocular structures and malignant melanomas and carcinomas from the skin of the eyelids and conjunctiva. Metastatic lesions may reach the orbit from the lung or breast. Neuroblastoma may also metastasize to the orbit in children. Meningiomas of the cranial nerves may invade the orbit through the optic canal.

Treatment and prognosis in all cases depend on the type of tumor.

LASER TREATMENTS FOR OCULAR DISEASE

The laser has many useful applications in ophthalmology. Using various gases, a single-wavelength beam can be produced that can be absorbed by selective tissues in the eye.

FOCAL DIABETIC TREATMENT

Macular edema occurs in the preproliferative stage of diabetic retinopathy and is characterized by retinal thickening with or without exudates within the central macular area. This procedure is performed with a slit-lamp delivery system with a contact lens and is aided by fluorescein angiography. Improvement may take up to 3 months to occur. Long-term studies by the National Institutes of Health have shown that treatment with an argon laser may improve visual outcome by up to 50%.

PANRETINAL PHOTOCOAGULATION

Panretinal photocoagulation is indicated for treatment of proliferative diabetic retinopathy. Using a contact lens and a slitlamp delivery system, extensive destruction of peripheral retina is undertaken to decrease production of vasoproliferative factors and increase retinal oxygenation, thus causing regression of abnormal blood vessels that lead to hemorrhage, scarring, and retinal detachment.

LASIK SURGERY FOR CORRECTION OF REFRACTIVE ERROR

Laser in-situ keratomileusis (LASIK) is a lamellar refractive surgical procedure, which involves creation of a partial-thickness corneal flap under high suction. The flap is then lifted and an ArF (argon-fluoride) excimer beam is used to ablate stromal tissue with minimal damaging thermal effect. The flap is then replaced and allowed to heal. The combination of accuracy, precision, minimal postoperative discomfort, and quick visual recovery has made this the most popular refractive technique.

PHOTODYNAMIC THERAPY

Photodynamic therapy is a laser procedure that allows selective treatment for wet exudative age-related macular degeneration in patients who have subfoveal choroidal neovascularization. The choroidal lesion must be predominantly "classic" in nature, which means more than half of it must be evident on fluorescein angiography. The procedure involves intravenous infusion of a photosensitizer, verteporfin, which collects only in abnormal tissue and is then photoactivated by a nonthermal laser light applied through a slitlamp delivery system. The theory is that photoactivation leads to cellular damage and subsequent vessel occlusion and regression of abnormal blood vessels without damage to surrounding normal tissue.

Rhee DJ, Pyfer M: *Wills Eye Manual,* 3rd ed. Lippincott Williams & Wilkins, 1999.

Yanoff M, Duker JS: *Ophthalmology,* 2nd ed. Mosby, 2004.

Urology 40

Christopher S. Cooper, MD, & Richard D. Williams, MD

EMBRYOLOGY OF THE GENITOURINARY TRACT

A basic understanding of genitourinary embryology facilitates the learning of many aspects of urology. Embryologically, the genital and urinary systems are intimately related. Associated anomalies of the two systems are commonly encountered.

The Kidneys

The kidneys pass through three embryonic phases (Figure 40–1): (1) The **pronephros** is a vestigial structure without function in human embryos that, except for its primary duct, disappears completely by the fourth week. (2) The pronephric duct gains connection to the **mesonephric tubules** and becomes the mesonephric duct. While most of the mesonephric tubules degenerate, the mesonephric duct persists bilaterally; from where it bends to open into the cloaca, the ureteral bud grows cranially to interact with the metanephric blastema. (3) This forms the **metanephros**, which is the final phase. The metanephros develops into the kidney. During cephalad migration and rotation, the metanephric tissue progressively enlarges, with rapid internal differentiation into the nephron and the uriniferous tubules. Simultaneously, the cephalad end of the ureteral bud expands and divides within the metanephros to form the renal pelvis, calices, and collecting tubules.

The Bladder & Urethra

Subdivision of the cloaca (the blind end of the hindgut) into a ventral (urogenital sinus) and a dorsal (rectum) segment is completed during the seventh week and initiates early differentiation of the urinary bladder and urethra. The urogenital sinus receives the mesonephric duct and absorbs its caudal end, so that by the end of the seventh week the ureteral bud and mesonephric duct have independent openings. The ureteral orifice migrates upward and laterally. The mesonephric duct orifice moves downward and medially, and the structure in between (the trigone) is formed by the absorbed mesodermal tissue, which maintains direct continuity between the two tubes (Figure 40–2).

The fused müllerian ducts also meet the urogenital sinus at Müller's tubercle. The urogenital sinus above Müller's tubercle differentiates to form the bladder and the part of the prostatic urethra proximal to the seminal colliculus in the male or the bladder and the entire urethra in the female (Figure 40–3). Below Müller's tubercle, the urogenital sinus differentiates into the distal part of the prostatic urethra and the membranous urethra in the male or the distal vagina and vaginal vestibule in the female. The rest of the male urethra is formed by fusion of the urethral folds on the ventral surface of the genital tubercle. In the female, the genital folds remain separate and form the labia minora.

The prostate develops at the end of the 11th week as several groups of outgrowths of urethral epithelium both above and below the entrance of the ejaculatory duct (distal vas deferens). The developing glandular element (seminal colliculus) incorporates the differentiating mesenchymal cells surrounding it to form the muscular stroma and capsule of the prostate. The seminal vesicles form as duplicate buds from the distal end of the mesonephric duct (vas deferens).

The Gonads

The potential to differentiate along male or female lines is present in every embryo initially. The development of one set of sex primordia and the gradual involution of the other are determined by the genetic sex of the embryo and differential secretion of numerous hormones. The *SRY* gene—or testis-determining factor—on the Y chromosome drives the gonad to differentiate into a testicle. Gonadal differentiation begins during the seventh week (Figure 40–3). If the gonad develops into a testis, the germinal epithelium progressively grows into radially arranged, cord-like seminiferous tubules. The production of müllerian inhibiting factor (MIF) by the testicle causes regression of the müllerian duct and acts in a local (paracrine) fashion so that only the ipsilateral müllerian duct is affected. The subsequent production of testosterone by the testicle leads to masculinization of the mesonephric (wolffian) duct

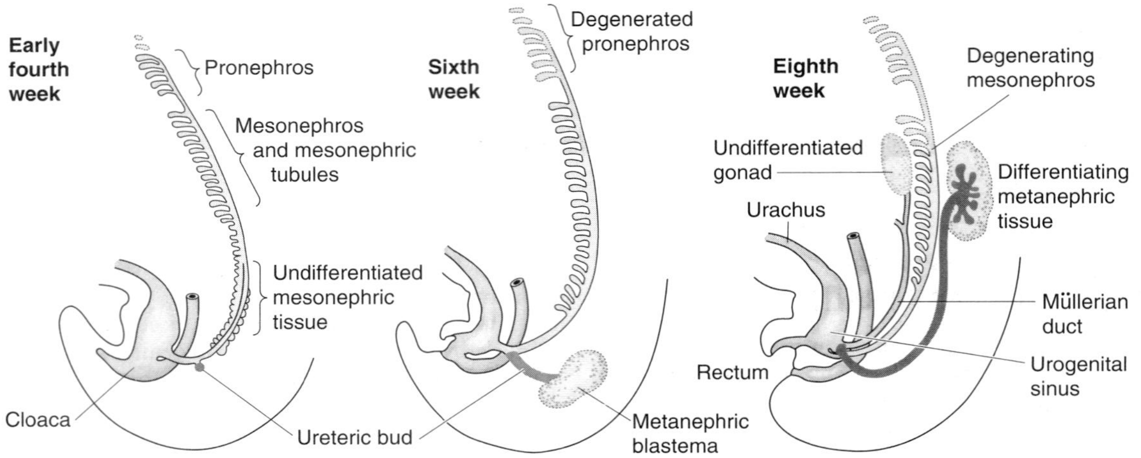

Figure 40–1. Schematic representation of the development of the nephric system. Only a few of the tubules of the pronephros are seen early in the fourth week, while the mesonephric tissue differentiates into mesonephric tubules that progressively join the mesonephric duct. The first sign of the ureteral bud from the mesonephric duct is seen. At 6 weeks, the pronephros has completely degenerated and the mesonephric tubules start to do so. The ureteral bud grows dorsocranially and has met the metanephric blastema. At the eighth week, there is cranial migration of the differentiating metanephros. The cranial end of the ureteral bud expands and starts to show multiple successive outgrowths (renal calices).

structures (ie, epididymides, vas deferens, seminal vesicles, and ejaculatory duct). If the gonad develops into an ovary, it becomes differentiated into a cortex and a medulla; the cortex later differentiates into ovarian follicles containing ova. The lack of testosterone leads to the disappearance of the mesonephric duct.

The testes remain in the abdomen until the seventh month and then pass through the inguinal canal to the scrotum, following the path of the gubernaculum. The mechanism of descent remains uncertain. Lack of complete testicular descent is known as cryptorchidism; descent to an abnormal site beyond the external inguinal ring is known as testicular ectopia.

The ovary, which is attached to ligaments, undergoes internal descent to enter the pelvis.

In the female, the genital duct system develops from the müllerian ducts, which fuse at their caudal ends and differentiate into the uterine tubes, the uterus, and the proximal two-thirds of the vagina.

The external genitalia start to differentiate by the eighth week. The genital tubercle and genital swellings develop into the penis and scrotum in the male and the clitoris and labia majora in the female. The external genitalia are masculinized by dihydrotestosterone (DHT), which is created from testosterone under the influence of 5α-reductase.

With the breakdown of the urogenital membrane in the seventh week, the urogenital sinus achieves a separate opening on the undersurface of the genital tubercle. The expansion of the infratubercular part of the urogenital sinus will form the vaginal vestibule and the distal third of the vagina. The two folds on the undersurface of the genital tubercle unite in the male to form the penile urethra; in the female, they remain separate to form the labia minora.

Patten RM et al: The fetal genitourinary tract. Radiol Clin North Am 1990;28:115.

ANATOMY OF THE GENITOURINARY TRACT: GROSS & MICROSCOPIC

The Kidneys

The kidneys lie retroperitoneally in the posterior abdomen and are separated from the surrounding renal fascia (Gerota's fascia) by perinephric fat. The renal vascular pedicle enters the renal sinus; the vein is anterior to the artery, and both are anterior to the renal pelvis. The renal artery divides just outside the renal sinus into anterior and posterior branches that undergo further subdivisions with variable extents of distribution. They are end arteries and thus result in segmental infarction when occluded. The venous tributaries anastomose freely and usually drain into one renal vein.

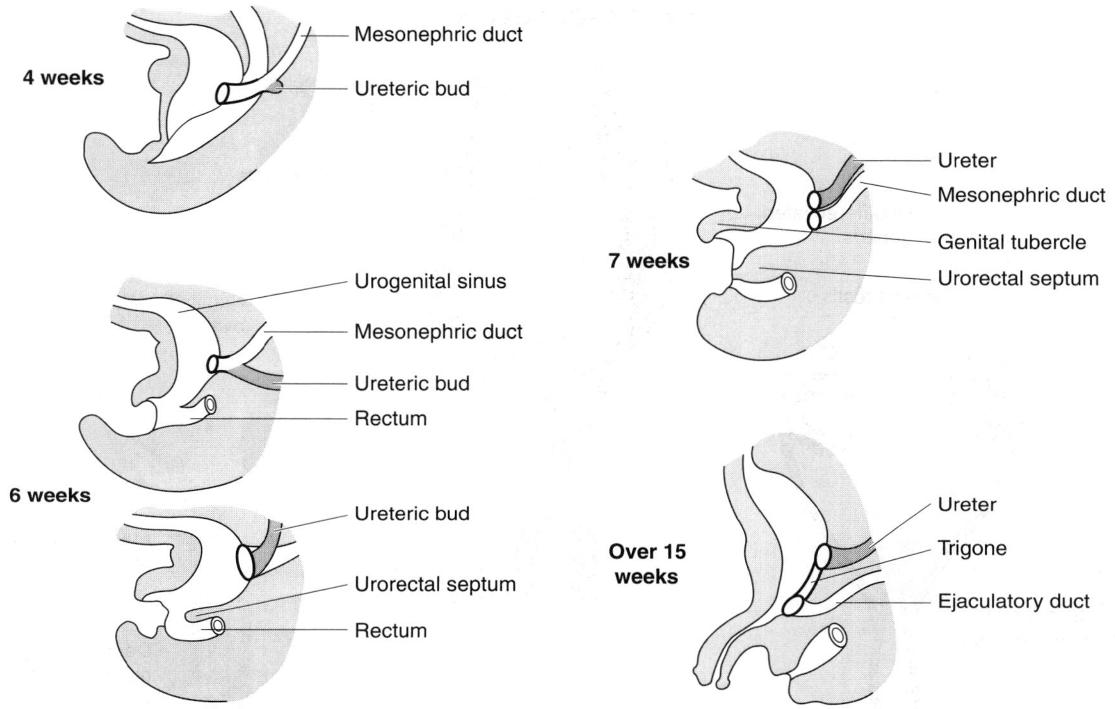

Figure 40–2. The development of the ureteral bud from the mesonephric duct and their relationship to the urogenital sinus. The ureteral bud appears at the fourth week. The mesonephric duct distal to this ureteral bud will be gradually absorbed into the urogenital sinus, resulting in separate endings for the ureter and the mesonephric duct. The mesonephric tissue that is incorporated into the urogenital sinus will expand and form the trigonal tissue. The mesonephric duct will form the vas deferens in the male and Gartner's duct (if present) in the female.

The Renal Parenchyma

The renal parenchyma consists of more than 1 million functioning units (nephrons) and is divided into a peripheral cortex containing secretory elements and a central medulla containing excretory elements. The nephron starts as Bowman's capsule, which surrounds the glomerulus and leads to elongated proximal and distal convoluted tubules with the loop of Henle in between, ending in a collecting duct that opens into a minor calix at the tip of a papilla.

The Renal Pelvis & Calices

The renal pelvis and calices are within the renal sinus and function as the main collecting reservoir. The pelvis, which is partly extrarenal and partly intrarenal (but occasionally is totally extra- or intrarenal), branches into three major calices that in turn branch into several minor calices. These calices are directly related to the tips of the medullary pyramids (the papillae) and act as a receiving cup to the collecting tubules. The pelvicaliceal system is a highly muscular structure; the fibers run in many directions and are directly continuous from the calices to the pelvis, allowing synchronization of contractile activity.

The Ureter

The ureter connects the renal pelvis to the urinary bladder. It is a muscularized tube; its muscle fibers lie in an irregular helical arrangement and function primarily in peristaltic activity. Ureteral muscle fibers are directly continuous from the renal pelvis cranially to the vesical trigone distally.

The blood supply to the renal pelvis and ureters is segmental, arising from multiple sources, including the renal, gonadal, and vesical arteries—with rich subadventitial anastomoses.

The Bladder

The bladder is primarily a reservoir with a meshwork of muscle bundles that not only change from one plane to

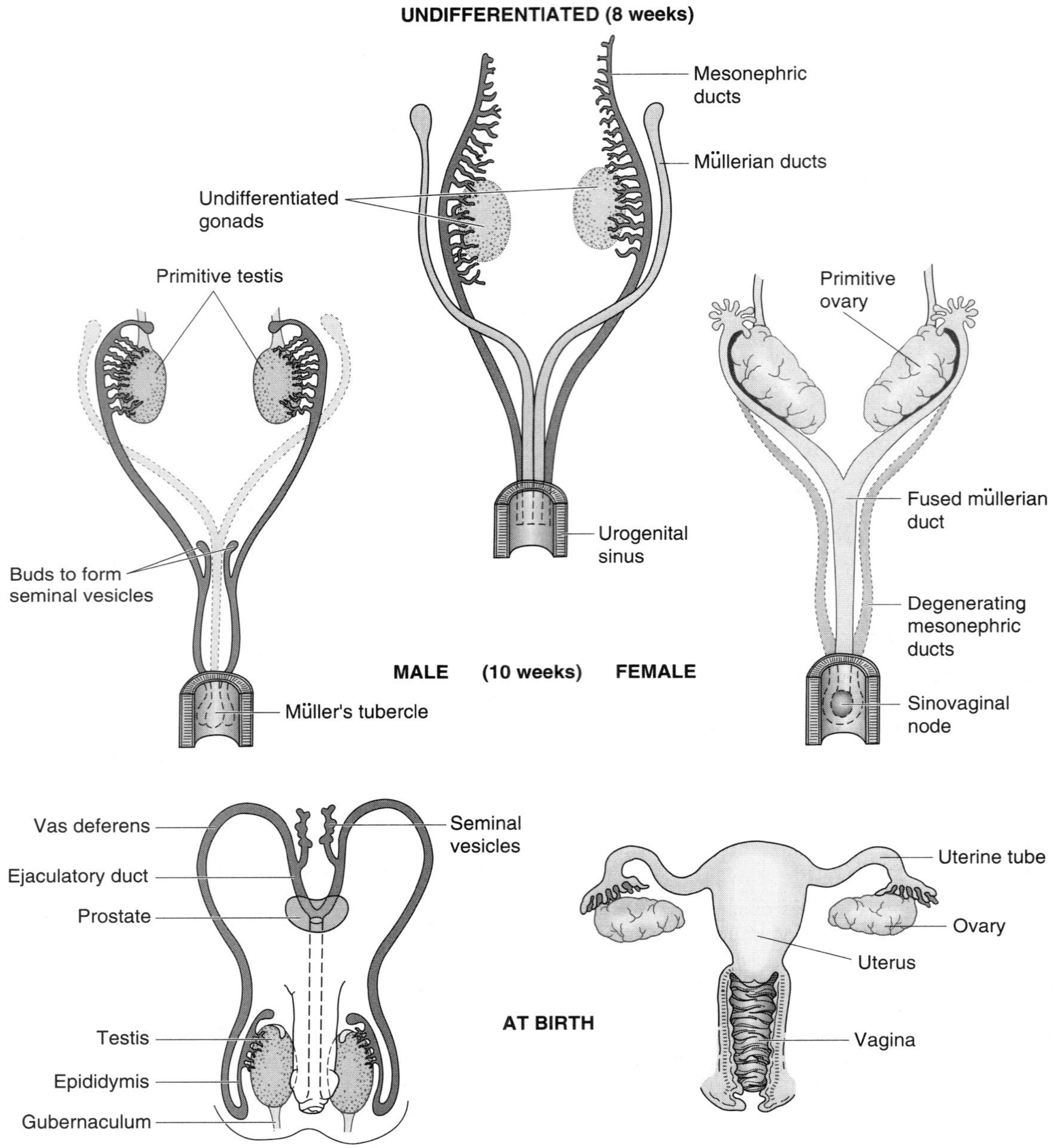

Figure 40–3. Transformation of the undifferentiated genital system into the definitive male and female systems.

another but also branch and join each other to constitute a synchronized organ. Its musculature is directly continuous with the urethral musculature and thus functions as an internal urethral sphincteric mechanism in spite of the lack of a true circular sphincter.

The ureters enter the bladder posteroinferiorly through the ureteral hiatus; after a short intravesical submucosal course, they open into the bladder and become continuous with the trigone, which is superimposed on the bladder base though deeply connected to it.

The Urethra

The adult female urethra is about 4 cm long and is muscular in its proximal four-fifths. This musculature is arranged in an inner longitudinal coat that is continuous with the inner longitudinal fibers of the bladder and an outer circular coat that is continuous with the outer longitudinal coat of the bladder. These outer circular fibers comprise the sphincteric mechanism. The striated external sphincter surrounds the middle third of the urethra.

In the male, the prostatic urethra is heavily muscular and sphincteric. The membranous urethra is within the urogenital diaphragm and is surrounded by the striated external sphincter. The penile urethra is poorly muscularized and traverses the corpus spongiosum to open at the tip of the glans.

The Prostate

The prostate surrounds the proximal portion of the male urethra; it is a fibromuscular, cone-shaped gland about 2.5 cm long and normally weighing about 20 g in the adult. It is traversed from base to apex by the urethra and is pierced posterolaterally by the ejaculatory ducts from the seminal vesicles and vas deferens that converge to open at the verumontanum (seminal colliculus) on the floor of the urethra.

The prostatic glandular elements drain through about 12 paired excretory ducts that open into the floor of the urethra above the verumontanum. The prostate is surrounded by a thin capsule, derived from its stroma, which is rich in musculature, and part of the urethral musculature and the sphincteric mechanism. A rich venous plexus surrounds the prostate, especially anteriorly and laterally. Its lymphatic drainage is into the hypogastric, sacral, obturator, and external iliac lymph nodes.

The Testis, Epididymis, & Vas

The testis is a paired organ surrounded by the tunica albuginea and subdivided into numerous lobules by fibrous septa. The extremely convoluted seminiferous tubules gather to open into the rete testis, where they join the efferent duct and drain into the epididymis. The epididymis drains into the vas deferens, which courses through the inguinal canal into the pelvis and is joined by the duct from the seminal vesicle to form the ejaculatory duct, which opens before opening into the prostatic urethra on either side of the verumontanum.

Arterial supply is via the spermatic, vas deferential, and external cremasteric arteries. Venous drainage is through the pampiniform plexus, which drains into the internal spermatic veins; the right spermatic vein joins the vena cava and the left joins the renal vein.

Testicular lymphatics drain into the retroperitoneal lymph nodes; the right primarily into the interaortocaval area, the left into the para-aortic area, both just below the renal vessels.

de Groat WC: Anatomy and physiology of the lower urinary tract. Urol Clin North Am 1993;20:383.

Preuss HG: Basics of renal anatomy and physiology. Clin Lab Med 1993;13:1.

PHYSIOLOGY OF THE GENITOURINARY TRACT

The Kidneys

The kidneys maintain and regulate homeostasis of body fluids by the following mechanisms:

A. Glomerular Filtration

This is dependent on glomerular capillary arterial pressure minus plasma colloid osmotic pressure plus Bowman's capsular resistance. The resultant glomerular filtration pressure (about 8–12 mm Hg) forces protein-free plasma through the capillary filtering surface into Bowman's capsule. Normally, about 130 mL of plasma is filtered every minute through the renal circulation; the entire volume of plasma recirculates through the kidney and is subjected to the filtration process once every 27 minutes.

B. Tubular Reabsorption

About 99% of the filtered volume will be reabsorbed through the tubules, together with all the valuable constituents of the filtrate (chlorides, glucose, sodium, potassium, calcium, and amino acids). Urea, uric acid, phosphates, and sulfates are also reabsorbed to varying degrees. The process of reabsorption is a combination of active and passive transport mechanisms. Reabsorption of water and electrolytes is under the control of adrenal, pituitary, and parathyroid hormones.

C. Tubular Secretion

This helps (1) to eliminate certain substances and thus maintain their plasma levels and (2) to exchange valuable ions from the filtrate for less desirable ions in the plasma (eg, a sodium ion from the urine for a hydrogen ion in the plasma). Failure of adequate secretory function leads to the acidosis commonly encountered in chronic renal disease.

The Ureteropelvicaliceal System

This system is one continuous tubular structure with a syncytial type of smooth musculature that is imperceptibly in motion from one segment to the other. Waves of peristaltic contractions start from the calices and are propagated along the smooth muscle cells to the renal pelvis. At normal urine flow rates, many of these contraction waves are terminated at the ureteropelvic junction; however, some are transmitted to the ureter and down toward the urinary bladder. These peristaltic waves occur at a rate of about 5–8/min, involve a 2- to 3-cm segment at a time, and usually proceed at the velocity of 3 cm/s. Frequency, amplitude, and velocity are influenced by urine output and flow rate. In a state of diuresis, there may be a 1:1 relationship between caliceal contractions and ureteral contractions. Ureteral filling is primarily passive and occurs by reception of a bolus of urine from a renal pelvis contraction. The ureteropelvic junction closes after passing a bolus of urine, preventing back pressure and back flow of urine unto the renal pelvis secondary to the elevated ureteral contraction pressure. A contraction ring forms in the proximal ureter, and as it migrates down the ureter it pushes the bolus of urine antegrade. In states of diuresis, the size of the bolus increases and the pressure in the bolus may be greater than the pressure in the contraction ring ahead of it. In this case, the ureteral walls cannot coapt, and urine is transported as an uninterrupted column of fluid.

The Ureterovesical Junction

The ureterovesical junction allows flow of urine from the ureter to the bladder and at the same time prevents retrograde flow. The continuity and the specific muscular arrangement of the intravesical ureter and the trigone provide a muscularly active valvular mechanism that can efficiently adapt itself to the variable phases of bladder activity during filling and voiding.

The normal resting pressure of the ureterovesical junction (10–15 cm H_2O) is greater than the more cephalad ureteral resting pressure (0–5 cm H_2O). Progressive bladder filling leads to firm occlusion of the intravesical ureter against retrograde urine flow and to increased resistance to antegrade flow resulting from trigonal stretching. During voiding, trigonal contraction completely seals the intravesical ureter against any antegrade or retrograde flow of urine.

The Urinary Bladder

The urinary bladder functions primarily as a reservoir that can accommodate variable volumes without increasing its intraluminal pressure. When the bladder reaches full capacity, the detrusor muscle voluntarily contracts following relaxation of the external sphincter and maintains its contraction until the bladder is completely empty. Funneling of the bladder outlet with progressive downward movement of the dome ensures complete emptying.

The vesical sphincteric mechanism is primarily a smooth muscle sphincter in the bladder neck and male prostatic urethra and in the proximal four-fifths of the female urethra. There is no purely circular sphincteric entity, but there are abundant circularly oriented smooth muscle fibers that are directly continuous with the outer coat of the detrusor muscles. The sphincter has an abundance of alpha receptors that respond to sympathetic neural input from the pelvic nerve to maintain urethral closure. Parasympathetic input from the pelvic nerve facilitates bladder contracture and voiding.

There is a voluntary striated muscle sphincter that is part of the urogenital diaphragm and surrounds the mid urethra in the female and the membranous urethra in the male. It responds to somatic neural input from the pudendal nerve. It is essential for continence when the internal sphincter is nonfunctional. Its pathologic irritability or spasticity can lead to obstructive manifestations.

DEVELOPMENTAL ANOMALIES OF THE GENITOURINARY TRACT

Genitourinary tract anomalies constitute about one-third of all congenital abnormalities and occur in over 10% of the population. The severity varies from lesions incompatible with life to insignificant findings detected during diagnostic studies for unrelated reasons. The anatomic abnormalities are often not intrinsically harmful, yet they may predispose to infection, stone formation, or chronic renal failure.

RENAL ANOMALIES

Bilateral absence of the kidneys is rare and is associated with oligohydramnios, Potter facies, and pulmonary hypoplasia. It occurs more often in males and results in death shortly after birth. Unilateral renal agenesis is seen more often but is not usually associated with illness. **Renal agenesis** is thought to be due to both lack of a ureteral bud and lack of subsequent development of the metanephric blastema. The trigone is absent on the affected side. Because adrenal gland development is unrelated to kidney development, both adrenals are usually present in the normal position. Rarely, more than two kidneys are seen, a condition clearly dissimilar to ureteral duplication, as described later.

Abnormal ascent of the metanephros leads to an **ectopic kidney**, which may be unilateral or bilateral. Lumbar, pelvic, and the less common thoracic and crossed ectopic varieties are seen. Ectopic kidneys are associated with genital anomalies in 10–20% of cases. Fusion abnormalities are also associated with failure of normal ascent and include fused pelvic kidneys and

horseshoe kidneys (the most common), which are typically fused at the lower poles. Intravenous urography typically establishes the diagnosis. The relationship of the kidneys to the psoas muscles is abnormal: instead of an oblique orientation with the medial border of the kidney parallel to the psoas muscle, the kidneys are vertical and the medial border intersects and crosses the psoas muscle (Figure 40–4). Horseshoe kidneys have an elevated incidence of vesicoureteral reflux and are at increased risk of ureteropelvic junction obstruction. The latter may be related to a high ureteral insertion in the renal pelvis, crossing of the ureter over the isthmus, or compression by one of many anomalous arteries. Failure of rotation during ascent results in "malrotated" kidneys and is rarely significant.

Polycystic Kidneys

Parenchymal anomalies include a variety of cystic and dysplastic lesions. Polycystic kidney disease is hereditary and bilateral. The autosomal recessive polycystic kidney disease (ARPKD), previously called "infantile" PKD, has numerous small cysts that only arise from the collecting ducts and result in bilateral symmetrical enlargement of the kidneys. The autosomal dominant PKD, previously called "adult" PKD, has cysts arising from all areas of the nephron, which are usually larger and more variable in size than the ARPKD cysts. ARPKD occurs in 1 in 40,000 births and may be detected in utero by the presence of enlarged hyperechogenic kidneys and oligohydramnios. Infants usually die of respiratory failure rather than renal problems; however, the 1-year survival probability after the first month is over 85%. These children have declining renal function as well as severe hypertension and hepatic periportal fibrosis with portal hypertension leading to hypersplenism and esophageal varices.

The genes mutated in ADPKD may include the *PKD1* gene (located on chromosome 16p13.3) in 85% of patients or the *PKD2* gene (on chromosome 4q21-23) in 12–15% of patients. These genes code for the polycystin-1 and -2 proteins, respectively. ADPKD occurs in 1:1000 individuals and is a major cause of end-stage renal disease in adults. Cysts may also be present in the liver, pancreas, and spleen, and cerebral arterial aneurysms may occur. Renal cystic enlargement exerts pressure on normal parenchyma, leading to its gradual destruction and glomerulosclerosis.

The diagnosis is often made during a workup for hypertension or uremia discovered in the third to sixth decades. Hematuria with or without flank pain is a common finding. An intravenous urogram will reveal the enlarged kidneys, with marked elongation of the calices, which are compressed by large cysts (Figure 40–5). Ultrasonography or CT scan will readily make the diagnosis.

Surgery is rarely warranted. Therapy is medical and ultimately includes dialysis. The median age for reaching end-stage renal disease (ESRD) is 54 years in PKD1 and 74 years in PKD2. Renal transplantation is often indicated, though potential family donors must be carefully screened to determine whether they have the same disorder. The leading cause of death in ADPKD is cardiovascular disease, which may relate to early untreated hypertension.

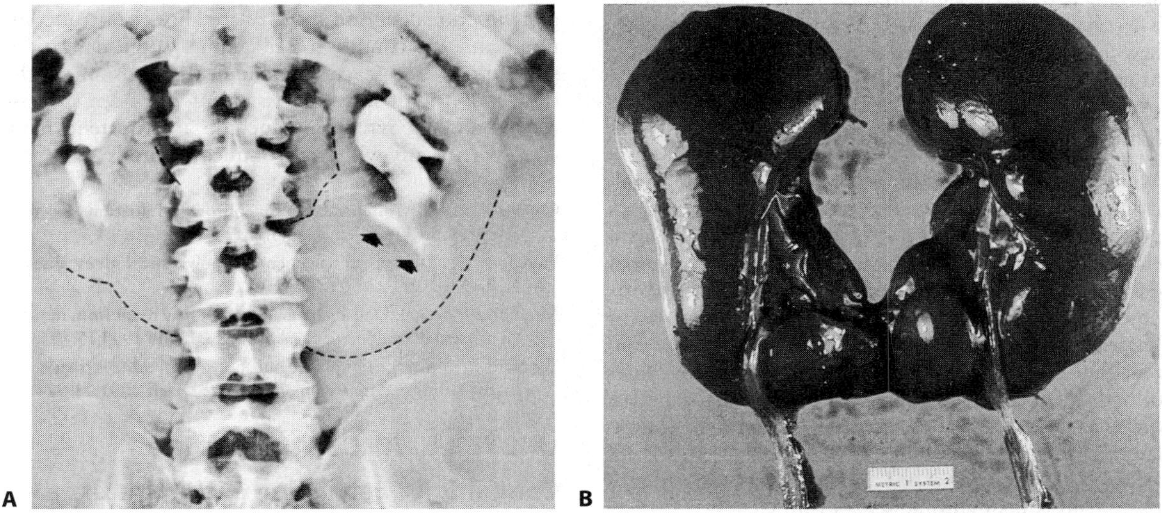

Figure 40–4. ***A:*** Excretory urogram showing horseshoe kidney with expansion of left side of isthmus and compression of lower left caliceal system. ***B:*** Gross pathology of horseshoe kidney.

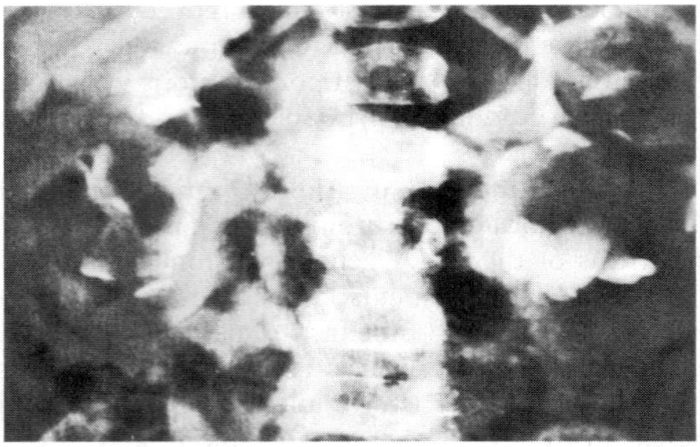

Figure 40–5. Polycystic kidneys. Excretory urogram in a child, showing elongation, broadening, and bending of the calices around cysts. Renal function was normal.

Medullary Sponge Kidney

Medullary sponge kidney results from collecting tubular ectasia (see Polycystic Kidneys) and is associated with recurrent urolithiasis and an increased incidence of infection in 50% of patients. The lesion is often bilateral and may involve all of the calices. Intravenous urograms reveal dilated collecting tubules as a "blush" in the renal papilla. Microscopic hematuria is common. Specific antibiotics should be given for documented infections, and prophylactic therapy for renal stones should be recommended, based on the results of metabolic stone evaluation.

Simple Renal Cysts

Simple renal cysts are common (approximately 50% after age 50) and are thought to arise from tubular dilation. They may be solitary or bilateral and multiple. They rarely have pathologic significance except in the differentiation from solid renal masses. (See Renal Adenocarcinoma.)

Multicystic Dysplastic Kidney

Multicystic dysplastic kidney is a congenital abnormality consisting of macroscopic cysts of variable sizes compressing dysplastic renal parenchyma. It is usually associated with an atretic proximal ureter. The disorder occurs in about 1:3000 live births and is frequently noted on prenatal ultrasound. Rarely, it may occur bilaterally and is associated with oligohydramnios and renal failure. It may be distinguished from other causes of hydronephrosis by the absence of any renal function on renal scan. There is an increased incidence of contralateral ureteropelvic junction obstruction (5–10%) and reflux (18–43%), either of which increases the patient's risk of subsequent chronic renal insufficiency.

The chance of developing a malignancy in multicystic dysplastic kidney appears to be no greater than 1:2000. There may also be an increased incidence of hypertension. These two factors constitute a rationale for treatment by nephrectomy. However, conservative management with routine ultrasound examinations at intervals of 6–12 months is reasonable practice, since about half involute within 5 years.

Renal Vascular Abnormalities

Multiple renal arteries occur in 15–20% of patients and are significant only when they cause ureteropelvic junction obstruction. Congenital **renal artery aneurysms** are infrequent; they are differentiated from acquired lesions by their location at the bifurcation of the main renal artery or at a distal branch point. The lesions are usually asymptomatic, but they can cause hypertension. They require surgical treatment only if hypertension is uncontrolled, if they are incompletely calcified, or if they have a diameter of more than 2.5 cm. **Congenital arteriovenous fistulas** are rare but may result in hematuria, hypertension, or cardiac failure necessitating operative treatment.

Renal Pelvis Anomalies

Ureteropelvic junction obstruction is the most common cause of antenatal hydronephrosis. The condition may be associated with compression by anomalous renal arteries or intrinsic stenosis of the junction. The diagnosis is not uncommonly made when gross hematuria follows minor trauma. Renal ultrasound provides a safe screening technique in patients suspected of ureteropelvic junction obstruction. Intravenous urography will suggest the diagnosis, and diuretic renal scan or retrograde pyelography, or both, may confirm it and suggest functional significance. Bilaterality is not uncommon, and the condition will require surgical repair if symptomatic or severe. Percutaneous incision of the obstruction with short-term stenting has been successful in adults. Symptoms include intermittent flank pain, particularly with orally induced diuresis.

Cooper CS et al: Antenatal hydronephrosis: evaluation and outcome. Curr Urol Rep 2002,3:131.

Hateboer N: Clinical management of polycystic kidney disease. Clin Med 2003;3:509.

Mesrobian HG et al: Unilateral renal agenesis may result from in utero regression of multicystic renal dysplasia. J Urol 1993;15:793.

Winyard P, Chitty L: Dysplastic and polycystic kidneys: diagnosis, associations and management. Prenat Diagn 2001;21:924.

URETERAL ANOMALIES

Congenital Obstruction of the Ureter

Congenital obstruction of the ureter may be due to ureterovesical and ureteropelvic junction obstruction or to neurologic deficits such as sacral agenesis or myelomeningocele. Functional ureteral obstruction—also known as **primary obstructive megaureter**—is not uncommon (Figure 40–6). Symptoms are renal pain during oral diuresis or those resulting from pyelonephritis. Excretory urograms depict dilation above the obstruction. Vesicoureteral reflux is uncommonly associated with megaureter. Milder forms without symptoms or significant hydronephrosis are the rule and do not require treatment if renal function is normal. When treatment is necessary, it consists of division of the ureter proximal to the obstruction and reimplantation of the ureter into the bladder often involving ureteral tapering or plication.

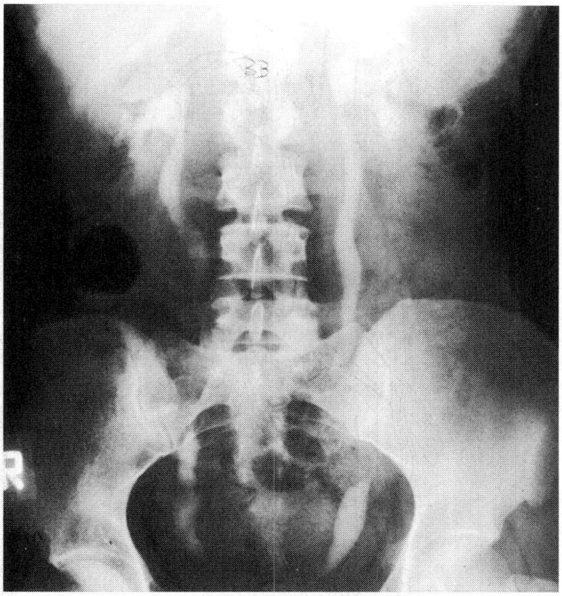

Figure 40–6. Excretory urogram showing bilateral megaureter.

Duplication of Ureters

Bifurcation of the ureteral bud before it interacts with the metanephric blastema results in incomplete ureteral duplication, commonly in the mid or upper ureter. A second ureteral bud from the metanephric duct leads to complete ureteral duplication (Figure 40–7A; right kidney) draining one kidney. This represents the most common ureteral anomaly, occurring in 1:125 people. It occurs twice as often in females. The presence of more than two ureters on each side is not common, but bilaterality of ureteral duplication occurs 40% of the time. Usually, all of the duplicated ureters enter the bladder; the ureter draining the upper pole of the kidney enters closest to the bladder neck (due to its later reabsorption into the bladder). Because of this relationship, the ureter draining the lower pole often has a short intramural tunnel and an inadequate surrounding musculature and is thus prone to vesicoureteral reflux. The ureter draining the upper pole may be ectopic (because of its late absorption) and thus empty into the bladder neck, urethra, or genital structures (vagina or vestibule in the female and seminal vesicle or vas deferens in the male [Figure 40–7A; left kidney]). The ureter draining the upper pole is prone to obstruction and may be associated with a ureterocele, which is a common cause of obstruction. Duplication becomes significant when hydronephrosis or pyelonephritis occurs. The diagnosis is made by intravenous urography (Figure 40–7B). Ureteral reimplantation to prevent recurrent infection is necessary in some cases. An anastomosis between the upper pole renal pelvis and the lower pole ureter or a low ureteroureterostomy are alternatives in selected cases. The upper pole of the kidney and its ureter may require removal if obstruction is severe and renal function of that segment is poor.

Ectopic Ureteral Orifice

Ureteral ectopia can occur in the absence of duplication and drain into any of the abnormal positions mentioned above. If the orifice lies proximal to the external urinary sphincter, no incontinence ensues, but vesicoureteral reflux is common. In contradistinction to the female, the ectopic orifice in the male never lies distal to the external sphincter, making incontinence an extremely rare presentation. Should the ectopic orifice in the female drain into the vagina or at the vestibule, there may be continuous leakage of urine apart from voiding. Most ectopic orifices involve the ureter draining the upper pole of a duplicated system, and most are observed in females. Hydroureteronephrosis of the involved segment frequently occurs due to ureteral obstruction as it traverses the muscle of the bladder neck.

An ectopic orifice may be seen beside the urethral orifice or in the roof of the vagina on endoscopy. Renal ultrasound or intravenous urograms will often demonstrate hydroureteronephrosis of the upper renal segment. Cystography may show reflux into the ectopic orifice but may require cyclic voiding first to decompress the obstructed segment with bladder neck relaxation and subsequently to permit reflux. In the rare case when there is significant upper pole renal function, the ureter can be divided and reimplanted into the bladder or lower pole ureter. Usually, however, heminephroureterectomy is necessary.

Ureterocele

A ureterocele is a ballooning of the distal submucosal ureter into the bladder. This structure commonly has a pinpoint orifice and therefore leads to hydroureteronephrosis. If large enough, it may obstruct the vesical

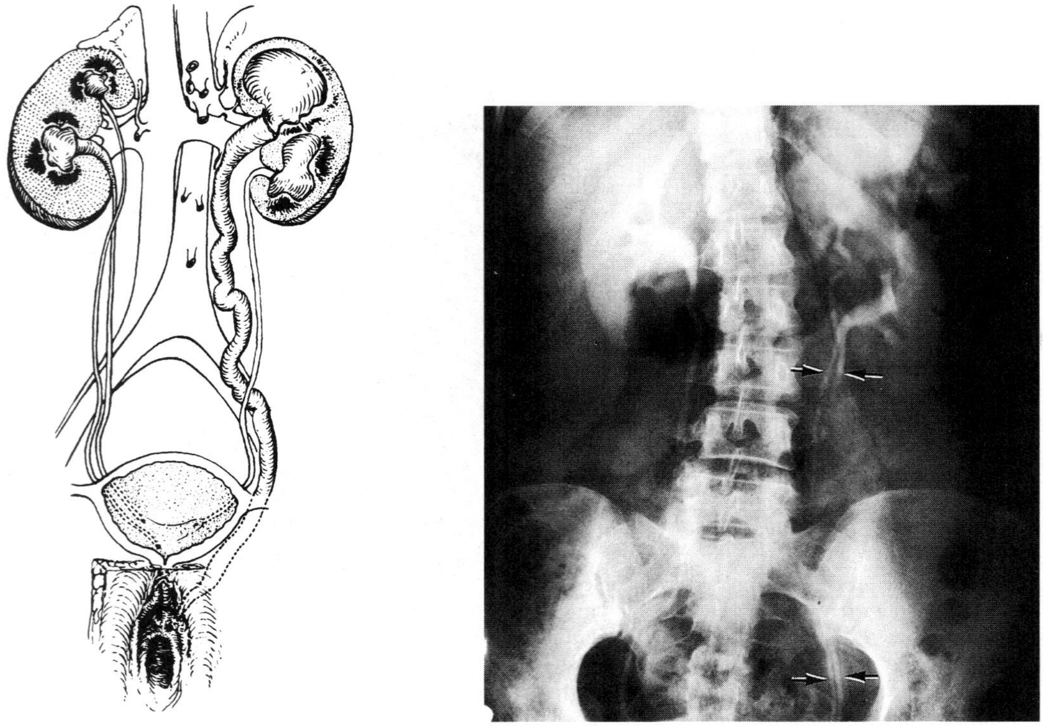

A B

Figure 40–7. ***A:*** Duplication of ureters and ectopic ureteral orifice. Complete duplication with obstruction to one ureter with ectopic orifice on left. The ureter with the ectopic opening always drains the upper pole of the kidney. ***B:*** Excretory urogram showing left complete ureteral duplication.

neck or the contralateral ureter. It is most common in females with ureteral duplication and always involves the ureter draining the upper renal pole.

Most ureteroceles are now detected by prenatal ultrasound. Symptoms are usually those of pyelonephritis or obstruction. Intravenous urograms may show a negative shadow in the bladder cast by the ureterocele (Figure 40–8). The ureter and renal calices may be normal or may reveal marked dilation or no excretory function at all. A cystogram may show reflux into the ipsilateral lower pole ureter.

Treatment of ureteroceles depends upon multiple factors, including the presence or absence of reflux in any or all of the ureters as well as whether or not the ureterocele is completely contained within the bladder (orthotopic) or if a portion is at the bladder neck or urethra (ectopic). A simple method of establishing drainage involves cystoscopy and puncture of the ureterocele. Associated reflux, if present, can be managed with prophylactic antibiotics until the child has grown larger, at which time a technically easier ureteral reimplant may be performed with a decompressed ureter. In the relatively uncommon situation when there is no associated reflux, an upper pole heminephrectomy is considered. Minimally obstructive ureteroceles within the bladder in adults do not require treatment.

Cooper CS et al: Long-term follow-up of endoscopic incision of ureteroceles: intravesical versus extravesical. J Urol 2000; 164:1097.

Fretz PC et al: Long-term outcome analysis of Starr plication for primary obstructive megaureters. J Urol 2004;172:703.

VESICOURETERAL REFLUX

The main function of the ureterovesical junction is to permit free drainage of the ureter and simultaneously prevent urine from refluxing back from the bladder. Anatomically, the ureterovesical junction is well equipped for this function, because the ureteral musculature continues uninterrupted into the base of the bladder to form the superficial trigone. Additionally, the terminal 4–5 cm of ureter are

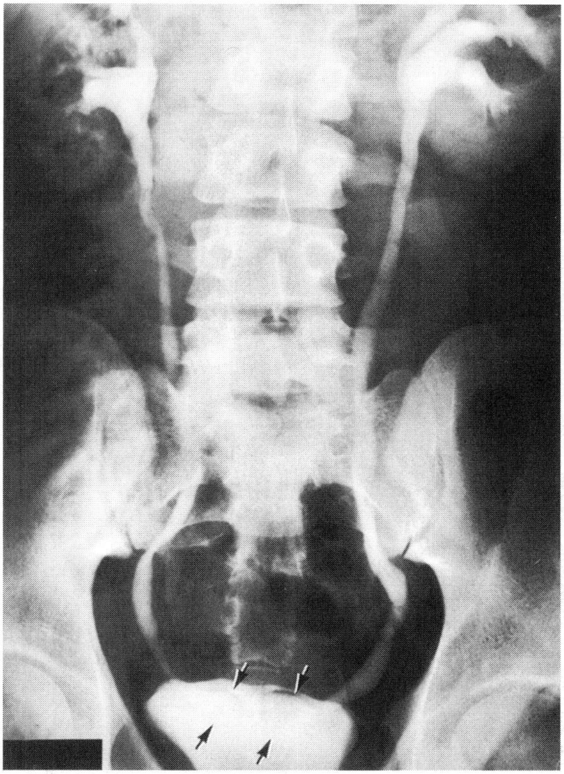

Figure 40–8. Ureterocele. Excretory urogram showing bilateral space-occupying lesions in the bladder caused by ureteroceles (arrows).

surrounded by a musculofascial sheath (Waldeyer's sheath) that follows the ureter through the ureteral hiatus and continues in the base of the bladder as the deep trigone (Figure 40–9).

Direct continuity between the ureter and the trigone offers an efficient, muscularly active, valvular function. Any stretch of the trigone (with bladder filling) or any trigonal contraction (with voiding) leads to firm occlusion of the intravesical ureter, thus increasing resistance to flow from above downward and sealing the intravesical ureter against retrograde flow (Figure 40–10).

Etiology & Classification

Vesicoureteral reflux may be classified as primary reflux due to developmental ureterotrigonal weakness or associated with ureteral anomalies such as ectopic orifice or ureterocele, and secondary reflux due to bladder outlet or urethral obstruction, neuropathic dysfunction, iatrogenic causes, and inflammation, especially specific infection (eg, tuberculosis). Primary reflux is associated with some degree of congenital muscular deficiency in the trigone and terminal ureter.

Reflux is associated with an increased incidence of pyelonephritis and renal damage. It also allows bacteria free access from the bladder to the kidney.

Reflux is the most common cause of pyelonephritis and is found in 30–50% of children presenting with urinary tract infection. It is present in over 75% of patients with radiologic evidence of chronic pyelonephritis and is responsible for end-stage renal disease in a large percentage of patients requiring chronic dialysis or renal transplantation.

In primary reflux, the child (on average, between 2 and 3 years of age) usually presents with symptoms of pyelonephritis or cystitis. Vague abdominal pain is not uncommon. Renal pain and pain with voiding are relatively uncommon. On rare occasions, the patient may present with advanced renal failure with bilateral renal parenchymal damage. Significant reflux and its sequelae are more common in females and are usually detected after a urinary tract infection. About one-third of the

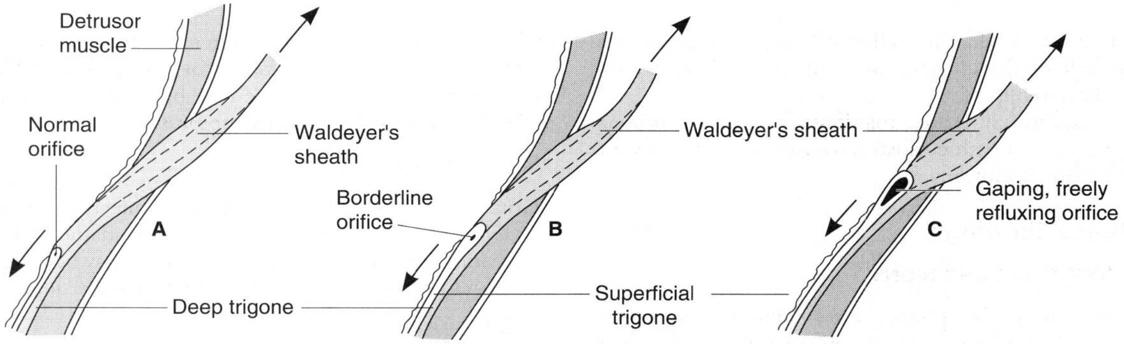

Figure 40–9. Vesicoureteral reflux. The length and fixation of the intravesical ureter and the appearance of the ureteral orifice depend upon the muscular development and efficiency of the lower ureter and its trigone. ***A:*** Normal structures. ***B:*** Moderate muscular deficiency. ***C:*** Marked deficiency results in a golf hole distortion of the submucosal ureter.

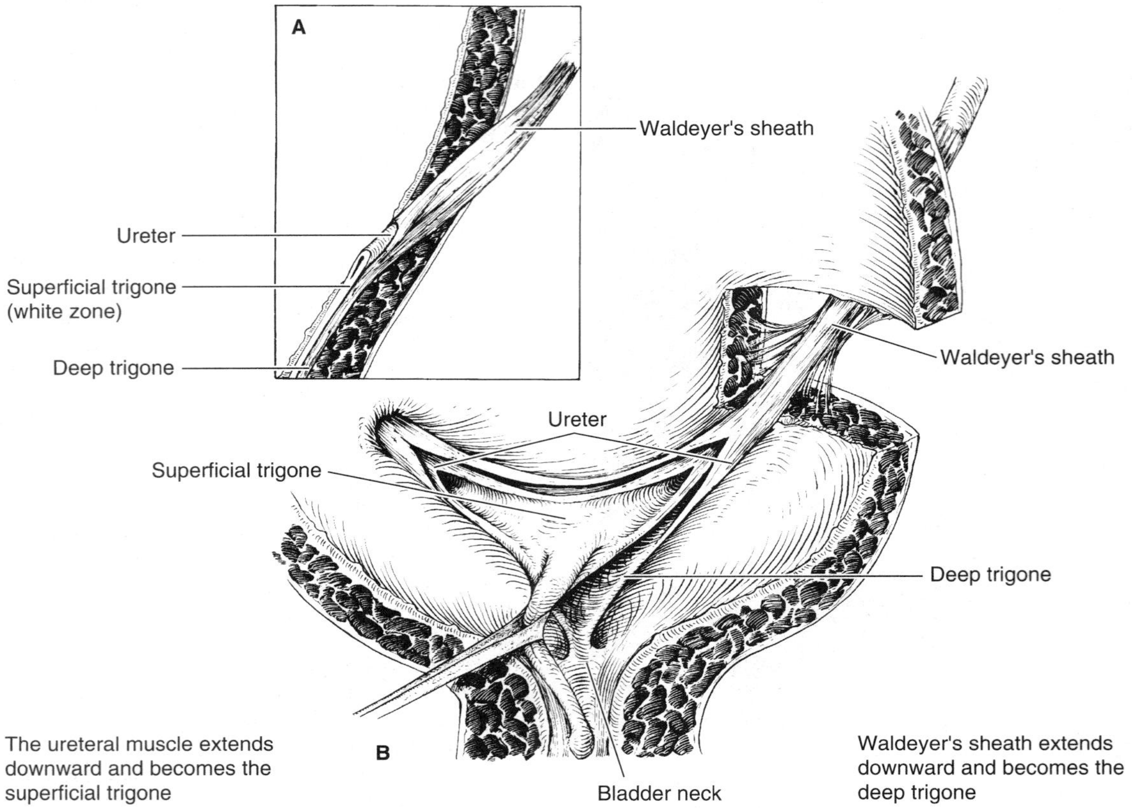

Figure 40–10. Normal ureterotrigonal complex. ***A:*** Side view of ureterovesical junction. Waldeyer's muscular sheath invests the juxtavesical ureter and continues downward as the deep trigone, which extends to the bladder neck. The ureteral musculature becomes the superficial trigone, which extends to the verumontanum in the male and stops just short of the external meatus in the female. ***B:*** Waldeyer's sheath is connected by a few fibers to the detrusor muscle in the ureteral hiatus. This muscular sheath, inferior to the ureteral orifices, becomes the deep trigone. The musculature of the ureters continues downward as the superficial trigone. (Adapted from Tanagho EA, Pugh RCB: Br J Urol 1963:35;151.) (Reproduced with permission of Blackwell Publishing, Ltd.)

siblings of a child with reflux will also have reflux, and one-half of the children of a mother with reflux will also have reflux.

In secondary reflux, manifestations of the primary disease (neuropathic, obstructive, etc.) are usually the presenting symptoms.

Clinical Findings

A. Symptoms and Signs

With acute pyelonephritis, fever, chills, and costovertebral angle tenderness may be present. Children usually do not have renal pain but may complain of vague abdominal pain. Occasionally, daytime frequency, incontinence, or enuresis may be caused by infection associated with reflux. In cases of obstruction or neuropathic deficit, a palpable hydronephrotic kidney or a distended bladder may be found. The diagnosis may be elusive in infants who present with ill-defined symptoms.

B. Laboratory Findings

Urinalysis will usually reveal evidence of infection (pyuria and bacteriuria). Urine cultures are mandatory when infection is suspected. Renal function tests may be abnormal if reflux and infection have caused renal scarring.

C. Imaging Studies

The most useful study for conclusive diagnosis of reflux continues to be voiding cystourethrography (Figure 40–11). This study demonstrates the grade of

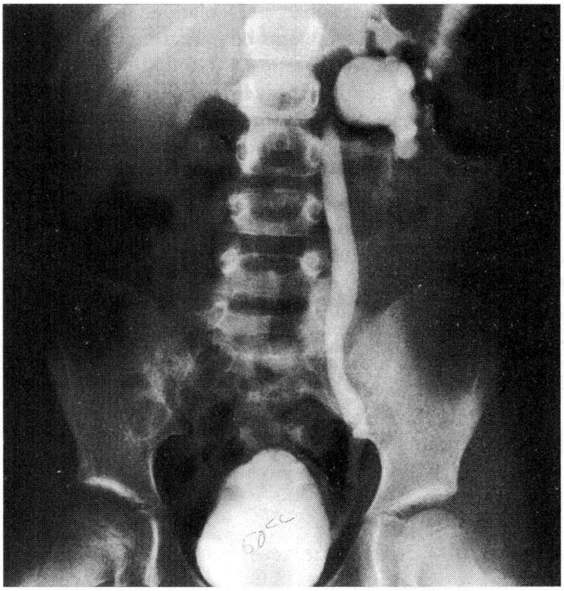

Figure 40–11. Voiding cystourethrogram showing total left vesicoureteral reflux.

reflux as well as the urethral anatomy. Radionuclide voiding studies are extremely sensitive at detecting reflux but do not demonstrate the anatomic detail seen with a voiding cystourethrogram. Radionuclide voiding studies are often performed as follow-up after an initial voiding cystourethrogram since they offer the advantage of decreased radiation exposure.

Radioisotopic renal scanning provides accurate differential renal function data and detection of renal scars. Ultrasound can provide accurate measurement of renal size and may demonstrate the presence of renal scarring and ureteral or caliceal dilation. In many cases, there may be no abnormality visible in the upper urinary tract, or only mild distal ureteral dilatation may be seen.

D. Urodynamic Considerations

A significant number of children with dysfunctional voiding present with urinary tract infections and are subsequently found to have reflux. These children contract the bladder against a closed external sphincter. Elevated voiding pressures associated with dysfunctional voiding may increase renal damage with an associated urinary tract infection and may also lessen the chance for either spontaneous or surgical resolution of reflux. When the history suggests the possibility of voiding dysfunction (incontinence, frequency, urgency), urodynamic studies are conducted to evaluate the voiding dynamics. Treatment of voiding dysfunction may result in resolution of the reflux.

Treatment

Although some children with reflux may not require antibiotics, the current standard of care requires that any child with reflux be maintained on prophylactic antibiotics. Prompt treatment of pyelonephritis prevents renal scar formation. Factors causing secondary reflux—such as dysfunctional voiding or obstruction—should be corrected.

In many children, reflux will resolve with time. Reflux is graded as seen on voiding cystourethrography as follows:

Grade I: Contrast enters ureter

Grade II: Contrast enters the renal collecting system

Grade III: Slight dilation of the calices or ureter

Grades IV and V: Progressively increased amounts of caliceal dilation and ureteral dilation or tortuosity

Reflux most likely to resolve is of lower grade or detected at a younger age. Over 70% of children with grades I, II, or unilateral grade III reflux will have resolution within 5 years. Resolution in children with grade V or bilateral grade IV reflux can be anticipated in less than 10% of cases.

In obstructive secondary reflux (eg, posterior urethral valves), release of obstruction may cure reflux. Occasionally, surgical reimplantation is still required. In neuropathic reflux, intermittent catheterization for control of infection may allow return of valvular competence. However, many cases will require bladder augmentation for a noncompliant bladder and ureteral reimplantation. In reflux associated with ectopic orifices, duplication with ureterocele, and other congenital malformations, reimplantation is generally required.

The aim of surgery is to correct the reflux. This is accomplished by the creation of a longer submucosal tunnel for the ureter. With bladder filling and increased pressure, the ureter is compressed between the mucosa and underlying detrusor muscle. This flap valve prevents reflux of urine. The necessary length of the tunnel to stop reflux depends upon the diameter of the ureter, with a 5:1 length-to-diameter ratio being ideal. One of three methods is used in most cases: (1) In suprahiatal repair (Politano-Leadbetter procedure), a new ureteral hiatus is developed about 2.5 cm above the original one and the ureter—after passing through a submucosal tunnel—is sutured to the cut edge of the trigone at the level of the original orifice. (2) In the cross-trigonal repair (Cohen procedure), the original hiatus is maintained, and the ureter is advanced through a submucosal tunnel, extending across the trigone to the contralateral bladder wall. (3) A totally extravesical ureteral advancement procedure (extravesical ureteroplasty) achieves results similar to those achieved with the intravesical methods described above, with a shorter hospital stay and shorter convalescence.

Injections of sub-ureteric bulking agents have also been used to increase submucosal support of the ureter. With proper placement beneath the ureteral orifice under endoscopic vision, these injections act to bolster the deficient antireflux mechanism. Concern regarding late sequelae of Teflon injections (eg, particle migration) has prevented use of this approach in the United States. Short-term success in stopping reflux with the injection techniques appears to be around 75%. The long-term success rates with agents other than Teflon remain to be determined.

Prognosis

The long-term prognosis is excellent for patients with mild to moderate reflux successfully treated with antibiotic prophylaxis. There are few instances of recurrent infection or renal insufficiency. Patients with more significant reflux or persistent urinary tract infections may benefit from sub-ureteric injection or surgical reimplantation; the success rate is approximately 95% with the open surgical technique (cessation of reflux, clearance of renal infection, and absence of obstruction). Unfortunately, for patients with advanced disease (irreversible ureteral decompensation and chronic pyelonephritis, which is now thought to be a self-perpetuating immune complex process), the prognosis is less favorable. These patients account for a significant proportion of patients with end-stage renal disease who ultimately require chronic dialysis, renal transplantation, or both.

Austin JC, Cooper CS: Vesicoureteral reflux: surgical approaches. Urol Clin North Am. 2004;31:543.

Bjorgvinsson E et al: Diagnosis of acute pyelonephritis in children: comparison of sonography and 99Tc-DMSA scintigraphy. AJR Am J Roentgenol 1991;157:539.

Cooper CS, Austin JC: Vesicoureteral reflux: who benefits from surgery? Urol Clin North Am 2004;31:535.

Cooper CS et al: Bladder pressure at the onset of vesicoureteral reflux determined by nuclear cystometrogram. J Urol 2003;170:1537.

Cooper CS et al: The outcome of stopping prophylactic antibiotics in older children with vesicoureteral reflux. J Urol 2000;163:269.

Elder JS et al: Pediatric Vesicoureteral Reflux Guidelines Panel summary report on the management of primary vesicoureteral reflux in children. J Urol 1997;157:1846.

Jodal U et al: Infection pattern in children with vesicoureteral reflux randomly allocated to operation or long-term antibacterial prophylaxis: the international reflux study in children. J Urol 1992;148:1650.

Koff SA: Relationship of dysfunctional voiding and reflux. J Urol 1983;130:1138.

Noordzij JW et al: A view on the anatomy of the ureterovesical junction. Scand J Urol Nephrol 1993;27:371.

BLADDER ANOMALIES

Anomalies of the bladder are infrequent and include the following: (1) **agenesis**, or complete absence, which results in a persistent cloaca; (2) bladder **duplication,** which may be complete, with separate ureteral openings drained by duplicated urethras, or incomplete, with a septum or hourglass deformity; and (3) **urachal anomalies**, which in the most severe forms appear as a patent opening at the umbilicus and are usually associated with some form of bladder outlet obstruction. In less severe forms, a **urachal diverticulum** may be present at the dome of the bladder or a **urachal cyst** along the course of the partially obliterated urachus. These latter conditions may cause abdominal pain and umbilical or bladder infection requiring surgical treatment. Occasionally, adenocarcinoma develops in a urachal remnant (see section on Tumors of the Bladder).

Failure of cloacal division results in a persistent cloaca. Incomplete division is more frequent (though still rare) and results in a rectovesical, rectourethral, or rectovestibular fistula (usually with imperforate anus or anal atresia).

Exstrophy of the Bladder

Exstrophy of the bladder is the most severe bladder anomaly—the result of a complete ventral defect of the urogenital sinus and the overlying inferior abdominal wall musculature and integument (Figure 40–12). The lower central portion is devoid of skin and muscle. The anterior bladder wall is absent, and the posterior wall is contiguous with surrounding skin. Urine drains onto the abdominal wall, the rami of the pubic bones are

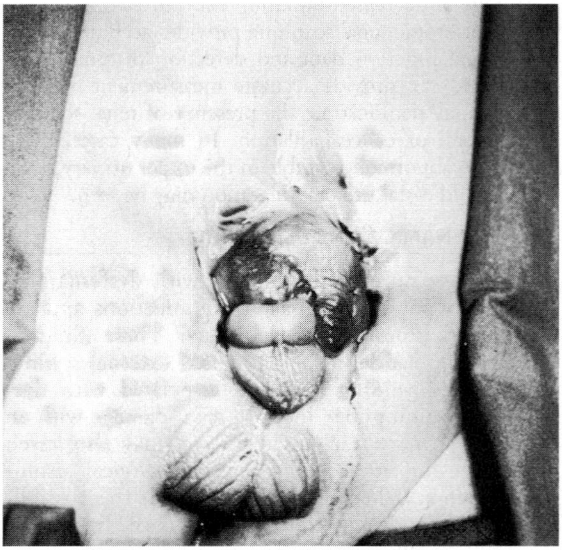

Figure 40–12. Photograph of male patient with bladder exstrophy.

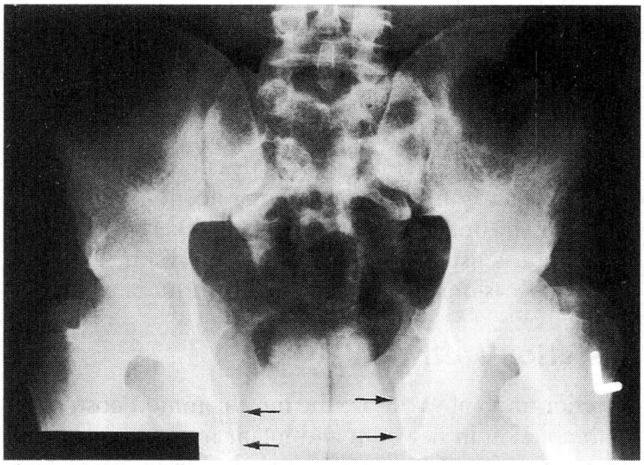

Figure 40–13. Roentgenogram of pelvis with widely separated pubes (arrows) in patient with exstrophy.

widely separated (Figure 40–13), and the open pelvic ring may affect gait. In males, the penis is shortened and the urethra is epispadiac. The exposed bladder mucosa tends to be chronically inflamed.

Currently, the favored treatment is bladder salvage, which includes closure of the bladder in the newborn period. Urethral closure and penile reconstruction have also been advocated at the time of the initial bladder closure. Ureteral obstruction or vesicoureteral reflux may develop and require ureteral reimplantation. The closed bladder may have a small capacity, and incontinence is often a complication. Patients frequently require multiple operations, including bladder augmentation and bladder neck reconstruction. Good results have been observed in more than half of all patients treated, with preservation of renal function and continence.

Cooper CS et al: Pediatric reconstructive surgery. Curr Opin Urol 2000;10:195.

Prune Belly Syndrome

Prune belly syndrome consists of a triad of abnormalities: deficient abdominal wall musculature, bilateral cryptorchidism, and variable amounts of dilation of the urogenital tract. The cause is not known. Almost all children with prune belly syndrome have reflux. The incidence of eventual renal failure is 25–30%. Risk factors for renal failure include bilateral abnormal kidneys on ultrasound or renal scan, a serum creatinine that never falls below 0.7 mg/dL, and clinical pyelonephritis. These children are managed with prophylactic antibiotics and frequent urine cultures, followed by prompt treatment of any urinary tract infections. Abdominoplasty may be performed to help correct the abdominal wall defect.

Noh PH et al: Prognostic factors of renal failure in children with prune belly syndrome. J Urol 1999;162:1399.

Congenital Neurovesical Dysfunction

Congenital neurovesical dysfunction frequently accompanies a posterior myelomeningocele or sacral agenesis, with associated spinal abnormalities. Both conditions may result in incontinence and recurrent urinary infection with late sequelae (ureteral reflux, pyelonephritis, and renal failure). These children require frequent evaluation of their kidneys and kidney function since high bladder storage pressures may harm the kidneys.

PENILE & URETHRAL ANOMALIES

Hypospadias

Hypospadias rates in the United States have doubled over the past 30 years. The condition results from failure of fusion of the urethral folds on the undersurface of the genital tubercle. The urethral meatus is ventrally displaced on the glans on the shaft of the penis or more proximal at the level of the scrotum or perineum. With more proximal displacement, chordee (ventral curvature of the penile shaft) frequently occurs and requires treatment or it will preclude straight erections and normal intercourse (Figure 40–14). The midscrotal hypospadiac

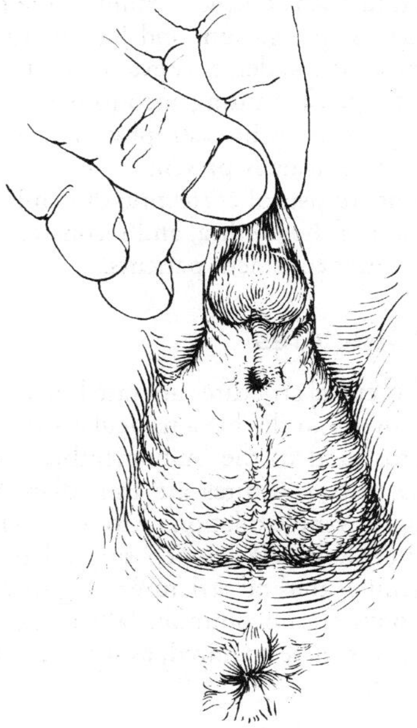

Figure 40–14. Hypospadias, penoscrotal type. Redundant dorsal foreskin that is deficient ventrally; ventral chordee.

penis may resemble female external genitalia with an enlarged clitoris and labia. Sexual assignment in these latter infants requires hormonal and chromosomal analysis.

In hypospadias with the meatus positioned proximal to the corona, the prepuce is abnormal—not forming a complete cylinder due to a ventral defect. Circumcision should not be done in these patients, as the prepuce can be used later in surgical repair.

The degree of hypospadias dictates the need for repair. If the opening is glandular or coronal (85% of patients), the penis is usually functional both for micturition and procreation, and repair is done primarily for cosmetic reasons. Openings that are more proximal on the shaft require correction to allow voiding while standing, normal erection, and proper sperm deposition during intercourse. Surgical plastic repair of hypospadias is currently accomplished by a variety of highly successful one-stage operations and is routinely performed between 6 and 19 months of age. The most common complications of hypospadias surgery include meatal stenosis and fistula formation; however, improved techniques have decreased the incidence of these complications.

Epispadias

Epispadias is a rare congenital anomaly that is commonly associated with bladder exstrophy. When it occurs alone, it is considered a milder degree of the exstrophy complex.

The urethra opens on the dorsum of the penis, with deficient corpus spongiosum and loosely attached corpora cavernosa. If the defect is extensive, it may extend to the bladder neck, causing incontinence. The pubic bones are separated, as in exstrophy. Marked dorsiflexion of the penis is usually present.

Treatment consists of correction of penile curvature, reconstruction of the urethra, and reconstruction of the bladder neck in incontinent patients.

Urethral Strictures

Congenital urethral strictures are rare but when present are most common in the fossa navicularis (just proximal to the meatus) and in the bulbomembranous urethra. Commonly, these strictures are thin diaphragms that may respond to simple dilation or to direct vision internal urethrotomy. Rarely is open surgical repair necessary. Congenital urethral strictures in girls and meatal stenosis in boys are uncommon. When the latter does occur, it appears to be acquired, as it is seen only in circumcised boys.

Urethral Diverticulum

In males, urethral diverticula are nearly always in the pendulous or bulbous urethra. They are often associated with an obstructive flap of the urethral mucosa (anterior urethral valve)—thought to represent incomplete closure of the urethral folds. Treatment by endoscopic unroofing is usually successful, though most diverticula are small and require no therapy. In females they occur in adult life and are usually manifested by irritative symptoms and recurrent infection. The cause is unknown, but the disorder is most likely congenital. Treatment is usually by transvaginal excision. Diverticula may occasionally harbor stones or tumors.

Posterior Urethral Valves

Posterior urethral valves are the most common obstructive urethral lesion in newborn and infant males and the most common cause of end-stage renal disease in boys. They consist of obstructive folds of mucosa, seen only in males, which originate at—or are attached at some point to—the verumontanum in the prostatic urethra. The embryologic derivation is indefinite. They are partially obstructive and thus lead to variable degrees of back pressure damage to the urinary bladder and upper urinary tract. Dilation and obstruction of the prostatic urethra are always present. Spontaneous urinary ascites from the kidneys is often seen in neonates. This clears when the obstruction is relieved.

About one-third of children with posterior urethral valves are now diagnosed by prenatal ultrasound. Another one-third are diagnosed in the first year of life, with the remaining third presenting later. Clinical manifestations consist of difficult voiding, a weak urinary stream, and a midline lower abdominal mass that represents a distended bladder. In some cases, the kidneys are palpable and the child may have signs and symptoms of uremia and acidosis. Urinary incontinence and urinary tract infection may occur. Laboratory findings include elevated serum urea nitrogen and creatinine and evidence of urinary infection. Ultrasound shows evidence of bladder thickening and trabeculation, hydroureter, and hydronephrosis. Demonstration of urethral valves on a voiding cystourethrogram establishes the diagnosis, as does endoscopic identification of valves. Up to 70% of children with valves may have vesicoureteral reflux.

Treatment consists of destruction of the valves by endoscopic incision. In a premature infant with a small urethra prohibiting transurethral resection, a temporary cutaneous vesicostomy may be required to provide drainage and improve impaired kidney function.

The prognosis depends upon the original degree of kidney damage and the success of efforts to prevent or treat infection. Rates of chronic renal failure or ESRD range from $^1/_4$ to $^2/_3$ of boys with valves. Poor prognostic factors include the presence of bilateral reflux or an elevated nadir serum creatinine in the first year of life. Many of these children have delayed development of urinary continence due to bladder changes and impaired urinary concentration.

Cooper CS et al: Preservation of urethral plate spongiosum: technique to reduce hypospadias fistulas. Urology 2001;57:351.

Kirsch AJ et al: Laser tissue soldering for hypospadias repair: results of a controlled, prospective clinical trial. J Urol 2001;165:574.

Paulozzi LJ et al: Hypospadias trends in two U.S. surveillance systems. Pediatrics 1997;100:831.

Ylinen E, Ala-Houhala M, Wikström S: Prognostic factors of posterior urethral valves and the role of antenatal detection. Pediatr Nephrol 2004;20:874.

SCROTAL & TESTICULAR ANOMALIES*

Testicular Torsion

Neonatal testicular torsion (extravaginal torsion) is an extremely rare condition. The entire testicle and the tunica vaginalis are twisted. No trigger mechanism associated with the torsion has been identified. Though the vast majority are necrotic and nonsalvageable, several studies have reported salvage of testicular tissue when torsion is detected immediately following birth. Any scrotal swelling in the neonate requires close follow-up. Intravaginal testicular torsion in adolescents is described later in this chapter.

Cooper CS et al: Bilateral neonatal testicular torsion. Clin Pediatr 1997;36:653.

Scrotal Lesions

Congenital scrotal lesions include hypoplasia of the scrotum (unilateral or bilateral) in association with cryptorchidism (see below) and bifid scrotum with extensive hypospadias. Midline inclusion cysts may also occur.

ACQUIRED LESIONS OF THE GENITOURINARY TRACT

OBSTRUCTIVE UROPATHY

Obstruction is one of the most important abnormalities of the urinary tract, since it eventually leads to decompensation of the muscular conduits and reservoirs, back pressure, and atrophy of renal parenchyma. It also invites infection and stone formation, which cause additional damage and can ultimately end in complete unilateral or bilateral destruction of the kidneys.

Both the level and the degree of obstruction are important to an understanding of the pathologic consequences. Any obstruction at or distal to the bladder neck may lead to back pressure affecting both kidneys. Obstruction at or proximal to the ureteral orifice leads to unilateral damage unless the lesion involves both ureters simultaneously. Complete obstruction leads to rapid decompensation of the system proximal to the site of obstruction. Partial obstruction leads to gradual progressive muscular hypertrophy followed by dilation, decompensation, and hydronephrotic changes.

Etiology

Acquired urinary tract obstruction may be due to inflammatory or traumatic urethral strictures, bladder outlet obstruction (benign prostatic hyperplasia or cancer of the prostate), vesical tumors, neuropathic bladder, extrinsic ureteral compression (tumor, retroperitoneal fibrosis, or enlarged lymph nodes), ureteral or pelvic stones, ureteral strictures, or ureteral or pelvic tumors.

Pathogenesis

Regardless of its cause, acquired obstruction leads to similar changes in the urinary tract, which vary depending on the severity and duration of obstruction.

A. Urethral Changes

Proximal to the obstruction, the urethra dilates and balloons. A urethral diverticulum may develop, and dilation and gaping of the prostatic urethra and ejaculatory ducts may occur.

B. Vesical Changes

Early detrusor and trigonal thickening and hypertrophy compensate for the outlet obstruction, allowing complete bladder emptying. This change leads to progressive development of bladder trabeculation, cellules, saccules, and, finally, diverticula. Subsequently, bladder decompensation occurs and is characterized by the above changes plus incomplete bladder emptying (ie, postvoid residual urine). Trigonal hypertrophy leads to secondary ureteral obstruction owing to increased resistance to flow through the intravesical ureter. With detrusor decompensation and residual urine accumulation, there is stretching of the hypertrophied trigone, which appreciably increases ureteral obstruction. This is the mechanism of back pressure on the kidney in the presence of vesical outlet obstruction (while the ureterovesical junction maintains its competence). Catheter drainage of the bladder relieves trigonal stretch and improves drainage from the upper tract.

A very late change with persistent obstruction (more frequently encountered with neuropathic dysfunction) is decompensation of the ureterovesical junction, leading to reflux. Reflux aggravates the back pressure effect

* Undescended testicles (cryptorchidism) and hydroceles in infants are discussed in Chapter 45.

on the upper tract by transmitting abnormally high intravesical pressures and favors the onset or persistence of urinary tract infection.

C. Ureteral Changes

The first change noted is a gradual increase in ureteral distention. This increases ureteral caliber and stimulates hyperactive ureteral contraction and ureteral muscular hypertrophy. Because the ureteral musculature runs in an irregular helical pattern, stretching of its muscular elements leads to lengthening as well as widening, causing the dilated ureter to assume a tortuous, serpiginous course, weaving back and forth across the relatively straight course of the ureteral vessels, which are unaffected by the ureteral obstruction. This is the start of ureteral decompensation, where tortuosity and dilation become apparent. These changes progress until the ureter becomes atonic, with infrequent, ineffective, or completely absent peristalsis.

D. Pelvicaliceal Changes

The renal pelvis and calices, subjected to increased volumes of retained urine, distend. First, the pelvis shows evidence of hyperactivity and hypertrophy, and then progressive dilation and atony. The calices show similar changes to a variable degree, depending on whether the renal pelvis is intrarenal or extrarenal. In the latter, caliceal dilation may be minimal in spite of marked pelvic dilation. In the intrarenal pelvis, caliceal dilation and renal parenchymal damage are maximal. The successive phases seen with obstruction are rounding of the fornices, followed by flattening of the papillae and finally clubbing of the minor calices.

E. Renal Parenchymal Changes

With continued pelvicaliceal distention, there is parenchymal compression against the renal capsule and, more importantly, compression of the arcuate vessels results in a marked drop in renal blood flow leading to parenchymal ischemic atrophy. With increased intrapelvic pressure, there is progressive dilation of the collecting and distal tubules, with compression and atrophy of tubular cells.

Clinical Findings

A. Symptoms and Signs

The findings vary according to the site of obstruction.

1. Infravesical obstruction—Infravesical obstruction (eg, due to urethral stricture, benign prostatic hypertrophy, bladder neck contracture) leads to difficulty in initiation of voiding, a weak stream, and a diminished flow rate with terminal dribbling. Burning and frequency are common associated symptoms. A distended or thickened bladder wall may be palpable. Urethral induration due to stricture, benign prostatic hypertrophy, or cancer of the prostate may be noted on rectal examination. Meatal stenosis and impacted urethral stones are readily diagnosed by physical examination.

2. Supravesical obstruction—Renal pain or renal colic and gastrointestinal symptoms are commonly associated. Supravesical obstruction (eg, due to ureteral stone, ureteropelvic junction obstruction) may be completely asymptomatic when it develops gradually over a period of months. An enlarged kidney may be palpable. Costovertebral angle tenderness may be present.

B. Laboratory Findings

Evidence of urinary tract infection, hematuria, or crystalluria may be seen. Impaired renal function may be noted in cases of bilateral obstruction. Postrenal azotemia (serum changes reflecting impaired renal function due primarily to obstruction) is suggested by elevation of serum urea nitrogen and serum creatinine with a ratio greater than 10:1.

C. Imaging Studies

Radiologic examination is usually diagnostic in cases of stasis, tumors, and strictures. Dilation and anatomic changes occur above the level of obstruction, whereas distal to the obstruction, the configuration is usually normal. This helps in localizing the site of obstruction. Combined antegrade imaging by intravenous urograms and retrograde imaging by ureterograms or urethrograms is sometimes needed to demonstrate the obstructed segment. In supravesical obstruction, demonstration of stasis and delayed drainage is essential to establish and quantitate the severity of obstruction.

1. Ultrasonography—This will reveal the degree of dilation of the renal pelvis and calices and allows for diagnosis of hydronephrosis even in the prenatal period. Color Doppler ultrasound can reveal blood flow and restrictive indices to help determine functional impairment.

2. Isotope studies—A technetium Tc 99m DTPA scan portrays the degree of hydronephrosis as well as renal function. Use of diuretics during the scan can provide specific data on the significance of the obstruction and the need for treatment. Multiple studies can reveal ongoing functional changes.

3. CT scan—This is of particular value in revealing the degree and site of obstruction as well as the cause in many cases. The use of contrast agents will allow estimation of residual renal function.

4. MR urogram—Magnetic resonance imaging provides anatomic images and identification of the site of obstruction. With dynamic contrast-enhanced MR urography functional information is also obtained without the use of ionizing radiation.

5. Antegrade urography—Antegrade urography via percutaneous needle or tube nephrostomy is valuable when the obstructed kidney fails to excrete the radiopaque material on excretory urography. The Whitaker test requires percutaneous catheter access to the collecting system above the site of suspected obstruction. This permits fluid introduction into the renal pelvis and simultaneous measurement of urine flow rate and pressures in the bladder and renal pelvis, thus providing a quantitative assessment of the degree and severity of obstruction. The fluid transport can be measured and the degree of obstruction estimated by the use of a pressure monitor.

Complications

The most important complication of urinary tract obstruction is renal parenchymal atrophy as a result of back pressure. Obstruction also predisposes to infection and stone formation, and infection occurring with obstruction leads to rapid kidney destruction.

Treatment

The first goal of therapy is relief of the obstruction (eg, catheterization for relief of acute urinary retention). Definitive therapy often requires surgery, but minimally invasive techniques are becoming utilized more often. Simple urethral stricture may be managed by dilation or internal urethrotomy (incision of the stricture under direct vision through the resectoscope). However, urethroplasty (open surgical graft or flap of skin or buccal mucosa to replace urethral diameter) may be required and have better long-term success. Benign prostatic hyperplasia and obstructing bladder tumors classically require excision, but thermal and laser techniques are providing satisfactory outcomes with less morbidity. Impacted ureteral stones may either be removed or bypassed by a catheter unless it is thought that they may pass spontaneously.

Ureteral or ureteropelvic junction obstruction requires surgical repair; however, endoscopic approaches within the ureter or by laparoscopy may be equal to open repair. Renal stones may be removed instrumentally via retrograde or antegrade percutaneous approach or by irrigation through a tube placed directly into the kidney.

Preliminary drainage above the obstruction is sometimes needed to improve kidney function. Occasionally, intestinal urinary diversion or permanent nephrostomy is required. If damage is advanced, nephrectomy may be indicated.

Prognosis

The prognosis depends on the cause, site, duration, and degree of kidney damage and renal decompensation. In general, relief of obstruction leads to improvement in kidney function except in seriously damaged kidneys, especially those destroyed by inflammatory scarring.

Barbagli G et al: Dorsal onlay graft urethroplasty using penile skin or buccal mucosa in adult bulbourethral strictures. J Urol 1998;160:1307.

Bauer SB, Joseph DB: Management of the obstructed urinary tract associated with neurogenic bladder dysfunction. Urol Clin North Am 1990;17:395.

Grattan-Smith JD et al: MR imaging of kidneys: functional evaluation using F-15 perfusion imaging. Pediatr Radiol 2003;33:293.

Rink RC, Mitchell ME: Physiology of lower urinary tract obstruction. Urol Clin North Am 1990;17:329.

URETEROPELVIC JUNCTION OBSTRUCTION

Stenosis of the renal pelvis outlet is commonly due to congenital narrowing of the junction or compression by anomalous vessels. However, the lesion may be acquired. Presentation in adults often includes the abrupt onset of flank pain usually following ingestion of large amounts of fluids. Presentation in childhood is now most often made following the diagnosis of hydronephrosis by prenatal ultrasonography.

The diagnosis may be confirmed with a diuretic nuclear renal scan or intravenous urography, which reveals hydronephrosis with a dilated renal pelvis and slow drainage of either radiotracer or contrast medium. Occasionally, patients present with intermittent hydronephrosis and normal urograms, except during attacks of pain, when x-rays show typical obstruction. These patients generally have normal renal parenchyma. Retrograde ureteropyelography is usually needed in patients with chronic moderate to severe obstruction to determine the extent of the lesion and to provide assurance that the distal ureter is normal (Figure 40–15). Marked obstruction may make it difficult to determine whether kidney function is surgically salvageable. In these cases, it may be necessary to perform either (1) differential radioisotope renography with use of a diuretic during the study or (2) percutaneous nephrostomy with flow measurement through the pelvic junction (Whitaker test) and differential creatinine clearance collection.

Severe obstruction with minimal remaining renal function is best treated by unilateral nephrectomy. If renal function is adequate (> 10% of total renal function or > 10 mL/min creatinine clearance), surgical repair of the stenosis, either by creation of a renal pelvis flap or by resection of the stenotic area and reanastomosis, is warranted. The use of ureteroscopy or percutaneous nephroscopy with endopyelotomy, incising the strictured ureteropelvic junction, offers an alternative method of therapy. This approach appears less successful in the presence of a crossing vessel, poor renal function, and significant hydronephrosis. Laparoscopic repair has proponents as well. The

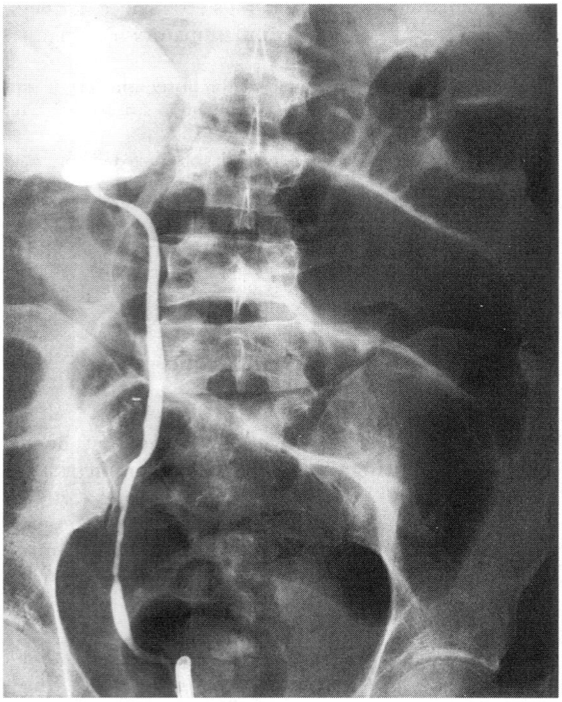

Figure 40–15. Retrograde ureteropyelogram showing right ureteropelvic junction obstruction.

surgical results of these methods are excellent in terms of functional preservation, improvement of urine flow, and relief of symptoms, but dilation of the calices may persist.

Gerber GS et al: Endopyelotomy: patient selection, results and complications. Urology 1994;43:2.

Tan BJ, Smith AD: Ureteropelvic junction obstruction repair: when, how, what? Curr Opin Urol 2004;14:55.

URETERAL STENOSIS

Acquired ureteral stenosis is less common than the congenital types. Causes include (1) ureteral injury (surgical, traumatic, radiation therapy), (2) compression of the ureter by lymph nodes harboring cancer, (3) prolonged compression by an anomalous blood vessel, (4) tuberculous or bilharzial ureteritis, (5) retroperitoneal fibrosis, (6) aneurysm of the aorta following aortofemoral bypass grafts, (7) ureteropelvic junction obstruction secondary to reflux, (8) occlusion of the ureterovesical junction by infiltrating cancer of the bladder or cervix, and (9) functional obstruction of the ureterovesical junction secondary to hypertrophy of the trigone developing from obstruction distal to the bladder neck.

Symptoms are usually those of obstruction to urine flow from the kidney, though many cases are asymptomatic. An unsuspected lesion is often discovered on excretory urography.

Therapy consists of treatment of the cause, eg, resection of the stenosed segment with end-to-end anastomosis. Endoscopy-guided ureteral dilation or incision may be curative. Ureteral stents may be beneficial for postoperative ureteral stricture or following injury due to radiation therapy.

RETROPERITONEAL FIBROSIS

See also Chapter 22.

One or both ureters may be compressed by a chronic inflammatory process, usually of unknown cause, which involves the retroperitoneal tissues of the lumbosacral area. Patients treated for migraine with methysergide may develop this fibrosis. Sclerosing Hodgkin's disease and fibrosis from metastatic cancer have also been implicated. Symptoms include renal pain, low backache, and those associated with uremia. Some patients present with complete anuria. Urinary infection is unusual. If both ureters are obstructed, the serum creatinine is elevated.

Excretory urograms show hydronephrosis and a dilated ureter down to the point of obstruction. The ureters are displaced medially in the lumbar area. Retrograde ureterograms show a long segment of ureteral stenosis, though a catheter passes easily through the ureter. Sonograms and CT scans may demonstrate fibrous plaques with proximal hydroureteronephrosis. If the patient is anuric, indwelling ureteral catheters or percutaneous nephrostomy should be done. When the patient's condition has improved, definitive therapy can be accomplished. If methysergide is suspected to be the causative agent, fibrosis may subside when the drug is discontinued. These patients may benefit from administration of corticosteroids. Chronic indwelling ureteral stents have also been used successfully. If these methods fail, ureterolysis must be performed to free the ureter from the fibrous plaque. The involved ureter should be dissected from the plaque, moved to a lateral position, and wrapped with omentum to prevent recurrent entrapment.

BENIGN PROSTATIC HYPERPLASIA

ESSENTIALS OF DIAGNOSIS

- *Prostatism: nocturia, hesitancy, slow stream, terminal dribbling, frequency.*
- *Residual urine.*
- *Acute urinary retention.*
- *Uremia in advanced cases.*

General Considerations

The cause of benign prostatic enlargement is not known but is probably related to hormonal factors. By upsetting the mechanism for opening and funneling the vesical neck at the time of voiding, hyperplasia of the prostate causes increased outflow resistance. Consequently, a higher intravesical pressure is required to accomplish voiding, causing hypertrophy of the vesical and trigonal muscles. This may lead to the development of bladder diverticula—outpocketings of vesical mucosa between the detrusor muscle bundles. Hypertrophy of the trigone causes excessive stress on the intravesical ureter, producing functional obstruction and resulting in hydroureteronephrosis in late cases. Stagnation of urine can lead to infection; the onset of cystitis will exacerbate the obstructive symptoms. The periurethral and subtrigonal prostate enlargement produces the most significant obstruction.

The prostate in young men has an anatomic capsule like an apple peel. In men with prostatic enlargement, there is a thick "surgical" capsule similar to an orange peel, composed of peripherally compressed true prostatic tissue ("peripheral zone"). The hyperplastic benign periurethral glands correspond to the "transition zone" and are the cause of the obstruction (Figure 40–16).

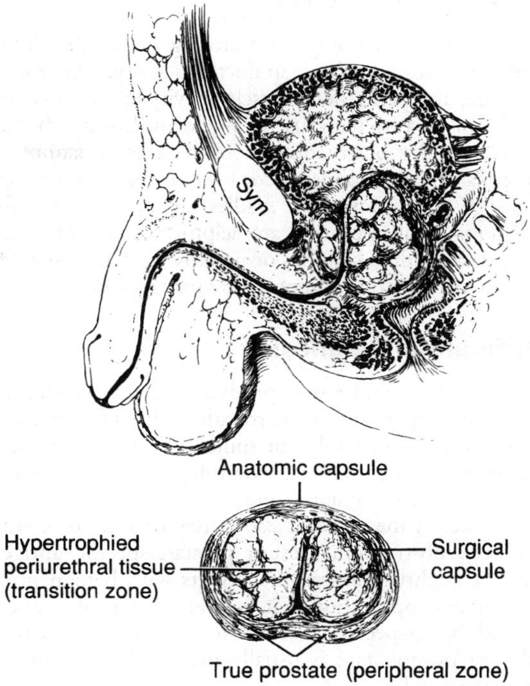

Figure 40–16. Benign prostatic hyperplasia. The enlarged periurethral glands are enclosed by the surgical capsule. The true prostate has been compressed.

Clinical Findings

A. Symptoms and Signs

Typically, the patient has lower urinary tract symptoms (LUTS) and notices hesitancy and loss of force and caliber of the stream. The urgent need to void when the bladder is nearly full may be an early sign. He may also be awakened by the urge to void several times at night (nocturia). Postvoid dribbling ("terminal dribbling") is particularly disturbing. The complication of infection increases the degree of obstructive symptoms and is often associated with burning on urination. Acute urinary retention may supervene. This is associated with severe urgency, suprapubic pain, and a distended, palpable bladder.

The size of the prostate rectally is not of primary diagnostic importance, since there is a poor correlation between the size of the gland and the degree of symptoms and amount of residual urine. The American Urological Association (AUA) developed a seven-item, self-administered questionnaire (AUA Symptom Score) that can assist the patient and physician in evaluating the patient's LUTS.

B. Laboratory Findings

Urinalysis may reveal evidence of infection. Residual urine is commonly increased (> 50 cc), and a timed urinary flow rate will be decreased (< 10–15 cc/s). The serum creatinine may be elevated in cases with prolonged severe obstruction.

C. Imaging Studies

Excretory urograms are often normal and not diagnostic, and are thus not required. In late-stage cases, the study may show hydroureteronephrosis if severe obstruction is present. This almost always resolves after prostatectomy. The enlarged gland may cause an indentation in the inferior surface of the bladder, which may result in a "J-hook" deformity of the distal ureter. The postvoiding film may reveal varying amounts of residual urine. Renal ultrasound examination may obviate the need for urograms; however, imaging is not required to make the diagnosis or to determine the need for or method of treatment. Pelvic ultrasound, commonly an office procedure using a small machine expressly for this purpose, can obviate bladder catheterization and can also accurately predict the amount of residual urine.

D. Cystoscopic Examination

Bladder cystoscopy will reveal secondary vesical changes (eg, trabeculation) and enlargement of the periurethral prostatic glands; however, cystoscopy is not required to make the diagnosis. It may identify other conditions such as bladder stones or tumors, in selected cases.

E. Urodynamic Studies

Simultaneous physiologic monitoring of bladder filling and emptying, urethral sphincter activity, abdominal pressure, and pelvic floor muscle activity (electromyography) can be extremely useful in documenting whether bladder outlet obstruction, poor bladder function, or other causes are responsible for lower urinary tract symptoms. While urodynamic studies are not required for diagnosis in all cases, they are helpful in cases with large post-void residual volumes or underlying neurologic disease to help determine appropriate management.

Differential Diagnosis

Neuropathic bladder may produce a similar syndrome. A history suggesting a neuropathic difficulty, such as diabetes mellitus, stroke, or spinal cord injury or compression, may be obtained. Neurologic deficit involving S2–4 is particularly significant.

Cancer of the prostate also causes symptoms of vesical neck obstruction. Serum prostate-specific antigen may be slightly elevated in patients with benign prostatic hypertrophy, but if it is over 10 ng/mL, cancer should be suspected (normal is < 4 ng/mL). Serum alkaline phosphatase is usually increased if the tumor has spread to bone.

Acute prostatitis may cause symptoms of obstruction, but the patient is septic and has infected urine. The prostate is exquisitely tender.

Urethral stricture diminishes the caliber of the urinary stream. There is usually a history of gonorrhea or local trauma. A retrograde urethrogram will show the stenotic area. A stricture blocks the passage of an instrument or catheter.

Complications

Obstruction and residual urine lead to vesical and prostatic infection and occasionally pyelonephritis; these may be difficult to eradicate.

The obstruction may lead to the development of bladder diverticula. Infected residual urine may contribute to the formation of calculi.

Functional obstruction of the intravesical ureter, caused by the hypertrophic trigone, may lead to hydroureteronephrosis.

Treatment

The indications for operative management are impairment of or threat to renal function and bothersome symptoms. Because the degree of obstruction progresses slowly in most patients, conservative treatment may be adequate. Drugs that relax the prostatic capsule and internal sphincter (α-adrenergic blocking agents) or decrease the volume of the prostate (5α-reductase inhibitors or antiandrogens) have been tried with considerable success.

A. Conservative Measures

Treatment of chronic prostatitis may reduce symptoms. The resolution of a complicating cystitis will usually afford some relief. In order to protect vesical tone, the patient should be cautioned to void as soon as the urge develops. Forcing fluids over a short time causes rapid vesical filling, and decreasing vesical tone; this is a common cause of sudden acute urinary retention and thus should be avoided. Patients with urinary obstructive symptoms should avoid the use of cold remedies including antihistamines, as this also is a common cause of urinary retention. These conservative measures are of only temporary help—if any—in patients with prostatic hyperplasia. There has been recent great interest, particularly by patients, in the use of phytotherapy for LUTS treatment, including saw palmetto, pumpkin seeds, and other plant extracts. Despite the claim of efficacy, however, adequate scientific studies have not been done.

Controversy surrounds choices in the treatment of benign prostatic hyperplasia. No treatment (watchful waiting) may be appropriate in patients who complain of mild to moderate symptoms and thus have low AUA symptom scores. Interest has also focused on nonoperative medical therapy for those with more significant symptoms. Alpha-adrenergic blocking agents relax the internal (bladder neck) sphincter and prostatic capsule. Selective agents that are long-acting and preferentially work for this purpose include doxazosin and tamsulosin. 5α-Reductase inhibitors block conversion of testosterone to dihydrotestosterone (the androgen active in promoting prostate growth) and are useful for large glands, particularly in combination with an alpha-blocker, which has been shown to best prevent urinary retention and other common progressive symptoms of prostatic obstruction.

Catheterization is mandatory for acute urinary retention. Spontaneous voiding may return, but a catheter should be left indwelling for 3 days while detrusor tone returns. If this fails, treatment is indicated.

B. Surgical Measures

There are four classic approaches used in prostatectomy: transurethral, retropubic, suprapubic, and perineal. The transurethral route is preferred in patients with glands weighing under 50 g because morbidity rates are lower and the hospital stay is shorter. Larger glands may require open surgery, depending on the preference and experience of the urologist. The death rate is low in each procedure (1–2%). Potency is at greatest risk when the transperineal exposure is used, but impotence occasionally results following transurethral resection of the prostate.

An alternative approach to the treatment of benign prostatic hyperplasia is transurethral incision of the prostate (TUIP). This procedure consists of incision of the prostate at the bladder neck up to the verumontanum, allowing expansion of the entire prostatic urethra. It is especially effective when the primary point of obstruction is caused by a "median bar" or high posterior lip of the bladder neck.

Additional alternative treatments are transurethral vaporization, laser prostatectomy, transurethral microwave thermotherapy, transurethral needle ablation, and high intensity focused ultrasound ablation of the prostate. Laser prostatectomy seems to have the most promise at present and recent data suggest that Holmium and KTP laser may have nearly the same efficacy as transurethral resection of prostate, with less morbidity. However, long-term results of randomized trials are pending.

Prognosis

Most patients with marked symptoms receive considerable relief and substantial improvement in urine flow following surgical treatment; however, those with milder forms may benefit from drug therapy.

Barry MJ, Fowler FJ Jr., O'Leary MP, et al: The American Urological Association symptom index for benign prostatic hyperplasia: The Measurement Committee of the American Urological Association. J Urol 1992;148:1549.

Lam JS, Cooper KL, Kaplan SA: Changing aspects in the evaluation and treatment of patients with benign prostatic hyperplasia. Med Clin North Am 2004;88:281.

McConnell JD, Barry MJ, Bruskewitz RC: Benign prostatic hyperplasia: diagnosis and treatment. Agency for Health Care Policy and Research. Clin Pract Guideline Quick Ref Guide Clin 1994:8:1.

McConnell JD et al: The effect of finasteride on the risk of acute urinary retention and the need for surgical treatment among men with benign prostatic hyperplasia. N Engl J Med 1998;338:557.

URETHRAL STRICTURE

Acquired urethral strictures in males may be due to external trauma or to prior instrumentation (most common). Strictures may be inflammatory, due to gonorrhea, tuberculous urethritis, or schistosomiasis, or may rarely be a complication of cancer. The common presenting symptoms are dysuria, weak stream, splaying of the urinary stream, urinary retention, and urinary tract infection. Evidence of scarring due to trauma or induration and perineal fistula may be seen. Urethroscopy reveals the degree of narrowing. A retrograde urethrogram will delineate the site and degree of stricture.

Urethral stricture must be differentiated from bladder outlet obstruction due to prostatism, impacted urethral stones, urethral foreign bodies, and tumors.

Initial treatment consists of transurethral direct vision internal urethrotomy (incision of the stricture). Successful results are obtained in 75% of patients. For long dense strictures or those failing to respond to an initial internal urethrotomy, open surgical repair is indicated. This is probably best achieved by the transpubic or perineal route if the lesion involves the membranous urethra. If the mid urethra is involved, the perineal approach is indicated; if the distal urethra is involved, the ventral penile approach is appropriate. End-to-end anastomosis is satisfactory, but a one-stage inlay patch graft, tube, or pedicle flap of preputial skin is currently favored for most strictures.

Andrich DE et al: Urethral strictures and their surgical treatment. BJU Int 2000;86:571.

Kavoussi LR et al: Laparoscopic pyeloplasty. J Urol 1993;150:1891.

Kessler TM et al: Long-term results of surgery for urethral stricture: a statistical analysis. J Urol 2003;170:840.

McAninch JW: Reconstruction of external urethral strictures: circular fasciocutaneous penile flap. J Urol 1993;149:488.

Wessels H et al: Current controversies in anterior urethral stricture repair: free-graft versus pedicled skin-flap reconstruction. World J Urol 1998;16:175.

URINARY TRACT INFECTIONS

Urinary tract infection is the second most common type of infection in humans and is frequently encountered by primary care physicians as well as urologists.

These infections are caused by a variety of pyogenic bacteria that typically produce a nonspecific tissue response. The most common organisms are gram-negative bacteria, particularly *Escherichia coli.* Less common are *Enterobacter aerogenes, Proteus vulgaris, Proteus mirabilis, Pseudomonas aeruginosa,* and *Enterococcus faecalis.*

Owing to the short length of the female urethra and bacterial colonization of the introitus, ascending infection is a common occurrence in young girls and in sexually active women. In males, ascending infection is usually a consequence of urethral instrumentation.

Though relatively uncommon, descending or hematogenous urinary tract infection is usually associated with local urinary tract disorders—most commonly, obstruction and stasis; less commonly, trauma, foreign bodies, or tumors.

Lymphatic spread occasionally occurs from the large bowel or from the cervix and adnexa in the female through the perivesical and periureteral lymphatics.

Direct extension to the urinary bladder of nearby inflammatory processes—eg, appendiceal abscess, enterovesical fistula, or pelvic abscess—may occur.

Predisposing Factors

Infection is usually initiated or sustained by predisposing factors. Predisposing systemic factors include diabetes mellitus, immunosuppression, and malnutrition; these disorders probably favor urinary tract infection by interfering with normal bladder and body defense mechanisms. Predisposing local factors include incontinence, constipation, organic or functional obstruction, stasis (residual urine), foreign bodies (especially catheters and stones), tumors, or necrotic tissue. Vesicoureteral reflux facilitates transport of bacteria from the bladder to the kidney, and this subsequently predisposes to pyelonephritis.

Classification of Urinary Tract Infection

Urinary tract infection is classified as (1) upper urinary tract infection (most commonly, acute or chronic pyelonephritis or infection due to renal abscess); (2) lower urinary tract infection (cystitis or urethritis); or (3) genital infection (prostatitis, epididymitis, seminal vesiculitis, or orchitis).

Urologic Instrumentation or Surgery & Urinary Tract Infection

In the absence of urinary tract infection, surgery of the upper urinary tract rarely requires prophylactic antibacterial therapy. In the presence of infection, one attempts to sterilize the system before operation. If stenting or tube drainage is required and there are no symptoms of infection, colonization by urea-splitting organisms such as *P mirabilis* or *Klebsiella pneumoniae* does not call for antibacterial therapy until the stent or tube is to be removed. Urine culture is obtained approximately 24 hours before removal, and specific antibacterial therapy is started at that time.

With lower urinary tract surgery, the situation is different. Even when the urine is sterile, antibacterial therapy is advised before operations involving the urethra and the bladder, especially for women in whom contamination from vaginal organisms is likely. Men undergoing prostatectomy for obstructive prostatism often have urinary tract infection, particularly when catheter drainage is used preoperatively. In these cases, antimicrobial therapy is necessary before and after surgery to prevent bacteremia.

In the presence of urinary tract infection, any urethral instrumentation poses a threat of bacteremia—more apt to occur in males than in females. Appropriate antibacterial coverage should be instituted before manipulation.

When the urinary tract cannot be sterilized, effective serum levels of antibiotic (eg, aminoglycoside plus ampicillin) should be achieved before instrumentation.

A. Principles of Catheterization

After a short-term single catheterization, the rate of infection is 1–5%. However, in certain patients—pregnant women, elderly or debilitated patients—and in the presence of urologic disease, the risk is much higher. An indwelling catheter often leads to colonization, especially in women. The incidence is proportionate to the duration of catheterization and reaches approximately 95% after 5 days.

Strict aseptic technique is of critical importance in catheterization. Proper cleansing of the genitalia is essential. Iodophor preparations may be used for cleaning the vaginal introitus or the glans penis. Many common urinary tract pathogens are present in normal colonic flora, and these organisms often gain access to the urinary tract of catheterized patients. Cross-contamination of urinary catheters (passive transmission of bacteria from patient to patient on the hands of hospital personnel) is a frequent mode of transfer of resistant organisms. Measures directed to the prevention of catheter cross-contamination are essential. Closed catheter drainage is probably the best way to reduce cross-contamination.

With sterile technique during catheterization and a closed drainage system, most catheters can be kept sterile for 48–72 hours. In a closed drainage system, an added airlock or one-way valve preventing reflux of urine from the collecting bag to the draining tubes also helps prevent infection. The general principles are as follows: (1) Indwelling catheters should be used only when absolutely necessary. (2) Catheters should be inserted with strict aseptic technique. (3) A closed drainage system, preferably with a one-way valve, is advisable. (4) Nonobstructed dependent drainage is essential. (5) Unnecessary irrigation of the system should be avoided. (6) If the catheter is needed for a prolonged period, it should be changed every 2–3 weeks to minimize encrustation and stone formation. (7) The urine of catheterized patients should be cultured before manipulation. (8) Catheterized patients with asymptomatic catheter colonization should be given antibiotics just before the catheter is removed—not during the period of catheterization unless symptomatic infection occurs.

B. Evaluation

Imaging of the urinary tract is recommended in every febrile infant or young child following the first urinary tract infection. Imaging includes a renal and bladder ultrasound and a voiding cystourethrogram. The renal ultrasound may detect hydronephrosis, duplication anomalies, stones, or abnormalities of the bladder wall and should be obtained at the earliest convenient time. A cystogram may be obtained by instillation of contrast medium with fluoroscopy or by instillation of a radionuclide. Radionuclide cystography has the advantage of decreased radiation, while the contrast-voiding cystourethrogram has the advantage of providing better anatomic detail, which may help detect bladder/urethral abnormalities. Either method should include a voiding phase since reflux is the most likely abnormality to be detected and may only occur with voiding. The cystogram should be obtained once the child is free of infection. Imaging recommendations in adults with a urinary tract infection vary depending on the patient's past history and present symptoms.

C. Antibacterial Therapy

The choice of antibiotics depends on the type of organism and its sensitivity, as determined by urine cultures. For uncomplicated infection, adequate urine concentrations of the antibiotic determine efficacy, but in cases of bacteremia and septic shock, serum concentrations are crucial. Commonly used oral medications are sulfonamides, nitrofurantoin, ampicillin, trimethoprim-sulfamethoxazole, fluoroquinolones, and oxytetracycline. For parenteral therapy, aminoglycosides and cephalosporins are effective against the most common organisms, ie, *P mirabilis, E aerogenes,* and *P aeruginosa.*

ACUTE PYELONEPHRITIS

ESSENTIALS OF DIAGNOSIS

- *Chills, fever, and flank pain.*
- *Frequency and urgency of urination; dysuria.*
- *Pyuria and bacteriuria.*
- *Bacterial growth on urine cultures.*

General Considerations

Except in the presence of stasis, foreign bodies, trauma, or instrumentation, pyelonephritis is an ascending type of infection. Pathogenic organisms usually reach the kidney from the bladder, often via an incompetent ureterovesical junction.

Clinical Findings

A. Symptoms and Signs

In acute attacks, pain is present in one or both flanks. Diagnosis in infants requires a high index of suspicion since they may present with nonspecific symptoms such as fever and failure to thrive. Young children commonly present with poorly localized abdominal pain; irritative lower urinary tract symptoms may be present. Chills and fever are common. Severe infection may produce hypotension, peripheral vasoconstriction, and acute renal failure. Gross hematuria is not common.

B. Laboratory Findings

Pyuria and bacteriuria are consistent findings. Leukocytosis with a shift to the left is common. Urine culture identifies the organism.

C. Imaging Studies

In acute attacks, only minimal changes such as delayed visualization and poor concentrating ability are noted on intravenous urography. CT scans may demonstrate zones of decreased enhancement in the renal parenchyma as well as perinephric fat stranding. Renal or ureteral calculi may be seen on plain abdominal x-rays or nonenhanced CT scans. Chest x-ray may show a small ipsilateral pleural effusion.

Differential Diagnosis

Pneumonia, acute cholecystitis, or splenic infarction can be confused with pyelonephritis. Acute appendicitis will sometimes cause pyuria and microhematuria. Any acute abdominal illness such as pancreatitis, diverticulitis, or intestinal angina can simulate pyelonephritis. Appropriate chest x-rays and urinalysis will usually make the distinction.

Complications

If the diagnosis is missed in the acute stage, the infection may become chronic. Both acute and chronic pyelonephritis lead to progressive renal damage.

Treatment

Specific antibiotic therapy should be given for at least 7 days to eradicate the infecting organism after proper identification and sensitivity determination. Symptomatic treatment is indicated for pain and irritative voiding symptoms. Adequate fluid intake to assure optimum urinary output is required. Failure to simultaneously identify and treat predisposing factors (eg, obstruction) is the principal cause of failure to respond to therapy, leading to chronic pyelonephritis.

Prognosis

The prognosis is good with adequate treatment of both the infection and its predisposing cause, depending on the degree of preexisting renal parenchymal damage.

EMPHYSEMATOUS PYELONEPHRITIS

Emphysematous pyelonephritis is a form of acute necrotizing pyelonephritis secondary to a gas-producing bacteria (*E coli in 66% of cases and Klebsiella in 26%*). It is commonly seen in patients with poorly controlled diabetes (over 90% of cases) or in patients with upper urinary tract obstruction. The diagnosis is made by the usual signs of acute pyelonephritis and by the presence of gas in the renal collecting system and parenchyma seen on plain films, ultrasound, or CT. The condition is life-threatening, with a mortality rate of 40–80% with intravenous antibiotics alone. Obstruction requires drainage either percutaneously or by stent placement. Operative treatment, including nephrectomy and drainage along with antibiotics, decreases the mortality rate to less than 20%.

CHRONIC PYELONEPHRITIS

Chronic pyelonephritis is the result of inadequately treated or recurrent acute pyelonephritis. The diagnosis is primarily made by x-ray, since patients rarely have signs or symptoms until late in the course, when they develop chronic flank pain, hypertension, anemia, or renal failure. Pyuria is not a consistent finding. Because chronic pyelonephritis may be a progressive localized immune response initiated by bacteria long since eradicated, urine cultures are usually sterile. Early cases may have no findings on intravenous urography, whereas in late cases it may reveal small kidneys with typical caliceal deformities (clubbing), with evidence of peripheral scarring and a thin cortex. Voiding cystourethrography may document vesicoureteral reflux as the cause. Complications include hypertension, stone formation, and chronic renal failure.

Antibiotic treatment is not helpful in these patients unless ongoing infection can be documented. The prognosis depends on the status of renal function but is generally not good, particularly when the disease is contracted in childhood. Progressive deterioration of renal function usually occurs.

Xanthogranulomatous pyelonephritis is a form of chronic pyelonephritis seen most frequently in middle-aged diabetic women and rarely in children. The disease is usually unilateral and is associated with prolonged obstructing nephrolithiasis. Patients often have nonspecific symptoms similar to those of acute pyelonephritis but have an enlarged kidney with calculi and a mass often indistinguishable from tumor. Proteus species are common causative agents. Nephrectomy is usually the treatment of choice, though a partial nephrectomy may be performed for focal disease. Histologic examination confirms the diagnosis following nephrectomy by the demonstration of foamy lipid-laden macrophages.

PAPILLARY NECROSIS

This disorder consists of ischemic necrosis of the renal papillae or of the entire pyramid. Excessive ingestion of analgesics, sickle cell trait, diabetes, obstruction with infection, and systemic conditions decreasing renal blood flow are common predisposing factors.

The symptoms are usually those of chronic cystitis with recurring exacerbations of pyelonephritis. Renal pain or renal colic may be present. Azotemic manifestations may be the presenting symptoms. In acute attacks, localized flank tenderness and generalized toxemia may occur. Laboratory findings consist of pyuria, hematuria, occasionally glycosuria, and acidosis. Impaired kidney function is shown by elevated serum creatinine and urea nitrogen. Intravenous urography usually shows impaired function and poor visualization in advanced cases. Evidence of ulceration, cavitation, or linear breaks in the base of the papillae and radiolucent defects due to sloughed papillae may be seen; the latter may become calcified. Retrograde urograms may be needed for proper imaging if kidney function is markedly impaired.

Preventive measures consist of proper management of diabetic patients with recurrent infections and avoidance of chronic use of analgesic compounds containing phenacetin and aspirin.

Intensive antibacterial therapy may be needed, though it is commonly unsuccessful in eradicating infection. Little can be done surgically except to remove obstructing papillae and correct predisposing factors (eg, reflux, obstruction) if identified.

In severe cases, the prognosis is poor. Renal transplantation may be required.

RENAL ABSCESS

While renal abscess is occasionally due to hematogenous spread of a distant staphylococcal infection, most abscesses are secondary to chronic nonspecific infection of the kidney, often complicated by stone formation. The onset may be acute, with high fever, but occasionally low-grade fever and general malaise are the presenting symptoms. Localized costovertebral angle tenderness and a palpable flank mass may be present. A mass may be evident on intravenous urograms, DTPA scans, sonograms, CT scans, or renal angiograms. If the abscess is due to hematogenous spread, the urine will not contain bacteria unless the abscess has broken into the pelvicaliceal system. More frequently, gram-negative organisms are found, as would be expected in light of the preponderance of ascending infection.

If organism sensitivity can be established by appropriate tests (blood and urine cultures and sensitivity tests), treatment with the proper antibiotic is indicated. Many infections have responded to percutaneous drainage and irrigation with antibiotic solutions, especially in cases of unilocular abscess cavity seen on either ultrasound or CT examination. In multilocular abscess or persistent bacteremia despite percutaneous drainage, surgical drainage or even heminephrectomy may be necessary.

When the abscess is found to be secondary to chronic renal infection, nephrectomy is usually indicated because of advanced destruction of the kidney.

PERINEPHRIC ABSCESS

Abscess between the renal capsule and the perirenal fascia most often results from rupture of an intrarenal abscess into the perinephric space. *E coli* is the most common causative organism. The pathogenesis usually begins with severe pyonephrosis secondary to obstruction, as with renal or ureteral calculi. Clinical findings are similar to those of renal abscess. A pleural effusion on the affected side and signs of psoas muscle irritation are common. Abdominal plain films may show obliteration of the psoas muscle shadow, and an intravenous urogram may show poor concentration of contrast medium and hydronephrosis. CT scan is the current study of choice for diagnosis.

Treatment involves prompt drainage of the abscess and use of appropriate systemic antibiotics, including coverage of anaerobes. Percutaneous drainage is often successful; however, open surgical drainage is necessary if percutaneous drainage is incomplete. Mortality ranges between 20% and 50% with antibiotics and drainage, whereas treatment with antibiotics alone increases this rate to 75–100%.

CYSTITIS

Cystitis is more common in females and is usually an ascending infection. In males, it usually occurs in association with urethral or prostatic obstruction, prostatitis, foreign bodies, or tumors. The urinary bladder is normally capable of clearing bacterial inoculation unless an underlying pathologic process interferes with its defensive mechanisms.

In the acute phase, the principal symptoms of cystitis are dysuria, frequency, urgency, and hematuria; low-grade fever and suprapubic, perineal, and low back pain may be present. In chronic cystitis, irritative symptoms are usually milder.

Evidence of prostatitis, urethritis, or vaginitis may be present. Laboratory findings, in addition to hematuria, consist of bacteriuria and pyuria. Leukocytosis is not common. Urine culture identifies the organism. Cystoscopy is not advisable in the acute phase. In chronic cystitis, evidence of mucosal irritation may be present.

In any documented recurrent lower urinary tract infection (particularly in males), a complete urologic workup is indicated. Instrumentation is contraindicated in the acute phase, but cystoscopy is essential to identify the predisposing factor in chronic or recurrent bacterial cystitis.

Specific antibacterial therapy is given according to sensitivity testing of recovered organisms (*E coli* in > 80% of cases). Sterilization of urine should usually be followed by a variable period of continuous antibiotic therapy (depending upon the predisposing factor or the chronicity and recurrence of the disease). Prolonged suppressive medication is usually indicated in cases associated with voiding dysfunction.

In women with recurrent postcoital cystitis, premedication (eg, sulfonamides, nitrofurantoin) on the night of intercourse and the following day in addition to immediate postcoital voiding decreases recurrences.

PROSTATITIS

Acute Bacterial Prostatitis

Acute bacterial prostatitis is a severe acute febrile illness caused by ascending coliform bacteria, which frequently colonize the male urethra. Symptoms include high fever; chills; low back and perineal pain; and urinary frequency and urgency, with diminished stream or retention. On examination, the prostate is extremely tender, swollen, and warm to the touch. A fluctuant abscess may be palpable. The prostate must be examined cautiously, because vigorous palpation may cause acute septicemia. Laboratory findings include pyuria, bacteriuria, and leukocytosis.

Transurethral manipulation by catheter or cystoscopy should be avoided; urinary retention should be treated by introducing a percutaneous suprapubic tube. Treatment with systemic antibiotics (fluoroquinolones or aminoglycosides and ampicillin-cephalosporin) should be started immediately and should be adjusted later when results of urine culture or blood culture (or both) and sensitivity tests are known. *E coli* is found in 80% of cases. Treatment with oral antibiotics for several weeks after the initial phase has subsided is necessary to eradicate the bacteria completely. A prostatic abscess usually requires open perineal drainage or transurethral unroofing. The prognosis is good if treatment is thorough and prompt.

Chronic Prostatitis

Chronic prostatitis is a common and complex problem. With differential diagnosis including urethritis, bacterial and nonbacterial prostatitis, prostatodynia (chronic pelvic pain syndrome [CPPS]), and seminal vesiculitis, assigning the correct diagnosis may challenge even the expert. The symptoms are varied and include suprapubic pain, low back pain, orchialgia, dysuria at the tip of the penis, and urinary frequency and urgency. The urinalysis may be normal. There may be a clear white urethral discharge. Prostate examination may reveal a soft, boggy prostate.

Expressed prostatic secretions may contain numerous leukocytes (> 10 per high-power field) in clumps as well as macrophages. Cultures of urine are usually sterile, but cultures of expressed prostatic secretions and urine obtained after prostatic massage are usually positive in bacterial prostatitis. Chlamydia or Ureaplasma may be an offending organism, particularly in males under age 35. Determination of the site of infection may require differential cultures. The first part of the voided urine stream is collected as VB_1 and the midstream specimen as VB_2. The prostate is then massaged to obtain expressed prostatic secretions (EPS), and the postmassage urine is collected as VB_3. The differential leukocyte and bacterial counts from each of these specimens can help localize the site of infection. If VB_1 has high levels of leukocytes and bacteria relative to the other specimens, urethritis is likely; if VB_2 has high levels, a site above the bladder neck is likely; and if the EPS, VB_3, or both have high counts, prostatitis is likely.

Treatment depends on culture results, but if there is no bacterial growth on culture, tetracycline, 250–500 mg four times a day for 14 days, may be curative. For chronic bacterial prostatitis, at least a 6-week course of a fluoroquinolone or trimethoprim-sulfamethoxazole is often given. Surgical treatment for prostatitis is rarely indicated or helpful. Some patients improve following discontinuation of caffeine and alcohol, and a few respond to repeated prostatic massage. Patients with no evidence of bacterial infection or obstructive findings and those who have recurrent pelvic pain in association with voiding dysfunction (eg, intermittent or weak urinary stream) may be treated with α-adrenergic blocking agents or biofeedback to decrease the internal and external sphincter tone. 5α-reductase inhibitors may be helpful, and phytotherapy has proponents but needs further study.

Nickel JC: Recommendations for the evaluation of patients with prostatitis. World J Urol 2003;21:75.

Schaeffer AJ: Etiology and management of chronic pelvic pain syndrome in men. Urology 2004;63(Suppl 3A):75.

ACUTE EPIDIDYMITIS

Acute epididymitis is most commonly a disease of young males, caused by bacterial infection ascending from the urethra or prostate. The disease is less common in older males, but when it does occur, it is most often due to infection secondary to urinary tract obstruction or instrumentation.

The symptoms are sudden pain in the scrotum, rapid unilateral scrotal enlargement, and marked tenderness that extends to the spermatic cord in the groin and may be relieved by scrotal elevation **(Prehn's sign)**. Fever is present. An acute hydrocele may result, and secondary orchitis with a swollen, painful testicle may occur. Laboratory studies reveal pyuria, bacteriuria, and marked leukocytosis.

Epididymitis must be differentiated from torsion of the testis, testicular tumor, and tuberculous epididymitis. A technetium Tc 99m pertechnetate scan reveals increased uptake with epididymitis but decreased uptake with torsion. Scrotal ultrasound will distinguish between the solid mass of a testicular tumor and an enlarged, inflamed epididymis and can also identify epididymal or testicular abscess, which will require operative treatment. Increased blood flow on Doppler ultrasound also helps distinguish epididymitis from torsion, though it is not completely reliable.

Cultured aspirates from inflamed epididymides of men under age 35 tend to show gonococci and chlamydiae; in men older than 35, *E coli* is most common. Epididymal aspiration for culture is not required routinely, however. Pyuria with a negative urine culture suggests the presence of chlamydial infection in both prostate and epididymis. (See also Tuberculosis, below.)

Treatment consists of antibiotics, usually ceftriaxone and doxycycline in men under age 35 and fluoroquinolones in those over age 35. In some patients, pain is relieved by scrotal hypothermia, and consideration should be given to infiltration of the spermatic cord by 1% bupivacaine. Nonsteroidal anti-inflammatory drugs are recommended to aid in pain relief. In most instances, prompt treatment will result in rapid resolution of pain, fever, and swelling. Patients must refrain from exertion for 1–3 weeks.

Exacerbations can be controlled by treating the predisposing factor. Chronic epididymitis rarely resolves completely; it has no consequences except, occasionally in bilateral cases, sterility due to scarring and obstruction of the delicate epididymal tubules. Rarely, epididymectomy is necessary.

TUBERCULOSIS

Tuberculosis is a commonly missed genitourinary infection that should be considered in any case of pyuria without bacteriuria or in any case of urinary tract infection that does not respond to treatment.

Genitourinary tuberculosis is always secondary to pulmonary infection, though in many cases, the primary focus has healed or is quiescent. Infection occurs via the hematogenous route. The kidneys and (less commonly) the prostate are the principal sites of urinary tract involvement, though any part of the genitourinary system can be affected.

Pathology

Renal tuberculosis usually starts as a tuberculoma that gradually enlarges, caseates, and finally ulcerates, breaking into the pelvicaliceal system. Caseation and scarring are the principal pathologic features of renal tuberculosis. In the ureter, tuberculosis usually leads to distal strictures, periureteritis, and mural fibrosis.

In the bladder, the infection is characterized by areas of hyperemia and a coalescent group of tubercles, followed by ulcerations. Bladder wall fibrosis and contraction are the end results.

Urethral involvement in the male is uncommon but when present leads to urethral stricture, usually in the bulbous portion. Periurethral abscess and fistula are possible complications.

Genital tuberculosis may involve the prostate, seminal vesicles, and epididymides, either separately or in association with renal involvement. Tubercle formation with later caseation and fibrosis is the basic pathologic feature. The prostate becomes enlarged, with palpable nodules and an irregular consistency. The affected seminal vesicle is fibrotic and distended. Induration and thickening of the epididymis and beading of the vas deferens are characteristic findings. The testicles are rarely involved.

Clinical Findings

A. Symptoms and Signs

The patient commonly presents with lower urinary tract irritation, usually with pyuria. Less common manifestations are hematuria, renal pain, and renal colic.

B. Laboratory Findings

"Sterile" pyuria is the rule, but 15% of cases have secondary bacterial infection (eg, *E coli*). *Mycobacterium tuberculosis* can be identified on an acid-fast stain of the centrifuged sediment of a 24-hour urine specimen or by culture of the first morning urine collected on 3 successive days (positive in 90% of cases).

C. Imaging Studies

Radiologic findings that suggest genitourinary tuberculosis include moth-eaten, caseous renal cavities or bizarre, irregular calices. Strictures in straight, rigid, moderately dilated ureters and a contracted bladder with vesicoureteral reflux are all suggestive evidence.

Treatment

A. Medical Treatment

Tuberculosis must be treated as a systemic disease. Once the diagnosis is established, medical treatment is indicated regardless of the need for surgery. Whenever possible, medical treatment should be continued for at least 3 months before surgery is considered.

Active medications against tuberculosis include rifampin, isoniazid, pyrazinamide, ethambutol, and streptomycin. Standard initial treatment is with rifampin, isoniazid, and pyrazinamide for 8 weeks. Pyridoxine, 100 mg/d, is given in divided doses to counteract the vitamin B_6 depletion effect of isoniazid. In patients with more severe infections, ethambutol or streptomycin may be added to the initial treatment. Following the initial 8 weeks of therapy, rifampin and isoniazid are continued in combination three times per week for another 8 weeks. Liver function tests must be followed in view of the hepatotoxicity of rifampin, isoniazid, and pyrazinamide.

B. Surgical Measures

If medical therapy fails to cure a unilateral lesion, nephrectomy may be necessary. However, this is rare. In bilateral disease that has seriously damaged one kidney and is in an early stage in the other, unilateral nephrectomy may be considered; in localized polar lesions, partial nephrectomy may be done.

In unilateral epididymal involvement, epididymectomy plus contralateral vasectomy is indicated to prevent descent of the infection to the prostate; bilateral epididymectomy should be done if both sides are involved.

For a severely contracted bladder, augmentation enterocystoplasty will increase vesical capacity following eradication of the infection.

Prognosis

In a high percentage of cases, cure is obtained by medical means. Unilateral renal lesions have the best prognosis.

Cooper CS et al: The outcome of stopping prophylactic antibiotics in older children with vesicoureteral reflux. J Urol 2000;163:269.

Eastham J et al: Xanthogranulomatous pyelonephritis: clinical findings and surgical considerations. Urology 1994;43:295.

Jones BF et al: Acute renal failure due to acute pyelonephritis. Am J Nephrol 1991;11:257.

Lang EK: Renal, perirenal, and pararenal abscesses: percutaneous drainage. Radiology 1990;174:109.

Loughlin KR: Management of urologic problems during pregnancy. Urology 1994;44:159.

Lucas MJ et al: Urinary infection in pregnancy. Clin Obstet Gynecol 1993;36:855.

Mokrzycki MH: Renal malacoplakia with papillary necrosis and renal failure. Am J Kidney Dis 1992;19:587.

Saw KC et al: Tuberculosis prostatitis: nodularity may simulate malignancy. Br J Urol 1993;72:249.

Stapleton A et al: Postcoital antimicrobial prophylaxis for recurrent urinary tract infection: a randomized, double-blind, placebo-controlled trial. JAMA 1990;264:703.

Talner LB et al: Acute pyelonephritis: can we agree on terminology? Radiology 1994;192:297.

Wise GJ, Marella VK: Genitourinary manifestations of tuberculosis. Urol Clin North Am 2003;30:111.

CALCULI

RENAL STONE

ESSENTIALS OF DIAGNOSIS

- *Flank pain, hematuria, pyelonephritis, previous stone passage.*
- *Costovertebral tenderness.*
- *Red cells in urine.*
- *Stone visualized on urography, ultrasonography, or spiral CT scan.*

General Considerations

Most stones are composed of calcium salts (oxalate, phosphate) or magnesium-ammonium phosphate—the latter secondary to urea-splitting organisms. Most calcium stones are idiopathic (ie, idiopathic hypercalciuria). In patients with hyperparathyroidism or those who ingest large amounts of calcium or vitamin D or in patients who are dehydrated or immobilized, hypercalciuria promotes stone formation. Recent evidence suggests that calcium stones may be initiated by cholesterol deposits in the vasa recta at the tip of the renal papilla due to repeated vascular injury, which eventually erodes into the calyx, forming a stone nidus.

The less common metabolic stones, cystine and uric acid, usually form secondary to hypersecretion of these substances or to a defect in urinary acidification. Owing to the radiodensity of sulfur, cystine stones are radiopaque (albeit less so than calcium stones), whereas uric acid stones are radiolucent. Stones that obstruct the ureteropelvic junction or ureter lead to hydronephrosis and infection.

Clinical Findings

A. Symptoms and Signs

If the stone acutely obstructs the ureteropelvic junction or a calix, moderate to severe renal pain will be noted, often accompanied by nausea, vomiting, and ileus. Hematuria is common. Symptoms of infection, if present, will be exacerbated. Nonobstructing calculi are usually painless. This includes staghorn calculi, which may form a cast of all calices and the pelvis. In the symptomatic patient, there may be costovertebral angle tenderness and a quiet abdomen. Infection secondary to obstruction may lead to high fever and a rigid abdomen.

B. Laboratory Findings

With acute infection, leukocytosis is to be expected. Urinalysis may reveal red and white blood cells and bacteria. A pH of 7.6 or higher implies the presence of urea-splitting organisms. A pH consistently below 5.5 is compatible with the formation of uric acid or cystine stones. If the pH is fixed between 6.0 and 7.0, renal tubular acidosis should be considered as a cause of nephrocalcinosis. Crystals of uric acid or cystine in the urine are suggestive. A 24-hour urine collection for calcium may reveal hypercalciuria, which occurs with hyperparathyroidism and idiopathic hypercalciuria.

Increases in urine calcium and phosphate plus hypercalcemia (and hypophosphatemia) suggest the presence of hyperparathyroidism. Measurement of serum parathyroid hormone is helpful in patients suspected of having hyperparathyroidism. Excessive urinary uric acid is compatible with uric acid stone formation.

A qualitative test for urinary cystine should be part of the routine evaluation. If levels are elevated, a 24-hour quantitative measurement should be made. Hyperchloremic acidosis suggests renal tubular acidosis with secondary renal calcifications. Total renal function will be impaired only if the stones are bilateral, and particularly if chronic infection complicates the clinical presentation.

C. Imaging Studies

About 90% of calculi are radiopaque (calcium, cystine). Excretory urography is necessary to verify their location within the urinary tract and also affords a qualitative measure of renal function (Figure 40–17). An acutely obstructed kidney may show only increasing density of the renal shadow without significant radiopaque material in the calices. A nonopaque stone (uric acid) will be seen as a radiolucent defect in the opaque contrast media. Calculi larger than 1 cm cast a specific acoustic shadow on ultrasonography. Spiral (helical) CT has become the study of choice in emergent situations, as the entire urinary tract can be scanned rapidly and without contrast injection. Calculi can be readily identified and distinguished from clot or tumor. Plain x-ray of the skeletal system may identify Paget's disease, sarcoidosis, or osteoporosis due to prolonged immobilization responsible for hypercalciuria.

D. Stone Analysis

If a stone has previously been passed or if one is recovered, its chemical composition should be analyzed. Such information may be useful when planning a preventive program.

Differential Diagnosis

Acute pyelonephritis may begin with acute renal pain mimicking that of renal stone. Urinalysis reveals pyuria, and urograms or CT fails to reveal a calculus.

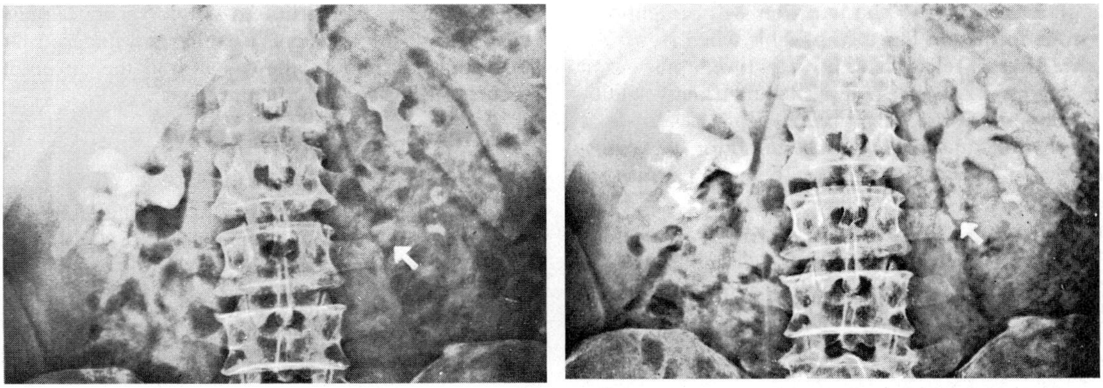

Figure 40–17. Bilateral staghorn calculi and left upper ureteral stone. *Left:* Plain film. Arrow points to ureteral stone. *Right:* Excretory urogram showing bilateral impaired function.

Renal adenocarcinoma may bleed into the tumor, causing acute pain mimicking that of an obstructing stone. Imaging can make the differentiation.

Transitional cell tumors of the renal pelvis or calices will mimic uric acid stone; both are radiolucent. CT scan without contrast or ultrasound will reveal the stone by virtue of increased density compared with adjacent soft tissues.

Renal tuberculosis is complicated by stone formation in 10% of cases. Pyuria without bacteriuria is suggestive. Urography reveals the moth-eaten calices typical of tuberculosis.

Papillary necrosis may cause renal colic if a sloughed papilla obstructs the ureteropelvic junction. Imaging (particularly CT) will settle the issue.

Renal infarction may cause renal pain and hematuria. Evidence of a cardiac lesion, nonfunction of the kidney on urography, and exclusion of a calculus help in differentiation. Infarction is confirmed by angiography, radioisotopic renography, or color Doppler ultrasound.

Complications

Acting as a foreign body, a stone increases the probability of infection. However, primary infection may incite stone formation. A stone lodged in the ureteropelvic junction leads to progressive hydronephrosis. A staghorn calculus, as it grows, may destroy renal tissue by pressure, and the infection that is usually present also contributes to renal damage.

Prevention

An effective preventive regimen depends upon stone analysis and chemical studies of the serum and urine.

A. General Measures

Ensure a high fluid intake (3–4 L/d) to keep solutes well diluted. This measure alone may decrease stone-forming potential by 50%. Combat infection, relieve stasis or obstruction, and advise the patient to avoid prolonged immobilization. For calcium stone formers, stop vitamin D supplements and foods and medications containing calcium salts.

B. Specific Measures

1. Calcium stones—Remove the parathyroid tumor, if present. Reduce dairy products (milk, cheese) in the diet. Calcium in the diet should be less than 400 mg/d. Dietary sodium may promote calcium absorption, and restriction to 100 meq/d may be helpful. Limitation of proteins and carbohydrates may also reduce hypercalciuria.

Oral orthophosphates are effective in reducing the stone-forming potential of urine by decreasing urine calcium and increasing inhibitor activity. Thiazide diuretics such as hydrochlorothiazide, 50 mg twice daily, decrease the calcium content in urine by 50%. If hyperuricosuria is coincident with calcium urolithiasis, then allopurinol and urinary alkalinization can reduce the formation of urate crystals, which may act as a nidus for calcium crystallization.

For a patient with primary absorptive hypercalciuria, cellulose sodium phosphate can be given. This substance will combine with calcium in the gut to prevent absorption.

2. Oxalate stones (calcium oxalate)—Prescribe phosphate or a thiazide diuretic (see above) and limit calcium intake. Elimination of excessive oxalate in coffee, tea, colas, leafy green vegetables, and chocolate may also be helpful. Vitamin C in excess of 1 g can be metabolized in some individuals to oxalate and thus should be avoided.

3. Magnesium-ammonium-phosphate stones—These stones are usually secondary to urinary tract infection due to bacteria that produce urease (primarily proteus species). Eradication of the infection will prevent further stone formation but is impossible when stones are present. After all calculi have been removed, prevention of stone growth is best accomplished by urinary acidification, long-term use of antibiotics, and, perhaps, use of acetohydroxamic acid, a urease inhibitor that maintains an acid urinary pH and may potentiate antibiotic action.

4. Metabolic stones (uric acid, cystine)—These substances are most soluble at a pH of 7.0 or higher. Give sodium-potassium citrate solution, 4–8 mL four times daily orally; monitor the urine pH with a paper indicator. For uric acid stone formers, limit purines in the diet and give allopurinol. Patients with mild cystinuria may need only urinary alkalinization, as described above. For severe cystinuria, penicillamine, 30 mg/kg/d orally, will reduce urinary cystine to safe levels. Penicillamine should be supplemented with pyridoxine, 50 mg/d orally. Propionyl glycine preparations have been used with similar results and fewer side effects.

Treatment

A. Conservative Measures

Intervention is not required for small nonobstructive, asymptomatic caliceal stones. Hydration and dietary management may be sufficient to prevent growth of existing or new calcium stones in patients without metabolic abnormalities. Those with identifiable metabolic disorders may benefit from the specific measures described previously. Patients with primary renal tubular acidosis and secondary stones can be treated with hydration and urinary alkalinization.

B. Percutaneous Intervention (Endourology)

In selected patients with symptomatic or large pelvic stones, percutaneous stone removal may be successful. A percutaneous tract enters the renal collecting system through an appropriate calix **(percutaneous nephrostomy)**. The tract is subsequently dilated, and endoscopic extraction of the stones **(percutaneous nephroscopy and percutaneous nephrolithotomy)** is done. Pulverization by means of ultrasonic, electrohydraulic, or laser probes passed through the nephrostomy tract may also be useful. Residual infection stones may be dissolved by percutaneous irrigation with hemiacidrin. For cystine and uric acid stones, alkaline or other irrigants that increase the specific crystal solubility may be used (eg, *N*-acetyl-L-lysine or propionyl glycine for cystine stones). Specific antibiotic treatment for infection must be given before irrigation to prevent sepsis.

Success with these endourologic methods approaches 100%. The advantages over surgical procedures include no incision, use of local anesthesia in many cases, and rapid recovery and return to employment. Disadvantages include the occasional need for multiple treatments to completely remove the calculi and the uncommon occurrence of significant hemorrhage.

C. Extracorporeal Shock Wave Lithotripsy (ESWL)

With this technique, patients are positioned in the path of shock waves focused on the renal calculi with the aid of fluoroscopy or ultrasound. General or regional anesthesia is required in selected patients, but sedation is sufficient in most cases. The shock waves (more than 1500 are usually given) pulverize the stones, and the small particles pass spontaneously over 2–5 days. Results are excellent. Calcium stones and magnesium-ammonium-phosphate stones have been treated successfully. Because of the physical properties of the crystal lattice, ESWL is not as effective in fragmenting cystine stones. Radiolucent uric acid stones, which can be "visualized" using contrast medium via intravenous pyelography or retrograde ureteropyelography, are amenable to ESWL treatment. Staghorn calculi are amenable to a combined approach: percutaneous nephrolithotomy to remove the major bulk of the stone followed by ESWL to pulverize any inaccessible fragments. Fewer than 10% of patients treated with ESWL have required subsequent endourologic or surgical treatment.

A variety of devices now effectively pulverize stones using less energy and thus can be used with only intravenous sedation; an increased number of pulses are required to obtain the same results as with previous higher-energy devices. Some instruments use ultrasound instead of x-rays for stone localization.

D. Open Surgical Removal of Stones

Endourologic intervention and ESWL have markedly decreased the indications for open surgery. Rarely, both percutaneous nephrolithotomy and ESWL will be contraindicated, and open nephrolithotomy will be necessary. The goal of any approach is to remove all stone fragments, and the approach chosen must allow for intraoperative localization by radiography or ultrasonography. Incisions into the renal pelvis (pyelolithotomy) or the renal parenchyma (radial nephrotomy or anatrophic nephrolithotomy) may be required for complete stone removal. Instillation of a mixture of thrombin and calcium into the kidney causes the fragments to become trapped in a dense clot, which is removed through a pyelotomy incision (coagulum pyelolithotomy). Operative nephroscopy allows a full view of all the calices and removal of all fragments. "Bench" surgery with autotransplantation of the kidney may be required in very few instances. Rarely, poorly functioning kidneys containing symptomatic stones require nephrectomy.

Prognosis

The recurrence rate of renal stone is high unless sufficient attention is paid to measures for prevention of stone formation. The danger of recurrent stone is progressive renal damage due to obstruction and infection.

URETERAL STONE

ESSENTIALS OF DIAGNOSIS

- *Severe ureterorenal colic.*
- *Hematuria.*
- *Nausea, vomiting, and ileus.*
- *Stone visible on excretory urography or spiral CT.*

General Considerations

Ureteral stones originate in the kidney. When symptoms occur, ureteral obstruction is implicit and renal function endangered. Complicating infection may occur. Most ureteral stones pass spontaneously.

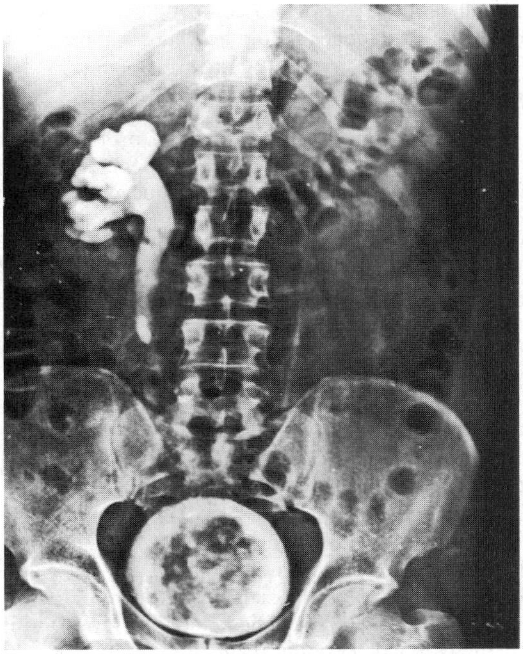

Figure 40–18. Excretory urogram showing right ureteral stone causing hydronephrosis. Large irregular filling defect from unsuspected vesical neoplasm.

Clinical Findings

A. Symptoms and Signs

The onset of pain is usually abrupt. Pain is felt in the costovertebral angle and radiates to the ipsilateral lower abdominal quadrant. Nausea, vomiting, abdominal distention, and gross hematuria are common. When the stone approaches the bladder, symptoms mimic cystitis. If the kidney is infected, acute ureteral obstruction exacerbates the infection.

The patient is usually in such agony that only parenteral opioids will give relief. Costovertebral angle tenderness and guarding may be evident. Absence of bowel sounds and abdominal distention signify ileus. Fever may occur as a result of complicating renal infection.

B. Laboratory Findings

Laboratory findings are the same as for renal stone.

C. Imaging Studies

Excretory urograms or spiral CT is essential. Plain films may reveal an opacity in the region of the ureter. Confirmation of ureteral location requires demonstration of confluence of stone and ureteral contrast (Figure 40–18). Spiral CT is diagnostic. This procedure depicts the degree of obstruction and the size and position of the stone, information that permits selection of appropriate treatment. A radiolucent stone will appear as a filling defect within a proximally dilated ureter—indistinguishable from a ureteral tumor or blood clot by intravenous urography. CT scan will discriminate between stone and tumor or clot density. Cystoscopy, ureteral catheterization, retrograde urography, and ureteroscopy may also be helpful.

Differential Diagnosis

A tumor of the kidney or renal pelvis may bleed, and passage of a blood clot may cause ureteral colic. Urograms may reveal a radiolucent area in the ureter surrounded by the radiopaque urine. A CT scan without contrast agents will reveal no radiopacity.

A primary tumor of the ureter may cause obstructing pain and hematuria. The urogram will reveal the ureteral filling defect, often with secondary obstruction. A CT scan will differentiate a stone from tumor. Urinary cytologic study may reveal malignant transitional cells.

Acute pyelonephritis may cause pain as severe as that seen with stone. Pyuria and bacteriuria are found but do not rule out stone. Stone is absent on urography.

A sloughed papilla (consequent to conditions such as diabetes mellitus) traversing the ureter may cause colic and will produce a urogram compatible with uric acid stone. Papillary sloughs should be evident, however.

Complications

If obstruction from the ureteral stone is prolonged, progressive renal damage may ensue. Bilateral stones may cause anuria, requiring immediate drainage of the proximal collecting system with indwelling ureteral catheters or percutaneous nephrostomy.

Infection may supervene, but many renal infections are iatrogenic, ie, introduced at the time of stone manipulation.

Prevention

See Renal Stone.

Treatment

A. General Measures

Most ureteral stones pass spontaneously—particularly those less than 0.5 cm in diameter. Once the diagnosis has been established, analgesics should be given and the patient hydrated. Periodic plain films should be taken to follow the progress of the stone and interval renal ultrasound studies obtained to assess the degree of hydronephrosis. The urine should be strained until the stone passes in order to recover the calculus for analysis. With larger stones, acute obstruction can be temporarily relieved by inserting an indwelling ureteral stent.

B. Specific Measures

If the stone causes intractable pain, progressive hydronephrosis, or acute infection, it should be removed. Obstructing stones in the upper two-thirds of the ureter can often be successfully treated by simultaneous ureteral catheterization and manipulation of the stone back to the renal pelvis, followed by ESWL or percutaneous nephrolithotomy, as described above. Ureteroscopy permits ultrasonic or laser fragmentation or stone basket retrieval under direct vision. Retrograde basket extraction under fluoroscopic control may be used to remove small distal ureteral stones. Open surgical removal (ureterolithotomy) is only very rarely required for ureteral stones. ESWL has been applied to ureteral stones in the proximal ureter but is more problematic in the distal ureter owing to bone interference by surrounding pelvis, which interferes with imaging and attenuates shock wave force.

Prognosis

About 80% of ureteral stones pass spontaneously. Periodic plain films of the abdomen or excretory urograms will portray progress of the stone and warn of ensuing renal damage that would prompt operative intervention.

VESICAL STONE

Primary vesical calculi are rare in the USA but are common in Southeast Asia and the Middle East. The cause is probably dietary. Secondary stones usually complicate vesical outlet obstruction with residual urine and infection; 90% of those affected are men. Other causes of bladder stasis such as neurogenic bladder and bladder diverticula also promote vesical stone formation. They are common in vesical schistosomiasis or in association with radiation cystitis. Foreign bodies in the bladder may act as a nidus for the precipitation of urinary salts. Most stones contain calcium; some are composed of uric acid.

Clinical Findings

A. Symptoms and Signs

Symptoms of bladder neck obstruction are elicited. There may be sudden interruption of the stream and urethral pain if a stone occludes the bladder neck during voiding. Hematuria is common. Vesical distention may be noted; evidence of urethral stricture or an enlarged prostate is usually found.

B. Laboratory Findings

Pyuria and hematuria are almost always present.

C. Imaging Studies

Vesical calculi are usually radiopaque. Excretory urograms will reveal that the stones are intravesical; residual urine is usually depicted on the postvoiding film. If nonopaque areas are noted, CT scan or ultrasound will differentiate between stones and vesical tumors or blood clots, but direct vision endoscopically is preferred.

D. Instrumental Examination

Inability to pass a catheter or sound into the bladder signifies urethral stricture. Catheterization may demonstrate residual urine. Cystoscopy will visualize the stones and may reveal an obstructing prostate.

Differential Diagnosis

A pedunculated vesical tumor may suddenly occlude the vesical neck during voiding. Excretory urograms, pelvic ultrasound, CT scan, or cystoscopy leads to definitive diagnosis.

Extravesical opacifications may simulate stones on a plain film.

Complications

Acting as foreign bodies, bladder stones exacerbate urine infection and foil antibiotic therapy given for the purpose of sterilizing the urine. Stones obstructing the urethra must be removed.

Prevention

Prevention requires relief of the primary obstruction, removal of the stones, and sterilization of the urine.

Treatment

A. General Measures

Analgesics should be given for pain and antimicrobials for control of infection until the stones can be removed.

B. Specific Measure

Small stones can be removed or crushed transurethrally **(cystolitholapaxy)**. Larger stones are often disintegrated by transurethral electrohydraulic lithotripsy (shock wave generating probe) or laser destruction, or they may require suprapubic transvesical removal (vesicolithotomy). The obstructive lesion must also be corrected.

Prognosis

Recurrent vesical stone is uncommon if the obstruction and infection are treated.

NEPHROCALCINOSIS

Nephrocalcinosis is a precipitation of calcium in the tubules, parenchyma, and, occasionally, the glomeruli. It always causes renal functional impairment, often severe. Stones may be found in the calices and pelvis. The common causes are primary or secondary hyperparathyroidism, excessive milk-alkali or vitamin D intake, or they may be found with severe renal damage associated with hyperchloremic acidosis, renal tubular acidosis, or sarcoidosis. Calcifications may also be seen in the skin, lungs, stomach, spleen, and corneas, or around the joints.

Clinical Findings

A. Symptoms and Signs

There are no specific symptoms. In childhood, the patient may merely fail to thrive. Stones or sand may be passed. The complaints are usually those of the primary disease. Physical examination may reveal an enlarged parathyroid gland, corneal calcifications, and pseudorickets.

B. Laboratory Findings

The urine may be infected. In renal tubular acidosis, the pH is fixed between 6.0 and 7.0. Urinary calcium is high in hyperparathyroidism, both primary and secondary. Tests of renal function are depressed; uremia is common. Hypercalcemia and hypophosphatemia are seen with primary hyperparathyroidism; secondary hyperparathyroidism may be associated with a low serum calcium and an elevated serum phosphate. Hyperchloremic acidosis and hypokalemia accompany renal tubular acidosis.

C. Imaging Studies

A plain x-ray will reveal punctate calcifications in the papillae of the kidneys. Caliceal or pelvic stones may also be noted. The pattern of calcification may have to be differentiated from renal tuberculosis and medullary sponge kidney.

Complications

Complications include renal damage caused by the calcifications and renal and ureteral calculi. Chronic renal infection may complicate the primary disease.

Treatment & Prognosis

The primary cause should be treated, if possible (eg, parathyroidectomy). Discontinue vitamin D, give a low-calcium diet, and force fluids. With hyperchloremic acidosis, alkalinize the urine with potassium citrate. Osteomalacia requires administration of vitamin D and calcium even though nephrocalcinosis is present.

If nephrocalcinosis is secondary to primary renal disease, the outlook is poor. If the cause is correctable and renal function is fairly good, the prognosis is more favorable.

Heneghan JP et al: Helical CT for nephrolithiasis and ureterolithiasis: comparison of conventional and reduced radiation-dose techniques. Radiology 2003;229;575.

Pak CYC: Southwestern Internal Medicine Conference: medical management of nephrolithiasis—a new, simplified approach for general practice. Am J Med Sci 1997;313:215.

Preminger GM: Is there a need for medical evaluation and treatment of nephrolithiasis in the "age of lithotripsy"? Semin Urol 1995;12:51.

Ramakumar S et al: Renal calculi: percutaneous management. Urol Clin North Am 2000;27:617.

Sarica K et al: 371 bladder calculi in a benign prostatic hyperplasia patient. Int Urol Nephrol 1994;26:23.

Segura JW et al: Nephrolithiasis Clinical Guidelines Panel summary report on the management of staghorn calculi. The American Urological Association Nephrolithiasis Clinical Guidelines Panel. J Urol 1994;151:1648.

Shokeir M: Transurethral cystolitholapaxy in children. J Endourol 1994;8:157.

Spencer BA et al: Helical CT and ureteral colic. Urol Clin North Am 2000;27:231.

Stanley KE, Winfield HN: Management of staghorn calculi: percutaneous nephrolithotripsy versus extracorporeal shock wave lithotripsy. Semin Urol 1994;12:15.

Stoller ML et al: The primary stone event: a new hypothesis involving a vascular etiology. J Urol 2004;171:1920.

Vieweg J et al: Unenhanced helical computerized tomography for the evaluation of patients with acute flank pain. J Urol 1998;160:679.

GENITOURINARY TRACT TRAUMA

INJURIES TO THE KIDNEY

ESSENTIALS OF DIAGNOSIS

- *History or evidence of trauma, usually local.*
- *Hematuria.*
- *Flank mass.*
- *Failure to opacify the kidney or extravasation of urine on excretory urography.*

General Considerations

Renal injury is uncommon but potentially serious and often accompanied by multisystem trauma. The most common causes are athletic, industrial, or automobile accidents. The degree of injury may range from contusion to laceration of the parenchyma or disruption of the renal pedicle.

Clinical Findings

A. Symptoms and Signs

Gross hematuria following trauma means injury to the urinary tract. Pain and tenderness over the renal area may be significant but could be due to musculoskeletal injury. Hemorrhagic shock may result from renal laceration and lead to oliguria. Nausea, vomiting, and abdominal distention (ileus) are the rule. Physical examination may reveal ecchymosis or penetrating injury in the costovertebral angle or flank. Extravasation of blood or urine may produce a palpable flank mass. Other injuries should be sought.

B. Laboratory Findings

Serial hematocrit determinations will give clues to persistent bleeding. Hematuria is to be expected, but the absence of hematuria does not exclude renal injury (as in renal vascular injury).

C. Imaging Studies

A plain film may reveal obliteration of the psoas shadow; this suggests the presence of a retroperitoneal hematoma or urinary extravasation. Bowel gas may be displaced from the area. Evidence of transverse vertebral process fractures or rib fracture may be noted. In the past the excretory urogram was used for evaluating renal trauma. Excretory urograms may show a normal kidney if it is mildly contused or may show extravasation of contrast medium if the kidney is lacerated. Nonfunction suggests injury to the vascular pedicle. The excretory urogram should demonstrate that the contralateral kidney is normal. CT scan with intravenous contrast medium is now the method of choice for staging a patient with hemodynamically stable renal trauma. CT scans may miss urinary extravasation if performed too rapidly following intravenous contrast administration—before the contrast is excreted into the collecting system and ureter. If renal vascular damage is suspected and the patient's condition is stable, preoperative renal angiography may facilitate planning of renovascular reconstruction or permit arterial stenting. In special circumstances, selective renal artery embolization may control segmental arterial bleeding. Renal imaging is indicated in any adult with gross hematuria or microscopic hematuria with shock. Imaging is also required with deceleration injuries and is indicated in children with any hematuria > 50 red blood cells per high-power field.

Differential Diagnosis

Bony fractures or contusion of soft tissues in the region of the kidney may cause confusion. Hematuria might be secondary to vesical injury. The absence of a perirenal mass (ie, hematoma or urinoma) or contrast extravasation on urograms or CT scan would rule out significant trauma.

Complications

A. Early

The most serious complication is continued perirenal hemorrhage, which may be fatal. Serial hematocrit, blood pressure, and pulse determinations are essential. Serial CT scans may also be useful. Evidence of an enlarging flank mass implies persistent bleeding. In most cases, bleeding stops spontaneously, probably as a result of tamponade by the perirenal fascia. Delayed bleeding 1 or 2 weeks later is rare. Infection of the perirenal hematoma may occur.

B. Late

Ultrasound should be obtained 1–3 months after surgery to look for progressive hydronephrosis from ureteral obstruction. The blood pressure should be checked at regular intervals, because hypertension may be a late sequela.

Treatment

Treat shock and hemorrhage with fluids and transfusion. Most patients with blunt renal trauma stop bleeding and heal spontaneously. Bed rest is indicated until hematuria resolves. If bleeding persists, laparotomy is indicated.

Penetrating renal trauma requires exploration. Lacerations may be sutured, the collecting system closed, and urinary extravasation drained. Nephrectomy or partial nephrectomy may be necessary to remove devitalized tissue and secure the collecting system.

Late complications may occur. Perinephric abscess should be drained. Hypertension due to renal ischemia requires vascular reconstruction or nephrectomy.

Prognosis

Most injured kidneys heal spontaneously, though the patient must be examined at intervals for the onset of hypertension due to renal ischemia or progressive hydronephrosis due to secondary ureteral stricture. Many patients with genitourinary trauma have associated injuries. In most cases, death is due to associated injury rather than renal injury.

INJURIES TO THE URETER

ESSENTIALS OF DIAGNOSIS

- *Anuria or oliguria; prolonged ileus or flank pain following pelvic operation.*
- *Onset of urinary drainage through wound or vagina.*
- *Demonstration of urinary extravasation or ureteral obstruction by urography.*

General Considerations

Most ureteral injuries are iatrogenic in the course of pelvic surgery. Ureteral injury may occur during transurethral bladder or prostate resection or ureteral manipulation for stone or tumor. Ureteral injury is rarely a consequence of penetrating trauma. Unintentional ureteral ligation during operation on adjacent organs may be asymptomatic, though hydronephrosis and loss of renal function will result. Ureteral division leads to extravasation and ureterocutaneous fistula.

Clinical Findings

A. Symptoms

If the ureteral injury is not recognized at surgery, the patient may complain of flank and lower abdominal pain on the injured side. Ileus and pyelonephritis may develop. Later, urine may drain through the wound (or through the vagina following transvaginal surgery). Wound drainage may be evaluated by comparing creatinine levels found in the drainage fluid with serum levels: urine exhibits very high creatinine levels when compared with serum. Intravenous administration of 5 mL of indigo carmine will cause the urine to appear blue-green; therefore, drainage from a ureterocutaneous fistula becomes blue, while serous drainage remains yellow. Anuria following pelvic surgery not responding to intravenous fluids means bilateral ureteral ligation until proved otherwise. Peritoneal signs may occur if urine leaks into the peritoneal cavity.

B. Laboratory Findings

Microscopic hematuria is usually found but may be absent. Tests of renal function may be normal unless both ureters are occluded.

C. Imaging Studies

Excretory urograms may show evidence of ureteral occlusion. Extravasation of radiopaque fluid may be seen in the region of the ureter. Retrograde ureterography will depict the site and nature (occlusion or division) of the injury.

Ultrasonography may reveal hydroureter and hydronephrosis or a fluid mass representing urinary extravasation. Radionuclide scanning will show delayed excretion, with an accumulation of counts in the pelvis and renal parenchyma resulting from ureteral obstruction; although urinary extravasation is detected, anatomic specificity for site of injury is not clearly defined.

Differential Diagnosis

Ureteral injury may mimic peritonitis if urine leaks into the peritoneal cavity. Excretory urography will reveal the ureteral involvement.

Oliguria may be due to dehydration, transfusion reaction, or bilateral incomplete ureteral injury. A survey of fluid and electrolyte intake and output, including serial body weights, should prove definitive. Total anuria implies bilateral ureteral injury and indicates the need for immediate urologic investigation.

Vesicovaginal and ureterovaginal fistulas may be confused. Methylene blue solution instilled into the bladder will stain the drainage of a vesicovaginal fistula. Cystoscopy may show the vesical defect. Retrograde ureterography should reveal a ureteral fistula. The presence of both injuries occurring simultaneously should also be considered and evaluated.

Complications

These include urinary fistula, ureteral obstruction or stenosis with hydronephrosis, renal infection, peritonitis, and uremia (with bilateral injury).

Prevention

Before operation for large pelvic masses, which may cause displacement of the ureters, catheters should be placed in the ureters to facilitate their identification at surgery. Although the catheters may not prevent injury, they facilitate recognition of a ureteral injury.

Treatment

A. Injury Recognized at Surgery

1. Ureteral division—Repair of a ureter inadvertently cut during surgery consists of anastomosis of the ends over an indwelling stent **(ureteroureterostomy)**, reimplanting the ureter into the bladder if the injury is juxtavesical **(neoureterocystostomy)**, or anastomosing the proximal segment of divided ureter to the side of the contralateral ureter **(transureteroureterostomy)**. The anastomosis must be tension-free and the area of repair must be drained.

2. Ureteral resection—Repair of a ureter from which a segment has been removed requires interposition of a ureteral substitute or mobilization of the proximal and distal ureter to provide a tension-free anastomosis. With loss of the distal ureter, the bladder may be hitched cephalad to the psoas muscle or a bladder flap may be created to facilitate a ureteral implant. In extreme cases, autotransplant of the kidney to the pelvis may be necessary.

B. Injury Discovered After Surgery

Early reoperation is recommended. Depending on the findings, the following procedures may be utilized: ureteroureterostomy, neoureterocystostomy, and transureteroureterostomy. A psoas hitch (as noted above) or a bladder flap may be used when the proximal ureter is short. If a long segment of ureter is not viable, an intestinal ureter may be constructed. If hydronephrosis is advanced or if sepsis develops, percutaneous nephrostomy should precede repair. When the patient's condition is stable, definitive repair can be accomplished. Nephrectomy may be indicated if the contralateral kidney is normal and there is a contraindication to transureteroureterostomy (such as calculi or upper tract transitional cell carcinoma).

Prognosis

In cases of iatrogenic injury, the results are best if the injury is recognized at the time of surgery. Late repair, if severe periureteral fibrosis has developed, is less likely to afford a good outcome.

INJURIES TO THE BLADDER

ESSENTIALS OF DIAGNOSIS

- *History of trauma (including surgical or endoscopic).*
- *Fracture of the pelvis.*
- *Suprapubic pain and abdominal muscle rigidity.*
- *Hematuria.*
- *Extravasation shown on cystogram.*

General Considerations

The most common cause of vesical injury is an external blow over a full bladder. Rupture of the organ is seen in 15% of patients with pelvic fracture. The bladder may be inadvertently opened during pelvic surgery or injured by cystoscopic maneuvers, eg, transurethral resection of bladder tumor. If the injury is intraperitoneal (40% of all bladder ruptures), blood and urine will extravasate into the peritoneal cavity, producing signs of peritonitis. If it is extraperitoneal (54% of all bladder ruptures), a mass will develop in the pelvis. About 6% of all bladder ruptures have a combination of both intra- and extraperitoneal extravasation.

Clinical Findings

A. Symptoms and Signs

There is usually a history of hypogastric or pelvic trauma. Hematuria and suprapubic pain and an inability to void are expected. Associated injury may cause hemorrhagic shock. There is suprapubic tenderness and guarding. Intraperitoneal extravasation causes peritoneal signs, while extraperitoneal extravasation results in formation of a pelvic urinoma.

B. Laboratory Findings

A falling hematocrit reflects continued bleeding. Hematuria is expected in patients who are able to void. A patient who cannot void should be catheterized unless pelvic fracture (and urethral injury) is suspected or blood is noted at the urethral meatus.

C. Imaging Studies

A plain film may reveal fracture of the pelvis. An extraperitoneal collection of blood and urine may displace the bowel gas laterally or out of the pelvis. If bladder trauma is suspected, cystography should precede excretory urography. Extravasation is most reliably demonstrated by a postdrainage cystogram film. If one suspects urethral trauma, a retrograde urethrogram should precede catheter insertion. The excretory urogram may suggest the diagnosis of bladder perforation but by itself is insufficient to exclude bladder injury. A CT cystogram can be used, but images of the bladder obtained by passive bladder filling after catheter clamping are not sufficient to exclude a bladder injury. The bladder should be filled to capacity by gravity with diluted contrast (350–400 mL).

Differential Diagnosis

Renal injury is also associated with trauma and usually presents with hematuria. Excretory urograms show changes compatible with renal trauma; the cystogram is negative.

Injury to the membranous urethra can mimic extraperitoneal rupture of the bladder. A urethrogram will reveal the site of injury. Urethral disruption is a contraindication to urethral catheterization.

Complications

Extraperitoneal extravasation may lead to pelvic abscess. Intraperitoneal extravasation will cause delayed peritonitis, oliguria, and azotemia.

Treatment

Treat shock, hemorrhage, and other life-threatening injuries. Marked extraperitoneal extravasation should be drained, the bladder decompressed by either a suprapubic or urethral catheter, and appropriate antibiotics administered. Small extraperitoneal extravasations are treated nonoperatively by urethral catheter.

Intraperitoneal extravasation of bladder urine requires exploratory laparotomy, midline cystotomy, bladder closure, and bladder catheter drainage. Penetrating injuries (ie, gunshot, stabbing) require exploration and closure of the bladder. The ureters should also be evaluated in all cases of bladder injury by preoperative imaging or intraoperative assessment, which may be done by injecting indigo carmine and looking for ureteral extravasation or retrograde passage of 5F feeding tubes through the ureteral orifice.

Prognosis

Early diagnosis minimizes morbidity and mortality rates. The prognosis depends chiefly upon the severity of associated injuries.

INJURIES TO THE URETHRA

Membranous Urethra

Injury to the membranous urethra is usually a consequence of pelvic fracture and thus is associated with hemorrhage and multi-organ injury. The mechanism of injury is blunt trauma and deceleration resulting in shearing forces applied to the prostate and urogenital diaphragm. Penetrating injuries result from external missiles or laceration by bone fragments acting as secondary projectiles.

If the urethral disruption is incomplete, the patient may be able to void, and hematuria would be inevitable. Urethral injury is suspected if blood is expressed from the urethral meatus. In cases of complete avulsion, extravasation causes a suprapubic mass. Rectal examination may reveal a nonpalpable or upwardly displaced prostate.

X-ray reveals a fractured pelvis; urethrography delineates any extravasation, and cystography identifies an associated bladder injury (Figure 40–19). An immediate excretory urogram or CT scan should be obtained in all cases to assess kidney and ureteral function.

Treatment must be coordinated with care of associated injury. Once a membranous urethral injury with urinary extravasation has been identified, suprapubic cystostomy should be performed either at the time of laparotomy or percutaneously before placement of external pelvic fixation. Definitive urethral repair may be delayed until the patient has recovered from the acute injury and pelvic fractures have healed. Occasionally, when urethral disruption is incomplete, late repair is unnecessary. Primary repair may be indicated in cases of severe prostatomembranous dislocation, major bladder neck laceration, or concomitant pelvic vascular or rectal injury.

Late sequelae are urethral stricture, impotence, and incontinence. Urethral stricture must be identified by retrograde urethrography and may be treated by transurethral incision of the stricture or urethroplasty. Impotence due to injury of nerves to the corpora cavernosa that course adjacent to the membranous urethra may resolve without treatment during the year following injury. Vascular injury of the hypogastric or pudendal arteries may cause impotence following trauma. Cavernosometry and arteriography will confirm the diagnosis; appropriate treatment may include vascular reconstruction. Incontinence depends upon the neurologic status of the patient. Medical or surgical therapy is utilized to increase bladder capacity and bladder outlet resistance.

Bulbous Urethra

The bulbous urethra may be injured as a result of instrumentation or, more commonly, falling astride an

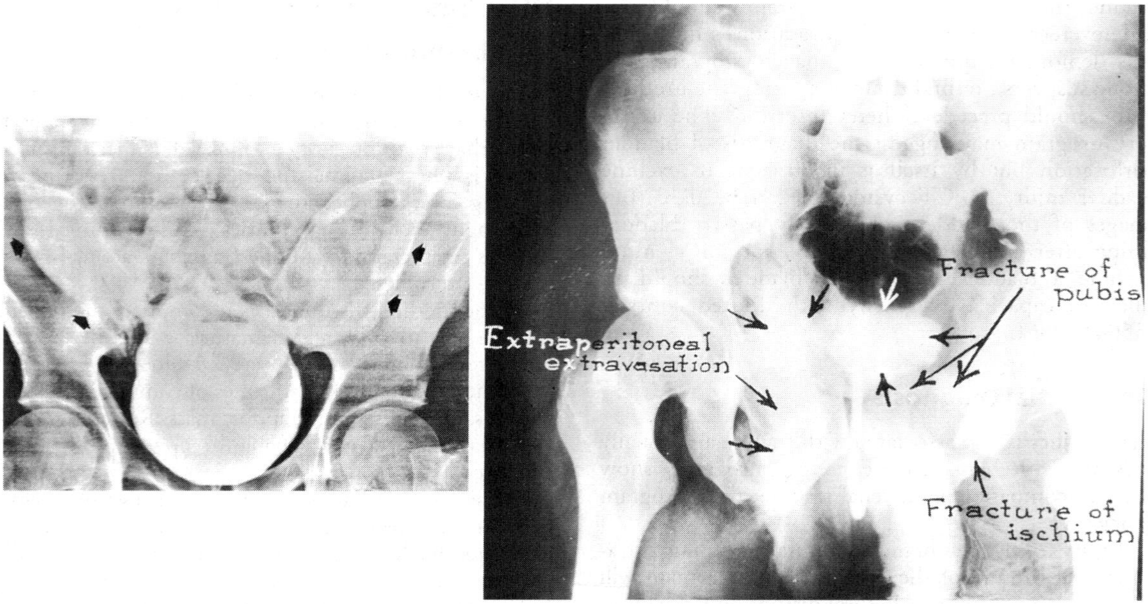

Figure 40–19. Vesical injuries. *Left:* Retrograde cystogram showing intraperitoneal extravasation. Note radiopaque material in both lumbar gutters. *Right:* Retrograde cystogram showing extraperitoneal rupture of the bladder secondary to fracture of the pelvis.

object (straddle injury). Urethral contusion may cause a perineal hematoma without injury to the urethral wall. Laceration will lead to urinary extravasation.

Perineal pain and some urethral bleeding are to be expected. Sudden swelling in the perineum may develop following attempted urination. Examination reveals a perineal mass; swelling due to extravasation of blood and urine involves the penis and scrotum and may spread onto the abdominal wall.

If the patient can void well and the perineal hematoma is small, no treatment is necessary. If urethrography reveals significant extravasation, suprapubic cystostomy should be performed. Minor injury without extravasation (contusion, compression by hematoma) may be managed by careful insertion of a urethral catheter (Figure 40–20).

The only serious complication is stricture, which requires internal urethrotomy or surgical repair.

Pendulous Urethra

External injury to this portion of the urethra is not common, since the penis is so mobile. The erect organ, however, is vulnerable. Most trauma to this area is secondary to instrumentation or sex play. As a rule, these injuries are mild, although a few may be complicated by stricture.

Urethral bleeding and penile swelling are to be expected. A urethrogram will reveal the site and severity of injury.

If voiding is normal, no treatment is required. A large hematoma may require drainage. If significant injury is present, a suprapubic tube should be inserted and delayed surgical repair performed after swelling and inflammation have resolved.

INJURIES TO THE PENIS

Mechanisms of penile injury include penetration, blunt trauma to the erect penis during sexual activity (eg, fracture of corpora cavernosa), avulsion of skin (also known as "power takeoff injury"), and amputation. Pendulous urethral injury is rare (discussed above).

Tourniquet injury is also uncommon; the circumferential compression may be due to a rubber band, a steel ring, string, or a hair and may be exacerbated by subsequent erection. The tourniquet may have been applied unintentionally, but child abuse cases have been reported in which the penis has been ligated as punishment for enuresis.

Treatment includes assessment and care of urethral injuries if present. Removal of tourniquet, split-thickness skin grafting of avulsion injuries, and primary closure of corporal lacerations are principles of therapy. The penis may be acutely reimplanted up to 16 hours following amputation using microsurgical techniques.

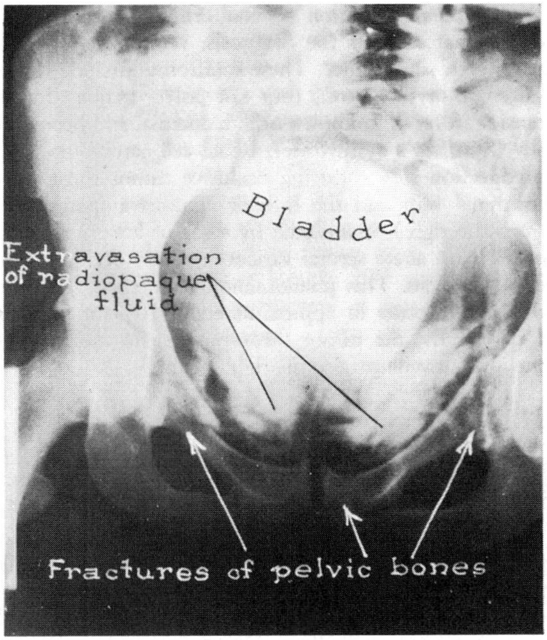

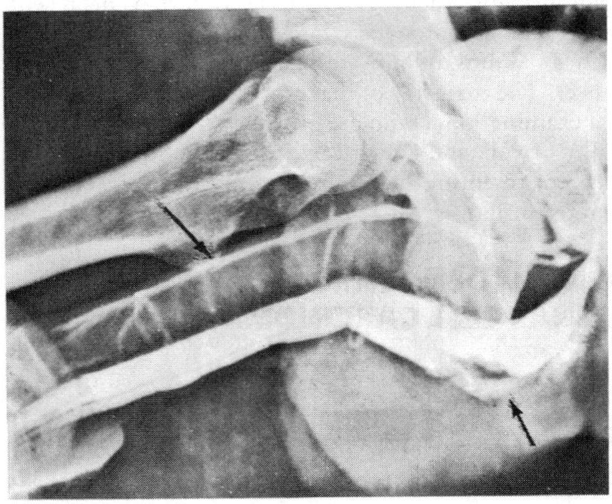

Figure 40–20. Injury to the membranous urethra. *Left:* Retrograde cystogram showing periprostatic extravasation; laceration of membranous urethra with fracture of pelvis. *Right:* Oblique urethrogram showing extravasation in region of bulbous urethra. Pressure injection caused radiopaque solution to enter venous system. (This is the mechanism for emboli if oily lubricants are injected into the urethra.)

INJURIES TO THE SCROTUM & TESTIS

Avulsion of the scrotal skin may require a meshed split-thickness skin graft. If the avulsion is severe, involving the skin and dartos muscle, then the testes may be implanted in the subcutaneous tissue of the thigh or left out and dressed with 0.25% acetic acid-soaked gauze. Scrotal reconstruction is performed at a later time, frequently by using skin grafts, as noted above.

Penetrating trauma rarely injures the mobile testes. Lacerations should be explored, debrided, and closed primarily. If hemorrhage into the tunica vaginalis is noted, drainage is indicated.

Blunt trauma to the testes may cause contusion or rupture. Rupture of the tunica albuginea may be demonstrated by ultrasonography as abnormal echotexture of the parenchyma. In cases of rupture, scrotal exploration allows debridement and closure of the tunica albuginea. The testes may ultimately undergo atrophy despite these efforts.

Brubaker LT, Wilbanks GD: Urinary tract injuries in pelvic surgery. Surg Clin North Am 1991;71:963.

Gomez RG et al: Consensus statement on bladder injuries. BJU Int 2004;94:27.

McAleer IM et al: Genitourinary trauma in the pediatric patient. Urology 1993;42:563.

Morey AF et al: Reconstruction of posterior urethral disruption injuries: outcome analysis in 82 patients. J Urol 1997;157;506.

Santucci RA et al: Evaluation and management of renal injuries: Statement of the Renal Trauma Subcommittee. BJU Int 2004;93:937.

Wessels H et al: Criteria for nonoperative treatment of significant penetrating renal lacerations. J Urol 1997;157:24.

TUMORS OF THE GENITOURINARY TRACT*

Tumors of the genitourinary tract are among the most common neoplastic diseases found in adults. Prostate cancer, for example, is the most common cancer in males (33%), and renal and bladder cancer account for nearly 10% of all malignant tumors in men, but only

* Wilms' tumor is discussed in Chapter 45.

about 3% in women. Even though excellent diagnostic methods are available, one-third of all genitourinary tumors are not found until regional or distant spread has occurred. Advances in diagnosis and treatment of genitourinary tract tumors have occurred in recent years, and the prognosis has improved in conditions such as Wilms' tumor, testicular cancer, and bladder cancer. The mainstay of diagnosis continues to be physical examination, complete urinalysis, intravenous urography or CT, and cystoscopy whenever indicated. Curative treatment of these tumors continues to be surgical in most instances.

RENAL ADENOCARCINOMA (RENAL CELL CARCINOMA)

ESSENTIALS OF DIAGNOSIS

- *Painless gross or microscopic total hematuria.*
- *Solid renal parenchymal mass on intravenous urography with nephrotomograms, renal ultrasound, or abdominal CT scan.*
- *Paraneoplastic syndromes common.*

General Considerations

Malignant tumors of the kidney account for approximately 3% of all tumors in adults. Often the diagnosis is suspected because of microscopic hematuria or manifestations of metastases such as pathologic fractures or superficial skin nodules. The cause is unknown, though a hormonal influence is suspected, as the disease occurs in males three times more commonly than in females. Tobacco use is also implicated. A suppressor gene on chromosome 3p has been shown to be present in von Hippel-Lindau renal cancers as well as in most sporadic renal adenocarcinomas. The cell of origin is in the proximal convoluted tubule, as determined by morphologic and cell surface antigen homology; thus, 85% of these tumors are adenocarcinomas. The tumor metastasizes commonly to the lungs (50–60%), adjacent renal hilar lymph nodes (25%), ipsilateral adrenal (12%), opposite kidney (2%), and lytic lesions in mainly long bones (30–40%).

There are numerous conditions that predispose to renal cell cancer, including adult polycystic kidney disease, von Hippel-Lindau syndrome (cerebellar hemangioblastomas, retinal angiomatosis, and bilateral renal cell carcinoma), and acquired renal cystic disease developing in patients with end-stage renal disease. Paraneoplastic syndromes are common in renal cell carcinoma and are often what suggests the diagnosis, yet they rarely have prognostic significance. These syndromes include hypercalcemia, erythrocytosis (but not polycythemia), hypertension, fever of unknown origin, anemia, and hepatopathy **(Stauffer's syndrome)**. Renal cell carcinoma has a predilection for producing occlusive tumor thrombi in the renal vein and the inferior vena cava (particularly from the right), manifested by signs of lower extremity edema and acute scrotal varicocele when occluding the left renal vein. This phenomenon of inferior vena cava thrombus occurs in approximately 5–10% of patients. Occasionally, the tumor thrombus reaches up through the inferior vena cava to the right atrium.

Clinical Findings

A. Symptoms and Signs

Painless gross or microscopic hematuria throughout the urinary stream ("total hematuria") occurs in 60% of patients. The degree of hematuria is not necessarily related to the size or stage of the tumor. Although a triad of hematuria, flank pain, and a palpable flank mass suggests renal cell carcinoma, fewer than 10% of patients will so present. Both pain and a palpable mass are late events occurring only with tumors that are very large or invade surrounding structures or when hemorrhage into the tumor has occurred. Symptoms due to metastases may be the initial complaint (eg, bone pain, respiratory distress).

B. Laboratory Findings

Microscopic urinalysis will reveal hematuria in most patients. The erythrocyte sedimentation rate may be elevated but is nonspecific. Elevation of the hematocrit and levels of serum calcium, alkaline phosphatase, and aminotransferases occur in less than 10% of patients. These findings nearly always resolve with curative nephrectomy and thus are not usually signs of metastases. Anemia unrelated to blood loss occurs in 20–40% of patients, particularly those with advanced disease.

C. Imaging Studies

The diagnosis of renal cell carcinoma is often made by intravenous urography or CT performed as an initial step in the workup of hematuria, an enigmatic metastatic lesion, or suspicious laboratory findings (Figure 40–21). Ultrasonography and CT scan often reveal incidental renal masses, which now account for 40% of the initial diagnoses of renal cancer in patients without manifestations of renal disease. Plain abdominal x-rays may reveal a calcified renal mass, but only 20% of renal masses contain demonstrable calcification. (Twenty percent of masses with peripheral calcification are malignant; over 80% with central calcification are malignant.)

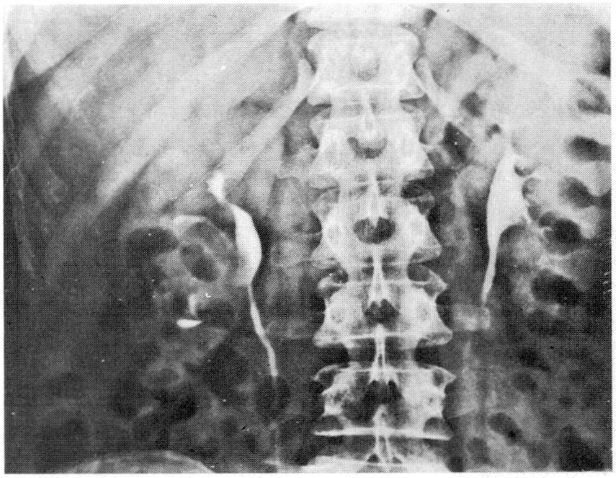

Figure 40–21. Adenocarcinoma of the kidney. Intravenous urogram. Distortion of the pelvis and the middle and lower calices of the right kidney. The left kidney is normal.

The initial technique for workup of hematuria is intravenous urography with nephrotomography or CT urography; intravenous urography alone will define only 75% of renal mass lesions. Differentiation of the most common renal mass (ie, a simple benign cyst) can be made by the finding of a radiolucent center with a thin wall and a sharp interface between the mass and the renal cortex (the typical "beak sign" of a cortical cyst).

1. Ultrasonography—Further definition of all renal masses seen on intravenous urography is required. Abdominal ultrasonography can define the mass as a benign simple cyst or a solid mass in 90–95% of cases (Figure 40–22D). Abdominal ultrasound can also identify a vena caval tumor thrombus and its cephalad extent in the cava.

2. Isotope scanning—Occasionally, a renal mass will be suspected on intravenous urography but is equivocal or not seen on ultrasound. In these cases, a renal cortical isotope scanning agent such as technetium Tc 99m DMSA will be helpful. Isotope scans of a renal tumor or cyst will show an area of decreased uptake, whereas an area of increased uptake indicates a renal "pseudotumor" or a hypertrophied column of Bertin.

3. CT scan—CT scan is the diagnostic procedure of choice when a solid renal mass is noted on ultrasound. CT scan accurately delineates renal cell carcinoma in over 95% of cases. Over 80% of tumors are enhanced by iodinated contrast medium, reflecting their high vascularity (Figures 40–22A and 22B).

CT scan is also helpful in local staging and can reveal tumor penetration of perinephric fat; enlargement of local hilar lymph nodes, indicating metastases; or tumor thrombi in the renal vein or inferior vena cava.

4. Magnetic resonance imaging (MRI)—MRI (Figure 40–22C) is not more accurate than CT and is much more expensive. It is, however, the most accurate noninvasive means of detecting renal vein or vena caval thrombi. With the further refinement of pulse sequencing and the use of paramagnetic contrast agents, MRI has become one of the primary techniques for staging solid renal masses. Magnetic resonance angiography (MRA) has become particularly useful for mapping the blood supply and the relationship to adjacent structures in candidates for partial nephrectomy.

D. Other Diagnostic or Staging Techniques

Isotopic bone scanning is useful in patients with bone pain, elevated alkaline phosphatase, or known metastases. Chest x-ray is sufficient if negative, but if equivocal then CT scan of the chest can be used to detect metastases. There are currently no tumor markers specific for renal cell carcinoma. Occasionally, aspiration cytology of the mass can be useful in an enigmatic case. Previously, such procedures were discouraged because of fear of disseminating the tumor along the needle tract, but this has proved to be rare, and the technique is safe. The diagnosis is most often made by noninvasive means, and needle aspiration is required only in indeterminate cases (< 10%).

Differential Diagnosis

A variety of lesions in the retroperitoneum and kidney other than renal cysts may simulate renal cancer. These include lesions due to hydronephrosis, adult polycystic kidney disease, tuberculosis, xanthogranulomatous pyelonephritis, angiomyolipoma or other benign renal tumors, or adrenal cancer and retroperitoneal lipomas, sarcomas, or abscesses. In general, the radiographic, MRI, or ultrasonographic techniques described above should make the differentiation. Hematuria may be caused by renal, ureteral, or bladder calculi; renal pelvis, ureteral, or bladder tumors; or many other benign conditions usually delineated by the studies described. Cystoscopy is obligatory in hematuric patients with a normal intravenous urogram to rule out disease of the bladder and to determine the source of the hematuria.

Complications

Occasionally, patients may present with acute flank pain secondary to hemorrhage within a tumor or colic secondary to obstructing ureteral clots. Tumor in the renal vein or vena cava may cause an acute left varicocele or lower extremity edema associated with proteinuria. Pathologic fractures due to osteolytic metastases in long bones are common, as are symptomatic brain metastases.

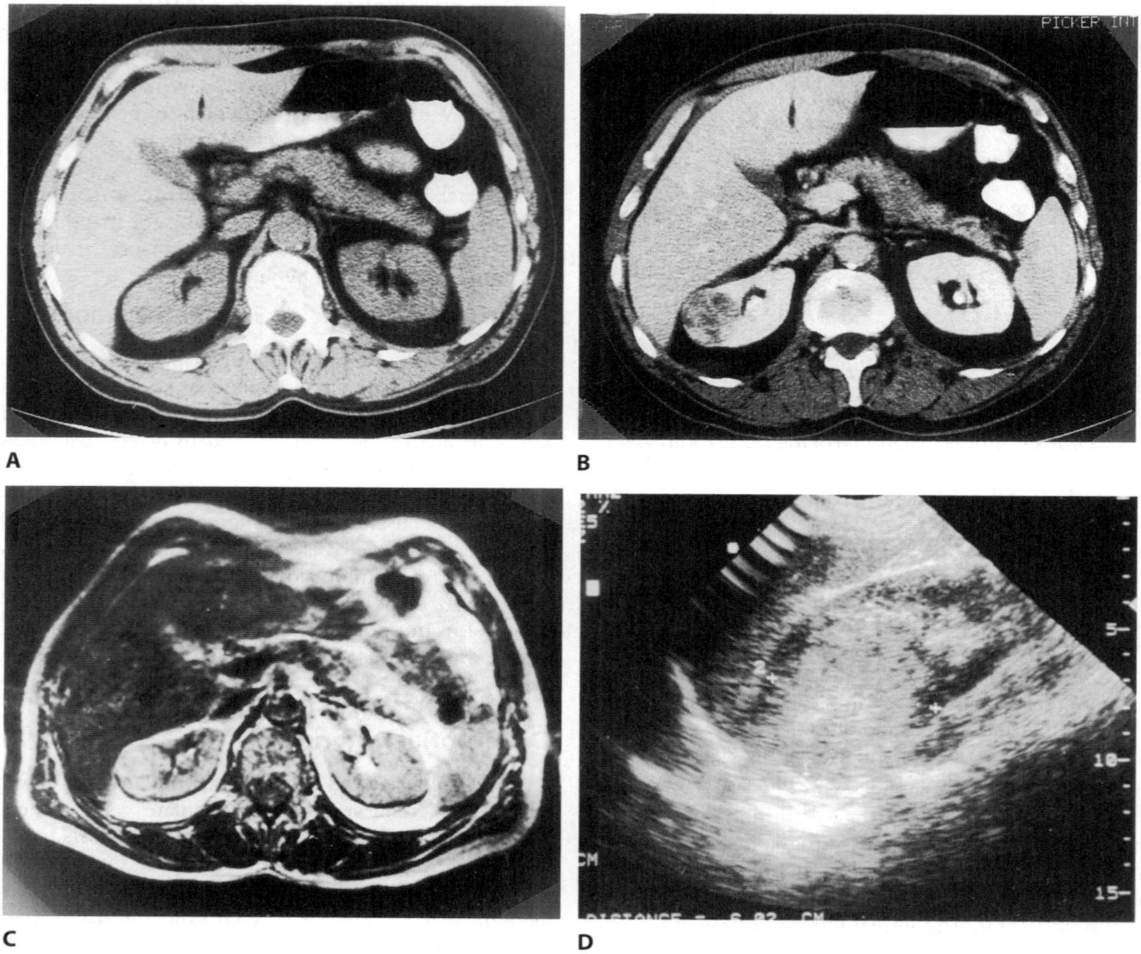

Figure 40–22. ***A:*** Nonenhanced CT scan showing renal cell carcinoma in the right kidney. The mass, which is difficult to identify, is lateral to the lower pole of the kidney. ***B:*** Contrast-enhanced CT scan in the same patient clearly shows heterogeneous enhancement of the tumor. ***C:*** T1-weighted magnetic resonance image (MRI) delineates an obvious mass in the same patient without contrast injection. ***D:*** Renal ultrasound shows a solid mass within the renal parenchyma of the left kidney in another patient.

Treatment

Staging is the key to designing the treatment plan (Table 40–1). Patients with disease confined within the renal fascia (Gerota's fascia) or limited to nonadherent renal vein or vena caval tumor thrombi (stages I, II, and IIIA) are best treated by radical nephrectomy. This involves en bloc removal of the kidney and surrounding Gerota's fascia (including the ipsilateral adrenal), the renal hilar lymph nodes, and the proximal half of the ureter. Para-aortic node dissection has not been proven beneficial and is not routinely recommended. In patients with very large tumors and a normal contralateral kidney, open radical nephrectomy is recommended. Patients with tumors in solitary kidneys, those with diabetes mellitus or renal insufficiency, and those with tumors under 4 cm (even with a normal opposite kidney) should be considered for partial nephrectomy because the prognosis in such cases (if negative surgical margins are obtained) is the same as that of radical nephrectomy. Laparoscopic radical or partial nephrectomy has been advocated as a method equal to the open approach with the advantages of less blood loss, shorter hospitalization, and earlier return to normal function. It is becoming the gold stan-

Table 40–1. TNM staging classification and prognosis of renal cell cancer.

Stage	T	N	M	Five-Year Survival (%)
I. Tumor confined by renal capsule	T1 (< 7.0 cm tumor) T2 (> 7.0 tumor)	N0 (nodes negative)	M0 (lack of distant metastases)	80–100
II. Tumor extension to perirenal fat or ipsilateral adrenal but confined by Gerota's fascia	T3a	N0	M0	50–60
IIIa. Renal vein or inferior vena cava involvement	T3b (renal vein involvement) T3c (renal vein and caval involvement below the diaphragm) T4b (caval involvement above the diaphragm)	N0	M0	50–60 (renal vein) 25–35 (vena cava)
IIIb. Lymphatic involvement	T1–3	N1 (single homolateral regional node involved) N2 (multiple regional, contralateral, or bilateral nodes involved) N3 (fixed regional nodes) N4 (juxtaregional nodes involved)	M0	15–35
IIIc. Combination of IIIa and IIIb	T3–4	N1–4	M0	15–35
IVa. Spread to contiguous organs except ipsilateral adrenal	T4a	N3–4	M0	0–5
IVb. Distant metastases	T1–4	N0–4	M1	0–5

dard in institutions with appropriate expertise. Laparoscopic or percutaneous cryoablation of renal cancer has also shown considerable promise. Alternatively, radiofrequency ablation has been utilized for small renal tumors, but this procedure requires more definitive study.

Nephrectomy has not been associated with improved survival rates in patients with multiple distant metastases (stage IV), and the procedure is not recommended unless patients are symptomatic or a promising therapeutic protocol is being studied. Flanigan and others have shown, however, that up to a 6-month improvement in survival can be achieved with nephrectomy—even with soft tissue metastasis—in selected patients who also receive interferon alfa. Patients with solitary pulmonary metastases have benefited from joint surgical removal of both the primary lesion and the metastatic lesion (30% at 5 years). Preoperative arterial embolization in patients with or without metastases does not improve survival rates, though it may be helpful as a single treatment measure in patients with symptomatic but nonresectable primary lesions. Radiation therapy is of little benefit except as treatment for symptomatic bone metastases. Medroxyprogesterone for metastatic renal cell carcinoma has given an equivocal 5–10% response rate of short duration. Vinblastine has also had a response rate of approximately 20%, again of minimal duration. There are no other cytotoxic chemotherapeutic agents of benefit.

Immunotherapy with interferon alfa has had a 15–20% response rate. Other interferons, alone (interferon beta, interferon gamma) or in combination with chemotherapeutic agents, have been less effective than interferon alfa. Adoptive immunotherapy—using lymphocytes (lymphokine-activated killer [LAK] cells) from exposure of the patient's own peripheral blood lymphocytes to interleukin-2 (IL-2) in vitro followed by reinfusion into the patient along with systemic IL-2 infusion—has shown up to 33% objective response rates. High-dose intravenous IL-2 causes a profound capillary leak syndrome and substantial toxicity. Subsequent studies have shown only a 16% response rate. Studies using lymphocytes isolated from the patient's own tumor (tumor-infiltrative lymphocytes [TIL]) expanded in IL-2 in vitro followed by reinfusion of the selected CD8 TIL and systemic IL-2 have shown limited response rates. Finally, clinical trials of combined IL-2 and interferon alfa show a 30% response rate with extended survival, and this is currently the best conventional method available.

Prognosis

Patients with localized renal cancer (stages I, II, and IIIA) treated surgically have 5-year survival rates of approximately 70–80%, whereas rates for those with local nodal extension or distant metastases are 15–25% and less than 10%, respectively. Most patients who present with multiple distant metastases succumb to disease within 15 months (Table 40–1).

RENAL SARCOMA

Renal sarcomas include rhabdomyosarcoma, liposarcoma, fibrosarcoma, and leiomyosarcoma; the latter is the most common, though all are very uncommon. Sarcomas are highly malignant and are usually detected at a late stage and thus have a poor prognosis. The diagnostic approach is similar to that of renal cell carcinoma. The histology of the lesion is rarely suspected preoperatively. These tumors have a tendency to surround the renal vasculature and do not exhibit neovascularity on magnetic resonance angiography (MRA).

Treatment is surgical, with wide local excision; however, local recurrence and subsequent distant metastases are the rule. There is no therapy of proved benefit for metastatic disease.

SECONDARY MALIGNANT RENAL TUMORS

Metastases to the kidney often develop from primary tumors of distant sites, most commonly the lung, stomach, and breast. It is rare for the diagnosis to be made before autopsy; this suggests that renal metastasis is a late event. There are usually no symptoms, though microscopic hematuria occurs in 10–20% of cases. Intravenous urograms may be normal, since the tumors are located peripherally in the parenchyma. Contiguous spread of a tumor adjacent to the kidney is not infrequent (eg, tumors of the adrenal, colon, and pancreas and retroperitoneal sarcomas). Tumors such as lymphoma, leukemia, and multiple myeloma may also infiltrate the kidney. Routine radiologic, hematologic, and chemical examinations should demonstrate the primary tumor in most cases.

BENIGN RENAL TUMORS

Renal Adenoma

Renal adenoma is the most common benign solid parenchymal lesion. Tumors less than 3 cm in diameter have been considered benign and those larger than 3 cm malignant; however, small lesions are not histologically distinguishable from renal adenocarcinomas, and the biology cannot be predicted preoperatively. These tumors should be considered malignant and should be treated aggressively.

Renal Oncocytoma

Renal oncocytoma is a subtype of adenoma. The tumors are generally asymptomatic, unassociated with the paraneoplastic syndromes often encountered in patients with renal adenocarcinoma. There commonly is a central stellate scar. However, because there is no other diagnostic finding specific enough to exclude malignancy preoperatively, total removal or aggressive cryotherapy is most often performed for these lesions.

Mesoblastic Nephroma

Mesoblastic nephroma is a benign congenital renal tumor seen in early childhood, which must be distinguished from the highly malignant nephroblastoma, or Wilms' tumor (see Chapter 45). Unlike Wilms' tumor, mesoblastic nephroma is commonly diagnosed within the first few months of life. Histologically, it is distinguished from Wilms' tumor by cells resembling fibroblasts or smooth muscle cells and by the lack of epithelial elements. The prognosis is excellent; complete surgical resection is curative, and neither chemotherapy nor radiotherapy is required.

Angiomyolipoma

Angiomyolipoma is a benign hamartoma seen most often bilaterally in adults with tuberous sclerosis (which also includes adenoma sebaceum, epilepsy, and mental retardation). The tumor is also common in middle-aged women, but only unilaterally. It is often detected following spontaneous retroperitoneal hemorrhage. The tumors may be quite large and are commonly multiple. CT scan defines these tumors; a negative CT number is seen in areas of fat within the mass. Occasionally, an angiomyolipoma will elude diagnosis preoperatively and will require nephrectomy. Asymptomatic patients with small (< 5 cm) tumors and typical findings on CT scan of fat within the tumor do not require surgery, as the prognosis is excellent without treatment. Those presenting with a retroperitoneal hemorrhage or a size greater than 5 cm should have the tumor removed surgically or via angioinfarction, which has recently been shown to be effective.

Other Benign Renal Tumors

Other benign renal tumors include the following: (1) **fibroma**, a renal parenchymal capsular or perinephric fibrous mass; (2) **lipoma**, an adipose deposit within or around the kidney, often perihilar or within the renal sinus; (3) **leiomyoma**, a common retroperitoneal tumor that may arise from the renal capsule or renal vascular walls; and (4) **hemangioma**, which is occasionally found to be the elusive cause of hematuria. Hemangiomas are generally quite small, and the diagnosis can be confirmed by direct vision of the lesion in the renal collecting system on ureteroscopy.

TUMORS OF THE RENAL PELVIS & CALICES

ESSENTIALS OF DIAGNOSIS

- *Gross or microscopic hematuria.*
- *Radiolucent filling defect in the renal pelvis or the calices on intravenous urography or CT.*
- *Malignant cells on urine cytologic study.*

General Considerations

In over 90% of cases, tumors involving the collecting system of the kidney are urothelial transitional cell carcinomas. Less than 5% of tumors in this location are squamous carcinomas (often in association with chronic inflammation and stone formation) or adenocarcinomas. The cause of transitional cell carcinoma of the upper urinary tract is similar to that of epithelial tumors in the ureter or bladder; there is a strong association with cigarette smoking and exposure to industrial chemicals. Excessive use of phenacetin-containing analgesics and the presence of Balkan nephritis are also predisposing factors.

Clinical Findings

A. Symptoms and Signs

Gross or microscopic painless hematuria occurs in over 70% of patients. The lesions are usually asymptomatic unless bleeding causes acute flank pain secondary to obstructing clots. Presenting symptoms can often be due to metastases to bone, the liver, or the lungs. Physical examination is not usually helpful.

B. Laboratory Findings

Microscopic hematuria on urinalysis is the rule. Pyuria is not seen. Cytologic examination of voided urine specimens may be diagnostic in high-grade tumors. Urine obtained from the ureter by retrograde catheterization or by brushing with specialized ureteral instruments can improve the diagnostic accuracy of cytologic examinations. Direct biopsy during ureteroscopy is the most accurate. There are no commonly associated paraneoplastic syndromes or diagnostic serum tumor markers in transitional cell carcinoma. A large number of urine markers are currently being studied, but only in situ hybridization studies identifying abnormalities in chromosomes 3, 7, 17 and 9p21 can be recommended at present.

C. Imaging Studies

The diagnosis is commonly made on intravenous urography and confirmed by retrograde pyelography, which reveals a radiolucent filling defect in the renal pelvis or calices (Figure 40–23). Renal ultrasound or CT scan can be used to rule out calculus. CT scan is also useful in local staging of the tumor. The tumors metastasize to the lungs, liver, and bone, so chest x-ray, CT scan of the lungs and liver, and a bone scan are useful to determine the presence of metastases. Transitional cell carcinoma tends to be multifocal in the urinary tract, involving the opposite kidney (1–2%), ipsilateral ureter, or bladder (40–50%). Surveillance of these potential sites is important.

D. Endoscopic Findings

Cystoscopy is necessary when gross hematuria is present to determine the location of the bleeding. Retrograde pyelography and ureteral cytologic studies or brushing as described above can be useful, though mildly abnormal cytologic findings may occur in patients with upper tract inflammation or calculi. Rigid or flexible ureteroscopes can be used to view the upper ureter and renal pelvis directly. Biopsy of upper tract lesions is possible through these

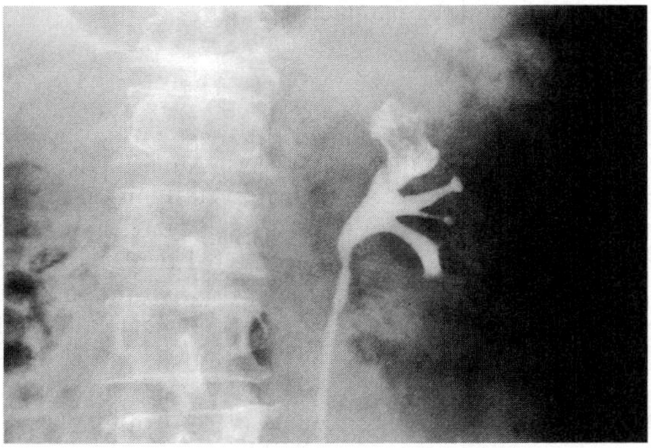

Figure 40–23. Retrograde pyelogram showing transitional cell carcinoma of left upper pole collecting system.

instruments. Although percutaneous approaches to the renal collecting system have been perfected, their use for diagnosis or treatment of suspected transitional cell carcinoma in routine cases is not recommended, because of the possibility of spreading tumor cells outside the kidney.

Differential Diagnosis

A variety of conditions may mimic transitional cell carcinoma of the renal pelvis, including calculi, sloughed renal papillae, tuberculosis, and renal cell carcinoma with pelvic extension of the tumor. These can usually be ruled out by the diagnostic studies described above.

Complications

Occasionally, bleeding may be severe enough to require immediate nephrectomy. Infection may develop, particularly when there is obstruction and hydronephrosis, requiring prompt use of systemic antibiotics.

Treatment

Renal transitional cell carcinoma is treated by nephroureterectomy (perifascial nephrectomy and removal of the entire ureter, down to and including the ureteral orifice within the bladder). Transureteral or percutaneous endoscopic techniques for resection of selected low-grade lesions have been successful. High recurrence rates and the potential for local tumor spread would argue against this approach in high-grade or extensive lesions. Laparoscopic nephroureterectomy has become common, but management of the distal ureter is still not optimum by this technique. Para-aortic lymphadenectomy has not been shown to improve survival rates and is not recommended. Because 50% of these patients will develop transitional cell carcinoma of the bladder, cystourethroscopy must be performed postoperatively; it is usually done quarterly during the first year, twice the second year, and then annually.

Prognosis

Because most of these tumors are low-grade and noninvasive, the 5-year tumor-free survival rate is higher than 90% for lesions treated with complete removal of the ipsilateral upper urinary tract. Survival rates are much lower for lesions that invade the renal parenchyma or are of histologic grade III or higher. A poor prognosis is associated with tumors having histologic features of squamous carcinoma or adenocarcinoma. These tumors are mildly radiosensitive, but pre- or postoperative radiotherapy has not been particularly helpful. Metastatic lesions are particularly problematic, and survivors are rare. Chemotherapy combinations, which have shown benefit in transitional cell carcinoma of the bladder (methotrexate, cisplatin, and vinblastine [CMV] or, with the addition of doxorubicin [Adriamycin], M-VAC), are also efficacious in transitional cell carcinoma of the upper urinary tract. Both VIG (vinblastine, ifosfamide, and gallium) and paclitaxel alone have achieved substantial responses as well.

TUMORS OF THE URETER

ESSENTIALS OF DIAGNOSIS

- *Gross or microscopic hematuria.*
- *Radiolucent filling defect in the ureter on intravenous urography, CT, or retrograde pyelography.*
- *Malignant cells on urine cytologic study.*

General Considerations

Ureteral tumors are rarely benign, but benign fibroepithelial polyps do occasionally occur within the ureter. More than 90% of ureteral tumors are transitional cell carcinomas. The cause is unknown, but tobacco smoking and exposure to industrial chemicals are known to be associated. Ureteral transitional cell carcinoma is often found in association with renal pelvis transitional cell carcinoma and slightly less often with bladder transitional cell carcinoma. The lesions develop in persons aged 60–70 years and are twice as common in men as in women. More than 60% of these tumors occur in the lower ureter.

Clinical Findings

A. Symptoms and Signs

Gross or microscopic hematuria is the rule (80% of cases). Because ureteral tumors grow slowly, they may not cause symptoms even though they completely obstruct the kidney. Occasionally, gross hematuria may cause acute obstruction because of clots. The initial presentation may be due to symptomatic metastases to bone, lungs, or liver.

B. Laboratory Findings

Urinalysis commonly reveals hematuria. There are no biochemical markers specific to the diagnosis, though patients with metastases may have abnormal liver function tests or anemia. Serum creatinine levels may be elevated with complete unilateral obstruction in elderly patients. Cytologic studies of voided urine or ureteral urine or brush studies may be diagnostic.

C. Imaging Studies

The diagnosis may be made on intravenous urography or CT, though the tumor often obstructs the ureter completely, so that cystoscopy and retrograde pyelography are required for definition of the lesion. These studies often reveal a filling defect in the ureter (classically described as a "goblet sign") (Figure 40–24). The ureter is dilated proximal to the lesion. CT scan is useful in ruling out nonopaque calculi and in abdominal tumor staging. Chest x-ray, CT scans, and bone scans are helpful in determining the presence of metastases.

D. Endoscopic Findings

Cystoscopy is necessary when gross hematuria is present to determine the site of bleeding. Retrograde pyelography may then be necessary. Ureteroscopy may provide a direct view of the tumor and access for biopsy.

Differential Diagnosis

Nonopaque calculi, sloughed renal papillae, blood clots, or extrinsic compression by retroperitoneal masses or nodes may all produce signs, symptoms, and x-ray findings similar to those with ureteral tumors. The radiographic, cytologic, and endourologic studies listed above should make the distinction, but surgical exploration will be required occasionally.

Treatment

Most ureteral transitional cell carcinomas are not associated with metastases and can be definitively treated with nephroureterectomy. Selected patients with noninvasive low-grade lesions may be treated by segmental ureteral resection with end-to-end anastomosis (ureteroureterostomy). In some patients carefully selected with low-grade noninvasive tumors, resection or laser ablation can be considered. Para-aortic lymphadenectomy has not been helpful. Pre- or postoperative radiation therapy appears to be of no benefit. As with renal pelvis and bladder transitional cell carcinoma, cystoscopy should be performed periodically postoperatively. Patients with metastases are rarely helped by removal of the primary tumor. These tumors are responsive to chemotherapy. A small series of metastatic ureteral cancer patients treated with CMV (cisplatin, methotrexate, and vinblastine) showed a 60% response rate; however, there are no reports of durable remissions or long-term survivors.

Prognosis

The 5-year survival rate for patients with low-grade noninvasive lesions treated surgically approaches 100%. Those with high-grade or invasive lesions have a poorer prognosis, and those with metastases have a 5-year survival rate of less than 10%.

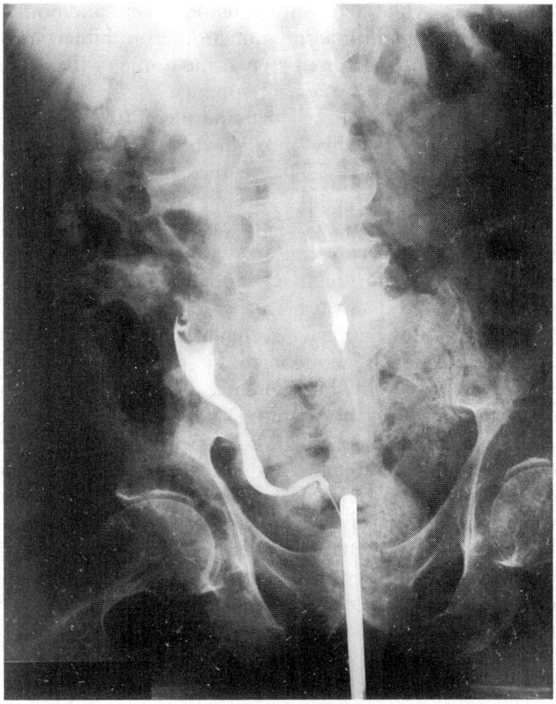

Figure 40–24. Retrograde ureterogram showing "negative" shadow caused by transitional cell carcinoma of the obstructed lower right ureter and the typical "goblet sign."

TUMORS OF THE BLADDER

ESSENTIALS OF DIAGNOSIS

- *Gross or microscopic hematuria.*
- *Malignant cells on urine cytologic study.*
- *Cystoscopic visualization of the tumor.*
- *Histologic confirmation of the lesions.*

General Considerations

Vesical neoplasms account for nearly 6% of all cancers in men and are the second most common cancer of the genitourinary tract in men. In women, these tumors account for 2% of all cancers and are the most common cancer of the genitourinary tract. Males are affected twice as often as females. More than 90% of tumors are transitional cell carcinomas, while a few are squamous cell carcinomas (associated with chronic inflammation, as in bilharziasis) or adenocarcinomas (often seen at the dome of the bladder in patients with a urachal remnant).

Most transitional cell carcinomas (70-80%) are superficial (not invasive into the bladder wall) when recognized. Only 10-15% of recurrent tumors will become invasive.

The cause of transitional cell carcinoma is unknown; there is a strong association with chronic cigarette smoking and exposure to chemicals prevalent in dye, rubber, leather, paint, and other chemical industries. Common use of artificial sweeteners such as cyclamates and saccharin was thought to be related to bladder tumor development, but evidence to substantiate this claim has not been forthcoming.

The treatment and prognosis depend entirely on the degree of anaplasia (grade) and the depth of penetration of the bladder wall or beyond (Table 40–2). Most of these tumors develop on the trigone and the adjacent posterolateral wall; thus, ureteral involvement with obstruction is common. Tumors tend to be multifocal within the bladder. Approximately 5% of patients develop upper urinary tract transitional cell carcinoma as well.

Clinical Findings

A. Symptoms and Signs

Gross hematuria is a common finding, though microscopic hematuria often leads to the diagnosis. Patients with diffuse superficial tumors, particularly carcinoma in situ, may have urinary frequency and urgency. Occasionally, large necrotic tumors become secondarily infected, and patients exhibit symptoms of cystitis. Pain secondary to clot retention, tumor extension into the bony pelvis, or ureteral obstruction may occur but are not frequent presenting complaints. When both ureters are obstructed, azotemia with attendant secondary symptoms may be the finding that requires diagnostic studies.

External physical examination is not generally revealing, though occasionally a suprapubic mass may be palpable. Rectal examination may reveal large tumors, particularly when they have invaded the pelvic side walls. Thus, bimanual examination is a necessary part of staging evaluation.

B. Laboratory Findings

Microscopic hematuria is the only consistent diagnostic finding. Patients with bilateral ureteral obstruction may have azotemia and anemia. Liver metastases may cause elevation of serum transaminases and alkaline phosphatase. There are no paraneoplastic syndromes or tumor markers consistently present in patients with transitional cell carcinoma. Urinary markers currently being studied are various tumor-associated antigens, growth factors, and nuclear matrix proteins, but none are proved to be accurate enough to obviate cystoscopy for diagnosis.

C. Imaging Studies

Small bladder tumors will not be seen on intravenous urography but may be seen on CT. Larger tumors will usually produce filling defects in the bladder on both urography or CT (Figure 40–25). Ureteral obstruction with hydroureteronephrosis may be seen as well. Invasion of the bladder wall may be predicted in patients with asymmetry or marked irregularity of the bladder wall. Noninvasive lesions seen on intravenous urography tend to be exophytic within the bladder, without evidence of bladder wall distortion.

Table 40–2. Treatment and prognosis of bladder tumors related to stage of disease.

Conventional Stage	TNM Stage	Tumor Involvement	Treatment	Five-Year Survival (%)
O	Ta	Mucosa only	Transurethral resection	85–90
A	T1	Submucosal invasion (lamina propria)	Transurethral resection and intravesical chemo-immunotherapy	60–80
B1	T2a	Superficial muscle invasion	Total cystectomy and pelvic lymphadenectomy	50–55
B2	T2b	Deep muscle invasion		30–50
C	T3	Perivesical fat invasion		30–40
D1	T3–4N+	Regional lymph node invasion	Systemic chemotherapy	6–35
D2	T3–4M1	Distant metastases		0–10

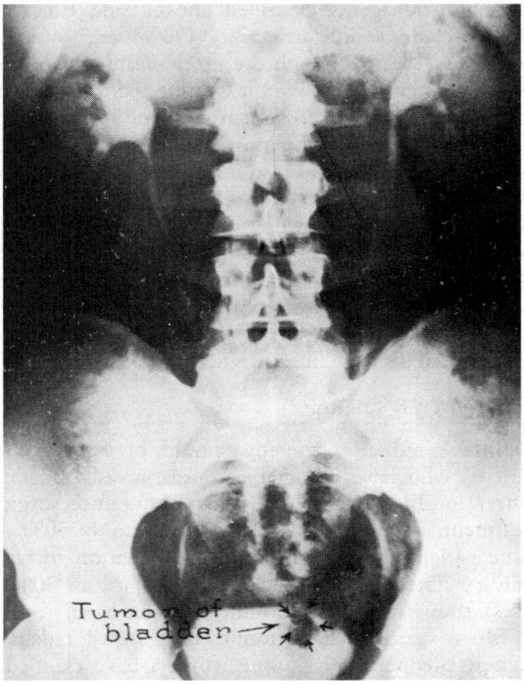

Figure 40–25. Excretory urogram showing space-occupying lesion (transitional cell carcinoma) on the left side of the bladder. The upper tracts are normal.

Ultrasonography by external, transrectal, or transurethral routes can accurately define moderate-sized bladder tumors and can often depict deep invasion.

CT scan can be useful for staging, but the depth of bladder wall penetration and delineation of tumor deposits in adjacent nonenlarged lymph nodes are not accurately defined. In patients with nodal metastases suspected on CT scans, fine-needle aspiration and cytologic studies may confirm the diagnosis and eliminate the need for surgical exploration. MRI is helpful in the pelvis, where motion artifacts are minor and the scant pelvic fat is just enough to provide organ differentiation. However, the information is not superior to that obtained with CT.

D. Urinary Cytologic Studies

Transitional cell tumors shed neoplastic cells into the urine in large numbers. Low-grade tumor cells may not appear abnormal on cytologic examination, but higher-grade tumor cells can be detected by cytologic study. These studies are most useful in checking for recurrence of transitional cell carcinoma. Flow cytometry (differential staining of DNA and RNA within urine cells to measure the amount of nuclear protein and thus the relative number of aneuploid [abnormal] cells) has been used to screen patients with some success. This technique may be useful for early diagnosis of recurrence. The urinary FISH assay is more sensitive and comparably specific for bladder cancer cells as compared to cytology.

E. Endoscopic Findings

Cystoscopy is mandatory in any adult patient with unexplained hematuria and a normal intravenous urogram. Many transitional cell carcinomas will not be seen on intravenous urography. Cystoscopic examination should detect nearly all tumors in the bladder (Figure 40–26). Only a few patients will have carcinoma in situ (superficial high-grade tumor) that is not visible. Any tumor seen should be biopsied. Superficial-appearing tumors can be diagnosed and removed transurethrally at the same time. The entire bladder, including the bladder neck, should be routinely scrutinized in all patients with microscopic hematuria. In patients without visible tumor and no other causes of hematuria, random biopsies may be diagnostic of carcinoma in situ. A bimanual examination should be done during cystoscopy in all patients with transitional cell carcinoma to be certain that the bladder is not fixed, signifying extensive extravesical extension.

F. Staging

Therapy depends on the stage of the tumor as seen on histologic sections and examinations for metastases. Table 40–2 sets forth the stage, treatment, and prognosis of patients with transitional cell carcinoma of the bladder. The histologic grade of the tumor is also important in determining treatment and prognosis, but

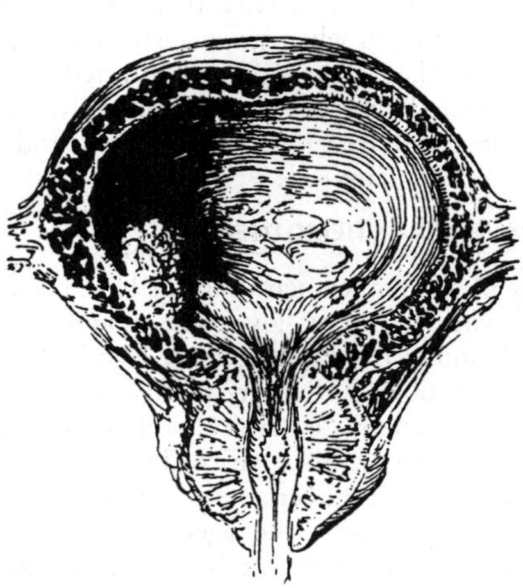

Figure 40–26. Transitional cell (papillary) carcinoma of the bladder with minimal invasion of the bladder wall.

in general, low- and high-grade histologic characteristics tend to occur in low- and high-stage tumors, respectively.

As previously discussed, CT scan, MRI, or both may be helpful in predicting the stage of the tumor. Isotope bone scanning, chest x-ray, and chest CT scan will eliminate the possibility of bone or pulmonary metastases and should be done before determining therapy in patients with invasive lesions.

Treatment

A. Transurethral Resection, Fulguration, and Laser Therapy

Endoscopic transurethral resection of superficial and submucosally invasive low-grade tumors can be curative. Nevertheless, because the tumor recurs in more than 50% of patients, cystoscopy should be performed periodically. Quarterly examinations are recommended during the first year following tumor resection, every 6 months during the second year, and annually thereafter. Periodic urinary cytologic examinations can be helpful as well. Intravenous urography is recommended yearly for the first 3–5 years but is not mandatory. Recurrent small tumors without obvious invasion may be treated by fulguration only, though biopsy is recommended to document the stage and grade.

Neodymium:YAG lasers have been used for desiccation of low-grade, low-stage tumors. There is as yet no proven advantage to this approach except that patients can be treated under local anesthesia as outpatients and perhaps that tumor cells are rendered nonviable and thus incapable of reimplantation elsewhere in the bladder or urethra. Biopsies for diagnosis and staging are still required, however. An alternative approach involves using photosensitizing agents that are preferentially taken up by tumors when given systemically. Selective wavelengths of laser light (630 nm) directed to the bladder transurethrally in patients previously given a photosensitizer can selectively destroy tumor cells and perhaps adjacent premalignant cells as well.

B. Intravesical Chemotherapy

A variety of chemotherapeutic agents have been used in patients with recurrent low-grade, low-stage (O–A) tumors. Thiotepa is instilled into the bladder by catheter (30–60 mg in 60 mL of water) and left indwelling for 2 hours. Patients are treated once a week for 1 month and then monthly for up to 2 years. Treatment results in decreased frequency of recurrence or no recurrence in nearly 50% of patients. Other agents include mitomycin C and doxorubicin. Immunotherapeutic drugs, which include BCG, are effective in prophylaxis (60%) of recurrent papillary tumors and curative (70%) in carcinoma in situ, a highly malignant lesion less responsive to the cytotoxic agents described above. Side effects of BCG include vesical irritability (90%) and systemic BCG-osis (1%). Although the mechanism of action of BCG is not entirely known, it is suspected to induce T-cell recruitment and subsequent cytokine release locally at the tumor site. It is the most effective agent currently used. Interferon alfa has also been studied and is effective (nearly 50% of cases) for carcinoma in situ, with less toxicity than BCG; however, its durability as a single agent is poor. The combination of BCG and interferon alfa has shown improved results over either agent used alone. Immediate postresection intravesical chemotherapy with either mitomycin C or Adriamycin has shown a substantial decrease in recurrence rates.

C. Radiation Therapy

Definitive radiation therapy should be reserved for patients who have inoperable muscle-invasive bladder cancer localized to the pelvis or who refuse surgical treatment, as the 5-year survival rate is only 30%. In some patients with recurrence after radiation therapy, "salvage cystectomy" can be curative (in at least 30% of cases), though surgical morbidity rates are high.

Much controversy surrounds the use of radiation therapy preoperatively. Some workers have claimed a down-staging effect with 2000 cGy given over 1 week or 4000 cGy given over 3–4 weeks. The studies were poorly controlled, however, and subsequent reports have not confirmed these findings. Currently, urologic oncologists rarely use preoperative radiation therapy.

D. Surgical Therapy

Occasional patients are seen with muscle-invasive lesions (T2) localized to an area in the bladder well away from the bladder base or orifices and without tumor in other sites of the bladder (proved by multiple biopsies) or beyond. Partial cystectomy (removal of the tumor and a 3-cm surrounding margin of normal bladder) is appropriate in these patients. Such tumors are rare, and patients must be selected carefully for partial cystectomy. Administration of one dose of 1000 cGy preoperatively to prevent tumor wound seeding may be considered. All other patients with high-grade or invasive (T2 and T3) lesions without distant spread or a fixed pelvis on bimanual examination are best treated by cystectomy and pelvic lymph node dissection. This includes removal of the bladder and the prostate in males. Removal of the entire urethra may be necessary in selected patients with tumors at the bladder neck or in the prostate or in those with diffuse carcinoma in situ in the bladder. In females, the uterus, the urethra, and the anterior vaginal wall are usually removed. Urinary diversion is required and is commonly accomplished by creation of an ileal diversion. Continent cutaneous urinary diversions requiring intermittent cutaneous catheterization rather than cutaneous bag drainage became popular in the late 1980s. The basic principles are large-volume reservoirs with detubularization of bowel to maintain low intrapouch pressures and construction of an intussuscepted or plicated ileal segment to provide cutaneous continence. Orthotopic reservoirs also have been devised using bowel configurations similar to those described above to connect directly to the membranous urethra in males and in the distal two-thirds of the female urethra, permitting the patient to void normally. These procedures are appropriate in both men and women and have been shown to be safe, with minimal increase in morbidity over cutaneous diversions. Recently, laparoscopic cystectomy and urinary diversion has been done in a few centers in the USA and Europe.

E. Systemic Chemotherapy

Chemotherapy in the form of CMV (cisplatin, methotrexate, vinblastine) or M-VAC (CMV plus doxorubicin [Adriamycin]) has been used precystectomy (neoadjuvant) or postcystectomy (adjuvant) for muscle-invasive tumors or as treatment of metastatic urothelial cancer. The neoadjuvant series all show an approximate 60% downstaging from clinical to pathologic stage and a 30% rate of complete tumor eradication. As with the prior preoperative radiation studies, however, there is no evidence as yet that these results will eventuate in a higher long-term survival rate. Adjuvant chemotherapy may be useful, but few patients have been studied and no definitive prospective randomized trials comparing adjuvant versus no adjuvant treatment have been reported. Several reports of efficacy with either CMV or M-VAC for treatment of metastatic disease have shown a 60% overall objective response rate with a 30% complete response rate. A few long-term survivors with apparent cure have been reported (10–15%), and either of these regimens thus appears to be a definite advance in the treatment of urothelial cancer. Newer approaches include paclitaxel, carboplatin, and gemcitabine in various regimens that appear to have similar efficacy with less toxicity. These results have caused a few investigators to study chemotherapy alone or in combination with radiation to attempt bladder salvage in patients with invasive bladder cancer, and this has become a viable alternative to cystectomy.

Prognosis

Approximately half of the low-grade superficial tumors will be controlled by transurethral surgery or intracavitary use of chemotherapeutic agents (Table 40–2). Following radical cystectomy, the 5-year survival rate varies with the extent, stage, and grade of the tumor, but with T2N0M0 tumors averages about 50–70%. The complications of urinary diversion (ureteral obstruction with hydronephrosis, pyelonephritis, and nephrolithiasis) also influence the outcome.

CARCINOMA OF THE PROSTATE

ESSENTIALS OF DIAGNOSIS

- *Palpable rock-hard nodule in the prostate on rectal examination.*
- *Serum PSA elevation.*
- *Histologic confirmation on needle biopsy.*
- *Osteoblastic bone metastases and in advanced cases.*

General Considerations

In adult males, prostate cancer is the most common neoplasm (after skin cancer) and the second most common cause of death due to cancer. The tumor is more prevalent in black males than in any other group in the USA. The tumor rarely occurs before age 40, and the incidence increases with age such that in the eighth decade, more than 60% of men have prostate cancer (at autopsy). In most of these older men, however, the disease is not clinically apparent; only 10% of men over age 65 develop clinical evidence of the disease. Ninety-five percent of tumors are adenocarcinomas. The tumor arises primarily in the peripheral zone (70%), an area that differs in embryologic derivation from the periurethral (transition) zone, which is the site of formation of benign prostatic hyperplasia. Thus, the causes of the two diseases are considered to be different; they may occur simultaneously but are not related. The cause of prostate cancer is unknown, but many factors appear to be involved, including genetic, hormonal, dietary (particular high-fat diets), and perhaps environmental carcinogenic influences.

Screening

Advances in transrectal ultrasound (TRUS) and prostate-specific antigen (PSA) monitoring have allowed for enhanced detection of nonpalpable tumors. Much controversy currently exists over whether men over age 50 should be encouraged to undergo screening. While available data show a decrease in the mortality rate of prostate cancer, there is as yet little evidence that screening has been the cause of this change. Even so, the realities of clinical practice are that the combination of digital rectal examination and serum PSA monitoring is the most effective screening protocol.

Clinical Findings

A. Symptoms and Signs

Incidental or stage A (T1) carcinoma of the prostate presents no physical signs (it is nonpalpable) and is only diagnosed by the pathologist when prostate tissue is removed as treatment for symptomatic bladder outlet obstruction presumed to be caused by benign prostatic hyperplasia or is found by an elevated PSA (T1c). Patients with stage B (T2) or higher disease have a hard nodule on the prostate that can be felt during rectal examination (Table 40–3). In over 60% of these men, the cancer causes obstructive symptoms, urinary retention, or urinary infection. Previously, 50% of patients presented with evidence of metastases, including weight loss, anemia, bone pain (commonly in the lumbosacral area), or acute neurologic deficit in the lower limbs. Today, however, fewer than 20% of patients present in this way because earlier diagnosis is the rule.

B. Laboratory Findings

Patients with extensive metastases may have anemia due to bone marrow replacement by tumor. Those with bilateral ureteral obstruction secondary to trigonal compression by tumor may exhibit azotemia and uremia. Serum alkaline phosphatase is often elevated in patients with bone metastases but not in those with localized disease.

Prostate-specific antigen is elevated in the serum of approximately 60% of men with prostate cancer. Levels above 4 ng/mL are abnormal and can be falsely elevated due to cystoscopy, prostate biopsy, or urethral catheterization but *not* by normal digital rectal examination.

Methods for enhancing PSA specificity include the following: (1) age-specific PSA (younger men [under age 55 years], normal < 2.5 ng/mL; older men [over age 65 years], normal > 6.5 ng/mL); (2) PSA density (PSA divided by prostate volume), where < 0.15 ng/mL suggests cancer; (3) percent-free PSA (total PSA minus complexed PSA), where when < 10%, the risk of prostate cancer is 60% (only useful with total PSA 2–10 ng/mL); and (4) complexed PSA (similar specificity to percent-free PSA). While total PSA is useful for staging, it is not absolute. PSA appears to be most helpful in following up on patients after treatment, as levels fall to almost nil with complete response and rise early.

C. Imaging Studies

Transrectal ultrasound (TRUS) has become very useful for evaluating tumor volume and guiding biopsy needles into the peripheral zone and other specific areas, such as the base, the apex, and the transition zone of the prostate. The study can also reveal typical hypoechoic peripheral zone lesions in 70% of patients with palpable lesions (Figure 40–27). Because many prostate cancers are not hypoechoic and not all hypoechoic lesions are cancer, TRUS alone for screening for prostate cancer is not rec-

Table 40–3. Treatment and prognosis of prostate cancer related to tumor stage.

Conventional Stage	TNM Stage	Clinical Findings	Treatment	Fifteen-Year Recurrence-Free Survival (%)
A1	T1a	Nonpalpable tumor; incidental finding at transurethral prostatectomy (low-grade cancer seen in < 5% of prostate).	Observation	100
A2	T1b	Same as above except tumor is high-grade, or > 5% of prostate is involved, or both.	Radical prostatectomy with pelvic lymphadenectomy	70–80
B1	T2a	Localized nodule 1–1.5 cm in diameter in one lobe.	External beam radiation	85
B2	T2b	Tumor is ≥ 1.5 cm in diameter or in more than one lobe.	Brachytherapy	60–70
C	T3, T4	Periprostatic extension.	Radiation with or without pelvic lymphadenectomy	20–60
D	N+ or M+	Pelvic lymph node involvement or distant metastases.	Hormonal therapy (orchiectomy or LHRH/antiandrogen) when symptomatic. Irradiation for isolated bone pain.	0–10

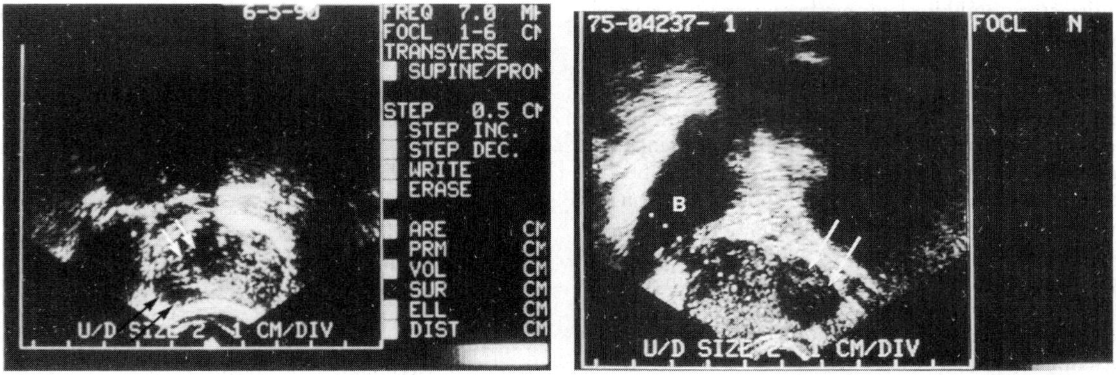

A B

Figure 40–27. Transrectal ultrasound of the prostate. ***A:*** Transaxial plane. Transition zone is shown at white arrows and hypoechoic prostate cancer in the peripheral zone at black arrows. ***B:*** Sagittal plane, showing large hypoechoic prostate cancer at white arrows. (B = bladder.)

ommended. An intravenous urogram or CT may reveal urinary retention or distal ureteral obstruction. Extensive lesions may exhibit a ragged-edged filling defect in the bladder base. A chest x-ray may help in identifying the uncommon lung metastases but more often shows typical osteoblastic metastases in the thoracic spine or ribs. An abdominal x-ray may reveal metastases in the lumbosacral spine or ilium. A CT scan of the pelvis may show an enlarged prostate and large pelvic or para-aortic lymph nodes; however, the study is rarely accurate for staging and is not routinely recommended unless the PSA is > 20 ng/mL or the Gleason sum of the tumor is ≥ 7, or the tumor is palpably outside of the prostate (stage C/T3). Fine-needle aspiration and cytologic studies of abnormal nodes may provide important staging data and perhaps obviate staging laparotomy. Endorectal and pelvic MRI appear to be more helpful than CT scan in pelvic staging of prostate cancer (Figure 40–28). A monoclonal antibody, Cyt-356 (which identifies the *intra*cellular epitope of prostate-specific membrane antigen), has been coupled with a radioisotope for diagnosis of soft tissue metastases. Results show that the Prostascint scan is 60% accurate but that it has a false-positive rate, which limits its usefulness. A new study using J-591 (which identifies the *extra*cellular epitope of PSMA) appears to be more accurate.

D. Biopsy

The diagnosis is established by TRUS-guided transrectal biopsies in most instances. Because the great majority of patients have biopsies due to an elevated serum PSA (stage T1c) and no abnormal findings on TRUS, symptomatic biopsies of the base, middle, and apex of the prostate—concentrating on the peripheral zone with six biopsies per side of the prostate—are required for accurate diagnosis.

Differentiation of the tumor is graded by the pathologist using the Gleason scale, which assigns a grade of 1–5 (low to high grade) for both the primary and secondary forms of the tumor. The two numbers are added, and the cancer can thus be Gleason sum 2–10, with 10 being the most poorly differentiated cancer. The likelihood of metastasis can be inferred from the Gleason sum, as 7 or more is an aggressive cancer.

E. Staging

Rectal examination can provide initial staging in patients with palpable tumors (Table 40–3). Needle biopsy is

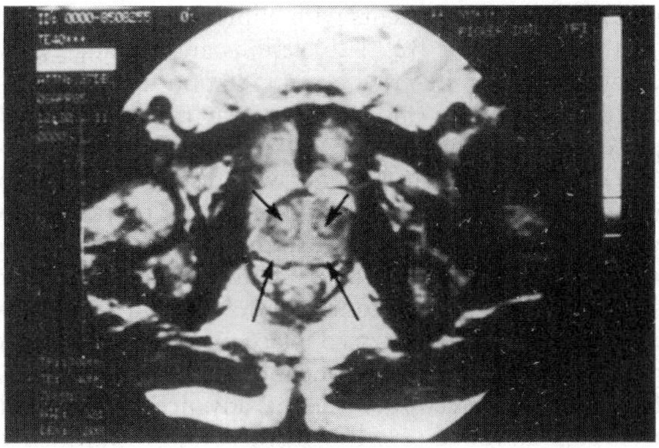

Figure 40–28. T2-weighted MRI in the transaxial plane showing transition zone at short arrows and peripheral zone at long arrows, with hypointense area in right posterior zone of prostate cancer.

confirmatory, and histologic grading can fairly accurately predict the metastatic potential of the tumor. A normal isotopic (technetium Tc 99m) bone scan will rule out bone metastases, but is not necessary if Gleason score is < 7 and/or PSA is < 20 ng/mL. A pelvic CT scan may be useful to define pelvic lymphadenopathy in patients with high-grade lesions, PSA > 20 ng/mL, or both. The laparoscopic approach to pelvic lymph node dissection has provided the same prognostic information as an open surgical procedure with less morbidity and a markedly reduced hospital stay. This approach is useful in patients with high-grade or high-stage lesions and those considered for radical perineal prostatectomy. Cystoscopy is not required except in large lesions suspected to involve the bladder neck and trigone.

Differential Diagnosis

Nodules caused by benign prostatic hyperplasia may be difficult to distinguish from cancer; benign nodules are usually rubbery, whereas cancerous nodules have a much harder consistency. Fibrosis following a prior prostatectomy or secondary to chronic prostatitis or prior biopsies may be associated with lesions indistinguishable from cancerous nodules and require biopsy for definition. Occasionally, phleboliths or prostatic calculi on the surface of the prostate may be confusing; however, TRUS can be helpful in the differentiation and for biopsy guidance.

Treatment

See also Table 40–3.

A. Curative Therapy

Patients with low-grade, low-stage incidental lesions (stage A1; T1a) have a prognosis similar to that of patients without cancer of the prostate and require observation only. Patients with clinical stage A2 (T2b), T1c, B1 (T2a), or B2 (T2b) lesions are candidates for curative therapy. External beam radiation therapy, radical prostatectomy, and transperineal radioactive seed placement all have similar 10- to 15-year recurrence-free survival figures in patients with disease localized to the prostate. Complete staging, including pelvic lymph node dissection, is important so that appropriate candidates will be selected. Patients with T3 disease are best suited for neoadjuvant androgen deprivation and external beam radiation or seed placement. Patients with grossly positive pelvic lymph nodes are not candidates for total prostatectomy. Recent advances in surgical technique have led to a low incidence of incontinence (1–4%) and preservation of potency in up to 70% of patients. Alternative procedures include external beam pelvic irradiation plus interstitial radiation (with ^{125}I, ^{103}Pd, and ^{192}Ir). Recently, laparoscopic and robotic radical prostatectomy has been reported to have decreased blood loss and length of hospital stay and more rapid return to normal activity than open surgery. It remains to be seen if long-term complications and efficacy will be improved as well.

B. Palliative Therapy

Patients with metastatic disease cannot be cured, but significant palliation can be offered. Androgen deprivation therapy in the form of oral estrogen (diethylstilbestrol, 1–3 mg/d) or bilateral orchiectomy is effective in 70–80% of symptomatic patients. Choice of therapy depends on patient preference (many patients find castration unacceptable) or coexistent disease (eg, estrogens have numerous side effects—about 25%—including congestive heart failure, thrombophlebitis, and myocardial infarction, and thus should not be used except in selected patients). These hormonal treatments are not additive, and use of both treatments simultaneously has no advantages over use of either alone. Luteinizing hormone-releasing hormone (LHRH) agonists have shown efficacy comparable to that of estrogen or orchiectomy, with reduced side effects. The drug must be given by injection every three to four months and is expensive. Studies have also shown that if an LHRH agonist is used, concomitant administration of an antiandrogen (flutamide or bicalutamide) slightly improves survival. Studies to determine if orchiectomy plus an antiandrogen is more effective than orchiectomy alone have not shown an advantage to the combination. Osteoporosis is a long-term side effect of either orchiectomy or LHRH agonist.

Controversy continues concerning whether to treat asymptomatic patients at the time of diagnosis or to wait until symptoms develop. Because either approach is palliative only and there are no definitive studies showing survival advantages with early treatment, it is recommended that treatment be withheld until symptoms occur except in patients who cannot accept a no-treatment philosophy. Recent studies do show that patients who have had a radical prostatectomy and have node-positive disease do have a slight survival advantage with each hormonal treatment.

Patients in whom hormonal therapy has failed can be treated by ketoconazole (which inhibits adrenal androgen production) with oral corticosteroids for short-term response. Radiation therapy for symptomatic bone lesions can be helpful, as can local irradiation for an obstructing or bleeding prostate tumor. A bone-seeking radioisotope (strontium) appears to have some efficacy in therapy of bone metastases. On occasion, transurethral prostatectomy will be required to relieve bladder outlet obstruction. Chemotherapy with docetaxel and estracyt or prednisone has recently shown a slight survival advantage in phase III trials.

Prostate Cancer Prevention

Because the etiology of prostate cancer is not known, prevention is difficult to determine. However, there is evidence that a low-fat diet, vitamin E, selenium, and lycopene (found in tomatoes) all decrease the growth of prostate cancer cells in vitro and in vivo in animals. Further large-scale epidemiologic studies appear to confirm a decrease in prostate cancer in humans who consumed vitamin E and selenium. However, these studies were not planned specifically for this purpose and thus are questionable. A current randomized trial comparing the two (SELECT) is in progress. The largest chemoprevention trial, with over 18,000 men, compared finasteride (5α-reductase) to placebo and found a 25% reduction in prostate cancer with finasteride, but also showed an increased risk of high-grade cancer in the finasteride-treated patients. These latter results have generated limited enthusiasm for recommending prevention therapy with finasteride routinely.

Prognosis

Radical prostatectomy cures 70–80% of the patients suitable for that operation, but its use should be limited to those with a reasonable life expectancy (Table 40–3). Currently, about 60–70% of patients with prostatic cancer are amenable to curative therapy when their disease is discovered. Careful annual rectal examination to check for suspicious areas of induration and serum PSA monitoring should be performed in all men over age 50—and over age 40 if there is a positive family history in a first-degree relative (father, brother) or in blacks—if this cure rate is to be improved.

SARCOMA OF THE PROSTATE

Sarcoma of the prostate is rare. Half of all cases occur in boys under age 5. The tumor is highly malignant and metastasizes to the pelvic and lumbar lymph nodes, lungs, liver, and bone. Symptoms of urinary tract obstruction are present. The prostate is enlarged. Cystography or excretory urography may show superior displacement of the bladder or encroachment of the tumor into the bladder. Endoscopy will reveal the mass and allow biopsy.

Total prostatocystectomy, postoperative radiotherapy, and chemotherapy have cured a few cases in adults. In children, combination chemotherapy with surgery for residual tumor has shown increasing success. The tumor is relatively radioresistant.

TUMORS OF THE URETHRA

Malignant tumors of the urethra are rare. The disease is more common in females than in males. Squamous cell types are seen most often in both sexes.

In females, urethral bleeding is the most common symptom. Distal urethral lesions of low grade and without extension can be treated by radiotherapy or wide local excision. Extensive or proximal lesions are best treated by preoperative irradiation and anterior exenteration (removal of the bladder, uterus, adnexa, and urethra with the anterior vaginal wall), including pelvic lymphadenectomy and urinary diversion. The prognosis is excellent for distal lesions without extension, but 5-year survival rates are less than 50% for those with proximal lesions.

In males, the lesion is most commonly in the bulbomembranous urethra and is associated with a history of chronic urethral strictures, often secondary to gonorrheal infection. Patients present with urethral bleeding, a weak urinary stream, and a perineal mass. The diagnosis is made by urethroscopy and biopsy. Distal penile urethral lesions can be treated by partial or total penectomy. Lesions in the bulbous urethra or more proximal lesions require extensive surgical resection, including en bloc removal of the penis, urethra, prostate, bladder with overlying pubis, pelvic lymph nodes, and urinary diversion. Preoperative radiation therapy (2000–4000 cGy) is recommended, although too few patients have been treated to determine the benefit. In both males and females with distal lesions, groin lymphatics may be involved, but node dissection is required only when gross disease is palpable. Prophylactic node dissection is controversial. Five-year survival rates are 60% for distal urethral tumors but less than 40% for the more common proximal lesions.

Primary irradiation—other than to distal lesions in the female—is rarely helpful. Patients with metastatic disease may respond to methotrexate or cisplatin alone or in combination, but objective remissions are usually of short duration.

TUMORS OF THE TESTIS

ESSENTIALS OF DIAGNOSIS

- *Painless, firm mass within the testicle in a man aged 18–40.*
- *Elevated serum levels of the beta subunit of human chorionic gonadotropin (β-hCG), alpha-fetoprotein (AFP), lactic dehydrogenase (LDH), or all three.*
- *Enlarged retroperitoneal nodes on abdominal CT scan.*
- *Palpable abdominal mass in advanced cases.*

General Considerations

Most testicular tumors are malignant germ cell tumors. Non-germ cell tumors such as Sertoli cell tumors and Leydig cell tumors are rare and usually benign. Germ cell tumors are categorized as either seminomatous (35%) or nonseminomatous (embryonal, 20%; teratocarcinoma, 38%; teratoma, 5%; choriocarcinoma, 2%). Cryptorchidism predisposes to testicular cancer, with the incidence increasing inversely with the level of testicular descent (ie, testicles remaining in the abdomen have a much higher incidence of cancer). Metastases first develop in the retroperitoneal nodes; right-sided tumors metastasize primarily to the interaortocaval region just below the renal vessels and left-sided tumors primarily to the left para-aortic area at the same level. Distant spread is to supraclavicular areas (left, primarily) and the lungs. Just under 50% of patients have metastases when first seen.

Clinical Findings

A. Symptoms and Signs

Testicular tumors present as a painless firm mass within the testicular substance. They often have been present for several months before the patient seeks consultation. Occasionally (10%), a hydrocele will be present, obscuring palpation of the mass. A few patients have spontaneous bleeding into the mass, causing pain. Patients with high serum levels of hCG may have gynecomastia. Patients with extensive abdominal metastases may present with abdominal pain, anorexia, and weight loss. Examination may reveal palpable retroperitoneal nodes when spread is extensive, or palpable supraclavicular nodes, particularly on the left side.

B. Laboratory Findings

In general, testicular tumors do not alter the usual laboratory parameters, but serum tumor markers are diagnostically helpful. Patients with extensive retroperitoneal metastases may have bilateral ureteral obstruction that causes azotemia and anemia.

Serum lactic dehydrogenase (LDH), particularly isoenzyme I, is elevated in approximately 60% of patients. β-hCG, a particularly sensitive marker, is a glycoprotein produced by 65% of nonseminomatous testicular tumors but only 10% of seminomas. The alpha subunit of the molecule is identical to luteotrophic hormone (LH), but the beta subunit is unique to testicular tumors in adult males. There is cross-reactivity in some assays between the alpha and beta subunits; treated patients who develop modest elevations should have simultaneous assay of LH to be certain the marker detected is β-hCG. Urinary β-hCG studies have been even more sensitive than serum levels but are useful only in selected patients with suspected early recurrences.

Alpha-fetoprotein (AFP) is elevated in 70% of patients with nonseminomatous testicular cancer but is *not* elevated in patients with seminoma. Patients in whom histologic study has shown seminoma but in whom serum AFP is elevated should be suspected of having nonseminomatous elements in the primary specimen or metastatic lesions.

Approximately 85% of patients demonstrate elevation of one of these markers at presentation. Serum levels decrease when the tumor is completely removed or regresses. Markers are used mainly to follow tumor regression or predict recrudescence, as even minute amounts of tumor may cause serum elevations; however, tumor may be present without elevation of serum markers.

C. Imaging Studies

An intravenous urogram, though not essential, may reveal deviated or obstructed ureters secondary to retroperitoneal metastases. Abdominal CT scan will define enlarged lymph nodes in approximately 90% of cases when they are present. Chest x-ray and CT scan will detect most pulmonary metastases.

Scrotal ultrasound is useful for identifying the typical hypoechoic lesion in the testicle. Regardless of the findings on ultrasound, however, a young man with an intratesticular mass on palpation requires surgical definition of the mass.

Differential Diagnosis

Testicular masses in men aged 18–40 are almost always malignant and should be treated accordingly. Confusion can occur with scrotal hydroceles, cord hydroceles, epididymal masses or cysts, or epididymitis. Most of these can be differentiated from masses within the testicle by palpation, but if not, scrotal ultrasound is usually helpful.

Treatment

See also Table 40–4.

Inguinal orchiectomy with high ligation of the cord at the internal ring is proper initial treatment for all kinds of testicular cancer. Rarely is incisional biopsy of the testicle advisable. Recommendations for further therapy (retroperitoneal dissection, chemotherapy, radiation therapy) are then based on the pathologic findings. A staging workup, including measurement of serum markers, chest x-ray and chest CT scan, and abdominal CT scan, is conducted to determine the extent of disease.

A. Nonseminomatous Tumors

Following orchiectomy, retroperitoneal lymph node dissection is recommended for all patients with nonseminomatous testicular cancer except in the presence of bulky abdominal or distant metastases. Patients with

Table 40–4. Treatment and prognosis of testicular cancer related to tumor stage.

Conventional Stage	TNM Stage	Clinical Findings	Treatment	Five-Year Survival (%)
I	T1	Confined to testicle	Inguinal orchiectomy; retroperitoneal lymphadenectomy (irradiation for seminoma)	> 95
IIA	N1–N2a	< 6 microscopic nodes	Adjuvant chemotherapy	> 90
IIB	N2b	> 6 microscopic nodes	Adjuvant chemotherapy	> 85
IIC	N3	Bulky abdominal nodes	Orchiectomy and chemotherapy followed by resection of residual disease	~70
III	M+	Distant metastases		

pure choriocarcinoma are an exception and do not usually require retroperitoneal surgery, because the disease in such cases is invariably systemic and requires multiagent chemotherapy. The extent of lymphadenectomy depends on the testicle involved but in general includes para-aortic and paracaval nodes from the renal vessels down to the aortic bifurcation and along the external iliac artery to the internal inguinal ring on the involved side. Seminal emission can be preserved; loss of this function was previously a complication of retroperitoneal lymph node dissection because of interruption of autonomic nerves crossing the aorta and near the aortic bifurcation.

Because of the associated morbidity, some have proposed that retroperitoneal lymph node dissection be withheld after orchiectomy in patients with normal serum markers and no evidence of retroperitoneal nodal disease on abdominal CT scan and lymphangiography and who have no findings of distant metastases on chest x-ray and CT scan. The rationale was that only 20% of these patients will develop recurrent disease, which could then be treated when it appeared. This approach should be discussed at length with the patient to ensure his or her reliable compliance with a program for frequent follow-up.

Patients with any nonseminomatous cell type who have extensive retroperitoneal or chest metastases are best treated after orchiectomy by multiagent chemotherapy followed by excision of persistent masses. Combination chemotherapy with bleomycin, etoposide, and cisplatin achieves over a 90% cure rate in stage II patients and a 70% cure rate in stage III patients. Patients who do not respond may be treated with ifosfamide, doxorubicin, or both, with some expectation of success.

B. Seminoma

In the absence of extensive distant spread, patients with pure seminoma should be treated with external beam radiation therapy (2500 cGy) to the abdomen following orchiectomy. In the presence of bulky abdominal disease or more distant metastases, survival rates are better with multiagent chemotherapy (described above) given initially in lieu of radiation therapy. Patients with substantial residual tumor (> 3 cm) after chemotherapy may benefit from surgical removal of the remaining tumor.

Prognosis

The prognosis for the various stages of testicular cancer is outlined in Table 40–4. Even in the presence of metastases, many of these patients can be cured. The only exception is patients with choriocarcinoma, who still have a poor survival rate (35% at 5 years) despite extensive chemotherapy.

TUMORS OF THE PENIS

Cancer of the penis is a rare disease occurring in the fifth to sixth decades. The cause is uncertain. The disease is rarely seen in circumcised men. The lesion commonly is on the glans penis or foreskin. Early cases may exhibit a painless red, velvety lesion, but most often the lesion is an exophytic nodular or wart-like growth with secondary infection. The initial diagnosis is made by a generous incisional biopsy of the lesion, which reveals squamous cell carcinoma in over 95% of cases. The tumors tend to metastasize to superficial or deep inguinal nodes, though the attendant infection may cause enlarged, tender nodes, which may be difficult to differentiate from metastatic cancer.

The differential diagnosis includes syphilitic chancre, soft chancre due to *Haemophilus ducreyi* infection, and simple or giant condyloma. Biopsy will usually differentiate between these conditions.

Small noninfiltrating lesions can be treated with fluorouracil cream, external beam radiation, or laser therapy. However, close follow-up is mandatory in patients so treated. Larger lesions not involving deep structures are treated by partial penile amputation at least 2 cm proximal to the lesion, leaving enough of the penis for adequate direction of the urinary stream. Deeply infiltrating lesions require total penectomy, with formation of a perineal urethrostomy.

Palpable inguinal nodes should be treated by antibiotics for 6 weeks following treatment of the primary lesion to eliminate infection. Persistently palpable nodes will require bilateral ilioinguinal lymphadenectomy. Prophylactic node dissection has not been associated with increased survival rates in patients without palpable nodal involvement. Even those who undergo delayed node dissection when the nodes become palpable can be cured. Radiation therapy for palpable nodes or as prophylaxis for nonpalpable nodes has been effective.

Patients with distant metastases (to the lungs or bone) have a poor prognosis, though cisplatin and methotrexate have shown objective but not durable responses. Five-year survival rates for patients with noninvasive lesions localized to the penis are 80%; for those with inguinal node involvement, 50%; and for those with distant metastases, nil.

Atkins MB et al: Randomized phase 11 trial of high-dose interleukin-2 either alone or in combination with interferon alfa-2b in advanced renal cell carcinoma. J Clin Oncol 1993;11:661.

Baselli EC et al: Intravesical therapy for superficial bladder cancer. Oncology 2000;14:719.

Canfield SE et al: Surveillance and management of recurrence for upper tract transitional cell carcinoma. Urol Clin North Am 2003;30:791.

Carter BS et al: Hereditary prostate cancer: epidemiological and clinical features. J Urol 1993;150:797.

Chodak GK et al: Results of conservative management of clinically localized prostate cancer. N Engl J Med 1994;330:242.

Cookson MS et al: Management of stage T_1 bladder cancer with intravesical bacillus Calmette-Guérin therapy. J Urol 1992;148:797.

Einhorn LH et al: Vinblastine, ifosfamide and gallium (VIG) combination chemotherapy in urothelial carcinoma. J Clin Oncol 1994;12:2271.

Elliott DS et al: If nephroureterectomy necessary in all cases of upper tract transitional cell carcinoma? Long-term results of conservative endourologic management of upper tract transitional cell carcinoma in individuals with a normal contralateral kidney. Urology 2001;58:174.

Epstein JI: PSA and PAP as immunohistochemical markers in prostate cancer. Urol Clin North Am 1993;20:757.

Flanigan RC et al: Cytoreductive nephrectomy in patients with metastatic renal cancer: a combined analysis. J Urol 2004;171:1071.

Fleischmann J, Goldberg G: Management of superficial transitional cell carcinoma of the bladder. Semin Urol 1993;11:193.

Fleming C et al: A decision analysis of alternative treatment strategies for clinically localized prostate cancer. JAMA 1993;269:2650.

Foster RS et al: Testicular cancer: what's new in staging, prognosis, and therapy. Oncology 1999;13:1689.

Garnick MB: Prostate cancer: screening, diagnosis and management. Ann Intern Med 1993;118:804.

Gill IS: Laparoscopic radical nephrectomy for cancer. Urol Clin North Am 2000;27:707.

Gill IS et al: Laparoscopic renal cryoablation: initial clinical series. Urology 1998;52:543.

Glas AS et al: Tumor markers in the diagnosis of primary bladder cancer. A systematic review. J Urol 2003;169:1975.

Gschwend JE et al: Radical cystectomy for invasive bladder cancer: contemporary results and remaining controversies. Eur Urol 2000;38:121.

Han M et al: Prostate-specific antigen and screening for prostate cancer. Med Clin North Am 2004;88:245.

Heidenreich A et al: Quality-of-life issues in the treatment of testicular cancer. World J Urol 1999;17:230.

Hernandez J, Thompson IM: Diagnosis and treatment of prostate cancer. Med Clin North Am 2004;88:267.

Jarrett TW et al: Endourologic management of upper tract transitional cell carcinoma. World J Urol 2000;18:243.

Jewett MAS et al: Management of recurrence and follow-up strategies for patients with nonseminoma testis cancer. Urol Clin North Am 2003;30:819.

Kahn D et al: Radioimmunoscintigraphy with 111In-labeled monoclonal antibody 7E11-C5 (CYT 356) in subjects with occult recurrent prostate cancer. J Urol 1994;152:1490.

Kamat AM et al: Intravesical therapy for bladder cancer. Urology 2000;55:161.

Kaufman DS et al: Selective bladder preservation by combination treatment of invasive bladder cancer. N Engl J Med 1993;329:1377.

Kirkali Z, Tuzel E: Transitional cell carcinoma of the ureter and renal pelvis. Crit Rev Oncol Hematol 2003;47:155.

Lamm DL: Complications of bacillus Calmette-Guérin immunotherapy. Urol Clin North Am 1992;19:565.

Litwin MS, deKernion J: Perspectives on the problem of prostate cancer. J Urol 1994;152:1680.

Lotan Y, Roehrborn CG. Sensitivity and specificity of commonly available bladder tumor markers versus cytology: results of a comprehensive literature review and meta-analyses. Urology 2003;61:109.

Matlaga BR et al: Radiofrequency ablation of renal tumors. Curr Urol Rep 2004;5:39.

Meuillet E et al: Chemoprevention of prostate cancer with selenium: an update on current clinical trials and preclinical findings. J Cell Biochem 2004;91:443.

Michaelson MD et al: Selective bladder preservation for muscle-invasive transitional cell carcinoma of the urinary bladder. Br J Cancer 2004;90:578.

Moinzadeh A, Gill IS: Laparoscopic radical cystectomy with urinary diversion. Curr Opin Urol 2004;14:83.

Nanus DM et al: Clinical use of monoclonal antibody HuJ591 therapy: targeting prostate specific membrane antigen. J Urol 2003;170:S84.

Pentyala SN et al: Prostate cancer: a comprehensive review. Med Oncol 2000;17:85.

O'Donnell MA: Combined bacillus Calmette-Guerin and interferon use in superficial bladder cancer. Expert Rev Anticancer Ther 2003;3:809.

Raghavan D: Testicular cancer: maintaining the high cure rate. Oncology 2003;17:218.

Rassweiler JJ et al: Laparoscopic partial nephrectomy: the European experience. Urol Clin North Am 2000;27:721.

Shelley MD et al: Intravesical bacillus Calmette-Guerin is superior to mitomycin C in reducing tumor recurrence in high-risk superficial bladder cancer: a meta-analysis of randomized trials. BJU Int 2004;93:485.

Steele GS et al: Management of low-stage nonseminomatous germ cell tumors of the testis. Compr Ther 2000;26:210.

Stenzl A, Höltl L: Orthotopic bladder reconstruction in women—what we have learned over the last decade. Crit Rev Oncol Hematol 2003;47:147.

Stockle M et al: Advanced bladder cancer (stages pT3b, pT4a, pN1 and pN2): Improved survival after radical cystectomy and 3 adjuvant cycles of chemotherapy: Results of a controlled prospective trial. J Urol 1992;148:302.

Studer UE et al: Orthotopic ileal neobladder. BJU Int 2004;93:183.

Taneja SS et al: Management of disseminated kidney cancer. Urol Clin North Am 1994;21:625.

Tierney AC et al: Laparoscopic radical and partial nephrectomy. World J Urol 2000;18:249.

van den Ouden D et al: Management of locally advanced prostate cancer. 1. Staging, natural history, and results of radical surgery. World J Urol 2000;18:194.

Vasey PA: Immunotherapy for renal carcinoma: theoretical basis and current standard of care. Br J Clin Pharmacol 2000;50:521.

Walther PJ: Contemporary chemotherapeutic approaches for the treatment of hormone-refractory prostate carcinoma. World J Urol 2000;18:216.

Whitmore WF Jr: Localized prostate cancer: management and detection issues. Lancet 1994;343:1263.

NEUROPATHIC (NEUROGENIC) BLADDER

A neuropathic bladder has abnormal activity secondary to a neurologic condition. To understand the variety of neuropathic bladder conditions, a basic understanding of the normal innervation and myoneurophysiology is required.

Myoneural Anatomy

The urinary bladder and its involuntary sphincter develop and differentiate from the tubular urogenital sinus. The differentiation of the encasing mesenchymal cells forms the musculature of the detrusor and urethral sphincter.

Innervation

The innervation of the bladder and its involuntary sphincter is via the autonomic nervous system. The parasympathetic supply to the bladder and the sphincter is via the pelvic nerves, which arise from S2–4. These fibers also carry the stretch sensory receptors to the same spinal cord center (S2–4).

The sensory supply for pain, touch, and temperature is carried via the sympathetic fibers arising from the thoracolumbar segments (T11–L2).

Motor and sensory supply of the trigone is via the thoracolumbar sympathetic fibers.

The striated external sphincter, as well as the entire urogenital diaphragm, receives its motor and sensory innervation from the somatic fibers arising from S2–4 (via the pudendal nerve).

It is clear that the S2–4 segment is the origin of the motor supply to the bladder musculature, to the involuntary sphincter, and to the striated external sphincter. The trigone is the only structure that is partly independent in its innervation. This is why segment S2–4 is called the spinal cord center for micturition. It is located at the level of the T12 and L1 vertebral bodies. There are connections between the spinal reflex center and the midbrain and cerebral cortex. Through these connections, inhibition and control of the spinal cord reflexes can be maintained. The micturition reflex is coordinated in the pontine micturition center.

Myoneurophysiology

The primary functions of the urinary bladder are to store and empty urine at a safe pressure and in a continent fashion. Intact myoneural elements are essential for these functions. The primary reservoir function is possible because of the specialized detrusor muscle arrangement and because of the bladder compliance phenomenon. The normal adult bladder can accommodate volumes up to 400 mL without increasing intravesical pressure. Bladder fullness is perceived through increases in stretching of bladder mechanoreceptors.

Distention and stretch initiate detrusor activity that can be controlled and inhibited by the high cortical centers or can be allowed to progress to active detrusor contraction and voiding. Normally during voiding, detrusor contraction continues until the bladder is completely empty unless voiding is voluntarily interrupted or inhibited.

Before voiding begins, the pelvic floor and the striated external sphincter relax, the bladder base descends, and the bladder outlet assumes a funnel shape. As a result, urethral resistance decreases. This is followed by detrusor muscle contraction and a rise in intravesical pressure to 20–40 cm of water, which results in a urine flow of about 15–30 mL/s. When the bladder is completely empty, the pelvic floor and striated external sphincter contract, elevating the bladder base, increasing urethral pressure, and ending voiding. Intact nerve pathways are essential for these synchronized activities to occur.

Cystometry

Cystometry is a simple method for testing the bladder's storage function and gives the following information: bladder capacity, extent of accommodation or compliance, the ability to sense bladder filling and temperature, and the presence of an appropriate detrusor muscle contraction. In addition, postvoid residual urine can be measured at the same time. A normal cystometrogram is shown in Figure 40–29.

Uroflowmetry

Uroflowmetry is the measurement of urine flow rate. If detrusor contraction is properly coordinated with sphincter relaxation, then the outlet resistance will fall as the bladder pressure increases, and the flow rate will be adequate. Normally, the flow rate changes with age but is > 20 mL/s in males under 60 and > 25 mL/s in females under 50 years of age. Any flow rate below 15 mL/s suggests obstruction or detrusor dysfunction. A flow rate under 10 mL/s strongly suggests underlying pathology.

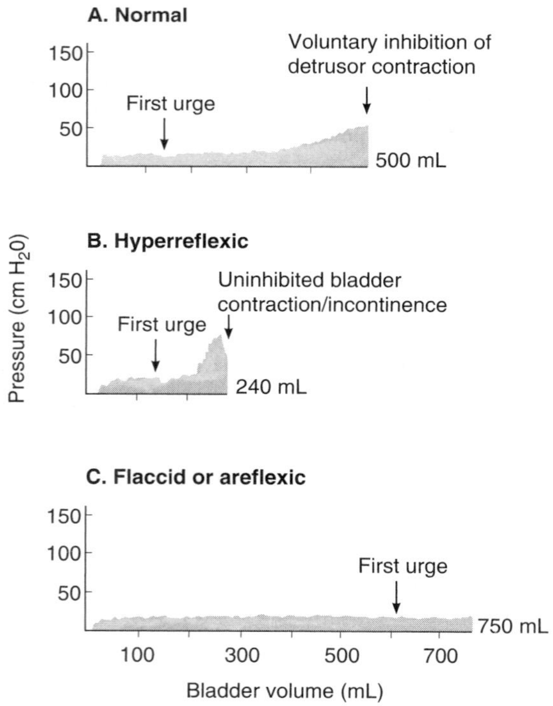

Figure 40–29. Cystometrograms. ***A:*** Normal cystometrogram. ***B:*** Cystometrogram in a patient with hyperreflexic bladder caused by transection of the spinal cord above S2. ***C:*** Cystometrogram in a patient with an areflexic flaccid neuropathic bladder caused by a myelomeningocele.

Urodynamics

Urodynamic studies require measurement of bladder pressure during micturition. The pressure measured within the bladder (intravesical pressure) is a combination of the intra-abdominal pressure and the pressure generated by the detrusor. To determine the detrusor pressure, the intra-abdominal pressure is measured with a rectal catheter and this pressure is subtracted from the total intravesical pressure (measured by the bladder catheter). The urine flow rates may then be assessed in light of the detrusor pressure. No consensus exists on a critical value for pressure and flow that is diagnostic of obstruction. Nomograms have been developed for evaluating the pressure-flow relationship and thus to categorize these values as obstructed, equivocal, or unobstructed.

Electromyographic Recording

Needle or patch electrodes may be employed to record the activity of the external sphincter. This information is useful when obtained during micturition. Increased activity in the sphincter after voiding begins suggests detrusor-sphincter dyssynergia.

Classification & Clinical Findings

Several classification systems exist that describe the variety of pathologic bladder conditions that develop secondary to neuropathies. Many bladder conditions are predictable based on the neurologic lesion. A lesion above the brain stem (ie, stroke) affecting micturition frequently results in involuntary bladder contractions (detrusor hyperreflexia) with coordinated (synergistic) sphincter relaxation. These patients will have urge incontinence.

A complete lesion of the spinal cord (ie, trauma) above the T12 vertebral body may leave the spinal reflex center intact. This often leads to what has been categorized as an upper motor neuron lesion. These patients have detrusor hyperreflexia and uncoordinated sphincter activity (detrusor-sphincter dyssynergia). Although detrusor contractions can generate abnormally high intravesical pressure, they are not effective in producing adequate urine flow because of the spastic external sphincter. Thus, there is residual urine. Bladder capacity is reduced. Detrusor contraction and mass reflexes can be initiated from certain trigger areas.

Figure 40–29B is a typical cystometrogram of a hyperreflexic bladder.

An injury to the spinal reflex center or below often leads to what has been categorized as a lower motor neuron lesion. These patients often develop detrusor areflexia. Trauma is the most common cause, but tumors, ruptured intervertebral disks, and meningomyelocele may also cause this type of neuropathic bladder. Both motor and sensory fibers are usually affected, and there is loss of sense of fullness (Figure 40–29C). These contractions are usually weak and unsustained, and bladder emptying is incomplete, resulting in large amounts of residual urine.

The bladder dynamics in a person with a neuropathic bladder often change over time. This may occur secondary to changes in innervation (ie, tethering of spinal cord, multiple sclerosis, recovery from spinal shock) or changes in the bladder. For example, a patient with a hyperreflexic bladder and dyssynergic sphincter often develops a trabeculated, noncompliant bladder over time. These changes require periodic reevaluation of all patients with neuropathic bladders regardless of the initial classification.

Differential Diagnosis

Cystitis, interstitial cystitis, and organic obstruction are occasionally confused with neuropathic bladder, but associated neurologic lesions usually make the diagnosis of neuropathic bladder easy. Psychosomatic disturbances can cause spasm of the external sphincter, incomplete voiding, retention, or incontinence.

Complications

Common complications include urinary tract infection, stone formation, and incontinence. The most serious consequences of these lesions are the hydrodynamic back pressure on the kidneys, hydronephrosis, infection, decompensation of the ureterovesical junction, and loss of renal function.

Treatment

Immediately following spinal cord injury, there is a shock phase that may last a few weeks to 2–3 years. The average time is 2–3 months. The bladder is completely dissociated from nervous control and thus has no sensation and is areflexic.

Treatment is aimed at avoiding the aforementioned complications in the hope of partial or complete recovery. During the shock phase, continuous closed drainage or, preferably, clean intermittent (every 4–6 hours) catheterization should be instituted until bladder activity is restored.

A. Hyperreflexic Bladder

In the hyperreflexic bladder, attaining a functional bladder depends upon mobilizing residual urine and increasing the bladder capacity. Residual urine volume can be decreased by reducing urethral resistance by several methods: transurethral prostatectomy, division of the external sphincter, pudendal nerve manipulation (ablation or electrical stimulation), or alpha-blocker pharmacologic therapy. Clean intermittent catheterization may also be required to evacuate the residual urine.

Functional capacity can be increased by decreasing detrusor instability with anticholinergic-parasympatholytic drugs (ie, oxybutynin or tolterodine), or by operative augmentation. This is often performed with small or large intestine (enterocystoplasty).

Conversion to a flaccid areflexic bladder can be achieved by cord rhizotomy. The storage function of the bladder is preserved, and the patient can be managed by clean intermittent catheterization.

Supravesical urinary diversion may be called for in patients with upper tract deterioration due to elevated storage pressures or female incontinence. Male incontinence may be controlled by a condom catheter.

B. Areflexic Bladder

Function of the flaccid bladder can be improved by measures that facilitate complete emptying; these include voiding by Credé's maneuver (suprapubic pressure), transurethral resection of the bladder neck to reduce outlet resistance, and timed voiding or timed clean intermittent catheterization. An indwelling urethral catheter or suprapubic cystostomy is required in a few cases, but chronic intubation should be avoided if possible.

Suprapubic urinary diversion (ileal or colon conduit, etc) can circumvent deterioration of upper tracts. Implantable prosthetic sphincters, periurethral bulking agent injections, or urethral slings may also improve urinary control.

Prognosis

Renal injury from elevated bladder pressure and infection are the most serious consequences of neuropathic bladder. When diversion or bladder augmentation is required, proper timing of the operation is essential for preservation of kidney function. Patients with a neuropathic bladder require close follow-up of their kidneys with renal ultrasound and serum creatinine determinations.

Appell RA: Collagen injection therapy for urinary incontinence. Urol Clin North Am 1994;21:177.

Cooper CS et al: Pediatric reconstructive surgery. Curr Opin Urol 2000;10:195.

Hollander JB et al: Urinary diversion and reconstruction in the patient with spinal cord injury. Urol Clin North Am 1993; 20:465.

Jensen JK et al: The role of patient history in the diagnosis of urinary incontinence. Obstet Gynecol 1994;83(5 Part 2):904.

Peggs JF: Urinary incontinence in the elderly: pharmacologic therapies. Am Fam Physician 1992;46:1763.

Perkash I: Long-term urologic management of the patient with spinal cord injury. Urol Clin North Am 1993;20:423.

Rousseau P et al: Urinary incontinence in the aged. Part 1: patient evaluation. Geriatrics 1992;47:22.

Rousseau P et al: Urinary incontinence in the aged. Part 2: management strategies. Geriatrics 1992;47:37. (Published erratum appears in Geriatrics 1992;47:87.)

Webster GD et al: Voiding dysfunction following cystourethropexy: its evaluation and management. J Urol 1990;144: 670.

OTHER DISEASES & DISORDERS OF THE GENITOURINARY TRACT

SIMPLE RENAL CYST

A simple renal cyst is usually unilateral and solitary but may be multiple and bilateral. The cause of this disorder is unclear. The cyst can compress and destroy adjacent parenchyma. Cysts contain fluid that resembles (but is not) urine. Most are diagnosed in patients after the fourth decade. Occasionally, what appears to be a simple cyst may in fact be a papillary cystadenocarcinoma—an uncommon form of renal cancer with both solid and cystic components. In those cases, however, ultrasound will usually demonstrate a complex mass with both cystic and solid components.

Flank pain may be a presenting symptom, though most renal cysts are found incidentally on urography done for other purposes. A mass may be felt in the flank or upper quadrant and must be distinguished from tumor. Urinalysis and tests of renal function are normal. Excretory urograms reveal a mass that distorts adjacent calices. Nephrotomography shows a radiolucent mass (in contradistinction to tumor). If the CT scan or ultrasound reveals an equivocal cystic mass, cyst aspiration may be performed, the fluid submitted for cytologic examination, and the cyst filled with contrast material to delineate its wall. A simple cyst must be distinguished from adenocarcinoma of the kidney; ultrasonography or CT scan usually makes that distinction.

Complications are rare, but bleeding into or infection of a cyst may occur.

If the diagnosis of cyst is established, surgery is not necessary unless the lesion causes pain or endangers renal function. Simple percutaneous aspiration with instillation of 95% ethanol may suffice. If sclerosis fails, laparoscopic or open excision may be performed.

RENAL ARTERY ANEURYSM

Aneurysm of the renal artery is relatively rare. It results from weakening of the artery wall by arteriosclerosis, poststenotic dilation, intimal or perimedial fibroplasia, or trauma. If the aneurysm causes stenosis of the artery, hypertension may ensue secondary to ischemia and activation of the renin-angiotensin system. A plain abdominal x-ray may reveal a ring-like calcification in the wall (Figure 40–30). Angiography or CT scan is diagnostic.

Surgery is indicated in the following situations: (1) secondary renal ischemia and hypertension, (2) dissecting aneurysm, (3) aneurysm associated with pain or hematuria, (4) anticipation of pregnancy, (5) aneurysm coincident with significant stenosis, (6) radiographic evidence of incomplete calcification or increase in size on serial films, and (7) aneurysm containing thrombus with evidence of distal embolization. If the aneurysm ruptures, emergency nephrectomy may be necessary.

RENAL INFARCTION

The common causes of renal artery occlusion include emboli due to subacute infective endocarditis, atrial or ventricular thrombi, arteriosclerosis, polyarteritis nodosa, trauma, and, in the neonate, umbilical artery catheterization. Multiple emboli are common and

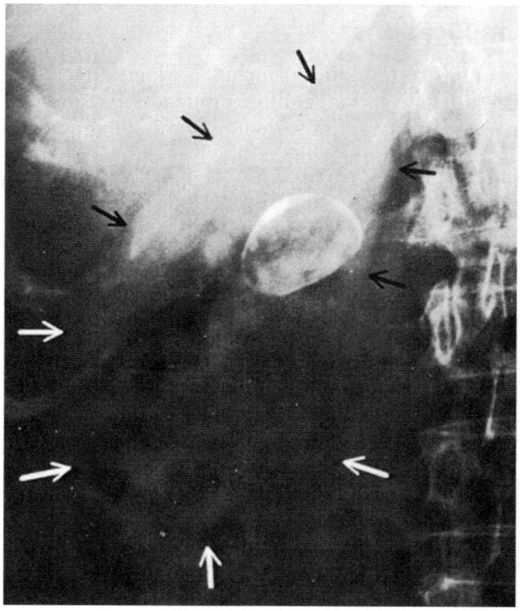

Figure 40–30. Intrarenal aneurysm of renal artery. Plain film showing calcified structure over the right renal shadow.

lead to patchy renal ischemia. Occlusion of a main renal artery will cause renal total infarction.

The patient may suffer from severe flank pain, or the lesion may be silent. Hematuria is common. Excretory urograms may reveal no excretion of radiopaque material or may only opacify a portion of the kidney. With complete acute occlusion of the main renal artery, a ureteral catheter will drain no urine, yet the retrograde urogram will reveal normal anatomy. Renal angiography, color Doppler ultrasound, or magnetic resonance angiography makes the diagnosis by revealing occlusion of the artery or arterioles; a renal scan will show similar findings. CT scan after the intravenous injection of radiopaque medium will show no concentration in the ischemic area. Ureteral stone may mimic renal infarction, but urograms, CT scan, or angiograms will distinguish one from the other. Following renal infarction, hypertension may develop secondary to renal ischemia; it may later resolve spontaneously.

If the diagnosis is made promptly (within 5–8 hours), thrombectomy or endarterectomy should be considered. Otherwise, anticoagulation therapy should be instituted (eg, heparin). Thrombolytic therapy (eg, streptokinase) may be used to lyse the clot. If permanent hypertension develops, definitive treatment of the arterial occlusion or nephrectomy (preferably laparoscopic) should be performed.

RENAL VEIN THROMBOSIS

Thrombosis of the renal vein affects both infants and adults and can be either acute or chronic. In children, thrombosis may be caused by severe dehydration (eg, due to ileocolitis and diarrhea or the nephrotic syndrome). In adults, it may be secondary to renal infection, ascending thrombosis of the vena cava, or caval occlusion due to tumor thrombus. There is usually flank pain and a palpable distended kidney. If renal vein thrombosis is secondary to infection, the patient is septic and urinalysis reveals pus cells and bacteria. In noninfectious cases, the urine may reveal microhematuria and mild proteinuria. The patient with bilateral involvement is azotemic. Nephrotic syndrome may develop. Excretory urograms show delayed opacification in an enlarged kidney. The calices are elongated. Later, the kidney may become atrophic. Renal angiography reveals stretching and bowing of arterioles. Selective renal venography will demonstrate the thrombus, as will renal ultrasound (Figure 40–31).

Treatment should attempt to eliminate the underlying cause whenever possible. If the diagnosis of unilateral infected renal vein thrombosis can be established, nephrectomy should be performed. In bilateral disease, anticoagulant or thrombolytic therapy (or both) is required.

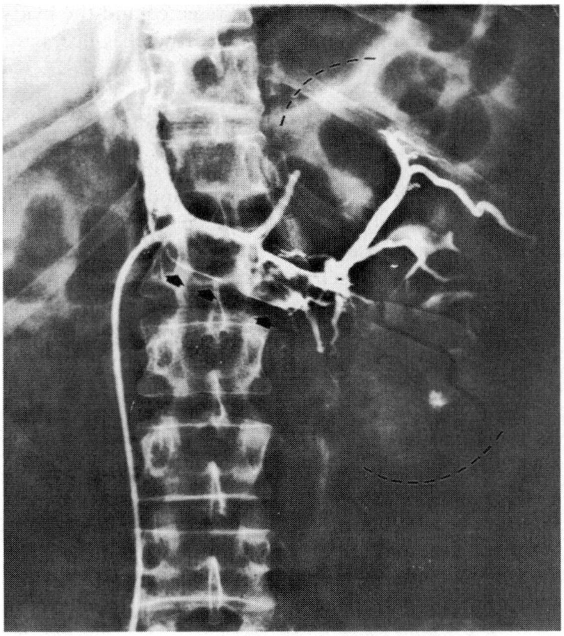

Figure 40–31. Thrombosis of renal vein. Selective left renal venogram showing almost complete occlusion of vein. Veins to lower pole failed to fill. Note large size of kidney.

VESICAL FISTULAS

Vesical fistulas may be congenital or acquired. Congenital fistulas usually involve the urachus. Acquired fistulas may be iatrogenic or due to trauma, tumor, or inflammation.

The most common types of vesical fistulas are vesicovaginal, vesicointestinal, and vesicocutaneous. Vesicovaginal fistulas are commonly secondary to gynecologic or birth trauma; rarely, they occur as a complication of infiltrating cervical carcinoma. Vesicointestinal fistulas are most often due to inflammatory bowel disease: Crohn's disease, diverticulitis, and appendicitis. Cystostomy in the presence of bladder outlet obstruction, bladder cancer, or foreign body may result in vesicocutaneous fistula.

Diagnostic maneuvers include cystoscopy, conventional cystography, barium enema or barium swallow, and CT scan with contrast infusion. Oral charcoal may be useful for detecting a urinary intestinal fistula, as the granules can be seen in spun urine under the microscope.

Therapy for vesicovaginal fistula requires surgical closure, with placement of an omental flap between the bladder and the vagina. For vesicointestinal fistula, the primary intestinal lesion must be resected and the bladder closed. An indwelling urethral catheter is necessary during the healing period.

INTERSTITIAL CYSTITIS

This lesion is most commonly found in middle-aged women. Urinary frequency both day and night is most often accompanied by suprapubic pain with bladder distention. The cause is uncertain, though some suggest an autoimmune collagen disease, while others have documented the presence of mast cells and mast cell mediators (histamine and prostaglandin) in bladder biopsy specimens of affected patients.

The diagnosis is based on the history and the results of cystoscopy under general anesthesia. Cystoscopy reveals a small-capacity bladder and punctate hemorrhage following forceful distention. (Studies suggest this is a nonspecific finding.) Biopsy may reveal lymphocytic infiltration, mast cell infiltration, and submucosal fibrosis. In patients suspected of having interstitial cystitis, one must rule out carcinoma in situ; urine cytologic study precedes cystoscopy and random bladder biopsy.

Treatment of established cases of interstitial cystitis often fails. Response has been obtained with hydraulic bladder overdistention, intravesical treatment with 50% DMSO, 0.4% oxychlorosene sodium, or sodium pentosanpolysulfate. Systemic corticosteroids have their proponents as well, and BCG has been tried with some success. Some patients require operative augmentation of bladder capacity by enterocystoplasty or, rarely, cystourethrectomy and permanent urinary diversion.

URINARY STRESS INCONTINENCE

Involuntary loss of urine during stress (coughing, sneezing, or physical strain) is a common complaint of postmenopausal women. The cause is related to pelvic relaxation with age, resulting in descent of the trigone and proximal urethra. There is obliteration, of the urethrovesical angle, which normally provides resistance at the bladder outlet. The diagnosis is made by the history and physical examination and urodynamic evaluation. When the bladder is full, the patient should be asked to cough while in both the supine and upright positions, producing incontinence. Digital pressure applied to the paraurethral tissues in an anterior direction through the vagina will reestablish the urethrovesical angle and prevent stress incontinence (Marshall's test).

Treatment in patients with normal bladder function and low residual urine is initiated with behavioral therapy and perineal exercises; if unsuccessful, pharmacologic methods include oxybutynin and ephedrine. Definitive management is surgical. Currently, the most effective surgical approach is a sling procedure with a piece of autologous or synthetic fascia attached to the rectus muscle or os pubis and surrounding the urethra at the bladder neck. Newer approaches include the use of collagen injection into the periurethral tissues, resulting in increased urethral outflow resistance.

FEMALE URETHRITIS & PERIURETHRITIS

Urethritis in the female may be acute or chronic. Acute urethritis can be gonorrheal in origin. Chemical urethritis is occasionally acquired from exposure to soap or bath oils. Chronic urethritis is a common problem in females, since the female urethra is exposed to pathogenic bacteria because of its anatomic location. Urethral trauma, instrumentation, and increase in the number of pathogenic organisms lead to infection and overt urethritis. Urethritis usually precedes cystitis.

Hormonal changes associated with menopause cause vaginal and urethral mucosal changes, leading to irritative symptoms and increased susceptibility to inflammation.

Urethritis usually causes irritative voiding symptoms similar to those of cystitis and, occasionally, functional obstructive symptoms. Examination may reveal urethral discharge, marked tenderness, or congested everted mucosa at the external meatus. Induration of the urethra may be associated with vaginitis and cervicitis. Endoscopy may reveal obstruction, mucosal congestion, and inflammatory polyps. Urethral calibration rarely reveals obstruction. Spasm of the external sphincter may be noted.

Treatment is directed to the underlying cause. Estrogen cream is indicated for senile vaginitis. Surgical treatment consists of urethral dilation and opening and draining infected periurethral ducts. Alpha-blockers given orally may also help decrease urethral resistance. Correction of vaginitis, cervicitis, and cervical erosions helps in ameliorating symptoms.

FEMALE URETHRAL CARUNCLE

Urethral caruncle, commonly seen after menopause, represents granulomatous overgrowth of the posterior lip of the external meatus. The caruncle is tender and causes pain with intercourse and urination. The primary concern is exclusion of urethral cancer. Treatment is complete excision.

FEMALE URETHRAL DIVERTICULUM

Urethral diverticulum in the female commonly presents as recurrent lower urinary tract infection. It should be suspected whenever urinary infection fails to resolve with treatment. Symptoms are urinary dribbling and cystic swelling in the anterior vaginal wall during voiding. If diverticulum is suspected, it can usually be identified during panendoscopy and opacified by contrast medium on a voiding cystourethrogram while occluding the external meatus. These lesions occasionally contain stones or tumors.

Treatment consists of transvaginal diverticulectomy.

SPERMATOCELE

Spermatocele is a retention cyst of a tubule of the rete testis or the head of the epididymis. The cyst is distended with a milky fluid that contains sperm. Located at the superior pole of the testis and caput epididymidis, the spermatocele is soft and fluctuant and can be transilluminated.

No treatment is needed unless the spermatocele is painful, in which case surgical excision may be performed.

VARICOCELE

Varicocele is due to incompetent valves in the testicular vein, permitting transmission of hydrostatic venous pressure; distention and tortuosity of the pampiniform plexus results. Varicocele is on the left side in 98% of cases, presumably because of venous drainage of the left testes to the left renal vein, causing increased retrograde venous pressure. The varicocele is bilateral in up to 50% of cases.

Mild varicoceles are commonly asymptomatic, but a dragging scrotal sensation may be noted. Varicocele may lead to infertility in some men (see Male Infertility).

Asymptomatic varicocele is best untreated unless it is a suspected factor in male infertility. Treatment then consists of operative ligation of the spermatic vein at or above the internal inguinal ring. In recurrent varicocele, transfemoral catheterization and occlusion or ablation of the spermatic vein may be performed with a detachable balloon or sclerosing agents. The technical success rate is high.

TORSION OF THE SPERMATIC CORD

Torsion of the spermatic cord (intravaginal torsion) is most common in adolescent boys. A twist in the spermatic cord interferes with testicular blood supply. If torsion is complete, testicular infarction may occur within 4–6 hours. The cause is unknown, but an underlying anatomic abnormality (spacious tunica vaginalis, loose epididymotesticular connection, undescended testis) is usually present.

Clinical findings consist of precipitous onset of lower abdominal and scrotal pain and scrotal swelling. There may be a history of previous attacks in young adolescents. The testis is swollen, tender, and retracted. The pain is not relieved by testicular support. The cord above the swelling is normal. The cremasteric reflex is usually absent on the affected side.

Torsion must be differentiated from orchitis, epididymitis, and pain due to testicular trauma. Technetium Tc 99m pertechnetate scan *may* differentiate orchitis-epididymitis from testicular torsion if performed early in the course of symptoms: the former will demonstrate increased blood flow, in contrast to the ischemic pattern of torsion. Color Doppler ultrasound is more definitive and less time-consuming and can delineate the lack of testicular blood flow. No radiologic study is completely accurate, and imaging should be used to confirm the clinical decision that the cause of the acute scrotum is not torsion. If the diagnosis cannot be established by examination, history, and imaging, exploration is required.

Torsion of the spermatic cord is a surgical emergency! Contralateral orchiopexy is always necessary because of frequent bilateral involvement—ie, the "bell clapper" deformity (lack of fixation of the cord structures by the testicular mediastinum)—and the high incidence of recurrent torsion and infertility in bilateral cases.

TORSION OF TESTICULAR APPENDAGES

The epididymis and the testicle often have a vestigial remnant of embryologic ducts known as an appendix testis or appendix epididymis. These structures can undergo spontaneous infarction usually in young boys, causing acute testicular pain and swelling that may be difficult to differentiate from testicular torsion. With torsion of the appendix testis or epididymis, physical examination will often demonstrate point tenderness at the site of the torsed appendage. Occasionally, the infarcted appendage can be seen through the scrotal wall as a "blue dot" sign on the scrotum. This sign is only visible early in the course, prior to hydrocele formation and onset of scrotal edema. Scrotal ultrasound occasionally delineates the enlarged appendage and a normal testicle, establishing the diagnosis. In most cases—and certainly in equivocal ones—immediate scrotal exploration and removal of the infarcted appendage is required to rule out testicular torsion. Although the appendages often occur bilaterally, appendiceal torsion does not; thus, removal of the opposite appendage is not indicated.

MALE INFERTILITY*

Male infertility accounts for 30–50% of infertile couples (10–15% of marriages). Both partners should be evaluated for causes of infertility.

The causes of male infertility include the following: congenital anomalies (genetic, such as Klinefelter's syndrome, or developmental, such as absent vas deferens); trauma (both testicular, resulting in atrophy, and neurologic, resulting in erectile or ejaculatory dysfunction);

---

* Female infertility is discussed in Chapter 41.

infections (either systemic or reproductive organ specific); endocrine disorders (pituitary insufficiency, androgen deficiency); acquired anatomic abnormalities (varicocele, vasectomy); or drug side effects (nitrofurantoin, estrogens, antineoplastic agents).

Diagnosis

The most important aspect of infertility evaluation is the history, which uncovers the cause in many patients. The physical examination is no less important and may reveal small testicles, a varicocele, or absence of the vas deferens.

A. Semen Analysis

Semen analysis is essential in evaluation of male factor infertility. At least three samples should be analyzed, since values may vary over time and with the method of collection. The specimen is produced by masturbation after 3 days of ejaculatory abstinence and collected in a clean wide-mouth container and examined within 2 hours. Determination of the volume, pH, liquefaction, sperm count, viability, abnormal forms, and motility constitutes a complete analysis. Normal values include volume of more than 1.5 mL, 20 million sperm per milliliter, 60% motile sperm, and 60% normal oval sperm heads.

B. Hormone Studies

Patients with no sperm in the ejaculate (azoospermia) or very low counts (oligospermia) should have serum FSH, LH, prolactin, and testosterone levels measured. Patients with elevated prolactin levels should be investigated for pituitary tumor; those with markedly elevated FSH levels have primary testicular abnormalities that are not amenable to therapy.

C. Testicular Biopsy

Testicular biopsies are indicated in azoospermic patients to distinguish obstructive versus parenchymal disease. Testicular biopsy should be performed in patients with unexplained oligospermia to establish a histologic diagnosis, to assess prognosis, and to direct treatment. If the serum FSH is more than two times normal, one may presume the presence of severe and irreversible testicular damage without confirmatory testis biopsy.

Vasography requires injection of contrast material into the vas. The purpose of this study is to delineate obstruction of the vas, epididymis, seminal vesicle, or ejaculatory duct. Vasography is used in patients who are azoospermic and have no evidence of retrograde ejaculation while demonstrating normal spermatogenesis on testicular biopsy. Seminal fructose levels should be obtained before operative exposure of the vas. Absence of fructose would indicate obstruction of the ejaculatory duct, and if this diagnosis is confirmed by vasography, the obstructing tissue may be resected by transurethral methods.

D. Other Diagnostic Studies

The **sperm penetration assay**, performed by incubation of sperm with hamster eggs whose zona pellucida has been enzymatically removed, offers an objective method of determining the ability of sperm to penetrate the ovum. The **cervical mucus penetration test** compares sperm motility in cervical mucus with a known standard. Although these two important parameters of sperm function can be evaluated, neither test alone can establish the cause of male factor infertility.

Antisperm antibodies can be measured in the serum of either the male or female partner, or in the seminal fluid. This assessment is indicated when spontaneous sperm agglutination or decreased sperm motility is noted on semen analysis. If antisperm antibodies are found, immunosuppressive therapy in the form of steroids may be effective in reducing agglutination (clumping) and increasing motility. Another method of treating autosperm antibodies is in vitro sperm washing with immunobeads coated by anti-human antibody. The sperm not bound by antibody remain in the supernatant and can be used for intrauterine insemination.

Studies to detect a nonpalpable varicocele include **venous Doppler, scrotal thermography, venography, and ultrasound with color Doppler**. Physical examination is the most effective method of detecting clinically significant varices. Venography is reserved for patients with recurrent varices, since identification of collateral venous channels would direct choice of therapy.

Transrectal ultrasound is used to support the diagnosis of ejaculatory duct obstruction in the azoospermic patient. Absence of the seminal vesicles or distention due to distal obstruction can be identified. This study should be preceded by measurement of fructose in the ejaculate (lack of fructose suggests obstruction of the ejaculatory duct) and examination of postejaculate urine (to determine the presence of sperm, suggesting retrograde ejaculation).

Treatment

A. Nonoperative Treatment

Primary male infertility may be caused by hypogonadotropic hypogonadism, diagnosed by demonstrating low serum levels of FSH, LH, and testosterone. Spermatogenesis may be stimulated by administration of hCG followed by FSH. Isolated absence of either FSH or LH is rare; the LH deficiency is overcome by administration of testosterone, and lack of FSH is treated by administration of menotropins. Hyperprolactinemia may contribute to male infertility and would be treated with bromocriptine.

Infection of the reproductive organs should be treated when found during evaluation of male infertility. Infection may cause infertility immediately by several mechanisms: decreased spermatogenesis due to hyperthermia, immune interaction with sperm causing agglutination and decreased motility, as well as later sequelae such as obstruction of the ejaculatory tract. Pyospermia suggests the diagnosis, and treatment should be designed to eliminate the common pathogens: *Neisseria gonorrhoeae, Chlamydia trachomatis,* and *Ureaplasma urealyticum* (all are sensitive to tetracycline).

If antisperm antibodies are found in either partner, steroids may be used to suppress the immune system. One must use steroids with caution and after thoroughly discussion of possible side effects with the patient; acne, hypertension, gastrointestinal bleeding, and avascular necrosis of the hip have been reported with steroid administration. Response to treatment is assessed by repeat semen analysis and measurement of antisperm antibodies in the patient's serum. Sperm washing in an attempt to remove cytotoxic antibodies may improve motility and decrease clumping; washed semen may then be instilled into the uterus (artificial insemination of the husband's semen, AIH) or used in conjunction with in vitro fertilization techniques.

Retrograde ejaculation or lack of seminal emission—usually due to spinal cord injury or sympathetic nerve injury during retroperitoneal surgery leading to bladder neck (ie, internal sphincter) incompetence—can be treated with α-adrenergic drugs or antihistamines to reestablish internal sphincter function and antegrade ejaculation. Alternatively, alkalinized postejaculate urine can be collected and centrifuged and the concentrated sperm instilled into the female partner's uterus.

Other medications under investigation include clomiphene and tamoxifen. Currently, these drugs have not been objectively shown to be effective.

B. Operative Therapy

Ligation of varicocele will yield pregnancy in 30–50% of patients. Several approaches are available, including inguinal and retroperitoneal. Transvenous occlusion of the spermatic vein by balloon is useful especially in cases of recurrent varicocele.

Obstruction of the epididymis-vas system may be amenable to vasovasostomy or vasoepididymostomy. Currently, these procedures are performed with the aid of the operating microscope, and patency is established in 50–90%.

Obstruction of the ejaculatory ducts is rare. When this diagnosis is made, transurethral resection of the ducts may establish patency.

C. Assisted Reproductive Techniques

These include the following: artificial insemination with husband's sperm (AIH), gamete intrafallopian transfer (GIFT), and in vitro fertilization (IVF) using intracytoplasmic sperm injection (ICSI) after retrieving eggs by transvaginal ultrasound guidance and sperm by testicular aspiration in selected partners. In cases of male factor infertility not amenable to treatment, artificial insemination by donor sperm is also available.

PRIAPISM

Priapism is a rare disorder in which prolonged, painful erection occurs, usually not associated with sexual stimulation. The blood in the corpora cavernosa becomes hyperviscous but not clotted. About 25% of cases are associated with leukemia, metastatic carcinoma, sickle cell anemia, or trauma. In most cases, the cause is uncertain.

If the erection does not subside, needle aspiration of the sludged blood of the corpora followed by lavage with alpha-adrenergic agents such as phenylephrine should be performed. Delayed or unsuccessful treatment may result in impotence. Unsuccessful treatment calls for the Winter procedure, in which a biopsy needle is passed through the glans into one of the corpora. A piece of tunica albuginea is removed, creating a fistula between corpora cavernosa and corpus spongiosum. This simple procedure is highly successful, and potency is usually maintained. Other procedures include cavernosal-glandular shunt, cavernosal-spongiosum shunt, and saphenous vein-cavernous shunt. If priapism persists, impotence results.

In sickle cell anemia, hydration and hypertransfusion often give relief and should constitute initial therapy.

PEYRONIE'S DISEASE (PLASTIC INDURATION OF THE PENIS)

Fibrosis of the dorsal covering sheaths of the corpora cavernosa occasionally occurs without known cause in men over age 45. The fibrosis will not permit the involved surface to lengthen with erection, thus leading to dorsal chordee. The disorder may be due to vasculitis in the connective tissues. Palpation of the penile shaft reveals a raised, firm plaque dorsally. There is an association with Dupuytren's contracture.

Controversy exists regarding treatment. Expectant therapy or medical treatment, including vitamin E and aminobenzoic acid, may limit or cure the disease in half of patients. Operative therapy is necessary for patients who do not respond or for impotent patients. In the potent patient, a Nesbit procedure—excision of an ellipse of tunica albuginea from the ventral convex aspect of the shaft and suture closure—or plaque excision and dermal grafting has been used successfully. If the patient is impotent, insertion of a penile prosthesis is the procedure of choice.

PHIMOSIS & PARAPHIMOSIS

Phimosis—inability to retract the foreskin to expose the glans—may be congenital but is more often acquired. At birth, the foreskin cannot be easily retracted, but by age 3, the prepuce becomes pliant and the glans can be exposed and cleansed. If the foreskin is then retractable, circumcision is not necessary. Acquired phimosis is usually a result of chronic and recurrent bacterial balanitis (infection of the prepuce), common in patients with diabetes or balanitis xerotica obliterans. These patients are best treated by circumcision.

Paraphimosis is the inability to reduce a previously retracted foreskin. The prepuce becomes fixed in the retracted position proximal to the corona. With prolonged retraction, lymphedema of the prepuce exacerbates the condition and increases the circumferential pressure of the shaft proximal to the glans. Manual reduction can usually be accomplished using the index fingers to pull the prepuce distally while pushing the glans into the prepuce. If this measure fails, the preputial cicatrix may be incised (dorsal slit) and the foreskin reduced with relative ease. Circumcision may be performed as an elective procedure once the edema has subsided.

CONDYLOMATA ACUMINATA

Condylomata acuminata are wart-like lesions that occur on the penis, scrotum, urethra, and perineum in men and the vagina, cervix, and perineum in women. They are caused by human papillomavirus and are usually transmitted by sexual contact. Pain and bleeding are common presenting complaints. Warts outside the urethra can be treated with excision, application of podophyllum resin, liquid nitrogen, or CO_2 laser. Urethroscopy is needed to determine the proximal extent of lesions in the urethra. Intraurethral fulguration, CO_2 laser treatment, injection of fluorouracil solution, or IFN-α can be curative.

IMPOTENCE

Impotence is the inability to obtain and sustain an erection satisfactory for sexual intercourse.

Causes of Impotence

Causes can be grouped into the following categories: neurologic, vascular, endocrine, systemic, pharmacologic, and psychologic. Treatment is directed accordingly.

A. Neurologic

Reflex erections are mediated by the afferent fibers of the pudendal nerve and efferent fibers of the parasympathetic outflow (S2–S4). Psychogenic erections are initiated via cerebral centers. Specific neurologic diseases that may cause impotence may be congenital (spina bifida), acquired (cerebrovascular accident, Alzheimer's disease, multiple sclerosis), iatrogenic (electroshock therapy), neoplastic (pituitary or hypothalamic tumors), traumatic (cord compression), infectious (tabes dorsalis), and nutritional (vitamin deficiency).

B. Vascular

Vascular causes of impotence may be cardiac (anginal syndromes, congestive failure), aortoiliac disease (Leriche's syndrome, atherosclerosis, other embolic phenomena), microangiopathy (diabetes, radiation injury), and abnormal venous drainage.

C. Endocrine

The accepted endocrine causes of impotence are hypogonadism, hyperprolactinemia, pituitary tumors, hypothyroidism, Addison's disease, Cushing's syndrome, acromegaly, and testicular feminizing syndrome.

D. Pharmacologic

Impotence is a common and often unsuspected complication of many therapeutic and illicit drugs. Major groups that may cause sexual dysfunction are the following: tranquilizers, antidepressants, antianxiety agents, anticholinergic drugs, antihypertensives, and many drugs with abuse potential. One should recognize that virtually all antihypertensives (including diuretics) can be associated with impotence or ejaculatory dysfunction. Drugs with abuse potential include alcohol (both as a direct affect and secondary to cirrhosis) and cocaine.

E. Psychogenic

Up to 50% of cases of impotence are related to psychogenic factors. Establishing an organic cause of impotence is important in choosing appropriate therapy. Factors that indicate a psychogenic cause are the following: selective erectile dysfunction (episodic, normal nocturnal erections, normal erections with masturbation), sudden onset, associated anxiety or external stress, affect disturbances (anger, anxiety, guilt, fear), and patient convinced of an organic cause.

Diagnosis

The history and physical examination suggest the cause in most cases. Confirmatory tests are necessary to ensure an appropriate choice of therapy.

In investigating a possible neurologic cause of impotence, the neurologic examination should include review of systems with respect to bladder and bowel function. More invasive studies would include a cystometrogram with bethanechol supersensitivity testing, electromyography of the external urethral sphincter, and bulbosphincteric reflex latency.

Vascular impotence is suggested by signs of peripheral vascular disease as well as a history of atherosclerotic heart disease. Noninvasive diagnostic testing is performed by Doppler penile-brachial index. A penile blood pressure to brachial blood pressure ratio less than 0.6 suggests a vascular cause. Venous leak requires cavernosography and cavernosometry. Arteriography is rarely required but may be indicated in patients with a history of pelvic trauma.

Endocrine evaluation mandates measurement of serum testosterone and prolactin; many investigators would include assessment of follicle-stimulating and luteinizing hormones. Routine automated chemical screening may suggest other hormonal abnormalities that require additional testing. These studies should also detect systemic disease capable of causing impotence: cirrhosis, renal failure, scleroderma, and diabetes.

Psychogenic impotence may be established by nocturnal penile tumescence monitoring or outpatient snap-gauge cuffs. Additional testing includes one of the following: Minnesota Multiphasic Personality Inventory, DeRogatis Sexual Function Inventory, and Walker Sex Form.

Treatment

A. Nonoperative Treatment

In patients without arterial-vascular causes of impotence, intracorporal injections of papaverine, phentolamine, or prostaglandin E_1 (or all three) offer a nonoperative means of restoring sexual function. Intractable psychogenic impotence may also respond to this treatment. Intraurethral pellets of alprostadil (prostaglandin E_1) can also be used; however, they often cause pain and are not favored by most patients. Sildenafil, a phosphodiesterase inhibitor, is the first successful oral agent for erectile dysfunction. It works in patients who have normal blood flow and neurologic innervation, but it is expensive and is contraindicated in men with heart disease. Finally, a vacuum erection device can be used to sustain erection.

Endocrine disturbances responsible for impotence include hypotestosteronemia and hyperprolactinemia. Testosterone deficiency is treated by replacement therapy using a depot testosterone intramuscular injection every 2–3 weeks. Hyperprolactinemia is currently treated by bromocriptine therapy; the patient should be evaluated to assess the presence of a pituitary tumor.

Pharmacologic causes of impotence require altering medical treatment to ameliorate or eliminate secondary impotence. The ability to change medications depends upon the severity of the underlying disease.

Psychogenic impotence is treated by a trained sex therapist, and response may be anticipated in a majority of cases. The importance of eliminating organic causes of impotence before embarking upon psychological therapy is obvious: the best psychological methods applied to organic impotence will not resolve the dysfunction but will serve to frustrate both the therapist and patient.

B. Operative Treatment

Penile prosthesis insertion is currently the most common operative method for treatment of impotence. Two categories of prosthesis are in use: semirigid and inflatable. The semirigid prostheses are composed of a rigid shaft and a flexible hinge at the penile-pubic junction or a malleable soft metal case within the prosthesis; the erection is constant and is satisfactory to effect vaginal penetration, but the penile circumference is not equal to that of a natural erection.

Inflatable prostheses offer erections more similar in size to those experienced by the patient prior to the onset of impotence when compared to those achieved by semirigid prostheses. Two types of inflatable prostheses are available: the standard inflatable prosthesis consists of two corporal inflatable rods, a reservoir situated in the retropubic space, and a pump placed in the scrotum; the new inflatable rods combine the simplicity of two corporal rods with the sophistication of a self-contained pump and reservoir system (Flexi-Flate and Hydroflex), permitting the convenience of inflation and deflation without tubing and multiple components.

Satisfactory results are achieved in 85% of patients. Complications common to both types of prostheses are infection and erosion of skin or urethra. The inflatable prostheses are also at risk for mechanical failure of the pump, tubing or reservoir leak, and aneurysm or rupture of the corporal cylinders.

Arterial revascularization of the penile arteries has met with limited success. Aortoiliac reconstruction improves erectile function in only 30% of cases. Microsurgical revascularization of the penile arteries (dorsal artery of the penis or deep corporal arteries) is successful in 60% of patients. While these methods avoid the risks of prosthetic infection and offer the advantage of reestablishing the natural physiologic mechanisms or erection, the mediocre success rate (when compared with the results of prosthetic insertion) would suggest that microsurgical penile revascularization be reserved for carefully selected cases.

Brubaker L: Surgical treatment of urinary incontinence in women. Gastroenterology 2004;126:S71.

Brugh VM III, Lipshultz LI: Male factor infertility. Evaluation and management. Med Clin North Am 2004;88:367.

Carrier S et al: Pathophysiology of erectile dysfunction. Urology 1993;42:468.

Chancellor MB, Yoshimura N: Treatment of interstitial cystitis. Urology 2004;63(Suppl 3A):85.

Chuang AT et al: Male infertility: evaluation and nonsurgical therapy. Urol Clin North Am 1998;25:703.

Diokno AC: Medical management of urinary incontinence. Gastroenterology 2004;126:S77.

Donovan JF et al: Laparoscopic varix ligation. J Urol 1992;147:77.

Erickson DR et al: Interstitial cystitis. Int Urogynecol J 1998;9:174.

Hansen SW et al: Long-term fertility and Leydig cell function in patients treated for germ cell cancer with cisplatin, vinblastine and bleomycin versus surveillance. J Clin Oncol 1990;8:1695.

Howards SS: Treatment of male infertility. N Engl J Med 1995;332:312.

Kamischke A et al: Analysis of medical treatment of male infertility. Hum Reprod 1999;14:1.

Lamb DJ et al: Male infertility: recent advances and a look towards the future. Curr Opin Urol 2000;10:359.

Martin-du Pan RC, Campana A: Physiopathology of spermatogenic arrest. Fertil Steril 1993;60:937.

Nickel JC: Interstitial cystitis. A chronic pelvic pain syndrome. Med Clin North Am 2004;88:467.

Ralph DJ, Minhas S: The management of Peyronie's disease. BJU Int 2004;93:208.

Sant GR et al: Interstitial cystitis. Curr Opin Urol 1999;9:297.

Schlesinger MH et al: Treatment outcome after varicocelectomy: a critical analysis. Urol Clin North Am 1994;21:517.

Seftel AD et al: Erectile dysfunction: etiology, evaluation and treatment options. Med Clin North Am 2004;88:387.

Sigman M: Assisted reproductive techniques and male infertility. Urol Clin North Am 1994;21:505.

Simon LJ et al: The Interstitial Cystitis Data Base Study: concepts and preliminary baseline descriptive statistics. Urology 1997; 49(Suppl 5A):64.

Gynecology 41

Edward C. Hill, MD, & Elena A. Gates, MD

CONGENITAL ANOMALIES OF THE FEMALE REPRODUCTIVE SYSTEM

Edward C. Hill, MD, & Elena A. Gates, MD

Congenital defects of the female reproductive system arise as a result of abnormal embryonic development of the müllerian ducts and urogenital sinus. The most common defects are imperforate hymen, septate or double vagina, transverse septum of the vagina, congenital absence of the vagina, and duplication defects of the uterus. Although most such defects are idiopathic, some result from in utero exposure to teratogenic agents such as diethylstilbestrol or androgenic progestins during the first $4^1/_2$ months of fetal development.

An adequate physical examination will detect or at least arouse suspicion of defective development. Careful examination of the genitalia of the newborn is especially important; errors have been made in gender assignment because of casual examinations. Imaging with ultrasound (or, preferably, MRI), pelvic examination under anesthesia, and laparoscopic or hysteroscopic examination can provide additional information. The urinary tract should be imaged as well because one-third to one-half of cases are associated with anomalies of the urinary tract such as absent kidney, horseshoe kidney, and duplication of the collecting system. Injury to the urinary tract can result from failure to recognize associated urinary tract anomalies during corrective surgery.

VAGINAL ANOMALIES

Imperforate Hymen

Imperforate hymen is often not recognized until puberty, when, despite the appearance of menstrual symptoms such as cramping, no bleeding is seen. Examination at this time will reveal the bulging imperforate hymen. Rectal examination may demonstrate a large cystic pelvic mass representing a distended vagina (hematocolpos) and even a cystically enlarged uterus (hematometra). Urinary obstruction has been reported as a result of a large hematocolpos from accumulation of menstrual fluid behind an imperforate hymen.

Imperforate hymen is treated by cruciate incisions (hymenotomy) or laser excision of the mucous membrane, releasing the trapped menstrual fluid and correcting the hematocolpos and hematometra. Antibiotics should be given when there is significant hematocolpos and hematometra in order to prevent secondary infection.

Duplication of the Vagina

Duplication of the vagina may occur with or without duplication of the uterine corpus. The duplication may be only partial and may take the form of a longitudinal septum, in which case excision may be required if soft tissue dystocia occurs in labor or if coitus is obstructed. Complete duplication of the vagina usually requires no treatment.

Occasionally, the duplication takes the form of a hemivagina, a rudimentary vagina that fails to communicate with the second vagina or the introitus. This may result in formation of hematocolpos at menarche, with an apparent paravaginal cystic mass as a presenting sign. Renal agenesis may occur ipsilateral to the hemivagina. Marsupialization of the rudimentary vagina with the primary vagina is the usual method of management.

Transverse Septum of the Vagina

A transverse vaginal septum usually is incomplete. If imperforate, it may be mistaken for congenital absence of the vagina. Transverse vaginal septa are treated by excision.

Absence of the Vagina

Absence of the vagina usually is associated with absence of the uterus as well. Often there is a very small lower vagina representing the portion that develops from the urogenital sinus. The condition is commonly not recognized until the physician is consulted because of primary amenorrhea in a teenager. Treatment is frequently desired in an attempt to achieve more satisfactory sexual function.

Congenital absence of the vagina is managed by creation of an artificial vagina. This should be deferred until the patient has a desire and a need for a functioning vagina. In a well-motivated patient, congenital absence of the vagina may be corrected by nonoperative dilation and elongation of the vulvar vestibule. Success has been reported with vaginal dilators, vaginal molds, and with intercourse alone. Should a conservative approach fail or seem inappropriate to the management of an individual patient, the condition can be managed by surgical construction of an artificial vagina. A variety of techniques have been described and typically involve segments of small or large bowel, skin graft, or vulvoperineal skin flaps placed in an artificially created channel between the bladder and the rectum.

DUPLICATION DEFECTS OF THE UTERUS

Duplication defects of the uterus are often detected in the course of investigation for habitual abortion or for repeated premature labor. While many women with uterine anomalies have normal pregnancy outcomes, these anomalies are associated with increased rates of first- and second-trimester loss, cervical incompetence, preterm labor, and malpresentation of the fetus. Conception rates do not appear to be affected. Anomalies may vary from a simple midline septum in a single uterus (septate uterus) to duplication of the uterine horns (bicornuate uterus) to complete duplication of the corpus and cervix (uterus didelphys). These types of uterine anomalies may be suspected after physical examination, especially during pregnancy. Diagnosis can be confirmed using MRI or hysterosalpingography. The latter should be combined with ultrasonography or laparoscopy to distinguish a large septum from a bicornuate state. A combined laparoscopic-hysteroscopic evaluation is also useful, particularly if operation is planned.

The principal indication for surgical correction of uterine anomalies is recurrent pregnancy loss. It is important to select surgical candidates carefully, as cervical incompetence can be associated with uterine anomalies and is best treated by cerclage. The septate uterus is most often treated by hysteroscopic metroplasty with transcervical incision or resection of the septum. If the septum cannot be successfully resected hysteroscopically, abdominal metroplasty may be warranted. Pregnancies occurring after abdominal metroplasty should be delivered by cesarean section as the risk of uterine rupture is increased. When uterine anomalies are responsible for a poor obstetric history with high fetal wastage, one can expect significant improvement following surgical correction.

Grimbizis G et al: Hysteroscopic septum resection in patients with recurrent abortions or infertility. Hum Reprod 1998;13:1188.

Heinonen PK: Reproductive performance of women with uterine anomalies after abdominal or hysteroscopic metroplasty or no surgical treatment. J Am Assoc Gynecol Laparosc 1997;4:311.

Hensle TW et al: Vaginal reconstruction. Urol Clin North Am 1999;26:39.

Li S et al: Association of renal agenesis and müllerian duct anomalies. J Comput Assist Tomogr 2000;24:829.

CORRECTION OF INFERTILITY DUE TO TUBAL ABNORMALITIES

Marcelle Cedars, MD

A couple may be considered infertile if a pregnancy does not occur after 1 year of normal coital activity (12 ovulatory exposed cycles) without contraceptives. About 15% of couples are infertile, and in approximately 40% of these there is a significant male factor (low sperm count, impaired motility, or anomalous forms). One-third of infertile couples have more than one problem. Anatomic abnormalities of the pelvic organs are the single most common cause of infertility in women. The list may include chronic salpingitis, endometriosis, and peritubal adhesions from previous appendicitis (with rupture). The bacteria involved with an inflamed appendix may be quite "toxic" to the female tube. Desire to reverse previous tubal sterilization may also be a reason for tubal surgery.

History

Specific questions should elicit information regarding any history of sexually transmitted disease, pelvic inflammatory disease, and any abdominal surgery. Patients should also be asked about worsening dysmenorrhea or deep dyspareunia that might suggest endometriosis.

Clinical Findings

Pelvic examination should always be performed. The size and mobility of the uterus should be assessed and the presence of adnexal masses excluded. Rectovaginal examination is required to evaluate the uterosacral ligaments for nodularity and tenderness (suggesting endometriosis). Ultrasound is often helpful. The ovaries can be evaluated for the presence of iso-echoic masses that might suggest endometriosis (endometriomas). A large hydrosalpinx may be easily seen on ultrasound and may modify treatment recommendations.

Even if the examination is normal, a hysterosalpingogram may reveal an obstruction at the cornu, a hydrosalpinx, partial fimbrial occlusion, or tubo-ovarian adhesions. For safety reasons, the procedure should always be performed first with a water-based dye; if the tubes are patent and there is no extravasation of the dye, an oil contrast medium may then be used. Data suggest that this procedure improves pregnancy rates in patients with unexplained infertility and minimal to mild endometriosis.

Laparoscopy with direct visualization of the pelvic organs may be warranted if the above findings are inconclusive. Evaluation of the pelvic organs, as well as therapeutic (corrective) measures, can be performed at the same time with this procedure. This treatment might involve lysis of adhesions or fulguration of endometrial implants. If the hysterosalpingogram is entirely normal, there is about a 30% chance that an abnormality will be found on laparoscopy. Almost 80% of these abnormalities will be minimal or mild (peritoneal) endometriosis. Only about 6% of patients will have adhesive disease not suspected on the hysterosalpingogram.

Treatment

Transvaginal tubal catheterization (much like an angioplasty) may be performed either by radiologic guidance (by the interventional radiologist) or by hysteroscopy (by the gynecologist) to relieve proximal tubal obstruction. This may avoid the need for more elaborate procedures such as tubal reimplantation.

Tuboplasty operations are designed to reestablish tubal patency or return pelvic anatomy to normal by lysis of adhesions. These surgical procedures are more successful if the damage is localized and there is little intrinsic damage to the tube (eg, with fimbrial adhesions or previous tubal ligation). Reestablishment and maintenance of tubal patency have been more successful with the development of microsurgical techniques that require gentle tissue handling. Salpingolysis, reimplantation of the tube into the uterus, end-to-end anastomosis, and fimbrial salpingostomy may be performed. The use of laparoscopy (avoiding exposure of the bowel and peritoneal surfaces to air and handling) decreases the chances for new adhesion formation. Minimizing manipulation to the tissues and minimizing bleeding and necrosis limit the re-formation of adhesions. Newer agents that act as barriers to separate tissues and prevent adhesion re-formation are under investigation.

Evaluation of the extent of tubal damage (damage to the fimbria and internal tubal structures) and of peritubal adhesive disease is critical to the estimation of expected success with any tubal repair. Tubal surgery statistics are generally quoted as the cumulative pregnancy rate over a 2-year period of time. Therefore, other infertility factors must be evaluated and will influence the likelihood of success following surgery. The female partner's age and the presence of other infertility factors (eg, ovulatory dysfunction, male factor) might make tubal surgery a less attractive option even when the anatomy would suggest the likelihood for a good anatomic repair.

In vitro fertilization is an alternative when tubal obstruction cannot be remedied or when multiple infertility factors exist. If a hydrosalpinx is visible on ultrasound, consideration should be given to its removal (or obstruction) prior to proceeding to in vitro fertilization as implantation rates are lower and miscarriage rates higher in their presence.

Prognosis

When the female partner is young (under 35) and only mild disease exists, pregnancy rates may reach 70%. With the most severe disease, this rate drops to < 15%. Ectopic (tubal pregnancy) rates are approximately 10%, and all tubal surgery patients should be followed closely until an intrauterine pregnancy is documented. Tubal reanastomosis rates may be as high as 80–90% for an isthmic-isthmic anastomosis. All rates for tubal surgery must be compared with the success of the local in vitro fertilization program to determine the best option for an individual patient.

Benadiva CA et al: In vitro fertilization versus tubal surgery: is pelvic reconstructive surgery obsolete? Fertil Steril 1995;64:1051.

Spielvogel K et al: Surgical management of adhesions, endometriosis, and tubal pathology in the woman with infertility. Clin Obstet Gynecol 2000;43:916.

Watson A et al: Techniques for pelvic surgery in subfertility. Cochrane Database Syst Rev 2000;(2):CD000221.

Watson A et al: Liquid and fluid agents for preventing adhesions after surgery for subfertility. Cochrane Database Syst Rev 2000;(2):CD001298.

ABNORMAL UTERINE BLEEDING

Abner Korn, MD

Abnormal uterine bleeding may occur at any age. In the newborn, it is frequently related to removal of the infant at birth from the influence of maternal estrogen, which has produced endometrial proliferation in the baby's uterus. During the reproductive years, it may occur as **hypermenorrhea** (or **menorrhagia**), excessive or prolonged bleeding at the normal time of menstruation; **polymenorrhea**, bleeding that occurs more frequently than every 3 weeks; or **intermenstrual bleeding** (or **metrorrhagia**), which occurs during the interval between normal menstrual periods.

Hypermenorrhea may be due to such organic conditions as uterine leiomyoma, endometrial polyps, and blood dyscrasias or it may be related to a functional disturbance such as irregular shedding of the endometrium, presumably resulting from faulty regression of the corpus luteum of the ovary. Polymenorrhea may be related to early ovulation with a shortened proliferative phase, which frequently is secondary to hypothyroidism. One of the most frequently encountered problems is the completely acyclic and sometimes heavy and prolonged bleeding of the anovulatory patient, leading to so-called **dysfunctional uterine bleeding**. This condition is seen most often in adolescents and in perimenopausal women and is due to a failure in regular ovulatory function. The endometrium is proliferative in type at a time in the menstrual cycle when it would show secretory changes if ovulation had occurred. In many instances there is, after a period of time, the development of endometrial hyperplasia owing to the prolonged stimulus of estrogen on the endometrium without the modifying influence of progesterone. Intermenstrual bleeding may be due to the slight drop in estrogen titer associated with ovulation, in which event it occurs quite regularly at about mid cycle. Other causes of intermenstrual bleeding that occurs at any time are polyps, submucous leiomyomas, blood dyscrasias, genital tuberculosis, and cancer of the cervix, uterine corpus, or uterine tube. Complications of pregnancy should not be overlooked as a cause of abnormal bleeding in women of reproductive age.

Postmenopausal bleeding—vaginal bleeding occurring a year or more after menopause—is of concern because it may be indicative of endometrial cancer. The exogenous administration of estrogenic substances, including their use in cosmetic preparations and herbal supplements, is also an important cause. Atrophic changes, polyps, trauma, blood dyscrasias, hypertensive cardiovascular disease, and estrogen-producing tumors of the ovary are less frequent causes. The bleeding may be represented by a scant brownish vaginal discharge, or it may be frank, profuse, bright red bleeding. Because it looms so large in the etiology of postmenopausal bleeding, cancer should be considered the cause until proved otherwise.

Clinical Findings

In the assessment of any type of menstrual disorder, the following points should be considered:

(1) Careful documentation of the menstrual history and a record of the temporal relationship of the abnormal bleeding to the menstrual cycle are necessary. A special menstrual calendar kept by the patient or a basal body temperature graph can be very helpful.

(2) A history of hormonal medication, herbal supplement, or hormone-containing cosmetic use.

(3) A general history and physical examination may lead to the correct diagnosis of hypothyroidism, blood dyscrasia (most commonly in adolescents), anticoagulant use, genital tuberculosis, etc.

(4) A carefully performed pelvic examination will often reveal vaginal, cervical, uterine, or adnexal disease.

(5) Cervical cytologic examination is essential in all patients, and the specimen should be collected prior to the introduction of lubricating jelly into the vagina.

(6) A complete blood count and measurement of red cell indices will reflect the degree of iron deficiency secondary to acute or chronic blood loss. Additional blood studies may be necessary when endocrine disorders or blood dyscrasias are suspected.

(7) Endometrial biopsy is often required to establish the cause of abnormal menstrual bleeding. Biopsy should be done at an appropriate time in the menstrual cycle—eg, after the 16th day of the cycle if anovulatory bleeding is suspected—but can be done at any time to evaluate for hyperplasia or carcinoma. Endometrial sampling with a disposable suction-device (Pipelle, Vabra, etc) can be accomplished in an office setting.

(8) Hysteroscopy may help establish the cause of bleeding and offers the opportunity for simultaneous treatment. Hysteroscopy can be accomplished in an office or outpatient surgical setting and is recommended when bleeding is recurrent or resistant to therapy or when structural abnormalities of the endometrium (eg, myomas) are suspected.

(9) Transvaginal ultrasound can show endometrial thickness and structural abnormalities of the uterus (such as polyps or myomas), especially when saline is introduced into the endometrial cavity (sonohysterogram). Using an endometrial thickness threshold of 5 mm, 96% of cancers are detected with a specificity of 92% when hormone replacement therapy is not being used and 77% when hormone replacement is used.

Treatment

Dilation and curettage is a most effective short-term method of controlling uterine bleeding. Longer-term treatment will generally be directed toward the cause of the abnormal uterine bleeding.

In chronic blood loss due to hypermenorrhea produced by leiomyomas, reduction in bleeding can be achieved by the administration of progestins. A gonadotropin-releasing hormone agonist will result in menstrual suppression and amenorrhea. Bleeding due to leiomyomas can be lessened by removal of the fibroid tumors (myomectomy) or cured by hysterectomy.

Dysfunctional bleeding due to chronic anovulation is treated with cyclic progestin therapy (medroxyprogesterone acetate, 10 mg/d for 10 days every 4 weeks), with oral contraceptive pills, or, for women who desire to become pregnant, with clomiphene for ovulation induction. Control of acute heavy bleeding may be achieved through the use of higher dose combination oral contraceptives (one pill four times a day for 3 or 4 days to control bleeding, then tapered to one pill a day over the ensuing week). An antiemetic is often needed when using high-estrogen therapy. A low-dose oral contraceptive is started and continued for 3 months or longer, if the patient desires. Intravenous conjugated estrogen, 25 mg every 4 hours, has been used also to control acute bleeding. Such a regimen must be followed by administration of a progestin to stabilize the endometrium. This can then be followed by daily use of an oral contraceptive pill for longer-term control. Termination of hormonal treatment will result in withdrawal bleeding. A 5-year intrauterine device (IUD) containing levonorgestrel produces amenorrhea in about 25% of women and light bleeding in the remainder.

Severe and intractable bleeding of a dysfunctional nature may rarely require hysterectomy. In the absence of other causes, hypermenorrhea associated with ovulatory cycles can be ameliorated with nonsteroidal anti-inflammatory drugs. Hysteroscopic endometrial ablation by Nd:YAG laser or electrosurgery may avoid hysterectomy in the premenopausal patient with intractable bleeding. These operations generally require a normal uterine cavity. About 20% of women have amenorrhea following endometrial ablation, but up to 35% will require hysterectomy within 5 years. Alternative methods of endometrial ablation developed recently (eg, thermal balloons) seem to have efficacy equal to hysteroscopic ablation but are technically simpler to perform. The levonorgestrel IUD has been shown in recent randomized, controlled trials to be nearly as effective as hysteroscopic ablation operations.

Postmenopausal bleeding of nonneoplastic origin may require estrogen therapy if it is due to atrophic changes. More commonly, it is seen as a side effect of hormone replacement therapy (HRT) and can be treated by discontinuing HRT or choosing an alternative regimen. Curettage is curative if the bleeding is due to endometrial polyps. Endometrial carcinoma is a contraindication to estrogen therapy and is treated by total abdominal hysterectomy and bilateral salpingo-oophorectomy with or without preoperative radiation therapy. Well-differentiated endometrial adenocarcinoma in young women who desire to maintain fertility has been successfully treated using high-dose progestins in about three-fourths of cases.

Randall TC: Progestin treatment of atypical hyperplasia and well-differentiated carcinoma of the endometrium in women under age 40. Obstet Gynecol 1997;90:434.

A randomised trial of endometrial ablation versus hysterectomy for the treatment of dysfunctional uterine bleeding: outcome at four years. Aberdeen Endometrial Ablation Trials Group. Br J Obstet Gynaecol 1999;106:360.

Smith-Bindman R et al: Endovaginal ultrasound to exclude endometrial cancer and other endometrial abnormalities. JAMA 1998;280:1510.

Stewart A: The effectiveness of the levonorgestrel-releasing intrauterine system in menorrhagia: a systematic review. Br J Obstet Gynaecol 2001;108:74.

CHRONIC PELVIC PAIN

Lee Learman, MD, PhD

Chronic pelvic pain is most often defined as 6–12 months of pain below the umbilicus producing a significant impact on a patient's quality of life. A 1994 Gallup Poll found that one in seven reproductive-age women had experienced chronic pelvic pain and estimated the annual cost of illness to be $882 million in outpatient visits alone. The evaluation and treatment of chronic pelvic pain accounts for 15–40% of all referrals to gynecologists, 40% of all laparoscopies, and 12% of all hysterectomies.

Diagnosis

The differential diagnosis and comorbidity of chronic pelvic pain make it one of the most challenging issues encountered in ambulatory practice. While many patients attribute their pain to a gynecologic cause, the physician must conduct a meticulous patient interview and physical examination to assess a wide range of nongynecologic diagnoses. The most common of these are irritable bowel syndrome and inflammatory bowel disease; nephrolithiasis and interstitial cystitis; abdominal wall hernia, muscle strain, or nerve injury; and depressive disorders or somatization. Patients may also have mood symptoms as a consequence of living with pain and are more likely to have suffered sexual assault as an adult or child.

The gynecologic causes of chronic pelvic pain are grouped into cyclic and continuous symptom patterns. Cyclic causes include primary dysmenorrhea, in which periods are painful but no pelvic pathology can be identified; and secondary dysmenorrhea due to endometriosis, adenomyosis, or perhaps chronic salpingitis. Midcycle ovulatory pain (mittelschmerz) occurs during oocyte release from an ovarian follicle and thus produces lateral pain that migrates from one side to the other from month to month. Gynecologic causes of continuous pain include later stages of endometriosis and adenomyosis, uterovaginal prolapse, and chronic salpingitis or pelvic adhesions. Ovarian remnant syndrome occurs after oophorectomy when residual ovarian tissue is trapped in a retroperitoneal location. Ovarian dystrophy occurs when an ovary undergoes progressive ischemic injury after ligation of the uterine circulation at hysterectomy or tubal surgery.

Clinical Findings

The pelvic examination for chronic pelvic pain proceeds in a slow and methodical fashion in which the patient remains fully informed of each step in the examination and is allowed to interrupt or terminate the examination at any time. The goal is first to determine what the background degree of tenderness is and then to identify focal tender areas that exceed this background level. The patient is instructed before the examination to indicate which maneuvers during the examination reproduce their pain. A rectovaginal examination should be conducted to evaluate cul-de-sac tenderness or mass and to palpate the uterosacral ligaments for evidence of endometriosis. A pelvic mass found on examination is usually further characterized by ultrasound into suspicious versus nonsuspicious for neoplasm, and surveillance, medical treatment, or surgical excision is then planned accordingly. An abnormal pelvic examination has about an 80% predictive value for pelvic abnormalities noted at laparoscopy but only about a 45% sensitivity and a 40% negative predictive value.

Treatment

After ruling out nongynecologic causes by history, physical examination, and appropriate studies and referrals, reproductive-age women are often offered treatment consisting of analgesics and ovulation suppression. A typical regimen would include low-dose combined oral contraceptives (to be used in patients over 35 years old only if they are nonsmokers) and nonsteroidal anti-inflammatory agents. When pain is refractory to medical management or when physical examination findings are abnormal, diagnostic laparoscopy is conducted. This procedure includes a survey of upper abdominal structures and meticulous inspection of the pelvic peritoneum, bladder, uterus, tubes, ovaries, appendix, rectum, and sigmoid colon. Approximately one-third of patients will have evidence of endometriosis, one-third will have adhesions or evidence of chronic salpingitis, and one-third will have a normal pelvis. The presence of abnormalities may not explain the pain, however. Among pain-free patients undergoing laparoscopy for other indications, about 30% will have abnormal findings.

Although the evidence for success of laparoscopic treatments is not strong, patient preference and clinical experience support correction of focal abnormalities and other procedures that could credibly lessen the patient's pain. These procedures include lysis of adhesions, destruction or removal of endometriotic implants and ovarian endometriomas, and interruption of the autonomic nerve tracts through which pain messages travel from the pelvis to the spinal cord (presacral neurectomy, uterine nerve ablation). The best available data indicate that laparoscopic treatments will produce a short-term improvement in pain in 62–82% of patients. The treatment success data come primarily from case series reports and thus are likely to overestimate real-world success. While the interventions to improve pelvic pain could also be performed via laparotomy, this is avoided out of a concern that laparotomy is more adhesiogenic than laparoscopy because there is greater peritoneal injury.

In nondepressed patients who have completed their childbearing or who wish definitive treatment, hysterectomy is a highly effective therapy with success rates of 75–95% if uterine pathology is present and 50–91% if no pelvic pathology is noted. The success rate plummets to less than 5% if the patient has any neurovegetative signs or symptoms of depression. Patients with endometriosis should also be offered bilateral ovarian removal to prevent stimulation of residual implants. Finally, patients with refractory pain after multiple medical regimens and surgical procedures should be referred to a multidisciplinary clinic where the myriad causes of pelvic pain can be systematically investigated and chronic pain management instituted.

Jamieson DF et al: The prevalence of dysmenorrhea, dyspareunia, pelvic pain, and irritable bowel syndrome in primary care practices. Obstet Gynecol 1996;87:55.

Mathias SD et al: Chronic pelvic pain: prevalence, health-related quality of life, and economic correlates. Obstet Gynecol 1996;87:321.

CONTRACEPTION

Philip D. Darney, MD

The majority of the world's people who want to avoid an unintended birth rely on methods of family planning that require some sort of operative procedure, including sterilization operations for men and women, the insertion of contraceptives into the uterine cavity or under the skin, and termination of unwanted pregnancies by therapeutic abortion. These family planning procedures are in fact the world's most commonly performed operations. In the United States, nearly one million sterilization operations and more than a million abortions are performed yearly. Nearly 40% of American women rely on their own tubal sterilization or the male partner's vasectomy for contraception. These common operations are simple, safe, and effective, but specialized equipment, knowledge of methods of pain relief, and training are required. It is beyond the scope of this chapter to provide more than an overview of these procedures. Texts listed in the bibliography provide technical details.

Americans use sterilization for contraception more than the people of most countries because temporary methods such as intrauterine and oral contraceptives have an undeservedly bad reputation in the United States. An increase in both female and male sterilization procedures occurred between 1973 and 1988, a period during which the use of intrauterine contraception declined and the use of oral contraception decreased substantially. Since the late 1980s, oral contraception has regained some of its popularity.

Sterilization by tubectomy was first proposed by James Blundell in lectures at Guy's Hospital in London, but the operation did not become common until the 1930s. Many methods of female sterilization were developed, including the Madelener, Irving, Uchida, and the still popular Pomeroy operations, but these all required laparotomy. Not until laparoscopic tubal occlusion was introduced did female sterilization become more common than the simpler male vasectomy. In laparoscopic procedures, the oviducts are occluded with Filshie titanium clips, Hulka spring-loaded clips, Yoon Silastic bands, or unipolar or bipolar electrocautery. A 10-year follow-up study has shown that long-term failure of all these operations is higher than expected, ranging from 2% to 4%—comparable to the failure rates of copper or hormonal intrauterine contraceptives and subdermal implants. This study did not demonstrate adverse health or menstrual effects of tubal occlusion operations. Because tubal occlusion reversal is difficult and expensive, 2–25% of women express regret at having had the operation. Both mini laparotomy for Pomeroy-type tubal excision and laparoscopic tubal occlusion are commonly performed under local anesthesia with conscious sedation in about 20 minutes.

Modern intrauterine contraceptives carry copper or progestational hormones to the uterine cavity where they inhibit sperm motility and block fertilization. They are packaged with disposable inserters that can usually be passed through the cervical canal without local anesthesia or cervical dilation. Both copper and progestin devices are highly effective and have long durations of action (less than 5% failure at 10 years of use). These modern intrauterine contraceptives do not increase the risk of pelvic infection. On the contrary, the levonorgestrel-containing system, like other hormonal contraceptives, actually decreases the risk of pelvic inflammatory disease. Ectopic pregnancy rates in users of these intrauterine contraceptives are reduced to a tenth of those reported in women not using contraception of any kind.

The principal side effect of intrauterine contraceptives is change in menstrual bleeding: the copper devices increase blood loss and the progestin devices decrease it to about half the normal flow. Because of this action, the levonorgestrel device has been shown to be as effective as uterine surgery for treatment of abnormal uterine bleeding as well as to protect the endometrium from precancerous hyperplasia during estrogen replacement therapy. The copper device is an effective postcoital (emergency) contraceptive, but progestin devices cannot be used in this way.

Despite the safety and efficacy of intrauterine contraceptives, they are much less used in the USA than in the rest of the world. For example, in Germany and Denmark, about 20% of women practicing contraception use intrauterine methods, while in the USA less than 1% do.

Subdermal implant contraception uses low serum concentrations of contraceptive progestins found in birth control pills to thicken cervical mucus and inhibit ovulation. These actions result in failure rates comparable to those reported following sterilization and intrauterine contraception. Their duration of action ranges from 1 year to 7 years depending on the number of implants, the progestin employed, and the delivery system. As with intrauterine contraceptives, the principal side effect is change in menstrual bleeding; the majority of users experience a diminution in blood loss but an increase in number of days of bleeding, sometimes at unpredictable intervals.

Contraceptive implants require subdermal insertion with a disposable trocar under local anesthesia. They are removed under local anesthesia with a scalpel and forceps. These procedures take only a few minutes, and pain and infections are rare. The 7-year system (Norplant) uses six capsules, requiring more time for insertion and removal. Newer single-rod systems (eg, Implanon and Uniplant) are easier to use, have a shorter life, and are associated with somewhat more acceptable bleeding patterns.

Although new contraceptives are safe and highly effective, they are not perfect. Unintended pregnancies result in the need for about one million abortions per year in the USA. In the past, contraceptive failure meant an unwanted birth or recourse to dangerous secret abortion services. Changes in the law and in abortion techniques have meant that in most countries of the world women need not risk their lives to limit family size. Uterine aspiration procedures using manual or electric sources of vacuum have led to safe induced abortions in the first trimester, with mortality rates of less than 1:200,000 procedures. Second-trimester terminations require more complex equipment and greater surgical skill: The principal determinant of the morbidity and mortality of abortion is the duration of gestation, with abortion at 20 weeks being ten times as risky as abortion at 10 weeks.

Medical methods of abortion using prostaglandins with or without progesterone antagonists (eg, mifepristone) are employed at gestations earlier than 9 weeks and beyond 20 weeks, but surgical abortion remains much more common and less expensive in both the first and second trimester. The principal complications are hemorrhage and uterine perforation (primarily with second-trimester operations), but the principal cause of death associated with abortion is anesthesia. Local anesthesia, with or without conscious sedation, is safer than general anesthesia.

Darney P et al: *Protocols for Ambulatory Gynecologic Surgery.* Blackwell Science, 1996.

Speroff L et al: *A Clinical Guide for Contraception,* 3rd ed. Lippincott Williams & Wilkins, 2001.

PELVIC ORGAN PROLAPSE & URINARY INCONTINENCE

Sharon Knight, MD, & Elaine Waetjen, MD

An understanding of pelvic floor relaxation requires a thorough knowledge of the anatomic relationship of the pelvic viscera and their supporting tissues. These conditions are thought to result initially from stretching and tearing of the muscles, nerves, and connective tissues of the pelvis during vaginal childbirth. Other factors thought to contribute to loss of support include chronic or repetitive increases in intra-abdominal pressure (eg, chronic cough, constipation, heavy lifting, obesity).

Anatomically, multiple factors play a role in pelvic support. The paired levator ani muscles collectively form the pelvic floor. The collagenous support of the pelvis includes the endopelvic fascia, which is continuous with the cardinal and uterosacral ligaments. The bladder, upper vagina, and rectum all rest horizontally upon and are supported by the levator ani muscles, which actively contract to maintain the position of those structures in the pelvis.

Obstetric injuries to the pelvic floor can involve damage (stretching or breaks) to the investing endopelvic fascia and the supporting ligaments of the uterus as well as muscular and neurologic injury, which may also contribute to loss of levator function and thus loss of support. Careful repair of lacerations occurring during delivery will avoid these problems.

Stress incontinence is involuntary loss of urine from the urethra with increases in intra-abdominal pressure (eg, Valsalva maneuver) in the absence of detrusor activity. It can be demonstrated clinically during pelvic examination by asking the patient to cough. Stress incontinence should be distinguished from other common types of urinary incontinence. With **urge incontinence**, the patient experiences the loss of urine with bladder filling and the desire to void. Stress and urge incontinence may occur simultaneously and are referred to as **mixed incontinence. Overflow incontinence** may present with symptoms of any of the other described types of incontinence. It can be ruled out by checking a postvoid residual urine volume during examination. Surgical correction of stress incontinence may produce a temporary urge incontinence that may persist in 10–15 % of patients.

The bladder and urethra are supported by the muscles of the pelvic floor and the endopelvic fascia. There are two primary mechanisms of stress incontinence. In women with normal pelvic support, the proximal urethra is held in a pelvic position and is subjected to the same intra-abdominal pressure changes as those affecting the bladder. Thus, increases in abdominal pressure (eg, during coughing) are distributed equally to the urethra and bladder and in this way the greater "closing pressure" of the urethra is maintained and the patient remains continent. In patients with anterior vaginal wall relaxation, however, increased abdominal pressure causes descent of the proximal urethra and bladder base into the vagina (hypermobile urethra). Thus, pressure is no longer equally distributed (intravesical pressure exceeds intraurethral pressure) and urinary leakage occurs.

The second mechanism of stress urinary incontinence, **intrinsic sphincter deficiency**, involves loss of integrity of the urethral sphincter. Risk factors include previous surgery to treat incontinence, a history of radiation therapy, and age over 50 years. This diagnosis is independent of pelvic support.

In cases of pelvic organ prolapse beyond the hymen, stress incontinence may be unmasked only after correcting the prolapse. This should be evaluated preoperatively with office cytometrics, formal urodynamic testing, or a pessary test.

Clinical Findings

Mild degrees of pelvic organ prolapse are found in many women without significant symptoms. Prolapse is measured in various ways. The Baden and Walker system is the most commonly used clinical method: Grade 0 indicates no prolapse. In grade 1, the leading edge of the prolapse is beyond the midvaginal line but above the vaginal hymen. In grade 2, the prolapse is no more than about 4 cm beyond the hymen. Grade 3 occurs with complete uterine (total procidentia) or vaginal prolapse.

Descent and bulging of the anterior vagina usually indicates the presence of a cystocele or, less commonly, an anterior enterocele. Similarly, an anatomic defect in the posterior vagina signifies that a rectocele or enterocele (or both) exists. All of these conditions can be demonstrated during examination with the patient in the lithotomy or standing position by asking her to bear down or strain.

The symptoms of pelvic organ prolapse may include: pelvic pressure or a sensation of "falling out" of the pelvic organs, a mass protruding from the vagina (which may be a cystocele, rectocele, cervix, or all of these), stress incontinence, fecal incontinence, and other difficulties with defecation.

Differential Diagnosis

There are few entities in the differential diagnosis of pelvic organ prolapse. Urethral diverticula may simulate cystocele and produce a bulge of the anterior vaginal wall. The diverticulum is usually palpable as a discrete mass, and pressure against the mass often expresses purulent material from the urethral meatus. Endoscopic and urethrocystographic examinations confirm the diagnosis.

With regard to urinary incontinence, urodynamic studies are helpful in distinguishing stress incontinence from urge incontinence and are used to rule out intrinsic sphincter deficiency.

Treatment

A. Nonoperative Treatment

The postmenopausal woman with mild to moderate anatomic defects may have some improvement of symptoms after the administration of a topical estrogen. Pelvic floor muscle (Kegel) exercises may improve symptoms in up to 60% of patients with stress or urge urinary incontinence. A pessary to support the descending pelvic structures often provides relief of symptoms, including those of urinary incontinence. Pessaries are good options for patients who do not want or cannot have surgery.

B. Surgical Treatment

There are many different surgeries to correct pelvic organ prolapse. The choice involves consideration of specific anatomic defects as well as the patient's age, health status, previous surgeries, and sexual activity. In cases of uterine prolapse, hysterectomy is often involved. Common procedures done for specific defects include the following: (1) for cystocele or anterior vaginal prolapse, anterior colporrhaphy and abdominal or vaginal paravaginal repair; (2) for rectocele, posterior colporrhaphy; (3) for vaginal apex or vault prolapse, vaginal procedures such as sacrospinous ligament fixation, uterosacral suspension, and iliococcygeus suspension, or abdominal sacrocolpopexy. In patients for whom sexual activity is not an issue, closure (colpocleisis) or removal (colpectomy) of the vagina is an option. Surgical correction of prolapse has variable results—up to one-third of patients require reoperation for recurrent prolapse. There is some suggestion that the abdominal approach (sacrocolpopexy) may be more durable.

Many surgeries have been described for the treatment of stress urinary incontinence. Retropubic urethropexy and suburethral sling procedures are the most commonly performed and most durable procedures. Success of these two procedures is approximately 85% at 5 years. Sling procedures are the operation of choice in patients with intrinsic sphincter deficiency with a hypermobile urethra. In patients who have intrinsic sphincter deficiency with a nonmobile urethra, transurethral collagen injection is a minimally invasive treatment option. Anterior repairs and transvaginal needle suspensions have much lower success rates and should not be done for urinary incontinence.

Benson JT et al: Vaginal versus abdominal reconstructive surgery for the treatment of pelvic support defects: a prospective randomized study with long-term outcome evaluation. Am J Obstet Gynecol 1996;175:1418.

Black NA et al: The effectiveness of surgery for stress incontinence in women: a systematic review. Br J Urol 1996;78:497.

Bump RC et al: Epidemiology and natural history of pelvic floor dysfunction. Obstet Gynecol Clin North Am 1998;25:723.

Olsen AL et al: Epidemiology of surgically managed pelvic organ prolapse and urinary incontinence. Obstet Gynecol 1997; 89:501.

FISTULAS

Robert Domush, MD

URINARY TRACT FISTULAS

Urinary tract fistulas to the vagina are of three kinds: vesicovaginal (most common), ureterovaginal, and urethrovaginal. They occur most often as a result of accidental injury to the urinary tract at the time of pelvic surgery or because of ischemic necrosis resulting from an impaired blood supply. The latter can occur either following radiation therapy for carcinoma of the reproductive organs (especially the cervix) or following prolonged impaction of the fetal head during labor. Fistulas may also occur as a result of tumor invasion of the vesicovaginal septum.

Total abdominal hysterectomy is the operation most often complicated by the development of vesicovaginal fistula. Fistulas caused by urinary tract injury can be prevented by skillful surgical technique. The surgeon should be alert for injuries, which should be repaired at the time of operation.

Clinical Findings

A. Symptoms and Signs

Constant urinary leakage is the cardinal symptom. Urine can usually be seen coming through an opening in the vagina. In vesicovaginal and ureterovaginal fistulas, the vaginal ostium is at or near the vault closure (post hysterectomy) whereas the urethrovaginal fistula opens along the anterior wall of the vagina. If the urethrovaginal fistula involves the distal urethra, the patient may remain continent and lose urine into the vagina only at the time of voiding.

A communication between the urinary bladder and the vagina can be demonstrated by instilling sterile milk or a dye (methylene blue or indigo carmine) into the bladder via a catheter and watching it pass through into the vagina on speculum examination. If leakage of urine into the vagina cannot be demonstrated in this fashion, the defect probably is ureteral and can be demonstrated by giving the patient methylene blue tablets by mouth and later finding a blue stain on a cotton pledget placed in the vagina.

B. Urologic Examination

Cystoscopy and x-ray studies of the urinary tract will localize the urinary tract opening of the fistulous tract. Occasionally, the fistulous tracts are branching or multiple.

Treatment

Urinary tract fistulas rarely close spontaneously. Most must be repaired surgically, but sufficient time should elapse after diagnosis to allow for resolution of edema and inflammatory reactions. Otherwise, attempts at repair are likely to be unsuccessful. The use of cortisone as an anti-inflammatory agent has been challenged, and surgical results are excellent without its use. Urinary tract infections should be treated and skin excoriation and infection resolved before surgical correction is attempted.

Ureterovaginal fistulas are repaired by performing a ureteroureterostomy or by implanting the severed ureter into the bladder (ureteroneocystostomy). Attempts at conservative measures to close vesicovaginal fistulas include prolonged Foley drainage or cauterization with silver nitrate or electrocautery. Surgery via both abdominal (suprapubic) and vaginal approaches is used to repair vesicovaginal fistulas, and a number of techniques are available (layered closure, partial colpocleisis). Regardless of the method used, the principles of repair are the same: meticulous technique, using fine suture material; approximation of broad surfaces without tension; and maintenance of bladder decompression postoperatively until healing can occur. Improvement in surgical outcomes will increase with the use of interpositioning grafts.

Radiation fistulas are more complex because of tissue ischemia. They may require the introduction of a new blood supply provided by bulbocavernosus or gracilis myocutaneous flaps for successful repair.

RECTOVAGINAL & SIGMOIDOVAGINAL FISTULAS

Rectovaginal fistulas can occur as a result of obstetric injury, surgical procedures, cervical cancer, radiation therapy, inflammatory bowel disease, or diverticulitis. The symptoms are those of incontinence of flatus or feces through the vagina. Foul vaginal discharge with or without blood may be the presenting sign. The vaginal ostium usually can be demonstrated by speculum examination, and a probe passed through the fistulous tract can be palpated by the rectal diagnosing finger. A sigmoidovaginal fistula may require colonoscopy or retrograde dye studies.

Low rectovaginal fistulas near the introitus should be repaired after the surrounding inflammatory reaction and edema have subsided. This may require 3–4 months from the time of diagnosis. Those found high in the vagina—particularly fistulas resulting from radiation therapy—are often best managed with an initial diverting colostomy which is then closed 2–3 months after a successful repair. Before surgical repair of a rectovaginal fistula, the bowel should be prepared with a low-residue diet, antibiotics, cleansing enemas, and oral bowel-emptying agents.

Fistulas that are related to inflammatory bowel disease (Crohn's disease) carry a very poor prognosis and usually will not heal when repair is attempted unless the disease is clearly in remission. Ileostomy and abdominoperineal resection are necessary in patients whose symptoms are unacceptable despite medical management. Fistulas that occur as a result of cancer are not amenable to surgical repair. A diverting colostomy may give the patient considerable comfort.

Tancer ML et al: Genital fistulas secondary to diverticular disease of the colon: a review. Obstet Gynec Surv 1996;51:67.

Woo HH et al: The treatment of vesicovaginal fistulae. Eur Urol 1996;29:1.

BENIGN TUMORS OF THE VULVA & VAGINA

Elena A. Gates, MD

Hidradenoma

Hidradenomas are small, discrete, firm, mobile structures in the subcutaneous tissues of the labia or perianal region. These sweat gland tumors are benign but may be mistaken for cancer because of an adenomatous microscopic pattern. Treatment consists of local excision.

Sebaceous Cysts

Sebaceous cysts are small, raised, discrete, white cystic structures in the skin of the labia majora or minora that contain white sebaceous material. They may become infected, producing small abscesses. Most sebaceous cysts require no therapy. If they cause discomfort, simple excision is indicated.

Bartholin Cyst

Bartholin cysts—typically cysts of the gland duct—occur secondary to inflammation and occlusion of the duct opening. Located deep to the posterior labium majus, they vary in size from 1 cm to several centimeters in diameter. The larger masses tend to bulge into the vestibule of the vulva and the lower vagina. They may be asymptomatic or may cause local pressure symptoms and dyspareunia. Secondary infection occurs frequently, producing a painful abscess.

Symptomatic cysts and low-grade abscesses can be drained using a small mushroom catheter or word catheter introduced through a stab incision in the fluctuant medial aspect of the mass just cephalad to the hymen. The catheter should remain in place for 2 weeks to allow the tract to epithelialize and act as a new duct opening. In the event of surrounding cellulitis, antibiotic therapy can be added. If drainage fails, the cyst can be marsupialized. Rarely, excision of the gland itself is required.

Solid nodules within a Bartholin cyst should be biopsied to evaluate for malignancy.

Gartner Duct Cysts

These occur as small round or fusiform cystic swellings beneath the mucosa of the anterolateral wall of the vagina. They arise from remnants of the vaginal portion of the mesonephric (wolffian) duct and contain a clear serous fluid. They are usually asymptomatic and are discovered in the course of routine physical examination. Occasionally, they reach 5–6 cm in size. Small asymptomatic cysts require no therapy. Larger masses should be excised.

ENDOMETRIOSIS

Marcelle Cedars, MD

Endometriosis is the presence of functioning endometrial tissue in extrauterine sites, most commonly the ovaries, the uterosacral ligaments, and the cul-de-sac peritoneum. Other sites are the uterine tubes, the serosal surface of the uterus, the rectovaginal septum, the sigmoid colon, the pelvic peritoneum, and the small intestine (Figure 41–1). Ectopic endometrium has been found in the umbilicus, in abdominal scars, and (rarely) in the breasts, the extremities, the pleural cavity, and the lungs.

Endometriosis is thought to occur by one or more of three mechanisms: (1) retrograde menstruation and implantation; (2) müllerian metaplasia of coelomic epithelium; and (3) lymphatic and venous dissemination. Retrograde menstruation through the uterine tubes is common. It is not known what favors the growth and development of these tissues in the peritoneal cavity in some women and its regression and resorption in others. In some women, menstrual endometrium implants on the surface of the ovaries and falls by gravity into the cul-de-sac (pouch of Douglas), where it implants and responds to the cyclic hormonal influences of the menstrual cycle, shedding and bleeding at the time of menstruation. Conditions favoring retrograde passage of

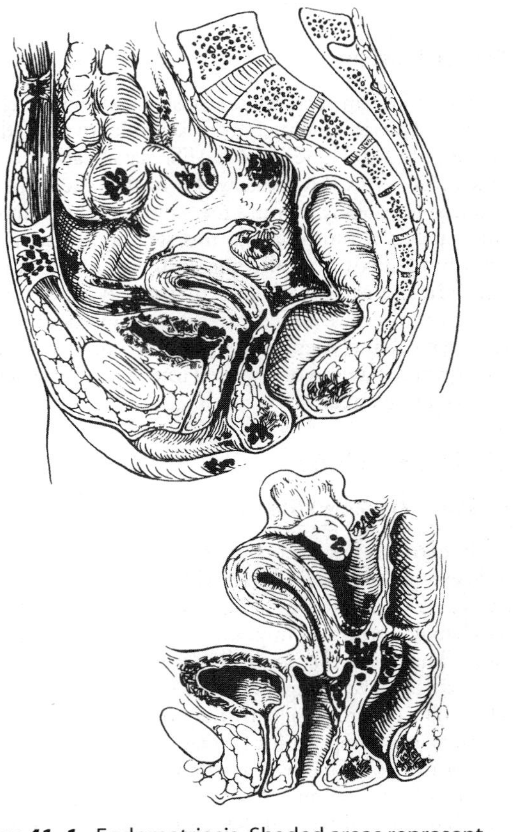

Figure 41–1. Endometriosis. Shaded areas represent frequent sites of endometriosis deposits.

menstrual flow—eg, cervical stenosis or congenital anomalies such as vaginal atresia or transverse vaginal septum—predispose to endometriosis.

The reported prevalence of endometriosis is generally accepted to be 10–20%. Diagnosis at the time of laparoscopy for infertility may be as high as 20–47% while patients undergoing laparoscopy for tubal sterilization have an incidence of only 1–5%. The incidence of endometriosis appears to increase with several social and environmental factors such as delayed childbearing, a family history of the disease, declining use of oral contraceptive pills, and exposure to some toxins (such as dioxin).

It has been claimed that teenagers do not have endometriosis, but newer information suggests otherwise. Endometriosis may rarely occur following menopause but almost always in response to hormonal replacement therapy.

Carcinoma has been known to develop in areas of endometriosis within the pelvis and usually takes the form of endometrioid adenocarcinoma. Adenoacanthomas and endometrial stromal sarcomas have been reported, but these also are quite rare.

Classification

A staging system for endometriosis has been developed by the American Society of Reproductive Medicine (Table 41–1). The Revised AFS classification system now accepted worldwide is useful in that the inspection required for staging requires meticulous evaluation of the entire pelvis. Unfortunately, this staging system is only broadly predictive of outcome with treatment and may not correlate at all with patient pain. A newer system that recognizes the varied presentation of endometriosis (eg, atypical and deep infiltrating implants) and reflects scientifically based scores as a marker for disease activity has been suggested.

Table 41–1. Staging of endometriosis.

Minimal, mild (stages I and II)
a. Scattered pelvic implants over the peritoneal surfaces of the pelvis (< 4 cm total).
b. Rare superficial implants on ovaries.
c. No significant adhesive disease.
Moderate (stage III)
a. Multiple implants or small endometriomas (< 3 cm) involving one or both ovaries.
b. Minimal periovarian or peritubal adhesions.
c. Scattered implants with scarring on other structures.
Severe (stage IV)
a. Large ovarian endometriomas (> 3 cm).
b. Significant periovarian or peritubal adhesions.
c. Tubal obstruction.
d. Obliteration of cul-de-sac.
e. Bowel or bladder adhesions.

Clinical Findings

A. Symptoms and Signs

Endometriosis has various presentations. Some patients with extensive disease—even with large bilateral ovarian endometriomas—may remain asymptomatic. Others with small peritoneal implants may be incapacitated by pain. The disease is typically first manifested as dysmenorrhea developing in the third or fourth decade. This may progress to pain that occurs not only with menstruation but also for several days preceding or following menses. This pain is often accompanied by dyspareunia and tenesmus. Some women complain of low back pain and of painful defecation associated with the menstrual period. This symptom is quite characteristic of cul-de-sac and rectovaginal septum involvement. Patients may also have pain in the buttock or radiating down the leg from involvement in the sciatic nerve.

Bladder involvement may cause a suprapubic pressure-type pain with or without dysuria and hematuria at the time of menstruation. Involvement of the bladder mucosa is quite rare. If an endometriotic implant involves the peritoneum overlying the ureter, the resulting tissue reaction may produce hydroureter and hydronephrosis with flank and lower abdominal pain.

Bowel obstruction may occur when endometrial implantation involves the small or large bowel. Mechanical ileus may result from the numerous dense adhesions that form as a result of the inflammatory reaction in response to cyclic bleeding from peritoneal implants.

Rupture of a large ovarian endometrial cyst occasionally causes symptoms of an acute abdominal emergency. Treatment is important to prevent pelvic adhesions and future infertility.

In some cases the only symptom is infertility. Endometriosis should be considered in all infertile patients.

B. Pelvic Examination

Bimanual pelvic examination is essential for assessment of the mobility of the uterus and the presence of adnexal masses. Rectovaginal examination is the only way the cul-de-sac, the uterosacral ligaments, and the posterior wall of the uterine corpus can be adequately palpated. The ovaries frequently are prolapsed and adherent to the posterior leaf of the broad ligament lateral to the cul-de-sac and are best felt by the rectal finger. Examination just preceding the menstrual period is the best time for palpation of the characteristic shotty nodules in the pouch of Douglas. Suspicious findings on pelvic examination should be further evaluated by ultrasound. The presence of isoechoic masses within the ovaries is highly suggestive of endometrioma.

C. Special Examinations

Serum concentrations of CA-125 are elevated (> 35 units/mL) in approximately one-third of patients with advanced disease. As a screening test, CA-125 lacks specificity and sensitivity, but in patients with advanced disease it may serve as a marker of recurrence of disease after treatment.

Laparoscopic examination is required to establish the diagnosis. A finding of characteristic raspberry or blueberry implants of ectopic tissue or the powder-burn marks of scarred endometrium is diagnostic. Endometriosis may also appear in "atypical" lesions recognized as red glandular excrescences, petechiae, white nodules (subperitoneal glands) or clear vesicular lesions. These may, in fact, be more active disease than the classic powder-burn bluish-gray lesions. Any questionable lesions should be biopsied and sent for pathologic diagnosis. The diagnosis requires the presence of glands and stroma in the ectopic site. Microscopic disease is sometimes evident as a ground-glass appearance of the peritoneum. Laparotomy is rarely necessary and may involve major resection of the pelvic organs or bowel.

Prevention

The early diagnosis and treatment of menstrual obstruction (dilation of the cervix, hymenotomy, metroplasty, removal of vaginal septum) may help to prevent or delay the development of endometriosis in those patients with outflow obstruction. Early multiparity appears to prevent the development of endometriosis. There is evidence that long-term contraceptive pill users are less likely to develop endometriosis, particularly if the pill contains a small amount of estrogen in combination with a potent progestin.

Treatment

Treatment should be tailored to fit the circumstances with respect to the age of the patient, her symptoms, her desire for children, and the extent of the disease. Therapy may vary, therefore, from mere observation, reassurance, and analgesia if necessary to complete surgical removal of the uterus, tubes, and ovaries. A conservative approach is recommended for the patient who is symptom-free or only mildly symptomatic and with minimal pelvic findings such as slightly tender cul-de-sac nodules. Regular examinations should be scheduled at intervals of not more than 6 months. Evidence of progression of the disease—in the form of either increasing symptomatology, infertility, or the development of pelvic masses—requires more specific treatment.

A. Medical Treatment

All medical treatment induces a remission and not a cure of endometriosis. Recurrence of symptoms is common when treatment is discontinued. Long-term suppression with oral contraceptive pills should be considered in all women, but particularly those who have had a recurrence of symptoms following prior successful treatment. Medical treatment is not indicated for endometriosis associated with infertility.

The induction of amenorrhea has been successful in bringing about regression in a high percentage of patients with endometriosis. This may be accomplished in several ways:

1. Danazol—This synthetic androgen derived from ethisterone has been found to be effective in the medical treatment of endometriosis. It acts by suppressing the secretion of gonadotropins. It is given in doses of 200–800 mg daily and continued without interruption for 6–9 months. Drawbacks are expense and androgenic side effects.

2. Progestins—Norethynodrel, norethindrone acetate, and medroxyprogesterone acetate are the agents most commonly used. Continuous progestins induce amenorrhea (although breakthrough bleeding may occur). Symptomatic improvement is reported in up to 80% of patients. Induction of decidualization and ultimately necrosis in the implants as well as cessation of menses seem to be important in the response. This treatment can be continued for 6–12 months or longer in some patients. Side effects include breakthrough bleeding, fluid retention, and headaches.

3. Oral contraceptive pills—The production of a pseudopregnancy state through hormonal therapy with combined estrogen and progestin is another alternative. Treatment with cyclic or continuous oral contraceptive pills for 6–12 months is effective in about 80% of patients. This treatment can be continued long-term until fertility is desired. The most frequent indication for prolonged use is recurrent endometriosis following a conservative operation or other medical therapies. Side effects are nausea, breast tenderness, fluid retention, and breakthrough bleeding.

4. GnRH analogues—The analogues of gonadotropin-releasing hormone (eg, leuprolide, nafarelin, goserelin) act by down-regulation of the GnRH receptor in the pituitary and elimination of FSH and LH secretion. Without gonadotropin secretion, estradiol levels fall to the castrate range. In the face of this hypoestrogenism, endometrial implants regress and about 80% of patients report symptomatic improvement. Side effects are those of menopause with vasomotor symptoms, vaginal dryness, sleep disturbances and moodiness, and bone loss with long-term treatment. So-called "add-back" therapy with either norethindrone acetate or combined hormone replacement therapy reduces side effects while not interfering with efficacy.

B. Surgical Treatment

The surgical approach to endometriosis may be designed to improve fertility, prevent further progression of the disease with preservation of the ovaries, or eliminate the disease by removal of the uterus and adnexal structures. Surgical treatment is required for large endometriomas (> 4 cm) as these will not respond to medical therapy. Their persistence may increase the risk for destruction of normal ovarian tissue and for premature development of diminished ovarian reserve.

1. Conservative surgery—Preservation of childbearing function by removal or cauterization of implants, freeing up of tubal adhesions, presacral neurectomy for the relief of pain, and perhaps by uterine suspension is indicated for the patient who desires to preserve childbearing capacity and has failed medical therapy. Conservative surgery in which an attempt to preserve a single ovary at the time of hysterectomy and oophorectomy for severe disease carries a 20% risk for a subsequent surgery to remove the remaining ovary. Laparoscopic surgery on an ambulatory basis has all but eliminated the need for laparotomy.

2. Definitive surgery—This requires the removal of the uterus and the tubes and ovaries. Since endometriosis is dependent upon ovarian function for its continued growth and development, total hysterectomy and bilateral salpingo-oophorectomy should be done in patients with extensive disease, particularly those with bowel involvement. It is critically important not to mistake bowel implants for cancer. Unnecessary abdominoperineal resections have been performed in young women for unrecognized endometriosis. Provided there has been a preoperative bowel preparation, bowel implants can be locally resected.

Oral estrogen replacement therapy in the form of conjugated estrogens, 0.625–1.25 mg/d, may be given without danger of exacerbating the endometriotic process. The use of estrogen-progestin combinations is not required. A 6-month course of continuous progestins may reduce vasomotor symptoms, protect the bone, and allow suppression of residual disease. Estrogen replacement therapy may then be instituted.

Henzl MR et al: Administration of nasal nafarelin as compared with oral danazol for endometriosis: a multicenter double-blind comparative clinical trial. N Engl J Med 1988;318:485.

Hoeger KM et al: An update on the classification of endometriosis. Clin Obstet Gynecol 1999;42:611.

Hughes E et al: Ovulation suppression for endometriosis. Cochrane Database Syst Rev 2000;CD000155.

Lebovic DI et al: Immunobiology of endometriosis. Fertil Steril 2001;75:1.

Moore J et al: Modern combined oral contraceptives for pain associated with endometriosis. Cochrane Database Syst Rev 2000;CD001019.

Reddy S et al: Treatment of endometriosis. Clin Obstet Gynecol 1998;41:387.

ADENOMYOSIS

Lee Learman, MD, PhD

Adenomyosis occurs when fingers of endometrium extend into the myometrium to a depth greater than two low-power microscopic fields. It may be a focal or a diffuse process and may involve the entire thickness of the myometrium. The pathogenesis is not known, but the theory of direct growth of the basal layer of endometrium into the myometrium is widely accepted. Estrogen has been implicated as a stimulus to the development of adenomyosis, and the symptomatic improvement that occurs with the onset of menopause supports this concept. The disease is seen most often in the decade preceding menopause.

Clinical Findings

The condition is most common in women between ages 35 and 50 and leads to hypermenorrhea, polymenorrhea, or intermenstrual bleeding with dysmenorrhea or dyspareunia. It may be associated with endometriosis. Examination will reveal a slightly to moderately enlarged symmetric, mobile uterus that may be tender to palpation, particularly in the premenstrual phase of the cycle.

The preoperative diagnosis of adenomyosis is very difficult. MRI is somewhat more effective than ultrasonography in suggesting the diagnosis. The use of needle biopsy of the uterus has been reported as a means of diagnosing the condition, though the sensitivity of this approach is only fair. The definitive diagnosis is made by pathologic examination of uterine tissue, generally after hysterectomy.

Differential Diagnosis

Adenomyosis must be distinguished principally from leiomyomas of the uterus. An analogous condition, endolymphatic stromal myosis (stromal endometriosis, low-grade stromal sarcoma), although histologically benign, clinically behaves as a low-grade cancer. Connective tissue cells resembling those of the endometrial stroma infiltrate the lymphatic and venous spaces of the myometrium, and the process may extend into the vessels of the broad ligament, in which event local recurrence is possible following hysterectomy. Metastases to the ovary, peritoneal surfaces, and lung have been reported in rare cases. This disease, usually of the postmenopausal years, is very rare and should not be confused with adenomyosis.

Treatment

Total hysterectomy with or without bilateral salpingo-oophorectomy is curative. Hormonal approaches that are successful in treating endometriosis are also useful. These include continuous progestin therapy administered orally, by depot injection, or as an intrauterine system, and gonadotropin-releasing hormone analogues.

Prognosis

Adenomyosis is a self-limited process that undergoes spontaneous regression, becoming asymptomatic after the menopause.

Fedele L et al: Treatment of adenomyosis-associated menorrhagia with a levonorgestrel-releasing intrauterine device. Fertil Steril 1997;68:426.

Vercellini P et al: Transvaginal ultrasonography versus uterine needle biopsy in the diagnosis of diffuse adenomyosis. Hum Reprod 1998;13:2884.

Vercellini P et al: Treatment with a gonadotropin releasing hormone agonist before endometrial resection: a multicentre, randomised controlled trial. Br J Obstet Gynaecol 1996;103:562.

LEIOMYOMAS OF THE UTERUS

Alison Jacoby, MD

Leiomyomas of the uterus are found in at least 20% of women over age 30. The true prevalence is unknown because most women with myomas have no symptoms. Black women have a threefold to ninefold higher incidence than white women. Myomas arise from proliferation of a single clone of uterine smooth muscle cells under the influence of estrogen, progesterone, and other growth factors. As a result, myomas often have an increased growth rate during pregnancy and a cessation of growth after menopause. They are usually multiple and can be located within the myometrium (intramural), beneath the external surface (subserous), or adjacent to the endometrium (submucous). Other types of myomas are intraligamentous (between the leaves of the broad ligament), parasitic (detached from the uterus and deriving blood supply from other abdominal organs), and cervical. Myomas may vary in size from tiny "seedlings" to massive tumors filling the entire pelvis and abdomen.

On cut section, leiomyomas are well-circumscribed, pearly-gray, solid tumors with a pseudocapsule and a whorled appearance. Microscopically, myomas are composed of fascicles of uniform, spindle-shaped smooth muscle cells. Mitotic figures are rare. Other common features include hyaline, cystic, and carneous degeneration, edema, calcifications, and focal hemorrhage.

Clinical Findings

A. Symptoms and Signs

The clinical presentation depends on the location, number, and size of the myomas. Although myomas are frequently discovered in the course of a routine pelvic examination, the majority of these women have no symptoms. The most common symptoms reported are heavy, prolonged menses, a sensation of pelvic pressure, abdominal distention, and urinary frequency. In addition, women can develop urinary retention, dyspareunia, low back pain, and constipation. When degenerative changes occur, mild symptoms may suddenly become severe and require treatment. Submucous and intracavitary myomas are liable to cause heavy, prolonged and frequent bleeding, at times alarmingly profuse. These myomas may become pedunculated and protrude through the cervix.

Palpation of the uterus reveals an irregular and enlarged structure that may be felt on abdominal examination. It is usually firm and nontender but may become soft and tender following an episode of degeneration. Hydronephrosis can occur from external compression of the ureters by the enlarged uterus.

B. Laboratory Findings

Anemia may result from acute or chronic blood loss. An endometrial biopsy should be performed in women with abnormal uterine bleeding to rule out endometrial hyperplasia and cancer.

C. Imaging Studies

Pelvic sonography is the most useful radiographic study for diagnosing leiomyomas. When a submucous myoma is suspected clinically, saline sonohysterography and hysteroscopy are useful for visualizing the contour of the uterine cavity. MRI is reserved for evaluation of a radiographically atypical leiomyoma and for the precise localization of myomas prior to myomectomy.

Differential Diagnosis

Before surgery, it can be difficult to distinguish a uterine myoma from a uterine sarcoma (leiomyosarcoma, endometrial stromal sarcoma, and mixed mesodermal tumor). However, the incidence of uterine sarcoma among women operated on for uterine myomas is extremely low (0.23%). Even rapidly growing myomas, defined as an increase by 6 weeks gestational size in 1 year, are unlikely to be malignant. However, a postmenopausal woman with an enlarging uterine mass, especially if accompanied by vaginal bleeding, should be evaluated for sarcoma.

Solid ovarian tumors and pedunculated subserous myomas may be difficult to differentiate on physical examination. Pelvic sonography is useful. MRI or laparoscopy is sometimes necessary to identify the origin of the mass. Enlargement of the uterus by a myoma may mimic a pregnant uterus or vice versa. A pregnancy test should be done in all suspected cases.

Complications

Hemorrhage from a submucous myoma or chronic menorrhagia often results in secondary iron deficiency anemia. Patients with torsion of a pedunculated subserous myoma present with severe pain and evidence of an acute abdomen.

Infertility may occur secondary to myomas, particularly if the uterine cavity is enlarged or distorted by a submucous myoma. Miscarriage, preterm labor, premature rupture of membranes, and postpartum hemorrhage can be caused by myomas. Rarely, a large myoma in the lower uterine segment can obstruct passage of the fetus during labor. The majority of women with myomas have uncomplicated pregnancies and deliveries.

Treatment

Asymptomatic myomas require no therapy. Reexamination is recommended every 6–12 months to assess symptoms and record the rate of growth. Women with heavy, prolonged, or frequent episodes of bleeding can benefit from a trial of cyclic or continuous birth control pills or progestins. GnRH agonists decrease myoma size and stop menstruation prior to surgery. Long-term use of GnRH agonists causes osteoporosis, and myomas regrow soon after the medication is discontinued.

For women with pelvic pressure or bleeding unresponsive to medical management, several surgical and nonsurgical treatment options are available. Women who have not completed childbearing usually undergo a myomectomy, though women who do not desire pregnancy often choose this option as well. Myomectomy can be performed by laparotomy, laparoscopy, or hysteroscopy depending on the location, number, and size of the myomas. Women who have completed childbearing and seek an alternative to hysterectomy may benefit from uterine artery embolization. This nonsurgical procedure involves diminishing blood flow to the uterus. Subsequently, the uterus and myomas decrease in size by 30–50% and symptoms such as heavy bleeding and pelvic pressure improve in 80–90% of women. Hysterectomy is definitive treatment for women with symptomatic myomas. Alternatives to total abdominal hysterectomy include vaginal hysterectomy, supracervical hysterectomy, and laparoscopic hysterectomy.

Prognosis

Myomas are benign neoplasms. There is no evidence that myomas can transform into sarcomas. Myomectomy results in symptom improvement in 80% of women. The risk of recurrence following myomectomy is approximately 25%, but only 10% of these women require a second operation. The outcome following uterine artery embolization appears favorable, but the duration of follow-up in the published literature is 3 years or less. Hysterectomy is definitive therapy for myomas.

Hurst BS et al: Uterine artery embolization for symptomatic uterine myomas. Fertil Steril 2000;74:855.

ADNEXAL MASSES

Lisa Everson, MD

Adnexal masses are abnormal structures found in the ovary, uterine tube, or broad ligament. It is often impossible to determine the origin of adnexal masses by physical examination or radiographically.

The differential diagnosis of adnexal masses is broad (see Table 41–2). The majority are benign, though the likelihood of malignancy increases significantly with age. It is estimated that approximately 13% of persistent adnexal masses are malignant in 13% of premenopausal women and in 45% of women who are postmenopausal.

MANAGEMENT OF ADNEXAL MASSES

Functional Cysts

The most common adnexal mass in a premenopausal woman is either a follicular or corpus luteum cyst. While these functional cysts typically measure 3 cm or less, they can reach sizes up to 8–10 cm. Functional cysts are usually self-limited and will regress over time. Follow-up examination with ultrasound after 4–6 weeks will reveal a decrease in size, and nearly all will ultimately resolve without treatment. Oral contraceptives are often initiated at the time of identification of a presumed functional cyst. While this practice may prevent development of a second functional cyst that could ultrasonographically mimic the original cyst—giving the impression that no reduction in size has taken

Table 41–2. Differential diagnosis of adnexal masses.

Follicular or corpus luteum cyst
Mature cystic teratoma
Immature teratoma
Cystadenofibroma
Endometrioma
Serous or mucinous cystadenoma
Epithelial ovarian carcinoma
Tumors of low malignant potential
Sertoli-Leydig cell tumor
Theca lutein cyst
Granulosa cell tumor
Fibroma
Thecoma
Endodermal sinus tumor
Choriocarcinoma
Uterine tube carcinoma
Paraovarian or paratubal cyst
Hydrosalpinx
Pedunculated leiomyoma

place—the clinical benefit of oral contraceptives in this setting has not been clearly demonstrated.

While the vast majority of functional cysts resolve without incident, they will occasionally rupture or cause torsion of the ovary, resulting in severe acute abdominal pain. Torsion requires prompt surgical intervention to untwist the vascular infundibulopelvic ligament before significant ischemia and necrosis of the ovary occurs so that the ovary can be preserved. This is frequently accomplished laparoscopically. Cyst rupture can occur spontaneously or at the time of sexual intercourse. Once a diagnosis of cyst rupture is made, the decision for inpatient or outpatient management depends on the degree of pain, the hemodynamic stability of the patient, and the certainty of the diagnosis. Typically, a woman will be observed in a hospital setting for 24 hours, allowing for the administration of intravenous analgesia and serial examinations and blood counts. Recovery is usually rapid. Occasionally, a ruptured functional cyst will demonstrate ongoing bleeding requiring operation to achieve hemostasis. This is usually accomplished by cautery via laparoscopic access. If this is unsuccessful, cystectomy is indicated.

Persistent Adnexal Masses

Adnexal masses that do not decrease in size over time are likely to be neoplasms. Differentiating benign from malignant masses is one of the challenges in women's health care. Benign masses can generally be removed effectively by the general gynecologic surgeon, often endoscopically, while malignancies are more effectively treated by specialists with training in appropriate surgical staging and maximal cytoreduction, which are important in optimizing the outcome.

Transvaginal ultrasonography is an important tool in evaluation of the uterine adnexa. It has been shown to have a sensitivity for identifying malignant neoplasms of about 90%. However, the specificity has been reported at about 60%. In an effort to improve specificity without sacrificing sensitivity, a number of diagnostic models based on combinations of ultrasonographic features, age, serum CA-125 measurements, and menopausal status have been devised. Unfortunately, attempts at prospective external validation of these models have found them to be less accurate than initially reported. MRI appears to have a promising role in the characterization of adnexal masses, but its sensitivity is somewhat less than that of ultrasound, in particular for early stage tumors of low-malignant potential.

Because it is difficult with radiographic and laboratory evaluation to determine conclusively if persistent adnexal masses are benign or malignant, persistent adnexal masses should generally be surgically removed either laparoscopically or via laparotomy. The size of the mass, its sonographic appearance, and one's level of concern about malignancy are all factors in choosing the operative approach. The decision to perform cystectomy or oophorectomy is typically based on the degree of concern for malignancy, as well as the age of the patient. Ovarian conservation is generally attempted in women under 45, as they can expect to have at least 5 more years of ovarian steroidogenesis prior to menopause. Masses with worrisome sonographic features should be removed by oophorectomy. This allows for complete histologic examination of the ovary. In addition, although intraoperative spillage of malignant cyst fluid into the peritoneal cavity has not been conclusively shown to worsen the outcome, it seems prudent to avoid rupture of the cyst during removal. Oophorectomy probably minimizes the risk of intraoperative cyst rupture.

If a menopausal woman with a cystic adnexal mass is not a good candidate for surgery or simply wants to avoid operation, one can cite several series demonstrating that simple unilocular cysts measuring less than 5 cm in women with low serum CA-125 levels have a very small likelihood of being malignant. However, occasional malignancies have been found even when these criteria are met. Carefully following these women and recommending operation if the cyst size or characteristics change considerably is a reasonable option in such cases.

Aslam N et al: Prospective evaluation of three different models for the pre-operative diagnosis of ovarian cancer. Br J Obstet Gynaecol 2000;107:1347.

Dottino PR et al: Laparoscopic management of adnexal masses in premenopausal and postmenopausal women. Obstet Gynecol 1999;93:223.

Gallup DG et al: Management of the adnexal mass in the 1990s. South Med J 1997;90:972.

Kinkel K et al: US characterization of ovarian masses: a meta-analysis. Radiology 2000;217:803.

ECTOPIC PREGNANCY

Mindy Goldman, MD

The incidence of ectopic pregnancy has increased with the use of advanced reproductive technologies, occurring in approximately two in every 100 pregnancies. Given that many ectopic pregnancies are now diagnosed and treated in clinicians' offices, the true incidence of ectopic pregnancy is probably underestimated. Death as a result of ectopic pregnancy has decreased because of earlier diagnosis and currently is about 0.3% of ectopic pregnancies. Risk factors for ectopic pregnancy include prior ectopic pregnancy, conditions that lead to tubal scarring such as pelvic inflammatory disease and prior pelvic surgery, a history of infertility, in vitro fertilization, current IUD use, smoking, diethylstilbestrol exposure, and increased age. The largest risk is felt to be due to salpingitis, with about a sevenfold increased risk of an ectopic pregnancy after acute pelvic inflammatory disease. Infertility patients who have undergone in vitro fertilization are at special risk.

Ninety-five percent of ectopic pregnancies occur in the uterine tube, usually in the ampullary portion. Less common locations include interstitial or cornual pregnancies, which can cause significant intraperitoneal bleeding if rupture occurs, and, more rarely, pregnancies in the abdomen, ovary, or cervix. In vitro fertilization has also increased the rate of heterotopic pregnancy, which is the occurrence of an intrauterine pregnancy with an ectopic, but this is rare.

Fertilization normally occurs in the outer third of the uterine tube, and anything that inhibits transport of the fertilized zygote can result in implantation within the wall of the tube. As the fertilized ovum implants within the tube, there is vascular engorgement and trophoblastic invasion that may weaken the wall of the tube. This can lead to rupture with marked blood loss into the peritoneal cavity. Early diagnosis can help prevent rupture and subsequent complications, including shock and death.

Clinical Findings

A. Symptoms and Signs

The clinical signs and symptoms of an ectopic pregnancy can be variable. Fortunately, because of earlier diagnosis, most women do not present with the classic signs of rupture, including severe abdominal pain and hemodynamic instability. Typically, patients present with amenorrhea and some degree of vaginal bleeding with or without pelvic pain. An adnexal mass may be present on pelvic examination, but findings may be as subtle as vaginal spotting without other clinical symptoms. The uterus is usually slightly enlarged because of decidualization of the endometrium resulting from increased estrogen and progesterone levels.

B. Laboratory Findings and Imaging Studies

Laboratory evaluation may show a low hematocrit, particularly if there are clinical signs of rupture. Because the clinical presentation can vary considerably, other tests such as transvaginal ultrasound and serum β-hCG are useful in distinguishing an ectopic from a threatened spontaneous abortion and a failed intrauterine pregnancy. In some cases, serum progesterone levels or findings on suction curettage may be helpful in diagnosis.

1. Human chorionic gonadotropin and transvaginal ultrasound—Trophoblastic cells of the chorionic villi produce β-hCG after implantation of the blastocyst. In early pregnancy, β-hCG typically rises in a curvilinear fashion, doubling approximately every 48 hours. For practical purposes, a rise of at least 66% should be observed every 48 hours until levels plateau at a gestational age of 7–8 weeks. In general, ectopic pregnancies have lower values of β-hCG and subnormal increases, but 15% of ectopics may have normal doubling times. An absolute β-hCG does not permit distinction between an ectopic and a nonviable intrauterine pregnancy. Another problem with β-hCG evaluation is the existence of different reference standards for β-hCG assays, so it is important to ensure that serial values are reported from the same standard.

The use of transvaginal ultrasound has allowed intrauterine pregnancies to be diagnosed at an earlier gestational age, usually within 5 weeks of the last menstrual period. In general, transvaginal sonography allows anatomic landmarks to be seen about 1 week earlier than transabdominal sonography. The concept of a "discriminatory β-hCG zone," defined as a threshold value above which an intrauterine gestational sac should be seen by endovaginal sonography, is highly predictive for diagnosing an ectopic pregnancy unless a multiple gestation is present. The discriminatory zone value varies depending on the β-hCG assay, the reference standard, and the quality of ultrasound resolution. For the First and Second International Reference Preparations (IRP), the value is usually between 1000 and 2000 mIU/mL. Institutions should determine their own discriminatory β-hCG level depending on the assay used and skills of the ultrasonographers. Other findings that ultrasound can detect include free fluid in the cul-de-sac and in some cases an adnexal gestational mass.

2. Serum progesterone—Serum progesterone levels increase during pregnancy, and viable intrauterine pregnancies tend to have higher levels than spontaneous abortions and ectopic pregnancies. In most studies, progesterone levels < 5 ng/mL are associated with abnormal pregnancies and levels > 25 ng/mL are consistent with viable pregnancies. Absolute values vary with ectopic pregnancies, and in many laboratories the assay is not immediately available, thus limiting the practical utility of this test.

3. Suction curettage—If the β-hCG value is less than the discriminatory zone and β-hCG titers have plateaued or are rising abnormally, suction curettage may be helpful in distinguishing between a nonviable intrauterine pregnancy and an ectopic gestation. In a woman without signs of spontaneous abortion the absence of chorionic villi on curettage in the presence of an elevated hCG is predictive of an ectopic pregnancy, though in very early gestations products may be missed by curettage.

Treatment

Treatment of ectopic pregnancy has been traditionally surgical, with procedures done to remove the ectopic gestation and preserve as much uterine tube as possible. Procedures include salpingostomy, where the ectopic pregnancy is removed through an incision in the antimesenteric aspect of the tube, leaving the remainder of the tube intact; and partial salpingectomy, where the involved portion of the tube is removed. In cases of extensive tubal damage, complete salpingectomy is recommended. In the past, laparotomy was required, but the laparoscopic approach is now preferred unless the patient is hemodynamically compromised. If conservative approaches such as salpingostomy are used, β-hCG titers should be followed after the procedure to make certain that no viable trophoblastic tissue remains.

For many patients, medical management with the folic acid antagonist methotrexate is a viable option. Criteria include a hemodynamically stable patient who is compliant and has no medical contraindication to methotrexate. Relative contraindications include an unruptured mass > 3.5 cm, fetal cardiac motion, or a β-hCG level > 15,000 mIU/mL, since these characteristics decrease the likelihood of success. Published success rates average 84% for single-dose therapy. There are algorithms for the use of methotrexate, though no standardized protocol has been defined. β-hCG levels are monitored until they fall to zero, and if levels have not fallen at a specified rate, a second dose may be required. Time to resolution can be quite variable and operation is needed for treatment failures. During methotrexate use, patients should discontinue folic acid supplements and refrain from sexual intercourse. They are instructed about ongoing risks of rupture. Patients who are Rh negative are given RH_0(D) immune globulin whether treated medically or surgically. Other developments in medical management include the use of other agents such as potassium chloride, prostaglandins, and mifepristone, but these have not been studied as well as methotrexate.

As with spontaneous abortions, some patients with ectopic pregnancies may actually have spontaneous resolution. Expectant management of a documented ectopic pregnancy may be an option if β-hCG levels are declining rapidly and the patient is stable. Patients need to be aware of the risks of rupture and hemorrhage, and emergency management must be readily available.

Most studies show similar success rates for methotrexate and conservative surgical therapy (mainly salpingostomy). Future conception rates are felt to be similar, but more studies are needed regarding the impact of methotrexate on future fertility. In general, the approach to ectopic pregnancy today is to achieve earlier diagnosis in the unruptured state to minimize morbidity and mortality as well as allow for more conservative treatment options.

ACOG Practice Bulletin. Medical management of ectopic pregnancy. Number 3, December 1998. In: 2001 Compendium of Selected Publications. American College of Obstetricians and Gynecologists, 1998.

Lehner R et al: Ectopic pregnancy. Arch Gynecol Obstet 2000;263:87.

Lipscomb GH et al: Nonsurgical treatment of ectopic pregnancy. N Engl J Med 2000;343:1325.

GYNECOLOGIC MALIGNANCIES

Lee-May Chen, MD, & Bethan Powell, MD

CARCINOMA OF THE VULVA

The vast majority (90–95%) of vulvar cancers are squamous cell carcinomas, and these tumors represent about 5% of all cancers of the female reproductive tract. Human papillomavirus (HPV) plays a role in etiology, but a relationship to invasive cancer has not been conclusively established. Vulvar intraepithelial neoplasia is considered precancerous and occurs more commonly in premenopausal women. Other types of vulvar cancer are Bartholin gland adenocarcinoma, Paget's disease of the vulva, basal cell carcinoma, malignant melanoma, and metastatic carcinoma from the cervix, endometrium, ovary, or elsewhere. Rarely, sarcomas are found arising primarily in the vulvar soft tissues.

The area most often involved is the labium majus (about 50% of cases). Approximately 25% of cases occur on the labium minus; the clitoris and Bartholin's gland are less common sites.

Metastasis to the regional lymph nodes (inguinal, femoral, iliac, and obturator) occurs in about 30% of operable lesions. Lymph node status is the most important factor predicting survival. Risk factors for node metastasis are clinical node status, age degree of differentiation, tumor stage, tumor thickness, depth of stromal invasion, and presence of capillary-lymphatic space invasion.

There is a high incidence of second primary cancers in vulvar cancer patients, particularly in the cervix, endometrium, and breast. Cancer of the vulva should be classified and clinically staged according to the recommendations of the Cancer Committee of the International Federation of Gynecology and Obstetrics (Table 41–3).

Clinical Findings

In situ squamous cell carcinoma of the vulva may be seen in women age 25–40 years as small, slightly raised or papillary (resembling condylomas) white, red, or brownish patches on the skin or mucosa. One-third of lesions are solitary, and two-thirds are multiple. The early invasive lesion is a small, elevated, superficial papillary or ulcerated lesion with underlying subcutaneous induration. Late cancers present either as large, fungating, infected tumors or as shallow ulcers with indurated margins. The larger the primary lesion, the greater the chance of lymph node involvement; but palpatory evidence is misleading, as regional node enlargement may be related to secondary infection in these tumors. Furthermore, metastatic disease in the lymph nodes may not be palpable. There may be submucosal spread of the tumor cephalad to involve the vagina and urethra—or there may be involvement of the posterior vulva with invasion of the anus and rectum. All suspicious lesions should be examined frequently by biopsy.

Differential Diagnosis

Chronic hypertrophic and atrophic skin conditions may or may not be associated with vulvar cancer. Multiple biopsies are necessary to establish the correct diagnosis. Granulomatous venereal lesions of the vulva may be clinically suspicious, and biopsy of the involved area is mandatory. The complement fixation test may be helpful, but it must be remembered that granulomatous disease and cancer of the vulva may occur simultaneously.

Prevention

Treatment of precancerous lesions is thought to reduce the subsequent development of invasive carcinoma. Vulvar intraepithelial neoplasia is diagnosed by colposcopic examination after treatment of the vulva with 3–5% acetic acid. Lesions usually will appear white. Elim-

Table 41–3. FIGO staging for vulvar cancer.

FIGO Stage	Description	TNM Class
Stage 0	Carcinoma in situ; intraepithelial carcinoma	T0
Stage I	Tumor confined to the vulva or perineum; 2 cm or less in greatest dimension; no nodal metastasis	T1
IA	Stromal invasion 1 mm	T1a
IB	Stromal invasion > 1 mm	T1b
Stage II	Tumor confined to the vulva or perineum; no more than 2 cm in greatest dimension; no nodal metastasis	T2
Stage III	Tumor of any size with adjacent spread to the urethra, vagina, or anus or with unilateral regional lymph node metastasis	T3, N0, or N1
Stage IVA	Tumor invades upper urethra, bladder mucosa, rectal mucosa, pelvic bone; or bilateral regional node metastases	T4, N0, or N1
Stage IVB	Any distant metastasis, including pelvic lymph nodes	M1

Benedet JL, Hacker NF, Ngan HYS (editors): Staging classifications and clinical practice guidelines of gynaecologic cancers. Int J Gynaecol Obstet 2000;70:207. http://www.figo.org/content/PDF/staging-booklet.pdf

inating cigarette smoking may also contribute to the reduction of vulvar cancer.

Treatment

Vulvar intraepithelial neoplasia, if localized, may be treated by wide excision or laser vaporization. Skinning vulvectomy with split-thickness skin grafting, if necessary, is done for diffuse, multifocal disease.

Microinvasive lesions (< 1 mm invasion) are adequately treated by wide local excision with 1 cm margins. All other stage 1 lesions, if well lateralized, can be treated with radical local excision with a 2-cm margin along with an ipsilateral inguinofemoral nodal dissection. Contralateral groin dissection is performed if ipsilateral positive nodes are found. Medial stage 1 lesions and more advanced stages that are operable are treated with radical vulvectomy plus bilateral inguinofemoral lymph node dissection. Radiation therapy with concurrent chemosensitization is required for inoperable lesions and for cases with close margins or positive nodes.

Prognosis

Adequate surgery is effective in a high percentage of patients, even when there is evidence of spread to the inguinal and femoral nodes. When the nodes are not involved, 5-year cure rates of 90% are reported, and a 50% salvage rate is possible in the presence of lymph node involvement.

Creasman WT et al: The National Cancer Data Base report on early stage invasive vulvar carcinoma. The American College of Surgeons Commission on Cancer and the American Cancer Society. Cancer 1997;80:505.

Grendys EC Jr et al: Innovations in the management of vulvar carcinoma. Curr Opin Obstet Gynecol 2000;12:15.

CARCINOMA OF THE VAGINA

Carcinoma in situ of the vagina occurs either as a direct extension of the process from the portio vaginalis of the cervix or as a separate area in a "neoplastic field." It should be suspected whenever carcinoma in situ or invasive carcinoma of the vulva or cervix is present, and it may appear in the vagina many months or years after successful treatment of either of those two conditions. Carcinoma in situ of the vagina is most often diagnosed by cytologic examination, colposcopy, and biopsy of acetic acid-staining or Schiller-positive lesions, ie, those that do not take up the iodine stain after application of Lugol's solution. As in carcinoma of the cervix and vulva, human papillomavirus is an etiologic factor.

Treatment is by local excision of involved areas when they are few and small. Electrocautery, laser therapy, and topical fluorouracil have been used; failure rates are 25–50%. Extensive involvement of the vaginal mucosa may require partial or complete vaginectomy with complete colpocleisis in the elderly, sexually inactive patient or with skin graft construction of an artificial vagina in the patient who wishes to retain coital function.

Invasive squamous cell carcinoma of the vagina, arising primarily from the vagina, is an unusual lesion, most cancers of the vagina being extensions from an epidermoid carcinoma of the cervix. The lesion is most often ulcerative, with a cauliflower configuration being less common. There is firm induration surrounding the ulcerative lesion, which is easily palpated, whereas a small, soft papillary lesion may be missed. The upper third of the vagina is the site in about 75% of patients. In many cases the only symptom is a bloody vaginal discharge, and the diagnosis is made by biopsy.

Treatment is by radiation therapy or radical surgery. Unfortunately, these tumors grow rapidly and insidiously, and in over 50% of patients they have penetrated the vaginal wall at the time of the initial examination. Involvement of the bladder and rectum is common. As a result, the overall 5-year survival figures are in the range of 20–30%.

Adenocarcinoma of the vagina has occurred in teenage girls, apparently arising in areas of vaginal adenosis (probably müllerian duct remnants). There appears to have been a relationship between the appearance of this tumor in these young patients and the administration of diethylstilbestrol to their mothers during the fetal life of the patient.

The classification and staging of carcinoma of the vagina is outlined in Table 41–4.

Metastatic carcinoma of the vagina is much more common than primary vaginal carcinoma, the most frequent sources being the cervix, vulva, bladder, urethra, rectum, endometrium, and ovary.

Rare primary tumors of the vagina are sarcoma (mixed mesodermal tumors, including sarcoma botryoides of infants, fibrosarcoma, leiomyosarcoma, and hemangiosarcoma), adenocarcinoma arising from mesonephric (Gartner's) duct or müllerian duct remnants, embryonal carcinoma, and malignant melanoma. Radical surgical removal offers the best hope of cure for the majority of these neoplasms.

Fine BA et al: The curative potential of radiation therapy in the treatment of primary vaginal carcinoma. Am J Clin Oncol 1996;19:39.

Manetta A et al: Primary invasive carcinoma of the vagina. Obstet Gynecol 1990;76:639.

CARCINOMA OF THE CERVIX

Carcinoma of the cervix is now the second most common invasive cancer of the female reproductive tract. Early sexual activity, multiple partners, multiparity, and

Table 41–4. FIGO staging for vaginal cancer.

FIGO Stage	Description	TNM Class
Stage 0	Carcinoma in situ; intraepithelial neoplasia grade 3	Tis N0 M0
Stage I	The carcinoma is limited to the vaginal wall	T1 N0 M0
Stage II	The carcinoma has involved the subvaginal tissue but has not extended to the pelvic wall	T2 N0 M0
Stage III	The carcinoma has extended to the pelvic wall	T1 N1 M0 T2 N1 M0 T3 N0 M0 T3 N1 M0
Stage IV	The carcinoma has extended beyond the true pelvis or has involved the mucosa of the bladder or rectum. Bullous edema as such does not permit a case to be allotted to stage IV.	
IVA	Tumour invades bladder and/or rectal mucosa and/or direct extension beyond the true pelvis	T4 any N M0
IVB	Spread to distant organs	Any T Any N M1

Benedet JL, Hacker NF, Ngan HYS (editors): Staging classifications and clinical practice guidelines of gynaecologic cancers. Int J Gynaecol Obstet 2000;70:207. http://www.figo.org/content/PDF/staging-booklet.pdf

chronic inflammation are associated factors. Herpesvirus hominis type 2 and human papillomavirus (HPV) have been found to be frequently associated with cervical cancer, and there is increasing evidence that HPV infections, particularly types 16, 18 and 31, are the most important risk factor for high-grade squamous intraepithelial lesions of the cervix and cervical cancer. The precancerous potential of low-grade squamous intraepithelial neoplasia has not been established.

The majority of cervical cancers are squamous cell (85%); the remainder consist of adenocarcinomas, mixed carcinomas (adenosquamous), and rare sarcomas (mixed mesodermal tumors, lymphosarcomas).

The earliest squamous cell carcinoma is confined to the epithelial layers (carcinoma in situ, intraepithelial carcinoma, preinvasive carcinoma), and it is thought that the disease remains confined to the mucous membrane for several years before invading the subjacent stroma. Carcinoma in situ occurs most frequently in the fourth decade, whereas invasive carcinoma is encountered most often in women between age 40 and age 50.

Following penetration of the basement membrane and involvement of the cervical stroma, the disease spreads by direct contiguity to the vagina and the adjacent parametrium and via the lymphatic channels (which are abundant in this area) to the regional lymph nodes of the pelvis (iliac and obturator) and to the periaortic lymph nodes. Estimating the extent of the malignant process is extremely important in determining the mode of therapy and in estimating the prognosis. This is judged clinically as shown in Table 41–5.

It is known from an examination of surgical specimens that the probability of lymph node metastasis increases according to the local extent of the disease, being approximately 15% in stage I, 30% in stage II, and 45% in stage III. About 80% of patients with stage IV cancer have lymph node involvement.

Clinical Findings

A. Carcinoma In Situ

High-grade squamous intraepithelial lesions and carcinoma in situ do not cause symptoms. Fifteen to 20 percent of patients with carcinoma in situ have no visible lesion. Cytologic examination (Papanicolaou) of a representative specimen collected from the squamocolumnar junction (transformation zone) of the cervix will demonstrate severely dysplastic or frankly malignant cells in 95% of women with this stage of disease.

The Schiller test, using Lugol's solution, is often helpful in demonstrating areas of abnormal epithelium—even in a cervix that appears normal on gross inspection—because the lack of glycogen in these cells makes them unable to take up the stain. The test is not specific for neoplasm, since areas of ectopy, cervicitis, atrophy, and dysplasia are also iodine-negative. A sharply demarcated border of nonstaining is more suggestive of epithelial neoplasia.

Table 41–5. FIGO staging for cervical cancer.

FIGO Stage	Description	TNM Class
Stage 0	Carcinoma in situ	Tis
Stage I	Cervical carcinoma confined to uterus (extension to corpus should be disregarded)	T1
IA	Invasive carcinoma, diagnosed only by microscopy. All macroscopically visible lesions—even with superficial invasion—are TIB/TIBI.	T1a
IAI	Measured stromal invasion 3 mm or less and 7 mm or less in horizontal spread	T1a1
IA2	Measured stromal invasion more than 3 mm and not more than 5 mm with a horizontal spread of 7 mm or less	T1a2
IB	Clearly visible lesion confined to the cervix or microscopic lesion greater than TIA2	T1b
IBI	Clearly visible lesion 4 cm or less in greatest dimension	T1b1
IB2	Clearly visible lesion more than 4 cm in greatest dimension	T1b2
Stage II	Tumor invades beyond uterus but not to pelvic wall or to the lower third of vagina	T2
IIA	Tumor without parametrial invasion	T2a
IIB	Tumor with parametrial invasion	T2b
Stage III	Cervical carcinoma extends to the pelvic wall and/or involves lower third of vagina or causes hydronephrosis or nonfunctioning kidney	T3
IIIA	Tumor involves lower third of the vagina, no extension to pelvic wall	T3a
IIIB	Tumor extends to pelvic wall or causes hydronephrosis or nonfunctioning kidney	T3b
Stage IV	Cervical carcinoma involving the mucosa of adjacent organs, or distant metastases	
IVA	Tumor invades mucosa of bladder or rectum and/or extends beyond true pelvis	T4
IVB	Distant metastasis	M1

Benedet JL, Hacker NF, Ngan HYS (editors): Staging classifications and clinical practice guidelines of gynaecologic cancers. Int J Gynecol Obstet 2000;70:207. http://www.figo.org/content/PDF/staging-booklet.pdf

Colposcopic examination of the cervix may define areas of dysplasia and carcinoma in situ and should be done in all women who have abnormal (dysplastic or malignant) epithelial cells unrelated to an inflammatory condition. This method is based primarily upon changes that occur in the capillary vascular pattern of the cervix associated with epithelial proliferation.

Punch biopsy is required in all cases in which there is a visible area of redness, an iodine-negative area, or an area of colposcopic abnormality. A cone biopsy and curettage should be done when cytologic examination reveals moderate or severe dysplasia, carcinoma in situ, or perhaps invasive carcinoma and (1) if colposcopy is not available and there is no visible lesion and no iodine-nonstaining area; (2) when colposcopy reveals no abnormalities of the exocervix or when an abnormal transformation zone is seen that extends into the endocervical canal; (3) when a colposcopically directed punch biopsy reveals microinvasive carcinoma; or (4) when colposcopically directed biopsies fail to explain the abnormal cytologic findings.

B. Invasive Carcinoma

With the exception of early stromal involvement, invasive carcinoma of the cervix usually produces symptoms. Intermenstrual or postcoital bleeding is often the first symptom. A watery vaginal discharge, occasionally blood-streaked, may be the only symptom. Pain is a manifestation of far-advanced disease. In most patients with invasive cancer, inspection of the cervix reveals an ulcerated or papillary lesion of the cervix that bleeds on contact. The cytologic examination almost always demonstrates exfoliated malignant cells, though it should be remembered that false-negative Papanicolaou smears are more frequent in the face of invasive carcinoma than in intraepithelial neoplasia. Biopsy usually reveals the invasive nature of the lesion. An occasional endocervical endophytic lesion will produce enlargement of the cervix without becoming evident on the portio vaginalis.

Differential Diagnosis

Chronic cervicitis can be distinguished from cancer of the cervix only by multiple negative cytologic and biopsy examinations. Polyps of the cervix should be examined by a pathologist to exclude malignant change.

Complications

The complications are those caused by spread of the disease or occurring secondary to treatment. Obstruction of the ureter, resulting in hydroureter, hydronephrosis, and uremia, occurs with advancing disease. Bilateral obstruction of the ureters leads to failure of kidney function and death. Involvement of the iliac and obturator lymph nodes may lead to lymphatic obstruction, with lymphedema of the lower extremity. The lumbosacral plexus may become infiltrated by tumor, causing pain in the low back, hip, and leg.

Vesicovaginal and rectovaginal fistulas occur as a result of tumor involvement of these structures or as complications of radiation therapy. A cloaca may result from massive slough of necrotic tumor tissue. Widespread metastases to lung, liver, brain, and bone may occur.

Complications of radiation therapy such as cystitis, colitis, and proctitis are not uncommon but are usually only transitory problems in modern treatment centers. Ovarian failure is an unavoidable complication of radiation therapy. Severe radiation damage to the bladder and rectum may result in hemorrhage, fistulas, and strictures. Radiation necrosis of the cervix and diffuse radiation pelvic fibrosis are rare complications.

The complications of surgery are hemorrhage, infection, thromboembolism, and fistula formation (ureterovaginal, vesicovaginal, and rectovaginal).

Prevention

Invasive cancer of the cervix can be prevented by detecting and properly treating chronic cervicitis, cervical dysplasia, and carcinoma in situ of the cervix. Regular pelvic examinations, with cervical cytologic examination every 1–3 years, have proved to be effective in the prevention of this disease. Cigarette smoking also contributes to the incidence of cervical cancer.

Treatment

The proper treatment of cervical cancer requires individualization of therapy for each patient according to the clinical circumstances. Cervical epithelial dysplasia is destroyed by cauterization or cryosurgery or by laser therapy.

A. Carcinoma In Situ

Carcinoma in situ and lesser degrees of cervical intraepithelial neoplasia are best treated by eradication of the entire transformation zone. This can be accomplished by cauterization, cryotherapy, laser vaporization, cone biopsy, electrosurgical loop excision, or cervicectomy. Hysterectomy may be done if there is another indication for removing the uterus. Regardless of the procedure, close follow-up is necessary in order to ensure that treatment has indeed been adequate.

B. Invasive Carcinoma

Stage 1A1 cases can be managed conservatively with cone excision (with negative margins) or hysterectomy. Radical hysterectomy with bilateral pelvic lymph node dissection is a treatment option in cases of small (stage 1A2, IB, IIA) disease in young women or invasive carcinoma complicating pregnancy. These women also have the option of radiation therapy with equal cure rates. More advanced invasive carcinomas are best treated by irradiation under the cooperative management of a radiotherapist and a gynecologist experienced in the treatment of cancer. Both internal sources (radium or cesium) and external sources (x-ray, ^{60}Co, betatron, linear accelerator) should be employed. Several randomized phase III trials have shown an overall survival advantage for cisplatin-based therapy given concurrently with radiation therapy. The risk of death from cervical cancer was decreased by 30–50% by concurrent chemoradiation. This is now recommended in most cases. Recurrent or persistent cancer following radiation therapy may require pelvic exenteration.

Prognosis

The earlier the disease is treated, the better the prognosis. Carcinoma in situ is almost 100% curable. The prevalence of invasive carcinoma of the cervix is decreasing, partly as a result of detection and treatment in the intraepithelial stage of the disease. The best results in stage I cancer of the cervix approach a 90% 5-year survival rate. For stage II, the figure drops to 60%; for stage III, to 30%; and for stage IV, to less than 10%.

Hricak H et al: Role of imaging in cancer of the cervix. American College of Radiology. ACR Appropriateness Criteria. Radiology 2000;215(Suppl):925.

Morris M et al: Pelvic radiation with concurrent chemotherapy compared with pelvic and para-aortic radiation for high-risk cervical cancer. N Engl J Med 1999;340:1137.

Rose PG et al: Concurrent cisplatin-based radiotherapy and chemotherapy for locally advance cervical cancer. N Engl J Med 1999;340:1144.

Sawaya GF et al: Current approaches to cervical-cancer screening. N Engl J Med 2001;344:1603.

ENDOMETRIAL CARCINOMA

Endometrial carcinoma is primarily a disease of postmenopausal women, with a peak incidence in the decade from 55 to 65 years of age. It also occurs in premenopausal women, particularly those with prolonged anovulation. Evidence suggests that prolonged unopposed (by progesterone) estrogen stimulation of the endometrium may be a predisposing factor in the development of endometrial carcinoma. The prolonged use of exogenous estrogens (and tamoxifen) in postmenopausal women multiplies the risk of endometrial cancer about seven times. There is also an association of obesity, hypertension, and diabetes with endometrial cancer.

Complex hyperplasia with atypia is a precursor of endometrial cancer. Well-differentiated (grade 1) tumors tend to be superficial, whereas higher-grade (2, 3) cancers are associated with deep myometrial invasion. Fortunately, deep myometrial penetration, extension beyond the corpus of the uterus, lymph node involvement, and distant metastases occur relatively late in the disease, so that most lesions are detected early. Anaplastic or high-grade tumors and the papillary serous, clear cell, and squamous cell variants behave more aggressively. Adverse prognostic factors include grade, histology, depth of myometrial invasion, cervical extension, tumor size, and extension beyond the uterus.

Endometrial cancer is now staged surgically as shown in Table 41–6.

Clinical Findings

Postmenopausal bleeding is the primary symptom and should be considered to be caused by cancer until proved otherwise. About 40% of women with vaginal bleeding following the menopause will have reproductive tract cancer, and in the vast majority of these cases the cancer is endometrial. Cervical stenosis with pyometra or hematometra is highly suggestive of endometrial carcinoma. Pain is not a common symptom but there may be mild uterine cramping, particularly if there is any degree of stenosis of the cervix. Vaginal cytology is positive in 40–80% of cases. Endometrial biopsy will almost always detect an endometrial carcinoma, as will cytologic sampling of the endometrial cavity. Curettage, first of the endocervix and then of the endometrial cavity, with careful examination under anesthesia is considered the most definitive method of diagnosing and clinically staging the disease. Myometrial involvement is suspected if the corpus is enlarged. MRI may be helpful in defining myometrial penetration.

Endometrial carcinoma that is histologically poorly differentiated, or high-grade, may disseminate relatively early in the course of the disease. Metastatic spread may

Table 41–6. FIGO staging for endometrial cancer.

FIGO Stage	Description	TNM Class
Stage 0	Carcinoma in situ	Tis
Stage I	Tumor limited to corpus uteri	T1
IA	Tumor limited to endometrium	T1a
IB	Invasion to less than half the myometrium	T1b
IC	Invasion to more than half the myometrium	T1c
Stage II	Tumor invades cervix but does not extend beyond uterus	T2
IIA	Endocervical glandular involvement only	T2a
IIB	Cervical stromal invasion	T2b
Stage III	Local and/or regional spread	T3 and/or N1
IIIA	Tumor invades serosa and/or adnexa and/or positive cytologic findings	T3a
IIIB	Vaginal involvement (direct or metastases)	T3b
IIIC	Metastases to pelvic and/or para-aortic lymph nodes	Any T N1
Stage IVA	Tumor invades bladder or bowel mucosa	T4
Stage IVB	Distant metastases, including intra-abdominal and/or inguinal lymph nodes	M1

Benedet JL, Hacker NF, Ngan HYS (editors): Staging classifications and clinical practice guidelines of gynaecologic cancers. Int J Gynecol Obstet 2000;70:207. http://www.figo.org/content/PDF/staging-booklet.pdf

occur to the vagina, regional pelvic and para-aortic lymph nodes, ovaries, lungs, brain, and bone. The most frequent site of recurrence following treatment for endometrial carcinoma is the vaginal vault.

Prevention

There is presumptive evidence that progesterone therapy will reduce the possibility of endometrial carcinoma in the anovulatory patient as well as in postmenopausal women receiving estrogen replacement therapy. Detection and adequate therapy of the precursors of the disease (hyperplasia with atypia and carcinoma in situ of the endometrium) will prevent the subsequent development of endometrial carcinoma.

Treatment

Total abdominal hysterectomy and bilateral salpingo-oophorectomy is definitive therapy for endometrial carcinoma. Washings of the peritoneal cavity for cytologic examination should be obtained at the time. Pelvic and para-aortic lymph node sampling should be done in most patients with endometrial cancer, with the exception of those with low-risk lesions, small grade 1 cancers without myometrial invasion.

If the cervix is grossly involved, patients should receive preoperative radiation followed by hysterectomy and node sampling or, if they are young, should undergo a radical hysterectomy with pelvic and para-aortic node sampling.

Adjuvant radiation therapy is administered to those with nodal disease, high-grade or deep myometrial involvement, and those with extension beyond the uterus. Radiation alone can be used in patients who are considered poor surgical risks. Poor-risk surgical patients with grade 1 tumors can also be treated with progestin therapy.

Disseminated endometrial carcinoma is treated with large-dose progestin therapy (hydroxyprogesterone caproate, medroxyprogesterone, or megestrol), which produces satisfactory remission of the metastatic disease in about 35% of cases, particularly in patients with tumors that are positive for progesterone receptors. Subjective improvement is noted in the majority of patients so treated. Cisplatin or carboplatin, doxorubicin, or paclitaxel is given to those with high grades, absent receptors, and disseminated disease.

Prognosis

Five-year survival rates of 70–90% are recorded in stage I disease. This drops to 60% in stage II. Histologic undifferentiation, deep myometrial penetration, and absence of estrogen and progesterone receptors all worsen the prognosis.

Kinkel K et al: Radiologic staging in patients with endometrial cancer: a meta-analysis. Radiology 1999;212:711.

Rose PG: Endometrial carcinoma. N Engl J Med 1996;335:640.

SARCOMAS OF THE UTERUS

Uterine sarcomas are relatively rare. They may arise from the myometrium itself, from the endometrial stroma, or, rarely, in preexisting leiomyomas. Mixed tumors (carcinosarcoma, mixed mesodermal tumors) containing both epithelial and connective tissue malignant cells are also encountered. Sarcomas of the uterus metastasize via the bloodstream and lymphatics and spread by contiguity. The lungs are a frequent site of metastatic disease.

In patients in whom the tumor is confined to the pelvic organs, treatment consists of total hysterectomy and bilateral salpingo-oophorectomy, with individualized postoperative radiation or chemotherapy (or both) for those with deep myometrial invasion.

The outlook for patients with uterine sarcoma is variable. Leiomyosarcomas with more than ten mitoses per ten high-power fields carry a poor prognosis, with recurrence within 5 years in about two-thirds of patients. About 40% of patients with malignant mixed müllerian tumors survive.

Doxorubicin has been reported to be effective in the treatment of some leiomyosarcomas. High-dose progestin therapy will bring about complete resolution of metastatic low-grade endometrial sarcoma in some patients. Unresectable or recurrent malignant mixed mesodermal tumors may respond to cisplatin and ifosfamide.

Gonzalez-Bosquet E et al: Uterine sarcoma: a clinicopathological study of 93 cases. Eur J Gynaecol Oncol 1997;18:192.

Levenback CF et al: Uterine sarcoma. Obstet Gynecol Clin North Am 1996;23:457.

TUMORS OF THE UTERINE TUBE (ADENOCARCINOMA)

Benign tumors of the uterine (fallopian) tubes are very rare. Primary carcinoma of the tube is the most common malignant lesion, but it is rarely encountered, constituting less than 1% of female reproductive tract cancers. Women with *BRCA12* mutations are at risk for uterine tube cancer as well as the more common breast and ovarian cancers.

Postmenopausal vaginal bleeding is the usual presenting complaint. There may be a history of intermittent and profuse, serous, yellow, or bloody vaginal discharge (hydrops tubae profluens). An adnexal mass may or may not be palpable.

The diagnosis of primary carcinoma of the uterine tube is rarely made preoperatively. Total abdominal hysterectomy and bilateral salpingo-oophorectomy constitute the treatment of choice in operable lesions. Tumors that are inoperable yet are confined to the pelvic structures should receive radiation therapy, followed by operation if there is a favorable response as judged by increased mobility and diminution in tumor size. Radical hysterectomy and bilateral pelvic lymph node dissection have been advocated as possibly a more curative procedure than simple hysterectomy and bilateral salpingo-oophorectomy.

If the disease is confined to the tube, the prognosis is quite good. Unfortunately, most of these tumors are advanced at the time of discovery, and the overall 5-year cure rate is in the range of 10–20%.

Early use of the laparoscope or the CT scanner may be of aid in the earlier diagnosis of this disease and should be considered in any postmenopausal woman with a vague adnexal mass, particularly if it is accompanied by a watery discharge or postmenopausal bleeding.

Uterine tube cancers are staged and treated as ovarian cancers.

Nikrui N et al: Fallopian tube carcinoma. Surg Oncol Clin N Am 1998;7:363.

OVARIAN CANCER

Ovarian malignancies may develop in the form of epithelial tumors, germ cell tumors, sex cord-stromal tumors, and various mixtures of these groups. Epithelial carcinomas arise from the coelomic epithelium and account for 85–90% of malignant ovarian neoplasms. The peak incidence of epithelial ovarian carcinoma is in the fifth and sixth decades of life, while malignant germ cell tumors are more likely to occur under the age of 30. Stromal tumors seem to be more evenly distributed among the age groups.

The common epithelial histologies are serous, mucinous, endometrioid, clear cell, transitional cell, and undifferentiated adenocarcinoma. Spread of disease is primarily by exfoliation of cells that implant in the peritoneal cavity, but lymphatic channels and hematogenous spread are also common. Serous histology is the most common, comprising approximately 40% of ovarian carcinomas. Mucinous tumors in particular may become very large and distend the entire abdomen. Endometrioid carcinomas are the second most frequent variety (24% of ovarian cancers) and sometimes are associated with endometriosis. Clear cell tumors are also associated with endometriosis but have a significantly more aggressive histologic appearance. Borderline tumors or atypical epithelial proliferation of low malignant potential are considered less aggressive histologic subtypes yet are still considered malignancies because of their risk for recurrence and metastasis.

Tumors of germ cell origin include dysgerminomas (the homolog of testicular seminomas), immature teratomas, endodermal sinus tumor, and choriocarcinoma. While benign cystic teratomas are among the most common benign ovarian tumors, malignant change occurs in rare instances; such tumors are usually squamous cell carcinomas and not immature teratomas.

Less common are the hormone-producing neoplasms. The granulosa-theca cell tumors are the most frequent of the hormonally active tumors, constituting about 4–6% of ovarian cancers. About two-thirds are benign in their clinical behavior. Sertoli-Leydig cell tumors are rare and usually manifest themselves first by producing defeminization (amenorrhea, atrophy of the breast) and then masculinization (deepening of the voice, hirsutism, clitoral hypertrophy). Like granulosa-theca cell tumors, the majority are benign, the reported incidence of cancer being about 20%. Metastatic carcinoma from the gastrointestinal tract (Krukenberg tumor), breast, pancreas, and kidney must always be considered as a possible diagnosis whenever there is bilateral malignant disease of the ovaries.

Although only 10–15% of ovarian cancers are thought to be hereditary, family history is one of the strongest risk factors for epithelial ovarian cancer. Genetic inheritance of a mutation in the *BRCA1* or *BRCA2* gene imposes a 20–40% lifetime risk of developing ovarian cancer along with a 60–80% lifetime risk of developing breast cancer. An increased risk has also been observed in women from families with a background of colorectal and endometrial cancer. Other reproductive factors associated with an increased risk include infertility, probably independent of the use of ovulation induction agents.

Clinical Findings

Despite the common belief that early-stage ovarian cancer is without symptoms, most women with ovarian cancer have vague symptoms such as lower abdominal pressure. The most important sign is the presence of a pelvic mass on physical examination. Any enlargement of the ovary in women of menopausal or postmenopausal age should be regarded as malignant until proved otherwise. A solid, irregular, fixed pelvic mass is highly suggestive of an ovarian malignancy, particularly in combination with an upper abdominal mass or ascites. The CA-125 tumor is helpful to differentiate between a benign or malignant process, though the marker may be negative in half of early-stage ovarian cancers. Although ultrasonography or CT scanning may be helpful, it is often impossible to determine the benign or malignant nature of an ovarian tumor until laparotomy. If an ovarian malignancy is suspected preoperatively, it is appropriate to refer the patient for surgical exploration, staging, and cytoreduction by a gynecologic oncologist.

On occasion, an ovarian malignancy is not detected until it is discovered at operation for another intra-abdominal disorders. Papillations of the external surface, adherence to surrounding structures, and peritoneal implants are signs of cancer. The tumor should be removed without spilling its contents into the peritoneal cavity and should be submitted to a pathologist in the operating room for gross examination and frozen-section microscopic analysis of any suspicious areas. These cystic enlargements may represent simple cysts, serous or mucinous cystadenomas, adenofibromas, or cystadenocarcinomas. Solid enlargements of the ovary may be benign fibromas or thecomas. If a malignancy is identified or suspected, a gynecologic or surgical oncologist should be consulted for thorough surgical staging.

Differential Diagnosis

Ovarian neoplasms may be benign, borderline, or malignant. Pelvic masses may arise from the uterus, adnexa, bowel, or occasionally the genitourinary tract. In most instances the correct diagnosis can be made if an accurate medical history is obtained, a careful physical examination performed, and judicious use made of ancillary diagnostic procedures such as ultrasound, CT scanning, and serum tumor markers. Surgery is often required in order to establish the definitive diagnosis of an ovarian mass and, if the mass is malignant, to accurately assess the extent of disease.

Prevention

Bilateral salpingo-oophorectomy at the time of hysterectomy for benign uterine disease in women over age 40—and after childbearing function has been completed in younger women with strong family histories—is advocated by many to prevent the development of ovarian cancer. To date, no effective screening test for ovarian cancer is applicable to the general population, though women with a strong family history should be considered for genetic counseling and close clinical surveillance. Known protective factors for ovarian cancer include childbearing and use of oral contraceptive pills. Even 6 months of pill use seems to decrease the relative risk for ovarian cancer, and the effects appear to remain protective for up to 10 years. For patients with genetic mutations predisposing them to increased risk, prophylactic oophorectomy may be performed with or without prophylactic mastectomy as well.

Treatment

Accurate pathologic evaluation and thorough surgical staging (Table 41–7) are essential to the management of early stage disease. When a complex adnexal mass is removed in the operating room, washings should be obtained first, and the mass should be removed intact. Laparoscopy may be considered for some lesions, but puncturing the ovarian mass in a bag before removal still risks the possibility of intraperitoneal spill and spread. Solid or papillary projections are particular areas of suspicion. A frozen section should be obtained to exclude malignancy. If an ovarian malignancy is confirmed or suspected, surgical staging includes removal of the uterus, the contralateral ovary, pelvic and para-aortic lymph nodes, and omentum. Peritoneal and bowel surfaces should be carefully inspected and suspicious areas biopsied. Even in ovarian malignancies clinically confined to the ovary, there can be occult metastatic disease in the lymph nodes or omentum. In women without any evidence of extra-ovarian disease who want to maintain future childbearing capacity, the uterus and contralateral ovary may be preserved, with consideration of later removal on completion of childbearing. Complete surgical staging gives the most accurate prognosis of disease, and if early-stage disease is confirmed it may obviate the need for additional chemotherapy. Patients with stage IA grade 1 or grade 2 tumors have a very good prognosis and usually are not treated with additional chemotherapy.

When the disease extends beyond the ovaries into the pelvis or abdomen, cytoreduction of all bulky disease contributes to an advantage in chemotherapy response and survival. Even in stage IV disease, tumor debulking improves survival if the intraperitoneal disease can be resected to minimal residual. A hysterectomy and bilateral salpingo-oophorectomy should be performed along with removal of the omentum. Intestinal resection, diaphragm resection, splenectomy, and other upper abdominal procedures may also be indicated if the patient can be left with minimal residual disease. In one series of patients resected to less than 0.5 cm disease, median survival was 40 months, compared with a median survival of 18 months for patients whose disease was only less than 1.5 cm. Successful cytoreductive surgery may be successful in over 70% of patients when performed by gynecologic oncologists, subspecialists trained in ovarian cancer surgery. The CA-125 tumor antigen is a poor marker for ovarian cancer screening but is elevated in over 75% of ovarian carcinomas and can serve as a marker in assessing the effectiveness of therapy.

Chemotherapy is very effective in ovarian cancer as adjuvant therapy and in achieving clinical remission. The current standard regimen for advanced epithelial ovarian carcinoma in the United States is a combination of a taxane and platinum agent for at least six cycles, usually using paclitaxel and carboplatin. Patients who are not surgical candidates may be considered for primary chemotherapy with these agents as well, and many will have a significant tumor response. The current standard regimen for malignant germ cell tumors is cisplatin, etoposide, and bleomycin.

Table 41–7. FIGO staging for ovarian cancer.

FIGO Staging	Description	TNM Class
Stage I	Tumor limited to the ovaries	T1
IA	Limited to one ovary, no tumor on external surface, capsule intact; negative peritoneal cytology	T1a
IB	Limited to both ovaries, no tumor on external surface, capsule intact; negative peritoneal cytology	T1b
IC	IA or IB tumor, but with surface tumor, ruptured capsule, or positive ascites or peritoneal cytology	T1c
Stage II	Tumor extending to the pelvis	T2
IIA	Metastasis to the uterus or tubes	T2
IIB	Metastasis to other pelvic tissues	T2b
IIC	IIA or IIB tumor, both with surface tumor, ruptured capsule, or positive ascites or peritoneal cytology	T2c
Stage III	Tumor extending outside the pelvis and/or retroperitoneal or inguinal nodes. Extension to small bowel, omentum, or superficial liver	T3 and/or N1
IIIA	Histologically confirmed microscopic disease of abdominal peritoneal surfaces; lymph nodes negative	T3a
IIIB	Implants of abdominal or peritoneal surfaces not exceeding 2 cm in diameter; lymph nodes negative	T3b
IIIC	Implants of abdominal or peritoneal surfaces greater than 2 cm in diameter, or positive retroperitoneal or inguinal lymph nodes	T3c and/or N1
Stage IV	Distant metastasis beyond the peritoneal cavity	M1

Benedet JL, Hacker NF, Ngan HYS (editors): Staging classifications and clinical practice guidelines of gynaecologic cancers. Int J Gynecol Obstet 2000;70:207. http://www.figo.org/content/PDF/staging-booklet.pdf

Prognosis

The prognosis for epithelial ovarian carcinoma is related primarily to stage and histologic grade. Because most ovarian cancers are of advanced stage at the time of initial diagnosis, the overall cure rate for ovarian cancer is approximately 50%. Five-year survival rates for patients with stage III or stage IV disease are around 20–35%. Nevertheless, significant disease-free remission can be achieved by combining accurate surgical staging and thorough surgical cytoreduction with chemotherapy. For stage I disease, 5-year survival rates can be over 80–85%, emphasizing the need for improved early detection.

Bomalaski JJ: The treatment of recurrent ovarian carcinoma: balancing patient desires, therapeutic benefit, cost containment and quality of life. Curr Opin Obstet Gynecol 1999;11:11.

Lynch HT et al: Genetics and ovarian carcinoma. Semin Oncol. 1998;25:265.

Marsden DE et al: Current management of epithelial ovarian carcinoma: a review. Semin Surg Oncol 2000;19:11.

Scully RE et al: *Tumors of the Ovary, Maldeveloped Gonads, Fallopian Tube, and Broad Ligament.* Armed Forces Institute of Pathology, 1998.

GESTATIONAL TROPHOBLASTIC DISEASE

Gestational trophoblastic neoplasms are chorionic tumors arising from placental tissue. Hydatidiform moles are related to the swelling of the villi in the absence of a fetal circulation and are accompanied by varying degrees of trophoblastic proliferation. There is a tendency for myometrial penetration that may progress to frank deep invasion of the uterine wall (chorioadenoma destruens, or invasive mole), and a small percentage (about 2–3%) of hydatidiform moles are followed by development of the highly malignant choriocarcinoma.

Hydatidiform moles can be classified as either complete or partial, based on cytogenetics and histopathology. Most complete moles have a 46,XX karyotype, with chromosomes entirely of paternal origin. Most partial moles have a triploid karyotype (69,XXY or 69,XYY), with extra chromosomes again derived from the father. Complete moles have a higher incidence of persistent gestational trophoblastic disease.

Staging of gestational trophoblastic tumors is outlined in Table 41–8.

The frequency of hydatidiform mole is about 1:2000–1:1500 pregnancies in the USA and about 1:650–1:240 pregnancies in the Far East and Mexico. Hydatidiform mole is also more common in women over 40 years of age.

Trophoblastic disease should be assessed for risk of persistent disease to determine optimal treatment and follow-up. (See Table 41–9.)

Table 41–8. FIGO staging of gestational trophoblastic tumors.

Stage I	Disease confined to uterus
A	No risk factors
B	1 risk factor
C	2 risk factors
Stage II	Disease extending outside uterus, limited to genital structures—adnexa, broad ligament, vagina
A	No risk factors
B	1 risk factor
C	2 risk factors
Stage III	Disease extending to lungs, with or without genital tract involvement
A	No risk factors
B	1 risk factor
C	2 risk factors
Stage IV	Disease involving other metastatic sites
A	No risk factors
B	1 risk factor
C	2 risk factors

Clinical Findings

The usual picture is one of a nonviable gestation or presumed threatened abortion. Often there is vaginal bleeding. This may go on for several weeks with little or no abdominal pain. Examination reveals a disproportionately large uterus for the duration of the pregnancy in about 50% of cases. There may be bilateral cystic enlargement of the ovaries (theca lutein cysts). Preeclampsia may develop in women with large moles, and molar pregnancy should be suspected in any patient who develops hypertension, edema, and proteinuria in the first half of pregnancy. Anemia is common.

Serum and urinary β-hCG levels are unusually high and persist at high levels beyond the 12th week, when in normal pregnancy there is usually a significant drop. Ultrasound is quite accurate in the diagnosis of molar pregnancy, with a characteristic appearance of multiple small sonolucencies due to the presence of hydropic villi. Correlating sonographic findings with hCG levels may differentiate the finding of a molar pregnancy from a missed abortion.

In many cases, the diagnosis is not made until the patient spontaneously aborts the molar pregnancy. Any products of conception in which hydropic change is suggested on gross examination should be formally examined by a pathologist. Care must be taken by the pathologist in distinguishing degenerating products of conception from hydropic villi with trophoblastic proliferation. Placental site trophoblastic tumor is a rare form of trophoblastic disease that can arise from any type of pregnancy. β-hCG is a less reliable tumor marker in this disease, and it is relatively insensitive to chemotherapy compared with other chorionic tumors.

Differential Diagnosis

A diagnosis of threatened abortion or missed abortion is often entertained in the presence of a mole. Multiple pregnancy must be considered because it may produce unusually high levels of chorionic gonadotropin. Ultrasound diagnosis is quite reliable in complete hydatidiform mole. There may be an aneuploid fetus in cases of partial hydatidiform mole; however, the presence of focal cystic spaces in the placenta is often diagnostic. There are rare cases of a normal fetus coexisting with a molar pregnancy.

Complications

About 15% of moles become locally invasive (chorioadenoma destruens) and impose a danger of hemorrhage owing to penetration of the vascular uterine wall or pelvic infection from perforation. About 2–3% of moles are followed by choriocarcinoma, a highly malignant tumor. Although this cancer may occur after normal pregnancy, abortion, or ectopic pregnancy, about half of cases develop from an antecedent hydatidiform mole. Metastases are found in the lungs, liver, central nervous system, bone, vagina, and vulva. Despite the highly aggressive nature of this tumor, gestational trophoblastic disease is one of the most curable forms of malignancy.

Treatment

Once the diagnosis of a molar pregnancy has been established, the uterus should be emptied. This is done

Table 41–9. WHO scoring system for risk of gestational trophoblastic tumors.

≤ 4 = low risk
5–7 = intermediate risk
> 7 = high risk

Score → / **Prognostic Factors**	**0**	**1**	**2**	**4**
Age	≤ 39	> 39		
Prior pregnancy	Mole	Abortion	Term	
Interval (months)	< 4	4–6	> 6	
β-hCG titer	< 1000	1001–10,000	10,000–100,000	> 100,000
ABO group	O, A, or A, O	B, AB		
Largest tumor (cm)	< 3	3–5	> 5	
Metastatic site		Spleen Kidney	Liver GI tract	Brain
Number of metastases		1–3	4–8	> 8
Prior chemotherapy			One drug	Two or more drugs

by both suction and sharp dilation and curettage. Larger moles are better evacuated with the simultaneous administration of intravenous oxytocin. All specimens are examined pathologically for evidence of proliferative activity of the trophoblast, which serves as an indication of the probability of malignant change.

Lutein cysts of the ovaries, which occur in about one-third of molar pregnancies, will regress following removal of the mole and should not be surgically excised.

All patients with hydatidiform mole should be followed weekly after evacuation of the uterus for the possible development of persistent gestational trophoblastic disease. Patients should be given effective contraceptive advice and counseled not to become pregnant for at least a year. Weekly serum β-hCG levels should be obtained until the titer is normal for 3 weeks; thereafter, monthly levels are measured until the titer is normal for 6–12 months. It may take as long as 14–16 weeks for hCG to reach normal levels following molar evacuation. A plateau or rising titer, particularly with the disappearance of the hormone followed by a later reappearance, is strongly suggestive of choriocarcinoma or invasive mole if pregnancy can be ruled out.

Patients with persistent gestational trophoblastic tumors should be evaluated with a metastatic workup and considered for chemotherapy based on their risk factors (Table 41–8). The workup should include a pelvic examination, pelvic ultrasound, chest x-ray, a complete blood count, and renal and liver function tests. If these tests are normal, other sites of metastasis are not likely to be present. If metastatic lesions are suspected, a CT scan of the head, chest, abdomen, and pelvis should be performed.

Single-agent chemotherapy is the preferred treatment for patients with stage I or low-risk disease who wish to maintain reproductive options. If future childbearing is not an issue, patients with invasive mole should be considered for hysterectomy and single-agent adjuvant chemotherapy. Prophylactic chemotherapy should be considered in older women with extremely high gonadotropin titers given their high risk of persistent disease after evacuation. Single-agent management with methotrexate or dactinomycin has resulted in similar response and remission rates for gestational trophoblastic tumors. Methotrexate competes with folic acid in cellular metabolism and is given either by weekly intramuscular injection or as infusions 5 days in a row given every other week. Dactinomycin is a vesicant agent but is also given as five daily infusions given every other week or as a single bolus infusion given every other week. Both of these regimens can be quite cytotoxic and should be administered under the guidance of a gynecologic oncologist or medical oncologist. Intermediate-risk gestational trophoblastic disease can be treated with combination chemotherapy: methotrexate, dactinomycin, and cyclophosphamide or chlorambucil. Even in high-risk patients, a combination regimen of etoposide, methotrexate, dactinomycin, cyclophosphamide, and vincristine is still effective in drug-resistant disease.

Prognosis

The prognosis for cure of gestational trophoblastic tumors is excellent. Before chemotherapeutic agents became available, the outlook for choriocarcinoma was very poor. Five-year remission rates in the range of 80% or better are now being reported even in the presence of metastatic disease. Follow-up of a reliable tumor marker and assessment of risk factors to select an efficacious chemotherapy regimen have made gestational trophoblastic disease one of the success stories in oncology. The risk in subsequent pregnancies for another molar pregnancy is slightly increased (about 1%), and early ultrasound is recommended to confirm normal gestation. The placenta or products of conception should be examined after delivery, and follow-up hCG levels should be obtained to exclude the possibility of persistent trophoblastic disease.

Berkowitz RS et al: Chorionic tumors. N Engl J Med 1990; 335:1740.

Bower M et al: EMA/CO (etoposide, methotrexate, actinomycin-D, cyclophosphamide, vincristine) for high-risk gestational trophoblastic tumours: results from a cohort of 272 patients. J Clin Oncol 1990;15:2636.

Newlands ES et al: Recent advances in gestational trophoblastic disease. Hematol Oncol Clin North Am. 1999;13:225.

Orthopedics

42

Bobby K-B Tay, MD, William W. Colman, MD, Sigurd Berven, MD, Roger Fontes, Jr, MD, Stephen Gunther, MD, William Holmes, MD, Hubert T. Kim, MD, PhD, Lisa Lattanza, MD, Edward Diao, MD, Serena S. Hu, MD, & David S. Bradford, MD

Orthopedic surgery and orthopedic medicine have evolved substantially over the last decade. Improvements in implant design and materials have been responsible for major breakthroughs in our ability to treat patients with complex orthopedic problems. The limitations on what we can achieve with engineering advances have motivated us to seek greater understanding of the biologic mechanisms that determine the optimal outcomes for our patients.

A Note on Terminology

In general, the use of eponyms to denote fractures or deformities is best avoided by the student and nonorthopedist. Although well-entrenched eponyms are included in this chapter, it is often less confusing to use anatomic terms.

Varus and **valgus** are descriptive terms frequently used in the characterization of angular musculoskeletal deformities. They refer to the direction of the apex of the deformity in relation to the midline of the body. If the apex points away from the midline, the deformity is varus; if toward the midline, the deformity is valgus. Knock-knees are an example of valgus deformity; the entire lower limb is abnormally angulated, with the apex of the deformity (the knee) pointing toward the midline. In bowlegs, the angle of deformity points away from the midline; this condition is called varus knees or genu varum. Similar designations apply to angular deformities of the elbow (cubitus varus or valgus) and the hip (coxa vara or valga).

When a long bone such as the femur or humerus is fractured, the limb may be visibly deformed. The relationship between the main fracture fragments, or the alignment, can be characterized by describing the angular deformity in the sagittal and coronal planes. In this case, the fracture itself constitutes the apex of the deformity and may be designated as varus or valgus. However, in practical use, the angulation of the fracture is more clearly described by noting the apex of the deformity (apex anterior, posterior, lateral, or medial). The fracture is said to be comminuted if the bones are fragmented. The fracture is displaced when the main bony fragments are translated or separated from each other. Fracture displacement is then subcategorized into minimally, moderately, and completely displaced.

If there is a wound overlying the fracture through which the fracture is either exposed or through which it may have communicated with the external environment, the fracture is described as **open.** In this situation, fracture contamination must be promptly addressed by surgically cleaning the wound and the underlying bone to minimize the likelihood of developing osteomyelitis.

Joint dislocations also warrant immediate treatment. The maneuver to restore proper alignment of a joint or fracture is called **reduction.** Vascular structures spanning the joint may be injured at the time of injury or may be compressed by malalignment of bony structures. The arterial pulses distal to the injury should be assessed and documented. Absent pulses are often restored after reduction of the joint. If the vessels are torn, early repair or reconstruction is often required to restore distal circulation to the limb.

Joint or fracture reduction may be performed by **open (surgical)** or **closed (nonsurgical)** techniques. A dislocation or fracture is described as unstable if there is a high likelihood of further deformation. Following reduction, unstable fractures or dislocations may be stabilized by closed or open techniques. Closed techniques involve traction, casts, splints, or braces; open techniques involve exposure of the fracture and reduction of the fracture fragments with maintenance of the reduction with some form of internal or external fixation device. The surgical management of an unstable fracture or dislocation is therefore described as "open reduction and internal or external fixation."

FRACTURES & JOINT INJURIES

FRACTURES & DISLOCATIONS OF THE SPINE

Demographics

In a survey of 165 trauma centers evaluating a total of 111,219 trauma patients, the incidence of cervical spine injury was 4.3%, with a 1.3% incidence of spinal cord injury. Most studies report an incidence of 3.2–5.3 new spinal cord injuries per 100,000 persons at risk in the United States. There is a bimodal distribution in the prevalence of spinal column injury, with peaks occurring in people between 15 and 24 years of age and in people 50 years of age and older. The percentage of the population over 50 years of age is constantly increasing as a result of longer life expectancies. The elderly are also more active, and as this subset of the population increases in number the incidence of spinal cord injury in the elderly will certainly increase as well. Improvements in emergency medical care and trauma care have reduced the mortality and morbidity associated with these injuries. The mortality from spinal cord injury also decreased from 20% to 9%.

Most patients with spinal column injury are young men. The most common causes in this age group are motor vehicle accidents, followed by falls, gunshot injuries, and sports injuries. In the pediatric population, motor vehicle accidents are the most common cause of injury; in the elderly, falls are the most common cause. Disturbingly, the proportion of spinal cord injuries from gunshot wounds is increasing, and controversy continues over optimal management of a patient with a bullet in the spinal canal.

As with internal fixation of extremity fractures, internal fixation of spine fractures has allowed early mobilization and rehabilitation, resulting in improvements in outcome. Internal fixation has also made it easier to achieve decompression of the neural elements.

Anatomy

The spinal column consists of multiple individual motion segments made up of the vertebral bodies and the intervertebral disks. Mobility is greatest in the cervical spine, least in the thoracic spine, and of intermediate range in the lumbar spine. Injuries may occur anywhere along the spinal column depending upon the mechanism of injury. However, most nonpathologic vertebral column fractures occur in the more mobile segments (cervical and lumbar spines) and at the junctions between flexible and less flexible segments (cervicothoracic junction, thoracolumbar junction, and lumbosacral junction).

The bony vertebral column also protects the neural elements from injury. In the cervical and thoracic spine, the spinal canal contains the spinal cord, nerve roots, and spinal nerves as they exit from the neural foramina. The spinal cord is composed of central gray matter (neuronal cell bodies) surrounded by white matter (axons). Within a cross section of the cord, several important anatomic structures can be identified. These include the lateral spinothalamic tracts that are responsible for transmitting pain and temperature sensation; the lateral corticospinal tracts, responsible for motor function at that level; and the posterior columns, which transmit position sense, vibratory sensation, and deep pressure sensation. The spinothalamic tracts cross to the opposite side of the spinal cord within three levels of entering the cord. In contrast, the corticospinal tracts and the posterior columns decussate at the craniocervical levels. The most central portions of the corticospinal tracts control the function of the more proximal areas of the body, and the more peripheral portions control the function of the distal areas.

The spinal roots exit the vertebral column through the intervertebral foramina. In the cervical spine, the C1 root exits above the C1 body; the C2 root exits below the C1 body; and the C8 root exits below the C7 body. In the thoracic and lumbar spine, each root exits under the pedicle with the same number.

During development, the spinal cord does not grow longitudinally as rapidly as the vertebra, so the terminal segment of the spinal cord (conus medullaris) ends near the lower border of the first lumbar vertebra. The dural sac distal to the L1 contains the spinal nerves for all the segments from L2 through S5.

Initial Management & Clinical Assessment of Spinal Injury

Treatment is initiated at the scene of the injury. Without exception, all victims of trauma are suspected of having a spinal column injury until such an injury has been ruled out. Cervical spine injury has been closely linked to the presence of severe head injury (odds ratio 8.5), a high-energy mechanism (odds ratio 11.6), or a focal neurologic deficit (odds ratio 58). Initial stabilization begins with the application of a rigid cervical collar, a spine board, and sandbags.

Careful evaluation and documentation of the patient's neurologic status will allow the physician to determine the appropriate treatment plan and estimate the prognosis for functional recovery. Once at the trauma center, clinical assessment of a suspected spine injury begins with evaluation of the patient's airway, breathing, and circulation. Significant retropharyngeal soft tissue swelling, especially in the upper cervical spine, may lead to upper airway obstruction. High cervical injuries causing diaphragmatic and chest wall muscle paralysis will result in respiratory failure. Neurogenic shock can cause significant hypotension and bradycardia. Sensory deficits caused by either cord or root level injuries can result in the rapid development of decubiti over insensate skin over high-pressure areas of the body (especially heels and ischium). Prompt assessment and removal of the patient from the spine board and onto an appropriate bed may help to prevent decubiti. Airway and breathing are ensured by intubation and mechanical ventilation. Nasotracheal intubation is the safest method of airway control in the acute setting because it causes less cervical spine motion than direct oral intubation. The diastolic pressure should be kept above 70 mm Hg to maximize spinal cord blood flow. In the polytrauma setting, this is initially done with fluid resuscitation. However, once the diagnosis of neurogenic shock is established, the blood pressure should be managed with vasopressors to prevent fluid overload. Methylprednisolone, if given within 8 hours after injury, improves motor function recovery after incomplete spinal cord injury. NASCIS-2 (National Acute Spinal Cord Injury Studies) and NASCIS-3 trials have demonstrated that an initial bolus of 30 mg/kg given over the first 15 minutes followed by 5.4 mg/kg/h over the following 24 hours (if steroids were started within 3 hours after injury) or 48 hours (if steroids were started within 3–8 hours after injury) were beneficial in improving long-term motor recovery.

After the initial resuscitation, the primary survey can be performed to evaluate for any life-threatening injuries. At this time, information from emergency medical personnel about the mechanism of injury and the accident scene may alert the physician to possible associated injuries. After the primary survey is complete, the secondary survey should include inspection and palpation of the entire spine. Ecchymosis, soft tissue swelling, tenderness, crepitance, and gaps between the spinous processes suggest underlying spinal column injury. Noncontiguous spinal injuries occur in 6% of patients, and these can easily be missed if there is associated head injury, upper cervical injury, or cervicothoracic injury.

In addition to spinal trauma, other injuries should be assessed since they may influence the treatment of the spinal lesion and may alter the outcome. Suspicion of associated injuries is dependent on the mechanism of the initial traumatic event that is responsible for the characteristic spinal injury pattern. In cervical spine trauma, much attention has been devoted to the investigation of possible vertebral artery injury. Reports indicate a 20–25% incidence of vertebral artery injury after cervical spine injury; the incidence increases with fractures extending into the transverse foramen. Bilateral or dominant vertebral artery injury can cause fatal ischemic damage to the brain stem and cerebellum. Delayed cortical blindness and recurrent quadriparesis can also occur from occult vertebral artery injury after cervical trauma. Despite the high incidence of vertebral artery injury with cervical trauma as well as the potential morbidity and mortality associated with vertebral artery injury, the great majority of these injuries are clinically silent. Up to 50% of all flexion-distraction injuries (seat-belt injuries) of the thoracolumbar spine are associated with intra-abdominal injuries. Axial loading injury mechanisms that are responsible for the majority of burst fractures in the lumbar spine are also responsible for axial loading injury patterns in the lower lumbar spine and lower extremities. These include fractures of the pars interarticularis of the L5 vertebra, the tibial plafond, and the calcaneus.

Classification of Injury

A. Classification of Bony Injury

The spinal column consists of four major components that contribute to its stability: (1) the vertebral bodies; (2) the posterior elements (pedicles, laminae, spinous process, and interlocking paired facets at each level); (3) the intervertebral disk; and (4) the ligamentous and musculoaponeurotic sleeves attached to the bone (interspinous ligaments, facet capsules, ligamentum flavum). In general, an injury disrupting only one of the three components will be relatively stable if protected, whereas if all three components are disrupted the spinal column will be significantly unstable at the level of injury, with risk of reinjury to the spinal canal contents. If injury is present in two of the components, the degree of instability will lie between these extremes. For example, the common mild anterior compression fracture at the thoracolumbar junction of the vertebral body is stable, whereas anterior dislocation of the cervical vertebrae is quite unstable. In the latter injury, there is complete anterior displacement of the facets, disruption of the posterior elements, rupture of the interspinous ligaments and the capsule of the facet joints, and disruption of the entire annulus fibrosus with or without a small fracture of the anterior vertebral body beneath the dislocation.

B. Classification of Neurologic Injury

The motor and sensory examination outlined by the American Spinal Injury Association (ASIA) is the most widely accepted and utilized system to assess the impact on the patient of spinal cord injury. It involves the use of a grading system to evaluate the remaining sensory and motor function. The system allows the patient to be assessed through scales of impairment and functional independence. A thorough neurologic examination should be performed and documented when the patient is initially seen and at frequent intervals thereafter both to ensure that there is no further neurologic deterioration and to document the resolution of spinal shock. Spinal shock is the initial period after spinal cord injury during which metabolic rather than structural derangements in the injured cord (depletion of adenosine triphosphate) result in spinal cord dysfunction characterized by paralysis, hypotonia, and areflexia. Once spinal shock has resolved, the motor and sensory examination allows the patient to be graded on a scale of functional impairment. Return of the bulbocavernosus reflex heralds the end of spinal shock. In most cases, this local reflex arc returns within 48 hours after injury. If a patient has a complete neurologic deficit after spinal shock has resolved, the chance for recovery of neurologic function below the level of injury is practically nonexistent. In contrast, patients with root level injuries (at or below the cauda equina) will recover from functionally complete injuries if they have not been transected and if initial compression by bone fragments, malalignment, disk material, etc, has been relieved.

Determination of Sensory Levels

The sensory level is determined by the patient's ability to perceive pinprick (using a disposable needle or safety pin) and light touch (using a cotton ball). Testing of a key point in each of the 28 dermatomes on the right and left sides of the body as well as evaluation of perianal sensation is required. The variability in sensation for each individual stimulus is graded on a 3-point scale:

0 = Absent
1 = Impaired
2 = Normal
NT = Not testable

In the cervical spine, the C3 and C4 nerve roots supply sensation to the entire upper neck and chest in a cape-like distribution from the tip of the acromion to just above the nipple line. The next adjacent sensory level is the T2 dermatome. The brachial plexus (C5–T1) supplies the upper extremities.

ASIA also recommends testing of pain and deep pressure sensation in the same dermatomes as well as evaluation of proprioception by testing the position sense of the both index fingers and both great toes.

Determination of Motor Levels

The motor level is determined by manual testing of a key muscle in the ten paired myotomes from rostral to caudal. The strength of each muscle is graded on a six-point scale:

0 = Total paralysis
1 = Palpable or visible contraction
2 = Full range of motion of the joint powered by the muscle with gravity eliminated
3 = Full range of motion of the joint powered by the muscle against gravity
4 = Active movement with full range of motion against moderate resistance
5 = Normal strength
NT = Not testable

For myotomes that are not clinically testable by manual muscle evaluation, the motor level is presumed to be the same as the sensory level (C1–4, T2–L1, S2–5).

ASIA also recommends evaluation of diaphragmatic function (via fluoroscopy; C4 level) and the abdominal musculature (via Beevor's sign, ie, upward migration of the umbilicus resulting from upper abdominal contraction in the absence of lower abdominal contraction due to paralysis at the T10 level). Evaluation of medial hamstring and hip adductor strength is also recommended but not required.

ASIA Impairment Scale

Once spinal shock has resolved, motor and sensory examination allows the patient to be graded on a scale of functional impairment. The grading system used is a modification of the Frankel classification system.

ASIA A (complete): No sensory or motor function is preserved below the level of injury, including the sacral segments S4–5.

ASIA B (incomplete): Sensory function is spared but there is no motor function below the level of injury except for the preservation of sacral segments S4–5.

ASIA C (incomplete): Motor function is preserved below the neurologic level, and more than half of the key muscles below the neurologic level have a muscle strength less than grade 3.

ASIA D (incomplete): Motor function is preserved below the neurologic level, and at least half of the muscles below the neurologic level have a muscle strength of at least grade 3.

ASIA E: No neurologic deficit.

Imaging Studies

A. Cervical Spine

Plain radiographs are used as the first imaging modality for the cervical spine. The standard series includes an anteroposterior, lateral, and an open-mouth view. Eighty-five percent of all significant injuries to the cervical spine will be detected on the lateral view of the cervical spine. If the standard lateral view does not adequately visualize the C7–T1 junction, further studies such as a swimmer's view, oblique views, or CT of this area are necessary.

B. Thoracolumbar Spine

All patients with significant injury and pain in the spinal area require anteroposterior and lateral x-rays of appropriate regions of the thoracic and lumbar spine. Overlying shadows (ribs, transverse processes, visceral soft tissue shadows) can make accurate interpretation of the fracture configuration difficult. CT scanning is useful in assessing the degree of bony injury as well as the amount of bony encroachment into the spinal canal. CT is helpful also for preoperative planning and optimizing the choice of spinal fixation necessary to reduce and stabilize the fracture. MRI is extremely helpful in assessing the degree of neural injury and helps in determining outcome. For example, the presence of intraparenchymal hemorrhage in the spinal cord implies a very poor prognosis for neurologic recovery after incomplete injuries.

Complications

Patients with cervical spine injury may have impaired pulmonary function secondary to intercostal nerve paralysis. Mobilization of secretions by chest physical therapy and frequent suctioning are critical in preventing atelectasis and pulmonary infections. All patients with sensory deficits and paralysis are at high risk of developing decubiti. Padding and suspension of high-risk pressure points (heels), frequent turning, and vigilant nursing care are necessary.

Patients with thoracolumbar spine fractures with or without spinal cord injury may have paralytic ileus secondary to sympathetic chain dysfunction. Oral intake should be limited to clear fluids initially, and gastric suction may be necessary if the degree or duration of ileus is significant.

The stress caused by the injury itself—in combination with systemic corticosteroid therapy—can increase the incidence of gastrointestinal ulceration and bleeding. High-dose corticosteroids can also contribute to the development of pancreatitis and infections.

Venous thromboembolic disease remains a significant problem in the management of patients with spinal injury. Pulmonary embolism is the most common cause of preventable death in hospitalized patients. After major trauma, the incidence of deep venous thrombosis has been estimated to be approximately 58%. The prevalence of deep venous thrombosis in patients with spinal cord injury approaches 100%. Symptomatic and fatal pulmonary embolism occurs in up to 6% of trauma patients despite improvements in trauma care and deep venous thrombosis prophylaxis. Fatal pulmonary embolism occurs in 1–2% of people with spinal cord injury.

Deep venous thrombosis typically occurs within the first 3 weeks after spinal cord injury. However, it can also occur late in the setting of a chronic spinal cord injury, with 83% of the events occurring within the first 6 months. In a recent study, Powell noted that 11.6% of all new spinal cord injury admissions to their rehabilitation unit were diagnosed with a new episode of deep venous thrombosis. Having had a previous deep venous thrombosis increases the risk of developing a subsequent episode by a factor of 2.4.

Optimal prophylaxis against thromboembolic disease in the spinal injury patient has not been determined. Early in the course of management, sequential compression devices and foot pumps are a reasonable alternative to pharmacologic anticoagulation. However, after the first few days of recovery from surgery, pharmacologic prophylaxis has the greatest promise for effective prevention of deep venous thrombosis and pulmonary thromboembolism in spinal cord injury. Low-molecular-weight heparins have shown the greatest promise for efficacy and safety in this population.

Treatment

A. Spine Fractures or Dislocations Without Neurologic Deficit

The goal of treatment is to maintain enough stability to protect the neural elements from further mechanical injury while allowing early mobilization and ameliorating pain.

1. Stable fractures—Fractures with a stable configuration, such as an anterior wedge compression, can be managed by external immobilization in a rigid brace that controls motion and maintains satisfactory alignment at the fracture site. Adult patients with anterior compression greater than 50% of normal vertebral height—especially in the lumbar spine with posterior ligamentous injury—are best treated with open reduction and short-segment posterior fusion and spinal instrumentation. This allows early mobilization and prevents late development of spinal deformity.

2. Unstable fractures or fracture-dislocations—These injuries require external immobilization (cast or brace), skeletal traction, or reduction and internal fixation. In most cervical spine fractures, skeletal traction in the long axis will achieve adequate reduction and restore canal integrity. If used as definitive treatment, 6–12 weeks of traction in recumbency is required, followed by bracing for another 6–12 weeks. Because of this, other forms of immobilization are preferable to extended periods of traction. Halo-vest or halo-cast immobilization may allow adequate control of the fracture with earlier ambulation. External immobilization alone is inadequate for significant ligamentous injuries, as these are less likely than fractures to heal with immobilization. Ligamentous disruptions with spinal instability are best managed with open reduction, internal fixation, and spinal fusion.

Unilateral and bilateral facet subluxations are flexion-distraction injuries that disrupt the posterior ligaments and facet capsules while leaving the intervertebral disk uninjured. A small amount of kyphosis (< 10 degrees) may be seen on lateral radiographs. These subluxations must be differentiated from more severe flexion-distraction injuries that have spontaneously reduced with neck extension.

Bilateral perched facets are at the next level of severity with the flexion-distraction mechanism. The inferior facets slide superiorly and anteriorly over the superior facet until the tips engage on each other. Perching of the facets creates a significant kyphotic deformity of the cervical spine. Disruption of the ligamentum flavum and the posterior annulus of the disk occurs in this injury. Treatment consists of reduction and stabilization with posterior fusion and instrumentation.

Unilateral facet dislocations are caused by adding a rotational force to the flexion-distraction mechanism. This results in attenuation of the interspinous ligament and disruption of the facet capsule and the posterolateral corner of the disk. The overall result of the injury mechanism is a rotational deformity of the spine.

Bilateral facet dislocations are the terminal stage of the flexion distraction injury. On lateral x-rays, there can be 50% anterior translation of the superior vertebra. Up to 60% of cases of bilateral facet dislocations will have associated disk disruption, and disk herniation can be present before reduction of facet dislocations in as many as 55% of cases. This is especially worrisome if the disk fragment is associated with the superior translated vertebra, since reduction of the dislocation is apt to push the herniated disk material into the spinal canal.

Controversy exists over the practicality of imaging the intervertebral disk at the level of the injury prior to reduction in an alert, awake, and neurologically intact patient. This debate is based upon several observations: Despite the alarming frequency of disk herniation associated with these injuries, a large proportion of these disk herniations will be clinically insignificant. In addition, most neurologic deficits have occurred during operative reduction under general anesthesia. Thus, several studies have concluded that immediate traction and reduction of facet dislocations in alert and awake patients can be done safely without the need for preliminary MRI. These studies also noted that immediate reduction leads to improved neurologic recovery as compared with delayed reduction. It is important to point out that these patients were treated at either a level I trauma center or a spinal cord injury unit with staff who have developed an expertise in the closed treatment of facet dislocations. Furthermore, the ability to perform a detailed neurologic examination between each incremental increase in cervical traction is a critical step in the technique. Any deterioration in neurologic function can be immediately addressed. Patients who present with severe spinal cord injury (Frankel grades A and B) should undergo immediate closed reduction of the dislocation. Patients who have worsening neurologic status, those who have a spinal cord injury not explained by CT scan, and those with dislocations not reducible with less than 40–60 lb of traction should be evaluated by MRI.

Thoracolumbar fractures may be reduced or maintained in an acceptable position using a rigid orthosis. Open reduction and internal fixation are justified when bracing fails to correct the position (increase in deformity, pain that prevents mobilization, development of a neuralgic deficit). Facet dislocation in the thoracolumbar spine is best treated with open reduction, short-segment instrumentation, and fusion. With the development of improved anterior and posterior spinal fixation systems (such as pedicle screws and rods), reduction and stable fixation can be achieved over fewer spinal segments. This has the advantage of preserving uninjured motion segments and minimizing the development of problems with the adjacent vertebral levels. The injured segment should be fused by placement of an onlay bone graft; the internal fixation device may be removed after the fracture and graft have healed.

B. Spine Fractures or Dislocations with Neurologic Deficit

1. Incomplete neurologic deficit—Patients with stable fractures can be treated in the same way as patients with no neurologic abnormalities if angulation is corrected and if MRI shows no evidence of bone or disk fragments significantly compromising the neural elements. This is with the caveat that the external brace is able to adequately immobilize the injured segment to prevent further neurologic injury. If a significant degree of canal compromise is demonstrated at the spinal cord level or if there is a neurologic deficit, surgical decompression is justified. This can be done either through an anterior approach (followed by strut graft) and internal fixation, a posterior costotransversectomy approach, or a combined anterior and posterior approach. The operative plan is individualized to the particular patient. In general, the anterior or combined approach allows easier decompression of the spinal canal and minimizes the number of levels that need to be included in the fusion (Figure 42–1).

Patients with incomplete neurologic deficits and unstable fractures or fracture-dislocations have the same stability requirements as patients without neurologic deficits. They are best managed with open reduction, instrumentation, and spinal fusion. Neural canal compromise should be managed as in the preceding paragraph.

2. Complete neurologic deficit—No operative procedure has been devised that will achieve recovery in cases of complete neurologic deficit that has persisted beyond the stage of spinal shock. However, surgical stabilization is often necessary (1) because spinal instability may interfere with early mobilization and rehabilitation training and (2) because it may result in loss of function at a higher level by causing mechanical injury on the root or cord segment just above the level of injury.

All stable bony injuries are treated in the same way as those that occur in neurologically intact patients except that any orthosis extending below the level of sensory loss can cause pressure ulcerations on insensate

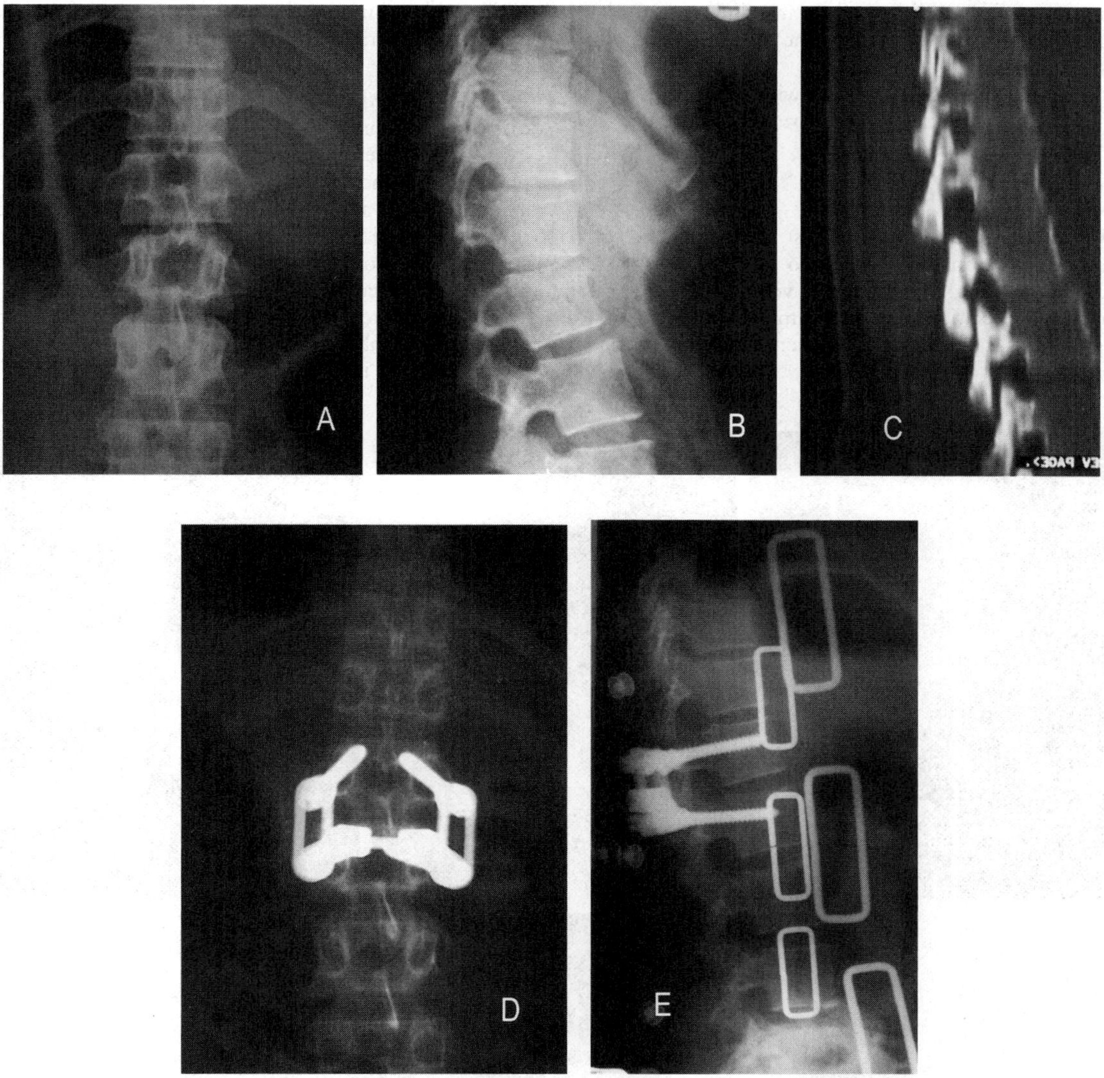

Figure 42–1. ***A:*** Anteroposterior radiograph of a 25-year-old woman who was a belted passenger in a motor vehicle accident, sustaining a duodenal injury and a flexion distraction injury at L1–L2. ***B:*** Lateral radiograph showing widening of the posterior elements and injury to the facet joints of L1–L2. ***C:*** CT scan showing subluxation of the inferior facet of L1. ***D and E:*** Anteroposterior and lateral radiographs after posterior stabilization with pedicle screws and plates and posterior spinal fusion..

skin. Patients with unstable injuries of the cervical spine can be managed with continuous traction for 6–12 weeks. Frequent turning—either in an ordinary hospital bed or on a turning frame—and good skin care are necessary to prevent pressure ulceration. However, halo-vest immobilization or internal fixation and spinal fusion is preferable to an extended period of traction.

Relatively early mobilization of patients with cervical spine injuries can be achieved using halo-vest immobilization. Cervical burst fractures with impingement on the spinal cord are best treated with anterior decompression of the spinal cord through removal of the fractured vertebra and anterior spinal fusion using autogenous structural graft, cadaveric strut graft, or a titanium fusion cage. The addition of an anterior cervical plate will allow early mobilization of the patient in a cervical collar.

Thoracolumbar spine injuries with neurologic injury are best treated with internal fixation and short-segment fusion (Figure 42–2).

C. External Support

1. Cervical spine—The halo vest or halo cast is constructed by connecting the halo to either a plaster body cast or a padded plastic vest. The body cast offers better fixation if properly molded over the iliac crests, but it cannot be used if sensory impairment is present.

In stable injuries of the cervical spine, cervical collars or cervical thoracic braces (four-poster) are adequate (Figure 42–3).

2. Thoracolumbar spine—In the thoracolumbar spine, cast or brace immobilization for fractures with potential instability must extend from the sternal notch to the symphysis pubica and should be molded to fit body contours. Thoracic braces are not able to immobilize injuries above the T7 level and must be modified to extend to the cervical spine. As noted above, if brace support is used in patients with sensory deficits, frequent monitoring for potential pressure necrosis of skin requires that the cast or brace be removable to permit inspection of all body surfaces at frequent intervals.

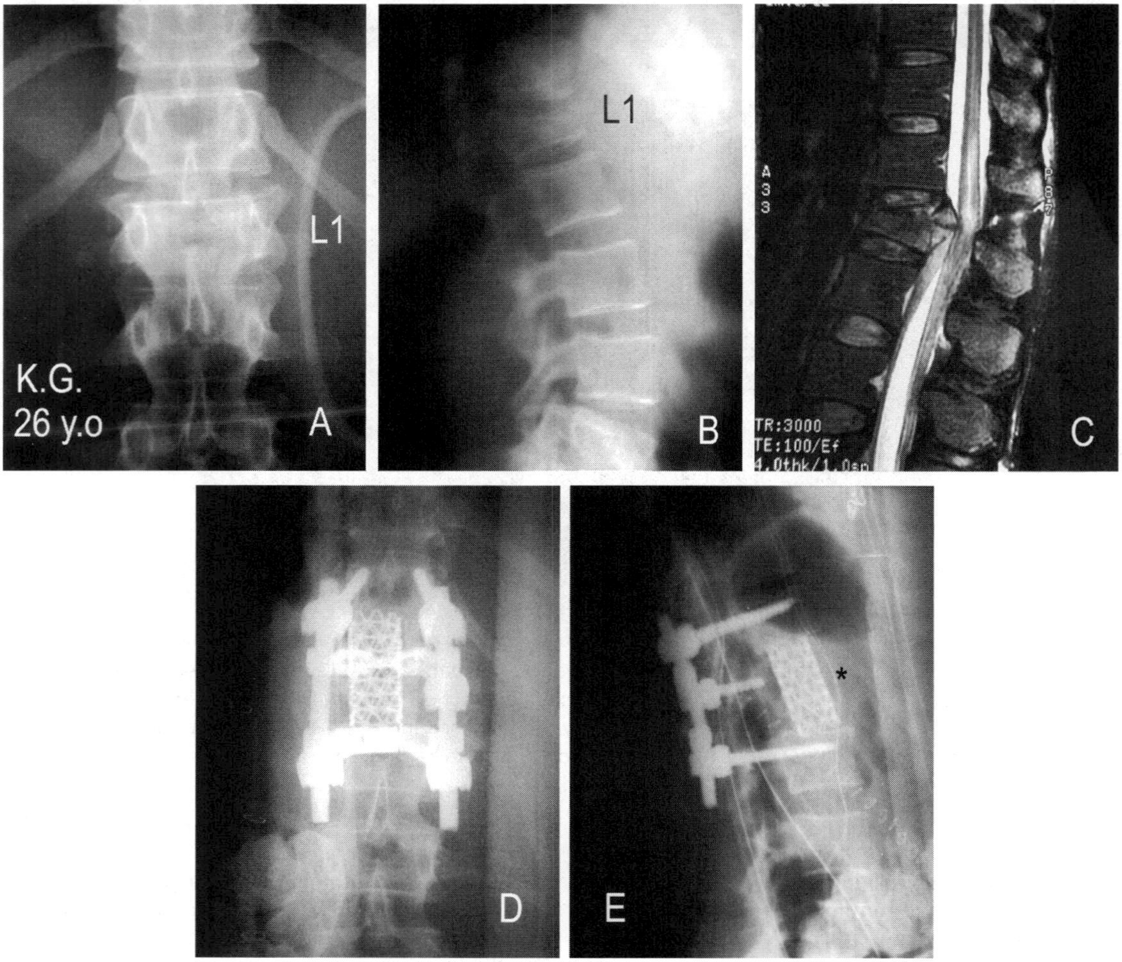

Figure 42–2. ***A*** and ***B:*** Anteroposterior and lateral radiographs of a severe burst fracture of L1 with canal retropulsion. ***C:*** Sagittal T2-weighted MRI showing injury to the conus medullaris and intraparenchymal hemorrhage. ***D and E:*** Anteroposterior and lateral images after L1 vertebrectomy and reconstruction with an anterior titanium cage and short segment posterior fusion.

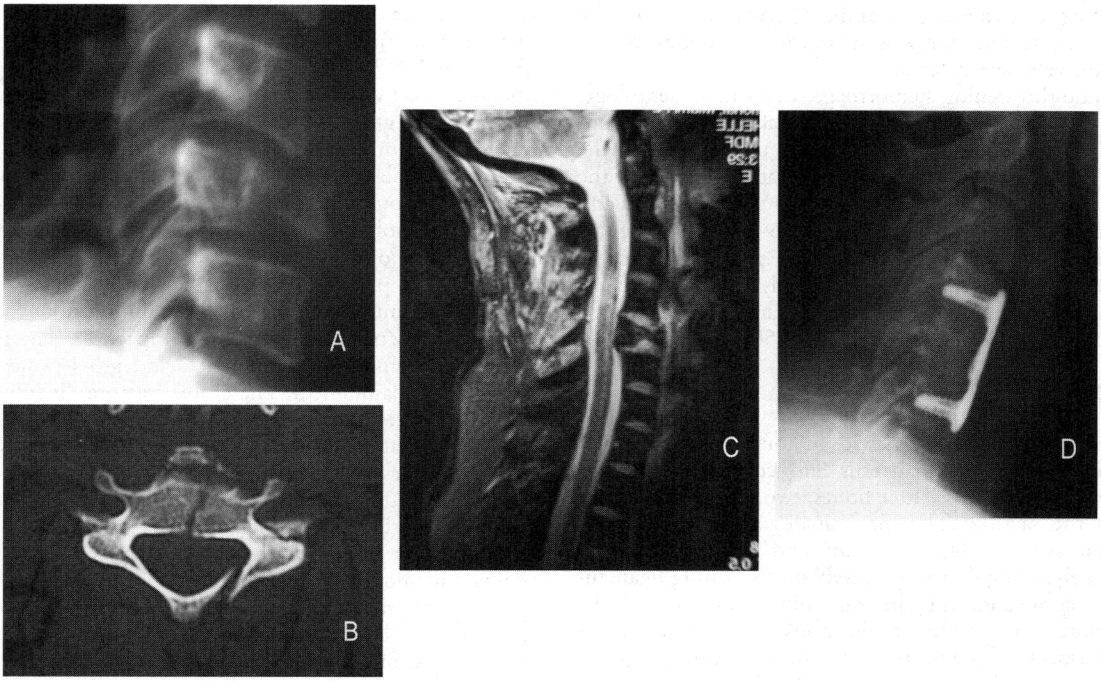

Figure 42–3. Thirty-year-old woman suffering a cervical burst fracture following a motor vehicle accident in which she hit her head on the windshield. ***A–C:*** Lateral radiograph, CT scan, and MRI showing burst fracture of C5. ***D:*** The burst fracture was treated with a vertebrectomy of C5 and fusion from C4 to C6 with a tricortical iliac crest bone graft and plate.

Anderson PA, Bohlman HH: Anterior decompression and arthrodesis of the cervical spine: Long-term motor improvement: part II—Improvement in complete traumatic quadriplegia. J Bone Joint Surg Am 1992;74:683.

Bohlman HH, Anderson PA: Anterior decompression and arthrodesis of the cervical spine: long-term motor improvement: part I—Improvement in incomplete traumatic quadriparesis. J Bone Joint Surg Am 1992;74:671.

Bracken MB et al: Administration of methylprednisolone for 24 or 48 hours or tirilazad mesylate for 48 hours in the treatment of acute spinal cord injury. Results of the Third National Acute Spinal Cord Injury Randomized Controlled Trial. National Acute Spinal Cord Injury Study. JAMA 1997;277:1597.

Carl AL, Tromanhauser SG, Roger DJ: Pedicle screw instrumentation for thoracolumbar burst fractures and fracture-dislocations. Spine 1992;17(8 Suppl):S317.

Cybulski GR et al: Complications in three-column cervical spine injuries requiring anterior-posterior stabilization. Spine 1992; 17:253.

Denis F, Burkus JK: Shear fracture-dislocations of the thoracic and lumbar spine associated with forceful hyperextension (lumberjack paraplegia). Spine 1992;17:156.

Ferree BA, Wright AM: Deep venous thrombosis following posterior lumbar spinal surgery. Spine 1993;18:1079.

Garvey TA, Eismont FJ, Roberti LJ: Anterior decompression, structural bone grafting, and Caspar plate stabilization for unstable cervical spine fractures and/or dislocations. Spine 1992;17(10 Suppl):S431.

Gertzbein SD: Scoliosis Research Society: multicenter spine fracture study. Spine 1992;17:528.

Heary RF et al: Acute stabilization of the cervical spine by halo/vest application facilitates evaluation and treatment of multiple trauma patients. J Trauma 1992;33:445.

Jeanneret B, Magerl F: Primary posterior fusion C12 odontoid fractures: indications, technique, and results of transarticular screw fixation. J Spinal Disord 1992;5:464.

Maynard FM Jr et al: International Standards for Neurological and Functional Classification of Spinal Cord Injury. American Spinal Injury Association. Spinal Cord 1997;35:266.

Roy-Camille R et al: Treatment of lower cervical spinal injuries—C3 to C7. Spine 1992;17(10 Suppl):S442.

Vaccaro AR et al: Neurologic outcome of early versus late surgery for cervical spinal cord injury. Spine 1997;22:2609.

FRACTURES & DISLOCATIONS OF THE PELVIS

Pelvic fractures are among the most serious injuries and account for 3% of all fractures. About 60% result from vehicular trauma (eg, automobile, motorcycle, bicycle), 30% from falls, and 10% from crush injuries, athletic injuries, or penetrating trauma. Pelvic fractures are the third most commonly seen injury in fatalities due to motor vehicle accidents.

Life-threatening hemorrhage, deformity, neurologic injury, and genitourinary injury are all potential complications that must be identified and treated early in the setting of a pelvic fracture. The literature shows that the mortality rate varied from 9% to 20% in the 1970s and seemed to decrease in the 1980s to 6–10%. Despite this apparent decrease, pelvic fractures pose a formidable clinical challenge. Hemodynamically unstable patients who present to the emergency department with pelvic fracture have a mortality rate of 40–50%.

Anatomy

An understanding of pelvic anatomy is essential for identifying fracture patterns and complications. The pelvis is made up of three bones: two innominate bones and the sacrum. The innominates are further subdivided into the ilium, ischium, and pubis. Stability of the pelvic ring depends entirely on the strong ligamentous connection of the innominate bones and the sacrum. A thick fibrocartilaginous disk joins the anterior aspects of the innominate bones to form the pubic symphysis. This joint acts as a supporting strut for the pelvis because the stability of the ring depends almost entirely upon the sacroiliac joints.

The posterior ligamentous structures can be divided into anterior and posterior complexes. The anterior sacroiliac joint ligaments are broad and flat and connect the iliac wing and the sacral ala. These ligaments primarily resist external rotation and torsional forces. However, posterior ligamentous stability is chiefly imparted by the tension band effect of the posterior sacroiliac ligament complex. Composed of the interosseous sacroiliac ligaments within the joint and the posterior sacroiliac ligaments spanning the sacrum between the posterior iliac spines, the posterior complex is considered to be the strongest ligament in the human body. The posterior sacroiliac complex resists shear forces between the sacrum and the ilium, clinically preventing displacement of the ilium onto the sacrum.

Finally, the pelvic floor contains two strong ligaments, the sacrospinous and the sacrotuberous ligaments. The sacrospinous ligament exerts strong restraint upon torsional forces while the sacrotuberous ligament resists torsion, shear, and flexion forces on the sacroiliac joint.

Stability

Pelvic stability can be defined as the ability of the pelvic ring to withstand physiologic forces without abnormal deformation. Pathologically, the pelvic ring fails under one or more of three basic modes. External rotation strains the pubic symphysis and the sacrotuberous, sacrospinous, and anterior sacroiliac joint ligaments. After roughly 2.5 cm of diastasis, the pelvic floor ligaments and the anterior sacroiliac ligaments begin to fail, giving rise to gross rotatory instability. Because the posterior ligament complex is largely intact, superior or posterior displacement of the involved hemipelvis does not occur. Combined external and shear forces are necessary to completely disrupt pelvic stability. Conversely, internal rotation places the pubic rami under compression and the posterior ligament complexes under tension. The rami often fail in their midportions with transverse fractures and sacral alar impaction. The pelvic floor ligaments remain intact, and gross posterior stability is maintained. Therefore, fractures involving torsional forces on the pelvis often have partial instability in the rotatory plane only, with maintenance of stability to other displacement.

Complete instability, however, disrupts both the anterior and the posterior ligamentous restraints. These injuries often present with widely displaced sacroiliac joints and multiaxial instability of the involved hemipelvis. Such fractures have components of superior and posterior displacement relative to the sacrum in addition to rotational displacement in the sagittal and horizontal planes.

Clinical Findings

Physical examination includes palpation of the pelvic bony landmarks, compression maneuvers to assess stability, and rectovaginal examination looking for bony spikes protruding through the mucosa representing an open fracture. The mortality rate of open pelvic fractures is as high as 50%—compared with 8–15% for closed fractures. Associated injuries should be assessed systematically—lower urinary tract injuries, distal vascular status—and a thorough neurologic examination should be performed.

The anteroposterior radiograph required in all patients with blunt trauma rapidly identifies the major pelvic injury. Inlet and outlet radiographs are often required to supplement the anteroposterior film and better define the position and degree of pelvic instability. Eventually, CT scanning will further delineate fracture stability.

Acute Management

Immediate care of the polytrauma patient with a pelvic fracture must address associated retroperitoneal hemorrhage, pelvic ring instability, and injuries to the genitourinary system and rectum as well as fractures open to the peritoneum. Cessation of blood loss, minimization of septic sequelae, and stabilization of the fracture, allowing early and safe patient mobilization, are the immediate treatment goals. Hemorrhage is the leading cause of death in patients with pelvic fracture, accounting for 60% of the deaths. Most of the blood loss is from the fracture site or injured retroperitoneal veins; only 20% of the deaths are associated with major arterial injury. An average blood replacement of 5.9 units has been reported.

General resuscitative principles are applied to stabilize the patient and provide adequate tissue perfusion. Once other sites of hemorrhage have been ruled out, active bleeding from a pelvic fracture may be controlled by the use of an external fixator device. Major fracture fragments are stabilized, and the pelvic and retroperitoneal space available for fluids is decreased or at least prevented from increasing. If this fails to control hemorrhage, arterial embolization is indicated. Definitive internal fixation is usually required after hemorrhage has been controlled and the patient has been stabilized.

Classification & Treatment

Fractures may be classified as type A (rotationally and vertically stable), type B (rotationally unstable and vertically stable, or type C (rotationally and vertically unstable). Common radiographic signs of pelvic instability include (1) displacement of the posterior sacroiliac complex more than 5 mm in any plane; (2) the presence of a posterior fracture gap rather than an impaction; and (3) the presence of an avulsion fracture of the transverse process of the fifth lumbar vertebra or the sacro-ischial end of the sacrospinous ligaments.

Type A fractures involve the pelvic ring in only one location and are considered stable. Type A1 fractures are avulsion fractures that usually occur at muscle origins such as the anterosuperior iliac spine, anteroinferior iliac spine, and ischial apophysis. These fractures most often occur in adolescents, and conservative treatment is usually sufficient. If displacement is minimal, prompt healing without disability is to be expected. If displacement is marked (ie, > 1 cm), reattachment by open operation is justifiable.

Rarely, symptomatic nonunions develop and are best treated surgically. Type A2 fractures are isolated fractures of the iliac wing without involvement of the hip or sacroiliac joints and are usually a result of direct trauma. Even with significant displacement, bony healing is expected and treatment is therefore symptomatic. Healing may be accompanied by ossification of the hematoma with exuberant new bone formation. Finally, type A3 fractures are isolated fractures of the obturator foramen and usually involve minimal displacement of the pubic or ischial rami. The posterior sacroiliac complex is intact, and the pelvis remains stable. Treatment is symptomatic, with early ambulation and weightbearing as tolerated.

Type B fractures involve breaks in the pelvic ring in two or more sites. This creates a pelvic fracture that is rotationally unstable but vertically stable. Type B1 fractures are open book fractures that occur from anteroposterior compression. Unless the anterior separation of the pubic symphysis is severe (> 6 cm), the posterior sacroiliac complex is usually intact and the pelvis is relatively stable to vertical forces. Significant associated injuries to the perineal and urogenital structures are often present and should always be looked for. For minimally displaced symphysial injuries (< 2.5 cm), only symptomatic treatment is needed. For more displaced fracture-dislocations, reduction is done by lateral compression using the intact posterior sacroiliac complex as the hinge on which the "book is closed." Reduction can be maintained with the use of an external fixator; however, internal fixation is currently favored. "Closing the book" decreases the space available for hemorrhage, increases patient comfort, facilitates nursing care, and allows early mobilization. The use of a sheet in the resuscitative period to tie the thighs together can provide temporary stability and help control hemorrhage.

Type B2 and B3 fractures involve a lateral force applied to the pelvis, causing inward displacement of the hemipelvis through the sacroiliac complex and ipsilateral (B2) or, more often, contralateral (B3) pubic rami fractures. The degree of involvement of the posterior sacroiliac ligament complex will determine the degree of instability. The hemipelvis is infolded, with overlapping of the pubic symphysis. Reduction can be accomplished with external fixation, with internal fixation, or with both. External fixation facilitates nursing care but is not strong enough for ambulation. Definitive care usually is accomplished with internal fixation of both the anterior and posterior aspects of the pelvic ring. Major hemorrhage is associated with these fracture types.

Type C fractures are both rotationally and vertically unstable. They often result from a vertical shear injury such as a fall from a height. Anteriorly, the pubic symphysis or pubic rami may be disrupted. Posteriorly, the sacroiliac joint may be disrupted and dislocated, or there may be a fracture through the sacrum or adjacent iliac wing. The hemipelvis is completely unstable, and there may be associated massive hemorrhage and injury to the lumbosacral pelvis. External fixation is insufficient to maintain reduction, but it may help to control hemorrhage and ease nursing care in the acute stage. Internal fixation is usually required as definitive treatment.

FRACTURES OF THE ACETABULUM

The acetabulum is the portion of the pelvic bone that articulates with the femoral head to form the hip joint. It results from closure of the Y or triradiate cartilage and is covered with hyaline cartilage.

Fractures of the acetabulum (Figure 42–4) occur through direct trauma on the trochanteric region or

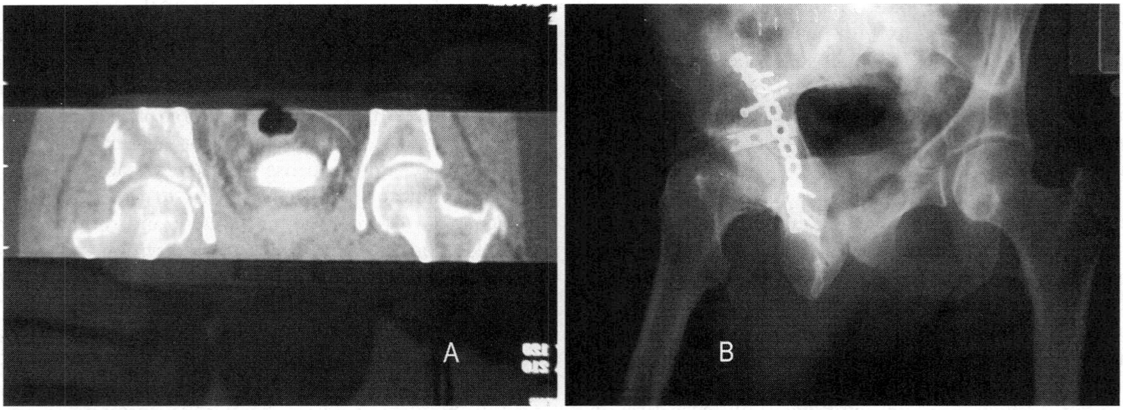

Figure 42–4. Forty-year-old man who fell from a height, sustaining a posterior hip dislocation and an acetabular fracture of the weightbearing dome. ***A:*** Coronal CT reconstructions showing large fragment of the superior dome of the right acetabulum. ***B:*** Oblique radiograph demonstrating concentric reduction of the hip and restoration of the articular surface after open reduction and internal fixation..

indirect axial loading through the lower limb. The position of the limb at the time of impact (rotation, flexion, abduction, or adduction) will determine the pattern of injury. Comminution is common.

Classification

Acetabular fractures are classified based on which column is involved. The anterior column comprises the anterior iliac crest, the anterior half of the acetabulum, and the pubic ramus. The posterior column includes the sciatic buttress and the sciatic notch, the posterior half of the acetabulum, and the ischial tuberosity. These two columns unite in an inverted Y pattern whose center articulates with the femoral head. Fractures may involve one or both columns in a simple or complex pattern.

Proper fracture classification requires x-rays of good quality. Two oblique views (Judet views) taken 45 degrees toward and away from the involved side complement the standard anteroposterior view of the pelvis. CT scanning gives further information on the fracture pattern, the presence of free intra-articular fragments, and the status of the femoral head and the rest of the pelvic ring.

Letournel has classified acetabular fractures into ten different types: five simple patterns (one fracture line) and five complex patterns (the association of two or more simple patterns). This is the most widely used classification system as it allows the surgeon to choose the most appropriate surgical approach.

Treatment

The goal of treatment is to achieve a spherical congruency between the femoral head and the weightbearing acetabular dome and to maintain it until the bones are healed. As with other pelvic fractures, acetabular fractures are frequently associated with abdominal, urogenital, and neurologic injuries, which should be systematically sought and treated. Significant bleeding is often present and should be stopped as soon as possible.

The stabilized patient should be put in longitudinal skeletal traction through a distal femoral or proximal tibial pin pulling axially in neutral position. A trochanteric screw for lateral traction is contraindicated as it will create a contaminated pin tract and thus preclude possible further surgical treatment. Postreduction x-rays are obtained. In general, a displaced acetabular fracture is rarely reduced adequately by closed methods. If the reduction is judged acceptable, traction is maintained for 6–8 weeks until bone healing is evident. Another 6–8 weeks is necessary before full weightbearing can be attempted. Most authors now feel that any residual displacement after traction is an indication for open reduction and internal fixation as there is a clear correlation between anatomic reduction and prognosis. The choice of approach is of primary importance, and more than one approach will sometimes prove necessary. Acetabular surgery uses extensile approaches and sophisticated reduction and fixation techniques and is best performed by pelvic surgeons. Other surgical indications include free osteochondral fragments, femoral head fractures, irreducible dislocations, or unstable reductions.

Complications

Complications inherent to the injury include posttraumatic degenerative joint disease, heterotopic ossification, femoral head osteonecrosis, deep vein thrombosis, and other complications related to conservative treatment. Surgery is performed to prevent or delay osteoarthritis, but it increases the possibility of complications such as infection, iatrogenic neurovascular injury, and increased heterotopic ossification. When the reduction is stable and fixation is solid, the patient can be mobilized after a few days with nonweightbearing ambulation, and weightbearing may begin as early as 6 weeks. Most pelvic surgeons now routinely use postoperative prophylactic anticoagulation and heterotopic bone formation prophylaxis with irradiation or indomethacin or both.

Lowe MA et al: Risk factors for urethral injuries in men with traumatic pelvic fractures. J Urol 1988;140:506.

McLaren AC, Rorabeck CH, Halpenny J: Long-term pain and disability in relation to residual deformity after displaced pelvic ring fractures. Can J Surg 1990;33:492.

Schafermeyer R: Pediatric trauma. Emerg Med Clin North Am 1993;11:187.

Siegel JH et al: Safety belt restraints and compartment intrusions in frontal and lateral motor vehicle crashes: mechanisms of injuries, complications, and acute care costs. J Trauma 1993; 34:736.

Sinnott R, Rhodes M, Brader A: Open pelvic fracture: an injury for trauma centers. Am J Surg 1992;163:283.

SHOULDER INJURIES

1. Clavicular Fracture

Fractures of the clavicle are commonly associated with a fall on the shoulder or outstretched hand. They may also be associated with a direct blow from high-energy trauma or contact sports. It is vital to evaluate these patients for associated injuries such as brachial plexus palsy, vascular injury, rib fracture, and pneumothorax, which are often more serious than the fracture. These fractures are divided into middle third fractures (most common), lateral third, and medial third fractures. The distal fragment is typically displaced downward by the weight of the arm, and the medial fragment is pulled superiorly by the trapezius and sternocleidomastoid muscles. Open fractures are rare. Anteroposterior and anteroposterior-lordotic x-rays (oblique cephalad projection) should be obtained.

Treatment

All nondisplaced clavicular fractures may be treated in a sling for 4–6 weeks if there is no open wound communicating with the fracture and no tenting of the skin. General indications for surgery are open fractures and fractures with significant displacement (especially if there is tenting of the skin). Neurovascular injuries requiring repair may also require surgical fixation. Fractures of the lateral third of the clavicle may require surgical treatment if they are displaced. Most fractures of the middle third heal with nonoperative treatment unless there is significant overlap of the fracture fragments. Most medial fractures are not significantly displaced and many are missed, since this area overlaps the ribs on x-ray. These are also usually treated with a sling or cuff and collar. Open reduction and internal fixation may be performed with an intramedullary screw or extramedullary plate. Complications of open reduction include infection, migration, or breakage of the fixation device; nonunion; and neurovascular injury (Figure 42–5).

Pyper JB: Non-union of fractures of the clavicle. Injury 1978; 9:268.

Zenni FJ, Krieg JK, Rosen MJ: Open reduction and internal fixation of clavicular fractures. J Bone Joint Surg Am 1981;63: 147.

2. Acromioclavicular Dislocation

Dislocation (separation) of the acromioclavicular joint is usually caused by a fall on the tip of the shoulder. The acromion is displaced downward by the weight of the arm, and the clavicle is pulled superiorly by the trapezius. These injuries can be classified by degree of displacement, which correlates with the force of injury. Type I acromioclavicular separation is a strain of the acromioclavicular ligament. Type II injury involves rupture of the acromioclavicular ligament and strain of the coracoclavicular ligament complex. This causes the clavicle to be displaced superiorly. Type III injury involves rupture of both the acromioclavicular and the coracoclavicular ligaments, which causes marked superior migration of the lateral end of the clavicle and a drooping appearance of the shoulder. Occasionally, the clavicle is violently ruptured through the deltotrapezial fascia, locked on the acromion, or displaced under the

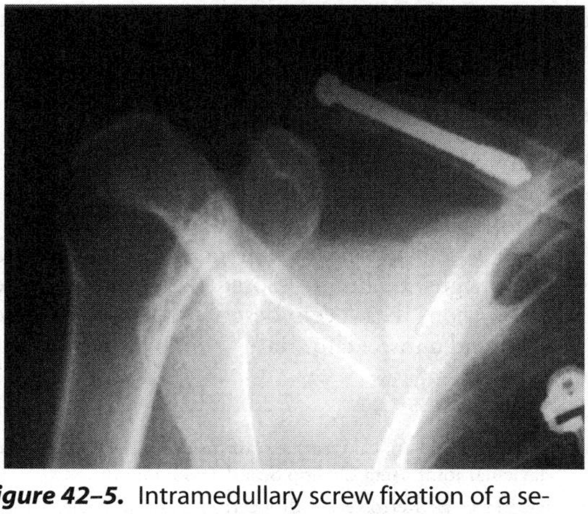

Figure 42–5. Intramedullary screw fixation of a severely displaced middle-third clavicular fracture.

coracoid process. Anteroposterior x-rays should be taken of both shoulders with the patient standing erect.

Treatment

Most acromioclavicular joint injuries are managed nonoperatively with a sling for approximately 4 weeks followed by gradual return to full activity. Most patients do not have significant dysfunction or any need to modify their activities. Surgical reconstruction may be indicated for severe injuries, especially in the population of young athletes.

Bjerneld H, Hovelius L, Thorling J: Acromio-clavicular separations treated conservatively. A 5-year follow-up study. Acta Orthop Scand 1983;54:743.

Galpin RD, Hawkins RJ, Grainger RW: A comparative analysis of operative versus nonoperative treatment of grade III acromioclavicular separations. Clin Orthop 1985;193:150.

Larsen E, Bjerg-Nielsen A, Christensen P: Conservative or surgical treatment of acromioclavicular dislocation: a prospective, controlled, randomized study. J Bone Joint Surg Am 1986; 68:552.

Smith MI, Stewart MJ: Acute acromioclavicular separations: a 20-year study. Am J Sports Med 1979;7:62.

3. Sternoclavicular Joint Dislocation

Dislocation of the sternoclavicular joint is rare. The mechanism of injury is usually a motor vehicle accident or sporting injury. Physical examination and anteroposterior and anteroposterior-cephalic tilt x-rays may demonstrate asymmetry. However, confirmation of the diagnosis with a CT scan is often necessary, especially with retrosternal displacement. It is important to identify the direction of displacement because posterior displacement can cause injury to the esophagus, trachea, great vessels, subclavian artery, carotid artery, and pneumothorax. Dislocations of the sternoclavicular joint in children are often associated with physial fractures.

Treatment

Most injuries to the sternoclavicular joint may be treated with a sling or figure-of-eight harness. Posterior dislocations may require emergent reduction if there is associated vascular compression or injury to the trachea, esophagus, or lungs. Closed reduction of posterior dislocations has been described using shoulder retraction and a towel clip. Rarely, open reduction may be necessary.

Barth E, Hagen R: Surgical treatment of dislocations of the sternoclavicular joint. Acta Orthop Scand 1983;54:746.

Selesnick FH et al: Retrosternal dislocation of the clavicle. J Bone Joint Surg Am 1984;66:287.

4. Scapular Fracture

Scapular fractures are classified by location. Scapular body fractures are often associated with other injuries such as subclavian vessel injury, aortic rupture, pneumothorax, rib fractures, brachial plexus injuries, and other soft tissue injuries associated with high-energy trauma. Fractures of the acromion and coracoid occur rarely. Glenoid fractures must be carefully evaluated for articular surface step-off and associated glenohumeral instability. These fractures may be caused by a blow on the shoulder or by a fall on the outstretched arm. Diagnosis with anteroposterior x-ray in the plane of the scapula and axillary x-ray may be supplemented by an axial view of the scapular body and transscapular Y-view. CT scan may also be helpful if surgery is being considered.

Treatment

Most scapular fractures are treated nonoperatively in a sling for 4–6 weeks. Associated injuries may need to be treated emergently and should not be overlooked. Surgical reconstruction of the scapular body or glenoid is indicated for joint surface malreduction and glenohumeral instability. Comminution of articular surface fragments is common, and surgical reconstruction is technically demanding.

Armstrong CP, Van der Spuy J: The fractured scapula: importance and management based on a series of 62 patients. Injury 1984;15:324.

Froimson AI: Fracture of the coracoid process of the scapula. J Bone Joint Surg Am 1978;60:710.

Wilber MC, Evans EB: Fractures of the scapula: an analysis of forty cases and a review of the literature. J Bone Joint Surg Am 1977;59:358.

5. Proximal Humerus Fracture

Fractures of the proximal humerus occur most commonly in elderly individuals with osteoporosis. The weakened bone and the propensity for falls in this population predispose to hip and shoulder fractures. Initial assessment should seek to determine the cause of any related fall as well as the fracture pattern. Prodromal symptoms related to a syncopal episode, myocardial infarction, stroke, transient ischemic attack, or seizure are not rare. Patients in this population are prone also to associated neurovascular injuries and rotator cuff tears. Careful evaluation is important.

Diagnosis is established by x-rays, occasionally supplemented with CT scan. The radiographic examination should consist of a high-quality anteroposterior x-ray in the plane of the scapula (approximately 30 degrees oblique to the frontal plane of the chest) and axillary x-ray. This may be supplemented with a trans-

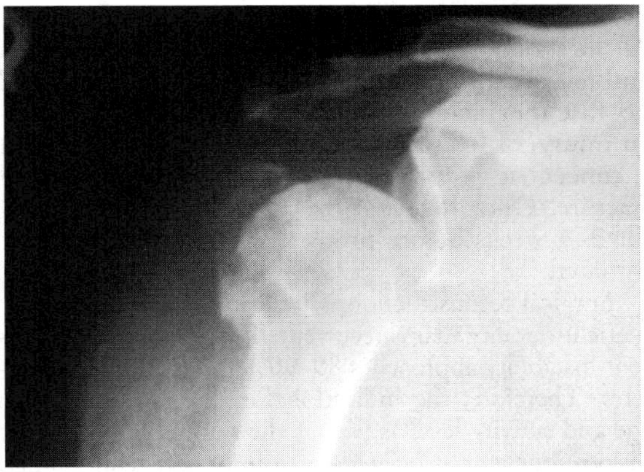

Figure 42–6. Four-part proximal humerus fracture, impacted on inferior glenoid rim.

scapular Y view, but this x-ray is usually less helpful than the axillary view.

Treatment

Most proximal humerus fractures are nondisplaced and can therefore be treated in a sling or cuff and collar and early gentle range of motion exercises. The most commonly used classification system of proximal humerus fractures defines displacement of more than 1 cm or 45 degrees of the humeral head, humeral shaft, greater tuberosity, or lesser tuberosity. Displaced fractures usually require operative reduction and fixation. Surgical reconstruction ranges from closed reduction alone or closed reduction and percutaneous fixation to open reduction and internal fixation or prosthetic arthroplasty (Figures 42–6 and 42–7). Patients do not invariably regain symmetric range of motion, but excellent pain relief and function can be attained. There are many potential complications both from the initial injury and from surgical reconstruction. Avascular necrosis of the humeral head can result from injury to the anterior humeral circumflex artery, and stiffness is common.

Neer CS II: Displaced proximal humeral fractures. 1. Classification and evaluation. 2. Treatment of three-part and four-part displacement. J Bone Joint Surg Am 1970;52:1077, 1090.

Paavolainen P et al: Operative treatment of severe proximal humerus fractures. Acta Orthop Scand 1983;54:374.

Weseley MS, Barenfeld PA, Eisenstein AL: Rush pin intramedullary fixation for fractures of the proximal humerus. J Trauma 1977;17:29.

6. Dislocation of the Shoulder Joint

The shoulder (glenohumeral) joint is the most commonly dislocated joint in the body because it is less constrained than other joints and motion is possible in multiple planes. The constraints that prevent instability include the concavity of the glenoid articular cartilage as it conforms to the humeral head and labrum, negative pressure of the joint, and check-rein glenohumeral ligaments. The rotator cuff also provides dynamic stability by compressing the humeral head against the glenoid. These static and dynamic stabilizers create a delicate balance between motion and stability.

Dislocations are usually related to overhead trauma when the arm is in abduction, extension, and external rotation—eg, when an athlete dislocates a shoulder by falling on an outstretched hand away from the body. This most common position causes a traumatic anterior dislocation. Most traumatic dislocations are anterior, but posterior dislocations can occur. Shoulder instability is classified by several factors such as traumatic versus atraumatic, initial versus recurrent, acute versus chronic, direction, and voluntary versus involuntary.

Anterior Dislocations of the Shoulder Joint

Anterior dislocations can be diagnosed by history and physical examination. The arm is usually extremely painful and held in a position of slight abduction and external rotation. The anterior shoulder area appears full, and there is a vacant sulcus in the posterior shoul-

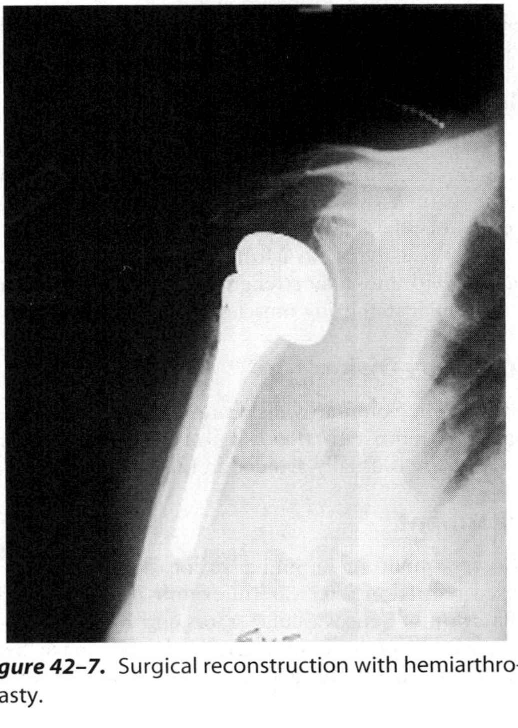

Figure 42–7. Surgical reconstruction with hemiarthroplasty.

der area. Anteroposterior x-ray in the plane of the scapula and axillary x-ray are necessary to determine the direction of the dislocation and the presence of fracture if any. Humeral head impression fractures and glenoid rim fractures are easily missed if the radiographs are inadequate. Dislocation may also be complicated by injury to the brachial plexus (most commonly the axillary nerve) and rotator cuff tear. The examiner should check particularly over the lateral aspect of the arm for sensory changes due to injury of the axillary nerve.

Posterior Dislocation of the Shoulder Joint

Posterior dislocation is characterized by fullness beneath the spine of the scapula, flattening of the anterior shoulder, prominence of the coracoid, and restriction of motion in external rotation. This injury is frequently missed even by experienced surgeons. The reported incidence of missed diagnosis is as high as 60%. The injury occurs either from direct or indirect force to the anterior shoulder, so that the humeral head is pushed out posteriorly. Common causes of posterior dislocation of the shoulder are indirect forces produced with convulsive seizures or electric shock. Anteroposterior x-rays of the chest may look deceptively normal with posterior dislocation, but an axillary view and an anteroposterior x-ray in the scapular plane will show the true position of the head in relation to the glenoid. This dislocation may also be reduced by longitudinal and gentle transverse traction. The reduction may be held in a sling for 3–6 weeks with some external rotation if necessary.

Multidirectional Instability

Patients with congenital or acquired laxity may develop symptomatic shoulder instability in multiple directions. These patients should be initially treated with 6–9 months of rehabilitation and strengthening monitored by a physical therapist. Most of these patients recover stability with muscular strengthening of the rotator cuff and scapular stabilizing muscles.

Voluntary Dislocators

Patients who voluntarily dislocate their shoulders have a high recurrence rate after surgical procedures. Therefore, surgery is usually avoided in this population.

Treatment

The treatment of shoulder dislocations consists of closed reduction after careful examination and documentation of neurovascular status and high-quality x-rays. Many methods of closed reduction have been described, including gentle traction in the prone position and traction-countertraction with a sheet. All methods of reduction rely on adequate analgesia and relaxation. Forceful reductions should be avoided because they may cause brachial plexus injury, vascular injury, or fracture. Postreduction x-rays document a concentric reduction and rule out any associated fracture. Once reduced, the arm is placed in a sling for 3–4 weeks before protected motion exercises are initiated.

Surgical reconstruction is indicated for anterior traumatic instability that is recurrent. The incidence of recurrent instability approaches 80–90% for active young athletes. Therefore, the indication for surgery depends on age and activity level as well as the number of traumatic dislocations and associated fracture or soft tissue injury. After operative repair, the shoulder is usually immobilized in a shoulder immobilizer for 3–6 weeks before active motion is begun. Open surgical repairs for anterior dislocation are successful in preventing further episodes of dislocation in 90–95% of patients. Arthroscopic repair may also be performed.

Aronen JG, Regan K: Decreasing the incidence of recurrence of first time anterior shoulder dislocations with rehabilitation. Am J Sports Med 1984;12:283.

Cisternino SJ et al: The trough line: a radiographic sign of posterior shoulder dislocation. AJR Am J Roentgenol 1978;130:951.

Engelhardt MB: Posterior dislocation of the shoulder: report of six cases. South Med J 1978;71:425.

Morrey BF, Janes JM: Recurrent anterior dislocation of the shoulder: long-term follow-up of the Putti-Platt and Bankhart procedures. J Bone Joint Surg Am 1976;58:252.

Rowe CR: Acute and recurrent anterior dislocations of the shoulder. Orthop Clin North Am 1980;11:253.

Rowe CR, Zarins B: Chronic unreduced dislocations of the shoulder. J Bone Joint Surg Am 1982;64:494.

7. Rotator Cuff Tears

Rotator cuff tears and rotator cuff impingement are common sources of shoulder pain. Four rotator cuff muscles (supraspinatus, infraspinatus, teres minor, and subscapularis) function to move the arm and stabilize the shoulder joint. There is a full spectrum of injury ranging from minor irritation (tendonitis, bursitis, strain) of the rotator cuff to bony impingement and rotator cuff tears. The most severe condition is a massive, chronic rotator cuff tear that subsequently leads to proximal migration of the humeral head, local osteopenia, and arthritic changes of the humeral head. This is rotator cuff arthropathy.

Patients with "rotator cuff syndrome" usually present with pain and weakness related to attempted overhead activities and active movements with the arm away from the body. Physical examination demonstrates impingement pain with certain overhead movements and sometimes significant rotator cuff weakness. Diagnosis is made by history and physical examination. Specific shoulder x-rays can be helpful to evaluate any bony impingement from the acromion, acromioclavicular joint, or coracoacromial ligament. MRI is the most useful test to evaluate rotator cuff tears and associated intra-articular pathology (Figure 42–8).

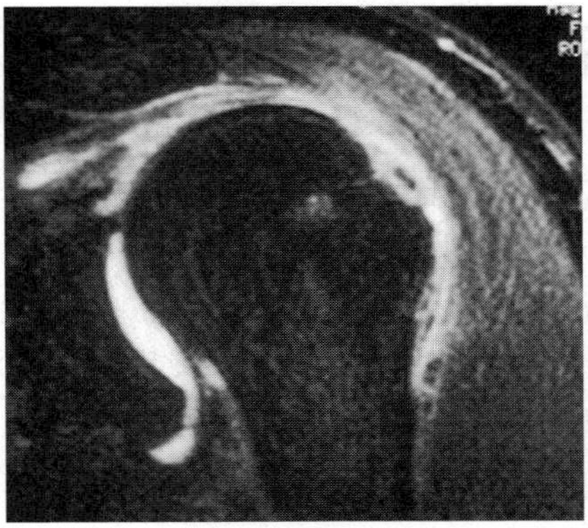

Figure 42–8. T2-weighted MRI showing a massive rotator cuff tear.

Treatment

The treatment of shoulder pain related to rotator cuff pathology (inflammation, degeneration, tear) depends on other patient variables such as age, activity level, hand dominance as well as the chronicity and level of pain and dysfunction. Tears may result from single event trauma (a fall on the outstretched hand), repetitive trauma (baseball pitchers), or degeneration of the rotator cuff in older patients.

Most cases of shoulder pain related to the rotator cuff are initially treated nonoperatively. Activity modification, NSAIDs, physical therapy, home exercises—all can be beneficial. Some patients require a subacromial lidocaine with corticosteroid injection to control inflammation and pain. Rotator cuff tears can also be treated with surgical reconstruction if they continue to be painful and disabling despite attempted nonoperative therapy. One exception to this general rule is the acute traumatic massive rotator cuff tear, which should be repaired acutely in order to prevent rotator cuff atrophy and retraction. Acromioplasty and distal clavicle excision are performed at the same time if coracoacromial arch impingement contributes to the rotator cuff tear.

Bassett RW, Cofield RH: Acute tears of the rotator cuff. Clin Orthop 1983;175:18.

Gore DR et al: Shoulder-muscle strength and range of motion following surgical repair of full-thickness rotator-cuff tears. J Bone Joint Surg Am 1986;68:266.

Hawkins RJ, Misamore GW, Hobeika PE: Surgery for full-thickness rotator-cuff tears. J Bone Joint Surg Am 1985;67:1349.

Neer CS, Marberry TA: On the disadvantages of radical acromionectomy. J Bone Joint Surg Am 1981;63:416.

Tibone JE et al: Shoulder impingement syndrome in athletes treated by an anterior acromioplasty. Clin Orthop 1985; 198:134.

8. Glenohumeral Arthritis

Arthritis of the glenohumeral joint may be caused by osteoarthritis, inflammatory disease, previous trauma, previous surgery, or arthritis of recurrent instability. Patients have pain with activities and rainy weather just as in arthritis in other joints. They also complain of stiffness, which is usually progressive over time. Physical examination discloses limited motion and usually crepitus with motion (even with the arm at the side). Examination by proper shoulder x-rays shows the characteristic joint space narrowing, humeral head osteophytes, and eburnation of the subchondral bone.

Before operative treatment is elected, a thorough course of conservative measures is indicated such as physical therapy, analgesics, and nonsteroidal anti-inflammatory drugs. An intra-articular lidocaine-steroid injection can be helpful for nonsurgical candidates with debilitating pain. Surgery becomes an option for patients with significant pain and limitation of activity because of their arthritis. Arthroscopic debridement can be helpful for some patients but may offer only a short term solution. Shoulder arthroplasty (hemiarthroplasty, total shoulder replacement) offers a longer-term solution with an excellent 10-year symptom-free function rate. Pain relief is consistent and function is usually improved. Contraindications to total arthroplasty are active or latent septic arthritis, paralysis of the shoulder musculature, and neuropathic joints. Another option for younger patients with severe bone destruction is surgical arthrodesis.

Cofield RH: Total shoulder arthroplasty with the Neer prosthesis. J Bone Joint Surg Am 1984;66:899.

Cofield RH, Briggs BT: Glenohumeral arthrodesis: operative and long-term functional results. J Bone Joint Surg Am 1979; 61:668.

Neer CS, Watson KC, Stanton FJ: Recent experience in total shoulder replacement. J Bone Joint Surg Am 1982;64:319.

Post M, Haskell SS, Jablon M: Total shoulder replacement with a constrained prosthesis. J Bone Joint Surg Am 1980;62:327.

Ranawat CS, Warren R, Inglis AE: Total shoulder replacement arthroplasty, Orthop Clin North Am 1980;11:367.

Rybka V, Raunio P, Vainio K: Arthrodesis of the shoulder in rheumatoid arthritis: a review of forty-one cases. J Bone Joint Surg Br 1979;61:155.

FRACTURES OF THE SHAFT OF THE HUMERUS

Most fractures of the shaft of the humerus result from direct trauma. X-rays in two planes are necessary to determine the configuration of the fracture and the direction of displacement of the fragments. The shoulder and elbow must be included on the initial x-rays to rule out the possibility of fracture or dislocation involving adjacent joints. Before definitive treatment is initiated, a careful neurologic examination should be performed in order to determine the status of the radial nerve and brachial vessels.

Treatment

Most midshaft humeral fractures can be treated nonoperatively in a cast, splint, or brace. The coaptation splint may be molded to improve reduction of the fracture. Alignment should be verified on anteroposterior and transthoracic x-rays with the patient standing. If stabilization has not taken place after 6–8 weeks, consideration of internal fixation and bone grafting is justified. About 5–10% of humeral fractures demonstrate radial nerve involvement. Fractures of the distal third of the humerus are especially vulnerable because the nerve is fixed to the proximal fragment by the intermuscular septum and is more easily injured at the time of displacement. Most radial nerve injuries are the result of stretching or contusion, and function will return in days or months. Open reduction of closed fractures may be indicated if adequate apposition of major fragments cannot be obtained by closed methods, the fracture communicates with an open wound, or arterial circulation has been interrupted.

Balfour GW, Mooney V, Ashby ME: Diaphyseal fractures of the humerus treated with a ready-made fracture brace. J Bone Joint Surg Am 1982;64:11.

Mast JW et al: Fractures of the humeral shaft: a retrospective study of 240 adult fractures. Clin Orthop 1975;112:254.

Pollock FH et al: Treatment of radial neuropathy associated with fractures of the humerus. J Bone Joint Surg Am 1981;63:239.

FRACTURES & DISLOCATIONS ABOUT THE ELBOW

Anatomy & Biomechanics

The elbow is a complex hinged joint that consists of three bony articulations: the radiocapitellar joint, the ulnohumeral joint, and the proximal radioulnar joint. The bony architecture lends stability to the elbow, but the soft tissue restraints play an important role as well. On the medial side of the elbow, the anterior band of the medial (ulnar) collateral ligament is the primary stabilizer to valgus stress. The lateral ulnar collateral ligament is the primary stabilizer on the lateral side of the elbow. Disruption of this portion of the lateral collateral ligament complex leads to posterolateral instability.

The normal range of motion of the elbow is up to 150 degrees of flexion. Normal pronation and supination are 75 degrees and 85 degrees, respectively. The carrying angle is the resting point of the elbow in full extension. In males, the carrying angle is generally 10–15 degrees valgus; in females, 15–20 degrees valgus.

When elbow injury is suspected, it is important to perform a thorough physical examination of the entire upper extremity including the shoulder and the wrist, looking for associated injuries. Inspections for swelling and deformity as well as palpation are important. Careful neurovascular examination is also critical prior to implementing treatment. Do not forget to assess components of the forearm and hand.

The type of fracture or dislocation sustained is dependent on the mechanism of the injury. A minimum of three x-ray views of the elbow should be obtained: anteroposterior, lateral, and oblique. If examination or subjective complaints indicate the possibility of an associated wrist or forearm injury, x-rays of these areas should also be obtained.

Probably the most useful classification system for distal humerus fractures is the AO system, based on the concept of column integrity and intra-articular involvement. Type A fractures are extra-articular and are further subdivided into A1–A3 fractures based on degree of comminution. This would include epicondylar, supracondylar, and transcondylar fractures. Type B fractures involve only a portion of the articular surface, as in unicondylar and intercondylar fractures. Type B1 fractures are lateral column fractures only; type B2 fractures are medial column fractures only; and type B3 fractures involve only the distal articular surface without either column. Type C fractures involve the entire distal articular surface and are subclassified as C1–3 based on the amount of metaphysial and articular comminution.

Supracondylar Fractures of the Humerus

A. In Children

Supracondylar fractures are much more common in the pediatric population, generally from a direct blow to the elbow from a fall. There are extension (96%) and flexion type fractures. In the extension type, the fragment is displaced posteriorly; in the much less common flexion type, the distal fragment is displaced anteriorly.

These are extra-articular fractures that occur proximal to the olecranon fossa. They are AO type A fractures. Understating normal radiographic anatomy of the elbow is crucial to diagnosing any elbow fracture, especially in the pediatric patient. They require emergent treatment. In the skeletally immature patient, stable and nondisplaced fractures can be treated in a posterior splint or long arm cast for 3–4 weeks with careful weekly x-ray follow-up.

Displaced A2 fractures with the posterior cortex intact can usually be reduced with gentle manipulation by applying longitudinal traction, an anteriorly directed force on the fragment, and flexing the elbow to 120 degrees under sedation or general anesthetic (Figure 42–9). If reduction can be obtained, this can be treated in a long arm cast or splint. However, close follow-up is imperative. Many surgeons will elect to do a closed reduction and percutaneous pinning with Kirschner wires in order to avoid complications of late loss of reduction and malunion or vascular compromise (Volkmann's ischemic contracture) if it is necessary to keep the elbow flexed > 90 degrees to hold the reduction.

Completely displaced, unstable A3 fractures require fixation. They are often associated with neurovascular injury, and this must always be evaluated. Closed reduction and percutaneous pinning is the first choice if the reduction can be achieved. Some surgeons prefer to make an incision on the medial side to visualize the ulnar nerve and avoid injury during pin placement. If closed reduction is unsuccessful, open reduction and pin placement are required.

If there is any question of vascular injury, angiography or open exploration should be undertaken to avoid vascular compromise. Careful postoperative monitoring is always indicated in these injuries.

Occasionally in the patient with multiple injuries, surgery is not an option. Under these circumstances, unstable fractures can be treated with olecranon pin skeletal traction.

B. In Adults

Supracondylar fractures are uncommon after the physes have closed. The transcondylar fracture is even less common but is more common in the older age group. As in the pediatric patient, there are both extension and flexion types, with the extension type being much more common.

Examination and diagnosis are the same as previously described for the pediatric patient. Treatment consists of closed manipulation with longitudinal traction and manipulation of the distal humeral fragment into position with the thumb. If reduction can be achieved, the patient is then splinted in the degree of flexion necessary to maintain the reduction. However, if extreme flexion is necessary and there are risks of vascular compromise, an alternative method of fixation must be used—closed reduction and percutaneous pinning, open reduction and fixation with screws or plates, or external fixation. Some advocate surgical fixation to prevent vascular compromise and allow earlier range of motion activity.

The rare flexion supracondylar fracture should be converted to an extension type if possible. If that cannot be done, the fracture is reduced by longitudinal traction on the humerus with the elbow flexed 90 degrees. The distal fragment is pushed posteriorly while the humerus is translated anteriorly. The same recommendations concerning immobilization versus surgery are followed as for the extension type.

Epicondylar Fractures of the Humerus

Lateral epicondylar fractures are rare, but medial epicondylar fractures are not uncommon especially in children and adolescents. If displacement is minimal < 2–3 mm), closed treatment is appropriate. However, if the

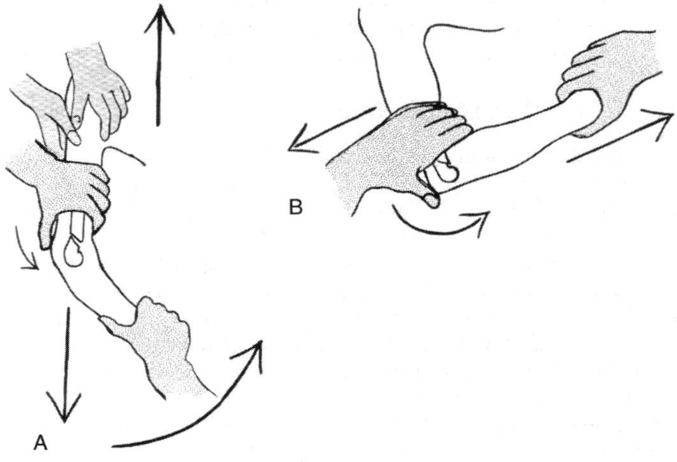

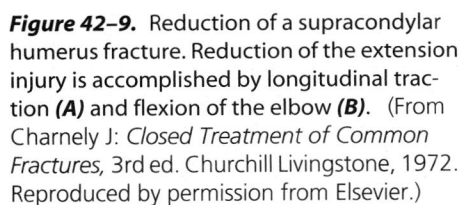

Figure 42–9. Reduction of a supracondylar humerus fracture. Reduction of the extension injury is accomplished by longitudinal traction ***(A)*** and flexion of the elbow ***(B)***. (From Charnely J: *Closed Treatment of Common Fractures,* 3rd ed. Churchill Livingstone, 1972. Reproduced by permission from Elsevier.)

fragment is displaced more than a few millimeters, open reduction and fixation with smooth pins or screws would be the recommended treatment. On the medial side, open treatment is preferred over percutaneous fixation so that the ulnar nerve can be visualized and protected. Occasionally, the fragment remains symptomatic or can cause ulnar nerve irritation after healing. If this occurs, the fragment can be excised.

INTRA-ARTICULAR FRACTURES OF THE HUMERUS

Condylar Fractures

These are uncommon fractures, accounting for only 3–5% of distal humeral fractures. Lateral condylar fractures are more frequent than medial condylar fractures and occur in the sagittal plane by one of two mechanisms. Avulsion fractures occur by indirect force, and the fragment ends up distal to its origin. An axial load causes a shear fracture and displaces the fragment proximally.

The classification system used is that described by Milch (Figure 42–10). A type I lateral condylar fracture involves part or all of the capitellum. A type II lateral condylar fracture extends into part or all of the trochlea. Type I medial condylar fractures do not extend beyond the trochlear groove, and type II fractures extend into the trochlear sulcus. Type II condylar fractures are unstable injuries and are technically fracture-dislocations.

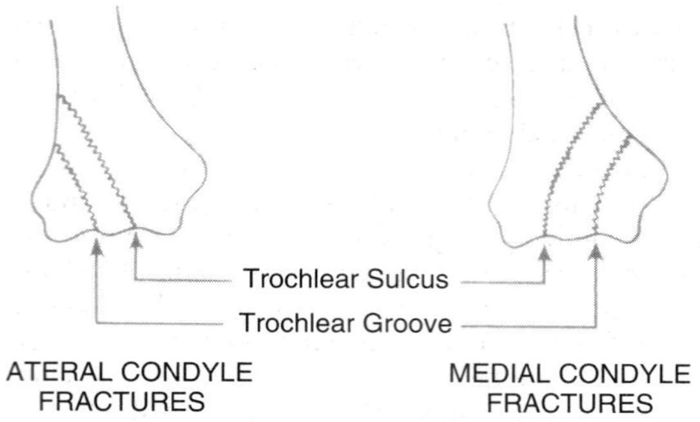

Figure 42–10. **Condyle fractures. Milch classification. The type II fracture involves the lateral lip of the trochlea—thus its inherent instability.** (Reproduced, with permission, from Milch H: Fractures and fracture dislocation of the humeral condyles. J Trauma, 1964.)

Undisplaced type I fractures can be treated with splint or cast immobilization and close follow-up to check for displacement. Displaced type I fractures can be treated with closed reduction and immobilization if reduction is successful. Type II fractures are inherently unstable and should be treated with open reduction and screw fixation. It is important to obtain joint congruity.

Malunion of type I lateral condylar fractures can lead to tardy ulnar nerve palsy. Malunion of type I lateral and medial condylar fractures can be treated with open wedge osteotomy. Type II malunions are more difficult to deal with secondary to the joint incongruity and subluxation.

Fractures of the Capitellum

This fracture accounts for less than 1% of all elbow fractures. It is important to distinguish it from the lateral condylar fracture. The most widely accepted classifications system is as follows (Figure 42–11): Type I (most common) involves most or all of the capitellum and sometimes part of the trochlea; type II involves a variable amount of articular surface, usually with very little subchondral bone attached; and type III is a comminuted compression fracture of the articular surface.

The mechanism of injury is usually a fall on the outstretched hand for type I and type III fractures and a shearing indirect force for type II fractures. There is often an associated radial head fracture. Diagnosis requires careful scrutiny of the radiographs and suspicion on physical examination. Tomograms may be necessary to see the fragment.

In general, with large fragments, an attempt should be made for open reduction and internal fixation. Small fragments should be excised.

Intercondylar Fractures

These are commonly described as T or Y condylar fractures and are among the most challenging to treat. The mechanism of injury is a wedge effect of the proximal ulna on the trochlear groove of the humerus causing a splitting of the humerus. Comminution is usually associated with these injuries. Classification systems used are the AO classification described earlier and a more succinct system described by Riseborough and Radin in 1969, as follows (Figure 42–12): Type I, nondisplaced fracture between the capitellum and trochlea; type II, separation of the capitellum and trochlea without appreciable rotation of the fragments in the frontal plane; type III, separation of the fragments with rotational deformity; and type IV, severe comminution of the articular surface with wide separation of the humeral condyles.

In the past, treatment consisted of closed reduction and casting or traction. Open reduction and internal fixation is now the treatment of choice for certain types of fractures. Type I fractures can be treated closed with early mobilization when swelling subsides and the fracture has had two weeks or so to consolidate. Most type II and type III fractures should be treated with open reduction and internal fixation with plates and screws. Type IV fractures are the most difficult to treat, especially in the older patient with osteopenia. With diffuse

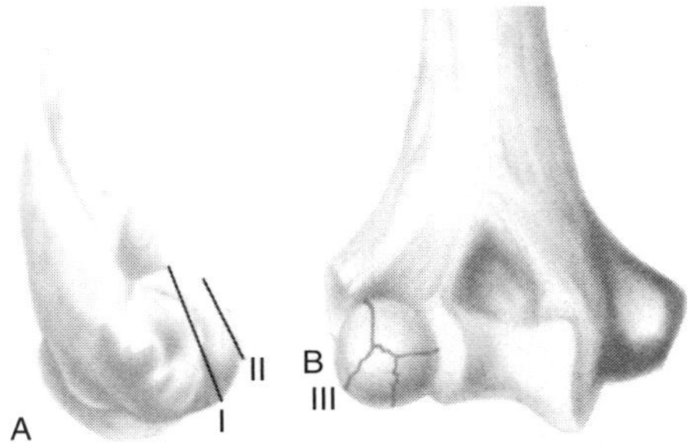

Figure 42–11. Fractures of the capitellum. The type I fracture involves a large portion of bone, often the entire structure. Type II is a shear fracture, often with minimal subchondral bone, and may displace posteriorly ***(A)***. A type III fracture is a comminuted fracture with varying amounts of displacement of the fracture fragments ***(B)***. (From Morrey B: *The Elbow and Its Disorders,* Saunders, 1985. Reproduced by permission of Mayo Foundation for Medical Education and Research. All rights reserved.)

osteopenia in the elderly, type IV fractures are probably best treated with the "bag of bones" technique—in other words, conscientious neglect. This means short-term immobilization and early range of motion exercises without trying to reduce the comminuted fragments. In the younger patient with good quality bone and a type IV fracture, it is reasonable to attempt reconstruction. Bone grafting of defects may be necessary.

It is important to realize that there are two distinct components that require reduction and fixation with intercondylar fractures: the intra-articular intercondylar component and the supracondylar one. Kirschner wires or, preferably, screw fixation can be used to stabilize the intercondylar component. This is the most important part of the reduction, reestablishing joint congruity. It is recommended then that the medial and lateral columns be stabilized with plates. The critical issue is to obtain rigid fixation if open reduction and internal fixation are undertaken. Early mobilization can then begin. Operation without obtaining rigid fixation is the worst option of all, as stiffness and joint ankylosis is accelerated.

FRACTURES OF THE PROXIMAL ULNA

Olecranon Fractures

The olecranon is the most proximal palpable portion of the ulna. It is located subcutaneously without much soft tissue coverage. The triceps has a broad insertion at this level.

Anteriorly, the olecranon forms the greater sigmoid (semilunar) notch of the ulna, which articulates with the trochlea. The most proximal anterior portion of the ulna is the coronoid process, which lends stability to the elbow joint.

Olecranon fractures usually occur with a direct blow or as an avulsion injury with forceful triceps contraction. They have been classified as undisplaced, displaced, transverse, oblique, and comminuted. Fracture type dictates appropriate treatment.

A true lateral radiograph of the elbow is essential to accurately assess fracture type. An anteroposterior view and an oblique view should be obtained as well. The goals of treatment are to restore articular congruity and stability, to preserve triceps function, to prevent stiffness, and to avoid complications.

Undisplaced fractures can be managed in a long arm splint or cast with the arm in mid flexion. Careful follow-up with radiographs should be done at weekly

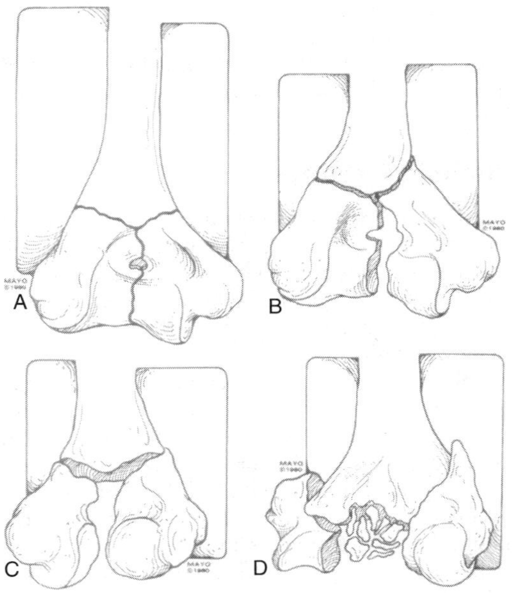

Figure 42–12. Intercondylar fractures. ***A:*** Type I undisplaced T-condylar fracture of the elbow. ***B:*** Type II displaced but not rotated T-condylar fracture. ***C:*** Type III displaced and rotated T-condylar fracture. ***D:*** Type IV displaced rotated and comminuted T-condylar fracture. (From Bryan RS: Fractures about the elbow in adults. In: *American Academy of Orthopaedic Surgeons: Instructional Course Lectures,* vol. 30. Mosby, 1981. Reproduced by permission of Mayo Foundation for Medical Education and Research. All rights reserved.)

intervals for at least 2 weeks. In general, there is sufficient stability at 3 weeks to allow early motion from full extension to 90 degrees of flexion, with progression of flexion at 6 weeks.

There are two options available for displaced fractures—again, depending on fracture pattern and demands of the patient: open reduction and internal fixation or excision.

The tension band wire technique with either longitudinal Kirschner wires or a 6.5 mm cancellous screw is the preferred method for most fractures with minimal comminution. Segmental fractures or comminuted fractures are often better addressed with plating.

External fixation is also an option for comminuted fractures and those with accompanying soft tissue disruption, as in open fractures.

If there is significant comminution or in the elderly patient with poor bone quality, excision of the fragment with reattachment of the triceps is acceptable treatment. Stability must be considered if excision is to be undertaken. If there is also anterior fracture (coronoid) or soft tissue disruption, simple excision could render the elbow unstable.

The most frequent complication of these fractures is prominent implants that must be removed after healing has occurred. Elbow stiffness and loss of fixation have also been reported.

Coronoid Fractures

The coronoid process is the anterior beak-shaped portion of the ulna, forming the buttress anteriorly of the greater sigmoid notch. The anterior portion of the medial collateral ligament attaches here, as well as a portion of the anterior capsule. It therefore contributes to elbow stability.

Isolated fractures of the coronoid are uncommon and are more frequently associated with elbow dislocations or other fractures about the elbow. The mechanism of injury is usually forced posterior displacement of the proximal ulna as with a dislocation or hyperextension force of the elbow. It is important to obtain oblique radiographic views in assessing these fractures as they are sometimes difficult to see on lateral and anteroposterior views.

These fractures have been classified by Regan and Morrey into three types as follows (Figure 42–13): Type I, avulsion of the tip of the coronoid; type II, a single or comminuted fragment involving 50% or less of the coronoid process; and type III, a single or comminuted fragment involving over 50% of the coronoid process.

Type I fractures can be treated with immobilization in flexion for 3 weeks (or less if the fragment and elbow are stable). Associated fractures should be treated as appropriate in each case with the goal of fracture stability for early range of motion. Isolated coronoid fractures without elbow instability can be treated in the same way as type I fractures. If there is associated elbow instability from soft tissue damage or other fractures, consideration should be given to open reduction and internal fixation. If there is one large fragment, this can be achieved with a screw, Kirschner wire fixation, or suture technique. With comminution, the best approach may be application of an external fixator. Type III fractures are most often associated with significant elbow instability. They are treated in the same way as unstable type II fractures. Excision of fragments is not recommended as this can lead to permanent elbow instability.

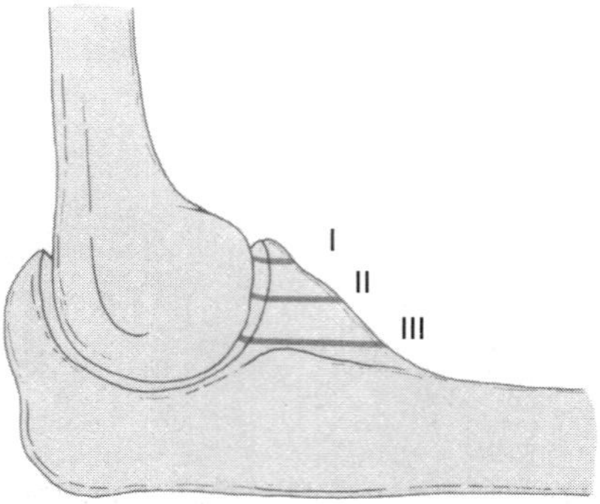

Figure 42–13. Coronoid fractures. The coronoid fracture has been classified into three types by Regan and Morrey. (From Browner B et al: *Skeletal Trauma.* Saunders, 1992. Reproduced by permission from Elsevier.)

FRACTURES OF THE PROXIMAL RADIUS

Radial Head Fractures

Radial head fractures are caused by an axial load on the pronated forearm. The fracture can be isolated or associated with elbow dislocation. Anteroposterior, lateral, and radial head view radiographs will show the fracture. There is usually a fat pad sign on the lateral x-ray.

The Mason classification system is the one most commonly used to describe these fractures. There are three types (Figure 42–14): Type I, nondisplaced; type II, displaced (often a single fragment); and type III, comminuted. Some also add a type IV, fractures associated with dislocation, as this calls for different treatment and implies a worse prognosis.

Other than amount of displacement and comminution, elbow motion is another important factor in considering appropriate treatment. Motion should be assessed acutely by aspirating the hematoma and inject-

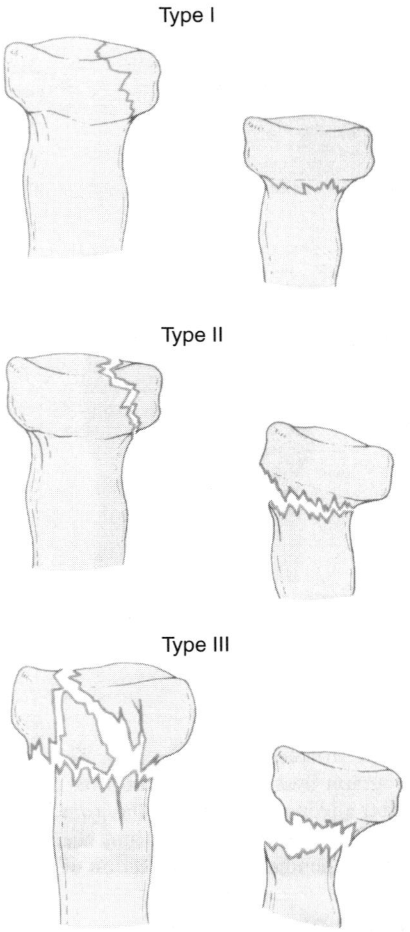

Figure 42–14. Radial head fractures. The modified Mason classification system for radial head fractures. (From Browner B et al: *Skeletal Trauma.* Saunders, 1992. Reproduced by permission from Elsevier.)

ing local anesthetic into the elbow joint. If full range of motion is present, treatment is based on the radiographic findings. However, if there is an obstacle to full range of motion, that must be considered in planning operative versus nonoperative intervention.

Type I (nondisplaced) fractures are treated with a brief period of immobilization in a sling followed by early motion at about 10–14 days after injury. This generally yields good results, with the most common complication being loss of full extension.

There is controversy and about what is the proper treatment of type II fractures. If displacement is minimal and range of motion is full, some would advocate treating with a period of immobilization. If the amount of displacement is unacceptable or there is bony block, operation is necessary. Options include open reduction with internal fixation and excision of part or all of the radial head. If the radial head is excised in its entirety, the decision must be made whether or not to replace it with an implant. If there is instability after removal of the head or if there is concomitant injury to the wrist, a radial head implant should be used. Titanium implants are preferable to Silastic.

Type III fractures are treated by excision of fragments with or without implant replacement, based on the same criteria as set forth above for type II fractures.

Type IV fractures are treated with reduction of the dislocation followed by treatment of the radial head based on its type as described above.

ACUTE INSTABILITY OF THE ELBOW JOINT

The elbow is the second most commonly dislocated joint in the adult (after the shoulder). It occurs when the load placed on the structures about the elbow exceed the intrinsic stability provided by the bony anatomy and ligamentous and muscular constraints. As with any other joint dislocation, the goal of treatment is expeditious reduction.

Dislocations are classified by the direction of displacement of the distal bone. Because there are two bones in the forearm, in addition to the anterior, posterior, medial, and lateral dislocation, one can also have a divergent dislocation when the radius and ulna are forced apart by the distal humerus (Figure 42–15). This is a rare situation. It is also possible to have partial dislocations in which only the radial head or the ulna alone is dislocated. Isolated radial head fractures are rare and are usually accompanied by a fracture of the ulna (Monteggia's fracture).

Standard anteroposterior, lateral, and oblique radiographs of the elbow should be obtained to determine the direction of dislocation as an aid in determining the appropriate reduction maneuver. If fracture about the elbow has occurred with the dislocation, overall treatment is usually dictated by the fracture. The elbow may not be rendered stable until the fractures are fixed. Adequate fracture care will usually cause secondary reduction of the dislocation. Careful neurovascular examination both before and after reduction is critical. Postreduction radiographs should always be obtained—not only to determine the success of the reduction but also to look for any other injury that may have been obscured on the initial x-rays or caused by the reduction maneuver. These patients should be observed for 24 hours to watch for the development of compartment syndrome.

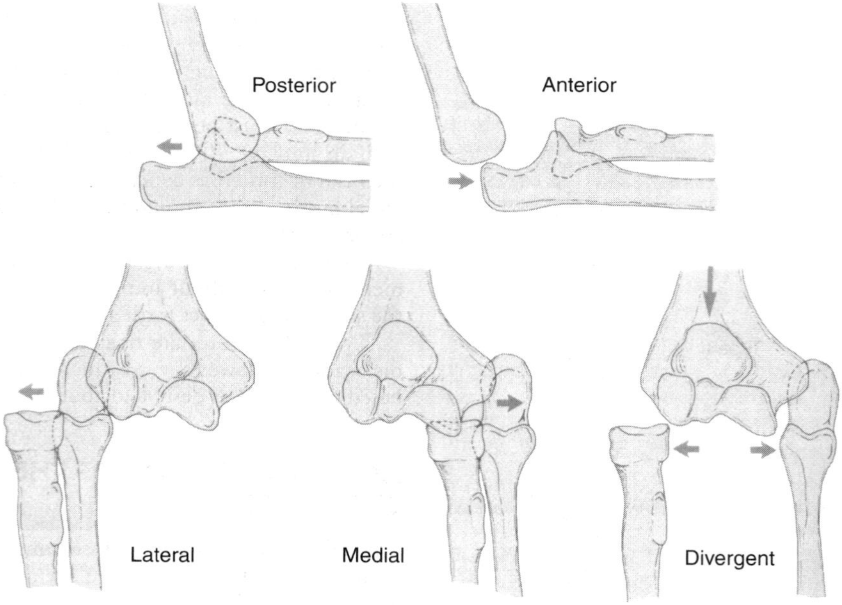

Figure 42–15. Elbow dislocations. An elbow dislocation is defined by the direction of the forearm bones. (From Browner B et al: *Skeletal Trauma.* Saunders, 1992. Reproduced by permission from Elsevier.)

Posterior Elbow Dislocations

This is by far the most common type of elbow dislocation. It results from an axial force being applied to the extended elbow. The extremity may appear to be shortened and the elbow flexed. Both collateral ligaments are disrupted regardless of whether the dislocation is posteromedial or posterolateral.

With adequate anesthesia (conscious sedation, local joint infiltration, or perhaps general anesthesia), traction is applied with the forearm flexed to 90 degrees, and the concomitant medial or lateral displacement is then corrected. This should be a gentle maneuver. A "clunk" is usually appreciated as the elbow is reduced back into position. The elbow is then taken through a full range of motion to check for bony block as well as instability. Repeat neurovascular examination and radiographs are obtained.

Anterior Elbow Dislocations

These are relatively rare. Treatment is similar to that of posterior dislocations except that the reduction maneuver is reversed.

Medial & Lateral Elbow Dislocations

With lateral dislocations, some joint motion may be maintained as the ulna may be displaced into the groove between the trochlea and capitellum. The anteroposterior radiograph best shows the direction of dislocation. Again, after adequate anesthesia, the joint is reduced by first applying a distraction force and then a medial or lateral force depending on the direction of dislocation.

Irreducible Dislocations

Rarely, it is not possible to reduce the elbow by closed reduction techniques. This may be due to delayed treatment, after the elbow has been dislocated for days to weeks, or by tissues being interposed in the joint and blocking the reduction. Another possibility is the extremely unstable elbow, in which case the elbow is reducible but the reduction cannot be maintained. In these instances, it may be necessary to do an open reduction to extract interposed tissues or repair damaged tissues that are contributing to the instability. Although most elbow dislocations can be treated closed, careful consideration should be given for open treatment of unstable dislocations. While it is better to have a stiff elbow than an unstable elbow, the worst outcome is the stiff and unstable elbow.

Postreduction Care & Rehabilitation

Once it has been established that the elbow is reduced and stable, the patient is placed in a long arm posterior splint with the elbow flexed 90 degrees. Patients should be observed for 24 hours for development of compartment syndrome. Range of motion exercises should be started when pain and swelling permit, usually within a few days after injury. Frequent radiographs should be taken to confirm that the elbow remains reduced during early rehabilitation. The splint is generally discontinued in 1 or 2 weeks if the elbow is stable.

Complications

Several complications can occur with this injury, both acutely and chronically. Acute complications are mainly those of nerve and vascular injury. Careful assessment is required both before and after treatment, with early intervention for the development of compartment syndrome. Other complications include continued instability or stiffness with loss of motion. Instability is addressed surgically in most cases. Stiffness can usually be avoided with early range of motion exercises, but if it does occur and is severe it can be addressed by surgical capsulectomy. Heterotopic ossification can also be seen—more commonly in the brain-injured or burn patient. It is generally recommended that areas of heterotopic ossification be excised not earlier than 6 months after injury. In high-risk patients, indomethacin or radiation can be used as prophylaxis.

Davidson PA, Moseley JB Jr, Tullos HS: Radial head fracture: a potentially complex injury. Clin Orthop 1993;(297):224.

Helfet DL, Schmeling GJ: Bicondylar intra-articular fractures of the distal humerus in adults. Clin Orthop 1993;(292):26.

Hotchkiss RN: Displaced Fractures of the Radial Head: internal Fixation or Excision. J Am Acad Orthop Surg 1997;5:1.

Jupiter JB, Mehne DK: Elbow trauma: fractures of the distal humerus. Orthopaedics 1992;15:825.

Kuhn JE, Louis DS, Loder RT: Divergent single-column fractures of the distal part of the humerus. J Bone Joint Surg Am 1995; 77:538.

McKee MD, Jupiter JB: A contemporary approach to the management of complex fractures of the distal humerus and their sequelae. Hand Clin 1994;10:479.

Morrey BF: Current concepts in the treatment of fractures of the radial head, the olecranon, and the coronoid. J Bone Joint Surg Am 1995;77:316.

O'Driscoll SW: Elbow instability. Hand Clin 1994;10:405.

O'Driscoll SW et al: Elbow subluxation and dislocation: a spectrum of instability. Clin Orthop 1992;280:186.

Otsuka NY, Kasser JR: Supracondylar fractures of the humerus in children. J Am Acad Orthop Surg 1997;5:19.

Sponseller PD: Problem elbow fractures in children. Hand Clin 1994;10:495.

Topping RE, Blanco JS, Davis TJ: Clinical evaluation of crossed-pin versus lateral pin fixation in displaced supracondylar humerus fractures. J Pediatr Orthop 1995;15: 435.

FRACTURES OF THE FOREARM

The anatomy of the forearm can be thought of as a closed ring, somewhat analogous to the pelvis. It is very difficult to break a ring (in this case, a ring composed of the radius and ulna and their intervening proximal and distal joints) in only one place. Isolated radial or ulnar fractures are therefore uncommon except as a result of a direct blow to that bone.

Fractures of both forearm bones simultaneously or of one bone with a concomitant joint injury to the elbow or wrist joint are more commonly seen than fracture of either bone in isolation.

It is important in evaluating these fractures to obtain anteroposterior, lateral, and oblique radiographs of the forearm that include the elbow and the wrist. In this way, distal radioulnar joint or radial head dislocations can be evaluated. As always, careful neurovascular evaluation and documentation both before and after reduction are critical.

FRACTURES OF THE SHAFT OF THE RADIUS

Isolated Radial Shaft Fractures

An isolated radial shaft fracture should arouse suspicion of a concomitant injury to the wrist or elbow. Closed treatment of this injury is acceptable practice only if very strict criteria are satisfied: There cannot be any displacement of the radius; the normal bow of the radius must be maintained; and there cannot be any concomitant injury to the elbow or wrist. In the adult, essentially no amount of displacement is acceptable as it may limit the return of forearm rotation. If there is displacement, open reduction and internal fixation are recommended.

Galeazzi's Fracture

This is a fracture of the shaft of the radius (most commonly the distal third) in conjunction with a distal radioulnar joint injury. Wrist pain on physical examination arouses suspicion. However, the diagnosis should be confirmed radiographically. The following radiographic findings are suggestive of a distal radioulnar joint disruption when an isolated radial shaft fracture is present: fracture at the base of the ulnar styloid, widening of the distal radioulnar joint space on the anteroposterior radiograph, dislocation of the radius relative to the ulna on a true lateral radiograph, and radial shortening greater than 5 mm relative to the distal ulna.

In adults, these fractures should always be addressed surgically. The recommendation is for open reduction with internal fixation of the radius fracture and then intraoperative evaluation of the stability of the distal radioulnar joint. If after fixing the radius the joint is stable through full pronation and supination, there is no need for immobilization (other than short-term until the incision is healed). If the joint can be reduced but is unstable with rotation, additional treatment is necessary. If there is a repairable ulnar styloid fracture, then open reduction with internal fixation of this piece will often render the distal radioulnar joint stable. If there is no ulnar styloid fracture but the distal radioulnar joint is reducible but unstable with rotation, then two 0.0625-inch Kirschner wires are used to pin the distal ulna to the radius in a reduced position (usually supination). With both open reduction with internal fixation of the ulnar styloid or the use of transfixing pins, the forearm should be immobilized in full supination in an above-elbow cast or brace for 4–6 weeks. The transfixing pins are removed prior to allowing forearm range of motion. Rarely, the distal radioulnar joint cannot be reduced. In this instance, a dorsal approach to the joint is used to extract interposed tissues blocking reduction. This is most commonly the extensor carpi ulnaris tendon.

Complications of this injury include malunion, nonunion, chronic distal radioulnar joint instability (usually only if this injury is missed and not treated initially) and nerve injury at the time of open reduction with internal fixation.

FRACTURES OF THE SHAFT OF THE ULNA

Isolated Ulnar Shaft Fractures (Nightstick Fractures)

This fairly common injury is caused by a direct blow to the ulna. Radiographic evaluation should include the elbow and wrist to rule out associated injuries. For the nondisplaced isolated fracture, some advocate long arm casting for 6–8 weeks. Functional bracing also gives good results. Some even advocate minimal (Ace bandage) or no bracing with isolated nondisplaced ulnar shaft fractures. In general, it is probably preferable to provide some immobilization until pain subsides. In isolated displaced ulnar shaft fractures, open reduction and internal fixation with plate and screws is the treatment of choice.

Monteggia's Fracture

Monteggia's fracture is fracture of the proximal third of the ulna with dislocation of the radial head. It was first described by Monteggia of Milan in 1814. Bado extended the description to include the entire spectrum of ulnar shaft fractures associated with radial head dislocations. They are classified as follows (Figure 42–16).

Type I: Fracture of the ulnar diaphysis with anterior angulation and anterior dislocation of the radial head (60% of cases).

Type II: Fracture of the ulnar diaphysis with posterior or posterolateral dislocation of the radial head (15% of cases).

Type III: Fracture of the ulnar metaphysis with lateral or anterolateral dislocation of the radial head (20% of cases).

Type IV: Fracture of he ulna and radius at the proximal third with anterior dislocation of the radial head (5% of cases).

If an isolated ulnar shaft fracture is noted on x-ray, adequate elbow radiographs must be taken to rule out Monteggia's fracture and careful neurovascular evaluation is required. Injury to both the radial nerve and the posterior interosseous nerve has been described with this injury.

In the child, closed reduction of ulnar shaft fracture usually also reduces the radial head dislocation. In the adult patient, open reduction and internal fixation of the ulnar shaft fracture with compression plating is the treatment of choice. Once the ulnar shaft fracture is anatomically reduced and fixed, the radial head usually reduces. Failure of the radial head to reduce is either secondary to malreduction of the ulna or due to interposed soft tissue, rarely requiring open reduction of the radial head for removal. After reduction, the stability of the radial head should be checked, preferably under fluoroscopy.

Complications include nerve palsy, malunion, nonunion, a stiff elbow, and occasional formation of a radioulnar synostosis. This is seen more often with type IV fractures.

Both-Bone Forearm Fractures

Fractures of both radius and ulna are caused by high-energy injuries such as motor vehicle accidents or falls from a height. The fractures are usually displaced. Careful examination to rule out neurovascular injury and compartment syndrome should be performed. Radiographs of the entire forearm including the elbow and wrist are necessary.

In children with open physes, closed reduction and long arm cast immobilization is usually adequate, since they have the potential to remodel small amounts of deformity. Bayonet apposition with 10–20 degrees of angular deformity and maintained interosseous space is considered acceptable depending on the age of the child. Frequent (weekly) radiographs are necessary to look for displacement. Older children close to skeletal maturity should be treated more like adults.

Treatment for both-bone forearm fractures in adults consists of open reduction and internal fixation with compression plating using 3.5 mm dynamic plates. This affords the best results by restoring normal anatomy and therefore rotation of the forearm. Bone grafting is recommended for comminuted fractures with bone loss.

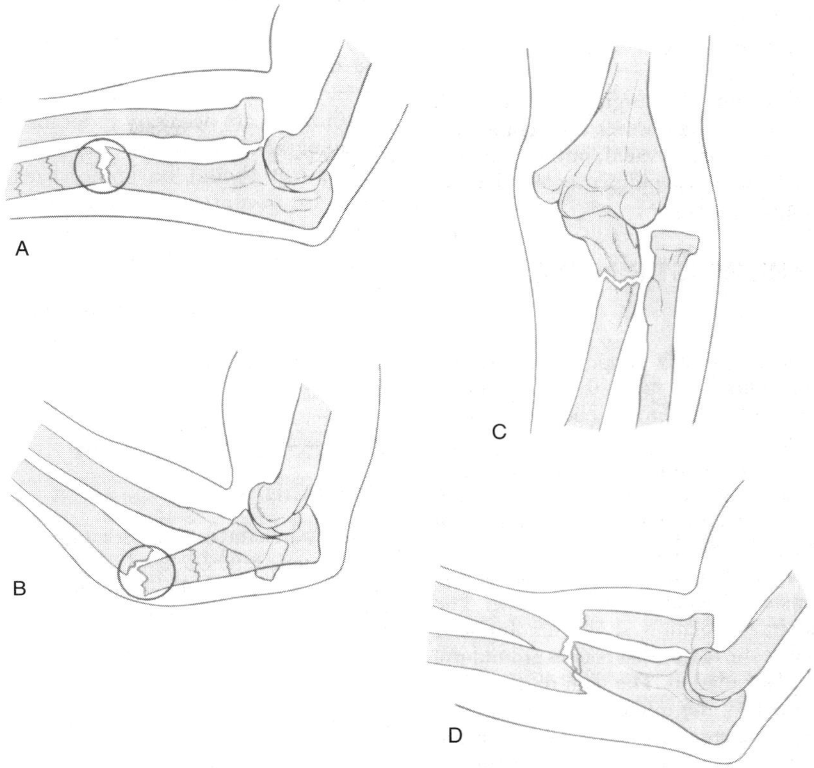

Figure 42–16. Monteggia's fractures. The classification of Monteggia lesions by Bado. ***A:*** Type I: anterior angulation of the ulnar fracture and anterior dislocation of the radial head. ***B:*** Type II: posterior angulation of the ulnar fracture and anterior dislocation of the radial head. ***C:*** Type III: fracture of the proximal ulna metaphysis and lateral dislocation of the radial head. ***D:*** Type IV: anterior dislocation of the radial head and fracture of the radial and ulnar shafts. (From Browner B et al: *Skeletal Trauma.* Saunders, 1992. Reproduced by permission from Elsevier.)

The radius can be approached through an anterior Henry incision regardless of the location of the fracture. Some prefer the dorsal Thompson approach for proximal third radius fractures. The ulna is approached dorsally on its subcutaneous border. To avoid development of a compartment syndrome postoperatively, the fascia is not closed after reduction and plating. Patients are splinted immediately postoperatively for comfort and to allow healing of the skin incisions. With solid fixation, active range of motion of the forearm and elbow can be started at 10–14 days. Open fractures can also be treated successfully with these methods. However, if there is excessive soft tissue damage or wound contamination, the use of an external fixator may be a preferable option.

Complications of this fracture include compartment syndrome, neurovascular injury, malunion, nonunion, synostosis, and loss of motion.

COMPARTMENT SYNDROME

Compartment syndrome is caused by increased pressure in an enclosed space that leads to compromise of circulation and function of tissues in that space. It can be the result of swelling from trauma or postsurgical swelling. It should be differentiated from primary nerve or vascular injury. Careful inspection after trauma or surgery is essential to prevent this devastating complication, especially in the obtunded patient. Pain with passive range of motion of the digits is thought to be the most sensitive early sign of compartment syndrome. Paresthesias and a tense swollen forearm are also signs of compartment syndrome. Pulselessness can occur but is a late sign and does not always occur.

Compartment syndrome is a surgical emergency. If it is suspected, compartment pressures should be measured immediately. If they are elevated, immediate forearm fasciotomy is indicated to avoid permanent damage to muscles, nerves, and vessels.

INJURIES OF THE WRIST REGION

Anatomy

The radius and ulna structurally support the forearm. The distal radius and ulna have specialized articulations with the carpus and with each other. The distal radius has three articular components: the scaphoid fossa, the lunate fossa, and the sigmoid notch. The scaphoid and lunate fossae articulate with their respective carpal bones (the scaphoid and lunate), making up the radiocarpal joint. The sigmoid notch articulates with the distal ulna, forming the distal radioulnar joint. The shafts of the radius and ulna are nearly parallel to one another. The ulnar shaft is fixed in its rotation at the ulnohumeral joint, and it is therefore the radius that rotates around the ulna in pronation and supination. The shaft of the radius and ulna are connected by the interosseous membrane, which is important in transmission of force between the two bones. It also provides muscular attachment for the flexors and extensors of the wrist and digits. The orientation of the distal radius is 5–10 degrees of volar tilt and 22 degrees of radial inclination. These become important parameters in interpreting adequate position of distal radius fractures.

In addition to the bony architecture, there is complex ligamentous and soft tissue anatomy of the wrist. The distal ulna has an ulnar styloid that provides attachment for the triangular fibrocartilage complex, the volar and dorsal ulnar carpal ligaments, and the ulnar collateral ligaments of the wrist. There are also volar and dorsal radiocarpal ligaments that attach to the radius along with the radial collateral ligaments. There are six dorsal compartments of the wrist that contain wrist and digital extensor tendons. On the volar surface, the pronator quadratus lies across the distal radius and ulna. Just anterior to the pronator quadratus are the contents of the carpal canal, containing nine digital flexor tendons and the median nerve. Anterior to the transverse carpal ligament lie the flexor carpi radialis, flexor carpi ulnaris, and palmaris longus muscles. Guyon's canal contains the ulnar nerve and artery. It is bounded by the volar retinacular ligament and flexor retinacular ligament, the hook of the hamate radially, and the pisiform ulnarly.

1. Wrist Sprain

The diagnosis of wrist sprain is made only after ruling out fractures and dislocations of the wrist. Radiographs should be taken at presentation. Careful palpation and examination are necessary to localize the area of injury. If radiographs are negative for fracture or dislocation, the patient should be immobilized in a volar wrist splint for comfort for a period of 2 weeks. If pain and swelling persist, x-rays should be repeated to look for more subtle occult fractures. MRI or an MR arthrogram may be necessary to discern ligamentous injury or damage to the triangular fibrocartilage complex of the wrist. If symptoms improve with a short period of immobilization, range of motion and strengthening exercises should be introduced in a graded fashion.

2. Distal Radius Fracture

Mechanism

Distal radius fractures most commonly occur from a fall on the outstretched hand. They are more common in the middle years and old age and in patients with osteoporosis. High-energy injuries such as motor vehicle accidents and falls from a height can produce this injury in young patients.

Classification of Fractures

In 1814—long before the availability of radiographs—Abraham Colles described the dorsally angulated and displaced distal radius metaphysial fracture. The term Colles fracture is often inappropriately used today to describe any distal radius fracture. Other names for distal radius fractures are Smith's fracture (reverse Colles fracture), an extra-articular metaphysial fracture with volar angulation and displacement; Barton's fracture, a displaced unstable articular fracture-subluxation of the distal radius with volar displacement of the carpus along with the articular fragment; Chauffeur's fracture, intra-articular fracture of the radial styloid; and "die punch" fracture, an intra-articular depression fracture of the lunate fossa. Although these terms are commonly used, more complete and descriptive classification systems are now available and preferred.

The Frykman classification system categorizes these fractures based on the presence or absence of ulnar styloid fractures and whether the fracture lines are extra-articular, intra-articular involving the radial carpal joint, intra-articular involving the distal radioulnar joint, or intra-articular involving both the radiocarpal and distal radioulnar joints (Figure 42–17).

The AO/ASIF classification separates distal radius fractures into three groups as shown in the accompanying box. It should be noted that injury to the distal radioulnar joint can occur with any of these fractures.

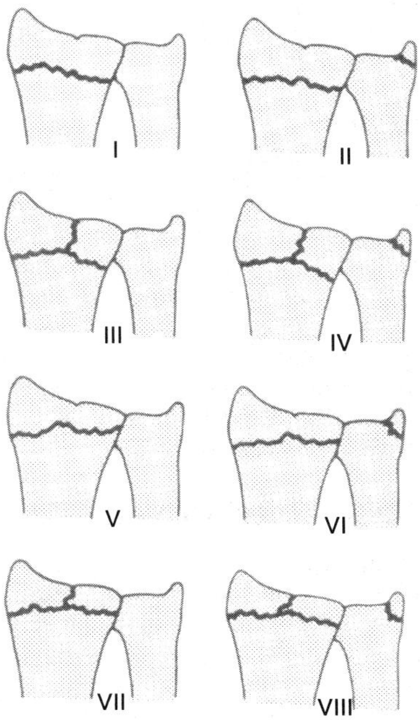

Figure 42–17. Frykman classification of distal radius fractures. Types I, III, V, and VII do not have an associated fracture of the distal ulna. Fractures III–VIII are intra-articular fractures. Higher-classification fractures have worse prognoses. (From Green D, Hotchkiss R, Pederson W: Green's Operative Hand Surgery. Churchill Livingstone, 1993.)

AO/ASIF CLASSIFICATION OF DISTAL RADIUS FRACTURES

Type A: Extra-articular fractures
1. Isolated distal ulnar fracture
2. Simple radius fracture
3. Radial fracture with metaphysial impaction

Type B: Intra-articular complex fracture
1. Radial styloid fracture
2. Dorsal rim fracture
3. Volar rim fracture

Type C: Intra-articular complex fracture
1. Metaphysial fracture with radiocarpal congruity preserved
2. Articular displacement
3. Diaphysial-metaphysial involvement

Treatment

Radiographs in the anteroposterior, lateral, and oblique planes should be obtained. If examination shows pain at the forearm or elbow, these radiographs should also be taken. The median nerve can be damaged by fracture fragments or compression from swelling and hematoma and the function of this nerve should be carefully documented both before and after reduction.

Treatment of distal radius fractures depends on many factors, including the amount of displacement and angulation, the degree of comminution, the age of the patient, the quality of the bone, and the functional demands required.

A. Nonoperative Treatment

Nondisplaced, stable fractures can be treated with cast immobilization. Displaced extra-articular fractures that can be reduced and are stable can also be treated in a cast or sugar-tong splint. Because it is often difficult to assess stability, once the fracture is reduced, radiographic evaluation should be done on a weekly basis for the first 2–3 weeks to make sure the alignment is maintained. Volar tilt, radial length, and radial inclination should be restored to acceptable parameters.

B. Indications for Surgical Management

Operation is warranted if reduction cannot be achieved or maintained by closed methods. Very comminuted fractures, even if they are extra-articular, often will shorten and displace in a cast. Fractures with intra-articular stepoff or gap of more than 2 mm require surgical fixation. Volar tilt should be restored to at least neutral in all but the very low demand wrist. Certain types of fractures such as the volar Barton's fracture are known to be unstable and always require volar buttress plating.

C. Techniques of Surgical Management

There are many techniques for surgical management of distal radius fractures. Choice is determined by the pattern of the fracture, the quality of the bone, and the surgeon's preference.

1. Closed reduction and percutaneous pinning— This is an effective method for securing large fragments to help prevent collapse after reduction of unstable fractures. In general, 0.0625-inch Kirschner wires are used in either an interfragmentary or an intrafocal pinning technique. With the interfragmentary technique, wires are passed across the fracture site after the fracture is reduced. With the intrafocal technique, the wire is placed in the fracture site, used there to achieve reduction, and then driven into the bone. These techniques can be used alone or in combination (Figure 42–18). Patients are placed in a cast or splint. The wires are gen-

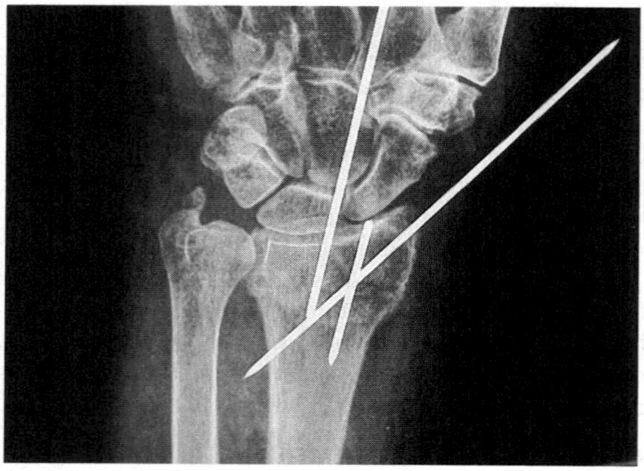

Figure 42–18. Closed reduction and percutaneous pinning of a distal radius fracture using a combination of intrafocal and interfragmentary techniques.

erally left in place for 6 weeks and then removed in the office after adequate healing has occurred.

2. External fixation—This is a very effective way of treating distal radius fractures. It is especially helpful in treating very comminuted fractures and intra-articular fractures where there are too many small pieces for pins or open reduction. External fixation devices take advantage of ligamentous tension and indirect reduction of the fracture fragments. External fixation is also used for open fractures with soft tissue compromise. It can be used in conjunction with percutaneous pins.

3. Open reduction and internal fixation with plates and screws—This is an effective technique in younger patients with good bone quality and large fragments. It has the added advantage of allowing early range of motion if the fixation is rigid. Many different plating systems are available, including a new Tri-Med system designed for treating intra-articular fractures by obtaining purchase on the intact proximal bone.

Disadvantages of open reduction and internal fixation with plates and screws include a potential for scarring, soft tissue stripping causing devascularization of small fragments, and the possibility of needing to have implants removed in the future.

4. Arthroscopic assisted reduction—The use of wrist arthroscopy to aid in reduction and also assess the quality of reduction is becoming more widely used for intra-articular fractures. It is often somewhat difficult to assess intra-articular fracture reduction with radiographs alone. With the use of wrist arthroscopy, the articular surface can be directly visualized and manipulated. It is also useful for identifying other concomitant pathology such as triangular fibrocartilage complex tear. This technique can be used in conjunction with percutaneous pins, external fixation, or plates and screws.

Complications

The most common complication of distal radius fractures is stiffness of the wrist and digits. Patients should be instructed to begin range of motion exercises for the digits immediately after the fracture is initially treated. Other complications include median nerve injury, unnoticed derangement of the distal radioulnar joint, infection (after operation), malunion, and late rupture of the extensor pollicis longus tendon after nondisplaced fractures. Stiffness of the shoulder and reflex sympathetic dystrophy can also occur.

FRACTURES OF THE ULNAR STYLOID

Fractures of the ulnar styloid are commonly seen in conjunction with distal radius fractures and but can also be seen in isolation. Fractures of the ulnar styloid are often too small to fix. However, large fragments (the entire styloid from its base) that are displaced should be treated by open reduction and internal fixation with small screws, pins, or tension band wires. If these large fragments are not fixed, the patient can go on to have chronic pain in this area as well as instability of the distal radioulnar joint.

DISTAL RADIOULNAR JOINT DISLOCATION

This is discussed earlier in conjunction with the Galeazzi fracture. It should be pointed out that this injury can also occur with a simple distal radius fracture. Careful examination of radiographs and the distal radioulnar joint will keep the clinician from missing this injury in the face of a distal radius fracture.

FRACTURES & DISLOCATIONS OF THE CARPUS

Most carpal bone fractures occur in the proximal carpal row. The scaphoid is the carpal bone most commonly fractured. Carpal bone fractures usually occur in younger people, often from high-energy falls on an outstretched wrist such as may occur while skiing, snowboarding, or rollerblading. Wrist radiographs can be difficult to interpret, and careful scrutiny is necessary so as not to miss these injuries. In addition to the standard anteroposterior, lateral, and oblique views of the wrist, special radiographic views such as a scaphoid view, clenched fist view, or carpal tunnel view can often be helpful.

1. Fracture of the Scaphoid

Treatment of scaphoid fractures can be difficult due in large part to the poor blood supply of this bone, which makes it susceptible to delayed union, nonunion, and avascular necrosis. Blood supply is from branches of the radial artery entering the distal aspect of the bone. Proximal pole blood supply is from retrograde flow. If a fracture occurs at the scaphoid waist or more proximally, the blood supply to this region is interrupted.

The most common area in the scaphoid for fracture is the scaphoid waist. Fractures can also occur in the distal tubercle and proximal pole. Patients present with pain in the radial side of the wrist, more specifically in the "anatomic snuffbox." If a patient has pain in this region, a scaphoid view radiograph of the wrist should be added to the wrist series. Nondisplaced fractures should be treated in a thumb spica cast. Nondisplaced fractures with more unstable oblique patterns should probably be treated in a long arm thumb spica cast for the first 3–4 weeks. Weekly radiographic follow-up for the first 3 weeks is necessary to look for displacement. The average time to healing is 12 weeks. Absence of clinical tenderness and bridging trabeculae on x-ray indicate healing. If no fracture is seen on initial x-ray examination but the patient has pain at the scaphoid, treatment should be as for nondisplaced scaphoid fracture. Scaphoid fractures are often not visible on initial x-ray. Radiographs out of plaster should be repeated in 2–3 weeks. If x-rays show no fracture and the pain has resolved, the cast can be left off. If the x-rays show no fracture and the patient continues to have pain, MRI should be done in a search for occult fracture.

Even with optimal cast treatment, some of these fractures will be complicated by delayed union or nonunion. Treatment in such cases consists of operation with bone grafting and internal fixation, usually with a screw (Figure 42–19). Some surgeons have advocated percutaneous screw fixation even for nondisplaced fractures. The advantages are shorter immobilization time and faster time to union (an average of 7 weeks versus 12 weeks in one study). This is somewhat controversial.

All displaced fractures should be treated with open reduction and internal fixation, either through a dorsal or a volar approach depending on the type of fracture. A bone graft from the distal radius or iliac crest is often used to increase healing potential or correct deformity, especially in the case of delayed union or late presentation. Most surgeons are using screw fixation, though under some circumstances pin fixation may be necessary.

Avascular necrosis of the proximal pole can occur even with adequate treatment but is more common when treatment is delayed. This is a difficult problem to treat. Some surgeons are using vascularized bone grafts to address this problem. In other cases, salvage procedures are necessary. Patients with long-standing scaphoid nonunions go on to develop early arthritis of the radioscaphoid joint secondary to altered mechanics of the wrist.

2. Fracture of the Lunate

The lunate is the carpal bone most likely to dislocate, but fractures are rare. Small dorsal or volar avulsion fractures can be treated in a splint or cast for 4 weeks.

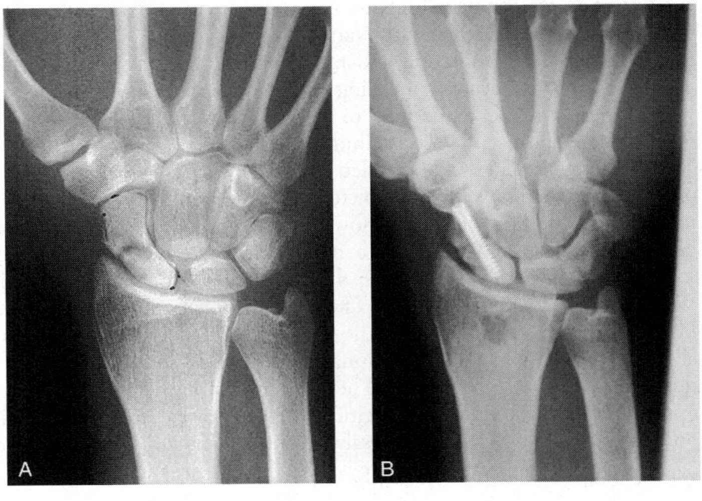

Figure 42–19. Scaphoid fracture. ***A:*** Scaphoid fracture nonunion. ***B:*** Open reduction and internal fixation of scaphoid nonunion.

The lunate has a tenuous blood supply and can also develop avascular necrosis, which is known as Kienböck's disease when it occurs in the lunate.

3. Fracture of the Hamate

This fracture generally occurs from a direct blow to the area such as occurs when swinging a baseball bat or golf club that suddenly comes to an abrupt stop as it encounters a firm surface. The fracture can occur through the body or proximal pole but by far the most common place is in the hook of the hamate. Patients present with ulnar-sided hand pain over the hamate hook. Fracture will often not be seen on routine wrist and hand radiographs. A carpal tunnel view should be obtained if this fracture is suspected. If the diagnosis is suspected clinically but the radiographs show no fracture, a CT scan should be obtained. Hook of the hamate fractures are best treated with excision as they do not heal with immobilization and remain painful.

4. Other Carpal Bone Fractures

Fractures can occur in any of the other carpal bones as well, but much less commonly. Triquetral avulsion or dorsal impaction fractures can occur from falls on the outstretched hand. Isolated fractures of the remaining carpal bones are rare and generally occur with high-energy trauma and other injuries.

5. Traumatic Carpal Instability

Severe injury to the wrist causing damage to the complex ligamentous structures may lead to carpal bone dissociation, carpal dislocations, and fracture dislocations.

Scapholunate dissociation secondary to disruption of the scapholunate ligament leads to altered kinematics of the wrist and early degenerative arthritis. Diagnosis is made by clinical examination and radiography. Patients will have a history usually of falling on an outstretched wrist. There will be tenderness to palpation over the scapholunate interval. If this injury is suspected, a "clenched fist view" should be added to the routine series of wrist radiographs. With a complete tear of the scapholunate ligament, this view will show abnormal gapping between the scaphoid and lunate bones. An increased scapholunate angle will be seen on the lateral projection. With partial tears there may be no radiographic changes. If the diagnosis is made acutely, the ligament can generally be repaired. Chronic scapholunate ligament disruptions do not do well with repair. There are reconstructive options prior to the onset of arthritic changes. However, once arthritis has developed, only salvage options exist.

In cases of severe high-energy trauma, perilunate dislocations, transscaphoid perilunate fracture-dislocations, and lunate dislocations can occur. Perilunate dislocations and lunate dislocations are on a continuum of the same type and mechanism of injury with increasing disruption of the ligamentous structures of the wrist. Patients present with severe wrist pain and swelling after trauma. Good-quality anteroposterior, lateral, and oblique radiographs must be obtained in order to make this diagnosis, which is missed sometimes even by experienced physicians. The relationship of the carpal bones to each other and to the distal radius must be carefully scrutinized. With lunate dislocation, on the lateral radiograph the lunate will be volar to the rest of the carpus and not in alignment with the distal radius. With a perilunate dislocation, the lunate remains in its normal position, articulating with the distal radius, but is angled volar ward, and the rest of the carpus is dislocated. On occasion these injuries occur and then reduce when the splint is applied in the field or when radiographs are taken. In this case, careful attention to the radiographs is necessary to make the diagnosis.

Immediate closed reduction under adequate anesthesia should be attempted. Even if closed reduction is successful, most surgeons feel that open reduction and fixation should be performed to restore the normal relationships of the carpal bones and distal radius. Closed reduction is sometimes not possible, and these patients should be taken emergently to the operating room for open reduction and fixation. If a scaphoid fracture is present with the dislocation, it should be repaired first—rigidly with a screw or pins—and attention then turned to restoring the carpal bone relationships and holding them with pins that will later be removed. Controversy exists as to whether these injuries should be approached volarly, dorsally, or via a combined approach.

Even with the best care, carpal bone and ligament injuries can be devastating, with long-term sequelae of pain, stiffness and early arthritis.

6. Management of Posttraumatic Arthritis of the Wrist

Arthritis of the wrist is treated in most cases only when it becomes painful. Intermittent splinting and anti-inflammatory medication can be helpful for mild cases in the low-demand wrist. There are many salvage options available depending on which joints are affected and how much pain the patient is having. If radioscaphoid arthritis is present and painful but the radiolunate joint is in good condition, a four-corner fusion can be a successful operation. The scaphoid is excised and the lunate, capitate, triquetrum, and hamate are fused. The uninvolved radiolunate joint now bears most of the force across the wrist. In cases of painful arthritis of multiple joints of the wrist, a total wrist arthrodesis provides a stable, pain-free wrist. However, the patient must be willing to accept the loss of motion. Proximal row carpectomy is a good option in the nonlaborer if the capitate is not involved. Total wrist arthroplasty has not gained wide acceptance because of its high reported failure rate over time.

Bond CD et al: Percutaneous screw fixation versus cast immobilization for non-displaced scaphoid fractures. J Bone Joint Surg Am 2001;83:483.

Cassidy C et al: Traumatic wrist disorders—what's in and what's out. AAOS 68th Annual Meeting Instructional Course, 2001.

Jupiter JB et al: Update on the management of traumatic and reconstructive problems of the scaphoid. AAOS 68th Annual Meeting Instructional Course, 2001.

Kozion SH: Peri-lunate injuries: diagnosis and treatment. J Am Acad Orthop Surg 1998;6:114.

Shin AY, Bishop AT, Berger RA: Vascularized pedicled bone grafts for disorders of the carpus. Techniques in Hand and Upper Extremity Surgery 1998;2:94.

Trumble TE et al: Intra-articular fractures of the distal aspect of the radius. AAOS Instructional Course Lecture, Vol 48, 1999.

FRACTURES & DISLOCATIONS ABOUT THE HAND

In evaluating any fracture of the metacarpals and phalanges, certain principles should be kept in mind. For suspected metacarpal fractures, anteroposterior, lateral, and oblique radiographs of the hand should be obtained. When a phalanx fracture of a specific digit is suspected, anteroposterior, lateral and oblique radiographs of just that digit will give better detail. Assessment of neurovascular status of the hand and digits must be done to rule out other injuries, including tendon injury. It is critical to assess rotation and angular deformity of the digit in both extension and flexion. The digit may look fine in extension but when the digits are flexed into a fist there can be rotational malalignment causing overlap of the digits. Fractures of the metacarpals and phalanges should not be immobilized for more than 3 weeks except under unusual circumstances. Fractures of the small bones of the hand heal more rapidly than fractures of larger bones, and prolonged immobilization can cause stiffness and loss of motion that can be difficult or impossible to regain. The safe position for splinting or casting of the hand is with slight wrist extension, the MP joints flexed 60–90 degrees, and the PIP and DIP joints extended.

1. Metacarpal Fractures

Metacarpal Neck Fractures

The most common metacarpal neck fracture is the "boxer's fracture" of the fifth metacarpal, usually caused by the fist striking a stationary object. Metacarpal neck fractures can occur in all of the metacarpals. There is controversy over what is an acceptable amount of angulation. Because there is less compensatory movement at the base of the second, third, and fourth metacarpals, less angulation is accepted in these digits. A general rule is that there should be no more than 10 degrees of dorsal angulation in the index metacarpal, 20 degrees in the middle metacarpal, 30 degrees in the ring metacarpal, and 40 degrees in the small finger metacarpal.

Stable, nondisplaced fractures can be treated in a cast that extends to the PIP joint of the involved digit. Unstable, displaced fractures may require closed reduction and pinning or open reduction with plates and screw. The advantage of open reduction and rigid fixation is that early range of motion exercises can be started almost immediately. The disadvantage is scarring and a possible need for later removal of the implants.

Metacarpal Shaft Fractures

These are described as transverse, oblique, or spiral. Angulations of more than 20 degrees in the ring metacarpal and 30 degrees in the small finger metacarpal should be reduced. Essentially no angulation is acceptable in the index and middle finger metacarpals since in would leave a cosmetically unacceptable prominence on the dorsum of the hand. Rotational deformity should be corrected and held with either percutaneous pins or plates and screws. Multiple metacarpal shaft fractures in the same hand are best treated by means of open reduction with internal fixation to prevent shortening and deformity.

Bennett's Fracture

This is an intra-articular fracture with subluxation at the base of the thumb metacarpal. The volar oblique ligament of the thumb remains attached to the small Bennett fragment (which lies volar and ulnar) and the trapezium. The remainder of the metacarpal slips radially, proximally, and dorsally as a result of the muscular and tendinous attachments. These injuries cannot be adequately treated with casting alone as they tend to slip. The treatment of choice is closed reduction and percutaneous pinning for reducible small fragments that are less than 25% of the joint surface. For larger fragments or those that cannot be reduced by closed means, open reduction and fixation with pins or a screw is preferable.

Fracture-Dislocation of the Small Finger Carpometacarpal Joint

Intra-articular fracture-dislocation of the small finger carpometacarpal joint is an inherently unstable fracture, difficult to assess on x-ray. Some say it is analogous to Bennett's fracture of the thumb. Most surgeons recommend either closed reduction and percutaneous pinning or open reduction and pinning. For extremely comminuted fractures where articular congruity cannot be restored, some advocate arthrodesis.

2. Phalanx Fractures

Fractures of the proximal and middle phalangeal shafts can be treated closed if they are nondisplaced and stable. Many of these fractures are unstable and require percutaneous pin fixation in order to avoid angular and rotational deformity. Intra-articular fractures with displacement pose a special challenge. Stiffness is always a problem, so that methods of fixation allowing immediate range of motion activity (such as rigid screw fixation, hinged external fixation; Figure 42–20) or traction splinting are recommended.

Distal phalanx tuft fractures do not usually cause much of a problem and require only a short period of splinting for comfort. Nail bed lacerations are often associated with these injuries and should be repaired. Unstable transverse fractures of the distal phalanx may require pin fixation. A special type of distal phalanx fracture is the bony mallet finger, which is avulsion of the terminal insertion of the extensor tendon. These can be treated with a dorsal extension splint of the DIP joint. If the joint is dislocated or if more than 50% of the articular surface is involved, surgical repair may be indicated.

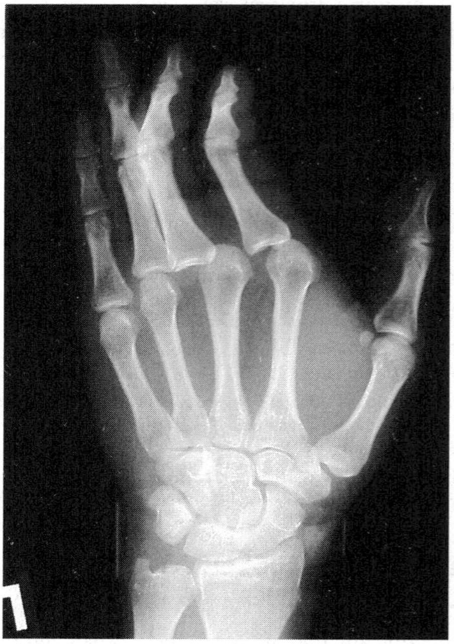

Figure 42–21. MP joint dislocation of the index and middle fingers.

3. Dislocations of the Digits

Dislocations of the PIP and MP joints are the most common dislocations in the digits. Painful swelling and deformity is the presentation, plus limited range of motion. Radiographs will confirm the diagnosis (Figure 42–21). Most often these injuries can be reduced closed by accentuating the deforming force and applying gentle pressure to reduce the joint. Dorsal MP joint dislocations sometimes cannot be reduced closed because of interposed volar plate. Distraction forces applied for reduction actually prevent reduction by causing a "noose effect" around the metacarpal neck. These dorsal MP dislocations require open reduction through either a dorsal or volar approach.

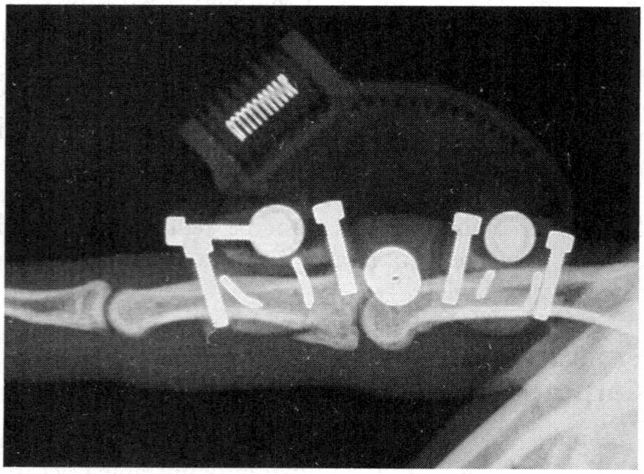

Figure 42–20. PIP hinged external fixation. Fixation of intra-articular fracture-dislocation of the PIP joint with a hinged external fixation device.

4. Ligamentous Injuries in the Digits

The ulnar collateral ligament of the thumb MP joint is the most commonly injured ligament in the digits. The acute injury is called skier's thumb, whereas chronic injury from repetitive trauma is referred to as gamekeeper's thumb. A sprain without instability can be treated with thumb spica casting or splinting for 4–6 weeks and then range of motion exercises. In the unstable situation, the ligament should be repaired—or reconstructed if adequate tissue is not available for repair.

The collateral ligaments of the other MP joints and the PIP joints can also be injured. In most cases these are treated with splinting or buddy taping to protect the ligament and early range of motion activity to prevent joint stiffness. In rare circumstances when instability remains, open repair may be in order.

Freeland AE, Benoist LA: Open reduction and internal fixation methods for fractures at the proximal interphalangeal joint. Hand Clin 1994;10:239.

Schuind F et al: Small external fixation devices for the hand and wrist. Clin Orthop 1993;293:77.

INJURIES OF THE HIP REGION

1. Fracture of the Femoral Neck

Fracture of the femoral neck occurs most commonly in patients over age 50. If displacement has occurred, the extremity is externally rotated and shortened. Motion of the hip causes pain. If the fragments are not displaced and the fracture is stable, pain at the extremes of passive hip motion may be the only significant finding. The fact that the patient can actively move the extremity often interferes with early diagnosis. Before treatment is instituted, anteroposterior and lateral films of excellent quality must be obtained. Gentle traction and internal rotation of the extremity while the anteroposterior film is exposed may provide a more favorable relation of fragments to demonstrate the fracture cleft.

Fractures may be classified as stable or unstable. Stable fractures include stress fractures and impacted fractures. The unstable category includes displaced and comminuted fractures.

Stable Fractures of the Femoral Neck

Patients with stress fractures or impacted fractures may have minimal groin pain and may be able to walk with some pain and a limp. No obvious deformity or shortening is apparent on physical examination, and for that reason the diagnosis may be elusive. If initial x-rays do not reveal the stress fracture, a repeat x-ray, radionuclide study, or MRI may be necessary to confirm the diagnosis. An impacted fracture is usually in valgus position. Impaction must be seen on both anteroposterior and lateral films for diagnosis.

Stress fractures can be treated by crutch ambulation to minimize weightbearing stress. The patient should be instructed not to place the leg in stressful positions or use it for leverage. If the fracture appears to be healing, partial weightbearing may be started at 6 weeks after injury, with progression to full weightbearing when the fracture is healed. Healing usually takes place in 3–6 months.

Impacted fractures may also be treated nonoperatively, but the tendency for displacement is much greater than in stress fractures. Most surgeons prefer to use internal fixation for impacted fractures to allow maintenance of reduction, earlier crutch ambulation, and earlier weightbearing. Multiple screw or pin fixation is in many cases the best treatment and should be secure enough to allow weightbearing immediately. Truly impacted fractures treated with internal fixation without disruption of the fracture have healing rates approaching 100%.

Unstable Fractures of the Femoral Neck

Displaced and comminuted femoral neck fracture can be a life-endangering injury, especially in elderly persons. Treatment is directed toward preservation of life and restoration of function to the hip joint. In most cases, reduction and internal fixation are the treatment of choice. Immobilization of this fracture by means of a plaster spica is unreliable. Definitive treatment by skeletal traction requires prolonged recumbency with constant nursing care and is associated with more numerous complications than early mobilization. Operative treatment usually consists of internal fixation or primary arthroplasty and should be done as soon as the patient is medically prepared for surgery. In general, the younger the patient, the more effort is justified to save the femoral head.

A. Internal Fixation

The goal of internal fixation is to preserve the femoral head fragment by providing a setting for bony healing of the fracture. The objective is to allow the patient as much general physical activity during healing as is compatible with the mechanics of fixation. To permit necessary preoperative evaluation of the patient when internal fixation is elected, initial treatment may be by balanced suspension, skeletal traction, and prompt closed reduction of the fracture. Persistent displacement may cause further compromise of the retinacular blood supply to the articular fragment.

Anatomic or near-anatomic reduction and firm fixation are desirable to provide optimal conditions for bone healing. Comminution at the fracture site, injury to the retinacular blood supply of the capital fragment, excessive stressing of the fracture site, and insecure fixation are some of the factors that lead to failure.

When the fragments are nondisplaced or minimally displaced, manipulation is unnecessary. Displacement may be corrected by closed reduction preliminary to fixation or by surgical exposure of the fragment site. Adequate closed reduction is usually obtained by traction and marked internal rotation of the extremity—frequently to 90 degrees. The fixation apparatus may consist of multiple screws applied percutaneously or more elaborate implants that require open operation. After operation, the patient does not require traction and may be mobilized immediately.

Depending upon the relative security of fixation, the extent of early weightbearing must be regulated until bone continuity is restored to the point where displacement of fragments is unlikely. Patients may be ambulatory on crutches or with a walker within a few days after operative treatment.

B. Primary Arthroplasty

In electing primary arthroplasty, the surgeon realizes that the main proximal fragment must be sacrificed because of injury to the blood supply, preexisting disease, or inability to obtain satisfactory reduction of the fracture for internal fixation.

When the acetabulum is undamaged or is not the site of preexisting disease, the commonly accepted technique is hemiarthroplasty using a femoral component (generally of the intramedullary type) that may or may not be stabilized by a grouting substance such as methylmethacrylate. In the rare circumstance when there is concomitant involvement of the acetabulum, total joint replacement may be justified. Primary head and neck resection may be indicated when there is preexisting infection or local tumor.

The most common sequelae of fracture of the femoral neck are redisplacement after reduction and internal fixation, failure of bone healing, and avascular necrosis of the head fragment. Avascular necrosis and associated collapse occur in 15–35% of these patients from interruption of the blood supply to the femoral neck at the time of injury. It is most likely to appear during the 2 years after fracture. Secondary osteoarthritis (posttraumatic arthritis) appears somewhat later and may be complicated by any of the common sequelae mentioned above. The most serious complication of any open operative treatment is infection.

2. Trochanteric Fractures

Fracture of the Lesser Trochanter

Isolated fracture of the lesser trochanter is quite rare but may develop as a result of the avulsion force of the iliopsoas muscle. It occurs commonly as a component of intertrochanteric fracture. Rarely, a symptomatic nonunion may require fragment fixation or excision. Avulsion fractures may also represent a pathologic fracture secondary to metastatic disease.

Fracture of the Greater Trochanter

Isolated fracture of the greater trochanter may be caused by direct injury or may occur indirectly as a result of the activity of the gluteus medius and gluteus minimus muscles. It occurs most commonly as a component of intertrochanteric fracture.

If displacement is less than 1 cm and there is no tendency to further displacement (determined by repeated x-ray examinations), treatment may be by bed rest with the affected extremity in balanced suspension until acute pain subsides. As rapidly as symptoms permit, activity can increase gradually to protracted weightbearing with crutches. Full weightbearing is permitted as soon as healing is apparent, usually in 6–8 weeks. If displacement is greater than 1 cm and increases on adduction of the thigh, extensive tearing of surrounding soft tissues may be assumed, and open reduction and internal fixation are indicated.

Intertrochanteric Fractures

These fractures occur most commonly among elderly persons, usually after a fall. The cleft of an intertrochanteric fracture extends upward and outward from the medial region of the junction of the neck and lesser trochanter toward the summit of the greater trochanter. Peritrochanteric fracture includes both trochanters and is likely to be comminuted (Figure 42–22).

It is important to determine whether comminution has occurred and the magnitude of displacement. These fractures may vary from fissure fracture without significant separation to severe comminution into four major fragments: head-neck, greater trochanter, lesser trochanter, and shaft. Displacement may be marked, with obvious extreme rotation and shortening of the extremity more severe than with femoral neck fractures.

These fractures are extracapsular and occur through cancellous bone that has a good blood supply. Healing occurs in 3–4 months, and lack of healing is uncommon.

Initial treatment of the fracture in the hospital can be by balanced suspension and, when indicated, by the addition of traction. The selection of definitive treatment—closed or operative techniques—depends in part upon the general condition of the patient and the type of fracture. Rates of illness and death are lower when the fracture is internally fixed, allowing for early mobilization. Operative treatment is indicated as soon as the patient is medically able to tolerate surgery.

If the patient is unable to tolerate anesthesia or if the fracture is too severely comminuted to permit internal fixation with good stability, the fracture may be treated by skeletal traction with a Kirschner wire through the proximal tibia. Within 3–4 months, healing is usually sufficient to allow the patient to be out of bed. Long-term traction is associated with many complications, including bedsores, pulmonary complications, deterioration of mental status, and varus position of the fracture.

Open reduction may be done electively or may be mandatory for optimal treatment. Reduction of the fracture can be accomplished by closed techniques or it can be an integral part of the open operation. Some surgeons do not prefer to anatomically reduce unstable fractures caused by comminution of the medial femoral cortex. It is argued by some authors that medial displacement of the upper end of the main distal fragment enhances mechanical stability (although it may cause concomitant varus deformity), and this advantageously permits earlier weightbearing and earlier healing. The chief objective of

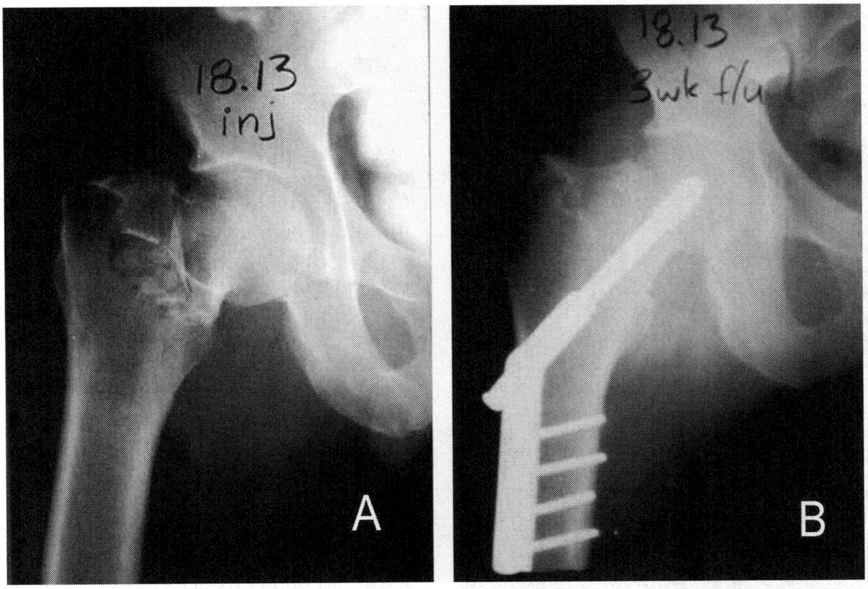

Figure 42–22. Comminuted intertrochanteric hip fracture. ***A:*** Anteroposterior radiograph. ***B:*** Anteroposterior radiograph after fixation with a compression hip screw and sideplate.

open operation is to provide sufficient fixation of the fragments by a metallic surgical implant so that the patient need not be confined to bed during the healing process.

The fixation most widely used is a sliding screw with a side plate. The screw can slide in the barrel of the side plate, allowing the fracture to impact. A fixed nail and side plate may cause the fracture to be "nailed apart" and contribute to lack of healing. As the fracture impacts, the nail cannot slide and may instead cut through the head of the femur.

Subtrochanteric Fracture

Subtrochanteric fracture due to severe trauma occurs below the level of the lesser trochanter at the junction of cancellous and cortical bone. It is most common in men during the active years of life. Soft tissue damage is extensive. The direction of the fracture cleft may be transverse or oblique. Comminution occurs, and the fracture may extend proximally into the intertrochanteric region or distally into the shaft.

Closed reduction should be attempted by continuous traction to bring the distal fragment into alignment with the proximal fragment. If comminution is not extensive and the lesser trochanter is not detached, the proximal fragment is often drawn into relative flexion, external rotation, and abduction by the predominant activity of the iliopsoas, gluteus medius, and gluteus minimus muscles.

Internal fixation, unless contraindicated, is now the treatment of choice. If conservative treatment is elected, the patient should be placed in distal femoral skeletal traction with the hip and knee flexed 90 degrees to counteract the deforming forces. Traction should be continued for 6–8 weeks in this position until the fracture is "sticky" and then progressively brought to a neutral position for another 6–8 weeks until clinical and radiographic signs of healing are present. Using a hip spica can be an alternative to traction.

Internal fixation is most widely favored. Temporary skeletal traction will maintain femoral length until definitive surgical treatment can be performed. This should be done early to allow mobilization and prevent malunion.

Closed intramedullary interlocking nails have gained popularity recently (Figure 42–23). Newer devices with intracephalic proximal interlocking allow fixation where conventional nails may be contraindicated. Fixation can also be obtained with nails of the Zickel type, blade plates or lag screws with long sideplates. Retrograde flexible nailing (Ender type) has also been used with less success in providing stability and rotational control.

The activity status after operative treatment depends upon the adequacy of internal fixation. If fixation is secure and the patient is agile and cooperative, ambulation on crutches (nonweightbearing or partial weightbearing) on

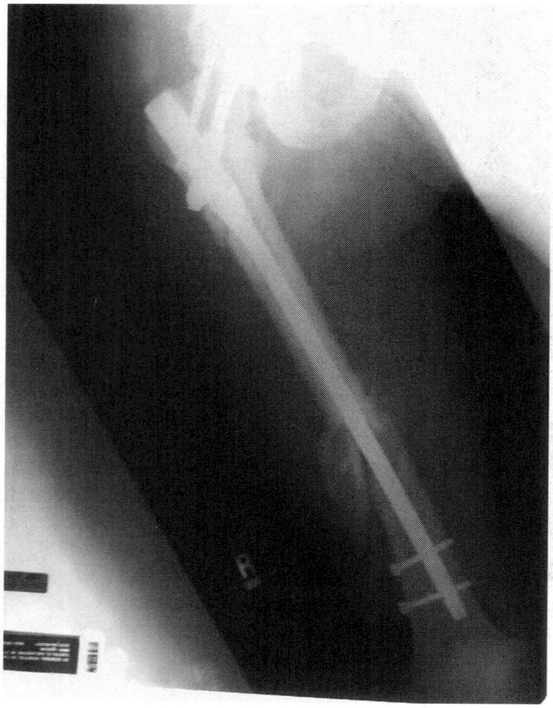

Figure 42–23. Subtrochanteric femur fracture with fracture of the distal third of the ipsilateral femoral shaft treated with a reconstruction type intramedullary nail.

the affected side may be allowed immediately after the operation. The fracture is usually healed at 3–4 months, but delayed union and nonunion are not uncommon. Hardware failure commonly occurs in these cases, requiring repeat internal fixation and bone grafting.

3. Traumatic Dislocation of the Hip Joint

Traumatic dislocation of the hip joint (Figure 42–24) may occur with or without fracture of the acetabulum or the proximal end of the femur. It is most common during the active years of life and is usually the result of severe trauma unless there is preexisting disease of the femoral head, acetabulum, or neuromuscular system. The head of the femur cannot be completely displaced from the normal acetabulum unless the ligamentum teres is ruptured or deficient from some unrelated cause. Traumatic dislocations can be classified according to the direction of displacement of the femoral head from the acetabulum.

Posterior Hip Dislocation

The head of the femur is usually dislocated posterior to the acetabulum while the thigh is flexed, as may occur in a head-on automobile collision when the driver's or passenger's knee is driven violently against the dashboard.

The significant clinical findings are shortening, adduction, and internal rotation of the extremity. Anteroposterior, transpelvic, and, if fracture of the acetabulum is demonstrated, oblique x-ray projections are required. Common complications are fracture of the acetabulum, injury to the sciatic nerve, and fracture of the head or shaft of the femur. The head of the femur may be displaced through a rent in the posterior hip joint capsule, or the glenoid lip may be avulsed from the acetabulum. The short external rotator muscles of the femur are commonly lacerated. Fracture of the posterior margin of the acetabulum can create instability.

If the acetabulum is not fractured or if the fragment is small, reduction by closed manipulation is indicated. General anesthesia provides maximum muscle relaxation and allows gentle reduction. Reduction should be achieved as soon as possible, preferably within the first few hours after injury as soon as the patient's general status has been adequately assessed. The main feature of reduction is traction in the line of deformity, followed by gentle flexion of the hip to 90 degrees with stabilization of the pelvis by an assistant. While manual traction is continued, the hip is gently rotated into internal and then external rotation to obtain reduction.

The success of reduction is determined immediately by anteroposterior and lateral x-rays. Interposition of capsule substance or bone fragments will be manifested by widening of the joint cleft. If x-rays are difficult to interpret, CT scan can be helpful in assessing concentricity of reduction. If reduction is adequate, the hip

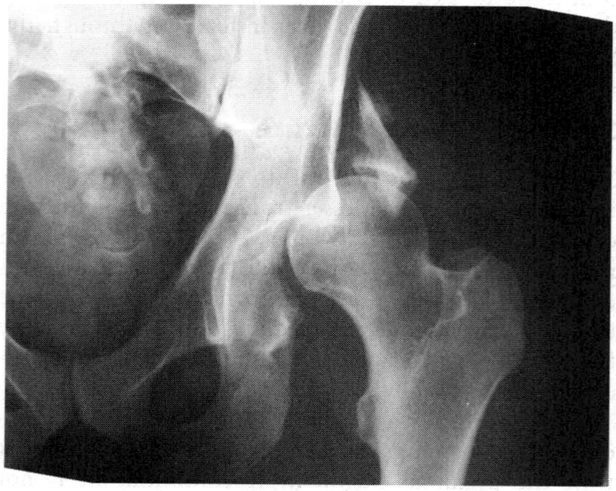

Figure 42–24. Posterior hip dislocation with concomitant fracture of the posterior wall and weightbearing dome of the acetabulum.

will usually be stable, with the extremity in extension and slight external rotation. Stability of the hip should be tested immediately after reduction by motion of the hip in flexion and adduction to assess the maximum limits of stability. A very easy manipulative reduction (eg, the hip "slides in" with very little effort) may suggest major instability and a potential for redislocation even though the hip is maintained in traction.

Postreduction treatment may be by immobilization in traction or balanced suspension or in a plaster spica cast. Since this is primarily a soft tissue injury, sound healing should occur in 4 weeks. Opinion differs on when unsupported weightbearing should be resumed. Some authors believe that disability caused by ischemic osteonecrosis of the femoral head is less likely when complete weightbearing is deferred for 6 months after injury; others believe that early loading is not harmful.

If the posterior or superior acetabulum is fractured, dislocation of the hip must be assumed to have occurred even though displacement is not present at the time of examination. Undisplaced fissure fractures may be treated initially by bed rest and avoidance of full weightbearing for 2 months. Frequent examination is necessary to make certain that the head of the femur has not become displaced from the acetabulum.

Minor fragments of the posterior margin of the acetabulum may be disregarded unless they are in the hip joint cavity. Larger displaced fragments often cannot be reduced adequately by closed methods. If the fragment is large and the hip is unstable following closed manipulation, open operation is indicated. The fragment is then placed in anatomic position and fixed with bone screws or a bone plate and screws.

After the operation, if fixation is tenuous because of severe comminution of the fracture, the patient is placed in bed with the extremity in balanced suspension with 5–8 kg of skeletal traction on the tibial tubercle for about 4–6 weeks until healing of the acetabular fracture is sound. If fixation is stable, the patient may be allowed out of bed in a few days with progression to ambulation on crutches that is nonweightbearing on the injured side. Full weightbearing is not permitted until healing is complete—a process that takes about 3–6 months.

Anterior Hip Dislocation

Anterior dislocation of the hip is much rarer than posterior dislocation. It usually occurs when the hip is extended and externally rotated at the time of impact. Associated fractures of the acetabulum and the femoral neck occur rarely. The femoral head usually remains lateral to the obturator externus muscle but can rarely be found beneath it (obturator dislocation) or under the iliopsoas muscle in contact with the superior pubic ramus (pubic dislocation).

The hip is classically flexed, abducted, and externally rotated. The femoral head is palpable anteriorly below the inguinal flexion crease. Anteroposterior and transpelvic lateral radiographic projections are usually diagnostic.

Closed reduction under general anesthesia is generally successful. Concentric reduction must be obtained. The patient starts mobilization within a few days when pain is tolerable. Active and passive hip motion, excluding external rotation, are encouraged, and the patient is usually fully weightbearing by 4–6 weeks.

Daum WJ: Traumatic posterior acetabular defects reconstructed with iliac crest autograft: a report of two cases. Clin Orthop 1993;291:188.

Desjardins AL et al: Unstable intertrochanteric fracture of the femur: a prospective randomised study comparing anatomical reduction and medial displacement osteotomy. J Bone Joint Surg Br 1993;75:445.

Eiskjaer S, Ostgard SE: Survivorship analysis of hemiarthroplasties. Clin Orthop 1993;286:206.

Hinton RY, Smith GS: The association of age, race, and sex with the location of proximal femoral fractures in the elderly. J Bone Joint Surg Am 1993;75:752.

Karachalios T et al: Reconstruction nailing for pathological subtrochanteric fractures with coexisting femoral shaft metastases. J Bone Joint Surg Br 1993;75:119.

Mullaji AB, Thomas TL: Low-energy subtrochanteric fractures in elderly patients: results of fixation with the sliding screw plate. J Trauma 1993;34:56.

Nilsson LT, Johansson A, Stromqvist B: Factors predicting healing complications in femoral neck fractures: 138 patients followed for 2 years. Acta Orthop Scand 1993;3;64:175.

Oransky M, Sanguinetti C: Surgical treatment of displaced acetabular fractures: results of 50 consecutive cases. J Orthop Trauma 1993;7:28.

Parfenchuck TA, Carter LW, Young TR: Ipsilateral fractures of the femoral neck and shaft. Orthop Rev 1993;22:356.

Pitsaer E, Samuel AW: Functional outcome after intertrochanteric fractures of the femur: does the implant matter? A prospective study of 100 consecutive cases. Injury 1993;24:35.

Ragnarsson JI et al: Instability and femoral head vitality in fractures of the femoral neck. Clin Orthop 1993;287:30.

Roffi RP, Matta JM: Unrecognized posterior dislocation of the hip associated with transverse and T-type fractures of the acetabulum. J Orthop Trauma 1993;7:23.

Schlickewei W et al: Hip dislocation without fracture: traction or mobilization after reduction? Injury 1993;24:27.

Shaw JA, Wilson S: Internal fixation of proximal femur fractures: a biomechanical comparison of the Gamma Locking Nail and the Omega Compression Hip Screw. Orthop Rev 1993;22:61.

Snorrason F, Karrholm J, Holmgren C: Fixation of cemented acetabular prostheses: the influence of preoperative diagnosis. J Arthroplasty 1993;8:83.

Swiontkowski MF: Intracapsular fractures of the hip: current concepts review. J Bone Joint Surg Am 1994;76:129.

Operations for Sequelae of Fractures & Dislocations of the Hip Region

A. Osteotomy

Osteotomy is usually performed in the predominantly cancellous intertrochanteric region, and the bone fragments are generally stabilized by a fixation device. An indication for osteotomy is correction of torsional or varus deformity. Supportive osteotomy is used to minimize displacing stresses at unhealed fracture sites. Abduction, adduction, or rotational osteotomy has been performed for relief of pain associated with ischemic osteonecrosis of the femoral head or secondary osteoarthritis. Although osteotomy preserves joint motion and provides stability, the prognosis for relief of pain is unpredictable.

B. Arthrodesis

Arthrodesis may be intra-articular, extra-articular, or a combination of both. Bone grafting to aid fusion and internal fixation to provide support at the coxofemoral relationship are elective supplemental features. Arthrodesis has been a favored operation as an adjunct in the control of chronic hip joint infection. When arthrodesis is bony—although articular pain is relieved and mechanical stability of the joint is ensured—added stress is placed on the lumber spine and knee joint. Pain from degeneration in those areas is a frequent result. The patient must also accept some disability because of loss of hip joint function.

C. Head & Neck Resection (Girdlestone Arthroplasty)

The indications for resection of the head and neck of the femur for treatment of fractures, dislocations, and fracture-dislocations have been frequently modified. This operation allows motion but causes significant shortening of the extremity and creates instability that usually requires one or two crutches for ambulation as well as a large shoe lift. Currently, its chief application is in the treatment of chronic hip joint infection. It is useful occasionally in the treatment of pathologic fracture of the proximal femur due to primary or metastatic tumors. Rarely is osteopenia or destruction of bone from causes other than those mentioned above so extensive that resection is preferable to an endoprosthesis

D. Total Hip Joint Replacement

Total hip joint replacement (Figure 42–25) has been widely accepted as an excellent operation to relieve the pain and dysfunction caused by arthritis of the hip. This technique implies substitution of at least the articular surfaces of both the acetabulum and the head of the femur by implants made of metal or plastic. The femoral component is usually made of cobalt-chrome alloy, stainless steel, or titanium. The acetabular constituent is usually made of polyethylene of very high molecular weight or a combination of a metal hemispherical shell that supports a liner of polyethylene, ceramic, or metal.

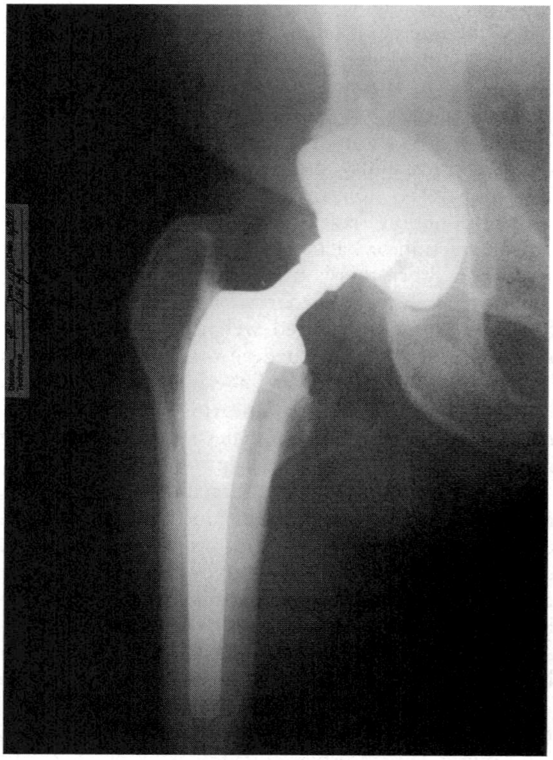

Figure 42–25. Hybrid total hip replacement with porous coated acetabular shell and cemented femoral stem performed for osteoarthritis.

The main indications for any type of hip arthroplasty are relief of incapacitating pain and restoration or improvement of joint function. The presence of joint sepsis is a contraindication to replacement arthroplasty.

Total hip joint replacement requires removal of the entire head of the femur and part of the femoral neck as well as extensive remodeling of the acetabulum. The femoral head and acetabular components are stabilized in bone either by a "press fit" or with polymethylmethacrylate cement. Total hip joint replacement has wider application in the treatment of posttraumatic arthritis resulting from fractures and dislocations of the hip joint in the adult than in their primary treatment. It is useful as a reconstructive procedure in the treatment of failure of the joint without infection. Success rates of over 90% have been reported. Because long-term reliability has not been established, the operation should be reserved for patients over age 50 unless specific factors warrant its use in younger persons.

Failure of total hip joint replacement can be caused by recurrent dislocation within the prosthesis complex, loosening of the components at the interface between the bone and the cementing substance, breakage of the femoral component, sepsis, and undetermined causes of disabling pain. The long-term effects of wear of the material and the effect of wear debris on the surrounding tissues have not been determined. Infection is the most serious complication; even if it is promptly discovered and vigorously treated, removal of the device complex may be necessary. Removal of the prosthesis leaves the patient with a severely shortened extremity and an unstable hip and necessitates indefinite use of crutch support for ambulation.

Many attempts have been made to develop prostheses that do not require such extensive removal of bone, so that if failure occurs major shortening and instability are less likely to develop. The younger the patient, the longer the time the prosthesis will be subjected to loading and wear. Thus, several revision arthroplasties over the patient's lifetime may be needed. Long-term failure of total hip arthroplasty has been linked to bony resorption around the implant from foreign particle wear debris (usually polyethylene) that causes activation of bone resorbing cells (osteoclasts). Newer formulations of polyethylene as well as alternative bearing surfaces and medical treatment (bisphosphonates) hold great promise to minimize endoprosthetic failure from these mechanisms.

E. Hemiarthroplasty (Endoprosthesis)

Hemiarthroplasty involves replacement of the femoral head and neck fragment and implies the presence of a normal or nearly normal acetabulum. The procedure is useful when the femoral head is extensively involved with a degenerative process or when treatment is required for unhealed femoral neck fracture. The femoral stem may be stabilized in the femoral canal by a "press fit" or with methylmethacrylate cement. The choice is dependent upon the patient's age and bone quality. The best results are obtained with patients who are motivated to participate in a vigorous rehabilitation program. Functional improvement continues over several years. Causes of failure include motion between the implant and cement or bone, acetabular deterioration secondary to wear, and postoperative infection.

F. Bipolar or Universal Endoprosthesis

These prostheses are intermediate steps between the conventional femoral head prosthesis (endoprosthesis) and the total hip joint prosthesis. The femoral head is removed and replaced with an endoprosthesis with the stem cemented or press-fit in the femoral intramedullary canal. A polyethylene liner is fixed in a metallic cup, and the edges of the liner are so fashioned that the socket "snap fits" on the head. The acetabulum is not altered. Motion occurs between the outer surface of the metallic cup and the articular surface of the acetabulum and between the head of the femoral prosthesis and the polyethylene liner. Theoretic advantages of this prosthesis are that there may be less erosion of the acetabulum than with an endoprosthesis alone, and if revision to the total hip joint is necessary later, only the cup may have to be replaced. One major disadvantage is that dislocation within the prosthetic complex is virtually impossible to reduce by closed manipulation. In addition, the polyethylene liner in a bipolar endoprosthesis may generate more polyethylene wear.

Gebhard JS et al: A comparison of total hip arthroplasty and hemiarthroplasty for treatment of acute fracture of the femoral neck. Clin Orthop 1992;282:123.

Jalovaara P et al: Treatment of hip fracture in Finland and Sweden: prospective comparison of 788 cases in three hospitals. Acta Orthop Scand 1992;63:531.

Kim YH, Oh JH, Koh YG: Salvage of neglected unstable intertrochanteric fracture with cementless porous-coated hemiarthroplasty. Clin Orthop 1992;277:182.

Moeckel BH et al: Modular hemiarthroplasty for fractures of the proximal part of the humerus. J Bone Joint Surg Am 1992;74:884.

Parker MJ: Internal fixation or arthroplasty for displaced subcapital fractures in the elderly? Injury 1992;23:521.

INFECTIONS ASSOCIATED WITH JOINT REPLACEMENTS

Infections that occur following joint replacement arthroplasty may be due to organisms introduced at surgery or may result from late hematogenous contamination. They are generally more serious than infections that follow fractures. The implanted prosthesis is intended to be a permanent substitute for a failed joint and not a temporary fixation, as is used for fracture healing. Removal of the prosthesis shortens the limb and produces instability unless arthrodesis is achieved, fusing the adjacent bones to prevent motion. Removal of a prosthetic joint without arthrodesis leaves a so-called "excisional arthroplasty," which may offer an acceptable salvage. Arthroplasty following removal of a total hip prosthesis is often called Girdlestone arthroplasty after the surgeon who proposed hip joint excision as primary treatment for certain disorders. While such a salvage procedure may be well tolerated, crutches are usually required and pain is a frequent problem. Furthermore, even removal of all of the implanted material may fail to cure the infection.

It is sometimes possible to control infection and repeat the prosthetic arthroplasty. However, early failure rates tend to be at least 15%, and questions remain about long-term results following revision arthroplasty for infection. Chronic oral antibiotic treatment—to suppress rather than cure infection—may be a reasonable alternative to removal or replacement of the prosthesis for appropriately selected patients.

Treatment of infected joint replacements depends upon the time of occurrence, the virulence of the infecting organism, and the mechanical stability of the prosthesis. Infection must be suspected whenever pain develops following prosthetic arthroplasty. Loosening of the prosthetic components within their bony seats may be due to infection, mechanical failure, or both. Either loosening or infection may cause pain. Relatively avirulent organisms cause infection with a low-grade smoldering course that slowly spreads through the bone adjacent to the prosthesis. Aspiration for culture and sensitivity testing is essential for early diagnosis. Treatment requires surgery and skillful antibiotic management. If the prosthesis is loose, it will require removal, which is necessary for adequate debridement of most chronic infections. All foreign material and infected granulation tissue must be debrided. Viable bone should be preserved. Currently, a hip spacer composed of antibiotic containing methylmethacrylate achieves high local antibiotic concentrations while preserving soft tissue tension around the joint. Wound closure over drains, 4–6 weeks of intravenous antibiotic treatment to achieve adequate serum bactericidal levels (usually 1:8 dilution or more), and adequate mechanical support of the limb are advised. Following removal of a total hip prosthesis, an antibiotic cement spacer, is often placed, and so traction is rarely needed. Decisions must be made about whether or not to replace the removed prosthesis and, if replacement is chosen, whether to proceed immediately or defer reimplantation for weeks or months until the wound is quiescent. Two-stage reimplantation of an infected total hip prosthesis may be more successful than single-stage reimplantation, but this remains controversial. Adding antibiotics to the acrylic cement used to seat prosthetic components is another adjunct that appears to improve the success rate of total hip revision for infection.

Beck-Sague CM et al: Outbreak of surgical wound infections associated with total hip arthroplasty. Infect Control Hosp Epidemiol 1992;13:526.

Fitzgerald RH Jr: Total hip arthroplasty sepsis: Prevention and diagnosis. Orthop Clin North Am 1992;23:259.

Schmalzried TP et al: Etiology of deep sepsis in total hip arthroplasty: the significance of hematogenous and recurrent infections. Clin Orthop 1992;280:200.

FRACTURE OF THE SHAFT OF THE FEMUR

Fracture of the shaft of the femur (Figure 42–26) usually occurs as a result of severe trauma. Indirect violence, especially torsional stress, is likely to cause spiral fractures that extend proximally or, more commonly, distally into the metaphysial region. Most are closed fractures; open fracture is often the result of compounding from within. Extensive soft tissue injury, bleeding, and shock are commonly present.

The most significant features are severe pain in the thigh and deformity of the lower extremity. Surgical shock is likely to be present, as several units of blood may be lost into the thigh with only moderate swelling becoming apparent. Careful x-ray examination in at least two planes is necessary to determine the exact site and configuration of the fracture cleft. The hip and knee should be examined and x-rays obtained to look for associated injury. A femoral neck fracture may occur in association with a femur fracture and if overlooked can increase patient morbidity.

Injuries to the sciatic nerve and to the superficial femoral artery and vein are not common but must be recognized promptly. Surgical shock and secondary anemia are the most important early complications. Later complications are those of prolonged recumbency, joint stiffness, malunion, nonunion, leg-length discrepancy, and infection.

Treatment

A. Closed Treatment

Treatment depends upon the age and medical status of the patient as well as the site and configuration of the fracture. Closed treatment of femoral shaft fractures in adults is rarely indicated. Skeletal traction is generally the most effective form of closed treatment. However, 2–3 months of traction are often required, followed by external plaster or brace support. Acceptable alignment may be difficult to maintain, and joint stiffness is frequent. Other complications of prolonged recumbency like pressure sores and deep vein thrombosis can have disastrous consequences. Fractures of the distal femoral shaft are more suitable for cast-brace treatment. After about 6 weeks in traction, the patient may be placed in a cast-brace (long-leg cast with a hinged knee) to allow early knee motion and progressive weightbearing.

B. Operative Treatment

Most fractures in the middle third of the femur can be internally fixed by an intramedullary rod. Intramedullary fixation of femoral shaft fractures allows immediate mobilization of the patient, more anatomic alignment, improved knee function by decreasing the time spent in traction, and a substantial decrease in the cost of hospitalization.

The procedure may be performed open or "blind." In open nailing, the fracture site is opened and the nail is driven retrograde from the fracture site into the proximal fragment. The fracture is then reduced and the

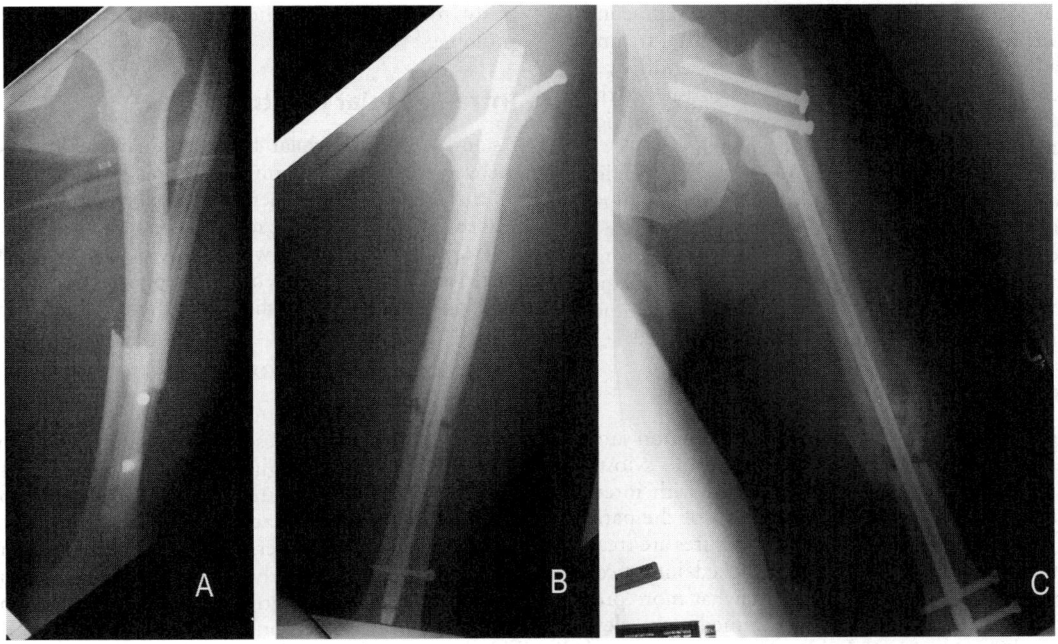

Figure 42–26. Femoral shaft fracture. ***A:*** Anteroposterior x-ray showing fracture of the midshaft of the femur. ***B:*** Anteroposterior x-ray after closed reduction and intramedullary fixation using an antegrade titanium locked nail. ***C:*** Anteroposterior x-ray showing fixation of a midshaft femoral fracture and ipsilateral femoral neck fracture with a retrograde intramedullary nail.

nail driven across the fracture into the distal fragment. This requires a large incision and major manipulation of the fracture fragments, with significant blood loss.

In blind nailing, the fracture is reduced by closed manipulation on the fracture table under fluoroscopic control. An 8-cm to 10-cm incision is made proximal to the greater trochanter, and the nail is inserted through the trochanteric notch down into the intramedullary canal. The fracture site is not opened. Blind nailing decreases the chance of infection and nonunion by decreasing the amount of soft tissue dissection necessary and by leaving the fracture site closed.

If the fracture is comminuted, interlocking nails can be used to maintain length by increased fixation proximally and distally. These may allow patients early mobilization even with comminuted femoral shaft fractures. If there is extensive soft tissue loss surrounding the fracture, stability of the bone fragments may be achieved with an external fixation device.

Complications of this procedure usually involve technical problems at the time of surgery, resulting in malalignment or shortening from choosing a rod that is too short or too narrow. Infection can occur after any open procedure but is very uncommon in blind nailing. Occasionally, a painful bursa may develop over the proximal end of the nail that causes discomfort when the patient sits or walks. The rod may be removed after healing is complete—usually after 1 year to $1^1/_2$ years. The healing rate of femoral shaft fractures in general is very high and approaches 100% after blind nailing.

Benirschke SK et al: Closed interlocking nailing of femoral shaft fractures: assessment of technical complications and functional outcomes by comparison of a prospective database with retrospective review. J Orthop Trauma 1993;7:118.

Hajek PD et al: The use of one compared with two distal screws in the treatment of femoral shaft fractures with interlocking intramedullary nailing: a clinical and biomechanical analysis. J Bone Joint Surg Am 1993;75:519.

Parfenchuck TA, Carter LW, Young TR: Ipsilateral fractures of the femoral neck and shaft. Orthop Rev 1993;22:356.

Wu CC et al: Treatment of segmental femoral shaft fractures. Clin Orthop 1993;287:224.

INJURIES OF THE KNEE REGION

1. Fractures of the Distal Femur

Supracondylar Fracture of the Femur

These fractures involve the distal metaphysis and epiphysis of the femur. It is important to distinguish between extra-articular and intra-articular supracondylar femur fractures (Figure 42–27). The distal fragment is usually rotated into extension from traction by the gastrocnemius muscles. The distal end of the proximal fragment is apt to perforate the overlying quadriceps and may penetrate the suprapatellar pouch.

The distal fragment may impinge on the popliteal neurovascular bundle, and an immediate thorough neurovascular examination is mandatory. Absence or marked decrease of pedal pulses is an indication for immediate reduction. If this fails to restore adequate circulation, an arteriogram should be obtained immediately and the vascular lesion repaired as indicated.

Extra-articular Fractures

For simple fracture patterns, closed reduction under general anesthesia is occasionally successful. Most of these fractures, however, are best treated with internal fixation, which allows early mobilization of the patient and of the neighboring joints. Most fractures are treated with internal fixation. Closed interlocked intramedullary nailing is recommended for somewhat more proximal fractures. An interlocked intramedullary device introduced in a retrograde fashion from the intercondylar notch has shown promising results. Most fractures are best treated with open reduction and internal fixation with screws and plates and screwplate devices. Skeletal traction is reserved for patients for whom surgery is contraindicated and is fraught with all the previously mentioned complications that can accompany prolonged recumbency.

Intra-articular Fractures

As for all intra-articular fractures, maximal functional recovery of the knee joint requires anatomic reduction of the articular components. Closed reduction of displaced fractures is almost never successful. Nondisplaced fractures can be treated with a cast brace for about 12 weeks or with percutaneous pinning or open internal fixation, which allows earlier mobilization of the joint.

Intercondylar Fractures

These comminuted fractures of the distal femoral epiphysis are classically described as T or Y fractures according to the configuration of the articular fragments. Displaced fractures are best treated by open reduction—to restore anatomic alignment of the articular surface—and by internal fixation using lag screws and plates to allow early motion. Even if anatomic alignment is achieved, joint stiffness, pain, and posttraumatic arthritis are not uncommon outcomes.

Condylar Fractures

Isolated fractures of the lateral or medial femoral condyles are rare. They usually result from varus or valgus stress to the knee joint with possible associated liga-

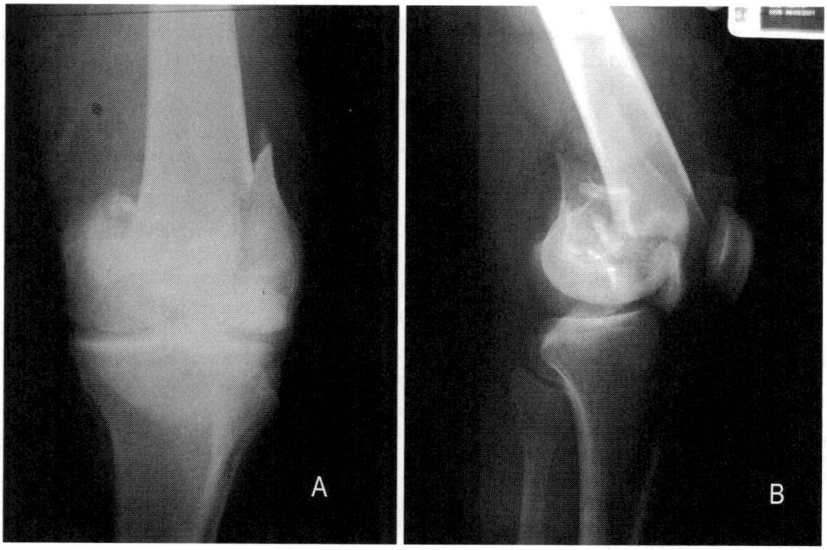

Figure 42–27. A: Anteroposterior radiograph demonstrating a comminuted supracondylar femur fracture with intra-articular extension. ***B:*** Lateral radiograph.

mentous injuries to the knee. Fractures of the posterior portion of one or the other condyle in the frontal plane can also be seen.

Closed reduction of displaced fragments is very rarely successful. Open reduction with screws is usually indicated. If fixation is solid, postoperative motion is started immediately. Weightbearing is allowed at 3 months when clinical and radiographic healing is present.

2. Fracture of the Patella

Transverse Fracture of the Patella

Transverse fracture of he patella is the result of indirect violence, usually with the knee in semiflexion. Fracture may be due to sudden voluntary contraction of the quadriceps muscles or sudden forced flexion of the leg when these muscles are contracted. The level of fracture is most often in the middle. The extent of tearing of the patellar retinacula depends upon the degree of force of the initiating injury. The activity of the quadriceps muscles causes displacement of the proximal fragment; the magnitude of displacement is dependent upon the extent of the tear of the quadriceps expansion.

Swelling of the anterior knee region is caused by hemarthrosis and hemorrhage into the soft tissues overlying the joint. If displacement is present, the defect in the patella can be palpated, and active extension of the knee is lost.

Open reduction is indicated if the fragments are offset or separated more than 2–3 mm. The fragments must be accurately repositioned to prevent early posttraumatic arthritis of the patellofemoral joint. If the minor fragment is small (no more than 1 cm in length) or severely comminuted, it may be excised and the rectus or patellar tendon (depending upon which pole of the patella is involved) sutured directly to the major fragment. If the fragments are approximately the same size, repair by wire cerclage or figure-of-eight wire is preferred. Accurate reduction of the articular surface must be confirmed by lateral x-rays taken intraoperatively.

Comminuted Fracture of the Patella

Comminuted fracture of the patella is caused only by direct violence. Little or no separation of the fragments occurs because the quadriceps expansion is not extensively torn. Severe injury may cause extensive comminution of the articular cartilages of both the patella and the opposing femur. If comminution is not severe and displacement is insignificant, immobilization for 8 weeks in a plaster cylinder extending from the groin to the supramalleolar region is sufficient.

Severe comminution requires excision of the patella and repair of the defect by imbrication of the quadriceps expansion. Excision of the patella can result in decreased strength, pain in the knee, and general restriction of activity.

Tear of the Quadriceps Tendon

Tear of the quadriceps tendon occurs most often in patients over age 40. Preexisting attritional disease of the tendon is apt to be present, and the causative injury may be minor. The tear commonly results from sudden deceleration, such as stumbling, or slipping on a wet surface. A small flake of bone may be avulsed from the superior pole of the patella, or the tear may occur entirely through tendinous and muscle tissue.

Pain may be noted in the anterior knee region. Swelling is due to hemarthrosis and extravasation of blood into the soft tissues. The patient is unable to extend the knee completely. X-rays may show avulsion of a bit of bone from the superior patella.

Operative repair is recommended for complete tear. If treatment is delayed until partial healing has occurred, the suture line can be reinforced by transplantation of the iliotibial band from the upper area of the tibia.

Tear of the Patellar Ligament

The same mechanism that causes tears of the quadriceps tendon, transverse fracture of the patella, or avulsion of the tibial tuberosity may also cause tear of the patellar ligament. The characteristic finding is proximal displacement of the patella. A bit of bone may be avulsed from the lower pole of the patella if the tear takes place in the proximal patellar tendon.

Operative treatment is necessary for complete tear. The ligament is resutured to the patella, and any tear in the quadriceps expansion is repaired. The extremity should be immobilized for 8 weeks in a tubular plaster cast extending from the groin to the supramalleolar region. Guarded exercises may then be started.

Dislocation of the Patella

Acute traumatic dislocation of the patella should be differentiated from episodic recurrent dislocation, since the latter condition is likely to be associated with occult organic lesions. When this injury occurs alone, it may be due to direct violence or muscle activity of the quadriceps, and the direction of dislocation of the patella is usually lateral. Spontaneous reduction is apt to occur if the knee joint is extended; if so, the clinical findings may consist merely of hemarthrosis and localized tenderness over the medial patellar retinaculum. Gross instability of the patella, which can be demonstrated by physical examination, indicates that injury to the soft tissues of the medial aspect of the knee has been extensive. Recurrent episodes require operative repair for effective treatment.

Dislocation of the Knee Joint

Traumatic dislocation of the knee joint is uncommon. It is caused by severe trauma. Displacement may be transverse or torsional. Complete dislocation can occur only after extensive tearing of the supporting ligaments and is apt to cause injury to the popliteal vessels or the tibial and peroneal nerves.

Signs of neurovascular injury below the site of dislocation are an absolute indication for prompt reduction, preferably under general anesthesia, since failure of circulation will undoubtedly result in gangrene of the leg and foot. Axial traction is applied to the leg to obtain reduction. If pedal pulses do not return promptly, patency of the popliteal vessels should be investigated immediately by angiography. Even if pulses do return, angiography is usually indicated to rule out an intimal tear of the vessel. Inadequate assessment and treatment of the vascular injuries can lead to an amputation rate of 50%. If a vascular injury is confirmed, repair should be started as soon as the patient's general status allows. Ischemia of more than 4 hours is associated with a poor prognosis for limb salvage. Prophylactic fasciotomy of the leg compartments should be performed at the time of vascular repair to eliminate the compartment syndrome caused by postischemic edema.

Anatomic reduction of uncomplicated dislocation should be attempted. If impinging soft tissue cannot be removed by closed manipulation, arthrotomy is indicated. After reduction, repair of the major ligamentous injuries may be performed, but this should not be done if the time and dissection necessary will further jeopardize survival of the limb. The extremity should be immobilized in a plaster cast extending from the inguinal region to the toes, with the knee in slight flexion. A window should be cut in the plaster over the dorsum of the foot to allow for frequent determination of dorsalis pedis artery pulsation. In anteroposterior dislocations, adequacy of reduction should be assessed at frequent intervals during the first 3–4 weeks to rule out posterior subluxation. If subluxation occurs, the knee joint must be reduced and placed in an external fixation device. After 8 weeks of immobilization, the knee can be protected by a long-leg brace. Intensive quadriceps exercises are necessary to minimize functional loss.

Appel MH, Seigel H: Treatment of transverse fractures of the patella by arthroscopic percutaneous pinning. Arthroscopy 1993;9:119.

Braun W et al: Indications and results of nonoperative treatment of patellar fractures. Clin Orthop 1993;289:197.

Rasul AT Jr, Fischer DA: Primary repair of quadriceps tendon ruptures: results of treatment. Clin Orthop 1993;289:205.

Schenck RC Jr, Heckman JD: Injuries of the knee. Clin Symp 1993;45:1.

Shrewing DJ, Meggitt BF: Fractures of the distal femur treated with the AO dynamic condylar screw. J Bone Joint Surg Br 1992;74:122.

Tucker JB, Corsetti J, Gregg JR: Arthroscopically assisted proximal quadricepsplasty for patellar instability. Clin Sports Med 1993; 12:81.

INJURIES TO THE LIGAMENTS, MENISCI, & CARTILAGE OF THE KNEE JOINT

Internal derangement of the knee joint mechanism is usually caused by trauma but can also result from overuse. Injuries to the ligaments, cartilage, and meniscus commonly occur as combined lesions.

X-rays are typically the first-line radiographic modality but are often normal in suspected ligament or cartilage injury. Arthroscopy and MRI are valuable adjuncts in diagnosis when the usual methods are inconclusive.

Arthroscopy is a valuable adjunct to the history, physical examination, and x-ray studies for evaluation of the knee joint. The arthroscope introduced into the knee joint through a small stab incision allows examination of most structures inside the knee without major surgical exploration.

Arthroscopy can be helpful in diagnosis of any confusing knee problem, but MRI has largely replaced arthroscopy for the diagnosis of injuries to the menisci and ligaments. MRI also assists with preoperative confirmation of a clinical diagnosis (eg, patients with anterior cruciate tears, meniscal tear, or chondromalacia) and for follow-up evaluation after therapy.

Surgical procedures such as meniscus repair, meniscectomy, synovial biopsy, or removal of loose bodies can be performed through the arthroscope with minimal postoperative morbidity compared with open procedures. However, this is a demanding technique and requires considerable experience for good results.

Injury to the Menisci

Injury to the medial meniscus is the most frequent internal derangement of the knee joint. Clinical findings after acute injury are swelling, pain, and varying degrees of restriction of flexion or extension. True locking (inability to fully extend the knee) is highly suggestive of meniscal tear. A marginal tear permits displacement of the medial fragment into the intercondylar region (bucket handle tear) and prevents either complete extension or complete flexion. Motion may cause pain over the anteromedial or posteromedial joint line. Tenderness can often be elicited at the point of pain. Forcible rotation of the foot with the knee flexed to a right angle may cause pain over the medial joint line. If symptoms have persisted for 2–3 weeks and the patient avoids weightbearing on the knee, weakness and atrophy of the quadriceps femoris may be present. Injury to the lateral meniscus is less common but may also cause mechanical blockage of joint motion. Pain and tenderness may be present over the lateral joint line, and MRI is the imaging modality of choice for diagnosing medial and lateral meniscus tears.

Initial treatment may be conservative. Swelling and pain can be relieved by aspiration, and younger patients usually prefer to be ambulatory on crutches. Isometric quadriceps exercises should be performed frequently throughout the day with the knee in maximum extension, and the emphasis should be placed on restoring range of motion. Physical therapy and nonsteroidal anti-inflammatory drugs are helpful.

Arthroscopy with either meniscectomy or meniscus repair is advisable for recurrent or persistent "locking," recurrent effusion, or pain. Isometric quadriceps exercises and range of motion exercises are started immediately and are gradually increased in frequency. As soon as the patient is able to perform these exercises comfortably, graded resistance maneuvers should be started. Exercises should be continued until motion and strength is equal to the other healthy knee.

Injury to the Ligaments

Ligaments in general prevent displacement or angulation beyond its normal envelope of motion. When the knee is in full extension, the collateral ligaments are taut; in flexion, only the anterior fibers of the tibial collateral ligament are taut.

A. Medial Collateral Ligament

This ligament—often referred to as the tibial collateral ligament—is the primary restraint to valgus. Forced abduction of the leg at the knee causes injury varying from complete rupture to tearing of a few fibers of the ligament. A bit of bone may be avulsed from its femoral or tibial attachment.

A history of a twisting injury at the knee with valgus strain can usually be obtained. Pain is present over the medial aspect of the knee joint. In severe injury, joint effusion may be present. Tenderness can be elicited at the site of the lesion. When only an isolated ligamentous tear is present, x-ray examination may not be helpful unless it is made while valgus stress is applied.

Treatment of an incomplete tear consists of protection from further injury while healing progresses in a brace that allows motion but protects the knee from valgus injury. It may be helpful to bend the brace into varus to take load off of the ligament.

Tear of the medial collateral ligament is frequently associated with other lesions, such as tear of the medial meniscus, rupture of the anterior cruciate ligament, or fracture of the lateral condyle of the tibia. Bony injury is more common in young patients.

B. Lateral Collateral Ligament

Tear of the lateral collateral ligament is often associated with injury to surrounding structures, eg, the popliteus muscle tendon or the iliotibial band. Avulsion of the apex of the fibular head may occur, and the peroneal nerve may be injured.

Pain and tenderness are present over the lateral aspect of the knee joint, and hemarthrosis may be present. X-rays may show bone avulsion from the fibular head.

The treatment of partial tear is similar to that described for partial tear of the medial collateral ligament. If complete tear is suspected, healing is rare without operative measures, and exploration and reconstruction will probably be required.

C. Anterior Cruciate Ligament

The function of the anterior cruciate ligament is prevention of anterior displacement of the tibia. Injury to the anterior cruciate ligament is often associated with injury to the menisci or the medial collateral ligament. The cruciate ligament may be avulsed with part of the tibial tubercle (Figure 42–28), but it usually ruptures within the substance of its fibers.

The characteristic clinical sign of tear of the anterior cruciate ligament is a positive anterior drawer sign: the knee is flexed to 90 degrees and pulled forward, and if excessive anterior excursion of the proximal tibia (in comparison with the opposite normal knee) occurs, tearing of the anterior ligament is suspected. Other tests include the Lachman test (anterior drawer with the knee flexed 20 degrees) and the pivot shift test. MRI is very accurate for the diagnosis of these injuries. Reconstruction is usually required for young active patients who wish to participate in sports that call for sudden cutting or twisting movements. Reconstruction is delayed until full range of motion is obtained.

With avulsion, displaced tibial bone is present, and attachment of the fragment in anatomic position by arthrotomy or arthroscopy is necessary. When the fragment of bone is large, displaced, and not treated until several weeks after injury, excision of the fragment and reinsertion of the ligament may be necessary to eliminate the blocking effect of the bone fragment and permit recovery of function.

D. Posterior Cruciate Ligament

Tear of the posterior ligament may occur within its substance or by avulsion of a fragment of bone at its tibial attachment. Tear of the posterior cruciate ligament can be diagnosed by the posterior "drawer" sign: The knee is flexed at a right angle, and the upper tibia is pushed backward; if excessive posterior excursion of the proximal tibia can be noted, tear of the posterior ligament is likely. MRI is very accurate for diagnosis of these injuries.

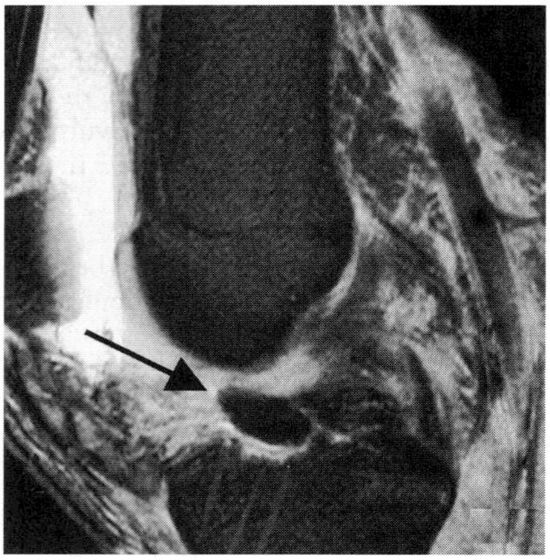

Figure 42–28. Lateral T1-weighted MRI image showing an acute rupture of the anterior cruciate ligament (arrow).

Treatment is directed primarily at the associated injuries and maintenance of competency of the quadriceps musculature. Primary repair of tears within the fibers is difficult and of dubious value. Open reduction and fixation of a fragment of tibia with the attached ligament is feasible and is apt to restore functional competency of the ligament.

Cartilage Injury

Damage to the cartilage is common with trauma to the knee and should be differentiated from osteoarthritis. Developments in cartilage transplantation, including autograft and allograft tissue, have greatly improved the prognosis for these injuries. Arthroscopy and MRI are required for accurate diagnosis (Figure 42–29). Cartilage is biopsied from the knee, cultured, and then reimplanted at a later date.

Ligamentous Reconstruction of the Knee

Knee joint instability may be (1) single plane (medial, lateral, posterior, or anterior), (2) rotatory, or (3) a combinations of the two. To speak of repair of ligaments denotes treatment of acute injuries, whereas the term reconstruction is reserved for treatment of ligamentous laxity several months after injury.

Reconstructive procedures to replace the function of the anterior and posterior cruciate ligament include use of a portion of autograft or allograft tendon introduced through drill holes in the proximal tibia and the posterior femur.

Indications for major reconstruction of knee ligaments depend on the patient's age and activity level and the status of the articular cartilage within the knee. Early results of these procedures are often excellent, but the integrity of the repair tends to deteriorate after 2–5 years.

Andriacchi TP, Birac D: Functional testing in the anterior cruciate ligament-deficient knee. Clin Orthop 1993;288:40.

De Smet AA et al: Diagnosis of meniscal tears of the knee with MR imaging: effect of observer variation and sample size on sensitivity and specificity. AJR Am J Roentgenol 1993;160:555.

DiStefano V: Anterior cruciate ligament reconstruction: autograft or allograft? Clin Sports Med 1993;12:1.

Frank CB, Jackson DW. The science of reconstruction of the anterior cruciate ligament. J Bone Joint Surg Am 1997;79:1556.

Gillquist J: Repair and reconstruction of the ACL: is it good enough? Arthroscopy 1993;9:68.

Halling AH, Howard ME, Cawley PW: Rehabilitation of anterior cruciate ligament injuries. Clin Sports Med 1993;12:329.

Jackson DW et al: Cartilage substitutes: overview of basic science and treatment options. J Am Acad Orthop Surg 2001;9:37.

Newman AP, Daniels AU, Burks RT: Principles and decision making in meniscal surgery. Arthroscopy 1993;9:33.

Woo SL, Livesay GA, Engle C: Biomechanics of the human anterior cruciate ligament: muscle stabilization and ACL reconstruction. Orthop Rev 1992;21:935.

FRACTURES OF THE PROXIMAL TIBIA

1. Fractures of the Tibial Plateau

Fractures of the tibial plateau (Figure 42–30) account for about 1% of all fractures. As with most orthopedic injuries, they occur primarily in two demographic groups: younger patients sustaining high-energy injuries and elderly patients as a result of minor trauma.

Mechanism of Injury

Fractures of the tibial plateau occur as a result of a combination of axial compression and strong valgus or varus

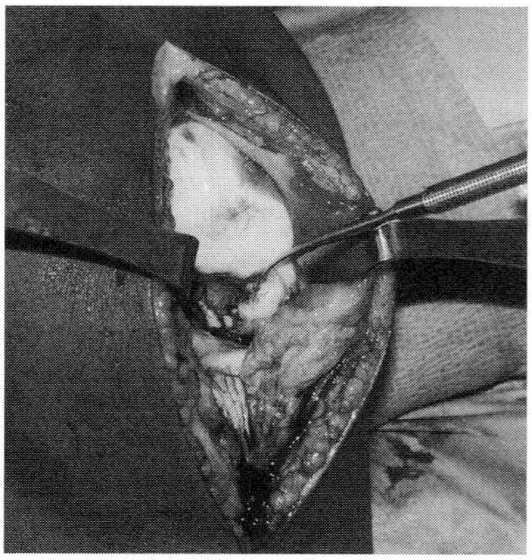

Figure 42–29. Intraoperative photograph showing a full-thickness cartilage injury.

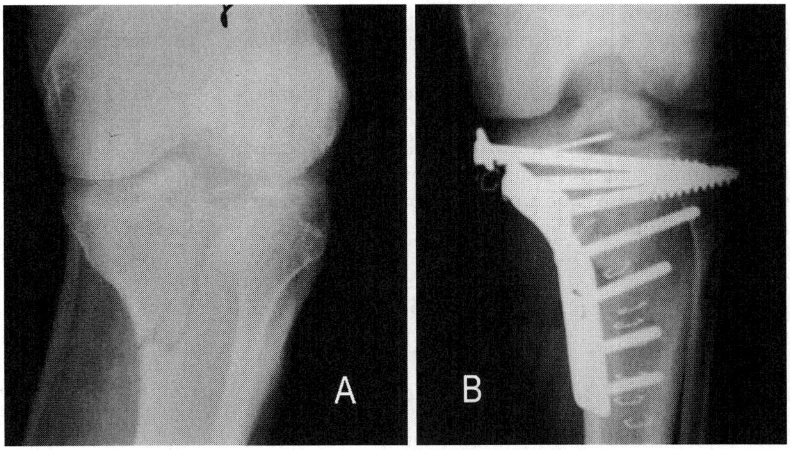

Figure 42–30. Schatzker II tibial plateau fracture. ***A:*** Anteroposterior radiograph. ***B:*** Radiograph after fixation with lateral plate and bone grafting.

load applied to the knee. A classic example is a pedestrian struck by a car in which the car bumper produces an extreme valgus or varus load on the knee while the leg is axially loaded and fixed by the foot to the ground. With this injury mechanism, the femoral condyle exerts both a compressive and shearing force on the corresponding tibial plateau. The fracture pattern may be a pure split, a pure compression, or a combination of both. Older patients with osteoporosis will usually have some component of bony compression.

It must be emphasized that injuries to the soft tissues about the knee are commonly associated with plateau fractures. One report identified injuries of the menisci (20%), medial collateral ligaments (20%), and anterior cruciate ligaments (10%) in 56 patients treated operatively for tibial plateau fractures.

Clinical Findings

A. Symptoms and Signs

Patients will invariably present with a painful and swollen knee. As with all intra-articular fractures, hemarthrosis will be present. Physical examination will show tenderness of the bone and soft tissues. Care should be taken to palpate both collateral ligaments and assess for tenderness. Active and passive range of motion of the joint will be painful and limited. Careful assessment of knee stability should be performed if the patient permits it. Intra-articular injection of lidocaine and aspiration of the hemarthrosis will often give enough pain relief to allow this examination in the emergency room.

B. Imaging Studies

Anteroposterior, lateral, and two oblique views centered on the proximal tibia are usually adequate to make the diagnosis. CT scans can be helpful to assess articular congruence and plan surgical approaches. MRI is increasingly being used because it has been shown to be as effective as CT at demonstrating the bony anatomy but has the added benefit of identifying injuries of the menisci and ligaments.

Treatment

The goal of treatment is to obtain a stable, congruent, mobile, and painless joint. While there are no accurate data on the amount of tibial articular surface depression necessary to produce posttraumatic arthritis, it has been shown that more than 3 mm of depression significantly increases joint reactive forces. This is now generally accepted as the maximum acceptable fracture displacement. However, treatment is determined as much by the characteristics of the patient as by the characteristics of the fracture. For this reason, the patient's age, functional status, and comorbidities along with fracture displacement, comminution, and associated soft tissue injuries must influence treatment options. Closed treatment usually consists of gentle reduction and placement in a locked hinged knee brace. Frequent follow-up radiographs are needed to assess fracture alignment, since malalignment can develop in the brace. Knee motion in the hinged brace is allowed once the fracture has healed sufficiently to avoid fracture displacement. Surgical treatment may consist of a variety of techniques, including open or arthroscopically assisted elevation of depressed joint fragments followed by internal fixation sufficient to allow early range of motion. Strict avoidance of weightbearing is maintained for 12 weeks regardless of the treatment utilized.

2. Fracture of the Tibial Tuberosity

Violent contraction of the quadriceps muscle may cause avulsion of the tibial tuberosity. When avulsion is complete, active extension of the knee is not possible. This injury may also occur in children through the apophysis of the proximal tibia.

If displacement is minimal, treatment is by immobilization in a cylinder cast extending from the inguinal to the supramalleolar region with the knee in full extension. Immobilization is maintained for 8 weeks or until sufficient healing has occurred to allow early protected range of motion activity.

A loose fragment that has been displaced more than 5 mm can be treated either by closed reduction and percutaneous fixation or by open reduction and internal fixation.

3. Fracture of the Tibial Eminence

This injury usually occurs in association with a comminuted fracture of the tibial plateau. The medial intercondylar tubercle may be avulsed with adjacent bone attached to the anterior cruciate ligament, and injury to this structure is of greater importance. In addition to avulsion of the anterior cruciate ligament, there may also be injury to the tibial collateral ligament and the medial knee joint capsule. Hemarthrosis is always present.

Isolated, nondisplaced fractures with a stable knee may be treated by immobilization of the extremity for 6 weeks in a long-leg plaster cast with the knee in 15–20 degrees of flexion to minimize tension on the anterior cruciate ligament. Displaced eminence fractures or fractures in unstable knees or those associated with other intra-articular injuries require surgical stabilization of the bony fragment if it is large enough or anterior cruciate ligament reconstruction if it is not.

Benirschke SK et al: Immediate internal fixation of open, complex tibial plateau fractures: treatment by a standard protocol. J Orthop Trauma 1992;6:78.

Bennett WF, Browner B: Tibial plateau fractures: a study of associated soft-tissue injuries. J Orthop Trauma 1994;8:183.

Honkonen SE, Jarvinen MJ: Classification of fractures of the tibial condyles. J Bone Joint Surg Br 1992;74:840.

Mallik AR, Covall DJ, Whitelaw GP: Internal versus external fixation of bicondylar tibial plateau fractures. Orthop Rev 1992;21:1433.

Kode L et al: The evaluation of tibial plateau fractures: efficacy of MR Imaging compared to CT. AJR Am J Roentgenol 1994; 163:141.

O'Dwyer KJ, Bobic VR: Arthroscopic management of tibial plateau fractures. Injury 1992;23:261.

TOTAL KNEE REPLACEMENT

Reconstructive surgery for the arthritic knee (Figure 42–31) has been characterized by the development of total replacement prostheses designed to compensate for varying degrees of cartilage, bone, or ligamentous destruction. Indications for knee replacement include intractable pain (with or without deformity) along with x-ray evidence of arthritis (rheumatoid, posttraumatic, or degenerative). The many designs of implants available vary in the degree to which they constrain knee motion. The unconstrained implants are mainly resurfacing replacements and require intact collateral and posterior cruciate ligaments. A minimum amount of bone is removed from the articular surfaces of the distal femur and proximal tibia and is replaced by metal on the femoral side and polyethylene (or a metal tray with a polyethylene insert) on the tibial side. The components are cemented in place with polymethylmethacrylate. The largest number of prostheses fall into the semiconstrained category and provide varying amounts of intrinsic stability. Fully constrained prostheses permit motion only in the sagittal plane and are used in joints with severe deformity or major ligamentous laxity. These prostheses require removal of a significant amount of bone to allow room for the device, to correct deformity, and to permit placement of the intramedullary stems.

Enthusiastic early short-term reports of total knee arthroplasty have been qualified by more thoughtful long-term studies, with reoperation rates of 15% and higher. The most common mechanism of failure has been loosening of the prosthetic components, usually on the tibial side. Factors contributing to loosening include inadequate fixation, less than optimal cementing techniques, and restricted rotation of the prosthesis. Obesity, overactivity, and insufficient bone stock are patient factors contributing to failure.

Patients with preoperative varus deformity appear to have a higher incidence of loosening. Other complications include peroneal nerve palsy, problems with wound healing, and deep infection, which frequently requires removal of the prosthesis and arthrodesis of the knee joint.

Pain relief is achieved in 80–90% of patients, and a mild to moderate increase in a range of motion of the knee can be expected. Patients must be motivated to participate in a vigorous rehabilitation program for maximum results.

If osteoarthritis involves one compartment of the joint only, unicompartmental replacement has been successful in elderly patients. In young active patients who have varus deformity of less than 10 degrees, no subluxation, and flexion of 80 degrees or more, high tibial osteotomy to correct varus deformity is advocated.

Cates HE et al: Intramedullary versus extramedullary femoral alignment systems in total knee replacement. Clin Orthop 1993; 286:32.

Edgerton BC, Mariani EM, Morrey BF: Distal femoral varus osteotomy for painful genu valgum: a five-to-11-year follow-up study. Clin Orthop 1993;288:263.

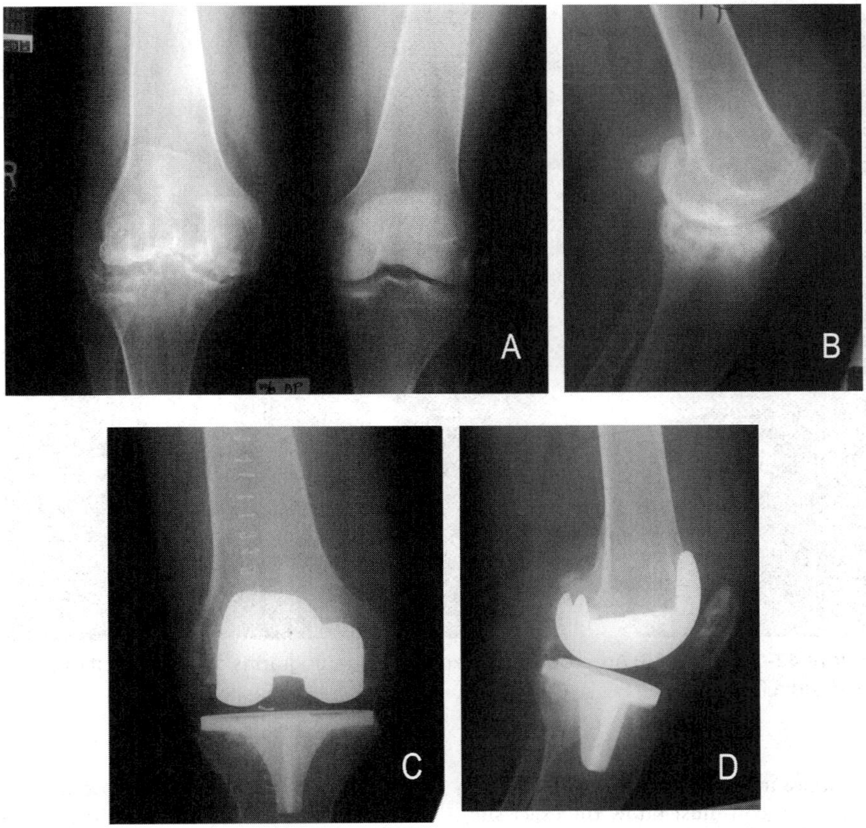

Figure 42–31. A–B: Patient with rheumatoid arthritis and severe joint destruction of the right knee. ***C–D:*** Patient was treated with a cemented right total knee replacement.

Skinner HB: Pathokinesiology and total joint arthroplasty. Clin Orthop 1993;288:78.

Whiteside LA: Correction of ligament and bone defects in total arthroplasty of the severely valgus knee. Clin Orthop 1993; 288:234.

FRACTURE OF THE SHAFTS OF THE TIBIA & FIBULA

Fracture of the shaft of the tibia or fibula (Figure 42–32) may occur at any age but is most common during adolescence and active adulthood. Fractures of the tibial shaft have the highest rate of nonunion of all long bone fractures and, in cases of open tibia fracture, the highest rate of infection. Injury mechanisms range from low-energy rotational injuries to violent, high-energy injuries such as those associated with motorcycle accidents. These are clearly different injuries with different types and incidences of complications, different rates of healing and in many cases very different goals of treatment.

Clinical Findings

A. Symptoms and Signs

Patients present with pain, swelling, and inability to bear full weight on the affected limb. The fracture will be tender to palpation, and crepitance may be present. The injury mechanism should be carefully documented. The condition of the soft tissue envelope surrounding the fibula and especially the almost entirely subcutaneous tibia should be carefully inspected. Any open wounds should be measured, cleaned of any gross contamination, and covered with a sterile saline-soaked gauze dressing. Gross malalignment should be corrected without delay and the limb splinted. As with all long bone fractures, examination of the joints above and below the fracture (knee and ankle) must be performed.

B. Imaging Studies

X-rays in the anteroposterior and lateral projection of the entire lower leg, including both the knee and ankle

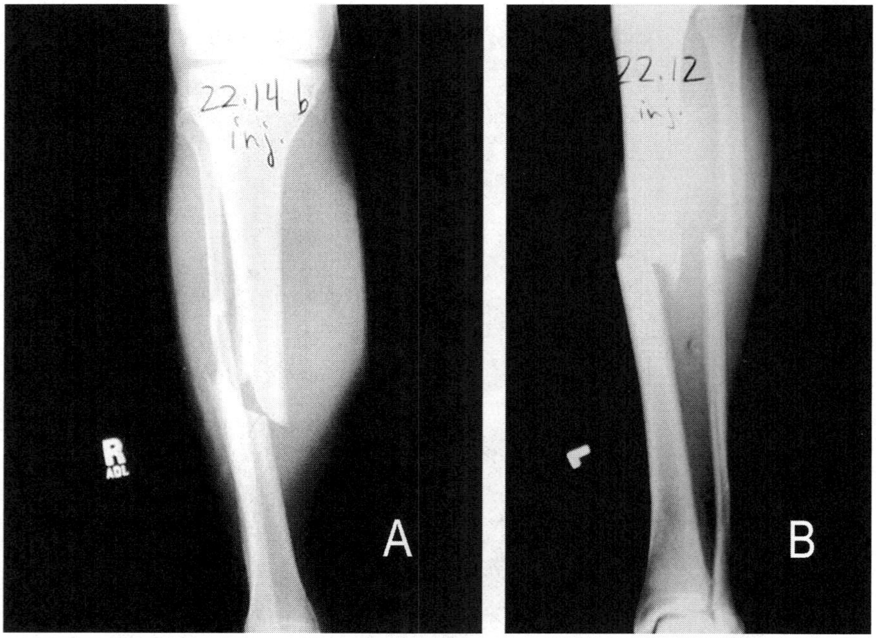

Figure 42–32. A and B: Anteroposterior and lateral radiographs of a displaced midshaft tibia fracture.

joints, are always necessary, and oblique projections are often desirable. The surgeon must know the exact site, configuration, and direction of displacement of the fragments. Inadequate x-ray examination can lead to incomplete diagnosis.

1. Fracture of the Shaft of the Fibula

Isolated fracture of the shaft of the fibula is uncommon though it can occur with a direct blow to the side of the lower leg. Particular attention should be given to clinical and radiographic examination of the ankle and knee to rule out ligamentous or other subtle bony injuries. If no other injury is present, immobilization is for comfort only. Three weeks or a month in a walking cast or removable cast boot is usually sufficient, and complete healing can be expected.

2. Fracture of the Shaft of the Tibia

Isolated fractures of the shaft of the tibia are not common and tend to be caused by indirect injury such as a torsional movement and can be recognized by the spiral fracture pattern produced. These low-energy injuries tend to be relatively stable because the periosteum around the tibia is typically intact and the fibula provides additional support.

The goal of treatment is to obtain fracture healing with less than 5 degrees of angulation in the coronal plane and 10 degrees of angulation in the sagittal plane. Closed reduction may be needed in cases exceeding these limits. Typically, isolated fractures of the tibia heal well with plaster cast or similar immobilization but may take up to 5 months before clinical and radiographic union is complete. Frequent radiographic follow-up is required during the early stages of fracture consolidation because the intact fibula can cause secondary varus angulation of the tibia. Operation is indicated if acceptable angulation cannot be achieved through closed reduction or if an acceptable reduction is lost during cast treatment.

3. Fracture of the Shafts of Both Bones in Adults

Simultaneous fractures of the shafts of the tibia and fibula are almost always unstable moderate-energy to high-energy injuries that tend to displace despite reduction. Treatment remains controversial though there is increasing support in the orthopedic literature for some form of surgical treatment for all displaced fractures of the tibia and fibula. However, many orthopedists still feel that an attempt at closed reduction and cast or fracture brace treatment should be considered in certain circumstances.

Absolute indications for surgical treatment include open fractures, fractures with associated nerve or vascular injury, and fractures with associated compartment syndrome. Relative indications for surgical treatment include multiply injured patients, head-injured patients, and patients with compromised soft tissue around the fracture site.

Closed treatment can be considered in those patients without the indications for open treatment listed above. The single most important determinant of fracture healing in an acceptable position is the position of the fracture at the time of presentation—ie, the more displaced or angulated a fracture is at presentation, the more likely it is that displacement or angulation will occur in the cast. Other factors increasing risk of displacement in the cast include high-energy injuries, comminuted and segmental fractures, and fracture patterns in which the fractures of the tibia and fibula are at the same level. If an acceptable position can be obtained, casting initially should be with a long-leg cast. Extreme vigilance on the part of the practitioner and the patient for signs of developing compartment syndrome in the cast is critically important for the first 4–5 days. Frequent radiographs are needed to verify that the fracture position remains acceptable in the cast. Six weeks in a long-leg cast is usually sufficient to allow conversion to a short leg cast or fracture brace and at least some protected weightbearing. Some form of external support is typically needed for 4–6 months until fracture healing is complete.

If surgical treatment is indicated—either because closed treatment failed or because indications for acute open treatment are present—treatment can be with intramedullary rodding, external fixation, or open reduction and internal fixation. The majority of tibia fractures are now treated with intramedullary fixation because this form of treatment allows early functional rehabilitation of the knee and ankle, permits early weightbearing, and imposes the lowest risk of infection and soft tissue complications.

Bone LB et al: Displaced isolated tibial shaft fractures treated with either cast or intramedullary nailing. J Bone Joint Surg Am 1997;79:1336.

Brumback RJ: Open tibial fractures: current orthopaedic management. Instr Course Lect 1992;41:101.

Dagher F, Roukoz S: Compound tibial fractures with bone loss treated by the Ilizarov technique. J Bone Joint Surg Br 1991;73:316.

Garcia-Cimbrelo E et al: Ilizarov technique: results and difficulties. Clin Orthop 1992;283:116.

Piecioni L, Guanche CA: Clinical experience with unreamed locked nails for open tibial fractures. Orthop Rev 1992; 21:1213.

Siebenrock KA, Schillig B, Jakob RP: Treatment of complex tibial shaft fractures: arguments for early secondary intramedullary nailing. Clin Orthop 1993;290:269.

Wiss DA, Johnson DL, Miao M: Compression plating for non-union after failed external fixation of open tibial fractures. J Bone Joint Surg Am 1992;74:1279.

ACUTE COMPARTMENT SYNDROME

Compartment syndrome is caused by increased pressure in a closed fascial space, compromising perfusion of nerves and muscles. The fascial compartments of the lower leg and forearm are most commonly involved. The syndrome can be caused by a fracture with subsequent hemorrhage and edema in the compartment, limb compression or crush, vigorous exercise, burns, or any other pathogenic factor that increases intra-compartmental pressures. While a large variety of inciting mechanisms exist, the essential feature of compartment syndrome is increased intracompartmental pressure leading to tissue ischemia. Severe ischemia for 6–8 hours or more leads to muscle and nerve death.

The late signs of arterial insufficiency are pain, pallor, paresthesias, paralysis, and pulselessness. However, these are usually late findings, and if nerve and muscle ischemia has been present long enough to result in paralysis and paresthesias, tissue damage has probably already occurred. Furthermore, compartment syndrome can occur at intracompartmental pressures well below arterial pressure, and compartment syndrome can therefore exist in a pink limb with normal pulses.

Clinical findings include swelling and palpable tenseness over a muscle compartment. Paresthesias, pallor, pulselessness, and paralysis should be sought and documented. However, the two most reliable early indicators of compartment syndrome are pain out of proportion to what is expected for a given injury and pain with passive stretch of the muscles in the compartment suspected of having compartment syndrome. Suspicion is perhaps the physician's best aid in diagnosis of this problem.

If compartment syndrome cannot be diagnosed clinically, intracompartmental pressure must be measured directly. This is performed by inserting a large-bore catheter into the compartment using sterile technique. The catheter is then connected to a pressure monitor via intravenous tubing filled with sterile saline solution. Another option is a commercially available self-contained compartment pressure-measuring system. Compartments with pressures above 30–40 mm Hg or within 30 mm Hg of the diastolic pressure should be considered for fasciotomy.

Fasciotomy should be performed with complete release of the skin and fascia of the involved compartments. Compartment pressures are rechecked after fasciotomy to make certain that decompression has been achieved. The wounds are usually left open and covered with sterile dressings and are then treated days later by delayed primary closure or skin grafting.

Cameron SE: Acute compartment syndrome of the triceps: a case report. Acta Orthop Scand 1993;64:107.

Fakhouri AJ, Manoli A 2d: Acute foot compartment syndromes. J Orthop Trauma 1992;6:223.

McQueen MM, Court-Brown CM: Compartment monitoring in tibial fractures: the threshold for decompression. J Bone Joint Surg Br 1996;76:99.

INJURIES OF THE ANKLE REGION

1. Ankle Sprain

Ankle sprain is most often caused by forced inversion of the foot, as may occur in stumbling on uneven ground. Pain is usually maximal over the anterolateral aspect of the joint; greater tenderness is apt to be found in the region of the anterior talofibular and talocalcaneal ligaments. Eversion sprain is less common; maximal tenderness and swelling are usually found over the deltoid ligament.

Sprain is differentiated from major partial or complete ligamentous tears by anteroposterior, lateral, and 30-degree internal oblique (mortise view) x-ray projections; if the joint cleft between either malleolus and the talus is greater than 4 mm, major ligamentous tear is probable. Occult lesions can be demonstrated by x-ray examination under inversion or eversion stress after infiltration of the area of maximal swelling and tenderness with 5 mL of 1% lidocaine.

If swelling is marked, elevation of the extremity and avoidance of weightbearing for a few days are advisable. The ankle can be supported with Gibney strapping, air cushion splints, or a cast for 2–3 weeks to relieve pain and swelling. Further treatment may be by warm foot baths and elastic bandages. Treatment should be continued until muscle strength and full joint motion are recovered. Tears of major ligaments of the ankle joint are discussed below.

Nyska M et al: Radiological assessment of a modified anterior drawer test of the ankle. Foot Ankle 1992;13:400.

Raatikainen T, Putkonen M, Puranen J: Arthrography, clinical examination, and stress radiograph in the diagnosis of acute injury to the lateral ligaments of the ankle. Am J Sports Med 1992;20:2.

2. Fractures of the Ankle Joint

Ankle trauma accounts for between 3% and 12% of all emergency room visits. The frequency and severity of ankle fractures has been increasing as our population ages yet remains active. In fact, ankle and foot fractures are among the most common fractures among elderly women. Obesity, intoxication, and high-heeled or platform shoes are also risk factors for ankle fracture. Motor vehicle accidents remain a common cause of high-energy injuries despite the development of secondary restraint systems such as airbags, which appear to provide little protection for foot and ankle injuries.

Although most patients who present to the emergency room with ankle pain will have radiographs taken, only 7–36% will have fractures. In an effort to reduce the number of unnecessary radiographs, the Ottawa clinical decision rule was developed to guide physicians in their use of radiographs in ankle and foot injuries. This rule states that radiographs need be obtained only if patients have pain near the malleoli and one of the following: (1) age over 54, (2) inability to bear weight immediately after the injury and for four steps in the emergency room, and (3) bony tenderness at the posterior edge or tip of either malleolus. The rule does not apply for patients with obvious ankle deformities or for patients who are obtunded or have impaired ability to communicate. The overall sensitivity of the Ottawa scale for predicting ankle fracture ranges from 93% to 100%. However, it should not replace sound clinical judgment when considering ordering radiographs.

Clinical examination will reveal swelling and point tenderness over damaged ligaments or fractured bones. The examining physician should palpate both tibia and fibula up to the knee as some ankle fracture patterns propagate the skeletal or soft tissue injury well up the lower leg. The skin should be carefully inspected for wounds that may communicate with the bone. A neurologic examination should also be performed. Radiographic examination should consist of a lateral and mortise view of the ankle. The standard anteroposterior view has been shown to add very little to the diagnostic workup. The mortise view is obtained by obtaining an anteroposterior view of the ankle with the leg internal rotated 20 degrees. This view, when obtained correctly in a noninjured ankle, should show an equal "clear space" between the talar dome and its articulations with the distal tibia, the medial malleolus, and the lateral malleolus.

Fracture of the Medial Malleolus

Fracture of the medial malleolus may occur as an isolated lesion of any part of the malleolus (including the tip) or may be associated with (1) fracture of the lateral malleolus, with medial or lateral dislocation of the talus; and (2) dislocation of the inferior tibiofibular joint, with or without fracture of the fibula. An isolated fracture of the medial malleolus does not usually cause instability of the ankle joint.

Nondisplaced isolated fractures of the medial malleolus should be treated by immobilization in a short leg cast with the ankle flexed to a right angle and the foot slightly inverted to decrease tension on the deltoid ligament. Immobilization without weightbearing should be continued for 6–8 weeks or until bone healing is demonstrated bother clinically and radiographically. The rate of nonunion in isolated medial malleolus fractures treated nonoperatively has been reported to be as high as 20%.

Displaced isolated fracture of the medial malleolus can be treated by closed manipulation under general or local anesthesia. The essential maneuver consists of anatomic realignment by digital pressure over the distal fragment followed by immobilization in a plaster cast (as for nondisplaced fracture) until bone healing occurs. If anatomic reduction cannot be achieved by closed methods, open reduction and internal fixation with one or two screws is required.

Fracture of the Lateral Malleolus & Combined Injury Patterns

A fracture of the lateral malleolus may occur as an isolated lesion or may be associated with a fracture of the medial malleolus, a tear of the deltoid ligament, or disruption of the syndesmotic ligaments between the distal tibia and fibula. If the structures on the medial side of the ankle (either bony or ligamentous) are injured, lateral subluxation or instability of the talus may be present.

When a lateral malleolus fracture is noted, particular care should be directed toward the physical and radiographic finding on the medial side of the ankle. Medial tenderness without a medial malleolus fracture suggests deltoid ligament injury. Medial clear space widening of more than 4 mm on the mortise view confirms deltoid or syndesmosis ligament disruption. In these cases, anatomic reduction may not be achievable or maintainable with closed manipulation and casting.

Isolated stable fractures of the lateral malleolus can be treated with a short leg cast. Weekly radiographs are obtained in the cast to verify that an acceptable position has been maintained. Casting normally needs to be continued for 4–6 weeks until fracture healing is sufficient to allow some weightbearing in a removable over-the-counter cast boot. Long-term results of this type of treatment have been shown to be quite satisfactory.

The vast majority of fractures that involve both malleoli or that consist of a lateral malleolar injury in conjunction with a deltoid or syndesmotic ligamentous disruption, will require open reduction and internal fixation to achieve anatomic reduction. In addition to the benefit afforded by anatomic reduction, open reduction with internal fixation typically allows the patient to begin weightbearing and physical therapy much sooner than is possible with closed reduction and casting.

Fractures of the Distal Tibia

Perhaps no other fracture in orthopedics offers such an astounding variety of injury mechanisms, fracture patterns, and treatment pitfalls as a distal tibia fracture (Figure 42–33). These injuries may consist of everything from very low energy avulsion fractures of the posterior or anterior distal tibial rim to high-energy fractures in which the distal tibia disintegrates within—

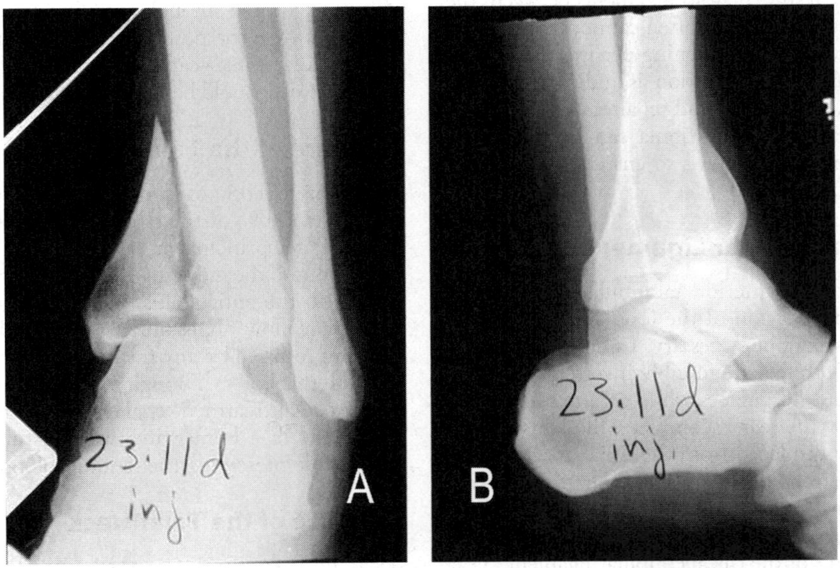

Figure 42–33. Axial loading injury to the ankle joint with the foot in dorsiflexion leading to a fracture of the tibial plafond. Anteroposterior ***(A)*** and lateral ***(B)*** radiographs.

and often through—the meager envelope of soft tissue surrounding it. Treatment is guided by the mechanism of injury, the fracture configuration, and, most importantly, the condition of the surrounding soft tissues.

Bonar SK, Marsh JL: Unilateral external fixation for severe pilon fractures. Foot Ankle 1993;14:57.

McFerran MA et al: Complications encountered in the treatment of pilon fractures. J Orthop Trauma 1992;6:195.

3. Dislocation of the Ankle Joint

Complete dislocation of the ankle joint is rare because the talus cannot be completely dislocated from the joint unless all ligaments are torn. Major ligamentous injuries in the region of the ankle joint with incomplete dislocations are usually associated with fracture.

Tear of the Deltoid Ligament

Complete tear of the talotibial portion of the deltoid ligament can permit interposition of the posterior tibial tendon between the medial malleolus and the talus. Associated injury is usually present, especially fracture of the lateral malleolus with lateral dislocation of the talus.

Pain, tenderness, swelling, and ecchymosis in the region of the medial malleolus without fracture suggest partial or complete tear of the deltoid ligament. If fracture of the lateral malleolus or dislocation of the distal tibiofibular joint is present, the cleft between the malleolus and the talus is likely to be widened. If significant widening is not apparent, x-ray examination under stress is necessary.

Interposition of the deltoid ligament between the talus and the medial malleolus often cannot be corrected by closed manipulation. If widening persists after closed manipulation, surgical exploration is indicated so that the ligament can be removed and repaired by suture.

Associated fracture of the fibula can be treated by fixation with a plate and screws to ensure maintenance of anatomic reduction.

Tear of the Talofibular Ligament

Isolated tear of the anterior talofibular ligament is caused by forced inversion of the foot. X-ray examination under stress may be necessary, using local or general anesthesia. Both feet are forcibly inverted and internally rotated about 20 degrees while an anteroposterior film is exposed. If the tear is complete, the talus will be seen to be axially displaced from the tibial articular surface (talar tilt). Up to 25 degrees of talar tilt has been reported in normal ankles without a history of injury.

Rupture of the anterior talofibular ligaments may be associated with tear of the calcaneofibular ligament. Tear of both ligaments may be associated with fracture of the medial malleolus and medial dislocation of the talus.

Instability of the ankle joint, characterized by a history of recurrent sprains, may result from unrecognized tears of the anterior talofibular ligament.

Recent isolated tear of the anterior talofibular ligament or combined tear of the calcaneofibular ligament should be treated by immobilization for 4 weeks in a plaster boot. Associated fracture of the medial malleolus creates an unstable mechanism. Unless anatomic reduction can be achieved and maintained by closed methods, open reduction of the malleolar fragment is indicated—followed by internal fixation of the fracture and repair of the ligamentous injury.

Toohey JS, Worsing RA: A long-term follow-up study of tibiotalar dislocations without associated fractures. Clin Orthop 1989; 239:207.

INJURIES OF THE FOOT

1. The Talus

Dislocation of the Subtalar & Talonavicular Joints

Dislocation of the subtalar and talonavicular joints without fracture occasionally occurs. Displacement of the foot can be by either inversion, in which case the calcaneus dislocates medially, or eversion, in which the calcaneus dislocates laterally. Inversion injuries are classically low-energy injuries and are frequently seen in situations in which a simple ankle sprain was initially suspected. Eversion injuries are classically high-energy injuries. Fortunately, both dislocation patterns are typically easy to reduce in the emergency room though occasionally incarceration of structures—eg, the posterior tibial tendon trapped in the talonavicular joint—can block reduction. After reduction, the extremity should be immobilized in a cast for 3 weeks.

Fracture of the Talus

The talus is composed of the body, neck, and head. More than 60% of the talus is covered by articular cartilage. Three principal arteries that form an anastomotic ring around the neck of the talus provide the blood supply to the entire talus, including the body through retrograde flow. This blood supply, while robust, can be compromised by any fractures of the neck or dislocation of the body. Though rare, fractures of the talus present dual treatment challenges—to restore anatomic alignment in a bone with seven distinct articular surfaces while preserving the tenuous blood supply.

Fracture of the Talar Neck

Talar neck fractures comprise over 50% of talus fractures and are thought to occur by forced dorsiflexion of the forefoot with axial loading. These are usually high-energy injuries, often seen in the brake foot of a driver involved in a high-speed motor vehicle accident. The injury begins as a simple talar neck fracture, but additional energy can propagate the injury to include dislocation of the subtalar, ankle, or talonavicular joints. Surprisingly, neurovascular compromise is rare. Open fractures are common, occurring in up to 25% of talus fractures, and have very high infection rates (38%) despite aggressive management.

An absolutely nondisplaced fracture of the neck can be treated adequately with a nonweightbearing cast for 8–12 weeks. Any displacement of the talar neck is an orthopedic emergency and requires immediate operation to restore the alignment and—to the extent possible—minimize any compromise in talar perfusion.

Fractures of the Talar Body & Head

Fractures of the body and head of the talus are rarely isolated injuries and are frequently associated with other injuries of the talus, calcaneus, or subtalar joint. Treatment is directed toward restoring anatomic alignment of articular surfaces. For fractures that are truly nondisplaced, cast immobilization and avoidance of weightbearing is acceptable treatment. Any measurable displacement requires operative treatment. Displaced talar body fractures have a high rate of avascular necrosis despite operative management.

Fractures of the Lateral Process of the Talus

This injury—now called "the snowboarder's fracture" because of its frequent association with that recreational activity—deserves separate mention only because of the frequency with which the diagnosis is initially missed. The mechanism of injury is thought to be forced inversion under axial loading. The physical finding is lateral ankle pain and swelling, often very difficult to differentiate from an ankle sprain. However, careful palpation may show the exact site of maximal tenderness to be slightly more distal and anterior to the tip of the lateral malleolus than a typical ankle sprain. Plain radiographs often miss this fracture. CT scan should be obtained if the diagnosis is uncertain. Early treatment gives the best result, with nondisplaced fractures treated with a nonweightbearing cast for 4–6 weeks. Displaced fractures require open reduction.

2. The Calcaneus

Fracture of the Calcaneus

The most common mechanism of injury for calcaneus fracture (Figure 42–34) is a fall from a height. Patients with calcaneus fractures frequently have other associated injuries, including fractures of the spine at the thoracolumbar junction. Comminution and impaction are general characteristics. While various classifications have been advocated, the key distinction that must be made is whether the fracture disrupts the subtalar and calcaneocuboid articulations. In general, fractures associated with involvement and displacement of the articular surfaces, are candidates for some type of surgical reduction. High-energy, comminuted, and open fractures of the calcaneus continue to have high rates of subtalar arthrosis despite more aggressive surgical management.

Fracture of the Calcaneal Tuberosity

Isolated fractures of the tuberosity are not common. They may occur in a horizontal or vertical direction. A horizontal fracture may be limited to the superior portion of the region of the former apophysis and represents an avulsion by the Achilles tendon. When the superior fragment is widely displaced proximally with the tendon, open reduction and fixation may be necessary to obtain the best functional result. Further extension of the fracture cleft toward the subtalar joint in the substance of the tuberosity creates a so-called beak fracture. The fragment may be displaced proximally by the action of the Achilles tendon. If displacement is significant, open reduction is advised.

Vertical fracture occurs near the sagittal plane somewhat medially through the tuberosity. Because the medial fragment normally is not widely displaced, immobilization is not required but will reduce pain.

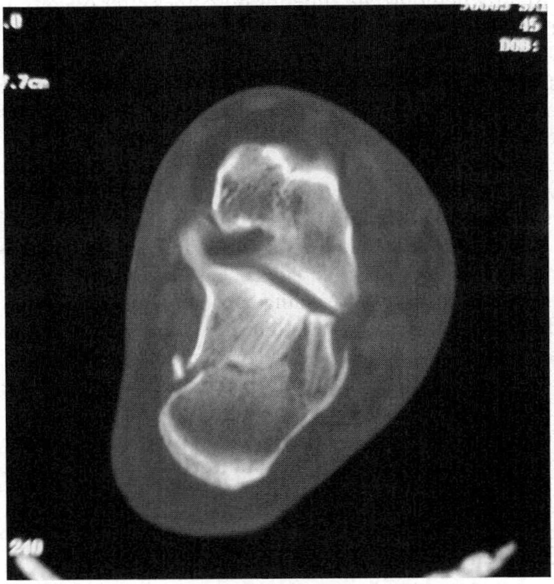

Figure 42–34. Axial CT section showing a fracture of the calcaneus caused by an axial loading mechanism.

Fracture of the Anterior Process of the Calcaneus

Fracture of the anterior process of the calcaneus is caused by forced inversion of the foot. It must be differentiated from midtarsal and ankle joint sprains. The firmly attached bifurcated ligament (calcaneonavicular and calcaneocuboid components) avulses its bony attachment on the calcaneus. Maximal tenderness occurs midway between the tip of the lateral malleolus and the base of the fifth metatarsal. The lateral x-ray view projected obliquely demonstrates the fracture cleft. Treatment is with a nonweightbearing cast with the foot in neutral position for 4 weeks.

Fracture of the Body of the Calcaneus

A. Nonarticular Fracture

Where fracture of the body occurs posterior to the articular surface, the direction of displacement of the tuberosity fragment is proximal. Since the subtalar joint is not disrupted, symptomatic posttraumatic degenerative arthritis is rare though some joint stiffness may persist permanently. Marked displacement can usually be corrected with percutaneous manipulation and pinning.

B. Articular Fracture

The management of intra-articular fractures continues to be controversial. The need for surgery or for closed reduction and the methods used with either approach have all been occasions for debate. The inability to consistently demonstrate superior outcomes after operation reflects this controversy.

Closed treatment continues to be favored by many surgeons. When closed treatment is selected, early range of motion is important to preserve as much ankle, subtalar, and calcaneocuboid motion as possible. A number of studies have shown inferior outcomes in fractures with displaced articular fragments owing to the inability to elevate these fragments with closed techniques.

A better understanding of the biomechanical consequences of articular incongruence is driving an increasing trend for operative management of these fractures. The goals of operation are to restore the calcaneal width and height and restore the articular surface congruence.

Persistent and disabling pain originating in the deranged subtalar joint may require subtalar arthrodesis for adequate relief. Concomitant involvement of the calcaneocuboid joint is an indication for the more extensive triple arthrodesis.

3. The Navicular

Minor avulsion fractures of the tarsal navicular may occur as a feature of severe midtarsal sprain and require neither reduction nor specific treatment. Avulsion fracture of the tuberosity near the insertion of the posterior tibialis muscle is uncommon and must be differentiated from a persistent ununited apophysis and from the supernumerary sesamoid bone, or os tibiale externum.

In general, the fracture occurs either through the middle of the navicular in a horizontal or, less commonly, in a vertical plane. Only noncomminuted fractures with displacement of the dorsal fragment can be satisfactorily reduced. Closed manipulation by strong traction on the forefoot and simultaneous digital pressure over the displaced fragment can restore it to its normal position. If the reduction is not stable, fixation with a percutaneously placed Kirschner wire or interfragmentary screw is needed. Fractures in which acceptable reduction cannot be achieved by closed means should undergo open reduction and fixation. Nonweightbearing immobilization in a plaster cast is required for a minimum of 6 weeks.

4. The Cuneiform & Cuboid

Because of their relatively protected position in the mid tarsus, isolated fractures of the cuboid and cuneiform bones are rarely encountered. Minor avulsion fractures occur as a component of severe midtarsal sprains. Extensive fracture usually occurs in association with other injuries of the foot and often is caused by severe crushing. The most important fracture is the "nutcracker" fracture, which is a compression injury of the lateral column. When more than 2–3 mm of cuboid shortening is present, lateral column lengthening and bone grafting are indicated.

5. Midtarsal Dislocations

Midtarsal dislocation through the cuneonavicular and calcaneocuboid joints or more proximally through the talocalcaneonavicular and calcaneocuboid joints may occur as a result of twisting injury to the forefoot. Fractures of adjacent bones are frequently present as well. When treatment is given soon after the accident, closed reduction by traction on the forefoot and manipulation is generally effective. If reduction is unstable and displacement recurs upon release of traction, stabilization for 4 weeks by percutaneously inserted Kirschner wires is recommended.

6. Fractures & Dislocations of the Metatarsals

Fractures of the metatarsals and tarsometatarsal dislocations are typically caused by a direct crush or indirect twisting injury of the forefoot.

Tarsometatarsal Dislocations

Dislocations of the tarsometatarsal (Lisfranc) joints may present as subtle midfoot sprains or obvious open fracture dislocations. The most common mechanism of injury is axial loading on a hyperplantarflexed midfoot. Midfoot swelling and pain with transverse midfoot compression are hallmarks of these injuries. Anteroposterior, lateral, and oblique radiographs should be obtained, preferably with weightbearing if tolerated by the patient. Careful review of the radiographs will reveal malalignment between the medial border of the second metatarsal and the medial cuneiform and the medial border of the fourth metatarsal and the medial border of the cuboid. CT scan is very sensitive for detecting subtle displacement of this three-dimensional joint.

The goal of treatment is to obtain and maintain anatomic reduction because long-term outcome has been found to correlate best with the quality of the reduction. For widely displaced dislocations, attempted closed reduction should not be deferred. Closed reduction and percutaneous pinning are recommended if perfect reduction can be achieved. The difficulty in achieving anatomic reduction—and particularly in verifying it—has led most authors to recommend open reduction when treating tarsometatarsal fracture-dislocations.

Fracture of the Metatarsal Shafts

Undisplaced fractures of the metatarsal shafts cause no permanent disability unless they fail to heal. Displacement is rarely significant in those fracture patterns in which the middle metatarsals are fractured but the first and fifth are uninjured because the peripheral metatarsals act as in situ splints.

Care should be taken to correct angular malposition in the longitudinal axis of the shaft. Untreated apex dorsal angulation causes plantar prominence of the head of the involved metatarsal, which can cause concentrated local plantar pressure and lead to painful callosities or even full-thickness pressure-induced ulceration. Every effort should be made to correct convex dorsal angulation by distraction of impacted fragments and appropriate manipulation. Closed reduction is best achieved by use of the Chinese fingertrap applied to the toes of the involved metatarsals. If closed reduction is not successful, open reduction with Kirschner wire fixation should be performed. If correction after closed manipulation is acceptable, a plaster cast should be well molded to the plantar aspect of the foot to minimize recurrence of deformity and to support the longitudinal and transverse arches.

Fatigue Fracture of the Metatarsal Shafts

Fatigue fracture of the shafts of the metatarsals has been given various names (eg, march, stress, and insufficiency fracture). Its protean clinical manifestations cause difficulty in precise recognition—even to the point of confusion with osteogenic sarcoma. It commonly occurs in active young adults—such as military recruits—who are unaccustomed to vigorous and excessive walking. A history of a single significant injury is lacking. Incipient pain of varying intensity in the forefoot that is accentuated by walking, swelling, and localized tenderness of the involved metatarsal is the cardinal manifestation. Depending upon the stage of development of the injury, x-rays may not demonstrate fracture, and extracortical callus formation may ultimately be the only clue. More striking findings may vary from an incomplete fissure to an evident transverse cleft. Persistent unprotected weightbearing may cause arrest of bone healing and even displacement of the distal fragment. The second and third metatarsals are most frequently involved near the junction of the middle and distal thirds. The lesion can occur more proximally and in other lesser metatarsals. Since weightbearing is likely to prolong and aggravate symptoms, treatment is by protection in either a walking cast or removable cast boot. Weightbearing should be restricted until pain subsides and bone continuity has been restored radiographically.

Fracture of the Tuberosity of the Fifth Metatarsal

Forced adduction of the forefoot may cause avulsion fracture of the tuberosity of the fifth metatarsal. If displacement of the fragment is minimal, adhesive strapping or a stiff-soled shoe is adequate treatment. If displacement is greater than 3–4 mm, treatment should consist of a walking boot until bone healing occurs. Nonunion is rare, but the time to radiographic union can often lag well behind clinical fracture healing.

7. Fractures & Dislocations of the Phalanges of the Toes

Fractures of the phalanges of the toes are caused most commonly by direct injury such as crushing or stubbing.

Comminuted fractures of the proximal phalanx of the great toe, alone or in combination with fracture of the distal phalanx, are the most disabling injuries. Since wide displacement of fragments is not likely, correction of angulation and support with an adhesive dressing and splint usually suffices. A weightbearing plaster cast may be useful for relief of symptoms arising from associated soft tissue injury. Spiral or oblique fracture of the proximal phalanges of the lesser toes can be treated adequately by binding the involved toe to an adjacent uninjured toe. Comminuted fracture of the distal phalanx is treated as a soft tissue injury.

Traumatic dislocation of the metatarsophalangeal joints and the uncommon dislocation of the proximal interphalangeal joint usually can be reduced by closed manipulation. These dislocations are rarely isolated and usually occur in combination with other injuries to the forefoot.

8. Fracture of the Sesamoids of the Great Toe

Fracture of the sesamoid bones of the great toe is rare, but it may occur as a result of a crushing injury. It must be differentiated from a bipartite sesamoid. Undisplaced fracture requires no treatment other than a foot support or a metatarsal bar. Displaced fracture may require immobilization in a walking plaster cast, with the toe strapped in flexion.

FRACTURES THAT FAIL TO UNITE

Delayed fracture healing and nonunion are most common in long bone fractures associated with severe soft tissue damage or infection. However, closed fractures with minimal displacement occasionally fail to unite for reasons that remain obscure. The long bone with the highest risk of nonunion is the tibia. Nonunions of the carpal scaphoid and the femoral neck are not uncommon and are thought to be associated with damage to the blood supply of the fractured area at the time of injury.

Differentiating a slowly healing fracture (delayed union) from a fracture that is never going to heal (nonunion) remains a clinical challenge. Most orthopedic traumatologists reserve the term nonunion for a fracture that is not healed within the average time for a typical fracture in that location to heal and, more importantly, has lost the ability to heal without some type of operative treatment. The treatment of nonunions is based on several factors, including the biology of the fracture, the mechanics of the fracture, the anatomy of the fracture, the patient, and the presence or absence of infection. In general, hypertrophic nonunions that are not infected can be treated successfully with some type of orthopedic construct, whether internal or external, to increase fracture stability. Uninfected atrophic nonunions result from poor healing potential due to absence of necessary biologic factors and require some type of bone grafting procedure to bring new healing potential to the fracture site. Infected nonunions require simultaneous treatment of the fracture and infection because eradication of infection is nearly impossible in the setting of an unstable fracture.

Burdeaux BD Jr: The medical approach for calcaneal fractures. Clin Orthop 1993;290:96.

Cameron HU et al: Repair of nonunion of tibial osteotomy. Clin Orthop 1993;287:167.

Marsh JL et al: Major open injuries of the talus. J Orthop Trauma 1995;9:371.

McCrory P et al: "Snowboarder's fracture": fracture of the lateral process of the talus. J Am Board Fam Pract 1994;7:130.

Mody BS et al: Nonunion of fractures of the scaphoid tuberosity. J Bone Joint Surg Br 1993;75:423.

Stephenson JR: Surgical treatment of displaced intraarticular fractures of the calcaneus: a combined lateral and medial approach. Clin Orthop 1993;290:68.

Swanson TV, Bray TJ, Holmes GB Jr: Fractures of the talar neck: a mechanical study of fixation. J Bone Joint Surg Am 1992; 74:544.

PEDIATRIC ORTHOPEDICS

CHILDREN'S FRACTURES & DISLOCATIONS

Children are not "small adults," and their skeletal injuries are different from those of adults in several significant ways. The most striking characteristic of immature bone is its potential for growth. Longitudinal growth occurs at the physis, or cartilaginous growth plate. Bones increase in diameter by appositional growth from the periosteum. Injuries can affect normal growth, usually by impeding it. However, growth may be accelerated, especially by femoral shaft fractures in mid childhood. Growth may help correct deformity of some but not all children's fractures. Such correction is greatest in young children with a lot of growing yet to be achieved. Growth tends to correct angulation in the plane of motion of an adjacent joint but improves varus or valgus deformities only in the very young and does not correct rotational malalignment. Children's bones heal rapidly, and nonunion is exceedingly rare. A child's periosteum is thick and strong. It surrounds a long bone like a sleeve and must be torn to permit displacement of a fracture. Usually the displaced fracture end protrudes through a rent in the periosteum, but the remaining intact portion of the sleeve bridges the fracture area to facilitate reduction and maintenance of alignment.

Any injury in a young child, especially one under 3 years of age, must be considered a sign of possible battered child syndrome (see Chapter 45). State law in all jurisdictions requires that suspected cases be reported to local authorities. Good patient care requires thorough pediatric and social service assessments.

Closed treatment is usually sufficient for children's fractures. Manipulative reduction under general anesthesia may be required for significant displacement. Open fractures, epiphysial fractures with articular surface displacement, and the very rare fracture that cannot be reduced satisfactorily by closed manipulation are the generally accepted indications for open treatment of fractures in children.

Although children's fractures do heal rapidly and pain soon ceases to interfere with function, it is important to recognize that callus bridging a fracture may deform plastically and angulate if the fracture is loaded too early. Immobilization rarely causes joint stiffness in children, so that casts can and should be left on until union is secure.

Because bone in children is mechanically different from that in adults, there are several unique fracture types in this age group. Immature bone is more porous and fails in compression as well as in tension. The result is the so-called buckle or torus fracture that occurs near the metaphysis. The distal forearm provides a typical example. This stable injury should be protected in plaster for 3 weeks to control symptoms and prevent further trauma to the weakened bone.

Immature bone is less brittle than that of adults, and children's bones may therefore bend significantly rather than fracture. Two potential injury patterns result. The first is traumatic bowing, in which the shaft of a bone is bent. Bowing may produce significant deformity—eg, bowing of the ulna may prevent reduction of an associated displaced fracture of the radius. Depending upon the age of the child, some correction of the deformity can occur, but osteotomy may be required for severe traumatic bowing.

Greenstick fracture, the second fracture type related to the plasticity of children's bones, incompletely disrupts a long bone, so that the bone fractures partially on the tension side but maintains continuity of a portion of the opposite cortex. The periosteum also remains intact on the concave side. Depending upon how much it has been bent, the intact cortex promotes persisting angulation. This can be prevented by briskly overcorrecting the deformity, thereby completing the fracture. The remaining periosteum prevents actual reversal of the deformity and facilitates maintenance of reduction. If angulation of a greenstick fracture exceeds 15 degrees, reduction should be carried out as described. Following reduction—or without it if angulation is minimal—the fracture is immobilized in a long plaster cast with three-point molding to keep tension on the intact periosteal hinge during healing.

1. Growth Plate Fractures (Epiphysial Fractures, Epiphysial Separations)

About 15% of children's fractures involve a growth plate—most commonly the distal radius, distal tibia or fibula (or both), and distal humerus.

Classification

Classification of physial injuries helps to distinguish patterns that may disturb growth and also provides some guidance for treatment. However, it should be recognized that even "benign" injuries of the distal femoral and tibial growth plates can have clinically significant consequences. Naturally, injuries to nearly mature physes have little effect on growth no matter what their type or location.

Physial injuries are classified according to the Salter and Harris system (Figure 42–35). A given injury may have different degrees of severity. For example, an apparent Salter-Harris type II fracture may have sustained sufficient compression adjacent to the metaphysial fragment so that a localized area of type V injury is present, with attendant growth abnormality.

A. Type I

Type I injuries have fracture lines that follow the growth plate, separating epiphysis from metaphysis. Unless the periosteum is torn, displacement cannot occur. Without displacement, radiographs appear normal, and only tenderness localized over the physis instead of an adjacent collateral ligament confirms that a growth plate injury

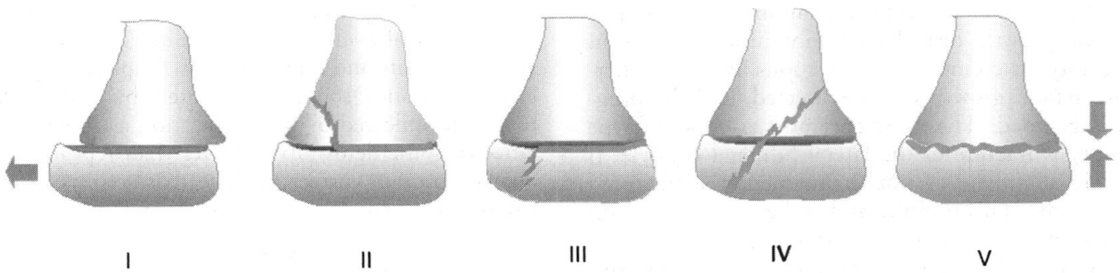

Figure 42–35. Salter-Harris classification of physial injuries occurring at the zone of provisional calcification of the growth plate.

has occurred. Healing occurs rapidly, usually within 2–3 weeks. Complications are rare.

B. Type II

In type II injuries, the fracture line separates epiphysis from metaphysis much as in type I injuries but also enters the metaphysis, so that a flake of metaphysial bone is carried with the epiphysis. This finding is known as the Thurston-Holland sign and is diagnostic of a growth plate injury. Type II injuries are the most common physial fractures. Gentle closed reduction should achieve satisfactory alignment. Healing is rapid, and growth is rarely disturbed. Type II injuries of the distal ends of the femur and the tibia may result in impaired growth that should be watched for.

C. Type III

Type III physial injuries are quite uncommon separations of a portion of the epiphysis along the physis, with the fracture line then passing through the epiphysis to the articular surface. This generally occurs when the growth plate is partially fused. Although growth disturbances are therefore rare, displacement of these injuries disturbs the joint surface and therefore may merit open reduction.

D. Type IV

Salter-Harris type IV fractures potentially interfere with normal growth. The fracture line crosses the physis, separating a peripheral fragment of bone that includes portions of epiphysis, physis, and metaphysis. Because it involves the articular surface, it may compromise normal joint mobility and long-term function. Anatomic reduction, maintained until healing, is essential to minimize the after-effects of type IV growth plate fractures. If they are displaced, open reduction and internal fixation are advisable. Very gentle technique is essential, with avoidance of unnecessary periosteal elevation. Fixation is best obtained with fine smooth Kirschner wires that do not cross the physis or do so temporarily through its most central portion, since screw threads and even peripherally placed smooth wires can interfere with physial growth. Unless anatomic reduction is obtained, growth disturbance, nonunion, and joint incongruity are common complications. Even with perfect reduction, growth may be affected, and the prognosis is guarded. The most common example of type IV injury is fracture of the lateral humeral condyle. If anatomic alignment is not maintained, the fractured lateral condyle fails to unite and makes no further contribution to elongation of the distal humerus. With relative overgrowth of the medial condyle, a progressive cubitus valgus deformity develops. As it becomes stretched around the medial epicondyle, the ulnar nerve develops a "tardy" palsy.

E. Type V

Type V growth plate injuries are due to severe axial loading. Some or all of the physis is so severely compressed that growth potential is destroyed. Since initial radiographs may appear normal, the history of a significant fall with swelling and tenderness over the physis should suggest the possibility of such an injury. Subsequent follow-up radiographs confirm it by demonstrating failure to grow, with premature closure of the physis, or progressive angular deformity from tethering of one side of the growth plate. The outlook for these rare injuries is poor. Progressive angulation can be stopped—if a third or less of the physis is involved—by resecting the bridging bone and filling the defect with autogenous fat or a Silastic spacer. This should allow normal growth to resume. An alternative, which stops growth, is to obliterate any remaining physial plate. Osteotomy may be required to correct significant angulation. Any resulting leg length inequality may require treatment.

Imaging Studies

Radiographs are essential but may be difficult to interpret. In addition to the usual anteroposterior and lateral views, oblique projections may be helpful to show displacement or a small Thurston-Holland fragment of metaphysis. Localized soft tissue swelling and signs of hemarthrosis should be heeded. Comparison views of the opposite normal limb may be helpful, especially if exactly symmetric projections are obtained. Epiphysial injuries that are undisplaced may be demonstrated by varus or valgus stress films, which are required for differentiating ligament disruptions from growth plate injuries in skeletally immature children.

Treatment

A. Conservative Treatment

Most fractures involving the physis may be managed nonoperatively. Undisplaced injuries of any type should be protected in plaster casts until healed. A cast for 3–6 weeks is usually sufficient depending upon the child's age and the site and type of injury. Displaced type I and type II injuries should be treated by gentle closed reduction followed by immobilization as above. Acceptance of some deformity is better than repeated vigorous attempts to correct it, since these efforts involve a risk of additional damage to the physis.

B. Operative Treatment

Displaced type III and type IV injuries usually require open reduction and internal fixation. Type V injuries should be protected in a cast or splint, but the poor outcome of these fortunately rare injuries cannot be improved by any early treatment.

Prognosis

All injuries that involve physes should be followed long enough to confirm that normal growth has not been disrupted. This may require several years, especially if the child is growing slowly or if interference is slight. If the child sustains a type III or type IV injury or any injury of the distal femoral physis, the parents should be warned of the possibility of altered growth. Close follow-up observation is required after growth plate injuries to permit timely diagnosis and treatment of any resulting growth abnormality. Progressive angular deformity may result from an incomplete bony bridge crossing and tethering one side of the physis. Such bridges can be resected, with interposition of a free fat graft, to restore normal growth. A number of techniques are now available to correct limb length inequality due to complete growth arrest. Traditionally, the most frequent has been epiphysiodesis to stop growth of the contralateral limb. Lengthening techniques are being developed that often permit restoration of the short limb to its normal length.

2. Upper Extremity Fractures & Dislocations

Proximal Humeral Fractures

An occasional birth injury causes separation of the unossified proximal humeral epiphysis. The child's failure to use the arm raises the possibility of brachial plexus palsy. Such pseudoparalysis resolves quickly, and radiographs in 10 days demonstrate abundant callus, confirming the nature of the original trauma. Older children usually sustain type II epiphysial fractures. Most are only slightly displaced and can be treated in a sling for 3 weeks. If more displacement is present, manipulation under anesthesia and skin or skeletal traction can improve alignment. There is so much potential for remodeling in the proximal humerus that the best obtainable closed reduction is preferable to open surgery. Deformity, nonunion, and restricted motion are almost never problems for children who sustain proximal humerus fractures.

Supracondylar Fractures of the Humerus

Hyperextension of a child's elbow may cause an undisplaced greenstick supracondylar fracture. There is elbow pain, swelling, and tenderness of both epicondylar ridges. Radiographs confirm swelling and usually show a positive fat pad sign, indicating elbow hemarthrosis. The fracture line is easily missed but may be found where it crosses the olecranon fossa transversely. Careful inspection of a lateral radiograph of the distal humerus shows loss of normal anterior angulation of the capitellum. Comparison to the other elbow may be useful. Closed reduction is advised if angulation is more than 20 degrees from normal. Whether or not closed reduction is performed, the fracture should be protected for 3 weeks in a long-arm cast or splint, with the elbow flexed above 90 degrees and the arm restrained to the chest with a secure sling or collar and cuff.

Rotation superimposed upon a hyperextended elbow produces a displaced supracondylar fracture of the humerus. A sharp corner of the proximal piece penetrates the periosteum but leaves an intact hinge on the side toward which the distal fragment is displaced. The anteroposterior radiograph shows the direction of displacement and thus the site of the periosteal hinge. Displaced supracondylar fractures of the humerus are serious injuries that threaten the neurovascular status of the involved limb and may result in unsightly deformity if reduction is not accurate. Before radiographs are taken, the elbow should be splinted in moderate extension rather than flexed to a right angle. The wrist pulses and the function of the radial, ulnar, and median (including anterior interosseous) nerves should be checked immediately. Ischemia may be present initially or may develop during early treatment. If left to progress, ischemia causes Volkmann's contracture, with loss of motor and sensory function and necrosis of some of the forearm flexor muscles. The involved muscles contract as they are replaced by scar, so that the wrist develops a flexion contracture and the fingers become clawed. Irreversible muscle necrosis begins after 4–6 hours of ischemia. Effective treatment requires prompt restoration of arterial flow and, if necessary, reduction of elevated compartmental pressure in the forearm. It is mandatory to recognize the signs of ischemia: pain in the forearm (rather than the elbow) and progressive loss of sensory and motor function. Ischemic pain is usually increased when the involved muscles are stretched, so that pain on extension of the fingers is a danger sign. Pulses may be felt at the wrist, and the skin may appear well perfused in spite of elevated compartmental pressure. Alternatively, the pulses may be diminished or absent without dangerously impaired perfusion as long as the forearm is comfortable and the hand warm and pink, with intact sensation and motion. If elevated compartmental pressure is suspected, prompt measurement of tissue pressures is indicated (see Acute Compartment Syndrome, above). Ischemia with supracondylar fractures may be due to (1) vascular injury, which requires surgical repair; (2) vascular entrapment, which usually resolves with reduction; or (3) compression from marked elbow flexion—in which position the elbow may have been placed to preserve fracture alignment—or from tight casts or bandages.

Prompt reduction of deformity is the next step toward restoration of normal perfusion and venous drainage. Acute flexion helps maintain closed reduction but is contraindicated if it impairs perfusion of the forearm. Ischemia that develops during treatment must be corrected by release or removal of any constricting bandages and by extension of the elbow as necessary to reestablish arterial flow. Prompt surgical exploration of the brachial artery and forearm musculature may be required if ischemia is evident. Arteriography usually adds little helpful information, and indirect attempts to restore flow (stellate ganglion blocks, anticoagulants, or vasodilators) waste time and are usually not successful.

Supracondylar humerus fractures can usually be managed without open operation. If displacement and soft tissue damage are mild to moderate, closed reduction is done under general anesthesia by manipulating the distal fragment into position and flexing the elbow to hold it. A bandage or cast that leaves the antecubital fossa free is applied, and the arm is secured to the chest to prevent rotation. If the fracture is badly displaced or unstable, if soft tissue swelling is marked, or if the amount of flexion required to hold the reduction obliterates the radial pulse, some other means must be chosen. Overhead skeletal traction with an olecranon pin or screw is effective. Dunlop's skin traction with the arm out to the side is less effective. The currently favored approach is to maintain the reduction with pins inserted percutaneously across the fracture with fluoroscopic guidance, following which the elbow can be splinted in sufficient extension to avoid interfering with perfusion.

The "gunstock deformity" of cubitus varus is the most common late problem after supracondylar fracture. It is caused by inadequate reduction or reduction that is not maintained during healing. Radiographic monitoring is difficult but must be done with care, since correction is much easier and safer before healing has occurred than with a late osteotomy.

Subluxation of the Radial Head (Pulled Elbow, Nursemaid's Elbow)

This common minor injury occurs in children under 4 years of age. It is caused by a sudden pull on the extended pronated arm, usually by an adult tugging on a reluctant toddler. The pronated radial head slips partially under the annular ligament, whose proximal portion displaces into the radiocapitellar joint. The distressed child suddenly stops using the arm, which is held flexed and pronated. Tenderness, usually mild, is well localized to the radial head region, and all motions are permitted except supination. After these physical findings are confirmed, the physician performs reduction by firmly supinating the forearm with one hand while the other supports the elbow in 90 degrees of flexion, feeling for a "click" near the radial head just as full supination is achieved. Radiographs, if obtained, show no abnormalities—in fact, positioning for elbow films will often reduce the subluxation. Promptly after reduction, the child becomes less apprehensive and soon resumes use of the limb. A sling may be applied for a few days. Recurrence is an occasional complication that may require more formal immobilization.

Other Elbow Region Fractures & Dislocations

It is essential to remember that "sprains" rarely occur and that swelling, tenderness, and difficulty in moving an injured elbow suggest a serious problem. Radiographic interpretation is difficult because many of the pertinent structures ossify late in childhood. However, precise early diagnosis is necessary to identify several exceptions to the general principle of nonoperative treatment of children's fractures. Surgery is needed for displaced lateral condylar fractures, displaced medial epicondylar fractures, and badly angulated radial neck fractures that resist closed manipulation. Displaced olecranon fractures, if not reduced by elbow extension, will also require internal fixation. Significant distortion of the elbow region by any fracture or dislocation raises the specter of vascular compromise and resulting Volkmann's contracture. Hospitalization for a day or so is advisable if swelling is severe, or if the parents cannot be relied on to bring the child in promptly for follow-up visits.

Forearm Fractures

Fractures of the shafts of both the radius and the ulna occur frequently in children. Neurovascular complications, including those due to constricting plasters, are always possible. Initial elevation of the limb and close observation are thus advisable, and children treated as outpatients must be supervised by an observant and informed adult. Forearm fractures in children unite reliably. The most common problem is malunion with angular or rotational deformity and limited supination-pronation. Closed reduction almost always corrects angulation. Greenstick fractures are reduced as described above. If displacement is complete, general anesthesia is advisable. Direct manipulation or traction can be used to align the fracture. End-on-end reduction is not essential. Side-by-side ("bayonet") apposition is acceptable in a growing child, but angulation must be minimal; the space between radius and ulna must be preserved; and rotational alignment must be correct. Radiographs are repeated weekly for 3 weeks to permit early remanipulation should a potentially unstable fracture displace in plaster. More distal fractures may involve the physis but rarely interfere with growth.

It is important to be aware of the possibility of dislocation of one forearm bone in association with an isolated displaced fracture of the other. With Monteggia's fracture, there is dislocation of the radial head at the elbow, associated with a broken or bent ulnar shaft. Galeazzi's fracture combines dislocation of the distal radioulnar joint with fracture of the radial shaft. Fracture lines attract attention on radiographs, but dislocations are not as obvious. To avoid missing these injuries, check for tenderness, swelling, and deformity at the wrist and elbow in any patient with trauma to the forearm. Look carefully at radiographs of the wrist and the elbow to ascertain whether the normal bony relationships are present. Children with these injuries, unlike adults, can usually be treated successfully with closed reduction of both the fracture and the joint dislocation. Open reduction is required if joint alignment cannot be restored by closed manipulation.

3. Lower Extremity Fractures & Dislocations

Traumatic Hip Dislocation

In children, traumatic dislocation is more common than fracture of the hip and has fewer complications. Prompt closed reduction under general anesthesia with good muscle relaxation is usually successful. Interposed soft tissue or bone fragments may necessitate open reduction. Following reduction, the hip should be protected for 4–6 weeks until soft tissue healing has occurred. Balanced suspension, traction, or a spica cast may be used. With prompt reduction, avascular necrosis is a rare problem.

Fractures of the Proximal Femur

Proximal femur fractures are rare in children. This is fortunate, as displacement and injury to the growth plate and blood supply predispose to frequent complications such as avascular necrosis, nonunion, and deformity that imperil the hip joint. The strength and resiliency of the proximal femur are such that a fracture in this region can only occur with severe trauma—another factor increasing the likelihood of complications.

Birth fractures, now quite unusual, may displace the proximal femoral epiphysis. Pain and swelling suggest septic arthritis, and the deformity raises fears of dislocation. Aspiration or arthrography yields no pus but demonstrates that the femoral head is located in a normal acetabulum and that deformity is at the neck-shaft junction. Splinting in abduction and flexion, a spica cast, or skin traction will maintain alignment during the 2–3 weeks required for healing. Remodeling may occur with any of these injuries, but nonunion, avascular necrosis, and deformity are possible.

In older children, most hip fractures involve the mid and lower portions of the femoral neck. If there is no displacement, spica cast immobilization maintains alignment during healing, but close radiographic monitoring is required for prompt identification and rectification of any displacement. Displaced fractures of the femoral neck should be treated with three or four small pins, preferably placed short of the physis. Postoperatively, a spica cast is advisable until healing is progressing. Satisfactory results are achieved in half or less of cases, with avascular necrosis, varus malunion, epiphysial arrest, nonunion, and postoperative wound infection the principal complications. Intertrochanteric and subtrochanteric fractures can generally be managed by use of traction for 3–4 weeks until early fracture stability is present, at which time a $1^1/_2$ hip spica is applied for 8–12 weeks. Late problems (eg, angular deformity, unequal limb lengths) are rare but do occur.

Femoral Shaft Fractures

Femoral shaft fractures are fairly common childhood injuries. They often result from significant trauma, so that other injuries may also be present. Radiographs of the hip are required to ensure that fracture or dislocation is not present. The knee should also be x-rayed. Alignment of a femoral shaft fracture is achieved with skin or (for older children) skeletal traction or immediate spica application. Rotational alignment should be corrected. Children 2–10 years of age will usually demonstrate transiently stimulated growth of a fractured femur. It is conventional to align their fractures with about a 1 cm overlap to compensate for this overgrowth. Protection must be continued until mature bony callus has developed, a process that takes roughly as many weeks as the child's age in years. So-called Bryant's skin traction, with both legs suspended vertically, may cause severe ischemia and Volkmann's contracture, even of the uninjured leg. This technique is dangerous for children over the age of 2 years. Femoral fractures in children who are closer to maturity are often most effectively managed with intramedullary nailing, especially if there is head trauma or if multiple injuries have been sustained.

Distal Femoral Growth Plate Fractures

Fractures of the distal femoral growth plate are potentially serious injuries that cause growth abnormalities in up to 45% of patients. They must be suspected whenever a child sustains a knee injury and are suggested by the finding of an intra-articular fat-fluid line on a cross-table lateral radiograph of the knee. Stress radiographs may be required to demonstrate instability. With marked displacement, the popliteal artery or peroneal nerve may be injured. Treatment must be individualized. Gentle anatomic reduction should be accomplished, and reduction should be maintained until healing is secure. A hip spica cast is often required to prevent displacement. If instability is marked, fixation with smooth pins may be required; if open reduction is necessary, such fixation is advisable. The distal femoral epiphysis is responsible for 70% of the growth of the femur and 35% of the growth of the entire lower extremity. Even small disturbances of growth can produce significant limb length inequality if the injured child is young enough. Follow-up of distal femoral growth mechanism injuries should be continued until skeletal maturity is achieved.

Fractures of the Tibia & Fibula

Fractures of the tibia and fibula are not unusual in childhood. An occult undisplaced spiral fracture may be the cause of an acute gait disturbance ("toddler's fracture"). Oblique radiographs may reveal this injury. Most are easy to manage and heal rapidly in a long-leg cast. The spectrum of injuries is quite wide, however, so that each must be evaluated carefully and treated according to its particular attributes. Nerve and vessel damage may be present, especially with displaced fractures of the proximal metaphysis. Nearly undisplaced valgus greenstick fractures of the proximal tibia are pernicious causes of deformity. The initial angulation may not be appreciated, or progressive medial overgrowth may follow apparently satisfactory healing. Fractures in this region with any valgus deformity should be completely reduced and held extended in a long-leg or single-spica cast molded into varus. In some cases, open reduction may be required to remove interposed soft tissues. Another cause of angular deformity is an intact fibula, which may have been bent by the original injury or may encourage collapse into varus by providing relatively more support to the lateral aspect of the leg. One must critically assess the postreduction and early follow-up radiographs following casting to permit timely treatment of angulation. Rotational alignment requires careful visual comparison with the other limb, as it is not obvious on radiographs.

Fractures of the Distal Epiphyses of the Tibia & Fibula

Fractures of the distal epiphyses of the tibia and the fibula occur frequently in children, often from trauma that would produce ligamentous injury in an adult. Suspicion, physical examination that localizes tenderness to a growth plate, and carefully evaluated radiographs will usually suggest the diagnosis. Additional radiographic views, including stress films, will occasionally be required for confirmation. Salter-Harris type I fractures, type II fractures of the fibula, and undisplaced (within 2 mm of anatomic position) type III and type IV fractures have little risk of growth disturbance. Type II fractures of the distal tibial epiphysis are unpredictable, with a higher risk of growth disturbance that does not correlate well with original displacement. Displaced type III and type IV injuries and comminuted epiphysial fractures have a 30% chance of growth disturbance.

If displaced, growth plate injuries of the ankle should be treated by gentle closed reduction, usually under general anesthesia. If this does not correct displacement, type III and type IV injuries should be treated by open reduction and internal fixation, whereas moderate deformity, especially in the sagittal plane, can generally be accepted in type I and type II fractures. Distal fibular growth plate injuries usually have few complications, but those of the distal tibia should be followed until skeletal maturity is achieved.

GAIT DISORDERS & LIMB DEFORMITY

Abnormalities of the lower extremities in children are often a source of parental concern and are frequently noticed when the child is first learning to walk. Rotational alignment—indicated by the orientation of the feet to the line of progression—and angulation at the knees are the two most common areas of concern.

1. Intoe Gait (Pigeon Toe)

Children normally walk with their feet rotated 10 degrees externally from the line of progression. Significant variation occurs from step to step, so that gait must be observed more than just briefly before a reliable conclusion can be made about whether a problem exists. Metatarsus adductus—medial deviation of the forefoot at the tarsometatarsal junction—is a deformity occasionally present at birth. If it persists beyond early childhood, gait appears intoed.

Tibial torsion, the relative rotational alignment of the ankle joint axis compared with that of the knee, increases in an outward direction during childhood. The ankle axis is a line connecting the tips of the medial and lateral malleoli. In a very young child whose leg is hanging freely with the knee flexed 90 degrees and the tibia in neutral rotation, the ankle axis is in the same plane as the knee axis. By adulthood, the transmalleolar axis is externally rotated about 20 degrees. Children 1–3 years of age with intoeing will frequently have relative internal tibial torsion, which almost always corrects spontaneously with growth. Treatment is necessary only if there is significant interference with gait and if spontaneous correction is not occurring. A Denis Browne splint is a metal bar that connects the shoes and holds them in external rotation. It is worn while the child sleeps. This treatment is usually effective. Only rarely—and only in children over 8 years of age—must tibial osteotomy be considered.

Excessive femoral anteversion is a common finding in older children who walk with their feet turned in. Observation reveals that the whole limb is internally rotated, so that the patella—as well as the foot—points medially. Anteversion is the normal anterior inclination of the femoral neck when the distal femur is positioned with the knee axis in a frontal plane. From about 40 degrees in the newborn, femoral anteversion decreases normally to about 15 degrees by adulthood. Excessive femoral anteversion also decreases, often to a normal range, although significant correction is unlikely to occur after age 8 years. Precise measurement of femoral anteversion requires complicated radiographic techniques, but a good clinical determination can be made by internally rotating the extended hip to produce maximal lateral prominence of the greater trochanter. The required amount of internal rotation is roughly equivalent to the degree of femoral anteversion. Significant anteversion is the usual cause of limited external rotation of the extended hip, with associated increase of the range of internal rotation. The normal newborn's hips have an external rotation contracture, presumably the result of intrauterine posture. This diminishes during the first 3 years of life independently of changes in anteversion of the femoral neck. Femoral anteversion can be corrected only by rotational osteotomy. If the limb can be externally rotated beyond neutral, osteotomy is rarely needed.

2. Angular Deformity of the Lower Extremities (Knock-Knees & Bowlegs)

The angle (varus denotes tibia deviated medially; valgus denotes tibia deviated laterally) between femur and tibia in the frontal plane is age-dependent. Bowlegs (genu varum) are normal in the newborn but progress toward valgus, passing through neutral at about age 18 months. Valgus becomes maximal between ages 2 and 3 years, gradually resolving so that the average leg appears straight by age 6 or 7 years. In young children, angular deformity of the knees requires x-ray evaluation (and perhaps measurement of serum calcium, phosphate, and alkaline phosphatase) if it is not symmetric; if it is associated with abnormally short stature; or if it is severe (more than 10 cm between the knees with the ankles touching in genu varum, or more than 10 cm between the ankles with the knees touching in genu valgum). Operative treatment may be considered in severe cases to improve function and appearance and perhaps to decrease the risk of degenerative joint disease in middle age. Angulation can be corrected by stapling one side of a physis to obtain asymmetric growth or by osteotomy with removal or addition of a wedge of bone.

Pathologic Genu Varum

It is important to distinguish symmetric infantile bowlegs, which should resolve by age 3–5 years, from varus deformity produced by rickets, Blount's disease, or skeletal dysplasias, in which involvement is often bilateral but usually asymmetric. Blount's disease (tibia vara) is a frequently bilateral disorder that has both infantile and adolescent types. Radiologic changes in the medial proximal tibial metaphysis consist of lucency, sclerosis, and fragmentation. Unilateral varus suggests a traumatic origin. In young patients, the metaphysial-diaphysial angle of the tibia helps to differentiate between physiologic bowing and infantile tibia vara prior to development of typical radiologic signs. The angle is formed between the line of the lateral tibial cortex and the line of the prominent medial and lateral metaphysial beaks. A metaphysial-diaphysial angle of greater than 11 degrees strongly suggests Blount's disease. Progressive tibia vara should be treated with corrective osteotomy of the proximal tibia and fibula to achieve physiologic valgus alignment of both knees.

SYSTEMIC DISORDERS AFFECTING BONES & JOINTS IN CHILDREN

1. Juvenile Rheumatoid Arthritis

Rheumatoid arthritis is an autoimmune disorder whose exact cause remains elusive. It is a systemic disease that in its most florid form is characterized by rash, fever, and enlargement of lymph nodes and spleen. There are three basic clinical types of juvenile rheumatoid arthritis. Pauciarticular arthritis generally involves the knee or the ankle but occasionally the hip or an upper extremity (mainly the elbow or the wrist). One joint or only a few joints are affected. Insidious onset of swelling, with effusion, synovial thickening, and often flexion contracture, are noted. Except for possible sedimentation rate elevation, systemic manifestations are absent. A serious complication of juvenile rheumatoid arthritis, most common in the pauciarticular form, is iridocyclitis—inflammation of the iris and ciliary body. This insidious process can lead to glaucoma and blindness if left untreated. Early diagnosis is essential and requires slit lamp examination every 3–6 months in these patients. The outlook for patients with pauciarticular juvenile rheumatoid arthritis is said to be good, but—even though residual involvement may be minimal—few patients remain truly asymptomatic.

Polyarthritis is characterized by multiple joint involvement and minimal evidence of systemic disease. Fingers and toes, the neck, and the temporomandibular joints are more likely to be involved. The course is persistent, with periods of exacerbation.

Polyarthritis with systemic rheumatoid disease (Still's disease) usually presents with multiple (more than five) involved joints, fever, lymphadenopathy, hepatosplenomegaly, rash, subcutaneous nodules, and pericarditis. The course may be remitting or relentless, causing severe permanent disability.

Inflamed joints develop synovial hypertrophy and pannus, which destroy articular cartilage. The associated hyperemia can stimulate the adjacent physes, with resulting overgrowth, or physial arrest may occur. Damage to underlying bone and ligament can produce severe deformity and joint subluxation. In polyarthritis, musculoskeletal involvement is more likely to include the cervical spine, typically with spontaneous fusion of the apophysial joints. C1–2 instability will occasionally occur, as in the adult with rheumatoid arthritis.

When a single joint is inflamed, it is necessary to exclude septic arthritis, foreign body synovitis, and transient synovitis of the hip. Polyarticular juvenile rheumatoid arthritis must be differentiated from rheumatic fever and leukemia. Lyme disease may present as joint inflammation.

Management is initially medical, with anti-inflammatory drugs, rest, splinting, and range of motion exercises, followed by strengthening as synovitis resolves and appropriate bracing to minimize deformity and allow function. Synovial biopsy—percutaneously with a needle, via arthroscopy, or with formal arthrotomy—may be helpful for diagnosis, especially to rule out infection. Synovectomy is controversial but may retard the progression of arthritis if medical measures fail. To be successful, it must be done before joint destruction has progressed too far. Contractures may require soft tissue releasing procedures. Osteotomy may be needed to correct bony deformity, and symptomatic destroyed joints can be treated by arthrodesis or arthroplasty. Extensive orthopedic surgery can often be avoided if the pediatrician and the orthopedist cooperate to provide maximal medical control and appropriate use of bracing and physical therapy.

2. Brachial Plexus Palsy

Brachial plexus palsy due to birth injury has three general patterns of involvement: (1) Erb's palsy, involving C5 and C6 roots; (2) Klumpke's paralysis, involving C8 and T1; and (3) whole arm paralysis, where the extent of involvement of individual roots may vary. Erb's palsy is most common and affects the shoulder, with loss of extension, abduction, and external rotation. Also affected are elbow flexion and forearm supination. Spontaneous improvement will occur and will level off by age $1^1/_2$ years. Initial treatment is directed at maintaining shoulder motion by positioning and passive stretching to prevent the characteristic contracture in adduction and internal rotation. If muscle imbalance persists at the shoulder, the pectoralis major and subscapularis muscles can be lengthened with posterior transfer of the latissimus dorsi and teres major muscles, so that they become external rotators. Humeral osteotomy may be preferable to tendon transfer when the shoulder joint is unstable. These procedures will position the hand where it can best be used, but a normal limb is not achieved.

SCOLIOSIS & SPINAL DEFORMITY

The spine has an important role in supporting erect posture, stabilizing the limbs relative to the trunk, supporting the abdominal and thoracic cavities, and in protecting neural elements. The spine is in balance when the head is aligned with the pelvis in the coronal and sagittal planes. Scoliosis is spinal curvature of more than 10 degrees in the coronal or frontal plane. An important component of scoliotic deformity is a concurrent rotational asymmetry around the vertical axis of the body. Deformity may also exist in the sagittal plane, with kyphosis, flexion of the spine anteriorly; and lordosis, extension of the spine posteriorly.

Spinal deformity in children may be caused by congenital anomalies, neuromuscular disorders, connective tissue abnormalities, or infection or injury to the developing spine. Most commonly, the cause is unknown, or idiopathic.

Clinical Findings

A. Symptoms and Signs

Spinal deformity may present in the perinatal period or during infancy in children with congenital anomalies of the spine. More commonly, deformity of the spine due to all causes is detected during the preadolescent growth spurt, when the spine is growing most rapidly. The cause of deformity is an important determinant of the natural history, treatment options, and the goals of management. The history should include age at initial presentation, family history, neuromuscular or connective tissue disorders, prior surgery to the spine or trunk, prior trauma or infection, coexisting skeletal, cardiac, renal, or pulmonary abnormalities, and information on growth and the progression of the deformity.

The initial detection of spinal asymmetry is variable between individuals and across communities. Spinal deformity is often detected by family members, friends, or patients with deformity. Routine screening for spinal deformity remains controversial because there is little evidence that routine screening reduces rates of surgery for spinal deformity or in any way improves outcomes of management. The Adams forward bending test is the most common method of screening for scoliosis. An angular measurement of a line connecting the rib prominences relative to horizontal demonstrates axial rotation of the spine, a characteristic of scoliosis. Angular measurements of greater than 7 degrees are associated with coronal deformity greater than 10 degrees and are therefore an indication for radiographic evaluation.

Physical examination of the patient with spinal deformity includes both examination of the spine and a comprehensive examination of the patient. Examination of the spine may include the location of the curve, curve magnitude, deviation of the trunk from the midline, shoulder asymmetry, pelvic obliquity, and flexibility of the spine. Examination of reflexes (including abdominal reflexes), strength, clonus, hamstring tightness, muscle weakness and contractures, and foot deformity may reveal abnormalities suggestive of intraspinal pathology, including tethering of the cord or a syrinx. Skin examination will include detection of dermal sinuses, hemangiomas, nevi, and hyperelasticity that may be associated with spinal deformity. Chest wall deformity, preauricular skin tags, cleft palate, radial dysplasia, scapular elevation, and thumb duplication or hypoplasia may be found on examination of a patient with congenital deformity of the spine. Scoliosis due to connective tissue pathology may present with joint hypermobility, ocular findings, and cardiac murmurs.

B. Imaging Studies

Spinal deformity occurs in three dimensions, and most imaging studies are limited by providing only a two-dimensional representation. Plain radiographs are useful for the detection of deformity and will provide an accurate quantification of progression of deformity. The Cobb technique is used to accurately measure deformity in the coronal and sagittal planes and is important in demonstrating changes in curve magnitude and pattern. The Cobb technique uses a standing or weightbearing film, and an angular measurement is made between the end-vertebrae that are most tilted from the horizontal at either end of the curve (Figure 42–36). Other plain radiographic measures may include trunk shift relative to the pelvis and overall sagittal and coronal balance of the spine measuring a plumbline between C7 and the sacrum.

MRI examination of the entire spine is an important imaging tool because of the association between intraspinal anomalies with certain types of spinal deformity. Congenital scoliosis may be associated with intraspinal abnormalities, including tethering of the cord, syringomyelia, diastematomyelia, diplomyelia, lipoma, teratoma, and neuroenteric cysts. MRI of the entire spine is indicated for congenital deformity, patients with abnormal neurologic findings on physical examination, and atypical curve patterns including left thoracic curves in females.

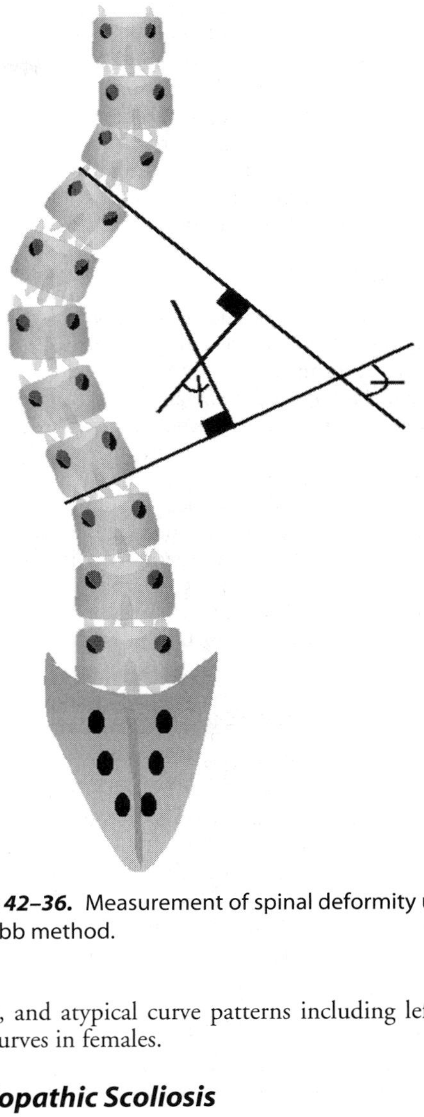

Figure 42–36. Measurement of spinal deformity using the Cobb method.

1. Idiopathic Scoliosis

Idiopathic scoliosis is the most common cause of spinal deformity in children and adolescents. The prevalence of adolescent idiopathic scoliosis, or deformity in the coronal plane measuring greater than 10 degrees, is 2–3% at age 16. Curves larger than 20 degrees are present in 0.3–0.5% of adolescents. The ratio of affected males to females is equal in curves less than 15 degrees. However, for curves larger than 20 degrees, females are seven times more likely to be affected than males.

Nonoperative management of adolescent idiopathic scoliosis is intended to prevent progression of deformity during the growing years. Bracing is the only nonoperative treatment that has demonstrated efficacy in the management of progressive idiopathic scoliosis. Exercises alone, electrical stimulation, and manipulation of the spine have not demonstrated efficacy relative to the natural history of curve progression. Bracing is recommended for curves of magnitude between 30 and 45 degrees. Curves measuring less than 30 degrees should demonstrate progression before initiation of bracing, while curves measuring greater than 50 degrees may not be managed effectively in a brace.

Treatment

Surgical management of adolescent idiopathic scoliosis is generally indicated to prevent the future consequences of progressive deformity. It is important that the patient, family, and care provider share an accurate understanding of the future consequences of adolescent scoliosis in order to participate in an informed decision regarding surgical care. Future consequences of concern include ongoing progression of deformity, cardiac or pulmonary compromise, neurologic deterioration, unacceptable appearance, and possible development of progressive pain. With information gained from studying the natural history of untreated idiopathic scoliosis, we have useful insight into predicting the future consequences of spinal deformity in general.

2. Neuromuscular Scoliosis

Neuromuscular scoliosis develops secondary to loss of muscular control of the trunk. The term encompasses a multitude of disorders all of which result in some compromise of the patient's ability to control posture and trunk position. The severity of deformity is related to the severity of weakness or spasticity, the patient's age at presentation of neuromuscular pathology, and the rostral or caudal level of involvement within the spinal cord. Spinal deformity may be the reason for initial presentation of a patient with a neuromuscular disorder. Therefore, a detailed history including birth circumstances, family history, and timing of developmental milestones is important in evaluating the child with spinal deformity. Similarly, neurologic examination including documentation of muscle tone, strength, reflex symmetry, and ataxia may reveal a neuromuscular cause of scoliosis. More commonly, a child will have a known neuromuscular disorder and the orthopedic surgeon will monitor the patient for the development of spinal deformity in concert with management of associated deformities, including involvement of the hips, feet, and upper extremities.

Neuromuscular scoliosis may present in patients with disorders involving upper motor neurons, lower motor neurons, or primary myopathies. Upper motor neuron disorders may include cerebral palsy, spinocerebellar degeneration (Friedreich's ataxia, Charcot-Marie-Tooth disease, Roussy-Levy disease), syringomyelia, spinal cord tumor, and spinal cord trauma. Lower motor neuron disorders include poliomyelitis, spinomuscular atrophy, myelodysplasia, dysautonomia, and trauma. Poliomyelitis was the most common cause of neuromuscular scoliosis before the development of vaccination and remains an important cause of neuromuscular deformity in many parts of the world. Primary myopathies that may lead to neuromuscular deformity of the spine include muscular dystrophy, arthrogryposis, and congenital hypotonia.

Neuromuscular scoliosis characteristically presents with long, sweeping patterns, involving more vertebrae than idiopathic curves, with fewer compensatory curves. This may result in imbalance of the trunk relative to the pelvis. Pelvic obliquity is common in neuromuscular scoliosis, resulting in poor sitting balance and skin breakdown. Pulmonary compromise may be an important feature of neuromuscular curves due to the combination of thoracic deformity with intercostal and accessory muscle weakness. Therefore, the child with neuromuscular spinal deformity presents with comorbidities and functional considerations that are distinct from the patient with idiopathic or congenital scoliosis.

Treatment

In the neuromuscular patient who sits and is nonambulatory, goals of surgery include restoration of sitting balance and lumbar lordosis, prevention of sacral and ischial skin breakdown, and improvement of the ability of caregivers to assist with patient transfers and mobility. In the patient with neuromuscular scoliosis that is ambulatory, management includes consideration of maintenance of truncal balance relative to the pelvis, pulmonary function, and functional ability in transfers and gait.

Orthotics—including molded body jackets and thoracolumbar orthoses—may be useful in preserving sitting balance and delaying surgical correction and stabilization. Orthotics do not appear to effectively slow curve progression. Surgical correction and stabilization of the spine is the most effective management. Indications for surgery include curve progression, poor sitting balance, respiratory compromise, and skin compromise. In the patient who is ambulatory, fusion of the spinal column to the pelvis may compromise functional independence.

3. Congenital Scoliosis

Congenital anomalies of the spine are caused by defects in the embryologic formation and segmentation of spinal elements. The formation of the spine begins during the third week of embryonic development with cells from the epiblast layer invaginating into the primitive pit and migrating cephalad to the prochordal plate. These epiblast cells form a notochordal process that separates ectoderm from mesoderm. Proliferation of notochordal cells creates a solid notochord that serves as a midline axis for the axial skeleton. During the fourth week of embryonic development, sclerotomal segments shift to surround the notochord and the neural tube. The process of formation and resegmentation of sclerotomes is induced by the notochord, and the formation of the posterior arch of the spine is induced by the neural tube. Abnormalities of either the notochord or the neural arch may cause congenital anomalies of the spine. Congenital anomalies may include unilateral failure of formation (hemivertebrae and wedge vertebrae), unilateral or bilateral failure of segmentation, rib fusion, and mixed or complex anomalies. Solitary anomalies of the spine appear sporadic and are not hereditary. Multiple congenital anomalies of the spine may have a heritable basis.

Progression of deformity in congenital scoliosis is related to the type of vertebral anomaly, the position of the vertebral anomaly, and the growth potential for that segment of the spine. Congenital anomalies of the spine have the potential for rapid progression and development of fixed deformity. Therefore, patients with congenital scoliosis warrant early identification and close observation. The patient with a congenital deformity of the spine may have associated intraspinal and systemic abnormalities. Intraspinal disorders associated with congenital scoliosis include tethering of the cord, syringomyelia, diastematomyelia, diplomyelia, lipoma, teratoma, and neuroenteric cysts. Extraspinal disorders, including tracheoesophageal fistula, esophageal atresia, renal anomalies, bowel malrotation, anal atresia, radial forearm and hand anomalies, and cardiac septal defects, may be detected in the child with congenital deformity of the spine.

Bracing the spine may delay surgery in the young child, and is appropriate for long flexible deformities. Most patients with congenital deformity of the spine detected before 10 years of age will require operative management for control of curve progression. The goal of surgery in young patients is to prevent the development of a severe rigid deformity. Timing of operation requires understanding of curve progression patterns.

SEPTIC ARTHRITIS OF THE HIP

ESSENTIALS OF DIAGNOSIS

- *Limited hip motion, with local swelling and tenderness.*
- *Variable signs of systemic illness.*
- *Purulent exudate in the hip joint, confirmed by aspiration or arthrotomy.*

General Considerations

See Figure 42–37.

Infection is usually hematogenous and more frequent in infants exposed to invasive measures likely to cause bacteremia. The joint can be primarily involved, or secondary involvement may occur by spread of hematogenous osteomyelitis from the proximal femur. Hip sepsis has also followed penetration of the joint during attempted blood aspiration from the femoral vein.

Staphylococcus aureus and *Streptococcus pyogenes* are the most common causative organisms.

Clinical Findings

A. Symptoms and Signs

Impaired voluntary and reflex motion of the entire involved limb—pseudoparalysis—is the most typical early finding. Fever is unlikely in very young children,

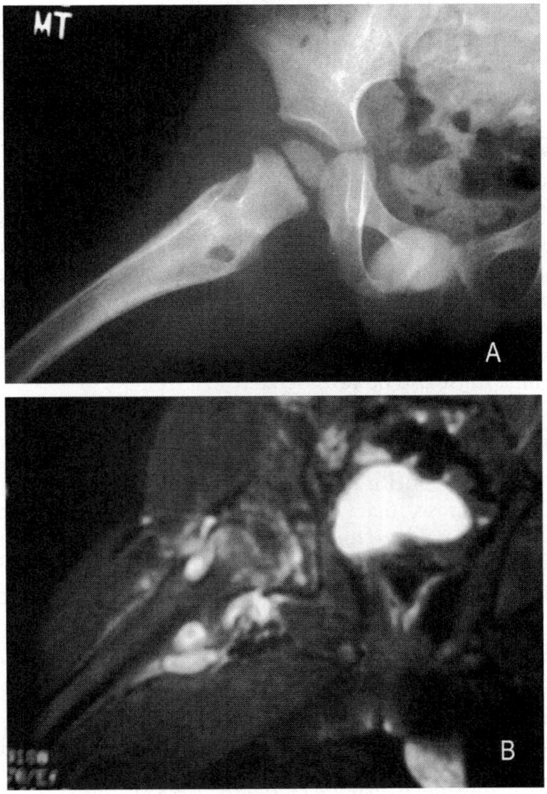

Figure 42–37. Septic arthritis of the hip in a 2-year-old boy. ***A:*** Lateral radiograph shows signs of proximal femoral osteomyelitis. ***B:*** T2-weighted MRI showing large effusion in the hip joint and edema of the proximal femur.

but sepsis may be suggested by irritability and failure to thrive. Another focus of infection should increase suspicion. The hip is held flexed in slight abduction and external rotation, with local swelling becoming evident as disease progresses. The area is tender, and attempts to move the hip are resisted and seem especially painful. If pathologic dislocation has occurred, hip asymmetry and instability may be noted.

B. Laboratory Findings

The sedimentation rate is elevated, but the white blood count may be normal. Leukocytes are abundant in the joint fluid, and Gram-stained smears of fluid show microorganisms as well. Bone scan may initially be negative, especially in children under 6 months of age, but usually shows increased uptake around the involved joint before radiographic changes become evident.

C. Imaging Studies

The early radiographic signs are subtle, with obliteration of soft tissue planes and a suggestion of capsular distention. Lateral subluxation and complete dislocation may occur. Decreasing bone density and periosteal erosion or new bone formation occur later. Ultrasound imaging provides an early indication of joint effusion.

Differential Diagnosis

Alternative diagnoses in the neonate are fractures of the femur occurring during birth and acute hematogenous osteomyelitis of the proximal femur that has not yet spread into the hip. Congenital hip dislocation is not painful and limits motion to a lesser extent. In older children, transient synovitis, rheumatoid arthritis, pelvic osteomyelitis, and acute hemarthrosis from hemophilia must also be considered.

Complications

Structural sequelae include pathologic dislocation; avascular necrosis that may cause total and irreversible destruction of the femoral head and neck; and leg length discrepancy, usually due to undergrowth of the involved femur. Chronic persisting infection may also result.

Treatment

Emergent surgical drainage is required. Side effects from negative arthrotomy are so few that exploration is warranted if the diagnosis is uncertain. Gram-stained smears of intra-articular pus guide the initial choice of parenteral antibiotic, which is modified if necessary according to the results of culture and sensitivity tests. Suction-irrigation tube drainage will maintain adequate decompression. Postoperatively, traction or a spica cast is used to rest and align the joint.

Course & Prognosis

If the diagnosis is made and surgical drainage performed within a few days after onset, the long-term results are good. Delay and nonoperative treatment are predictably followed by the complications mentioned above.

TRANSIENT SYNOVITIS OF THE HIP (IRRITABLE HIP SYNDROME, TOXIC SYNOVITIS, "OBSERVATION HIP")

This syndrome of unknown origin is the most common cause of painful hip in young children. A respiratory illness often precedes the complaint of pain, which may be localized in the knee, thigh, or hip. The short duration of symptoms, absence of diagnostic radiographic signs, and nearly normal laboratory studies suggest a benign process. Children of any age may be affected, though the average age is 6 years. Perhaps the most important aspect of transient synovitis is to recognize it appropriately and not confuse it with more serious causes of hip joint inflammation.

Clinical Findings

A. Symptoms and Signs

When first evaluated, the child has rarely been symptomatic for more than a week. Pain in the lower extremity with activity (or even with rest) is the most common complaint. Limp and refusal to walk are also common. Localization of pain to the hip region is not reliable, and a specific provocative test of hip motion must always be part of the physical examination of a child with lower extremity complaints. Passive range of motion of the hip must be checked and compared carefully with the opposite side. Normally, the child should be able to relax and motion should be free and easy without "guarding," which is especially noticeable on rotation or at extremes of flexion or extension. Low-grade fever may be present, but the child does not appear ill.

B. Laboratory Findings

Although the white blood cell count and erythrocyte sedimentation rate may be somewhat elevated, they are usually normal. Bone scan often shows increased activity in the hip joint, without the decreased femoral head uptake suggestive of early avascular necrosis. Hip aspiration, if performed to help clarify a confusing case, reveals clear synovial fluid with a low white cell count, no organisms on Gram-stained smears, and negative cultures for all types of organisms.

C. Imaging Studies

Radiographs are essential to rule out other diagnoses. X-rays are usually normal with transient synovitis of the hip.

Shadows adjacent to the femoral neck sometimes suggest "hip effusion," but the significance is questionable, since they can be produced by abduction and external rotation of a normal hip. Occasionally, the joint space will be widened.

Differential Diagnosis

Pyogenic or tuberculous sepsis is the primary concern. Legg-Perthes disease (avascular necrosis), slipped capital femoral epiphysis, and, rarely, other forms of inflammatory joint disease such as rheumatoid arthritis or rheumatic fever must be considered.

Treatment

Hospitalization is often advisable to ensure that an infection is not missed. The hip is placed at rest in 4–5 lb of Buck's or Russell's skin traction. This almost always relieves symptoms promptly and also helps confirm the diagnosis. A few days of rest may be required to regain normal hip motion. A week or so of protection from weight-bearing with bed rest at home or with crutches is usually advised. The child should then be reexamined to make certain that normal hip motion and comfort have been achieved. Anteroposterior and lateral x-rays are repeated in 2–3 months to ensure that avascular necrosis has not developed. Occasionally, signs of systemic reaction are more pronounced or the child continues to guard the hip longer than usual. In such cases, needle aspiration confirmed by arthrogram should be performed to rule out infection.

Prognosis

Recurrent symptoms may develop after release from the hospital and resumption of activity but usually resolve with more rest. Permanent (but usually unnoticeable) limitation of motion is present in about 18% of cases. A small number of patients develop other abnormalities and may represent errors in initial diagnosis.

CONGENITAL DYSPLASIA & DISLOCATION OF THE HIP

ESSENTIALS OF DIAGNOSIS

- *Mechanical instability of the hip.*
- *Persistent limitation of abduction.*
- *Shortening or other asymmetry of the hip if unilateral.*
- *Widening of buttocks and perineum if bilateral.*
- *Abnormal gait once walking begins.*

General Considerations

Congenital hip dysplasia may be manifested by dislocatability, dislocation, or inadequate joint development that results in early degenerative arthritis of the hip. True dislocation is not necessarily present at birth but develops early in life in some infants with dislocatable hips. The incidence of dislocation is 1 in 1000 infants. Both hips may be involved. Congenital hip dysplasia is more common in females and in patients with other congenital deformities. It is neither painful nor disabling in children but causes significant symptoms in adults if successful atraumatic closed reduction is not achieved in early childhood. If atraumatic reduction is not possible, surgical release of the obstructing or limiting soft tissues should be performed.

Clinical Findings

A. Symptoms and Signs

The physical signs of congenital hip dislocation are the key to diagnosis. They may be subtle, however, and can be missed by the most experienced examiner. This emphasizes the need for repeated evaluation of the hips during routine "well baby" checks.

1. Dislocatable hip—The examiner attempts to displace the infant's femoral head posterolaterally from the acetabulum by means of the subluxation provocation test (Figure 42–38). In a positive test, the femoral head is felt to displace with a jerk, which is repeated as the femur slides back into the acetabulum upon release of the displacing force. Mechanical instability—not a "click"—is the essential finding. Dislocatability is most easily demonstrated shortly after birth and should resolve within a few days.

2. Dislocated hip—Ortolani described the sign of "snapping" produced by relocation of a dislocated femoral head when the examiner abducts the flexed hip and lifts the greater trochanter anteriorly. This test can appear normal in the presence of congenital hip dysplasia if the soft tissues surrounding the joint are not lax enough to permit reduction. Diagnosis then rests upon other signs: limitation of abduction, asymmetry with apparent shortening, and deeper skin creases (if the dislocation is unilateral). As the child begins to walk, an abnormal gait becomes apparent. Trendelenburg's sign is positive, the contralateral side of the pelvis drooping when the child stands on the affected limb. If dislocation is bilateral, the diagnosis is more challenging. The perineum and buttocks are widened, and abduction limitation is bilateral. Gait is "waddling," and lumbar lordosis is prominent.

B. Imaging Studies

Until the cartilaginous acetabulum and femoral head become substantially ossified, x-rays may fail to indicate

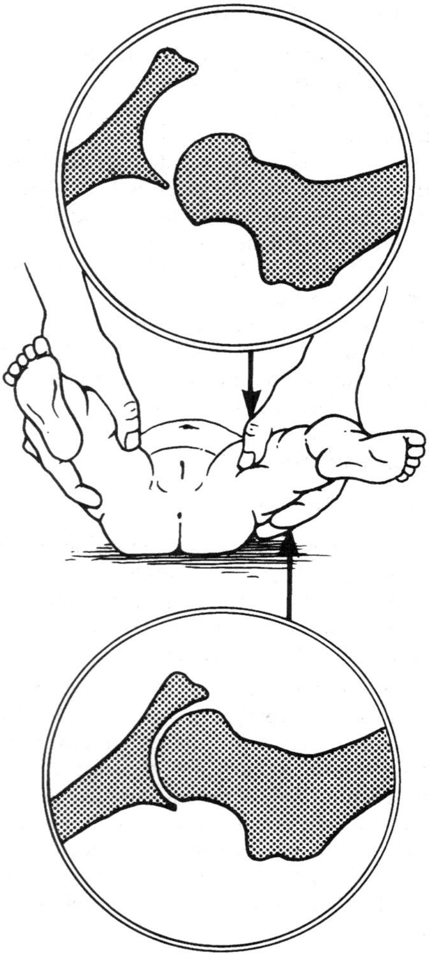

Figure 42–38. Upper window: Subluxation provocation test. Holding the thighs of the relaxed infant as illustrated, the examiner stabilizes the pelvis with one hand while gently but firmly trying to displace the opposite femoral head posteriorly out of the acetabulum. Adduction of the thigh aids this maneuver. If mechanical instability of the femoral head is present, a "jerk" will be felt, indicating that the hip is subluxable. ***Lower window:*** In Ortolani's test, abduction and lifting with the fingers produces a corresponding jerk when the dislocated femoral head slides back into the acetabulum.

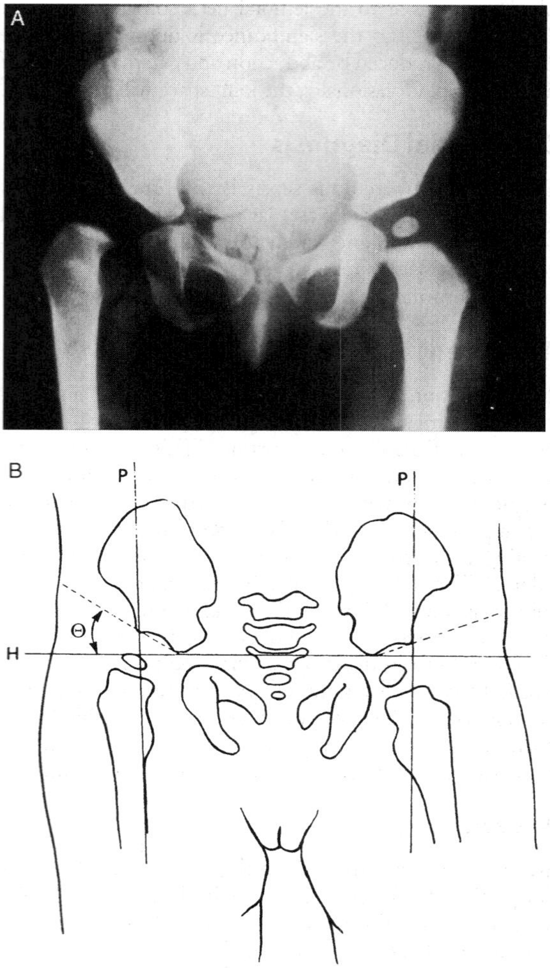

Figure 42–39. A: X-ray of congenital dislocation of the right hip. ***B:*** Analysis of hip radiographs presupposes adequately exposed films of a properly positioned patient. Hilgenreiner's horizontal line is drawn through both triradiate cartilages (H), and Perkins's vertical line is drawn through the outer margin of each acetabulum (P). If the hip is located, the proximal femoral epiphysis will lie in the inferomedial quadrant formed by the two intersecting lines. Proximal or lateral displacement indicates dislocation. Abnormal acetabular development is suggested by lack of obvious concavity and by an acetabular index (Θ) greater than 30 degrees.

the true condition of the hip joint. Obvious abnormalities must be considered significant, but apparently normal radiographs do not exclude congenital hip dysplasia until a well-ossified femoral head is adequately contained by the acetabulum. Femoral head ossification is usually present by 6 months of age but is often delayed in dislocated hips. Figure 42–39 shows several of the many radiographic relationships that are important for

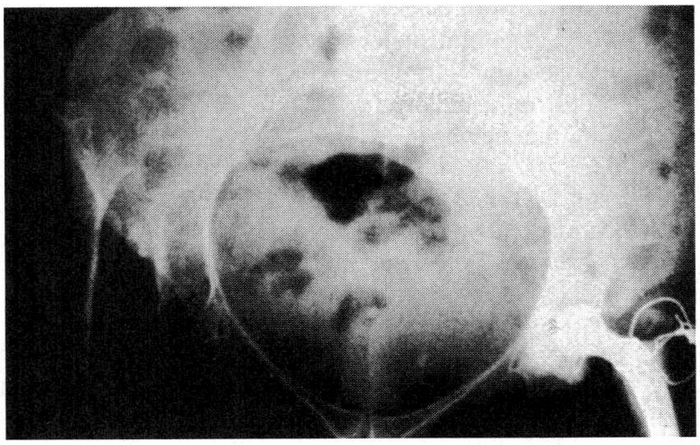

Figure 42–40. Adult with left total hip arthroplasty and persistent dislocation of the right hip caused by bilateral congenital hip dislocations.

evaluation of the hip joint in infants. In older children, the femoral head should be adjacent to the radiolucent triradiate cartilage that forms the medial wall of the acetabulum. Displacement of the femoral head confirms dislocation. A shallow acetabulum that poorly covers the femoral head is termed dysplastic. Hip arthrography or CT scans help evaluate reduction of the unossified hip joint. Ultrasonography is gaining popularity as a technique for assessing the infant's hip prior to calcification of the cartilaginous joint structures. Congenital hip disease in the adult is shown in Figure 42–40.

Differential Diagnosis

Congenital abduction contracture of the hip is not unusual in neonates. Proximal femoral focal deficiency and congenital coxa vara are rare conditions that produce shortening or instability in the hip region. Pathologic dislocation can occur rapidly in infected hips; the femoral head is displaced from a radiographically normal acetabulum. Hip dislocation may be caused by muscle imbalance in some children with cerebral palsy or myelomeningocele.

Complications

Complications include inability to gain or maintain a stable reduction, avascular necrosis of the femoral head following operative or nonoperative treatment, and limitation of motion.

Treatment

A. Dislocatable Hip

Neonates with confirmed dislocatable hips should be treated by means of abduction splinting (Pavlik harness, Frejka cushion, etc) until stability and normal radiographic development are confirmed. It is important to flex the hips and abduct them no more than 60 degrees to avoid interfering with the blood supply, so that avascular necrosis does not occur.

B. Dislocated Hip

1. Birth to 18 months—In this age group, closed reduction is usually possible. Reduction can be maintained with removable splints as mentioned above if the parents are reliable and careful medical supervision can be continued. A plaster spica cast is often safer. If closed reduction is not possible or cannot be maintained, open reduction is required. X-rays to confirm reduction and its maintenance are essential to any form of treatment.

2. Eighteen months to 4 years—Preliminary traction and open reduction are more likely to be required in this group. If adequate reduction is obtained, more than 90% of patients should have satisfactory results.

3. Older children and adults—Treatment of newly diagnosed congenital hip dysplasia in this age group is difficult. Acetabular remodeling through growth is slight. Mere achievement of a concentric reduction does not ensure a stable pain-free hip. Choices of treatment are operation or no treatment at all. Several osteotomies of the innominate bone have been described for improving acetabular coverage of the femoral head. Pain and limitation of motion will eventually necessitate total hip arthroplasty for many of these individuals.

SLIPPED CAPITAL FEMORAL EPIPHYSIS

During the period of rapid growth in early adolescence, the normal relationship of the femoral head with the femoral neck may become distorted by a shearing displacement through the growth plate—so-called slipped capital femoral epiphysis. The head remains within the acetabulum, while the femoral neck shifts anteriorly and laterally. This displacement may occur rapidly, often in response to minor trauma, or it can be gradual, as indicated by reactive bone formation and remodeling of the femoral neck adjacent to the growth plate. An acute slip may be superimposed upon a gradual "chronic" one. An acute slip is not a traumatic injury to a normal growth plate but is a "pathologic fracture" through a plate that is abnormally weak. Boys are more likely to be affected than girls. Involvement is bilateral in at least 25% of cases. The condition is progressive and can lead to severe deformity and limitation of hip motion if untreated. Marked deformity may cause early degenerative joint disease and is associated with increased risk of avascular necrosis and chondrolysis, though it is difficult to differentiate between the natural history of the disease and the complications of its treatment.

Clinical Findings

A. Symptoms and Signs

The patient reports pain in the knee or groin, limps, and has limited hip motion, especially flexion, internal rotation, and abduction.

B. Imaging Studies

Radiographs are diagnostic in all but the most minimal slips (Figure 42–41). The epiphysis is not centered on the neck, as is normally the case, but is relatively posterior and medial. Since posterior displacement is often more marked, the deformity may not be as evident on the anteroposterior view as on the lateral view. Bony callus, or widening of the metaphysis adjacent to the growth plate, indicates a chronic slip. A significant slip produces a bony prominence on the anterolateral femoral neck, restricting hip motion.

Treatment

Surgical stabilization of the proximal femoral epiphysis is advised. As soon as the diagnosis is made, the patient is hospitalized and placed in skin traction. An internal rotation strap may help reduce an acute slip; this is preferable to forceful manipulation under anesthesia, which increases the risk of avascular necrosis. In situ pinning of the epiphysis is then performed. The surgeon should make sure that pins do not enter the joint space. Gradual mobilization with protected weightbearing follows. The goal of pinning is to prevent further slip and gain closure of the physis. The opposite side must be watched until it closes because of the significant risk of its slipping as well. If severe deformity prevents normal motion, a subtrochanteric osteotomy or excision of the bony hump may be considered. Interference with function rather than abnormality on radiographs is the indication for such procedures.

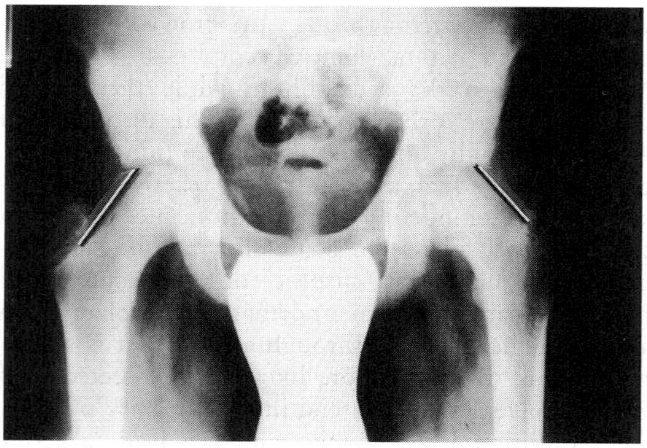

Figure 42–41. Left slipped capital femoral epiphysis. Note that a line extended along the lateral side of the femoral neck misses the capital epiphysis. On the normal right side, this line enters the femoral head, which should overlap the neck on both anteroposterior and lateral views.

LEGG-PERTHES DISEASE

(Legg-Calve-Perthes Disease; Coxa Plana)

Legg-Perthes disease is an uncommon hip affliction that occurs in about one in 2000 children, generally between the ages of 4 and 10. Boys are affected five times as often as girls, who tend to have more severe involvement. About 10–15% of patients have bilateral disease. The process is self-limited and of unknown cause. Its hallmark is avascular necrosis of the capital femoral epiphysis. When avascular necrosis of the femoral head occurs in adults, little potential exists for reconstitution of dead bone; however, the growing child with Legg-Perthes disease is able to completely replace the necrotic bone with new live bone. Some patients achieve normal hip development. Others acquire permanent deformity of the femoral head, with limited motion and degenerative joint disease becoming symptomatic in middle age.

Determinants of Final Outcome

A. Stage of Illness

The earliest signs are an apparent increase in density of the capital epiphysis and thickening of the surrounding cartilage. As revascularization occurs, femoral head density increases, a subchondral crescent-shaped radiolucent fracture appears transiently, and the metaphysis may widen. The epiphysis itself appears irregular and flattened. Gradually, living bone replaces cartilage and fibrous tissue, so that the femoral head is completely ossified. The ultimate shape will depend upon the molding of the malleable head during replacement of the necrotic epiphysis. A spherical head correlates well with good long-term results.

B. Age of Patient

Younger patients have a better prognosis. They are lighter in weight, have more rapid healing of necrotic bone, and have more growth time in which remodeling of residual deformity may occur.

C. Severity of Involvement

Catterall has classified patients with Legg-Perthes disease into four groups—according to the extent of involvement of the epiphysis—from group I, with only the anterior part of the epiphysis involved, to group IV, with involvement of the entire head. The extent of involvement is an indicator of the likelihood that the femoral head will deform and thus helps suggest the outcome for a given patient.

D. The "Head at Risk"

Catterall also proposed certain clinical and radiographic criteria for determining whether the femoral head might deform in the course of the disease. The clinical criteria are (1) obesity, (2) decreasing range of motion of the involved hip, and (3) adduction contracture. The radiographic criteria are (1) lateral subluxation of the femoral head, (2) Gage's sign (widening of the lateral part of the growth plate, so that the superior portion of the femoral neck appears convex), (3) calcification lateral to the epiphysis in the cartilaginous femoral head, (4) diffuse metaphysial reaction, and (5) a horizontal growth plate. Others agree that these signs are helpful indications of which patients are likely to have a poor outcome and might thus benefit from treatment aimed at maintaining a spherical femoral head.

Clinical Findings

A. Symptoms and Signs

Insidious development of limp and sometimes pain in the groin, anterior thigh, or knee eventually bring the patient to a physician. An occasional case presents as acute synovitis. Examination shows antalgic gait, decreased hip motion (especially abduction and internal rotation), and sometimes flexion-adduction contracture. Passive motion is guarded rather than free.

B. Laboratory Findings

Bone scan may help with early diagnosis and assessment of the extent of head involvement.

C. Imaging Studies

Well-exposed radiographs in both anteroposterior and frog-leg lateral views are essential. If synovitis significantly limits hip motion, a period in traction may be required before adequate positioning can be achieved. Findings will depend upon the stage and severity of disease, as discussed above, but initial films usually show increased density and deformity of the femoral head epiphysis, which may be flattened or fragmented (Figure 42–42).

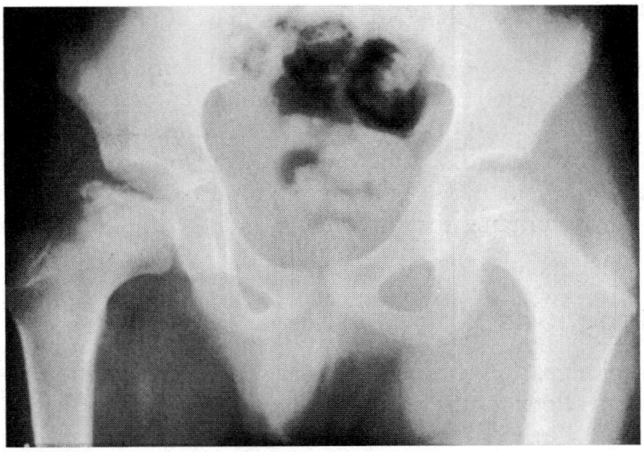

Figure 42–42. X-ray of Legg-Perthes disease, with significant deformity of right femoral head.

Differential Diagnosis

The early inflammatory stage of Legg-Perthes disease can be confused with toxic synovitis, septic (including tuberculous) arthritis, and rheumatoid arthritis. The epiphysial abnormalities are similar to those seen in epiphysial dysplasias, hypothyroidism, and avascular necrosis from other causes, notably sickle cell anemia, Gaucher's disease, and chronic use of corticosteroid drugs.

Treatment

Rational treatment requires categorization according to the stage of disease, the extent of head involvement, and the condition of the hip joint at the time of presentation. The mobility of the involved joint must be determined and then followed as an important indicator of prognosis.

A. Observation

Treatment is unnecessary and contraindicated for the following patients: children with involvement of less than half the femoral head, young children (under 5 years of age) without "at risk" signs, and children who already show radiologic evidence of healing. If significant deformity exists and insufficient growth time remains for remodeling, only symptomatic treatment is appropriate.

B. Rest and Traction

If joint motion is limited, bed rest and traction are employed to decrease synovitis and muscle spasm. Muscle releasing procedures may be required if contractures have developed. Once the hip is mobilized, containment of the femoral head within the acetabulum is necessary to maintain its spherical shape. If it is allowed to extrude laterally from the acetabulum, it will become deformed.

C. Bracing

Containment can be achieved with bracing, which should be maintained until reossification is under way; an average of 18 months is required.

D. Surgical Treatment

An alternative to prolonged bracing is surgery to reorient the acetabulum or the proximal femur to achieve containment. Both innominate osteotomy and varus proximal femoral osteotomy have advocates. Surgical containment properly achieved appears to be as effective as containment by bracing and to be much more expeditious.

Prognosis

Prolonged follow-up is necessary to determine the outcome. Poor results on x-rays do correlate positively with pain, limited motion, and disability. However, the affected hip may not be symptomatic for years. If Legg-Perthes disease of all degrees of severity is untreated, 55% of patients report good results and 45% report fair and poor results. If group I patients are excluded, the figures can be reversed. Following osteotomy of selected patients with more severe disease, two-thirds or more are reported to have a favorable outcome.

FOOT DEFORMITIES IN CHILDREN

Positional deformities of the foot are described with the following specific terms. Equinus refers to plantar flexion. Calcaneus is the opposite position, or dorsiflexion. Varus indicates angulation in the frontal plane, with inversion of the involved part. The forefoot alone may be in varus, or the deformity may be present in the hindfoot as well. Valgus is the opposite of varus and implies eversion of the involved part. Inversion and eversion of the forefoot (metatarsus) describe rotation about the long axis of the foot. Adduction of the forefoot is the term used to distinguish deviation of the metatarsals toward the medial side of the foot without the rotational component suggested by the term varus.

The goal of treatment of foot deformity is a pain-free, flexible, plantigrade foot—ie, a foot whose plantar surface is level with the ground during normal gait.

1. Clubfoot

Talipes equinovarus, or clubfoot, is most commonly an idiopathic congenital condition affecting approximately one in 1000 children. It occurs twice as often in boys and is bilateral half the time. There is a familial tendency, with a 5% chance that a sibling will also be affected.

Clinical Findings

A. Symptoms and Signs

In congenital clubfoot, there is more or less rigid inversion of the hindfoot, adduction of the forefoot, and limited dorsiflexion—an equinovarus deformity. While the cause is not certain, the deformity involves medial subluxation of the navicular and calcaneus on the talus. The joints principally involved are thus the subtalar and talonavicular joints. The adjacent ankle and midtarsal joints are affected to a lesser degree. The overlying soft tissues are contracted, and the longer the subluxation remains, the more deformed become the involved bones, which are composed largely of malleable cartilage. Successful treatment requires early reduction of joint subluxations and maintenance of correction throughout growth.

B. Imaging Studies

X-rays are useful primarily for assessing the adequacy of correction rather than for establishing the diagnosis of clubfoot. At birth, only the ossific nuclei of the calcaneus, talus, and metatarsals are present. Navicular ossification does not begin until about age 4. Therefore, radiographs of the newborn foot provide less information than the clinical examination. A good photograph documents the deformity more adequately. By 2–3 months of age, the ossification centers of the talus and calcaneus have elongated sufficiently to indicate their long axes, so that radiographs can provide helpful data about interosseous relationships. An anteroposterior view of a normal foot shows divergence of the talus and calcaneus, the former directed along the first ray and the latter along the fifth ray. In clubfoot, the talus usually points more laterally and may actually appear superimposed upon the calcaneus. On a lateral radiograph of a normal foot in maximal dorsiflexion, the calcaneus is dorsiflexed, so that its axis crosses that of the navicular, and the anterior ends of their shadows overlap. Clubfoot prevents this dorsiflexion and overlapping. Full calcaneal dorsiflexion is a valuable radiographic indicator of adequate treatment.

Treatment

Initial treatment is always nonoperative and should be started as soon as possible, preferably the day the infant is born.

A. Manipulation

Gentle manipulation into a corrected position should be done in order to stretch the contracted soft tissues—specifically, to align the calcaneus and navicular relative to the talus. Gentleness is required to avoid tissue trauma and to prevent overcorrection of the forefoot relative to persisting tarsal deformity.

B. Casting

After several minutes of manipulation, a plaster cast is applied and molded to maintain the maximally corrected position. Manipulation and cast application should be repeated weekly.

Casts are advisable for at least 6 months, followed by a Denis Browne bar with attached out-flare shoes. Similar shoes are worn when the child begins to walk, but the Denis Browne bar splinting should be continued at night and during nap times for several more years. During this time, close follow-up is required, with immediate use of a plaster cast if deformity recurs. Correction achieved by age 7 years is usually permanent. Carefully and conscientiously pursued, nonoperative treatment has been sufficient to correct clubfoot deformity in 35–90% of cases in large series. If satisfactory correction has not been achieved by age 3 months, operative management should be considered.

C. Surgical Treatment

Operations for clubfoot are many and varied. The present trend is toward a single combined procedure to release all of the posteromedial contracted tissues and permit open realignment of the talonavicular and talocalcaneal joints. Temporary percutaneous wire fixation is advocated by some surgeons. Postoperative care requires persistent follow-up and prolonged support in a plaster cast, splints, and special shoes. Satisfactory results from posteromedial release are reported in 75–85% of patients. Triple arthrodesis and other surgical procedures provide salvage for symptomatic patients in whom posteromedial release does not provide good results.

2. Metatarsus Adductus

The terms "metatarsus varus" and "metatarsus adductus" are used more or less interchangeably for deformity characterized by medial "hooking" of the forefoot. The adduction is at the tarsometatarsal joint, and the hindfoot is either in neutral position or in valgus. Metatarsus adductus is somewhat commoner than clubfoot and seems to have a stronger familial tendency. The deformity is often quite mobile. If passively correctable, there is an 85% chance of spontaneous correction by age 3 years. No treatment is required if stroking of the lateral border of the foot provokes active correction. Easy passive correction also suggests that treatment is unnecessary. If the forefoot cannot readily be returned to a normal position, restoring a concave lateral border to the foot, treatment is advisable. The surgeon stabilizes the hindfoot with one hand while manipulating the forefoot to correct the deformity with the other hand. A well-molded plaster cast is applied to maintain this position. The cast is changed every 1–2 weeks for 6–8 weeks, followed by night splints for several months. Only a very rare severe deformity will require surgical release or osteotomy and fusion of the tarsometatarsal joints.

Cook DA et al: Observer variability in the radiographic measurement and classification of metatarsus adductus. J Pediatr Orthop 1992;12:86.

3. Flatfoot

The normal newborn foot appears flat because subcutaneous fat fills the longitudinal arch. This fat deposit recedes over the first 4 years of life to reveal the typical adult appearance of a medial arch under the midfoot, which does not touch the floor with weightbearing. An inadequate bony arch, which permits the medial portion of the midfoot to bear weight, is the essential feature of true flatfoot. This deformity is classified as rigid or flexible.

Rigid flatfoot is identified by the absence of normal mobility of the foot. Obvious deformity with convexity of the sole is present in congenital convex pes valgus, where congenital dorsal dislocation of the talonavicular joint is the cause. Early open reduction is advisable. Rigid flatfoot presenting later in childhood is usually due to coalition of the tarsal bones. Associated episodic foot pain and spasm of the peroneal muscles are typical. Depending on the child's age and symptoms and the site of coalition, resection may be advisable or nonoperative treatment may suffice.

In flexible flatfoot, weightbearing obliterates the medial arch and also produces obvious valgus alignment of the calcaneus. Standing on tiptoes or sitting with the feet hanging free will restore the arch and substantially correct heel valgus. Some patients with flexible flatfoot develop foot pain with weightbearing. Pain may range from minimal to severely incapacitating and is not clearly related to the severity of the deformity.

Treatment of asymptomatic flexible flatfoot in children is controversial. Parents distressed by the foot's appearance or by abnormal shoe wear often request treatment, but there is little evidence that treatment prevents future symptoms, and many young children with flexible flatfoot have minimal deformity or symptoms in adulthood.

The child with painful flexible flatfoot deformity deserves treatment. Exercises to stretch tight gastrocsoleus muscle groups or to strengthen intrinsic plantar muscles are usually advised, and external support for the mediolongitudinal arch can be provided if necessary by flexible or rigid arch supports or shoe modifications. If nonoperative treatment fails to control symptoms or if deformity precludes use of normal footwear, surgery may be considered. Many procedures have been proposed. If present, an accessory navicular may be excised, with transposition of an abnormally inserted tibialis posterior tendon. Ligament reconstructions, arthrodeses, and osteotomies may be used separately or in combination to attempt restoration of the arch. A major risk of all such procedures is that a flexible deformity will be exchanged for a potentially more painful rigid one.

Briggs TW, Orr MM, Lightowler CD: Isolated tibial fractures in children. Injury 1992;23:308.

Caine D et al: Stress changes of the distal radial growth plate: a radiographic survey and review of the literature. Am J Sports Med 1992;20:290.

Heath CH, Staheli LT: Normal limits of knee angle in white children: genu varum and genu valgum. J Pediatr Orthop 1993;13:259.

Heinrich SD et al: Stabilization of pediatric diaphyseal femur fractures with flexible intramedullary nails (a technique paper). J Orthop Trauma 1992;6:452.

Henderson RC, Kemp GJ, Campion ER: Residual bone-mineral density and muscle strength after fractures of the tibia or femur in children. J Bone Joint Surg Am 1992;74:211.

Hennrikus WL et al: The function of the quadriceps muscle after a fracture of the femur in patients who are less than seventeen years old. J Bone Joint Surg Am 1993;75:508.

Hope PG, Cole WG: Open fractures of the tibia in children. J Bone Joint Surg Br 1992;74:546.

Kling TF Jr et al: Distal tibial physeal injuries in children that may require open reduction. J Bone Joint Surg Am 1984;66:647.

Krueger-Franke M, Siebert CH, Pfoerringer W: Sports-related epiphyseal injuries of the lower extremity: an epidemiologic study. J Sports Med Phys Fitness 1992;32:106.

Krueger-Franke M, Siebert CH, Pfoerringer W: Sports-related epiphyseal injuries of the lower extremity: an epidemiologic study. J Sports Med Phys Fitness 1992;32:106.

Levy J, Ward WT: Pediatric femur fractures: an overview of treatment. Orthopedics 1993;16:183.

Marcinko DE, Azzolini TJ, Mariash SA: Enigma of pediatric vertical talus deformity. J Foot Surg 1990;29:452.

Meyers MC et al: Delayed treatment of a malreduced distal femoral epiphyseal plate fracture. Med Sci Sports Exerc 1992;24:1311.

Oestreich AE, Ahmad BS: The periphysis and its effect on the metaphysis: I: definition and normal radiographic pattern. Skeletal Radiol 1992;21:283.

Salo JM et al: Congenital flat foot: different clinical forms. Acta Orthop Belg 1992;58:406.

Salter RB, Best TN: Pathogenesis of progressive valgus deformity following fractures of the proximal metaphyseal region of the tibia in young children. Instr Course Lect 1992;41:409.

PAIN SYNDROMES

PAIN SYNDROMES OF THE SHOULDER

1. Painful Arc Syndrome (Rotator Cuff Tendinitis, Subacromial Bursitis)

ESSENTIALS OF DIAGNOSIS

- *Pain over the anterior or lateral shoulder, most severe during abduction.*
- *Restriction of joint motion.*

General Considerations

Inflammation within the glenohumeral joint is the most frequent cause of shoulder pain and limitation of motion. The patient is typically middle-aged. Repeated minor trauma from occupational or sports activity is the cause, and the most common site of inflammation at onset is the rotator cuff, particularly the supraspinatus tendon. The location of the supraspinatus tendon between the greater tuberosity of the humeral head and the overhanging acromion process renders it particularly vulnerable to mechanical compression. Rotator cuff inflammation will often spill over into the subacromial bursa, and subdeltoid soreness frequently radiates along the lateral humerus to the deltoid insertion.

Clinical Findings

Active abduction becomes especially painful when the shoulder moves between 60 and 120 degrees because the inflamed rotator cuff and overlying bursa are compressed beneath the acromion. Because of this characteristic feature, the condition is known as painful arc syndrome. The range of active abduction may be extended if the patient is instructed to rotate the arms so that the palms face upward. This rotates the greater tuberosity posteriorly, so that the attached rotator cuff tendons pass behind the acromion, resulting in diminished pain with continued abduction.

Treatment

Treatment of rotator cuff tendinitis and subacromial bursitis is with analgesics such as aspirin or nonsteroidal anti-inflammatory agents (naproxen, ibuprofen), and local application of cold packs. Physical therapy may be useful in preserving full range of motion. Slings and shoulder immobilization should not be used for more than a few days, since capsular adhesions and prolonged stiffness may result. Gentle passive range-of-motion exercises by a therapist or family member should be started as soon as tolerated, followed by active pendulum exercises consisting of circular swinging motions of the dangling arm while leaning forward. Active exercise is gradually increased while passive range of motion is extended with exercises such as pulley-enhanced abduction using a bath towel over a shower curtain rod.

If pain does not respond to oral anti-inflammatory agents, prolonged relief may be obtained by injecting 40 mg of methylprednisolone acetate (or equivalent) and 1–2 mL of lidocaine into the subacromial bursa. The patient should be warned that injection may produce a brief exacerbation of pain before relief is noted and should be provided with analgesic medications. When full function has been recovered, reduction of stressful activities should be advised.

2. Calcific Tendinitis

ESSENTIALS OF DIAGNOSIS

- *Excruciating shoulder pain.*
- *Severe restriction of joint motion.*

General Considerations

Calcium deposition in the degenerative rotator cuff may lead to a variant form of tendinitis in the shoulder region. Asymptomatic bilateral calcium deposits in the shoulder tissues are a common finding in persons over age 40. The pathogenesis is unclear. The deposits may enlarge or rupture into the subacromial bursa.

Clinical Findings

A. Symptoms and Signs

The presentation of acute calcific tendinitis or bursitis is dramatic, with excruciating pain and severe restriction of shoulder motion. The patient may refuse even the gentlest examination for fear of motion-induced muscle spasm.

B. Imaging Studies

X-rays reveal either focal calcium deposits within the rotator cuff or a large "cap" of calcium overlying the humeral head, which represents dissemination of calcium into the subacromial bursa.

Treatment

Treatment of acute calcific tendinitis includes immediate injection of a corticosteroid and lidocaine solution into the tendon near the calcium deposit or into the bursa if calcium has entered that structure. Multiple needle punctures into the calcium deposit may break up the deposit and provide dramatic relief. Mobilization of the shoulder should proceed as described in the preceding section.

3. Biceps Tendinitis

ESSENTIALS OF DIAGNOSIS

- *Localized tenderness over the bicipital groove.*
- *Pain during supination of the forearm against resistance.*

General Considerations

A common inflammatory lesion producing shoulder pain involves the biceps tendon in the bicipital groove. Biceps tendon inflammation usually affects individuals whose occupation involves repetitive biceps flexion against resistance or whose recreational activities include forceful throwing of a ball. Pain is prominent over the anterior aspect of the arm and is aggravated by shoulder motion. Symptoms are worse at night and improve with rest. Deltoid muscle spasm may be present and may limit both active and passive motion.

Clinical Findings

Biceps tendinitis can be distinguished from rotator cuff tendinitis by localization of tenderness to the bicipital groove. Forearm supination against resistance with the elbow flexed at the patient's side elicits extreme tenderness in the region of the bicipital groove when the tendon is palpated near the shoulder. Instability of the tendon in the groove is occasionally manifested by a snapping sensation as the arm is abducted and externally rotated. Subluxation of the tendons can be provoked for diagnostic verification by Yergason's maneuver, in which the patient actively flexes the elbow against resistance while the physician rotates the humerus externally. An unstable tendon will "pop" out of the groove.

Treatment

Treatment of bicipital tendinitis includes cessation of offending activities and short-term immobilization of the shoulder in a sling; a trial of aspirin or nonsteroidal anti-inflammatory agents; and, occasionally, local injection of corticosteroids. Repeated corticosteroid injections may result in tendon attrition or rupture and should be avoided. Surgery is occasionally required to stabilize a subluxating tendon.

When discomfort has subsided, progressive mobilization is begun with exercises similar to those described in the section on rotator cuff tendinitis.

4. Adhesive Capsulitis (Frozen Shoulder)

ESSENTIALS OF DIAGNOSIS

- *Diffuse shoulder tenderness.*
- *Restriction of shoulder joint motion.*

General Considerations

A common cause of shoulder pain in middle-aged and elderly patients is adhesive capsulitis, or so-called frozen shoulder. This disorder may complicate other inflammatory shoulder ailments, particularly in individuals immobilized for prolonged periods. It may also occur without any identifiable inciting trauma and has been associated with cardiovascular disease, rheumatoid arthritis, and degenerative cervical spine disease. Though the exact pathogenesis is unknown, the end result is a chronically inflamed, contracted fibrotic capsule densely adherent to the humeral head, the acromion, and the underlying biceps and rotator cuff tendons. Normal bursae are obliterated by scarring.

Clinical Findings

A. Symptoms and Signs

The onset of symptoms is usually gradual and heralded by complaints of diffuse tenderness with disproportionately severe restriction of active and passive motion. Motion is not improved by lidocaine or corticosteroid injection.

B. Imaging Studies

Arthrography reveals a contracted joint capsule and no bursal filling. X-rays may reveal severe osteoporosis of the humeral head.

Treatment

The success of various treatments is difficult to assess, as the natural history of adhesive capsulitis is spontaneous resolution. Subsidence of pain and return of nearly full motion can be anticipated, though the process may persist for 6 months to several years. Efforts to speed return of function have included intensive physical therapy, oral corticosteroids and anti-inflammatory agents, and a procedure called infiltration brisement, which consists of pressure injection of the joint with 50 mL of saline and corticosteroid solution in order to break the adhesions binding the capsule to the surrounding structures.

Clearly, the best treatment of this condition is prevention. Prolonged disuse or immobilization of a painful shoulder must be avoided. Early mobilization is stressed, with initiation of gentle range of motion exercises and persistent encouragement and guidance by the physician and the physical therapist.

Ekelund AL, Rydell N: Combination treatment for adhesive capsulitis of the shoulder. Clin Orthop 1992;282:105.

PAIN SYNDROMES OF THE ELBOW

1. Tennis Elbow (Humeral Epicondylitis)

ESSENTIALS OF DIAGNOSIS

- *Tenderness over the lateral humeral epicondyle.*
- *Pain at the elbow with flexion or extension of the wrist.*

General Considerations

Though far more common in nonathletes, humeral epicondylitis is commonly termed tennis elbow. This overuse syndrome is uncommon before age 18 years and most frequent in the fourth and fifth decades. Though frequently blamed on faulty backhand motion, tennis elbow is occasionally seen in professional players but is far more common in nonathletes performing activities that require frequent rotary motion of the forearm, such as gardening, use of screwdrivers or wrenches, turning of doorknobs, and even operation of vehicles without power-assisted steering.

Clinical Findings

Tennis elbow is characterized by tenderness and pain at the humeral epicondyle provoked by extension or flexion of the wrist, depending on which epicondyle is involved. The lateral aspect of the elbow is far more often involved, and the origin of the inflamed common extensor muscle is the source of discomfort. Underlying synovitis may accompany the tendinitis. The pain is readily reproduced with traction on the extensor muscles by passive flexion of the fingers and wrist with the elbow extended.

Though the pathogenesis of tennis elbow is unknown, symptoms are usually attributed to inflammation of the origin of the common extensor muscle and, in some cases, to a tear in the origin of the extensor carpi radialis brevis. The tears are thought to be the result of repeated stress on degenerated tendon fibers. Elbow motion remains normal.

Differential Diagnosis

Differential diagnosis includes radial nerve irritation at the elbow, which may often be delineated by electromyography.

Treatment

A. Medical Treatment

Most patients with tennis elbow respond favorably to a brief period of rest and administration of analgesics followed by a program of gradually increasing exercise to strengthen the forearm muscles. Anti-inflammatory drugs or subtendinous injection of soluble corticosteroids with lidocaine may be required in more severe cases. Repeated injections may further weaken tendons and should be avoided.

After the acute symptoms subside, a nonelastic forearm band is prescribed to be worn near the elbow during occupational or recreational activities that aggravate the condition. The band is thought to be effective either because it limits full contraction of the tender muscles or because it slightly alters the position of the extensor tendons. Tennis players are advised to warm up slowly. Changes in the tension of racket strings and racket size or composition may also be of benefit.

B. Surgical Treatment

Some patients with severe or refractory symptoms may require operative treatment. Most surgeons repair the origin of the torn wrist extensor tendon after excision of granulation tissue and any rough subjacent bone. Lengthening of the short wrist extensor has also been advocated, though loss of strength has been reported with this procedure.

2. Olecranon Bursitis

ESSENTIALS OF DIAGNOSIS

- *Tenderness and swelling over the olecranon.*
- *Limitation of elbow flexion.*

General Considerations

Olecranon bursitis is a common cause of periarticular elbow pain. Like epicondylitis, this condition is often related to occupational activities, in this case prolonged periods of leaning on the elbow while studying ("student's elbow"), gardening, working on plumbing, or carpentry.

Clinical Findings

A. Symptoms and Signs

The subcutaneous olecranon bursa becomes distended, sometimes to dramatic proportions. The skin of the extensor surface of the forearm may be edematous and pitted. Traumatic bursitis is often only mildly painful despite marked swelling.

B. Laboratory Findings

Because of the tenderness of the skin over the bursa, elbow motion is limited only in extreme flexion. Fluid obtained by aspiration demonstrates a predominance of mononuclear cells, with fewer than 1000 white cells per microliter. Red cells are numerous, and mucin clot formation is poor. Strict aseptic technique is advised during aspiration of the bursa, as superinfection is common after multiple aspirations. Penetration of the inner wall of the cavity must be avoided; in septic olecranon bursitis, penetration may result in inoculation of bacteria into the underlying triceps tendon, leading to disastrous extension of infection into the posterior aspect of the arm.

Differential Diagnosis

Laboratory findings will differentiate septic olecranon bursitis, in which aspiration fluid demonstrates a predominance of PMNs in far greater numbers. Gout may affect the olecranon bursa, but urate crystals are present.

Treatment

Treatment of idiopathic or traumatic olecranon bursitis consists of protecting the bursa from further pressure or irritation. Aspiration and compression dressings may be necessary if symptoms are prolonged. Recurrence is not uncommon. Water-soluble corticosteroid injection may be helpful once infection has been ruled out as a possible cause. Excision of the bursa may be required for rare persistent cases. The bursa must be totally excised and the overlying skin sutured to the olecranon periosteum to ensure obliteration of the space.

Labelle H et al: Lack of scientific evidence for the treatment of lateral epicondylitis of the elbow: an attempted meta-analysis. J Bone Joint Surg Br 1992;74:646.

Wittenberg RH, Schaal S, Muhr G: Surgical treatment of persistent elbow epicondylitis. Clin Orthop 1992;278:73.

PAIN SYNDROMES OF THE HIP

1. Bursitis & Tendonitis of the Hip

Bursitis and tendonitis are frequent causes of pain around the hip area. These conditions most commonly affect middle-aged and elderly patients. Patients with a history of prior hip surgery, such as hip replacement or fixation of a hip fracture, may be especially prone to these conditions.

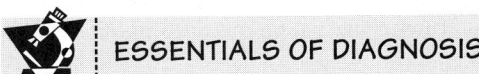

Clinical Findings

A. Symptoms and Signs

A common complaint is the inability to sleep or rest on the affected side. The painful area is localized over the prominence of the greater trochanter, and the pain is reproduced by firm palpation. Hip bursitis may be associated with tendonitis of the hip abductors that insert onto the greater trochanter. Pain due to tendonitis may be reproduced with active hip abduction against resistance.

It is important to differentiate extra-articular sources of hip pain such as bursitis and tendonitis from intra-articular sources such as osteoarthritis. Intra-articular pathology is suggested by pain localized to the groin or buttock, decreased passive internal rotation, and reproduction of the patient's pain at the limits of rotation.

B. Imaging Studies

Plain radiographs are extremely useful in the evaluation of hip joint disorders.

Treatment

Trochanteric bursitis often responds to rest, oral anti-inflammatory medications, and ice. Corticosteroid injection is highly effective in refractory cases. Typically, a mixture of lidocaine and corticosteroid is injected into the areas of maximal tenderness. This often requires a spinal needle to reach the trochanteric bursa that lies just superficial to the trochanter itself. Rapid relief of symptoms confirms injection of the proper area. Treatment of hip abductor tendonitis should include stretching exercises in addition to anti-inflammatory medication and ice. Direct injection of steroid into the tendon should be avoided.

2. The Snapping Hip

The painful snapping hip is most commonly caused by the iliotibial band snapping over the prominence of the greater trochanter. Less commonly, the iliopsoas tendon may be the cause of pain as it snaps over the hip joint capsule.

Snapping due to the iliotibial band can be reproduced with passive flexion of the hip starting from an adducted position. Snapping of the iliopsoas tendon may be reproduced with passive extension and internal rotation of the hip starting from a flexed and externally rotated position. Fluoroscopy after injection of the iliopsoas bursa with contrast can help to confirm this diagnosis.

Treatment usually consists of stretching and strengthening exercises. In rare circumstances, surgical release may be indicated for refractory cases.

3. Avascular Necrosis of the Femoral Head

Avascular necrosis of the femoral head is a disease process that results in focal areas of bone death within the femoral head. Subsequent collapse and flattening of the head may occur. The usual area of involvement is the subchondral bone in the anteromedial portion of the femoral head. The precise cause is not fully understood, but it appears that the final common pathway is disruption of the microcirculation that supplies the cancellous bone within the femoral head.

The most frequent cause of avascular necrosis is prior trauma to the hip. In particular, hip dislocation and fractures of the femoral neck are associated with a high incidence of subsequent avascular necrosis. These types of trauma often result in disruption of the retinacular vessels that are the primary blood supply to the femoral head. Avascular necrosis may also occur in the absence of trauma. In many cases, a predisposing factor or factors can be identified. Known risk factors include the use of systemic steroids (even a single dose), alcohol abuse, blood dyscrasias such as sickle cell disease, Gaucher's disease, and radiation therapy.

Clinical Findings

A. Symptoms and Signs

Patients present with hip or groin pain that typically worsens with activity and weightbearing. On clinical examination, the patient may limp and have increased discomfort with passive internal rotation of the hip. The earliest stage of the disease may be asymptomatic. Because this disease is often bilateral (up to two-thirds of cases), careful evaluation of the opposite hip is essential.

B. Imaging Studies

Plain radiographs serve as the basis for staging the extent of disease and to monitor its progression. MRI is extremely useful in identifying patients with the earliest stages of avascular necrosis, before abnormalities can be detected with plain radiographs.

Treatment

The treatment of avascular necrosis depends on the stage of the disease and the age of the patient. Patients identified with early stage disease, before collapse of the femoral head, may benefit from "core decompression," a procedure in which a reamer is used to create a channel into the affected area of the femoral head. The use of vascularized fibular grafts has also been advocated. However, these procedures are not uniformly successful, and the specific indications remain somewhat controversial.

Patients with more advanced disease, particularly elderly patients, may be good candidates for joint replacement surgery. Replacement may involve either the femoral side alone or both the femoral side and the acetabular side depending on the condition of the acetabular cartilage. Some surgeons prefer to replace both sides in all cases because of more consistent pain relief. Because of the limited durability of prosthetic hip joints, joint replacements in young patients should be reserved for those who have exhausted all conservative measures.

4. *Osteoarthritis*

ESSENTIALS OF DIAGNOSIS

- *Joint pain and stiffness.*
- *Pain increases with activity.*
- *Tenderness along joint line.*
- *Joint space narrowing and osteophytes on x-ray.*

General Considerations

Osteoarthritis is commonly referred to as "wear and tear" arthritis. Patients present with complaints of joint pain and stiffness. Pain due to osteoarthritis constitutes the most common joint complaint for which patients seek medical attention. The onset of symptoms may be insidious or may be associated with mild trauma. It is common for patients to experience a waxing and waning course, but gradual progression is expected. The severity of symptoms, particularly pain, typically increases with activity. As the disease progresses, night pain becomes a more frequent complaint. Osteoarthritis affecting an otherwise normal joint is termed primary osteoarthritis, while disease that is the sequela of a specific event or condition, such as trauma or infection, is termed secondary osteoarthritis.

Osteoarthritis is the most common of all arthropathies. Onset of symptomatic disease is typically in the sixth decade. Most people over the age of 55 have some radiographic evidence of osteoarthritis, though less than half develop joint symptoms. Genetic factors may play a role in the development of osteoarthritis, but only a small fraction of patients have been found to carry genetic markers known to be associated with the disease.

Mechanical factors that result in abnormally high loads across joint surfaces are associated with the development of osteoarthritis. Such predisposing factors include limb malalignment, joint instability, damaged or resected menisci, and malreduced intra-articular fractures. At a cellular level, osteoarthritic chondrocytes exhibit abnormal responses to anabolic and catabolic signaling molecules. They also express increased levels of proteolytic enzymes that lead to extracellular matrix degradation. The matrix of osteoarthritic cartilage is characterized by alterations in the structure and relative abundance of its key structural components, collagen and proteoglycans. These changes make osteoarthritic cartilage a less effective bearing surface and contribute to a vicious cycle of cartilage degeneration and an ineffective repair response.

Clinical Findings

A. Symptoms and Signs

Patients with osteoarthritis complain of a painful joint or joints, particularly with increased levels of activity. The pain is often reproduced with passive motion and loading of the involved joint. Commonly, both active and passive ranges of motion are decreased. Crepitation and mild swelling may also be present. Associated findings include juxta-articular prominences from bone spurs and angular deformities, particularly varus or valgus deformities of the knee. Examination of an arthritic knee often reveals pain along the affected joint line, due either to the arthritis itself or to an associated degenerative meniscal tear.

B. Imaging Studies

Plain radiographs are the primary imaging tool used in the evaluation of osteoarthritis. Weightbearing films are essential for complete evaluation of weightbearing joints. Special views, such as a bent knee posteroanterior projection, are often requested. Early findings include joint space narrowing, subchondral sclerosis, and early osteophyte formation. Later findings include progressive loss of joint space to the point of bone-on-bone contact, subchondral cyst formation, large osteophytes, joint subluxation, and even severe bone erosion.

Treatment

A. Bracing

Bracing may be effective treatment for a subset of patients with osteoarthritis. The benefits of bracing can be derived from immobilization of a painful joint (such as the use of an molded ankle support) or by decreasing the load across a joint (such as the use of an "unloader brace" for medial compartment arthritis of the knee).

B. Medical Treatment

Nonsteroidal anti-inflammatory drugs remain the mainstay for the pharmacologic treatment of osteoarthritis. The risk of gastrointestinal bleeding is of great concern, particularly with long-term use that is common for these patients. The recent introduction of COX-2 selective agents may decrease this complication. Acetaminophen may also be helpful. The role of nutritional supplements such as glucosamine and chondroitin sulfate remains unclear.

C. Surgical Treatment

Operation is indicated once more conservative measures prove inadequate in providing a level of function acceptable to the patient. Surgical options include joint debridement (either open or arthroscopic), osteotomy, joint fusion, joint reconstruction or resection, and joint replacement.

Joint debridement can be effective in delaying or preventing the need for more aggressive operative management. Joints such as the knee are particularly suitable for arthroscopic debridement, which is associated with minimal morbidity and, in some cases, lasting improvement.

Osteotomies are most commonly performed around the knee to treat isolated medial or lateral compartment degeneration. Osteotomies of the hip are performed to prevent progression of joint degeneration, particularly in patients felt to be too young for joint replacement.

Joint fusion can provide excellent pain relief at the expense of joint motion. Fusion of small joints, such as the interphalangeal joints, is well tolerated whereas fusion of large joints, such as the hip or knee, is often unsatisfactory. Nevertheless, fusion may be the procedure of choice, particularly in the case of active infection.

Some arthritic joints are amenable to reconstructive procedures that can provide effective and durable results. One example is reconstruction of the carpal-metacarpal joint of the thumb using a rerouted tendon and partial or total resection of the trapezium. In other cases, resection of the diseased joint itself may be an effective option, such as removal of the proximal row of carpal bones to treat wrist arthritis.

Prosthetic joint replacement has revolutionized the management of severe and disabling osteoarthritis. Hip, knee, or shoulder arthroplasty provides excellent pain relief and improved function and with current implants and techniques lasts 10 years or more in over 90% of cases. New bearing surfaces hold significant promise in extending the life of these implants even further. Replacements of the elbow, wrist, and ankle are performed less commonly. In general, these surgeries are not as consistently successful as the replacement of larger joints.

5. Rheumatoid Arthritis

ESSENTIALS OF DIAGNOSIS

- *Joint pain and swelling.*
- *Morning stiffness improving with activity.*
- *Elevated rheumatoid factor and ESR.*
- *Periarticular erosions and osteopenia on x-ray.*

General Considerations

Rheumatoid arthritis is a chronic systemic inflammatory, disease characterized by joint pain, swelling, and joint destruction. The incidence is 0.5–3% worldwide, increasing with age with a peak in the fifth decade. Women are affected three times as commonly as men. Rheumatoid arthritis in many cases results in partial or total disability and is associated with a shortened life expectancy.

The cause of rheumatoid arthritis is not known. However, the molecular and cellular basis of the disease is becoming clearer. The fundamental mechanism is characterized by dysregulation of the immune system with activation of inflammatory cells, including T cells, B cells, monocytes, and macrophages. These activated immune cells secrete factors that lead to chronic inflammation, cartilage destruction, and soft-tissue damage.

Clinical Findings

A. Symptoms and Signs

The onset and clinical course of rheumatoid arthritis are variable. A gradual onset with polyarticular involvement is the most common clinical presentation. About 20% of patients have disease that will abate within 2 years, and perhaps 5% will remain in long-term remission. The remainder will have either multiple flares or a progressive course. Major clinical features of active disease include symmetric polyarthritis with joint swelling, tenderness, and morning stiffness lasting an hour or longer. Involvement of the synovium and soft tissues precedes erosion of the cartilage and bone. The hands and feet often are the first sites to be affected with inflammation, joint and tendon subluxation, and, in later stages, joint destruction and tendon rupture. Rheumatoid arthritis affects mainly small and medium-sized joints. The joints most frequently involved are the metacarpophalangeal, proximal interphalangeal, and metatarsophalangeal joints. Less commonly affected joints include the wrist, elbow, shoulder, hip, knee, and mid foot. In addition, the upper cervical spine is frequently involved.

B. Laboratory Findings

Although no specific laboratory test can be used to make the diagnoses of rheumatoid arthritis, a high titer of rheumatoid factor is present in 80% of patients. The acute-phase reactants, markers, erythrocyte sedimentation rate, and C-reactive protein are also commonly elevated. Antinuclear antibodies are often present in patients with severe rheumatoid arthritis, but their presence is not specific for the disease. Joint aspiration during an acute flare typically reveals 500–25,000 leukocytes/μL.

C. Imaging Studies

The typical radiographic findings in rheumatoid arthritis include periarticular erosions and osteopenia. Joint space narrowing occurs in later stages of the disease. Advanced changes include bone resorption, deformity, dislocation, and fragmentation. In addition, protrusio acetabuli (medial migration of the femoral head into the pelvis) is not uncommonly seen in rheumatoid arthritis as well as in other forms of inflammatory arthritis.

Differential Diagnosis

Rheumatoid arthritis is usually easily distinguished from osteoarthritis based upon presentation, physical examination, and radiographic findings. Other inflammatory arthritides that may mimic rheumatoid arthritis include psoriatic arthritis, Reiter's syndrome, and arthritis associated with systemic lupus erythematosus, hepatitis, and inflammatory bowel disease. The differential diagnosis is more difficult in early stages of rheumatoid arthritis when joint involvement may be monoarticular and relatively mild. Joint aspiration to rule out infectious arthritis and crystal-induced arthritis may be indicated.

Treatment

A. Splinting

When acute inflammation is present, rest and splinting of joints can decrease symptoms and limit deformity. In particular, splinting small joints of the hand may prevent the development and progression of finger flexion and hyperextension deformities.

B. Medical Treatment

1. Nonsteroidal anti-inflammatory drugs (NSAIDs)—NSAIDs reduce inflammation and pain but rarely eliminate altogether the symptoms of active rheumatoid arthritis. Both nonselective and COX-2 selective agents are utilized. Although COX-2 selective drugs have a more favorable safety profile, their efficacy is not substantially different from that of the nonselective agents. There is no convincing evidence that these drugs affect long-term progression of the disease.

2. Corticosteroids—Corticosteroids are potent suppressors of inflammation and are highly effective in controlling severe polyarticular disease. However, the detrimental effects of systemic corticosteroids are well described and they should be used sparingly. Intra-articular steroid injection can provide temporary relief of joint symptoms without associated systemic effects.

3. Disease-modifying antirheumatic drugs (DMARDs)—DMARDs are a diverse class of agents that target the mechanisms responsible for tissue destruction in rheumatoid arthritis. Their use is associated with reduced morbidity and mortality in patients with rheumatoid arthritis. Combination therapy is often employed for better disease control. The most commonly used agent in the United States is methotrexate. Other DMARDs include hydroxychloroquine, sulfasalazine, cyclosporine, and azathioprine. Some traditional agents, such as penicillamine and gold, are now less frequently used with the advent of more effective agents that have better-understood mechanisms of action.

4. Anticytokine agents—This new class of drugs (infliximab, etanercept) shows great promise in the treatment of rheumatoid arthritis. These agents specifically target cytokines that are key mediators of the inflammatory response.

C. Surgical Treatment

1. Synovectomy—In early stages of the disease, synovectomy of tendon sheaths can be effective in preventing or delaying some tendon ruptures. Open or arthroscopic synovectomy of affected joints may have a limited role in providing symptomatic relief but does not affect the long-term prognosis.

2. Joint fusion—Joint fusion is effective in providing pain relief and correction of joint deformity at the expense of joint motion. In many cases, joint motion is already severely restricted by the disease. Fusion is commonly performed for joints of the hand and wrist with good long-term results.

3. Joint replacement—Joint replacement for patients with advanced rheumatoid arthritis can provide excellent pain relief and function. Joints that are commonly replaced include the hip, knee, shoulder, elbow, and metacarpophalangeal joints. Because patients with rheumatoid arthritis generally are not as active as patients with osteoarthritis, the question of implant durability in younger patients is less of a concern.

Howie DW, Cornish BL, Vernon-Roberts B: The viability of the femoral head after resurfacing hip arthroplasty in humans. Clin Orthop 1993;291:171.

Lafforgue P et al: Early-stage avascular necrosis of the femoral head: MR imaging for prognosis in 31 cases with at least 2 years of follow-up. Radiology 1993;187:199.

Sadat-Ali M: Avascular necrosis of the femoral head in sickle cell disease: an integrated classification. Clin Orthop 1993;290:200.

Swiontkowski MF et al: The effect of fracture on femoral head blood flow: osteonecrosis and revascularization studied in miniature swine. Acta Orthop Scand 1993;64:196.

Takatori Y et al: Avascular necrosis of the femoral head: natural history and magnetic resonance imaging. J Bone Joint Surg Br 1993;75:217.

PAIN SYNDROMES OF THE NECK

1. Cervical Strain

ESSENTIALS OF DIAGNOSIS

- *Paraspinous neck pain with or without radiation to the shoulder.*
- *Limitation of neck rotation.*

General Considerations

Neck pain is a common complaint in most outpatient clinics. It has been estimated that at any given time in the general population, one of every ten persons is suffering from neck and arm pain. Taking all ages together, 40% of all persons have suffered from neck and arm pain at some time. In most cases, symptoms are mild and self-limited.

Cervical muscle strain is perhaps the most frequent cause. Patients are usually in their forties or fifties. Symptoms typically appear within 24 hours after an episode of overexertion or in response to prolonged tension or poor posture.

Clinical Findings

A. Symptoms and Signs

Pain is most intense in the paraspinous muscles, within the superior trapezius fibers between the spine and the scapula, or at the periosteal site of muscle attachments in the scapula or occiput. Discomfort is characterized as deep aching or a boring sensation, and pain may occasionally radiate to the posterior shoulder or upper arm. This symptom complex is often difficult to differentiate from radicular pain. Discrete "trigger points"—specific points of deep tenderness—may be present. Spasm within the trapezius, levator scapulae, or paraspinous muscles may be palpable as a firm "knot." The neck is held in a guarded position with the head slightly flexed. Active and passive motion of the neck are often limited by voluntary splinting of the painful muscles. Rotation of the head away from the afflicted side is often resisted. The patient may also complain of headache or dizziness. The neurologic examination is always normal.

B. Imaging Studies

X-ray examination may show some straightening of the cervical spine. Mild or severe degenerative changes may be present, including osteophytes of the vertebral bodies or posterior facets. Radiographs are often normal.

Differential Diagnosis

The differential diagnosis includes cervical spondylosis or herniated cervical disk. A patient with a herniated cervical disk will complain of radicular symptoms in a specific dermatomal distribution corresponding to the affected disk level. These patients will often exhibit abnormalities in the neurologic examination such as muscle weakness in the corresponding myotomes, diminished reflexes, and diminished sensation or paresthesias. Pain arising from cervical spondylosis is often indistinguishable from that due to cervical strain. Whatever the precise anatomic source of pain, distinguishing cervical muscle sprain from early degenerative disk symptoms is of little importance, since both conditions are usually self-limited and are best managed conservatively.

Treatment

Treatment of acute cervical spine pain consists primarily of rest and immobilization. If pain is severe, mild halter traction may help to alleviate some of the pain arising from paraspinous muscle spasm. Halter traction with 2.5–3.5 kg (5–7 lb) may be used conveniently at home by most patients. Hospitalization is rarely required or indicated in the treatment of these patients. Analgesics and muscle relaxants are prescribed as needed to facilitate rest. Limited use of a soft collar to keep the head in a slightly flexed position may be helpful for daily function. To prevent both cervical muscle atrophy and psychologic dependence, the collar should not be used for more than 1–2 weeks. Injection of trigger points with 0.5% lidocaine, acupuncture, or electrical stimulation may help to alleviate spasm. Ice or heating pads may also diminish discomfort.

Severe neck pain from cervical strain often subsides within 1 week. When acute pain has subsided, the patient should begin exercises to strengthen cervical muscles and improve posture. Exercises are isometric and may be performed at home after instruction by the therapist. When all pain has resolved, range of motion exercises are added to improve flexibility.

Prevention of flare-ups also depends upon maintenance of good posture with avoidance of overhead work, long automobile rides, or prolonged cervical flexion and extension posture. Patients are cautioned to avoid sleeping in the prone position, which places the neck in excessive extension. A cylindric pillow (cervical pillow) may help to keep the neck in neutral position during sleep.

Course & Prognosis

The prognosis in cervical pain syndrome not associated with disk degeneration is good if the above measures are undertaken. Symptoms may recur, but early institution of home traction and avoidance of offending activities greatly limit the duration of pain.

2. *Whiplash Injury*

ESSENTIALS OF DIAGNOSIS

- *Pain in paraspinous muscles radiating to arms.*
- *Occipital headache.*
- *Limitation of neck rotation.*

General Considerations

A well-known type of soft tissue injury of the neck is the acceleration-deceleration injury called **whiplash**. The most common cause is rear-end automobile collision during which the trunk of the victim's body is rapidly accelerated by the force of impact and the head is "left behind" because of lack of head contact with the seat. Head acceleration (which is an angular acceleration) is always greater than vehicle acceleration. In experimental models, a 10 mph impact produced 11 *g* of angular acceleration of the head. Acute hyperextension injures the anterior soft tissue structures of the neck, including the anterior longitudinal ligament, the intervertebral disk, the strap muscles, and the esophagus. The longus colli and sternocleidomastoid muscles are particularly vulnerable. The cervical sympathetic plexus may also be injured. The hyperextension movement also overloads and injures the posterior facet joints. When acceleration of the vehicle stops, the head recoils into flexion, leading to injuries to the facet capsules, posterior ligaments, and paraspinal musculature.

Clinical Findings

A. Symptoms and Signs

The symptom complex following whiplash injury is highly variable. Onset of pain may be delayed as long as 24 hours. Neck pain and stiffness are the most common symptoms. Occipital headaches and retro-ocular pain are also frequently noted. The presence of numbness in the medial hand and forearm has been attributed to scalenus muscle spasm. Visual blurring may result from stretch injury to the cervical sympathetic plexus, and Horner's syndrome may rarely occur. Dysphagia may represent retropharyngeal hematoma or swelling. Vertebral artery spasm occasionally causes tinnitus, dizziness, and vertigo. When the neck is rotated at the time of injury, symptoms are more pronounced on the side toward which the head is turned.

Physical findings are usually attributable to muscle spasm and only rarely to nerve root compression or disk herniation. Spasm is manifested by diminished neck motion and predominant anterior paracervical tenderness to palpation. Posterolateral pain may occur if articular facet joint damage is present. Neurologic examination, including testing of reflexes and muscle strength, is often normal.

B. Imaging Studies

X-rays are usually normal. Care must be taken to avoid overlooking subtle hyperextension injuries such as widening of an anterior disk space, avulsion fractures of the anterior vertebral body, retropharyngeal swelling, or fracture of the posterior facet. Loss of cervical lordosis may imply spasm but may also be artifactual. Reversal of cervical lordosis, resulting in an S-shaped (swan-neck) deformity, signifies damage to the posterior joints. The kyphosis is most often seen at the C4–5 and C5–6 levels.

Treatment

Management of whiplash injuries is as for other soft tissue injuries—analgesics, rest, and immobilization in a soft cervical collar until the pain is controlled, followed by gradual mobilization. Isometric strengthening exercises are initiated when range of motion normalizes. Occasionally, facet injections may be both therapeutic and diagnostic.

Course & Prognosis

Most patients respond well to conservative measures, though anticipated litigation may complicate management. However, up to 45% of patients continue to have symptoms at 2 years even if their litigation has been settled. Degenerative changes in the cervical spine and minor neck discomfort are more common following whiplash injuries, but persistent pain and prolonged disability are unusual.

3. *Degenerative Cervical Disc Disease (Cervical Spondylosis)*

ESSENTIALS OF DIAGNOSIS

- *Neck pain radiating down the arm.*
- *Muscle weakness.*
- *Dermatomal sensory changes.*

General Considerations

The degenerative changes typically associated with aging are collectively termed spondylosis of the cervical spine. Men and women are affected equally. Among persons over age 50, radiologic signs of degeneration of the cervical spine are extremely common. It is estimated that by the seventh decade, 75% of individuals demonstrate such degeneration, though most are asymptomatic. Disk degeneration is therefore considered a natural aging phenomenon.

Cervical spondylosis is characterized initially by tears in the posterior annulus followed by softening and fragmentation of the disk. The weakest area of the annulus is the posterolateral region, which is the most common site of bulging of the disk. The hydrostatic support provided by the degenerating disk steadily diminishes, and the adjacent vertebral bodies converge. The longitudinal ligaments become lax and are stripped from their bony attachments by the bulging disks. Degenerative calcification of the ligaments produces the familiar bony spurs. The ligamentum flavum also becomes lax and may bulge into the spinal canal. The posterolateral regions of the vertebral bodies become closely approximated and ultimately form an area of friction. These so-called uncovertebral joints of Luschka become increasingly hypertrophic, creating prominent spurs that may encroach onto the neural foramen and spinal canal.

As the vertebral bodies converge because of loss of disk support, the facet joints become subluxated as the superior facet slides posteriorly. Mechanical dysfunction of the joints results in osteoarthritic degeneration and osteophyte formation. Osteophytes about the facets may project into the intervertebral foramina and impinge upon the exiting nerve roots.

Clinical Findings

A. Symptoms and Signs

Clinical symptoms may or may not accompany the degenerative changes of cervical spondylosis. Neurologic compromise may result from nerve root compression (cervical spondylotic radiculopathy) or compression of the cord itself (cervical spondylotic myelopathy). Very rarely, vertebral artery and radicular artery stenosis may occur from osteophyte formation. This may cause vertebrobasilar insufficiency or cervical cord ischemia.

1. Cervical spondylotic radiculopathy—Cervical spondylotic radiculopathy results from pressure on a nerve root as it emerges from the cord to pass peripherally through the intervertebral foramen. A bulging or herniated disk or osteophytes are usually the cause of the compression. The onset of symptoms may be acute or insidious. Patients will usually complain of neck pain with radiation into the infrascapular area.

2. Cervical spondylotic myelopathy—Cervical spondylotic myelopathy is the most common form of spinal cord dysfunction in people over the age of 55. Patients over age 60 are more likely to have multisegmental disease. Spinal cord compression is caused by a combination of factors, including anterior and posterior osteophytes, bulging or herniated intervertebral disks, and a buckled ligamentum flavum. In the Japanese population, ossification of the posterior longitudinal ligament is a common cause of multisegmental cervical compression and myelopathy.

In addition to the mechanical compression of the spinal cord, vascular insufficiency from compression of the anterior spinal artery and the radicular arteries contributes to the neurologic injury. The severity of the myelopathy is dependent upon three factors: (1) the degree of initial compression on the spinal cord, (2) the length of time over which the compression occurs, and (3) the constancy or intermittency of the compressive force. The average space available for the spinal cord in the subaxial cervical spine is between 17 mm and 18 mm. Cervical stenosis is felt to exist if the space available for the spinal cord is less than 13 mm (Figure 42–43). It is important to note that these measurements are taken using the lateral cervical spine radiograph with the neck in neutral position. In the case of multisegmental disease, the actual space available for the cord may be much smaller when the neck is extended.

The symptoms of cervical myelopathy occur and progress very gradually, with functional losses occurring over many years in a "stepladder" type distribution. Radicular pain is often absent, and it may be a long time before the patient seeks medical attention. A few patients demonstrate steadily progressive deterioration leading to spastic paraplegia or quadriplegia.

The patient usually complains of "numbness" in the arms and legs and often of clumsiness and burning in the hands and difficulty in handling small objects. Walking is difficult initially because of balance problems and later due to loss of motor strength. Diffuse, nonlocalized "pins and needles" in the forearm and anterior thigh are also typical. Neck pain may be present or absent, but neck motion is frequently limited.

When myelopathy is precipitated by trauma, symptoms are similar to those described above. Hyperextension injuries in the presence of preexisting cervical stenosis cause the classic central cord syndrome with quadriparesis. Limb involvement is usually more symmetric, with more weakness in the arms and hands than in the lower extremities. The acute injury generally subsides, though neurologic deficits frequently persist.

Physical examination of patients with spondylotic myelopathy is characterized by marked motor findings and relatively few sensory changes. Spasticity is present

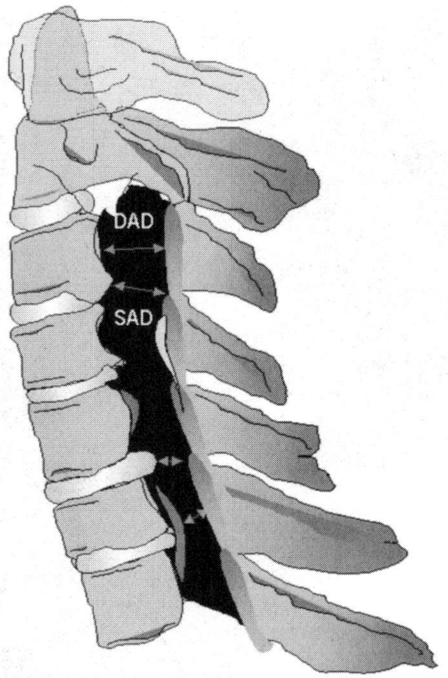

Figure 42–43. The space available for the spinal cord in the subaxial cervical spine can be measured as the developmental anterior-posterior diameter (DAPD) in patients with developmental spinal stenosis and as the spondylolytic anterior-posterior diameter (SAPD) in patients with cervical spondylosis.

in the upper and lower extremities. Clonus and hyperreflexia are common though often asymmetric. An inverted radial reflex and a scapulohumeral reflex may also be seen. Long tract signs, including positive Babinski and Hoffman signs, may be present. Fine motion of the fingers is often lacking, and intrinsic muscle wasting may be profound. The patient may have an abnormal gait characterized by wide-based, shuffling movements. Generalized muscle wasting and weakness are less common. Sphincter control is generally preserved, though mild difficulty with micturition is common. Erectile dysfunction is a frequent complaint. Vibration sensation in the lower extremities may be diminished.

B. Imaging Studies

The roentgenographic changes in cervical spondylosis include narrowing of the disk space, seen most clearly on a lateral projection (Figure 42–44). Osteophyte formation at the vertebral body margins and in particular at the posterolateral uncovertebral joints is best observed on an anteroposterior projection. Arthritic degeneration of the facet joints with osteophyte formation is best demonstrated in oblique views. The highest incidence of degeneration is observed in segments C5–6 because of the concentration of mechanical forces in this region. C6–7 is the next most common level. In the lateral projection, the size of the spinal canal can be measured to assess the degree of cervical stenosis.

MRI has improved our ability to determine the levels that are affected by the compression. Electromyography may be useful to demonstrate generalized motor impairment resulting from motor neuron involvement.

Differential Diagnosis

A. Cervical Spondylotic Radiculopathy

The syndrome is difficult to distinguish from cervical muscle strain unless there are objective radicular signs such as muscle atrophy and sensory changes in a dermatomal distribution.

B. Cervical Spondylotic Myelopathy

Differential diagnosis includes tumors and vascular malformations of the spinal cord, syringomyelia, amyotrophic lateral sclerosis, subacute combined degeneration, and multiple sclerosis. In advanced stages, radiculopathy is commonly seen in association with myelopathy. At this point the syndrome is referred to as a myeloradiculopathy. Upper motor neuron involvement producing spasticity in the extremities distinguishes myelopathy with radiculopathy from isolated radiculopathy, in which pain and weakness in the extremity are limited to the specific

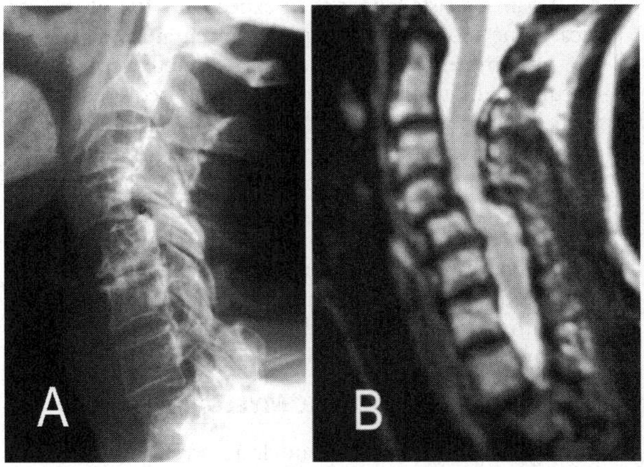

Figure 42–44. ***A:*** Lateral radiograph of a 50-year-old man with neck pain and myelopathy. ***B:*** Sagittal T2-weighted MRI showing spinal cord compression at C4–5 at the level of the spondylolisthesis.

neural segment involved. Radiculopathy is aggravated by neck motion and is associated with more profound dermatomal sensory loss. Multiple sclerosis tends to occur in younger patients, with a peak onset between ages 20 and 40 years, and seldom appears for the first time after age 50 years. Though many of the motor signs are similar, onset in multiple sclerosis is usually more abrupt. Cranial nerve palsies are common in multiple sclerosis, as is cerebellar dysarthria, giving rise to characteristic "scanning speech" (speech punctuated by long, regularly occurring pauses). Elevated cerebrospinal fluid IgG levels and abnormal visual evoked responses also accompany multiple sclerosis. Remission in multiple sclerosis is frequently more complete than in spondylotic myelopathy.

Neoplasm of the cervical cord is usually more profound and progressive. The segmental level is more discrete with spinal tumor, and cerebrospinal fluid protein is elevated. Loss of sphincter control is rare in spondylotic myelopathy and extremely common with neoplasms. MRI is the diagnostic test most useful for differentiating tumor from a degenerative process.

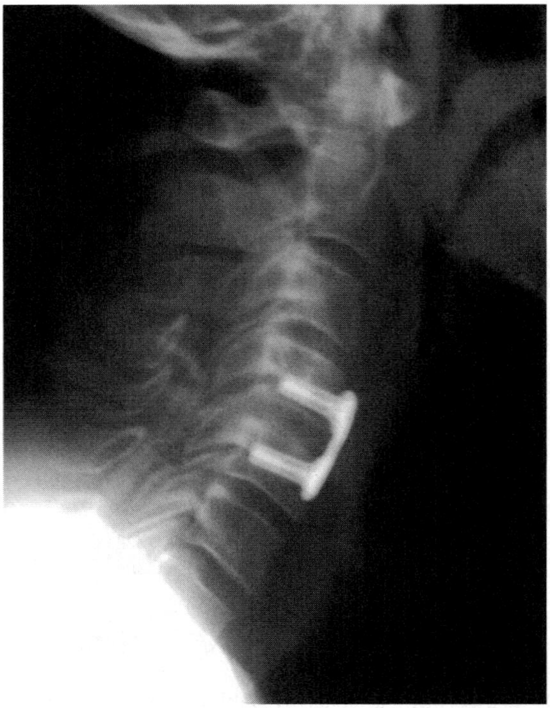

Figure 42–45. Lateral postoperative radiograph of a patient who underwent C4–C5 anterior cervical discectomy and fusion with a titanium plate and tricortical iliac crest bone graft.

Treatment

A. Cervical Spondylotic Radiculopathy

Most patients with acute onset of cervical spondylotic radiculopathy have regression of symptoms over 4–6 weeks. Progression to myelopathy is rare, and most patients require only rest, analgesics, and immobilization to relieve pain. Paresthesias and slight sensory changes may persist after neck and arm pain have subsided. Chronic symptoms may involve an element of nerve root inflammation that may require vigorous anti-inflammatory drug therapy.

If pain persists longer than expected, MRI of the cervical spine should be performed to accurately localize the site of compression. Only when a discrete herniation is documented is surgical decompression required, either with foraminotomy through a posterior approach or by complete removal of the involved cervical disk and osteophytes through an anterior approach followed by anterior interbody fusion. Patients with significant neck pain, kyphosis, bilateral symptoms, or a central disk herniation should be treated by an anterior approach (Figure 42–45). Young patients with little or no neck pain and pure radiculopathy with unilateral disk herniation can be managed by either approach.

B. Cervical Spondylotic Myelopathy

Management of cervical spondylotic myelopathy depends upon the course and severity of symptoms.

1. Medical measures—The management of slowly progressive disease in elderly patients is conservative, and judicious use of a cervical collar for support is generally sufficient. Cyclooxygenase 2 inhibitors (celecoxib, rofecoxib) are newer NSAIDs with less tendency to cause gastrointestinal ulceration with chronic use, although there may be increased cardiovascular risk.

2. Surgical treatment—When symptoms are more severe or progressive despite use of a collar and when they occur in younger patients, operative treatment may be necessary. The choice of treatment depends upon the nature of the compression (disk, vertebral body, posterior osteophytes, hypertrophied ligamentum flavum, ossified posterior longitudinal ligament), the sagittal alignment of the cervical spine (kyphotic, neutral, or lordotic), and the number of levels involved. Compression confined to the intervertebral disks can be relieved by means of single-level or multiple-level anterior discectomies and fusion. When the disease is limited to two vertebral body levels or if there is a preexisting kyphosis greater than 15 degrees, anterior vertebrectomy, foraminotomy, and fusion with a strut graft allows excellent decompression and stabilization of the degenerative segments. When the compression involves more than two vertebral body levels, the morbidity asso-

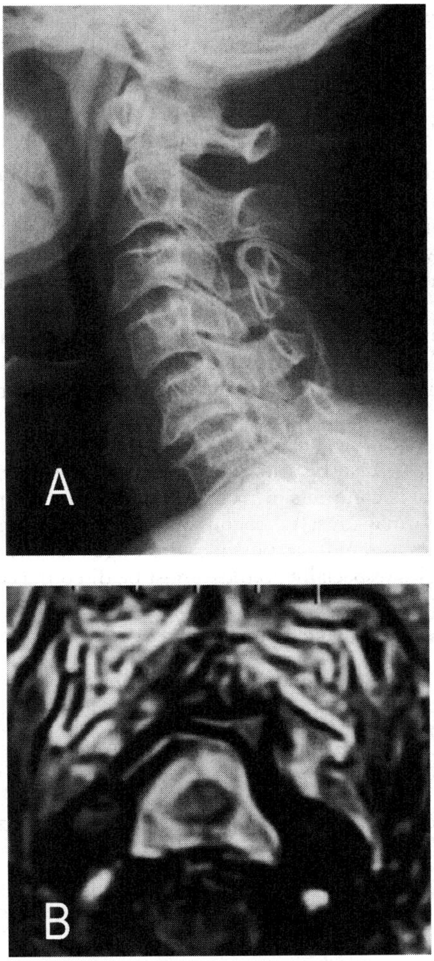

Figure 42–46. A: Lateral postoperative radiograph of a patient who had multisegmental cervical stenosis and myelopathy treated with canal expansive cervical laminoplasty from C3 to C7. ***B:*** Postoperative axial MRI image showing significant canal expansion after the procedure.

ciated with the anterior approach increases significantly. In this case, a posterior decompression via multilevel laminectomy with or without fusion or laminoplasty is preferred (Figure 42–46).

Course & Prognosis

A. Cervical Spondylotic Radiculopathy

The course is benign. Most cases resolve in 4–6 weeks with conservative management.

B. Cervical Spondylotic Myelopathy

In general, the results of surgical management of spondylotic myelopathy are better when symptoms are mild and of relatively shorter duration. However, complete postoperative resolution of symptoms is rare even in these cases. It is noteworthy that the natural evolution of spondylotic myelopathy will often produce at least partial spontaneous remission. Chronic myelopathy and multiple-level involvement are associated with poorer surgical results, particularly in elderly individuals who have lost the ability to ambulate.

Evans RW: Some observations on whiplash injuries. Neurol Clin 1992;10:975.

Poggi JJ et: Cervical spondylolysis. J Spinal Disord 1992;5:349.

Yoshida M et al: Indication and clinical results of laminoplasty for cervical myelopathy caused by disc herniation with developmental canal stenosis. Spine 1998;23:2391.

PAIN SYNDROMES OF THE BACK

1. Low Back Pain

ESSENTIALS OF DIAGNOSIS

- *Paraspinous low back pain aggravated by exertion.*
- *Radiation of pain into the buttock or thigh.*

General Considerations

In the United States, 400,000 workers are disabled by back pain each year. It has been estimated that 80% of the population suffers low back pain at some time. All physicians are called on at least occasionally to advise patients with this complaint, and a systematic approach is necessary to differentiate the numerous possible causes. Diagnosis and management can be frustrating because the precise cause of most cases of low back pain is uncertain and no cure is known. The first task is to identify the relatively few cases with specific causes that can be treated. The less rewarding and more demanding task is to provide long-term guidance and management for patients for whom specific remedies are unavailable.

Clinical Findings

A. Symptoms and Signs

The most common cause of low back pain is mechanical strain. Patients complain of pain related to overexertion. Pain may immediately follow lifting or other forms of exertion or may have a more insidious onset after prolonged physical activity. Many patients in this group demonstrate generally poor conditioning, with poor abdominal muscle tone and poor posture.

Pain from lumbar strain is exacerbated by bending or lifting and relieved by rest. Pain is often described as a deep-seated ache that is dull and somewhat diffuse. Pain is most severe in the lumbosacral area and may radiate into the buttocks. Palpation reveals tenderness in the paraspinous area, with "trigger points" or "knots" in the erector spinae muscle. Spasm of the paraspinous muscles is a common finding, and the patient may have a slight list toward the nonpainful side. Motion of the lumbar spine is limited by pain.

The neurologic examination is often normal. Deep tendon reflexes are present and symmetric. Motor power and sensation in the lower extremities are normal. Rectal tone is normal. Provocative tests such as straight leg raising and the crossed straight leg raising are negative. The former is performed with the patient supine on the examining table. The examiner then lifts the patient's leg, which is extended at the hip and knee. This maneuver passively stretches the sciatic nerve and results in transmission of tension to the lumbosacral roots that contribute to the nerve. Absence of radicular leg pain associated with straight leg raising reduces the likelihood of spinal nerve compression as the source of symptoms.

B. Imaging Studies

X-ray examination may reveal changes such as lumbar disk space narrowing and osteophytosis or may be entirely normal. Because x-ray signs are nonspecific, many clinicians avoid x-ray studies during the initial evaluation. X-rays should be obtained for persons over age 50, in whom metastatic tumors are more likely to be present, and those under age 20, in whom symptomatic congenital or developmental anomalies may be present. For other patients, x-rays may be obtained during subsequent visits if symptoms do not resolve within several weeks.

Treatment

Management of lumbar strain includes analgesics and rest during the acute phase. A firm board beneath the patient's mattress provides support for tender spinal muscles. Abdominal conditioning and spinal muscle strengthening exercises are prescribed only when the pain subsides. Typical exercises include bent-knee sit-ups and hamstring and spinal muscle stretching. Lumbosacral corsets with steel stays provide mechanical support for the spine by compressing and reinforcing the flaccid abdominal wall. Proper body mechanics should be discussed with the patient, especially the correct manner of lifting objects while bending the legs rather than the spine. Postural exercises may be useful and are most effectively taught by physical therapists.

Course & Prognosis

The usual course of lumbar strain is spontaneous remission with time. Relapses of pain are commonly precipitated by stressful activity, though months may pass without symptoms. Some patients complain of constant pain. Probing inquiry frequently reveals profound depression in these individuals, for whom illness and disability have become dominant elements in their lives. When strain is attributed to working conditions, the clinical course may be complicated by considerations of secondary gain.

Patients who fail to respond to rest and supportive measures must be carefully reexamined to assess for neurologic compression. Those judged to be neurologically normal must be encouraged to return to normal activities as rapidly as possible. Prolonged reliance upon analgesics (especially opioids) must be discouraged.

2. Lumbar Disk Syndrome

ESSENTIALS OF DIAGNOSIS

- *Low back pain radiating into the thigh, leg, and foot.*
- *Paresthesia in the affected dermatome.*

General Considerations

Relapse of low back pain may or may not be associated with leg pain. Patients who present with low back and leg pain frequently recall earlier episodes of postexertional pain limited to the low back. Though specific evidence is lacking, the pattern of leg pain developing secondarily has led many clinicians to attribute the initial episode of localized low back pain to early degeneration of the annulus fibrosus. With annulus degeneration, the nucleus pulposus bulges into the defect, causing further concentration of stress on the damaged fibers. The annulus is richly innervated with pain fibers, and further degeneration tends to be associated with more frequent and episodes of more severe pain. Locking and stiffness characterize the pain-free periods. Degeneration continues with alteration in the collagen structure of both the annulus and the nucleus, culminating in fibrosis and nuclear fragmentation. The shock-absorbing capacity of the nucleus is diminished, and forces are transmitted in a progressively irregular fashion. Fragments of the deteriorating nucleus are pushed outward against or through the weakened annulus, which tends to be weakest at the posterolateral margin of the annulus fibrosus. The protrusion begins as a posterolateral bulge that causes variable compression and irritation of neural structures.

The dural sac below L1 contains only nerve rootlets. Each nerve root emerges below its respective vertebra, hugging the inferomedial border of its respective pedicle, and enters the neural foramen just above the intervertebral disk of that level. A paracentral disk herniation just misses the exiting nerve root at the specific spinal level and compresses the traversing root to the lower adjacent level. Thus, an L4–5 paracentral disk herniation will compress the traversing L5 nerve root. In contrast, a far lateral disk herniation occurs near the exit zone of its respective neural foramen and therefore is most likely to compress the exiting root at that level. The L4–5 and L5–S1 disk levels correspond to the region of maximal mechanical stress in the lumbar spine. Lesions affecting the L5 and S1 nerve roots account for over 90% of disk-mediated nerve root lesions.

Clinical Findings

A. Symptoms and Signs

Sciatica (pain radiating down the posterior leg) is the most common presentation. Prolonged compression results in nerve root inflammation and pain referred in a specific dermatomal distribution. The onset of leg pain is usually insidious, but pain may begin acutely when sudden disk herniation follows injury.

Pain is piercing, burning, or electrical in nature and typically radiates from the thigh into the leg and foot. Activity, such as coughing, sneezing, or bearing down during bowel movements, increases intra-abdominal pressure. This is directly transmitted to intraspinal structures, provoking or exacerbating pain.

When nerve root compression results from annular bulging, it is often accentuated by prolonged sitting or standing and relieved at least partially by rest. A patient usually prefers to sleep on one side in the fetal position and when sitting prefers a straight-backed chair. When disk extrusion occurs, pain may be less responsive to rest.

Compression of nerve roots often produces objective sensory changes early, with paresthesia and loss of sensation detectable in the affected dermatome. With continued root compression, motor weakness may develop. Motor weakness corresponds to the specific myotomes innervated by the compressed nerve root. With involvement of the L4 root, the patellar tendon reflex may be diminished and slight quadriceps weakness may be observed. Sensation may be diminished over the medial calf. Since the foot dorsiflexors are innervated by L4 and L5, slight weakness of the foot dorsiflexors may also be noticed on side-to-side testing. With involvement of the L5 root, weakness is frequently manifested by loss of strength in great toe dorsiflexion. Pain and numbness are present in the anteromedial leg and foot. First sacral root involvement affects the calf muscles, and the Achilles tendon reflex may be lost on the involved side. Weakness is best demonstrated by the patient's inability to rise on the toes repeatedly. Sensory findings include pain and numbness in the posterolateral leg and foot. Muscle atrophy may accompany sensory and motor changes.

Occasionally, acute posterior midline disk prolapse at the L2–3 level may cause compression of many nerve roots in the cauda equina. This is known as acute cauda equina syndrome. Symptoms include intense leg pain in one or both extremities, with severe muscle weakness or paralysis. Compression of sacral roots results in acute urinary retention. An MRI of the lumbar spine will reveal the site of compression, which is best treated by urgent decompression.

In the presence of severe disk space degeneration and spondylosis, a generalized narrowing of the lumbar spinal canal occurs. Lumbar spinal stenosis occurs as a consequence of the degenerative process of aging. It is a multifactorial narrowing of the spinal canal from facet joint hypertrophy, disk degeneration and loss of disk height, and hypertrophy and buckling of the ligamentum flavum. Spinal stenosis afflicts people in their mid to late fifties and early sixties. There is no clear gender predominance. Early symptoms include generalized backache and stiffness. Narrowing of the lateral recess occurs early in the process, causing unilateral nerve root symptoms. Neurogenic claudication becomes the chief complaint once the central spinal canal becomes narrowed.

B. Diagnostic Tests

With less well defined signs of root compression, several tests may help to detect the presence of lumbar disk disease. The straight leg raising test is performed by lifting the extended leg of the supine patient. The test produces tension in the lumbosacral roots and frequently reproduces sciatica in the presence of inflamed or irritated lumbosacral roots.

The straight leg raising test can also be performed on the leg without symptoms. The crossed straight leg raising test is positive if it produces sciatica in the symptomatic leg. Many clinicians believe that a positive test is strong evidence of disk herniation.

Laségue's test is performed with the patient lying supine. The hip and knee are flexed 90 degrees. The knee is then slowly extended, producing sciatic stretch as in the straight leg raising maneuver.

In patients with spinal stenosis, extension typically exacerbates the symptoms. Flexion of the spine improves the symptoms. Typical physical findings include diminished or asymmetric reflexes in the lower extremities. The extensor hallucis longus is most often found to be weak.

C. Imaging Studies

X-ray examination may reveal degenerative changes, such as disk space narrowing and osteophytosis, or the results may be entirely normal. A myelogram, CT scan, or MRI will confirm the diagnosis.

Differential Diagnosis

Whether nerve root signs are present or not, the main differential concern with back pain is spinal tumor or infection. In addition, palpation of the distal pulses and abdominal aorta is necessary to rule out the presence of aortic aneurysm.

The most common extradural tumors in adults are metastatic, most often from carcinoma of the breast in women and of the prostate in men. Lung, thyroid, and uterine tumors are less common sources of metastases. Multiple myeloma also frequently involves the spine and often causes pain by weakening of bony structures, causing pathologic fractures. Intradural spinal tumors are less common than metastases in adults and include neurofibromas, meningiomas, and ependymomas. Diagnosis of these slow-growing tumors is often quite difficult, as symptoms may mimic discogenic pain and may appear to improve with conservative measures. Metastatic tumors of bone are often detected on routine x-ray studies.

The history may suggest the possibility of spinal tumor. A history of primary tumors elsewhere should immediately arouse this suspicion. A complaint of pain that is more severe at night than during the day is also strongly suggestive of spinal tumor. The reasons for this phenomenon are unclear but may be related to nocturnal increase in cerebrospinal fluid pressure. Persistent bilateral leg pain with no history of back pain also suggests spinal tumor. Both primary and metastatic tumors are easily detected by MRI.

Discitis and vertebral osteomyelitis can cause back pain in the absence of significant neurologic symptoms. Pyogenic vertebral osteomyelitis is due to bacterial infection of the vertebra that can arise from a number of sources, including direct inoculation, contiguous spread from a local infection, and hematogenous seeding. Local spread of bacteria or fungi can occur following intra-abdominal and retroperitoneal abscesses. Direct inoculation results from penetrating injuries and from surgical procedures performed on the intervertebral disk (chemonucleolysis, discography, discectomy). Although local spread from direct inoculation of bacteria into the spine is becoming more prevalent, hematogenous seeding of infection is by far the most common mechanism by which these infections occur. The sources of pathogenic organisms include skin and soft tissue infections, infected vascular access sites, and the urinary tract.

Once the infection is established in the metaphysis, it can then rupture through the end plate into the adjoining disk and infect the adjacent vertebral body. The disk material is relatively avascular and is rapidly destroyed by the bacterial enzymes. Infection in the cervical spine can extend into the mediastinum or into the supraclavicular fossa with disastrous sequelae. In the lumbar spine, abscess formation may occur in the psoas muscle, the buttock (piriformis fossa), the perianal region, the groin, or even the popliteal fossa. Extension of infection into the spinal canal can result in an epidural abscess or bacterial meningitis. Destruction of the vertebral body and intervertebral disk can lead to instability and collapse of the vertebral body. In addition, retropulsion of infected bone and granulation tissue into the spinal canal can cause neural compression or vascular occlusion. If a spinal infection is suspected, the pathogenic organism must be identified before appropriate treatment with antibiotics (with or without surgical debridement) can be instituted. An MRI with gadolinium will clearly delineate the location of the infection as well as the presence of an epidural abscess (Figure 42–47).

Treatment

Management of acute lumbar dilsk disease is controversial.

A. Conservative Management

If symptoms are produced by bulging rather than by extrusion of the herniated disk, conservative measures such as bed rest, analgesics, and anti-inflammatory medications often result in complete resolution of symptoms.

B. Percutaneous Discectomy

If pain becomes intractable or if neurologic symptoms progress or fail to respond to conservative measures, laminotomy and removal of the herniated disk may be required. This can be performed via standard microdiscectomy techniques or though a "minimally invasive" endoscopic approach that is done through a paramedian muscle splitting exposure.

C. Laminectomy

If free fragments are present in the spinal canal, laminectomy is clearly indicated if pain or neurologic symptoms fail to respond to conservative measures. However, if the symptoms are tolerable, free fragments have a higher likelihood of spontaneous resorption over time than the classic herniated disk. Complications of laminectomy for disk removal include recurrence of pain due to reherniation of residual disk fragments or scar formation involving the nerve roots; damage of nerve

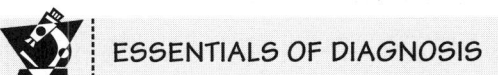

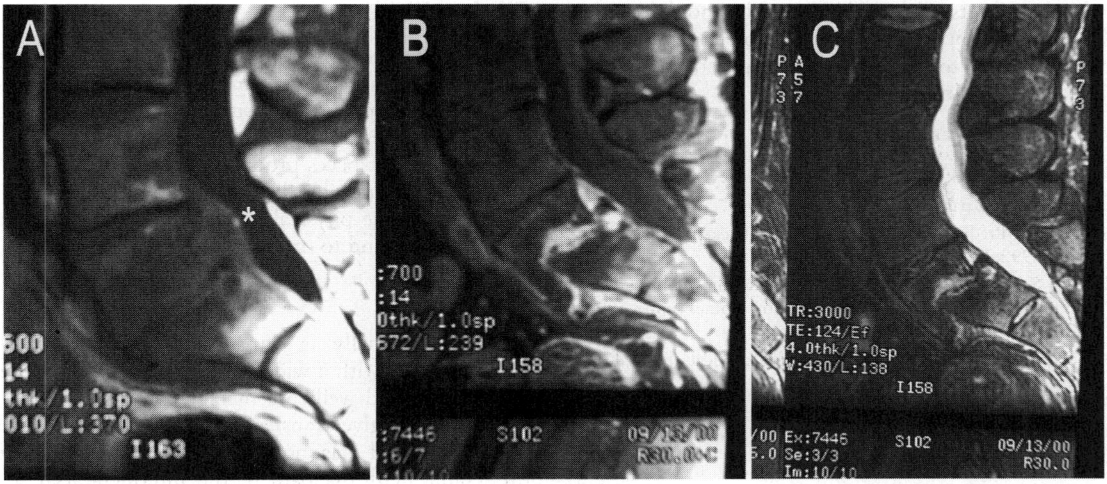

Figure 42–47. Sagittal MRI images of a patient with low back pain due to L5–S1 discitis, vertebral osteomyelitis, and a small anterior epidural abscess. ***A:*** T1-weighted image. ***B:*** T1-weighted image with gadolinium vascular contrast. ***C:*** T2-weighted image.

roots, resulting in neurologic deficit; tear of the dura, with resulting dural leak of cerebrospinal fluid; and penetration of the anterior annulus during diskectomy, with damage to the great vessels lying anterior to the spine. Hemorrhage in this situation may be catastrophic owing to difficulties in detection and control.

In the patient with persistent neurogenic claudication that fails to respond to conservative measures, decompressive laminectomy is very effective in relieving symptoms and improving function. If spinal instability (degenerative spondylolisthesis) of deformity is also present, the spine should also be stabilized and fused over the affected levels.

3. Mechanical Back Pain (Facet Syndrome)

ESSENTIALS OF DIAGNOSIS

- *Pain in the low back.*
- *"Locking" of back during bending.*

General Considerations

People with long-standing lumbar disk disease may develop numerous degenerative changes in the involved segments (facet syndrome). Collapse of the disk results in abnormal motion anteriorly between the vertebral bodies and posteriorly between the intervertebral facets. Osteophytes form as a result of abnormal stress on the annulus and the joint capsules of the facets.

Clinical Findings

Symptoms may arise from inflammation surrounding the abnormal facets and generally include diffuse aching that may or may not radiate into the buttock or posterior thigh.

The mechanical nature of the pain is reflected by postural discomfort and by locking of the low back during stooping or attempts to straighten the back after forward bending. Abnormal motion is the presumed cause of irritation that leads to reflex muscular inhibition and spinal "locking."

Differential Diagnosis

Experimental injection of hypertonic saline into normal facet joints has been noted to cause low back pain associated with sciatica as well as limitation of straight leg-raising. These experimentally induced symptoms are eradicated by injection of the facets with lidocaine. These observations make it clear that sciatica without weakness or sensory deficit is insufficient evidence on which to base a diagnosis of nerve root compression.

Treatment

Patients demonstrating symptoms suggestive of facet syndrome may respond well to systemic anti-inflammatory agents or to fluoroscopically guided injection of the lumbar facets with corticosteroids and lidocaine. Lumbar fusion by anterior or posterior techniques has been advocated to eliminate abnormal motion, but results have been inconsistent.

Fischgrund JS, Montgomery DM: Diagnosis and treatment of discogenic low back pain. Orthop Rev 1993;22:311.

Frank A: Low back pain. Br Med J 1993;306:901.

Frymoyer JW: Predicting disability from low back pain. Clin Orthop 1992;279:101.

Haldeman S, Rubinstein SM: Cauda equina syndrome in patients undergoing manipulation of the lumbar spine. Spine 1992; 17:1469.

Lang IM et al, MR imaging appearances of cervical epidural abscess. Clin Radiol 1995;50:466.

Omarini LP, Garcia J: CT-guided percutaneous puncture-biopsy of the spine. Review of 104 cases. Schweiz Med Wochenschr 1993;123:2191. (In French.)

PAIN SYNDROMES OF THE FOOT

1. Morton's Neuroma

The interdigital nerve to the third and fourth toes is formed by the third digital branch of the medial plantar nerve and a connecting branch from the lateral plantar nerve. In 1876, Morton described a painful condition of the forefoot that he attributed to neuritis of this digital nerve. The symptoms included pain centered around the fourth metatarsophalangeal joint and in the third intermetatarsal space. Pain is exacerbated by weightbearing, particularly while wearing shoes, and in some cases is steadily progressive. Neuroma pain is distinguishable from simple structural forefoot pain by the fact that it is constant and not relieved by rest. Structural metatarsalgia is experienced almost exclusively during weightbearing and is relieved by rest. The incidence of Morton's neuroma is eight to ten times higher in women than in men.

Interdigital nerve neuroma has been attributed to the course the nerves follow on the way to their destinations in the skin of the toes. Each nerve passes beneath the deep intermetatarsal ligament and then changes its course in a dorsal direction. The more dorsally situated digital branches then enter adjacent toes and provide cutaneous sensation. Dorsiflexion of the toes produces constant friction along the edge of the intermetatarsal ligament. Friction causes fibrosis and enlargement of the nerve sheath, which in turn increase the potential for impingement. The third and fourth interdigital nerves are most commonly involved. This predilection is attributed to the peculiar mobility of the fourth metatarsal, which is least rigidly anchored at its base. The second and third interdigital nerves are sometimes affected, and the first nerve is only rarely involved. The disease very rarely involves two digital nerves simultaneously in the same foot.

Clinical Findings

Diagnosis is based on the history and physical examination. A complaint of unremitting pain in the interspaces of the toes is highly suggestive. Palpation of the space reproduces sharp, stabbing pain, as does compression of the interspaces produced by squeezing the forefoot circumferentially. Simple metatarsalgia should be ruled out by the physical examination. Neuroma pain will rarely respond to orthotics alone.

Treatment

Treatment initially is nonsurgical, emphasizing the need for shoes with a wide toe box and low heel. Some patients respond well to a metatarsal pad. Corticosteroid injections give transient relief in many cases, but long-term relief has not been consistently achieved. Intractable neuroma pain in the intermetatarsal space unresponsive to conservative measures requires operative treatment. Treatment consists of excision of the nerve through a longitudinal incision in the dorsal web space. The neuroma is usually located at the bifurcation into digital branches. The excision must be made well proximal to the intermetatarsal ligament to prevent subsequent adhesion of the cut nerve end and the ligament, with recurrence of pain. Denervation of the digits with sensory loss has proved inconsequential to patients, who usually describe dramatic relief of symptoms immediately after surgery.

2. Metatarsalgia

ESSENTIALS OF DIAGNOSIS

- *Pain beneath the metatarsal heads with weightbearing.*
- *Plantar callosities.*

General Considerations

Metatarsalgia is a descriptive term denoting a group of disorders causing pain beneath the metatarsophalangeal joints. Mechanical factors are perhaps the chief cause. Laxity of the transverse intermetatarsal ligament permits collapse of the transverse metatarsal arch, resulting in loss of the concavity beneath the central metatarsal heads. The normal concentration of weightbearing by the first and fifth metatarsal heads is dispersed, with relatively greater loads delivered to the second and third metatarsals.

Clinical Findings

Plantar keratoses (callosities) form in areas of excessive stress and are particularly common beneath the second metatarsal head. This is in part due to the prominence of the condyle on the fibular aspect of the central metatarsal heads. Constant irritation of hypertrophic callosities results in inflammation and pain with weightbearing. Symptoms vary from intermittent discomfort to severe and disabling pain.

Collapse of the transverse arch may result from laxity of the intermetatarsal ligament. Ligamentous laxity may exist as a congenital deformity or may result from obesity, prolonged standing, injury, or aging. Intramuscular paralysis may also permit collapse of the arch, and shoes that crowd the toes also create abnormal stress concentration beneath the metatarsal heads.

Differential Diagnosis

Diagnosis is easily made if callosities are evident. Reactive keratoses are occasionally mistaken for plantar warts, but the latter are rarely located beneath metatarsal heads.

Treatment

A. Orthotics

Therapy is directed toward relieving pressure beneath the metatarsal heads by placing felt or rubber pads into the shoe behind the central metatarsal heads. Shoes that comfortably accommodate the padded forefoot are mandatory.

B. Surgical Treatment

In cases where pain is intractable despite conservative measures, operative treatment is required. Procedures designed to relieve metatarsal pressure include excision of the plantar condylar prominence, osteotomy to shorten the metatarsal, resection of the metatarsal head, and, in particularly resistant cases, excision of the entire offending metatarsal. The latter procedures may cause increased disability and should be undertaken only after failure of less radical procedures, such as condylectomy.

3. Hallux Valgus

ESSENTIALS OF DIAGNOSIS

- *Prominence of the medial first metatarsal.*
- *Lateral deviation of the great toe.*

General Considerations

Hallux valgus is subluxation of the first metatarsophalangeal joint, which results in lateral deviation (valgus) of the great toe and formation of a medial prominence by the first metatarsal head. The cause is a topic of controversy, though a number of factors are involved.

Anatomic factors predisposing to hallux valgus include varus alignment of the first metatarsocuneiform joint. The medially directed first metatarsal widens the angle between the first and second metatarsal beyond the normal 5–8 degrees. This so-called metatarsus varus adds mechanical advantages to the adductor hallucis tendon insertion on the proximal phalanx of the great toe, with resulting lateral deviation of the toe. Ligamentous laxity may also aggravate the imbalance.

The most significant extrinsic causative factor in development of hallux valgus is improper footwear. The predominance of women in all reports of this deformity has been interpreted as a strong indictment of women's shoe styles. Bunching up of the toes in a pointed shoe buckles the first metatarsophalangeal joint by forcing the great toe into a marked valgus deformity. The first metatarsal is levered medialward. With prolonged use of offending footwear, the medial joint capsule becomes attenuated, further lowering the resistance to deformation. The abductor hallucis tendon is pulled plantarward, and its ability to resist great toe adduction is lost. The long flexor and extensor tendons are pulled laterally with the great toe. When the displaced tendons contract, they create a bowstring effect, further exacerbating the deformity.

Clinical Findings

The "bunion" of hallux valgus represents a prominence of the medial first metatarsal head, which results when the great toe becomes progressively laterally subluxated. True exostosis is uncommon, though the ligamentous structures overlying the medial eminence may be thickened, and an adventitial bursa may form over the prominent medial metatarsal head. Pain from irritation of the bursa and the overlying skin occurs as these tissues are compressed between the shoe and underlying bone.

Treatment

A. Orthotics

Conservative measures for treatment of hallux valgus emphasize selection of footwear of proper size and shape to accommodate the deformed forefoot. The pain associated with irritation of the bunion can in many cases be minimized by this simple measure. Night splints have also been recommended, though hallux valgus may progress despite their use. Only when the pain significantly interferes with the patient's lifestyle should surgery be recommended.

B. Surgical Treatment

Over 50 operations have been advocated for the correction of hallux valgus, which is by way of saying that there is no perfect bunion operation. The main indications for surgery include intractable pain and inability to find comfortable shoes. The elements of surgical correction include excision of the medial prominence of the metatarsal head (bunionectomy), release of the deforming adductor hallucis tendon, excision of the lateral sesamoid bone if it is widely displaced, and reefing of the medial capsular structures to reinforce static resistance to recurrence of the deformity. When the varus deformity of the first metatarsal is excessive, sutures are placed between the capsules of the first and second metatarsal heads or corrective osteotomy of the metatarsal is performed.

Recurrence of the deformity and overcorrection creating hallux varus deformity are the major complications of surgery. Both problems are more apt to occur when correction of severe hallux valgus deformity has been attempted. Some loss of first metatarsophalangeal joint motion can be expected in most cases. Adequate vascularity must be confirmed prior to any correction procedure. The complication rates are low when surgery is performed by experienced surgeons. Ambulation is usually possible shortly after surgery. Careful attention must be paid to postoperative dressings, which should immobilize the great toe and thus reinforce the surgical repair.

Coughlin MJ: Treatment of bunionette deformity with longitudinal diaphyseal osteotomy with distal soft tissue repair. Foot Ankle 1991;11:195.

Schoenhaus HD, Cohen RS: Etiology of the bunion. J Foot Surg 1992;31:25.

ORTHOPEDIC INFECTIONS

OSTEOMYELITIS DUE TO EXTENSION OF ADJACENT SOFT TISSUE INFECTION

Infections that develop in the soft tissues of the fingers or toes can extend into and destroy adjacent bone. Septic arthritis from puncture wounds may have a similar result. Prompt treatment of the initial infection will prevent this complication and avoid the need either for amputation or for joint resection and fusion to salvage some function. A more common form of osteomyelitis due to extension from an established infected site is that which occurs beneath trophic ulcers associated with arterial insufficiency, diabetes mellitus, or neuropathy due to other causes. Such chronic soft tissue ulcers inevitably become infected, usually with a mixture of organisms that frequently includes anaerobes. Persisting infection may spread to involve adjacent bone, but usually only its surface unless septic arthritis develops or the infection is of exceptionally long duration. The possibility of osteomyelitis is raised by radiographs of the involved area. Focal demineralization may be present without bone infection. Cortical erosion and periosteal new bone formation are more suggestive, but only the presence of necrotic sequestered bone is convincing evidence of osteomyelitis. MRI has been found to be very sensitive for detecting osteomyelitis.

In fact, persistence of such trophic ulcers rarely results from osteomyelitis but instead from inadequate debridement of soft tissues, continuing mechanical trauma, or inadequate blood supply. Treatment should be directed at these factors. Ray resection or amputation may be necessary to achieve soft tissue healing. Superficially involved bone at the base of an ulcer may require only superficial debridement. Prolonged antibiotic treatment is not necessary in such cases if healing is progressing and will be insufficient if it is not.

Joints adjacent to pressure sores (decubitus ulcers) or neurotrophic or ischemic ulcers may develop septic arthritis that is easily overlooked without synovial fluid aspiration or arthrography. Without adequate joint drainage and debridement, there is little hope for controlling these serious infections it is important to be aware of the marked radiographic abnormalities produced by neuropathic joint destruction in diabetes mellitus as well as other causes of peripheral neuropathy. These can be confused with infection or can coexist with it.

CHRONIC OSTEOMYELITIS

The foregoing discussions should suggest that there is often no clear division between acute and chronic osteomyelitis. From a practical viewpoint, however, the concept of chronic osteomyelitis is valuable because it emphasizes the persisting, recurring nature of infections involving bone and because it is usually associated with more or less easily definable areas of necrotic bone that harbor the causative microorganisms and thus provide a source for recurrences. Chronic osteomyelitis will not be cured without removal of this sequestered and necrotic bone.

Clinical Findings

A. Symptoms and Signs

Chronic osteomyelitis may recur as apparent cellulitis in the region of previously infected bone or as an obvious soft tissue abscess. This may "point" and rupture to produce a sinus tract that persists or drains periodically. Persistent or recurring serous or purulent wound drainage from an area of previous osteomyelitis is highly suggestive, if not diagnostic, of chronic osteomyelitis.

B. Laboratory Findings

Cultures of a draining sinus usually yield organisms but rarely differentiate the true pathogenic bacteria from bacterial soup colonizing a chronic wound. Tissue biopsy or deep aspiration is necessary for reliable bacteriologic diagnosis, which is the key to appropriate antibacterial therapy. Chronic bone infections may be caused by mycobacteria or fungi, so stains and cultures appropriate for these microorganisms are always required. When tissue is obtained for culture, an adjacent specimen should also be sent for histopathologic study.

C. Imaging Studies

Radiographs demonstrate both destructive and reactive bone changes, with more or less circumscribed areas of lucency, sclerosis, and often periosteal or appositional new bone formation. Involucra and sequestra may be obvious or may require CT scans or MRI for demonstration. A sinogram obtained after gentle injection of iodinated soluble contrast medium will delineate the area of involvement and may indicate the source of recurring infection. Occasionally, a sinus that appears to arise from the pelvis communicates with infection originating in the gastrointestinal tract or genitourinary tract.

Differential Diagnosis

Chronic osteomyelitis must be differentiated from benign and malignant bone tumor, bone dysplasia, and traumatic lesions, including fatigue fracture.

Complications

Failure to eradicate the infection is common. Infection may spread systemically or locally. Pathologic fracture may occur, especially after bone debridement. Bone deformity or shortening, nonunion, malunion, and stiffness or ankylosis of adjacent joints may cause significant loss of function. Amputation may be necessary to control infection or to provide a more functional limb than would remain after prolonged infection and repeated surgery. After years of drainage, malignant degeneration may occur in the sinus tract. This should be suspected if increasing pain or drainage develops with long-standing osteomyelitis.

Treatment

A. Conservative Treatment

When chronic osteomyelitis is quiescent, no treatment is necessary, and the patient may live an essentially normal life. Dressing changes alone may be sufficient for minor exacerbations with drainage.

B. Medical Treatment

If symptoms are more severe, rest with elevation of the involved limb, analgesics as needed, and systemic antibiotics are advisable. The choice of antibiotic may be aided by culture and sensitivity test results from prior symptomatic episodes; by aspiration or biopsy of the involved area; or, least desirably, by a more or less educated guess at the infecting organism and its antibiotic sensitivities. In the early phases of recurrence, without abscess or sinus tract, these measures alone may produce a prompt—though usually temporary—clinical resolution. The optimal duration of antibiotic treatment for chronic osteomyelitis remains unclear. Some authors recommend only brief usage, during acute exacerbations and surgical procedures. Current opinion among infectious disease experts supports a 4- to 6-week course, though the results of this regimen are not well documented. It is clear that antibiotics are adjuncts to adequate debridement and are not in themselves sufficient treatment. Adjunctive oral antibiotic coverage for at least 6 months appears to be beneficial for treatment of chronic staphylococcal osteomyelitis due to susceptible organisms.

C. Surgical Treatment

Surgical treatment will be necessary if rest and antibiotics do not result in prompt improvement or if significant drainage, bone destruction, or sequestration is evident. Soft tissue abscesses require incision and drainage. The resulting wound may be left open or closed over suction-irrigation tubes. Tubes can be managed in several ways. Continuous flow systems are complicated. Doses of antibiotics delivered by continuous flow may be too large, and toxicity may occur. Scrupulous sterile precautions must be followed with all techniques, and tubes should generally be removed within a few days to minimize the risk of superinfection.

The following regimen has been effective: Periodic irrigation is performed with small volumes of antibiotic solution, followed by prolonged suction to prevent fluid accumulation and minimize soft tissue dead space. As a rule, no more than 10–20 mL of solution (eg, 0.1% gentamicin in normal saline) is injected every 12 hours, allowed to stay in the wound for a few hours, and then withdrawn by suction applied to the tube via a three-way stopcock that also permits irrigation. A single tube is used for small wounds, but double tubes may be needed for larger ones (Figure 42–48). Suction-irrigation tube systems are not a substitute for adequate surgical drainage of pus and adequate debridement of poorly vascularized, chronically infected tissue. Neither do they replace systemic antibiotic treatment with appropriate drugs. They

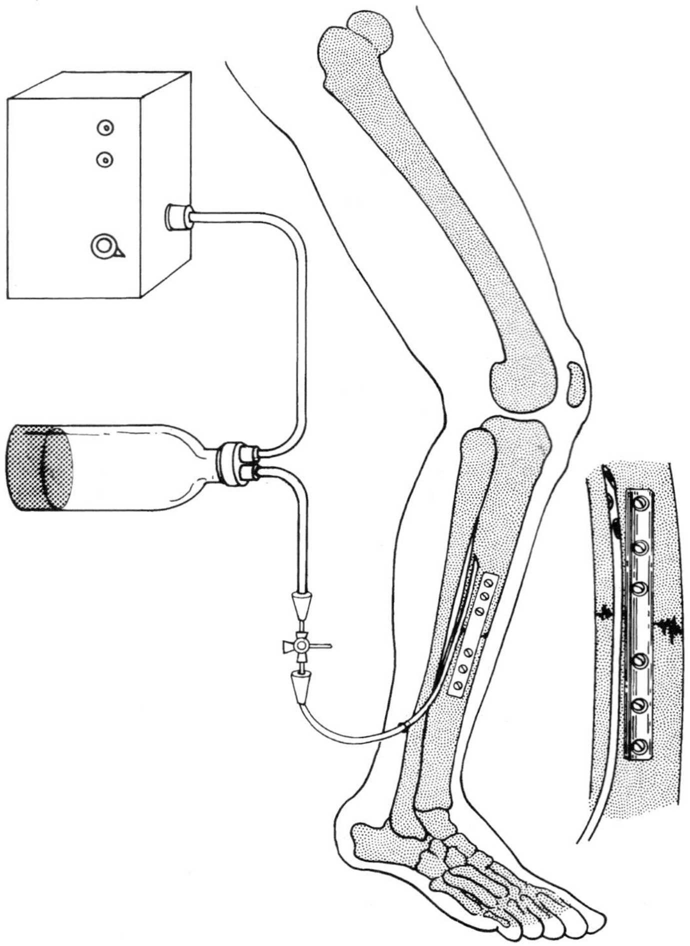

Figure 42–48. Jergesen tube system for periodic suction-irrigation. A tube with several openings near the end is positioned in the area to be drained and brought out obliquely through the soft tissues and skin. The tube is attached to a sterile three-way stopcock and sterile trap bottle. Small volumes of irrigating solution containing antibiotics are injected via the stopcock wi to remain in the wound for a few hours before the stopcock is opened for suction for several more hours. The process is then repeated.

do offer an effective means of obtaining early closure of an infected wound that would otherwise require open management.

Removal of bone may be necessary to extract a sequestrum or to unroof an intraosseous abscess. The resulting cavity acts as a "dead space," which fills with hematoma rather than healthy, well-perfused tissue and leaves a potential focus for recurrence of infection. Saucerization and then exteriorization of the cavity may be followed by split-thickness skin grafting or open cancellous bone grafting once the defect is lined with healthy granulation tissue. A better alternative is to fill the defect with a muscle graft, either with its own local blood supply or as a free microvascular transfer. Coverage of adequately debrided chronic osteomyelitis with a well-perfused muscle pedicle appears to be the most effective surgical treatment for significantly symptomatic chronic osteomyelitis. Extensive bone debridement is often required, resulting in a need for bone grafts if function and structural integrity are to be preserved. Free vascularized muscle grafts make adequate debridement and reconstruction possible when the involved area is too large to be managed with locally available tissue resources.

Prognosis

Whatever the initial cause, once an infection involving bone has become well-established, with focally necrotic bone and scar tissue and microabscesses scattered through the involved area, the long-term outlook must remain guarded. Although infection may be controlled with adequate debridement and prolonged treatment with antibiotics, there is always a risk of late recurrence, even after many years of quiescence.

SEPTIC ARTHRITIS

ESSENTIALS OF DIAGNOSIS

- *Joint pain.*
- *Limitation of motion.*
- *Joint swelling, effusion, warmth, and tenderness.*
- *Pus and organisms in aspirate of synovial fluid.*

General Considerations

Septic arthritis is an inflammatory joint disease caused by bacteria or fungi. Primary infection is caused by direct inoculation of the joint by trauma, including surgery. Secondary infection occurs hematogenously or by extension from adjacent osteomyelitis. Septic arthritis characteristically involves a single joint. This disease must always be considered in the differential diagnosis of monarticular arthritis.

Occasionally, septic arthritis will develop in a joint already involved by another form of arthritis. This possibility must be considered whenever an arthritic joint "flares" or an arthritic patient becomes systemically ill. Septic arthritis is more common in children and debilitated elderly individuals except when gonococci are the cause.

Septic arthritis destroys articular cartilage. The initial reaction to joint infection is acute synovitis, with effusion that develops an increasing concentration of PMNs. The fluid tends to coagulate, producing loculations within the joint cavity. Inflammatory cells infiltrate the synovium, and the overlying tissues become edematous. With continuing infection, the cartilage matrix is destroyed, collagen is lost, and chondrocytes are killed. The damaged cartilage is susceptible to mechanical trauma and is eroded at points of loading. Continued infection may destroy synovial and capsular components as well as cartilage and bone. Spread to adjacent bone produces osteomyelitis. Following successful treatment of early infections, there may be no permanent sequelae, but extensive tissue destruction rarely resolves completely. Fibrous or complete bony ankylosis may result, as well as painful postinfectious degenerative arthritis.

Gonococci are probably the most common cause of septic arthritis at present, at least in sexually active individuals, and must be considered whenever a seemingly sterile pyarthrosis is encountered. *Staphylococcus aureus* is by far the next most common pathogen. Septic joints in children 6 months to 2 years of age are often due to *Haemophilus influenzae.* Gram-negative bacilli have recently become a more frequent cause of septic joints, especially in adults with chronic debilitating illness. However, almost every bacterial pathogen has been reported to cause septic arthritis, and the clinical presentation is not helpful for determining the causative organism.

Clinical Findings

A. Symptoms and Signs

In acute hematogenous arthritis, the larger joints (knee, hip, elbow, shoulder, and ankle) are more commonly involved. Infections of other organ systems (skin, respiratory tract, genitourinary tract, etc) are possible sources of blood-borne infections. Although infections in adults usually involve only one joint, multiple joint involvement occurs occasionally in children. Any joint may be involved secondarily by spread of a nearby acute or chronic infection. Systemic disease or another serious infection may divert attention from the infected joint. Systemic symptoms usually include fever, chills, and malaise—and, occasionally, misleading migratory polyarthralgia. Pain is progressive and accentuated by joint motion. Local tenderness and warmth are accompanied by soft tissue swelling, and an effusion is palpable if the joint is superficial.

B. Laboratory Findings

Examination of joint fluid is crucial. By the time infection is clinically apparent, the fluid is usually turbid or purulent. The white cell count is often over 50,000/μL, with more than 90% PMNs. Synovial fluid glucose is decreased, usually to 50 mg/dL below a simultaneously obtained blood glucose level. Gram-stained smears and cultures are essential. The stain will often dictate the choice of first antibiotic pending sensitivity confirmation. Pyarthrosis without visible organisms on a Gram-stained smear is usually gonococcal in origin. Culture specimens for this fastidious organism must be conveyed promptly to the bacteriology laboratory for proper plating on a selective medium and incubation in 5% carbon dioxide. The erythrocyte sedimentation rate is almost always elevated, and the white count may be. Blood cultures are sometimes positive even when organisms are not recovered from joint fluid.

C. Imaging Studies

The appearance of significant x-ray findings depends upon the duration and virulence of infection. X-ray changes lag behind the clinical and pathologic process. During the first 2 weeks, the joint capsule may appear distended, the overlying soft tissues swollen, and fat planes obscured. In infants especially, increased intra-articular pressure from effusion may cause widening of the radiologic "joint space," with possible progression to pathologic dislocation. Comparative x-rays of the opposite normal joint can aid in identification of subtle changes. With persistent hyperemia and disuse, demineralization of subchondral bone occurs and extends proximal and distal to the joint. Trabecular detail is progressively lost, and the compact subchondral bone appears accentuated. Destruction of cartilage is reflected by narrowing of the width of the joint space until subchondral bone is in apposition, a finding accentuated by x-rays taken during weightbearing.

Complications

Complications consist of joint destruction, osteomyelitis, and direct or hematogenous spread to other sites. The risk of complication is increased by delayed diagnosis.

Differential Diagnosis

Acute pyogenic arthritis must be differentiated from other acute arthropathies (reactive arthritis, systemic lupus erythematosus, rheumatoid arthritis, gout, pseudogout, neurogenic arthropathy, etc). Hematogenous osteomyelitis (especially of the proximal femur), rheumatic fever, and epiphysial trauma may mimic acute septic arthritis in childhood. Lyme disease must also be considered.

Acute pyogenic arthritis may complicate almost any type of preexisting joint disease, especially rheumatoid arthritis and neuropathic arthropathy. Concomitant or recent treatment with locally injected or systemic corticosteroids may both predispose to infection and interfere with diagnosis. Polyarthralgia occurs in systemic viral infections and allergic reactions, but the other features of septic arthritis are lacking. Acute infections or inflammations of periarticular structures (eg, septic bursitis and tenosynovitis, osteomyelitis, cellulitis, and acute calcific tendinitis) may be especially difficult to differentiate. Aspiration, examination, and culture of joint fluid are essential to establish or rule out infection of a joint. Occasionally, synovial biopsy is helpful in diagnosing obscure cases of synovitis.

Treatment

A. General Measures

Analgesics and splinting of the involved joint in the position of maximal comfort alleviate pain. Other foci of infection and any coexisting medical conditions must be identified and treated appropriately. Fluid replacement and nutritional support may be required.

B. Specific Measures

Definitive treatment requires drainage of the pyarthrosis and prompt institution of effective antibiotic therapy. The technique of drainage depends upon the joint involved, the stage of infection, and the response of the patient. Although many infected joints can be drained satisfactorily with repeated needle aspiration, the hip—and perhaps other joints that are difficult to aspirate—will require arthrotomy as soon as possible after identification of joint sepsis. Other indications for surgical drainage of septic arthritis are inability to aspirate loculated pus, lack of prompt response to nonoperative management, long-standing infection, and joint infections after surgery or penetrating wounds.

Parenteral antibiotics are indicated for septic arthritis. If organisms are not seen on Gram-stained smears and the patient is a previously healthy adult, gonococcal arthritis is an appropriate working diagnosis, and penicillin should be started as outlined below. Children under 4 years of age have a significant incidence of *H influenzae* arthritis. Preliminary antibiotic treatment in this age group must be effective against this organism, which also may be difficult to see on Gram-stained smears. In adults with negative results on Gram-stained smears and a suspected cause of infection other than gonococci, treatment should be started with a cephalosporin or a beta-lactamase-resistant penicillin and an aminoglycoside.

When organisms are seen, initial antibiotic therapy should be based on that finding. Culture results and clinical response must subsequently be used to ensure an appropriate antibiotic regimen. Parenteral antibiotics are continued at high doses until inflammation resolves significantly. Ten to 14 days of treatment is usually required. An additional 3–4 weeks of oral antibiotic therapy is often advised after parenteral treatment. Briefer treatment usually suffices for gonococcal arthritis. Intravenous penicillin G, 10 million units/24 h, should be continued until significant improvement is achieved. While the response is often prompt, several days of treatment may be required. Once local signs resolve, the antibiotic can be changed to oral ampicillin, 500 mg four times daily, to complete a 7-day course.

Prognosis

Satisfactory results are achieved in 70% or more of patients with septic arthritis if early diagnosis and treatment are provided. Joint destruction—especially of the hip in infants—and joint stiffness in the elderly are the most common causes of failure. Deaths are rare.

Chaudhuri K et al: Septic arthritis of the shoulder after mastectomy and radiotherapy for breast carcinoma. J Bone Joint Surg Br 1993;75:318.

Dagan R: Management of acute hematogenous osteomyelitis and septic arthritis in the pediatric patient. Pediatr Infect Dis J 1993;12:88.

Ostrum RF: Nocardia septic arthritis of the hip with associated avascular necrosis; a case report. Clin Orthop 1993;288:282.

Rankin KC, Rycken JM: Bilateral dislocation of the proximal humeral epiphyses in septic arthritis: a case report. J Bone Joint Surg Br 1993;75:329.

BONE TUMORS

Primary tumors of bone are relatively uncommon in comparison with secondary or metastatic neoplasms. However, they are of great clinical significance because of the possibility of cancer and because some grow rapidly and metastasize widely. Persistent skeletal pain, localized tenderness, and an enlarging mass with or without limitation of motion of adjacent joints or spontaneous fracture are indications for prompt clinical, radiographic, laboratory, and perhaps biopsy examination. Histologic characteristics generally provide the best information about the nature of the lesion, but they must be correlated with all other related facts. The diagnosis of bone tumors is most precise when made by the clinician, the radiologist, and the pathologist in close consultation.

Operative Technique

There are several surgical approaches to the treatment of bone tumors. With intralesional excision (curettement, debulking), the tumor is entered, but gross as well as microscopic tumor may remain. Excision indicates local removal of a tumor following visualization of the capsule or pseudocapsule to establish the plane of dissection. Tumor cells may be left in the wound even if the capsule is not grossly violated. Wide excision indicates a margin of normal tissue between the capsule or pseudocapsule and the planes of dissection. Radical resection implies removal of the entire anatomic compartment containing the tumor. Amputation may be any of these depending on the margin, but it is usually "wide excision" or "radical resection."

Radiologic Characteristics

A. Benign Characteristics

1. Cystic expansion of a diaphysis or metaphysis with mature cortex around the area of expansion.
2. The presence of a definable though thin cortical end plate (capsule) around an intraosseous area from which cancellous or cortical bone has been lost, sometimes referred to as a "geographic lesion."
3. No periosteal new bone formation.

B. Malignant Characteristics

1. Permeative destruction of either cancellous or cortical bone, manifest by gradual transition from a region of gross destruction with loss of bony continuity to a region of lesser destruction and normal bone. There is no clear line of demarcation between abnormal and normal bone.
2. Gross bone destruction with cortical defects, manifested by loss of large areas of bony substance without encapsulation.
3. Periosteal or bone formation within the tumor or at its margins may be manifested by multiple layers of parallel periosteal reaction (onionskin formation) or sunburst (spiculated, hair-on-end) linear areas of calcification. The latter generally parallel the expansile direction of the tumor as it breaks through bone.
4. A few metastatic tumors (breast, prostate) incite local reactive new bone formation and are classified as osteoblastic rather than osteolytic tumors (the latter are more common in metastatic cancer).

Grading & Staging of Bone Tumors

Some tumor categories can be subclassified into varying degrees of malignancy (grading) according to histologic criteria, radiologic appearance, and clinical course. Grade 0 is benign; grade 1 is low-grade malignancy; and grades 2 and 3 indicate increasingly higher degrees of malignancy. Grading reflects the biologic behavior of the lesion.

The size of the tumor, the presence or absence of local invasion of adjacent compartments or lymph nodes, and the presence or absence of distant metastases can be combined with the surgical grade to establish stage categories that reflect prognosis. When grading and staging are possible, treatment options may be more realistically chosen.

Among musculoskeletal neoplasms, chondrosarcomas lend themselves to grading, though in tumors occurring secondary to osteochondroma, size is of less significance than it is with other sarcomas. Grading and staging of soft tissue sarcomas by histologic criteria, intra- or extracompartmental location, and metastatic spread have prognostic value and aid in planning treatment.

In osteogenic sarcoma and Ewing's sarcoma, the prognosis is not easily determined from the histologic pattern, and grading is therefore not as useful as in soft tissue sarcomas or chondrosarcomas.

Biopsy

The possibility of cancer exists in almost every lesion prior to histologic examination. Therefore, the choice of excision and the extent of exposure for biopsy should be planned to avoid unnecessary contamination of tissue planes with tumor cells, which would complicate subsequent local resection. This consideration takes precedence over more standard surgical approaches used for trauma and reconstruction. In the extremities, biopsy incisions should be longitudinal and placed where minimal dissection is needed to reach the tumor. Frozen section guidance should be obtained. This may permit immediate definitive diagnosis and operation. Even when this is not so, the surgeon can be assured that an adequate and representative sample has been examined and may occasionally be forewarned that the lesion is inflammatory rather than neoplastic. For the latter reason, it is also advisable to take appropriate culture specimens of some of the tissue removed at biopsy even though the clinical picture and x-ray appearance may seem typical of a neoplastic lesion.

Chemotherapy

Adjunctive chemotherapy following appropriate management of the primary lesion delays the appearance and lowers the incidence of metastases and the 2-year death rates for osteogenic sarcoma, Ewing's sarcoma, and primary lymphoma of bone. Alterations in drug combinations, dosage, and frequency continue to be made. For this reason, specific protocols for chemotherapy will not be set forth here. The reader is referred to reports of the appropriate cancer study groups of the National Cancer Institute for current guidelines.

Radiation Therapy

Radiation therapy combined with chemotherapy has become standard treatment for Ewing's sarcoma and primary lymphoma of bone. Radiation therapy used alone sometimes produced dramatic initial control of primary lesions, but 5-year survival rates for these tumors did not improve significantly until chemotherapy was added.

Radiation therapy plus chemotherapy has a less well defined role in the treatment of primary osteogenic sarcoma. Irradiation alone will produce a temporary response manifested largely by brief cessation of the prior rapid rate of growth. However, even when chemotherapy is added, sufficient control of the primary lesion is not achieved.

Radiation therapy of benign lesions of bone is undesirable if the primary can be controlled surgically, since radiation-induced sarcoma of bone occurs with an incidence of 0.2% in normal bone (ie, in radiation fields in patients treated for other lesions). The risk appears to be greater in growing bone than adult bone. Certain benign but locally aggressive tumors of bone with high local recurrence rates necessitate consideration of radiation therapy if the anatomic location makes the risk of morbidity and death associated with surgical removal unacceptable (spine, skull, or facial bones).

METASTATIC BONE TUMORS

The most common form of cancer affecting the skeleton is metastatic tumor deposits from primary lesions elsewhere in the body. Eighty percent of these metastatic lesions are from primary carcinomas—particularly of the breast, prostate, lung, kidney, thyroid, pancreas, or stomach, in that order of frequency.

The presenting symptom is usually pain. Pathologic fracture may be present and is more common in the lower than the upper extremity.

The presenting radiologic finding is destruction of bone—usually osteolytic but in the case of breast or prostate metastasis either partly or solely osteoblastic. The size of an individual lesion is usually less than what is seen in primary tumors of bone at the time of first diagnosis.

In a patient with a known primary malignant tumor presenting with a painful lytic lesion of bone, a diagnosis of metastatic deposit can be made with some assurance; but there are individuals in whom the primary is not yet recognized at the time the early metastatic lesion becomes painful. Bone scan or skeletal survey will aid the prebiopsy workup since there is a high probability of more than one area of skeletal involvement. The most common primary source of solitary skeletal metastases at the time of first diagnosis is carcinoma of the kidney. Therefore, an excretory urogram should be part of the prebiopsy workup of solitary metastases with no obvious primary. Metastases from carcinoma of the kidney are extremely vascular—an important point to remember when planning biopsy.

The treatment of metastatic cancer has two goals: management of the neoplasm and management of the symptoms produced by the local lesion.

Management of the neoplasm at the metastatic site depends upon the type and prognosis in each case but usually involves radiation therapy, chemotherapy, hormone therapy, or a combination of these treatment methods.

Operative treatment with internal fixation for pathologic fracture is often desirable in metastatic tumors of long bones, particularly in the lower extremities, so that the patient can remain ambulatory and more comfortable during the months or even years of life that remain. Although less commonly indicated because of the nonweightbearing function of the upper extremity, internal fixation may be necessary for pain control or to improve the patient's ability to manage crutches. In addition to the usual techniques for fracture fixation, methylmethacrylate supplementation frequently is necessary to substitute for bone loss and possible lack of healing response.

MYELOMA

In one sense, multiple myeloma is the most common malignant tumor affecting bone, but since it arises from the hematopoietic marrow, it is not, strictly speaking, a tumor "of bone." Its incidence is about equal to that of all malignant tumors of bone combined. Pain is the principal presenting symptom, and local swelling is uncommon. Pathologic fractures do occur but are not a common initial symptom. The lesions can occur in any bone, but small bone involvement is infrequent. There is a slightly higher incidence in males than females, with peak incidence in the sixth and seventh decades. The bony lesions are manifested radiologically by osteolytic areas of bone destruction, with little or no reactive bone.

As indicated by the term multiple myeloma, there frequently are multiple lesions at the time of initial diagnosis.

The treatment strategy is essentially the same as that outlined above for metastatic tumors.

MALIGNANT BONE TUMORS

1. Osteogenic Sarcoma

Osteogenic sarcoma is the most common primary malignant tumor of bone, with an incidence of 0.25 cases per 100,000 population per year. It usually occurs in the distal femoral metaphysis, proximal tibial metaphysis, proximal humeral metaphysis, pelvis, or proximal femur, in that order of frequency. Most patients are in the adolescent age group, and males predominate in a 3:2 ratio.

The usual presenting manifestations are pain, tenderness, and swelling near a joint. Some limitation of motion may be present.

X-rays show a permeative destructive lesion in the metaphysis that rarely crosses the epiphysial plate and is commonly accompanied by periosteal elevation. Periosteal new bone frequently presents in the form of Codman's triangle at the diaphysial end of the lesion (Figure 42–49). The more central area will show evidence of tumor extension beyond the confines of the cortex and contains sunburst or hair-on-end radially oriented filaments of calcification and bone formation. There is considerable variation in the degree of osteolytic versus osteoblastic activity in these lesions.

The natural history of this tumor is one of relentless growth, early metastasis to the lungs, and death if appropriate treatment is not given. Lymphatic involvement is not common. Treatment by resection (usually amputation) of the primary lesion in past years produced a 5-year survival rate of 15–20%. Most deaths occurred in the first 2 years. With adjunctive chemotherapy following amputation or other local complete resection of the tumor, the appearance of pulmonary metastases has been significantly delayed, and the projected 5-year survival rate currently is about 60%. The apparent ability of adjunctive chemotherapy to destroy microscopic metastases suggests

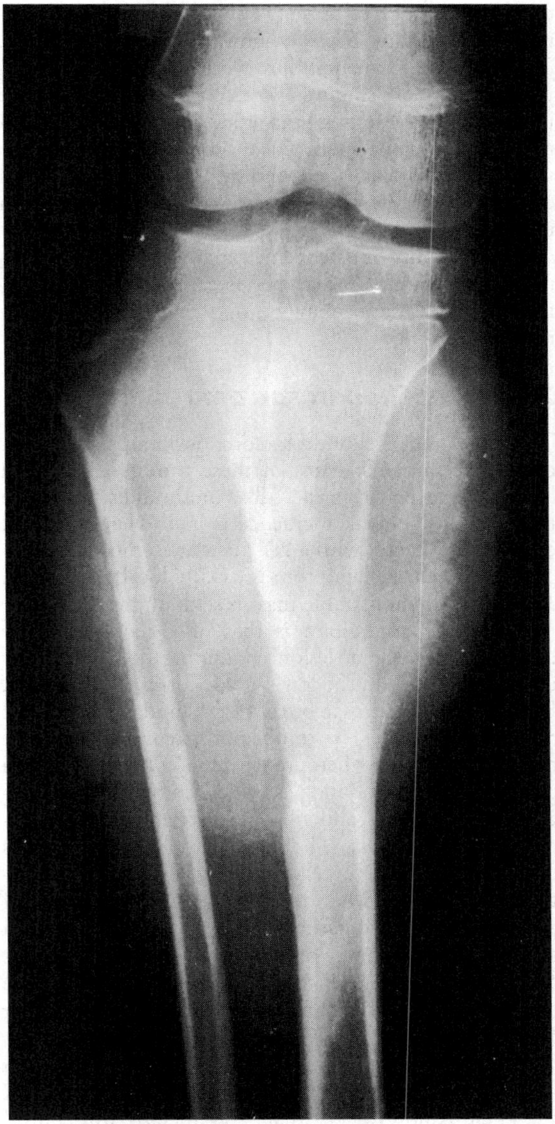

Figure 42–49. Osteosarcoma with Codman's triangle.

that local resection of primary lesions followed by adjunctive chemotherapy may be substituted for amputation. This is still experimental, however, since at this time 5-year rates for both survival and absence of local recurrence in a suitably functioning limb are not available. Lesions in the pelvis or spine might have boundaries too close to vital structures and hence should be treated with local excision, adjunctive chemotherapy, and perhaps radiation therapy.

Rare variants of osteogenic sarcoma with a less ominous history are parosteal, periosteal, and central sarcomas. These variants may be more amenable to local resection.

2. Primary Chondrosarcoma

The incidence of chondrosarcoma is about half that of osteogenic sarcoma. Most of these tumors are located either in the pelvic girdle, ribs, or shoulder girdle, in that order. The peak incidence is in the late fifth and early sixth decades, with a 2:1 male predominance.

The presenting symptom is usually local discomfort. A visible or demonstrable mass is seldom present.

The x-ray appearance is that of a central, slightly expansile, radiolucent lesion containing flocculent areas of calcific density in the lower-grade forms of the tumor. High-grade chondrosarcomas may simulate osteogenic sarcoma on x-rays. The tumor occurs commonly in the metaphysial region when present in long bones but has a predilection for flat bones, as evidenced by the high incidence in the pelvis and ribs and a relatively high incidence in the scapula. The gross pathologic anatomy is that of firm, translucent, usually gritty gray tissue of cartilaginous density with demonstrable fine sediment of calcific density. The natural history is one of continued growth, with a high rate of local recurrence if all tumor is not removed. Metastases to distant sites—particularly the lungs—occur much later than is the case with most other bone sarcomas.

The treatment of chondrosarcoma is individualized in terms of how radical the attempt at surgical removal must be. There is no evidence that x-ray therapy will control the lesion or that chemotherapy will affect the outcome. Complete surgical removal will result in cure at 5 years in almost all grade 1 tumors and a significant percentage of grade 3 tumors. When these tumors are graded, it is important to be certain that all of the tumor has been well sampled, since there may be considerable variation in different geographic areas within the tumor.

3. Ewing's Tumor (Ewing's Sarcoma)

Ewing's sarcoma occurs with an incidence of 0.1 cases per 100,000 population per year. The male:female ratio is 3:2. The tumor occurs most commonly in the second decade. Patients tend to be slightly younger than those with osteogenic sarcoma. Ewing's tumor is most common in the extremities, particularly the lower extremities and pelvic girdle. The symptoms and signs are pain, local swelling, and occasionally fever, with an elevated white blood count.

The x-ray appearance is that of a permeative destructive lesion, usually in the metaphysis but also in the diaphysis more often than osteogenic sarcoma. Periosteal new bone formation is common. The gross pathologic picture is nonspecific, with neoplastic tissue permeating bone and muscle with a consistency varying from firm gray connective tissue to liquefaction necrosis. The latter has at times mimicked purulence secondary to bacterial infection and may be confused with osteomyelitis. These facts reinforce the general wisdom of routinely obtaining material both for culture and for histopathologic examination whether the clinical diagnosis is infection or neoplasm.

The early history is one of progressive local growth, early distant metastases, and death if proper treatment is not given. Metastasis is most commonly to the lung but may occur in other tissues (including bone) more frequently than is the case with osteogenic sarcoma. Radiation therapy to the primary tumor combined with multiple-drug chemotherapy has improved the 5-year survival rate to about 60%.

Treatment of Ewing's sarcoma of the pelvis has a significantly higher failure rate following such combination therapy. Anatomically feasible resection or wide excision following initial tumor response to combined treatment should therefore be considered. If the primary tumor is in an expendable bone, wide excision or resection may be considered after an initial course of combined treatment.

4. Fibrosarcoma

The incidence of fibrosarcoma is about 0.05 cases per 100,000 population per year. Males and females are equally affected. More than half of cases occur in the long bones, and the distal femur and proximal tibia are the most common sites. The humerus and scapula together have been reported as representing perhaps the second or third most common site. These tumors have been reported in every decade through the ninth but are most common in the third and fourth decades. If fibrosarcoma in Paget's disease or other preexisting disease is included, the mean age at diagnosis is the mid 50s.

The signs and symptoms are those of pain and, at times, local swelling. The incidence of pathologic fracture is relatively high.

X-rays show a destructive lesion of bone, almost universally osteolytic, with little or no calcification within the tumor mass but with periosteal reactions at the margins, which may be horizontal (onionskin) in character or spiculated (hair-on-end). The periosteal reaction is less prominent than in osteogenic sarcoma. The lesions are usually quite large at first presentation. The gross pathologic anatomy is nonspecific, and the tumor itself consists of tissue of connective tissue density and is seldom accompanied by liquefaction necrosis.

The natural history is one of progressive growth, frequent pathologic fracture, and distant metastases usually to the lung, with death if appropriate treatment is not given. Treatment consists of local removal of the primary tumor, which in most situations requires amputation. Neither radiation therapy nor chemotherapy has been helpful. The 5-year survival rate is 30–35%.

5. Malignant Lymphoma (Reticulum Cell Sarcoma of Bone)

This tumor occurs with an estimated incidence of 0.1 case per 100,000 population per year. There is a slight (3:2) male predominance. The tumor is most common between the third and sixth decades. It is relatively rare in the forearm, hand, and foot.

The usual presenting signs and symptoms are pain, local tenderness, and, occasionally local swelling. The x-ray appearance is usually that of a permeative diffuse, destructive lesion with minimal or absent periosteal reaction, even in the case of rather large lesions. The gross pathologic picture is nonspecific.

If systemic generalized involvement is excluded by appropriate staging, the treatment of choice is radiation, which is associated with a 5-year survival rate of 35–50%. The generalized disease, which may be present with localized symptoms initially, requires combined radiation therapy and chemotherapy and has a reported 5-year survival rate of 23%.

BENIGN BONE TUMORS

1. Osteochondroma

Osteochondromas (bony exostoses) comprise at least 45% of benign bone tumors. These tend to occur at the metaphyses of long bones but may also occur in the spine and ribs. The most common sites are the distal ends of the femur and the proximal ends of the humerus. The patients are usually under 20 years of age at the time of initial excision. Since these are very slow-growing tumors, the time of diagnosis or excision does not coincide with the time of onset.

The x-ray appearance is that of a bony stalk with a cartilaginous cap extending from the metaphysial region near the epiphysial plate and usually inclined away from the joint. These lesions rarely enlarge after childhood. The usual reasons for operation are local mechanical problems related to tumor size or perhaps pressure against musculotendinous structures operating in the vicinity. Sarcomatous degeneration occurs in 1% of cases. Thus, a sudden increase in size or a change in symptomatology warrants exploration and biopsy.

Multiple congenital osteochondromas (exostoses) occur as a heritable autosomal dominant characteristic. There is usually some growth retardation and bowing deformity of the long bones. The incidence of sarcomatous degeneration is variously reported to be 5–15% in this group, but this may simply reflect the larger number of lesions present.

The treatment of symptomatic lesions is by surgical excision, which should include the entire stalk and its base. Secondary chondrosarcoma requires complete removal (resection, with some anatomic areas requiring amputation).

2. Enchondroma (Chondroma)

Enchondroma is most commonly in the hand, including the metacarpals and phalangeals, and next most commonly in the proximal end of the humerus. It is equally distributed between males and females and accounts for about 10% of benign tumors. It may occur from the first decade through the seventh, with the mean age in the mid thirties. The x-ray appearance is that of a cystic, slightly expansile lesion in the shaft of a long bone, with some scalloping of the cortex but without periosteal new bone formation. A speckled, calcific series of shadows within the cystic lesion is characteristic. The gross pathology is that of firm, translucent gray-white granular material.

The natural history is one of slow growth and a low incidence of pathologic fracture. Pain is often present. Except for lesions in the clavicle or small bones of the hand or foot, visible or palpable masses are uncommon.

Treatment consists of curettement and bone grafting.

3. Giant Cell Tumor of Bone

Giant cell tumor (Figure 42–50) is most common around the knee, the sacrum, the distal radius, and the proximal humerus. It occurs with a female:male ratio of 3:2. It is almost never seen before closure of the epiphysial plate. It tends to be centered in the epiphysial area and to extend eccentrically beyond the epiphysial plate boundary. The chief symptom is pain. Pathologic fracture is rare, and the pain usually leads to diagnosis before there is visible or palpable external swelling.

X-rays show a cystic expansion of the involved bone. The area of destruction has a soap bubble appearance, with normal trabeculae and little reactive bone at the margins. Grossly, the lesion is filled with an orange and brown soft tumor mass without calcification. Ninety-eight percent of cases are benign and the remainder are malignant, with potential for metastatic spread. The neoplastic portion of the tumor is the mesenchymal stromal cell rather than the giant cell element. Benign giant cell tumor may recur and become malignant.

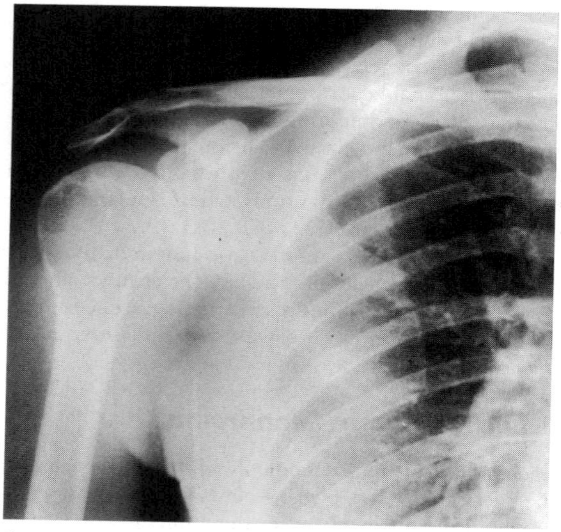

Figure 42–50. Giant cell tumor of proximal humerus.

The natural history without treatment is one of continuous growth resulting in an enormous tumor, pathologic fracture, and in some cases necrosis of overlying skin. Treatment is by operative removal, and complete cure can be expected if the lesion is completely resected. Since it is most common in nonexpendable bones, thorough curettement and grafting is the standard initial treatment. This form of treatment carries a risk of recurrence as high as 40%. If tumor recurs, biopsy should be performed again to verify the absence of malignant change. If malignant change has not taken place, resection followed by allograft, arthrodesis, or prosthetic replacement has the greatest probability of preventing recurrence. But curettement—followed by filling the cavity with methylmethacrylate—is not inappropriate.

In addition to a high recurrence rate, this lesion also carries a higher rate of postoperative wound infection than comparable operations in the same anatomic region.

Radiation therapy is probably not justified because of a risk of later postradiation sarcoma—except in the spine or sacrum, where complete surgical removal is not possible.

4. Aneurysmal Bone Cyst

Aneurysmal bone cyst is most common in the metaphyses of long bones and in the vertebrae, particularly the posterior elements. The peak incidence is in the second decade. The male:female incidence is equal. The most common symptoms and signs are pain and swelling. Pathologic fractures are rare.

The x-ray appearance is that of an eccentric metaphysial lesion containing expansile cysts with septa. A large thin shell portion protrudes beyond the normal confines of the bony anatomy. Grossly, the tumor is a blood-filled cavity with a soft membrane lining the bony margins.

These tumors are locally destructive by expansile growth but do not metastasize.

Treatment consists of operative removal. Radiation therapy is justified only for lesions in areas where local resection (or thorough curettement) is not feasible (eg, the spine). A recurrence rate ranging from 30% to 60% has been reported following curettement. Several factors relating to recurrence are (1) the adequacy of surgical removal; (2) the age of the patient (risk is much greater in patients under age 15); and (3) tumor size (large tumors in young patients have a high recurrence rate). There may also be a correlation between the frequency of mitotic figures and an increased risk of recurrence.

Resection is the treatment of choice where location permits. Some giant cell tumors and some osteogenic sarcomas will have an aneurysmal cystic element, and diagnosis therefore requires a representative sample.

5. Unicameral Bone Cyst

The incidence of unicameral bone cyst in the general population is not clearly defined, since this is a benign lesion with a tendency to be self-limited and possibly self-healing. Most patients are children, usually between the ages of 5 and 15 years, with a slight (3:2) male preponderance. These tumors are usually asymptomatic until pathologic fracture produces pain.

The roentgenographic appearance is that of a multilocular expansile, cystic lesion, principally radiolucent, with its proximal end at or near the epiphysial plate (Figure 42–51). The overlying cortex is attenuated, but no periosteal new bone formation is present. The central portion is rarefied, and undisplaced fracture is the most common initial symptom.

Grossly, the cyst is predominantly a fluid-filled space with a thin capsule. The fluid may vary from serous to sanguineous. The lesions are of varying size, from moderately large to small, and are occasionally seen in x-rays taken for other reasons in asymptomatic patients. At first presentation, however, they classically encompass the entire diameter of the metaphysis. Recognition that these tumors are seen in asymptomatic patients permits the assumption that some are self-healing. Spontaneous regression has been documented following fracture in about 15% of these lesions.

In the past, the usual treatment was curettement and autogenous bone graft to fill the space. The recurrence rate following this treatment varies from 20% to 50% and is reported to be twice as high in patients under age 10 compared with those over age 10. Subtotal resection techniques, with excision of most of the cyst wall including the bony shell, both with or without grafting, have been associated with a recurrence rate of 5–9%,

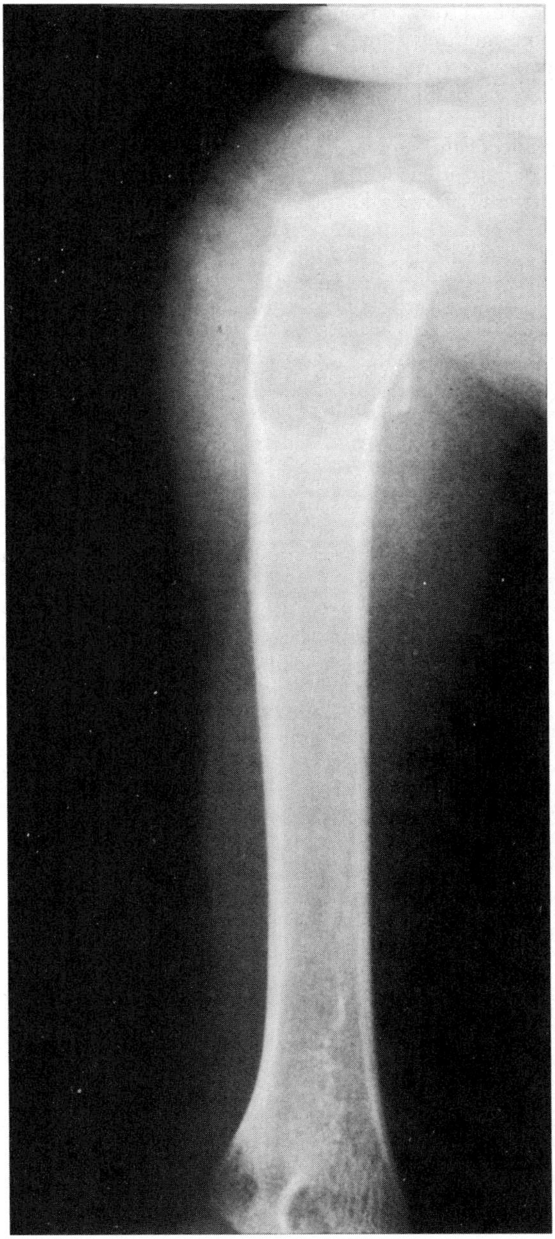

Figure 42–51. Unicameral bone cyst with fracture.

but the number of cases from which these figures are derived is small. If the proximal end of the cyst is in contact with the epiphysial plate, the cyst is classified as "active"; if the cyst is separated from the plate by normal cancellous metaphysial bone, it is classified as "latent." Active cysts carry the greater risk of recurrence following curettement and grafting and also (owing to the proximity to the epiphysial plate) carry a higher risk of damage to the plate at the time of operation. Intracystic injection of methylprednisolone is a safe alternative to surgical treatment of these lesions. Results of this procedure show a recurrence rate of 5–10% with few complications.

Expectant treatment can be offered until the pathologic fracture is healed, at which time needle biopsy should be done. Although details of classification are sometimes difficult with needle biopsy because of the small sample, this procedure will clearly separate the classic cyst from solid tumor lesions simulating unicameral bone cyst. If the mass is identified as cystic, consideration of operative removal can be postponed (particularly if the patient is under 10 years of age) and the progress of the cyst merely observed. If a second pathologic fracture occurs and the cyst does not show signs of resolution, either curettement with grafting or steroid injection may be tried.

Oppenheim WL, Gallend H: Operative treatment versus steroid injection in the management of unicameral bone cysts. J Pediatr Orthop 1984;4:1.

6. Eosinophilic Granuloma

Eosinophilic granuloma is a solitary lytic lesion of bone that is classified with disorders of the reticuloendothelial system and may not be a true neoplasm. It is relatively rare, and the most common site is the skull. The male:female ratio is 3:2, and the peak incidence is between 7 years and 8 years of age. Most cases occur before age 30.

Pain is the principal presenting complaint. There is almost never any demonstrable tumor mass on physical examination.

The radiologic appearance is that of a lytic defect, which in long bones frequently expands the shaft and may be accompanied by periosteal new bone formation, usually of the horizontal (onionskin) type. In flat bones, the lesion is also lytic but tends to be flattened to conform to the shape of the host bone.

Grossly, the tissue is soft (sometimes semigelatinous) and gray or yellow. Hemorrhagic areas are occasionally seen.

If the systemic variants of histiocytosis X (Hand-Schüller-Christian disease, Letterer-Siwe disease) are excluded, the lesions are probably self-limited and may run through a rapid growth cycle followed by spontaneous healing. There is evidence that they heal following biopsy with or without bone grafting. Low-dose irradiation has been used for treatment, particularly for symptomatic spine lesions, but it is more appropriate to merely observe the patient following biopsy in the hope that spontaneous healing will occur. If pathologic fractures are present, they should be treated by cast or fixation.

7. Chondroblastoma

Chondroblastoma is a relatively rare lesion that characteristically occurs in the epiphysis prior to closure of the epiphysial plate. This location is a rare site of other primary or secondary tumors in growing bone. Ninety percent of cases occur between the ages of 5 and 25 years. The male:female ratio is 2:1. The epiphyses around the knee and the proximal humerus are the common locations. Pain and joint effusion are common, with associated local tenderness and limitation of motion of the adjacent joints.

The x-ray appearance is that of a lytic lesion in the epiphysial body or, if the plate is closed, in its former location. The lesions are usually not expansile and seldom as large as giant cell tumors. They rarely extend significantly across the old epiphysial plate in patients whose physial lines are closed. The lesions tend to be eccentric in the epiphysis and have a mottled appearance compatible with calcification within the tumor. Pathologic fracture and subperiosteal reaction are uncommon. The gross pathologic anatomy is that of granular tissue of cartilaginous density containing foci of calcification. A chondroblastoma grows slowly and lacks malignant characteristics, although a few cases of metastases have been reported.

The most common treatment is curettement and bone grafting, since the location frequently does not permit resection. The recurrence rate varies from 10% to 40% in different series. If recurrence does occur, recurettement with grafting is still the treatment of choice if the site is one that does not permit resection. There is no evidence that radiation therapy or chemotherapy has any value in these lesions.

Conway WF, Hayes CW: Miscellaneous lesions of bone. Radiol Clin North Am 1993;31:339.

Caso Martinez J et al: En-bloc resection of the distal fibula for aneurysmal bone cyst. Acta Orthop Belg 1993;59:87.

Hudson TM, Stiles RG, Monson DK: Fibrous lesions of bone. Radiol Clin North Am 1993;31:279.

McCarthy CS, Becker JA: Multiple myeloma and contrast media. Radiology 1992;183:519.

Mercuri M et al: The management of malignant bone tumors in children and adolescents. Clin Orthop 1991;264:156.

Pennington DG, Marsden W, Stephens FO: Fibrosarcoma of metacarpal treated by combined therapy and immediate reconstruction with vascularized bone graft. J Hand Surg Am 1991;16:877.

Simon MA, Finn HA: Diagnostic strategy for bone and soft-tissue tumors. J Bone Joint Surg Am 1993;75:622.

Steiner RM et al: Magnetic resonance imaging of diffuse bone marrow disease. Radiol Clin North Am 1993;31:383.

Plastic & Reconstructive Surgery 43

Henry C. Vasconez, MD, Robert E. H. Ferguson, Jr, MD, & Luis O. Vasconez, MD

Plastic surgery, although thought of as a technique-oriented specialty, is in fact a problem-solving field. The training of a plastic surgeon allows him or her to see surgical problems in a different light and select from a variety of options to solve these surgical problems. Plastic surgeons have received broad training, and most have completed residencies in other fields such as general surgery, otolaryngology, orthopedics, urology, or neurosurgery. Other modalities of training have more recently integrated these and other surgical subspecialties into a more comprehensive program.

The basic principles of plastic surgery are careful analysis of the surgical problem, careful planning of procedures, precise technique, and atraumatic handling of tissues. Alteration, coverage, and transfer of skin and associated tissues are the most common procedures performed. Plastic surgery may deal with the closure of surgical wounds—particularly recalcitrant wounds such as those occurring post radiation or poorly healing wounds in immunocompromised patients. Plastic surgery also deals with the removal of skin tumors, repair of soft tissue injuries including burns, correction of acquired or congenital deformities, or enhancement of undesirable cosmetic features. Craniofacial and hand surgery, also within the realm of plastic surgery, may require additional surgical training.

In the past quarter century, increased knowledge of anatomy and the development of many new techniques have brought about important changes in plastic surgery. It is now known that in many areas the blood supply of the skin is derived principally from vessels arising from underlying muscles and larger perforating blood vessels rather than solely from vessels of the subcutaneous tissue, as was formerly thought. One-stage transfer of large areas of skin, fascia, and muscle tissue can be accomplished if the axial pedicle of the underlying fascia or muscle is included in the transfer. With the use of microsurgical techniques, musculocutaneous units or combinations of bone, fascia, muscle, and skin can be successfully transferred and vessels and nerves less than 1 mm in size can be repaired. These so-called free-flap transplantations are a major advance in the treatment of defects that were previously untreatable or required lengthy or multistaged procedures. More sophisticated knowledge of the blood supply to the skin has introduced the concept of perforator flaps whereby one perforating vessel is identified that may supply a large segment of overlying skin and tissues. Similarly, the concept of neurocutaneous flaps has given rise to the design of additional flap territories such as the so-called sural flap in the lower leg and the sensate radial flap in the forearm.

The plastic surgeon, as a member of the craniofacial surgical team, is able to dramatically improve the appearance and function of children with severe congenital deformities. Children of normal intelligence who previously had been social outcasts are now able to lead relatively normal lives. Improved understanding of facial growth and abnormal development and diagnostic techniques such as the CT scan, MRI, and three-dimensional computer-assisted imaging enable the reconstructive surgeon to develop a complex strategy for remodeling the deformed craniofacial skeleton. This may involve remodeling or repositioning of part or all of the cranial vault, the orbits, the mid face, and the mandible. These complex and at times formidable reconstructions, which were performed by moving the skeletal units and adding autogenous bone grafts, have now more recently been simplified with the use of miniplate fixation as well as certain bone substitutes that may serve as a scaffold upon which normal bone can regrow.

A recent notable advance in craniofacial surgery has been the introduction of distraction osteogenesis, which borrows from the Ilizarov principle of distraction. Here, one makes a cortical cut in the bone and then applies a distraction apparatus so that in measured amounts (usually 1 mm per day) the bone is either stretched to offset a length discrepancy or transported to bridge a gap. In craniofacial surgery it is more commonly brought to bear to enlarge or cause overgrowth of areas such as an underdeveloped mandible.

Additional areas of involvement for the plastic surgeon entail allotransplantation, particularly with the increasing number of clinical limb allotransplants, which unfortunately at present still require immunosuppression. It is hoped that immunotolerance will some day become a reality, thus allowing transplantation of nonessential organs. Transplantation of the hand has been performed but still requires a great deal of immunosuppression. Face transplants are on the horizon, but a number of ethical issues still need to be resolved. Thus, as of this writing, centers poised to perform face transplantation have not yet received full approval from their respective institutional ethics committees.

Tissue engineering of bone, cartilage, and nerve is an area of ongoing research for plastic surgeons. Although encouraging experimental results have been reported in anatomic areas difficult to reconstruct such as the external ear, there are as yet no clinical applications.

Fetal surgery for cleft disorders and scar considerations, an area pioneered by a number of plastic surgeons, appears to be in a quiescent stage, particularly because of technical advances in the treatment of cleft lip and cleft palate in the newborn and infant.

Jones JW et al: Successful hand transplantation. One-year follow-up. Louisville Hand Transplant Team. N Engl J Med 2000; 343:468.

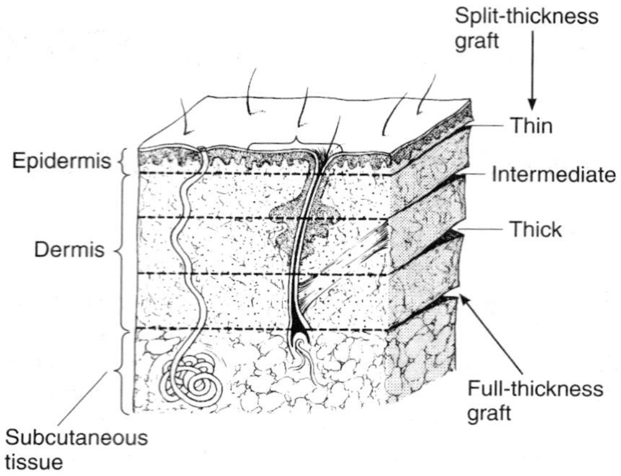

Figure 43–1. Depths of full-thickness and split-thickness grafts.

I. GRAFTS & FLAPS

SKIN GRAFTS

A graft of skin detaches epidermis and varying amounts of dermis from its blood supply in the **donor area** and is placed in a new bed of blood supply from the base of the wound, or **recipient area**. The way a skin graft survives or "takes" is first by diffusion of nutrient elements from the graft bed, known as "imbibition"; then after a period of 2–5 days the graft actually revascularizes from the bed, a process known as "inosculation." Although the technique is relatively simple to perform and generally reliable, definite considerations about the donor area and adequacy of the recipient area are important. Skin grafting is a quick, effective way to cover a wound if vascularity is adequate, infection is not present, and hemostasis is assured. Color match, contour, durability of the graft, and donor morbidity must be considered.

TYPES OF SKIN GRAFTS

Skin grafts can be either split-thickness or full-thickness grafts (Figure 43–1). Each type has advantages and disadvantages and is indicated or contraindicated for different kinds of wounds (Table 43–1).

A. Split-Thickness Grafts

Thinner split-thickness grafts (0.01–0.015 inch) become vascularized more rapidly and survive transplantation more reliably. This is important in grafting on less than ideal recipient sites, such as contaminated wounds, burn surfaces, and poorly vascularized surfaces (eg, irradiated sites). A second advantage is that donor sites heal more rapidly and can be reused within a relatively short time (7–10 days) in critical cases such as major burns.

In general, however, the disadvantages of thin split-thickness grafts outweigh the advantages. Thin grafts exhibit the highest degree of postgraft contraction, offer the least amount of resistance to surface trauma, and are least like normal skin in texture, suppleness, pore pattern, hair growth, and other characteristics. Hence, they are usually aesthetically unacceptable.

Thicker split-thickness skin grafts (> 0.015 inch) contract less, are more resistant to surface trauma, and are more similar to normal skin than are thin split-thickness grafts. They are also aesthetically more acceptable but not as acceptable as full-thickness grafts.

The disadvantages of thick split-thickness grafts are relatively few but can be significant. They are less easily vascularized than thin grafts and thus result in fewer successful takes when used on less than ideal surfaces. Their donor sites are slower to heal (requiring 10–18 days) and heal with more scarring than donor sites for thin split-thickness grafts—a factor that may prevent reuse of the area.

Meshed grafts are usually thin or intermediate split-thickness grafts that have been rolled under a special cutting machine to create a mesh pattern. Although grafts with these perforations can be expanded from one and one-half to nine times their original size, expansion to one and one-half times the unmeshed size is the most useful. Meshed grafts are advantageous because they can be placed on an irregular, possibly contaminated wound bed and will usually take. Also, complications of hemostasis are fewer because blood and serum exude

Table 43–1. Advantages and disadvantages of various types of skin grafts.

Type of Graft	Advantages	Disadvantages
Thin split-thickness	Survive transplantation most easily. Donor sites heal most rapidly.	Fewest qualities of normal skin. Maximum contraction. Least resistance to trauma. Sensation poor. Aesthetically poor.
Thick split-thickness	More qualities of normal skin. Less contraction. More resistant to trauma. Sensation fair. Aesthetically more acceptable.	Survive transplantation less well. Donor site heals slowly.
Full thickness	Nearly all qualities of normal skin. Minimal contraction. Very resistant to trauma. Sensation good. Aesthetically good.	Survive transplantation least well. Donor site must be closed surgically. Donor sites are limited.

through the mesh pattern. The disadvantage is poor appearance following healing (alligator hide look).

Donor sites for split-thickness grafts heal spontaneously by epithelialization. During this process, epithelial cells from the sweat glands, sebaceous glands, or hair follicles proliferate upward and spread across the wound surface. If these three structures are not present, epithelialization will not occur.

B. Full-Thickness Grafts

Full-thickness skin grafts include the epidermis and all the dermis. They are the most aesthetically desirable of the free grafts since they include the highest number of skin appendage elements, undergo the least amount of contracture, and have a greater ability to withstand trauma. There are several limiting factors in the use of full-thickness grafts. Since no epidermal elements remain to produce epithelialization in the donor site, it must be closed primarily, and a scar will result. The size and number of available donor sites is therefore limited. Furthermore, conditions at the recipient site must be optimal in order for transplantation to be successful.

Areas of thin skin are the best donor sites for full-thickness grafts (eg, the eyelids and the skin of the postauricular, supraclavicular, antecubital, inguinal, and genital areas). Submammary and subgluteal skin is thicker but allows camouflage of donor area scars. In grafts thicker than approximately 0.015 inch, the results of transplantation are less reliable, except on the face, where vascularity is usually superior.

C. Composite Grafts

A composite graft is also a free graft that must reestablish its blood supply in the recipient area. It consists of a unit with several tissue planes that may include skin, subcutaneous tissue, cartilage, or other tissue. Dermal fat grafts, hair transplant grafts, and skin and cartilage grafts from the ear fall into this category. Obviously, composite grafts must be small or at least relatively thin and will require recipient sites with excellent vascularity. These grafts are generally used in the face.

D. Cultured Epithelial and Dermal Grafts

Epithelial cells, grown or cultured in a special medium in vitro, will coalesce into thin sheets that can be used to cover full-thickness wounds. Although these cultured epithelial sheets were first used in the treatment of burns, the result was somewhat unsatisfactory because the coverage was very fragile and disfiguring. More recently, success has been obtained with artificial dermis which when placed in an appropriate bed will revascularize and can then be covered by a very thin (0.05 cm) split-thickness skin graft, cultured or otherwise. This artificial dermis is increasingly being used in the treatment of burns. Modifications of this concept have also been applied to the care of chronic ulcers, particularly in the leg. The artificial dermis is made out of a collagen matrix and has very low or no antigenicity.

Obtaining Skin Grafts

Instruments used for obtaining skin grafts include razor blades, skin grafting knives (Blair, Ferris Smith, Humby, Goulian), manual drum dermatomes (Padgett, Reese), and electric or air-powered dermatomes (Brown, Padgett, Hall, Zimmer). The electric and air-powered dermatomes are the most widely used because of their reliability and ease of operation. A surgeon, even with only limited experience, can successfully obtain sheets of split-thickness skin grafts, using the electric dermatomes.

The Skin Graft Recipient Area

To ensure survival of the graft, there must be (1) adequate vascularity of the recipient bed, (2) complete contact between the graft and the bed, (3) adequate immobilization of the graft-bed unit, and (4) relatively few bacteria in the recipient area.

Since survival of the graft is dependent upon growth of capillary buds into the raw undersurface of the graft, vascularity of the recipient area is of prime importance. Avascular surfaces that will not generally accept free grafts are tissues with severe radiation damage, chronically scarred ulcer beds, bone or cartilage denuded of periosteum or perichondrium, and tendon or nerve without their paratenon or perineurium, respectively. For these surfaces, a bed capable of producing capillary buds must be provided; in some cases, excision of the deficient bed down to healthy tissue is possible. All unhealthy granulation tissue must be removed, since bacterial counts in granulation tissue are often very high. If bone is exposed, it can be decorticated down to healthy cancellous bone with the use of a chisel or power-driven burr, and a meshed split-thickness skin graft can be applied. If an adequate vascular bed cannot be provided or if the presence of essential structures such as tendons or nerves precludes further debridement, skin or muscle flaps are generally indicated for coverage.

Inadequate contact between the graft and the recipient bed can be caused by collection of blood, serum, or lymph fluid in the bed; formation of pus between the graft and the bed; or movement of the graft on the bed.

After the graft has been applied directly to the prepared recipient surface, it may or may not be sutured in place and may or may not be dressed. Whenever the maximum aesthetic result is desired, the graft should be cut exactly to fit the recipient area and precisely sutured into position without any overlapping of edges. Very large or thick split-thickness grafts and full-thickness grafts will usually not survive without a pressure dressing. In areas such as the forehead, scalp, and extremities, adequate immobilization and pressure can be provided by circular dressings. Tie-over pressure stent dressings are advisable for areas of the face, where constant pressure cannot be provided by simple wraparound dressings, or areas where movement cannot be avoided, such as the anterior neck, where swallowing causes constant motion; and areas of irregular contour, such as the axilla. The ends of the fixation sutures are left long and tied over a bolus of gauze fluffs, cotton, a sponge, or other suitable material (Figure 43–2).

Grafts applied to freshly prepared or relatively clean surfaces are generally sutured or stapled into place and dressed with pressure. A single layer of damp or other nonadherent fine-mesh gauze is applied directly over the graft. Immediately over this are placed several thicknesses of flat gauze cut in the exact pattern of the graft. On top of these is placed a bulky dry dressing of gauze fluffs, cotton, a sponge, or other material. Pressure is then applied by wraparound dressings, adhesive tape, or a tie-over pressure stent dressing. An alternative dressing is to place a nonadherent fine-mesh gauze atop the graft followed by a negative-pressure dressing. The vacuum-

Figure 43–2. Tie-over stent dressing.

assisted dressings may be useful for irregular contours, such as around digits and webspaces or joint surfaces, by maintaining wound-to-graft interface, immobilizing the grafted area, suctioning serosanguinous fluid, and possibly promoting neovascularization.

In many cases, it is permissible—and sometimes even preferable—to leave a skin graft site open with no dressing. This is particularly true in slightly infected wounds, where the grafts tend to float off in the purulent discharge produced by the wound. These wounds are best treated with meshed grafts, so that liquid forming between the graft and the wound bed can exude and be removed without disturbing the graft. This treatment can also be used for noninfected wounds that produce an unusual amount of serous or lymphatic drainage, as occurs following radical groin dissections.

In severely ill patients, such as those with major burns, where time under anesthesia must be kept to a minimum, large sheets of meshed split-thickness skin grafts are rapidly applied but not sutured. Skin staples may be used to fix the graft rapidly. Grafts need not be dressed if the area is small, but if the area is large or circumferential, a dressing should be applied. Meshed grafts should generally be covered for 24–48 hours to prevent dryness, since their dermal barrier has been partly disrupted.

Various biologic adhesives, in particular autologous fibrin glue, is being used to immobilize skin grafts. This is especially useful in the face or hands, or areas where bandaging is difficult or cumbersome.

Skin graft dressings may be left undisturbed for 5–7 days after grafting if the grafted wound was free of

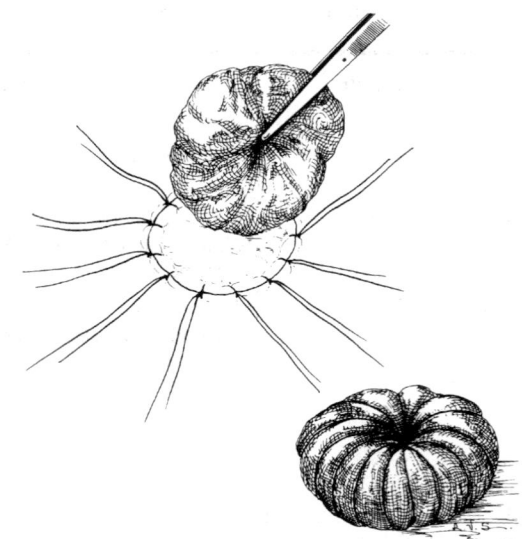

infection, if complete hemostasis was obtained, if fluid collection is not expected, and if immobilization is adequate. If any one of these conditions is not met, the dressing should be changed within 24–48 hours and the graft inspected. If blood, serum, or purulent fluid collection is present, the collection should be evacuated—usually by making a small incision through the graft with a scalpel blade and applying pressure with cotton-tipped applicators. The pressure dressing is then reapplied and changed daily so that the graft can be examined and fluid expressed as it collects.

The Skin Graft Donor Area

The ideal donor site would provide a graft identical to the skin surrounding the area to be grafted. Since skin varies greatly from one area to another as far as color, thickness, hair-bearing qualities, and texture are concerned, the ideal donor site (such as upper eyelid skin to replace skin loss from the opposite upper eyelid) is usually not found. However, there are definite principles that should be followed in choosing the donor area.

A. Color Match

In general, the best possible color match is obtained when the donor area is located close to the recipient area. Color and texture match in facial grafts will be much better if the grafts are obtained from above the region of the clavicles. However, the amount of skin obtainable from the supraclavicular areas is limited. If larger grafts for the face are required, the immediate subclavicular regions of the thorax will provide a better color match than areas on the lower trunk or the buttocks and thighs. When these more distant regions are used, the grafts will usually be lighter in color than the facial skin in Caucasians. In people with dark skin, hyperpigmentation occurs, producing a graft that is much darker than the surrounding facial skin.

B. Thickness of the Graft and Donor Site Healing

Donor sites of split-thickness grafts heal by epithelialization from the epithelial elements remaining in the donor bed. The ability of the donor area to heal and the speed with which it does depends upon the number of these elements present. Donor areas for very thin grafts will heal in 7–10 days, whereas donor areas for intermediate-thickness grafts may require 10–18 days and those for thick grafts 18–21 days or longer.

Since there is a normal anatomic variation in the thickness of skin, donor sites for thicker grafts must be chosen with the potential for healing in mind and should be limited to regions on the body where the skin is thick. Infants, debilitated adults, and elderly people have thinner skin than healthy younger adults. Grafts that would be split-thickness in the normal adult may be full-thickness in these patients, resulting in a donor site that has been deprived of the epithelial elements necessary for healing.

C. Management of the Donor Site

The donor site itself can be considered a clean open wound that will heal spontaneously. After initial hemostasis, the wound will continue to ooze serum for 1–4 days, depending on the thickness of the skin taken. The serum should be collected and the wound kept clean so that healing can proceed at a maximal rate. The wound should be cared for as described above for clean open wounds in either of two ways.

The more common method is the open (dry) technique. The donor site is dressed with porous sterile fine-mesh or nonadherent gauze. After 24 hours, the dry gauze is changed but the nonadherent gauze is left on the wound and exposed to the air, a heat lamp, or a blow dryer. A scab will form on the gauze and will peel off from the edges as epithelialization is completed underneath. This method has the advantage of simple maintenance once the wound is dry.

The second method is the closed (moist) technique. Studies have demonstrated that the rate of epithelialization is enhanced in a moist environment. In contrast to the dry technique, pain can be reduced or virtually eliminated. Moist-to-moist gauze dressings that require frequent wetting have been replaced by newer synthetic materials. A gas-permeable membrane (OpSite, Tegaderm) that sticks to the surrounding skin provides an artificial blister over the wound. Occasionally there is a break in the protective seal covering leakage of serum collected under the membrane. This increases the risk of infection, especially in a contaminated zone. Newer hygroscopic dressings actually absorb and retain many times their weight in water. They are permeable to oxygen yet impervious to bacteria. Infection is still a concern, however, because of occasional exposure of the wound during healing. Newer dressings with silver-impregnated ions are being used that control bacterial contamination and may hasten healing and reepithelialization. Silver ion is exquisitely antimicrobial and is used for burn dressing care as well as skin graft sites.

Demling RH, DeSanti L: The rate of re-epithelialization across meshed skin grafts is increased with exposure to silver. Burns 2002;28:264.

van Zuijlen PP et al: Graft survival and effectiveness of dermal substitution in burns and reconstructive surgery in a one-stage grafting model. Plast Reconstr Surg 2000;106:615.

Wang JC, To EW: Application of dermal substitute (Integra) to donor site defect of forehead flap. Br J Plastic Surg 2000;53:70.

FLAPS

The term "flap" refers to any tissue used for reconstruction or wound closure that retains part or all of its original blood supply after the tissue has been raised and moved to a new location. That part still connected through which the blood supply enters and exits is referred to as the flap base, or pedicle. With local skin flaps, a section of skin and subcutaneous tissue is raised from one site and moved to a nearby area, with the base remaining attached at its original location.

Flaps can be classified according to the pattern of blood supply to the skin into random or axial pattern. Flaps can further be classified according to their tissue content into muscle, musculocutaneous, fasciocutaneous, and others.

Random Pattern Flaps

Random pattern flaps consist of skin and subcutaneous tissue cut from any area of the body in any orientation, with no distinct pattern or particular relation to the blood supply of the skin of the flap. Such flaps receive their blood supply from vessels in the subdermal tissue. Although commonly used, this is the least reliable type of flap, and except when cut from facial and scalp skin the ratio of length to width cannot safely exceed 1.5:1. Its use should be minimized. Presently, in any reconstructive effort, one should use a flap with known reliability and a predictable blood supply.

Axial Pattern Flaps

The axial pattern flap has a well-defined arteriovenous system running along its long axis. Because of good vascular supply, it can be made comparatively long in relation to width. Foremost among the axial flaps are the deltopectoral and the forehead flaps, which are based on perforating branches of the internal mammary artery and supraorbital and supratrochlear or superficial temporal vessels, respectively. Other axial flaps are the groin flap, based on the superficial circumflex iliac artery; the dorsalis pedis flap, based on the artery of the same name; the radial forearm flap; the scapular flap; the lateral upper arm flap; and various scalp and face flaps.

Muscle & Musculocutaneous Flaps

Musculocutaneous flaps consist of skin and underlying muscle, which provide reliable coverage with usually one operation. The use of musculocutaneous units has developed as surgeons have gained more knowledge of the way in which blood is supplied to the skin. The technique has revolutionized reconstructive surgery.

The subdermal plexus of vessels from which skin flaps derive their blood supply is augmented or directly supplied in many areas by sizable perforating vessels arising from underlying muscles. Many muscles receive their blood supply from a single axial vessel, with only minor contributions from other sources (Figure 43–3). The skin over these muscles can be completely circumscribed and elevated in continuity with the underlying muscle up to its major vascular pedicle. If the vessels in the pedicle are preserved, the unit can be moved in wide arcs to distant areas of the body while normal or near normal blood flow is continued to the skin island as well as to the muscle. The donor sites of such flaps can often be closed primarily.

Knowledge of the anatomy of muscles and their nerve and blood supply is necessary for the successful design of musculocutaneous flaps. Although almost any skeletal muscle can be used, muscles with a dominant arterial pedicle and reliable perforating vessels to the skin are most useful.

In addition to their reliability, musculocutaneous flaps clean up recipient sites that are heavily contami-

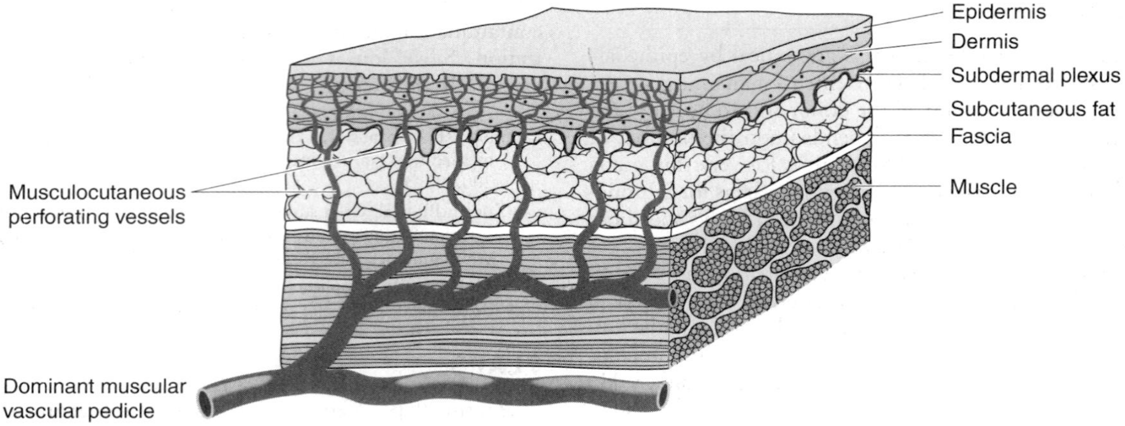

Figure 43–3. Arterial supply to skin from main artery supplying muscles, as occurs in musculocutaneous flaps.

nated with bacteria better than skin flaps do. This is why muscle-containing flaps are the best choice for coverage of wounds caused by radiation or osteomyelitis or those that have a high probability of infection.

The most commonly used muscles and musculocutaneous flaps are the latissimus dorsi, pectoralis major, tensor fasciae latae, rectus femoris, rectus abdominis, trapezius, temporalis, serratus anterior, gluteus maximus, gracilis, and gastrocnemius muscles.

A. Latissimus Dorsi

The latissimus dorsi musculocutaneous unit is supplied by the thoracodorsal vessels. Use of this unit has been widely applied in the one-stage reconstruction of the breast following radical or modified radical mastectomy (see rectus abdominis muscle below). The entire latissimus dorsi muscle can be detached from its origin and transposed to the anterior chest. An island of skin can also be included in the center of the muscle to restore the skin lost on the anterior chest wall. Refinements in technique utilize only enough muscle to carry the skin island, thus leaving intact a good portion of innervated, functional muscle. This unit is also useful for coverage of defects on the anterior chest, shoulder, head and neck, and axilla and even for restoration of flexion of the elbow. It is a popular muscle for free tissue transfer due to its long and relatively large and reliable vascular pedicle.

B. Pectoralis Major

The pectoralis major musculocutaneous unit obtains its vascular supply from the thoracoacromial axis of the subclavian artery just medial to the medial border of the pectoralis minor. It derives a dual blood supply from medial intercostal perforators branching from the internal mammary artery. The entire unit may be transposed medially, especially after disinsertion from the humerus, to cover defects of the sternum, neck, and lower face. Also, an island of skin can be outlined low on the chest and made to reach intraoral defects following cancer excision.

C. Trapezius

The trapezius musculocutaneous unit, based on the descending branch of the transverse cervical artery, is useful for covering defects in the neck, face, and scalp. When skeletonized as an island, the flap will reach the top of the head. When it is used in conjunction with a neck dissection, the transverse cervical artery must be preserved. Functional preservation of shoulder elevation may be accomplished by selectively sparing the transverse, superior fibers of the muscle.

D. Temporalis

The temporalis muscle extends from the temporal fossa to the coronoid process of the mandible. It is supplied by the deep and superficial temporal systems. It is commonly used to fill orbital defects. However, it can cover neighboring cranial, maxillary, palatal and pharyngeal regions.

E. Tensor Fasciae Latae

The tensor fasciae latae musculofascial unit is supplied by the lateral femoral circumflex artery, a branch of the profunda femoris. It has a wide arc of rotation anteriorly and posteriorly. It is elevated with the fascia lata and thus can be used to reconstruct the lower abdominal wall. It has been used to cover defects following excision of osteoradionecrotic ulcers of the pubis or groin. It is also the method of choice for coverage of greater trochanteric pressure ulcers.

F. Rectus Femoris

The rectus femoris, a more robust flap than the tensor fasciae latae with a shorter arc of rotation, has supplanted the latter for reconstruction of the lower abdominal wall and for coverage to postradiation ulcers in the pubis and groin. It has a dual blood supply: a muscular branch from the profunda femoris and an axial branch from the superficial femoral artery to the overlying skin and fascia.

G. Rectus Abdominis

The rectus abdominis is supplied by the deep superior and inferior epigastric vessels that run in the undersurface of the muscle and anastomose with the segmentally arranged intercostal vessels to form the epigastric arcade. These vessels send perforating branches throughout the length of the muscle, perforating the anterior rectus sheath and supplying the overlying skin. The transverse rectus abdominis myocutaneous (TRAM) flap, when based on the superior epigastric vessel and including the infraumbilical skin, has become a workhorse for autologous tissue breast reconstruction. In situations of marked deformity such as a radical mastectomy associated with radiation therapy or previous abdominal surgery, reconstruction of the breast can be accomplished reliably with infraumbilical skin and adipose tissue based on both rectus muscles. This superiorly based TRAM flap involves an abdominoplasty as well as reconstruction of the breast. It is a technically demanding operation but gives a very satisfying result. When based on the deep inferior epigastric vessel and using the supraumbilical skin (the "flag" flap), the flap can cover defects of the abdominal wall, flank, groin, and thigh. Using the inferior epigastric vessels to transport the skin and adipose tissue by means of microvascular surgery (see Free Flaps) has become a popular method of breast reconstruction. A small portion of the rectus muscle is taken or just a main perforator vessel that supplies the overlying fat and skin. This flap is known as the deep inferior epigastric perforator flap, or DIEP flap (see Perforator Flaps and Breast Reconstruction).

H. Gluteus Maximus

The gluteus maximus is useful as a muscle or musculocutaneous unit for covering pressure sores or traumatic defects over the sacrum and ischium. The muscle has a double blood supply from the superior and inferior gluteal arteries to the respective halves of the muscle. In ambulatory patients, it is advisable to perform a function-preserving operation by advancing the muscle medially and preserving its insertion laterally.

I. Gracilis

The gracilis muscle receives its dominant blood supply proximally from the medial femoral circumflex artery. Its arc of rotation makes it an excellent source of coverage for ischial pressure sores and vaginal reconstruction. Other recent uses have included transportation of the muscle alone for repair of a persistent perineal sinus following abdominal-perineal resection.

J. Gastrocnemius

The gastrocnemius musculocutaneous unit is based on either the medial or lateral head of the muscle. Each head is supplied by a sural artery, a branch of the popliteal artery that enters the muscle at its most proximal third near its origin. The flap is most useful to cover defects of the knee and proximal anterior tibia. Coverage of exposed bone in the middle and lower leg, where this unit cannot reach, can be accomplished by use of local muscle flaps such as the soleus. Complex bone and soft tissue injuries of the middle and lower leg may require reconstruction with free muscle flaps.

Fasciocutaneous Flaps

A plexus of vessels is located on top of the muscular fascia and is supplied from vessels that run within the intermuscular septa. These vessels tend to run axially along the fascia, sending perforators to the skin at intervals. Flaps can be designed that are safer than random flaps and that need not contain an entire muscle unit for their transfer. Furthermore, it is possible to make fasciocutaneous or septocutaneous flaps that safely exceed the traditional limits of a 1.5:1 ratio between length and width. Examples of fasciocutaneous flaps are those overlying the gastrocnemius, quadriceps, and rectus abdominis muscles. Other commonly used flaps are the radial forearm, lateral arm, scapular, and deltopectoral flaps.

Neurocutaneous Flaps

Anatomic studies have confirmed the presence of an arterial pedicle accompanying a sensory nerve such as the sural nerve. Consequently, one may be able to outline a skin territory over the trajectory of a sensory nerve with good viability of the overlying skin.

Free Flaps

Free flaps involve tissue transplantation using microvascular surgery. The term is actually incorrect, since the blood supply from the main axial pedicle of the flap is completely detached and then reattached at a distance to recipient vessels near the wound area.

An operating microscope with two viewing binocular lenses, specialized instruments, and swaged-on needles of 60–80 μm are required for microsurgery; 8-0, 9-0, and 10-0 suture is used to anastomose vessels as small as 0.5 mm in diameter.

Examples of free flaps in current use are axial pattern skin and fasciocutaneous flaps, such as scapular, groin, radial forearm, and anterolateral thigh, which are used when only skin and subcutaneous tissue are needed, and muscle and musculocutaneous flaps, such as latissimus dorsi, gracilis, and rectus abdominis flaps, which are used when the bulk and vascularity of muscle are needed. Composite free flaps such as the fibular flap with its overlying skin are most helpful free flaps for reconstruction of the mandible as well as the floor of the mouth following head and neck tumor extirpations.

The vascular pedicle areas of some flaps contain functional nerves, which can also be reattached with microscopic guidance. Examples are inferior gluteal, thigh, and tensor fasciae latae flaps, which contain sensory nerves. Attempts using sensory flaps to provide protective sensation in critical areas such as the feet or the ischium in paraplegic patients have so far been clinically unsuccessful. More encouraging is the work being done to provide sensibility to the floor of the mouth with a sensory innervated radial forearm flap. Motor flaps can restore functions such as forearm flexion or facial expression.

Bone and functional joints can be transplanted as free flaps. Flaps from the ribs, fibula, and iliac crest have all been successfully transferred to areas such as the mandible and tibia. The toe-to-thumb transfer is an example of a complex transplantation, which includes bone with a functional joint, tendons, and nerves as well as skin.

Perforator Flaps

A sophisticated variation on the use of the musculocutaneous principle has been the development of perforator flaps. This usually entails taking a branch from the major vascular pedicle that may perforate the muscle to arborize and form a subcutaneous vascular plexus that will supply a considerable amount of overlying skin. Perhaps the greatest benefit from a perforator flap is decreased donor site morbidity. Structures such as the fascia, muscle, and associated nerves may be preserved while allowing the skin to be used for reconstruction.

The deep inferior epigastric perforator (DIEP) flap exemplifies this well for autologous tissue breast reconstruction. While maintaining the same skin territory as the TRAM flap, the perforating vessels are carefully dissected away from the rectus abdominis. By sparing the muscle, there is potentially a reduction in excessive abdominal wall weakness at the donor site.

The anterolateral thigh flap has become the mainstay for cutaneous flaps at some institutions. Based on musculocutaneous perforators from the vastus lateralis, it can be used when a relatively thin cutaneous flap is needed, such as in head and neck reconstruction. The donor site may be closed primarily depending on the flap width.

The perforator concept has been applied to further territories of skin over the perforator segments of the gluteal, thoracodorsal, and medial plantar arteries among others.

Blondeel N et al: The donor site morbidity of free DIEP flaps and free TRAM flaps for breast reconstruction. Br J Plast Surg 1997;50:322.

Coskunfirat OK et al: Reverse neurofasciocutaneous flaps for soft-tissue coverage of the lower leg. Ann Plast Surg 1999;43:14.

de Almeida OM et al: Distally based fasciocutaneous flap of the calf for cutaneous coverage of the lower leg and dorsum of the foot. Ann Plast Surg 2000;44:367.

Gill PS et al: A 10-year retrospective review of 758 DIEP flaps for breast reconstruction. Plast Reconstr Surg 2004;113:1153.

Imanishi N et al: Venous drainage of the distally based lesser saphenous-sural veno-neuroadipofascial pedicled fasciocutaneous flap: a radiographic perfusion study. Plast Reconstr Surg 1999;103:494.

Song YG et al: The free thigh flap: a new free flap concept based on the septocutaneous artery. Br J Plast Surg 1984;37:149.

Wei FC et al: Have we found an ideal soft-tissue flap? An experience with 672 anterolateral thigh flaps. Plast Reconstr Surg 2002;109:2219.

II. PRINCIPLES OF WOUND CARE

There are many types of wounds and many factors to consider when choice of coverage procedure is made. Skin type and color, glandular association, and hair-bearing characteristics must be considered. Avascular wound beds, such as exposed bone, cartilage, or tendon, will not accept skin grafts unless viable periosteum, perichondrium, or paratenon (respectively) is present. Other areas with poor vascularity are joint capsules, radiation-damaged tissue, and heavily scarred tissue. Exposed or implanted alloplastic material cannot be used as a graft bed. Such areas must be covered with tissue that is attached to its own blood supply. Skin flaps can be used but are sometimes inadequate because their blood supply is tenuous and the layer of subcutaneous fat is even less reliably vascular and may not attach to the underlying avascular surface. Muscle or musculocutaneous flaps are generally required for avascular areas.

The coverage tissue may need to have more bulk than the original tissue. Areas such as bony surfaces and prominences, weight-bearing surfaces, densely scarred areas, and areas of potential pressure breakdown may require thick, durable covering. Again, skin grafts or skin flaps may not be of adequate thickness even though they may survive and cover the wound. Musculocutaneous flaps are more successful. Bulkiness may be undesirable in areas such as the scalp, face, neck, or hand. Defects in these areas that for other reasons require a musculocutaneous flap for coverage may need to be debulked in a secondary procedure. Axial skin flaps or free axial pattern flaps may be a better choice than musculocutaneous flaps in some areas.

Contraction begins during the proliferative phase of healing and continues to a large degree in wounds covered only by split-thickness skin grafts. The grafted area may shrink to 50% of its original size, and both the graft and surrounding tissue may become distorted. Splinting of the area for 10 days or longer may favorably alter contraction. Full-thickness skin grafts rich in dermis, attached to a fresh wound bed, will considerably reduce contraction, and skin flaps will eliminate it altogether. In an orifice or tubular passageway, such as the nasal airway, pharynx, esophagus, or vagina, absence of contraction is critical.

The effects of atrophy and gravity should also be considered when technique of coverage is chosen. A denervated muscle will atrophy up to 60% of its regular size. The muscle tissue in a musculocutaneous flap will atrophy even when the nerve to the muscle is preserved in the pedicle, because the muscle's functional tension is generally not restored. Gravity will cause sagging of any tissue that does not have enough plasticity or muscle dynamics to counteract gravitational pull. Reconstructions in the face often tend to sag.

Wounds at risk for or known to have bacterial contamination also require certain types of coverage (eg, pressure sores, lower extremity defects, and wounds resulting from incision and drainage of abscesses). If the area can be skin grafted, meshed split-thickness grafts are most effective, since bacterial exudate will not collect under these grafts. Musculocutaneous flaps are associated with fewer residual bacteria over time than are random pattern skin flaps. This is probably due to the vastly superior vascularity of musculocutaneous flaps.

Contaminated wounds or wounds that are exuding a considerable amount of fluid can be treated by negative-pressure or vacuum wound dressings. This entails the application of a sponge-like material connected to a suction device that keeps the wound dry as it suctions the excess exudates. The negative pressure on the wound also appears to have a positive effect on healing and increased revascularization. It has become a popular method of preparing a wound for definitive closure.

Wounds associated with nearby injuries that will probably require further surgery (eg, injuries to tendons or nerves) should be covered with flaps, because the flaps can be incised or undermined to allow for additional surgery. Skin grafts do not have sufficient vascularity to allow for these procedures.

Choice of Coverage

Table 43–2 shows some of the indications for choice of coverage in various types of wounds.

Once a given type of flap is chosen, there are still at least two major considerations in the selection of the exact flap to be used. The most significant consideration is the degree of injury that will occur in the donor area. There is always a trade-off when tissue is taken from one area and used in another. This trade-off is minimal when a well-designed, well-placed skin flap leaves a donor defect that can be closed primarily, but the trade-off is great when the donor defect is as severe as the original wound (eg, skin graft donor sites that become infected or musculocutaneous donor sites that fail to heal).

The patient can often participate in the choice of donor locations and should certainly be made aware of potential donor site scars and complications. The tendency has been to use muscle flaps instead of musculocutaneous flaps to permit easy primary closure of the donor site. The muscle can then be resurfaced with a split-thickness skin graft during the same procedure to give a satisfactory result. This provides for an acceptable donor site scar rather than risking disruption of a tight closure or an otherwise ugly donor site.

The second consideration in selection of a flap is that some or all of the graft or flap may be lost. In general, if the patient's overall condition is poor or the loss of a flap would result in a devastating defect, a very reliable type of flap should be chosen. For example, a microvascular anastomosis can be performed on a leg with one remaining arteriosclerotic vessel to the foot, but if the anastomosis fails, the vessel may thrombose and the leg may be lost. In this case, a flap that is safer, although more time-consuming to place, may be chosen, such as a cross-leg flap.

Table 43–2. Indications for various types of tissue coverage.

Type of Wound	Type of Coverage	Reason for Choice
Mildly (< 10^5) infected wounds (including burns)	Thin split-thickness or meshed	Difficulty in obtaining successful take of thicker grafts. Donor sites may be reused sooner.
Significantly (> 10^5) infected wounds (osteomyelitis)	Thin split-thickness or meshed skin grafts or muscle or musculocutaneous flaps	Rich muscle vascular supply can sterilize an infected wound.
Wounds with poorly vascularized surfaces	Thin split-thickness skin grafts or flaps	Difficulty in obtaining successful take of thicker grafts. Flap with intrinsic blood supply may be required.
Small facial defects	Full-thickness skin graft or local flap	Produces best aesthetic result.
Large facial defects	Thick split-thickness skin grafts or flaps	Cannot use full-thickness graft, because of limited size of donor sites.
Full-thickness eyelid loss	Local flap or composite graft	Repair requires more than one tissue element.
Deep loss of nasal tip	Local flap or composite graft	Repair requires thicker tissue than present in split- or full-thickness grafts.
Avulsive wounds with exposed tendons and nerves	Flap	Requires thick protective coverage without graft adherence to tendons and nerves.
Exposed cortical bone or cartilage	Skin or muscle flap	Free grafts will not survive on avascular recipient site.
Wounds resulting from radiation burns	Muscle or musculocutaneous flap	Free grafts will not survive on avascular recipient site. Damaged tissue extends deeper than may be apparent.

Elevation & Transposition of Flaps

Additional considerations in reconstructive surgery involve the technique of elevating and transposing flaps. For random skin flaps, these considerations include proper length-to-width ratio, careful planning to allow for transposition with minimal tension and adjustments at the recipient site, accurate dissection in the subcutaneous plane to avoid injury to the subdermal plexus, and avoidance of folding or kinking of the flap. Surgical technique must be atraumatic, and hemostasis must be achieved. With axial pattern flaps, the surgeon must have knowledge of the important underlying blood vessels as well.

Closure Technique

Closure technique is as important as elevation and transposition technique. Flaps should not be allowed to dry out. The wound bed should be irrigated. Closed-system, nonreactive suction drains are routinely used in both the wound bed and the donor defect for most flaps of any significant size. Suction evacuates blood or serum that may accumulate and keeps the flap firmly pressed against the wound bed. External pressure is both ineffective and detrimental for these purposes. Sutures should accurately and completely appose skin edges without strangulating the epithelium, particularly on the flap side. Buried half-mattress (flap) sutures are recommended (Figure 43–4). Dressings over flaps should be minimal and should not cause pressure or constriction. Emollient dressings, such as petrolatum gauze, antibiotic ointment, or silver sulfadiazine cream, have been shown to aid in preventing desiccation and subsequent necrosis of areas of marginal vascularity.

After a flap is at least temporarily tacked into its final position, adequacy of vascularity can be determined by intravenous injection of fluorescein dye, 10–15 mg/kg, and examination under ultraviolet light (Wood's light). Areas that fluoresce within 10 minutes following dye injection can be expected to survive. Areas that do not fluoresce usually lack arterial inflow, which may be due to temporary arterial spasm but is often due to insufficient perfusion that will result in necrosis. A good clinical evaluation of the flap on the operating table is usually sufficient. Any sign of mottling or cyanosis or flap congestion that indicates a degree of venous obstruction warrants serious consideration of reexploration.

Excision & Primary Closure

The ideal type of wound closure is primary approximation of the skin and subcutaneous tissues immediately adjacent to the wound defect, producing a fine-line scar and the optimal aesthetic result in skin texture, thickness, and color match.

All excisions and wound closures should be planned with this ideal in mind. Obviously, large lesions cannot be excised and closed primarily. With invasive cancers, such as sarcomas, the primary goal is performance of adequate en bloc resection, with the type of wound closure being of secondary importance. Nevertheless, even larger excisions, such as mastectomies, can be planned with definite consideration for closure and subsequent reconstruction.

In most cases, minimal scars can be achieved only if the line or lines of incision are placed in, or parallel to, the skin lines of minimal tension. These lines lie perpendicular to the underlying muscles. On the face, they are obvious as wrinkles or lines of facial expression that become more pronounced with age, since they are secondary to repeated muscle contraction (Figure 43–5). On the neck, trunk, and extremities, the lines of minimal tension are most noticeable as horizontal lines of skin relaxation on the anterior and posterior aspects of areas of flexion and extension.

So-called Langer's lines, which were determined by cadaver study, probably show the direction of fibrous tissue bundles in the skin and are no longer considered accurate guides for placing skin incisions.

If the lines of expression cannot be followed, the line of incision should (if possible) be placed at the junction of unlike tissues such as the hairline of the scalp and the forehead, the eyebrow and the forehead, the mucosal and skin junction of the lips, or the areolar and skin margins of the breast. Scars will be partially hidden if incisions are placed in inconspicuous areas such as the crease of the nasal ala and cheek, the auricular-mastoid sulcus, or the submandibular-neck junction. Lines of incision should never purposely cross flexor surfaces such as the neck, axilla, antecubital fossa, or popliteal space or the palmar skin creases of the fingers and hand, because of the risk of contracture formation. A transverse oblique or S incision should be incorporated when crossing these sites.

If a lesion is to be excised, an elliptic incision placed parallel to the skin lines of minimal tension will give the best result if the amount of tissue to be excised does not preclude primary closure.

If the ellipse is too broad or short, a protrusion of skin, commonly called a "dog-ear," will occur at each pole of the wound closure (Figure 43–6). This is most easily corrected by excising the dog-ear as a small ellipse.

A dog-ear may also be present if one side of the ellipse is longer than the other (Figure 43–7). In this case, it may be easier to excise a small triangle of skin and subcutaneous tissue from the longer side.

A. Z-Plasty

One of the most useful and commonly used techniques in primary wound closure is the Z-plasty. The procedure

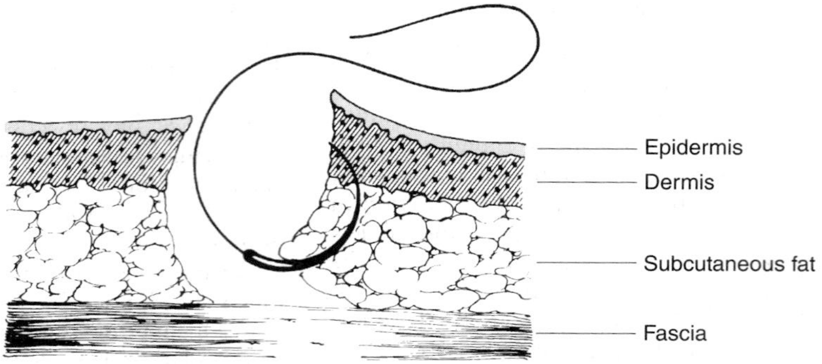

A. The strength of the closure lies in the dermis. Occasionally, the subcutaneous fat is incorporated to obliterate dead space.

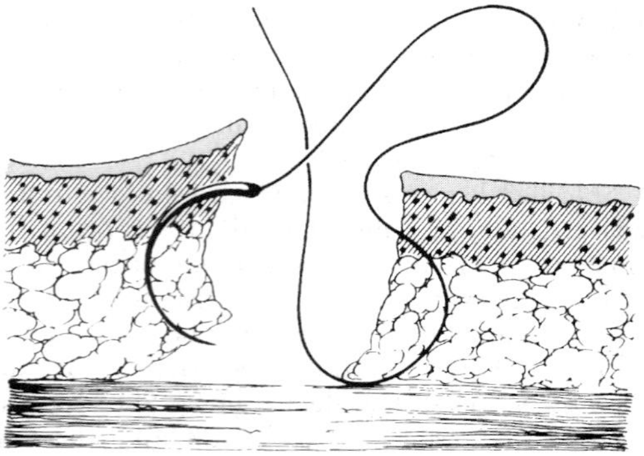

B. The suture is placed so that the knot will lie in the deepest part of the wound. Take care to avoid incorporating the epidermis with this suture, since epithelial cysts will form and result in suture extrusion.

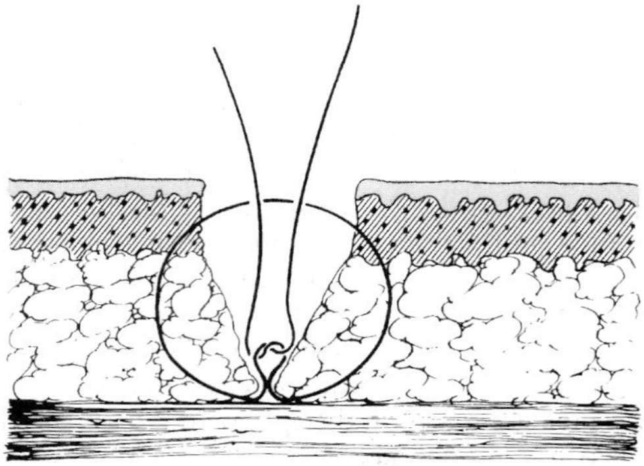

C. The dermal suture is tied just tightly enough to approximate the wound margins. Synthetic absorbable sutures are most commonly used for closure of the dermis.

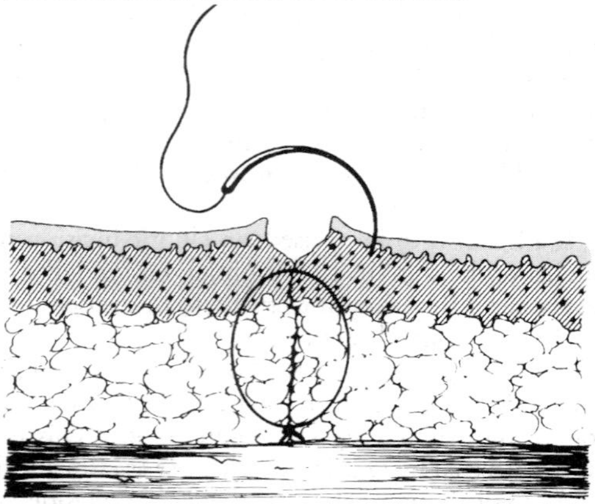

D. After the dermis is approximated, a fine "epidermal" suture is placed to align the wound edges. This suture adds little to the tensile strength of the wound closure.

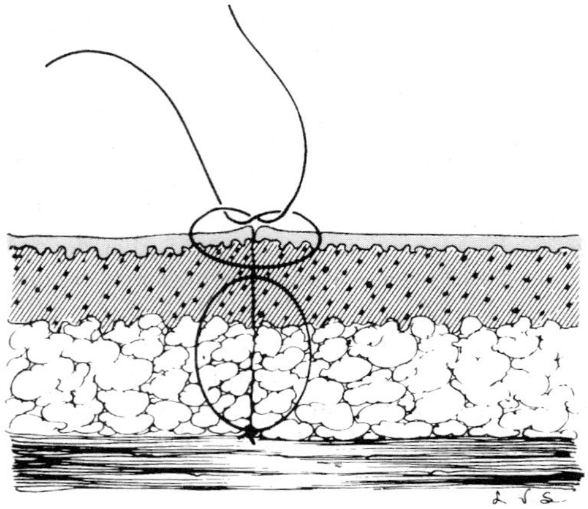

E. The epidermal suture is tied just tightly enough to approximate the epidermal edges of the wound. Since the strength of this closure lies in the dermis, the epidermal suture can be removed after 2–3 days. Skin tapes are often used to support the wound for an additional 7–10 days.

Figure 43–4. Layered cutaneous closure (buried half-mattress [flap] sutures). (Reproduced, with permission, from Ho MT, Saunders CE [editors]: *Current Emergency Diagnosis & Treatment,* 4th ed. Originally published by Appleton & Lange. Copyright © 1992 by The McGraw-Hill Companies, Inc.)

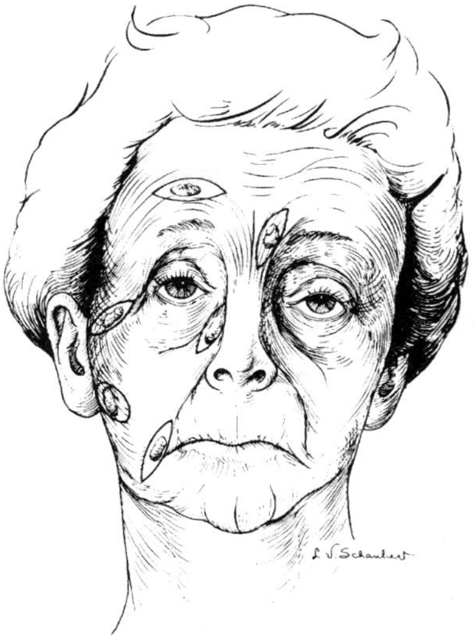

Figure 43–5. Sites of elliptic incisions corresponding to wrinkle lines on the face.

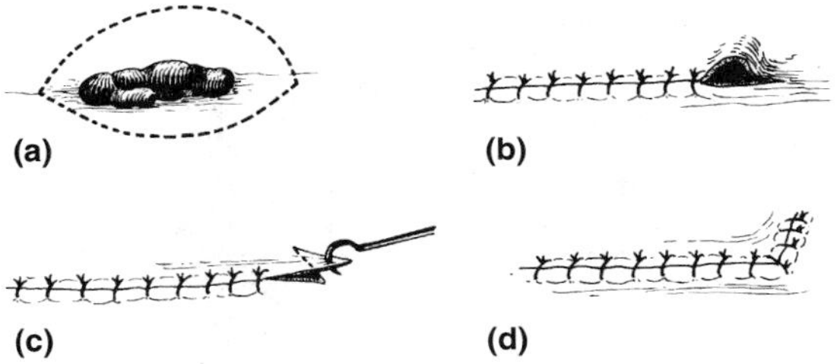

Figure 43–7. Alternative method of correction of dog-ear.

is illustrated in Figure 43–8. The angles formed by the Z-shaped incision are transposed as shown, in order (1) to gain length in the direction of the central limb of the Z or (2) to change the line of direction of the central limb of the Z. Ninety-degree angles would provide the greatest gain in length of the central limb, but smaller angles, such as 60-degree angles, are usually used, because the incision is easier to close and significant gain in length is still achieved. The Z-plasty is used for scar revision and reorientation of small wound incisions so that the main incision will be in a more ideal location. The lengthening function is used for the release or breakup of scar contractures across flexion creases. Frequently, many small Z-plasties in series rather than one large one are done. Occasionally, incisions will be placed under excessive vertical tension after the release of an underlying contracture, such as Dupuytren's contracture in the hand.

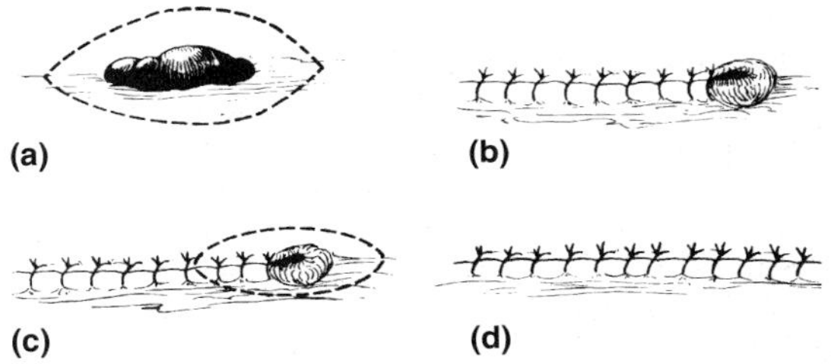

Figure 43–6. Correction of dog-ear.

B. Suture Technique

Suture technique in primary closure is important but will not compensate for poorly planned flaps, excessive tension across the incision, traumatized skin edges, bleeding, or other problems. Sometimes even a skillfully executed closure may result in an unsightly scar because of healing problems beyond the control of the surgeon.

The goal of closure is level apposition of dermal and epithelial edges with minimal or no tension across the incision and no strangulation of tissue between sutures. This is usually accomplished by placement of a layer of interrupted or running absorbable sutures in the superficial fascia and subdermal level at the base of the dermis. This suture prevents tension from forming in the upper dermis and epithelium and also causes the surface planes to be level. The epithelial edges can then be opposed with interrupted or running monofilament sutures of absorbable or permanent material. The absorbable suture is placed in the subcuticular or intradermal plane and is left in place. The permanent sutures are removed quickly according to the region of the body (within 3–4 days in the face), so the suture tracks can be avoided. Sterile adhesive tape (Steri-Strips) placed across the incision will also prevent surface marks and can be used either primarily or after surface sutures have been removed. Taping will not correct errors in suturing that have resulted in uneven edges or tension across the incision. Tape burns may occur if there is excessive tension or swelling around the incision.

The size and even the type of suture material are less important than careful suture placement and observance of previously mentioned factors. Almost any suture properly placed and removed early enough will provide closure without leaving suture marks. The use of monofilament nylon or polypropylene suture material is advised, however, since these types of sutures cause the fewest reactions of currently available suture materials, excluding stainless steel. Running subcuticular, pullout type monofilament sutures may be left in for up to 3 weeks without causing reactions. Even bur-

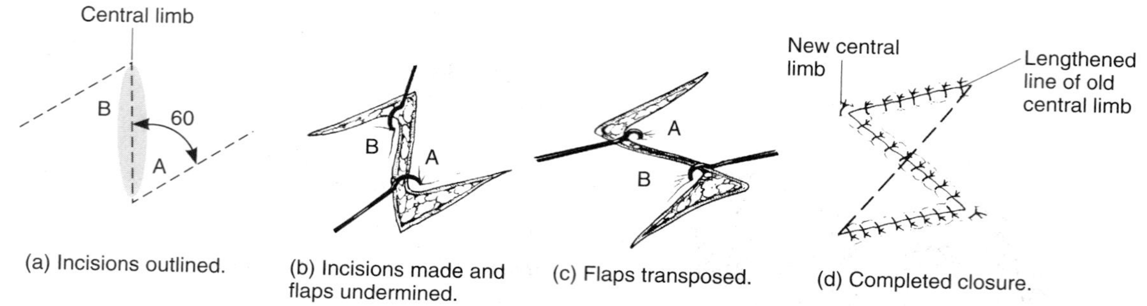

Figure 43–8. Z-plasty.

ied nylon sutures are well tolerated and generally cause fewer problems than braided or absorbable sutures.

An alternative to sutures is the use of skin adhesives such as 2-octylcyanoacrylate (Dermabond). It works well in small areas without much tension or shearing. It is also advisable in children. Further studies are needed to evaluate its wider applicability.

Avery C et al: Clinical experience with the negative pressure wound dressing. Br J Oral Maxillofac Surg 2000;38:343.

Switzer EF et al: Subcuticular closure versus Dermabond: a prospective randomized trial. Am Surg 2003;69:434.

III. SPECIFIC DISORDERS TREATED BY PLASTIC SURGERY

DISORDERS OF SCARRING

HYPERTROPHIC SCARS & KELOIDS

In response to any injury severe enough to break the continuity of the skin or produce necrosis, the skin heals with scar formation. Under ideal circumstances a fine, flat hairline scar will result. The details of wound healing are presented in Chapter 6.

However, hypertrophy may occur, causing the scar to become raised and thickened, or a keloid may form. A keloid is a true tumor arising from the connective tissue elements of the dermis. By definition, keloids grow beyond the margins of the original injury or scar; in some instances, they may grow to enormous size.

The tendency should be resisted to regard all thickened scars as keloids and to label as keloid formers all patients with unattractive scars. Hypertrophic scars and keloids are distinct entities, and the clinical course and prognosis are quite different in each case. The overreactive process that results in thickening of the hypertrophic scar ceases within a few weeks—before it extends beyond the limits of the original scar—and in most cases, some degree of maturation occurs and gradual improvement takes place. In the case of keloids, the overreactive proliferation of fibroblasts continues for weeks or months. By the time it ceases, an actual tumor is present that typically extends well beyond the limits of the original scar, involves the surrounding skin, and may become quite large. Maturation with spontaneous improvement does not usually occur.

Hypertrophic scars and keloids can be differentiated by histopathologic methods. Clinical observation of the course of the scar is also a practical means of differentiation.

Treatment

Since nearly all hypertrophic scars undergo some degree of spontaneous improvement, they do not require treatment in the early phases. If the scar is still hypertrophic after 6 months, surgical excision and primary closure of the wound may be indicated. Improvement may be expected when the hypertrophic scar was originally produced by excessive endothelial and fibroblastic cell proliferation, as is present in open wounds, burns, and infected wounds. However, little or no improvement can be anticipated if the hypertrophic scar followed uncomplicated healing of a simple surgical incision. Improvement of hypertrophic scars across flexion surfaces such as the antecubital fossa or the fingers requires a procedure such as a Z-plasty to change the direction of the scar.

Pressure may help flatten a potentially hypertrophic scar. It is particularly useful for burn scars. A measured elastic garment or face mask (Jobst) is applied to the scarred area and provides continued pressure that causes realignment and remodeling of the collagen bundles. Pressure should be applied early, continuously, and for 6–12 months. Use of intermittent pressure (eg, only at night) or after the hypertrophic scar is established (6–12 months) is of little value.

Additional methods of decreasing the thickness of hypertrophied scars include silicone sheeting applied early and continuously for weeks or months. More recently, early use of the potassium-titanyl-phosphate (KTP) laser or the vascular pulsed-dye laser have been advocated to decrease scar redness as well as hypertrophy. These instruments appear to work by decreasing capillary supply to the scar. They appear to have a good effect on the pruritus of the scar, but more studies are needed to determine their effects on scar modification.

The treatment of choice for keloids and intractable hypertrophic scars is still injection of triamcinolone acetonide, 10 mg/mL (Kenalog-10 Injection), directly into the lesion. This will also help control itching associated with these lesions. In the case of larger lesions, injection is made into more than one site. There is evidence that keloids may respond better to early than to late treatment.

Lesions are injected every 3–4 weeks, and treatment should not be carried out longer than 6 months. The following dosage schedule is used:

Size of Lesion	Dose per Injection
1–2 cm^2	20–40 mg
2–6 cm^2	40–80 mg
6–10 cm^2	80–110 mg

For larger lesions, the maximum dose should be 120 mg. The maximum doses for each treatment for children are as follows:

Age Maximum	Dose
1–2 years	20 mg
3–5 years	40 mg
6–10 years	80 mg

There is a tendency to inject the drug into the scar too often or in too high a dosage—or into the subjacent tissue, which may produce too vigorous a response, resulting in excessive atrophy of the skin and subcutaneous tissues surrounding the lesion and in depigmentation of darker skins. Both of these adverse responses may improve spontaneously in 6–12 months, but not necessarily completely. The response varies greatly; some lesions become flat after two or three injections, and some fail to respond at all. Topical corticosteroid therapy is of no value.

Before the advent of corticosteroid injection therapy, surgical excision and radiation therapy were the only methods of treatment of keloids. Both methods are disappointing; surgical resection usually leads to recurrence of a larger lesion; with very few exceptions, radiation therapy produces an unpredictable result and has obvious potential side effects, including neoplastic degeneration. At present, surgical excision is used only in conjunction with intralesional corticosteroid therapy. Excision is usually confined to the larger lesions in which steroid therapy would exceed safe dosages. (The wound is injected at the time of surgery and then postoperatively according to the schedule recommended above.) Care should be taken so that surgical incisions are not extended into the normal skin around the keloid, since the growth of a new keloid may occur in these scars. It has been reported that intramarginal excisions yield better results than extramarginal excisions.

Allison KP et al: Pulsed dye laser treatment of burn scars: alleviation or irritation? Burns 2003;29:207.

Niessen FB et al: On the nature of hypertrophic scars and keloids: a review. Plast Reconstr Surg 1999;104:1435.

Niessen FB et al: The use of silicone occlusive sheeting (Sil-K) and silicone occlusive gel (Epiderm) in the prevention of hypertrophic scar formation. Plast Reconstr Surg 1998;102:1962.

Ziegler UE: International clinical recommendations on scar management. Zentralbl Chir 2004;129:296.

CONTRACTURES

Contraction is a normal process of wound healing. Contracture, on the other hand, is a pathologic end stage related to the process of contraction. Generally, contractures develop when wounds heal with too much scarring and contraction of the scar tissue results in distortion of surrounding tissues. Although scar contractures can occur in any flexible tissue, such as the eyelids or lips, contractures usually occur across areas of flexion, such as the neck, axilla, or antecubital fossa. The contracted scar brings together the structures on either side of the joint space and prevents active or even passive extension. Exceptions to this pattern of flexion contractures are extension contractures of the toes and MP (metacarpophalangeal) joints of the digits. Contraction is thought to occur via smooth muscle contractile elements in myofibroblasts, but the mechanism is not well understood. In one vertical abdominal scar there may be an area of normal scar formation and an area of hypertrophic scar formation with visible contracture. Contracture can occur in response to the presence of foreign material such as Silastic or saline breast implants. Overall, there is a 10% incidence of some form of breast capsular contracture. Myofibroblasts are thought to play an important role, but the actual cause is not known. Some patients have a soft, excellent result on one side but significant contracture on the other. Clinical practice with a newer-type of implant by changing the surface from smooth to textured have yielded unclear results as to whether there is a decrease in capsular contracture with the textured surface. Polyurethane-coated silicone implants, which did show a decrease in the rate of capsular contracture, are no longer available for clinical use.

The best treatment of contractures is prevention. Incisions should not be made at right angles to flexion creases or should be reoriented by Z-plasties. Wounds in areas of flexion can be covered with flaps or grafted early with thick split-thickness or full-thickness grafts to stop the process of contraction. Such wounds should also be splinted in a position of extension during healing and for 2–3 weeks after healing is complete. Vigorous physical therapy may also be helpful.

Once a contracture is established, stretching and massage are rarely beneficial. Narrow bands of contracture may be excised and released with one or more Z-plasties. Larger areas must be incised from the medial to the lateral axis across the flexion surface and completely opened up to full extension. The resulting defect can be extensive and must be resurfaced with a skin flap or skin graft. In recurrent contractures a fasciocutaneous flap is the treatment of choice. If a skin graft is used, the area must be splinted in extension for approximately 2 weeks after the graft has healed. Less aggressive surgery is likely to result in recurrence.

Achauer GM, Spenler CW, Gold ME: Reconstruction of axillary burn contractures with the latissimus dorsi fasciocutaneous flap. J Trauma 1988;28:211.

Collis N et al: Ten-year review of a prospective randomized controlled trial of textured versus smooth subglandular silicone gel breast implants. Plast Reconstr Surg 2000;106:786.

SKIN TUMORS*

Tumors of the skin are by far the most common of all tumors in humans. They arise from each of the histologic structures that make up the skin—epidermis, connective tissue, gland, muscle, and nerve elements—and are correspondingly numerous in variety. Skin tumors are classified as benign, premalignant, and malignant.

BENIGN SKIN TUMORS

The many benign tumors that arise from the skin rarely interfere with function. Since most are removed for aesthetic reasons or to rule out malignancy, they are quite commonly treated by the plastic surgeon. The majority are small and can be simply excised under local anesthesia following the principles of elliptical excision and wound closure discussed above. General anesthesia may be necessary for larger lesions requiring excision and repair by skin grafts or flaps or those occurring in young children.

When the diagnosis is not in doubt, most superficial lesions (seborrheic keratoses, verrucae, squamous cell papillomas) can be treated by simple techniques such as electrodesiccation, curettage and electrodesiccation, cryotherapy, and topical cytotoxic agents.

Seborrheic Keratosis

Seborrheic keratoses are superficial noninvasive tumors that originate in the epidermis. They appear in older people as multiple slightly elevated yellowish, brown, or brownish-black irregularly rounded plaques with waxy or oily surfaces. They are most commonly found on the trunk and shoulders but are frequently seen on the scalp and face.

Since the lesion is raised above the epidermis, treatment usually consists of shave excision. Care should be exercised to avoid shaving a melanoma because if that is done it will interfere with the determination of the depth of invasion by the Breslow or Clark classifications. If there is any question about a pigmented lesion, it is preferable to do an excisional biopsy rather than to shave it.

Verrucae

Verrucae (common warts) are usually seen in children and young adults, commonly on the fingers and hands. They appear as round or oval elevated lesions with rough surfaces composed of multiple rounded or filiform keratinized projections. They may be skin-colored or gray to brown.

Verrucae are caused by a virus and are autoinoculable, which can result in multiple lesions around the original growth or frequent recurrences following treatment if the virus is not completely eradicated. They may disappear spontaneously.

Treatment by electrodesiccation is effective but is frequently followed by slow healing. Repeated applications of bichloroacetic acid, liquid nitrogen, or liquid CO_2 are also effective. Surgical excision is not recommended, since the wound may become inoculated with the virus, leading to recurrences in and around the scar.

Because recurrences are common despite thorough treatment, it is reasonable to delay treatment of asymptomatic lesions for several months to determine if they will disappear spontaneously.

Cysts

A. Epidermal Inclusion Cyst

Although sebaceous cyst is the commonly used term, these lesions more properly should be called epidermal inclusion cysts, since they are composed of thin layers of epidermal cells filled with epithelial debris. True cysts arising from sebaceous epithelial cells are uncommon.

Epidermal inclusion cysts are soft to firm, usually elevated, and are filled with an odorous cheesy material. Their most common sites of occurrence are the scalp,

* Melanoma is discussed in Chapter 46.

face, ears, neck, and back. They are usually covered by normal skin, which may show dimpling at the site of skin attachment. They frequently present as infected cysts.

Treatment consists of surgical excision.

B. Dermoid Cyst

Dermoid cysts are deeper than epidermal cysts. They are not attached to the skin but frequently are attached to or extend through underlying bony structures. They may appear in many sites but are most common around the nose or the orbit, where they may extend to meningeal structures, necessitating CT scans to determine their extent.

Treatment is by surgical excision, which may necessitate sectioning of adjacent bony structures.

Pigmented Nevi

Nevocellular nevi are groups of cells of probable neural crest origin that contain melanocytes that form melanin more rapidly upon stimulation than surrounding tissue. These cells migrate to different parts of the skin to give different types of nevi. They may also be distinguished by their clinical presentation.

A. Junctional Nevi

Junctional nevi are well-defined pigmented lesions appearing in infancy. They are usually flat or slightly elevated and light brown to dark brown. They may appear on any part of the body, but most nevi seen on the palms, soles, and genitalia are of the junctional type. Histologically, a proliferation of melanocytes is present in the epidermis at the epidermal-dermal junction. It was formerly thought that these nevi give rise to malignant melanoma and that all junctional nevi should be excised for prophylactic reasons. However, most investigators now feel that the risk is very slight. If there is no change in their appearance, treatment is unnecessary. Any change such as itching, inflammation, darkening in color, halo formation, increase in size, bleeding, or ulceration calls for immediate treatment.

Surgical excision is the only safe method of treatment.

B. Intradermal Nevi

Intradermal nevi are the typical dome-shaped, sometimes pedunculated, fleshy to brownish pigmented moles that are characteristically seen in adults. They frequently contain hairs and may occur anywhere on the body.

Microscopically, melanocytes are present entirely within the dermis and, in contrast to junctional nevi, show little activity. They are rarely malignant and require no treatment except for aesthetic reasons.

Surgical excision is nearly always the treatment of choice. Pigmented nevi should never be treated without obtaining tissue for histologic examination.

C. Compound Nevi

Compound nevi exhibit the histologic features of both junctional and intradermal nevi in that melanocytes lie both at the epidermal-dermal junction and within the dermis. They are usually elevated, dome-shaped, and light- to dark-brown in color.

Because of the presence of nevus cells at the epidermal-dermal junction, the indications for treatment are the same as for junctional nevi. If treatment is indicated, surgical excision is the method of choice.

D. Spindle Cell-Epithelioma Cell Nevi

These nevi, formerly called benign juvenile melanomas, appear in children or adults. They vary markedly in vascularity, degree of pigmentation, and accompanying hyperkeratosis. Clinically, they simulate warts or hemangiomas rather than moles. They may increase in size rapidly, but the average lesion reaches only 6–8 mm in diameter, remaining entirely benign without invasion or metastases. Microscopically, the lesion can be confused with malignant melanoma by the inexperienced pathologist. The usual treatment is excisional biopsy.

E. Blue Nevi

Blue nevi are small, sharply defined, round, dark blue or grayish-blue lesions that may occur anywhere on the body but are most commonly seen on the face, neck, hands, and arms. They usually appear in childhood as slowly growing, well-defined nodules covered by a smooth, intact epidermis. Microscopically, the melanocytes that make up this lesion are limited to (but may be found in all layers of) the dermis. An intimate association with the fibroblasts of the dermis is seen, giving the lesion a fibrotic appearance not seen in other nevi. This, together with extension of melanocytes deep into the dermis, may account for the blue rather than brown color.

Treatment is not mandatory unless the patient desires removal for aesthetic reasons or fear of cancer. Surgical excision is the treatment of choice.

F. Giant Hairy Nevi

Unlike most nevi arising from melanocytes, giant hairy nevi are congenital. They may occur anywhere on the body and may cover large areas. They may be large enough to cover the entire trunk (bathing trunk nevi). They are of special significance for several reasons: (1) Their large size is especially deforming from an aesthetic standpoint; (2) they show a predisposition for developing malignant melanoma; and (3) they may be associated with neurofibromas or melanocytic involvement of the leptomeninges and other neurologic abnormalities.

Microscopically, a varied picture is present. All of the characteristics of intradermal and compound nevi may be seen. Neurofibromas may also be present within the lesion. Malignant melanoma may arise anywhere within the large lesion; the reported rate of occurrence ranges from 1% to as high as 13.7% in one study. Malignant melanoma with metastases rarely arises in childhood or infancy.

The only full treatment is complete excision and skin grafting. Large lesions may require excision and grafting in stages. Some lesions are so large that excision is not possible and the most effective approach is using tissue expansion in combination with flaps. Split-thickness excision or dermabrasion has been successful when done in infancy.

The use of cultured epithelial autografts has been advocated for extensive lesions associated with multiple satellite nevi. Additionally, some have reported the use of laser photothermolysis of pigmented lesions that cannot be excised with favorable reconstructive outcomes. However, there is still concern over malignant transformation of remaining melanocytes, and close long-term follow-up is recommended when laser ablation is used.

Gur E, Zuker R: Complex facial nevi: a surgical algorithm. Plast Reconstr Surg 2000;106:25.

Hemangioma

It is confusing to attempt to classify hemangiomas on the basis of their histology. For example, the histologic term capillary hemangioma is used for both the common involuting hemangioma of childhood that disappears by age 7 and the port wine stain that persists into adulthood. The term cavernous is used to designate several types of hemangiomas that behave quite differently. Some hemangiomas are true neoplasms arising from endothelial cells and other vascular elements (such as involuting hemangiomas of childhood, endotheliomas, and pericytomas). Others are not true neoplasms but rather malformations of normal vascular structures (eg, port wine stains, cavernous hemangiomas, and arteriovenous fistulas).

A simple classification based upon whether or not the hemangioma undergoes spontaneous involution is proposed in Table 43–3.

Table 43–3. Proposed classification of hemangiomas based on appearance and clinical course of lesion.

Proposed Term	Terms in Common Use[1]
Involuting hemangioma	
Superficial	Strawberry nevus Nevus vasculosus Capillary hemangioma
Combined superficial and deep	Strawberry nevus Capillary hemangioma Capillary and cavernous hemangioma
Deep	Cavernous hemangioma
Noninvoluting hemangioma	
Port wine stain	Port wine stain Capillary hemangioma Nevus flammeus
Cavernous hemangioma	Cavernous hemangioma
Venous racemose aneurysm	Cavernous hemangioma
Arteriovenous fistula	Arteriovenous fistula

[1]Confusing because different terms are used to denote the same lesion and because the same term is sometimes used to denote different lesions.

A. Involuting Hemangioma

Involuting hemangiomas are the most common tumors that occur in childhood and constitute at least 95% of all the hemangiomas that are seen in infancy and childhood. They are true neoplasms of endothelial cells but are unique among neoplasms in that they undergo complete spontaneous involution.

Typically, they are present shortly after birth or appear during the first 2–3 weeks of life. They grow at a rather rapid rate for 4–6 months; then growth ceases and spontaneous involution begins. Involution progresses slowly but is complete by 5–7 years of age.

Involuting hemangiomas appear on all body surfaces but are seen more often on the head and neck. They are seen twice as often in girls as in boys and show a predisposition for fair-skinned individuals.

Three forms of involuting hemangioma are seen: (1) superficial, (2) combined superficial and deep, and (3) deep. Superficial involuting hemangiomas appear as sharply demarcated, bright-red, slightly raised lesions with an irregular surface that has been described as resembling a strawberry. Combined superficial and deep involuting hemangiomas have the same surface characteristics, but beneath the surface, a firm bluish tumor is present that may extend deeply into the subcutaneous tissues. Deep involuting hemangiomas present as deep blue tumors covered by normal-appearing skin.

The histologic findings in involuting hemangiomas are quite different from those seen in other types of hemangiomas. There is a constant correlation between the histologic picture and the clinical course. During the growth phase, the lesion is composed of solid fields of closely packed round or oval endothelial cells. As would be expected during the growth phase, cellular division with mitotic figures is seen, so that the lesion is sometimes called a hemangioendothelioma by the pathologist. This term must not be used, however, since it is commonly used to denote the highly malignant angiosarcoma that is seen in adults.

As the phase of involution progresses, the histologic picture changes, with the solid fields of endothelial cells breaking up into closely packed, capillary-sized, vessel-like structures composed of several layers of soft endothelial cells supported by a sparse fibrous stroma. These vascular structures gradually become fewer and spaced more widely apart in a loose, edematous fibrous stroma. The endothelial cells continue to disappear, so that by the time involution is complete the histologic picture is entirely normal, with no trace of endothelial cells.

Treatment is not usually indicated, since the appearance following spontaneous regression is nearly always superior to the scars that follow surgical excision. Complete surgical excision of lesions that involve important structures such as the eyelids, nose, or lips results in unnecessary disfigurement that is difficult to repair.

Partial resection of a portion of a hemangioma of the brow or eyelid is indicated when the lesion is large enough to prevent light from entering the eye—a condition that will lead to blindness or amblyopia. The same type of treatment may be necessary for lesions of the mucosal surfaces of the lips when they project into the mouth and are traumatized by the teeth. In these cases, surgery should be very conservative—only enough of the lesion should be resected to alleviate the problem, and the remaining portions should be allowed to involute spontaneously.

In approximately 8% of cases, ulceration will occur. This may be accompanied by infection, which is treated by the use of compresses of warm saline or potassium permanganate and by the application of antibiotic powders and lotions. Bleeding from the ulcer is not common; when it does occur, it is easily controlled by the application of pressure. In rare cases, the platelet trapping of these lesions leads to the clinical picture of disseminated intravascular coagulopathy called **Kasabach-Merritt syndrome**.

After involution of large lesions, superficial scarring may be present or the involved skin may be thin, wrinkled, or redundant. These conditions may require conservative plastic surgery procedures.

The application of local agents such as dry ice to the surface of these lesions has been popular. This type of treatment has no effect on the deep portions of the hemangioma. It will destroy superficial lesions but results in severe scarring. Injections of sclerosing agents have minimal effect. There is no place for radiation therapy in the treatment of these benign lesions. Corticosteroids given systemically or intralesionally have been used with varying success. Anecdotal evidence exists in favor of compression to speed up the involution process and give a better final result. Innovative treatments have recently been proposed for the most serious hemangiomas. They include the insertion of a laser probe deep into the lesion so that the heat generated by the laser produces contracture of the hemangioma. Systemic interferon treatment of life-threatening hemangiomas of the head and neck area obstructing the airway or vision that are resistant to corticosteroids have produced dramatic albeit varying results.

Ezekowitz RA et al: Interferon alfa-2a therapy for life-threatening hemangiomas of infancy. N Engl J Med 1992;326:1456.

B. Noninvoluting Hemangioma

Most noninvoluting hemangiomas are present at birth. In contrast to involuting hemangiomas, they do not undergo rapid growth during the first 4–6 months of life but grow in proportion to the growth of the child. They persist into adulthood and may cause severe aesthetic and functional problems. Some, such as arteriovenous fistulas, may cause death due to cardiac failure.

Unfortunately, treatment of noninvoluting hemangiomas is difficult and usually far from satisfactory.

Port wine stains are by far the most common of the noninvoluting hemangiomas. They may involve any portion of the body but most commonly appear on the face as flat patchy lesions that are reddish to purple in color. When present on the face, they are located in areas supplied by the sensory branches of the fifth cranial nerve. They usually start off light red in color yet have a propensity to deepen in color, as their name implies. Their growth is variable, but they persist into adulthood if not treated and become raised and thickened with nodules appearing on the surface.

Microscopically, port wine stains are made up of thin-walled capillaries that are arranged throughout the dermis. The capillaries are lined with mature flat endothelial cells. In the lesions that produce surface growth, groups of round proliferating endothelial cells and large venous sinuses are seen.

Results following treatment of the port wine stain were uniformly disappointing. Since most lesions occur on the face or neck, patients seek treatment for aesthetic reasons. The simplest and still most effective method of treatment is camouflaging. Unfortunately, this is difficult because the port wine stain is darker than the surrounding lighter skin.

Tattooing with skin-colored pigments may offer some measure of disguise in the lighter lesions but generally is unsatisfactory because the pigment deposited in the skin looks artificial and tends to be absorbed unevenly, producing a mottled appearance.

Superficial methods of treatment such as dry ice, liquid nitrogen, electrocoagulation, and dermabrasion are ineffective unless they destroy the upper layers of the skin, which can produce severe scarring.

Radiation therapy, including the use of x-rays, radium, thorium X, and grenz x-rays, is to be condemned. If it is administered in doses high enough to destroy the vessels involved, it also destroys the surrounding tissues and the overlying skin and the cancer incidence after radiotherapy for skin hemangioma increases.

The best treatment to date for early and intermediate port wine stains is with the pulsed-dye laser. The pulsed dye laser produces a light with a specific wavelength of 585 or 595 nanometers. The method of treatment is termed selective photothermolysis. The beam is selectively absorbed by red-pigmented material such as hemoglobin in the blood vessels of the lesion. This produces selective heat destruction of these structures and the treated area becomes whiter. When started early, these treatments can be very effective. Multiple treatments are necessary to obtain a satisfactory result. In darker and more advanced nodular lesions, the laser is less effective because of the severe scarring and hyperpigmentation that may develop.

If the lesion is small, surgical excision with primary closure is possible. Unfortunately, most lesions are large. Sometimes the best choice is no treatment. Certain fast-growing capillary or primarily arterialized hemangiomas have been managed successfully with superselective embolization, either alone or in conjunction with surgery. This is performed under fluoroscopic control and with an expert team. There have been reports of slough of large portions of the face as a result of misdirected embolizations.

C. Cavernous Hemangioma

Cavernous hemangiomas are bluish or purplish lesions that are usually elevated. They may occur anywhere on the body but, like other hemangiomas, are more common on the head and neck. They are composed of mature, fully formed venous structures that are present in tortuous masses that have been described as feeling like a bag of worms.

Cavernous hemangiomas are usually present at birth but do not usually grow except to keep pace with normal body growth. In many cases, growth occurs later in life and may interfere with normal function.

Microscopically, cavernous hemangiomas are made up of large dilated, closely packed vascular sinuses that are engorged with blood. They are lined by flat endothelial cells and may have muscular walls like normal veins.

Treatment is difficult. In only a few cases is the lesion small enough or superficial enough to permit complete surgical excision. Most lesions involve deeper structures—including muscle and bone—so that complete excision is impossible without radical surgery. Since most lesions are no more than aesthetic problems, radical surgery is rarely indicated. Occasionally, the injection of sclerosing agents directly into the venous channels may lead to some involution or may make surgical excision easier. Great care must be used so that areas of overlying skin do not slough.

Mulliken JB, Fishman SJ, Burrows PE: Vascular anomalies. Curr Probl Surg 2000;37:517.

PREMALIGNANT SKIN LESIONS

Actinic (Solar) Keratoses

Actinic keratoses are the most common of the precancerous skin lesions. They usually appear as small, single or multiple, slightly elevated, scaly or warty lesions ranging in color from red to yellow, brown, or black. Since they are related to sun exposure, they occur most frequently on the face and the backs of the hands in fair-skinned Caucasians whose skin shows evidence of actinic elastosis.

Microscopically, actinic keratoses consist of well-defined areas of abnormal epithelial cells limited to the epidermis. Approximately 15–20% of these lesions become malignant, in which case invasion of the dermis as squamous cell carcinoma occurs.

Since the lesions are limited to the epidermis, superficial treatment in the form of curettement and electrodesiccation or the application of chemical agents such as liquid nitrogen, phenol, bi- or trichloroacetic acid, or fluorouracil is curative. The application of fluorouracil (5-FU) cream is of particular benefit in preventive treatment in that it will destroy lesions of microscopic size—before they can be detected clinically—without causing damage to uninvolved skin.

Chronic Radiation Dermatitis & Ulceration

There are two distinct types of radiation dermatitis. The first and most common follows the acute administration of relatively high dosages of ionizing orthovoltage radiation over relatively short periods—almost always for the treatment of cancer. Dermatitis is characterized by an acute reaction that begins near the third week of therapy, when erythema, blistering, and sloughing of the epidermis start to occur. Burning and hyperesthesia are commonly present. This initial reaction is followed by scarring characterized by atrophy of the epidermis and dermis along with loss of skin appendages (sweat glands, sebaceous glands, and hair follicles). Marked fibrosis of the dermis occurs, with gradual endarteritis and occlusion of the dermal and subdermal vessels. Telangiectasia of the surface vessels is seen, and areas of both hypo- and hyperpigmentation occur.

The second type of radiation dermatitis follows chronic exposure to low doses of ionizing radiation over prolonged periods. It is usually seen in professional personnel who handle radioactive materials or administer x-rays or in patients who have been treated for dermatologic conditions such as acne or excessive facial hair. Therefore, the face and hands are most commonly involved. The acute reaction described above does not usually occur, but the same process of atrophy, scarring, and loss of dermal elements occurs. Drying of the skin becomes more pronounced, and deepening of the skin furrows is typically present. Fortunately, this second type of radiation dermatitis is rarely seen today.

In both types of radiation dermatitis, late changes such as the following may occur: (1) the appearance of hyperkeratotic growths on the skin surface, (2) chronic ulceration, and (3) the development of either basal cell or squamous cell carcinoma. Ulceration and cancer, however, are seen much less commonly in the first type of radiation dermatitis than in the second. When malignant growths appear, basal cell carcinomas are seen more frequently on the face and neck and squamous cell carcinomas more frequently on the hands and body.

Newer radiotherapeutic methods using megavoltage and electron beam techniques have a sparing effect on the skin. However, marked scarring and avascularity of deeper, more extensive areas may present more difficult problems.

Surgical excision is the treatment of choice. Excision should include all of the irradiated tissue including the area of telangiectasia, whenever possible, and the defect should be covered with an appropriate axial or musculocutaneous flap to provide a new blood supply.

Primary wound closure is feasible for only the smallest lesions, and even so at some risk. Free skin grafting is usually unsuccessful because of the damage to the vascular supply of the subcutaneous structures. Adjacent random flaps are unreliable because they depend upon blood supply from the surrounding irradiated area.

MALIGNANT LESIONS

1. Intraepidermal Carcinoma

Intraepidermal carcinoma includes Bowen's disease and erythroplasia of Queyrat.

Bowen's Disease

Bowen's disease is characterized by single or multiple, brownish or reddish plaques that may appear anywhere on the skin surface but often on covered surfaces. The typical plaque is sharply defined, slightly raised, scaly, and slightly thickened. The surface is often keratotic, and crusting and fissuring may be present. Ulceration is not common but when present suggests malignant degeneration with dermal invasion.

Histologically, hyperplasia of the epidermis is seen, with pleomorphic malpighian cells, giant cells, and atypical epithelial cells that are limited to the epidermis.

Treatment of small or superficial lesions consists of total destruction by curettement and electrodesiccation or by any of the other superficially destructive methods (cryotherapy, cytotoxic agents). Excision and skin grafting are preferred for larger lesions and for those that have undergone early malignant degeneration and invasion of the dermis.

Erythroplasia of Queyrat

Erythroplasia of Queyrat is almost identical to Bowen's disease both clinically and histologically but is confined to the glans penis and the vulva, where the lesions appear as red, velvety, irregular, slightly raised plaques. Treatment is as described for Bowen's disease.

2. Basal Cell Carcinoma

Basal cell carcinoma is the most common skin cancer. The lesions usually appear on the face and are more common in men than women. Since exposure to ultraviolet rays of the sun is a causative factor, basal cell carcinoma is most commonly seen in geographic areas where there is significant sun exposure and in people whose skin is most susceptible to actinic damage from exposure, ie, fair-skinned individuals with blue eyes and blond hair. It may occur at any age but is not common before age 40.

The growth rate of basal cell carcinoma is usually slow but nearly always steady and insidious. Several months or years may pass before the patient becomes concerned. Without treatment, widespread invasion and destruction of adjacent tissues may occur, producing massive ulceration. Penetration of the bones of the facial skeleton and the skull may occur late in the course. Basal cell carcinomas rarely metastasize, but death can occur because of direct intracranial extension or erosion of major blood vessels.

Typical individual lesions appear as small, translucent or shiny ("pearly") elevated nodules with central ulceration and rolled, pearly edges. Telangiectatic vessels are commonly present over the surface, and pigmentation is sometimes present. Superficial ulceration occurs early.

A less common type of basal cell carcinoma is the **sclerosing** or **morphea carcinoma**, consisting of elongated strands of basal cell cancer that infiltrate the dermis, with the intervening corium being unusually compact. These lesions are usually flat and whitish or waxy in appearance and firm to palpation—similar in appearance to localized scleroderma.

The superficial **erythematous basal cell cancer** ("body basal") occurs most frequently on the trunk. It appears as reddish plaques with atrophic centers and smooth, slightly raised borders. These lesions are capable of peripheral growth and wide extension but do not become invasive until late.

Pigmented basal cell carcinomas may be mistaken for melanomas, because of the large number of melanocytes present within the tumor. They may also be confused with seborrheic keratoses.

Treatment

There are several methods of treating basal cell carcinoma. All may be curative in some lesions, but no one method is applicable to all. The special features of each basal cell cancer must be considered individually before proper treatment can be selected.

Since most lesions occur on the face, aesthetic and functional results of treatment are important. However, the most important consideration is whether or not therapy is curative. If the basal cell carcinoma is not eradicated by the initial treatment, continued growth and invasion of adjacent tissues will occur. This will result not only in additional tissue destruction but also in invasion of the tumor into deeper structures, making cure more difficult. Adequate treatment of basal cell carcinoma by different modalities achieves a cure rate of approximately 95%.

The principal methods of treatment are curettage and electrodesiccation, surgical excision, and radiation therapy. Chemosurgery, topical chemotherapy, and cryosurgery are not often used but may have value in selected cases.

A. Curettage and Electrodesiccation

Curettage plus electrodesiccation is the usual method of treatment for small lesions. After infiltration with suitable local anesthetic, the lesion and a 2- to 3-mm margin of normal-appearing skin around it are thoroughly curetted with a small skin curette. The resultant wound is then completely desiccated with an electrosurgical unit to destroy any tumor cells that may not have been removed by the curette. The process is then repeated once or twice if necessary. The wound is left open and allowed to heal secondarily.

When used as treatment for superficial basal cell carcinoma, curettage and electrodesiccation is a simple, quick, and inexpensive procedure that will cure nearly all superficial lesions. However, this method of treatment should not be used in the deeper infiltrative and morphea type lesions. These lesions should be treated by surgical excision, x-ray therapy, or chemosurgery.

B. Surgical Excision

Surgical excision, following the principles outlined earlier in this chapter, offers many advantages in the treatment of basal cell carcinoma: (1) Most lesions can be quickly excised in one procedure. (2) Following excision, the entire lesion can be examined by the pathologist, who can determine if the tumor has been completely removed. (3) Deep infiltrative lesions can be completely excised, and cartilage and bone can be removed if they have been invaded. (4) Lesions that occur in dense scar tissue or in other poorly vascularized tissues cannot be treated by curettage and desiccation, radiation therapy, or chemosurgery, since healing is poor. Excision and flap coverage may be the only method for treatment in these conditions. (5) Recurrent lesions in tissues that have been exposed to maximum safe amounts of radiation can be excised and covered.

Small to moderate-sized lesions can be excised in one stage under local anesthesia. The visible and palpable margins of the tumor are marked on the skin with marking ink. The width of excision is then marked 3–5 mm beyond these margins. If the margins of the basal cell carcinoma are vague, the width of excision will have to be wider to ensure complete removal of the lesion. The lines of incision are drawn around the lesion as a circle. This tissue is excised, taking care to leave a margin of normal-appearing subcutaneous tissue around the deep margins of the tumor. Frozen sections may be obtained at the time of excision to aid in determining whether tumor-free margins have been obtained. This is minimized with experience. It is better to err on the side of removing more normal tissue than necessary rather than to run the risk of including tumor at the margins. Closure of the wound is accomplished in the direction of minimal skin tension, usually along the skin lines. The dog-ears are removed appropriately.

Wounds resulting from the excision of some moderate-sized tumors and nearly all large tumors may necessitate for optimum reconstruction of function and appearance, the use of local, regional and free flaps. This can nearly always be performed in one stage.

The disadvantages of surgical excision are as follows: (1) Specialized training and experience are necessary to master the surgical techniques. (2) Whereas curettage and desiccation may be performed in the office, surgical excision requires specialized facilities. (3) In lesions with vague margins, an excessive amount of normal tissue may have to be excised to ensure complete removal. (4) Structures that are difficult to reconstruct, such as the eyelids, nasal tip, and lips, have to be sacrificed when they are extensively infiltrated and immediate reconstruction to cover vital structures is indicated.

To overcome some of these objections, Mohs described in 1941 a new technique that allows for serial excisions and microscopic examination of chemically fixed tissue. Newer developments have obviated the cumbersome fixation techniques, but it may still take several hours to scan an area for suspected malignant cells. The procedure is nevertheless quite useful for recurrent lesions and in areas in which maximal preservation is desirable. Nonetheless, there are no prospective comparative studies to indicate that the so-called microscopically controlled removal of tumor by the Mohs technique, which amounts to excision of the lesion with serial review by fresh frozen section, is superior to surgical excision. An additional problem is that there is no quality control because the excising physician is also the one who evaluates the pathology slides. Some of the lesions treated with the Mohs technique do require secondary reconstruction.

C. X-Ray Therapy

X-ray therapy is as effective as any other in the treatment of basal cell carcinoma. Its advantages are as follows: (1) Structures that are difficult to reconstruct, such as the eyelids, tear ducts, and nasal tip, can be preserved when they are invaded by but not destroyed by tumor. (2) A wide margin of tissue can be treated around lesions with poorly defined margins to ensure destruction of nondiscernible extensions of tumor. (3) It may be less traumatic than surgical excision to elderly patients with advanced lesions. (4) Hospitalization is not necessary.

The disadvantages are as follows as follows: (1) Only well-trained, experienced physicians can obtain good results. (2) Expensive facilities are necessary. (3) Improperly administered radiation therapy may produce severe sequelae, including scarring, radiation dermatitis, ulceration, and malignant degeneration. (4) In hair-bearing areas, epilation will result. (5) It may be difficult to treat areas of irregular contour (ie, the ear and the auditory canal). (6) Repeated treatments over a period of 4–6 weeks may be necessary.

X-ray therapy should not be used in patients under age 40 except in unusual circumstances, and it should not be repeated in patients who have failed to respond to radiation therapy in the past.

3. Squamous Cell Carcinoma

Squamous cell carcinoma is the second most common cancer of the skin in light-skinned racial groups and the most common skin cancer in darkly pigmented racial groups. As with basal cell carcinoma, sunlight is the most common causative factor in whites. The most common sites of occurrence are the ears, the cheeks, the lower lip, and the backs of the hands. Other causative factors are chemical and thermal burns, scars, chronic ulcers, chronic granulomas (tuberculosis of the skin, syphilis), draining sinuses, contact with tars and hydrocarbons, and exposure to ionizing radiation. When a squamous cell carcinoma occurs in a burn scar, it is called a **Marjolin ulcer**. This lesion may appear many years after the original burn. It tends to be aggressive, and the prognosis is poor.

Since exposure to the sun is the greatest stimulus for the production of squamous cell carcinoma, most of these lesions are preceded by actinic keratosis on areas of the skin showing chronic solar damage. They may also arise from other premalignant skin lesions and from normal-appearing skin.

The natural history of squamous cell carcinoma may be quite variable. It may present as a slowly growing, locally invasive lesion without metastases or as a rapidly growing, widely invasive tumor with early metastatic spread. In general, squamous cell carcinomas that develop from actinic keratoses are more common and are of the slowly growing type, whereas those that develop from Bowen's disease, erythroplasia of Queyrat, chronic radiation dermatitis, scars, and chronic ulcers tend to be more aggressive. Lesions that arise from normal-appearing skin and from the lips, genitalia, and anal regions also tend to be aggressive.

Early squamous cell carcinoma usually appears as a small, firm erythematous plaque or nodule with indistinct margins. The surface may be flat and smooth or may be verrucous. As the tumor grows, it becomes raised, and, because of progressive invasion, becomes fixed to surrounding tissues. Ulceration may occur early or late but tends to appear earlier in the more rapidly growing lesions.

Histologically, malignant epithelial cells are seen extending down into the dermis as broad, rounded masses or slender strands. In squamous cell carcinomas of low-grade malignancy, the individual cells may be quite well differentiated, resembling uniform mature squamous cells having intercellular bridges. Keratinization may be present, and layers of keratinizing squamous cells may produce typical round "horn pearls." In highly malignant lesions, the epithelial cells may be extremely atypical; abnormal mitotic figures are common; intercellular bridges are not present; and keratinization does not occur.

As with basal cell carcinomas, the method of treatment that will eradicate squamous cell carcinomas and produce the best aesthetic and functional results varies with the characteristics of the individual lesion. Factors that determine the optimal method of treatment include the size, shape, and location of the tumor as well as the histologic pattern that determines its aggressiveness.

Treatment consists of surgery or irradiation. The advantages and disadvantages of each type of therapy are discussed above. Since basal cell carcinomas are relatively nonaggressive lesions that rarely metastasize, failure to eradicate the lesion may result only in local recurrence. Although this may result in extensive local tissue destruction, there is rarely a threat to life. Aggressive squamous cell carcinomas, on the other hand, may metastasize to any part of the body, and failure of treatment may have fatal consequences. For this reason, total eradication of each lesion is the imperative goal of treatment.

Because the overall incidence of lymph node metastasis is relatively low, most authorities agree that node resection is not indicated in the absence of palpable regional lymph nodes except in the case of very aggressive carcinomas of the genitalia and anal regions.

Alam M, Ratner D: Cutaneous squamous-cell carcinoma. N Engl J Med 2001;344:975.

Arbuckle HA, Morelli JG: Pigmentary disorders: update on neurofibromatosis-1 and tuberous sclerosis. Curr Opin Pediatr 2000;12:354.

Kanzler MH, Mraz-Gernhard S: Treatment of primary cutaneous melanoma. JAMA 2001;285:1819.

Lentsch EJ, Myers JN: Melanoma of the head and neck: current concepts in diagnosis and management. Laryngoscope 2001;111:1209.

Stadelmann WK et al: Cutaneous melanoma of the head and neck: advances in evaluation and treatment. Plast Reconstr Surg 2000;105:2105.

SOFT TISSUE INJURY

The plastic surgeon is often involved in emergency room assessment and treatment of soft tissue injuries. Many aspects of wound management must be considered in even a relatively simple facial laceration.

Careful analysis of the soft tissue injury should include: (1) the type of wound or wounds (abrasion, contusion, etc); (2) the cause of injury; (3) the age of the injury; (4) the location of injured tissues; (5) the degree of contamination of the injured area before, during, and after trauma; (6) the nature and extent of associated injuries; and (7) the general health of the patient (eg, any chronic or acute illnesses or any allergies; any medications being taken).

The location of the wound must be noted because different healing characteristics are present in various types of skin. The face and scalp are highly vascular and therefore resist infection and heal faster than other areas, but there are many important structures in and around the face, and scars and defects are noticeable. Skin of the trunk, upper arms, and thighs is fairly thick and heals more slowly than facial or scalp skin and is more susceptible to infection. Scarring is less noticeable. The hands are a critical area because there are important structures near the surface, and the destruction caused by infection can be devastating. The lower legs are a particular problem area because the relatively poor blood supply can cause skin loss, and infection is more likely to occur.

Treatment

The type of wound must be determined so that proper treatment can be given. Contusions and swelling require ice packs for 24 hours, rest, and elevation. Abrasions should be cleaned and dressed in a sterile manner as for a skin graft donor site or must be washed daily until a dry scab forms or healing takes place. Ground-in dirt or gravel must be entirely scrubbed out or picked out with a small blade within 24 hours after injury, or foreign material will be sealed in and traumatic tattooing will result. Extensive local anesthesia may be required to accomplish this. Imbedded particulate matter from an explosion must be removed in a similar manner. Hematomas may be treated with ice bags and pressure until stable. Evacuation is then indicated if vital structures such as the ear or nasal septal cartilage are in danger of being injured or destroyed. Lacerations over bony prominences and various types of cuts require special care that will be detailed below. Treatment must be meticulous if optimal results are to be achieved. Puncture wounds and bites are notoriously innocuous in appearance but may result in severe destruction or tetanus or gas gangrene. Antibiotic coverage, irrigation, open treatment, and observation are indicated. Most bites on the face, however, can be cleaned and safely closed. Wounds that create flaps of skin or avulsions are difficult to manage. Careful debridement and judicious use of full- or split-thickness grafts from the avulsed tissue are recommended. Timing is the first factor to consider.

Wound contamination can be caused by bacteria on the surface of the wounding agent, such as rust on a nail or saliva on a tooth, or bacteria that enter the wound when the skin is broken. Bacteria driven into tissue become more established as time passes, and it is therefore important to know the age of the wound at the time of the presentation for treatment. Other injuries associated with cuts almost always take precedence in treatment. In general, wounds other than those on the face or scalp should not be closed primarily if they occurred 8–12 hours or longer before presentation unless they were caused by a very clean agent and have been covered by a sterile bandage in the interim. Delayed primary closure as described previously is an excellent and safe alternative. Nearly any facial wound up to 24 hours old can be safely closed with careful debridement, irrigation, and antibiotic coverage.

The surgeon must decide whether or not antibiotic treatment is indicated. In general, wounds treated appropriately and early do not call for antibiotic therapy. Antibiotics should be given for wounds with delayed presentation or those for which treatment is delayed by choice (eg, wounds with known contamination; wounds in compromised patients, such as very young or old persons, debilitated persons, or persons with general ill health; wounds in areas where infection may have serious consequences, such as the lower legs and the hands; and wounds in persons in whom bacteremia might have serious sequelae, such as those with prosthetic heart valves or orthopedic appliances). Antibiotics should be started before debridement and closure. Only a few days of coverage are necessary—usually until the wound is checked at 2–3 days and found to be free of infection. Penicillin or a substitute is appropriate for wounds involving the mouth, such as through-and-through lip lacerations and bites. Other wounds are usually contaminated by *Staphylococcus aureus,* and an antibiotic effective for penicillin-resistant *S aureus* is therefore appropriate. If gram-negative or anaerobic contamination is suspected, wound closure is risky, and hospitalization of the patient for treatment with parenteral antibiotics should be considered. Tetanus prophylaxis should be routinely given for patients who have not received current immunizations or who have wounds likely to lead to tetanus. Guidelines for this are detailed in Chapter 8.

Anesthesia is an important part of adequate soft tissue wound care and closure. Local anesthesia with either 0.5% or 1% lidocaine with epinephrine 1:200,000 or 1:100,000 is recommended for all wounds. Smaller amounts of lidocaine and epinephrine may be used in areas of appendages, such as earlobes, toes, and the penis. The injection may be given through the wound edge before debridement and irrigation for maximum patient comfort. Complete epinephrine vasoconstrictor effect occurs within 7 minutes. Overdose of epinephrine and lidocaine injection into vessels or use of the drugs in patients sensitive to these agents should be avoided.

The importance of irrigation cannot be overstated. Over 90% of bacteria in a recently sustained and superficially contaminated wound can be eliminated by adequate irrigation. Ideally, a physiologic solution such as lactated Ringer's solution or normal saline should be forcefully ejected from a large syringe with a 19-gauge needle or from other equipment designed for this purpose such as a water-jet apparatus. The wound is irrigated once to remove surface clots, foreign material, and bacteria and is then debrided and irrigated again. Detergents and antiseptic solutions are toxic to exposed tissue and should not be used.

Debridement must include removal of all obviously devitalized tissues. In special areas such as the eyelids, ears, nose, lips, and eyebrows, debridement must be done cautiously, since the tissue lost by debridement may be difficult to replace. Where tissues are more abundant, such as in the cheek, chin, and forehead areas, debridement may be more extensive. Small irregular or ragged wounds in these areas can be excised completely to produce clean, sharply cut wound edges which, when approximated, will produce the finest possible scar. Because the blood supply in the face is plentiful, damaged tissues of questionable viability should be retained rather than debrided away. The chances for survival are good.

Following adequate anesthesia, debridement, and irrigation, the wound is ready for final assessment and closure. Lighting must be adequate, and appropriate instruments should be available. The patient and the surgeon must be positioned comfortably. The skin surrounding the wound is prepared with an antiseptic solution, and the area is draped. A final check of the depth and extent of the wound is made, and vital structures are inspected for injury. Hemostasis must be achieved by use of epinephrine, pressure, cautery, or suture ligature. Important structures in facial wounds include the parotid duct, lacrimal duct, and branches of the facial nerve. These should be repaired in the operating room by microsurgical techniques.

Layers of tissue—usually muscle—in the depth of the wound should be closed first with as few absorbable sutures as possible, since sutures are foreign material within the wound. If possible, dead space should be closed with judicious use of fine absorbable sutures. If dead space cannot be closed, external pressure or small drains are sometimes effective. Skin closure should begin at the most important points of the laceration (eg, the borders of the ears and nose; the vermilion border or margins of the lip; the margins of the eyebrow [which should never be shaved]; and the scalp hairline). Subcuticular sutures are very helpful. Skin edges can be approximated without tension or strangulation with 5-0 or 6-0 monofilament suture material as outlined earlier under wound closure.

Complicated lacerations, such as complex stellate wounds or avulsion flaps, often heal with excessive scarring. Because of the associated subcutaneous tissue injury, U-shaped or trap-door avulsion lacerations almost always become unsightly as a result of wound contracture. Small lacerations of this type are best excised and closed in a straight line initially; larger flaps that must be replaced usually require secondary revision. Extensive loss of skin is generally best treated by initial split-thickness skin grafting followed later by secondary reconstruction. Primary attempts to reconstruct with local flaps may fail because of unsuspected injury to these adjacent tissues. The decision to convert avulsed tissues to free grafts that may not survive and thus delay healing requires sound surgical judgment.

Small or moderate-sized closures on the face may be dressed with antibiotic ointment alone. The patient may cleanse the suture lines with hydrogen peroxide to clear away crusts and dirt and then reapply the ointment. Elsewhere, closures benefit from the protection of a sterile bandage. Pressure dressings are useful in preventing hematoma formation and severe edema that may result in poor wound healing. Dressings should be changed early and the wound inspected for hematoma or signs of infection. Hematoma evacuation, appropriate drainage, and antibiotic therapy based on culture and sensitivity studies may be required. Removal of sutures in 3–5 days, followed by splinting of the incision with sterile tape, will minimize scarring from the sutures themselves.

The final result of facial wound repair depends on the nature and location of the wounds, individual propensity to scar formation, and the passage of time. A year or more must often pass before resolution of scar contracture and erythema results in maximum improvement. Only after this time can a decision be made regarding the desirability of secondary scar revision.

In wounds involving the major joints the extracapsular soft tissue and the intracapsular structures should be considered individually to assess accurately the magnitude of the injury and to provide a prognosis. Open joint injuries that are single penetrating and without extensive soft tissue damage, permit uncomplicated joint and wound closure. Injuries that are single or multiple penetrations with extensive soft-tissue disruption (flaps, avulsions, degloving) often require secondary operations to attain closure. In injuries which show open periarticular fractures with extension through the adjacent intra-articular surface and with associated nerve or vascular injury requiring repair, the cornerstone for successful management is debridement, antibiotic therapy properly timed and performed, joint closure and aggressive treatment of the bony injury. Newer techniques such as free tissue transfer can expedite wound care, decrease morbidity and spare some limbs from amputation.

FACIAL BONE FRACTURES

Because of the aesthetic and functional importance of the face, fractures of the facial bones—though rarely life-threatening—are best treated by surgeons who have extensive experience with facial injuries and reconstruction. Operation is most successful when performed in the acute setting, usually within the first week, because reconstruction becomes much more difficult if surgery is delayed.

Facial bone fractures are usually caused by trauma from a blunt instrument, such as a fist or club, or by violent contact with the steering wheel, dash-board, or windshield during an automobile accident. Particularly in the latter case, the patient should be assessed for associated injuries. For example, cervical spine injuries are present in up to 12% of automobile accident patients and should be treated or stabilized before facial bone injuries are attended to. Injuries to the brain, eyes, chest, abdomen, and extremities must also be assessed and may require earlier treatment.

The diagnosis of facial fractures is made primarily on clinical examination. Ideally, the examination should be done immediately, so that swelling will not obscure the findings. The mechanism and the line of direction of injury are important. If conscious, the patient should be asked about previous facial injuries, areas of pain and numbness, whether the jaw opens properly and the teeth come together normally, and whether vision in all quadrants is normal.

Most facial fractures can be palpated, or at least the abnormal position of bones can be noted. Beginning along the mandibular rims, one can feel for irregularities of the facial bones. The dental occlusion is noted. With bimanual palpation, placing the thumbs inside the mouth, one can elicit bony crepitus if there is an associated fracture. The maxilla and mid face can be rocked forward and backward between the thumb and the index finger in the presence of a midfacial fracture. Nasal fractures may be detected by palpation. Irregularities and step-offs along the infraorbital border, lateral orbital rim, or zygomatic arch regions indicate a depressed zygomatic fracture.

Radiologic studies are additional aids to the proper diagnosis of facial fractures. Rarely is a significant fracture seen on x-ray that is not also clinically evident. Helpful views include the Waters and submentovertex projections and oblique views of the mandible. The Panorex view of the mandible is very useful to look at the condyles. CT scans of facial bones, with appropriate biplanar and three-dimensional reconstructions so that bones can be viewed through several planes, have essentially supplanted regular radiographs in the workup of the facially injured patient. They are helpful in assessing the extent of fractures, in particular in more posterior areas such as the ethmoid area, medial and inferior orbit, pterygoid plates, and base of the skull.

The bones of the nose are the most commonly fractured facial bones. Next in frequency are the mandible, the zygomatic-malar bones, and the maxilla.

NASAL FRACTURES

Fractures may affect the nasal bones, cartilage, and septum. Fractures occur in two patterns, caused by lateral or head-on trauma.

With lateral trauma, the nasal bone on the side of the injury is fractured and displaced toward the septum; the septum is deviated and fractured; and the nasal bone on the side away from the injury is fractured and displaced away from the septum, so that the upper part of the nose, as a whole, is deviated. Depending upon the degree of violence, one or more of these displacements will be present, and the degree of comminution is variable.

Head-on trauma gives rise to telescoping and saddling of the nose and broadening of its upper half as a result of the depression and splaying of the fractured nasal bones. This of course produces severe damage to the septum, which usually buckles or actually suffers a fracture. The diagnosis of a fractured nose is made on clinical grounds alone, and x-rays are unnecessary except for medical-legal reasons.

Nasal fractures requiring reduction should be treated with a minimum of delay, for they tend to become fixed in the displaced position in a few days. The surgical approach depends on whether the fracture has resulted in deviation or collapse of the nasal bones. Local anesthesia is preferred; either topical tetracaine or cocaine intranasally or lidocaine for infiltration of the skin can be used. The nasal bones may be disimpacted with intranasal forceps or a periosteal elevator and aligned by external molding or pressure. Collapsed nasal fractures can be repositioned with Walsham's nasal forceps, introduced into each nostril and placed on each side of the septum, which is then elevated to its proper position. A septal hematoma should be recognized and drained to prevent infection and subsequent necrosis of the cartilaginous septum with associated collapse of the entire nose. Compound fractures of the nose require prompt repair of the skin wound and, if possible, early reduction of the displaced nasal bones.

External splinting, which is essentially a protective dressing, and intranasal packing using nonadhering gauze are appropriate after reduction. The intranasal packing provides support for the septum in its reduced position and helps prevent development of a hematoma. It also provides counter pressure for the external splint immobilizing the nasal bones and prevents them from collapsing. The packing is usually removed within 48 hours.

In severe comminuted nasal fractures, the medial canthal ligaments, which are easily felt by applying lateral traction to the upper eyelid, may have dislodged. If they have been avulsed, they should be reattached in position to prevent late deformities. For these severe fractures involving the entire naso-orbital and ethmoid complex, the coronal approach, which offers wide exposure, allows for proper anatomic reduction of all small nasal fragments as well as repositioning of the canthal ligaments and correction and elevation of the telescoped bone fragments at the root of the nose and glabella.

The lacrimal apparatus is commonly disrupted in these injuries and should be repaired and stented appropriately.

MANDIBULAR FRACTURES

Mandibular fractures are most commonly bilateral, generally occurring in the region of the mid body at the mental foramen, the angle of the ramus, or at the neck of the condyle. A frequent combination is a fracture at the mental region of the body with a condylar fracture on the opposite side. Displacement of the fragments results from the force of the external blow as well as the pull of the muscles of the floor of the mouth and the muscles of mastication. The diagnosis is suggested by derangement of dental occlusion associated with local pain, swelling, and often crepitation upon palpation. Appropriate x-rays confirm the diagnosis. Special views of the condyle, including tomograms, may be required. Sublingual hematoma and acute malocclusion are usually diagnostic of a mandibular fracture.

Restoration of functional dental occlusion is the most important consideration in treating mandibular fractures. In patients with an adequate complement of teeth, arch bars or interdental wires can be placed. Local nerve block anesthesia is preferable for this procedure, though certain patients may require general anesthesia. Intermaxillary elastic traction will usually correct minor degrees of displacement and bring the teeth into normal occlusion by overcoming the muscle pull. When the fracture involves the base of a tooth socket with suspected devitalization of the tooth, extraction of the tooth should be considered. Particularly in the incisor region, such devitalized teeth may be a source of infection, leading to the development of osteomyelitis and nonunion of the fracture.

Patients with more severe mandibular injuries require anatomic reduction and fixation of the fracture by the open, direct technique. These include compound, comminuted, and unfavorable fractures. An unfavorable fracture is one that is inherently unstable because muscle pull distracts the fracture segments. In this situation, intermaxillary fixation alone is insufficient. Edentulous patients also benefit from the open technique, although proper dentures or dental splints are useful to maintain normal occlusion.

Metal wire fixation of fractured segments and intermaxillary fixation for 6 weeks was a proven and popular method of fracture treatment. The more recent resurgence in popularity of the screw-plate system is due to a number of advantages over wiring. The screw plate usually achieves rigid fixation in three dimensions, providing adequate stability; it eliminates the need for intermaxillary fixation in most cases; it is useful in complex, comminuted fractures; and it is quite easy to use after familiarity with the technique has been acquired.

With bilateral parasymphysial fractures, anterior stabilization of the tongue may be lost, so that it may fall back and obstruct the airway. Anterior stabilization and splinting must be accomplished early in these cases.

Open reduction is rarely advised in condylar fractures; simple intermaxillary fixation for 4–6 weeks is sufficient. Indications for open reduction are severely displaced fractures, which may prevent motion of the mandible because of impingement of the coronoid process on the zygomatic arch. In children, the fracture may destroy the growth center of the condyle, resulting in maldevelopment of the mandible and gross distortion.

ZYGOMATIC & ORBITAL FRACTURE

Fractures of the zygomatic bones may involve just the arch of the zygomatic bone or the entire body of the zygoma (the malar eminence) and the lateral wall and floor of the orbit. The so-called tripod fracture characteristically occurs at the frontozygomatic and zygomaticomaxillary sutures as well as at the arch. It should be referred to as a tetrapod fracture since the anterior or posterior buttress of the maxilla is also involved in the fracture. Displacement of the body of the zygoma results in flattening of the cheek and depression of the orbital rim and floor.

Important diagnostic signs are subconjunctival hemorrhage, disturbances of extraocular muscle function (which may be accompanied by diplopia), and loss of sensation in the upper lip and alveoli on the involved side as a result of injury to the infraorbital nerve. Reduction of a displaced zygomatic fracture is seldom an emergency procedure and may be delayed until the patient's general condition is satisfactory for anesthesia. Local anesthesia will suffice only for reduction of fractures of the zygomatic arch. More extensively displaced fractures usually require general anesthesia. At least two-point fixation with direct interosseous wiring is necessary for these fractures. Here again, delicate miniplates have been used with success, providing anatomic reduction and rigid fixation.

Simple depressed fractures of the zygomatic arch can best be elevated using the Gillies technique. Through a temporal incision above the hairline, an instrument is passed beneath the superficial layer of the deep temporalis fascia and under the arch and the body of the zygoma. The fracture can also be elevated percutaneously with a hook or screw in conjunction with overlying palpation to achieve accurate reduction. If the fracture is complex or comminuted, as is often the case with high-velocity injuries, repair through a coronal scalp approach may be necessary to obtain an anatomic and stable result.

Extensive disruption should be suspected in conjunction with the zygomatic fracture when significant diplopia and enophthalmos and posterior displacement of the globe are present. Orbital fat and extraocular muscles may herniate through the defect and become entrapped, giving rise to the signs and symptoms. A "blowout" fracture is similar disruption of the orbital floor due to blunt trauma to the globe but not associated with a fracture of the zygoma or orbital rim. Treatment in both cases demands exploration, reduction of herniated contents, and repair of the floor. The most direct approach is through a lower lid subciliary incision, which provides excellent visualization. A buccal transantral (Caldwell-Luc) approach can be used, and blind antral packing for support has been described. This is quite hazardous, because bony spicules may be pushed into the ocular globe and perhaps cause injury or blindness. In cases where there is extensive communication or loss of bony fragments of the floor, use of local autogenous bone or cartilage as a scaffold may be performed. At times, in cases of extensive injuries to the floor, alloplastic material in the form of titanium mesh may be necessary.

Even with careful anatomic reduction and repair of the orbital floor, ocular problems—particularly enophthalmos—may persist. This may be due to an undiagnosed fracture, especially a medial ethmoidal blowout fracture. These can be properly evaluated with CT scanning. Treatment requires reduction and repair of the defect. The injury can at times cause ischemia of herniated soft tissue and subsequent atrophy and scarring. This may result in enophthalmos, which is almost impossible to resolve completely.

MAXILLARY FRACTURES

Maxillary fractures range in complexity from partial fractures through the alveolar process to extensive displacement of the midfacial structures in conjunction with fractures of the frontonasal bones and orbital maxillary region and total craniofacial separation. Hemorrhage and airway obstruction require emergency care, and in severe cases, tracheostomy is indicated. Mobility of the maxilla can be elicited by palpation in extensive fractures. "Dish-face" deformity of the retrodisplaced maxilla may be disguised by edema, and careful x-ray studies are necessary to determine the extent and complexity of the midfacial fracture. Treatment may have to be delayed because of other severe injuries. A delay of as long as 10–14 days may be safe before reduction and fixation, but the earliest possible restoration of maxillary position and dental occlusion is desirable to prevent late complications.

In the case of unilateral fractures or bilateral fractures with little or no displacement, splinting by intermaxillary fixation for 4 weeks may suffice. Fractures are usually displaced inferiorly or posteriorly and require direct surgical disimpaction and reduction and proper fixation with appropriate plates and screws. Early reduction may help control bleeding, as torn, stretched vessels are allowed to reestablish their normal tension. In certain severe cases, external traction may be necessary. Manipulation is directed toward restoring normal occlusion and maintaining the reduction with intermaxillary fixation to the mandible in association with direct plate fixation. Complicated fractures may require external fixation utilizing a head cap and intraoral splints in conjunction with multiple surgical incisions for direct plate fixation. Coexisting mandibular fractures usually necessitate open reduction and fixation at the same time.

Antonyshyn O, Gruss JS: Complex orbital trauma: the role of rigid fixation and primary bone grafting. Plast Reconstr Surg 1988;7:61.

Krsarai L et al A biomechanical analysis of the orbital zygomatic complex in human cadavers: examination of load sharing and failure patterns after fixation with titanium and bioresorbable systems. J Craniofac Surg 1999;10:400.

Thaller SR, Kawamoto HK: A histologic evaluation of fracture repair in the midface. Plast Reconstr Surg 1990;85:196.

Thaller SR, Mabourakh S: Pediatric mandibular fractures. Ann Plast Surg 1991;26:511.

Yaremchuk MJ: Vascularized bone grafts for maxillofacial reconstruction. Clin Plast Surg 1989;16:29.

CONGENITAL HEAD & NECK ANOMALIES

CLEFT LIP & CLEFT PALATE

Cleft lip, cleft palate, and combinations of the two are the most common congenital anomalies of the head and neck. The incidence of facial clefts has been reported to be 1 in every 650–750 live births, making this deformity second only to clubfoot in frequency as a reported birth defect.

The cleft may involve the floor of the nostril and lip on one or both sides and may extend through the alveolus, the hard palate, and the entire soft palate. A useful classification based on embryologic and anatomic aspects divides the structures into the primary and the secondary palate. The dividing point between the primary palate anteriorly and the secondary palate posteriorly is the incisive foramen. Clefts can thus be classified as partial or complete clefts of the primary or secondary palate (or both) in various combinations. The most common clefts are left unilateral complete clefts of the primary and secondary palate and partial midline clefts of the secondary palate, involving the soft palate and part of the hard palate.

Most infants with cleft palate present some feeding difficulties, and breast-feeding may be impossible. As a rule, enlarging the openings in an artificial nipple or using a syringe with a soft rubber feeding tube will solve difficulties in sucking. Feeding in the upright position helps prevent oronasal reflux or aspiration. Severe feeding and breathing problems and recurrent aspiration are seen in Pierre Robin sequence, in which the palatal cleft is associated with a receding lower jaw and posterior and cephalic displacement of the tongue, obstructing the naso-oropharyngeal airway. This is a medical emergency and is a cause of sudden infant death syndrome (SIDS). Nonsurgical treatment includes pulling the tongue forward with an instrument and laying the baby prone with a towel under the chest to let the mandible and tongue drop forward. Insertion of a small (No. 8) nasogastric tube into the pharynx may temporarily prevent respiratory distress and may be used to supplement the baby's feedings. Placement of an acrylic obturator or appliance has proved quite successful in alleviating the breathing difficulties by bringing the tongue down and permitting a better nasal airway. Several surgical procedures that bring the tongue and mandible forward have been described but should be employed only when conservative measures have been tried without success. Recently, the use of distraction of the mandible has shown some beneficial effects. However it should be done with great caution in the neonate.

Treatment

Surgical repair of cleft lip is not considered an emergency. The optimal time for operation can be described as the widely accepted "rule of ten." This includes body weight of 10 lb (4.5 kg) or more and a hemoglobin of 10 g/dL or more. This is usually at some time after the 10th week of life. In most cases, closure of the lip will mold distortions of the cleft alveolus into a satisfactory contour. In occasional cases where there is marked distortion of the alveolus, such as in severe bilateral clefts with marked protrusion of the premaxilla, preliminary maxillary orthodontic treatment may be indicated. This may involve the use of carefully crafted appliances or simple constant pressure by use of an elastic band.

General endotracheal anesthesia via an orally placed endotracheal tube is the anesthetic technique of choice. A variety of techniques for repair of unilateral clefts have evolved over many years. Earlier procedures ignored anatomic landmarks and resulted in a characteristic "repaired harelip" look. The Millard rotation advancement operation that is now commonly used for repair employs an incision in the medial side of the cleft to allow the cupid's bow of the lip to be rotated down to a normal position. The resulting gap in the medial side of the cleft is filled by advancing a flap from the lateral side. This principle can be varied in placement of the incisions and results in most cases in a symmetric lip with normally placed landmarks. Bilateral clefts, because of greater deficiency of tissue, present more challenging technical problems. Maximum preservation of available tissue is the underlying principle, and most surgeons prefer approximation of the central and lateral lip elements in a straight line closure, rolling up the vermilion border of the lip (Manchester repair).

Secondary revisions are frequently necessary in the older child with a repaired cleft lip. A constant associated deformity in patients with cleft lip is distortion of the soft tissue and cartilage structures of the ala and dome of the nose. These patients often present with deficiency of growth of the structures of the mid face. This has been attributed to intrinsic growth disturbances and to external pressures from the lip and palate repairs. Some correction of these deformities, especially of the nose, can be done at the initial lip operation. More definitive correction is done after the cartilage and bone growth is more complete. These may include scar revisions and rearrangement of the cartilage structure of the nose. Recent approaches involve degloving of the nasal skin envelope with complete exposure of the abnormal cartilage framework. These are then rearranged in proper position with or without additional grafts. Maxillary osteotomies (Le Fort I with advancement) will substantially correct the midfacial depression. A tight upper lip due to severe tissue deficiency can be corrected by a two-stage transfer of a lower lip flap known as an Abbe flap.

Palatal clefts may involve the alveolus, the bony hard palate, or the soft palate, singly or in any combination. Clefts of the hard palate and alveolus may be either unilateral or bilateral, whereas the soft palate cleft is always midline, extending back through the uvula. The width of the cleft varies greatly, making the amount of tissue available for repair also variable. The bony palate, with its mucoperiosteal lining, forms the roof of the anterior mouth and the floor of the nose. The posteriorly attached soft palate is composed of five paired muscles of speech and swallowing.

Surgical closure of the cleft to allow for normal speech is the treatment of choice. The timetable for closure depends on the size of the cleft and any other associated problems. However, the defect should be closed before the child undertakes serious speech, usually before age 2. Closure at 6 months usually is performed without difficulty and also aids in the child's feeding. If the soft palate seems to be long enough, simple approximation of the freshened edges of the cleft after freeing of the tissues through lateral relaxing incisions may suffice. If the soft palate is too short, a pushback type of operation is required. In this procedure, the short soft palate is retrodisplaced closer to the posterior pharyngeal wall utilizing the mucoperiosteal flaps based on the posterior palatine artery.

Satisfactory speech following surgical repair of cleft palate is achieved in 70–90% of cases. Significant speech defects usually require secondary operations when the child is older. The most widely used technique is the pharyngeal flap operation, in which the palatopharyngeal space is reduced by attaching a flap of posterior pharyngeal muscle and mucosa to the soft palate. This permits voluntary closure of the velopharyngeal complex and thus avoids hypernasal speech. Various other kinds of pharyngoplasties have been useful in selected cases.

CRANIOFACIAL ANOMALIES

These are congenital deformities of the hard and soft tissues of the head. Particular problems of the brain, eye, and internal ear are treated by the appropriate specialist. The craniofacial surgeon often needs the collaboration of these specialists when operating on such patients.

Serious craniofacial anomalies are relatively rare, although mild forms often go undiagnosed or accepted as normal variants. A classification is therefore difficult, although many have been proposed. Tessier has offered a numerical classification based on clinical presentation. He considers a cleft to be the basis of the malformation, which involves both hard and soft tissues. Other classifications are based on embryologic and etiologic features. With greater understanding and continued investigation, classification efforts will no doubt be more satisfactory.

There are well-known chromosomal and genetic aberrations as well as environmental causes that can lead to craniofacial deformity. The cause in most cases, however, is unknown. Arrest in the migration and proliferation of neural crest cells and defects in differentiation characterize most of these deformities. We will describe some of the more common ones in brief terms.

Crouzon's syndrome (craniofacial dysostosis) and **Apert's syndrome** (acrocephalosyndactyly) are closely related, differing in the extremity deformities present in the latter. Both are autosomal dominant traits with variable expression. Both present with skull deformities due to premature closure of the cranial sutures. The cranial sutures most affected will determine the type of skull deformity. Exophthalmos, midfacial hypoplasia, and hypertelorism are also features of these two syndromes.

The facial organs and tissues proceed in great measure from the first and second branchial arches and the first branchial cleft. Disorders in their development lead to a spectrum of anomalies of variable severity. **Treacher-Collins syndrome** (mandibulofacial dysostosis) is a severe disorder characterized by hypoplasia of the malar bones and lower eyelids, colobomas, and antimongoloid slant of the palpebrae. The mandible and ears are often quite underdeveloped. The presentation is bilateral and is an autosomal dominant trait. A unilateral deformity known as **hemifacial microsomia** presents with progressive skeletal and soft tissue underdevelopment. The Goldenhar variant of hemifacial microsomia is a severe form associated with upper bulbar dermoids, notching of the upper eyelids, and vertebral anomalies.

Some of these patients show mental retardation, but in most cases intelligence is not affected. The psychosocial problems are serious and most often related to how the patients look. Within the past 2 decades, craniofacial surgery has progressed so that previously untreatable deformities can now be corrected. With the anatomic work of Le Fort as a basis—and guided by the incomplete attempts of Gillies and others—Paul Tessier, in the late 1960s, proposed a set of surgical techniques to correct major craniofacial deformities. Two basic concepts soon emerged from his work: (1) Large segments of the craniofacial skeleton can be completely denuded of their blood supply, repositioned, and yet survive and heal; and (2) the eyes can be translocated horizontally or vertically over a considerable distance with no adverse effect on vision. The tendency today is to operate at approximately 6–9 months of age (not later than 9 months) for cranial vault remodeling and fronto-orbital advancement.

A bicoronal scalp incision is utilized to expose the skull and facial bones with an intra- or extracranial approach. The cut bones are then reshaped, repositioned, and fixed with a combination of wires or miniplates and screws. The latter have the advantage of rigid fixation and less need to maintain large movements with bone grafts. Autogenous inlay and onlay bone grafts can be used to improve contour. The entire operation is usually completed in one stage, and complications are surprisingly few. Miniplates have been used extensively in the last few years. In infants, fixation with absorbable suture material or the newer absorbable plates and screws can replace the usual steel wires and avoid any radiologic tracks. They also seem to have less impairment of craniofacial growth and development.

Craniofacial surgery has improved the treatment not only of major congenital deformities but also of major complex facial fractures, chronic sequelae of trauma, isolated exophthalmos, fibrous dysplasia, and aesthetic facial sculpturing.

MICROTIA

Microtia is absence or hypoplasia of the pinna of the ear, with a blind or absent external auditory meatus.

The incidence of significant auricular deformity is about one in 8000 births and is usually spontaneous. Ten percent of these defects are bilateral, and boys are afflicted twice or three times as commonly as girls. Because the ear arises from the first and second branchial arches, the middle ear is always involved, and many patients have other disorders of the first and second arches. The inner ear structures are usually spared.

Generally, correction of conductive hearing by an otologist has not been long-lasting or helpful, and surgery for this problem is reserved for bilateral cases.

Reconstruction of the external ear usually involves a multistage procedure beginning at preschool age. Autogenous rib cartilage or cartilage from the opposite ear is used to construct a framework to replace the absent ear. The cartilage is imbedded under the skin in the appropriate area, and after adjustments are made in local tissue to reposition or recreate the earlobe and conchal cavity, the framework is elevated posteriorly and the resulting sulcus grafted to obtain projection. In cases where local tissue is poor or unavailable, the neighboring superficial temporalis fascia is dissected and placed over the cartilage framework. This is then skin-grafted with adequate tissue. The opposite (normal) ear is occasionally altered to provide better symmetry. Excellent results have been achieved. Silastic frameworks for ear cartilage have also been used, and although their use eliminates donor site problems, rates of infection and extrusion have been unacceptable. More recently, a porous polyethylene construct has been used with better long-term results. A temporalis fascia flap is rotated to cover the allograft and then a full-thickness skin graft is placed. They are quite useful in bilateral cases or when sufficient cartilage is not available.

Lesser deformities, such as overly large, prominent, or bent ears, are corrected by appropriate resection of skin and cartilage, "scoring" of the cartilage to alter its curve, and placement sutures to aid in contouring.

Cohen SR: Craniofacial distraction with a modular internal distraction system: evolution of design and surgical techniques. Plast Reconstr Surg 1999;103:1592.

McCarthy JG: The timing of surgical intervention in craniofacial anomalies. Clin Plast Surg 1990;17:161.

Nocini PF et al: Vertical distraction of a free vascularized fibula flap in a reconstructed hemimandible: case report. J Craniomaxillofac Surg 2000;28:20.

ANOMALIES OF THE HANDS & EXTREMITIES

The most common hand anomaly is syndactyly, or webbing of the digits. This may be simple, involving only soft tissue, or complex, involving fusion of bone and soft tissue. The fusion may be partial or complete. Surgical correction involves separation and repair with local flaps and skin grafts. Correction should be done before growth disturbance of the webbed digits takes place. Other anomalies such as extra digits (polydactyly), absence of digits (adactyly), and cleft hand also exist.

Flexion contractures of the hands or digits may require surgical release and appropriate skin grafting. Congenital ring constriction of the extremities may be associated also with congenital amputation. The ring constrictions are best treated by excision and Z-plasty.

Poland's syndrome consists of a variable degree of unilateral chest deformity—usually absence of the pectoralis major muscle—associated with hand symbrachydactyly. The hand deformity is treated according to the severity. The latissimus dorsi muscles can be transposed to replace the absent pectoralis major, simulating the sites of origin and insertion. In more severe cases and in women requiring breast and chest reconstruction, the transverse rectus abdominis island flap can be used to replace the deficit.

POSTABLATIVE RECONSTRUCTION

HEAD & NECK RECONSTRUCTION

Many of the tumors discussed in Chapter 14 require surgical excision as a primary form of therapy. This often involves removal of large areas of composite tissue, such as the floor of the mouth, the maxilla, part of the mandible, or the lymph-bearing tissue of the neck. Reconstruction after such resections can be very challenging and may require special skill.

A salient advance in the complete treatment of the patient with a head or neck tumor is reconstruction, usually done in the same setting. Free flaps with microvascular techniques are the most appropriate methods even though they require a high level of skill and are time-consuming. The free flaps most commonly used following ablative procedures in the head and neck include the anterolateral thigh flap or the radial forearm flap for resurfacing the floor of the mouth; and the composite fibular flap, which includes fibula as well as skin to reconstruct the mandible and the floor of the mouth. For larger defects, judicious use of the rectus abdominis muscle, latissimus dorsi, or other musculocutaneous flaps have also been helpful. For pharyngoesophageal reconstruction, either the tubed radial forearm flap or the free jejunum is most successful.

Since no two surgical resections for tumor in the head and neck are identical, the key to effective treatment is preoperative planning. Probable extent of resection, areas that will require pre- or postoperative radiation therapy, incision and flaps created by neck dissections, and available donor areas must all be carefully assessed. Tissue attached to an adequate blood supply must be used to ensure early and watertight healing in the mouth and oropharynx, in areas of radiation injury, and over metal or other alloplastic implants.

Useful musculocutaneous flaps in the head and neck are the sternocleidomastoid, platysma, trapezius, pectoralis major, and latissimus dorsi muscles. Useful axial skin flaps can be obtained from the forehead, deltopectoral, and cervicohumeral areas. When these flaps are insufficient or unavailable for the reconstructive needs of the patient, free tissue transfer must be used. Many flaps with acceptable donor sites exist. The fibula and the iliac crest provide an osteocutaneous flap quite useful in mandible reconstruction. The forearm and scapular areas are also good sites for composite free flaps. Healing is quick, so that radiation, if necessary, may be started as early as one month after surgery.

Pearl RM et al: An approach to mandibular reconstruction. Ann Plast Surg 1988;21:401.

Santamaria E et al: Sensation recovery on innervated radial forearm flap for hemiglossectomy reconstruction by using different recipient nerves. Plast Reconstr Surg 1999;103:450.

Yamamoto Y et al: Superiority of end-to-side anastomosis with the internal jugular vein: the experience of 80 cases in head and neck microsurgical reconstruction. Br J Plastic Surg 1999;52:88.

BREAST RECONSTRUCTION

Reconstruction of the female breast after mastectomy is available to all patients in the USA and new techniques continue to be developed providing women with more options. The insurance carriers now pay for this procedure as part of the treatment for breast cancer, and this includes symmetry surgery of the contralateral breast. Even women with significant defects in the anterior chest wall as a result of radical mastectomy and radiation therapy can undergo reconstructive surgery if they are otherwise appropriate candidates.

Heightened awareness of breast cancer along with well-established screening guidelines has affected surgical treatment of the cancer and, subsequently, approaches to reconstruction of the breast. A skin-sparing, modified radical mastectomy, for example, may allow for an immediate reconstruction with autologous tissue that results in an aesthetically pleasing breast mound. Lumpectomy followed by irradiation, initially indicated for relatively small tumors, has now expanded to larger tumors and may thus result in considerable distortion and concavity in the treated breast. In the appropriate patient, concomitant bilateral reduction mammaplasty may allow for a large lumpectomy while maintaining symmetry.

The methods of reconstruction include the use of saline implants, tissue expanders, autologous tissue, or a combination of these methods. Following mastectomy, simple placement of an implant is usually unsatisfactory except in a few thin patients with relatively small contralateral breasts. The implant is usually placed in the submuscular position, utilizing the remaining pectoralis major muscle and occasionally the serratus anterior muscle for adequate muscle coverage. This results in a firm, rounded type of reconstruction and does not simulate the soft "teardrop" appearance of the normal breast. Even when adequate skin has been saved following a skin-sparing mastectomy, placement of an implant is unsatisfactory because of the high rate of complications due to skin necrosis of the saved overlying skin, which results in exposure of the implant. When doing an immediate reconstruction with implant following a skin-sparing mastectomy, it is preferable to transpose the latissimus dorsi muscle to provide another layer of cover for the implant so that if there is necrosis of the skin from the skin-sparing mastectomy, the implant will not be exposed.

The latissimus dorsi myocutaneous flap is used most often for reconstruction of the breast with an implant. The myocutaneous unit is outlined with a skin island transversely so that the scar will be transverse and covered by the brassiere. The unit is freed up completely except for its insertion at the humerus, thus preserving the neurovascular pedicle. It is transposed as a pendulum through the anterior chest wall. The superior portion of the latissimus dorsi is sutured to the pectoralis major muscle and the lower edge is secured to the lower skin flap as far down as it will reach. The implant is then inserted, having been covered by the latissimus dorsi inferiorly and by two layers of muscle superiorly—the latissimus dorsi and the pectoralis major. The skin island is utilized in its entirety, if necessary, or is deepithelialized appropriately, maintaining only the skin portion that is needed. This method is most suitable for patients who do not have a large amount of abdominal skin, are relatively thin, and do not object to the use of implants, which sometimes may even be inserted in the opposite breast in an effort to achieve symmetry.

The use of tissue expanders is also a popular method of breast reconstruction. A partially filled silicone envelope with a separate valve is inserted under the chest skin and muscle, and at intervals over a period of 6 weeks to 3 months the bag is progressively inflated with saline percutaneously. The expander is inflated at least 25% more than the desired volume. A period of time—approximately 3 months—is advisable as a waiting period to prevent the "recall phenomenon," which is the shrinking that may occur following removal of the expander as it is replaced by a permanent implant. The disadvantages of this method include the rare occurrence of the hemispheric expansion of the skin, which may result in a hard, rounded breast mound; the necessity for a second operation; and problems with infection, deflation, exposure of the prosthesis, and occasional skin necrosis when expansion is too rapid.

The transverse rectus abdominis myocutaneous (TRAM) flap based on the superior epigastric vessel has been successfully used to provide adequate tissue so that an implant is not required in reconstructing the breast. This is the most versatile method of reconstruction in that one can usually obtain as much tissue as necessary to match the opposite breast and to contour it and position it to simulate the shape as well as the size of the opposite breast. The incision at the donor site is similar to that of an abdominoplasty operation along the lower abdomen. This method of reconstruction produces the most normal and natural breast in appearance and feel, but it requires a longer operating time as well as a longer period of hospitalization than reconstruction with tissue expanders and implants alone.

If the superior epigastric system has been violated (from surgery or trauma) or if there are other factors that would question the reliability of these vessels to adequately supply the volume and region of tissue required for the reconstruction, the surgeon may favor using the inferior epigastric system and transferring the TRAM as a free flap. Typical recipient vessels are the internal mammary or the thoracodorsal vessels. Again, past surgical history, previous (or planned) radiation, and anatomic variance may dictate reconstructive strategy regarding recipient vessels and whether to use the ipsilateral or contralateral inferior epigastric system.

Because successful breast reconstruction is common, many surgeons have sought to refine autologous reconstruction by decreasing donor site morbidity. Modifications of the free TRAM flap have been made so that the rectus abdominis muscle is mostly spared (muscle-sparing TRAM) or spared in its entirety. This latter technique is referred to as a deep inferior epigastric perforator (DIEP) flap. The same skin territory as the TRAM flap is used; however, the musculocutaneous branches that supply the skin are dissected away from the rectus abdominis muscle. In this manner the muscle itself is spared and left in situ in an effort to preserve muscular function and reduce abdominal wall weakness. The deep inferior epigastric vessels are then divided and the flap is inset into the thoracic defect, and the flap vessels are anastomosed to recipient vessels along the chest wall. Both techniques that spare the rectus abdominis and its innervation require more operative time and careful dissection. However, to some degree they seem to have a similar decrease in donor site morbidity with regard to avoiding an abdominal bulge and maintaining more muscle function.

In addition to reconstruction of the affected breast, many patients undergo procedures that alter the contralateral (noncancerous) breast so that volume and ptosis are comparable. Such symmetry procedures are considered stages in postoncologic breast reconstruction. The nipple-areola complex can also be reconstructed. Current techniques for nipple reconstruction utilize adjacent flaps from the area where the nipple is to be positioned, taking skin and variable amounts of underlying fat if a TRAM flap has been used or elevating skin and lesser amounts of subcutaneous tissue if an implant (with or without the latissimus dorsi flap) was used. The areola may be reconstructed with a full-thickness skin graft followed by tattooing at a later date for color match.

Bostwick J III: Breast reconstruction after mastectomy. Semin Surg Oncol 1988;4:274.

Hartrampf CR Jr: The transverse abdominal island flap for breast reconstruction: a 7-year experience. Clin Plast Surg 1988; 15:703.

Lejour M, Jabri M, Deraemaecker R: Analysis of long-term results of 326 breast reconstructions. Clin Plast Surg 1988;15:689.

Nahabedian MY et al: Breast reconstruction with the DIEP flap or the muscle-sparing (MS-2) free TRAM flap: is there a difference? Plast Reconstr Surg 2005;115:436.

LOWER EXTREMITY RECONSTRUCTION

Probably one of the most difficult areas for which to provide wound coverage and closure is the lower extremity, particularly the distal leg and foot areas. Tenuous and unstable skin grafts or poorly vascularized local or cross-leg skin flaps were once the only tissues available for resurfacing of these parts of the body. When large segments of bone were exposed or missing or when infection had become established, these grafts or flaps often were inadequate and amputation was the only recourse. Use of musculocutaneous flaps, and particularly free flaps, has greatly improved coverage in the lower extremities.

Generally, wound problems in the lower leg, ankle, and foot involve orthopedic injuries, such as compound tibial or ankle fractures. Incisions and metal screws and plates associated with open reduction and fixation of fractures may lead to increased scarring and make coverage more difficult. Other injuries requiring reconstruction are avulsion loss of the skin of the leg, heel, or sole of the foot and ischemic or venous stasis skin loss.

Treatment depends on the extent of tissue loss and the depth of the wound. Fairly extensive wounds around the knee and upper third of the leg can be reconstructed with a gastrocnemius muscle flap (usually the medial head) and a split-thickness skin graft. Soft tissue defects of the middle third of the leg can be reconstructed in a similar manner by the soleus muscle in many cases. Large middle third and distal third soft tissue defects are more difficult to reconstruct. When they are complicated by extensive bone and soft tissue loss, free tissue transfer may be necessary. Although there are small muscles that end in tendons in the foot, such as the peroneus brevis, flexor hallucis longus, and extensor digitorum muscles, they can provide only limited coverage. If there is a suitable recipient artery remaining in the leg, better coverage is generally provided by a free muscle flap such as the gracilis muscle for small and medium-sized defects or the latissimus dorsi or rectus abdominis muscle for larger defects.

Large areas of the heel or the sole of the foot are difficult to replace because skin in these regions is specially adapted to bear the weight of the body without shearing or breaking down. Free muscle flaps surfaced with skin grafts have proven to be adequate, but protective sensation is missing. The use of free neurovascular axial skin flaps, such as the inferior gluteal thigh flap and the deltoid flap, may help provide coverage with some gross sensation. Neurosensory flaps—and specifically the sural flap, distally based on one of the lower septocutaneous perforators from the lateral aspect of the leg and supplied by the sural artery, which accompanies the sural nerve—have been used to resurface defects around the ankle and heel. The procedure provides good skin and fascia for a weight-bearing area such as the heel, but it usually does not provide protective sensibility.

Segmental defects of the tibia may be reconstructed with bone grafts or, if the gap is large, free bone flaps such as the contralateral fibula or iliac crest. It is also possible to reconstruct the soft tissue defect and then reconstruct the bony gap with a distraction osteogenesis technique (Ilizarov bone transport). This bone transport method consists of performing a cortical osteotomy proximal to the site of injury and then applying a distraction apparatus, which in effect lengthens the bone 1 mm per day by appropriate adjustment screws. Such lower extremity reconstruction requires a well-coordinated, cooperative effort between the plastic and orthopedic surgeons. While such limb salvage is possible, amputation may be recommended in cases where a constellation of complications are present, such as bony gaps greater than 8 cm, extensive vascular injury, greater than 6 hours of warm ischemia time, an insensate limb, loss of plantar flexion, or an overall medically unstable patient.

Osteomyelitis of the tibia or bones in the foot may be devastating and often uncontrollable. Probably because of poor vascularity in the area, even long-term antibiotic treatment has often failed to control bone infections in the leg. Recently, effective surgical treatment for bone infections has been developed. The bone is surgically debrided and covered with a microvascular free muscle flap such as the gracilis or rectus abdominis muscle. Apparently, the muscle tissue with its excellent blood supply not only covers the exposed bone but assists natural defenses in controlling infection. Antibiotics are also used, but the well-vascularized muscle flap appears to be the deciding factor in control of infection. Reconstruction of bony defects may be accomplished at a latter date.

Erdmann MW, Court-Brown CM, Quaba AA: A five-year review of islanded distally based fasciocutaneous flaps on the lower limb. Br J Plastic Surg 1997;50:421.

Kuran I et al: Comparison between sensitive and nonsensitive free flaps in reconstruction of the heel and plantar area. Plast Reconstr Surg 2000;105:574.

May JW Jr et al: Foot reconstruction using fee microvascular muscle flaps with skin grafts. Clin Plast Surg 1986;13:681.

Vasconez HC et al: Management of extremity injuries with external fixator or Ilizarov devices: cooperative effort between orthopedic and plastic surgeons. Clin Plast Surg 1991;18:505.

PRESSURE SORES

Pressure sores—often less precisely called bedsores or decubitus ulcers—are another example of difficult wound problems that can be treated by plastic surgery. Pressure sores generally occur in patients who are bedridden and unable or unwilling to change position; patients who cannot change position because of a cast or appliance; and patients who have no sensation in an area that is not moved even though they may be ambulatory. The underlying cause of sores in these patients is ischemic necrosis resulting from prolonged pressure against the soft tissue overlying bone. There is also some evidence that local factors in denervated skin predispose to pressure breakdown because there is atrophy of the skin and subcutaneous tissue.

Absence of normal protective reflexes must be compensated for. Prevention is clearly the best treatment for pressure sores. Casts and appliances must be well padded, and points of pressure or pain should be relieved. Bedridden patients must be turned to a new position at least every 2 hours. Water and air mattresses, sheepskin pads, and foam cushions may help relieve pressure but are not substitutes for frequent turning. The introduction of the flotation bed system, which distributes pressure uniformly over a large surface area, has greatly aided in the management of these patients. The pressure on the skin at any time is less than the capillary filling pressure, avoiding many ischemic problems. Paraplegics should not sit in one position for more than 2 hours. Careful daily examination should be made for erythema, the earliest sign of ischemic injury. Erythematous areas should be freed from all pressure. Electrical stimulations, biomaterials, and growth factors are additional modalities to expedite wound repair, but the results are variable.

Once pressure necrosis is established, it is important to determine whether underlying tissues such as fat and muscle are affected, since they are much more likely than skin to become necrotic. A small skin ulcer may be the manifestation of a much larger area of destruction below. If the area is not too extensive and if infection and abscess due to external or hematogenous bacteria are not present, necrotic tissue may be replaced by scar tissue. Continued pressure will not only prevent scar tissue from forming but will also extend the injury. A surface eschar or skin may cover a significant abscess.

If the pressure sore is small and noninfected, application of drying agents to the wound and removal of all pressure to the area may permit slow healing. Wounds extending down to bone rarely heal without surgery. Infected wounds must be debrided down to clean tissue. The objectives at operation are to debride devitalized tissue, including bone, and to provide healthy, well-vascularized padded tissue as a covering. All of the original tissue that formed the bed of the ulcer must be excised.

When the patient's nutritional status and general condition of health are optimal, definitive coverage can be performed. Coverage is usually accomplished with a muscle, musculocutaneous, or, sometimes, an axial flap. Well-vascularized muscle appears to help control established low-grade bacterial contamination. The muscle flaps used for the more common bedsores are as follows: greater trochanter—tensor fasciae latae; ischium—gracilis, gluteus maximus, or hamstrings; sacrum—gluteus maximus. Occasionally, it is possible to provide sensibility to the area of a pressure sore with an innervated flap from above the level of paraplegia. The most common example is the tensor fasciae latae flap with the contained lateral femoral cutaneous nerve from L4 and L5, which is used to cover an ischial sore. Rarely, an innervated intercostal flap from the abdominal wall may be used to cover an insensible sacrum. Unfortunately, attempts to provide protective sensibility with sensory flaps have not had good results. The tissue expansion techniques should not be the primary surgery treatment of decubitus ulcers but can be used in difficult cases where available tissue is insufficient to close the wound.

Postoperatively, the donor and recipient areas must be kept free of pressure for 2–3 weeks to allow for complete healing. This puts significant demands on other areas of the body that may be equally at risk or may already have areas of breakdown. The use of the air-fluidized bed has greatly aided such situations.

In spite of excellent padding provided by musculocutaneous flaps, recurrence of pressure sores is still a major problem, because the situation that caused the original breakdown usually still exists. Prevention of sores is even more important for these patients.

Bruck JC et al: More arguments in favor of myocutaneous flaps for the treatment of pelvic pressure sores. Ann Plast Surg 1991;25:85.

Goodman CM et al: Evaluation of results and treatment variables for pressure ulcers in 48 veteran spinal cord-injured patients. Ann Plast Surg 1999;42:665.

AESTHETIC SURGERY

Aesthetic surgery is an integral part of plastic surgery. In fact, the two terms have become almost synonymous even though aesthetic surgery is only one band in a broad spectrum. Increased interest and curiosity about the specialty results in part from increased demands for its services by an aging population but also from the development of more predictable, lasting, and safer techniques. A number of specialists other than plastic surgeons have also performed and contributed to cosmetic surgery. A skilled surgeon can perform such cosmetic operations safely and with maximum benefit to the patient.

Patient selection is probably as important as any other factor. Not all patients are good candidates for aesthetic procedures, and such operations are contraindicated in others. Age or poor general health of the patient may be a reason for delay or avoidance of purely elective procedures. Two other major factors must be considered. The first factor is the anatomic feasibility of the procedure. Can the alterations be made successfully and safely? Which technique will best accomplish the goal? The second factor is the psychologic makeup of the patient. Does the patient fully understand the nature of the proposed procedure and its risks and consequences? Are the patient's expectations realistic? Cosmetic changes in appearance will generally not save a failing marriage, help to procure a new job, or substantially improve a person's station in life, and persons with such expectations should not undergo aesthetic surgery. Surgery should be postponed for persons experiencing severe stress, such as is associated with divorce, death of a loved one, or other periods of emotional instability.

The ideal candidate for cosmetic surgery is an adult or mature younger person who has a realistic idea of what is to be accomplished, is not under pressure from others to have the operation done, and does not expect major changes in interpersonal relations or career potential following surgery. Personal satisfaction is a valid reason for seeking aesthetic refinements.

The more common aesthetic procedures are discussed below. Some procedures involve correction of functional problems as well and are therefore not always considered purely cosmetic procedures.

RHINOPLASTY

Surgical alterations of nasal structures are done for relief of airway obstruction (usually secondary to trauma) and to reshape the nose because of undesirable characteristics, such as a prominent dorsal hump, bulbous or drooping tip, or overly large size. There is often a combination of problems.

Procedures are generally performed through intranasal incisions. The nasal skin is usually temporarily freed from its underlying bony and cartilaginous framework, so that the framework can be altered by removal, rearrangement, or augmentation of bone or cartilage. The skin is then redraped over the new foundation. The nasal septum and lower turbinate can also be altered to reestablish an open airway. A better understanding of nasal physiology has enabled surgeons to correct internal valve dysfunction by inserting spreader grafts—often following modification of the bony radix of the nose. Spreader grafts are small pieces of cartilage placed next to the septum and under the upper lateral cartilages. They serve to open up the internal valve in somewhat the same was as the external "breathe easy" appliances utilized by athletes.

Surgery can be done under local or general anesthesia; in either case, topical and injectable vasoconstrictors and anesthetic agents are commonly used. Hospitalization may or may not be indicated. Nasal packing is often used for hemostasis and support of the nasal mucosa during initial healing, as incisions are usually only minimally sutured with absorbable sutures. External nasal splints are placed to control swelling and provide some protection, particularly if osteotomy of the nasal bones is performed.

Convalescence requires 10–14 days before most swelling and periorbital ecchymosis subside; however, several months are often required before completely normal sensation returns, and all swelling resolves.

Nasal procedures are very commonly performed, generally quite safe, and usually effective. Complications include bleeding, internal scarring, recurrence of airways obstruction, and irregularities of contour. Infections are rare except with the use of alloplastic nasal implants.

RHYTIDECTOMY (FACELIFT)

The combined effects of gravity, sun exposure, and loss of elasticity due to aging result in varying degrees of wrinkles and sagging of skin along the cheeks, jawline, neck, and elsewhere in the facial area. These natural signs of aging can be removed to a great extent by a facelift procedure. Not all wrinkles can be removed, however; those in the forehead, around the eyes, in the nasolabial area, and around the lips are not significantly corrected without additional procedures.

Rhytidectomy is a major procedure requiring extensive incisions hidden in the scalp and in front of and behind the ears and occasionally in the submental region. The first such operations consisted of freeing up the skin and then stretching it and resuturing as it was drawn cephalad and laterally. This gave a mask-like and unnatural appearance. In the last few years, there has been a significant change in the concept of the facelift procedure, so that now it consists of elevation of the soft tissues—particularly the jowls and malar fat pads—to where they were at a younger age, giving more prominence to the cheek bones and better delineating the jawline. Undermining of the skin is done only to approach the soft tissues to be elevated, and the excess skin is now removed and reapproximated without tension. This approach to the mid face has given more natural and lasting results and provides also a three-dimensional type of restoration of the soft tissues, giving a more youthful appearance.

For the double neck, extensive freeing up of the skin over the neck from the jawline down to the hyoid is performed, and the fat overlying the platysmal muscle is removed either by suctioning or directly with scissors. The platysma itself is tightened laterally as well as centrally to provide an effect similar to a hammock that will give a more defined neck and jaw angle.

Drains are used particularly in the neck, as well as a padded circumferential dressing to protect the face and provide light pressure during healing. The introduction of fat aspiration procedures (liposuction) has been adapted to the neck but is not recommended for the face since it may produce abnormal lines ("railroad tracks of demarcation"). In appropriate patients, liposuction in the neck does give fine definition to the chin and jawline and may substantially correct the double chin appearance.

Either local or general anesthesia may be used for this often lengthy (3–4 hours) procedure. Local vasoconstrictors are routinely used.

Complications include hematoma, skin slough, injuries to branches of the facial nerve or greater auricular nerve, scars, and asymmetry. Signs of aging often recur years later.

Endoscopy

Endoscopy has become an integral part of plastic surgery, particularly for procedures involving the face or the breast. Smaller endoscopes are now utilized as well as different methods of achieving a desired optical field other than by distention of natural cavities with fluid or gases. In the face and in the breast, the optical cavity is usually obtained by tractioning the skin with appropriate elevators or sutures.

Endoscopy has been most effective for the forehead, where it has replaced the coronal incision, which goes from ear to ear, peeling the scalp down to the supraorbital rims. By means of endoscopy, the forehead lift becomes a more physiologic operation in that one frees up the forehead skin at the subperiosteal level, dividing the periosteum at the supraorbital rim and then removing the depressors of the eyebrows (the procerus and corrugator muscles in the glabella region), thus allowing the frontalis muscle to act unopposed to elevate the eyebrows. The key to the procedure appears to be the division of the periosteum, which by itself frees up the eyebrows and elevates them for at least 5–10 mm. In addition, removal of the glabellar muscles seems to ameliorate in a lasting way the vertical wrinkles in the glabella region. For suspension of the elevated eyebrows, different methods have been advocated that include soft tissue to bony anchoring, the use of temporary screws in the skull as well as miniplates, or, most simply, by providing external traction tied in between staples with nylon sutures. It appears that it is only necessary to maintain that elevation for a short period of time (3–5 days) until the periosteum reattaches at the higher level.

Endoscopy has also been effectively utilized to do a midface lift, and this procedure is applicable to younger patients where there is no excess skin in the face or neck and where scars will be unattractive.

Endoscopy is also utilized for the breasts—particularly for insertion of breast implants in the submammary or subpectoral plane through an axillary incision. An endoscope attached to a right-angle retractor allows perfect visualization of the cavity where the implant is to be inserted, and it allows the development of a pocket inferiorly down to—and if necessary below—the submammary fold and also the division of the lower portion of the origin of the pectoralis major muscle from the sternum to permit insertion of a saline implant and to provide acceptable cleavage. Appropriate instruments for dissection as well as hemostasis have been developed for this procedure, which recently has gained in popularity.

BLEPHAROPLASTY

Blepharoplasty involves removal of redundant skin of the upper and lower eyelids and removal of periorbital fat protruding through sagging orbital septa. It is done alone or as part of a facelift procedure.

Incisions are made in the upper lids surrounding previously marked redundant skin, which is removed. A subciliary incision is generally used in the lower lids. The orbicularis oculi muscle may be altered if necessary. The periorbital fat compartments are opened, and protruding fat is removed. The extent of redundant skin in the lower lid is gauged, and the skin is resected. External sutures are used. Minimal or no dressing is required.

Local anesthesia in the form of lidocaine with epinephrine is usually adequate. Swelling and ecchymosis subside in 7–10 days, and sutures are removed in 3–4 days.

Complications include bleeding, hematoma formation, epidermal inclusion cysts, ectropion, and asymmetry. Patients are usually satisfied with the results. Recurrence is much less of a problem than with facelift procedures.

In recent years there have been changes in the concept of the blepharoplasty procedure. For the upper lids, the change consists of the recognition of senile ptosis due to either disruption or stretching of the levator mechanism. This can be corrected by imbrication of the levator mechanism with sutures.

The second concept is with respect to the orbicularis muscle, which is disrupted when doing the traditional blepharoplasty. In an effort to avoid any injury to the orbicularis muscle, subconjunctival removal of fat has been advocated and is particularly applicable to young patients with congenital fat hernias. The subconjunctival approach is also utilized in conjunction with the laser, which has the effect of tightening the skin of the lower lid and ameliorating the periorbital wrinkles.

However, the most important change in the concept of blepharoplasty is the recognition that due to gravity the skin of the lid, which is distinct from the cheek skin, has dropped down below the infraorbital rim. With the midface procedure, the skin of the lid is restored to its youthful position above infraorbital rim, thus necessitating on occasion the removal of skin only and tightening of the uninjured and undivided orbicularis muscle.

MAMMOPLASTY

Aside from procedures related to breast cancer, surgery of the female breast is generally done for one of the following reasons: to increase the size of the breasts (augmentation mammoplasty), or to lift the breasts (mastopexy). Augmentation, lifting of the breasts, and correction of asymmetry are nearly always done for cosmetic reasons. Reduction of hypertrophied breasts may, however, be done for functional reasons, since such breasts can cause poor posture, back and shoulder pain, and discomfort due to grooves from brassiere straps.

Augmentation Mammoplasty

In procedures for augmentation of the breasts, a silicone bag filled with saline solution, air, or a combination of saline and air is placed beneath the breast tissue in the submammary or subpectoral plane. Incisions are concealed in the periareolar margin, inframammary fold area, or axilla. Dissection is then carried out above or below the pectoralis major muscle, and the implant is placed in the pocket created. Drains are not generally used, and a padded dressing providing light pressure is applied. The subpectoral plane is preferred by most surgeons for augmentation mammoplasty because it does not interfere with mammography, but it does necessitate division of the lower portion of the origin of the pectoralis major muscle up to approximately 3 o'clock in relation to the nipple to provide adequate cleavage.

The procedure can be done on an outpatient basis with local anesthesia, although this may not be satisfactory when subpectoral implants are used. General anesthesia is often used for augmentation procedures.

Although patient satisfaction is excellent in most cases, a significant rate of capsular contracture remains a problem in about 10%. Scar tissue around the implant may contract in variable degrees even in the same patient. Control of this process is difficult even though the best possible environment for healing is provided (ie, appropriate implants are used, infection is controlled, bleeding is not present, debris is removed, and movement is restricted). Implants placed in the subpectoral position appear to be associated with a lesser degree of capsular contracture and less severe deformity if contracture occurs. Deflation of saline implants occurs at a rate of 1% per year.

Other complications include hematoma, infection, exposure of the implant, deflation or rupture of the implant, asymmetry of the breasts, and external scars. Breast function and sensation are usually not altered in any way.

Silicone gel was used as an implant material for 30 years. Although the matter has recently become controversial, there is no definitive scientific evidence that silicone gel is carcinogenic or that it produces collagen type diseases. In fact, there is now sufficient evidence to warrant it as a safe substance, but even so its use is at present limited to investigational status.

Mastopexy

Mastopexy is another common procedure used for correction of sagging or ptotic breasts. Although some breasts develop in a ptotic manner, most cases are caused by normal relaxation of aging tissues, gravity, and atrophy after pregnancy and lactation. It is not clear whether use of a brassiere alters this process in any significant manner. The degree of deformity is defined by the relationship of the areola to the inframammary fold and the direction of the nipple. A ptotic breast will have a nipple that is below the inframammary line and pointing down towards the toes.

Correction may be done with simultaneous reduction or augmentation. An incision must be made around the areola, and the breast tissue itself is imbricated or, better still, an inferiorly based flap of breast tissue is designed and placed underneath the remnant superior part of the breast and over the pectoralis major muscle, serving as an autoaugmentation as one brings the lateral breast columns together. This procedure gives a more lasting effect than merely decreasing the skin envelope. Attempts at making more lasting corrections of ptosis of the breasts through the periareolar incision, which decreases the scarring, have included wrapping the breast with prosthetic material such as polyglycolic meshes or, more recently, by wrapping it around with segments of pectoralis major muscle.

Nonetheless, significant scarring may occur, particularly around the periareolar incision.

General anesthesia is usually necessary, and recovery from mastopexy may take 7–10 days. Complications include bleeding, infection, tissue loss, altered sensation or loss of function of the nipple and areolar areas, scars, and asymmetry of the breasts.

Patient satisfaction with the results is often not as great as with other procedures. Satisfaction often depends on how well the patient is prepared to accept the resulting scars.

Reduction Mammoplasty

Reduction mammoplasty is similar to mastopexy, since nearly all hypertrophic breasts are ptotic and must be lifted during correction. Enlargement can occur during puberty or later in life. Massive breasts can become a significant disability to the patient.

Although various techniques have been developed for breast reduction, nearly all require a pedicle to carry the nipple areola to its new position and a circumareolar incision as well as an inverted T incision beneath the areola. In gigantomastia, the nipple-areola is often removed as a free full-thickness graft and positioned appropriately. Most tissue is removed from the center and lower poles of the breast.

Vertical reduction mammoplasty has aroused considerable recent interest because of the decrease in amount of scarring. It can be accomplished through an incision made circumferentially around the areola and then a vertical incision that extends to and sometimes slightly below the inframammary fold. Resection of the breast tissue is done from below as well as from the lateral aspect of the breast. Considerable wrinkling of the skin occurs in an effort to avoid "T-ing off" the incision at the inframammary fold, but pleating of the skin usually resolves over a period of weeks. General anesthesia is nearly always required because dissection is considerable, but blood loss can be minimized by the use of epinephrine as a vasoconstricting agent. Transfusions are rarely indicated, and postoperative drains are often not used. The procedure can be done on an outpatient basis.

Although problems with nipple-areola loss, bleeding, infection, asymmetry of breasts, and scarring may occur; these women are generally among the most satisfied and appreciative of patients.

ABDOMINOPLASTY & OTHER AESTHETIC PROCEDURES

Other procedures usually classified as aesthetic are abdominoplasty and other operations for removal of excess tissue from the lower trunk, thighs, and upper arms. Patients with sagging tissue due to aging, pregnancies, multiple abdominal operations, or significant weight loss are usually good candidates for body contour procedures. Surgery can benefit the occasional patient with an isolated excessive deposit of fat below the lower abdominal skin, in the thighs (trochanteric lipodystrophy), or elsewhere. The typical case of generalized obesity, however, is not amenable to surgical correction of contour deformity.

Abdominoplasty usually involves removal of a large ellipse of skin and fat down to the wall of the lower abdomen. Dissection is carried out in the same plane up to the costal margin. The naval is circumscribed and left in place. After the upper abdominal flap is stretched to the suprapubic incision, excess skin and fat are excised. The fascia of the abdominal wall midline can be plicated and thus tightened. The umbilicus is exteriorized through an incision in the flap at the proper level, and the wound is closed over drains with a long incision generally in an oblique line or W shape just above the os pubis and out to the area below the anterior iliac crests (so-called bikini line).

Spinal anesthesia is used in some cases. Hospitalization may be required for a few days. Blood transfusions are sometimes necessary.

Complications involve blood or serum collections beneath the flap, infection, tissue loss, and wide scars. Results are generally very good, with excellent patient satisfaction in properly selected cases.

Various surgical procedures have been devised to remove excess skin and fat from the upper arms, buttocks, and thighs. Unfortunately, nearly all of these procedures result in significant scarring, and there may be difficulty in achieving a smooth transition between the end point of the contour alteration and normal tissue. The use of a suction apparatus fitted with appropriate cannulas to remove localized excess fat deposits has become widespread. It is clear, however, that patient selection and judicious use of liposuction are necessary to avoid complications, including hypovolemia due to blood loss, hematoma formation, skin sloughs, and waviness and depressions in the operative site. Used with discretion, liposuction can offer definition to areas of the abdomen, flanks, thighs, and buttocks.

SUCTION-ASSISTED LIPECTOMY

Suction-assisted lipectomy, or liposuction, has now become the most common cosmetic procedure performed in the United States. As presently practiced, it consists of infiltration of a solution of Ringer's lactate with the addition of 1 mg of epinephrine per 1000 mL of Ringer's and 250 mg of lidocaine—the former to provide vasoconstriction and the lidocaine to provide a certain amount of anesthesia and thus reduce the depth of general anesthesia. Some surgeons perform the entire operation under local anesthesia, necessitating the use of larger amounts of lidocaine.

Once the solution has been infiltrated sufficiently to produce tumescence, a small cannula is introduced through a small incision and suction is applied either with a syringe or with a suction machine. The fat that has been enlarged by the injection of tumescent solution dislodges easily and disrupts much faster than the blood vessels and the nerves.

Suction-assisted lipectomy is effective in removing abnormal bulges throughout the body, particularly in the trochanters or the abdomen and flanks, but it is not considered a weight reduction technique.

The procedure is safe when done by well-trained surgeons respecting sterility and in adequately equipped operating rooms. Safety in the use of up to 35 mg of lidocaine per kilogram has been established by clinical studies. Although fatalities have been reported with suction-assisted lipectomy—which is almost unacceptable in an entirely elective procedure—they are due to pulmonary embolization, perforation of the intestines, or severe infections of the abdominal wall. Fortunately, fatalities have markedly decreased since the American Society of Plastic and Reconstructive Surgeons established safety guidelines requiring that suctioning not exceed 5000 mL at a setting and that combined procedures should be cautiously undertaken.

Complications of suction-assisted lipectomy include irregularities of contour, dimpling, and, rarely, local infection at the entrance points.

Ultrasonic liposuction, external and internal, has also been advocated. External ultrasonic liposuction has the effect of a massage to disperse the infiltrated tumescent solution. Internal liposuction, on the other hand, dilutes the fat with ultrasonic energy, which produces heat, so that this diluted fat needs to be suctioned with standard suctioning equipment. The problems with ultrasonic liposuction include seroma formation, the need for larger portals of entrance, the possibility of burns of the skin if the cannula accidentally touches the skin, and, more importantly, problems with postoperative pain due perhaps to demyelinization of the sensory nerves as an effect of the ultrasonic energy.

Burk RW 3rd, Guzman-Stein G, Vasconez LO: Lidocaine and epinephrine levels in tumescent technique liposuction. Plast Reconstr Surg 1996;97:1379.

Cardoso de Castro C: The changing role of platysma in face lifting. Plast Reconstr Surg 2000;105:764.

Chajchir A: Fat injection: long-term follow-up. Aesthetic Plast Surg 1996;20:291.

Matarasso A, Hutchinson OH: Evaluating rejuvenation of the forehead and brow: an algorithm for selecting the appropriate technique. Plast Reconstr Surg 2000;106:687.

Pitanguy I: Facial cosmetic surgery: a 30-year perspective. Plast Reconstr Surg 2000;105:1517.

TELANGIECTASIAS (SPIDER VEINS)

When there is no trace of primary or secondary varicosities, most telangiectasias, or spider veins, are viewed as a cosmetic problem. However, one should be aware that in some cases spider veins may be an indication of deep venous valvular insufficiency. Factors that may play a role in the formation of spider veins include venostasis with decreased flow rate due to atony of the venous wall, chronic venous inflammation, hormonal influences, or venous compression at the saphenofemoral valve.

Treatment of spider veins is with sclerosing agents, which may include hypertonic saline, sodium tetradecyl, and hydroxypolyethoxydodecan (Sclerovein). These agents are injected directly into the spider veins with the objective of creating intimal damage that will result in fibrosis and obliteration of the lumen. The technique is simple and effective, but when the sclerosing agent extravasates it might produce superficial skin necroses.

Hand Surgery

44

Scott L. Hansen, MD, Mahesh Mankani, MD, & David M. Young, MD

Both in industry and in the home, the hand is the most commonly injured part of the body. A disorder of the hand rarely jeopardizes life but can significantly affect the ability to function.

Introduction

The prime functions of the hand are feeling (sensibility) and grasping. Sensibility is important on the radial sides of the index, long, and ring fingers and on the opposing ulnar side of the thumb, where one must feel and be able to pinch, pick up, and hold objects. The ulnar side of the small finger and its metacarpal, upon which the hand usually rests, must register the sensations of contact and pain to avoid burns and other trauma.

Mobility is critical for grasping. The upper extremity is a cantilevered system extending from the shoulder to the fingertips. It must be adaptable to varying rates and kinds of movements. Stability of proximal joints is essential for good skeletal control distally.

The specialization of the thumb has allowed humans to have superior aptitudes for defense, work, and dexterity. The thumb has exquisite sensibility and is a highly mobile structure with well-developed adductor and thenar (pronating) musculature. It is the most important digit of the hand, and every effort must be made to preserve its function.

The **position of function** of the upper extremity favors reaching the mouth and perineum and achieves a comfortable, forceful, and unfatiguing grip and pinch. The elbow is held at or near a right angle, the forearm neutral between pronation and supination, and the wrist extended 30 degrees with the fingers flexed to almost meet the opposed (pronated) tip of the thumb (Figure 44–1A). This is the desired position of the extremity if stiffness is likely to occur, and it should be maintained when joints are immobilized by splinting, arthrodesis, or tenodesis.

Opposite to the position of function is the **position of rest**, in which the flexed wrist extends the digits, making grip and pinch awkward, uncomfortable, weak, and fatiguing (Figure 44–1B). The forearm is usually pronated, and the elbow may be extended. This habitus is assumed, without intention, after injury, paralysis, or the onset of a painful stimulus. For that reason, it is also called the **position of the injury**. Immobility in this position jeopardizes function.

ANATOMY

All references to the forearm and hand should be made to the radial and ulnar sides (not lateral and medial) and to the volar (or palmar) and dorsal surfaces. The digits should be identified as the thumb, index finger, long finger, ring finger, and small finger.

Skin is the elastic outer sleeve and glove of the arm and hand. Sacrifice of its surface area or elasticity by debridement and fibrosis can severely diminish the range of motion and constrict circulation. In the adult hand, the dorsal skin stretches about 4 cm in the longitudinal and in the transverse planes when the palm is flattened and spread. The long finger can have as much as 48 cm^2 of skin cover, and the whole hand (exclusive of digits) has 210 cm^2.

Fascia anchors the palmar skin to bone to make pinch and grip stable; the midlateral fibers of Cleland's and Grayson's ligaments keep the skin sleeve from twisting around the digit (Figure 44–2). In the form of sheaths and pulleys, fascia holds tendons in the concavity of arched joints to convey mechanical efficiency and power. The fascial sleeve of the forearm, hand, and digits must sometimes be released along with skin to prevent or relieve congestion (eg, compartment syndrome). Any fascial compartment of the hand provides a space for infection or an avenue for its dissemination.

Each finger has three joints, the distal interphalangeal joint (DIP), the proximal interphalangeal joint (PIP), and the metacarpophalangeal joint (MCP). The thumb contains the interphalangeal joint (IP), the metacarpophalangeal joint (MCP), and the carpometacarpal joint (CMC). The position of the wrist stretches and governs the efficiency of extrinsic muscle contraction. The wrist is the "key joint" of the hand, governing motion of the digits, and must be included in the immobilization required for any major digital problem. The wrist is composed of a proximal and distal row of carpal bones. The proximal row contains the scaphoid, lunate, triquetrum, and pisiform, while the distal row contains the trapezium, trapezoid, capitate, and hamate. The stability of the digital joints and their planes of motion are governed by the length of the ligaments and the anatomy

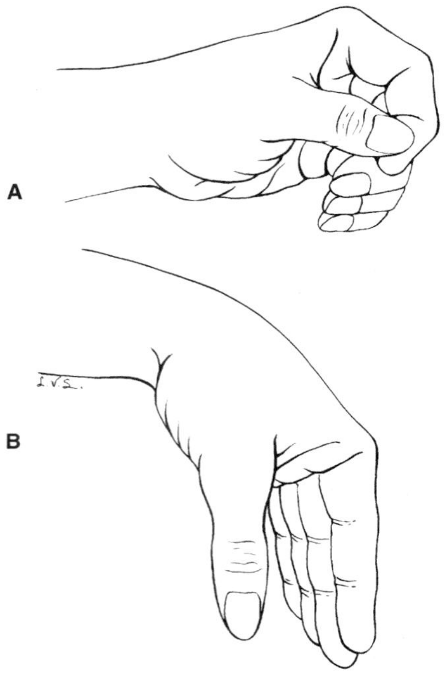

Figure 44–1. Positions of function (***A***) and rest (injury) (***B***).

of their articulating surfaces. The longitudinal and transverse arches of the hand (Figure 44–3) are architectural prerequisites to gripping, pinching, and cupping and are maintained by the active contraction and passive tone of intact muscles. The arches create the position of function. When the arches are collapsed, the hand assumes the position of injury. Loss of these arches is most often

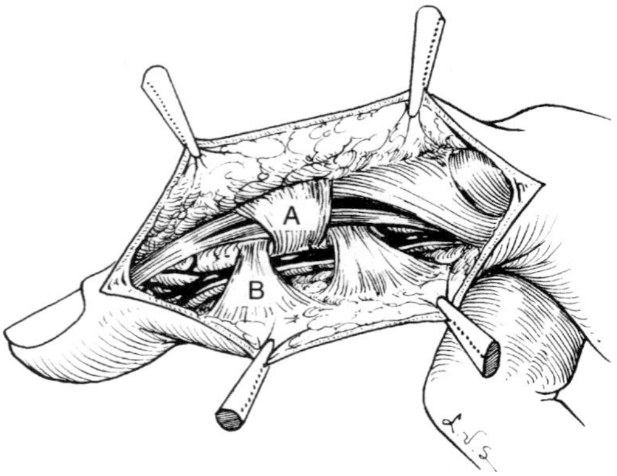

Figure 44–2. A: Cleland's ligament. ***B:*** Transverse retinacular ligament.

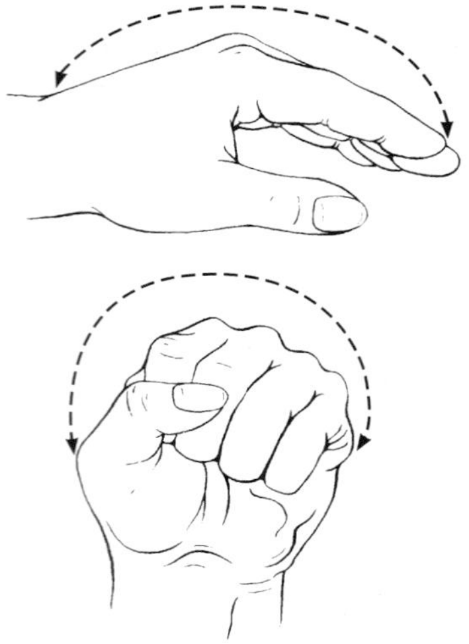

Figure 44–3. Longitudinal (*top*) and transverse (*bottom*) arches.

initiated by edema. They may be preserved by splinting in the position of function, elevation without constriction, and early restoration of active joint motion.

Each MCP and PIP joint has a distally anchored volar plate (Figure 44–4) in addition to collateral ligaments stabilizing the joint on either side (Figure 44–5). The

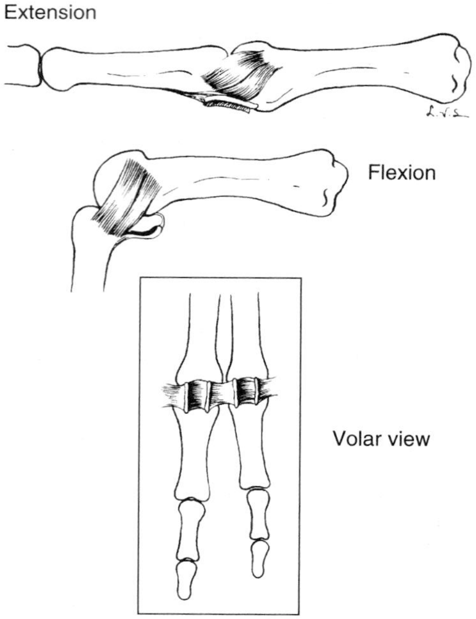

Figure 44–4. Volar plate.

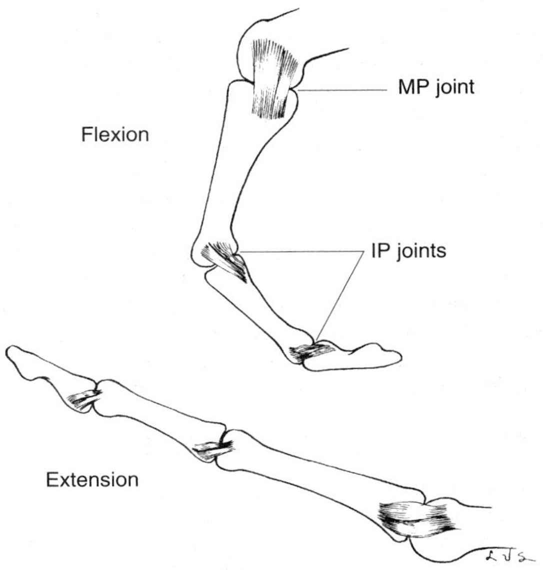

Figure 44–5. Collateral ligaments.

thickened lateral portions of the volar plate form the checkrein ligaments, which prevent IP hyperextension.

The extrinsic flexor tendons are contained in fibrous **sheaths** to prevent bowstringing and preserve mechanical efficiency as the digits flex into the palm. Pulleys (hypertrophied sections of the sheath) resist the points of greatest tendency to bowstring. The retinacular pulley system contains five annular bands and three cruciform bands. Sheaths are inelastic and relatively avascular. Therefore, they crowd and congest any swollen, inflamed, or injured tendons and curtail glide by friction, constriction, and the generation of inelastic adhesions. Five flexor tendon zones have been described. Zone II, or **"no man's land,"** is the zone from the middle of the palm to just beyond the PIP joint, wherein the superficialis and profundus tendons lay ensheathed together and where recovery of glide is difficult after wounding (Figure 44–6).

Across the wrist, the dense volar transverse carpal ligament closes the bony carpal canal (**carpal tunnel**) through which passes all eight finger flexors as well as the flexor pollicis longus and median nerve (Figure 44–6). The **ulnar bursa** is the continuation of the synovium around the long flexors of the small finger through the carpal tunnel, encompassing the other finger flexors, which interrupted their separated bursa at the mid palm level. The **radial bursa** is the synovium around the flexor pollicis longus contained through the carpal tunnel. These two bursas may intercommunicate. **Parona's space** is the tissue plane over the pronator quadratus in the distal forearm deep to the radial and ulnar bursas.

The extensor tendons are ensheathed in six individual compartments at the wrist beneath the extensor retinaculum (Figures 44–7 and 44–8), which predisposes to adhesions. Its role as a pulley is not vital and can be dispensed with.

The nerves of greatest importance to hand function are the musculocutaneous, radial, ulnar, and median nerves. The importance of the musculocutaneous and radial nerves combined is forearm supination and of the radial nerve alone is innervation of the extensor muscles. The ulnar nerve innervates 15 of the 20 intrinsic muscles. The median nerve, by its sensory innervation, is "the eye of the hand"; through its motor innervation, it maintains most of the long flexors, the pronators of the forearm, and the thenar muscles. Figure 44–9 shows the sensory distribution of the ulnar, radial, and median nerves.

CLINICAL EVALUATION OF HAND DISORDERS

The presenting complaint must be recorded in complete detail with egard to its mechanisms of onset, evolution,

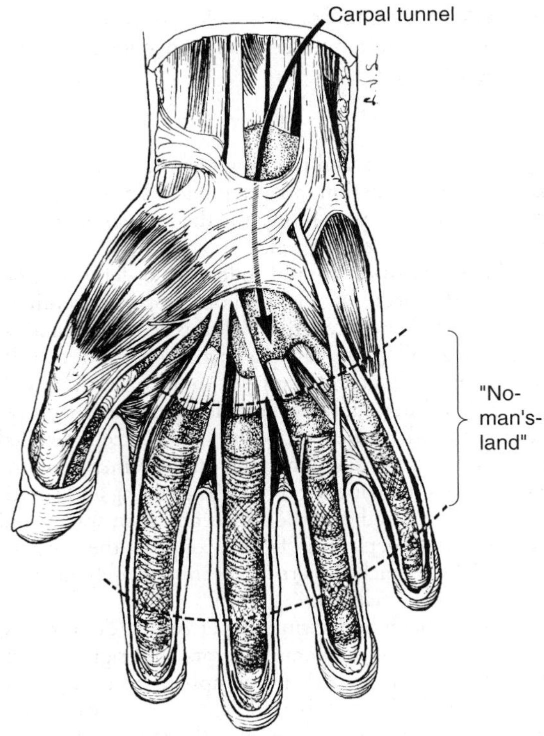

Figure 44–6. Carpal tunnel and no-man's-land.

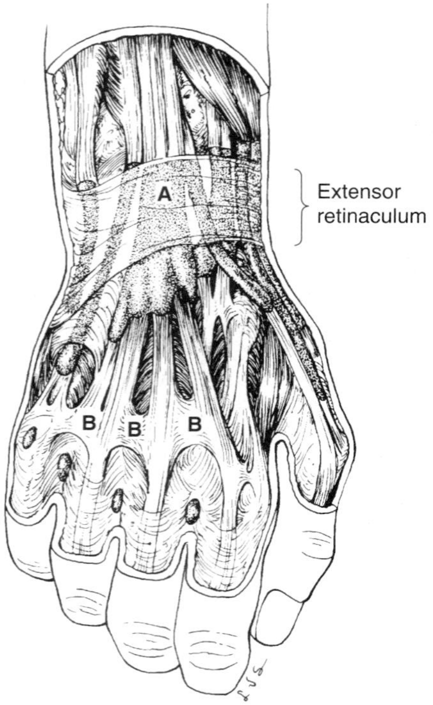

Figure 44–7. ***A:*** Extensor retinaculum over six tendon compartments. ***B:*** Juncturae tendinum (conexus intertendineus).

aggravating factors, and relieving factors. Age, sex, hand dominance, occupation, preexisting hand problems, and relevant matters pertaining to the patient's general health must also be recorded.

The examination should follow an orderly routine. Observe the neck, shoulders, both upper extremities, and the action and strength of all muscle groups, and be certain that all parts can pass painlessly and coordinately through a normal range of motion, starting with the head and neck and working down to the fingertips. Compare both upper extremities, and keep detailed immediate notes, diagrams, and measurements of the case. Having the patient reach for the ceiling and simultaneously open and close both fists and then spread and adduct the fingers and, finally, oppose the thumbs sequentially to each fingertip will immediately demonstrate any abnormalities.

Observe habitus, wasting, hypertrophy, deformities, skin changes, skin temperature, scars, and signs of pain (including when the patient attempts to bear weight on the palms). Feel the wrist pulses and the sweat of the finger pads, and test reflexes and the sensibility of the median, ulnar, and radial nerves.

Serial x-rays and laboratory studies may clarify a problem with an indolent evolution (eg, Kienböck's aseptic necrosis of the lunate, causing unexplained wrist pain). Contralateral and multiple-view x-rays in different planes are often helpful. In addition, CT scans, MRI, bone scans, or all of these may aid in diagnosis. This is especially true in patients who have persistent bone and joint pain or limited motion or in patients who have not attained adult growth. In the case of wrist problems, arthrograms and arthroscopy may be of diagnostic value. MRI can be quite helpful in the diagnosis of subtle carpal bone problems.

The diagnosis is often made by noting the response to therapy. This is particularly true in the case of local corticosteroids injected at the site of noninfectious inflammatory conditions (eg, carpal tunnel syndrome, trigger finger).

GENERAL OPERATIVE PRINCIPLES

A bloodless field (eg, by tourniquet ischemia) is essential for accurate evaluation, dissection, and management of tissues of the hand. This is achieved by elevating or exsanguinating the extremity and then inflating a padded blood pressure cuff around the arm to 100 mm Hg above systolic pressure. This is readily tolerated by the unanesthetized arm for 30 minutes and by the anesthetized arm for 2 hours.

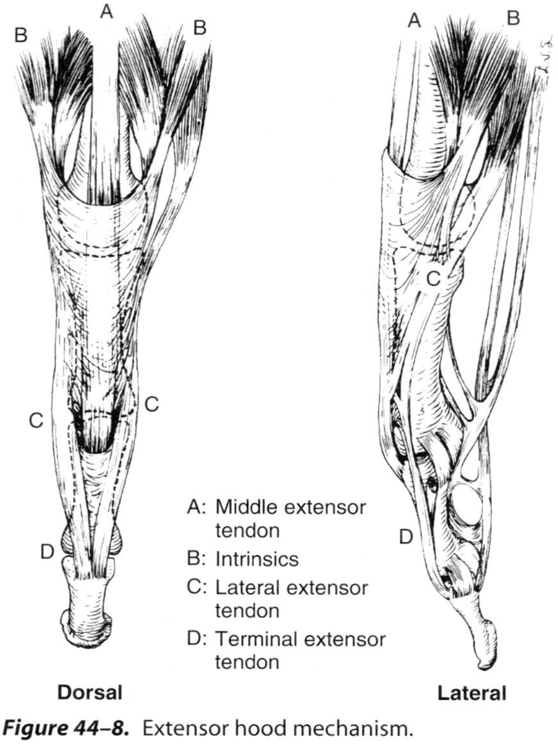

Figure 44–8. Extensor hood mechanism.

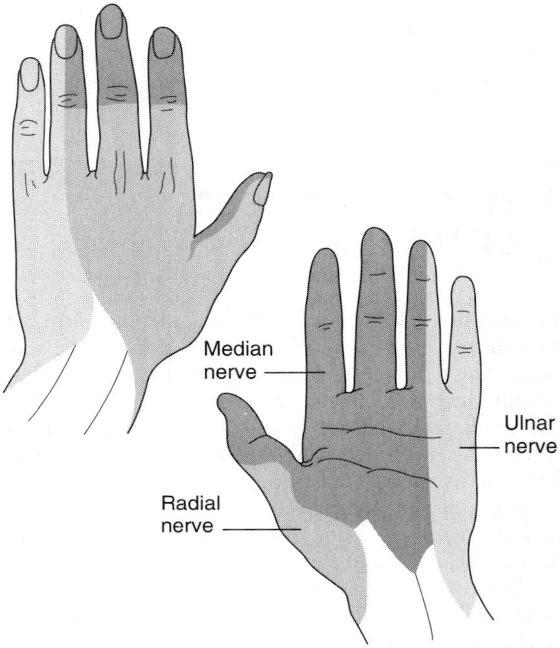

Figure 44–9. Sensory distribution in the hand. Dotted area, ulnar nerve; diagonal area, radial nerve; darker area, median nerve.

Incisions (Figure 44–10) must be either zigzagged across lines of tension (eg, must never cross perpendicularly to a flexion crease), termed Brunner's incisions, or run longitudinally in "neutral" zones (eg, connecting the lateral limits of the flexion and extension creases of the digits); and, whenever possible, must be designed so that a healthy skin-fat flap is raised over the zone of repair of a tendon, nerve, or artery.

Proper evaluation and treatment of an acute injury often requires extension of the wound. Normal structures can then be identified and traced into the zone of injury, where blood and trauma can make their identification difficult or impossible.

Constriction and tension by dressings must be avoided. The dressing should be applied evenly to the skin without wrinkles. The wound should be covered with a single layer of fine-mesh gauze followed by a wet spongy medium (fluffs, Rest-On, Kling, or Kerlix). Wetness facilitates the drainage of blood into the dressing, which should be applied with gentle pressure to restrict dead space.

Splinting and immediate elevation are paramount in controlling swelling and pain and favoring healing. In general, plaster (fast-setting) or fiberglass is preferred because of its adaptability to specific requirements. More often than not, the wrist requires immobilization along with any other part of the hand (Figures 44–11 and 44–12).

It must be appreciated that effective immobilization of a finger most often requires concomitant immobilization of one or more adjacent fingers, usually in the position of function. Straight splints such as tongue blades involve a hazard of digital stiffness and distortion and should not be used across the MP joint.

Persistence of pain signifies inadequate immobilization and, if throbbing is present, congestion. Congestion must be promptly relieved by elevation and sectioning of the cast and dressing and, if necessary, the skin and fascia.

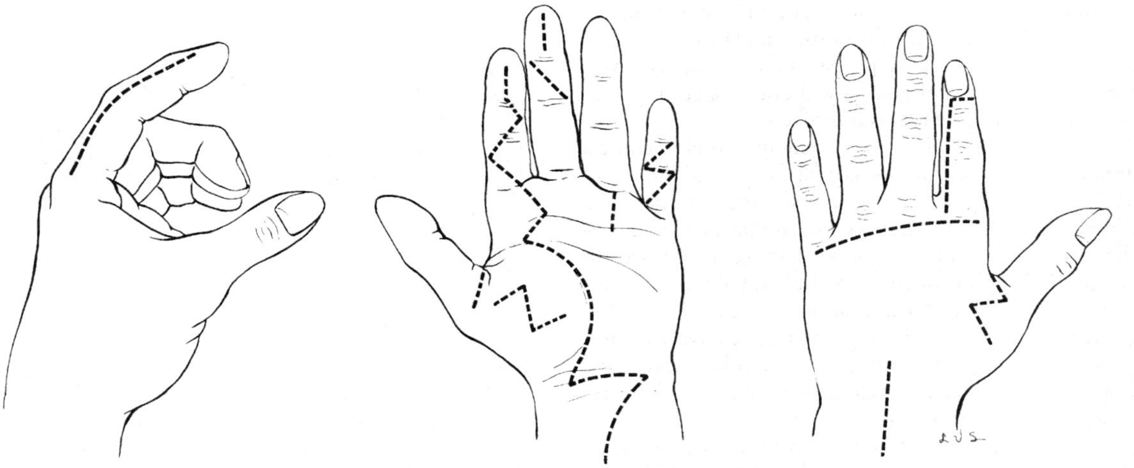

Figure 44–10. Proper placement of skin incisions.

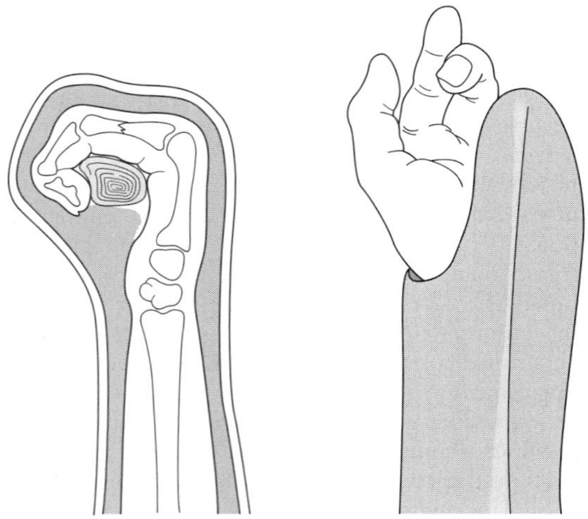

Figure 44–11. Casting.

CONGENITAL ANOMALIES OF THE HAND

Major congenital hand anomalies are not rare, with approximately one in 700 live births affected. When minor deformities are included, approximately 3% of all births are affected. Camptodactyly (bent finger), polydactyly (more than five fingers), and syndactyly (two or more fingers are joined together) are the most common malformations. Newborns with hand anomalies should be carefully examined for other malformations because multisystem syndromes can be present in 5% of patients (eg, VACTERL syndrome with radial head dysphasia).

Anomalies may be inherited, caused by environmental factors (drugs, viral infections, irradiation, alcohol), or may be idiopathic. Major genetic or major environmental causes are infrequently found, suggesting that the cause of most defects is multifactorial.

In order to simplify an extremely complex clinical problem, the American Society for Surgery of the Hand (ASSH) and all major international hand societies have adopted a single classification system that divides anomalies into six main categories: failures of formation (absent digits, phocomelia [seal limb]), failures of differentiation (syndactyly), duplication (polydactyly), undergrowth (brachydactyly), overgrowth (macrodactyly), and constriction ring syndrome (focal necrosis, intrauterine amputation). There is considerable overlap in the categories, as might be expected.

Ideally, surgery is performed early in the first two years of life, but timing is individually tailored to the problem.

McCarroll HR: Congenital anomalies: a 25-year overview. J Hand Surg [Am] 2000;25:1007.

Watson S: The principles of management of congenital anomalies of the upper limb. Arch Dis Child 2000;83:10.

TENDON DISORDERS OF THE HAND

Movement of the muscles of the hand and arm are transmitted into finger and wrist motion by the tendons. The tendons are strong, compact units that glide within their individual compartments. Disruption of the tendon by trauma or loss of tendon gliding by inflammation hinders tendon excursion and therefore limits active motion of the joints. Passive motion of the joint is still possible with an isolated tendon problem and distinguishes tendon disorders from joint disorders, when both active and passive motion are limited.

Tendon disruption can result from any penetrating injury and can be diagnosed by physical examination. A tendon injury should be suspected when the patient is unable to actively move a joint. Certain tendon lacerations, such as an isolated flexor digitorum superficialis disruption, may be masked because the profunda tendon can still move the entire finger. Blocking of profunda function by blocking flexion in the neighboring fingers (the profunda tendons are joined in the palm) reveals the injury to the superficialis when the injured PIP joint cannot be flexed.

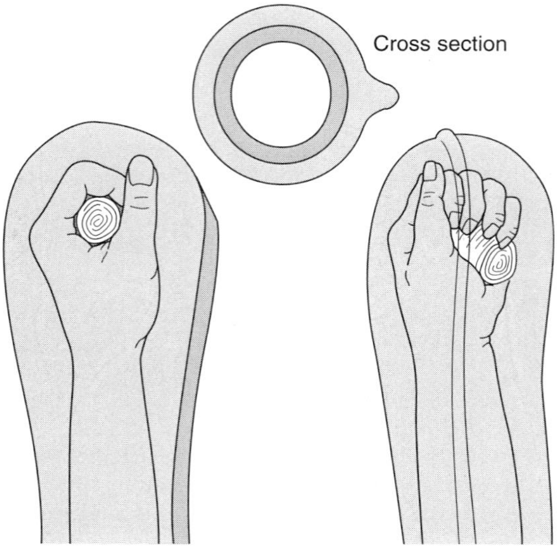

Figure 44–12. Casting.

The state of the wound and the complexity of the injury are the principal issues the hand surgeon must weigh in choosing between a primary or secondary tenorrhaphy. Tidy wounds generally favor primary tenorrhaphy. Primary tenorrhaphy is defined as one that is done within 24–72 hours after injury. When wounds are untidy, contaminated, or complicated by fracture or ischemia, formal tenorrhaphy may have to be delayed for weeks or months until the tendon bed is more favorable to healing and glide. However, interim tacking of the tendons—together, to tendon sheaths, or to bone—to maintain the fiber length of a muscle may be done as a preliminary procedure.

Preoperative treatment of fresh lacerations consists of wound closure, immobilization, and prophylactic antibiotics. Such cases can be deferred for definitive primary repair for 24 hours or more. The timing of delayed secondary procedures depends upon the resolution of wound edema and fibrous callus (ie, how soft and pliable it is). After 6–8 weeks, tendons that retract over 2.5 cm may defy full excursion because muscle elasticity has been lost or because the tendon is recoiled and congealed in scar.

Tenorrhaphy must be done without surface trauma along the tendon or its bed. The repair is made end-to-end or by weaving one tendon with the other, using nylon or wire sutures. A flexor tendon graft is anchored distally to bone (Figure 44–13). Tenodesis will occur if the surface of the tendon and the surface where adherence is desired are roughened. The position of immobilization should relieve tension on the tendon juncture. The duration of immobilization after tenorrhaphy is generally no more than 3–4 weeks. Controlled early passive or active mobilization after tenorrhaphy may be initiated to minimize excessive tendon scarring. This requires a very cooperative patient and close supervision by the hand therapist to avoid rupture of the repaired tendon.

Adhesions invariably form wherever tendons are even slightly inflamed or injured and can severely limit tendon function. Even so, adhesions are necessary for a tendon to reestablish continuity. With much active and passive movement over many months, tendon glide can be increased with maturation and molding of the collagen in the adhesions. If the adhesions remain thick and tendon excursion is limited, surgical release of the tendon adhesions (tenolysis) needs to be performed. Successful surgery requires the release of all adhesions limiting tendon glide without rupturing the tendon repair. Movement of the tendon as soon as possible after surgery under the guidance of the hand therapist is critical to avoid recurrence of adhesions.

The access to tenolysis should be through an incision offering effective exposure and placed where the immediate active and passive joint motion that must

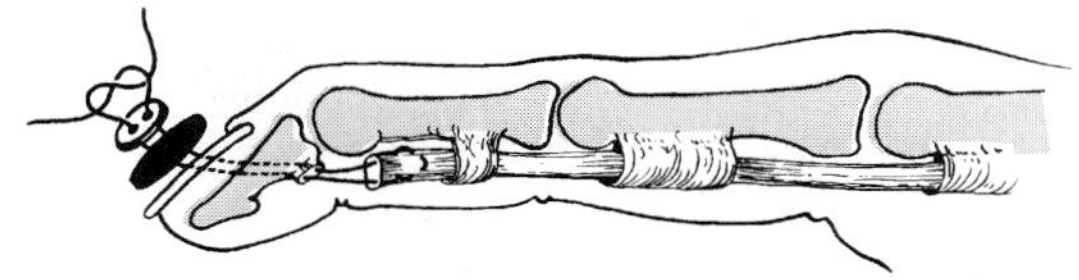

Figure 44–13. Flexor tenorrhaphy by advancement or graft. Pulleys are saved.

follow will not jeopardize healing of the wound by undue stretching or direct pressure. Performing a concomitant procedure requiring immobilization such as a neurorrhaphy should be avoided. The patient must understand that joint mobilization after tendon surgery is a time-consuming process, often taking many weeks or months to achieve maximum recovery.

"Mallet" finger ("baseball" or "drop" finger) (Figure 44–14) is due to disruption of the extensor tendon to the distal phalanx. A distal joint that can be passively but not actively extended is diagnostic. The injury most commonly results from sudden forceful flexion of the digit when it is held in rigid extension. Either the extensor is partially or completely ruptured or the dorsal lip of the bone is avulsed. Less frequently, the injury is due to direct trauma such as a laceration. An x-ray should be taken to determine the presence and extent of any fracture.

Treatment requires 6 weeks of continuous splinting in full distal joint extension (not hyperextension) with or without 40 degrees of PIP joint flexion. Joint fixation internally with a percutaneous Kirschner wire or externally with padded aluminum, plastic, or plaster splints is equally effective. A lacerated tendon should be repaired. When a significantly displaced fracture fragment represents one-third or more of the surface of the joint, it should be reduced by wiring or pinning. If there is sufficient articular surface disruption, one may consider joint fusion.

Swan-neck deformity (Figure 44–14) is a frequent complication of mallet finger, but it may also be the result of disparity of pull between the extrinsic flexors and extensor hood with or without attenuation of the DIP joint extensor. It is seen in congenitally hypermobile joints, spastic and rheumatoid states, and following resection of the superficialis tendon. The dorsal hood acts to extend the distal joint but is held back by its insertion at the base of the middle phalanx, which it therefore hyperextends. This in turn increases the tension on the profundus, which hyperflexes the DIP joint. If the mallet deformity is 25 degrees or less and there is some active distal joint extension, it may be treated by undermining and elevating the extensor hood at the PIP joint and severing its insertion on the base of the middle phalanx. Otherwise, the deformity

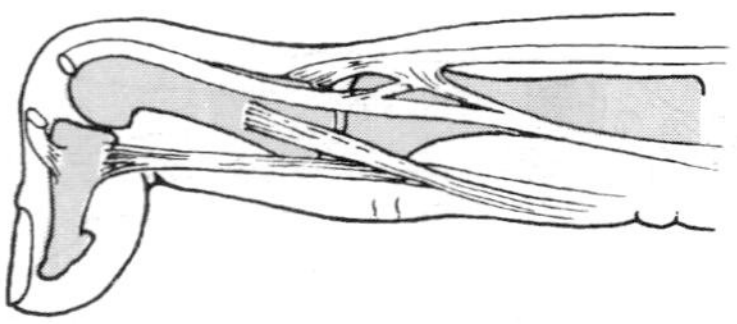

Figure 44–14. Mallet finger with swan-neck deformity.

may be corrected by tethering PIP joint extension with one slip of the flexor digitorum superficialis threaded through the flexor pulley of the proximal phalanx with the PIP joint flexed 20 degrees.

The **"buttonhole," or "boutonnière," deformity** (Figure 44–15) appears as the opposite of the swan-neck deformity: hyperextension of the DIP joint and flexion of the PIP joint. There is attenuation or separation of the dorsal hood, so that the middle extensor tendon becomes ineffective and the lateral extensor tendons shift volar to the PIP joint axis and the joint buckles dorsally. The entire extrinsic-intrinsic force on the hood passes onto the lateral extensor tendons, which flex the PIP joint and hyperextend the DIP joint. This deformity may develop suddenly or, more often, insidiously after closed blunt or open trauma over the dorsum of the PIP joint.

To avoid this complication, sutured extensor tendon lacerations and severe contusions over the PIP joint should always have the PIP joint alone splintered in extension for 3–4 weeks. Established deformities can be treated by such immobilization but more often require operative correction.

STENOSING TENOSYNOVITIS

In stenosing tenosynovitis there is a disproportion between the clearance inside a tendon pulley or tunnel and the diameter of the tendon or tendons that must glide through it. Any pulley or tunnel may be implicated. The more common sites are as follows:

(1) The proximal digital (A1) pulleys in the distal palm, causing **trigger finger** or thumb. There is local tenderness of the pulley; pain, which may be referred to the PIP joint; and (usually but not always) locking of the digit in flexion with a painful jog as it goes into extension (ie, as the bulge in the tendon or tendons passes through the tight pulley).

(2) The pulley over the radial styloid housing the abductor pollicis longus and extensor pollicis brevis, causing **De Quervain's tenosynovitis**. Local tenderness and pain occur if these tendons are actively stretched (eg, Finkelstein's test).

Relief of the symptoms can be achieved by local injections of triamcinolone mixed with lidocaine. Immediate surgery is justified if the constriction is so tight that the tendon is locked. Surgical section of the constricting tendon sheath is also indicated if symptoms persist or recur. When releasing the flexor tendon, care is taken not to resect more than the section of sheath restricting the tendon or else the tendon will pull away from the finger like a bowstring and weaken the grip.

Anderson B, Kaye S: Treatment of flexor tenosynovitis of the hand ("trigger finger") with corticosteroids. Arch Intern Med 1991;151:153.

Chan DY: Management of simple finger injuries: the splinting regime. Hand Surg 2002;7:223.

Finsen V, Hagen S: Surgery for trigger finger. Hand Surg 2003;8: 201.

Ingari JV, Pederson WC: Update on tendon repair. Clin Plast Surg 1997;24:161.

Rockwell WB, Butler PN, Byrne BA: Extensor tendon: anatomy, injury, and reconstruction. Plast Reconstr Surg 2000;106: 1592.

Thien T, Becker J, Theis JC: Rehabilitation after surgery for flexor tendon injuries in the hand. Cochrane Database Syst Rev 2004;CD003979.

SKELETAL INJURIES OF THE HAND

Injuries to the bones and joints of the hand are the most common skeletal injuries treated by physicians. Recognition of the injury, appropriate diagnostic tests, and timely treatment are essential for minimizing the complications of these injuries. Some patients may neglect obvious fractures and dislocations in hope of spontaneous recovery. More subtle injuries to the wrist are more often neglected by the patient and sometimes even missed by physicians until further damage is done. The use of the fluoroscope, found in many offices, greatly enhances the surgeon's ability to diagnose fractures. The machine allows real-time assessment of the bones as part

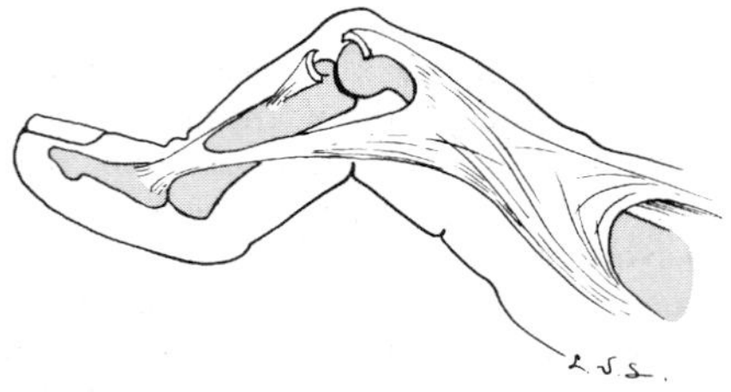

Figure 44–15. Buttonhole deformity.

of the physical examination. A common late sequela of skeletal injury at the articular surfaces is osteoarthritis, which is difficult to treat. Patients with symptoms related to the hand or wrist but without a discernible cause should be referred early to a hand specialist.

METACARPALS & PHALANGES

Fractures

Fractures of the metacarpal and phalangeal bones such as distal phalanx tuft of the fingers caught in closing doors and metacarpal shaft fractures of the ulnar side of the hand (boxer's fractures) create an obvious deformity and are easy to diagnose. Adequate x-rays of the specific site of the fracture with frontal, lateral, and oblique views are essential for developing a treatment plan.

Fractures of the shaft can usually be treated with closed reduction and a cast or splint holding the hand in the position of function (Figure 44–1) for 3–4 weeks. Residual angulation of a metacarpal shaft fracture of up to 30 degrees in the fifth finger and 20 degrees in the fourth finger is functionally well tolerated, although a dorsal bump may be aesthetically unpleasant. However, even a small rotational misalignment of the fracture at the metacarpal bone results in crossing of the fingers in flexion and causes severe dysfunction.

When fractures do not remain reduced, fixation with Kirschner pins placed through the skin is required. Placement of more than one pin is usually needed to keep the fracture reduced. The pins are removed after the fracture is healed. Displaced and comminuted fractures may require opening of the fracture site and reduction under direct visualization. Pins and, more recently, very small and thin metal plates and screws are used to maintain reduction. Metal plates provide strong support to the fracture site and allow earlier mobilization of the hand. However, plates are more difficult to place in small bones and occasionally interfere with tendon function.

Fractures through an articular surface need to be carefully evaluated. Nondisplaced fractures can be treated by casting. Displaced fractures require open reduction and accurate pin or lag screw fixation since discrepancies of the articular surface will eventually result in degenerative arthritis.

Fractures of the distal phalanx from crush injuries require attention to the disrupted nail bed. The nail is removed to decompress the painful subungual hematoma and provide irrigation of the open fracture and careful reapproximation of the nail matrix. Large disruptions in the nail matrix may result in deformity of the regenerating nail. The nail is replaced under the nail fold as a splint. A protective splint is placed over the finger to hold the distal fragment in extension.

An intra-articular fracture of the base of the thumb metacarpal bone with subluxation (displacement) of the metacarpal leaving a volar pyramidal shaped fragment attached to the trapezium is called a **Bennett fracture**. The anterior oblique ligament, responsible for stability of the thumb base, is left attached to the pyramidal fragment. The remainder of the thumb metacarpal is unstable and limits use of the thumb. The fracture must be reduced and stabilized with Kirschner pins or a lag screw. Accurate reduction of the articular surface is crucial in reducing complications. Even despite adequate treatment, most patients eventually develop arthritis.

Dislocations

Dislocations are most common in the PIP joint. Injuries are classified according to the position of the distal digit as hyperextension, dorsal displacement, or volar displacement. The type of dislocation determines which structures, such as the volar plate, collateral ligaments, and extensor tendon, are likely to be disrupted.

The MP and MC joints are better protected by surrounding soft tissue but can still be dislocated. The MP joint of the thumb is most frequently injured by forced abduction. The ulnar collateral ligament is torn, as occurs with forced use of a ski pole or as historically described in gamekeepers when twisting the neck of birds ("gamekeeper's thumb"). Of the MC joints, the fifth is most commonly injured. A fracture analogous to Bennett's fracture can occur. Examination to determine injury to the deep motor branch of the ulnar nerve in this area should be done.

Radiographs are occasionally useful for diagnosis, but the physical examination is most important. Since pain often limits the extent of the examination, regional anesthesia with a wrist or finger block allows a more detailed examination. Partial tears of ligaments without dislocation or instability are treated by splints. Dislocations can usually be reduced, and the need for surgical therapy is determined by the stability of the joint after reduction. Stable reductions are treated with early mobilization to decrease stiffness.

Fracture dislocations usually require surgical repair. Instability after reduction can be treated by repair of the torn collateral ligament or volar plate. Severe dislocations of the PIP and MP joints can result in interposition of disrupted soft tissue in the joint, making closed reduction impossible. The joint must be opened and the trapped soft tissue removed and repaired to correct the dislocation. A complete disruption of the ulnar collateral ligament in a gamekeeper's thumb injury can result in interposition of the adductor aponeurosis between the torn ends of the ulnar collateral ligament. The ends of the ligament must be reduced and repaired under direct vision.

WRIST & FOREARM INJURIES

Fractures

Fractures in the wrist and forearm usually result from falls on the outstretched hand. The distal radius is most commonly fractured. Many classification systems and eponyms have been used based on the extent and displacement of the fracture and involvement of the articular surface. The hyperextended wrist also exposes the scaphoid bone to injury in a fall. Since the scaphoid is crucial to wrist motion, displacement of the fracture is poorly tolerated. In addition, the blood supply enters the distal part of the bone and makes ischemic necrosis of the proximal fragment a problem.

Diagnosis of distal radius fractures is not difficult, but scaphoid fractures can easily be missed. Special radiographic views of the wrist or CT or MRI scans may be needed in difficult cases. If the clinical picture is suspicious but the radiographs are inconclusive, the wrist should be immobilized. Repeat radiographs in 2 weeks may demonstrate the fracture. Untreated scaphoid fractures lead to debilitating arthritis of the wrist.

Distal radius fractures are treated by reduction and immobilization. As with other fractures, articular irregularities and unstable fractures need to be treated by open reduction and internal fixation. Use of bone grafting and external fixation devices to initially treat the fracture has been advocated. Scaphoid fractures require careful and prolonged immobilization. Displaced fractures or nonhealing fractures require operative treatment with screw immobilization, bone grafts, or scaphoid replacement.

Dislocations & Sprains

Dislocations and ligamentous (sprain) injuries of the wrist are the most difficult hand injuries to diagnose and treat. Wrist injuries often present as a painful wrist after minor trauma. Routine radiographs are often normal, and physical findings can be unimpressive. Still, these injuries can lead to chronic problems. Special stress radiographs, fluoroscopy, and physical maneuvers (scaphoid shift test) help delineate the injury.

The scaphoid lunate ligament is most often injured. Instability of the joint is best treated by repair or reconstruction of the ligament. Injury of the ligaments of the radiocarpal-radioulnar joint is likewise difficult to determine. Surgical treatment involves repair of the disrupted ligament.

Bhandari M, Hanson BP: Acute nondisplaced fractures of the scaphoid. J Orthop Trauma 2004;18:253.

Cohen MS: Fractures of the carpal bones. Hand Clin 1997;13:587.

Corley FG Jr, Schenck RC Jr: Fractures of the hand. Clin Plast Surg 1996;23:447.

Divelbiss BJ, Baratz ME: The role of arthroplasty and arthrodesis following trauma to the upper extremity. Hand Clin 1999;15:335.

Kozin SH, Thoder JJ, Lieberman G: Operative treatment of metacarpal and phalangeal shaft fractures. J Am Acad Orthop Surg 2000;8:111.

Mack MG et al: Clinical impact of MRI in acute wrist fractures. Eur Radiol 2003;13:612.

Pao VS, Chang J: Scaphoid nonunion: diagnosis and treatment. Plast Reconstr Surg 2003;112:1678.

Wolf JM, Weiss AP: Portable mini-fluoroscopy improves operative efficiency in hand surgery. J Hand Surg [Am] 1999;24:182.

NERVE DISORDERS

Nerve disorders of the hands are conveniently organized into compression neuropathies, injuries of peripheral nerves, and various problems located more proximal to the upper extremities (spinal cord or central nervous system). For nerve dysfunction due to strokes, cerebral palsy, and spinal cord injury, readers are referred to more specific textbooks on hand surgery.

Compression Neuropathies

Compression of the nerves of the upper extremities due to an increase in surrounding tissue pressure occurs in specific locations and causes predictable signs and symptoms. Tissue edema from a variety of causes such as crushing injuries, vascular disorders, and prolonged repetitive hand motions can compress nerves traveling within tight compartments of the arm and produce nerve ischemia. Prolonged ischemia results in axonal destruction and sensory and motor dysfunction.

The median nerve can be compressed by local structures at the elbow (pronator syndrome), the anterior interosseous branch, and the wrist (carpal tunnel syndrome). Compression of the median nerve at the elbow causes forearm pain and sensory changes in the radial four fingers. The anterior interosseous branch of the median nerve is purely a motor nerve, and lesions produce only weakness of thumb and index finger flexion and no pain. Carpal tunnel syndrome presents with weakness in the hand, sensory abnormalities of the fingers sparing the little finger, and exacerbation of symptoms on forced flexion of the wrist (Phalen's sign) or tapping the nerve at the wrist (Tinel's sign). Shoulder, elbow, and forearm pain is also common. Atrophy of thenar muscles occurs in long-standing cases.

The ulnar nerve can be compressed at the elbow (cubital tunnel syndrome) or the wrist (Guyon's canal). Sensory abnormalities in the little finger and weakness of intrinsic hand muscles occur with compression in either area. Segmental nerve conduction velocity tests help to localize the abnormality to one site or the other. Compression of the radial nerve occurs most frequently from fractures of the humerus. Compression of the nerve along the proximal radius (radial tunnel syndrome) causes diffuse pain around the elbow but occurs rarely.

Abnormal findings on nerve conduction studies and clinical manifestations of nerve compression are adequate for diagnosis. Electromyography (EMG) demonstrating denervation patterns in the corresponding muscles or slowing of nerve conduction velocities indicates injury to the nerve. Although helpful, these tests only complement the physical examination, since electrodiagnostic tests can occasionally be inaccurate.

Early or mild cases of compression are treated by controlling tissue swelling. Resting the extremity with splints and using nonsteroidal anti-inflammatory medications and local injection of steroids often resolves the problem. If repetitive motions, such as typing, are thought to be the cause, changing the motion or hand position should help. If clinical manifestations are severe or if nonsurgical therapy fails, surgical decompression of the nerve is advocated.

Carpal tunnel syndrome is the most common type of compression neuropathy and one of the most common hand disorders. Surgical therapy of median nerve entrapment in the carpal tunnel or any of the compression neuropathies requires detailed knowledge of the anatomy. Division of the constricting structures results in partial or complete reversal of the abnormalities. In the carpal tunnel, the median nerve is surrounded on three sides by carpal bones. Incision of the transverse carpal ligament, which forms the roof of the tunnel, decompresses the nerve. Occasionally, internal fibrosis of the nerve occurs and internal neurolysis is required to allow the nerve to recover. Endoscopic release of the carpal tunnel through a smaller skin incision has been advocated.

Nerve Injuries

Injury to individual peripheral nerves of the arm results in predictable and defined deficits. More proximal injuries to the brachial plexus have more variable manifestations. Nerve conduction can be disrupted in the absence of structural changes due to compression, blunt injury, or ischemia (neuropraxia). More severe injury results in disruption of the axon with preservation of the epineurial covering of the nerve (axonotmesis). Both types of injury are followed by spontaneous recovery of function of good quality. Complete disruption of the nerve (neurotmesis), as with a laceration, requires surgical repair. Wallerian degeneration of the distal nerve occurs in both neurotmesis and axonotmesis, and recovery depends upon the growth of the cut axon to the end organ. However, with neurotmesis, orientation of the proximal and distal axons are lost and recovery may be incomplete, especially in mixed motor and sensory nerves. Methods to differentiate sensory from motor fascicles have been used during repairs with some benefit.

A patient with loss of the radial nerve is unable to extend the fingers or wrist, and a wrist drop is noticeable. The sensory loss to the dorsum of the hand is well tolerated. Median nerve dysfunction causes problems with opposition of the thumb and grip of the fingers. Sensory loss is to the radial four digits and can significantly impair use of the hand. An ulnar neuropathy causes dysfunction of the intrinsic muscles of the hand, clawing of the ulnar two digits, and weakness in gripping a key. Sensation is lost along the ulnar side of the hand.

Diagnosis of nerve injury is mainly by the physical examination. Understanding the functional anatomy of the peripheral nerves allows adequate evaluation of nerve loss. Electrodiagnostic studies are used to distinguish between partial and complete lesions and to follow functional recovery.

Obvious and complete disruption of the nerve is treated best by early surgical exploration and repair. An incomplete lesion or questionable disruption of nerve integrity is best treated with close observation, splinting to prevent contractures, and surgical exploration if no recovery occurs. Segmental loss of nerves requires nerve grafts, usually taken from a minor sensory nerve, such as the sural nerve, to bridge the gap. Results of primary repair are better than the results of grafts, and repairs done soon after injury are better than delayed repairs. Recovery of protective sensation of the hand is crucial for good functional recovery.

Motor dysfunction due to nerve damage can be treated by arthrodesis (stabilization of flail joints) and tendon transfers. Tendon transfers work best when the transferred muscle is unaffected by the nerve injury, has direction of force and excursion similar to those of the damaged muscle, and produces no further deficits due to loss of the donor muscle. For radial nerve palsy, the pronator teres to extensor carpi radialis transfer provides wrist extension, flexor carpi radialis to extensor digitorum communis transfer gives finger extension, and the palmaris longus or flexor digitorum superficialis of the fourth finger transfer to the extensor pollicis longus extends the thumb. Restoration of thumb opposition is most important with median nerve palsies, and the use of several donor muscles to achieve this result has been described. Tendon transfers to control claw deformity and strengthen key pinch are used for ulnar nerve palsies.

Brandsma JW, Ottenhoff-De Jonge MW: Flexor digitorum superficialis tendon transfer for intrinsic replacement. Long-term results and the effect on donor fingers. J Hand Surg [Br] 1992;17:625.

Dvali L, Mackinnon S: Nerve repair, grafting, and nerve transfers. Clin Plast Surg 2003;30:203.

Hentz VR: Surgical strategy: matching the patient with the procedure. Hand Clin 2002;18:503.

Richards RR: Tendon transfers for failed nerve reconstruction. Clin Plast Surg 2003;30:223.

Tung TH, Mackinnon SE: Brachial plexus injuries. Clin Plast Surg 2003;30:269.

Verdugo RJ et al: Surgical versus non-surgical treatment for carpal tunnel syndrome. Cochrane Database Syst Rev 2002;CD001552.

HAND INFECTIONS

Small breaks in the skin or nails of the hand can lead to widespread infection and abscess. The original injury can oftentimes not be identified. Poor venous and lymphatic drainage of the upper extremity, especially when held in a dependent position, aggravate the situation. Immunocompromised patients (diabetics, AIDS patients) are prone to develop extensive infections very quickly and should be treated more carefully.

The hallmark of infection (pain, swelling, and erythema) may be widespread in the hand and make localizing the infection difficult. Swelling of the dorsum of the hand is common even with palmar infections, and knowledge of the tissue planes of the hand is crucial to understanding how infections spread. Lymphatic streaks (lymphangitis) extending up the arm indicate rapid extension of the infection and must be treated urgently.

Oral antibiotics effective against staphylococcus and common anaerobic organisms (ie, first-generation cephalosporins and penicillin) are adequate to treat most infections. Infections from animal bites (*Pasteurella multocida*) and human bites (oral flora) also respond to penicillin. The intravenous route is reserved for severe infections or for those not responsive to oral antibiotics. Once the situation improves, oral antibiotics are given for 7–10 days. Equally as important, the infected hand needs to be immobilized and elevated. Pillows and trapezes help to elevate the arm, but slings aggravate the dependent position of the arm and should not be used. The best results are obtained when the patient is convinced that elevation of the extremity is beneficial.

Once treatment of a hand infection is begun, improvement within 24 hours is expected. If prompt improvement does not occur, an occult abscess may be present. Obvious abscesses should be drained at the point of maximum tenderness or the point of maximum fluctuation, where the overlying tissues are thinnest. The drainage wound should run parallel to and not across the paths of nerves, arteries, and veins. Wounds should be made long enough and should be zigzagged, when necessary, to avoid secondary contractures. Ultrasonography may be useful when a definite abscess cannot be located.

Pyogenic Granuloma

Pyogenic granuloma is a mound of granulation-like tissue 3–20 mm (or more) in diameter. It usually develops under a chronically moist dressing and may form around a suture. A small granuloma (6–7 mm in diameter) exposed to the air will soon dry up and epithelialize, whereas larger ones should be scraped flush with the skin under local anesthesia and covered with a thin split-thickness skin graft. If the granuloma is adjacent to the nail and the nail is acting as a foreign body aggravating the reaction, the nail must be removed.

Nail Infections

The nail fold is often traumatized and becomes secondarily inflamed, leading to a **paronychia** on the radial or ulnar side. The lesion is called an **eponychia** if it involves the base of the nail, although the entire fold can be involved; and a **subungual abscess** if pus develops and extends under the nail plate. Because of the early and unrelenting tissue tension that develops, these entities are quite painful. Early treatment before abscess formation is by means of soaking, elevation, immobilization, and antibiotics. Most abscesses can be drained painlessly with a scalpel without drawing blood; the insensible necrotic skin cap should be cut through where it points (Figure 44–16). Sagittal incisions, which form a "trapdoor" of the eponychium, should be reserved for the long-standing case in which a dense fibrous callus of the nail fold must be excised. Occasionally the nail must be basally excised or totally avulsed, after which the eponychial fold should be separated from the nail matrix by a thin, loose pack. Chronically wet nails of dishwashers may develop tissue changes and nail deformities, which are best treated by removing the nail plate. Fungal infections should be diagnosed and treated, and the fingers should be protected from water or excessive sweating.

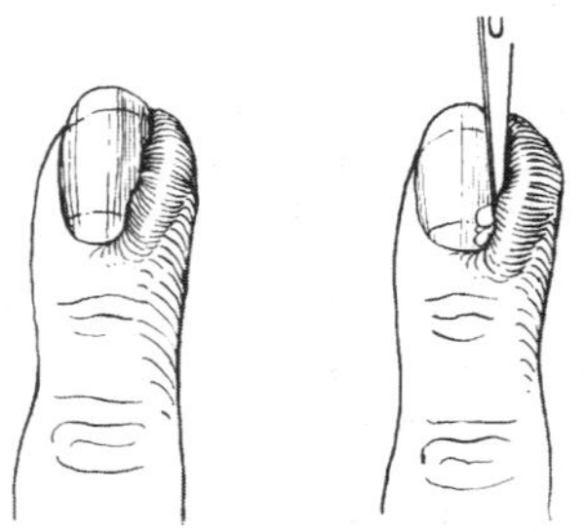

Figure 44–16. Incision and drainage of paronychia.

Deep Space Abscess

A **felon** is an abscess in the pulp of the fingertip and is often deep and very painful. Untreated or inadequately drained abscesses may lead to osteomyelitis of the distal phalanx. Wide incision and drainage with disruption of the many vertical fibrous septa of the pulp space are required to adequately drain the abscess (Figure 44–17). The traditional fishmouth incision is no longer recommended for drainage since it may expose the underlying bone and because it often heals in a tender scar. Instead, lateral through-and-through incisions or direct incisions on the pulp, where the abscess points, have better results (Figure 44–18).

The **web spaces** are the path of least resistance for pus from infected distal palm calluses, puncture wounds, and infections of the lumbrical canals. Infection and abscess formation in the dorsum of the thumb web may be the result of extension from the volar thenar space (collar button). A dorsal incision is usually made between the fingers to drain both spaces. A dorsal incision in the web of the thumb may be zigzagged to prevent contracture (Figure 44–10).

The **midpalmar space** becomes infected by direct puncture or by extension of infections from the flexor sheaths of the 2nd, 3rd, or 4th digit (Figure 44–6). Only the skin should be incised over the point of fluctuation. The rest of the dissection should be carried out by gentle spreading with a blunt clamp to avoid injury to arteries, nerves, and tendons. Infection spreads easily from this space along the lumbrical canals and to the thenar space.

A hypothenar space abscess is usually a product of a penetrating wound and should be drained where it points. The same is true for a thenar space abscess, which may point in the palm rather than the thumb web.

Infection within the synovium of the flexor tendon is difficult to diagnose. **Pyogenic tenosynovitis** spreads easily down the tendon sheath to affect the other fingers. Untreated, the infection causes adhesions of the tendon to the surrounding soft tissues and permanently limits movement of the fingers.

The signs of flexor tendon infection described by Kanaval include fusiform swelling of the digit, severe pain on passive finger extension, a fixed flexed position of the finger, and, most importantly, tenderness over the extent of the tendon sheath into the palm. Ultrasonography of the distal palm can also be helpful when the diagnosis is unclear. The probe is held across the palm and reveals swelling of the involved tendon and fluid around the tendon at the proximal flexor sheath.

Only unresponsive, tensely swollen, and toxic cases need immediate incision and drainage. With rest, elevation, and antibiotics, it is safe to observe most cases for several hours. The most common method of incision and drainage (Figure 44–19) is to make a short sagittal midline distal wound immediately over the tendon and introduce a small plastic catheter into the synovial bursa for irrigating with an antibiotic solution. The catheter should pass through the sheath and exit by a counterincision in the palm to allow for drainage of the fluid. Not all surgeons advocate placement of an irrigation catheter, however. These incisions do not cross flexion creases. The hand should then be elevated and immobilized in the position of function and covered by a dressing. Phlegmonous tenosynovitis usually requires opening of the entire synovial sheath (often through a lateral mid axial digital incision, or longitudinally across the wrist for extensor sheath infections) and, frequently, excision of necrotic tendon and sometimes amputation of a digit.

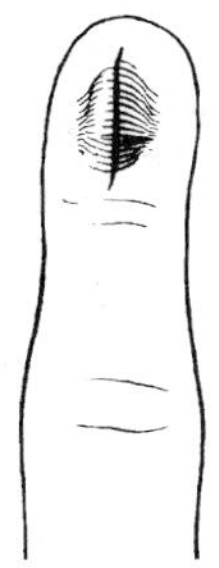

Figure 44–18. Incision of felon (distal fat pad infection).

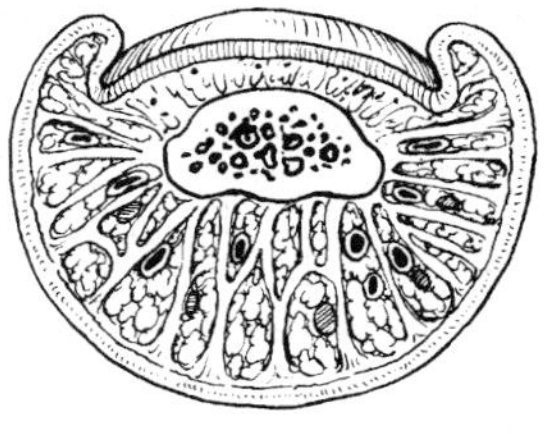

Figure 44–17. Cross section of distal phalanx.

Other Infections

Necrotizing soft tissue infections of the upper extremity are rare but devastating when they occur. The condition has been called many different names such as necrotizing fasciitis, Meleney's ulcer, and streptococcal gangrene. The organisms responsible include clostridium species, *Streptococcus pyogenes,* and mixed infections. The hallmarks are the rapid spread of infection and the extensive necrosis of soft tissue. Treatment includes wide debridement of the necrotic tissue and intravenous antibiotics.

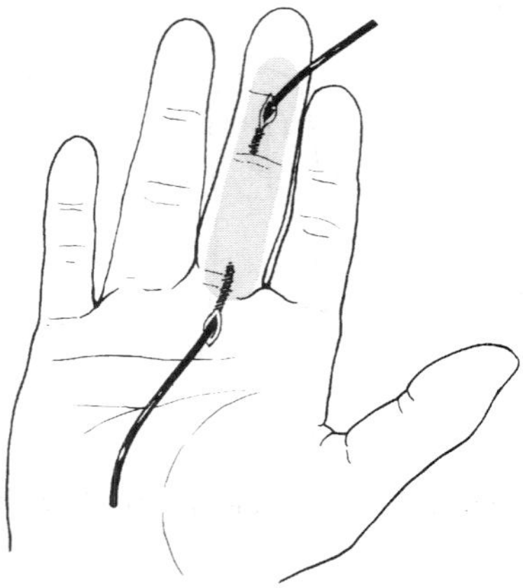

Figure 44–19. Drainage and irrigation for septic tenosynovitis. The antibiotic solution drips in through the distal catheter and drains out through the proximal one.

Human bite wounds of the hand occur most often during altercations when the fist strikes an opponent's tooth. The MP joint can be entered. The injury is often ignored by the patient until infection of the joint has begun. The joint must be explored and cleaned and the patient treated with antibiotics to cover oral flora (penicillin). Once the infection reaches the joint, destruction of the cartilage often occurs despite all therapy.

An inordinate amount of pain, with little or no swelling or induration, predating and accompanying the appearance of multiple tiny vesicles, suggests **herpes simplex (herpetic whitlow)**. The vesicles may appear cyclically. They contain clear fluid and not pus and should be distinguished from paronychias. Antibiotics are not indicated in this self-limited viral infection. Acyclovir 5% ointment applied topically for 7 days decreases the severity and duration of symptoms but is of no value in prophylaxis.

Tuberculous infection of the hand is usually chronic and may be relatively painless. Some cultures take months to become positive. Tuberculosis commonly involves only one hand, which may be the only focus of infection in the body. Bones and joints may be infected, but the process more commonly involves the tendon synovium, which becomes matted to the tendons. Treatment is by synovectomy and antituberculous drug therapy for 6–12 months.

Leprosy causes neuritis of the median and ulnar nerves, resulting in sensory and motor loss to the hand. Crippling claw deformities develop as a result of intrinsic muscle palsy. Open sores appear on the hands as a result of trauma to anesthetic digits. Reconstructive surgery and occupational training are required.

Fungal infections involve primarily the nails. Tinea unguium (onychomycosis) may be caused by many organisms, including *Epidermophyton floccosum,* trichophyton, and *Candida albicans.* Prolonged treatment with antifungal drugs—griseofulvin systemically or nystatin topically—may be necessary, along with daily applications of fungicidal agents such as tolnaftate. Removal of the nail is advocated for chronic intractable cases.

Jebson PJ: Infections of the fingertip. Paronychias and felons. Hand Clin 1998;14:547.

Lille S et al: Continuous postoperative catheter irrigation is not necessary for the treatment of suppurative flexor tenosynovitis. J Hand Surg [Br] 2000;25:304.

Perron AD, Miller MD, Brady WJ: Orthopedic pitfalls in the ED: fight bite. Am J Emerg Med 2002;20:114.

Spann M, Talmor M, Nolan WB: Hand infections: basic principles and management. Surg Infect (Larchmt) 2004;5:210.

INFLAMMATORY DISORDERS OF THE HAND

DUPUYTREN'S CONTRACTURE

(Palmar Fasciitis)

The cause of Dupuytren's contracture, which is common particularly among white populations of Celtic origin, is not known. It occurs in one of three types (acute, subacute, and chronic), predominately in males over 50 who have been in sedentary occupations, and is bilateral in about half of cases. There is a hereditary influence, and the incidence is higher among idiopathic epileptics, diabetics, alcoholics, and patients with chronic illnesses. The contracture may develop in people who do not work and (in laborers) in the hand that does the least work, so that it is not considered work-related. It is frequently found in the plantar fascia of the instep and occasionally in the penis (Peyronie's disease).

Dupuytren's contracture manifests itself most commonly in the palm by thickening, which may be nodular, and therefore mistaken for a callosity; or cord-like, and therefore mistaken for a tendon abnormality because it passes into the digits and restricts their extension. This process typically involves the longitudinal and vertical components of the fascia but at times seems to exist apart from anatomically distinct fascia. The skin may fuse with the underlying fascia and become raised and hard, or it may be greatly shrunken and sometimes drawn into a deeply puckered crevasse. The disorder invades the palm at the expense of fat but is never adherent to vessels, nerves, or musculotendinous structures (though it may be adherent to flexor tendon sheaths). It has an unpredictable rate of progression, but the earlier it starts in life, the more destructive and recurrent it is apt to be.

Dupuytren's fasciitis may involve any digit or web space, but it affects predominantly the ring and small fingers. In long-standing cases the fingers may be drawn tightly into the palm, resulting in secondary contracture of joint capsule and ligaments, flexor sheaths, and atrophic muscles.

Surgery is indicated when the disorder has progressed sufficiently, especially when it causes more than 30 degrees of flexion at the MP joint or any flexion contracture of the PIP joint. The patient must be warned about the increasing technical difficulty with progressive flexion and adduction contractures and the potential for recurrence after surgery. Fasciectomy is the surgical procedure that gives the best long-term results. In selected cases where only the longitudinal pretendinous fascial band is involved and the skin moves freely over it, subcutaneous fasciotomy done through a small longitudinal incision may release a contracture quite well with only a few days of postoperative disability. In the occasional case with acute and rapid onset of a tender nodule, local triamcinolone may be used for not only subjective but even objective relief.

Depending upon the amount of cutaneous shrinkage, skin grafts may be required for wound closure after fasciectomy. The overlying dermis has been implicated as an inductive mechanism in this process. Thus, skin grafting may diminish the recurrence rate in severe cases. The hopelessly contracted little finger must sometimes be amputated.

Motion should be started within 3–5 days after surgery. Dynamic splints and postoperative injection of corticosteroids into joints and the zone of surgery may help the well-motivated patient.

The complications of surgery are digital infarction and ischemic skin flaps, hematoma formation, fibrosis and stiffness, anesthesia (secondary to digital nerve injury) or neuromatous pain, and recurrence of contractures. Reflex sympathetic dystrophy, a painful debilitating neurologic disorder of the hand, can occur after surgery and must be treated aggressively. In general, the functional reward of the patient is great at any age.

Draviaraj KP, Chakrabarti I: Functional outcome after surgery for Dupuytren's contracture: a prospective study. J Hand Surg [Am] 2004;29:804.

Skoff HD: The surgical treatment of Dupuytren's contracture: a synthesis of techniques. Plast Reconstr Surg 2004;113:540.

DEGENERATIVE & RHEUMATOID ARTHRITIS

Arthritis of the hand is divided into two categories. **Degenerative changes** are usually due to some trauma resulting in damage to the bone or cartilage or to the supporting ligamentous structures. The increased wear to the joint results in inflammation and damage to the cartilage or underlying bone followed by reactive new bone formation (spurs). The wrists, hips, and knees are most commonly affected. **Rheumatoid arthritis** is a systemic disease characterized by synovial inflammation. The diseased synovium destroys adjacent tendons and joints in a specific way, leading to characteristic deformities in the hand.

Patients with degenerative arthritis complain of pain, aching, and stiffness in the area of the affected joint. Progression of the problem leads to immobility of the joint that affects the entire hand. Radiographic studies demonstrate joint narrowing and periosteal thickening early in the problem, progressing to bone spurs, loss of the articular surface, and bone destruction later. Patients with rheumatoid arthritis often present with very severe deformities without pain. Nodules around the olecranon and dorsum of the hand are often found. Both flexor and extensor tendons at the wrist can be inflamed, limiting tendon movement and resulting in rupture of the tendon. Involvement of the tendons and ligaments at the digits and MP joints results in ulnar deviation of the digits, MP joint destruction and dislocation, and swan-neck and boutonnière deformities. Destruction of the wrist joint is also common.

Arthritis is common among older patients and usually treated by primary care physicians and rheumatologists with anti-inflammatory medications and modification of the patient's activities. In most cases it is only when symptoms greatly hinder the patient's lifestyle that they are referred to a hand surgeon. Physical therapy, splints, and medications are often no longer effective for these patients.

Surgical treatment of painful joints includes replacement with a prosthetic joint and partial or full fusion. Prosthetic joints of metal or Silastic permit near-normal movement but can become unstable and dislocate or degenerate over time. For a durable solution to the problem, fusion of the joint is recommended. Motion is severely limited, but pain relief is complete. There are more therapeutic options for the wrist, such as replacement, local fusion of only the affected carpal bone, or complete excision of the proximal row of carpal bones, leaving motion and stability to the distal carpal bones and ligaments.

Therapy for synovial inflammation in rheumatoid disease includes excision of the synovium to increase tendon excursion and prevent rupture, repair of ruptured tendons, and excision of painful nodules. Tendon balancing procedures can help ulnar deviation of the MP joints and improve joint movement. The most important concept of treating patients with rheumatoid hand disease is that often the patients have adapted well to their functional deficits. Correcting a physical deformity in a well-compensated patient may actually result in more problems for that patient.

Adamson GJ et al: Flexible implant resection arthroplasty of the proximal interphalangeal joint in patients with systemic inflammatory arthritis. J Hand Surg [Am] 1994;19:378.

Alderman AK et al: Effectiveness of rheumatoid hand surgery: contrasting perceptions of hand surgeons and rheumatologists. J Hand Surg [Am] 2003;28:3.

Ferlic DC: Rheumatoid flexor tenosynovitis and rupture. Hand Clin 1996;12:561.

Murphy DM et al: Comparison of arthroplasty and arthrodesis for the rheumatoid wrist. J Hand Surg [Am] 2003;28:570.

Wilson RL, DeVito MC: Extensor tendon problems in rheumatoid arthritis. Hand Clin 1996;12:551.

SCLERODERMA & LUPUS ERYTHEMATOSUS

These systemic diseases of unknown cause have distinctive—though not necessarily pathognomonic—manifestations in the hands.

Scleroderma initially produces joint stiffness, hyperhidrosis, and Raynaud's phenomenon. Unchecked, it leads to marked tautness of skin and rigidity of joints with associated osteoporosis (even atrophy and ultimate resorption of the distal phalanges) and soft tissue calcifications.

Lupus erythematosus, which may be initiated or aggravated by certain drugs, foreign proteins, or psychic states, often causes polyarthritis indistinguishable from that of rheumatoid arthritis. It does not usually lead to similar joint destruction. Vasospasm in both lupus and scleroderma can cause severe ischemia of the hand and digits and may require therapy to prevent gangrene.

GOUT

Gout is a metabolic disorder of uric acid metabolism that affects about 1% of the population; approximately 50% of patients with gout have **cheiragra** (gouty hands).

The diagnosis is suggested by a rapid onset of severe pain and inflammatory signs about the joints and musculotendinous structure, simulating a phlegmonous infectious cellulitis with marked induration (most dramatically seen about the elbow). The usual duration of an attack is 5–10 days. The serum uric acid is elevated in 75% of cases. Gout may coexist with rheumatoid disease. The diagnosis is confirmed by identification of uric acid crystals in joint fluid or tissue biopsy.

In time, typical tophi form, consisting of toothpaste-like infiltrates of urate crystals, arising in multilobulated form about soft tissue structures that have been invaded. X-rays show characteristic punched-out lesions at the margins of articular cartilage.

Prophylactic treatment of gouty arthritis consists of diet, colchicine, allopurinol (a urate-blocking agent) or probenecid (a uricosuric agent), and avoidance of stress. Colchicine, 0.6 mg/h with a glass of water for 6–8 doses or to the point of gastrointestinal distress, is the time-honored means of interrupting an attack, but phenylbutazone, topical corticotropin gel, and systemic corticosteroids are also of value.

Surgical measures consist of drainage of abscessed tophi (seldom needed) and tophectomy. The latter procedure is more often of cosmetic rather than functional value. Tophectomy consists of removal of as much tophaceous material as can be fairly easily recovered. The surgeon should be careful not to destroy ligaments, tenoretinacular structures, nerves, and vessels in the process.

Gilbart MK et al: Surgery of the hand in severe systemic sclerosis. J Hand Surg [Br] 2004;29:599.

Nalebuff EA: Surgery of systemic lupus erythematosus arthritis of the hand. Hand Clin 1996;12:591.

Schuind FA et al: Gouty involvement of flexor tendons. Chir Main 2003;22:46.

BURNS & FROSTBITE OF THE HAND

Thermal Burns

The hands are a common site of thermal (including frictional), electrical, chemical, and radiation burns. Function is imperiled in all instances by swelling and scar formation. Prompt measures to preserve existing function are often urgently required. Burns over other areas of the body may be more life threatening and require more urgent attention, but burns of the hand should never be neglected. Delay in therapy leads to irreversible impairment and deformity that are impossible to correct later.

As in other areas of the body, thermal burns are grouped into three degrees. Superficial (first-degree) burns are red and painful; partial-thickness (second-degree) burns develop blisters; and full-thickness (third-degree) burns are insensate and appear like leather or charred tissue. The prognosis and therapy depend upon the location, depth, and extent of the burn.

All burns to the hand cause swelling of the tissues, and the need for elevation of the arm to relieve pain and prevent stiffness cannot be overemphasized. Tetanus immunization should be given. Cold compresses may help alleviate the pain in first-degree burns. Second-degree burns must be watched more carefully. Large blisters restricting motion are broken. Otherwise, since they are sterile, they should be left intact. Treatment with thrice-daily washing and silver sulfadiazine is usually adequate. Patients with third-degree burns or superficial burns that fail to heal and patients unable to care for their burns at home should be admitted to the hospital.

Deeper burns require close observation and more extensive treatment. In the first few hours after injury, circumferential or near-circumferential burns may cause ischemia in the extremity. Since evaluation of sensory function and capillary refill is nearly impossible in these limbs, escharotomies should be performed if compartment syndrome is suspected. If done correctly, escharotomies have few complications since these burns usually require surgical debridement anyway. Incisions are placed to avoid exposure of neurovascular structures.

Partial-thickness burns heal spontaneously. Deeper burns on the dorsum of the hand are best treated with early excision of the eschar and placement of skin grafts to prevent contractures. Palmar burns are best left to heal spontaneously since skin grafts function very poorly in this area. Some hand surgeons believe that excision and grafting of superficial burns should be performed to prevent contractures. This is true in cases where adequate therapy has not been available. In burn units with good rehabilitation services, surgeons are treating superficial second-degree burns without surgery and obtaining results as good as with skin grafting. Pigskin, cadaver homografts, or a number of commercially available biologic dressings can be used to cover the wounds temporarily, decreasing pain and keeping the wound moist until autologous skin grafts are placed.

Neglected burns of the hands result in contracture deformities that often require extensive surgery to restore function. Delayed healing and wound contractures often result in a claw hand with MP hyperextension and fusion of the digits with loss of the web space (syndactyly). Burns on the volar surface leave flexion contractures. Some contractures can be treated with release and skin grafting of the tissue gap. Web space contractures and released contractures with exposed tendons or nerves must be covered with skin or muscle flaps. Web space release is done with skin flaps from the dorsum folded down to create the space. Large flaps can be obtained by attaching the hand to the groin, allowing the tissue to adhere and vascularize before cutting the flap away from the groin. Recently, free tissue transfer from other parts of the body using microsurgical techniques has allowed more extensive reconstruction of severely burned hands.

Electrical Burns

Electrical burns of the upper extremity may not appear extensive on initial inspection. The skin may be burned only in a very small area of the entry point of the current or by ignited clothing. The current tends to spare the skin but damage underlying muscles, vessels, and nerves. Often the extent of dead tissue is not evident for several days.

Initial treatment is the same as for thermal burns. Since muscle damage may be extensive, it is important to prevent renal failure from myoglobinuria by maintaining a high output of alkaline urine. Arteriography, fluorescein injections, and radionuclide studies may help delineate the extent of necrosis. Examination of the patient in the operating room is still the most accurate method of assessing the extent of tissue damage. All obviously dead tissue should be removed during the initial evaluation. Two or three days later, the patient is reexamined in the operating room and any additional debris is removed. The wounds are closed when only clearly viable tissue remains.

Frostbite

Frostbite occurs most often in people under the influence of alcohol or with psychiatric illness. The lower extremity is affected more often than the upper. Freezing tissue causes cellular death and vascular thrombosis. Hypothermia of the entire body must first be treated. The frozen part should be quickly rewarmed by immersion in warm water (40 °C). Elevation of the extremity minimizes edema. Skin wounds are treated like burns with silver sulfadiazine cream. The extent of necrosis may not be obvious for several weeks, and debridement or amputation should be delayed until demarcation of the injury occurs. Sympathectomy may help ameliorate the sequelae of frostbite such as cold sensitivity and pain. Children with frostbite may develop premature closure of phalangeal epiphyses, which creates growth disturbances of the bone.

Smith MA, Munster AM, Spence RJ: Burns of the hand and upper limb—a review. Burns 1998;24:493.

Su CW, Lohman R, Gottlieb LJ: Frostbite of the upper extremity. Hand Clin 2000;16:235.

Tredget EE, Shankowsky HA, Tilley WA: Electrical injuries in Canadian burn care. Identification of unsolved problems. Ann N Y Acad Sci 1999;888:75.

Umraw N et al: Effective hand function assessment after burn injuries. J Burn Care Rehabil 2004;25:134.

MASSES OF THE HAND

Only 2% of all masses in the hand are malignant lesions; the majority are benign neoplasms, cysts, or a myriad of other masses. Though the clinician must be ever vigilant to identify malignancy, a mass of the hand is highly likely to be benign—excisional biopsies are thus reserved for subcutaneous lesions that are rapidly growing or for skin lesions that may be carcinomas. Otherwise, masses can be observed over a period of time to determine that they are not growing. They may be removed for functional or cosmetic reasons.

Ganglions are formed by herniation of the synovial lining of joints or tendons into the surrounding soft tissue. These cysts are filled with a viscous fluid thought to be modified joint fluid. Trauma to the wrist or hand may cause extrusion of the synovium, but it is more likely that the ganglion was already present and that trauma to that area merely brought the lesion to the surgeon's attention.

Ganglions can arise from any joint of the hand but most commonly appear on the dorsal wrist over the scapholunate ligament and the volar wrist near the radial artery. Tendon ganglions are most common on the flexor sheath at the metacarpal head (A1 pulley). Pain and tenderness are due to compression of adjacent nerves by the mass.

Ganglions have a typical appearance, and diagnosis is simple. If any doubt exists, aspiration with a large-bore needle of the viscous fluid confirms the diagnosis and occasionally cures the lesions. Injection of the empty sac with steroids and lidocaine may help to keep the mass from reappearing, but the majority recur. Ganglions need not be treated unless they cause pain or interfere with hand function. Often, it is enough just to reassure the patient that the mass is benign.

Operative removal of ganglions should be done using loupe magnification and a tourniquet. The entire ganglion should be removed, including all attachments to the joint capsule and the underlying ligament, without injuring the surrounding structures. Prolonged splinting after removal of ganglions does not decrease recurrence rates but does cause hand stiffness. Unfortunately, despite careful surgical removal of the lesion, recurrence of ganglions is relatively common.

Epidermal cysts are rests of epidermis located in the subcutaneous tissue. Many are thought to be due to traumatic disruption of epidermal cells into the soft tissue (inclusion cyst). The cells proliferate just as skin does and form a cyst filled with creamy keratin, the remains of dead epidermal cells that usually desquamate from the skin. Infected cysts become inflamed and form abscesses. Removal of the entire cyst wall is required to prevent abscess formation.

Pyogenic granuloma may form in any chronic wound. Histologically, it consists of vascular tissue identical to granulation tissue. Just as for hypertrophic granulation tissue elsewhere on the body, excision or cautery of the material flush to skin level allows epidermis to migrate over the wound.

Giant cell tumors are benign, multilobulated, solid masses found on the lateral aspects of the finger. They are often attached to the tendon sheath. The mass may be quite complex and extend throughout the adjacent nerves, vessels, tendons, and ligaments. The entire lesion should be removed, but recurrence is relatively common.

The most common bone tumors are **enchondromas**. Multiple enchondromas (Ollier's disease) are associated with other skeletal deformities. The lesion appears on x-ray as thinned cortical bone with speckled calcifications. Fractures through the tumors usually do not heal spontaneously. The tumor should be removed with a curette. Bone graft taken from the distal radius is used to fill the gap if needed.

A **carpal boss** is due to abnormal bone formation at the base of the second or third metacarpal bones and presents as a hard mass on the dorsum of the hand. The excess growth of bone can be removed if symptomatic.

Glomus tumors are composed of blood vessels and unmyelinated nerves of a heat-regulating arteriovenous malformation. They are usually found in the fingertip or under the fingernail and can be extremely painful. Local excision of the tumor is curative. Occasionally, when the tumor is large and disrupts the nail matrix, a split-thickness nail graft from another digit is needed to reconstruct the defect.

The most common malignant tumor of the hand is **squamous cell carcinoma**, though **basal cell carcinomas** and **melanomas** also occur. Subungual melanomas are often difficult to diagnose because they are difficult to examine. These tumors should be treated just the same as elsewhere on the body. Particular care should be taken to examine for spread of tumor in the lymphatic drainage at the supratrochlear and axillary nodes.

Other tumors include lipomas, fibromas, hemangiomas, arteriovenous malformations, neurofibromas, sarcomas, and various skin lesions. These tumors act no differently in the hand than elsewhere in the body. However, because of the close proximity of the nervous and vascular structures within the small spaces of the hand, these tumors cause compressive signs and symptoms sooner. CT scans or MRI help delineate the extent of soft tissue tumors and may help in preoperative planning.

Nahra ME, Bucchieri JS: Ganglion cysts and other tumor related conditions of the hand and wrist. Hand Clin 2004;20:249.

Peterson JJ, Bancroft LW, Kransdorf MJ: Principles of bone and soft tissue imaging. Hand Clin 2004;20:147.

Trigg SD: Biopsy of hand, wrist, and forearm tumors. Hand Clin 2004;20:131.

COMPLEX HAND INJURIES

Crush Injuries & Amputations

Recent advances in microvascular surgery have greatly increased our ability to treat complex hand injuries. Mangled and amputated digits, hands, and even entire upper extremities have been replanted or repaired. Complex nerve repairs, microvascular free tissue transfers of muscle flaps, and toe-to-hand reconstructions have made it possible to restore more function to severely injured hands. The end result must be a sensate, painless, and useful extremity. Patients who undergo multiple surgical procedures and prolonged rehabilitation with only marginal results would have benefited from early amputation. A surgeon with extensive experience can best assess the patient's injuries, occupational requirements, and psychosocial needs to determine if salvage is worthwhile.

Complex hand injuries often result from improper use or malfunction of machinery. Heavy machinery in the workplace or motorized cutting tools at home, such as rotary saws, are often cited as the mechanism of injury. Sharply amputated or partially devascularized parts are most likely to be saved. Severe crushing or avulsion of the part produces wider nerve and vessel injury. The extent of this type of damage is difficult to determine and often impossible to repair.

The decision to try to salvage a damaged part must be individualized to each situation, but some general principles apply. The thumb is crucial to hand function, and all efforts are made to save the entire digit or as much length as possible. When multiple digits or half of the hand is damaged or amputated, a greater effort is made to repair the part. Children can recover function in badly damaged extremities far better than adults, and any amputated parts in children should be replanted. Replantation of the entire arm at the elbow and above is controversial. The usefulness of these replanted limbs is limited by the slow nerve regeneration, and some hand surgeons believe that amputations in these cases result in better function.

Patients with complex hand injuries should be immediately referred to a regional center with the staff and facilities to manage the problems. Occasionally, in the rush to transfer patients with these very obvious injuries, intra-abdominal, neurologic, and other less obvious injuries have been overlooked. The entire patient must be evaluated and stabilized prior to transfer. A clean moist dressing should be placed on the wound and the extremity elevated. The amputated part is wrapped in a plastic bag and placed in ice water. The amputated part should never be frozen.

The accepting hand surgeon evaluates the patient's overall condition, potential for rehabilitation, and personal wishes before coming to a decision. To revascularize or replant a part, the patient must be taken urgently to the operating room. Ischemia over 6 hours is often associated with failure of revascularization, but—depending on the metabolic needs of the constituent tissues—extremities that have undergone periods of ischemia longer than this can be successfully replanted.

Bone must first be stabilized with Kirschner wires or metal plates before vascular repairs are performed. Arterial and venous repairs are done with microscopic magnification, and the ischemic tissue is reperfused. Failure of a replanted part is more often due to venous outflow problems than arterial inflow. Systemic and local anticoagulants help to maintain perfusion but are not always needed. Leeches placed on the part release a potent local anticoagulant and can decrease venous congestion. Nerve and tendon repairs must also be performed. When there is inadequate local soft tissue to cover the repaired structures, muscle or skin flaps from a distant site must be transferred using microsurgical methods to the area. Although these operations are not life-threatening, blood loss can be extensive and transfusions are sometimes required.

Secondary procedures to free tendon adhesions, reduce bulky flaps, and transfer tendons in motor nerve injuries may need to be done. Reconstruction of unsuccessful replantations is being done more often. The original method using toes to reconstruct thumbs has also been used to make fingers. These reconstructions give patients the ability to grasp objects. Because these digits are sensate, they can even perform fine movement tasks not possible with prosthetic devices. Patients with loss only of the thumb are better treated with transfer of the index finger to the thumb position (pollicization).

Partial or total loss of a single digit is less critical. Hand function is better without a stiff or painful digit. When a decision is made to amputate a digit, care must be taken to leave a painless stump with good sensate soft tissue coverage. The flexor tendon must not be sutured to the extensor tendon for soft tissue coverage since this will cause the tendons to pull each other rather than move the joint. Local flaps to cover the stump are preferred to skin grafts or cross finger flaps since they usually provide better sensation. A short amputation stump on the long or ring finger is often bothersome since small objects such as coins tend to fall out of the palm, and a ray amputation eliminates the problem. For cosmetic purposes, ray amputations are far less noticeable than partial amputations. The loss of hand breadth with a ray amputation can decrease grip strength, however.

The loss of part of all of the hand can be compensated both functionally and cosmetically by a variety of prostheses. Their use involves careful adaptation to the requirements of the patient, who must receive appropriate training to ensure success.

INJECTION INJURIES OF THE HAND

High-pressure devices used in industry to apply material such as air, grease, paint, and oil cause a unique hand injury. The typical case is injection of the material into the index finger of the nondominant hand of a factory worker. A pinpoint injection site may be the only external evidence of injury, and the hand appears discolored or pale, or swollen due to the injected material.

The examination should include a careful hand evaluation and an x-ray to demonstrate the distribution of material or gas in the hand. All such cases require continued unrelenting scrutiny, even if the part seems completely normal. If there is any evidence of retained foreign material, swelling, or ischemia, early surgical exploration is advocated to release the tourniquet effect of the skin and fascia and to remove as much of the material as possible without injuring healthy tissue. Prophylactic antisludging agents (dextran 40), corticosteroids, and antibiotics may help.

Often the pressure forces the material to spread along the tendon sheaths throughout the hand and even into the forearm. Expansion of the foreign material in a closed space and the chemical irritation cause congestion, inflammation, vascular thrombosis, and gangrene. The injected material is difficult to remove completely, and a foreign body response leads to fibrosis so extensive that it often destroys the function of the hand.

Buncke HJ Jr: Microvascular hand surgery—transplants and replants—over the past 25 years. J Hand Surg [Am] 2000;25:415.

Chen HC, Tang YB: Replantation of the thumb, especially avulsion. Hand Clin 2001;17:433.

Christodoulou L et al: Functional outcome of high-pressure injection injuries of the hand. J Trauma 2001;50:717.

Del Pinal F et al: Acute hand compartment syndromes after closed crush: a reappraisal. Plast Reconstr Surg 2002;110:1232.

Freeland AE, Lineaweaver WC, Lindley SG: Fracture fixation in the mutilated hand. Hand Clin 2003;19:51.

Woo SH, Kim JS, Seul JH: Immediate toe-to-hand transfer in acute hand injuries: overall results, compared with results for elective cases. Plast Reconstr Surg 2004;113:882.

MINIMALLY INVASIVE HAND SURGERY

The goal of reconstructive hand surgery is return of normal function, including pain-free movement, normal active and passive range of motion, premorbid strength, and intact sensation. Yet the process of incising, dissecting, and sewing is associated with significant scarring and pain. Scarring is especially troublesome in the hand since it leads to stiffness, ligamental tightening, and arthritis. As a result, any procedure in the hand that minimizes postoperative scarring or pain will contribute to an improved result.

Surgical care in the past decade has been revolutionized by the introduction and incorporation of minimally invasive surgical techniques. Laparoscopies and thoracoscopies have permitted the resection of hollow and solid organs through 1-cm incisions, reducing the need for laparotomies and thoracotomies. Likewise, urologists have employed cystoscopy for evaluation and treatment of bladder and kidney disorders, while orthopedic surgeons have used arthroscopy to similar effective ends in the knee, ankle, elbow, and shoulder.

Two areas of hand surgery incorporate minimally invasive techniques: Wrist arthroscopy has expanded the options for evaluating the chronically painful wrist, and endoscopic carpal tunnel release (ECTR) provides a less invasive method than open release for decompressing the median nerve. While ECTR theoretically allows for a faster recovery, it may in fact offer only limited advantages.

WRIST ARTHROSCOPY

Diagnostic wrist arthroscopy was first successfully used in 1970. Over the past 3 decades, it has taken its place among traditional imaging techniques as a low-morbidity method for evaluating chronic wrist pain. As the hardware for examining the wrist has become more sophisticated and as hand surgeons have become more familiar with the arthroscopic view of the wrist, increasingly aggressive attempts have been made to use the arthroscope to treat as well as to diagnose wrist problems.

Indications & Contraindications

Diagnostic wrist arthroscopy is a useful technique to evaluate patients with wrist pain, whether chronic or acute. In patients with chronic pain, this technique can be used to augment information offered by plain radiographs, CT, MRI, or wrist arthrography. It can confirm an uncertain diagnosis or be used to reevaluate a patient who has failed other treatments. In contrast, patients with acute symptoms—such as those suffering from mechanical wrist pain—may complain of pain localized over the joint, catching and popping sensations, and relief with rest. Here, the wrist can be manipulated during arthroscopy to localize the source of the symptoms. In general, the technique is useful for evaluating articular cartilage, ligaments, the triangular fibrocartilage complex (TFCC), and the synovium. Interestingly, diagnostic wrist arthroscopy may provide too comprehensive an examination. Only some of the lesions that are visualized during an examination may be responsible for a patient's symptoms. The hand surgeon must critically correlate arthroscopic findings with the patient's examination to arrive at the appropriate diagnosis.

Therapeutic wrist arthroscopy is useful for the treatment of ligament tears, TFCC lesions, articular cartilage lesions, subtle distal radius and carpus fractures, dorsal wrist ganglions, removal of isolated carpal bones up to and including the proximal carpal row, and disorders of the distal radioulnar joint. It is useful also in the management of lesions arising from rheumatoid arthritis. It has been successfully used in completing synovectomies, proximal row carpectomies in the case of scaphoid nonunion or scapholunate collapse, radial styloidectomy, and isolated symptomatic chondral defects.

Procedure

Equipment for diagnostic wrist arthroscopy includes an apparatus for elevating and distracting the wrist, an arthroscopic telescope, a video camera, a fluid infusion system, and both manual and powered instruments.

Either general or regional anesthesia may be used. A tourniquet is placed at the mid arm to provide a blood-free field during the operation. The distal forearm, wrist, and hand are prepared into the operative field. Traction is applied to the hand, usually via sterile finger traps, and a distraction force is applied across the wrist.

Individual skin incisions are then made at standard portal sites determined by the goal of the operation. Portal sites are described according to their relationship with the radius and ulna, the carpal bones, and the extensor tendons. The relationship to the extensor tendons is indicated by listing the extensor compartments on either side of the incision. Typical portals include the 3–4 radiocarpal, through which the scaphoid and lunate facets can be visualized; the 4–5 radiocarpal, through which the TFCC and the ulnocarpal ligaments can be seen; and the 6R radiocarpal, through which the extensor carpi ulnaris tendon and ulnar wrist are approached. The midcarpal joint is approached through any of three portals, including the midcarpal ulnar, the midcarpal radial, and the scaphotrapezial-trapezoid.

Once abnormalities are identified, therapeutic wrist arthroscopy can be used to effect repairs. Partial ligament tears and tears of the TFCC can be debrided arthroscopically using knife blades and motorized shavers. Carpal bone resections can be completed with miniature osteotomes and powered saw blades.

Outcomes

Operations employing diagnostic and therapeutic wrist arthroscopy typically result in less swelling, less postoperative pain, and less stiffness than comparable open wrist procedures. There is a concomitant earlier return to function and work. Therapeutic wrist arthroscopy even of dorsal wrist ganglia, the most superficial of wrist abnormalities, is followed by fewer—or no more—recurrences than the open technique.

Complications

The rate of complications associated with diagnostic and therapeutic wrist arthroscopy is estimated to be 2% and is due to a variety of causes. The continuous traction necessary to properly distract the wrist can cause problems, including ligamental strain at the MCP joints with concomitant joint edema and stiffness and stretching of peripheral nerves. Establishment of the operative portals can damage articular cartilage, ligaments, tendons, cutaneous nerves, the radial artery, and cutaneous and deep veins. Such injuries include abrasions, contusions, lacerations, and transections. A high proportion of complications of therapeutic wrist arthroscopy are associated with inadequate relief of symptoms or a diminished return of function. A now less common complication of therapeutic wrist arthroscopy results from the fluid infusion. Forearm compartment syndromes have resulted from extravasation of infusion fluid during endoscopic repair of distal radius fractures; this problem is now avoided by circumferential compression of the forearm during the procedure.

ENDOSCOPIC CARPAL TUNNEL RELEASE

Endoscopic release of the transverse carpal ligament is an increasingly popular method of treating carpal tunnel syndrome. Advocates of the procedure claim that it is associated with decreased postoperative morbidity and earlier return to work. Others caution that there is little if any short-term difference between endoscopic and open carpal tunnel release, no long-term difference, and that endoscopic carpal tunnel release is associated with an increased likelihood of significant nerve injury.

Indications & Contraindications

Endoscopic carpal tunnel release is easier to perform in patients with larger wrists. Ease of access to the carpal tunnel correlates with the wrist circumference and the height and age of patients. Surgeons should be aware that the procedure is likely to be more difficult in small patients with small wrists and are advised to maintain a lower threshold for conversion to the open technique to avoid neurologic complications.

Absolute contraindications to endoscopic carpal tunnel release include masses in the carpal canal and other space-occupying lesions, abnormalities in canal anatomy, and wrist stiffness that precludes proper positioning.

Procedure

In the United States, most surgeons use one of two techniques—either Chow or Agee. The two differ primarily in the number of incisions, or portals, needed to gain access. The Chow technique, first described in 1989, employs two portals while the Agee technique requires only one.

Either operation can be performed under local anesthesia with a brachial tourniquet. An initial transverse incision is made proximal to the wrist flexion crease between the palmaris longus and flexor carpi ulnaris tendons. The space between the transverse carpal ligament and the flexor tendons is defined with a dissector. In the Agee procedure, the endoscope is advanced under the transverse carpal ligament, radial to the hook of the hamate along the axis of the ring finger. The ligament is incised along its entire length, with care taken to avoid Guyon's canal and the superficial palmar arch. In the Chow operation, a second transverse incision is made just distal to the transverse carpal ligament along the axis of the ring finger. The wrist is dorsiflexed and a slotted cannula is advanced into the proximal incision, deep to the transverse carpal ligament, and out the distal incision. The endoscope is then used to visualize the ligament while the knife divides it. The wounds are closed, and the patient's wrist placed in dorsiflexion.

Outcomes

Several studies have compared open versus endoscopic carpal tunnel release, focusing upon the incidence of recovery from symptoms, the time span until the patient returns to work, and the incidence of recurrence of symptoms. Overall, both techniques have equivalent outcomes.

Many of the most convincing studies are prospective randomized trials. One such study, comparing open and endoscopic carpal tunnel release among 32 hands in 29 patients, found no difference in postoperative recovery time or surgical result. The only significant difference noted by the authors was transient numbness on the radial side of the ring finger in three endoscopic carpal tunnel release patients.

In another study, the authors compared in a prospective randomized manner the early outcome of carpal tunnel release using either a conventional open carpal tunnel release procedure in 40 patients or a two-portal endoscopic release in 56 patients. They found no statistically significant difference between the groups in postoperative pain, recovery from paresthesias, or time taken to return to work. However, the endoscopic group demonstrated better grip strength recovery at 1 and 3 months. No surgical complications were observed in either group.

Nonrandomized studies have supported this trend. An analysis of 191 consecutive patients undergoing carpal tunnel release with an average 2-year follow-up showed that none of the patients undergoing open release had a recurrence, while 7% of patients undergoing endoscopic release had recurrences. Another study observed a higher incidence of incomplete release of the carpal tunnel with endoscopic techniques than with standard open releases.

The factors identified with poor outcomes in endoscopic carpal tunnel release are similar to those seen in open release. Less satisfactory results were present in workers' compensation cases; patients with normal motor latencies on nerve conduction studies; patients with preoperative hand weakness, widened two-point discrimination, myofascial pain syndrome, or fibromyalgia; and patients involved in litigation, those with multiple compressive neuropathies, and those with abnormal psychologic factors.

Complications

Only a limited number of studies include a sufficient number of patients to compare complication rates and type between endoscopic and open carpal tunnel release. Overall, the types and rates of complications between the two forms of release are similar. Nonetheless, isolated but severe complications from endoscopic release over the past decade tend to dramatize its risk.

The study by Boeckstyns and Sorensen is perhaps the most comprehensive to date. These authors analyzed 54 published series of endoscopic and open releases comprising 9516 and 1203 patients, respectively. Irreversible nerve damage from the procedure occurred in 0.3% of endoscopic and 0.2% of open releases, including such injuries as transection of the median nerve. While reversible nerve injuries were more common with endoscopic release than with open release (4.4% versus 0.9%, respectively, among prospective controlled and randomized studies), tendon lesions, reflex sympathetic dystrophy, hematoma, and wound problems were equally common with either technique.

A less compelling analysis—a retrospective survey of hand surgeons who had performed either open or endoscopic carpal tunnel release over the preceding 5 years—found major complications with either approach, including median nerve lacerations, ulnar nerve lacerations, digital nerve lacerations, vessel lacerations, and tendon lacerations. While the authors could not reach a conclusion about the rate of complications for one procedure versus the other, their results demonstrate the potentially devastating sequelae of carpal tunnel release even in experienced hands.

Carpal tunnel symptoms may persist or recur following either open or endoscopic release. In patients who have persistent symptoms following endoscopic release, many authors recommend open carpal tunnel release as definitive therapy.

Beredjiklian PK et al: Complications of wrist arthroscopy. J Hand Surg [Am] 2004;29:406.

Shih JT et al: Arthroscopically-assisted reduction of intra-articular fractures and soft tissue management of distal radius. Hand Surg 2001;6:127.

Slutsky DJ: Wrist arthroscopy through a volar radial portal. Arthroscopy 2002;18:624.

Thoma A et al: A systematic review of reviews comparing the effectiveness of endoscopic and open carpal tunnel decompression. Plast Reconstr Surg 2004;113:1184.

Pediatric Surgery

45

Craig T. Albanese, MD, & Karl G. Sylvester, MD

Pediatric surgical patients are not merely small adults. The surgical care of children differs markedly from that of adults in many respects, including unique physiologic demands that vary according to age and development. The neonate's physiologic development is closer to that of a fetus, while adolescents are similar to adults, and infants or children have problems unique to their chronologic and developmental age. Infants and children also suffer from congenital abnormalities and diseases not seen in adults, and their management requires an intimate understanding of the relevant embryology and pathogenesis.

NEWBORN CARE

Neonatal Intensive Care

The newborn infant with a surgically correctable lesion often has other disorders that threaten survival. The care of these babies—particularly the premature and small-for-gestational-age babies, has improved with the emergence of the intensive care nursery. Dramatic advances have been made in the technology of infant monitoring and respiratory support. Low-birth-weight infants can now receive ventilatory support from sophisticated infant respirators for prolonged periods in a precisely controlled microenvironment. Surfactant therapy and high-frequency ventilation has allowed a population of extremely premature infants to survive. Temperature is controlled by servoregulation, while pulse and blood pressure are continuously recorded. Ventilation is monitored by transcutaneous O_2 and CO_2 electrodes or by indwelling arterial catheters. The metabolic consequences of prematurity and intrauterine growth retardation are monitored by frequent measurement of glucose, calcium, electrolytes, and bilirubin in microliter quantities of blood. Nutritional requirements for growth and development can be provided by enteral or parenteral routes. This kind of specialized care of critically ill newborns requires trained personnel and specialized equipment. The care of such babies is best accomplished in designated regional centers capable of providing pediatric surgical and neonatal intensive care.

Phibbs CS et al: The effects of patient volume and level of care at the hospital of birth on neonatal mortality. JAMA 1996;276:1054.

Classification

Newborn infants can be classified according to their level of maturation (weight) and development (gestational age). A normal full-term infant has a gestational age of 37–42 weeks and a body weight greater than 2500 g. The gestational age of the infant is calculated from the date of the last normal menstrual period. However, clinical assessment of gestational age by morphologic and neurologic examination of the small infant can be more accurate than calculation from the menstrual history.

Four signs may be useful in assessing gestational age. Infants less than 37 weeks' gestational age have (1) fine fuzzy hair with thin, semitransparent skin, (2) ears that lack cartilaginous support, (3) a breast nodule less than 3 mm in diameter, and (4) few transverse creases on the balls of the feet anteriorly. In males, the testicles are incompletely descended and reside in the inguinal canal, and the scrotum is small with few rugae. In females, the labia minora are relatively enlarged and the labia majora are small.

Preterm infants are those born before 37 weeks' gestation. Several physiologic abnormalities may coexist in preterm infants. Apneic and bradycardiac episodes are common and may represent an immature central nervous system or, conversely, may represent signs of physiologic instability, most notably with sepsis. The lungs and retinas of preterm infants are very susceptible to high oxygen levels. Retinopathy of prematurity from oxygen toxicity may lead to blindness. Relatively brief exposures to high oxygen concentrations, often coupled with barotrauma from the mechanical ventilator, may damage the lungs, resulting in hyaline membrane disease and respiratory distress syndrome. Shunting across a patent ductus arteriosus is not uncommon and may lead to pulmonary hemorrhage and congestive heart failure. The preterm infant has a friable choroids plexus and is thus susceptible to intraventricular hemorrhage when stressed in the first week of life. The premature infant may be unable to tolerate oral feeding due to a weak suck reflex. Tube feeds or total parenteral nutrition may be required. Preterm infants have increased requirements for glucose, calcium, and sodium as well as a propensity for hypothermia, impaired bilirubin metabolism, polycythemia, and metabolic acidosis. These problems are accentuated in very low-birth-weight infants or "micropremies"(birth weight less than 1000 g).

A small-for-gestational age (SGA) infant is one who is less than the tenth percentile in weight for their gestational age. An SGA infant is the product of a pregnancy complicated by any one of several placental, maternal, or fetal abnormalities. Although body weight is low, their body length and head circumference are age-appropriate. Compared with the premature infant of equivalent weight, the SGA infant is developmentally more mature and faces different physiologic problems. Intrauterine malnutrition results in reduced body fat and decreased glycogen stores. Their relatively large surface area and high metabolic rate predisposes them to hypothermia and hypoglycemia. SGA infants also have an increased risk of meconium aspiration syndrome. Polycythemia (which may lead to complications of hyperviscosity syndrome) is common and necessitates close monitoring of their hematocrit. Due to their relatively mature organ development and function (compared to preterm infants), retinopathy of prematurity, intraventricular hemorrhage, and hyaline membrane disease are uncommon.

Temperature Regulation

Infants and children are susceptible to heat loss because they have a relatively greater body surface area and a thinner subcutaneous fat layer compared with adults. Heat loss occurring by conduction, convection, evaporation, and radiation may be four times that of the adult and is further increased in the preterm infant. Infants are homeotherms and will expend metabolic energy to stay warm at the cost of other functions. Heat is generated not by shivering but by metabolizing brown fat reserves (nonshivering thermogenesis) in response to norepinephrine. This has practical consequences since brown fat may be rendered inactive by some medications (pressors and anesthetic agents) and may be depleted by poor nutrition. Exposure to cold environments increases metabolic work and caloric consumption. Due to limited energy reserves and thin skin, prolonged exposure may rapidly cause hypothermia. Resultant catecholamine secretion increases the metabolic rate (particularly in the myocardium) and produces vasoconstriction with impaired tissue perfusion and increased lactic acid production.

Thus, it is important to maintain the sick newborn in an optimal thermal environment (thermoneutrality). This is the ambient temperature in which a baby, at a minimal metabolic cost, can maintain a constant and normal body temperature by vasomotor control. To attain such an environment, the gradient between the skin surface and the environmental temperature must be less than 1.5 °C. As the skin surface temperature averages 35.5 °C, the optimal environmental temperature is 34 °C (slightly higher for premature infants). The neonate's environmental temperature is best controlled by placing the infant in an enclosed incubator. An open radiant warmer is used when the infant is sick and frequent access is necessary. Either the ambient temperature of the incubator can be monitored and maintained at thermoneutrality, or a servo system can be used. The latter regulates the incubator temperature according to the infant's skin temperature. Heat loss may be further reduced by wrapping the head, extremities, and as much of the trunk as possible in wadding, plastic wrap, plastic sheets, or aluminum foil.

In the operating room, the temperature of the infant must be continuously recorded by placing a thermistor in the rectum or esophagus. Body heat may be conserved by a heating pad, circulated warm air around the child (bear-hugger), infrared lamp, and warm irrigation fluids. The operating room should be prewarmed and the temperature kept at 20–27 °C. Wet sponges and drapes exaggerate evaporative heat losses. Plastic drapes contain body heat and keep the skin dry. One of the most effective means of regulating body temperature is to heat and humidify the inhalational anesthetic gases.

Albanese CT, Nour BM, Rowe MI: Anesthesia blocks nonshivering thermogenesis in the neonatal rabbit. J Pediatr Surg 1994; 29:983.

Nesher N et al: A novel thermoregulatory system maintains perioperative normothermia in children undergoing elective surgery. Paediatr Anaesth 2000;11:555.

Sauer PJ, Dane HJ, Visser HK: New standards for neutral thermal environment of healthy very low birth weight infants in week one of life. Arch Dis Child 1984;59:18.

Ventilation

Assisted ventilation is often necessary because of underlying disease (eg, persistent fetal circulation and pulmonary hypertension), medications (eg, opioids, PGE_2), or physiologic changes imposed by a surgical procedure (eg, closure of an abdominal wall defect or diaphragmatic hernia). At birth, the pharynx should be aspirated of mucus, amniotic fluid, or meconium. Inadequate respiration should be assisted with a bag and mask or endotracheal tube. The diameter of an endotracheal tube (uncuffed) should approximate that of the 5th digit or the nares, usually between 2.5 and 4 mm. The full-term newborn usually requires a 3.0-mm tube. An orotracheal tube is preferred to a nasotracheal one to minimize trauma and subsequent infection in the nasal passages. The trachea from the glottis to the carina in the newborn is 7.5 cm long, and placement of the tube into the right or left bronchus must be avoided. For infants, optimal tube placement can be estimated as follows: 7 cm from the lips in a 1 kg infant; 8 cm in a 2 kg infant; and 9 cm in a 3 kg infant. Once placed, the endotracheal tube is firmly fixed in place and connected to an infant ventilator. A small air leak between the endotracheal tube and the airway is necessary to minimize laryngeal and tracheal trauma.

Most infant ventilators are time-cycled flow generators capable of delivering both continuous positive airway pressure (CPAP) and intermittent mandatory ventilation (IMV). IMV is a synthesis of simple mechanical ventilation and CPAP breathing that allows the baby to breathe independently between mandatory breaths provided by the ventilator while a continuous positive pressure is maintained on the airway. CPAP breathing helps keep the terminal airways open and is particularly useful when alveolar collapse develops, such as in hyaline membrane disease or with persistent atelectasis.

The gas mixture flowing into the system should be carefully controlled by an air-oxygen mixing device, and the inspired oxygen concentration should be regulated to maintain the arterial PO_2 at 60–80 torr. The gas should be humidified by using a heated nebulizer. Absorption of fluid in the lung may be considerable, and parenteral fluid may have to be restricted. When the arterial PO_2 exceeds 80 torr, the inspired oxygen concentration is gradually lowered toward room air; the end-expiratory pressure is incrementally lowered, as is the IMV rate. In this way, the baby is gradually weaned from oxygen and mechanical ventilation. Upon removal of the tube, the inspired oxygen concentration should be increased during the transition period.

In severe respiratory compromise (eg, congenital diaphragmatic hernia, meconium aspiration syndrome), more complex ventilatory strategies are needed. High-frequency ventilation (jet and oscillatory modes) utilizes low tidal volumes at high rates (up to 600 breaths/min) to minimize the deleterious effects of high airway pressure. Inhaled nitric oxide can be administered via the ventilatory circuit and may help relax the small airways and pulmonary vasculature. There is a trend toward allowing higher pCO_2 levels (permissive hypercarbia) and lower pO_2 levels in order to lessen pulmonary trauma from pressure and oxygen. This has been termed "gentle ventilation." If gentle ventilation, permissive hypercapnia, and the high-frequency modes of ventilation are ineffective, oxygenation and gas exchange can be accomplished using extracorporeal membrane oxygenation. This temporary bypass unit oxygenates the blood through an external circuit as the lungs are left to mature or recover from the underlying disease process.

Gerstmann DR, deLemos RA, Clark RH: High-frequency ventilation: issues of strategy. Clin Perinatol 1991;18:563.

Hemmila MR, Hirschl RB: Advances in ventilatory support of the pediatric surgical patient. Curr Opin Pediatr 1999;11:241.

Fluids & Electrolytes

Effective fluid and electrolyte management involves (1) calculating the fluid and electrolyte requirements for maintaining metabolic functions, (2) replacing losses (evaporative, third space, external), and (3) considering preexisting fluid deficits or excesses. Taking these factors into consideration, a tentative program is devised for fluid and electrolyte administration. The patient's response is monitored, and the program is adjusted accordingly.

Monitoring fluid status and acid-base balance can be accomplished by both noninvasive and invasive means. Commonly used noninvasive devices include pulse oximetry, urine output, transcutaneous CO_2 monitoring, and sphygmomanometry. For critically ill infants, more invasive means are necessary to assess homeostasis. Blood gas analysis via heelstick (venous) or arterial catheter is frequently employed. Polyvinyl catheters may be placed via an umbilical artery into the distal aorta, with the tip positioned at the level of L4 (confirmed radiographically). Indwelling arterial catheters can also be placed in the radial, femoral, or temporal arteries, either percutaneously or by incision. Central venous access may assist in cases where prolonged venous access is needed or parenteral nutrition is necessary or when blood is frequently sampled. It may be obtained via the umbilical vein; a percutaneously inserted central catheter (PICC) via the saphenous, cephalic, median basilic, or temporal veins; or using a Broviac catheter via the femoral, internal jugular, facial, or subclavian veins.

A. Calculating Maintenance Needs

In the newborn infant, the basic maintenance requirement of water is the volume required for growth and replacement of losses from the skin, lungs, and stool. Requirements during the first day of life are unique because of the greatly expanded extracellular fluid volume in the newborn baby, which decreases after 24 hours. For example, infants born with intestinal obstruction (eg, intestinal atresia) are initially not hypovolemic as a result of fluid adjustments across the placenta. Up to 10% of a newborn infant's birth weight is lost in the first 3–7 days; the majority is water loss, with minor contributions from meconium and urine. During the first 24 hours of life, basic maintenance fluid should not exceed 90 mL/kg/d in preterm infants weighing less than 1000 g or of less than 32 weeks' gestation, or 65 mL/kg/d in larger infants. This requirement gradually increases to a minimum 80 mL/kg/d by 4 days of life in normal infants. For children and adolescents, the most commonly used method of calculating fluid requirements is based on body weight (Table 45–1). However, because of the many factors affecting maintenance requirements, there is no close or constant relationship between body weight and fluid and electrolyte needs.

Table 45–1. Calculation of maintenance fluid requirements.[1]

Body Weight	Fluid Volume per 24 h
1–10 kg	100 mL/kg
11–20 kg	1000 mL + 50 mL for each kg over 10 kg
> 20 kg	1500 mL + 20 mL for each kg over 20 kg

[1]Reproduced with permission from Albanese CT: Pediatric surgery. in: *Surgery*. Norton JA (editor). Springer, 2000.

B. Perioperative Fluid Management

In the surgical patient, fluid, serum electrolyte, and acid-base abnormalities are corrected before operation, when feasible. Intraoperative fluid requirements consist of the estimated maintenance requirement plus replacement of preexisting deficits (if uncorrected) plus replacement of intraoperative losses, including blood.

Postoperatively, losses from intestinal drainage and fistulas are directly measured and replaced with an appropriate electrolyte solution (Table 45–2). In neonates, it is wise to measure the electrolytes in the fluid to more accurately guide replacement, especially for proximal intestinal stomas or fistulas. Protein-rich losses (eg, chest tube drainage of a chylothorax) can be replaced with colloid such as an albumin solution or fresh frozen plasma. Internal losses into body cavities or tissues (third space losses) cannot be measured; adequate replacement of these losses depends on careful monitoring of the patient's vital signs and urine output. Following an operation such as a laparotomy or thoracotomy, the fluid requirement may exceed 150 mL/kg/d for several days postoperatively.

C. Electrolyte Considerations

Basic electrolyte and energy requirements are provided by sodium, 2–3 meq/kg/d (up to 5 meq/kg/d for preterm infants) in 5% or 10% dextrose, with the addition of potassium, 2–3 meq/kg/d, once urine production has been established. Calcium gluconate (200–400 mg/kg/d) may be added, especially in preterm infants. Additional electrolytes such as bicarbonate and magnesium are added, as needed.

Many stressed newborn infants develop low blood levels of potassium, calcium, magnesium, and glucose. A deficiency of any one of these will produce such signs as vomiting, abdominal distention, poor feeding, apneic spells, cyanosis, lethargy, eye rolling, high-pitched cry, tremors, or convulsions. Convulsions and tetany due to hypocalcemia should be treated with intravenous 10% calcium solution given at a rate of 1 mL/min while the ECG is carefully monitored. Although hypocalcemia can be largely eliminated by adding calcium salts to intravenous solutions, caution is required since subcutaneous infiltration may produce severe vasoconstriction and skin necrosis. If there is no response to correction of a documented calcium deficiency, hypomagnesemia should be suspected and a serum magnesium level obtained.

Table 45–2. Replacement of abnormal losses of fluids and electrolytes.

Type of Fluid	Electrolyte Content				Replacement
	Na^+ (meq/L)	K^+ (meq/L)	Cl^- (meq/L)	HCO_3^- (meq/L)	
Gastric (vomiting)	50 (20–90)	10 (4–15)	90 (50–150)	. . .	5% dextrose in half-normal (0.45%) saline plus KCl, 20–40 meq/L
Small bowel (ileostomy)	110 (70–140)	5 (3–10)	100 (70–130)	20 (10–40)	Lactated Ringer's
Diarrhea	80 (10–140)	25 (10–60)	90 (20–120)	40 (30–50)	Lactated Ringer's with or without HCO_3^-
Bile	145 (130–160)	5 (4–7)	100 (80–120)	40 (30–50)	Lactated Ringer's with or without HCO_3^-
Pancreatic	140 (130–150)	5 (4–7)	80 (60–100)	80 (60–110)	Lactated Ringer's with or without HCO_3^-
Sweat					
Normal	20(10–30)	4(3–10)	20 (10–40)	. . .	. . .
Cystic fibrosis	90(50–130)	15(5–25)	90 (60–120)	. . .	. . .

Table 45–3. Caloric requirements of various age groups per 24 hours.[1]

Age	kcal/kg per 24 hours
Newborn term (0–4 days)	110–120
Low birth weight	120–130
3–4 months	100–106
5–12 months	100
1–7 years	75–90
7–12 years	60–75
12–18 years	30–60

[1]Reproduced, with permission, from Albanese CT: Pediatric surgery. In: *Surgery*. Norton JA (editor). Springer, 2000.

Rapid determination of the blood glucose level can be done in the neonatal unit with blood glucose reagent strips. This may be correlated at intervals with serum glucose determinations, the frequency depending on the stability of the infant. Intravenous fluids should contain a minimum of 10% dextrose, and if non-dextrose-containing solutions such as blood or plasma are being administered, close monitoring of the blood glucose level is essential. The treatment of hypoglycemia consists of giving 50% glucose, 1–2 mL/kg intravenously, followed by a continuous infusion of 10–15% glucose solutions at a rate equivalent to that needed for maintenance water requirements.

Coran A, Drongowski R: Body fluid compartment changes following neonatal surgery. J Pediatr Surg 1989;24:829.

Statter MB: Fluids and electrolytes in infants and children. Semin Pediatr Surg 1992;1:208.

Nutrition

Newborns require a relatively large caloric intake because of their high basal metabolic rate, caloric requirements for growth and development, energy needs to maintain body heat, and limited energy reserve. An infant requires calories at a rate of 100–130 kcal/kg/d and protein at a rate of 2–3 g/kg/d to achieve a normal weight gain of 10–15 g/kg/d (Table 45–3). Thirty percent to 40% of the total nonprotein calories should be provided as fat. These requirements decline with age but increase with sepsis, stress, and trauma. Caloric requirements are increased 10–25% by surgery, more than 50% by infection, and 100% by burns.

A. Enteral Alimentation

The best means of providing calories and protein is through the gastrointestinal tract. If the gastrointestinal tract is functional, standard infant formulas, blenderized meals, or prepared elemental diets can be given by mouth, through nasogastric or nasojejunal feeding tubes, or through gastrostomy or jejunostomy tubes placed surgically. Gastric feeding is preferable because it allows for normal digestive processes and hormonal responses, a greater tolerance for larger osmotic loads, and a lower incidence of dumping. The use of nasoduodenal or nasojejunal tubes is reserved for infants who cannot tolerate intragastric feeding (eg, delayed gastric emptying, gastroesophageal reflux, depressed gag reflex).

The availability of nutritionally complete liquid diets of low viscosity allows continuous feeding through small-diameter catheters. Elemental diets made by mixing crystalline amino acids, oligosaccharides, and fats can be completely absorbed in the small intestine with little residue. Their use is limited because they cause diarrhea as a result of the high osmolality of full-strength formulas. This can be avoided by administering dilute solutions by continuous drip. Initially, the volume of dilute solution is gradually increased, and the concentration is then progressively increased in a stepwise fashion—ie, half strength, three-fourths strength, and full strength. Formulas that remain below 500 mosm are best.

Small Silastic or polyethylene catheters such as those used for intravenous infusion can be passed through the nose or mouth into the stomach or jejunum. In more complex cases, a surgically placed gastrostomy or jejunostomy may be necessary for postoperative feeding. A variety of techniques and methods are employed in their construction. In the case of a gastrostomy, either a balloon catheter is used (ie, Foley) or a low-profile gastrostomy button is placed. Silastic is superior to other plastics because it does not become rigid when exposed to intestinal contents. Parenteral nutrition combined with enteral feeding is often necessary for infants with short bowel syndrome until intestinal adaptation occurs.

B. Parenteral Alimentation

The indications for parenteral alimentation include the following: (1) expected period of prolonged ileus (eg, following repair of gastroschisis or high jejunal atresia); (2) intestinal fistulas; (3) supplementation of oral feedings, as in intractable diarrhea, short bowel syndrome, or various malabsorption syndromes; (4) intrauterine growth retardation; (5) catabolic wasting states such as infections or tumors when gastric feedings are inadequate or not tolerated; (6) inflammatory bowel disease; (7) severe acute alimentary disorders (pancreatitis, necrotizing enterocolitis); and (8) chylothorax.

Concentrated solutions (12.5% glucose or more) thrombose peripheral vessels. Placement of a central venous catheter (PICC or Broviac) into the superior or inferior vena cavae allows the large blood flow to dilute the solution immediately, allowing more concentrated

Table 45–4. Total parenteral nutrition requirements.[1]

Component	Neonate	6 mo to 10 yr	>10 yr
Calories (kcal/kg/d)	90–120	60–105	40–75
Fluid (mL/kg/d)	120–180	120–150	50–75
Dextrose (mg/kg/min)	4–6	7–8	7–8
Protein (g/kg/d)	2–3	1.5–2.5	0.8–2.0
Fat (g/kg/d)	0.5–3.0	1.0–4.0	1.0–4.0
Sodium (meq/kg/d)	3–4	3–4	3–4
Potassium (meq/kg/d)	2–3	2–3	1–2
Calcium (mg/kg/d)	80–120	40–80	40–60
Phosphate (mg/kg/d)	25–40	25–40	25–40
Magnesium (meq/kg/d)	0.25–1.0	0.5	0.5
Zinc (μg/kg/d)	300	100	3 mg/d
Copper (μg/kg/d)	20	20	1.2 mg/d
Chromium (μg/kg/d)	0.2	0.2	12 mg/d
Manganese (μg/kg/d)	6	6	0.3 mg/d
Selenium (mg/kg/d)	2	2	10–20 mg/d

[1]Reproduced, with permission, from Albanese CT: Pediatric surgery. In: *Surgery.* Norton JA (editor). Springer, 2000.

sugar solutions (15–30% glucose) to be administered. The catheter may be placed percutaneously through the subclavian or internal jugular vein or inserted by cutdown into the external jugular, anterior facial, internal jugular, cephalic, brachial, or saphenous veins. For long-term use, Broviac (single lumen) or Hickman (double lumen) catheters, with Dacron cuffs positioned near the exit site of the skin, are preferred to minimize infection and to prevent accidental dislodgment.

Intravenous alimentation solutions containing an amino acid source (2–5% crystalline amino acids or protein hydrolysate), glucose (10–40%), electrolytes, vitamins, and trace minerals are used. The electrolyte composition of the protein solution should be known so that the desired composition of the final solution can be adjusted by appropriate additives according to the individual patient's requirements. A standard solution suitable for infants and young children must contain calcium, magnesium, and phosphate to allow for growth. Trace minerals are also added to the basic solution (Table 45–4). These solutions should be infused at a constant rate with an infusion pump to avoid blood backing up the catheter and clotting and to prevent wide fluctuations of blood glucose and amino acid concentrations. If it is necessary to restrict the volume of infusion, more concentrated glucose solutions can be used to increase the caloric intake.

Complications of prolonged intravenous alimentation are numerous. The most frequent problem is catheter sepsis. Although catheter removal will quickly treat the problem, a trial of antibiotics effective against gram-positive and gram-negative pathogens is indicated. Catheter removal is indicated in the presence of worsening sepsis, three positive blood cultures, or documented yeast infection (with antifungal treatment after catheter removal). Clotting in the catheter may be controlled by adding 1 unit of heparin per milliliter of solution. Emphasis on a constant rate of infusion will minimize hyper- or hypoglycemia. Analysis of serum electrolytes (including calcium and phosphate) may be necessary several times a week initially, but the interval is decreased to once a week when the patient is stable. Patients must be observed for hyperammonemia and for vitamin or trace mineral deficiency. Progressive hepatomegaly and jaundice of uncertain origin can occur after prolonged parenteral alimentation. This syndrome may subside when the parenteral solution is discontinued or when it is infused for a period of 12–16 hours and then the infusion is stopped for 8–12 hours (cycling) or when augmented with enteral feeding.

Amii LA, Moss RL: Nutritional support of the pediatric surgical patient. Curr Opin Pediatr 1999;11:237.

Holcomb GW 3d, Ziegler MM Jr: Nutrition and cancer in children. Surg Annu 1990;2:129.

Pereira GR: Nutritional care of the extremely premature infant. Clin Perinat 1994;22:61.

Winthrop A et al: Analysis of energy and macronutrient balance in the postoperative infant. J Pediatr Surg 1989;24:686.

Blood Loss

Total blood, plasma, and red blood cell volumes are higher during the first few postnatal hours than at any other time in an individual's life. Several hours after birth, plasma shifts out of the circulation, and total blood and plasma volume decrease. The high red blood cell volume persists, decreasing slowly to reach adult levels by the seventh postnatal week. Age-related estimations of blood volume are summarized in Table 45–5.

Although not clinically significant, both the prothrombin time and the partial thromboplastin time may be slightly prolonged at birth due to relative deficiencies of clotting factors. Defects in the coagulating mechanism may occur in newborn infants as a result of vitamin K deficiency, thrombocytopenia, inherited disorders, and temporary hepatic insufficiency due to immaturity, asphyxia, or infection. It is standard to administer 1.0 mg of vitamin K intramuscularly to all newborns.

The blood lost during operation varies greatly according to the complexity of the operative procedure, the underlying disease, and the effectiveness of hemostasis. Mild blood loss, amounting to less than 10% of the blood volume, usually does not require transfusion. It is imperative to develop methods for closely monitoring the amount of blood lost during operations since significant blood loss is often underestimated in the newborn, especially the preterm infant. Dry sponges should be used and weighed shortly after use to minimize error from evaporation. The suction line, connected to a calibrated trap on the operating table, should be short to diminish the dead space of the tubing and to provide immediate data about accumulated blood loss. Visual observation may be used as a rough guide, but it tends to give a falsely low estimate of the loss.

Before operation, newborn infants should receive vitamin K, 1.0 mg intravenously or intramuscularly, if not already administered. If an extensive surgical procedure is anticipated, the patient's blood should be typed and crossmatched in case transfusion is required. In infants with hematocrits greater than 50%, blood loss may be replaced by infusing lactated Ringer's solution or fresh frozen plasma to compensate for losses of up to 25% of total blood volume. Greater blood losses should be replaced with fresh (< 3 days old) whole blood or packed red blood cells. A transfusion of packed red blood cells at a volume of 10 mL/kg usually raises the hematocrit 3–4%. The transfused blood should be prewarmed to body temperature by running it through coiled tubing immersed in water at 37 °C. With excessive blood loss, clotting factors and platelets can be depleted rapidly, and fresh frozen plasma and platelets of identical blood type should be available. A transfusion of 0.1 unit/kg of platelets raises the platelet count by approximately 25,000/μL.

Table 45–5. Blood volume based on age

Preterm infants	85–100 mL/kg
Term infants	85 mL/kg
Age > 1 month	75 mL/kg
Age 3 months to adult	70 mL/kg

Perioperative Considerations

A. Gastrointestinal Decompression

The importance of gastric decompression in the surgical newborn cannot be overemphasized. The distended stomach carries the risk of aspiration and pneumonia and may also impair diaphragmatic excursion, resulting in respiratory distress. For example, oxygenation and ventilation in a neonate with congenital diaphragmatic hernia may become progressively impaired as the herniated intestine becomes distended with air and fluid. With gastroschisis, omphalocele, and diaphragmatic hernia, the ability to reduce the prolapsed intestine into the abdominal cavity is impaired by intestinal distention. It is critical to avoid bag-mask ventilation in these patients. A double-lumen (sump) tube, such as a 10F Replogle or Anderson tube, is preferred, utilizing low continuous suction. If a single-lumen tube is used, intermittent aspiration by syringe or machine is required. The correct position of the tube in the stomach is confirmed by carefully measuring the tube prior to insertion and by radiographs. Careful taping of the tube is essential to avoid displacement.

B. Preoperative Blood Sampling

Blood analyses should be restricted to those studies essential for diagnosis and management. The volume of blood drawn for laboratory tests should be documented as these small volumes cumulatively represent significant blood loss in a small infant. Generally, the only "routine" preoperative blood analyses for a neonate consist of a complete blood count and a blood specimen for type and crossmatch (in the case of major newborn surgery). Electrolytes in the first 12 hours of life simply reflect the mother's electrolytes. Coagulation studies (eg, PT, PTT, ACT) are rarely indicated.

C. Preoperative NPO Guidelines

1. Patients younger than 6 months—No solids, breast milk, or formula 4 hours prior to the procedure. Infants may have clear liquids (water, oral electrolyte mixtures, glucose water, or apple juice) until 2 hours prior to the procedure.

2. Patients from 6 months to 18 years—Nothing to eat or drink after midnight except clear liquids (water, apple juice, oral electrolyte mixtures, gelatin dessert, white grape juice), which can be continued until 2 hours prior to the procedure.

3. Patients older than 18 years—Nothing to eat or drink after midnight except clear liquids (water, apple juice, plain gelatin desserts) until 4 hours prior to the procedure.

D. Bowel Preparation Instructions

The bowel is mechanically cleansed for elective bowel resection. Opinion varies about whether a bowel preparation is needed for certain procedures as well as about what to use to accomplish it and whether to do it at home or in the hospital. An inpatient regimen begins the day prior to surgery and consists of polyethylene glycol-electrolyte solution (GoLYTELY), 25 mL/kg/h for 4 hours or until the effluent is clear. Metoclopramide (0.1 mg/dose IV) is given 1 hour before the GoLYTELY. Pedialyte can be given ad lib until the time to have nothing by mouth.

Outpatient preparations are reserved for patients over 1 year of age. Clear liquids are given the day before surgery. Bisacodyl (Dulcolax) suppositories and 8-oz lukewarm tap water enemas are given the morning and in the evening the day before surgery. For children over 5 years of age, magnesium citrate is added (1 oz per year of age up to a maximum of 8 oz) is given orally in the morning and evening the day before surgery, along with 16-oz tap water enemas.

LESIONS OF THE HEAD & NECK

DERMOID CYSTS

Dermoid cysts are congenital inclusions of skin and skin appendages commonly found on the scalp and eyebrows and in the midline of the nose, neck, and upper chest. They present as painless swellings that may be completely mobile or fixed to the skin and deeper structures. Dermoid cysts of the eyebrows and scalp may produce a depression in the underlying bone that appears as a smooth, punched-out defect on radiographs of the outer table of the skull. They do not extend intracranially. In contrast, cysts of the face and scalp that are located in the midline can extend intracranially so it is imperative to obtain an MRI or CT scan preoperatively. Dermoid cysts of the midline neck may be confused with thyroglossal duct cysts. However, dermoids do not move with swallowing or protrusion of the tongue since they are not deep to the strap muscles, unlike thyroglossal cysts. All dermoids contain a cheesy material that is produced by desquamation of the cells of the epithelial lining. They should be excised intact, since incomplete removal will result in recurrence. Those arising near the eyebrows should be excised through an incision adjacent to the hairline. The eyebrows should not be shaved nor should the incision go through any eyebrow follicles since a permanent glabrous area will develop. There are reports of removing facial dermoids using an endoscope via an incision in the scalp, thus avoiding a facial scar.

McAvoy JM, Zuckerbraun L: Dermoid cysts of the head and neck in children. Arch Otolaryngol 1976;102:529.

Steele MH et al: Orbtiofacial masses in children: An endoscopic approach. Arch Otolaryngol Head Neck Surg 2001;128:409.

BRANCHIOGENIC ANOMALIES

During the first month of fetal life, the primitive neck develops four external clefts and four pharyngeal pouches that are separated by a membrane. Between the clefts and pouches are branchial arches. The dorsal portion of the first cleft becomes the external auditory canal; the other clefts are obliterated. The pharyngeal pouches persist as adult organs. The first pouch becomes the auditory tube, the middle ear cavity, and the mastoid air cells. The second pouch incompletely regresses and becomes the palatine tonsil and the supratonsillar fossa. The third pouch forms the inferior parathyroid glands and thymus; the fourth forms the superior parathyroid glands. Branchial anomalies are remnants of this fetal branchial apparatus.

A tract of branchial origin may form a complete fistula, or one end may be obliterated to form an external or internal sinus, or both ends may resorb, leaving an aggregate of cells forming a cyst (Figure 45–1). Fistulas that arise above the hyoid bone and communicate with the external auditory canal represent persistence of the first branchial cleft. These tracts are always lined by squamous epithelium. Cysts and sinuses of second or third branchial origin are lined by squamous, cuboidal, or ciliated columnar epithelium. Fistulas that communicate between the anterior border of the sternocleidomastoid muscle and the tonsillar fossa are of second branchial origin, and those that extend into the piriform sinus are derived from the third branchial pouch. Cysts developing from branchial structures usually appear later in childhood as opposed to sinuses and fistulas. Branchiogenic anomalies occur with equal frequency on each side of the neck, and 15% are bilateral. Second branchial cleft abnormalities are most common, occurring six times more frequently than first cleft anomalies.

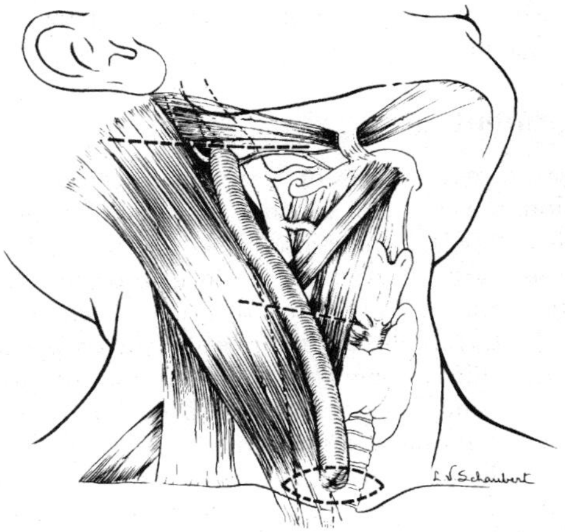

Figure 45–1. Branchiogenic fistula from second branchial cleft origin. The fistula extends along the anterior border of the sternocleidomastoid muscle and courses between the internal and external carotid arteries and cephalad to the hypoglossal nerve to enter the tonsillar fossa.

Clinical Findings

A sinus or fistulous opening along the anterior border of the sternocleidomastoid muscle may be noted at birth and usually discharges a mucoid or purulent material. The patient may complain of a foul-tasting discharge in the mouth upon massaging the tract, but the internal orifice is rarely recognized. Some may present with an acute infection. The cysts are characteristically found anterior and deep to the upper third of the sternocleidomastoid muscle, or they may be located within the parotid gland or pharyngeal wall, over the manubrium, or in the mediastinum. Sinuses and cysts are prone to become repeatedly infected, producing cellulitis and abscess formation. Incomplete branchial sinuses appear as a dimple that contain cartilage and do not drain or communicate with the deep structures of the neck.

Differential Diagnosis

Granulomatous lymphadenitis due to mycobacterial infections may produce cystic lymph nodes and draining sinuses, but these are usually distinguishable by the chronic inflammatory reaction that precedes the purulent discharge. Suppurative lymphadenitis, most commonly due to *Staphylococcus aureus,* may resemble an infected branchial remnant. However, treatment and complete healing of the lymphadenitis is curative, whereas an identifiable branchial remnant will persist after the infection resolves. Hemangiomas and lymphangiomas are soft, spongy tumor masses that might be confused with branchial cysts, but the latter have a firmer consistency. Lymphangiomas may transilluminate, while branchial cysts do not. Carotid body tumors are quite firm, are located at the carotid bifurcation, and occur in older patients. Lymphomas produce firm masses in the area where branchial remnants occur, but multiple matted nodes rather than a solitary cystic tumor distinguish these lesions. Mucoid material may be expressed from the openings of branchial sinuses or fistulas, and a firm cordlike tract may be palpable along its course.

Treatment

Nearly all branchial abnormalities should be excised early in life since repeated infection is common, making resection more difficult. Asymptomatic, small cartilaginous remnants may be watched, but they are usually removed for cosmetic reasons as well as the smaller risk of infection, compared to the true cyst/fistula. Infected sinuses and cysts require initial incision and drainage. Excision of these tracts is staged and usually performed approximately 6 weeks later, when the acute inflammatory reaction has subsided. Every effort should be made to excise the entire cyst wall or fistula tract (including the skin punctum, if present) since recurrence and infection are common with incomplete removal. Excision should be undertaken cautiously, as the tracts may lie adjacent to the facial, hypoglossal, and glossopharyngeal nerves as well as the carotid artery and internal jugular vein.

Roback SA, Talendar RL: Thyroglossal duct cysts and branchial cleft anomalies. Semin Pediatr Surg 1994;3:142.

PREAURICULAR LESIONS

Preauricular sinuses, cysts, and cartilaginous rests arise from anomalous development of the auricle and are unrelated to branchial anomalies. The sinuses are often short and end blindly. They can be cosmetically unappealing and often become infected. Superficial skin tags and cartilaginous rests are easily excised without risk to other structures. Preauricular sinus tracts, however, may be very deceptive in their extent, and one should be prepared to proceed with extensive dissection that risks damage to branches of the facial nerve.

Currie AR et al: Pitfalls in the management of preauricular sinuses. Br J Surg 1996;83:1722.

LYMPHANGIOMA (CYSTIC HYGROMA)

Lymphangiomas are benign multilobular, multinodular cystic masses lined by endothelial cells. They result from maldevelopment and obstruction of the lymphatic

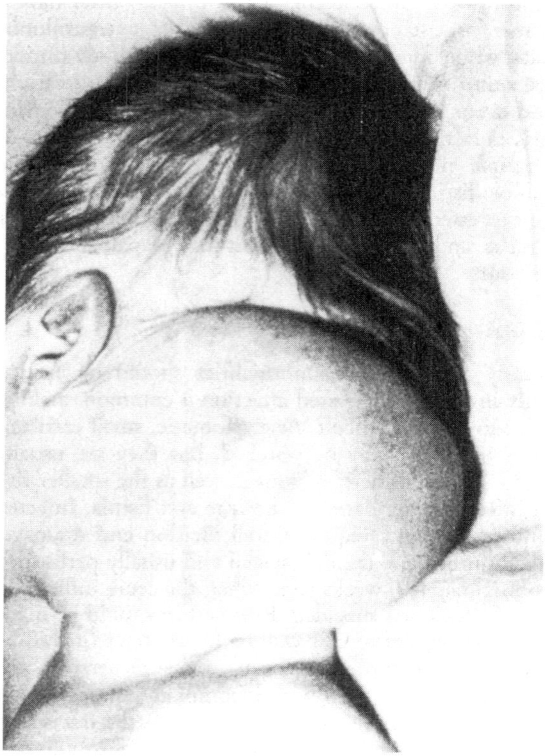

Figure 45–2. Typical neonatal lymphangioma arising from the posterior cervical triangle. (From Filston HC: Hemangiomas, cystic hygromas, and teratomas of the head and neck. Semin Pediatr Surg 1994;3:147. Reprinted with permission from Elsevier.)

system. Eventually, sequestrations of lymphatic tissue that do not communicate with the normal lymphatic system develop. Fifty to 65 percent appear at birth and 90% by the second year of life. They are located most commonly in the posterior triangle of the neck (75%) (Figure 45–2) and axilla (20%), with the remainder located in the mediastinum, retroperitoneum, pelvis, and groin.

Clinical Findings

Neck lymphangiomas may communicate beneath the clavicle with an axillary hygroma, mediastinal hygroma, or, rarely, both. The majority are asymptomatic, though large lesions invading the floor of the mouth may cause symptoms referable to pharyngeal or upper airway obstruction. The skin is never involved, although the lesion may be densely adherent to the undersurface of the dermis. These lesions grow along fascial planes and around neurovascular structures; they are invasive but not infiltrative. Large lesions may be recognized prenatally using ultrasound or MRI examination.

Treatment

There are two modes of treatment, sclerotherapy or excision, the choice of which is based on imaging studies (CT, MRI). Intralesional injection of a sclerosing agent is most effective for unilocular or macrocystic lesions. Examples of agents that have been used are OK-432 (a lyophilized mixture of *Streptococcus pyogenes* and penicillin G potassium), bleomycin, and doxycycline. Excision is carried out with bipolar cautery to ensure a hemostatic dissection and decrease the incidence of lymph leak and nerve injury. Nevertheless, postoperative lymph leak is common and is treated by closed suction drainage for days to weeks. Intraoperative cyst rupture increases the difficulty of the dissection since the thin-walled cyst is difficult to identify and the margins are obscured. The recurrence rate following surgery is 50%.

Brown RL, Azizkhan RG: Pediatric head and neck lesions. Pediatr Clin North Am 1998;45:899.

Fonkalsrud EW: Congenital malformations of the lymphatic system. Semin Pediatr Surg 1994;3:62.

Ogita S et al: OK-432 therapy in 64 patients with lymphangioma. J Pediatr Surg 1994;29:784.

THYROGLOSSAL DUCT REMNANT

During the fourth week of gestation, the thyroid gland develops from an evagination in the floor of the primitive pharynx located between the first pair of pharyngeal pouches. If the anlage of the thyroid does not descend normally, the gland may form at the base of the tongue or remain as a mass anywhere in the midline of the neck along its truncated path of descent. If the thyroglossal duct persists, the epithelial tract forms a cyst that usually communicates with the foramen cecum of the tongue. The thyroglossal duct descends through the second branchial arch anlage, which becomes the hyoid bone, prior to its fusion in the midline. Because of this, the tract of a persistent thyroglossal duct often extends through the hyoid bone (Figure 45–3).

Clinical Findings

The most common physical finding is a rounded cystic mass of varying size in the midline of the neck just below the hyoid bone. The acute inflammatory reaction of an infection may herald the presence of a cyst. The fluid in the cyst is usually under pressure and may give the impression of being a solid tumor. Cysts and aberrant midline thyroid glands move up and down with swallowing and with protrusion of the tongue since

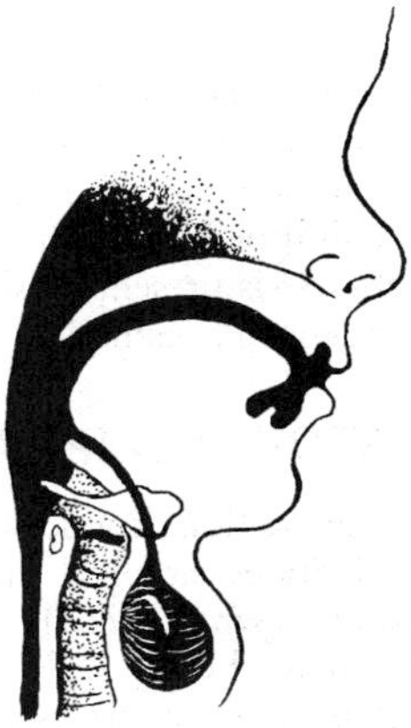

Figure 45–3. Thyroglossal cyst and duct course through the hyoid bone to the foramen cecum of the tongue.

they are deep to the cervical strap muscles. In contrast, lingual thyroid tissue is a rare clinical entity and may produce dysphagia, dysphonia, dyspnea, hemorrhage, or pain.

Differential Diagnosis

Lymph nodes, dermoid cysts, and enlarged Delphian nodes containing tumor metastases may be confused with thyroglossal remnants in the midline of the neck. Dermoid cysts do not move with swallowing. Lingual thyroids may be confused with a hypertrophied lingual tonsil or with a ranula, fibroma, angioma, sarcoma, or carcinoma of the tongue. These lesions and thyroglossal cysts may be distinguished from aberrantly located thyroid glands by needle aspiration or by radioiodine scintiscan.

Complications

Thyroglossal cysts are prone to infection, and spontaneous drainage or incision and drainage of an abscess will often result in a chronically draining fistula. Excision of an ectopic thyroid may remove all thyroid tissue, producing hypothyroidism. There is a malignant potential of the dysgenetic thyroid tissue located in a thyroglossal duct cyst; carcinoma develops more frequently in ectopic thyroid tissue than in normal thyroid glands.

Treatment

Complete excision is indicated because of the risk of infection and the possibility of the development of papillary carcinoma later in life. Acute infection in thyroglossal tracts should be treated with local heat and antibiotics. Abscesses should be incised and drained. After complete subsidence of the inflammatory reaction (approximately 6 weeks), a thyroglossal cyst and its epithelial tract should be excised. The mid portion of the hyoid bone should be removed en bloc with the thyroglossal tract to the base of the tongue (Sistrunk procedure). Recurrences occur when the hyoid is not removed and when the cyst was previously infected or drained.

Housawa M et al: Anatomical reconstruction of the thyroglossal duct. J Pediatr Surg 1991;26:766.

Roback SA, Telander RL: Thyroglossal duct cysts and branchial cleft anomalies. Semin Pediatr Surg 1994;3:142.

TORTICOLLIS

Torticollis presents with a hard, nontender, fibrotic mass within the sternocleidomastoid muscle. It may be present at birth but is usually not noticed until the second to sixth weeks of life. The mass appears with equal frequency in both sexes and on each side of the neck. Rarely, there is more than one mass in the muscle or both sternocleidomastoid muscles are involved. A history of breech delivery is present in 20–30% of these children.

Clinical Findings

Torticollis is manifested when the sternocleidomastoid muscle is shortened and the mastoid process on the involved side is pulled down toward the clavicle and manubrium. As a result, the head is abducted to the ipsilateral side and rotated to the contralateral side (toward the opposite shoulder). The shoulder on the affected side is raised, and there may be cervical and thoracic scoliosis. Passive rotation of the head to the side of the involved muscle will be resisted and limited to varying degrees, and the muscle will appear as a protuberant band. Because of persistent pressure when the patient is recumbent, the ipsilateral face and contralateral occiput will be flattened. Facial hemihypoplasia and plagiocephaly (flattening of the ipsilateral posterior skull) occurs in untreated cases, usually within 6 months.

Treatment

Surgery is rarely necessary for this disorder. Torticollis is treated with active range of motion exercises. The child's shoulders are held flat to a table and the head is tilted and rotated in a full range of motion. This procedure should be performed at least four times a day, usually for 2–3 months. The firm "tumor" often disappears well before the torticollis is cured. If the muscle continues to become progressively shortened, with facial and occipital skull deformity, both heads of the sternocleidomastoid muscle should be divided through a small transverse incision just above the clavicle. This procedure does not reverse the bony changes that have already developed but prevents progression of the process. Recurrence is rare.

Binder H et al: Congenital muscular torticollis: results of conservative management with long-term follow-up in 85 cases. Arch Phys Med Rehabil 1987;68:222.

Celayir AC: Congenital muscular torticollis: early and intensive treatment is critical. A prospective study. Pediatr Int 2000; 42:504.

CERVICAL LYMPHADENOPATHY

SUPPURATIVE LYMPHADENITIS

Infections in the upper respiratory passages, scalp, ear, or neck produce varying degrees of secondary lymphadenitis. Most of the causative organisms are streptococcal or staphylococcal species. In infants and young children, the clinical course of the suppurative lymphadenitis may greatly overshadow a seemingly insignificant or inapparent primary infection. Scalp or ear infections produce pre- or postauricular and suboccipital lymph node involvement; submental, oral, tonsillar, and pharyngeal infections affect the submandibular and deep jugular nodes.

Clinical Findings

With significant lymphadenitis, the regional lymph nodes become greatly enlarged and produce local pain and tenderness. Enlargement of cervical nodes is most common, followed by occipital and submandibular nodes. Fever is high initially and then becomes intermittent and may persist for days or weeks. The regional nodes may remain enlarged and firm for prolonged periods, or they may suppurate and produce surrounding cellulitis and edema. Subsequently, the nodes may involute or a fluctuant abscess may form, resulting in redness and thinning of the overlying skin. Infected, matted nodes may become so hard as to be indistinguishable (on palpation) from a solid mass.

Differential Diagnosis

A smoldering lymphadenitis that neither resolves nor forms an abscess can be confused with granulomatous lymphadenitis, lymphoma, or metastatic tumor. Excisional biopsy is required to differentiate these lesions. After several weeks, there will usually be a reduction in the size and firmness of suppurative adenitis, especially after antibiotic treatment has been started.

Treatment

In the acute phase, the patient should be treated with oral or intravenous antistaphylococcal antibiotics. In the subacute or chronic phase, the presence of pus in the node may be confirmed by needle aspiration of the mass. When an abscess is present, it should be incised and drained under general anesthesia.

GRANULOMATOUS LYMPHADENITIS

Although typical tuberculous cervical adenitis is very rare in the United States, atypical mycobacteria (eg, *Mycobacterium avium-intracellulare*) frequently cause chronic suppuration in the cervical (most common), axillary, and inguinal lymph nodes. Granulomatous lymphadenitis and caseation may occur in the regional nodes draining the inoculation site of BCG. Cat-scratch disease causes a caseating lymphadenitis in regional lymph nodes (eg, epitrochlear and axillary nodes enlarge after an upper extremity cat scratch).

Clinical Findings

Children under age 6 are most frequently affected. The initial manifestation is a painless, progressive enlargement of the lymph nodes in the deep cervical chain and the parotid, suboccipital, submandibular, and supraclavicular nodes. The duration of lymphadenopathy is usually 1–3 months or longer. The nodes may be large and mobile or, with progressive disease, may become matted, fixed, and finally caseate to form an abscess. Incision or spontaneous overlying skin breakdown will result in a chronically draining sinus. In tuberculosis, both sides of the neck or multiple groups of nodes are infected, and the chest radiograph indicates pulmonary involvement. In atypical mycobacterial lymphadenitis, pulmonary disease is rare and the cervical adenitis is unilateral. The tuberculin skin test is weakly positive in over 80% of patients with atypical mycobacterial infection. Skin test antigens from the various strains of atypical mycobacteria are available. A positive skin test helps differentiate granulomatous adenitis from malignant lymphadenopathy. A fluctuant node can be confused with a branchial cleft remnant or a thyroglossal duct cyst.

Cat-scratch disease is usually acquired by a bite or scratch from a kitten. It is caused by a pleomorphic gram-negative bacillus *(Bartonella henselae)* that is detected in tissues by a silver stain. It is an acute illness characterized by fever, malaise, and occasionally a pustular lesion at the site of the scratch. Tender lymph node enlargement usually develops. Two to 4 weeks later, regional lymphadenitis persists, producing painful, fixed suppurative nodes that may develop into a chronically draining sinus.

Treatment

Atypical tuberculous lymphadenitis may be treated with rifampin (10 mg/kg/d), though definitive treatment usually requires nodal excision. Trimethoprim-sulfamethoxazole may shorten the course of cat-scratch disease and prevent suppuration. When antibiotics are ineffective, the procedure of choice is excision of involved nodes before caseation occurs. Once the nodes become fluctuant or a draining sinus forms, a wedge of involved skin should be excised and the underlying necrotic nodes should be curetted out (rather than excised), taking care not to injure neighboring nerves. The wound edges and skin should be closed primarily. The value of continuing chemotherapy is influenced by sensitivity tests on the cultured material. Excision and primary closure usually result in excellent healing with good cosmetic results.

Beiler HA et al: Specific and nonspecific lymphadenitis in childhood: etiology, diagnosis, and therapy. Pediatr Surg Int 1997;12:108.

Bodenstein L, Altman RP: Cervical lymphadenitis in infants and children. Semin Pediatr Surg 1994;3:134.

Flint D et al: Cervical lymphadenitis due to non-tuberculous mycobacteria: surgical treatment and review. Int J Pediatr Otorhinolaryngol 2000;53:187.

Holley HP: Successful treatment of cat-scratch disease with ciprofloxacin. JAMA 1991;265:1563.

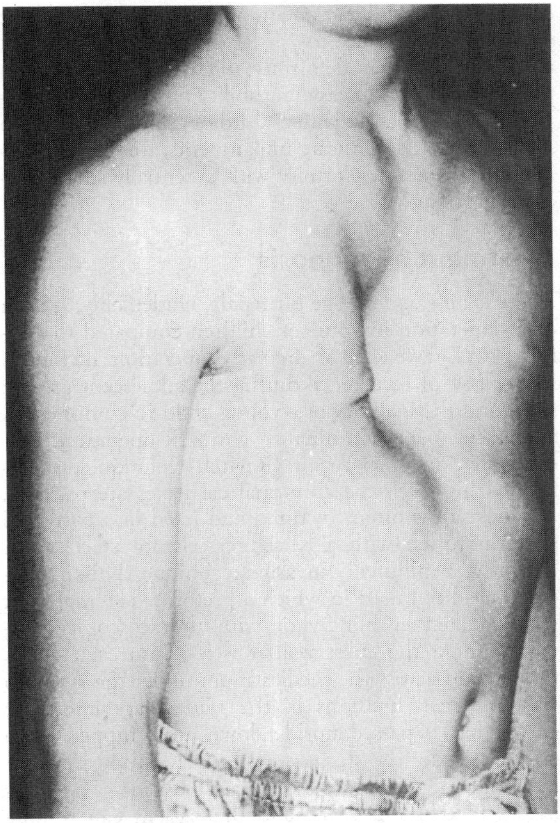

Figure 45–4. Adolescent with a pectus excavatum deformity. Note that the most pronounced sternal curvature is in the lower half.

CONGENITAL CHEST WALL DEFORMITIES

STERNAL CLEFT

Failure of fusion of the two sternal bars during embryonic development produces congenital sternal cleft, which may involve the upper, lower, or entire sternum. In its severe form, this defect is usually associated with protrusion of the pericardium and heart (ectopia cordis) and congenital heart lesions. Defects may be associated with extracardiac anomalies, including cleft lip, cleft palate, hydrocephalus, and other central nervous system disorders, or may be one component of the pentalogy of Cantrell. Operative correction is performed in the neonatal period since the chest wall is so pliable; it consists of simple suture approximation of the two sternal halves. More complex defects associated with ectopia cordis are often incompatible with life.

PECTUS EXCAVATUM

This depression deformity is the most common congenital chest wall abnormality, occurring in one in 300 live births, with a 3:1 male predominance. It is associated with other musculoskeletal disorders (Marfan's syndrome, Poland's syndrome, scoliosis, clubfoot, syndactyly), and 2% have congenital heart disease. There is a familial form. It results from the unbalanced posterior growth of costal cartilages that are often fused, bizarrely deformed, or rotated. The body of the sternum secondarily exhibits a prominent posterior curvature, usually involving its lower half (Figure 45–4). Commonly, the xiphoid is the deepest portion of the depression. The third, fourth, and fifth costal cartilages are usually affected, though the second to eighth costal cartilages may be involved. The severity of the defect varies greatly from a mild, insignificant depression to an extreme where the xiphoid bone is adjacent to the vertebrae. The depression may be symmetrical or asymmetrical with varying degrees of sternal rotation.

Clinical Findings

These patients are typically round-shouldered, with stooped posture, relative abdominal prominence, flared costal margins, and an asthenic appearance. They may be withdrawn and refuse to participate in sports activities, particularly if their deformity might be exposed. Few patients complain of easy fatigability or inability to compete in exertional activities. Cardiopulmonary function studies rarely demonstrate impairments; this is predominantly a cosmetic deformity with potentially severe psychosocial sequelae.

Treatment & Prognosis

There is no standard age for repair. Undeniably, it is an easier operation in younger children compared to adolescents. Drawbacks of an early operation include a higher risk of recurrence during the adolescent growth spurt and the inability of a young child to comprehend and assent to a predominantly cosmetic operation. Traditionally, an open repair (Ravitch technique) is performed in which the abnormal cartilages are resected; the sternum is often fractured and fixed in a corrected position (often with a Kirschner wire or steel strut). Recently, a minimally invasive technique (Nuss procedure) has been used in which a preformed sternal strut is passed, either blindly or with thoracoscopic assistance, under the chest wall muscles, into each hemithorax, and across the mediastinum under the sternum via two small incisions in the midaxillary line. The curved bar is passed upside down and "flipped" into position under the sternum, effectively lifting the sternum and chest wall into a corrected position. The bar is left in place for 2 years, and the patient can resume activity in 3 months. The recurrence rate for the open procedure is less than 3%; at present there is not enough long-term follow-up to assess the Nuss technique. In general, there is no cardiopulmonary benefit after chest wall repair except in rare instances when the deformity is excessive. Otherwise, the repair is performed solely to improve appearance. However, the psychosocial benefits of repair of this often embarrassing deformity cannot be minimized.

PECTUS CARINATUM

This is a protrusion deformity, also referred to as pigeon breast or chicken chest. It is approximately ten times less frequent than pectus excavatum. It results from the overgrowth of costal cartilages, with forward buckling and secondary deformation of the sternum (Figure 45–5). Atypical and asymmetric forms with rotation are common. There is a familial form. It is associated with Marfan's disease, neurofibromatosis, Poland's syndrome, and Morquio's disease. Unlike pectus excavatum, the deformity is typically mild or nearly imperceptible in early childhood and becomes increasingly prominent during the rapid growth in early puberty.

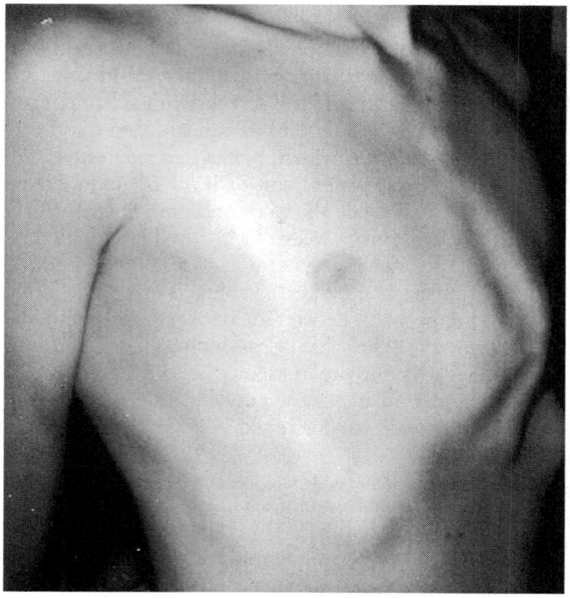

Figure 45–5. Severe pectus carinatum deformity. (Reproduced, with permission, from Albanese CT: Pediatric surgery. In: *Surgery.* Norton JA [editor]. Springer, 2000.) (Originally published in Shamberger R: Congenital chest wall deformities. In: *Pediatric Surgery,* 5th ed. O'Neill JA, Rowe MI, Grosted JL [editors]. © 1998 Mosby Co.)

Treatment & Prognosis

As with pectus excavatum, there is no cardiorespiratory compromise with this deformity, and repair is performed solely to achieve an improved cosmetic appearance. Mild deformities should be left alone and the patient followed to observe for progression. Moderate to severe defects should be repaired, particularly when the patient indicates a desire for improvement. The deformed cartilages are resected, leaving the costochondral membranes (perichondrium) intact. Sternal fracture is usually not necessary. To ensure that the costal cartilages grow back on a straighter line, "reefing" sutures are placed in the perichondrium to shorten them. The costal cartilages regenerate within 6 weeks. A thorough procedure will provide an excellent cosmetic result in nearly all cases. Recurrences are rare.

Fonkalsrud EW, Beanes S: Surgical management of pectus carinatum: 30 years' experience. World J Surg 2001;25:898.

Miller KA et al: Minimally invasive repair of pectus excavatum: a single institution's experience. Surgery 2001;130:652.

Nuss D et al: A 10-year review of a minimally invasive technique for the correction of pectus excavatum. J Pediatr Surg 1998;33:545.

Shamberger RC: Cardiopulmonary effects of anterior chest wall deformities. Chest Surg Clin N Am 2000;10:245.

SURGICAL RESPIRATORY EMERGENCIES IN THE NEWBORN

Certain aspects of respiration peculiar to the infant must be appreciated. Except during periods of crying, the newborn baby is an obligate nasal breather. The ability to breathe through the mouth may take weeks or months to acquire. Inspiration is accomplished chiefly by diaphragmatic excursion; the intercostal and accessory muscles contribute little to ventilation. Impaired inspiration results in retraction of the sternum, costal margin, and neck fossae; the resulting paradoxical motion may contribute to respiratory insufficiency. The airway is small and flaccid, so that it is readily occluded by mucus or edema, and it collapses readily under slight pressure. Dyspneic infants swallow large volumes of air, and the distended stomach and bowel may further impair diaphragmatic excursion.

Classification

A. Upper Airway Disorders

1. Micrognathia—Pierre Robin syndrome
2. Macroglossia—Muscular hypertrophy, hypothyroidism, lymphangioma, Beckwith-Wiedemann syndrome
3. Anomalous nasopharyngeal passage—Choanal atresia, Treacher-Collins syndrome, Apert's syndrome, and Crouzon's syndrome
4. Tumors, cysts, or enlarged thyroid remnants in the pharynx or neck
5. Laryngeal or tracheal stenosis, webs, cysts, tumors, or vocal cord paralysis
6. Epiglottitis
7. Tracheomalacia
8. Tracheal stenosis with or without complete tracheal rings

B. Intrathoracic Airway Disorders

1. Atelectasis
2. Pneumothorax and pneumomediastinum
3. Pleural effusion or chylothorax
4. Pulmonary cysts, sequestration, and tumors
5. Congenital lobar emphysema
6. Diaphragmatic hernia or eventration
7. Esophageal atresia with or without tracheoesophageal fistula
8. Anomalies of the great vessels (eg, double aortic arch, aberrant left subclavian artery, anomalous origin of left pulmonary artery)
9. Mediastinal tumors and cysts (foregut duplications, thymomas, substernal goiter, lymphoma)

PIERRE ROBIN SYNDROME

Pierre Robin syndrome is a congenital defect characterized by micrognathia and glossoptosis, often associated with cleft palate. The small lower jaw and strong sucking action of the infant allow the tongue to be sucked back and occlude the laryngeal airway and may be life-threatening.

Infants with mild cases should be kept in the prone position during care and feeding. A nasogastric or gastrostomy tube may be necessary for feeding. Nasohypopharyngeal intubation is effective in preventing occlusion of the larynx. If conservative measures fail, prompt attention to maintaining an open airway by tracheostomy is indicated. Surgical treatment involves tongue placation in which the tongue is sutured forward to the lower jaw, but this frequently breaks down. In time, the lower jaw develops normally. These infants eventually learn how to keep the tongue from occluding the airway.

CHOANAL ATRESIA

Complete obstruction at the posterior nares from choanal atresia may be unilateral and relatively asymptomatic. It may be membranous (10%) or bony (90%). When it is bilateral, severe respiratory distress is manifested at birth by marked chest wall retraction on inspiration and a normal cry.

There is arching of the head and neck in an effort to breathe, and the baby is unable to eat. The diagnosis is confirmed by the inability to pass a tube through the nares to the pharynx. With the baby in a supine position, radiopaque material may be instilled into the nares and lateral x-rays of the head taken to outline the obstruction. A CT scan of the nasopharynx will define bony occlusion.

Emergency treatment consists of maintaining an oral airway by placing a nipple, with the tip cut off, in the mouth. The membranous or bony occlusion may then be perforated by direct transpalatal excision, or it may be punctured and enlarged with a Hegar dilator. The newly created opening must be stented with plastic tubing for 5 weeks to prevent stricture.

CONGENITAL TRACHEAL STENOSIS & MALACIA

There are three main types of congenital tracheal stenosis: generalized hypoplasia; funnel-like narrowing, usually tapering to a tight stenosis just above the carina; and segmental stenosis of various lengths that can occur at any level. Tracheomalacia is a functional obstruction in a "soft" trachea that collapses with inspiration. It is often secondary to external compression by vascular anomalies or tumors or from a chronically dilated upper esophageal pouch in those with esophageal atresia.

Diagnosis

The diagnostic approach to an infant with respiratory distress and possible distal tracheal obstruction must be carefully integrated with plans for management of the airway, since the compromised infant airway is easily occluded by edema or secretions. This is especially true in distal tracheal lesions, where an endotracheal or tracheostomy tube may not relieve the distal obstruction. The diagnostic value of every procedure must be weighed against the threat of precipitating airway obstruction. Tracheal lesions can be visualized using esophagography, angiography, or CT/MRI scans. Dynamic lesions such as tracheomalacia and vascular compression syndromes are best defined by videotape fluoroscopy or cineradiography with barium in the esophagus. Angiography may be necessary. Flow-volume curves can define the level of obstruction (intrathoracic versus extrathoracic) and the type of obstruction (stenosis versus malacia).

Although bronchoscopy often provides the best delineation of tracheobronchial lesions, it is an invasive procedure that can precipitate acute obstruction from edema or inflammation. A ventilating infant rigid bronchoscope with Hopkins optics should be kept above the critical area to avoid precipitating obstruction. Flexible transnasal awake bronchoscopy is most useful in demonstrating functional abnormalities (eg, malacia).

Treatment

Noncritical stenotic and malacic lesions in infants and children should be managed as conservatively as possible, preferably without intubation. "Temporary" stenting of these lesions is seldom temporary, since the presence of the tube itself ensures continued trauma and irritation such that the tube cannot be removed without airway obstruction. If an infant or child cannot be managed without intubation, surgical correction must be considered. Tracheal reconstruction via resection or a variety of tracheoplasty techniques has proved to be the treatment of choice for tracheal lesions. Severe tracheomalacia is treated by addressing the underlying cause. Aortopexy or an endotracheal stent is often necessary. Tracheostomy is a last resort.

Backer CL et al: Tracheal surgery in children: an 18-year review of four techniques. Eur J Cardiothorac Surg 2001;19:777.

deLorimier AA et al: Tracheobronchial obstructions in infants and children: experience with 45 cases. Ann Surg 1990;212:277.

Rutter MJ, Hartley BE, Cotton RT: Cricotracheal resection in children. Arch Otolaryngol Head Neck Surg 2001;127:289.

Acosta AC et al: Tracheal stenosis: The long and short of it. J Pediatr Surg 2000;35:1612.

CONGENITAL DIAPHRAGMATIC HERNIA

Congenital diaphragmatic hernia is a highly lethal or morbid disease that affects 1 in 2000 live births (Figure 45–6). Anatomically, congenital diaphragmatic hernia results from an embryologic fusion defect, allowing herniation of intra-abdominal contents into the chest. Fusion of the transverse septum and pleuroperitoneal folds normally occurs during the eighth week of embryonic development. If diaphragmatic formation is incomplete, the pleuroperitoneal hiatus (foramen of Bochdalek) persists. Intestinal nonrotation is common as the bowel herniates into the thorax rather than undergoing its normal sequence of rotation and fixation. Severe defects cause pulmonary hypoplasia, pulmonary hypertension, and cardiac dysfunction. The larger the hernia and the earlier it occurs, the more severe the pulmonary hypoplasia.

Clinical Findings

A. Symptoms and Signs

Infants with large diaphragmatic defects are usually symptomatic in the delivery room, with tachypnea, grunting

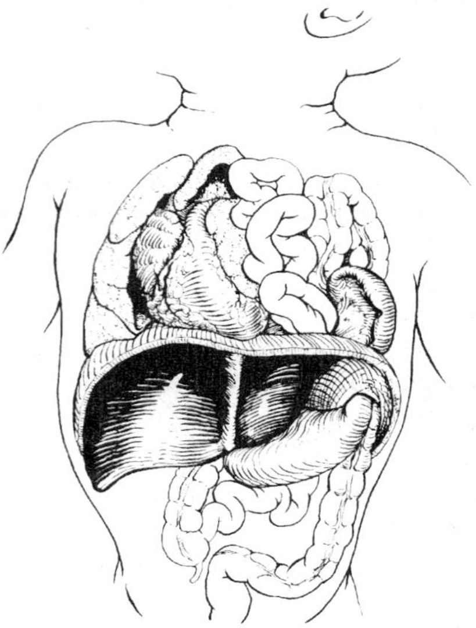

Figure 45–6. Congenital posterolateral (Bochdalek) diaphragmatic hernia. Bowel, spleen, and liver sometimes herniate into the chest and severely compromise lung development in utero and ventilation after birth. (Reproduced, with permission, from Schrock TR: *Handbook of Surgery,* 6th ed. Jones, 1978.)

respirations, retractions, and cyanosis, and may require urgent intubation. Smaller defects may not become symptomatic until the infant is several days or months old. Typically, the abdomen is scaphoid since much of the abdominal viscera is in the hemithorax. The chest on the side of the hernia may be dull to percussion, but bowel sounds are not usually appreciated. The left side of the diaphragm is affected four or five times as frequently as the right, with a rate of associated anomalies of 20% (chromosomal abnormalities, neural tube defects, and congenital heart disease). When the hernia is on the left, the heart sounds may be heard best on the right side of the chest.

The development of symptoms with CDH correlates with the degree of pulmonary hypoplasia and pulmonary hypertension. Prenatal diagnosis is occurring more and more frequently and allows the mother and the fetus to be referred to an institution where sophisticated perinatal and pediatric surgical units are available.

B. Imaging Studies

A chest radiograph may demonstrate the following: a paucity of gas within the abdomen, radiopaque hemithorax if the bowel does not contain a significant amount of gas or if the left lobe of the liver occupies the majority of the hemithorax, loss of normal ipsilateral diaphragmatic contour, bowel in the thorax, contralateral mediastinal shift, and a coiled nasogastric tube in the hemithorax. Right-sided hernias can be difficult to distinguish from a diaphragmatic eventration. This can be differentiated by an MRI scan. MRI or CT scan can also distinguish between CDH and a cystic lung lesion (eg, congenital cystic adenomatoid malformation).

Treatment

A nasogastric tube should be placed in the stomach to aspirate swallowed air and to prevent distention of the herniated bowel, which would further compress the lungs. Repair of the diaphragmatic defect is not a surgical emergency and should be performed once the infant has stabilized and has demonstrated minimal to no pulmonary hypertension. Early reduction (before 48 hours postnatally) and repair has been shown to transiently worsen pulmonary function by decreasing pulmonary compliance and increasing airway reactivity. A subcostal abdominal incision should be made and the herniated bowel reduced from the pleural space. Some surgeons prefer a thoracic approach, particularly for right-sided defects. The negative pressure between the bowel and the chest wall may make reduction difficult. This negative pressure may be broken by inserting a tube along the pleura and injecting air through it. Following reduction of the bowel, placement of a chest tube in the pleural space is optional; if used, it is connected to a water seal and not to vacuum. The diaphragmatic defect should be closed by nonabsorbable sutures. In many instances, a synthetic material is required to close large defects. The abdominal cavity may be too small and underdeveloped to accommodate the intestine and permit closure of the abdominal wall muscle and fascial layers. In such cases, abdominal wall skin flaps should be mobilized and closed over the protruding bowel or a silo created to allow for gradual visceral reduction with concomitant abdominal domain expansion and staged closure of the abdominal wall.

Respiratory support and treatment of hypoxemia, hypercapnia, and acidosis are required before and often after repair. Persistent pulmonary hypertension may result in right-to-left shunt and produce severe hypoxemia in the lower aorta. Nitric oxide added to the ventilation gases can induce pulmonary vasodilation, improve pulmonary perfusion, and reverse the right-to-left shunt. The persistent fetal circulation physiology may be treated successfully in many cases by extracorporeal membrane oxygenation and permissive ventilatory strategies (high-frequency ventilation). Hypoxemic myocardiopathy may require infusion of dopamine to enhance cardiac output. Prenatal treatment for severe CDH (temporary fetal tracheal occlusion to promote lung growth) has been extensively studied and presently offers no advantage over maximal postnatal care.

Prognosis

The death rate for infants with congenital diaphragmatic hernia depends upon the severity of pulmonary hypoplasia, the presence or absence of associated anomalies, and the quality of care provided for these critically ill infants. When diagnosed in utero, prognosis depends on the presence or absence of liver herniation into the left hemithorax, the gestational age at diagnosis, and an ultrasonographic estimation of lung size (the lung-to-head ratio). Long-term, there are a number of probably clinically insignificant physiologic abnormalities such as a reduction in total lung volume, restrictive or obstructive lung disease, and abnormal lung compliance. However, a small subset of patients will survive as "pulmonary cripples" and remain oxygen-dependent or ventilator-dependent, often requiring tracheostomies. Since there may be deficient periesophageal muscular tissue or an abnormal orientation of the gastroesophageal junction, gastroesophageal reflux is common. It is most commonly treated nonoperatively, but refractory cases may require a surgical antireflux procedure. Recurrent diaphragmatic hernia occurs in 10–20% of infants and should be considered in any child with a history of congenital diaphragmatic hernia who presents with new gastrointestinal or pulmonary symptoms. Recurrence is most common when a prosthetic patch is used for the repair.

Surgical units that are immediately adjacent to obstetric services report death rates as high as 80%, because infants with severe pulmonary hypoplasia will be recognized and treated immediately. Infants who survive transfer to surgical centers remote from the delivery area usually have less severe disease, and the death rates reported from these facilities are usually under 40%.

With improvements in prenatal ultrasonographic imaging, many of these defects can be appreciated early enough so that planned delivery at a tertiary facility is possible. Excluding those infants with severe associated anomalies, the overall survival rate using maximal medical therapy has been increasing over the past several years due to "gentle" ventilation strategies and is well over 70%.

FORAMEN OF MORGAGNI HERNIA

The foramen of Morgagni occurs at the junction of the septum transversum and the anterior thoracic wall. This anterior, central diaphragmatic defect accounts for only 2% of diaphragmatic hernias. It may be parasternal, retrosternal, or bilateral. Unlike Bochdalek hernias, children are typically asymptomatic and the defect is discovered later in life on a chest radiograph taken for reasons unrelated to the hernia. The lateral chest radiograph demonstrating an air-filled mass extending into the anterior mediastinum is pathognomonic. Repair is indicated in the asymptomatic patient due to the risk of bowel obstruction. The viscera are reduced and any associated hernia sac excised. The defect is closed by suturing the posterior rim of diaphragm to the posterior rectus sheath since there is no anterior diaphragm. Rarely, a prosthetic patch closure is required. There is no associated pulmonary hypoplasia or hypertension. This defect, when noted in newborns, can be associated with the pentalogy of Cantrell, a disorder with considerable morbidity and mortality that consists of the anterior diaphragmatic defect, distal sternal cleft, epigastric omphalocele, apical pericardial defect, and congenital heart disease (usually a septal defect). Excluding patients with the pentalogy of Cantrell, survival is nearly 100%.

EVENTRATION OF THE DIAPHRAGM

Diaphragmatic eventration is an abnormally elevated or attenuated portion of the diaphragm (or both). It may be congenital (usually idiopathic, but can be associated with congenital myopathies or intrauterine infections) or acquired (as a result of phrenic nerve injury during forceps delivery or surgery). In the congenital form, there is variable thinning or absence of diaphragmatic muscle, at which point its distinction from congenital diaphragmatic hernia with a persistent hernia sac is obscure. The elevated hemidiaphragm may produce abnormalities of chest wall mechanics with impaired pulmonary function. Respiratory distress and pneumonia are frequent presenting symptoms, although gastrointestinal symptoms such as vomiting or gastric volvulus have been reported.

The diagnosis is made by chest radiograph. It is confirmed by fluoroscopy or ultrasound, which demonstrate paradoxical movement of the diaphragm during spontaneous respiration. Incidentally discovered small, localized eventrations do not need repair. Eventrations that are associated with respiratory symptoms should be repaired by plicating the diaphragm using interrupted nonabsorbable sutures.

Harrison MR et al: A randomized trial of fetoscopic tracheal occlusion for severe fetal congenital diaphragmatic hernia. New Engl J Med 2003;349:1916.

Kizilcan F et al: The long-term results of diaphragmatic plication. J Pediatr Surg 1993;28:42.

Nobuhara K et al: Long-term outlook for survivors of congenital diaphragmatic hernia. Clin Perinatol 1996;23:873.

Pokorny W, McGill C, Halberg F: Morgagni hernia during infancy: Presentation and associated anomalies. 1984;19:394.

Puri P: Congenital diaphragmatic hernia. Curr Probl Surg 1994;31:785.

CONGENITAL LOBAR EMPHYSEMA

Congenital lobar emphysema results from hyperinflation of a single lobe; rarely, more than one lobe is affected. The upper and middle lobes are most frequently involved. Pathologically, there are three forms; hypoplastic emphysema, polyalveolar lobe, and bronchial obstruction.

Hypoplastic emphysema is distinguished by a segment, lobe, or whole lung that has a reduced number of bronchial branches with a diminished number and smaller size of blood vessels. The number of alveoli is abnormally decreased, but the air spaces are too large. The hyperlucent region seen on chest radiograph is normal or small in volume, and since it does not affect the surrounding normal lung, surgical treatment is unnecessary.

Polyalveolar lobe is characterized by a normal size and number of bronchial branches, but there is an abnormal number of alveoli from each respiratory unit. These alveoli are prone to expand excessively, producing emphysema, which encroaches on the surrounding normal lung and therefore requires removal.

Bronchial obstruction may occur from deficient bronchial cartilage support, redundant mucosa, bronchial stenosis, mucous plug, or bronchial compression by anomalous vessels or other mediastinal lesions. With inspiration, the bronchus opens to allow air into the lung; but on expiration the bronchus collapses, trap-

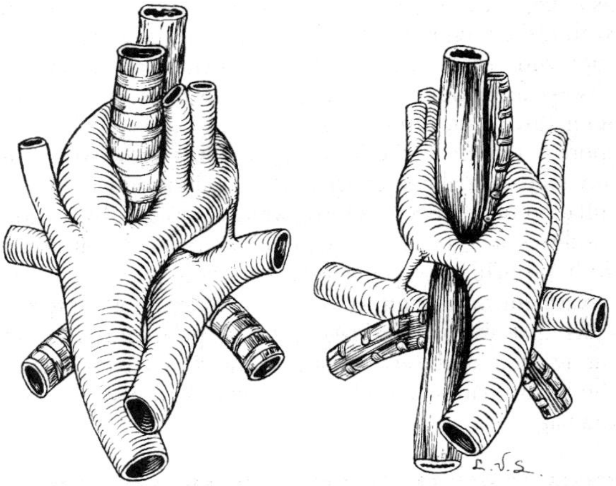

Figure 45–7. Anterior (left) and posterior views of double aortic arch constricting the trachea and esophagus.

ping the air, and with each respiratory cycle there is progressive expansion of the lobe.

Clinical Findings

In one-third of patients, respiratory distress is noted at birth; in only 5% of cases do symptoms develop after 6 months. Males are affected twice as frequently as females. The signs include progressive and severe dyspnea, wheezing, grunting, coughing, cyanosis, and difficulty feeding. An increased anteroposterior dimension of the chest and retractions may be seen. The chest is hyperresonant, and decreased breath sounds may be noted over the affected lobe. A chest radiograph may demonstrate radiolucency of the emphysematous lobe, with bronchovascular markings extending to the lung periphery. Compression atelectasis of the adjacent lung, shift of the mediastinum, depression of the diaphragm, and anterior bowing of the sternum can be seen. The emphysematous lobe may continue to expand, compressing adjacent lung and airways, producing progressively severe respiratory distress.

Treatment & Prognosis

Occasionally, the emphysema may be due to a mucous plug in the bronchus that may be aspirated by bronchoscopy. Compression of the bronchus by mediastinal masses may be relieved by removal of the tumor or repair of anomalous vessels. Treatment of mildly symptomatic cases may not be necessary.

Many patients with lobar emphysema are severely symptomatic, and pulmonary lobectomy is necessary. For those who are breathing spontaneously prior to operation, anesthesia should not be started until all personnel are ready for a rapid thoracotomy since positive-pressure ventilation may acutely enlarge the emphysematous lobe, thereby compressing the normal lung tissue and heart. The prognosis following surgical relief of the lobar emphysema is excellent. Rarely patients may show residual disease in the remaining lung. At long-term follow-up, lung volumes are normal, but the airflow rates are diminished.

Martinez-Frontanilla LA et al: Surgery of acquired lobar emphysema in the neonate. J Pediatr Surg 1984;19:375.

Olutoye OO et al: Prenatal diagnosis and management of congenital lobar emphysema. J Pediatr Surg 2000;35:792.

GREAT VESSEL ANOMALIES

Tracheobronchial and esophageal compression by the great vessels may occur as a result of anomalies of the aortic arch or of abnormally located or enlarged pulmonary and subclavian arteries. While the most common abnormality is an aberrant right subclavian artery, the most important is the double aortic arch, as it often causes serious respiratory distress in young infants (Figure 45–7). Affected infants have a characteristic inspiratory and expiratory wheeze, stridor, or croup-like cough. Echocardiography, CT, and MRI can demonstrate the anomalous anatomy. Esophagoscopy and bronchoscopy may be helpful in assessing the degree and level of compression. The surgical approach is through the left hemithorax. Following removal of the thymus, the aortic arch and its branches are skeletonized and the anatomy is identified. For the double aortic arch, the smallest arterial component is divided; an anomalous right subclavian artery is divided at its origin. The accompanying fibrous bands and sheaths constricting the trachea and esophagus must also be divided. The ductus arteriosus (or its fibrous remnant) is also divided.

Sebening C et al: Vascular tracheobronchial compression syndromes—experience in surgical treatment and literature review. Thorac Cardiovasc Surg 2000;48:164.

Woods RK et al: Vascular anomalies and tracheoesophageal compression: a single institution's 25-year experience. Ann Thorac Surg 2001;72:434.

MEDIASTINAL MASSES

Mediastinal masses are relatively common in infants and children and can be classified according to the compartment of the mediastinum from which they arise. The mediastinum is classically divided into anterior, middle, and posterior compartments. Anatomically, the anterior mediastinum consists of the area between the sternum and the anterior aspect of the trachea and pericardium. The middle compartment contains the trachea, major bronchi, and paratracheal spaces. The posterior segment extends from the posterior aspect of the trachea to the spine.

Anterior masses make up one-third and are most commonly teratomas and lymphomas. Teratomas may be cystic or solid and may also be found within the pericardium (middle compartment). Approximately 20% are malignant. Other masses include thymic cysts, thymomas, substernal goiters, and lymphangiomas. Middle mediastinal masses are rare but when present are most likely to be bronchogenic cysts. Sixty percent of mediastinal masses are located within the posterior compartment. Neurogenic tumors are most common and include neuroblastoma, ganglioneuroblastoma, ganglioneuroma, neurofibroma, and neurofibrosarcoma. Common symptoms include respiratory distress (via tracheal or lung compression), Horner's syndrome, and pain. Enterogenous cysts or duplications are also commonly seen in the posterior compartment. They are termed neurenteric when there is an associated cervical or thoracic vertebral anomaly.

Grosfeld JL et al: Mediastinal tumors in children: experience with 196 cases. Ann Surg Oncol 1994;1:121.

CONGENITAL LUNG LESIONS

Congenital lung lesions, which arise from anomalous development of the foregut, are classified as follows: (1) bronchogenic cyst, (2) cystic adenomatoid malformation, (3) pulmonary sequestration, and (4) bronchopulmonary foregut malformation. Embryonic tissues that are destined to form bronchi and lung become anomalous isolated structures within or outside of the lung. These lesions produce symptoms from their size and position, resulting in compression of bronchi or lung parenchyma, or from infection and abscess formation within the cyst and surrounding normal lung.

BRONCHOGENIC CYST

Bronchogenic cysts are lined by cuboidal or ciliated columnar epithelium and are filled with mucoid material. Repeated infection in the cyst may produce squamous epithelial metaplasia. About half arise in the mediastinum and do not communicate with the bronchi. They appear as radiopaque masses on chest radiographs. When located within the lung parenchyma, the cysts usually communicate with the airways and consequently are prone to abscess formation. Bronchogenic cysts arise in the right lung three times more often than in the left. They are more common in the lower lobes but may be found in any lobe. Partial compression of bronchi produces hyperinflation of the involved lung, while complete obstruction produces atelectasis. Rupture of a cyst that communicates with bronchi may present as a tension pneumothorax. Treatment of a noninfected cyst is by excision. Infected cysts first require drainage (usually percutaneous) and intravenous antibiotic therapy followed by resection after the inflammation subsides (no sooner than 6 weeks after drainage).

CONGENITAL CYSTIC ADENOMATOID MALFORMATION

This lesion is considered a hamartoma in which multiple cysts are lined by a polypoid proliferation of bronchial epithelium surrounded by striated muscle and elastic tissue, but there is an absence of mucous glands and cartilage. They are most often lobar and are classified radiologically based on cyst size: type I are large (> 2 cm) cysts, type II are smaller cysts (< 2 cm), and type III have cysts that are so small as to import a solid appearance. These malformations occur with equal frequency in both lungs, with a slight predominance in the upper lobes. Associated renal and nervous system anomalies may be present.

Clinical Findings

A large lesion can compress the fetal lung, resulting in pulmonary hypoplasia at birth, or may distort or obstruct the esophagus, producing polyhydramnios. In addition, compression of venous return to the heart with exudation of protein into the lung fluid may cause fetal congestive heart failure, hydrops fetalis, and death in utero. Large lesions that do not cause fetal hydrops can remain stable or involute during fetal life, producing little or no symptoms of respiratory distress at birth.

Treatment

If prenatal ultrasound can recognize the presence of this disorder in association with hydrops, resection in utero is an option for select cases. Children in whom hydrops did not occur before birth may be born asymptomatic (small lesions) or may have variable degrees of respiratory distress due to compression of the ipsilateral normal lung. Asymptomatic children may be observed, but resection (pulmonary lobectomy) is recommended since these lesions often become infected and there are case reports of malignant transformation occurring in untreated, long-standing cysts. Often the plain chest radiograph does not demonstrate the small, asymptomatic lesion. A CT scan is indicated for those patients.

PULMONARY SEQUESTRATION & BRONCHOPULMONARY FOREGUT MALFORMATION

A sequestration consists of normally developed bronchioles and alveoli supplied by systemic rather than pulmonary arteries. Sequestrations occur in the lower chest, most commonly on the left, adjacent to the mediastinum. Rarely, sequestrations may occur in the upper or middle lobes or even below the diaphragm. They usually have a systemic arterial blood supply from the aorta, either above or below the diaphragm. On rare occasions, a sequestration will communicate with the esophagus or stomach, a condition termed bronchopulmonary foregut malformation. Sequestrations may be intralobar (typically in older children) or extralobar. Intralobar lesions drain through the pulmonary veins, are in communication with the tracheobronchial tree, and are prone to infection and lung abscess formation. Extralobar lesions drain into the azygous venous system, do not communicate with the lung, and are commonly asymptomatic. They are often found in association with congenital diaphragmatic hernia. Histologic evidence suggests that these lesions have embryologic origin similar to that of bronchogenic cysts and congenital cystic adenomatoid malformations. However, unlike the latter, sequestrations rarely grow large enough to produce hydrops and demise in utero. Treatment is by excision of the extralobar sequestration or lobectomy in cases of intralobar sequestration.

Adzick NS et al: Fetal lung lesions: management and outcome. Am J Obstet Gynecol 1998;179:884.

Cass DL et al: Cystic lung lesions with systemic arterial blood supply: a hybrid of congenital cystic adenomatoid malformation and bronchopulmonary sequestration. J Pediatr Surg 1997;32:986.

Neilson IR et al: Congenital adenomatoid malformation of the lung: current management and prognosis. J Pediatr Surg 1991;26:975.

Nuchtern JG, Harberg FJ: Congenital lung cysts. Semin Pediatr Surg 1994;3:233.

■ CONGENITAL GASTROINTESTINAL LESIONS

ESOPHAGEAL ANOMALIES

The trachea and esophagus are derived from the primitive foregut. Initially, they appear as a common ventral diverticulum at about the nineteenth day of gestation. Beginning several days later, elongation and separation of the diverticulum into the airway and esophagus occurs in a caudal to cephalad direction. Errors in this process result in esophageal atresia, tracheoesophageal fistula, and their variants (Figure 45–8).

Classification

A. WITH ESOPHAGEAL ATRESIA

1. There is a blind proximal pouch and a fistula between the distal end of the esophagus and the distal one-third of the trachea (type C, 85% of cases).

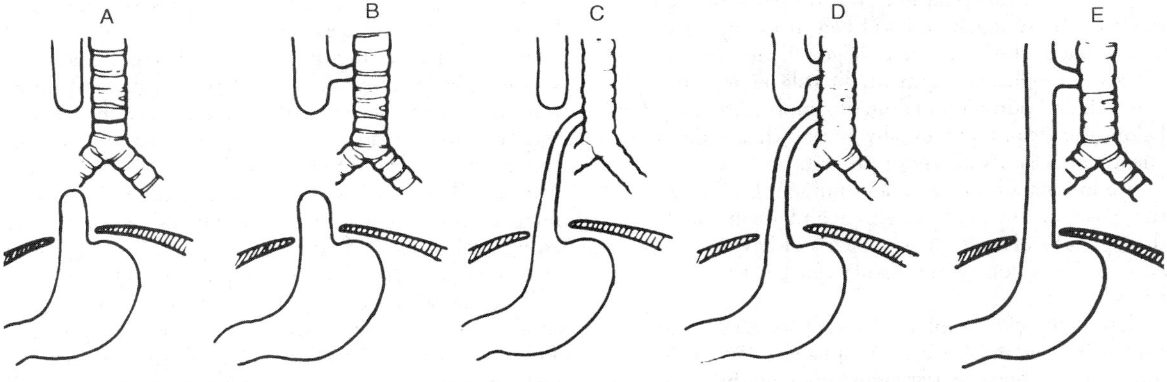

Figure 45–8. **A:** Pure (long gap) esophageal atresia. **B:** Esophageal atresia with proximal tracheoesophageal fistula. **C:** Esophageal atresia with distal tracheoesophageal fistula. **D:** Esophageal atresia with proximal and distal fistulas. **E:** Tracheoesophageal fistula without esophageal atresia. (From Grosfeld JL: Pediatric surgery. In: *Textbook of Surgery.* Sabiston DC [editor]. Saunders, 1991. Reproduced by permission from Elsevier.)

2. There is a blind proximal esophageal pouch, no tracheoesophageal fistula, and a blind, short distal esophagus (Type A, 10% of cases). This is referred to as "pure or long gap" atresia.
3. There are fistulas between both proximal and distal esophageal segments and the trachea (Type D, 2% of cases).
4. There is a fistula between the proximal esophagus and the trachea and a blind distal esophagus without fistula (Type B, 1% of cases).

B. Without Esophageal Atresia

1. There is an "H" type tracheoesophageal fistula that is usually present in the low cervical region (Type E, 4–5% of cases).
2. There is esophageal stenosis consisting of a membranous occlusion (often containing cartilage) between the mid and distal third of the esophagus (rare).
3. There is a laryngotracheoesophageal cleft of varying length, consisting of a linear communication between these structures (very rare).

Clinical Findings

Shortly after birth, the infant with esophageal atresia is noted to have excessive salivation and repeated episodes of coughing, choking, and cyanosis. Attempts at feeding result in choking, gagging, and regurgitation. Infants with tracheoesophageal fistula in addition to esophageal atresia will have reflux of gastric secretions into the tracheobronchial tree, with resulting pneumonia. Pulmonary infiltrates are usually noted first in the right upper lobe.

A size 10F catheter should be passed into the esophagus by way of the nose or mouth; if esophageal atresia is present, the tube will not go down the expected distance to the stomach and will coil in the upper esophageal pouch. If a tracheoesophageal fistula connects to the lower esophageal segment, air will be present in the stomach and bowel on plain radiographs. Absence of air below the diaphragm usually means that a distal tracheoesophageal fistula is not present.

Abdominal distention is a prominent finding because the Valsalva effect of coughing and crying forces air through a fistula into the stomach and bowel. The presence and position of the fistula can be determined by bronchoscopy.

Laryngotracheoesophageal cleft produces symptoms similar to those of tracheoesophageal fistula but of much greater severity. Laryngoscopy may show the cleft between the arytenoids extending down the larynx. Bronchoscopy is the best means of outlining the cleft.

There is a 50% incidence of associated anomalies: cardiac (patent ductus arteriosus, septal defects), gastrointestinal (imperforate anus, duodenal atresia), genitourinary, and skeletal. The VACTERL association (*v*ertebral, *a*norectal, *c*ardiac, *t*racheo*e*sophageal, *r*enal, and *l*imb anomalies) is present in 25% of cases. Isolated esophageal atresia has been associated with various genetic abnormalities, including trisomy 18 and trisomy 21.

Treatment

A sump suction catheter should be placed in the upper esophageal pouch and the head of the bed elevated. An echocardiogram is required to determine the position of the aortic arch since a right-sided arch makes the standard right thoracotomy (or thoracoscopic) repair difficult and is present in 5% of infants. If possible, aspiration pneumonia is treated before repair.

The goal of operative therapy is to divide and ligate the fistula and repair the atresia in one stage, if possible. This is usually performed using a right posterolateral thoracotomy with an extrapleural dissection, although a transpleural thoracoscopic approach is gaining popularity for those stable, full-term infants. In those with an H type tracheoesophageal fistula, the fistula is located above the thoracic inlet in two-thirds of cases. These fistulas may be divided through a left transverse cervical incision. A feeding gastrostomy tube is no longer routinely inserted except when the esophageal repair is under extreme tension, when there is long gap atresia not amenable to single-stage repair, and when there are severe associated anomalies (eg, congenital heart disease). A transanastomotic feeding tube is placed for postoperative feeding pending demonstration of a leak-free anastomosis by esophagogram obtained 7 days after surgery.

Staged operations are reserved for extremely premature babies, those who have severe aspiration pneumonitis, and those with severe anomalies or long gaps between the esophageal pouches. There are several strategies for repairing these defects. These include cervical esophagostomy, division of the fistula, and insertion of a gastrostomy tube. Several months later a staged reconstruction by esophageal replacement with colon or stomach interposition can be undertaken. Another alternative is a gastrostomy tube alone with intermittent bougienage and stretching of the upper esophageal pouch, followed by primary esophageal anastomosis and immediate interposition grafting.

Esophageal narrowing or webs in the distal esophageal segment readily respond to esophageal dilation. This is usually accomplished with Hurst or Maloney mercury-weighted bougies. Dilations are repeated until healing occurs without recurrence of the web. Esophagoscopy and excision of portions of a tough or thick web, using biopsy forceps or the endoscopic laser, may be required in addition to dilation. A lower esophageal stricture containing cartilage will require excision and anastomosis.

Prognosis

The survival rate for a full-term infant without associated anomalies is excellent. However, deaths occur as a result of pulmonary complications, severe associated anomalies, prematurity, and sepsis due to anastomotic disruption. Anastomotic leaks occur because of tension or poor blood supply. In performing the anastomosis, the extrapleural approach prevents the development of empyema and confines a leak and possible infection to a small localized area.

Swallowing is a reflex response that must be reinforced early in infancy. If establishment of esophageal continuity is delayed for more than 4–6 weeks, it may take many months to overcome oral aversion and learn to swallow. Babies with cervical esophagostomies should be encouraged to suck, eat, and swallow during gastrostomy feedings.

Dysphagia may occur for months or years following successful repair of esophageal atresia and is multifactorial. An anastomotic stricture is not uncommon and may require one or more dilations under anesthesia. Swallowed foreign bodies will lodge at the site of anastomosis and require removal with esophagoscopy. Another cause of dysphagia is poor peristalsis of the distal esophageal segment. This frequent problem improves with age.

Most of these infants have an alarming, barking cough and rattling sound on respiration from tracheomalacia. This results from in utero compression of the trachea by the dilated proximal esophageal pouch. This frequently improves with age and is rare after 5 years of age. Gastroesophageal reflux is common after successful repair and may result in recurrent aspiration pneumonitis, dysphagia, failure to thrive, and recurrent anastomotic stricture. A surgical antireflux procedure may be necessary.

Choudhory SR et al: Survival of patients with esophageal atresia: influence of birth weight, cardiac anomaly, and late respiratory complications. J Pediatr Surg 1999;34:70.

McKinnon LJ, Kosloske AM: Prediction and prevention of anastomotic complications of esophageal atresia and tracheoesophageal fistula. J Pediatr Surg 1990;25:778.

Rothenberg SS: Thoracoscopic repair of tracheoesophageal fistula in newborns. J Pediatr Surg 2002;37:869.

INTESTINAL OBSTRUCTION IN THE NEWBORN

Since fetuses continually swallow amniotic fluid into their gastrointestinal tracts and excrete it in their urine;, intestinal obstruction may be noted on prenatal ultrasound by the presence of polyhydramnios (increased amniotic fluid level). The presence of polyhydramnios correlates with the level of the obstruction; it is most common with proximal gastrointestinal tract obstruction (eg, esophageal and duodenal atresia), is rarely noted with ileal atresia, and is never noted in association with anorectal obstruction.

After birth, vomiting is the principal symptom, and it is bile-stained if the obstruction is distal to the ampulla of Vater. It is important to note that bilious vomiting in the newborn is pathologic until proved otherwise. On physical examination, the presence and degree of abdominal distention depends on the level of the obstruction and should be noted. For example, there is no significant distention with duodenal obstruction versus massive distention with colonic obstruction (eg, Hirschsprung's disease). A careful perineal examination should be performed to determine whether the anus is present, patent, and in the normal location. Meconium, the first newborn stool, passes in the first 24 hours of life in 94% of normal full-term infants and by 48 hours in 98%. Failure to pass meconium may be indicative of lower gastrointestinal tract obstruction. However, 30–50% of newborn infants with intestinal obstruction will pass meconium.

Depending on the pathology, the plain abdominal radiograph may demonstrate dilated bowel loops, air-fluid levels, calcifications (if in utero perforation occurred), or a gasless abdomen. Unlike in adult patients, one cannot differentiate small from large bowel by their usual markings on a plain radiograph of the newborn's abdomen. If a lower GI tract obstruction is suspected, a contrast (usually water-soluble contrast) enema is the most useful study since it can be both diagnostic and therapeutic in the majority of cases (see below). An upper GI series is rarely indicated unless malrotation is to be ruled out. The CT, MRI, or ultrasound scans are virtually never indicated in the workup of newborn intestinal obstruction.

HYPERTROPHIC PYLORIC STENOSIS

Pyloric stenosis is the most common surgical disorder producing emesis in infancy. It results from hypertrophy of the circular and longitudinal muscularis of the pylorus and the distal antrum of the stomach with progressive narrowing of the pyloric canal (Figure 45–9). The cause is not known. The male:female incidence is 4:1. The disorder is more common in firstborn infants and occurs four times more often in the offspring of mothers who had the disease as infants than in those whose fathers had the disease. If one monozygotic twin is affected, the other will also have the disorder in two-thirds of cases. A seasonal variation is noted in the occurrence of symptoms, with peaks in spring and fall.

Clinical Findings

A. Symptoms and Signs

Typically, the affected infant is full-term when born and feeds and grows well until 2–4 weeks after birth, at

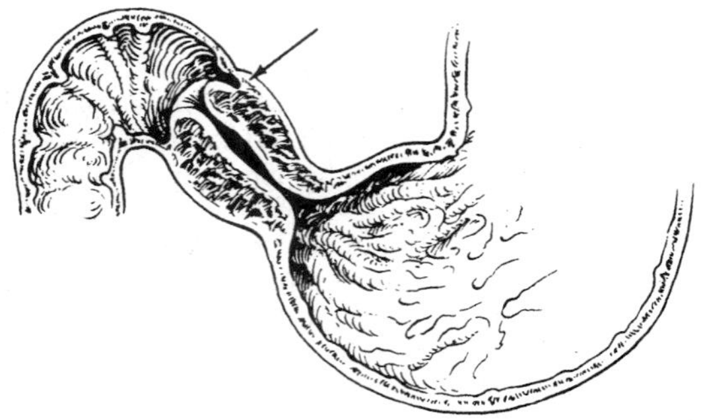

Figure 45–9. Hypertrophic pyloric stenosis. Note that the distal end of the hypertrophic muscle protrudes into the duodenum (arrow), accounting for the ease of perforation into the duodenum during pyloromyotomy.

which time occasional regurgitation of some of the feedings occurs. Several days later, however, the vomiting becomes more frequent and forceful. The vomitus contains the previous feeding and no bile. Blood may be seen in the vomitus in 5% of cases, and coffee-grounds or occult blood is frequently present. Shortly after vomiting, the infant acts starved and will feed again. The stools become infrequent and firm in consistency as dehydration occurs. With dehydration, infants often have sunken fontanelles, dry mucous membranes, and poor skin turgor. Weight loss follows progressive feeding intolerance. Jaundice with indirect hyperbilirubinemia occurs in fewer than 10% of cases. Gastric peristaltic waves can usually be seen moving from the left costal margin to the area of the pylorus. In over 90% of cases, the pyloric "tumor," or "olive," can be palpated when the infant is relaxed. Abdominal relaxation may be accomplished by sedating the infant or by feeding clear fluids and simultaneously aspirating the stomach contents with a gastric tube.

B. Imaging Studies

An imaging study is indicated when the pyloric tumor cannot be palpated. Abdominal ultrasound, the most sensitive and specific test, will identify hypertrophic pyloric stenosis when the muscle thickness is greater than 4 mm and the length of the pylorus is greater than 16 mm. A contrast upper gastrointestinal series is indicated if an experienced ultrasonographer is unavailable or if there is a reasonable chance that the patient's symptoms are not due to pyloric stenosis (eg, a premature, 1-week-old baby) since this examination can demonstrate other entities in the differential, whereas the ultrasound can simply comment on the presence or absence of a hypertrophied pyloris. A positive upper GI series can include the following diagnostic signs: (1) outlining of the narrow pyloric channel by a single "string sign" or "double track" owing to folds of mucosa; (2) a pyloric "beak" where the pyloric entrance from the antrum occurs; (3) the "shoulder" sign, in which the pyloric mass bulges into the antrum; and (4) complete obstruction of the pylorus.

Differential Diagnosis

Repeated nonbilious vomiting in early infancy may be due to overfeeding, intracranial lesions, pylorospasm, antral web, gastroesophageal reflux, pyloric duplication, duodenal stenosis, malrotation of the bowel, or adrenal insufficiency.

Complications

Repeated vomiting with inadequate intake of formula results in hypokalemic hypochloremic alkalosis, dehydration, and starvation. Gastritis and reflux esophagitis occur frequently. Aspiration of vomitus may produce pneumonia.

Treatment & Prognosis

The operative treatment is the Fredet-Ramstedt pyloromyotomy, in which the pylorus is incised along its entire length, spread widely exposing but not breaching the underlying mucosa. Surgery should be undertaken only after dehydration and the hypokalemic hypochloremic alkalosis have been corrected, heralded by a normal serum chloride and a urine output greater than 1 cc/kg/h. There are three approaches to the pyloromyotomy: a right upper quadrant transverse skin incision, a circumumbilical or intraumbilical skin incision, or a laparoscopic approach with the telescope in the umbilicus and the two working instruments placed directly through the abdominal wall. If, during the pyloromyotomy, the mucosa is inadvertently entered (usually on the duodenal side), it is closed with fine nonabsorbable sutures and an omental patch is placed. Large perforations are managed by closing the pyloromyotomy, rotating the pylorus 90 degrees, and repeating the myotomy. Successful repair is evident when the submucosa is seen to herniate out of the myotomy site.

Multiple postoperative feeding schedules have been described, ranging from immediate full feeds to delayed feeds with incremental advances in volume. This has stemmed from the observation that nearly all patients with pyloric stenosis vomit after surgery, presumably due to gastric ileus, gastritis, gastroesophageal reflux, or all of the above. An incomplete pyloromyotomy (usually on the antral side) is suspected when vomiting persists beyond 2 weeks postoperatively. This stems from a short myotomy or incomplete division of the muscle.

Pyloric stenosis never recurs, and there is a uniformly excellent outcome.

Forman HP et al: A rational approach to the diagnosis of hypertrophic pyloric stenosis. J Pediatr Surg 1990;25:262.

Leinwald MJ, Shaul DB, Anderson KD: The umbilical fold approach to pyloromyotomy: is it a safe alternative to the right upper-quadrant approach? J Am Coll Surg 1999;189:362.

Rothenberg SS: Laparoscopic pyloromyotomy: The slice and pull technique. Pediatr Endosurg Innov Tech 1997;1:39.

CONGENITAL DUODENAL OBSTRUCTION

The various causes of duodenal obstruction are atresia, stenosis, mucosal web (complete or variably perforate), annular pancreas, preduodenal portal vein, and peritoneal bands (Ladd's bands) from malrotation. Duodenal atresia is distinguished from more distal gastrointestinal atresias since it is due to failure of recanalization of the duodenum early in gestation rather than due to mesenteric vascular abnormality late in gestation. Atresia of the duodenum is twice as common as in the jejunum or ileum. In about half of cases, multiple congenital anomalies are present, including Down's syndrome in 30% and congenital heart disease in 20%. Birth weight is less than 2500 g in half of these infants. Mucosal webs or stenoses occur as often as pure atresia. Annular pancreas is almost always associated with hypoplasia of the duodenum at the level of the ampulla. The cause is a developmental defect characterized by circumferential persistence of the gland around the duodenum at the site of the embryonic ventral anlage, leading to duodenal obstruction and an accessory pancreatic duct.

Clinical Findings

In 75% of cases, duodenal obstruction occurs distal to the ampulla of Vater, causing bile to be diverted to the proximal duodenum and stomach. Bilious emesis occurs shortly after birth and during attempted feedings. The upper abdomen is rarely distended. Meconium is passed in over 50% of cases.

The plain abdominal radiograph demonstrates an air-distended stomach and duodenum ("double bubble" sign). Gas in the small and large intestine indicates incomplete obstruction. Contrast upper gastrointestinal series is used to identify the presence or absence of malrotation in those cases with incomplete obstruction since obstruction from intestinal malrotation is a surgical emergency.

Treatment

Surgery is performed using a right upper transverse abdominal incision or via laparoscopy. A Kocher maneuver should be performed, with complete mobilization of the third and fourth portions of the duodenum. Obstruction from Ladd's bands requires simple division of the bands and correction of the malrotation (see below). Duodenoduodenostomy is performed for duodenal atresia and annular pancreas. A mucosal web is excised, taking care to avoid injury to the adjacent ampulla. Commonly, the duodenum is hugely dilated above the obstruction, which results in impaired aboral progression of ingested feedings. This problem is resolved by excision or plication of a portion of the antimesenteric wall of the bowel to make the lumen diameter normal (tapered duodenoplasty). Gastrojejunostomy should not be done because the blind duodenal pouch may cause repeated vomiting. In all cases, the distal bowel must be irrigated and assessed for associated intrinsic obstruction and atresia (1–3% incidence). Mortality is related to prematurity and associated anomalies.

Grosfeld JL, Rescorla FJ: Duodenal atresia and stenosis: reassessment of treatment and outcome based on antenatal diagnosis, pathologic variance, and long-term followup. World J Surg 1993;17:301.

Spigland N, Yazbeck S: Complications associated with surgical treatment of congenital intrinsic duodenal obstruction. J Pediatr Surg 1990;25:1127.

ATRESIA & STENOSIS OF THE JEJUNUM, ILEUM, & COLON

Atresia and stenosis of the jejunum, ileum, and colon are caused by a mesenteric vascular accident in utero, which may result from hernia, volvulus, or intussusception, producing aseptic necrosis and resorption of the necrotic bowel. Although atresia may occur in any portion of the intestine, most cases occur in the distal ileum or proximal jejunum. Colonic atresia is very rare, accounting for no more than 1% of all intestinal atresias. A short area of necrosis may produce only stenosis or a membranous web occluding the lumen (type I) (Figure 45–10). A more extensive infarct may leave a fibrous cord between the two bowel loops (type II), or the proximal and distal bowel may be completely separated with a V-shaped defect in the mesentery (type IIIa). Multiple atresias occur in 10% of cases (type IV). A type III variant (type IIIb) is commonly called apple-peel or Christmas tree atresia, in which there is a blind-ending proximal jejunum, absence of a long length of mid small bowel, and a terminal ileum coiled around its tenuous blood supply from an ileocolic vessel.

Clinical Findings

Vomiting of bile, abdominal distention, and failure to pass meconium indicate intestinal obstruction. The plain abdominal radiograph will give an estimate of how far along the intestine the obstruction exists. A contrast enema may be indicated to detect the level of obstruc-

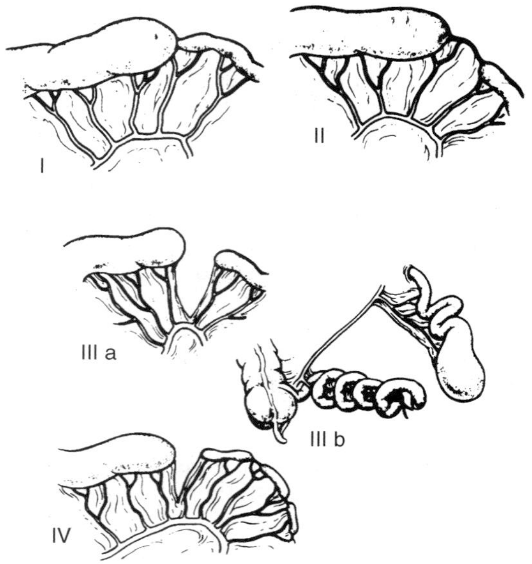

Figure 45–10. The anatomic spectrum of intestinal atresia. Type I is a stenosis or mucosal web. Type II, a fibrous cord between two bowel ends. Type IIIa, blind-ending proximal and distal bowel loops with a V-shaped mesenteric defect. Type IIIb (apple peel deformity, Christmas tree deformity) consists of a blind ending proximal jejunum, absence of a large portion of the midgut, and a terminal ileum that is coiled around its ileocolic blood supply. Type IV, multiple atresias of any kind. (From Grosfeld JL: Pediatric surgery. In: *Textbook of Surgery.* Sabiston DC [editor]. Saunders, 1991. Reproduced by permission from Elsevier.)

tion. In obstructions that occur in the distal bowel and appear relatively early in gestation, the colon is empty of meconium and appears abnormally narrow. When the obstruction is proximal or when it occurs late in pregnancy, meconium is passed into the colon. The contrast enema will then outline a more generous-sized colon with its contents (meconium). In older children with evidence of partial intestinal obstruction, a small bowel series may be indicated to identify intestinal stenosis.

Treatment

There are three main goals of operation: (1) to restore the continuity of the bowel; (2) to preserve as much intestinal length as possible; and (3) to retain the ileocecal valve if possible (the minimum length of bowel needed to sustain full enteral nutrition doubles in the absence of the ileocecal valve). A transverse upper abdominal incision is preferred. Infants with jejunal or ileal atresia usually have a segment of the proximal bowel adjacent to the atresia that is dilated out of proportion to the rest of the proximal bowel. This is referred to as the "club" and it lacks normal peristaltic activity. If left in or not tapered, it may become a source of persistent functional obstruction. It is tapered when it is a very proximal bowel segment, near the ligament of Treitz; otherwise it should be resected. A great discrepancy between the diameter of the segments of intestine proximal and distal to the atresia is the rule. Atresia of the proximal colon should be treated by resection of the dilated bowel and ileocolostomy. Atresia of the distal colon may be treated by proximal end colostomy or by a side-to-side colostomy. Later, the continuity of the distal colon may be established by end-to-end anastomosis.

Infants born with extensive small bowel loss may benefit from a Bianchi procedure, where the entire greatly dilated bowel is divided longitudinally into two lengths of bowel. The end of the jejunum in continuity with the duodenum is anastomosed to the proximal end of the divided bowel.

In contrast to duodenal atresia, associated anomalies are unusual in small bowel and colon atresia. Following repair, return of gastrointestinal function is prolonged (up to 10 days) with proximal atresia due to the overdistention of the duodenum.

Bianchi A: Autologous gastrointestinal reconstruction. Semin Pediatr Surg 1995;4:54.

Puri P, Fujimoto T: New observations on the pathogenesis of multiple intestinal atresias. J Pediatr Surg 1988;23:221.

Sato S et al: Jejunoileal atresia: a 27 year experience. J Pediatr Surg 1998;33:1633.

Thompson JS et al: Experience with intestinal lengthening for the short-bowel syndrome. J Pediatr Surg 1991;26:721.

DISORDERS OF INTESTINAL ROTATION

The fetal intestine begins as a somewhat straight tube that grows faster than the abdominal cavity and thus herniates out into the body stalk (future umbilicus) at about 4–6 weeks' gestation. At 10–12 weeks, the bowel returns to the abdominal cavity, rotates, and becomes fixed to the retroperitoneum along a long diagonal axis extending from the level of the left of the T12 vertebra to the level of the right of the L5 vertebra. The duodenojejunal portion of gut rotates posterior (counterclockwise) to the superior mesenteric vessels for 270 degrees and becomes fixed at the ligament of Treitz and located to the left of and cephalad to the superior mesenteric artery. The cecocolic portion of the midgut also rotates 270 degrees, but clockwise (anterior) to the superior mesenteric artery. The cecum becomes fixed in the right lower abdomen (L5 level).

Classification

Anomalies of rotation and fixation are twice as common in males as in females. They may be classified as (1) nonrotation, (2) incomplete rotation, (3) reversed rotation, and (4) anomalous fixation of the mesentery.

A. Nonrotation

With nonrotation, the midgut is suspended from the superior mesenteric vessels; the small bowel is located predominantly on the right side of the abdomen and the large bowel in the left abdomen. No fixation occurs, and adhesive bands are not present. This is the fetal anatomy prior to 10 weeks' gestation. Because its base is so short, the mesentery is narrow, which predisposes to volvulus, with clockwise twisting of the bowel about the superior mesenteric vessels. This anomaly is usually found in patients with omphalocele, gastroschisis, and congenital diaphragmatic hernia.

B. Incomplete Rotation

Incomplete rotation (commonly called malrotation) may affect the duodenojejunal segment, the cecocolic segment, or both. Adhesive bands (Ladd's bands) are usually present. In the most common form, the cecum stopped rotating and fixed near the origin of the superior mesenteric vessels, and dense peritoneal bands extend from the right flank to the cecum and obstruct the second or third portion of the duodenum or other segments of the small bowel. The duodenojejunal segment also only partially rotates, usually stopping at or to the right of the vertebral bodies. The intestinal mesentery is fixed posteriorly, but is very narrow, only extending the distance between the cecum and the duodenojejunal segment. This predisposes to volvulus (Figure 45–11).

C. Reversed Rotation

In reversed rotation, the bowel rotates varying degrees in a clockwise direction about the superior mesenteric axis. The duodenojejunal loop is anterior to the superior mesenteric artery. The cecocolic loop may be prearterial or may be rotated clockwise or counterclockwise in a retroarterial position. In either case, the cecum may be right-sided or left-sided. The most frequent anomaly is retroarterial clockwise rotation, which causes obstruction of the right colon.

D. Anomalous Fixation of Mesentery

Anomalies of mesenteric fixation account for internal mesenteric and paraduodenal hernias, a mobile cecum, or obstructing adhesive bands in the absence of anomalous bowel rotation. Excessive rotation of the duodenojejunal junction may result in superior mesenteric artery compression of the third portion of the duodenum.

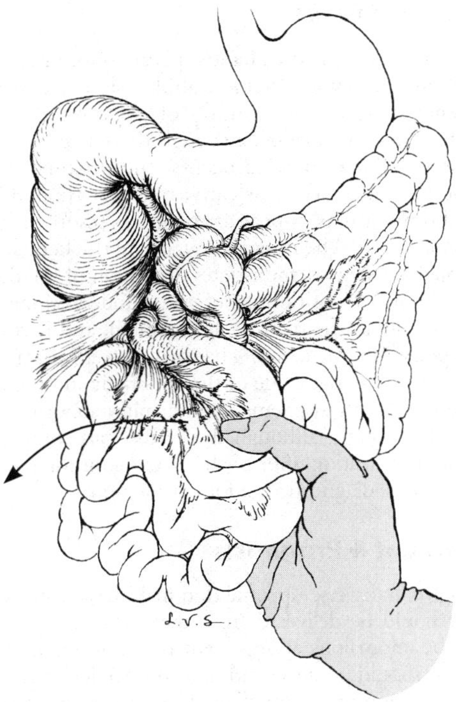

Figure 45–11. Malrotation of the midgut with volvulus. Note cecum at the origin of the superior mesenteric vessels. Fibrous bands cross and obstruct the duodenum as they adhere to the cecum. Volvulus is untwisted in a counterclockwise direction.

Clinical Findings

A. Symptoms and Signs

Anomalies of intestinal rotation may cause symptoms related to intestinal obstruction, peptic ulceration, or malabsorption. The majority of patients who develop intestinal obstruction are infants. Older patients may develop intermittent obstruction. The obstruction is in the duodenum or upper jejunum as a result of adhesive bands or midgut volvulus, respectively. Vomiting of bile occurs initially. Older patients may be thin and underweight because of chronic postprandial discomfort or malabsorption. Malabsorption with steatorrhea may result from partial venous and lymphatic obstruction, which is associated with coarse rugal folds in the small bowel. With duodenal obstruction from bands, abdominal distention is not prominent. Midgut volvulus, however, produces marked abdominal distention. Bloody stools and signs of peritonitis are manifestations of intestinal infarction. Peptic ulcer occurs in 20% of patients, presumably as a result of antral and duodenal stasis.

B. Imaging Studies

With obstructing Ladd's bands, plain abdominal radiographs may show a "double bubble" sign that mimics duodenal stenosis. Distribution of gas throughout the intestines may be normal, although there may be a paucity of it. When volvulus occurs, the proximal bowel will be distended with gas early, but over time, a "gasless" abdomen may appear as the gas is resorbed in the ischemic bowel. The intestinal walls are thickened.

Upper GI series demonstrates distention of the duodenum, abnormal positioning of the duodenojejunal segment (usually to the right of the midline), and narrowing at the point of obstruction. The small bowel is commonly visualized on the right side of the abdomen and the colon on the left. Contrast enema demonstrates abnormal position of the cecum, although the cecum can complete its rotation and fixation after birth, so the contrast enema is not a valuable diagnostic test for malrotation.

Treatment & Prognosis

Through a transverse upper abdominal incision, the entire bowel should be delivered from the abdominal cavity to assess the anomalous arrangement of the intestinal loops. Volvulus should be untwisted in a counterclockwise direction. The Ladd procedure is used for incomplete rotation with obstruction of the duodenum by congenital bands. It consists of division of the bands between the proximal colon and the lateral abdominal wall that cover and compress (obstruct) the duodenum. The mesentery is often folded upon itself due to intermesenteric adhesions, and these are incised. The appendix is removed. The cecum is then placed in the left lower quadrant, and the duodenum dissected and straightened as much as possible with a final position to the right of the midline. In essence, one is creating nonrotated intestinal anatomy much like the anatomic situation in early fetal life (prior to 10 weeks' gestation). The Ladd procedure has increasingly been performed using laparoscopic techniques for those cases without suspected volvulus.

About 30% of infants treated for volvulus die of complications of midgut ischemia and gangrene. If the anomaly is corrected before irreversible bowel damage occurs, the long-term results are good. Some patients tend to form adhesions that cause recurrent intestinal obstruction. Recurrent volvulus is rare after the Ladd procedure.

Bass KD, Rothenberg SS, Chang JH: Laparoscopic Ladd's procedure in infants with malrotation. J Pediatr Surg 1998;33:279.

Prasil P et al: Should malrotation in children be treated differently according to age? J Pediatr Surg 2000;35:756.

Rescorla F et al: Anomalies of intestinal rotation in childhood: analysis of 447 cases. Surgery 1990;108:710.

Torres AM, Ziegler MM: Malrotation of the intestine. World J Surg 1993;17:326.

MECONIUM ILEUS

In 10–20% of infants born with cystic fibrosis, the thick mucous secretions of the small bowel produce obstruction by inspissated meconium. This usually occurs in the terminal ileum. Although there is no clear correlation between pancreatic insufficiency and the development of inspissated meconium, meconium ileus also occurs in patients with pancreatic duct obstruction and pancreatic aplasia. Meconium obstruction with no apparent cause has also been described in newborn infants.

Clinical Findings

A. Symptoms and Signs

The infant typically has a normal birth weight and very distended abdomen. No meconium is passed, and bilious emesis occurs early. Loops of thick, distended bowel may be seen and palpated.

B. Imaging Studies

Plain abdominal radiographs show loops of bowel that vary greatly in diameter; the thick meconium gives a ground-glass appearance. Air mixed with the meconium produces the "soap bubble" sign, which is usually located in the right lower quadrant. Radiographs taken shortly after the infant has been placed in an upright position may fail to show air-fluid levels because the thick, viscid meconium fails to layer out rapidly. Contrast enema will show microcolon with rare meconium flecks. Reflux of contrast medium through the ileocecal valve demonstrates a small terminal ileum containing "pellets" of inspissated mucus; more proximally, the bowel is progressively distended with packed meconium. Antenatal perforation may be detected by the presence of abdominal calcifications since the meconium becomes saponified.

Complications

Meconium ileus may be complicated by a segmental (not midgut) volvulus due to the heavy, distended loops of distal ileum. If this occurs early in fetal life, the volvulus may progress to gangrene of the bowel segment. This can heal completely, with abdominal calcifications as the only clue that it occurred. Conversely, it may heal in such a way that an intestinal atresia is formed. Perforation late in gestation may lead to meconium peritonitis or a large meconium pseudocyst at birth.

Other common complications of meconium ileus are related to the almost universal presence of cystic fibrosis. These infants are susceptible to repeated pulmonary infection with chronic bronchopneumonia, bronchiectasis, atelectasis, and lung abscess. Malabsorption due to pancreatic insufficiency requires pancreatic enzyme replacement. Rectal prolapse and intussusception may be produced by strained passage of inspissated stools. Nasal polyps and chronic sinusitis are frequent. Biliary cirrhosis and bleeding varices from portal hypertension are late manifestations of bile duct obstruction by mucus.

Treatment & Prognosis

Nonoperative treatment is successful in 60–70% of cases. A nasogastric tube should be inserted and connected to suction. A contrast enema can be both diagnostic and therapeutic. It should be performed with a slightly hypertonic water-soluble contrast agent (never barium). The addition of *N*-acetylcysteine, which is mucolytic, may be necessary to disperse the meconium in uncomplicated cases. The infant must be well hydrated, and intravenous fluids must be continued during and after the procedure in order to prevent hypovolemia from the effects of the hypertonic contrast solution. If this fails to relieve the obstruction, laparotomy is indicated. The ileum is opened and, if possible, flushed clear. The bowel can be reanastomosed or brought out as a double-barrel stoma. Alternatively, a T-tube may be placed in the bowel and brought out of the anterior abdominal wall for postoperative irrigations. Compromised intestine is resected, and appendectomy is performed because of the high rate of appendicitis in patients with cystic fibrosis.

All patients should be evaluated for cystic fibrosis. Pancreatic enzyme replacement may be required. A formula low in long-chain fatty acids and high in medium-chain triglycerides may give better absorption and growth than standard formulas. The patient must be placed in an environment with high humidity to keep tracheobronchial secretions fluid. Ultrasonic mist is preferable. Postural drainage with cupping of the chest should be taught to the parents so that they will continue to maintain tracheobronchial toilet indefinitely. Long-term prophylactic antibiotics are not indicated, since infection with antibiotic-resistant pseudomonas and klebsiella organisms usually develops. Older children and adolescents may develop a meconium ileus-like syndrome termed distal ileal obstruction syndrome. This is ileal obstruction due to inspissated stool. It can occur when patients are not compliant with their medications or become dehydrated. Most often, it is successfully treated with hypertonic contrast enemas.

Mak GZ et al: T-tube ileostomy for meconium ileus: four decades of experience. J Pediatr Surg 2000;35:349.

Ziegler MM: Meconium ileus. Curr Probl Surg 1994;31:731.

HIRSCHSPRUNG'S DISEASE

Hirschsprung's disease is due to failure in the cephalocaudal migration of the parasympathetic myenteric nerve cells into the distal bowel. Therefore, the absence of ganglion cells always begins at the anus and extends a varying distance proximally. The aganglionic bowel produces functional obstruction because the bowel fails to relax in response to distention. Short-segment aganglionosis involving only the terminal rectum occurs in about 10% of cases; the disease extends to the sigmoid colon in 75%; more proximal colon in 10%; and the entire colon with small bowel involvement in 5%. Extensive involvement of the small bowel is rare.

Males are affected four times more frequently than females when the disease is limited to the rectosigmoid. Females tend to have longer aganglionic segments. A familial association occurs in 5–10% of cases—more frequently when females are affected. The length of involvement tends to be consistent in familial cases. Down's syndrome occurs in 10–15% of patients.

Clinical Findings

A. Symptoms and Signs

The absence of ganglion cells results in a functional obstruction since the affected area fails to relax due to unopposed sympathetic tone. The symptoms vary widely in severity but almost always occur shortly after birth. The infant passes little or no meconium within 24 hours. Thereafter, chronic or intermittent constipation usually occurs. Progressive abdominal distention, bilious emesis, reluctance to feed, diarrhea, listlessness, irritability, and poor growth and development follow. A rectal examination in the infant may be followed by expulsion of stool and flatus, with remarkable decompression of abdominal distention. In older children, chronic constipation and abdominal distention are characteristic. Passage of flatus and stool requires great effort, and the stools are small in caliber. Children with constipation from Hirschsprung's disease do not exhibit soiling of their diapers or undergarments, distinguishing this form of constipation from idiopathic constipation (encopresis). These children are sluggish, with wasted extremities and flared costal margins. Rectal examination in older children usually reveals a normal or contracted anus and a rectum without feces. Impacted stools in the greatly dilated and distended sigmoid colon can be palpated across the lower abdomen.

B. Imaging Studies

Plain abdominal radiographs in infants show dilated loops of bowel, but it is difficult to distinguish small and large bowel in infancy. A contrast enema should be performed. There should be no attempt to clean out the stool before the fluoroscopic examination, for this will obscure the change in caliber between aganglionic and ganglionic bowel. The contrast enema often demonstrates a contracted (aganglionic) segment that appears relatively narrow compared with the dilated proximal bowel. The proximal aganglionic intestine can be dilated by impacted stool or enema, giving a false impression of the level of the normal colon. Irregular, bizarre contractions (saw-toothed pattern) that do not encircle the aganglionic portion of the bowel may also be recognized. The dilated proximal bowel may have circumferential, smooth, parallel contractions (similar in appearance to those of the jejunum) that are exaggerated contraction waves. The contrast enema may not show a transition zone in the first 6 weeks after birth, since the liquid stool can pass into the aganglionic bowel and the proximal intestine may not be dilated. Lateral projection radiographs should be taken to demonstrate the rectum, the transition zone, and the irregular contractions that may otherwise be obscured by a redundant sigmoid colon on anteroposterior views. Normally, the neonatal rectum is wider than the rest of the colon (including the cecum), and when the rectum is seen to be narrower than the proximal colon, then Hirschsprung's disease is suspected. Radiographs of the abdomen and lateral pelvis should be repeated after 24–48 hours. The contrast agent will be retained for prolonged periods, and saline enemas may be required to evacuate it. The delayed film may show the transition zone and the bizarre irregular contractions more clearly than the initial study.

C. Laboratory Findings

Definitive diagnosis is made by rectal biopsy. Mucosal and submucosal biopsies may be taken from the posterior rectal wall with a suction biopsy capsule without anesthesia at the bedside. Serial sections may demonstrate the characteristic lack of ganglion cells and proliferation of nerve trunks in Meissner's plexus. If the findings are equivocal, it is necessary to remove a 1-cm or 2-cm full-thickness strip of mucosa and muscularis from the posterior rectum proximal to the dentate line under anesthesia. A sample of this size is sufficient for the pathologist to determine the presence or absence of ganglion cells in Meissner's plexus or in Auerbach's plexus. Manometric studies will show a failure of relaxation of the internal sphincter following rectal distention by a balloon, although this test is rarely performed except in older children.

Differential Diagnosis

Low intestinal obstruction in the newborn infant may be due to rectal or colonic atresia, meconium plug syndrome (see below), or meconium ileus as well as a variety of functional causes such as hypermagnesemia, hypocalcemia, hypokalemia, and hypothyroidism. Hirschsprung's disease in patients who develop enterocolitis and diarrhea may mimic other causes of diarrhea. Chronic constipation due to functional causes may suggest Hirschsprung's disease. Although functional constipation may occur early in infancy, the stools are normal in caliber, soiling is frequent, and enterocolitis is rare. In functional constipation, stool is palpable in the lower rectum, and a contrast enema shows uniformly dilated bowel to the level of the anus. However, short segment Hirschsprung's disease may be difficult to differentiate, and rectal biopsy may be necessary. Segmental dilation of the colon is a rare entity that causes constipation similar to that found in Hirschsprung's disease.

Treatment

Traditionally, the surgical treatment was staged and consisted of a leveling colostomy followed several months later by resection of the aganglionic bowel and performance of a pull-through procedure. The trend recently has been toward performing a single-stage procedure (no colostomy) in the newborn period. This paradigm is as follows: bowel obstruction and enterocolitis (if present) may be relieved by placement of a large (30F) rectal tube and repeated warmed saline irrigations in 10 mL/kg aliquots preoperatively. Infants with moderate to severe enterocolitis should be treated with a diverting colostomy. At the time of surgery, frozen section analysis of the colonic muscle is required in order to establish the correct (ganglionic) level for the stoma. Infants who are not ill may undergo any one of three effective operative procedures: Swenson operation, Duhamel operation, or Soave operation. The main operative principles for these procedures are removal of most or all of the aganglionic bowel—while preserving the surrounding nerves to the pelvic organs—and anastomosing ganglionic bowel (confirmed by frozen section analysis) to the rectum 0.5 cm above the dentate line. In contrast to the Swenson and Soave procedures, the Duhamel operation leaves a cuff of aganglionic rectum along which the ganglionic bowel is stapled, creating a mini-reservoir. Historically, these operations have been performed via a low transverse abdominal incision. However, the laparoscopic approach is the method of choice. A solely transanal mucosectomy has been used for those babies with short-segment disease. In total aganglionic colon, ileostomy is necessary. Conservative treatment with enemas is ineffective because it does not prevent further obstruction and enterocolitis.

Prognosis

The death rate for untreated aganglionic megacolon in infancy may be as high as 80%. Nonbacterial, nonviral enterocolitis is the principal cause of death. This tends to occur more frequently in infants but may appear at any age. The cause is not known but seems to be related to the high-grade partial obstruction, poor motility in the "normal" bowel, a frequently competent ileocecal valve, and hypertonic rectal sphincters. There is no correlation between the length of aganglionosis and the occurrence of enterocolitis. Perforation of the colon and appendix may result from distal bowel obstruction. Atresia of the distal small bowel or colon secondary to bowel obstruction due to Hirschsprung's disease in utero has been reported.

Anastomotic leak with perirectal and pelvic abscess is the most serious complication following the pull-through procedure. This complication should be treated immediately by proximal colostomy until the anastomosis has healed. Necrosis of the pulled-through colon may occur if the bowel has not been mobilized sufficiently to prevent tension on the mesenteric blood supply.

Long-term patients who are properly treated for Hirschsprung's disease do well. Incontinence and soiling may occur in a few cases despite a prompt diagnosis and a perfect operation. Episodic constipation and abdominal distention are more common, since the aganglionic internal anal sphincter is intact. Patients with these symptoms can respond to anal dilation. Occasionally, an internal sphincterotomy may be necessary. Smaller children may still develop enterocolitis after definitive treatment, and they should be treated with a large rectal tube and enemas. It is rare after age 5 years. Postoperative enterocolitis is more common in children with Down's syndrome.

Albanese CT et al: Perineal one-stage pull-through for Hirschsprung's disease. J Pediatr Surg 1999;34:377.

Coran AG, Teitelbaum DH: Recent advances in the management of Hirschsprung's disease. Am J Surg 2000;180:382.

Georgeson KE et al: Primary laparoscopic-assisted endorectal colon pull-through for Hirschsprung's disease: a new gold standard. Ann Surg 1999;229:678.

Langer JC et al: One-stage versus two-stage Soave pull-through for Hirschsprung's disease in the first year of life. J Pediatr Surg 1996;31:33.

NEONATAL SMALL LEFT COLON SYNDROME (MECONIUM PLUG SYNDROME)

This problem of newborn infants consists of low intestinal obstruction associated with a left colon of narrow caliber and a dilated transverse and right colon. The infants are in most cases otherwise normal, though approximately 30–50% are born to diabetic mothers and are large for gestational age. Most are over 36 weeks' gestational age and have normal birth weights. Two-thirds are male. Hypermagnesemia has been occasionally associated when the mother has been treated for eclampsia by intravenous magnesium sulfate.

Clinical Findings

Rectal examination may be normal or may reveal a tight anal canal. Little or no meconium is passed, and progressive abdominal distention is followed by vomiting. After thermometer or finger stimulation of the rectum, some meconium and gas may be evacuated. Contrast enema shows a very small left colon, usually to the level of the splenic flexure. Proximal to this point, the colon and commonly the small bowel are greatly distended. In about 30% of cases, a meconium plug is present at the junction of the narrow and dilated portion of the bowel, and the enema (using water-soluble contrast) will dislodge it.

Differential Diagnosis

The small left colon syndrome may be confused with Hirschsprung's disease or meconium ileus. These lesions rarely cause obstruction at the level of the splenic flexure, and when the colon readily decompresses without further obstruction, Hirschsprung's disease is unlikely.

Treatment

A nasogastric tube should be inserted and intravenous fluids started. A contrast enema is required to differentiate the various causes of low intestinal obstruction. When the left colon is narrow and contrast material refluxes into the dilated proximal colon, the diagnosis is most likely the small left colon syndrome. The contrast enema is usually followed by evacuation of copious meconium and decompression of the bowel. Incomplete evacuation of the meconium or persistent symptoms after the enema mandates a suction rectal biopsy to rule out Hirschsprung's disease.

INTUSSUSCEPTION

Telescoping of a segment of bowel (intussusceptum) into the adjacent segment (intussuscipiens) is the most common cause of intestinal obstruction in children between 6 months and 2 years of age (Figure 45–12). The process of intussusception may result in gangrene of the intussusceptum. The most common form is intussusception of the terminal ileum into the right colon (ileocolic intussusception). In 95% of infants and children it is idiopathic. The disease is most common in midsummer and midwinter, and there is a correlation with adenovirus infections. In most cases, hypertrophied Peyer's patches are noted on the leading edge of bowel. Mechanical factors such as Meckel's diverticulum, polyps, hemangioma, enteric duplication, intramural hematoma (Henoch-Schönlein purpura), and intestinal lymphoma are present with increasing frequency in patients over 2 years old. Postoperative intussusception can occur at any age, is usually ileoileal or jejunojejunal, and is due to differential return of bowel motility, often after retroperitoneal surgery. The ratio of males to females is 3:2. The peak

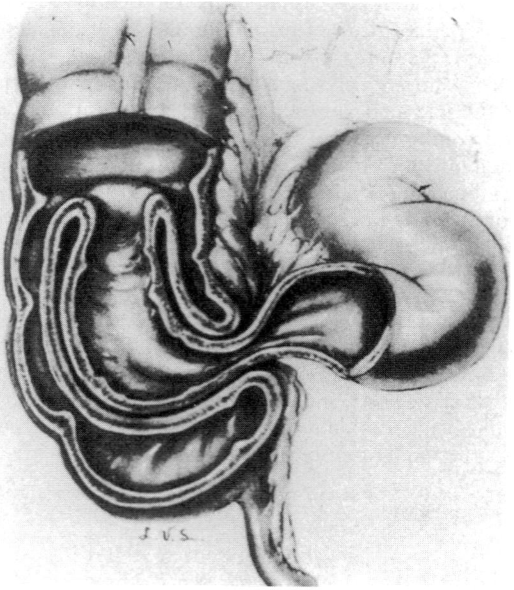

Figure 45–12. Intussusception.

age is in infants 5–9 months of age; 80% of patients are under the age of 2 years.

Clinical Findings

The typical patient is a healthy child who suddenly begins crying and doubles up because of abdominal pain. The pain occurs in episodes that last for about 1 minute, alternating with intervals of apparent well-being. Reflex vomiting is an early sign, but vomiting due to bowel obstruction occurs late. Blood from venous infarction and mucus produce a "currant jelly" stool. In small infants and in postoperative patients, the colicky pain may not be apparent; these babies become withdrawn, and the most prominent symptom is vomiting. Pallor and sweating are common signs during colic. Repeated vomiting and bowel obstruction will produce progressive dehydration. A mass is usually palpable along the distribution of the colon, most commonly in the right upper quadrant of the abdomen. Occasionally, intussusception is palpable on rectal examination. Prolonged intussusception produces edema and hemorrhagic or ischemic infarction of the intussusceptum.

Treatment & Prognosis

The contrast enema is diagnostic as well as therapeutic in 60–80% of cases (Figure 45–13). Contrast enema (using either barium or air) should not be attempted until the patient has been resuscitated enough to allow an operative procedure to be performed safely. It is contraindicated if peritonitis is present. If barium is used, the column of contrast should not stand more than 100 cm above the patient in order to minimize the risk of perforation. Air is pumped into the colon at a pressure of 60–80 mm Hg (never more than 120 mm Hg). A successful study reduces the intussusceptum and demonstrates reflux of barium or air into the terminal ileum. Several attempts should be made before taking the child to surgery. A contrast enema will not reduce gangrenous bowel.

Operation is required for unsuccessful enema reduction or signs of bowel perforation and peritonitis. The procedure may be performed either by laparotomy or laparoscopically. In the absence of gangrene, reduction is accomplished by gentle retrograde compression of the intussuscipiens, not by traction on the proximal bowel. Resection of the intussusception is indicated if the bowel cannot be reduced or if the intestine is gangrenous.

Intussusception recurs after 3% of barium enema reductions and 1% of operative reductions. Deaths are rare but occur if treatment of gangrenous bowel is delayed.

DiFiore JW: Intussusception. Semin Pediatr Surg 1999;8:214.

Meyer JS et al: Air and liquid contrast agents in the management of intussusception: a controlled, randomized trial. Radiology 1993;188:507.

Ong NT, Beasley SW: The leadpoint in intussusception. J Pediatr Surg 1990;25:640.

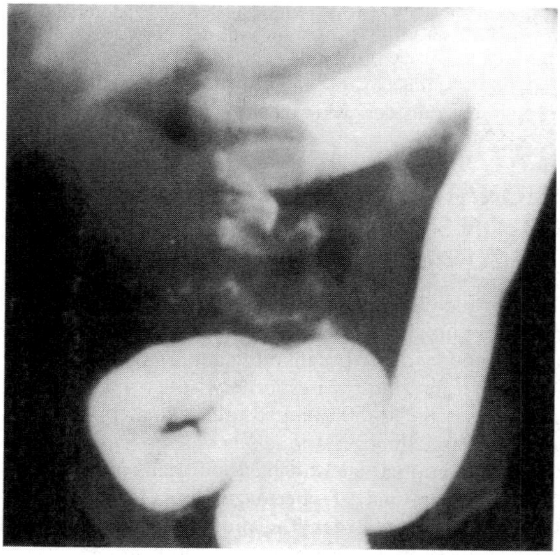

Figure 45–13. Contrast enema demonstrating obstruction to retrograde flow of barium by a filling defect (intussusceptum) in the mid transverse colon. (Reproduced with permission from Albanese CT: Pediatric surgery. In: *Surgery,* Norton JA [editor]. Springer, 2000.)

ANORECTAL ANOMALIES (IMPERFORATE ANUS)

The normal continence mechanism for bowel control consists of an internal sphincter composed of smooth muscle and the striated muscle complex from the levator ani and external sphincter. The striated muscles assume a funnel shape, originating from the pubis, pelvic rim, and sacrum. These muscles converge at the perineum while interdigitating with the internal and external sphincters. Most of the striated muscle complex consists of horizontal muscles that contract against the wall of the rectum and anus while longitudinal muscle fibers run in a cephalocaudal direction and elevate the anus.

Anomalies of the anus result from abnormal growth and fusion of the embryonic anal hillocks. The rectum is normally developed, and the sphincter mechanism is usually intact. With proper surgical treatment, the sphincter will function normally. Anomalies of the rectum develop as a result of faulty division of the cloaca into the urogenital sinus and rectum by the urorectal septum. In these anomalies, the internal sphincter and striated muscle complex are hypoplastic. Therefore, surgical repair results in varying degrees of continence.

Classification

Physical examination of the perineum and imaging studies determine the extent of malformation of the anus or rectum. When an orifice is evident at the perineum or distal vagina, the anomaly is referred to as a low imperforate anus; the absence of an obvious orifice at the perineal level suggests a high imperforate anus (see Figures 45–14 to 45–17). In most instances, with high imperforate anus, there is a communication (fistula) of the rectum with the urethra or bladder in the male or with the upper vagina in the female. Distinguishing between a high and low anomaly may be possible radiologically by determining the position of the rectum in relation to the levator ani or pubococcygeal line.

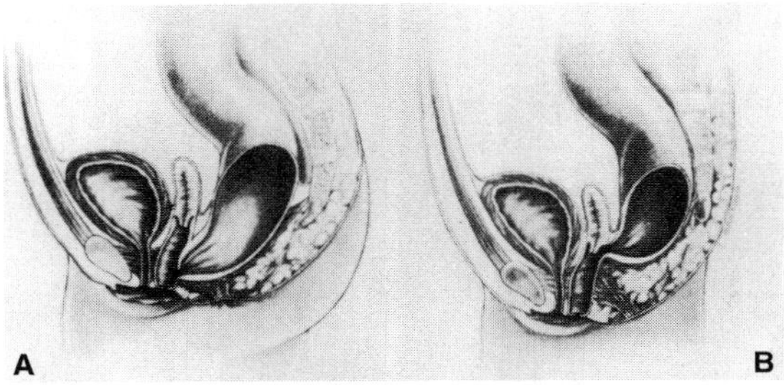

Figure 45–15. ***A:*** High female anatomic anomaly. Low vaginal fistula. ***B:*** High female anomaly. High vaginal fistula. (Reproduced, with permission, from Pena A: *Surgical Management of Anorectal Malformations.* Springer-Verlag, 1992.)

A. Low Anomalies

In low anomalies, the anus may be ectopically placed anterior to its normal position or it may be in the normal position with a narrow outlet due to stenosis or an anal membrane. There may be no opening in the perineum, but the skin at the anal area is heaped up and may extend as a band in the perineal raphe completely covering the anal opening. A small fistula usually extends from the anus anteriorly to open in the raphe of the perineum, scrotum, or penis in the male or the vulva in the female. These babies often have well-developed perineal and gluteal musculature and rarely have sacral vertebral anomalies.

B. High Anomalies

In high anomalies the rectum may end blindly (10%), but more commonly there is a fistula to the urethra or

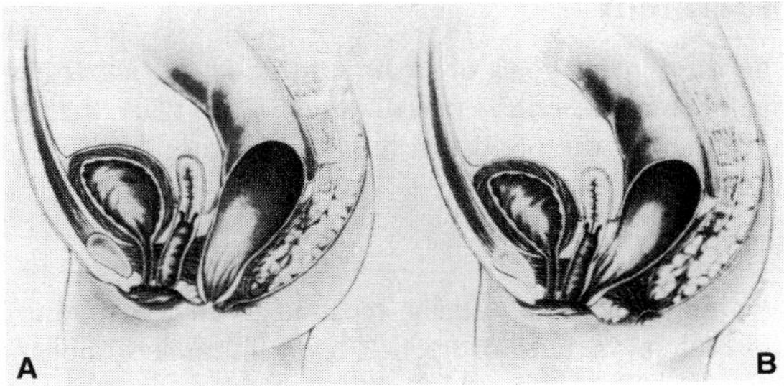

Figure 45–14. ***A:*** Low female anomaly. Perineal fistula. ***B:*** Low female anomaly. Fourchette/vestibule fistula. (Reproduced, with permission, from Pena A: *Surgical Management of Anorectal Malformations.* Springer-Verlag, 1992.)

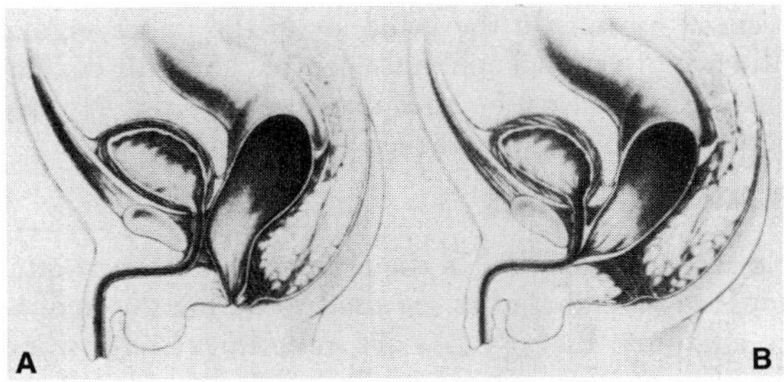

Figure 45–16. ***A:*** Low male anomaly. Perineal fistula. ***B:*** Low male anomaly. Rectobulbar urethra fistula. (Reproduced with permission from Pena A: *Surgical Management of Anorectal Malformations.* Springer-Verlag, 1992.)

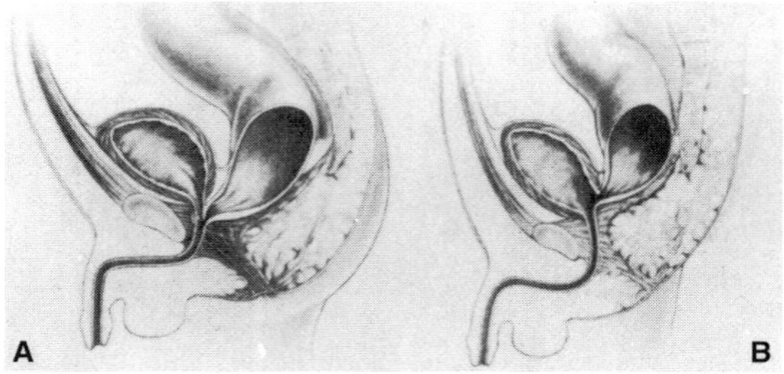

Figure 45–17. ***A:*** High male anomaly. Rectoprostatic urethra fistula. ***B:*** High male anomaly. Rectovesical neck fistula. (Reproduced, with permission, from Pena A: *Surgical Management of Anorectal Malformations.* Springer, 1992.)

bladder in the male or the upper vagina in the female. In the female, a very high fistula may extend between the two halves of a bicornuate uterus directly to the bladder. Patients with high imperforate anus often have deficient pelvic and gluteal innervation and musculature, a high incidence of sacral anomalies, and a poor prognosis for continence after surgical repair. The most severe of the high deformities is a cloacal anomaly in which there is a common channel between the poorly developed pelvic structures (urogenital sinus and rectum) with a single perineal opening.

Clinical Findings

A. Signs

The best means of establishing the type of anorectal anomaly is by physical examination. In low anomalies, an ectopic opening from the rectum can be detected in the perineal raphe in males or in the lower vagina, vestibule, or fourchette in females. A high anomaly exists when no orifice or fistula can be seen upon examination of the perineum or when meconium is found at the urethral meatus, in the urine, or in the upper vagina. Absence of external sphincter contraction with cutaneous stimulation of the anus may also help differentiate between high and low lesions.

B. Imaging Studies

No single test is ideal in the evaluation of imperforate anus, so several studies are used to define the neonatal anatomy. Radiographs are sometimes useful when the clinical impression is unclear. A lateral film of the pelvis with the baby inverted (Wangensteen invertogram), once commonly used, is an inaccurate method of establishing the lower extent of the rectum because swallowed air may not have completely displaced the meconium from the rectum; or the striated muscle complex may be contracted, which obliterates the lumen and makes it look as if the gas in the rectum ends high in the pelvis. With crying or straining, the puborectalis muscle and rectum may actually descend below the ischium, giving a falsely low estimate of rectal height. Gas in the bladder clearly indicates a rectourinary fistula. Lower abdominal and perineal ultrasound, CT, and MRI have been used to define the pelvic anatomy and location in relation to the rectal musculature. Anomalies of the vertebrae and the urinary tract occur in two-thirds of all patients with high anomalies and in one-third of male patients with low anomalies. Vertebral abnormalities in females invariably indicate a high imperforate anus. Anomalies of the sacrum warrant MRI of the lumbosacral area to identify spinal cord anomalies such as a tethered filum terminale.

Complications

Associated anomalies occur in up to 70% in those with a high anomaly. Imperforate anus is associated with the VACTERL syndrome (see Esophageal Anomalies). The possible constellation of anomalies includes esophageal atresia, anomalies of the gastrointestinal tract, hemivertebrae or agenesis of one or more sacral vertebrae (agenesis of S1, S2, or S3 is associated with corresponding neurologic deficits, resulting in neuropathic bladder and greatly impaired continence), genitourinary anomalies (up to 50% incidence with high imperforate anus), and anomalies of the heart and upper limbs/digits.

Delay in diagnosis of imperforate anus may result in excessively large bowel distention and perforation. The presence of a rectourinary fistula allows reflux of urine into the rectum and colon, and absorption of ammonium chloride may cause acidosis. Colon contents will reflux into the urethra, bladder, and upper tracts, producing recurrent pyelonephritis.

Treatment

The three main goals of treatment are (1) to allow passage of stool (ie, relieve obstruction), (2) to place the rectal pouch on the perineum in good position, and (3) to close the fistula.

A. Low Anomalies

Low anomalies are usually repaired from the perineal approach in the newborn period using a muscle stimulator to precisely determine the location of the sphincter complex. The anteriorly placed anal opening is completely mobilized and transferred to the normal position. After healing, the anal opening must be dilated daily for 3–5 months to prevent stricture formation and to allow for growth.

B. High Anomalies

Traditionally, a high deformity was treated by a three-stage repair consisting of colostomy and mucous fistula formation, a posterior sagittal anorectoplasty 4–6 weeks later, and closure of the colostomy several months after that. Recently, the staged approach has been challenged and a one-stage repair has been performed by both posterior sagittal and a laparoscopic approaches. Because the anal sphincters are poorly developed—especially the internal sphincter—continence is most dependent upon a functioning striated muscle complex, which requires conscious voluntary contraction. Care must be taken to preserve the afferent and efferent nerves of the defecation reflex arc as well as the existing sphincter muscles. In all cases, the surgically created anus must be dilated for several months to prevent circumferential cicatrix formation.

Prognosis

Surgical complications include damage to the nervi erigentes, resulting in poor bladder and bowel control and failure of erection. Division of a rectourethral fistula some distance from the urethra produces a blind pouch prone to recurrent infection and stone formation, while cutting the fistula too short may result in urethral stricture. Erroneously attempting to repair a high anomaly from the perineal approach may leave a persistent rectourinary fistula. An abdominoperineal pull-through procedure performed for a low anomaly invariably produces an incontinent patient who might otherwise have had an excellent prognosis. Injury to the vas deferens and ureter is possible during repair of high anomalies.

Patients with imperforate anus tend to have varying degrees of constipation as an inherent part of the defect, believed to be due to poor inherent motility of the rectosigmoid. Patients with low anomalies usually have good sphincter function. Children with high anomalies do not have an internal sphincter that provides continuous, unconscious, and unfatiguing control against soiling. However, in the absence of a lower spine anomaly, perception of rectal fullness, ability to distinguish between flatus and stool, and conscious voluntary control of rectal discharge by contraction of the striated muscle complex can be achieved. When the stools become liquid, sphincter control is usually impaired in patients with high anomalies.

Albanese CT et al: One-stage repair of high imperforate anus in the newborn male. J Pediatr Surg 1999;34:834.

Georgeson KE, Inge TH, Albanese CT: Laparoscopically assisted anorectal pull-through for high imperforate anus—a new technique. J Pediatr Surg 2000;35:927.

Hendren WH: Management of cloacal malformations. Semin Pediatr Surg 1997;6:217.

Pena A, Hong A: Advances in the management of anorectal malformations. Am J Surg 2000;180:370.

GASTROINTESTINAL TRACT ABNORMALITIES

GASTROESOPHAGEAL REFLUX

Studies of esophageal motility, including manometric measurements of the cardioesophageal junction, show absence of the high-pressure zone (lower esophageal sphincter) in the terminal esophagus in most normal newborns. Evolution to the normal adult pattern of peristalsis and cardioesophageal sphincter function occurs after several months. Until this happens, many infants experience varying degrees of regurgitation after feeding. Rarely, repeated gastric reflux may produce peptic esophagitis and interfere with the development of a competent sphincter. Unlike adults, children rarely have a hiatal hernia as a cause of gastroesophageal reflux (GER).

Clinical Findings

A. Symptoms and Signs

Symptoms consist of repeated effortless regurgitation of feedings, particularly when the baby is placed in a recumbent position. The baby will be hungry and will readily feed after regurgitating. Persistent regurgitation may result in poor weight gain (failure to thrive), peptic esophagitis with appearance of blood in the vomitus, or occult bleeding, producing anemia. One cause for apnea and sudden infant death syndrome (SIDS) is GER and aspiration. Lesser degrees of aspiration, particularly during sleep, may produce recurrent pneumonia. Stricture formation of the lower esophagus and metaplasia of the esophageal mucosa, producing Barrett's esophagus, are possible late effects. Almost half of infants and children with GER have neurologic disorders related to perinatal asphyxia or congenital nervous system anomalies; seizure disorders are very common in this population. Abnormal motility of the esophagus and gastric dysmotility and impaired gastric emptying are frequently present. Gastroesophageal reflux is associated with esophageal atresia, congenital diaphragmatic hernia, and abdominal wall defects.

B. Imaging Studies

The standard diagnostic test is lower esophageal 24-hour pH monitoring. An upper gastrointestinal series is less sensitive but is useful to rule out other disorders (eg, intestinal malrotation) and to assess for esophageal stricture. Gastric emptying may be assessed by technetium pertechnate scan. There is virtually no role for esophageal manometric studies in young children except for those in whom one suspects the relatively rare achalasia or diffuse esophageal spasm.

Treatment

Nonoperative treatment is successful in most cases. Feedings should be thickened with rice cereal, and GER is lessened if the baby is maintained upright in an infant seat or in a prone position after feeding. Persistent symptoms mandate drug therapy with an antacid (eg, H_2 blocker or proton pump inhibitor) with or without a prokinetic agent (eg, metoclopramide). If a prolonged trial of nonoperative therapy fails or if complications of reflux can be documented (ie, esophagitis, stricture, asthma, recurrent aspiration pneumonia, failure to thrive), an antireflux procedure such as the Nissen or Thal fundoplication procedure is indicated. The open operation has been virtually replaced by the more cosmetic and better visualized laparoscopic procedure. Pyloroplasty may be required when there is associated impaired gastric emptying, though there is accumulating evidence suggesting that the "funneling" effect of the fundoplication promotes gastric emptying even in the face of documented delayed emptying.

Georgeson KE: Laparoscopic fundoplication and gastrostomy. Semin Laparosc Surg 1998;5:25.

Johnson DG: The past and present of antireflux surgery in children. Am J Surg 2000;180:377.

Kazerooni NL et al: Fundoplication in 160 children under 2 years of age. J Pediatr Surg 1994;29:677.

ACUTE APPENDICITIS

Acute appendicitis is one of the most common causes of an acute abdomen in childhood. This diagnosis must be considered in all age groups, but it is most common between the ages of 4 and 15 years.

Clinical Findings

The diagnosis is most often made by obtaining a careful clinical history and performing a thorough physical examination. In some patients, observation and periodic reexamination by the same physician may be necessary to confirm or exclude the diagnosis. In young children, the diagnosis of appendicitis can be difficult to arrive at, as the clinical history may be difficult to elicit. The classic presentation includes the onset of epigastric or periumbilical pain followed by anorexia, nausea, and vomiting. Anorexia is a significant finding, as the child will often refuse favorite foods. A fever will usually develop, and the pain then localizes to the right lower quadrant. Rovsing's sign (right lower quadrant pain during palpation of the left lower quadrant), localized right lower quadrant tenderness, and involuntary spasm of the right hemirectus muscle indicate the presence of peritonitis.

A white blood count with differential and urinalysis should be obtained. The white blood cell count is greater than 10,000/μL (often with a left shift) in more than 80% of patients with appendicitis. Radiologic evaluation should include a chest film to exclude right lower lobe pneumonia. Findings on flat and erect abdominal radiographs are often nonspecific, though they may infrequently demonstrate the presence of a fecalith. Ultrasound (particularly in females) and CT scans are being used with increasing frequency, especially for those without the classic history and physical examination results.

Differential Diagnosis

Gastroenteritis is often confused with appendicitis. Vomiting follows periumbilical pain in appendicitis but often precedes abdominal pain in gastroenteritis. In addition, the patient with gastroenteritis commonly has diffuse abdominal pain and frequent copious watery diarrhea. Intussusception, intestinal obstruction and volvulus, mesenteric adenitis, Meckel's diverticulitis, Henoch-Schönlein purpura, ruptured ovarian cyst, and Crohn's disease must also be considered in the differential diagnosis for children. In adolescent girls, information regarding the menstrual cycle, previous episodes of pelvic inflammatory disease, and an accurate sexual history is important to exclude gynecologic causes of an acute abdomen.

Treatment

Once the diagnosis is made, fluid resuscitation is performed and antibiotics are administered. Appendectomy is accomplished through a right lower quadrant incision or using the laparoscope. In cases of perforation, the peritoneal cavity is irrigated and aspirated dry but drainage is not performed, unless there is a mature abscess cavity. The wound is closed in all cases. Antibiotics are continued for 3–7 days or until the white blood cell count and fever normalize. The morbidity and mortality of appendicitis in children have gradually decreased even though the incidence of ruptured appendix at diagnosis remains high. Perforation is present in 25% of children at 24 hours after onset of symptoms, in 50% at 36 hours, and in 80% at 48 hours. Most deaths are noted in the very young when the diagnosis is not considered and long delays in treatment occur and in those with a ruptured appendix who are not prepared properly for operation and develop renal failure and sepsis.

Madonna MB, Boswell WC, Arensman RM: Acute abdomen. Outcomes. Semin Pediatr Surg 1997;6:105.

Pearl RH et al: Pediatric appendectomy. J Pediatr Surg 1995; 30:173.

DUPLICATIONS OF THE GASTROINTESTINAL TRACT

Duplications may occur at any point along the gastrointestinal tract from the mouth to the anus. Duplications occur (in order of decreasing frequency) in the ileum (50% of cases), mediastinum, colon, rectum, stomach, duodenum, and neck. Intrathoracic and small bowel duplications are usually spherical; colonic duplications are commonly long and tubular (Figure 45–18). Characteristically, the intra-abdominal duplications are within the mesentery and have a common wall with the intestine.

Based on embryology, duplications have been categorized as foregut, midgut, and hindgut. Foregut duplications include the pharynx, respiratory tract, esophagus, stomach, and the first portion and proximal half of the second portion of the duodenum. Midgut duplications include the distal half of the second part of the duodenum, the jejunum, ileum, cecum, appendix, the ascending colon, and the proximal two-thirds of the transverse colon. The hindgut is composed of duplications of the distal third of the transverse colon, the descending and sigmoid colon, the rectum, anus, and components of the urologic system. Combined thoracoabdominal duplications also occur in which the thoracic saccular component extends through the esophageal hiatus or a separate diaphragmatic opening to empty into the duodenum or jejunum. A thoracic duplication, associated with a cervical or thoracic vertebral anomaly, in which the duplication communicates with the subarachnoid space, is called a neurenteric cyst. Associated cardiovascular, neurologic, skeletal, urologic, and gastrointestinal anomalies occur in more than a third of cases. Carcinoma may arise within duplications of the colon.

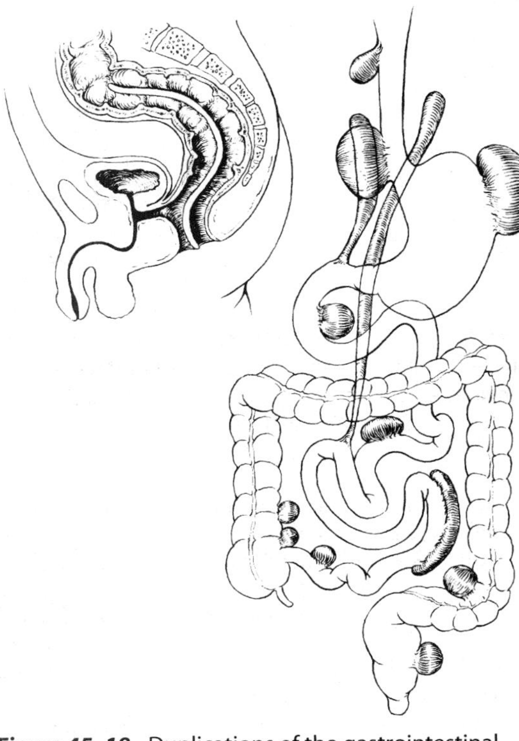

Figure 45–18. Duplications of the gastrointestinal tract. Duplications may be saccular or tubular. They usually arise within the mesentery, having a common wall with the intestine. Thoracoabdominal duplications arise from the duodenum or jejunum and extend through the diaphragm into the mediastinum.

Clinical Findings

A. Symptoms and Signs

Two-thirds of patients with duplications are symptomatic in the first year of life. Duplications of the neck and mediastinum produce respiratory distress by compression of the airway. Thoracic duplications may ulcerate into the lung and lead to pneumonia or hemoptysis. Intestinal duplications usually produce abdominal pain owing to spastic contraction of the bowel, excessive distention of the duplication, or peptic ulceration and bleeding resulting from ectopic gastric mucosa in the duplication. Intestinal obstruction due to intussusception, volvulus, or encroachment on the lumen by an intramural cyst also occurs. An isolated asymptomatic mass may be the only finding. Sixty percent of duplications are diagnosed by 6 months of life and 85% by 2 years.

B. Imaging Studies

Studies include radiographs of the chest and thoracolumbar spine, CT scan of the chest and abdomen, contrast enema, esophagography, and upper GI series. If an intraspinal extension of a duplication is suspected, MRI is indicated. Ultrasonography may show a cystic or tubular mass within the mediastinum or abdomen.

Treatment

Duplications not intimately adherent to adjacent organs should be excised. Isolated spherical duplications can be excised with the adjacent segment of bowel and an end-to-end anastomosis of the bowel performed. Long tubular duplications can be decompressed by establishing an anastomosis between the proximal and distal ends of adjacent bowel. Noncommunicating duplications, which would require radical resection of surrounding structures, should be drained by a Roux-en-Y technique. Duplications that cannot be removed completely and which contain gastric mucosa should be opened (without jeopardizing the blood supply of the normal bowel) and the mucosal lining excised. Extension of a mediastinal duplication into the spine or abdomen should be resected. An intra-abdominal extension is closed at the level of the diaphragm, and complete excision by laparotomy is accomplished.

Iyer CP, Mahour GH: Duplications of the alimentary tract in infants and children. J Pediatr Surg 1995;30:1267.

Merry C, Spurbeck W, Lobe TE: Resection of foregut-derived duplications by minimal access surgery. Pediatr Surg Int 1999;15:224.

Stern LE, Warner BW: Gastrointestinal duplications. Semin Pediatr Surg 2000;9:135.

Wilkinson CC et al: Fetal neurenteric cyst causing hydrops: case report and review of the literature. Prenat Diagn 1999;19:118.

OMPHALOMESENTERIC DUCT ANOMALIES

The omphalomesenteric (vitelline) duct is a remnant of the embryonic yolk sac. When the entire duct remains intact postnatally, it is recognized as an omphalomesenteric fistula. When the duct is obliterated at the intestinal end but communicates with the umbilicus at the distal end, it is called an umbilical sinus. When the epithelial tract persists but both ends are occluded, an umbilical cyst or intra-abdominal enterocystoma may develop. The entire tract may be obliterated, but a fibrous band may persist between the ileum and the umbilicus (Figure 45–19).

The most common remnant of the omphalomesenteric duct is Meckel's diverticulum, which is present in 1–3% of the population. Meckel's diverticulum may be lined wholly or in part by small intestinal, colonic, or gastric mucosa, and it may contain aberrant pancreatic tissue. Heterotopic tissue is found in 5% of asymptomatic and 60% of symptomatic cases. In contrast to duplications and pseudodiverticula, Meckel's diverticulum is located on the antimesenteric border of the ileum, 10–90 cm from the ileocecal valve. Meckel's diverticulum occurs with equal frequency in both sexes. It is usually asymptomatic and is seen as an incidental finding during operation for other disease. Of those with Meckel's diverticulum, the lifelong risk of complications is 4%, and 40% of these cases occur in children under 10 years of age.

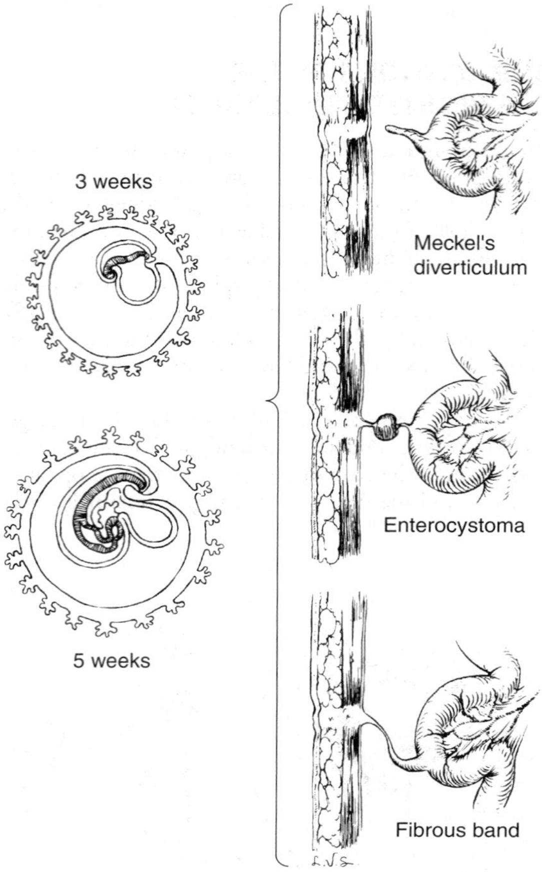

Figure 45–19. Omphalomesenteric duct anomalies arise from the primitive yolk sac. Remnants include Meckel's diverticulum, enterocystoma, and a fibrous band or fistulous tract between the ileum and the umbilicus.

Clinical Findings

Symptomatic omphalomesenteric remnants (male:female incidence 3:1) produce rectal bleeding in 40%, intussusception in 20%, diverticulitis or peptic perforation in 15%, umbilical fistula in 15%, intestinal obstruction in 7%, and abscess in 3% of cases. Rectal bleeding associated with Meckel's diverticulum is due to peptic ulceration of the adjacent ileum caused by ectopic gastric mucosa. Over 50% of these patients are under 2 years of age. The blood is mixed with stool and is most often dark red or bright red; tarry stools are unusual. A history of a previous episode of bleeding may be elicited in 40% of cases. Occult bleeding from Meckel's diverticulum is very rare. Younger patients tend to bleed quite briskly and may exsanguinate rapidly. Diverticulitis or free perforation will present with abdominal pain and peritonitis similar to acute appendicitis. The pain and tenderness occur in the lower abdomen, most commonly near the umbilicus. Periumbilical cellulitis may be present.

Intestinal obstruction may develop as a result of volvulus of the bowel about a persistent band between the umbilicus and the ileum or as a result of herniation of bowel between the mesentery and a persistent vitelline or mesodiverticular vessel. Obstruction is the most common presentation in adults. An infected umbilical sinus or omphalomesenteric fistula may present with mucoid, purulent, or enteric discharge, recurrent cellulitis, or a deep abdominal wall abscess about the umbilicus. This can be diagnosed by cannulation and contrast injection via the umbilical tract.

Upper and lower contrast studies rarely outline the primary defect. Technetium Tc 99m pertechnetate may localize in gastric mucosa lining Meckel's diverticulum and may identify the source of hematochezia or melena. Retention of dye in the mucous and parietal cells is enhanced by giving cimetidine, 30 mg/kg intravenously, 30 minutes before administration of the radiotracer nuclide.

Treatment

Resection is accomplished by laparotomy or laparoscopy. An omphalomesenteric remnant with a narrow base may be treated by amputation and closure of the bowel defect (usually with a surgical stapler). In cases where the anomaly has a wide mouth with ectopic tissue or where an inflammatory or ischemic process involves the adjacent ileum, intestinal resection with the diverticulum and anastomosis may be necessary.

Fa-Si-Oen PR, Roumen RM, Croiset van Uchelen FA: Complications and management of Meckel's diverticulum and intestinal duplication—a review. Eur J Surg 1999;165:674.

Moore TC: Omphalomesenteric duct malformations. Semin Pediatr Surg 1996;5:116.

NECROTIZING ENTEROCOLITIS

Necrotizing enterocolitis (NEC) is the most serious and frequent gastrointestinal disorder of predominantly premature infants, with a median onset of 10 days after birth. The incidence is increasing given the therapeutic advances in neonatal intensive care that have allowed ever more premature smaller and smaller babies to survive. It is characterized by necrosis, ulceration, and sloughing of intestinal mucosa, which frequently progresses to full-thickness necrosis and perforation. This process progresses from the submucosa through the muscular layer to the subserosa. Gas-producing bacteria in the intestinal wall may lead to pneumatosis, a finding that may be noted on gross examination as well as on plain abdominal radiographs. The terminal ileum and right colon are usually affected first, followed in descending order of frequency by the transverse and descending colon, appendix, jejunum, stomach, duodenum, and esophagus. The most extreme case, pannecrosis, is defined as necrosis of 75% or more of the bowel. Eighty percent of cases occur in premature infants weighing less than 2500 g at birth, and 50% are under 1500 g. However, the disorder may also occur in full-term infants. Contrary to earlier impressions, there is no established relationship between NEC and stressful perinatal events such as premature rupture of membranes with amnionitis, breech delivery, intrauterine bradycardia, umbilical vessel catheterization with or without exchange transfusion, respiratory distress syndrome, sepsis, omphalitis, and congenital heart disease. An associated patent ductus arteriosus is common. In older infants and children, NEC is usually preceded by malnutrition and gastroenteritis. The clustering of cases in nurseries suggests that an infectious agent may be responsible.

Clinical Findings

Clinical findings include increased gastric residual, bilious vomiting, abdominal distention, bloody stools, lethargy, and poor skin perfusion. When intestinal perforation occurs, guarding is evident on abdominal examination, but in weak premature infants this may not be obvious. There are a variety of nonspecific clinical findings that suggest physiologic instability such as apnea, bradycardia, hypoglycemia, and temperature instability. On examination, abdominal distention and fixed loops of intestine may be appreciated. The presence of abdominal wall erythema, edema, and crepitus may be a sign of bowel necrosis. Laboratory evaluation is nonspecific since the white blood cell count may be low or high, but thrombocytopenia and acidosis develop with perforation and sepsis.

Supine and cross-table lateral abdominal radiographs show small bowel distention early, followed by pneumatosis intestinalis. Gas within the portal venous system can be seen but it is fleeting. Serial examinations may show a loop or loops of bowel that are fixed in position and dilated. Perforation with peritoneal air develops in 20% of cases. Infants who develop ascites without pneumoperitoneum should have paracentesis and examination of the fluid for bacteria, which would signify perforation. Contrast studies are hazardous and contraindicated, as they may easily lead to perforation.

Treatment

Treatment includes cessation of feedings, orogastric suction, systemic antibiotics, and correction of hypoxemia, hypovolemia, acidosis, and electrolyte abnormalities. The only absolute indication for operation is pneumoperitoneum. Relative indications are portal vein air, clinical deterioration, a fixed intestinal loop on serial radiographs, erythema of the abdominal wall, an abdominal mass, and a paracentesis demonstrating bacteria. At laparotomy, necrotic bowel is resected and the proximal bowel is made into a stoma. Rarely is primary anastomosis safe. Severe disease may not be amenable to operation or require extensive bowel resection, resulting in short bowel syndrome. An alternative treatment option in very low birth weight infants (< 1500 g) that is gaining acceptance for documented perforation is bedside drainage of the peritoneal cavity in the right lower quadrant using local anesthesia.

In one-third of cases, the disorder resolves without further treatment, and the overall survival rate is more than 50%. Intestinal stricture may occur as a late complication following healing. For this reason, a contrast enema is used to evaluate the defunctionalized distal bowel before closing the stoma.

Andorsky DJ et al: Nutritional and other postoperative management of neonates with short bowel syndrome correlates with clinical outcomes. J Pediatr 2001;139:27.

Ladd AP et al: Long-term follow-up after bowel resection for necrotizing enterocolitis: factors affecting outcome. J Pediatr Surg 1998;33:967.

Noble HG, Driessnack M: Bedside peritoneal drainage in very low birth weight infants. Am J Surg 2001;181:416.

GASTROINTESTINAL BLEEDING

Significant gastrointestinal bleeding in children is rare. When it occurs, it can be alarming and anxiety-provoking for caregivers and parents. The diagnostic approach used in the evaluation of these children is similar to that used in adults, but the causes vary depending on the age of the child. Rarely is the gastrointestinal bleeding massive, and the majority of causes are benign. A diagnosis can be established in over 85% of cases. Usual presenting symptoms include hematemesis, hematochezia, and melena. Depending on the amount of bleeding, the child may have sunken fontanelles, dry mucous membranes, and cool skin. Tachycardia, oliguria, and hypotension may be present. Intravenous access should be obtained, fluid and blood administered as needed, and an evaluation begun. Laboratory tests include serial hematocrit measurements and coagulation studies. Following stabilization and physical examination, evaluation should then proceed to the appropriate diagnostic tests.

Upper Gastrointestinal Bleeding

Upper gastrointestinal bleeding originates above the ligament of Treitz. The presence of melena and the presence of blood on passage of an orogastric tube can help differentiate between upper and lower gastrointestinal bleeding. Upper gastrointestinal bleeding in infants and young children is most often associated with stress ulcers or erosions, but in older children it may also be caused by duodenal ulcer, esophagitis, and esophageal varices in children with underlying liver disease. The majority of these diseases are benign. Evaluation following stabilization of the child begins with flexible esophagoduodenoscopy. Once the diagnosis is made, treatment is usually amenable to antacids (H_2-blockers, proton pumpl inhibitors) and sucralfate. Variceal hemorrhage may require more aggressive intervention, including the use of octreotide, endoscopic varix sclerosis or band ligation, and, in extreme cases, transjugular intrahepatic portocaval shunt (TIPS), mesocaval shunt, or liver transplantation.

Lower Gastrointestinal Bleeding

Although diverticulitis, cancer, and angiodysplasia are the most common causes of lower gastrointestinal bleeding in adults, those diseases are not present in children. The causes of lower gastrointestinal bleeding in infants and children can be categorized in diagnostic age groups where the age of the patient, the amount of bleeding, and the color of the blood passed provide some guidance to the probable source of bleeding.

Bleeding in the neonate may be caused by swallowing maternal blood at delivery, an anorectal fissure, upper gastrointestinal bleeding secondary to gastritis or ulceration, necrotizing enterocolitis, volvulus, and an incarcerated hernia. The Apt test for maternal blood, physical examination of the rectum and inguinal canal, and evaluation of the upper gastrointestinal tract can quickly rule out most of these causes. Bleeding from necrotizing enterocolitis is rarely life-threatening, and the diagnosis is commonly made based on the premature delivery of the infant and radiologic evaluation. If bleeding from malrotation with midgut volvulus is suspected, prompt laparotomy is indicated.

In infants, anal fissures continue to be the most common cause of rectal bleeding. Other causes include intestinal volvulus, intussusception, intestinal duplication, Meckel's diverticulum, and infectious diarrhea. Contrast studies and appropriate stool cultures guide treatment. Children have a differential diagnosis similar to that of infants with the addition of rectal prolapse and a variety of polyps of the colon (juvenile, Peutz-Jeghers, polypoid lymphoid hyperplasia, and, rarely, adenomatosis). These entities are diagnosed by physical examination and proctosigmoidoscopy. If no source of bleeding is identified, colonoscopy is indicated. Juvenile polyps are the single most common cause of lower gastrointestinal bleeding in children (20–30%). Most juvenile polyps are single (80%) and often pass spontaneously without treatment. However, when bleeding continues to occur, the polyp can be snared and excised endoscopically. Adolescents may manifest signs and symptoms of inflammatory bowel disease (ulcerative colitis, Crohn's disease), familial adenomatous polyposis, and small vascular lesions such as telangiectasias.

Diagnosis is made by colonoscopy, and treatment is disease-specific.

Arain Z, Rossi TM: Gastrointestinal bleeding in children: an overview of conditions requiring nonoperative management. Semin Pediatr Surg 1999;8:172.

Oldham KT, Lobe TE: Gastrointestinal hemorrhage in children: a pragmatic update. Pediatr Clin North Am 1985;32:1247.

GASTROINTESTINAL FOREIGN BODIES

Children aged 9 months to 2 years are at particular risk for the ingestion or aspiration of foreign bodies given their newly acquired mobility, curiosity, and the tendency to place objects in their mouths. The type of foreign body and the location in the airway or gastrointestinal tract dictate management.

Esophagal Foreign Bodies

Typical foreign bodies found in the esophagus include coins, food, and small toys. The three most common sites of obstruction are at the level of the cricopharyngeus muscle, at the level of the aortic arch, and at the gastroesophageal junction. Previous areas of repair/anastomosis or injury predispose to obstruction due to scar and narrowing. Common symptoms include drooling, feeding intolerance, dysphagia, and pain. Perforation is rare but is dictated by the ingested object's shape, composition, and time in the esophagus. The diagnosis is easily obtained by anteroposterior chest or lateral neck radiography if the ingested object is radiopaque. Otherwise, esophagoscopy or an upper gastrointestinal series is needed.

Because of the risk of erosion, aspiration, perforation, and late stricture, impacted objects should be removed. Extraction can be performed using balloon catheter retrieval under fluoroscopic control or under direct visualization using esophagoscopy with general anesthesia. The latter technique is generally preferred if the nature of the object is unknown, or is sharp, or the ingestion was 24–48 hours previously. A Hopkins rod lens endoscopy system allows visualization of the object and retrieval with specially designed forceps for grasping small objects.

Ninety-five percent of foreign bodies that pass beyond the gastroesophageal junction proceed uneventfully through the gastrointestinal tract. Operative retrieval is reserved for batteries, which must be removed, and for cases where ingested objects cause obstruction (bezoars) or intestinal injury or have been in place for more than 1 week.

Tracheal Foreign Bodies

Children, particularly those 1–2 years of age, can occlude the airway by aspiration of a foreign body. The most common objects are peanuts and pieces of popcorn. Obstruction tends to occur at the level of the laryngeal inlet, the subglottis, or the right main stem bronchus. Because this can be a life-threatening problem, witnessed events should be treated with back blows, abdominal thrusts, or the Heimlich maneuver, which may dislodge the object.

Symptoms include coughing, choking, wheezing, dyspnea, and fever. Unilateral wheezing and rhonchi may be present. Air trapping may result when the foreign body forms a ball-valve obstruction leading to hyperinflation of the affected lung and mediastinal shift away from the affected side. On the other hand, complete obstruction may lead to loss of air volume with atelectasis and mediastinal shift to the ipsilateral side. Inspiratory and expiratory radiographs or bilateral decubitus films in infants may demonstrate air trapping; the foreign body is rarely noted on radiographs.

With a worrisome history, a foreign body suggested on a radiograph, or any symptoms, the child should undergo bronchoscopic evaluation under general anesthesia. Working in tandem with the anesthesiologist to allow ventilation during rigid endoscopy, the foreign body can be readily identified. Lighted grasping forceps made specifically for foreign body extraction are placed through the sheath of the bronchoscope; the foreign body is grasped; and the forceps, foreign body, and sheath are removed as one unit. Rarely, an unrecognized aspirated foreign body presents as chronic lung infection and can require removal of the affected lung.

Baharloo F et al: Tracheobronchial foreign bodies: presentation and management in children and adults. Chest 1999;115:1357.

Kaiser CW et al: Retained foreign bodies. J Trauma 1997;43:107.

LIVER & BILIARY TRACT DISORDERS

Jaundice in the first 2 weeks of infancy is usually due to indirect (unconjugated) hyperbilirubinemia. The causes include (1) "physiologic jaundice" due to immaturity of hepatic function (eg, that associated with breast-feeding); (2) Rh, ABO, and rare blood group incompatibilities, which produce hemolysis; and (3) infections. Jaundice that persists beyond the first 2 weeks in which the indirect and conjugated bilirubin levels are elevated should prompt a more thorough workup aimed at diagnosing potential surgical disorders. The most frequent cause (60%) of prolonged jaundice in infancy is biliary atresia; various forms of hepatitis occur in 35%; and choledochal cyst is found in 5% of cases of obstructive jaundice. Mild indirect hyperbilirubinemia occurs with pyloric stenosis and quickly disappears after pyloromyotomy. Intestinal obstruction can intensify jaundice by increasing the enterohepatic circulation of bilirubin. Finally, jaundice is an early and important sign of septicemia in the newborn.

BILIARY ATRESIA

Biliary atresia is the absence of patent bile ducts draining the liver. Familial cases and frequent association with the polysplenia syndrome indicate a congenital onset. However, biliary atresia probably develops after birth because jaundice is not usually remarkable in the newborn period but becomes evident more than 2 weeks later. Furthermore, conjugated bilirubin is not cleared by the placenta as unconjugated bilirubin is, and jaundice due to conjugated hyperbilirubinemia with biliary obstruction has not been recognized in newborn infants. The atretic ducts consist of solid fibrous cords that may contain occasional islands of biliary epithelium.

The extent of duct involvement varies greatly. There are three anatomic patterns of obstruction: (1) the proximal extrahepatic bile ducts are patent and the ducts distal to the cystic duct are obliterated; (2) the gallbladder, cystic duct, and common bile duct are patent and the proximal hepatic ducts are occluded; and (3) the entire extrahepatic ductal system is obstructed. Liver biopsy demonstrates proliferation of the bile canaliculi containing inspissated bile. Over time, the failure to excrete bile out of the liver results in progressive periportal fibrosis and obstruction of the intrahepatic portal veins, resulting in biliary cirrhosis.

Clinical Findings

A. Symptoms and Signs

The infant with biliary atresia often has an uneventful neonatal course until jaundice is noted at 2–3 weeks of age. Stools may be normal or clay-colored, and the urine may be dark. The stools contain an increased quantity of fat but are of normal consistency and not frothy. The liver may be of normal size early, but it becomes enlarged with time. A hard liver may develop as a consequence of progressive cirrhosis. Splenomegaly usually develops. Ascites and portal hypertension do not become manifest for several months.

B. Laboratory Findings

The workup of biliary atresia consists of analysis of liver function tests, complete blood count, and metabolic and serologic screening. The bilirubin levels may vary considerably from day to day, but direct bilirubin levels over 3 mg/dL are common. Alkaline phosphatase levels are often elevated to 500–1000 units/L, and γ-glutamyltranspeptidase levels are greater than 300 units/L.

C. Imaging Studies

Ultrasonography may demonstrate absence or inability to visualize a contracted gallbladder. Radionuclide scanning using technetium Tc 99m-labeled iminodiacetate compounds (IDA, HIDA, PIPIDA, DISIDA) to observe the intensity of uptake within the liver and evidence of secretion into the bowel is valuable, usually preceded by a 2- to 3-day course of phenobarbital to promote tracer uptake. Needle biopsy of the liver may be safely performed at any age if the clotting tests are normal. A diagnosis based on needle biopsy is accurate in 60%, equivocal in 16%, and erroneous in 24% of cases. Unless the workup has conclusively diagnosed another entity, all children suspected of having biliary atresia should undergo operative cholangiography with the intention of proceeding to exploration of the porta hepatis.

Other Causes

Other causes of obstructive jaundice are choledochal cyst, inspissated bile syndrome, and any one of several neonatal hepatitides. A choledochal cyst is identified by the presence of a palpable mass in the right upper quadrant and ultrasonographic confirmation. Inspissated bile syndrome follows a hemolytic process in which a large bilirubin load is excreted into the bile ducts, where it becomes coalesced and impacted, or may occur after a prolonged period of bowel rest with total parenteral nutrition. The syndrome is recognized by abdominal ultrasound. Hepatitis is most commonly of unknown cause. It may be due to a variety of infections, often of maternal origin, such as toxoplasmosis, cytomegalovirus, rubella syndrome, herpes simplex, coxsackievirus, and varicella. Serum should be tested for elevated antibody titers to these agents. Neonatal physiologic jaundice is self-limited and also responds to phototherapy.

Genetic metabolic diseases producing jaundice include α_1-antitrypsin deficiency, galactosemia, and cystic fibrosis. Other rare causes include sepsis, parenteral alimentation cholestasis, Gilbert's disease, and Alagille's syndrome.

Treatment

Surgical exploration for neonatal jaundice is indicated as early in infancy as possible, when biliary atresia is the likely cause. Delayed treatment will result in progressive cirrhosis. Fluoroscopy should be available in the operating room. The gallbladder is cannulated through a transverse abdominal incision or via laparoscopy. Water-soluble contrast should be gently instilled into the biliary tree. If the image shows a patent common bile duct but no reflux into the liver, a rubber-shod bulldog clamp may be placed on the distal common duct and the cholangiogram repeated. During development of the radiograph films, a core needle biopsy of each lobe is obtained.

Confirmed biliary atresia requires hepatic portoenterostomy (Kasai procedure). The scarred bile ducts and gallbladder are removed, and a Roux-en-Y limb of jejunum is sutured to an area of the hilum bounded laterally by the hepatic artery branches. A number of variations to this procedure, including use of an intussuscepted antireflux valve using the appendix or jejunal limb, have been used to minimize postoperative cholangitis, although this approach is falling out of favor. The appendix may also be used as a conduit between the porta hepatis and the duodenum.

Prognosis

A good long-term outcome is related to a meticulously performed procedure, age at operation less than 2 months, absence of cirrhosis at the time of operation, and establishment of adequate bile flow. In general, one-third of the infants will have excellent bile flow and do not develop liver failure; one-third never have bile flow and require early liver transplantation; and one-third have initially good bile flow but months to years later develop progressive biliary cirrhosis requiring liver transplantation. The average life span for infants with uncorrectable biliary atresia without transplantation is 19 months. Death is due to progressive liver failure, bleeding from esophageal varices, or sepsis. For those with established bile flow postoperatively, the most common complication is cholangitis, and this may recur. Most often, the cause is unknown and not readily correctable by surgical means.

Delarue A et al: Is the appendix graft suitable for routine biliary surgery in children? J Pediatr Surg 2000;35:1312.

Narkewicz MR: Biliary atresia: an update on our understanding of this disorder. Curr Opin Pediatr 2001;13:435.

Nio M, Ohi R: Biliary atresia. Semin Pediatr Surg 2000;9:177.

Tagge DU et al: A long-term experience with biliary atresia: reassessment of prognostic factors. Ann Surg 1991;214:590.

CHOLEDOCHAL CYST

A choledochal cyst is a dilation or diverticulum of all or a portion of the common bile duct. Estimates of incidence range from 1:2,000,000 to 1:13,000. There is a female predominance (3:1), and the lesions are more common in Asians, with a large majority of the reported cases from Japan. Numerous theories exist as to the cause of this abnormality, including infectious agents, reflux of pancreatic enzymes into the bile duct via a long common channel, genetic factors, and biliary autonomic dysfunction.

Choledochal cysts are classified into one of five subtypes. Type I is a fusiform dilation of the extrahepatic bile duct. Type II is a saccular outpouching of the common bile duct. Type III is referred to as a choledochocele and is a wide-mouth dilation of the common bile duct at its confluence with the duodenum. Type IV is cystic dilation of both the intra- and extrahepatic bile ducts. Type V consists of lakes of multiple intrahepatic cysts with no extrahepatic component and, when associated with hepatic fibrosis, is termed Caroli's disease. Type I and type IV are the most common lesions, with type I cysts accounting for 85% of these abnormalities. Caroli's disease appears to be a congenital syndrome and often follows an autosomal recessive pattern of inheritance in association with various other anomalies such as polycystic kidney disease and renal tubular ectasia.

If left untreated, a choledochal cyst may cause cholangitis and cholangiocarcinoma. The risk of cholangiocarcinoma in the first decade of life is only 0.7%; however, this increases to 14% at 20 years and is postulated to increase even further throughout life. It has been suggested that type III cysts, or choledochoceles, represent a form of duodenal duplication and therefore do not share the malignant potential of other bile duct cysts.

Clinical Findings

The clinical manifestations of a choledochal cyst are recurrent abdominal pain, episodic jaundice, and a right upper quadrant mass, though in most cases one of these features is missing. As children grow older, the cyst may become painful or infected. On rare occasions, children have been described with bile peritonitis secondary to perforation of a cyst. In adults, an abdominal mass is rarely appreciated, and patients present more commonly with symptoms of cholangitis or pancreatitis. Gallstones and cholangitis may develop due to biliary stasis.

The diagnosis is most often established by the clinical presentation and abnormal ultrasonography. Technetium Tc 99m-labeled IDA scan, CT and MRI scans, endoscopic retrograde cholangiopancreatography, and operative cholangiography may be necessary. Ultrasonography is increasingly responsible for detecting choledochal cysts in the fetus.

Treatment

In the past, the cysts were not removed but drained into a limb of intestine. However, many of these patients developed carcinoma in the cyst years later. Presently, the treatment is complete excision with Roux-en-Y hepaticojejunostomy. The duodenal end of the bile duct should be oversewn without injury to the anomalous entry of the pancreatic duct, limiting the amount of residual biliary tissue at risk for malignancy. Side-to-side choledochoduodenostomy is not recommended because it is followed by a high incidence of stricture of the anastomosis and recurrent cholangitis. Cholecystectomy is always performed. Biliary cirrhosis and portal hypertension, occurring from prolonged ductal obstruction, may be assessed with liver biopsy. The results of choledochal cyst excision with hepaticojejunostomy reconstruction are consistently excellent, but these children do require lifelong follow-up because of the risk of anastomotic stricture and intrahepatic stone formation.

Han S et al: Acquired choledochal cyst from anomalous pancreaticobiliary duct union. J Pediatr Surg 1997;32:1735.

Lipsett PA et al: Choledochal cyst disease: a changing pattern of presentation. Ann Surg 1994;220:644.

Miyano T, Yamataka A: Choledochal cysts. Curr Opin Pediatr 1997;9:283.

O'Neill J: Choledochal cyst. Curr Probl Surg 1992;29:365.

INGUINAL & SCROTAL DISORDERS

INGUINAL HERNIA & HYDROCELE

Inguinal hernia is a common condition in infancy and childhood, occurring in 1–3% of all children. Unlike hernias in adulthood, these nearly always result from a patent processus vaginalis (indirect hernia) and not from a weakness in the floor of the inguinal canal (direct hernia). The processus vaginalis follows the descent of the testis into the inguinal canal. Failure of obliteration of the processus may lead to a variety of anomalies, including hernia, communicating hydrocele, noncommunicating hydrocele, hydrocele of the spermatic cord, and hydrocele of the tunica vaginalis (Figure 45–20).

The processus vaginalis remains patent in over 80% of newborn infants. With increasing age, the incidence of patent processus vaginalis diminishes. At 2 years, 40–50% are open, and in adults 25% are persistently patent. Actual herniation of bowel into a widely patent processus vaginalis develops in 1–4% of children; 25% occur within the first year of life. Indirect inguinal hernia occurs four to six times more frequently in males. Direct and femoral hernias occur in children but are very rare.

Hernias are found on the right side in 60% of cases, on the left side in 30%, and bilaterally in 10%. Conditions associated with an increased risk of inguinal hernia include prematurity, family history, history of an abdominal wall defect (eg, gastroschisis), cryptorchidism, intersex anomalies, connective tissue disorders, and ascites. The processus vaginalis may be obliterated at any location proximal to the testis or labium.

Clinical Findings

The incidence of a clinically detectable inguinal hernia varies with gestational age: 9–11% in preterm infants and 3–5% for full-term infants. The diagnosis of hernia in infants and children can be made only by the demonstration of an inguinal bulge originating from the internal ring. The bulge can be elicited during times of Valsalva (crying, coughing, straining). Having an assistant hold the infant's arms over his or her head and legs straight will often elicit crying and straining that will aid in the physical examination. Indirect signs, such as a wide external ring and the "silk glove" sign (palpable thickening of the spermatic cord) are not dependable. One must always locate the position of the testis during examination for a hernia since an inguinal bulge due to an undescended or retractile testis may be mistaken for a hernia.

Incarcerated inguinal hernia accounts for approximately 10% of childhood hernias, and the incidence is highest in infants. In the majority of girls with incarcerated hernia, the sac contains the ovary and portion of the tube. These structures are usually a sliding component of the sac. In boys, small bowel, colon, or appendix can be within the sac.

A hydrocele is fluid within the remnant processus vaginalis. It is characteristically an oblong, nontender soft mass. It may be around the testicle only (testicular hydrocele), extend up from the testicle into the inguinal region (inguinoscrotal hydrocele), or be contained within a segment of the processus adjacent to the spermatic cord (hydrocele of the cord) or communicated with the peritoneal cavity (communicating hydrocele). With a noncommunicating hydrocele (the first three hydroceles described above), the processus vaginalis has closed proximally. The normal spermatic cord can usually be palpated above the level of the hydrocele. Transillumination is not reliable in the newborn since intestine and fluid transilluminate equally well. A communicating hydrocele is suspected by a history of size variation (smallest in the morning after sleep, largest during the day after the upright posture or repeated straining).

Differential Diagnosis

A hydrocele under tension may be confused with an incarcerated inguinal hernia. The sudden appearance of fluid confined to the testicular area may represent a noncommunicating hydrocele secondary to torsion of the testis or testicular appendage, epididymo-orchitis, pan-serositis from a recent viral syndrome, or idiopathic scrotal edema. Rectal examination and palpation of the peritoneal side of the inguinal ring may distinguish an incarcerated hernia from a hydrocele or other inguinoscrotal mass, but this is only reliable in the first 2–3 months of age as the internal ring is difficult to reach thereafter.

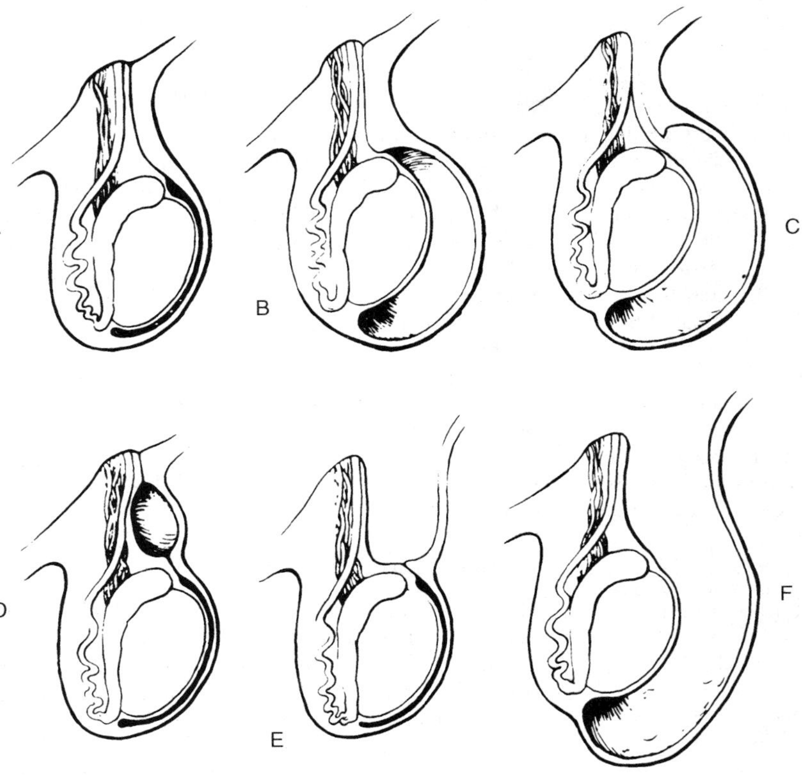

Figure 45–20. Spectrum of inguinoscrotal disorders. ***A:*** Normal anatomy. The processus vaginalis is obliterated and there is a small remnant, the tunica vaginalis, adjacent to the posterior surface of the testis. ***B:*** Scrotal hydrocele. ***C:*** Communicating hydrocele. Note the proximal patency of the processus vaginalis. ***D:*** Hydrocele of the spermatic cord. ***E:*** Inguinal hernia. ***F:*** Inguinoscrotal hernia. (From Sheldon CA: Inguinal and scrotal disorders. In: *Essentials of Pediatric Surgery.* Rowe MI et al [editors]. Mosby, 1995. Reproduced by permission from Elsevier.)

Complications

The principle risk of not treating an inguinal hernia is incarceration (viscus stuck in sac) and subsequent strangulation (ischemia of said viscus, usually the bowel, not the ovary). Compression of the spermatic vessels by an incarcerated hernia may produce hemorrhagic infarction of the ipsilateral testicle.

Treatment

In general, hydroceles that do not communicate with the peritoneal cavity are physiologic and the vast majority resolve by 18 months of age. Those that persist after 1 year or those that demonstrate changes in size (communicating hydroceles) should be repaired.

Inguinal hernia in infancy and childhood should be repaired; they never resolve spontaneously. In premature infants under constant surveillance in the hospital, hernia repair may be deferred until the baby is ready to be discharged. High ligation of the hernia sac by obliteration of the internal ring (leaving enough space for the spermatic cord) is all that is required. Historically, it was recommended that all boys under 2 years of age and all girls under 5 years undergo operative exploration of the contralateral inguinal canal in search of a clinically silent patent processus vaginalis. This approach has been replaced, in large part, by laparoscopic exploration. This is performed either through the ipsilateral hernia sac, through the umbilicus, or in-line with the internal ring (at the lateral border of the rectus muscle) using a needlescope. If a patent processus vaginalis is demonstrated, a second inguinal incision is made and the procedure is repeated as described above. Recently, a completely laparoscopic repair has been advocated, which has the advantage of simultaneous exploration of the contralateral side and virtually no manipulation of the spermatic cord. The incidence of complications from uncomplicated inguinal hernia repair (recurrence, wound infection, and damage to the spermatic cord) should be 2% or less.

An incarcerated hernia in an infant can usually be reduced initially before operation. This is accomplished by sedation and by elevation of the foot of the bed to keep intra-abdominal pressure from being exerted against the inguinal area. When the infant is well-sedated, the hernia may be reduced by gentle constant pressure over the internal ring in a manner that milks the bowel into the abdominal cavity. This is a two-handed maneuver in which one hand "squeezes" the incarcerated mass while the other directs it posteriorly into the internal ring. If the bowel is not reduced within an hour, operation is required. If the hernia is reduced, operative repair should be delayed for 48 hours to allow edema in the tissues to subside. An incarcerated ovary may not be able to be reduced but is usually asymptomatic, and repair at the next available operating room time is sufficient since torsion is rare and the blood supply, unlike that of the intestine, is not compromised by being trapped in the canal. Bloody stools and edema and red discoloration of the skin around the groin suggest a strangulated hernia, and reduction of the bowel should not be attempted. Emergency repair of incarcerated inguinal hernia is technically difficult because the edematous tissues are friable and tear readily. When gangrenous intestine is encountered, the bowel should be resected and an end-to-end intestinal anastomosis performed.

Fuenfer MM et al: Laparoscopic exploration of the contralateral groin in children: an improved technique. J Laparoendosc Surg 1996;1:S1.

Kapur P, Caty MG, Glick PL: Pediatric hernias and hydroceles. Pediatr Clin North Am 1998;45:773.

Yerkes EB et al: Laparoscopic evaluation for a contralateral patent processus vaginalis: part III. Urology 1998;51:480.

UNDESCENDED TESTIS (CRYPTORCHIDISM)

In the seventh month of gestation, the testicles normally descend into the scrotum. A fibromuscular band—the gubernaculum—extends from the lower pole of the testis to the scrotum, and this band probably acts by guiding the path for descent during differential growth of the fetus rather than by pulling the testes down. Undescended testis (cryptorchidism) is a form of dystopia of the testis that occurs when there is arrested descent and fixation of the position of the testis retroperitoneally, in the inguinal canal, or just beyond the external ring. Continued descent of the testes may progress after birth, but descent comes to a halt before 2 years of age.

Another form of dystopia is ectopic testis, in which the gubernaculum may have guided the testis near the pubis, penis, perineum, or medial thigh or to a subcutaneous position superficial to the inguinal canal. In these instances, the testis has descended beyond the external ring of the inguinal canal, and the vascular supply is sufficiently developed so as to pose little difficulty in operative repair.

Normal spermatogenesis requires the cooler temperature range provided in the scrotum. When the testis remains undescended and subjected to normal body temperature, degenerative changes in the seminiferous tubules occur in which the lining cells become progressively atrophic and hyalinized, with peritubular fibrosis. The degenerative changes begin to occur at 2 years of age. Unless the disorder is corrected, all bilaterally cryptorchid adult males become sterile.

The incidence of undescended or partially descended testis is 1–2% in full-term infants and up to 30% in premature babies. The right testis is affected in 45% of cases, the left testis in 30%, and both testes in 25%. A patent processus vaginalis is present in 95% of patients with cryptorchidism, and approximately 25% develop a clinical hernia.

Anomalies associated with cryptorchidism occur in about 15% of cases and include a wide variety of syndromes such as Klinefelter's syndrome, hypogonadotropic hypogonadism, the prune belly syndrome, horseshoe kidneys, renal agenesis or hypoplasia, exstrophy of the bladder, ureteral reflux, gastroschisis, and cloacal exstrophy.

Clinical Findings

Physical examination demonstrates an "empty hemiscrotum" with absent rugae. Cryptorchidism must be differentiated from a retractilie testis. Because of the very active cremaster of children under 3 years of age and the small size of the testis, the gonad can retract into the external inguinal ring or within the inguinal canal—this is called a retractile testis—and it is a variant of normal. The retractile testis can be manually manipulated into the mid to lower scrotum and no therapy is required.

Treatment

Operation is indicated after 12–18 months since degenerative changes begin to take place in these testes that may impair spermatogenesis and lead to malignant transformation. Additionally, cryptorchid testes are more susceptible to trauma and torsion, often have an associated inguinal hernia, and may cause adverse psychosocial effects. The incidence of testicular cancer in a cryptorchid testis is 30 times higher than in the normal population and is not lessened by repair. The role of repair is to allow reliable examination for a testicular mass later in life.

Orchidopexy is the surgical method for mobilizing the testis—based on the testicular vessels and the vas deferens—from its ectopic location into the scrotum. When the dystopic testis is not palpable preoperatively, 17% are absent, 33% are intra-abdominal, and 50% are in the inguinal canal or just beyond the inguinal ring. If the testis is not palpable when the child is anesthetized, laparoscopy should be performed before making an inguinal incision. Increasingly, the complete operation (diagnosis and intra-abdominal mobilization) is performed laparoscopically. This will allow for identification of an abdominal testis or the diagnosis of an absent testis (usually due to in utero torsion). Very high testes with a short blood supply can be brought into the scrotum by a two-stage repair (dividing the spermatic artery and vein with clips or laser followed by positioning in the scrotum 6–8 weeks later) based on collateral blood supply via the vas deferens and the gubernaculum. Testes confined in the inguinal canal (25% of cases) can usually be brought into the scrotum in one stage. Ectopic testicles located outside the inguinal canal, such as in the subcutaneous inguinal pouch, occur in over 50% of cases, and the testicular vessels are so well developed that scrotal placement is rarely a problem. The prognosis for fertility following orchidopexy in unilateral maldescent is 80%, whereas fertility after bilateral orchidopexy is about 50%. Due to variable degrees of tension and tenuous blood supply, the testis after an orchidopexy is often smaller than the contralateral one.

Docimo SG: The results of surgical therapy for cryptorchidism: a literature review and analysis. J Urol 1995;154:1148.

Humke U et al: Pediatric laparoscopy for nonpalpable testes with new miniaturized instruments. J Endourol 1998;12:445.

Mayr JM, Lawrenz K, Berghold A: Undescended testicles: an epidemiologic review. Acta Paediatr 1999;88:1089.

Pillai SB, Besner GE: Pediatric testicular problems. Pediatr Clin North Am 1998;45:813.

TESTICULAR TORSION

Testicular torsion is most frequent in late childhood and early adolescence, though the range can include the fetus and the adult. Anatomically, there are two forms of testicular torsion depending on where the spermatic cord is twisted with respect to the tunica vaginalis: intravaginal torsion (bell-clapper deformity), the most common form, and extravaginal torsion that occurs principally in neonates and in children with an undescended testis. Rarely, the testis may twist on a long epididymal mesentery. In children and adolescents, testicular torsion is either idiopathic or occurs after activity or trauma.

Clinical Findings

Acute scrotal or testicular pain that may radiate to the lower abdomen is usually present. Progressive swelling, edema, and erythema of the hemiscrotum occur. The testis is exquisitely tender to palpation. The testicle may be foreshortened, the epididymis may lie anteriorly, and the cremasteric reflex may be absent—though these signs are difficult to elicit. Fetal or neonatal torsion is probably responsible for the "absent" testis noted during laparoscopy.

The diagnosis of testicular torsion is based mainly on clinical examination. Although one may utilize Doppler ultrasonography and radionuclide scanning to aid in the diagnosis, these tests are time-consuming and, in the case of ultrasound, operator-specific.

Differential Diagnosis

Torsion of the testicular appendices (vestigial müllerian duct structures) and epididymitis may mimic testicular torsion. With epididymitis, there is often pyuria, voiding symptoms, and fever. Torsion of the testicular appendices often has a gradual onset, and careful palpation may reveal point tenderness rather than diffuse tenderness. There may be a visible necrotic lesion on scrotal transillumination (blue dot sign).

Treatment

If the diagnosis is strongly suspected, the best "test" is operative scrotal exploration. The testicular salvage rate if detorsion is performed within 6 hours after onset of symptoms is up to 97%, versus less than 10% if delayed more than 24 hours. At operation, the torsion is corrected and the gonad, if viable, is fixed to the hemiscrotum in three places. Because the paired testicle is at risk for torsion since the testicular anatomy tends to mirror itself, contralateral orchiopexy (suture fixation) should be performed in all cases. Torsion of the testicular appendices tends to be self-limiting since necrosis and autoamputation usually occur. Treatment is with warm baths, limited activity, and an anti-inflammatory agent. If significant pain persists after 2–3 days and the appendix has not autoamputated, excision is indicated. Testicular salvage after neonatal testicular torsion is very rare.

Kass EJ, Lundak BL: The acute scrotum. Pediatr Clin North Am 1997;44:1251.

ABDOMINAL WALL DEFECTS

UMBILICAL HERNIA

A fascial defect at the umbilicus is frequently present in the newborn, particularly in premature infants. The incidence is highest in African-American children. In most children, the umbilical ring progressively diminishes in size and eventually closes. Fascial defects less than 1 cm in diameter close spontaneously by 5 years of age in 95% of cases. When the fascial defect is greater than 1.5 cm in diameter, it seldom closes spontaneously. Unlike inguinal hernias, protrusion of bowel through the umbilical defect rarely results in incarceration in childhood. Surgical repair is indicated if the intestine becomes incarcerated, when the fascial defect is greater than 1.5 cm, and in all children over 4 years of age.

OMPHALOCELE

This is a midline abdominal wall defect noted in 1:5000 live births. The abdominal viscera (commonly liver and bowel) are contained within a sac composed of peritoneum and amnion from which the umbilical cord arises at the apex and center (Figure 45–21). When the defect is less than 4 cm, it is termed a hernia of the umbilical cord; when greater than 10 cm, it is termed a giant omphalocele. Associated abnormalities occur in 30–70% of infants and include, in descending order of frequency, chromosomal abnormalities (trisomy 13, 18, 21), congenital heart disease (tetralogy of Fallot, atrial septal defect), Beckwith-Wiedemann syndrome (large-for-gestational-age baby; hyperinsulinism; visceromegaly of kidneys, adrenal glands, and pancreas; macroglossia, hepatorenal tumors, cloacal extrophy), pentalogy of Cantrell, and prune belly syndrome (absent abdominal wall muscles, genitourinary abnormalities, cryptorchidism). Small omphaloceles are most often linked to chromosomal defects and Beckwith-Wiedemann syndrome, especially when the liver is not in the hernia sac.

Treatment

The primary goal of surgery is to return the viscera to the abdominal cavity and close the defect. With an intact sac, emergency operation is not necessary, so a thorough physical examination and workup for associated anomalies is performed. An orogastric tube should be placed on suction to minimize intestinal distention.

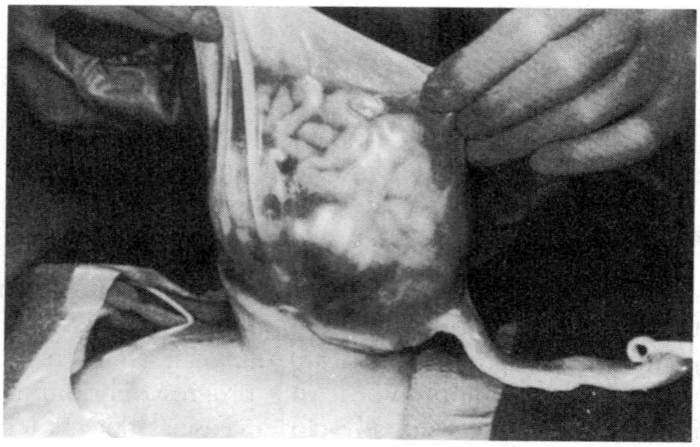

Figure 45–21. Neonate with omphalocele. The liver and bowel herniated through a midline abdominal wall defect and are surrounded by a sac of amnion and chorion from which the umbilical cord emanates. (Reproduced, with permission, from Albanese CT: Pediatric surgery. In: *Surgery,* Norton JA [editor]. Springer, 2000.)

The success of primary closure depends on the size of the defect and of the abdominal and thoracic cavities as well as the presence of associated problems (eg, lung disease). It is wise to leave the sac in situ since primary closure may not be possible, and in this way one has maintained the best biologic dressing for the viscera. Supplemental coverage with plastic wrap or a bowel bag can be used to prevent heat loss. If the viscera reduce but abdominal wall closure is not possible, there are two options: staged repair and prosthetic patch repair. A staged repair aims to create a protective extra-abdominal extension of the peritoneal cavity (termed a silo), allowing gradual reduction of the viscera and gradual abdominal wall expansion using two parallel sheets of reinforced Silastic sheeting sutured to the fascial edges or a preformed one-piece silo with a collapsible ring at its base for ease of insertion. A prosthetic patch repair bridges the fascial gap with a synthetic material (eg, polytetrafluoroethylene) and the skin is closed over the patch. The silo is progressively compressed to invert the amniotic sac and its contents into the abdomen and to bring the edges of the linea alba together by stretching the abdominal wall muscles. This usually requires 5–7 days, after which the defect is then primarily closed. The intra-abdominal pressure produced by the silo should not exceed 20 cm H_2O to avoid impairing venous return from the bowel and kidneys. When abdominal relaxation is sufficient to allow the rectus muscles to come together, the silo is removed, the amnion is left inverted into the abdominal cavity, and the defect is closed.

In rare cases, nonoperative management is advised for infants with severe associated anomalies or a giant omphalocele. The amnion is allowed to dry and form an eschar. The membrane becomes vascularized beneath the eschar, and contraction of the wound with skin growth covers the defect. A ventral hernia results, which is repaired electively when the patient is stable. The survival rate for infants with small omphaloceles is excellent. Deaths associated with larger omphaloceles are principally from wound dehiscence with subsequent and ensuing infection or and from associated anomalies.

GASTROSCHISIS

Gastroschisis is a defect in the abdominal wall that usually occurs to the right of a normal insertion of the umbilical cord (Figure 45–22). It is believed to arise at the site of involution of the right umbilical vein, though a less popular theory holds there is some evidence that it results from rupture of an omphalocele sac in utero. It is twice as common as omphalocele and the defect is usually smaller. The remnants of the amnion are usually reabsorbed. The skin may continue to grow over the remnants of the amnion, and there may be a bridge of skin between the defect and the cord. The

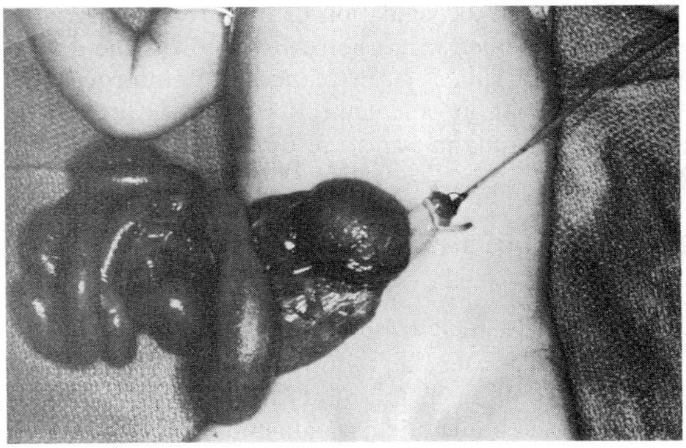

Figure 45–22. Neonate with a gastroschisis. The defect is to the right of the umbilical cord, and the bowel has no investing sac. Note edema of the bowel wall and the dilated stomach adjacent to the umbilical cord. (Reproduced, with permission, from Albanese CT: Pediatric surgery. In: *Surgery.* Norton JA [editor]. Springer, 2000.

small and large bowel, stomach, and often the fallopian tube/ovary/testis herniate through the abdominal wall defect. Unlike an omphalocele, the liver is virtually never present in the defect. Having been bathed in the amniotic fluid and with compression of the mesenteric blood supply at the abdominal defect, the bowel wall is edematous and has a very thick, shaggy membrane ("peel") covering it. The loops of intestine are usually matted together, and the intestine appears to be abnormally short.

Complications

Since the bowel has not been contained intra-abdominally, the abdominal cavity fails to enlarge, and it frequently cannot accommodate the protuberant bowel. Over 70% of infants with this disorder are premature, but associated anomalies occur in fewer than 10% of cases. Nonrotation of the midgut is present. Associated intestinal atresia occurs in approximately 7% because segments of intestine that have herniated through the defect become infarcted in utero.

Treatment & Prognosis

Unlike omphalocele, urgent repair is necessary. Small defects may be closed primarily after manually stretching the abdominal cavity. A staged approach is frequently required using a silo as described above (under Omphalocele). As bowel wall edema subsides, the bowel will readily reduce into the abdominal cavity. Reduction is aided by having the infant paralyzed and receiving endotracheal ventilation to relax the abdominal wall and allow it to stretch and accommodate the bowel. When the bowel has been completely reduced (usually 5–7 days), the silo is removed and the abdominal wall is closed.

The death rate for infants with gastroschisis is less than 5%. Poor gastrointestinal function and episodes of sepsis, presumably from compromised bowel, may occur. Prolonged postoperative ileus (more than 2 weeks) is the rule, and total parenteral nutrition is necessary. Primary repair of an associated intestinal atresia is rarely safe and possible. Either a proximal stoma is created or the atretic ends are reduced and repaired 6 weeks later when the intra-abdominal inflammation has subsided.

Langer JC: Gastroschisis and omphalocele. Semin Pediatr Surg 1996;5:124.

Lunzer H, Menardi G, Brezinka C: Long-term follow-up of children with prenatally diagnosed omphalocele and gastroschisis. J Matern Fetal Med 2001;10:385.

Molik KA et al: Gastroschisis: a plea for risk categorization. J Pediatr Surg 2001;36:51.

CUTANEOUS VASCULAR ANOMALIES

Cutaneous vascular anomalies comprise a group of congenital and acquired vascular malformations of the skin. They are present in 2.6% of all newborns. These anomalies are broadly divided into two categories: hemangiomas and vascular malformations. They are most precisely classified by the biologic activity of the endothelium.

HEMANGIOMAS

Hemangiomas demonstrate endothelial hyperplasia and are seen in children and adults but behave differently at different ages. Hemangiomas are much more common than vascular malformations. In the neonatal period, hemangiomas can be subclassified according to their growth phase. A rapid proliferating phase is usually seen during the first few years of life followed by an involuting phase that may last several years.

Clinical Findings

The clinical appearance depends on the depth of the lesion. Superficial dermal lesions (capillary hemangiomas, strawberry hemangiomas) are raised and profoundly erythematous, with an irregular texture; deep lesions (cavernous hemangiomas) are smooth and slightly raised, with a bluish hue or a faint telangiectatic pattern on the overlying skin. Mixed lesions are often noted (capillary-cavernous hemangiomas). Twenty percent of patients have multiple lesions. Complications from hemangiomas consist of ulceration (during the proliferative phase), bleeding, thrombocytopenia (Kasabach-Merritt syndrome), consumptive coagulopathy, high-output heart failure, visual field encroachment, airway obstruction, and minor skeletal distortions.

Treatment

Fifty percent of hemangiomas will involute without treatment by age 5 years and 70% by 7 years. The remainder will slowly resolve by age 10–12 years. Steroid therapy hastens the rate of proliferation of hemangiomas by 30–90% and is indicated for complicated lesions (ie, those causing severe physiologic or anatomic abnormalities).

CUTANEOUS VASCULAR MALFORMATIONS

Vascular malformations, in contrast to hemangiomas, have normal endothelial cell turnover and tend to grow proportionally with the child. These lesions are structural anomalies that are considered errors in vascular morphogenesis. They are usually visible at birth but may take years or even decades to become manifest. They are separated into low-flow and high-flow variants and further classified according to the type of vascular channel abnormality: capillary, venous, arterial, and mixed malformations. Capillary and venous malformations are low-flow variants; arterial and mixed arterial and venous ones are high-flow variants.

Capillary Malformations

Capillary malformations are nevus flammeus (port wine stain), nevus flammeus neonatorum (angel's kiss), nevus flammeus nuchae (stork bite, salmon patch), angiokeratomas, and telangiectasias [spider, hereditary hemorrhagic telangiectasia (Rendu-Osler-Weber syndrome)]. They are prone to infection and are treated aggressively with intravenous antibiotics. A compression garment should be used if anatomically feasible. Some lesions can be excised or injected with a sclerosing solution.

Venous Malformations

Venous malformations have a wide spectrum of appearances ranging from simple varicosities to complex lesions that may be located in deeper tissues (eg, bone, muscle, salivary gland). Pain is often related to thrombosis within the lesion. Radiographic imaging delineates the nature and extent of the lesion (angiogram, CT, MRI). Photocoagulation or Nd:YAG laser may be effective for superficial lesions. Resection is the definitive treatment since it can reduce bulk, improve contour and function, and control pain. It is limited by anatomic boundaries, and multiple, staged procedures may be required.

Arterial Malformations

Arterial and arteriovenous malformations are associated with multiple small fistulas surrounded by abnormal tissues and can cause high-output cardiac failure. They are most common in the head and neck region (especially intracerebral). There is pain and overlying cutaneous necrosis. Adjacent osseous structures are often destroyed. Selective embolization is used either as palliation or presurgically to limit hemorrhage. Excision, when possible, is the treatment of choice.

Combined Malformations

Combined vascular malformations and hypertrophy syndromes consist of Klippel-Trenaunay-Weber syndrome (combined capillary-lymphatic venous malformation associated with lower limb hypertrophy), Parkes-Weber syndrome (upper limb arteriovenous shunting), Maffucci's syndrome (low-flow vascular malformations and multiple extremity enchondromas with hypoplastic long bones), and Sturge-Weber syndrome (upper facial port wine stain and vascular anomalies of the choroid plexus and leptomeninges).

Low DW: Hemangiomas and vascular malformations. Semin Pediatr Surg 1994;3:40.

Mulliken JB, Fishman SJ, Burrows PE: Vascular anomalies. Curr Probl Surg 2000;37:517.

TUMORS IN CHILDHOOD

NEUROBLASTOMA

Of all childhood neoplasms, neuroblastoma is exceeded in frequency only by leukemia and brain tumors. Approximately 60% of cases occur within the first 2 years of life and 97% within the first 20 years. This tumor is of neural crest origin and may originate anywhere along the distribution of the sympathetic chain. The most common site for primary disease is in the abdomen (adrenal), followed by the thorax, pelvis, and occasionally the head and neck. Neuroblastomas originate in the retroperitoneal area in 75% of cases; 55% arise from the adrenal gland. They may reach massive size and violate tissue planes such that they envelop major blood vessels, their branches, and other important structures (eg, ureters), making initial primary resection potentially hazardous. The biologic behavior varies with the age of the patient, the site of primary origin, and the extent of the disease.

Clinical Findings

A. Symptoms and Signs

Symptoms are site-specific. The most common symptom is pain (from primary or metastatic disease). Nonspecific symptoms include growth retardation, malaise, fever, weight loss, and anorexia. Children frequently appear ill at the time of diagnosis. Constipation and urinary retention are signs of pelvic disease. Orbital metastases commonly present with periorbital ecchymoses and proptosis ("raccoon eyes"). Spinal canal involvement may present with acute paralysis due to compression. Opsomyoclonus syndrome is an acute cerebellar encephalopathy characterized by ataxia, opsoclonus ("dancing eyes"), myoclonus, and dementia. It occurs in association with approximately 3% of all neuroblastomas and is usually associated with a good prognosis, though the neurologic abnormalities tend to persist after successful treatment of the primary tumor. Interestingly, it is not due to CNS metastases of neuroblastoma and is believed to be immune-mediated. Infants with stage IV-S disease (see below) may display cutaneous metastases ("blueberry muffin" lesions) or respiratory embarrassment secondary to massive hepatomegaly from tumor infiltration. Palpable lesions are often hard and fixed.

In infants, metastases confined to the liver or subcutaneous fat are frequent and cortical bone metastases unusual. In older children, metastases to lymph nodes and bone are found in over 70% of cases at diagnosis. Pain in areas of bony involvement and in joints with associated myalgia and fever mimics rheumatic fever. Eighty-five to 90 percent secrete high levels of the catecholamine metabolites vanillylmandelic acid and homovanillic acid. Hypertension and diarrhea may occur as a result of catecholamine and vasoactive intestinal peptide secretion.

B. Imaging Studies

Imaging is aimed at defining the extent of the tumor and determining the presence of metastases to distant sites (most commonly lymph nodes, bone, lung, and liver). Neuroblastoma is the most common abdominal tumor to demonstrate calcifications (50%) prior to chemotherapy. CT scan of the area of tumor involvement helps to identify the relationship to surrounding structures and determine resectability. MRI is useful in assessing tumor within the spinal canal and spinal cord compression. MRI is as sensitive as CT scanning in terms of assessing tumor size and resectability but has the added advantage of being superior to CT in assessing vessel encasement, vessel patency, and spinal cord compression. MRI can also demonstrate bone marrow involvement in selected cases. Metaiodobenzylguanidine (MIBG) scintigraphy is very sensitive in detecting tumors that concentrate catecholamines and has been useful in the diagnosis of primary, residual, and metastatic disease in patients with neuroblastoma. For retroperitoneal tumors, an intravenous urogram may show displacement or compression of the adjacent kidney without distortion of the renal calices. Bone scans may be useful in detecting osseous metastases.

Prognostic Factors

Favorable prognostic factors include diagnosis before age 1, a thoracic primary lesion, and low stage. In addition, several molecular and cellular characteristics of neuroblastic tumors are prognostically important. The most important is the high incidence of amplification of the proto-oncogene N-*myc,* seen in approximately 30% of tumors. Amplification of N-*myc* (more than 10 copies) adversely correlates with prognosis independently of clinical stage. Using the histologic Shimada index, well-differentiated, stroma-rich tumors have a favorable prognosis. An elevated ratio of vanillylmandelic acid to homovanillic acid correlates with an improved outcome in patients with advanced disease. Other biochemical indicators of advanced disease include neuron-specific enolase, serum ferritin, and serum lactate dehydrogenase. Staging systems are surgically and anatomically based and have prognostic value. The most recent is the International Neuroblastoma Staging System (Table 45–6).

Table 45–6. Staging of neuroblastoma.

	Survival
I. Tumor confined to site of origin	100%
IIa. Unilateral tumor completely excised. Nodes negative.	80%
IIb. Unilateral tumor, complete or incomplete excision. Nodes positive.	70%
III. Tumor infiltrating across the midline, or a unilateral tumor with contralateral nodes positive.	40%
IV. Remote disease in bone, soft tissue, distant nodes.	15%
IVs. Infants with stage I or stage II primary and remote spread to liver, skin, or bone marrow. ("Special" case.)	85%

Treatment

Diagnosis depends upon demonstration of immature neuroblastic tissue obtained by tissue or bone marrow aspirate and biopsy. Tissue is obtained by biopsy (either by laparotomy or laparoscopically), which allows accurate determination of resectability and ensures that adequate tissue (1 g or 1 cm^3) is available for determination of tumor markers, cytologic studies, and the special stains required for accurate diagnosis and staging.

A localized neuroblastoma should be excised, and the local area of the tumor should be irradiated only when gross tumor remains. Unresectable neuroblastomas should be biopsied and treated initially by chemotherapy and radiation therapy and then by surgical resection for residual tumor. Removal of all residual disease is the goal, and a more radical approach is warranted. Most neuroblastomas are radiosensitive and respond to 3000 cGy or less of radiation. Patients with disseminated disease should be treated with a combination of chemotherapeutic agents such as cyclophosphamide, vincristine, dacarbazine, doxorubicin, cisplatin, and teniposide. Patients with stage III or stage IV tumors who are at high risk by virtue of their age or of the stage and biologic characteristics of the tumor benefit from total body irradiation followed by either allogeneic or, more commonly, purged autologous bone marrow transplantation.

Chamberlain RS et al: Complete surgical resection combined with aggressive adjuvant chemotherapy and bone marrow transplantation prolongs survival in children with advanced neuroblastoma. Ann Surg Oncol 1995;2:93.

Grosfeld JL: Risk-based management: current concepts of treating malignant solid tumors of childhood. J Am Coll Surg 1999;189:407.

Matthay KK: Neuroblastoma: a clinical challenge and biologic puzzle. CA Cancer J Clin 1995;45:179.

Shimada H et al: International neuroblastoma pathology classification for prognostic evaluation of patients with peripheral neuroblastic tumors: a report from the Children's Cancer Group. Cancer 2001;92:2451.

WILMS' TUMOR (NEPHROBLASTOMA)

Renal neoplasms account for about 10% of malignant tumors in children. Nephroblastoma (Wilms' tumor), which accounts for 80% of these, consists of a variety of embryonic tissues such as abortive tubules and glomeruli, smooth and skeletal muscle fibers, spindle cells, cartilage, and bone. Seventy-five percent of children with nephroblastoma are under 5 years of age; the peak incidence is at 2–3 years. With current multimodality treatment, the survival rate exceeds 85%.

The left kidney is affected in 50% of cases of Wilms' tumor and the right kidney in 45%. In 5% of cases, the tumors are bilateral; 60% are synchronous and 40% are metachronous. Associated anomalies and their incidence per 1000 cases are aniridia, 8.5; hypospadias, 18; hemihypertrophy, 25; and cryptorchidism, 28. Beckwith-Wiedemann syndrome and neurofibromatosis occur together occasionally, and renal tumors may also occur in families. The constellation of Wilms' tumor, aniridia, genitourinary anomalies, and mental retardation (WAGR syndrome) is associated with deletion of 11p13.

Clinical Findings

A. Symptoms and Signs

In contrast to those with neuroblastoma, children are usually healthy-appearing. Symptoms consist of abdominal enlargement in 60%; pain in 20%; hematuria in 15%; malaise, weakness, anorexia, and weight loss in 10%; and fever in 3%. Hypertension is noted in over half of patients. An abdominal mass, palpable in almost all cases, is usually very large, firm, and smooth, and it does not ordinarily extend across the midline.

B. Imaging Studies

Imaging is required to determine the extent of the mass; to assess for bilateral disease, venous invasion, and metastases; and to confirm contralateral renal function. This is accomplished with abdominal ultrasound (to assess venous invasion) and a CT scan of the chest and abdomen.

Differential Diagnosis

Abdominal masses may also be caused by hydronephrotic, multicystic, or duplicated kidneys and by neuroblastoma, teratoma, hepatoma, and rhabdomyosarcoma. Ultrasonography and CT scanning can usually distinguish nephroblastoma from these other tumors. Calcification occurs in 10% of cases of nephroblastoma and tends to be more crescent-shaped, discrete, and peripherally situated than the calcifications of neuroblastoma, which are finely stippled.

Treatment & Prognosis

Surgical excision is often accomplished without any preoperative treatment unless significant inferior vena caval thrombus is present. The aim of surgery is to completely remove the tumor (nephrectomy) and ureter without spill and to determine the tumor stage by virtue of its extent and the presence of lymph node involvement (Table 45–7). Stage I is tumor confined to a kidney that has been completely excised; stage II is tumor extending beyond the kidney (perirenal tissues, renal vein or vena cava, biopsy or local spill in the flank) and completely excised; stage III is residual, nonhematogenous tumor confined to the abdomen (lymph

Table 45–7. Wilms' tumor staging system.

Stage I: Tumor limited to kidney and completely excised. The surface of the renal capsule is intact and the tumor was not ruptured prior to removal. There is no residual tumor.

Stage II: Tumor extends through the perirenal capsule but is completely excised. There may be local spillage of tumor confined to the flank, or the tumor may have been biopsied. Extrarenal vessels may contain tumor thrombus or be infiltrated by tumor.

Stage III: Residual nonhematogenous tumor confined to the abdomen: lymph node involvement, diffuse peritoneal spillage, peritoneal implants, tumor beyond surgical margin either grossly or microscopically, or tumor not completely removed.

Stage IV: Hematogenous metastases to lung, liver, bone, brain, etc.

Stage V: Bilateral renal involvement at diagnosis; each kidney should be staged separately.

node metastases, preoperative or intraoperative diffuse peritoneal deposits, residual tumor at the surgical margins, or unresectable tumor); stage IV is hematogenous metastases (lung, liver, bone, and brain); and stage V is bilateral renal involvement.

Irradiation of the tumor bed is indicated if the tumor has extended beyond the capsule of the kidney to involve adjacent organs or lymph nodes or if intraoperative tumor spillage has occurred. Very large tumors may be treated with radiation therapy and chemotherapy preoperatively to reduce their size. A significant reduction in size usually occurs in 7–10 days, after which nephrectomy can be readily performed. Nephrectomy is accomplished through a long transverse or thoracoabdominal incision.

Palpation of the renal veins and inferior vena cava is performed to detect tumor thrombus. The contralateral kidney must be examined and palpated. Bilateral disease (6%) mandates "nephron-sparing" surgery. The treatment of bilateral disease is individualized with the goal of eradicating tumor while preserving the maximal amount of functional renal mass. It is a contraindication to primary nephrectomy. Suspicious lesions in the opposite kidney are biopsied. If the tumor is too large for safe resection, it is biopsied along with regional lymph nodes. Chemotherapy with or without radiation therapy will usually result in a significant reduction in tumor size and allow subsequent resection. Metastatic foci in the lung or liver may be resected or treated with radiation therapy. Any residual tumor following radiation therapy, including multiple lesions, should be resected.

Overall survival is 85%, and most patients are cured. Survival correlates with stage and histology. The 4-year survival with respect to stage and histology is shown in Table 45–8. Tumor rupture with gross spillage portends a sixfold increase in risk of local recurrence and requires the use of postoperative external beam radiation.

Capra ML et al: Wilms' tumor: a 25-year review of the role of preoperative chemotherapy. J Pediatr Surg 1999;34:579.

Green DM et al: Wilms tumor. CA Cancer J Clin 1996;46:46.

Haase GM, Ritchey ML: Nephroblastoma. Semin Pediatr Surg 1997;6:11.

RHABDOMYOSCARCOMA

Rhabdomyosarcoma is a childhood malignancy that arises from embryonic mesenchyme with the potential to differentiate into skeletal muscle. It is the most common pediatric soft tissue sarcoma and is the third most common solid malignancy. It accounts for 4–8% of all malignancies and 5–15% of all solid malignancies of childhood.

The age distribution is bimodal, the first peak is between 2 years and 5 years, and the second peak is between 15 years and 19 years. Fifty percent present before 5 years, and 6% present in infancy. There is an increased incidence in patients with neurofibromatosis, Beckwith-Wiedemann syndrome, and Li-Fraumeni cancer-family syndrome.

Rhabdomyosarcoma is divided into distinct histologic groups: favorable, intermediate, and unfavorable. Favorable types (5%) include the sarcoma botryoides and spindle cell variants. Botryoid tumors typically present in young children from within visceral cavities (eg, vagina), while spindle cell types have a predilection for paratesticular sites. Intermediate-prognosis tumors (50%) are of the embryonal type. Unfavorable-prognosis tumors (20%) include alveolar and undifferentiated tumors. Alveolar tumors arise from the extremities, trunk, and perineum. Undifferentiated tumors arise from the extremity and head and neck sites. Thirteen percent cannot be adequately characterized and are labeled "small, round cell sarcoma, type indeterminate."

Clinical Findings

The clinical presentation varies with the site of origin of the primary tumor, the patient's age, and the presence or

Table 45–8. Four-year survival for Wilms' tumor.

Stage I/FH:	98%
Stage I–III/UH:	68%
Stage II/FH:	90–95%
Stage III/FH:	85–90%
Stage IV/FH:	78–86%
Stage IV/UH:	52–58%

FH: Favorable histology
UH: Unfavorable histology

absence of metastatic disease. The majority of symptoms are secondary to the effects of compression by the tumor or by the presence of a mass. The most common site is the head and neck region (35%). These are subdivided into orbital (10%), parameningeal (15%), and nonparameningeal (10%) sites. They are usually embryonal and present as asymptomatic masses or functional deficits. Genitourinary rhabdomyosarcoma (26%) are divided into two groups: bladder and prostate (10%) and non-bladder and prostate, including paratesticular sites, perineum, vulva, vagina, and uterus (16%). The most common histologic type is embryonal, though botryoid tumors and spindle cell tumors are seen more frequently here than in any other site. These tumors may be so massive as to make determination of the primary tumor site impossible. There is a propensity for early lymphatic spread in genitourinary primary tumors. Bladder and prostate tumors frequently present with urinary retention or hematuria, while vaginal and uterine tumors present with vaginal bleeding or discharge or with a mass exiting the vagina. Extremity rhabdomyosarcoma (1%) are more common in the lower than in the upper extremity. These are usually alveolar varieties with a high incidence of regional nodal involvement and distal metastases. "Other" sites account for 20%. The most common are the thorax, diaphragm, abdominal and pelvic walls, and intra-abdominal or intrapelvic organs.

Staging is determined by the histologic variant, the primary site, and the extent of disease since each has an important influence on the choice of treatment and on prognosis. CT scanning or MRI is essential to evaluate the primary tumor and its relationship to surrounding structures. A clinical grouping system was designed by the Intergroup Rhabdomyosarcoma Study Group to stratify different extents of disease in order to compare treatment and outcome results (Table 45–9). It is based on pretreatment and operative outcome and does not account for the biologic differences or the natural history of tumors arising from different primary sites.

Table 45–9. Intergroup Rhabdomyosarcoma Study Clinical Group staging system.[1]

Group I: Localized disease, completely removed
- a. Confined to muscle or organ of origin
- b. Infiltration outside organ or muscle of origin; regional nodes not involved.

Group II: Total gross resection with evidence of regional spread
- a. Grossly resected tumor with microscopic residual
- b. Regional disease with involved nodes, completely resected with no microscopic residual
- c. Regional disease with involved nodes, grossly resected, but with evidence of microscopic residual and/or histologic involvement of the most distal regional node in the dissection

Group III: Incomplete resection, or biopsy with presence of gross disease

Group IV: Distant metastases

[1]Reproduced, with permission, from Neville HL et al: Preoperative staging, prognostic factors, and outcome for extremity rhabdomyosarcoma: a preliminary report from the Intergroup Rhabdomyosarcoma Study IV (1991–1997). J Pediatr Surg 2000;35:317.

Treatment & Prognosis

The surgical management is site-specific and includes complete wide excision of the primary tumor and surrounding uninvolved tissue while preserving cosmetic appearance and function. Incomplete excision (beyond biopsy) or tumor debulking is not beneficial, and severely mutilating or debilitating procedures should not be performed. Tumors not amenable to primary excision should be amply biopsied and then treated with neoadjuvant agents; secondary excision is then performed and is associated with a better outcome than partial or incomplete excisions. Clinically suspicious lymph nodes should be excised or biopsied, while excision of clinically uninvolved nodes is site-specific. Primary reexcision has been shown to improve outcome in patients where microscopic margins are positive, where the initial procedure was not a formal "cancer" resection, or where malignancy was not suspected preoperatively.

The 5-year survival for stage I tumors is 90%; for stage II, clinical group I or II, it is 77%; for stage II, clinical group III, it is 65%; and for stage III lesions (group I, II, or III), it is 55%. Stage IV tumors arising from favorable sites of origin are curable, while those from unfavorable sites have a very poor prognosis. The prognosis for recurrent disease is poor.

Andrassy RJ: Rhabdomyosarcoma. Semin Pediatr Surg 1997;6:17.

Neville HL et al: Preoperative staging, prognostic factors, and outcome for extremity rhabdomyosarcoma: a preliminary report from the Intergroup Rhabdomyosarcoma Study IV (1991–1997). J Pediatr Surg 2000;35:317.

Wiener ES: Rhabdomyosarcoma: new dimensions in management. Semin Pediatr Surg 1993;2:47.

TERATOMA

Teratomas are embryonal neoplasms derived from pluripotent cells containing tissue from at least two of three germ layers (ectoderm, endoderm, mesoderm). Approximately 80% are found in females. They are typically midline or para-axial tumors and are distributed in the following regions: sacrococcygeal (57%), gonadal (29%), mediastinal (7%), retroperitoneal (4%), cervical (3%), and intracranial (3%). Other sites are rare. Nongonadal teratomas present in infancy; gonadal ones, in adolescence. Twenty-one percent are malignant.

The serum alpha-fetoprotein (AFP) level is elevated in tumors containing malignant endodermal sinus (yolk sac) elements. Serial AFP levels are markers for recurrence. Beta-human chorionic gonadotropin (β-hCG) is produced from those containing malignant choriocarcinoma tissue. Rarely, enough β-hCG is produced to cause precocious puberty. Elevated AFP and β-hCG levels in histologically benign tumors indicate an increased risk of recurrence and malignant transformation, particularly with "immature" benign teratomas.

Sacrococcygeal Teratoma

The majority of sacrococcygeal teratomas present in the newborn period and can be detected by prenatal ultrasound. Females predominate; a history of twins is common. Pregnancy may be complicated by fetal high-output cardiac failure via arteriovenous shunting within the tumor, maternal polyhydramnios, and hydrops fetalis leading to fetal demise. Fetal surgery has been utilized successfully in those with hydrops. The tumors are classified according to location: Type I, predominantly external (46%); Type II, external mass and presacral component (35%); Type III, visible externally, but predominantly presacral (9%); and Type IV, entirely presacral, not visible externally (10%).

Treatment is excision of the tumor and coccyx; Type I and II lesions are resected from the perineal approach, and Type III and IV lesions require a combined intra-abdominal and perineal resection. The majority (97%) of newborn sacrococcygeal teratomas are benign and do not require adjuvant therapy. Follow-up requires serial AFP levels and physical examinations, including digital rectal examination. Recurrent tumors are excised. The greatest risk factor for malignancy is age at diagnosis. The malignancy rate is approximately 50–60% after 2 months of age. Malignant tumors are often treated with surgery and chemotherapy. The 5-year survival for malignant germ cell tumors arising from a sacrococcygeal teratoma is approximately 50%.

Mediastinal Teratoma

Mediastinal teratomas account for approximately 20% of all pediatric mediastinal tumors. They usually arise in the anterior mediastinum, though intrapericardial and cardiac lesions have been reported. Symptoms include respiratory distress, chronic cough, chest pain, and wheezing. Males with β-hCG-producing tumors may display precocious puberty. Cardiac failure may develop from compression or pericardial effusion. The chest radiograph demonstrates a calcified anterior mediastinal mass in over one-third of cases. Ultrasonography delineates cystic and solid components. General anesthesia should not be induced until a CT scan evaluation of the airway has been obtained since the supine position coupled with a loss of airway tone from anesthetic agents may allow the anterior mass to obstruct the distal trachea, making rapid establishment of an airway all but impossible. If significant airway compression is present, an awake needle biopsy under local anesthesia followed by radiation therapy or chemotherapy is indicated. Complete resection is definitive treatment.

Cervical Teratoma

Cervical teratomas are rare neonatal neck masses that by virtue of their large size frequently cause respiratory distress. Calcifications may be seen on a plain radiograph and a mixed cystic and solid appearance on ultrasound. These tumors are most commonly benign. The most common malignant type is the yolk sac tumor (endodermal sinus tumor). Serum AFP and β-hCG levels can be monitored to detect the presence of recurrent germ cell tumors. The rapid establishment of an endotracheal airway may be necessary. Tracheostomy is hazardous because of the distortion of landmarks by the large mass. Treatment is complete excision. Some malignant tumors respond to radiation therapy. Regardless of the stage of disease, these tumors behave aggressively and should be treated adjunctively with a combination of cisplatin, vinblastine, and bleomycin or with dactinomycin, cyclophosphamide, and vincristine.

Altman RP, Randolph JG, Lilly JR: Sacrococcygeal teratoma: American Academy of Pediatrics Surgical Section Survey-1973. J Pediatr Surg 1974;9:389.

Kerner B et al: Cervical teratoma: prenatal diagnosis and long-term follow-up. Prenat Diagn 1998;18:51.

Rescorla FJ et al: Long-term outcome for infants and children with sacrococcygeal teratoma: a report from the Children's Cancer Group. J Pediatr Surg 1998;33:171.

Tapper D, Lack EE: Teratomas in infancy and childhood: a 54-year experience at the Children's Hospital Medical Center. Ann Surg 1983;198:398.

LIVER NEOPLASMS

Tumors of the liver are uncommon in childhood (2% of all pediatric malignancies). More than 70% of pediatric liver masses are malignant. The majority of hepatic malignancies are of epithelial origin, while most benign lesions are vascular in nature.

1. Hepatoblastoma

Hepatoblastomas account for nearly 50% of all liver masses in children and approximately two-thirds of malignant tumors. The majority are seen in children under 4 years of age, and two-thirds are noted prior to 2 years of age. Beckwith-Wiedemann syndrome, hemihypertrophy, fetal alcohol syndrome, and parenteral nutrition administration in infancy all increase the risk of hepatoblastoma.

Clinical Findings

A. Symptoms and Signs

The most common finding is an asymptomatic abdominal mass or diffuse abdominal swelling in a healthy-appearing child. There may be obstructive gastrointestinal symptoms secondary to compression of the stomach or duodenum or acute pain secondary to hemorrhage into the tumor. Physical examination reveals a nontender, firm mass in the right upper quadrant or midline that moves with respiration. Advanced tumors present with weight loss, ascites, and failure to thrive. Approximately 10% of males present with isosexual precocity secondary to tumor secretion of β-hCG.

B. Laboratory Findings

Laboratory studies reveal nonspecifically elevated liver function tests and a mild anemia. Thrombocytosis of unknown cause is occasionally seen. AFP is significantly elevated in 90–95%. This marker is also associated with other malignant lesions such as germ cell tumors, but levels are lower. Serial serum AFP measurements are used to monitor patients for tumor recurrence. Levels fall to normal after curative resection.

C. Imaging Studies

Abdominal ultrasound demonstrates a solid, usually unilobar (right lobe most common) lesion of the liver but lacks sufficient detail to determine resectability. Abdominal CT scan using intravenous contrast is currently the imaging procedure of choice both for diagnosis and for planning therapy. The CT scan demonstrates the tumor's proximity to major vascular and hilar structures. The typical CT appearance is a solid solitary mass with lower attenuation levels than those of the surrounding liver. A novel technique, CT arterioportography, holds promise as a reliable means of assessing vascular invasion along with gross tumor distribution. MRI has proved to be very useful in defining the patency of vascular structures.

Differential Diagnosis

One major management problem is the inability to differentiate adenomas from hepatocellular carcinoma. Because of this, hepatic adenoma, despite being a benign lesion, is often excised. Focal nodular hyperplasia is a well-circumscribed, nonencapsulated nodular liver mass. Ultrasonography and CT scan demonstrate a solid mass, but one cannot differentiate it from adenoma or malignancy without a biopsy. If the diagnosis can be made by biopsy (percutaneous or open), no further treatment is needed. Mesenchymal hamartoma is an uncommon benign lesion presenting in the first year of life as an asymptomatic large solitary mass usually confined to the right lobe of the liver. CT scan demonstrates a well-defined tumor margin and minimal to no contrast enhancement. The treatment is surgical wedge resection; lobectomy is rarely required.

Table 45–10. Hepatic tumor staging.

Stage I: Tumor localized and completely resected
Stage II: Tumor resected with microscopic residual disease
Stage III: Unresectable tumor or gross residual disease
Stage IV: Metastatic disease

Treatment

The definitive diagnosis of hepatoblastoma requires tissue biopsy. Although this can be performed percutaneously, there are reports of "seeding" of the biopsy tract. It is preferable to perform open biopsy of the lesion with assessment of resectability. If the lesion is not primarily resectable, vascular access is obtained during the same anesthetic interval for subsequent chemotherapy. Table 45–10 outlines the surgical staging system for childhood hepatic malignancies.

Complete surgical resection is the major objective of therapy and represents the only chance for cure. Approximately 60% of patients will have primarily resectable lesions. Lobectomy or extended lobectomy (trisegmentectomy) is usual, but segmental (nonanatomic) resection of small isolated tumors may be possible. Careful preoperative evaluation and planning have made liver resection in children a safe procedure, with a mortality rate of less than 5%. Adequate exposure can be obtained via an extended subcostal or bilateral subcostal incision, although bulky lesions may require extension into the right hemithorax to gain adequate vascular control during dissection. Ascitic fluid is obtained for cytologic examination. If the lesion is deemed unresectable, the tumor is biopsied. If the lesion is made resectable following chemotherapy, lobectomy or trisegmentectomy is performed. Intraoperative cholangiography is helpful to verify the integrity of the remaining biliary tree.

Postoperative complications include bleeding, biliary fistula, subphrenic fluid collections or abscess, and inadvertent injury to the biliary tree. Hepatic regeneration occurs quickly, and hepatic insufficiency is rare if 25% or more of the liver parenchyma remains. Hepatic transplantation is used for unresectable disease when chemotherapy has failed to allow complete resection but no demonstrable metastases exist.

The overall survival for all children with hepatoblastoma is approximately 50%. The best survival (90%) is seen in patients with stage I tumors who receive adjunctive chemotherapy after complete excision. Survival decreases as the surgical stage increases, though long-term survival approaches 60–70% in patients with unresectable disease who receive chemotherapy.

Tagge EP et al: Resection, including transplantation, for hepatoblastoma and hepatocellular carcinoma: impact on survival. J Pediatr Surg 1992;27:292.

Wheatley JM, LaQuaglia MP: Management of hepatic epithelial malignancy in childhood and adolescence. Semin Surg Oncol 1993;9:532.

2. Hepatocellular Carcinoma

Hepatocellular carcinoma is less common than hepatoblastoma and typically presents in older children and adolescents (median age, 10 years). It is associated with preexisting chronic hepatitis, cirrhosis due to hepatitis B virus, and other causes of childhood cirrhosis (tyrosinemia, biliary cirrhosis, α_1-antitrypsin deficiency, type 1 glycogen storage disease, and long-term parenteral nutrition). Signs and symptoms consist of an abdominal mass or diffuse swelling, abdominal pain, weight loss, anorexia, and jaundice. The serum AFP level is elevated in 50%, though the absolute levels are lower than in patients with hepatoblastoma. Diagnostic studies, staging, and treatment are somewhat the same as for hepatoblastoma. Because of multicentricity, bilobar involvement, portal vein invasion, and lymphatic metastases, only 15–20% of hepatocellular carcinomas are resectable. Fibrolamellar hepatocellular carcinoma in younger patients is associated with a high rate of resectability and a better prognosis. The overall long-term survival is poor (15%), even for resectable disease. The role of liver transplantation is unclear.

3. Liver Hemangioma

This is the most common benign pediatric hepatic lesion. These tumors are solitary (cavernous hemangioma) or multiple (infantile hemangioendothelioma), involving the bulk of the liver. Isolated cavernous hemangiomas are not often associated with cutaneous hemangiomas, whereas infantile hemangioendotheliomas are commonly associated with hemangiomas in other parts of the body or integument. Patients with a solitary hemangioma frequently have no symptoms or present with a mass. Infrequently there is intratumor hemorrhage or rupture resulting in abdominal pain. Infants with hemangioendothelioma commonly present with massive hepatomegaly and high-output cardiac failure from arteriovenous shunting. Approximately 40% develop Kasabach-Merritt syndrome (thrombocytopenic coagulopathy due to platelet sequestration within the tumor). The diagnosis is made by red blood cell-labeled radionuclide or dynamic abdominal CT scanning. CT scan demonstrates increased filling and a rapid venous phase from arteriovenous shunting. Angiography is unnecessary, and percutaneous biopsy is contraindicated.

Treatment is not necessary in an asymptomatic child. Patients with congestive heart failure or thrombocytopenia are treated with corticosteroids, digoxin, and diuretics. Refractory patients benefit from hepatic artery embolization. External beam radiation reduces hepatic size and controls symptoms. Their large size and diffuse involvement often preclude resection. Indications for surgery include ruptured lesions with hemorrhage, masses with uncertain diagnoses, symptomatic lesions, or disease limited to one lobe. Hemangioendotheliomas may undergo malignant degeneration into angiosarcoma.

Newman KD: Hepatic tumors in children. Semin Pediatr Surg 1997;6:38.

Reynolds M: Pediatric liver tumors. Semin Surg Oncol 1999; 16:159.

Stringer MD: Liver tumors. Semin Pediatr Surg 2000;9:196.

BATTERED CHILD SYNDROME

Child abuse is any nonaccidental injury inflicted by a parent, guardian, or other supervising adult. It may be passive, in the form of emotional or nutritional deprivation, but is most readily recognized in the active form, characterized as "battered, bruised, beaten, broken, and burned." It is estimated that 1 million children per year in the United States suffer injuries that qualifying for reporting to the National Center on Child Abuse and Neglect. About 20–50% of children are rebattered after the first diagnosis, resulting in death in 5% and permanent physical damage in 35% when the syndrome is not recognized.

The child abuser is usually a young, insecure, unstable person who had an unhappy childhood and who has unrealistic expectations of the child. Most of these individuals are of low socioeconomic status. The abuser may be a parent, guardian, babysitter, neighborhood child, or other close associate. Active traumatic abuse is usually perpetrated by the father, but passive neglect with failure to thrive from nutritional or emotional deprivation is usually attributable to the mother.

Clinical Findings

In most cases, the battered child is under 3 years of age and is the product of a difficult pregnancy or premature labor, usually unwanted or born outside of a stable parental relationship. Many battered children have congenital anomalies or are hyperkinetic and colicky. In most cases there is a discrepancy between the history supplied and the magnitude of the injury—or else a reluctance to give a history. Contradictory histories or delay in bringing the child to medical attention—or taking the child to many different emergency room visits in different hospitals for unusual reasons—should be regarded with suspicion. A past injury in the child or sibling and almost any injury in an infant under 1 year of age should trigger a consideration of child abuse. The parents may be evasive or hostile. They may have open guilt feelings or may be capable of complete concealment. The innocent spouse is usually more protective of the abuser than of the child.

The child is usually withdrawn, apathetic, whimpering, and fearful and shows signs of neglect or growth retardation. Multiple forms of injury may be noted at varying stages of healing. The child should be completely disrobed to enable the clinician to look for welts, bruises, lacerations, bite or belt wounds, stick or coat hanger marks on the head, trunk, buttocks, or extremities, and similar evidence of mistreatment. Cigarette, hot plate, match, or scalding burns may be evident. Subgaleal hematomas may be caused by pulled hair. Retinal hemorrhage or detachment may follow blows to the head. Abdominal injuries may produce laceration to the liver, spleen, or pancreas or bowel perforation. Sexual abuse should be identified by determining whether the vaginal introitus or anus is bruised, lacerated, or enlarged and whether aspirated fluid contains sperm or prostatic acid phosphatase.

Even though no obvious fracture may be present, a skeletal radiographic survey should be performed. The bone most commonly fractured is the femur, followed by the humerus in the region of the diaphysis. Rib fractures and periosteal reactions in various stages of healing will be seen. Skull fractures are most commonly seen in infants less than 1 year old. Suture separation of the skull may indicate subdural hematoma. Neurologic injury may require a CT or MRI scan.

Treatment

The child should be admitted to hospital to be protected until the home environment can be evaluated. Injuries should be documented radiographically and with photographs. The presence of sperm in the vagina or anal canal should be confirmed. Bleeding disorders should be evaluated by a platelet count, bleeding time, prothrombin time, and plasma thromboplastin test to make certain that multiple bruises are not due to coagulopathy. A serologic test for syphilis may be indicated as well as cultures (including pharyngeal) for gonorrhea.

Injuries should be treated. Consultation with ophthalmologists, neurologists, neurosurgeons, orthopedic surgeons, and plastic surgeons may be required.

It is required by law in every state for both the hospital and the physician to report child abuse (suspected as well as documented) to local child protection services, usually via the hospital's social work department. The physician is the protector of the child and a consultant to the parents and must not assume the role of prosecutor or judge. The most difficult task is to notify the parents without confrontation, accusation, or anger that battering or neglect is suspected. The physician must tell the parents that the law requires reporting injuries that are unexplained or inadequately explained in view of the nature of the injury. A written referral should then be made to other professionals, such as child welfare personnel, hospital social workers, or psychiatrists. The referral should describe the history of past injuries and the nature of current injuries, results of physical examination and laboratory and x-ray studies, and a statement about why nonaccidental trauma is suspected.

Prognosis

The abuser may require careful evaluation for possible psychosis by a psychiatrist. Child welfare personnel and social workers will have to assess the home environment and work with the parents to prevent future abuse. It may be necessary to place the child in a foster home, but approximately 90% of families can be reunited.

Berkowitz CD: New patterns of injury. Emerg Med Clin North Am 1995;13:321.

Duhaime AC et al: Nonaccidental head injuries in infants—the "shaken-baby syndrome". N Engl J Med 1998;338:1822.

REFERENCES

Andrassy RJ (editor): *Pediatric Surgical Oncology.* Saunders, 1998.

Ashcraft KW et al (editors): *Pediatric Surgery,* 3rd ed. Saunders, 2000.

Burg FD et al (editors): *Gellis & Kagan's Current Pediatric Therapy.* Saunders, 1999.

Gray SW, Skandalakis JE: *Embryology for Surgeons: The Embryological Basis for Treatment of Congenital Defects,* 2nd ed. Williams & Wilkins, 1994.

Harrison MR et al: *The Unborn Patient: The Art and Science of Fetal Therapy,* 3rd ed. Saunders, 2001.

Oldham KT, Colombani PM, Foglia RP (editors): *Surgery of Infants and Children. Scientific Principles and Practice*, Lippincott-Raven, 1997.

O'Neill JA et al (editors): *Pediatric Surgery,* 5th ed. Mosby, 1998.

Rowe MI et al (editors): *Essentials of Pediatric Surgery,* Mosby, 1995.

Rudolph C, Rudolph AM, Hostetter MK (editors): *Rudolph's Pediatrics,* 21st ed. McGraw-Hill, 2002.

Oncology

46

Michael S. Sabel, MD, FACS

Over 1.3 million individuals in the United States are diagnosed with invasive cancer each year. Currently, 1 in 4 deaths in the United States is due to cancer, ranking second only to heart disease as the leading cause of mortality in this country. Before age 65, among men and women combined, cancer is the leading cause of death.

The surgeon is intimately involved in the care of cancer patients, since nearly 90% of patients with malignancies require surgical therapy at some time. Surgical resection is the initial curative treatment for nearly three-quarters of cancer patients. Since surgeons are often the first specialists to see newly diagnosed cancer patients, they will often be the ones responsible for orchestrating the patient's care. It is imperative that they have an in-depth knowledge of the different types of cancer and the different modalities available for treatment.

TUMOR NOMENCLATURE

Neoplasms may be defined as benign or malignant based on the clinical behavior of the tumor. Benign tumors have lost normal growth regulation but tend to be surrounded by a capsule and do not invade surrounding tissues or metastasize.

Benign tumors are generally designated by adding the suffix *-oma* to the name of the cell of origin. Examples include lipoma or adenoma. The term "cancer" normally refers to malignant tumors, which possess the capability to invade surrounding tissues or metastasize to distant sites in the host. The nomenclature of malignant tumors is typically based on the cell's embryonal tissue origins. Malignant tumors derived from cells of mesenchymal origin are called "sarcomas." These include cancers that derive from muscle, bone, tendon, fat, cartilage, lymphoid tissues, vessels, and connective tissue. Neoplasms of epithelial origin are called "carcinomas." These may be further categorized according to the histologic appearance of the cells. Tumor cells that have glandular growth patterns are referred to as adenocarcinomas, and those that resemble squamous epithelial cells are called squamous cell carcinomas. Cancers composed of undifferentiated cells that bear no resemblance to any tissues are designated as "poorly differentiated" or "undifferentiated carcinomas."

Tumor Grade

Beyond the type of cancer, it is important to classify tumors by their behavior and prognosis in order to determine appropriate therapy as well as evaluate different treatment modalities. Grading of a tumor is a histologic determination and refers to the degree of cellular differentiation. Separate pathologic grading systems exist for each histologic type of cancer. Depending on the type of tumor, these systems are based on nuclear pleomorphism, cellularity, necrosis, cellular invasion, and the number of mitoses. Increasing grades generally denote increasing degrees of dedifferentiation. While the grade of the tumor typically has less prognostic value than its stage, tumor grade has great clinical significance in soft tissue sarcoma, astrocytoma, transitional cell cancers of the genitourinary tract, and Hodgkin's and non-Hodgkin's lymphoma.

Tumor Stage

Tumor staging establishes the extent of disease and has important prognostic and therapeutic implications in most types of cancer. Clinical staging is based on the results of a noninvasive evaluation, including physical examination and various imaging studies. Pathologic staging is based on findings in surgical tumor specimens and biopsies and allows for the evaluation of microscopic disease undetectable by imaging techniques. Pathologic staging may reveal more extensive tumor spread than the clinical evaluation and is the more reliable information. Clinicians must be careful when attempting to compare clinically and pathologically staged patients, as the two groups may have dramatically different outcomes.

As with grading, the staging systems vary with different tumor types. Two major staging systems are currently in use, one developed by the Union Internationale Contre le Cancer (UICC), and the other by the American Joint Committee on Cancer (AJCC). The UICC system is based on the TNM classification. T refers to the primary tumor and is based on the size of the tumor and invasion of surrounding structures. Tumors are characterized as T1 to T4 cancers, with the higher T stages for larger and more invasive tumors. N refers to regional lymph nodes, and classifications of N0 to N3 denote increasing degrees of lymph node involvement. Finally, M refers to distant metastatic disease, with M0 signifying no distant metastases and M1 and M2 indicating the presence of blood-borne metastatic disease. The AJCC system divides cancers into stages 0 to IV, with higher stages representing more widespread disease and a poorer prognosis. Regardless of the staging system or the tumor type, higher stages correlate with decreased survival.

AJCC Cancer Staging Manual, 6th ed. Springer Verlag, 2002.

Cotran CS, Kumar V, Robbins SL (editors): *Robbins Pathologic Basis of Disease,* 6th ed. Saunders, 1999.

Jemal A et al: Cancer statistics, 2004. CA Cancer J Clin 2004;54:8.

ROLE OF THE SURGICAL ONCOLOGIST

The surgeon is often the first specialist to see a patient with suspected or newly diagnosed cancer, and in many cases assumes responsibility for orchestrating the overall management of the cancer patient's care. The role of the surgeon involves not only the curative resection of the tumor, but also obtaining tissue for diagnosis and staging, debulking tumors as part of multimodality therapy, providing palliation for incurable patients, and preventing cancer by the surgical removal of nonessential organs. With improving imaging technologies, expanded use of neoadjuvant therapies, molecular staging, and increasing knowledge of genetic predisposition to cancer, the role of the surgical oncologist is continuously evolving. It is therefore imperative for surgical oncologists to remain current on the newest approaches to cancer therapy and be prepared to adapt to the changing role of surgery.

Diagnosis & Staging

A tissue diagnosis is critical to the care of all cancer patients. Depending on the type of tumor and its location, the method of biopsy will vary. Common diagnostic techniques include needle aspiration biopsy, core needle biopsy, incisional biopsy, and excisional biopsy.

Fine-needle aspiration biopsy (FNAB) is a rapid and minimally invasive technique for the biopsy of palpable superficial tumors. Deeper, nonpalpable lesions may also be sampled by this technique when FNAB is combined with various imaging modalities, such as ultrasonography or CT. FNAB involves aspiration of cells from a suspicious mass, followed by cytologic examination of the stained smear. FNAB is particularly useful in the diagnosis of enlarged lymph nodes, breast lumps, thyroid masses, and lung nodules. FNAB cytology, however, does not demonstrate architecture, and so does not allow the pathologist to accurately grade tumors or reveal the extent of invasion of a tumor.

If this information is necessary, FNAB may be inadequate. Sampling errors commonly lead to false-negative results, so a negative FNAB should be interpreted cautiously. In addition, though rare, false-positive results can occur, so confirmation may be needed before definitive surgical intervention. For example, a mastectomy should never be performed on the basis of an FNAB of a breast lump without confirming the diagnosis by either preoperative core biopsy or frozen section analysis at the time of surgery.

Core needle biopsy utilizes a needle that cuts a sliver of tissue for analysis. This technique provides more histologic information than FNAB because it allows the pathologist to see the histologic architecture of the sample rather than just the cellular characteristics. False-positive results are extremely rare. Although less so than with FNAB, sampling errors may occur and a negative result must be weighed against clinical judgment. Core biopsies are frequently used for prostate, breast, and liver masses. Again, ultrasound and radiographic imaging may enable the clinician to sample deep-seated or nonpalpable masses. The technique may also be used during surgery to biopsy suspicious masses encountered at operation.

When a larger tumor sample is necessary for accurate grading or staging, an incisional or excisional biopsy is required. **Excisional biopsy** is defined as the surgical removal of an entire gross lesion, while **incisional biopsy** involves sampling a representative portion of a suspicious lesion. In general, excisional biopsy is recommended whenever it is possible to excise the entire lesion without damage to surrounding structures. For large (> 5 cm), deep soft tissue masses, incisional biopsy is the preferred method.

Although biopsy techniques are usually simple, the surgeon must adhere to some specific principles when performing a biopsy for a suspected malignancy. The positioning of the needle tract or scar should be such that if further surgery is required, the biopsy site will be easily included in the excised specimen. Excisional biopsies of the breast should consider the possibility of a subsequent mastectomy, and the excision of skin or subcutaneous lesions on the extremities should be oriented in a way that allows for the following wide excision if malignancy is discovered. Meticulous hemostasis is imperative, as the formation of a wound hematoma may make subsequent operation more difficult. The surgeon should also pay careful attention to the orientation of the pathologic specimen, as it may prove important in curative surgical procedures. Finally, if radiation therapy is anticipated following the biopsy or staging of a lesion, the surgeon should place radiopaque clips at the margin of resection to guide the radiation oncologist.

Surgeons are often called upon to perform operations that provide staging information for various types of cancer. Such procedures are necessary when the clinical extent of the disease has a direct bearing on the choice of treatment modalities. Examples include laparoscopy for gastric or pancreatic cancer, a staging laparotomy for ovarian cancer, or mediastinoscopy for lung and esophageal cancer. Staging procedures can often help to avert highly morbid procedures in cases where there is little chance for cure.

Curative Surgery

Surgical resections with curative intent can be divided into three categories: resection of a primary lesion, resection of isolated metastases, and the resection of metastatic deposits. In each of these cases, the clinician must strive to reach a balance between the chance for cure and the morbidity of the procedure. Each situation must be evaluated individually, and the patient's wishes must be paramount.

In the resection of a primary lesion, the tumor type guides the extent of the resection. Various tumors require different disease-free margins in order to achieve optimal chances for a cure. It is important that the surgeon have knowledge of other modalities that may be integrated into the management plan to allow for a less ablative surgical procedure. Radiation and chemotherapy are commonly used in combination with surgery and are referred to as adjuvant therapies if used after complete resection with no demonstrable local or systemic disease. If these modalities are used in the preoperative setting, they are called neoadjuvant therapies.

The regional lymph nodes represent the most prevalent site of metastases for solid tumors. For most cancers, involvement of the regional lymph nodes represents the most important prognostic factor. For this reason, the removal of the regional lymph nodes is often performed at the time of resection of the primary cancer. Besides staging information, a regional lymphadenectomy provides "regional control" of the cancer.

More controversial is whether the removal of regional lymph nodes can improve survival. These controversies have related to both the extent of the procedure as well as the timing of the procedure. For example, the extent of lymphadenectomy at the time of gastrectomy for stomach cancer has been hypothesized to have an impact on improving overall survival. This has not, however, been borne out in prospective randomized trials; the more extended lymphadenectomy appears to result in more accurate staging of patients at a cost of increased morbidity and minimal if any effect on overall survival.

For many nonvisceral solid tumors such as melanoma, breast cancers, and head and neck squamous cancers, the "elective" removal of clinically negative lymph nodes at the time of primary tumor resection has been postulated to result in better survival outcomes compared to performing a lymphadenectomy only when the patient relapses in a nodal basin (a therapeutic lymph node dissection). Prospective randomized clinical studies have yet to demonstrate a clear survival advantage for performing elective lymph node dissections, and this approach exposes a large number of node-negative patients to the morbidity of a dissection. The adoption of "selective lymphadenectomy" based upon the concept of the "sentinel lymph node" has dramatically improved our ability to stage the regional lymph nodes of certain cancers (helping guide adjuvant therapy decisions) and select patients who may benefit from a complete lymph node dissection.

The surgeon plays a much more limited role when the patient has metastatic disease; nonetheless, the resection of "isolated" metastases in patients with solid malignancies is sometimes a consideration when technically feasible. The selection of candidate patients for surgical resection requires a thorough evaluation of the extent of disease, medical status of the patient, and the feasibility of resecting the metastatic site with a negative margin. When all is said and done, this process ends up identifying a small subset of patients that would be surgical candidates. Although there are no prospective randomized trials documenting the survival benefit of surgical resection of metastatic disease, there is considerable retrospective evidence indicating that this approach can result in long-term benefit. The resection of lung metastases in patients with osteogenic or soft tissue sarcomas has been associated with an approximately 20–25% overall survival rate greater than 5 years. There is also a large body of retrospective evidence documenting the benefit of resecting colorectal metastases to the liver, resulting in a 25-40% overall 5-year survival rate, depending upon the extent of liver involvement. Other examples include an aggressive surgical approach to metastatic melanoma and the resection of isolated breast cancer metastases to the lung. One of the roles of the surgical oncologist is to know when it is appropriate to offer this option.

Palliation

Surgical intervention is sometimes required in the patient with unresectable advanced cancer for palliative indications such as pain, bleeding, obstruction, malnutrition, or infection. The decision to operate must balance several factors, including the likelihood of adding significantly to the quality of life of the patient, the expected survival of the individual, the potential morbidity of the procedure, and whether there are alternative methods of palliation.

Malnutrition is a common problem in the cancer patient, especially one with advanced, unresectable disease. Commonly, the surgeon is involved in placement of vascular access for hyperalimentation, or if the gastrointestinal tract is functional, the placement of gastrostomy or jejunostomy tubes for enteral nutrition. Occasionally, the surgeon is involved in palliating pain due to a metastatic lesion compressing upon an organ or adjacent nerves. Examples include cutaneous or subcutaneous melanoma metastases, a large ulcerating breast cancer, or a recurrent intra-abdominal sarcoma mass. The surgeon needs to assess the relative risk to benefit ratio in resecting a symptomatic mass knowing that it will not impact on the overall survival of the patient. If the quality of life of the individual can be improved at an acceptable operative risk, then the surgical intervention is warranted.

Finally, the surgeon may be called upon to manage oncologic emergencies. Acute hemorrhage or obstruction of a hollow viscus represent the most common potential oncologic emergencies. In these cases, surgeons may be called on to emergently intervene in the care of a cancer patient, or in certain instances, use nonsurgical approaches (such as stents or angiography) that can be effective.

Prophylaxis

With our improved understanding of inherited genetic mutations and the identification of patients who are predisposed to cancer, surgical therapy has expanded beyond the therapy of established tumors and into the prevention of cancer. Prophylaxis is not a new concept in surgical oncology. Patients with chronic inflammatory diseases are known to be at high risk of subsequent malignant transformation. This typically prompts close surveillance and surgical resection at the first identification of premalignant changes. One of the earliest examples of this is the recommendation for total proctocolectomy for subsets of patients with chronic ulcerative colitis.

The ability to perform genetic screening for relevant mutations has allowed for prophylactic surgery to be implemented prior to the onset of symptoms or histologic changes. Familial adenomatous polyposis coli (FAP) syndrome, defined by the diffuse involvement of the colon and rectum with adenomatous polyps, almost always predisposes to colorectal cancer if the large intestine is left in place. With the identification of the gene responsible for FAP, the adenomatous polyposis coli (APC) gene, members of families in which an APC mutation has been identified can have genetic testing prior to polyps becoming evident and be considered for prophylactic proctocolectomy. Medullary thyroid cancer (MTC) is a well-established component of multiple endocrine neoplasia syndrome type 2a (MEN 2a) or type 2b (MEN 2b). Mutations in the RET proto-oncogene are present in almost all cases of MEN 2a and 2b. Family members of MEN patients can be screened for the presence of a RET mutation, and those with the mutation should undergo total thyroidectomy at a young age (6 years for MEN 2a, infancy for MEN 2b). The role of prophylactic mastectomies has been greatly expanded with the identification of BRCA1 and BRCA2, which can be associated with a lifetime probability of breast cancer of between 40% and 85%. Other prophylactic surgeries are listed in Table 46–1. However, potential benefits of prophylactic surgeries must be weighed against quality of life issues and the morbidity of the surgery. A detailed discussion must be held with each patient considering prophylactic surgery regarding the risks and benefits, so today's surgical oncologist needs a clear understanding of genetics and inherited risk.

Miltenburg DM, Conklin L, Sastri S: The role of genetic screening and prophylactic surgery in surgical oncology. J Am Coll Surg 2000;190:619.

CYTOTOXIC CHEMOTHERAPY

The goal of chemotherapeutic regimens is to deliver pharmacologic agents systemically to eradicate all tumor cells. The ideal tumor drug would kill cancer cells without harming normal tissues. No such agent exists, and most drugs affect normal cells to some extent. The success of chemotherapy relies on the normal cell's greater capacity for repair and survival relative to tumor cells.

Even a single cancer cell can potentially reproduce to form a lethal tumor. For this reason, the goal of curative

Table 46-1. Prophylactic surgeries in surgical oncology.

Prophylactic Surgery	Potential Indications
Bilateral mastectomy	BRCA1 or BRCA2 mutation Atypical hyperplasia or lobular carcinoma in situ Familial breast cancer
Bilateral oophorectomy	BRCA1 mutation Familial ovarian cancer Hereditary nonpolyposis colorectal cancer Hysterectomy for endometrial cancer Colon resection for colon cancer
Thyroidectomy	RET proto-oncogene mutation Multiple endocrine neoplasia type 2A (MEN 2A) Multiple endocrine neoplasia type 2B (MEN 2B) Familial non-MEN medullary thyroid carcinoma (FMTC)
Total proctocolectomy	Familial adenomatous polyposis (FAP) or APC mutation Ulcerative colitis HNPCC germ-line mutation

chemotherapy must be the complete eradication of all tumor cells. Tumor burden is important in chemotherapy. A large cancer may harbor more than 10^9 tumor cells. If a tolerable dose of an effective drug killed 99.99% of these cells, the tumor burden would still be 10^5 cells. The remaining cells, while clinically undetectable, are likely to continue to grow and lead to a clinical recurrence of cancer. For this reason, most chemotherapy protocols rely on repeated administrations of drugs in order to achieve maximal cell killing. Tumor cells may avoid the cell-killing effects of a particular drug because of their stage in the cell cycle, residence in an area protected from the drug (central nervous system), or an inherent resistance to the drug.

Drug resistance plays a large role in chemotherapy failures. Several mechanisms of tumor resistance are known. The multidrug resistance (MDR) gene encodes a protein that actively pumps drugs out of tumor cells. This gene confers resistance on a variety of antitumor drugs, including the antibiotics and plant-derived compounds. Other tumor mechanisms of resistance include the alteration of target enzymes, increased production of a target enzyme to overwhelm the drug, and an increased capability for DNA repair. Tumor resistance to a given chemotherapeutic agent can often be overcome by the administration of multiple drugs.

Principles of Chemotherapy Use

A. Curative Chemotherapy

Hematologic malignancies are typically treated by chemotherapy, radiation, or both, with surgery used primarily for diagnosis and staging. On the other hand, surgery is the primary treatment for nonhematologic malignancies, although there are some exceptions. Anal cancer is cured in approximately 80% of patients with the Nigro protocol; 5-FU/mitomycin-C and radiation therapy, as first-line treatment. Testicular cancer, even when metastatic, is curable with bleomycin/etoposide/cisplatin in approximately 85% of patients.

B. Adjuvant Treatment

Although all visible tumor may be removed at the time of surgery, microscopic tumor deposits may still be present locally or may have spread to distant locations. Chemotherapy is most effective against very small tumors and microscopic tumor deposits. Therefore, adjuvant chemotherapy is often given to improve the likelihood of cure after surgical resection.

The benefit gained from adjuvant chemotherapy can be thought of in terms of absolute benefit or relative benefit (Figure 46–1). For example, after colectomy for stage III colon cancer, the chance of cure is approximately 50%. This can be increased to approximately 70% by adjuvant 5-FU/leucovorin. This represents a 40% relative benefit (40% more patients are cured with chemotherapy than without chemotherapy), but a 20% absolute benefit (20% of the patients who take the chemotherapy will have altered their outcome). Another way to look at this is that with a 20% absolute benefit, 80% of patients experience the inconvenience and side effects of chemotherapy without gaining any improvement themselves. The decision to receive adjuvant chemotherapy is a balance between the expected benefit of treatment, the patient's comorbid conditions and general health, and the patient's wishes.

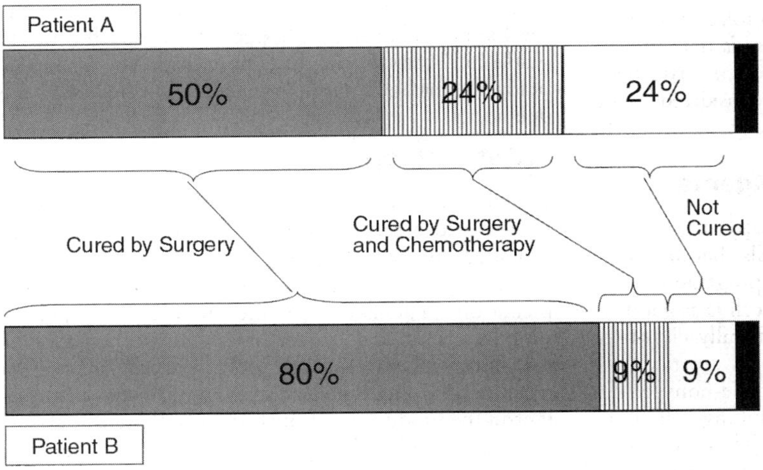

Figure 46–1. Benefits of adjuvant chemotherapy. For 100 patients treated with adjuvant chemotherapy, some will be cured by surgery alone (grey bar), some will die of other causes (black bar), and some will die of their cancer (white bar). Adjuvant therapy will prevent a cancer death in a portion of those patients (striped bar). Adjuvant chemotherapy will result in a relative benefit of 50% for both patient A and patient B, meaning treatment will reduce the likelihood of dying of cancer by 50%. However, the absolute benefit is different for both patients. For patient A, who has a high likelihood of dying of disease, the absolute benefit is 24%. For patient B, who has a good prognosis, the absolute benefit is only 9%.

C. Neoadjuvant Treatment

Neoadjuvant chemotherapy is usually given to facilitate surgical resection by shrinking the primary tumor, or it may convert an unresectable tumor into a resectable tumor. In some cases, this has been shown to prolong survival. Another advantage to neoadjuvant chemotherapy is that it allows the oncologist to observe the primary tumor to determine if it is sensitive to a particular chemotherapeutic regimen. During the course of cancer treatment, it is important to define the progress and outcomes resulting from therapy. The terms complete and partial response are often used as end points to evaluate the efficacy of a particular therapeutic regimen. A **complete response** is defined as the absence of demonstrable cancer. A **partial response** refers to a reduction of tumor mass by greater than 50%. The patient's response to neoadjuvant chemotherapy can be an important predictor of outcome.

D. Chemotherapy for Metastatic Disease

The majority of patients who are receiving chemotherapy have metastatic disease that is not curable. For these patients, treatment with chemotherapy is intended to prolong survival, improve quality of life, or both. Response rates range from 20% to 75%, depending on the tumor type and chemotherapy regimen. However, even a complete remission is rarely durable. Most partial or complete remissions last only months.

As with all therapies, the decision to use chemotherapy must balance the potential benefits with the risks, toxicities, and the patient's general health and condition. There is little to be gained by treating an asymptomatic patient if no prolongation of survival is expected. A detailed discussion must be held with each individual patient; some patients are more willing than others to tolerate the side effects of chemotherapy. Since the disease is not curable, treatment with single agents, which are less toxic than combination chemotherapy, are often considered, with more willingness to reduce doses for toxicity.

Classes of Chemotherapeutic Agents

With all forms of curative chemotherapy, the goal is elimination of all tumor stem cells. Cells that are incapable of further division cannot cause progression of a tumor, and the sterilization of a tumor cell is as good as a kill. Chemotherapeutic drugs are generally classified as cell cycle-specific (CCS) drugs, which are toxic to actively proliferating cells; or cell cycle-nonspecific (CCNS) drugs, which are capable of killing cells that are not dividing during drug exposure. These two classifications are not absolute, and many drugs may overlap between the two categories.

In order to achieve maximal cell killing, most therapeutic protocols use combination chemotherapy. Agents with differing mechanisms of action and different toxic side effects are used, allowing for relatively high doses of multiple agents. This method of combining agents helps to combat tumor cell resistance and increase the tumor cell killing while avoiding the compounding of toxic effects.

A. Alkylating Agents

These agents exert their effects by the transfer of alkyl groups to various cellular components, most importantly by the alkylation of DNA. Alkylators can cause DNA strand breaks, cross-linking of DNA strands, or miscoding of DNA during replication. The alkylating agents are considered cell cycle-nonspecific agents but tend to have their greatest effect on proliferating cells. Normal cells are able to avoid many of the lethal affects of alkylating agents because of their ability to repair DNA. The alkylating agents are effective in treatment of the hematologic malignancies and in a variety of solid tumors such as breast, melanoma, lung, and endometrial cancers. Included in this class are the nitrosoureas (eg, carmustine, semustine, lomustine), cyclophosphamide, chlorambucil, mechlorethamine, dacarbazine, and procarbazine.

B. Platinum Analogues

The platinum analogues are similar to the alkylating agents. They bind DNA to form inter- and intra-strand cross-links, leading to inhibition of DNA synthesis and transcription. The mechanisms of cancer cell resistance are also similar to those of alkylating agents: decreased cellular uptake of the drugs, increased activity of DNA repair enzymes, and increased thiol-containing proteins. In addition, resistance to both cisplatin and carboplatin has been associated with a deficiency of mismatch repair genes (MMR). It is not known why this mechanism of resistance appears to be specific to cisplatin and carboplatin, but the efficacy of the newest platinum analogue, oxaliplatin, is not affected by MMR deficiency.

C. Antimetabolites

Rapidly dividing cells require increased synthesis of nucleic acid precursors. This increased synthesis can be exploited pharmacologically by the antimetabolites. These drugs are analogues of nucleic acids or nucleic acid precursors. The antimetabolites may be incorporated into the nucleic acids of a cell and serve as a false messenger. Antimetabolites can shut down the cellular synthetic machinery by binding to and inhibiting enzymes important in the production of nucleic acids. Since this class of drugs affects all rapidly proliferating cells, they are relatively toxic to normal tissues that have a high rate of cell turnover. Antimetabolites are most effective in the hematologic malignancies but are also used in the treatment of solid tumors such as breast and gastrointestinal cancers.

They include methotrexate, mercaptopurine, thioguanine, fluorouracil, and cytarabine.

D. Antimicrotubule Agents

A variety of antitumor drugs are derived from natural plants (and are also known as plant alkaloids). Vincristine, vinblastine, docetaxel, and paclitaxel work by binding tubulin and poisoning the assembly of microtubules in the mitotic spindle. This leads to mitotic arrest in metaphase, and these compounds are effective only on rapidly dividing cell populations. The plant alkaloids are most useful for hematologic malignancies and breast, renal, testicular, and head and neck cancers.

E. Topoisomerase Inhibitors

These plant derivatives exert their antitumor effects by binding to and inhibiting various forms of the enzyme topoisomerase. Topoisomerases are responsible for the maintenance of DNA structure and are also important in the cleavage and re-ligation of DNA strands. Inhibition of these enzymes leads to DNA strand breakage and structural damage. The topoisomerase inhibitors are also cell cycle-specific agents and have their greatest activity against rapidly proliferating cells. Examples include etoposide, teniposide, and topotecan. These drugs are used in the treatment of hematologic malignancies and lung, bladder, prostate, and testicular cancers.

F. Antibiotics

The majority of the drugs in this class are derived from the soil fungus streptomyces. All the antibiotics exert their antitumor effects by interference with the synthesis of nucleic acids. Most of the drugs in this class intercalate in DNA; blocking DNA synthesis and inducing strand breakages. The antibiotics are considered cell cycle-nonspecific, and they have antitumor activity against a wide variety of solid tumors. Included in this class of drugs are doxorubicin, dactinomycin, plicamycin, mitomycin, and bleomycin.

Side Effects of Chemotherapy

Most side effects from chemotherapeutic regimens are the result of toxicities to rapidly dividing normal cell populations—particularly bone marrow and epithelial cells. Bone marrow suppression is an adverse effect of many of these drugs, resulting in neutropenia, thrombocytopenia, and even anemia. Mucosal ulcerations and alopecia also occur in patients treated with cell cycle-specific agents. Intractable nausea and vomiting is another common side effect that can severely affect quality of life. Testicular or ovarian failure can result from chemotherapy, leading to sterility. Many of these drugs also are powerful teratogens and should be avoided in pregnant patients. Finally, many of the alkylating agents have been implicated in the development of secondary cancers, especially hematologic malignancies.

REGIONAL THERAPY

Systemic chemotherapy is limited by toxicity to the host. Regional delivery of chemotherapeutic agents via arterial cannulation allows for high levels of drugs in the region of the primary tumor while decreasing systemic toxicity.

Isolated limb perfusion is a technique for the delivery of chemotherapeutic agents to an extremity with locally advanced cancer, and is of benefit primarily in the treatment of extremity melanoma and sarcoma. In this approach, a tourniquet is applied to the extremity to occlude venous outflow. The major artery perfusing the limb is then isolated, cannulated, and perfused with hyperthermic chemotherapeutic agents using a pump oxygenator as for cardiopulmonary bypass. The perfusion is done in the operating room and lasts for approximately 1 hour. The cannula is then removed. Most protocols involve only a single treatment. Melphalan, an alkylating agent, is the most common agent used today in the treatment of both sarcomas and melanomas. In patients with extensive in-transit melanoma confined to an extremity, ILP can provide regional control and palliation. In patients with unresectable extremity sarcomas, preoperative limb perfusion can often shrink the tumor and allow for a limb-sparing resection. While improving regional control, this therapy has yet to show a definitive survival benefit.

Another approach is isolated hepatic artery infusion for the treatment of colorectal cancer metastatic to the liver. Metastatic tumors derive nearly all of their blood supply from the hepatic artery, while the normal liver parenchyma derives more than two-thirds of its blood supply from the portal system. This permits the delivery of higher doses of chemotherapeutic agents to the tumor relative to the normal hepatocytes. The drug most commonly used in this protocol is floxuridine, which is almost completely extracted on its first pass through the liver, resulting in relatively low systemic toxicity. Hepatic artery infusion requires the surgical placement of a catheter into the hepatic artery, which is connected to an implanted or external infusion pump for continuous treatment. Hepatic artery infusion has been used for unresectable colorectal metastases as well as an adjuvant to hepatic resection. While there are clearly improved tumor responses in comparison to systemic therapy, the data is less clear on overall survival benefits. Some studies, however, have suggested an improved survival and have stimulated further investigation.

Chu E, DeVita VT: *Physicians' Cancer Chemotherapy Drug Manual.* Jones and Bartlett Publishers, 2003.

Dizon DS, Kemeny NE: Intrahepatic arterial infusion of chemotherapy: clinical results. Semin Oncol 2002;29:126.

Fraker DL: Hyperthermic regional perfusion for melanoma and sarcoma of the limbs. Curr Probl Surg 1999;36:841.

HORMONAL THERAPY

Hormones are normally involved in the differentiation, stimulation, and control of certain tissues, including but not limited to lymphoid tissue, the uterus, the prostate, and the mammary glands. Tumors arising from these tissues may also be stimulated or inhibited by hormones, and so manipulation of the hormonal balance can be beneficial in the systemic therapy of these cancers. In some cases, hormones themselves are used as cancer therapies. For example, the administration of estrogen to a man ultimately suppresses the production of testosterone, which is useful in the treatment of prostate cancer. Corticosteroids, particularly the glucocorticoids, have a powerful suppressive effect on lymphoid cells, making them useful in the treatment of acute leukemias, lymphomas, myeloma, and other myeloproliferative disorders. In most cases, however, hormonal therapy involves blocking the effects of hormones that stimulate proliferation.

Estrogen & Androgen Inhibitors

One approach to hormonal therapy is to block the hormone receptor on the cell. Selective estrogen receptor modulators (SERM) are medications that mimic the structure of estrogen. Because the estrogen-receptor complex varies among tissue types, SERMs can have different effects on different tissues, sometimes inhibiting the actions of estrogen while sometimes behaving like estrogen. The most well-known SERM is tamoxifen, which is used not only to treat estrogen-sensitive breast cancer but also to prevent breast cancer in high-risk individuals. Because it also has some pro-estrogen properties, side effects of tamoxifen can include an increased risk of uterine cancer and deep vein thrombosis. Raloxifene is a newer SERM that has been approved for prevention and treatment of postmenopausal osteoporosis and is presently being studied in the chemoprevention of breast cancer. Research is ongoing to identify related compounds that act like estrogen in desirable ways but do not act like estrogen in undesirable ways.

Flutamide is a testosterone antagonist used in the treatment of prostate cancer. It works by blocking translocation of the androgen receptor to the nucleus. Although hormonal therapy for prostate cancer is palliative, it can be quite effective in slowing the progression of disease. Hormonal therapy can add several years to the life expectancy of patients with unresectable or metastatic disease. Flutamide is most effective when used in combination with surgical or pharmacologic castration.

Gonadotropin-Releasing Hormone Analogues

The most definitive way to block the production of testosterone and estrogen is by surgical castration. The pharmacologic equivalent of castration can be accomplished with leuprolide, an analogue of gonadotropin-releasing hormone (GnRH). Normally, GnRH leads to the production of LH and FSH, the physiologic stimulators of sex hormone production. Constant stimulation with leuprolide actually inhibits LH and FSH release and leads to decreased synthesis of the sex steroids. Leuprolide is commonly used to decrease testosterone levels in the treatment of unresectable prostate cancer. In premenopausal women, estrogen levels fall to postmenopausal values with leuprolide administration. For this reason, the drug can be useful in the treatment of estrogen receptor-positive breast cancers in premenopausal women.

Aromatase Inhibitors

Postmenopausal women have functionally inactive ovaries; however, estrogens are still produced to a lesser extent in extragonadal tissues, primarily the conversion of adrenal steroids in fat cells by the enzyme aromatase. Aromatase inhibitors can eliminate functional estrogen in this population of women and may be an effective hormonal treatment of breast cancer. The selective aromatase inhibitor, anastrozole, is approved for the treatment of metastatic breast cancer and appears promising as adjuvant therapy for postmenopausal women whose tumors possess estrogen or progesterone receptors. Another aromatase inhibitor, letrozole, has been shown to be beneficial as continued hormonal therapy in women who have completed 5 years of adjuvant therapy with tamoxifen.

RADIATION THERAPY

Radiation therapy may be used alone or in combination with surgery and chemotherapy and may be given with curative or palliative intent. Some tumors, such as head and neck cancers, prostate cancer, and Hodgkin's disease, can often be cured by irradiation alone, eliminating the need for surgical resection or chemotherapy. More commonly, locoregional control of tumors often involves surgical resection combined with localized radiation. The theoretical advantage of combining these two therapies is based on the mechanisms by which they fail to achieve their purpose. Surgical failures occur at the margins of tumors, while radiation therapy fails in the center of tumors, where the malignant cells are numerous and hypoxic conditions exist. Radiation failures are rare at the periphery of tumors, where cell numbers are low and oxygenation is high. Depending on tumor histology and location, radiation therapy can be used as a surgical adjunct either preoperatively or postoperatively. Preoperative radiation can shrink tumors and increase the chances for complete surgical resection in cancers such as sarcomas, rectal cancers, and superior sulcus lung cancers.

Principles of Radiation Therapy

Ionizing radiation is defined as energy with sufficient strength to cause the ejection of an orbital electron from an atom when the radiation is absorbed. Ionizing radiation can take either an electromagnetic form, as high-energy photons, or particulate forms, such as electrons, protons, neutrons, alpha particles, or other particles. Most radiation therapies utilize either photons or electrons. Electrons interact directly with tissue, causing ionization, in contrast to photons, which affect tissues by the electrons that they eject. Electron beams deliver a high skin dose and exhibit a rapid fall-off after only a few centimeters, and are therefore commonly used to treat superficial targets such as skin cancers or lymph nodes within a few centimeters of the surface of the body. More commonly, electromagnetic radiation (high energy photons) is used to treat cancer. This consists of either gamma rays (photons created from the decay of radioactive nuclei) or x-rays (photons created by interaction of accelerated electrons with electrons and nuclei of atoms in an x-ray tube target).

To quantify the interaction of radiation on tissues, one must first measure the ionization produced in air by the beam of radiation. This quantity is known as **exposure**, and is measured in roentgens (R). One can then correct for the presence of soft tissue, and calculate the **absorbed dose**; the amount of energy absorbed per unit mass. This was previously measured in rads, but today is typically measured as joules per kilogram, or gray (Gy) units; 100 rad = 100 cGy = 1 Gy. As photons enter tissue, the dose increases at first and then begins to fall off as a result of the fact that radiation falls off with the square of the distance from the source (a law of physics known as the Inverse Square Law).

The effect on biological tissues when they encounter ionizing radiation comes from ejected electrons either interacting directly with target molecules within the cell, or indirectly with water to produce free radicals (such as hydroxyl radicals) that subsequently interact with target molecules. During their brief life span, electrons and free radicals interact with molecules in a random fashion. If they interact with molecules that are not crucial to cell survival, the effect of the radiation will be harmless. If they react with biologically important molecules, the effect will be detrimental. Molecular oxygen prolongs the life of reactive radicals, increasing the likelihood that it will have a detrimental effect. This is why tumor hypoxia tends to increase resistance to radiation.

While ionizing radiation may damage many molecules with the cell, the most critical injury with respect to cell death appears to be DNA damage in the form of single- or double-strand breaks. Cells have relatively efficient repair mechanisms for single-strand breaks in DNA, but double-strand breaks in DNA are much more difficult for cells to repair, although not impossible. Therefore, the ability of ionizing radiation to kill cells is dependent not only on the generation of enough DNA double-strand breaks to overwhelm repair pathways but also on the time the cell has to repair those breaks prior to the next mitotic cell division.

This phenomenon is known as **sublethal damage repair**, in which increased cell survival is observed if a dose of radiation is divided into two fractions separated by a time interval. As the time interval between the fractions increases, the surviving fraction of the cells also increases as the cells are able to repair double-strand DNA breaks. Of course, in clinical radiation therapy, the goal is to kill the cancer cells but spare the normal cells. Delivering a single large dose of radiation will have a high rate of tumor cell killing, but the concordant killing of the normal tissue cells may limit the clinical utility due to normal tissue toxicity. This has led to the development of multi-fraction regimens commonly used today, typically delivering daily fractions of 1.8–2.5 Gy. *Fractionation* of radiation dose spares normal tissues because of their greater ability to repair sublethal damage between dose fractions and repopulate with cells if the overall time is sufficiently long.

Modes of Delivery

A. Teletherapy

Radiation is administered by two methods: an external machine (teletherapy) or the implantation of radioactive sources in or around the tumor (brachytherapy). In the past, teletherapy radiation was delivered using cobalt 60, a radioisotope produced in nuclear reactors. Although cobalt machines were very reliable, their usefulness is restricted by limited penetration to deep tumors without significant skin toxicity and difficulty in confining the dose to normal tissues. Today, external radiation is most often administered using a linear accelerator, capable of producing higher energy photons without the geometric disadvantages associated with cobalt 60 units.

No matter the source, the beam of radiation needs to be modified to get optimal delivery of the desired dose to the tumor while minimizing dose to the normal tissues. Typically, the beam of radiation is rectangular. Collimators are thick shielding devices made from materials with a high atomic number. Primary collimators at the head of the machine create a rectangular beam, and additional devices such as wedges, compensators, blocks, or multileaf collimators are used to further modify the beam to desired specifications. Wedges or compensators can optimize the dose distribution if the treatment surface is curved or irregular in shape. The beam can also be shaped using individually fashioned blocks custom-made for each patient's anatomy and tumor size and shape. In modern linear accelerators, multileaf collimators have replaced handmade blocks and allow automated and precise field-shaping without the use of cumbersome handmade blocks.

B. Brachytherapy

Brachytherapy involves the placement of radioactive sources into or next to the target tissue. It takes advantage the inverse square law, which states that the intensity of electromagnetic radiation dissipates as the inverse square of the distance from the source. Thus, if radioactive sources can be placed so that the tumor is within a centimeter of the sources, the dose received by normal tissues just 2 cm distant from the source and 1 cm distant from the tumor would be one quarter of the dose received by the tumor. This can allow delivery of a high dose to the tumor with only a modest dose to normal tissue.

There are many implantation techniques for brachytherapy. The surgical approach to the target volume may be interstitial (such as prostate seed implantation), intracavitary (such as gynecologic applicators), transluminal (such as endoscopic applications), or surface mold techniques (such as eye plaques for ocular melanoma). The implants may be permanent or temporary and the dose may be delivered using low, medium, or high dose rates. Many modern applications use afterloading techniques that place treatment applicators and load radioactive sources afterwards to reduce radiation exposure for therapy personnel.

COMPLICATIONS OF RADIATION THERAPY

A. Acute Radiation Effects

Acute radiation effects refer to those toxicities that occur within a few weeks to months of radiation therapy. They occur mainly in self-renewing tissues that are characterized by actively proliferating stem cells producing progeny that divide and differentiate into mature functioning cells. This includes bone marrow, skin and its appendages, and mucosal surfaces of the oropharynx, esophagus, stomach, intestines, rectum, bladder, and vagina. Once the normal life span of the mature cells expires, the normal turnover and replacement with new cells does not occur because of radiation killing of the dividing stem cells. Acute toxicity is influenced by both fraction size and the time interval between fractions. The more rapidly a given dose is delivered during the overall treatment period, the more severe the acute effects will be. A decrease in fraction size or prolongation of the interval between fractions allows the cell populations to repair and repopulate, decreasing the severity of acute toxicity.

Head and neck irradiation is among the most toxic in the acute period due to significant mucositis of the oral cavity, oropharynx, larynx, and cervical esophagus. Skin and the salivary glands are also affected. Mucositis, yeast superinfection, desquamation, pain, xerostomia, odynophagia, dysphagia, dehydration, and malnutrition are all common clinical scenarios that radiation oncologists manage when delivering head and neck radiotherapy. Other common acute effects observed during radiation therapy directed at other anatomic sites include dysphagia and cough from thoracic radiation, nausea, vomiting and diarrhea from abdominal radiation, and dysuria, proctitis, and perineal desquamation and pain from pelvic radiation.

B. Late Radiation Effects

Late effects refer to those toxicities that occur months to years after radiotherapy and are more commonly permanent. Mitotically inactive tissues without the capacity for self-renewal are commonly involved. The mechanism causing late effects may include direct damage to the parenchymal cells within an organ or indirect effects due to microvascular damage. Each organ is characterized by a **tolerance dose**, a radiation dose above which the risk of organ complications increases rapidly. These normal tissue tolerances are the true dose-limiting factors in clinical radiation therapy, because late complications can be permanent and in some cases, life-threatening.

The types of late complications induced by radiation can vary. For the brain, late toxicity may mean necrosis of the brain tissue, while in the kidney it may mean nephrotic syndrome and organ failure. The tolerance doses for different organs vary over a large range, ranging from a few Gy for sterility from testicular irradiation to over 100 Gy for necrosis or perforation of the uterus. Late complications may include fibrosis, necrosis, ulceration and bleeding, chronic edema, telangiectasias and pigmentation changes, cataract formation, nerve damage, lung pneumonitis and fibrosis, pericarditis, myocardial damage, bone fracture, liver or kidney failure, sterility, intestinal obstruction, and fistula and stricture formation.

Perez CA, Brady LW (editors): *Principles and Practice of Radiation Oncology,* 4th ed. Lippincott Williams & Wilkins, 2003.

Tobias JS, Thomas PRM (editors): *Current Radiation Oncology,* vol 3. Oxford Univ Press, 1998.

IMMUNOTHERAPY

Principles of Antitumor Immune Responses

Immunotherapy refers to treatments designed to kill tumor cells through immune mechanisms. There are two broad types of antitumor immune responses; one involving the humoral arm of the immune system and the other involving the cellular arm. Humoral immunity involves antibody production by mature B lymphocytes. Cell-mediated immunity involves stimulation of cytotoxic (CD8+) T cells through a major histocompatibility complex (MHC) class I-restricted process and stimulation of helper (CD4+) T cells through an MHC class II-restricted process. The humoral and cell-mediated immune responses overlap in that the activation of a B cell response usually requires the presence of helper T cells. Whether a humoral or a cell-mediated immune response is more important in generating antitumor immunity is still debated; however, patients who exhibit both responses appear to fare better than those who demonstrate only one type of response or no response.

Essential to the generation of an immune response through either arm of the immune system is the ability of antigen presenting cells (APCs), such as monocytes, macrophages, B cells, and dendritic cells (DC), to process and present tumor-related peptide antigens. Proteins are phagocytosed by APCs and partially digested into smaller polypeptides. These small peptide antigens are then bound to MHC molecules on the cell surface. These unique antigen: MHC complexes can then be recognized by naïve T lymphocytes through the T-cell receptor (TCR). When a naïve helper (CD4+) T cell recognizes the antigen being expressed on the MHC class II molecule and also recognizes costimulatory molecules present on the APC, it becomes activated, resulting in proliferation and differentiation. There are two types of helper T cells. The Th1 helper T cells produces cytokines to promote a cellular response (IL-2, IFN-γ, TNF-α, GM-CSF). In the presence of these cytokines, naïve cytotoxic (CD8+) T cells that recognize antigen being presented on MHC class I molecules on the surface of an APC become activated. Once activated, cytolytic T cells destroy tumor cells via T-cell receptor recognition of tumor-specific antigen presented on MHC class I molecules at the tumor cell surface. Antigen-specific T cells bind to the MHC I receptor-tumor antigen complex and destroy the tumor cell via the release of granules containing granzyme B and perforin and via induction of the FAS/FAS ligand apoptosis. Cytotoxic T cells can only recognize antigen expressed on the tumor surface in the context of the MHC class I molecule.

The second type of helper T cell (Th2) secretes B-cell stimulatory cytokines (IL-4, IL-5, IL-10), which results in the proliferation and differentiation of plasma cells. As opposed to a cellular response, for an antibody response the antigens do not have to be presented on class I MHC receptors. Tumor cells can then be killed by a variety of methods. Antibody-dependent cell mediated cytotoxicity (ADCC) involves the attachment of tumor-specific antibodies to tumor cells and the subsequent destruction of the tumor cell by the natural killer (NK) cell. Complement-dependent cell-mediated cytotoxicity involves the recognition and attachment of complement-fixing antibodies to tumor-specific surface antigens followed by complement activation. A third mechanism of tumor destruction, opsonization, results when tumor-specific antibodies attach to their target antigens on tumor cell surfaces, thus marking them for engulfment by macrophages.

There are several methods by which the immune system may be incorporated into cancer therapy. Immunotherapy can be categorized as either active or passive. With passive immunotherapy, the host need not mount an immune response; the therapeutic agent will directly or indirectly mediate tumor killing. Examples of passive immunotherapy include the use of monoclonal antibodies or adoptive (cellular) immunotherapy. Active immunotherapy, on the other hand, refers to the delivery of materials designed to elicit an immune response by the host. This can further be broken down to nonspecific and specific active immunotherapies. Nonspecific agents are those that stimulate the immune system globally but do not recruit tumor-specific effector cells. Active specific immunotherapy is designed to elicit an immune response to one or more tumor antigens, the prime example being the use of vaccines.

Passive Immunotherapy (Monoclonal Antibodies)

The development of monoclonal antibodies with unique specificity to tumor antigens has allowed for multiple attempts to utilize them as cancer therapy. In addition to their relative selectivity and minimal toxicity, they are easily mass-produced for widespread application. Rituximab (Rituxan) is an anti-CD20 monoclonal antibody that is approved for the treatment of relapsed or refractory low-grade or follicular non-Hodgkin's lymphoma (NHL). Trastuzumab (Herceptin) is the first monoclonal antibody to be effective against solid tumors. Trastuzumab binds to HER-2/neu, a transmembrane glycoprotein receptor that is overexpressed in 25–30% of human breast cancers. It is FDA approved for the treatment of metastatic breast cancer and is being studied in the adjuvant setting. Antibodies directed against CEA and 17-1A/EpCAM are presently being evaluated as adjuvant therapies in colorectal cancer.

Adoptive Immunotherapy

Adoptive immunotherapy refers to the passive administration of cells with antitumor activity to the tumor-bearing host. Tumor-infiltrating lymphocytes (TIL) are lymphocytes that infiltrate growing tumors and can be isolated by growing single-cell suspensions from the tumor in the presence of IL-2. They have been isolated from virtually all types of tumors and are capable of recognizing tumor-associated antigens. Lymphokine-activated killer (LAK) cells can be obtained by growing human peripheral blood lymphocytes with high doses of IL-2. LAK cells have properties similar to both NK cells and cytotoxic T lymphocytes and appear capable of lysing tumor cells but not normal cells. Adoptive immunotherapy is presently under active investigation, primarily as a treatment of metastatic melanoma and renal cell carcinoma.

Nonspecific Active Immunotherapy

A. Immunostimulants

Before the mechanism by which the immune system can eradicate tumor cells was fully understood, early attempts at immunotherapy involved nonspecific stimulation of the immune system. The idea was that any increase in immune reactivity would be associated with a concomitant increase in the antitumor immune response. Probably the most widely embraced immunostimulant investigated has been the use of bacille Calmette-Guérin (BCG), a modified form of the tubercle bacillus. Initial trials suggested a possible benefit, but multiple prospective, randomized trials in various malignancies have failed to substantiate a survival benefit of BCG, either alone or in combination with other therapeutics. Local therapy with BCG in the bladder eliminates superficial bladder cancers and prevents tumor recurrences. It is one of several standard therapies for patients with bladder cancer. It is also being studied as an adjuvant to other immunotherapies, such as vaccines. Levamisole is an antihelminthic drug that was reported to have several immunomodulatory properties. Although the exact mechanism of action is unknown, it has been effective in the adjuvant therapy of colorectal cancer.

B. Cytokines

Cytokines are naturally occurring soluble proteins produced by mononuclear cells of the immune system that can affect the growth and function of cells through interaction with specific cell-surface receptors. There have been over 50 cytokines isolated to date, and several have subsequently been approved by the FDA for clinical use, including interferon-α and IL-2.

The interferons (IFN-α, IFN-β, IFN-γ) were originally described as proteins produced by virally infected cells that serve to protect against further viral infection through a variety of effects. These include the increased antigen presentation via increased expression of MHC and antigens, enhancement of NK cell function, and the enhancement of ADCC. In addition, the interferons exert direct antiangiogenic, cytotoxic, and cytostatic effects. While the anticancer effects of IFN-β and IFN-γ have been disappointing, several hematologic and solid tumors have proved responsive to IFN-α, including chronic myelogenous leukemia, cutaneous T-cell lymphoma, hairy cell leukemia, melanoma, and Kaposi's sarcoma. It is unclear whether the predominant effect of interferon is the direct antiproliferative activity or the immunologic actions.

IL-2 was originally described as the "T-cell growth factor" because it is required for the differentiation and proliferation of activated T cells. As such, it seems like an ideal choice for immunotherapy. The major drawback of IL-2 is the significant dose-related toxicity. IL-2 leads to significant interstitial edema and vascular depletion and lymphoid infiltration into vital organs. This can lead to severe hypotension and resultant ischemic damage to the heart, liver, kidneys, and bowel, which limits the use of IL-2 to patients with excellent performance status, normal pulmonary and cardiac function, and no active infections. Despite these limitations, IL-2 has proved to be an effective therapy in patients with metastatic melanoma and metastatic renal cell carcinoma.

Specific Active Immunotherapy (Vaccines)

The goal of cancer vaccines is to generate a host immune response to known or unknown tumor-associated antigens. Many different vaccine strategies are under investigation, each with advantages and disadvantages in regard to clinical feasibility, cost, the number of antigens available, and the mechanism of response (cellular, humoral, or both). Some vaccine strategies use specific peptide antigens. These are highly purified and, therefore, are easy to standardize, distribute, and administer. Unfortunately, immunizing a patient against a single antigen has several drawbacks that limit the potential clinical benefit. If a peptide vaccine does stimulate a response, it may not be the "right" peptide for many patients. Even commonly expressed tumor antigens are not present on all patients' tumors, or they may be present in varying degrees. In addition, the T cell's recognition of an antigen depends on the presentation of that antigen on a specific MHC molecule. Only certain human lymphocyte antigen (HLA) phenotypes can present any given peptide to induce an immune response, so they will only function on a limited subset of patients. A classic example is that of the MART-1/Melan-A antigen in melanoma. The antigen is expressed by 80% of melanomas, but the peptide only binds to HLA-A2. Because only about 45% of Caucasians have HLA-A2, only 36% (80% of 45%) of Caucasian melanoma patients given a MART-1/Melen-A vaccine would see a benefit. Finally, a cancer can escape immune recognition rather simply if a population of cells stops expressing that antigen or the MHC molecule.

For many cancers, only a few tumor-associated antigens have been defined; these may not be present on a large percentage of patients. Using the patient's cancer as the vaccine precludes the need to identify specific antigens. Autologous tumor cell vaccines are created from cancer cells harvested from the patient, altered to be more immunogenic, and irradiated, before being returned to the patient to stimulate a tumor-specific immune response. This approach is limited to individuals with sufficient tumor to prepare a vaccine. This has restricted trials to patients with bulky nodal or accessible distant metastatic disease who have a poor overall prognosis to begin with. Furthermore, the technical complexities inherent in procuring tumor and preparing a vaccine have made it difficult to conduct multi-institutional trials to test the efficacy of these vaccines.

Since many tumor-associated antigens are shared among a large number of patients, it is possible that one could create a vaccine from cultured cell lines that would stimulate an antitumor immune response in any patient who shared some of those antigens. This is the principle behind allogeneic tumor cell vaccines. This approach offers several advantages over autologous vaccines: Allogeneic vaccines are readily available, even for patients who lack sufficient tumor to produce an autologous tumor cell vaccine, and can be standardized, preserved, and distributed in a manner akin to any other therapeutic agent. Several allogeneic vaccines are being studied as adjuvant therapies in melanoma, including Canvaxin and Melacine.

Abbas AK, Lichtman AH, Pober JS (editors): *Cellular and Molecular Immunology,* 5th ed. Saunders, 2003.

Janeway C et al (editors): *Immunobiology,* 5th ed. Garland Science, 2003.

Ribas J et al: Current developments in cancer vaccines and cellular immunotherapy. J Clin Oncol 2003;21:2415.

SPECIFIC TYPES OF MALIGNANT NEOPLASMS

SOFT TISSUE SARCOMA

Soft tissue sarcomas account for approximately 1% of all new cancer diagnoses. Almost half of all patients diagnosed with the disease eventually die as a result of the cancer. Soft tissue sarcomas can occur anywhere in the body, but most originate in an extremity (59%), the trunk (19%), the retroperitoneum (15%), or the head and neck (9%). Soft tissue sarcomas originate from a wide variety of mesenchymal cell types and include malignant fibrous histiocytoma, liposarcoma, rhabdomyosarcoma, leiomyosarcoma, and desmoid tumors. While the histopathology of these tumors is highly variable, with some exceptions they tend to behave in a fashion dictated by tumor grade rather than the cell of origin.

Most soft tissue sarcomas arise de novo, and rarely do they result from malignant degeneration of a benign lesion. There are several familial syndromes in which patients are genetically predisposed to the formation of soft tissue sarcomas, including Li-Fraumeni syndrome, Recklinghausen's disease, and Gardner's syndrome. Other proven risk factors exist that may increase the chances of sarcoma formation. External radiation therapy can increase the incidence of sarcomas by 8- to 50-fold. Chronic extremity lymphedema also increases the risk for lymphangiosarcoma. A classic example is the development of upper extremity lymphangiosarcomas in the lymphedematous arm of women treated for breast cancer (Stewart-Treves syndrome). Other less clear associations link chronic tissue trauma and occupational chemical exposures with an increased risk for sarcoma formation.

The major features of the staging system for soft tissue sarcomas (Table 46–2) are the grade of the tumor, its size, and the presence of metastatic disease. Although the site of the tumor is not considered in staging, patients with retroperitoneal tumors tend to have a worse prognosis. Sarcomas generally metastasize by the hematogenous route, and the metastatic sites of sarcomas are related to the location of the primary tumor. The vast majority of metastases from extremity sarcomas are to the lung, while the majority of retroperitoneal tumors metastasize to the liver. Lymph node involvement is rare with most soft tissue sarcomas, although this may occur with epithelioid sarcoma, clear cell sarcoma, angiosarcoma, rhabdomyosarcoma, or synovial sarcoma.

The most important prognostic variables for patients with soft tissue sarcoma are the size and grade of the primary tumor. Since grading is based on the cellular architecture and invasive nature of the tumor, FNAB is not a typically useful biopsy technique for the initial diagnosis of a sarcoma. If a tumor is small (< 3 cm) and superficial, excisional biopsy should be performed. All extremity biopsy incisions should be oriented longitudinally, as the biopsy incision scar should be excised in a subsequent definitive resection of the tumor. Core needle biopsies may be performed for large, palpable superficial tumors. For large deep tumors or those adjacent to vital structures, incisional biopsy is usually the diagnostic method of choice. The incision should be centered over the mass, tissue flaps should not be raised, and

Table 46–2. AJCC staging system for soft tissue sarcoma.

Primary Tumor (T)		
T1	Tumor 5 cm or less	
	T1a	Superficial tumor
	T1b	Deep tumor
T2	Tumor more than 5 cm	
	T2a	Superficial tumor
	T2b	Deep tumor
Regional Lymph Nodes (N)		
N0	No regional lymph node metastasis	
N1	Regional lymph node metastasis	
Distant Metastasis (M)		
M0	No distant metastasis	
M1	Distant metastasis	
Histopathologic Grade (G)		
G1	Well differentiated	
G2	Moderately differentiated	
G3	Poorly differentiated	
G4	Undifferentiated	
Stage Grouping		
Stage IA	G1-2, T1a-1b, N0, M0	
Stage IB	G1-2, T2a, N0, M0	
Stage IIA	G1-2, T2b, N0, M0	
Stage IIB	G3-4, T1a-1b, N0, M0	
Stage IIC	G3-4, T2a, N0, M0	
Stage III	G3-4, T2b, N0, M0	
Stage IV	Any G, any T, either N1 or M1	

meticulous hemostasis should be ensured, all to prevent the dissemination of tumor cells into adjacent tissue planes.

Treatment of Extremity Sarcomas

MRI is the imaging modality of choice for any suspected extremity sarcoma, as it is most accurate in defining the extent of the tumor and invasion of surrounding structures. MRI is also used for follow-up imaging to assess response in patients undergoing therapy, as well as for local and regional recurrence. A chest x-ray or chest CT should be obtained in order to evaluate for pulmonary metastases in patients with high-grade tumors.

Surgery remains the primary therapy for localized extremity sarcomas, but multimodality therapy is recommended to minimize the likelihood of recurrence or the need for amputation. Historically, amputation was the only form of curative surgical therapy for large extremity sarcomas, but multimodality therapy has allowed for a high rate of limb preservation. Today, fewer than 5% of patients with extremity soft tissue sarcoma require amputation, generally reserved for patients whose tumors do not respond to preoperative therapy and cannot be resected adequately, have no evidence of metastatic disease, and have a good prognosis for rehabilitation.

A pseudocapsule composed of tumor cells surrounds sarcomas, and local invasion along fascial planes and neurovascular structures is common. It is important not to dissect along the pseudocapsule, as this is associated with high local recurrence rates, but rather obtain a wide (2-cm) margin of normal tissue. This may need to be compromised in the immediate vicinity of functionally important neurovascular structures. If the tumor involves these structures, nerve grafts and arterial reconstruction with autologous or prosthetic conduits may be required. Large soft tissue defects often require the construction of myocutaneous flaps to improve function and cosmesis. Soft tissue sarcomas rarely invade bone or skin, and wide resections of these structures are infrequently necessary.

Following wide local excision, metal clips should be placed at all margins of the resection in order to guide subsequent radiotherapy. For patients with T1 tumors that are located superficially in an area where it is not difficult to obtain widely negative margins, postoperative radiation therapy may not be necessary. For most other lesions, postoperative radiation is almost always recommended, with either external beam radiation (EBRT) or brachytherapy. Radiation should be started 4–8 weeks after surgery, as delay can result in a lower local control rate. Preoperative radiotherapy may have some advantages in patients with large tumors. Lower doses can be delivered to an undisturbed tumor bed, which may also have better oxygenation, and larger tumors may decrease in size, allowing for limb-sparing procedures. Preoperative radiation is associated with an increase in short-term wound complications but a decrease in long-term tissue fibrosis and edema. The optimal mode and sequence for treatment has yet to be defined, and often requires a multidisciplinary approach.

Adjuvant chemotherapy remains controversial. Chemotherapy can be given either preoperatively or postoperatively. The three drugs most effective in sarcoma are doxorubicin, dacarbazine, and ifosfamide. Preoperative chemotherapy is sometimes recommended in that in addition to the early treatment of micrometastatic disease, it allows for assessment of tumor response, which helps avoid prolonged therapy in patients not responding. However, while disease-free survival may be improved, there are conflicting data on overall survival. A recent meta-analysis of randomized trials suggested there may be a small survival benefit for extremity sarcomas, and so its use has increased. Subsequent randomized trials have yielded conflicting results, and the evidence remains inconclusive.

The vast majority of localized recurrences in soft tissue sarcomas occur in the first 2 years after resection, necessitating close follow-up during that period. A local recurrence is not indicative of systemic disease and, in the absence of evidence of metastases, should be treated aggressively in the same manner as a primary tumor. The resection of pulmonary metastases should be considered in patients who have fewer than four radiographically detectable lesions and who have achieved apparent local control following resection of the primary tumor. In such circumstances, disease-free survival can approach 25–35%.

Treatment of Retroperitoneal Sarcomas

Retroperitoneal sarcomas comprise approximately 15% of all soft tissue sarcomas, with liposarcoma, malignant fibrous histiocytoma, and leiomyosarcoma the three most common types. They most commonly present as a large abdominal mass. Nearly half are over 20 cm in size at diagnosis. Once they compress or invade contiguous structures, they can cause symptoms such as abdominal pain or nausea and vomiting. Workup should include CT of the abdomen and pelvis to evaluate the mass, as well as lung and liver to look for metastases. CT-guided core biopsy is the sampling technique of choice, with open or laparoscopic incisional biopsy reserved for inconclusive core biopsies.

As with extremity sarcomas, surgery represents the primary treatment, with the goal being en bloc resection with a rim of normal tissue. Although retroperitoneal tumors are generally large at presentation and often invade vital structures, the majority of these tumors are resectable. Retroperitoneal sarcomas rarely invade surrounding organs, but an intense desmoplastic reaction makes it difficult to assess the extent of tumor, so often these organs need to be resected rather than risk positive margins. The kidney, colon, pancreas, and spleen are the most commonly resected organs.

While adjuvant radiation therapy is standard in extremity sarcoma, evidence supporting its use in retroperitoneal sarcoma is less convincing. Because of the low tolerance to radiation of the abdominal and retroperitoneal organs, delivery of adequate radiotherapy is often difficult. There is encouraging evidence for intraoperative radiation therapy to the tumor bed, but this technique is still considered investigational and can only be performed in select centers. Although complex, preoperative radiation may be beneficial, as it uses lower radiation doses, has less injury to the small bowel, and can increase respectability by shrinking the tumor and creating a thickened capsular structure around the lesion.

Karakousis CP: Surgery for soft tissue sarcomas. In: *Atlas of Surgical Oncology.* Bland KI, Karakousis CP, Copeland EM (editors). Saunders, 1995.

Tierney JF: Adjuvant chemotherapy for localized respectable soft-tissue sarcoma of adults: meta-analysis of individual data. Lancet 1997;350:1647.

Weiss SW, Goldblum JR, Franz M (editors): *Enzinger and Weiss's Soft Tissue Tumors,* 4th ed. Mosby, 2001.

MELANOMA

The incidence of melanoma is rising faster than any other cancer. The reasons for this are not clear, but are most likely related to an increased exposure to ultraviolet radiation from sunlight. Individuals whose first sunburn occurred at an early age have an increased incidence of melanoma. Other risk factors include freckles, a fair complexion, reddish or blond hair, blue eyes, a first-degree relative with melanoma, and the presence of multiple or dysplastic nevi.

The best approach to melanoma is to prevent it from occurring, through sun avoidance and sun protection with sunscreens with a sun protection factor (SPF) of 30 or higher. Second to prevention, the most significant impact on melanoma will come from early recognition and diagnosis. The prognosis of melanoma is inversely and dramatically related to the depth of invasion at diagnosis (Breslow thickness), emphasizing the importance of early diagnosis of this disease. Lesions that are suspicious for melanoma can be identified by their clinical characteristics, often referred to as the ABCDs of melanoma. (Table 46–3). Diagnosed early, well over 90% of primary melanomas can be cured with surgical excision alone. Patients presenting with thicker lesions or regional nodal metastases have a significantly poorer prognosis. The AJCC and UICC staging system is presented in Table 46–4.

There are four distinct categories of melanoma: superficial spreading, nodular, lentigo maligna, and acral lentiginous melanoma.

Superficial spreading melanoma is the most common presentation, accounting for nearly 70% of all melanomas. These usually occur in sun-exposed areas of the body or in individuals with multiple dysplastic nevi. They generally arise in preexisting nevi and can occur at any age after puberty. The superficial spreading subtype tends to grow in a radial pattern during the earlier stages and converts to a vertical growth pattern during the later stages of development.

Table 46–3. Clinical identification (ABCD) of melanoma.

Asymmetry: Asymmetric shape, color, or contour
Borders: Irregular or ill-defined borders
Color: Black, brown, blue, red, gray, or white
Diameter: Larger than 5 mm *or*
Difference: Any lesion that has changed

Table 46–4. AJCC staging system for cutaneous melanoma.

TNM Classification

T1	1.0 mm	a) Without ulceration and level II/III b) With ulceration or level IV/V
T2	1.01–2.0 mm	a) Without ulceration b) With ulceration
T3	2.01–4.0 mm	a) Without ulceration b) With ulceration
T4	> 4.0 mm	a) Without ulceration b) With ulceration
N0	No lymph node metastasis	
N1	Metastasis in 1 lymph node	a) Micrometastasis b) Macrometastasis
N2	Metastasis in 2–3 lymph nodes	a) Micrometastasis b) Macrometastasis c) In-transit metastasis with no nodal involvement
N3	Metastasis in 4 lymph nodes or matted lymph nodes or in-transit metastasis with nodal involvement	
M0	No distant metastasis	
M1	Distant metastasis	a) Skin, subcutaneous tissue, or lymph node metastasis, normal LDH b) Lung metastasis, normal LDH c) All other visceral or any distant metastasis with elevated LDH

Stage Groupings

IA	T1a N0 M0
IB	T1b N0 M0
	T2a N0 M0
IIA	T2b N0 M0
	T3a N0 M0
IIB	T3b N0 M0
	T4a N0 M0
IIC	T4b N0 M0
IIIA	T1–4a N1a, 2a M0
IIIB	T4b N1a, 2a M0
	T1–4a N1b, 2b M0
	Any T N2c M0
IIIC	T4b N1b, 2b M0
	Any T N3 M0
IV	Any T any N M1

Nodular melanomas account for between 15% and 25% of all melanomas. These tend to occur in older individuals and are more common in men. Nodular melanomas generally develop de novo, not in a preexisting nevus. They usually are dome shaped with distinct borders and often resemble a blood blister. Nodular melanomas occur most commonly on the head, neck, and trunk. They lack a significant horizontal growth phase and tend to be deep at the time of diagnosis.

Lentigo maligna melanoma has less propensity to metastasize and thus has a more favorable prognosis relative to the other subtypes. However, it can be locally aggressive, with high recurrence rates after excision. These lesions account for 4–10% of melanomas and occur in an older population. Lentigo maligna lesions almost always develop in sun-exposed areas. They have a long horizontal growth phase and often have very convoluted borders.

Acral lentiginous melanomas account for between 2% and 8% of melanomas in Caucasians but for 30–60% of melanomas in blacks, Asians, and Hispanics. These lesions do not occur in sun-exposed areas; instead, they occur on the sole of the foot, the palm, beneath the nail beds, and in the perineal region. Acral lentiginous melanomas are often large, with an average diameter of 3 cm at the time of diagnosis. They develop relatively rapidly over the course of months to several years and tend to behave very aggressively. The clinical characteristics of these melanomas are often unmistakable, with variegations in color and convoluted borders. Ulceration of these lesions is common.

Treatment of Primary Melanoma

Any suspected melanoma should be removed by punch or excisional biopsy. Given the importance of Breslow thickness, shave or curette biopsies are contraindicated. If the biopsy specimen reveals melanoma, a formal excision with adequate margins is required. Because microscopic tumor cells frequently surround primary melanomas, excision with narrow margins is associated with an unacceptably high rate of local recurrence. The current standard for lesions less than 1 mm in depth is excision with 1-cm margins. Melanomas between 1 mm and 4 mm in thickness should be excised with 2-cm margins. Those deeper than 4 mm should be excised with a 2- to 3-cm margin. The resection should be carried down to the underlying fascia.

Melanoma generally metastasize by the lymphatic route in a predictable and orderly fashion. Any palpable nodes must be considered suspicious for metastatic involvement, easily verified with a fine-needle aspiration biopsy. About 10% of patients have clinical evidence of nodal metastases upon initial presentation and should undergo a therapeutic lymph node dissection (TLND) at the time of their wide excision. Many patients will have microscopic disease in the lymph nodes that will not be apparent on physical examination. In the past, there was substantial controversy regarding elective lymph node dissection of the draining nodal basin for melanoma. This changed dramatically with the advent of the sentinel lymph node biopsy (SLNB), which is based on the anatomic concept that lymphatic fluid from defined regions of skin drains specifically to an initial node or nodes ("sentinel nodes") prior to disseminating to other nodes in the same or nearby basins. Sentinel node biopsy allows for a more detailed histologic examination of the sentinel lymph nodes and helps avoid the morbidity of lymph node dissection in patients who are pathologically node-negative. Patients with a negative sentinel node are over 6 times more likely to survive than those with a positive sentinel lymph node, making the predictive impact of sentinel node status much greater than any other prognostic factor.

The SLNB has become the standard of care in the staging and treatment of melanoma and should be performed at the time of the wide excision for primary melanomas thicker than 1.0 mm. It should be selectively applied for tumors between 0.75 mm and 1.0 mm, when other worrisome features are present, such as ulceration or a high mitotic rate. Melanomas less than 0.75 mm are very unlikely to have regional metastases and do not require SLNB. The dominant drainage basins can be identified by lymphoscintigraphy, which involves intradermal injection of technetium-99m sulfur colloid in the area around the tumor and a gamma camera to image the sites of lymph node drainage. In the operating room, isosulfan blue dye is injected in a similar fashion. Any lymph nodes that have evidence of Tc-99m uptake on a handheld gamma probe, have evidence of blue dye, or are clinically suspicious should be excised. After removal of the nodes, they are analyzed by serial thin-sectioning, routine H&E staining, and immunohistochemical staining. Using these methods of analysis, the pathologist is able to detect even minute numbers of metastatic melanoma cells in the sentinel node. Patients with a positive SLNB should undergo formal lymph node dissection of the entire drainage basin.

Traditional chemotherapy regimens have proved largely ineffective in the treatment of melanoma; however, the cytokine interferon alfa-2b has been shown to improve disease-free and overall survival in high-risk patients with no evidence of systemic metastases. This is not without controversy, however, as the duration of therapy is long (12 months), the toxicities are substantial, and some of the data regarding the overall survival benefit are conflicting. Even so, interferon alfa-2b remains the only approved adjuvant therapy of melanoma, and all patients with high-risk melanoma (node-positive melanoma or thick, node-negative melanoma) should have a balanced discussion of the potential risks and benefits. A large body of research investigating the use of vaccines in the treatment of high-risk melanoma patients has shown great promise, but such therapies are still in the experimental stage. While melanoma is relatively radioresistant, there may be some benefit to regional control after node dissection with radiation in patients with gross extracapsular extension or multiple involved lymph nodes.

Local Recurrence & In-Transit Metastasis

Although rare with appropriate surgery, an isolated local recurrence can be treated with a repeat wide excision with 2-cm margins. Approximately 2–3% of melanoma patients will develop in-transit metastasis, which is the appearance of metastasis along the path from the primary tumor to its regional nodal basin, and is lymphatic in nature. The management of in-transit metastasis is dictated by the number and the size of the lesions. If few in number, surgical excision with a margin of surrounding normal cutaneous and subcutaneous tissue is appropriate; however, this becomes unlikely with multiple lesions. Intralesional therapy with granulocyte-macrophage colony-stimulating factor (GM-CSF) can result in significant regression of melanoma deposits. Although melanoma is relatively radiation-resistant, this therapy can provide palliation in unresectable lesions in many cases. Radiation therapy should be considered in those patients with a smaller volume of cutaneous or subcutaneous metastases.

Hyperthermic isolated limb perfusion (HILP) is a way of isolating the blood circuit to the extremity and administering chemotherapeutic agents regionally at a concentration 15–25 times higher without resulting in systemic side effects. Melphalan has been used as a standard drug for HILP secondary to its efficacy and low regional toxicity. While this has not been shown to improve survival, the use of HILP provides a significant palliation of locoregional symptoms when other options are not available.

Regional and systemic recurrence of melanoma can be latent, and recurrence 10 years after the original diagnosis is not uncommon. This fact necessitates close lifelong follow-up of these patients. Patients with a past history of melanoma have a dramatically increased risk of developing a second primary lesion and require diligent screening for other lesions.

Balch CM et al: *Cutaneous Melanoma,* 4th ed. Quality Medical Publishing, 2003.

Balch CM et al: Efficacy of 2-cm surgical margins for intermediate-thickness melanomas (1 to 4 mm). Results of a multi-institutional randomized surgical trial. Ann Surg 1993;218:262.

Leong SP: Selective sentinel lymphadenectomy for malignant melanoma. Surg Clin North Am 2003;83:157.

Sabel MS, Sondak VK: Pros and cons of adjuvant interferon in the treatment of melanoma. Oncologist. 2003;8:451.

Table 46–5. Classic subtypes of Hodgkin's lymphoma.

Subtype	Characteristics
Lymphocyte-predominant	Uncommon (6% of Hodgkin's lymphomas), diffuse lymphocytic infiltrate with few Reed-Sternberg cells, excellent prognosis
Lymphocyte-depleted	Rare (2% of Hodgkin's lymphoma), abundant Reed-Sternberg cells, paucity of lymphocytes, occurs in older males, aggressive clinically
Mixed cellularity	Common (20–25% of Hodgkin's lymphoma), histologically intermediate between above two forms, often presents with disseminated disease
Nodular sclerosis	Most common form (70% of Hodgkin's lymphoma), fibrosis with Reed-Sternberg and lymphoid cells, more common in young women, presents with cervical or mediastinal disease

LYMPHOMA

Lymphomas are malignant neoplasms that originate from the lymphoid tissues. Two distinct categories of lymphoma exist: Hodgkin's and non-Hodgkin's. The two types not only have different morphologic characteristics but differ also in their clinical behavior and their response to various therapeutic regimens. It is not possible to differentiate Hodgkin's and non-Hodgkin's lymphoma on clinical grounds, but only by surgical biopsy. In the diagnosis of a suspected lymphoma, excisional biopsy of the entire lymph node or nodes is imperative, as the architecture has a bearing on the diagnosis and the subsequent treatment of the tumor.

1. Hodgkin's Lymphoma

Hodgkin's lymphoma may occur at any age but is generally a disease of young adults. Prevalence in women peaks in the third decade and then falls, while it remains fairly constant in men after this time. The diagnosis of Hodgkin's lymphoma is based on the finding of Reed-Sternberg cells in an appropriate cellular background of reactive leukocytes and fibrosis. It is the pattern of the lymphocytic infiltrate that determines the classic subtypes of Hodgkin's disease (see Table 46–5). All subtypes of classical Hodgkin's lymphoma are presently treated in the same way, and modern therapy has allowed for cure of over 70% of patients with this malignancy.

The cause of Hodgkin's disease is not well understood; however, epidemiologic studies have revealed certain patterns of disease clustering. The incidence appears to be higher with a lower number of siblings, early birth order, siblings with Hodgkin's disease, a decreased number of playmates, certain HLA antigens, single-family dwellings, and patients who have undergone tonsillectomy. The incidence is increased also in persons with immunodeficiencies and autoimmune disorders. This pattern suggests that an oncogenic virus may cause Hodgkin's. Nuclear proteins of the Epstein-Barr virus (EBV) have been detected in about 40% of classical Hodgkin's lymphoma, and alternative lymphotropic viruses may be involved in the pathogenesis of cases negative for EBV.

Most patients present with enlarged but painless lymph nodes, typically in the lower neck or supraclavicular region. On occasion, mediastinal masses are associated with cough or dyspnea or discovered on routine chest x-ray. About 25% of patients will have systemic symptoms, called B symptoms, including weight loss, pruritus, fever, and drenching night sweats.

Staging

With regard to therapy, the most important prognostic factor in Hodgkin's lymphoma is the disease stage. The currently accepted classification for Hodgkin's is the Ann Arbor staging system (Table 46–6).

As discussed earlier, excisional lymph node biopsy is essential to the diagnosis of Hodgkin's lymphoma. Once the diagnosis is made, disease staging begins with a detailed history and physical examination, with attention to all lymph node beds, B symptoms, and symptoms related to extranodal involvement. CT of the chest, abdomen, and pelvis is the major means of staging intrathoracic and

Table 46–6. Modified Ann Arbor staging system of Hodgkin's lymphoma.

Stage I	Involving one lymph node group or structure or extends locally to involve a single adjacent site (stage IE)
Stage II	Involving two or more lymph node groups on the same side of the diaphragm or involves one or more lymph node groups on the same side of the diaphragm and there is localized involvement of the node(s) to one organ or site on the same side of the diaphragm (stage IIE)
Stage III	Involves lymph node groups on both sides of the diaphragm, or has extended to an organ or site next to the lymph nodes and/or spleen (stage IIIE)
Stage III 1	With/without involved nodes of the spleen, hilum, abdomen, or liver
Stage III 2	With involved nodes of the aorta, iliac or mesenteric arteries
Stage IV	Spread throughout the bloodstream to one or more organs or sites outside of the lymphatic system, with or without associated lymph node involvement

intra-abdominal disease. Bone marrow biopsy is also part of the staging evaluation of patients with bony symptoms or cytopenias. Positron emission tomography may prove to be more accurate than CT, but is not yet standard.

Clinical studies attempting to detect disease below the diaphragm may be falsely positive or negative in 25–33% of patients. Occasionally, a staging laparotomy is recommended if the anatomic extent of disease in the abdomen is important in guiding therapy. The staging laparotomy includes splenectomy, wedge liver biopsy, and dissection of the para-aortic, iliac, splenic hilar, and hepatic portal lymph nodes. If a female patient is likely to receive pelvic radiotherapy, an oophoropexy is performed. However, staging laparotomy is associated with potential morbidity and mortality and delays the initiation of therapy for several weeks. Therefore, the indications for staging laparotomy have been narrowed significantly in recent years. Only patients whose clinical stage is IIA or less and in whom mantle radiation is planned should be considered, and most oncologists forgo the staging laparotomy unless the procedure is absolutely necessary to guide therapy.

Treatment

In patients with localized (stage I or stage II) disease, external beam radiotherapy alone is the standard treatment. Wide field radiation rather than irradiation of involved areas is the current standard. Depending on the extent of disease, mantle, subtotal, or total lymphoid irradiation is performed. Mantle radiation consists of irradiation of the cervical, axillary, mediastinal, and hilar lymph nodes. Subtotal lymphoid irradiation (STLI) is treatment of the mantle plus the upper abdominal, para-aortic, and splenic bed lymph nodes. Total lymphoid irradiation (TLI) refers to irradiation of the pelvic field in addition to STLI.

Complete remission rates are high with wide field radiation, but relapse is frequent, as high as 20–30%. Relapse risk can be reduced by use of combined treatment with radiation and chemotherapy, although there is little evidence this improves survival. The most commonly used regimens include MOPP (mechlorethamine, Oncovin [vincristine], procarbazine, and prednisone) and ABVD (doxorubicin [Adriamycin], bleomycin, vinblastine, and dacarbazine). It is debatable whether it is better to use a more extensive treatment initially to cure as many individuals as possible, or use a less aggressive therapy upfront, followed by more aggressive salvage therapy in patients who relapse. Patients with bulky mediastinal disease or multiple areas of extranodal involvement have the highest risk of relapse, and combined-modality therapy is indicated.

In addition to the subgroups discussed above, several other clinical scenarios require combined chemotherapy and radiotherapy. Patients with unfavorable disease stages (stage III and stage IV) or extensive splenic involvement by staging laparotomy should be treated by both modalities. Another group of patients who can benefit from combined therapy are children whose growing bones and muscles cannot tolerate radiation therapy in full doses.

Although the current therapeutic regimens for Hodgkin's lymphoma are quite efficacious, a subset of patients will fail to undergo remission, or their disease may recur after multimodality therapy. Patients with a long first remission may be considered for further standard-dose chemotherapy. Otherwise, high-dose chemotherapy with stem cell transplant (bone marrow transplant) should be considered.

Investigational immunotherapeutic regimens also appear to have potential in preventing relapse of higher-stage disease. In contrast to normal cells, Reed-Sternberg cells express large numbers of the surface antigen CD30. Radioimmunotherapy with ^{131}I-labeled antiCD30 monoclonal antibodies is presently being investigated, and preliminary results of trials using this immunotoxin appear very promising in decreasing the rate of relapse. Other approaches to immunotherapy under investigation for Hodgkin's disease include bispecific antibodies against CD30 and CD3, CD28 or CD25, and dendritic cell vaccines against EBV antigens.

2. Non-Hodgkin's Lymphoma

Non-Hodgkin's lymphoma encompasses a wide spectrum of lymphoid-derived tumors. This heterogeneous group of diseases includes more than ten distinct tumor subtypes with variable biologic behavior and responses to treatment. As opposed to Hodgkin's lymphoma, the prevalence of non-Hodgkin's lymphoma rises with age. The incidence has been rising steadily over the past 20 years by about 3–5% per year, for unknown reasons. Several risk factors have been identified that predispose patients to the development of disease. Patients with congenital disorders such as ataxia-telangiectasia, Wiskott-Aldrich syndrome, and celiac disease have an increased incidence of lymphoma. Certain acquired conditions also predispose patients to lymphoma, including prior chemotherapy or radiotherapy, immunosuppressive therapy, EBV infection, HIV infection, HTLV-1 infection, *Helicobacter pylori* gastritis, Hashimoto's thyroiditis, and Sjögren's syndrome.

Non-Hodgkin's lymphoma may originate from B cells, T cells, or histiocytes. Morphologically, the tumors may appear as nodular clusters or diffuse sheets of lymphoid cells.

Classically, non-Hodgkin's lymphoma presents as nontender enlargement of lymph nodes, but nearly one-third of all cases originate outside the lymph nodes. These extranodal malignancies develop in organs that normally have nests of lymphoid tissue (mucosal surfaces, bone marrow, and skin).

Staging & Classification

Although the Ann Arbor system was developed for Hodgkin's disease, this staging system is also used in non-Hodgkin's lymphoma. The goal of the staging evaluation is to distinguish patients who have localized disease from those with disseminated disease. After pathologic diagnosis, the staging evaluation for non-Hodgkin's lymphoma consists of a detailed history and physical examination, routine laboratory tests, a bone marrow biopsy, and a CT scan of the neck, chest, abdomen, and pelvis. Although helpful in assessing the anatomic extent of disease, the Ann Arbor system is of minimal clinical value in non-Hodgkin's lymphoma. Instead, prognosis and treatment are more dependent on the grade and type of the malignancy.

Scientists have made countless attempts at developing a universal, clinically relevant classification system for the subtypes of non-Hodgkin's lymphoma, and the merits of the various classifications are an area of hot debate. The most widely accepted classification system is the Revised European-American Lymphoma/World Health Organization (REAL/WHO) Classification (Table 46–7).

In determining the therapeutic approach to patients with non-Hodgkin's lymphoma, a simpler classification system can be utilized. For treatment purposes, these lymphomas can be functionally divided into two groups: indolent (low-grade) and aggressive (high-grade) lymphomas (Table 46–8). Smaller, differentiated cells characterize the indolent lymphomas, and this class tends to have a follicular architecture. Although the course of these lymphomas is not very aggressive, they are very difficult to cure, and most patients eventually die of their disease. The natural history of indolent lymphomas often involves progression of the tumor cells to a more aggressive subtype. This progression is sometimes heralded by the onset of B symptoms and portends a dismal prognosis.

The aggressive lymphomas behave differently from the indolent ones and demand a different therapeutic approach. Histologically, the aggressive lymphomas spread more diffusely throughout the lymph nodes and consist of larger, less differentiated cell types. This class of lymphomas demonstrates a very rapid growth rate and an increased rate of early mortality. Despite this malignant behavior, this class of non-Hodgkin's lymphoma is more often curable. The extranodal lymphomas develop outside of the lymph nodes and are not amenable to conventional classifications, so they are generally regarded as a separate entity. They can involve any organ but most commonly affect the oropharynx, paranasal sinuses, thyroid, gastrointestinal tract, liver, testicles, skin, and bone marrow.

Table 46–7. REAL/WHO classification of non-Hodgkin's lymphoma.

B-cell
Precursor B-cell cancers (neoplasms)
Lymphoblastic lymphoma (LBL)
Peripheral B-cell neoplasms
B-cell chronic lymphocytic leukemia/small lymphocytic lymphoma
Lymphoplasmacytic lymphoma/immunocytoma
Mantle cell lymphoma
Follicular lymphoma
Extranodal marginal zone B-cell lymphoma of MALT type
Nodal marginal zone B-cell lymphoma
Splenic marginal zone lymphoma
Plasmacytoma/plasma cell myeloma
Diffuse large B-cell lymphoma
Burkitt's lymphoma
T-cell and Natural Killer-cell (NK)
Precursor T-cell neoplasm
Lymphoblastic lymphoma (LBL)
Peripheral T-cell and NK-cell neoplasms
T-cell granular lymphocytic leukemia
Mycosis fungoides/Sézary's syndrome
Peripheral T-cell lymphoma, not otherwise characterized
Hepatosplenic gamma/delta T-cell lymphoma
Angioimmunoblastic T-cell lymphoma
Extranodal T-/NK-cell lymphoma, nasal type
Enteropathy-type intestinal T-cell lymphoma
Adult T-cell lymphoma/leukemia (HTLV1+)
Anaplastic large cell lymphoma, primary systemic type
Anaplastic large cell lymphoma, primary cutaneous type

Table 46–8. Indolent versus aggressive classification of non-Hodgkin's lymphoma.

Indolent lymphomas
Follicular lymphoma
Small lymphocytic lymphoma
Lymphoplasmacytic lymphoma (Waldenström's macroglobulinemia)
Extranodal marginal zone B-cell lymphoma (MALT lymphoma)
Nodal marginal zone B-cell lymphoma (monocytoid B-cell lymphoma)
Aggressive lymphomas
Diffuse large cell lymphoma
Burkitt's lymphoma
Precursor B- or T-cell lymphoblastic lymphoma
Primary CNS lymphoma
Adult T-cell lymphoma
Mantle cell lymphoma
Polymorphic post-transplantation lymphoproliferative disorder (PTLD)
AIDS-related lymphoma
True histiocytic lymphoma
Blastic NK-cell lymphoma

Treatment

A. Indolent Lymphoma

Patients with localized disease, although this is the minority, can be treated with radiation therapy only. Most patients have disseminated disease, which tends to be chronic relapsing and remitting. The current therapies for systemic indolent lymphomas are rarely curative, and the goal of treatment is generally directed at palliation of symptoms. At present, a "watch and wait" approach to treatment is recommended. After diagnosis, asymptomatic patients are followed up clinically until they have progression to more aggressive disease, major symptoms, or organ dysfunction. Withholding chemotherapy does not reduce survival in patients with non-Hodgkin's lymphoma, and it probably improves quality of life. A promising new treatment is Rituximab, a monoclonal antibody that binds to the B-cell surface antigen CD20. CD20 is a cell-surface protein involved in the development and differentiation of normal B cells. It is found on the vast majority of B-cell lymphomas. Rituximab is well tolerated and has remission rates of 40–50% when used as single-agent therapy for relapsed indolent lymphoma. Studies of Rituximab in combination with chemotherapy are ongoing. In younger patients with systemic indolent disease, high-dose chemotherapy with autologous bone marrow transplant is currently under clinical investigation.

B. Aggressive Lymphomas

Despite their aggressive nature, these lymphomas have a better chance for cure than their more indolent counterparts. The consensus therapy for stage I and II disease is radiation alone for localized disease, or more often chemotherapy with a doxorubicin-containing regimen, with or without radiation. Systemic disease (stages II–IV) is treated by combination CHOP (cyclophosphamide, doxorubicin, Oncovin [vincristine], and prednisone) chemotherapy. Radiotherapy may be added following chemotherapy for areas of bulky disease. Disease-free survival after CHOP is 30% at 12 years. Methods of improving this, including the addition of Rituximab or escalated doses of chemotherapy using growth-factor support, are presently being investigated.

Patients who relapse after aggressive treatment have a poor prognosis, with less than 10% long-term survival rates. Currently, high-dose cytotoxic therapy and bone marrow transplant should be considered for patients who relapse or fail to enter remission after induction chemotherapy. The treatment-related mortality from bone marrow transplant is approximately 10%—high enough to restrict its use to patients who have failed conventional therapy. Another promising immunotherapy is tositumomab, an anti-CD20 monoclonal antibody bound to ^{131}I. This can kill cells by antibody-mediated cellular cytotoxicity, activation of complement-mediated tumor cell lysis, and the tumor-specific delivery of radiation. More studies are needed to determine long-term effects and their role in the therapy of aggressive non-Hodgkin's lymphoma.

C. Nonlymphoid Disease

There is no consensus about the proper management of localized nonlymphoid lymphomas since large-scale studies of therapy for this disease have not been conducted. With few exceptions, nonlymphoid disease is managed somewhat in the same way as systemic aggressive lymphomas, using combination CHOP therapy.

The CHOP regimen has the disadvantage of poor penetration of the blood-brain barrier and is thus ineffective in the treatment of primary central nervous system lymphomas. These lymphomas are sensitive to radiation, and current regimens utilize whole brain radiation with some form of adjuvant chemotherapy. Methotrexate is the most common adjuvant treatment in this patient population, and it can be effective when delivered either systemically or intrathecally. Central nervous system lymphomas have a poor prognosis, with approximately 20% 5-year survival rates in treated patients. The combined modalities, while providing modest survival benefits, have significant neurotoxicities, and as many as 50% of patients develop severe dementia. Given this morbidity, clinicians are currently attempting to improve the therapy for this disease, with most efforts directed toward using chemotherapy as the sole modality in the treatment of patients with primary central nervous system lymphomas. Extranodal lymphomas that have a predilection for metastases to the central nervous system, such as testicular, paranasal, and AIDS-related lymphomas, require systemic CHOP therapy combined with prophylactic intrathecal methotrexate treatments.

The treatment of gastric lymphomas in particular—and organ-isolated lymphomas in general—is controversial. The data supporting resection of these tumors are debatable; however, many centers continue to perform gastric resections for gastric lymphomas to prevent chemotherapy-related perforation or hemorrhage. Although some studies support gastrectomy as the sole treatment of isolated gastric tumors, many centers treat these patients with adjuvant regimens of radiotherapy or combination chemotherapy (or both). When these tumors are not isolated to the stomach, systemic treatment is required. Splenectomy in patients with lymphomatous splenic involvement has no demonstrated therapeutic benefit and should be reserved for patients with symptomatic splenomegaly, pain from recurrent splenic infarctions, and hematologic depression from hypersplenism.

Evans LS, Hancock BW: Non-Hodgkin lymphoma. Lancet 2003;362:139.

Mounier N et al: A multivariate analysis of the survival of patients with aggressive lymphoma. Cancer 1998;82:1952.

Specht L et al: Influence of more extensive radiotherapy and adjuvant chemotherapy on long-term outcome of early-stage Hodgkin's disease: a meta-analysis of 23 randomized trials involving 3,888 patients. J Clin Oncol 1998;16:830.

Stephens J, Smith J: Treatment of primary gastric lymphoma and gastric mucosa-associated lymphoid tissue lymphoma. J Am Coll Surg 1998;187:312.

Yung L, Linch D: Hodgkin's lymphoma. Lancet 2003;361:943.

PARANEOPLASTIC SYNDROMES

Many tumors develop the ability to elaborate hormones or cytokines that can have deleterious consequences for the host. Host antibodies to tumor antigens are also thought to play a role in the development of paraneoplastic syndromes. These immune effects probably result from cross-reaction with normal tissue antigens and immune complex deposition. Paraneoplastic syndromes can be systemic or can affect only a single organ system. Included in the paraneoplastic syndromes are the common cancer sequelae of hypercoagulopathy, cachexia, fevers, and anemia of chronic disease. More specific effects are summarized in Table 46–9.

Table 46–9. Paraneoplastic syndromes.

Syndrome	Associated Cancers	Suspected Causal Mechanisms
Cushing's syndrome	Lung, pancreatic, adrenal and neural tumors	ACTH or ACTH-like molecules
Syndrome of inappropriate ADH secretion	Lung and intracranial tumors	ADH secretion
Hypercalcemia	Lung, breast, parathyroid, renal, myeloma, prostate, and ovarian cancers	Osteolytic metastases or parathyroid hormone-related peptide
Hypoglycemia	Sarcomas, islet cell tumors, hepatocellular carcinoma	Insulin or insulin-like peptides
Myasthenia	Thymomas and lung cancer	Autoimmune
Encephalomyelitis	Lung, ovarian, and breast cancer	Autoimmune
Neuropathies	Myeloma, lung, breast, and ovarian cancer	Autoimmune
Cerebellar atrophy	Breast and ovarian cancer	Autoimmune
Acanthosis nigricans	Gastric, lung, and uterine cancer	Autoimmune
Dermatomyositis	Lung and breast cancer	Autoimmune
Venous thrombosis	Multiple cancers	Tumor products that activate clotting factors
DIC	Pancreas, lung, stomach, and prostate cancer	Tumor products that activate and consume clotting factors
Hypertrophic osteoarthropathy	Lung cancer	Unknown

Organ Transplantation 47

Jeffrey D. Punch, MD

The ability to transplant human organs successfully has developed in the span of a single generation of physicians and surgeons. This remarkable achievement is an excellent example of how animal models may be used to understand and develop treatments for human disease. Organ transplantation is now the preferred treatment modality for a variety of different types of organ failure. Transplantation not only offers improved long-term survival, but also improved quality of life for many patients afflicted by renal, hepatic, cardiac, and pulmonary failure.

Enormous effort is currently being expended to develop methods of artificially replacing vital organ functions. Despite these efforts, the ability to replace organ function with mechanical or biomechanical devices remains elusive. While hemodialysis can replace renal function effectively, it offers neither a normal quality of life nor a normal life span. Despite major advances in artificial heart technology, current systems have not reached the point where they can be used routinely to restore normal cardiac function. To date, there are no effective replacements for hepatic or pulmonary function that are suitable for long-term use. Organ transplantation is frequently the only treatment modality that offers a normal lifestyle for patients with advanced organ failure. This chapter will discuss the indications for organ transplantation as well as the limitations to the current state of the art.

KIDNEY TRANSPLANTATION

With the exception of organs from a genetically identical twin **(isografts)**, all organs from genetically dissimilar individuals **(allografts)** will naturally be subjected to immunologic rejection. This fundamental biologic limitation has largely been overcome by the development of targeted immunosuppression therapies. These therapies are able to suppress the immunological reactivity that produces graft rejection while leaving intact sufficient immune competency to allow recovery from most infectious diseases. The same degree of success has not been reached when transplanting organs between species (xenografts).

Once it was realized that allografts failed due to an active immunologic attack of the recipient's immune system on the donor organ, methods of suppressing the immune system were investigated. Early attempts at immunosuppression with substances such as nitrogen mustard and total lymphoid irradiation were unsuccessful due to the toxicity of the therapy. The first practical immunosuppressant was azathioprine, an antimetabolite inhibitor of DNA synthesis. When used in combination with corticosteroids, the first successful combination of immunosuppressants was born and the first boom in the number of transplants occurred. This combination remained the state of the art until it was realized that the cell type that exerts primary control over allograft rejection is the T lymphocyte. This led to the later development of agents able to specifically inhibit activation and proliferation of T cells. The result was immunosuppressants that were both more effective and much less toxic than the azathioprine/corticosteroids combination. These agents ushered in a further acceleration in the number of transplants occurring, as now it was possible to transplant organs between individuals who did not share human leukocyte antigens.

Almost all renal diseases responsible for renal failure can be treated by transplantation. Diabetes is the most common cause of chronic renal failure in adults and accounts for 45% of all renal failure in the United States. The second most common cause is hypertensive nephropathy (27%), followed by chronic glomerulonephritis (11%). The causes of renal failure in children are somewhat different, with congenital causes predominating, including both nonobstructive and obstructive uropathies.

IMMUNOLOGIC RESPONSES

HLA Histocompatibility Antigens

The **major histocompatibility** (MHC) antigens are the most antigenic proteins on donor organs, meaning that they cause the most intense immune responses when the donor and recipient do not share the same antigens. The MHC genes are coded by a single chromosomal complex of closely linked genes on the short arm of the sixth chromosome. This complex consists of at least seven loci that code for genes involved with histocompatibility: HLA-A, HLA-B, HLA-C, HLA-D, HLA-DR, HLA-DQ, and HLA-DP. Each HLA gene locus is highly polymorphic, so that as many 50 or more discrete antigens are controlled by each locus. The collection of HLA genes in an MHC complex is termed a **haplotype**.

Histocompatibility antigens are grouped into class I (A, B, and C) and class II (DR, DQ, DP) antigens. Class I antigens are composed of a 45kDa heavy chain with three globular extracellular domains (α1, α2, α3) that confers HLA specificity, a transmembrane portion, and an intracellular domain. Class I antigens are stabilized by β_2-microglobulin, a 12 kDa protein that is not encoded in the MHC complex. Class I antigens are expressed on all nucleated cells and interact primarily with CD8+ T cells. Class II antigens are composed of two noncovalently linked chains: a 33 kDa α chain and a 28 kDa β chain. Each chain has two extracellular domains that confer HLA specificities. Class II antigens are only constitutively expressed on B cells and antigen presenting cells (macrophages, monocytes, dendritic cells) but can be induced on activated T cells and endothelial cells. Class II antigens interact primarily with CD4+ T cells. The three most important antigens clinically in solid organ transplantation are A, B, and DR. Since each person has two MHC complexes, one on each copy of chromosome 6, everyone has a total of six HLA antigens that are relevant to organ transplantation.

The three-dimensional structures of both class I and II molecules are similar. The extracellular domains form a β-pleated sheet with two looping α-helices that creates a groove facing away from the cell. Following ribosomal synthesis, during assembly of the HLA antigens, peptides are added to this groove. Intracellularly derived peptides are added to class I antigens in the endoplasmic reticulum, while extracellularly derived proteins are added to class II antigens. The end of the groove on class II antigens is open, allowing class II antigens to accommodate longer peptides. Antigenic determinants are found predominantly on the α1 and α2 chains of the class I molecule and on the β chain of the class II molecule. Some antigenic determinants are shared by many different HLA allotypes. These common determinants are called **public specificities**. Antigenic determinants that are only found on a unique HLA antigen are termed **private specificities**.

Lymphocytes are categorized as either B or T cells. B cells are responsible for antibody production. T cells are categorized into two functional subsets: helper cells that are CD4+ and cytotoxic T cells that are CD8+. Helper T cells preferentially recognize peptides displayed in the groove of class II antigens, while cytotoxic T cells preferentially recognize peptides displayed by class I antigens. A third type of T cell called regulatory T cells has recently been identified and may be either CD4+ or CD8+. Helper T cells direct both the formation of cytotoxic T cells, which are able to cause graft destruction directly, and the maturation of B cells. Helper T cells can be further subdivided based on their cytokine secretion profile into type 1 and type 2 cells. Type 1 helper T cells secrete IL-2, IFN-γ, IL-12, and TNFα. These cytokines stimulate delayed-type hypersensitivity, cytolytic activity, and the development of complement-fixing IgG antibodies. Type 2 helper T cells secrete IL-4, IL-5, IL-10, and IL-13. These cytokines activate eosinophils and cause the production of IgE antibodies.

Allograft rejection begins when foreign antigen is taken up by an antigen presenting cell, processed, and presented to helper T cells. The T cell is activated in response to properly presented antigen and secretes cytokines that in turn recruit and activate additional lymphocytes and cause them to begin to clonally proliferate. Cytokines released in the allograft milieu by other cells including macrophages contribute to the generation of the immune response as well. Helper T cells also stimulate the differentiation and proliferation of cytotoxic T cells and B cells.

B-cell activation induces the production of specific antibodies directed against donor antigens. This response is important, especially for class I antigens. Recipients who develop a primary immunological response to a particular antigen and produce cytotoxic antibodies directed against the donor HLA will often retain memory B cells and maintain the ability to produce antibodies that are directed against that particular HLA allotype. Upon reexposure to the same antigens an immediate destructive reaction to the graft—called hyperacute rejection—occurs. Antibody directed against the donor vascular endothelium triggers fixation of complement, direct cellular damage, and the formation of platelet and fibrin plugs, leading to microvascular thrombosis and ischemic necrosis of the organ. Transplantation in the presence of cytotoxic anti-HLA antibody directed against a donor organ is prevented in practice by performing a complement-mediated cytotoxic crossmatch with pretransplant recipient sera against lymphocytes from the potential donor.

Histocompatibility Testing, Cross-Matching, & Blood Group Compatibility

Grafts between identical twins are rare, but very successful because immunosuppressive therapy is not required when there is no antigenic difference between the donor and recipient. Grafts between HLA-identical siblings that share two HLA haplotypes give the next best results. One-fourth of any given sibling pair will share both HLA haplotypes and thus share all of the same HLA antigens. Despite sharing HLA, immunosuppression is still required because of incompatibilities at minor histocompatibility loci. Parents, offspring, and half of siblings share one HLA haplotype. One-fourth of siblings will not share an HLA haplotype, and will therefore only share antigens by chance. The same is true for genetically unrelated donor/recipient pairs such as spouses and friends. At one time, HLA compatibility was considered to be crucial because there were large differences between graft survival depending on the degree of histocompatibility. Transplants between individuals who shared many HLA antigens were much more likely to avoid graft loss compared to donor/recipient pairs who did not share HLA antigens. This has changed due to the ability of modern immunosuppression to provide for excellent immunological outcome even in the setting of complete HLA mismatch. HLA testing is now of much lesser value than it once was. HLA histocompatibility testing is now primarily of value in determining which of several donors has the best histologic match to the intended recipient. Kidney allocation from deceased donors was once heavily influenced by HLA matching. This has now changed because of the realization that the degree of HLA match has a relatively unimportant effect on the odds of successful outcome. The newest allocation strategy relies more on waiting time and less on the degree of HLA match. Kidneys from donors that share all six HLA antigens with a recipient on the waiting list are still allocated first to any recipient that happens to be a "perfect match." This situation is uncommon, affecting fewer than 10% of the kidneys from deceased donors.

Regardless of the results of tissue typing and antigen matching, it is essential to determine whether a recipient has preformed antibodies against donor antigens, since their presence would result in an hyperacute rejection of the graft as described above. Preexisting antibodies may develop because of prior exposure to foreign histocompatibility antigens in the form of blood transfusion, pregnancy, or previous organ transplants. These antibodies are identified by performing a crossmatch between the patient's serum against the donor's lymphocytes. Multiple methods of performing the crossmatch are available with varying degrees of sensitivity and specificity. It is difficult to find an appropriate donor with a negative crossmatch for patients who have antibodies directed against multiple HLA specificities. Some of these patients can be treated with desensitization strategies to reduce their burden of circulating antibodies. Methods being currently investigated include plasmapheresis, infusion of random donor immune globulin, and anti-B cell monoclonal antibodies. Experience is accumulating with desensitization protocols suggesting that donor/recipient pairs with positive crossmatches can sometimes be successfully transplanted. The long-term outcome for these kidneys is unclear.

The ABO blood group antigens behave as strong histocompatibility antigens for kidney transplantation; therefore, ABO-incompatible kidney transplants have generally been considered an absolute impossibility. It is certainly true that ABO-incompatible kidneys will fail rapidly if nothing is done to reduce the amount of antibody directed against the incompatible antigen in the recipient's serum. Success is now being reported for AB-incompatible kidney transplants using combinations of anti-B cell therapy and plasmapheresis.

Klein J, Sato A: The HLA system. (Two parts.) N Engl J Med 2000;343:702, 782.

Immunosuppressive Drug Therapy

Multiple immunosuppressive strategies are effective at preventing acute allograft rejection. Most strategies involve the use of more than one agent. Conceptually this has the effect of blocking multiple targets in the immune response cascade, which allows relatively low doses of each drug to be used, thus avoiding toxicity associated with high doses of these powerful drugs. Thus, many patients are treated with "triple therapy" using corticosteroids, a calcineurin inhibitor, and either an antimetabolite or a TOR (target of rapamycin) inhibitor. A variant of this strategy, termed "quadruple therapy," involves the initial use of a very potent antilymphocyte agent and chronic administration of the same drugs used for triple therapy. The antibody treatment has two effects: it decreases the likelihood of rejection in the critical first few months after the transplant, and it allows there to be a delay before the introduction of the calcineurin inhibitor. This is advantageous because of the associated nephrotoxicity of calcineurin inhibitors. Since the risk of rejection is highest immediately after the transplant, it is typical to begin with relatively high doses of each agent and gradually taper down to a maintenance level over several weeks to months.

Rejection is diagnosed by biopsy. Patients are followed up with serial measurements of renal function in the form of serum creatinine. When a transplanted kidney begins to function, the serum creatinine will fall gradually over several days to reach a nadir level that becomes a new baseline for the patient. Any significant elevation above the baseline should prompt evaluation as to the cause, and once obstruction, dehydration, and infection have been ruled out, it is usually appropriate to biopsy the kidney graft. Rejection may be treated with high-dose "pulse" corticosteroid therapy over several days or with antilymphocyte antibodies. Rejection therapy is effective in more than 90% of cases.

Many drugs are available today for immunosuppression. All of these drugs share the common side effect of increasing susceptibility to infectious diseases. This is an intrinsic feature of currently available therapy, which aims to suppress natural immune responses against all foreign antigens. When the transplant recipient develops an infection, it is vital that a physician with experience prescribing immunosuppression is involved with the patient's care. In many cases, it is appropriate to temporarily reduce the degree of immunosuppression in order to allow recovery from the infection. Precisely how this is accomplished varies widely among practitioners, but it generally involves lowering the dosage or withholding one or more of the agents being used for maintenance immunosuppression. When the infection has resolved, immunosuppression is restored to an acceptable maintenance regimen. It is appropriate to individualize therapy because different individuals have different propensities to develop both rejection and infection.

Many long-term immunosuppressive therapies are associated with the development of malignancy, especially skin cancer and lymphomas. Patients receiving chronic immunosuppression should pay particular attention to minimizing direct exposure to ultraviolet radiation. Since many skin cancers are treatable with simple resection, it is also important that transplant physicians are careful to monitor for and treat skin lesions that develop in transplant recipients.

In the future it may be possible either to modify the graft so that it is not viewed as foreign to the recipient's immune system, or to modify the recipient's immune system so that it will not reject the graft without altering the immune response to other foreign antigens.

A. Antimetabolites

The antimetabolite drugs include azathioprine, cyclophosphamide, mycophenolate, and leflunomide. These drugs inhibit nucleic acid synthesis, which in turn limits the ability of activated lymphocytes to rapidly clonally expand. In general, these drugs are used to prevent rejection but are not effective at reversing active acute rejection.

Azathioprine, a purine analogue, is the original member of this family. The effects of this drug are not specific to lymphocytes; therefore, the drug also frequently causes decreased levels of circulating neutrophils and platelets. This side effect is dose dependent.

Cyclophosphamide is an alkylating agent that is a common component of chemotherapy protocols. It is an effective immunosuppressant when given in high doses, but it has been used only very infrequently in clinical transplantation.

Mycophenolate is an inhibitor of inosine monophosphate dehydrogenase, a critical enzyme in the de novo synthesis pathway of purines. Lymphocytes uniquely depend on the de novo pathway to synthesize purines, while other cells are able to utilize a salvage pathway for synthesis. Mycophenolate is therefore more specific for lymphocytes than the other antimetabolites. It has largely replaced azathioprine for use in combination with a calcineurin inhibitor and corticosteroids due to well-designed studies that showed it to have a superior ability to prevent rejection. Side effects are primarily gastrointestinal in nature.

Leflunomide is a selective inhibitor of de novo pyrimidine synthesis. It is thought to work by inhibiting the enzyme dihydroorotate dehydrogenase. It is used widely for treatment of rheumatoid arthritis. Clinical trials have demonstrated it to be efficacious in terms of preventing rejection, but it is difficult to use clinically because of its long half-life (15–18 days).

B. Corticosteroids

Corticosteroids used in combination with azathioprine was the first combination of immunosuppressants with the ability to prevent the development of allograft rejection, and high doses of corticosteroids was the first practical and effective means of reversing established rejection. Hence, over the past 40 years, corticosteroids have been a component of most successful immunosuppressive protocols. Typically a high dose of intravenous corticosteroids is given at the time of engraftment, and the dose is tapered over weeks to months down to a maintenance dosage of 0.1–0.2 mg/kg of oral prednisone. In the recent past, there has been strong interest in discontinuation of corticosteroids—and even more recently, in developing protocols that do not require the administration of any corticosteroids. The evidence is accumulating that this treatment is appropriate and effective for some low-risk renal transplant recipients, but the use of corticosteroid-free protocols for higher-risk candidates—including those with known sensitization to HLA and patients undergoing second renal transplants—is more controversial.

Corticosteroid therapy is associated with many different side effects, including infection, weight gain, cushingoid features, hypertension, increased bruisability, hyperlipidemia, hyperglycemia, and acne. Daily corticosteroid therapy in children may inhibit somatic growth. This may be circumvented to some degree by alternate-day treatment, administering the drug once in the morning every other day.

Corticosteroids are standard therapy for a rejection episode, typically consisting of three or more daily doses of between 100 mg and 500 mg of intravenous methyl-prednisolone ("steroid pulses"). Depending on the severity of the rejection, steroid pulses will resolve 50–80% of allograft rejection episodes.

C. Calcineurin Inhibitors

Transplantation was revolutionized by the introduction of the first calcineurin inhibitor, cyclosporine, into clinical practice in the early 1980s. Cyclosporine is a cyclic undecapeptide isolated from a fungus. It is a potent immunosuppressant and the first compound identified that can inhibit immunocompetent lymphocytes specifically and reversibly. Cyclosporine was followed by the introduction of tacrolimus, another compound derived from a fungus that also inhibits calcineurin. The primary mechanism of these agents appears to be inhibition of the production and release of IL-2 by helper T cells. In addition, it also interferes with the release of interleukin-1 by macrophages as well as with proliferation of B lymphocytes. Blood levels must be carefully monitored because both drugs are nephrotoxic and neurotoxic at higher levels. They also both have chronic effects on renal function and lead to significant long-term renal dysfunction in many patients who take them chronically. Both cyclosporine and tacrolimus are also associated with an increased incidence of neoplasms, particularly lymphomas.

D. Inhibitors of Mammalian Target of Rapamycin (mTOR)

Sirolimus is a macrocyclic triene antibiotic produced by a species of *Streptomyces.* It was originally developed as an antifungal and antitumor agent but was found to have significant immunosuppressive properties. The effect of sirolimus is believed to relate to inhibition of lymphocyte transduction pathways through binding to the mammalian target of rapamycin. It functions as an antiproliferative and prevents not only expansion of lymphocyte clones but also smooth muscle proliferation. It is known to effectively prevent rejection in combination with a calcineurin inhibitor. The major advantages of this drug are that it does not cause renal dysfunction and its antiproliferative properties suggest that it will not be associated with the same risk of developing long-term malignancy. Side effects, in addition to the infections associated with immunosuppression, include oral ulcerations, wound healing problems associated with its ability to inhibit smooth muscle proliferation, and significant hyperlipidemias.

E. Polyclonal Antithymoblast or Antilymphocyte Globulin (ALG) and Antithymocyte Globulin (ATG)

Antilymphoblast globulin and antithymocyte globulin are polyclonal antibody preparations derived by immunizing animals against some type of human lymphocytes and collecting and purifying the antibodies that animals develop in response to the foreign antigenic proteins. They are potent drugs that deplete circulating lymphocytes, an effect that can be measured and followed by flow cytometry or by simply following the complete blood count with differential. Because they are polyclonal, they are effective not only against T cells but may also have important effects against circulating B cells and natural killer cells.

These agents are particularly effective in induction of immunosuppressive therapy and in the treatment of established rejection that is either severe or is resistant to pulse corticosteroid therapy. Therapy is typically given daily for 5–7 days. The effect of these agents is profound immunosuppression that lasts for weeks to months. They are associated with increased incidence of viral infections due to their effects on cellular immunity, and also with a higher lifetime risk of developing malignancy, particularly B-cell lymphoma.

Side effects are many and include fevers and chills, neutropenia, and thrombocytopenia. Fever, chills, and malaise occur because of mediator release by T cells and circulating mononuclear cells, especially TNFα, IL-1, and IL-6, that occurs when the antibody is bound to certain cell surface receptors. The symptoms are very similar to those associated with an acute viral infection. These effects are usually transient, often lasting less than 12 hours. They occur primarily following the first or second dose of the treatment and can be attenuated markedly by pretreatment with corticosteroids, acetaminophen, and diphenhydramine. Neutropenia and thrombocytopenia occur because of direct antibody binding to these cell types, causing depletion. This effect is also transient and tends to resolve in 24–48 hours. It is necessary to monitor neutrophil and platelet counts during therapy and withhold doses of the treatment if the counts drop to dangerously low levels.

F. Monoclonal Antibody Therapy

The knowledge that the T cell is central to the development of allograft rejection led to the development of agents that selectively inhibit or deplete T cells, or both. The first example of such an agent is the monoclonal antibody OKT3 (muromonab-CD3), which is secreted by a hybridoma in culture. This agent may have some advantages over ALG or ATG preparations in management of rejection in that it specifically blocks T-cell generation and function. Because it is a monoclonal antibody and reacts with a defined antigen, it can be consistently produced with a defined activity and without unwanted reactivities against other cells like neutrophils and platelets. OKT3 is most effective in the treatment of steroid-resistant rejection, where more than 90% of rejection episodes are reversed, thus obviating further high-dose steroids. The downside of this antibody treatment is that since it is a murine monoclonal antibody, it may induce recipient antibody directed against the murine antibody molecule. This effect occurs in 5–10% of patients treated with OKT3 and may decrease the efficacy of the treatment if given a second or third time. Like the polyclonal antilymphocyte preparations, treatment is usually given daily for 5–7 days. Side effects due to cytokine release are typically more severe than that seen with polyclonal agents, but may also be attenuated with appropriate pretreatment. Since the antibody does not bind to epitopes other than the CD3 molecule, which is found only on T cells, it does not cause cytopenias.

The success of OKT3 led to the development of two drugs, Daclizumab and basiliximab, that bind to CD25, the high-affinity subunit of the T-cell receptor for IL-2. Since IL-2 is necessary for T-cell activation and proliferation, these agents have the ability to selectively inhibit the expansion of T-cell clones that are activated at the time of transplantation, without effecting existing T-cell immunity to other antigens. Existing cellular immunity to viruses, for example, is left intact. A second advantage of both of these agents is that the monoclonal antibody molecule has been modified by genetic engineering to avoid the side effects seen with OKT3. The genetic code directing the production of the antibody molecule by the hybridoma has been modified by replacing most of the murine portion of the sequence with human antibody sequence. The antibody is thus chimeric, or "humanized," since only the highly variable portion of the antibody that binds to the antigenic epitope is foreign to the human recipient. Cytokine release therefore does not occur when the antibody is administered, nor is it likely that the recipient will develop neutralizing antibodies against the monoclonal preparation. Because the antibodies so closely resemble human immunoglobulin, they also have a long circulating half-life. Induction treatment with anti-CD25 antibodies at the time of engraftment has been shown to reduce the incidence of future rejection episodes.

Carpenter CB: Immunosuppression in organ transplantation. N Engl J Med 1990;322:1224.

Krieger NR, Emre S: Novel immunosuppressants. Pediatr Transpl 2004;8:596.

Mourad G et al: Induction versus noninduction in renal transplant recipients with tacrolimus-based immunosuppression. Transplantation 2001;72:1050.

SOURCES OF DONOR KIDNEYS

The two sources of kidneys for renal transplantation are living donors and deceased donors. Approximately one-third of patients who are acceptable candidates for transplantation will have a willing and medically suitable living donor. ABO-compatible donors are not absolutely required today because of the availability of treatments that can reduce the amount of antidonor antibody in the recipient. However, ABO-compatible donors are greatly preferred, because antibody reduction treatments are expensive and associated with infectious risk due to the depletion of protective antibodies.

At one time, only related living donors were acceptable because it was necessary to have closely matched HLA antigens between the donor and recipient in order to achieve acceptable graft survival rates. The graft survival rate for donor/recipient pairs that do not share any HLA antigens is now greater than 90%, leading transplant programs to begin accepting more and more donors that are not genetically related to the recipients. It is now common practice to accept volunteer donors that are spouses, in-laws, friends, coworkers, and even members of the same community who may be only acquaintances.

Living donors should be in good health both physically and psychologically. Above all, the living donor should be a volunteer and must clearly understand the nature of the procedure so that informed consent to the operation can be given. Donors should generally be of legal age, but reasonable exceptions have been made in extenuating circumstances, particularly when an identical twin donor is available. In these circumstances it is wise for the program to use an outside advocate for the donor who has no relationship with either the recipient or the remainder of the family to ensure that the minor is not coerced into proceeding.

Living Donors

Live kidney donors are now as common as deceased donors, although since each deceased donor can donate two kidneys, the total number of kidneys from deceased donors still far exceeds that obtained from living donors. Because of the biological ability of the body to compensate for the loss of one kidney, renal function tends to stabilize at approximately 75–80% of the original renal function a few months following donation. Follow-up studies on donors show that they have good renal function and do not appear to suffer ill effects from the procedure, either physically or psychologically. Women with one kidney do not have an increased incidence of urinary infections during pregnancy.

There are at least two methods of performing donor nephrectomy in common practice: open nephrectomy and laparoscopic nephrectomy. Open nephrectomy, long the standard method, involves a flank incision about 15 cm long below the twelfth rib. The peritoneum is retracted medially and the kidney is removed along with its vessels and ureter without disturbing the intra-abdominal contents. More recently, laparoscopic techniques have been developed to allow the removal of a kidney for transplantation. The donor is placed under general anesthesia and the abdomen is insufflated with carbon dioxide to allow visualization of the abdominal structures. Some surgeons use a large port in the midline, just above the umbilicus, to insert their hand into the abdomen. The kidney is then withdrawn through the hand port once it has been dissected free from surrounding tissues and the vessels and ureter have been divided. It is also possible to remove the kidney using purely laparoscopic techniques without inserting a hand port. The kidney is removed by placing it in a bag inside the abdomen and withdrawing the bag through a low transverse incision. Laparoscopic nephrectomy tends to take longer than a nephrectomy through an open approach, but it is associated with somewhat less postoperative pain and a briefer period of convalescence. Prospective donors should be informed about the options for nephrectomy and the advantages and disadvantages of each technique as well as the associated risk and the known complications.

The main risk to a donor is the anesthesia and the operation itself. The mortality rate is estimated to be 0.03%, and most deaths are not judged to be preventable, but appear to be intrinsic risks of having a major operation. The most common significant complications following nephrectomy are wound related, including infection and hernia formation. These complications occur in less than 1–3% of cases. Wound infections typically respond to dressing changes, and hernias require operative repair.

The evaluation of a living donor must be thorough and complete. It is first necessary to make sure that the donor is truly a volunteer and is not being coerced or unfairly influenced by the recipient or other family members. This often involves a careful evaluation by an individual with excellent understanding of the transplant process as well as excellent communication skills. It is advisable that this portion of the interview be conducted in private, so that donors can be honest about their feelings. Transplant social workers, psychologists, and psychiatrists are typically involved with this aspect of donor selection. Once it is clear that the donor is genuinely seeking to donate on their own accord, a detailed history is taken, and a physical examination is performed. Factors that may affect operative risk as well as future risk of renal failure are carefully sought out. The routine workup includes chest x-ray, electrocardiography, urinalysis, complete blood count, fasting blood glucose, serum bilirubin, hepatic transaminases, serum creatinine, and blood urea nitrogen. If these are normal, the kidneys are imaged radiographically to make sure that two kidneys are present, to rule out intrinsic or structural renal disease, and to evaluate the vasculature of the kidneys. Angiography, computed tomography, and magnetic resonance imaging are all methods that can be used. Kidneys with multiple renal arteries may be transplanted, but care must be taken in the anastomosis of small accessory vessels, particularly when they come from the lower pole and may therefore provide the sole vascular supply to the ureter. When there are multiple renal veins, the smaller veins can often be ligated since there is free communication of the veins within the kidney.

Deceased Donors

Two-thirds of eligible kidney recipients do not have a suitable living donor. These patients are placed on a waiting list for a kidney from a deceased donor. Since more patients are added to the list each year, the number of patients waiting for a kidney from a deceased donor grows longer each year, and will exceed 100,000 in the United States by 2010.

Kidneys can be successfully transplanted from donors who are declared dead on the basis of brain death, or from donors that die of cessation of spontaneous cardiovascular activity.

Brain death is now widely accepted in principle in the United States, and all hospitals have protocols to be followed to ensure that the diagnosis of brain death is confirmed without any doubt.

Consent for donation should always be obtained by individuals with training in how to approach the family of the donors. In this way the family can be given time to grieve and express the inevitable sorrow and anger that accompanies the death of a loved one. Individuals who are not part of the team caring for the patient are best able to provide the emotional support that families need during this time. The discussion regarding donation can then occur separate from the discussion where the family learns that their loved one has died.

Kidneys from brain-dead donors are removed operatively. The excision of the kidneys occurs operatively following in situ cold perfusion and exsanguination of the kidneys, often in concert with the removal of other transplantable abdominal and thoracic organs. The kidneys are perfused with specially designed preservative solutions and kept cold. Successful transplantation has been reported following cold storage of more than 72 hours, but optimal results are achieved if the kidney is transplanted as soon as possible following removal from the donor, preferably within 24 hours.

Kidneys may also be transplanted from deceased donors following cardiopulmonary death, a practice termed "donation following cardiac death." The most common circumstance where this occurs in the United States is when medical therapy that is judged to be futile is withdrawn from an individual. Typically patients have suffered profound, irreversible brain injury and have essentially no conscious awareness and no potential for meaningful recovery. Standard medical practice in this circumstance is to recommend withdrawal of life-sustaining support such as mechanical respiration and intravenous infusions, since the vast majority of people state that they would not want to be kept alive in such a hopeless state. Withdrawal of support always occurs with the consent and understanding of the family. The decision to donate organs should be made separate from the decision to withdraw medical therapy. Once consent is obtained and preparation for donation is completed, support is withdrawn by the primary care team. When cardiopulmonary activity ceases, the primary physician team declares death and the organs are then excised as with brain-dead donors.

SELECTION OF RECIPIENTS

Patients with chronic renal failure should be considered for transplantation. Acute renal failure on the basis of acute tubular necrosis can usually be managed with temporary dialysis, and therefore kidney transplantation is not appropriate in this setting. It is not necessary for patients to be on dialysis at the time of transplantation. In fact, results for patients who receive kidney transplants prior to beginning dialysis have the best chance of graft survival, while patients who had long-term dialysis prior to transplantation have poorer success rates. It is therefore important to begin consideration for renal transplantation as soon as dialysis appears to be inevitable and imminent within the next year.

During the early years of renal transplantation, most of the patients accepted for transplantation were in the age group from 15 to 45 years. In recent years, the age range has been extended in both directions—children younger than age 1 and adults who are over 70 years old have received transplants. For many years the success rates for transplanting young children was inferior to that achieved with adults, but this problem has now been corrected. Even children younger than 1 year of age at the time of transplantation can be expected to have an excellent chance of graft survival.

Historically there has been reluctance to perform renal transplants in the elderly. However, as the practice of renal transplantation continues to improve, with less toxic and more effective immunosuppression and more effective methods of preventing post-transplant infections, this unwillingness appears less and less justified. Elderly individuals naturally have a shorter life span, but to date patients that are over 60 years old who receive transplants appear to enjoy approximately the same degree of improvement in life expectancy as do younger patients.

This benefit has been quantified by comparing the mortality rate of suitable candidates awaiting kidney transplantation with the mortality rate following transplantation. Life expectancy appears to be approximately doubled by kidney transplantation in all age ranges that have been studied to date. The improved life expectancy following kidney transplantation is particularly dramatic for diabetic patients. Today, patients tend to be judged based more on their physiologic functional status rather than their chronological age. It is nevertheless true that elderly patients are more commonly found to be poor candidates for transplantation either because of coexisting disease or poor functional status.

Candidates must be free of active infections at the time of transplantation. Chronically infected tissues such as chronic pyelonephritis or chronic osteomyelitis should be definitively treated prior to consideration for transplantation. Patients with active viral or bacterial infection at the time an organ is available for transplantation should usually be deferred until the infection has resolved. This is because it is unwise to initiate immunosuppression during an active infection, particularly given that the highest doses of immunosuppression are given around the time of the procedure.

Recipients with almost all types of primary renal disease have been successfully transplanted: glomerulonephritis, hypertensive nephropathy, chronic pyelonephritis, polycystic kidney disease, reflux pyelonephritis, Goodpasture's syndrome, congenital renal hypoplasia, renal cortical necrosis, Fabry's syndrome, and Alport's syndrome. Successful transplants have been achieved in patients with certain systemic diseases in which the kidney is one of the end organs affected (cystinosis, systemic lupus erythematosus, and diabetic nephropathy). Renal transplantation is generally inadvisable in patients with oxalosis if high serum levels of oxalate are present because the disease recurs in the transplant quickly. However, liver transplantation corrects the enzymatic defect that leads to excessive oxalate accumulation. Therefore, combined liver-kidney transplantation may be an acceptable treatment option for these patients.

Patients who do not have normal bladder function may be acceptable kidney transplant candidates, but a plan for ureteral drainage should be made before transplantation occurs. Many patients with long-term defunctionalized bladders can still undergo ureteral reimplantation and then be treated with intermittent catheterization if necessary post-transplant. If the bladder is congenitally or surgically absent, a defunctionalized loop of small bowel can be created, brought out as a stoma, and used for a urinary conduit. Care must be taken in planning the positioning of the conduit so that the ureter from a transplanted kidney will reach it.

Transplant patients must be compliant with post-transplant care to achieve successful outcome. Patients with a history of poor compliance may be candidates for transplantation if they are regretful of past behavior and have established a compliant pattern. In some cases, especially in the adolescent age group, it is wise for the patient to experience dialysis prior to receiving a kidney transplant in order to foster a complete understanding of the differences in lifestyle that are afforded by a successful kidney transplant. It is also necessary that patients have a support network to help them manage following the transplant. They will need a way to reliably obtain immunosuppressive therapy as well as transportation to and from the Transplant Center that is continuously and reliably available. Fortunately, support services are often available to patients who lack social support, and it is rare to deny transplantation solely on the basis of inadequate social support.

In the early years of kidney transplantation, it was common to perform bilateral nephrectomy prior to transplantation, but this has recently become very uncommon. Most patients who have native nephrectomy have polycystic kidney disease with profound pain, recurrent infections, or recurrent hemorrhage. Other indications for native nephrectomy include recurrent infection, especially when associated with ureteral reflux and occasionally profound hypertension attributable to an ischemic native kidney.

Wolfe RA et al: Comparison of mortality in all patients on dialysis, patients on dialysis awaiting transplantation, and recipients of a first cadaveric transplant. N Engl J Med 1999;341:1725.

OPERATIVE TECHNIQUES

The surgical technique of renal transplantation involves anastomoses of the renal artery and vein and ureter (Figure 47–1). The transplant kidney is placed in the iliac fossa through an oblique lower abdominal incision. The dissection is carried out by retracting the peritoneum medially so the kidney will lie in an extraperitoneal position. The iliac arteries and veins are mobilized as indicated for the proposed specific anastomoses. An end-to-side anastomosis is performed between renal vein and iliac vein; an end-to-side anastomosis is then performed between the renal artery and the iliac artery. An alternative technique is to connect the renal artery end-to-end to the internal iliac artery, but this technique is more difficult in most patients. When multiple arteries are present there are several options. If the artery is very small (less than 2 mm), it can often be ligated, especially if it is an upper pole branch. If the kidney is from a deceased donor, it is often possible to use a large "Carrell" patch of donor aorta that encompasses all of the arteries. Other options include reimplanting multiple renal arteries into the iliac artery using multiple anastomoses; reimplanting a smaller artery into the side of the dominant renal artery and then using the larger artery for anastomoses to the iliac; and spatulating the ends of the two arteries together to form a single lumen for anastomosis.

In small children and infants, the kidney transplant can either be performed through a midline abdominal incision or by making a very large flank-type incision extending from the pubic symphysis to the costal margin and exposing the aorta and vena cava by reflecting the peritoneal contents medially and superiorly. End-to-side anastomoses of the renal vessels may be made to the iliac vessels if they are large enough, but often it is necessary to use the infrarenal vena cava and aorta for the anastomotic site.

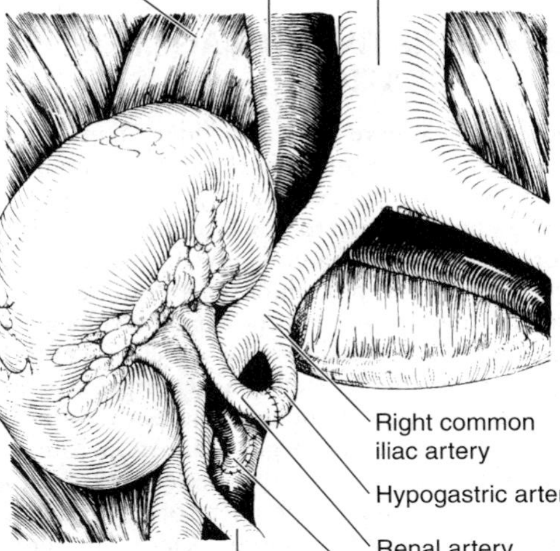

Figure 47–1. Technique of renal transplantation.

Kidneys from small pediatric deceased kidneys function poorly when transplanted into small pediatric recipients. However, many pediatric kidneys have often been transplanted en bloc with the donor aorta and vena cava anastomosed to the recipient's iliac vessels along with double ureteral anastomoses. The exact age at which it is best to transplant kidneys as a single unit is unclear, but certainly kidneys from children as young as 6 will function well and last a long time when transplanted into adults.

Urinary tract continuity can be established by pyeloureterostomy, ureteroureterostomy, or ureteroneocystostomy. The most common technique is ureteroneocystostomy. This technique can be performed by bringing the ureter into the bladder through a submucosal tunnel and suturing the mucosa of the ureter to the mucosa of the bladder from the inside of the bladder through a large cystotomy (Politano-Leadbetter method). Other techniques include an external neocystostomy, which avoids the need for a large cystotomy, and the "one stitch" technique, whereby the mucosa of the ureter is not directly sutured to the bladder mucosa, but rather the ureter is fixed into place in the interior of the bladder with a suture that traverses the full thickness of the bladder wall. A ureteral stent may be placed with any of the techniques discussed above. A 6Fr pediatric ureteral stent with a J shape at each end fits nicely across the anastomosis and goes from the interior of the renal pelvis into the bladder or other urinary conduit. The stent should be removed in the first month or two following the transplant to prevent stone formation and bladder infection.

POSTOPERATIVE MANAGEMENT & COMPLICATIONS

Recipients who have received a kidney transplants usually produce urine immediately and the serum creatinine falls over the next 3–7 days. The magnitude of urine output is related to how hydrated the patient was before transplantation and to how much fluid is administered during the procedure. It is important that the patient is fully hydrated at the time the kidney is revascularized in order to achieve the best chance of immediate transplant kidney function. Transplanted kidneys frequently will have an obligate diuresis for a period of hours to days after they begin to function. During this phase it may be necessary to replace urinary output in order to prevent the development of hypovolemia as a result of excess urinary output. Once this phase has passed, intravenous fluid can be discontinued. However, patients are encouraged to maintain generous fluid intake to prevent dehydration in the future, as transplanted kidneys appear to have a greater susceptibility to hypovolemia than native kidneys. Patients are usually able to eat the morning following the transplant procedure and should be encouraged to get out of bed with assistance. The urinary catheter can be removed as early as 2 days following the procedure, depending on the technique used for ureteral anastomosis. Some programs prefer to leave the urinary catheter in place for a longer period of time to allow sufficient healing of the anastomosis. Most recipients are able to be discharged from the hospital on the second or third postoperative day if there are no complications in their postoperative course once they are able to maintain oral hydration, they have learned how to properly take their medications, and they have received training about what to do, what not to do, and what to watch out for in the next few weeks.

Kidney transplantation can be followed by a variety of postoperative complications that must be recognized and treated early for optimal results. The most frequent complications are infection and rejection, reflecting the natural tension between too much and too little immunosuppression. Urinary infection is one of the most common complications and usually responds to antibiotic therapy. Bacterial pneumonia is the most common pulmonary complication and may be very serious if not promptly diagnosed and treated. Current immunosuppression protocols that focus on the T lymphocyte are associated with unusual, opportunistic types of infections including herpesviruses, the parasite *Pneumocystis carinii,* and fungal infections. These infections are seen much less often than previously because it is standard to prescribe prophylactic anti-infective therapy aimed at preventing the common types of infection. In particular, the availability of agents that are effective against cytomegalovirus (CMV) infection has almost eliminated clinical CMV infections. At one time, CMV infections were frequent, expensive, and exceedingly unpleasant occurrence after many transplants.

In approximately 20% of kidney transplants from deceased donors, the kidney will fail to function immediately. This complication is termed delayed graft function and is due to acute tubular necrosis of the kidney. In some cases there is a modest urinary output, but the serum creatinine does not fall. In other cases, there is profound oliguria. Delayed graft function can also occur following living donor transplantation, but it is much less common (less than 3%). Delayed graft function is associated with older donors and donors who had a rising creatinine at the time of donation. Long ischemic times are also known to increase the chance of delayed graft function. In most cases the acute tubular necrosis will resolve and the renal function will recover. Most recovery happens within a week, but in some cases the kidney will require several weeks before renal function is sufficient to support the patient without dialysis. Treatment is supportive with dialysis as necessary. If recovery takes more than a week, it may be wise to biopsy the kidney to rule out silent rejection.

Vascular complications of kidney transplants are uncommon, affecting 1–2% of renal transplants. Either renal artery or venous thrombosis of the kidney is devastating and almost uniformly results in graft loss. The incidence of acute graft thrombosis is higher in patients with high levels of circulating anti-HLA antibodies, suggesting that some of these cases related to accelerated acute rejection. The incidence of graft thrombosis is also higher in patients with Factor V Leiden and other physiologic derangements that cause a hypercoagulable state. Patients should be screened for Factor V Leiden if they have a history of unusual thrombotic events and receive anticoagulation perioperatively when it or other known hypercoagulable states are known. Renal artery stenosis, which may be associated with rejection involving the renal artery, is also a rare complication. It can present with severe hypertension. It may be treated surgically or in some cases by percutaneous transluminal balloon angioplasty.

Urologic complications occur in about 4% of patients, most often urinary extravasation from the cystotomy closure or ureteral obstruction. These complications can almost always be managed with percutaneous placement of a nephrostomy tube by an interventional radiologist and are not associated with a higher risk of graft loss.

A complication relatively unique to kidney transplantation is formation of a pelvic lymphocele in the transplant bed. Lymphatic fluid may come from either lymphatics in the hilum of the kidney or from lymphatics disrupted during exposure of the iliac vessels. Careful ligation of the adjacent lymphatics during preparation of the recipient blood vessels may decrease the incidence of this complication. Large lymphoceles may obstruct the ureter or the vasculature of the transplanted kidney, and they occasionally become infected. Sterile lymphoceles may be drained into the peritoneal cavity, while infected lymphoceles need to be drained externally.

Gastrointestinal complications may affect all levels of the intestine, but upper GI symptoms including nausea and abdominal pain are most common. In many cases, the culprit is the large number of medications that the patient must take. Peptic ulceration was once a major problem for transplant recipients, but this complication has virtually disappeared because of routine usage of medications like H_2 blockers and proton pump inhibitors to inhibit the production of gastric acid.

GRAFT REJECTION

Despite advances in immunosuppressive management, rejection is still a major hazard for the postoperative allograft recipient. Most episodes of rejection occur within the first 3 months. There are three basic kinds of rejection:

(1) Hyperacute rejection is due to preformed cytotoxic antibodies against donor antigens. Pretransplant crossmatch testing is designed to prevent this type of rejection. This reaction begins soon after completion of the anastomosis, and complete graft destruction occurs in 24–48 hours. Initially, the graft is pink and firm, but it then becomes blue and soft, with evidence of diminished blood flow. There is often no effective method of treating hyperacute rejection, but treatment with plasmapheresis and immunoglobulin infusion may be effective if the diagnosis is made immediately.

(2) Acute rejection is the most common type of rejection episode during the first 3 months after transplantation. It is primarily an immune cellular reaction against foreign antigens. The reaction may be predominantly cellular, or there may be a component of antibody-mediated inflammation. Typically the patient is asymptomatic and the diagnosis of rejection is suspected based on serial measurement of serum creatinine levels. In severe cases symptoms may include oliguria, weight gain, and worsened hypertension. Fever and tenderness and enlargement of the graft are uncommon with modern immunosuppressive protocols, but used to be seen when only azathioprine and corticosteroids were available. This type of rejection process is usually treated with pulse steroid therapy. If this is unsuccessful, or in very severe cases of acute rejection, either a polyclonal or monoclonal depleting antilymphocyte preparation is used. The vast majority of acute rejection episodes are successfully reversed. Currently grafts are only lost to rejection when patients are noncompliant, or when rejection occurs together with a life-threatening infection, since it is unsafe to enhance the degree of immunosuppression in this setting.

(3) Chronic rejection is a late cause of renal deterioration. It is unclear precisely what causes chronic rejection, but the absence of cellular elements on biopsy and the association of antidonor antibodies with chronic graft loss have led to the assumption that it is mediated by humoral factors. It is most often diagnosed on the basis of slowly decreasing renal function in association with proteinuria and hypertension. Chronic rejection is resistant to all known methods of therapy and graft loss will eventually occur, though perhaps not for several years after renal function begins to deteriorate. It is unclear what the relationship is between this pathologic process and the damage produced by chronic calcineurin inhibitor use, which is seen in nonrenal transplant recipients as well. It has recently been uncovered that chronic graft loss is accelerated in patients who experienced rejection in the first year after a transplant, in patients who had delayed graft function, and in patients who received kidneys from marginal donors.

Differential Diagnosis of Renal Allograft Dysfunction

An unexpected elevation in serum creatinine above baseline levels in a renal transplant recipient has a broad differential diagnosis list. Dehydration should be ruled out by history and physical examination. The medication the patient is taking should be reviewed, paying attention to over-the-counter medications, especially nonsteroidal anti-inflammatory drugs and herbal remedies. These drugs can cause renal dysfunction or can alter the metabolism of immunosuppressant medications and result in blood levels that are either too high or too low. Urinary infection should be ruled out with a urinalysis. If these simple evaluations do not disclose the cause of renal dysfunction, the next step is usually a renal ultrasound to rule out ureteral obstruction, followed by a renal allograft biopsy. This last step is crucial to arriving at the correct diagnosis. A biopsy may disclose acute rejection, or it may show calcineurin inhibitor toxicity. Since the treatment for these conditions is opposite, a biopsy is very important to guide appropriate therapy.

HEART TRANSPLANTATION

The first successful human heart allograft was performed in 1967 by Christiaan Barnard. At that time, however, the only available immunosuppressive therapy was azathioprine and steroids. This regimen was inadequate to safely prevent rejection in these patients. As a result, the procedure remained experimental and was limited to a small number of institutions worldwide. The introduction of cyclosporine in 1981 resulted in dramatically improved survival. As a result, heart transplantation was federally designated as no longer experimental in 1985. In 2003, there were about 2000 heart transplants performed in the United States at more than 100 centers. The 1-year survival rate is now over 85%, and the 3-year survival rate is over 75%.

SELECTION OF DONORS

At one time, deceased donors were only considered suitable for cardiac donation if they were men aged 40 years or younger or women 45 or younger. The large waiting list and the increasing number of patients who die on the waiting list has led surgeons to accept hearts from donors as old as 60, and more than one-third of current donors are older than 40. Cardiac donors must be ABO-compatible with the recipient and should be within 20% of the recipient's ideal body weight. Ideally, there should be no history of preexistent or intercurrent cardiac disease. It is routine to obtain echocardiography to determine cardiac function, even in young donors. At many programs it is routine to obtain cardiac catheterization in older donors to rule out silent coronary artery disease. Ideally, there should be no history of cardiac arrest, but if cardiac function is good, this factor alone does not usually rule out a cardiac donor. The donor should be receiving only moderate doses of pressor drugs.

At the donor operation, the chest is opened and the heart is inspected for evidence of contusion and observed to determine its overall function. If the heart is suitable, this information is relayed to the recipient operating team so that the timing of the recipient operation can be carefully coordinated. The heart is removed following cross-clamping of the aorta and infusion of cold cardioplegia, which results in cessation of electrical and mechanical cardiac activity. The heart is typically removed first, prior to the excision of kidney, liver, or pancreas. It is flushed with a preservative solution and stored aseptically at 4 °C. Optimal function is obtained when the heart is implanted within 4 hours of procurement. For recipients who have previously had cardiac procedures through a sternotomy, it is sometimes necessary to delay the procurement of the donor heart to make sure that the recipient will be ready to receive the heart when it arrives at the transplant hospital. The same is true when recipients have left ventricular assist devices implanted and extra time is necessary to prepare the recipient to receive the donor heart.

SELECTION OF RECIPIENTS

Patients for cardiac transplantation should have end-stage cardiac disease for which there is no other surgical option and should have received maximal medical treatment. Most heart transplant candidates have idiopathic dilated cardiomyopathy or ischemic cardiomyopathy. Most patients are younger than 55 years of age, but successful transplantation has been reported on more elderly patients. Patients should not have systemic disease that will be worsened by the immunosuppressive regimen (infection, type 1 diabetes, severe peripheral vascular disease, poorly controlled hypertension), nor should they have underlying renal insufficiency that cannot be attributed to low cardiac output.

Patients should have pulmonary vascular resistance of less than 5 Wood units, since levels above this or a pulmonary artery systolic pressure of greater than 50 mm Hg or a transpulmonary gradient (mean pulmonary artery pressure—pulmonary capillary wedge pressure) of greater than 15 mm Hg are associated with inadequate donor heart function. As with other organs, a history of compliance with a complex medical regimen and a strong social support system are necessary for long-term success.

If the recipient has circulating antibodies directed against HLA antigens, it is necessary to perform a cross-match between the recipient's serum and the donor lymphocytes to make sure that hyperacute rejection of the cardiac graft does not occur. Patients who have left ventricular assist devices in place may be particularly difficult to obtain hearts for, due to the sensitizing effect that the device has on the immune system.

OPERATIVE TECHNIQUE

The operative technique originally developed by Lower and Shumway continues to be used and is shown in Figure 47–2. A median sternotomy is performed and the patient is placed on cardiopulmonary bypass. The recipient heart is removed, and the atrial cuffs trimmed. The left atrial anastomosis is performed first and then the right, each with one continuous suture. Prior to closing the left atrium it is filled with saline to avoid air embolism. The aortic and then pulmonary artery anastomoses are then performed. Topical cooling may be continued, and the addition of blood cardioplegia after the atrial anastomoses may be done in order to improve graft function. The implant time is generally 45–60 minutes. It is frequently necessary to provide chronotropic support for the denervated heart in the form of atrial pacing or isoproterenol.

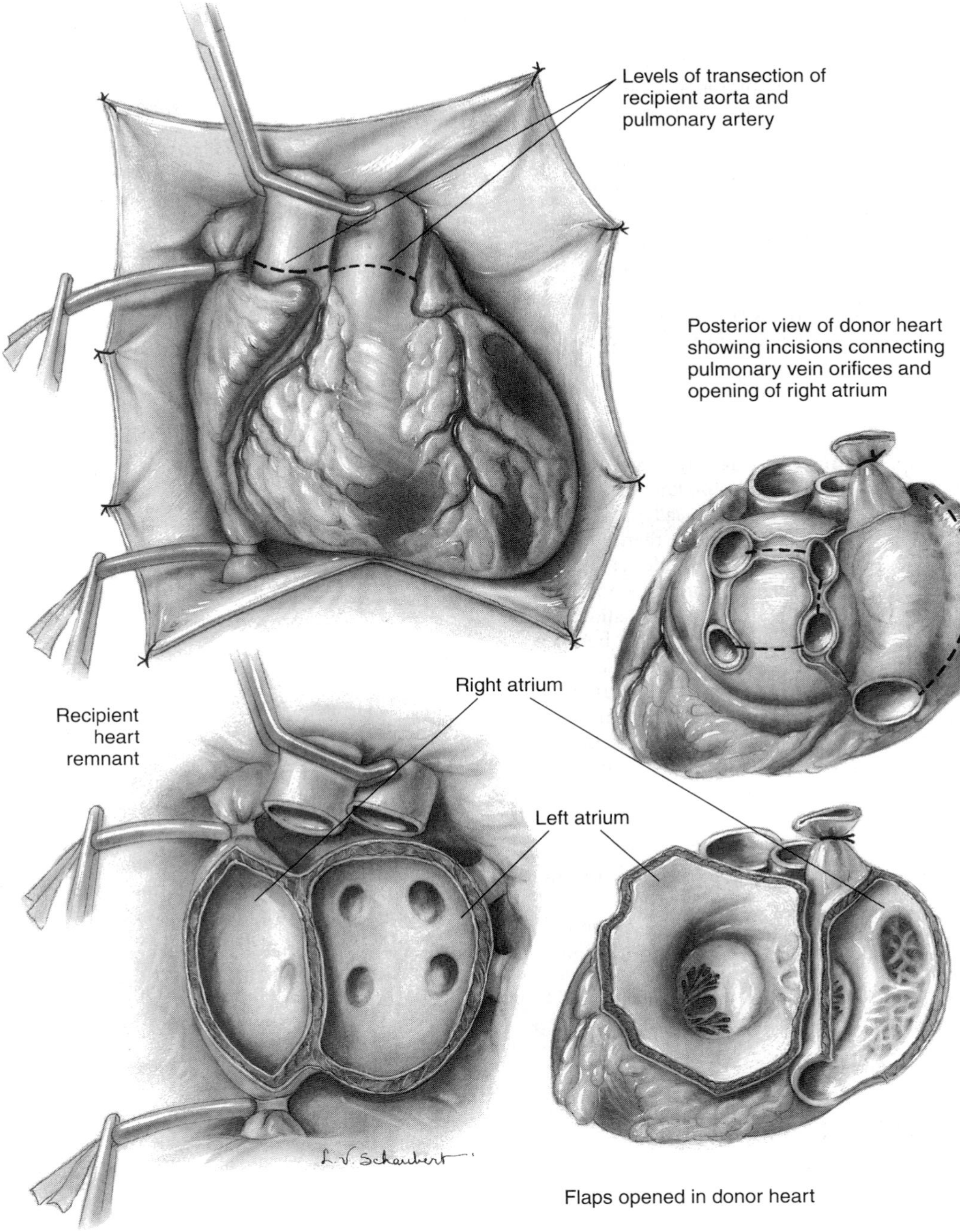

Figure 47–2. *Top left:* Recipient heart showing levels of transection across aorta and pulmonary artery. *Lower left:* Implantation site with recipient heart removed. *Top right:* Posterior view of donor heart showing lines of incision connecting pulmonary vein orifices and opening the right atrium in preparation for implantation. *Lower right:* Flaps opened in donor heart in preparation for implantation.

IMMUNOSUPPRESSION

Triple immunosuppression with a calcineurin inhibitor, antimetabolite, and corticosteroids is typical of the standard immunosuppressive protocol at most heart transplant programs. Perioperative induction immunosuppressive therapy with either polyclonal or monoclonal antibody therapy directed at lymphocytes is sometimes used in order to avoid the renal toxicity associated with early high-dose calcineurin inhibition and to reduce the risk of later rejection. Rejection is diagnosed on endomyocardial biopsy, which is performed regularly, since rejection may occur in the absence of clinical symptoms. Rejection is treated with 3 days of pulse steroids and resistant rejection with antilymphocyte therapy.

FOLLOW-UP CARE

Transplant recipients must be carefully monitored for infection and rejection. Protocols for endomyocardial biopsies vary by center, but are typically performed every other month for the first year, then every 3 months. The incidence of rejection episodes is 0.5–1.5 per patient for the first year. The major infection rate is 1.5 episodes per patient for the first year and then declines. Accelerated coronary atherosclerosis, believed to be a manifestation of chronic graft rejection, occurs in 30–40% of patients within 5 years after transplantation. There is no effective therapy for this condition except for retransplantation in highly selected, usually younger, patients. Progressive renal dysfunction may occur over time due to the cumulative effect of calcineurin inhibitor therapy.

Goldstein DJ, Oz MC, Rose EA: Implantable left ventricular assist devices. N Engl J Med 1998;339:1522.

Morrow WR: Cardiomyopathy and heart transplantation in children. Curr Opin Cardiol 2000;15:216.

Taylor DO: Immunosuppression therapies after heart transplantation: best, better and beyond. Curr Opin Cardiol 2000;15:108.

COMBINED HEART-LUNG TRANSPLANTATION

Combined heart-lung transplantation was first performed in 1981. Initially it was felt that rejection of both organs would be evident in the myocardial biopsy. However, experience has shown that rejection is dissimilar in the two organs, with heart rejection occurring infrequently and lung rejection, evidenced by obliterative bronchiolitis and arteritis, being a more severe problem. Heart-lung transplantation is currently performed with gradually decreasing frequently. In 1994 there were 71 heart-lung transplants in the United States. This number had declined to 28 in 2003. The main indication for heart-lung transplantation is end-stage disease in both organs or end-stage disease in one with poor function in the other prohibiting single-organ transplantation. Examples are primary pulmonary hypertension, congenital heart disease with Eisenmenger's physiology, fibrotic lung disease and cor pulmonale, and cystic fibrosis.

The operation consists of en bloc heart-lung transplantation with anastomosis of the trachea, right atrium, and aorta of the donor.

Immunosuppression parallels that of heart transplantation with the exception that steroids are avoided initially in order to promote tracheal wound healing. Heart-lung transplantation currently results in a 70% 1-year survival rate.

LUNG TRANSPLANTATION

Single lung transplantation became clinically successful through a systematic approach by the Toronto Lung Transplant Group to the problem of bronchial disruption, which had made previous attempts unsuccessful. The addition of an omental wrap to the bronchial anastomosis and the avoidance of steroids during the first 3 weeks allowed bronchial healing and clinical success. Lung transplantation is currently performed for a myriad of indications including emphysema, cystic fibrosis, idiopathic pulmonary fibrosis, α_1-antitrypsin deficiency, primary pulmonary hypertension, and congenital diseases. Candidates for lung transplantation have irreversible end-stage disease for which there is no other therapy, are oxygen dependent, and are likely to die of their disease within 12–18 months. Lung donors are scarce, but the use of one lung for transplantation does not preclude using the heart for another recipient. Long-distance procurement of lungs has been possible since institution of a regimen consisting of pulmonary artery flush with cold preservative solution following alprostadil (PGE_1) via the central venous line to promote pulmonary vasodilatation.

Patients with bilateral pulmonary sepsis, such as cystic fibrosis or bronchiectasis, or patients with emphysema and normal heart function may sometimes be eligible for double lung transplantation. The advantage is that the patient does not have the potential complications of heart transplant and rejection. Another innovative approach to the lung transplant patient with a normal heart is the operation where a heart-lung block is placed in a patient with end-stage lung disease and a normal heart, and the recipient's heart is extracted and donated to a patient in need of an isolated heart transplantation.

Immunosuppressive management of lung transplant recipients is very similar to that of heart recipients in that the cornerstone of therapy is a calcineurin inhibitor. The major difference is that steroids are omitted for several weeks in order to promote healing of the bronchial anastomosis. Postoperative management focuses on prevention of sepsis and detection and treatment of rejection. Bronchoscopy is performed liberally and transbronchial lung biopsy is used to diagnose lung transplant rejection. Acute rejection may be effectively treated with corticosteroid pulse therapy, or by enhancing the existing immunosuppressive regimen. The major long-term complication in lung transplant recipients is the development of bronchiolitis obliterans syndrome (BOS). BOS is felt to be the lung manifestation of chronic rejection. Episodes of acute rejection are risk factors for the development of BOS in the future. There is currently no effective therapy for BOS. A promising development that is currently experimental is aerosolized delivery of immunosuppression. It is hoped that directing immunosuppression preferentially to the lung itself may allow enhanced protection from rejection without increasing the risk of infection.

Tralock EP: Lung transplantation for COPD. Chest 1998;113:269S.

Yankaskas JR, Mallory GB: Lung transplantation and cystic fibrosis: consensus conference statement. Chest 1998;113:217.

LIVER TRANSPLANTATION

After many years of experimental effort, Dr. Thomas Starzl performed the first successful human liver transplantation in 1967. Over the next decade and a half the procedure was only done in low volumes and outcomes were generally poor. As with other organs, the introduction of cyclosporine in the 1980s resulted in marked improvement in survival rates. Today more than 5000 liver transplants are performed annually in the United States, and 1-year patient survival rates are more than 85%.

Since the introduction of clinical liver transplantation, the list of indications has rapidly expanded and the list of contraindications has diminished. The most common indication for liver transplantation is currently cirrhosis due to chronic hepatitis C infection. Other diseases for which liver transplant is indicated include cirrhosis due to hepatitis B, alcoholic cirrhosis, primary biliary cirrhosis, sclerosing cholangitis, autoimmune hepatitis, and cirrhosis secondary to nonalcoholic fatty liver disease. Less common indications are Wilson's disease, α_1-antitrypsin deficiency, Budd-Chiari syndrome, and hemochromatosis. In children the most common indication is biliary atresia. Other common diagnoses include α_1-antitrypsin deficiency, tyrosinemia, and other inborn errors of metabolism.

Alcoholic cirrhosis was once a subject of considerable controversy because of the self-induced nature of the disease. The world community rejected the notion that lifesaving therapy should be withheld from patients that could benefit from it merely because their disease is self-induced. It was pointed out that many, if not most, diseases are to some degree self-induced, whether it is diabetes and high blood pressure due to obesity, or cancer and heart disease due to smoking. It is now recognized that alcoholic cirrhosis is an accepted indication for liver transplant if the patient has demonstrated the ability to abstain from alcohol and is clearly committed to continued abstinence. Overall results in alcoholic recipients have shown that patients transplanted for alcoholic cirrhosis fare at least as well as patients transplanted for most other diagnoses.

Chronic active hepatitis B was formerly considered to be a controversial indication for liver transplantation because recurrence was quite frequent and tended to result in rapid graft failure. This changed when effective strategies to prevent recurrence of hepatitis B using high-dose hepatitis B hyperimmune globulin infusions post-transplant were reported. Now hepatitis B is considered to be a standard indication and results are equal to that obtained for other diagnoses. In contrast, the outcome for patients transplanted for hepatitis C was once considered to be equal to that of other diagnoses. Recent data, however, suggest that recurrence of hepatitis C in the new liver graft is virtually universal following transplantation and 25% of patients will have developed cirrhosis in the graft within 5 years. It is not surprising that longer-term data are now appearing showing that the 10-year survival for patients transplanted for hepatitis C is significantly worse than for other diagnoses.

As with transplantation for hepatitis B and C, the consensus opinion has gone back and forth in recent years regarding whether liver transplantation should be used for the treatment of hepatocellular carcinoma in adults. Patients with cirrhosis are at risk for development of primary hepatocellular cancer. Since these patients usually die of liver failure, unlike patients with other forms of malignancy that usually succumb to widespread metastatic disease, it was reasoned that transplantation would be a curative therapy. Unfortunately, the initial results with transplantation for hepatoma were disappointing due to a high rate of tumor recurrence. These poor results prompted many programs to stop doing transplants for hepatoma because of the poor results. The group from Barcelona, Spain, then reported that survival rates are good if the tumor is small (less than 5 cm in diameter), but poor if the tumor was large or showed evidence of large vessel invasion. Numerous reports have confirmed this finding, and currently liver transplantation is considered to be a standard treatment for patients with small hepatomas. Results for liver transplantation for other malignancies remains poor, with the exception of several encouraging reports of reasonable survival rates for highly selected patients with cholangiocarcinoma who receive adjuvant radiation and chemotherapy.

Current contraindications are few and are primarily related to evidence of cardiopulmonary disease that prohibits safe liver transplantation. Examples would be significant, uncorrected coronary artery disease, pulmonary hypertension with pulmonary artery systolic pressures greater than 70 mm Hg, and FEV_1 of less than 1 L on pulmonary function testing. Active substance abuse is also an absolute contraindication to transplantation. Diabetes increases the risk of transplantation and the incidence of post-transplant complications, but is not an absolute contraindication to liver transplantation. Even infection with HIV, long considered a contraindication to transplantation, is no longer an absolute contraindications at some centers that are reporting good results in small numbers of carefully selected HIV-positive patients. Portal vein thrombosis, which at one time was a contraindication to transplant, is now managed by either performing thrombectomy on the portal vein, by using vein grafts to bypass thrombosed vessels, or by using the infrahepatic cava for portal inflow.

Donor Selection

The number of patients listed for liver transplantation continues to grow larger and larger each year. This has led to a gradual increase in the number of patients who die while waiting and consequently to a relaxation of past standards for liver graft suitability. Livers are currently being transplanted from donors more than 80 years old with acceptable outcomes. It is important that the liver is a rough size match for the donor, but there is much leeway in this regard. Blood type compatibility is preferred, but not an absolute requirement. Matching of tissue antigens does not appear to be relevant for liver transplantation, and a positive crossmatch is not a contraindication to proceeding with transplantation because it is not associated with a worse outcome post-transplant.

The technique of preserving the liver grafts after removal from the donor is based on decreasing metabolic requirements by keeping the graft cold. Blood is flushed from the organ to prevent vascular occlusion; preservation solution is infused; and the organ is kept on ice at 4 °C. Multiple preservative solutions are in common usage across the world. Most contain inert high-molecular-weight molecules that do not diffuse into the cell to prevent cellular swelling. Also free oxygen radical scavengers, which are thought to prevent injury upon reperfusion of the graft, are frequently included. The introduction of Viaspan solution in the late 1980s revolutionized liver transplantation by extending the period of safe in vitro liver preservation from 10 hours to more than 24 hours. Despite this advance, it is clear that prolonged cold ischemia is bad for the liver graft, particularly if the graft contains a large amount of intracellular fat or is from an older donor. Transplant programs therefore continue to strive to minimize the cold ischemic time to whatever degree is feasible.

Operative Technique

In general, liver transplantation is an orthotopic procedure: The host liver is removed and the donor organ placed in an orthotopic position. The operation is performed in three phases: the dissection phase, during which the attachments of the diseased liver are dissected and the vascular structures are prepared for resection; the anhepatic phase, which extends from the time the host liver is removed until the time the donor liver is revascularized; and the reperfusion phase, during which blood is circulating through the new organ and the biliary tree is reconstructed.

Several techniques are available for handling the retrohepatic vena cava. Historically, the liver was removed en-bloc with the vena cava and hemodynamic instability was avoided by using venovenous bypass to overcome decreased venous return when vena caval and portal vein flow is interrupted. The new liver is then sutured into place using a bicaval technique with end-to-end caval anastomoses being performed from donor to recipient both above and below the new liver. With careful anesthetic technique and preloading with fluid, venovenous bypass may be avoided in many cases. An alternative method of handling the retrohepatic cava is to dissect the liver off the cava and sequentially ligate the hepatic venous branches that enter the cava directly from the right and caudate lobes. This allows the liver to be removed by clamping the main hepatic veins without occluding the vena cava. The new liver is then sutured into place by connecting the suprahepatic cava of the donor to a common orifice created by connecting the right, middle, and left hepatic veins. This technique is called the piggyback technique because the donor cava sits directly on top of the recipient cava. The infrahepatic cava of the donor is occluded with either sutures or a vascular stapler. This method avoids the need for venovenous bypass because caval flow is usually not completely interrupted. A third option for caval reconstruction is to connect the donor cava to the recipient cava using a side-to-side technique by making longitudinal incisions from the hepatic veins caudally, creating a very wide anastomosis. This technique is difficult when the donor liver is large relative to the size of the recipient's hepatic fossa.

The current methods of biliary reconstruction include primary choledochocholedochostomy (when the recipient duct is intact) or roux-en-y choledochojejunostomy if the recipient bile duct is not intact or if anatomically the donor and recipient duct cannot be approximated without creating tension on the anastomosis. It was once standard to place a T-tube or another type of biliary stent across the biliary anastomosis, but many programs have now discontinued this practice because it is not clear that the presence of a stent influences the rate of biliary complications.

Although the liver can function normally with only portal venous flow, the bile duct is dependent on hepatic arterial flow. For this reason, the hepatic arterial anastomosis is crucial to postoperative graft survival. The arterial supply of the liver is quite variable, with nearly half of the patients having some form of aberrant circulation. The most common aberrancies are replacement of the right hepatic artery to the superior mesenteric artery and the presence of an accessory left hepatic artery that derives from the left gastric artery. When aberrant arterial vessels are identified on a deceased donor, it is important that they are carefully preserved so that reconstruction can occur when the liver has been perfused and cooled and is sitting in sterile ice slush. Multiple methods of reconstruction of aberrant vessels are available and if necessary, a conduit of donor iliac artery may be used in the reconstruction.

Living Donor Liver Transplantation & Split Liver Transplantation

The shortage of organs for small children in the late 1980s prompted the development of techniques to reduce the size of an adult liver graft by performing an anatomic resection of one or more lobes and transplanting the reduced-size graft. In this way it was possible to transplant a child with the left lobe, or the left lateral segment from an adult liver. This technique was successful and rapidly became a standard method of obtaining grafts for small children. The natural evolution of this technique was to apply the method used to reduce the size of a deceased donor liver graft to adult living donors. Broelsch at the University of Chicago popularized the transplantation of the left lateral segment from an adult into a child and showed that this technique could be at least as effective as using full-size grafts from small children. It was hoped that living related liver transplantation would offer an immunologic advantage as it does with kidney transplantation, but this did not turn out to be the case. The major advantage of living donor liver transplantation appears to be the ability to allow transplant to occur prior to the deterioration of the recipient's condition into a poor state of health that is associated with a higher risk for transplantation.

The success of living donor liver transplantation from adult donors into children, together with the shortage of suitable adult donors, led to the development by Marcos and Tanaka of techniques to utilize the right lobe from a living donor to transplant another adult. The donor operation is a major undertaking and is associated with appreciable morbidity as well as a mortality rate of approximately 0.5%. Nevertheless, living donor liver transplants have become a standard option in areas where timely deceased donor liver transplantation is not possible.

By applying the living donor technique to deceased donors, it is also possible to transplant two recipients from a single adult liver from a deceased donor. This has been termed a split liver transplant. Typically the lateral segment of the left lobe is used for a child or very small adult, while the remainder of the liver consisting of the right lobe plus the medial segment of the left lobe is used to transplant an adult. Less commonly the liver from an adult deceased donor can also be split into a right lobe graft and a left lobe graft and used to transplant two adults.

Immunosuppressive Therapy

The mainstay of immunosuppression for liver transplant recipients is a calcineurin inhibitor. An antimetabolite, and/or corticosteroids, or both may also be included but are not absolutely necessary. Induction therapy with antilymphocyte preparations was once considered standard but has now been abandoned by many liver transplant programs because it appears unnecessary.

Despite being one of the largest organs transplanted in terms of mass, the liver seems to require less immunosuppression for maintenance therapy compared to other organs. Corticosteroids can frequently be safely discontinued. Typically monotherapy with a low dose of a calcineurin inhibitor is all that is required to suppress rejection long term. Spontaneous tolerance with normal graft function despite complete discontinuation of all immunosuppressants occurs in approximately 10–20% of liver transplant recipients. The liver is unique in this regard, since rejection is almost universal if immunosuppression is discontinued in recipients of renal, cardiac, pulmonary, and pancreatic grafts.

Complications

Complications following liver transplantation are common, but most can be treated effectively. Coagulopathy is routinely present during liver transplant procedures, particularly during the anhepatic phase. For this reason, bleeding is common following the procedure, and 5–10% of liver transplant recipients will require reoperation because of continued bleeding following the procedure.

One of the most devastating complications is primary nonfunction of the liver. Primary nonfunction refers to a condition where the new liver does not function and death results unless a second transplant is performed. Patients with primary nonfunction typically have profoundly elevated serum transaminases together with severe coagulopathy and acidosis. The incidence of this complication is between 5% and 10%. The cause of primary nonfunction is poorly understood, but multiple donor factors are known to be associated. Long cold ischemic times, poor perfusion of the graft with preservative solution, severe hepatic steatosis, and elevation of the donor serum sodium level above 165 meq/L are all known risk factors for primary nonfunction.

Vascular complications occur in 5–10% of transplant recipients. The hepatic artery is particularly prone to thrombosis, especially in children. If this is detected early, it is frequently possible to perform thrombectomy and restore hepatic arterial flow. If flow cannot be reestablished, necrosis of the intra- and extrahepatic biliary tree usually occurs, resulting in death from sepsis if retransplantation is not performed.

The bile duct has been called the Achilles' heel of the liver transplant because it is so prone to anastomotic leakage or stricture. Fortunately, while as many as 20% of liver transplant recipients will experience a bile duct complication, it is uncommon for this complication to be lethal. Leaks tend to occur early and can often be managed by placing a biliary stent using endoscopic retrograde cholangiopancreatography (ERCP). If a large collection of bile develops because of a bile leak, it is usually necessary to drain the area either operatively or by placing a percutaneous suction drain. Biliary stenosis can occur early or late. Unlike the native liver, the transplanted liver will not always develop intrahepatic biliary dilatation when the bile duct is obstructed. It is therefore necessary to have a high index of suspicion. Patients with elevated bilirubin or elevated serum alkaline phosphatase levels (or both) should be evaluated with either ERCP or magnetic resonance cholangiography. Strictures can often be managed noninvasively with biliary stents and balloon cholangioplasty, but in some cases, operative correction is required. Patients who develop multiple intrahepatic strictures usually require retransplantation.

Rejection is a frequent complication of liver transplantation—it occurs in about 20–50% of patients. Rejection should be suspected whenever serum transaminases or bilirubin levels or both worsen or fail to gradually normalize following a liver transplant. The diagnosis of rejection is made histologically by the finding of a mixed portal cellular infiltrate together with injury to bile duct epithelium and inflammation of the central vein endothelium (endotheliitis). When the condition is diagnosed early and treated aggressively, rejection rarely culminates in a need for retransplantation. Because the principal rejection target is the bile duct epithelium, severe unrelenting rejection is often manifested by destruction and disappearance of bile ducts (vanishing bile duct syndrome). The treatment for rejection depends on its severity. Mild rejection is treated with either corticosteroid pulse therapy or by increasing the dosage of maintenance immunosuppressive therapy. Rejection that does not respond to these measures may require treatment with an antilymphocyte preparation.

Cytomegalovirus is a member of the herpes family of viruses. Prior to the availability of prophylaxis against this virus, as many as one-half of liver transplant recipients developed clinical CMV infection. Symptoms of this infection typically include fever, leukopenia, and malaise, but a more serious clinical syndrome with pneumonitis or hepatitis is possible. Patients at greatest risk for severe CMV disease are those without previous CMV exposure who receive a liver from a CMV-positive donor, but reactivation of CMV infection is possible in any patient with prior exposure to the virus. In order to prevent CMV infection, most liver transplant programs prescribe either ganciclovir or valganciclovir for a period of months following liver transplantation to all patients at risk for CMV infection.

Epstein-Barr virus (EBV) is another common viral pathogen in these patients. Although the systemic illness with EBV infection is usually mild, it may be associated with development of a lymphoproliferative disorder known as "post-transplant lymphoma." This disorder can progress to frank malignancy and the mortality rate is high. In many cases, the lymphoproliferation resolves merely be reducing immunosuppression. If the lymphoproliferative tissue expresses CD-20, treatment with the monoclonal antibody Rituximab may be helpful. Patients with lymphoproliferation that does not respond to these measures may require chemotherapy.

Immunosuppression predisposes to fungal infections, especially esophageal *Candida albicans* ("thrush"). The incidence of this infection is reduced by the use of prophylactic nystatin to decrease gastrointestinal fungal colonization.

Bussutil RW, Goss JA: Split liver transplantation. Ann Surg 1999;229:313.

Edwards EB et al: The effect of the volume of procedures at transplantation centers on mortality after liver transplantation. N Engl J Med 1999;341:2049.

Gridelli B, Remuzzl G: Strategy for making more organs available for transplantation. N Engl J Med 2000;343:404.

Neuberger J: Liver transplantation. QJM 1999;92:547.

PANCREATIC TRANSPLANTATION

Although pancreatic transplantation involves transplantation of a nonessential organ as compared with the liver, heart, or kidney, it has enormous potential in the management of patients with insulin-dependent diabetes. In many patients with type I diabetes—even though insulin and diet are carefully controlled—the complications of the disease progress relentlessly. Many patients develop severe retinopathy at an early age, leading to blindness and renal disease as well as severe neuropathy and peripheral vascular disease that ultimately results in limb loss. The goal of pancreas transplantation is primarily to prevent or delay end-organ damage by the complications of diabetes. Another important indication for pancreas transplantation is hypoglycemic unawareness. Diabetic nephropathy can cause loss of the autonomic nervous pathways that allow patients to sense hypoglycemia. These patients can lapse into a coma at any moment. For patients with severe hypoglycemic unawareness, pancreas transplantation can truly be a lifesaving procedure.

Currently, most pancreas transplants are whole-organ grafts from deceased donors. The pancreas is procured along with a cuff of the first, second, and third portion of the duodenum attached. The graft can be placed into the pelvis with the iliac artery supplying arterial supply to the pancreas and the iliac vein used for portal venous drainage of the graft. Alternatively, the graft can be placed in the mid abdomen and connected to the infrarenal aorta and the superior mesenteric vein. This allows insulin secreted by the pancreas to enter the portal circulation rather than the systemic circulation, which is more physiologic. The pancreatic exocrine secretions may be managed by anastomosing the duodenum to the bladder or to a loop of small bowel.

If the pancreas graft is successful, the patient will quickly become normoglycemic. As long as the graft functions normally, the patient will no longer require exogenous insulin. This is because the pancreas graft responds normally by secreting insulin in response to rising blood glucose levels that occur following eating and ceasing insulin secretion when blood glucose levels fall to normal.

Much research has dealt with the transplantation of isolated pancreatic islet cells, which make up only about 2% of the pancreatic mass. This procedure is intuitively very attractive because it does not require an abdominal incision or general anesthesia. A team from Edmonton has reported on successful transplantation of islets into the liver using a transhepatic injection into the portal vein. The patients in the original report all achieved insulin independence, although this often required more than one infusion of islets from more than one deceased donor pancreas. Immunosuppression consisted of rapamycin, tacrolimus, and induction treatment basiliximab, an inhibitor of IL-2R. The success at Edmonton has led to increased enthusiasm worldwide for islet transplantation, but to date no other center has achieved the same degree of success. The critical factor appears to the isolation procedure of the islets themselves. Nevertheless, it seems likely that in the long run, islet transplantation will eventually replace whole-organ pancreas transplantation.

Shapiro AM et al: Islet transplantation in seven patients with type 1 diabetes mellitus using a glucocorticoid-free immunosuppressive regimen. N Engl J Med 2000;343:230.

Sutherland DG et al: Lessons learned from more than 1000 pancreas transplants at a single institution. Ann Surg 2001;233:463.

Index

Page numbers followed by *t* and *i* indicate tables and illustrations, respectively. Drugs are listed under their generic names; when a trade name is listed, the entry is cross-referred to the generic name.